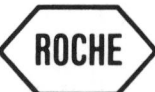

Principles of
Ambulatory
Medicine

SECOND EDITION

Principles of Ambulatory Medicine

SECOND EDITION

Edited by

L. Randol Barker, M.D.
Associate Professor of Medicine,
The Johns Hopkins University School of Medicine;
Director, Division of General Internal Medicine,
Francis Scott Key Medical Center
Baltimore, Maryland

John R. Burton, M.D.
Associate Professor of Medicine,
The Johns Hopkins University School of Medicine;
Deputy Director, Department of Medicine,
Francis Scott Key Medical Center
Baltimore, Maryland

Philip D. Zieve, M.D.
Professor of Medicine,
The Johns Hopkins University School of Medicine;
Chairman, Department of Medicine,
Francis Scott Key Medical Center
Baltimore, Maryland

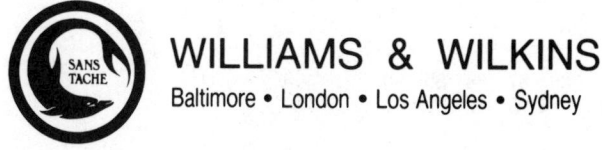

WILLIAMS & WILKINS
Baltimore • London • Los Angeles • Sydney

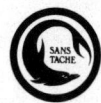

Editor: John N. Gardner
Associate Editor: Victoria M. Vaughn
Copy Editor: Deborah K. Tourtlotte
Design: Bert Smith
Illustration Planning: Lorraine Wrzosek
Production: Anne G. Seitz

Library of Congress Cataloging in Publication Data

Main entry under title:

Principles of ambulatory medicine.

Includes bibliographies and index.
1. Family medicine. 2. Ambulatory medical care. I. Barker, L. Randol (Lee Randol),
1939–   II. Burton, John R. (John Russell), 1937–   III. Zieve, Philip D.,
1932–   . [DNLM: 1. Ambulatory Care. WX 205 P957]
RC46.P894 1986   616   85-6554
ISBN 0-683-00436-0

Composed at the
Waverly Press, Inc.   86 87 88 89 90
                                    10 9 8 7 6 5 4 3 2 1

Preface to the Second Edition

Since publication of the first edition of *Principles of Ambulatory Medicine*, the locus of patient care has continued to shift from the hospital bed to the physician's office: hospitalized patients are discharged earlier, and many conditions for which patients were traditionally hospitalized are now managed entirely in the ambulatory setting. These facts, plus the increase in knowledge important in ambulatory care, are the reasons for preparing a second edition of this book. The objectives and the format for the book are identical to those described in the preface to the first edition. This edition is approximately 350 pages longer, due to the addition of several new chapters and to expansion in the scope of many chapters. Every chapter has been revised to incorporate new information. There are a number of new contributors, all with current or previous affiliations with the Francis Scott Key Medical Center (formerly Baltimore City Hospital) and/or the Johns Hopkins University School of Medicine.

New chapters in this edition are Chapter 3: The Doctor-Patient Relationship: Communication and Patient Education; Chapter 31: Ambulatory Care for Selected Subacute Infections: Osteomyelitis, Lung Abscess, and Endocarditis; and Chapter 33: Medical Advice for the International Traveler. In addition, the new version of Chapter 6, Geriatric Patients: Special Considerations, describes in greater depth the practical approach to urinary incontinence, comprehensive evaluation of functional status, and

other aspects of this important area of practice; a detailed chapter on Alcoholism, by new contributors, replaces the brief chapter on this subject from the first edition; chapters on a number of other psychiatric and behavioral topics (e.g., evaluation of psychosocial problems, office psychotherapy, psychosomatic syndromes, adjustment disorders, anxiety syndromes, and tobacco abuse) have been revised extensively; the chapter on infectious mononucleosis has been expanded to include a number of other conditions that affect lymphocytes (the acquired immune deficiency syndrome, chronic lymphocytic leukemia, and undiagnosed lymphadenopathy), the chapters on Rheumatoid Arthritis and Plasma Lipids and Hyperlipidemia have been largely rewritten; and the chapters on musculoskeletal problems cover additional conditions and include useful new illustrations and information on the examination of the musculoskeletal system.

To a great extent, the preparation of the second edition of *Principles of Ambulatory Medicine* has been guided by the responses of the book's readers. Uniformly, readers cited the practical details regarding patient management as the feature which set *Principles of Ambulatory Medicine* apart from other textbooks. In addition, they pointed out important conditions that were omitted from the first edition, and these conditions have been included in this edition.

Preface to the First Edition

This book is directed primarily to the general physician who cares for ambulatory adult patients. The purposes of the book are (a) to provide an in-depth account of the evaluation, management, and long term course of those common clinical problems which are handled by the generalist in the ambulatory setting, and (b) to provide guidelines for recognizing those problems which require either hospitalization or referral for specialized care and for appreciating the expected course of those problems.

For over 60 years, Baltimore City Hospital has offered education to medical students, residents, fellows, and practicing physicians. During the past decade, the full time professional staff of the hospital has developed major teaching and practice initiatives in ambulatory care. The recognition of the need for a clinical textbook which focused upon the ambulatory patient grew directly out of these initiatives. All of the contributors to this text have a present or recent affiliation with Baltimore City Hospital and/or with The Johns Hopkins University School of Medicine. All have had substantial experience caring for ambulatory patients in their areas of expertise. The editors have worked very closely with all contributors to assure that the material they prepared was focused upon the ambulatory patient.

Three principles have guided the preparation of each chapter.

1. That the physician working in a busy office practice needs to know a great deal about *probabilities* related to his patients' conditions. To address this need, the following types of information are emphasized throughout the book:
   a. Relative frequencies of the conditions which underlie common symptoms.
   b. Distribution of conditions in major subgroups of the population.
   c. The sensitivity, specificity, and predictive value of diagnostic tests and procedures.
   d. The expected course of conditions, in both treated and untreated patients.
   e. The frequency of the complications of treatment.
2. That the patient, in fact, makes most decisions in ambulatory care and that the physician should emphasize the following aspects of *patient education* to assure that the patient's decisions are appropriate:
   a. Information about the short and long term prognosis of the patient's condition, with special emphasis on the implications of the condition for the patient's usual occupational and recreational activities.
   b. Information about the treatment: *i.e.,* how much the treatment usually helps, the expected duration, the correct schedule for treatment (including options adapted to the patient's life style), common side effects, and cost of the treatment.
   c. Information about the experience the patient will undergo when he is referred for care by a specialist or for diagnostic procedures which require his cooperation.
3. That the physician and the patient should incorporate a *preventive point of view* into all of the actions which they take in dealing with a condition. For example, there should be:
   a. Primary prevention of certain conditions, in all patients.
   b. Risk reduction, in those patients who already have certain risk factors.
   c. Optimum maintenance of the patient's health, after a symptomatic condition has developed.
   d. Anticipation of and prevention of problems associated with an established condition or with the treatment prescribed for that condition.

In planning the scope of the book, we selected those conditions which most office-based general internists and general or family practitioners encounter in caring for adult patients from the general population. It was clear that the book should include all of the common conditions of the major organ systems which have been the focus of internal medicine. It was equally clear that a large group of conditions outside of the traditional scope of internal medicine should be included because of the importance they assume in everyday office practice. For all of the conditions included, we agreed that there is a special body of information needed for care of the ambulatory patient, as defined in the three principles named above.

An introductory chapter, entitled The Distinctive

Characteristics of Ambulatory Medicine, defines the domain of ambulatory medicine and delineates the knowledge and the skills which are particularly important in the care of ambulatory patients.

There are a limited number of specific references and a few general references at the end of each chapter. These references are included so that interested readers can pursue in greater depth problems of interest to them. Because we have striven to provide the practical information needed to deal with each of the clinical problems included in this book, readers should be able to make practical decisions for their patients without often having to consult the references.

The book is extensively cross-referenced in order both to avoid redundancy and to facilitate access to useful information contained elsewhere in the book.

In addition, for easy reference, the key topics in each chapter are presented in outline form at the beginning of the chapter.

Acknowledgments

The editors wish to acknowledge the helpful suggestions of many colleagues, both generalists and specialists, who provided feedback on the first edition and who reviewed chapters for this edition. We are greatly appreciative of the excellent help provided by Mrs. Margorie Gregerman and her staff in the Department of Art as Applied to Medicine. Two persons, Mrs. Carole Messman and Ms. Susan McFeaters, provided excellent administrative and typographic assistance throughout the preparation of both editions of the book.

Contributors

Unless otherwise indicated, hospital appointments are at the Francis Scott Key Medical Center (formerly Baltimore City Hospitals), Baltimore, Maryland and faculty appointments are at the Johns Hopkins University School of Medicine

Richard P. Allen, Ph.D.
Co-Director, Baltimore Regional Sleep Disorders
  Center
Assistant Professor of Neurology

Frank C. Arnett, Jr., M.D.
Professor of Internal Medicine
Director, Rheumatology Division
University of Texas Medical School
Houston, Texas

Walter F. Baile, M.D.
Associate Professor of Psychiatry
University of Maryland School of Medicine
Baltimore, Maryland

L. Randol Barker, M.D., Sc.M.
Chief, Division of General Internal Medicine
Associate Professor of Medicine

Edward Bartlet, B.A., M.P.H., D.R.P.H.
Assistant Professor of Health Education and Health
  Behavior
University of Alabama-Birmingham School of
  Public Health
Birmingham, Alabama

John G. Bartlett, M.D.
Chief, Division of Infectious Diseases
Stanhope Bayne-Jones Professor of Medicine
Johns Hopkins Hospital
Baltimore, Maryland

Barbara B. Bell, M.D.
Director, Heart Station
Assistant Professor of Pediatrics

George E. Bigelow, Ph.D.
Director, Behavioral Pharmacology Research Unit
Associate Professor of Behavioral Biology
Assistant Professor of Psychology

Marc R. Blackman, M.D.
Staff Endocrinologist
Assistant Professor of Medicine

Eugene R. Bleecker, M.D.
Chief, Division of Pulmonary Medicine
Associate Professor of Medicine

Margit L. Bleecker, M.D., Ph.D.
Chief, Department of Neurology
Assistant Professor of Neurology
Joint Appointment in Medicine

John C. Breitner, M.D.
Associate Chief of Staff for Education
Bronx Veterans Administration Medical Center
Bronx, New York
Assistant Professor of Psychiatry
Mt. Sinai School of Medicine
New York, New York

Gary R. Briefel, M.D.
Staff Nephrologist, Director of Satellite Dialysis Unit
Assistant Professor of Medicine

Andrew F. Brooker, Jr., M.D.
Chief, Adult Orthopedics
Associate Professor of Orthopedic Surgery
Johns Hopkins Hospital
Baltimore, Maryland

John R. Burton, M.D.
Deputy Director, Department of Medicine
Chief, Geriatric Division
Associate Professor of Medicine

Ronald P. Byank, M.D.
Chief, Orthopedic Surgery
Assistant Professor of Orthopedic Surgery

Nisha Chibber Chandra, M.D.
Director, Coronary Care Unit
Associate Professor of Medicine

Peter E. Dans, M.D.
Director, Office of Medical Practice Evaluation
Associate Professor of Medicine
Johns Hopkins Hospital
Baltimore, Maryland

John E. Davis, Ph.D.
Clinical Assistant Professor
Department of Family Medicine
University of Maryland School of Medicine
Baltimore, Maryland

Mahlon R. DeLong, M.D.
Associate Professor of Neurology
Associate Professor of Neuroscience
Johns Hopkins Hospital
Baltimore, Maryland

J. Raymond DePaulo, M.D.
Director, Affective Disorders Clinic
Associate Professor of Psychiatry
Johns Hopkins Hospital
Baltimore, Maryland

Burton D'Lugoff, M.D.
Director, Community Medicine
Associate Professor of Medicine
Associate Professor of Psychiatry

Calvin B. Ernst, M.D.
Chief, Division of Vascular Surgery
Henry Ford Hospital
Detroit, Michigan
Professor of Surgery
University of Michigan Medical School
Ann Arbor, Michigan

Robert S. Fisher, M.D., Ph.D.
Assistant Professor of Neurology
Johns Hopkins Hospital
Baltimore, Maryland

Andrew P. Goldberg, M.D.
Director, Geriatric Clinical Research
Associate Professor of Medicine

Archie S. Golden, M.D.
Chief, General Pediatrics
Associate Professor of Pediatrics
Associate Professor of International Health
Johns Hopkins University School of Hygiene and
Public Health
Baltimore, Maryland

Barry Gordon, M.D., Ph.D.
Assistant Professor of Neurology

Sheldon H. Gottlieb, M.D.
Clinical Director, Cardiology Division
Assistant Professor of Medicine

Marsha Grayson, M.A.
Communication Skills Preceptor
General Internal Medicine Residency Program
Instructor in Medicine

Robert I. Gregerman, M.D.
Chief, Endocrinology Division
Associate Professor of Medicine

Richard J. Gross, M.D.
Assistant Professor of Medicine and Public Health

Carol S. Haines, M.D., M.P.H.
Postdoctoral Fellow
Department of Behavioral Science and Health
Education
Johns Hopkins University School of Hygiene and
Public Health
Baltimore, Maryland

Nobel M. Hansen, M.D.
Formerly Assistant Professor of Orthopedic Surgery

S. Mitchell Harman, M.D., Ph.D.
Staff Endocrinologist
Associate Professor of Medicine

James Hawthorne, Ph.D.
Director, Southeast Baltimore Drug Treatment
Program
Assistant Professor of Medical Psychology

William R. Hazzard, M.D.
Director, Division of Internal Medicine
David J. Carver Professor of Medicine
Johns Hopkins Hospital
Baltimore, Maryland

Lorraine F. Josifek, M.D.
Assistant Professor of Neurology

Kripa S. Kashyap, M.D.
Assistant Professor, part time
Department of Psychiatry

Gregory B. Kelly, M.D.
Director, Greater Dundalk Medical Center
Baltimore, Maryland
Instructor in Medicine

James P. Keogh, M.D.
Chief, Division of Occupational Medicine
Assistant Professor of Medicine

David E. Kern, M.D.
Associate Director, Division of General Internal
Medicine
Assistant Professor of Medicine

Earl D. R. Kidwell, Jr., M.D.
Chief, Division of Ophthalmology
Assistant Professor of Ophthalmology

Frederick Koster, M.D.
Associate Professor of Medicine
Division of Infectious Diseases
University of New Mexico School of Medicine
Albuquerque, New Mexico

Stanford I. Lamberg, M.D.
Chief, Department of Dermatology
Associate Professor of Dermatology

Bruce S. Lebowitz, D.P.M.
Director, Podiatry Clinic

Douglas K. MacLeod, D.M.D.
Formerly Chief, Department of Dentistry

Raymond L. Malamet, M.D.
Formerly Instructor in Medicine

Esteban Mezey, M.D.
Professor of Medicine
Johns Hopkins Hospital
Baltimore, Maryland

Hamilton Moses, III, M.D.
Deputy Director, Department of Neurology
Assistant Professor of Neurology
Johns Hopkins Hospital
Baltimore, Maryland

Andrew Munster, M.D.
Director, Baltimore Regional Burn Center
Associate Professor of Surgery and Plastic Surgery

Nathaniel F. Pierce, M.D.
Diarrheal Disease Research Program
World Health Organization
Geneva, Switzerland
Professor of Medicine

Thomas J. Preziosi, M.D.
Associate Professor of Neurology
Johns Hopkins Hospital
Baltimore, Maryland

Robert M. Quinlan, M.D.
Chief of Surgery
Memorial Hospital
Worchester, Massachusetts
Associate Professor of Surgery
University of Massachusetts School of Medicine
Worcester, Massachusetts

Peter V. Rabins, M.D.
Director, T. Rowe and Eleanor Price Teaching
    Service
Associate Professor of Psychiatry
Johns Hopkins Hospital
Baltimore, Maryland

J. Courtland Robinson, M.D., M.P.H.
Medical Director
Planned Parenthood of Maryland
Baltimore, Maryland
Assistant Professor of Gynecology and Obstetrics
Lecturer, Population Dynamics
Johns Hopkins University School of Hygiene and
    Public Health

Warren Rothman, M.D.
Chief, Otolaryngology
Assistant Professor of Otolaryngology-Head and
    Neck Surgery

W. Robert Rout, M.D.
Chief of Surgery
Veterans Administration Medical Center
Gainesville, Florida
Associate Professor of Surgery
University of Florida
Gainesville, Florida

R. Bradley Sack, M.D., Sc.D.
Chief, Division of Geographic Medicine
Professor of Medicine

Larry N. Scherzer, M.D., M.P.H.
Northeast Permanente Medical Group
East Hartford, Connecticut
Assistant Professor of Pediatrics
University of Connecticut
Farmington, Connecticut

Chester W. Schmidt, Jr., M.D.
Psychiatrist-in-Chief
Associate Professor of Psychiatry

Marvin M. Schuster, M.D.
Chief, Division of Digestive Diseases
Professor of Medicine
Joint Appointment in Psychiatry

Stephen D. Sears, M.D., M.P.H.
Chief, Division of Infectious Diseases
Assistant Professor of Medicine

Edward P. Shapiro, M.D.
Director of Non-Invasive Cardiology Services
Assistant Professor of Medicine

Philip L. Smith, M.D.
Co-Director, Baltimore Regional Sleep Disorders
    Center
Associate Professor of Medicine
Instructor of Anesthesiology

James K. Smolev, M.D.
Assistant Professor of Urology

David T. Sowa, M.D.
Chief Resident in Orthopedic Surgery
Johns Hopkins Hospital
Baltimore, Maryland

Everett K. Spees, M.D., Ph.D.
Director, Renal Transplant Program
Presbyterian-St. Luke's Hospital
Denver, Colorado

Kerry J. Stewart, Ed.D.
Director, Human Performance Laboratories
Assistant Professor of Medicine

Maxine L. Stitzer, Ph.D.
Investigator, Behavioral Pharmacology Research
 Unit
Associate Professor of Behavioral Biology

Mahmud A. Thamer, M.D.
Director, Cardiac Rehabilitation Program
Assistant Professor of Medicine

Alexander S. Townes, M.D.
Chief, Medical Services
Veterans Administration Medical Center
Memphis, Tennessee
Professor of Medicine
University of Tennessee School of Medicine
Memphis, Tennessee

Harold J. Tucker, M.D.
Assistant Professor of Medicine

Martin D. Valentine, M.D.
The Center for Allergic Diseases
The Good Samaritan Hospital
Baltimore, Maryland
Associate Professor of Medicine

Gustav C. Voigt, M.D.
Director, Emergency Medicine
Associate Professor of Medicine
Assistant Professor of Emergency Medicine

Larry Waterbury, M.D.
Chief, Division of Hematology-Oncology
Associate Professor of Medicine

Charles L. Whitfield, M.D.
Associate Professor of Medicine and Family
 Medicine
Assistant Professor of Psychiatry
Director, Alcohol and Drug Abuse Medical
 Education
University of Maryland School of Medicine
Baltimore, Maryland

Fredrick M. Wigley, M.D.
Chief, Division of Rheumatology
Assistant Professor of Medicine

Philip D. Zieve, M.D.
Physician-in-Chief
Professor of Medicine

Contents

SECTION 10: Metabolic and Endocrinological Problems

SECTION 11: Neurological Problems

SECTION 12: Selected General Surgical Problems

SECTION 13: Gynecological Problems

SECTION 14: Problems of the Eyes and Ears

SECTION 15: Miscellaneous Problems

SECTION 1

Issues of General Concern in Ambulatory Care

CHAPTER ONE

Distinctive Characteristics of Ambulatory Medicine

L. RANDOL BARKER, M.D.

The fundamental tenet of this book is that ambulatory medicine has a number of distinctive characteristics that should shape physicians' approaches to their ambulatory patients. This chapter describes the present domain of ambulatory care in the United States and defines the goals and the basic knowledge and skills that are central to the practice of ambulatory medicine.

THE DOMAIN OF AMBULATORY MEDICINE

Who are the physicians providing ambulatory care? Which patients visit physicians in their offices? What are the problems that these patients present to their physicians? What is the ambulatory care provided for these problems? In order to answer these questions, the United States National Ambulatory Medical Care Survey (NAMCS), started in 1973, has collected information periodically from a representative sample of physicians' offices.

Office-Based Physicians

Table 1.1 shows the distribution by physician specialty of the 585 million office visits to physicians in the United States during 1981. Of these visits roughly 33% were to general and family practition-

ers and 13% were to internists, the two groups of generalists to whom this book is directed primarily.

Ambulatory Patients

The age and sex distribution of the patients who visit these two groups of generalists is shown in Table 1.2. Approximately 60% of visits to all generalists are made by female patients. The principal differences shown in Table 1.2 are that adolescents and young adults account for a larger proportion of visits to general and family physicians than to internists, and that visits by older patients make up a larger proportion of the practice of internists.

The NAMCS definition of an ambulatory patient is "an individual presenting himself for personal health services who is neither bedridden nor currently admitted to any health care institution." The author would add to this definition that an ambulatory or homebound patient (or a member of the household) *has most of the responsibility for his own care;* that is, he must administer most or all of his treatments, he must monitor his symptoms and

Table 1.1.
Number and Percentage Distribution of Office Visits by Physician Specialty and Type of Practice: United States, 1981[a]

Physician Specialty and Type of Practice	No. of Visits in Thousands	Percentage Distribution
All visits	585,177	100.0
Physician specialty		
General and family practice	189,966	32.5
Medical specialties	183,136	31.3
Internal medicine	74,691	12.8
Pediatrics	64,539	11.0
Other	43,906	7.5
Surgical specialties	183,635	31.4
General surgery	32,697	5.6
Obstetrics and gynecology	53,912	9.2
Other	97,026	16.6
Other specialties	28,440	4.8
Psychiatry	15,954	2.7
Other	12,486	2.1
Type of practice		
Solo	321,688	55.0
Partnership	110,330	18.9
Other[b]	153,159	26.2

[a] From *1981 Summary: National Ambulatory Medical Care Survey.* Advance data, no. 88, March 16, 1983.
[b] Includes group practice and other.

Table 1.2.
Percentage Distribution of Visits to General and Family Physicians and to Internists by Age and Sex of Patient, United States, 1980[a]

Age and Sex of Patient	Percentage Distribution	
	General and Family Practice	Internal Medicine
All ages	100.0	100.0
Under 15 years	13.9	2.5
15–24 years	14.9	7.1
25–44 years	27.4	21.4
45–64 years	24.4	36.4
65 years and over	19.4	32.7
Sex		
Female	60.5	59.2
Male	39.5	40.8

[a] Adapted from *Drug Utilization in Office Visits to Primary Care Physicians: National Ambulatory Medical Care Survey, 1980.* Advance data, no. 86, October 8, 1982.

functional status, he must adapt his activity to his degree of illness, and he must decide how to deal with new problems when they arise. These characteristics of an ambulatory patient have important implications for the physician, as discussed below.

Problems of Ambulatory Patients

What types of problems are seen in ambulatory practice? This question was asked from the point of view of the patient and the physician in a large sample of office visits to generalists participating in the NAMCS. Thus, patients were asked to name the principal reasons for their visits, and physicians were asked to name the principal diagnoses (using the *International Classification of Diseases*) for the problems addressed at the same visits. Tables 1.3 and 1.4 list the most common responses given in 1975 in the offices of internists and of general and family physicians, respectively. Three points bear emphasis: (*a*) For internists, 20 diagnoses or problems and for generalists 25 problems or diagnoses accounted for approximately 50% of total visits. (*b*) There are important differences in the frequency of problems reported by patients and physicians; for example, abdomimal pain is fifth among the problems reported by the patients of both types of physicians but does not appear as one of the most common problems reported by either group of physicians. (*c*) A number of the problems named by patients are symptoms for which a specific diagnosis often cannot be determined (abdominal pain, fatigue, nervousness).

In this study, physicians were also asked to rate the extent of impairment that might result if no care were available for the patient. The internists rated 70% of problems and the general and family physicians rated 80% of problems as either not serious or only slightly serious in terms of preventable impairment.

Ambulatory Care

The NAMCS defined ambulatory care as "health services rendered to individuals under their own cognizance, any time when they are not in a hospital or other health care institution." Table 1.5, from the 1975 NAMCS report, shows the percentage distribution of diagnostic and therapeutic services ordered or provided by internists and general or family physicians for their ambulatory patients. The table also shows the frequency distribution of duration of visit and the prior visit status of patients.

The majority of visits included some type of diagnostic service (for example, over half of the visits included a limited history or physical examination), and the majority of visits included some form of therapy (most commonly a prescription for medicine). At about 18% and 12% of visits, respectively, internists and general/family practitioners devoted a significant part of the visit to medical counseling defined as advice or counsel about diet, change of habit, or behavior. These data tend to underestimate the amount of time devoted to education of the patient. Observation of office practice has shown that generalists devote about 25% of their patient contact time to patient education and that some patient education in fact occurs during most visits (1).

At 66% of visits to internists and 56% of visits to general and family practitioners, the patient had been seen before for the same problem, and at only 13% (for both groups of physicians) was the patient seen for the first time. These findings point out another distinctive feature of ambulatory medicine—that the decisions made by the generalist usually concern problems already known to him in patients whom he has seen before.

Telephone encounters and *home visits* are two aspects of ambulatory care which have not been studied quantitatively. Nonetheless, both play an important role in the care of ambulatory patients—telephone encounters because they enable physicians and patients to handle many problems efficiently, and home visits, for selected patients, because they are necessary in providing care to patients who are too frail to make office visits or they enable the physician to learn facts about patients' home conditions that may facilitate management of their problems at future office visits. The roles of house calls and home health services in ambulatory medicine are discussed in Chapters 6 (Geriatric Patients) and 9 (Selected Special Services).

The Domain of Self-Care

Before making visits to physicians, patients usually attempt to diagnose and treat their own symp-

Table 1.3.
Reasons for Ambulatory Visits to Internists: United States, January to December 1975[a]

	Reasons Named by Patients				Principal Diagnoses Named by Physicians			
Rank	20 Most Frequent Patient Problems, Complaints, or Symptoms and NAMCS Code[b]		Percentage of Visits	Cumulative Percentage of Visits	Rank	20 Most Common ICDA 3-Digit Categories and Code[c]		Percentage of Visits	Cumulative Percentage of Visits
1	General and required physical examinations	900, 901	5.6	5.6	1	Essential benign hypertension 401		9.3	9.3
2	Pain in chest	322	4.6	10.2	2	Chronic ischemic heart disease 412		7.9	17.2
3	Problems of lower extremity	400	4.4	14.6	3	Diabetes mellitus	250	4.5	21.7
4	Fatigue	004	4.0	18.6	4	Medical or special examination Y00		4.1	25.8
5	Abdominal pain	540	3.7	22.3	5	Acute upper respiratory infection 465		2.6	28.4
6	High blood pressure	205	2.9	25.2	6	Neuroses	300	2.3	30.7
7	Problems of back region	415	2.8	28.0	7	Osteoarthritis and allied conditions 713		2.3	33.0
8	Cough	311	2.7	30.7	8	Symptomatic heart disease	427	2.0	35.0
9	Problems of upper extremity	405	2.4	33.1	9	Medical and surgical aftercare Y10		1.8	36.8
10	Vertigo-dizziness	069	2.3	35.4	10	Rheumatoid arthritis and allied conditions 712		1.6	38.4
11	Shortness of breath	306	2.2	37.6	11	Obestiy	277	1.6	40.0
12	Headache	056	2.0	39.6	12	Observation, without need for further medical care 793		1.3	41.3
13	Throat soreness	520	1.8	41.4	13	Emphysema	492	1.3	42.6
14	Diabetes mellitus	991	1.7	43.1	14	Hay fever	507	1.2	43.8
15	Cold	312	1.6	44.7	15	Other eczema and dermatitis 692		1.2	45.0
16	Visits for medication	910	1.4	46.1	16	Other nonarticular rheumatism 717		1.2	46.2
17	Nervousness	810	1.3	47.4	17	Synovitis, bursitis, and tenosynovitis 731		1.1	47.3
18	Problems of face, neck	410	1.2	48.6	18	Arthritis, unspecified	715	1.0	48.3
19	Allergic skin reactions	112	1.2	49.8	19	Symptoms referable to respiratory system 783		1.0	49.3
20	Other symptoms referable to cardiovascular system	220	1.1	50.9	20	Bronchitis, unqualified	490	1.0	50.2

[a] Adapted from *Office Visits to Internists: National Ambulatory Medical Care Survey, United States, 1975.* Advance data, no. 16, February 7, 1978.
[b] Symptomatic groupings and code number inclusions are based on a symptom classification developed for use in the NAMCS.
[c] Diagnostic groupings and code number inclusions are based on the *Eighth Revision International Classification of Diseases, Adapted for Use in the United States.*

toms. Studies of the domain of self-care have shown that at any one time approximately 30% of persons are taking nonprescribed medications or are engaged in self-care for a problem for which they have not consulted a physician (4). The frequency distribution of conditions managed by self-care has been estimated by Fry (3) on the basis of many years of general practice in a community well known to him: 25% upper respiratory infections, 20% musculoskeletal symptoms, 20% emotional problems, 10% acute gastrointestinal symptoms, 5% skin rashes, and 20% miscellaneous other symptoms.

The time interval between the onset of symptoms and the decision to go to the physician (i.e., the duration of self-care) is shown for a number of common conditions in Table 1.6, adapted from NAMCS. Not surprisingly, acute infections for which self-care failed were mostly seen within a

few days, while a majority of subacute problems such as headache and back symptoms were seen after at least 1 week of self-care.

The physician sees only the failures from this informal system of care. As part of his approach to each new problem, he should inquire about the patients' "working diagnosis" and etiological hunches. Such inquiry is often the most efficient way to learn about the roots of a problem, particularly a chronic problem.

Self-care *before* professional care is an important way in which the patient, not the physician, makes the decisions in the domain of ambulatory medicine. The patient's primary role in carrying out the plan of care *after* visiting the physician has already been emphasized in the expanded definition of the ambulatory patient given above. These two features combined confirm the primacy of the patient's de-

Table 1.4.
Reasons for Ambulatory Visits to General and Family Practitioners: United States, January to December 1975[a]

Rank	Reasons Names by Patients Most Frequent Patient Problem, Complaint, or Symptom and NAMCS Code[b]	Percentage of Visits	Cumulative Percentage	Rank	Principal Diagnoses Given by Physicians Most Common Principal Diagnosis and ICDA Code[c]	Percentage of Visits	Cumulative Percentage
1	General and required physical examinations 900, 901	4.9	4.9	1	Medical or special examination Y00	6.3	6.3
2	Problems of back 415	4.1	9.0	2	Essential benign hypertension 401	5.9	12.2
3	Throat soreness 520	3.8	12.8	3	Acute upper respiratory infection, site unspecified 465	3.6	15.8
4	Problems of lower extremity 400	3.8	16.6	4	Diabetes mellitus 250	2.5	18.3
5	Abdominal pain 540	3.1	19.7	5	Medical and surgical aftercare Y10	2.4	20.7
6	Problems of upper extremity 405	3.1	22.8	6	Acute pharyngitis 462	2.2	22.9
7	Cough 311	3.0	25.8	7	Chronic ischemic heart disease 412	2.2	25.1
8	Visit for medication 910	2.7	28.5	8	Other eczema and dermatitis 692	2.2	27.3
9	Fatigue 004	2.7	31.2	9	Influenza, unqualified 470	2.1	29.4
10	Cold 312	2.6	33.8	10	Obesity 277	2.1	31.5
11	Headache 056	2.5	36.3	11	Neuroses 300	1.8	33.3
12	Pregnancy examination 905	2.4	38.7	12	Bronchitis, unqualified 490	1.7	35.0
13	Pain in chest 322	2.1	40.8	13	Acute tonsillitis 463	1.7	36.7
14	Allergic skin reaction 112	2.0	42.8	14	Arthritis, unspecified 715	1.5	38.2
15	Wounds of skin 116	2.0	44.8	15	Cystitis 595	1.4	39.6
16	High blood pressure 205	1.9	46.7	16	Otitis media 381	1.3	40.9
17	Surgical aftercare 986	1.9	48.6	17	Osteoarthritis 713	1.2	42.1
18	Weight gain 010	1.6	50.2	18	Synovitis, bursitis 731	1.2	43.3
19	Vertigo-dizziness 069	1.5	51.7	19	Other nonarticular rheumatism 717	1.2	44.5
20	Problems of face, neck 410	1.4	53.1	20	Diarrheal disease 009	1.2	45.7
21	Earache 735	1.3	54.4	21	Menopausal symptoms 627	1.1	46.8
22	Fever 002	1.3	55.7	22	Chronic sinusitis 503	1.1	47.9
23	Gynecologic examination 904	1.2	56.9	23	Hay fever 507	1.1	49.0
24	Shortness of breath 306	1.1	58.0	24	Sprains, strains of sacroiliac region 846	1.0	50.0
25	Flu 313	1.1	59.1	25	Inoculations and vaccinations Y02	1.0	51.0

[a] Adapted from *National Ambulatory Medical Care Survey of Visits to General and Family Practitioners, January–December 1975.* Advance data, no. 15, December 14, 1977.
[b] Symptomatic groups and code number inclusions are based on a symptom classification developed for use in the NAMCS.
[c] Diagnostic groupings and code number inclusions are based on the *Eighth Revision International Classification of Diseases, Adapted for Use in the United States.*

Table 1.5.
Percentage Distribution of Visits to Office-based Generalists, by Diagnostic and Therapeutic Services Ordered or Provided, Duration of Visit, and Prior Visit Status: United States, January to December 1975[a]

Diagnostic and Therapeutic Services Ordered or Provided[b]	Percentage of Visits	
	To internists	To General and Family Practitioners
No services provided	1.3	1.7
Diagnostic services provided		
Limited history or examination	61.4	55.6
General history or examination	20.1	12.6
Clinical laboratory test	38.5	21.6
X-ray	13.1	6.2
Blood pressure check	61.4	40.2
EKG	14.0	2.3
Hearing test	1.5	0.8
Vision test	2.4	1.4
Endoscopy	1.6	0.6
Therapeutic services provided		
Drug administered or prescribed[c]	49.5	55.6
Injection	11.6	21.5
Immunization or desensitization	2.6	3.7
Office surgery	1.5	5.2
Physiotherapy	1.1	3.3
Medical counseling	17.8	11.7
Psychotherapy or therapeutic listening	2.7	2.9
Other sevices provided	1.7	3.6
Duration of visit[d]		
0 min (no face-to-face encounter with physician)	0.7	1.7
1–5 min	5.6	20.5
6–10 min	24.8	34.1
11–15 min	35.6	24.9
16–30 min	24.6	17.0
31 min or more	8.7	1.9
Prior visit status		
Patient seen for the first time	13.1	12.7
Patient seen before for another problem	20.9	30.5
Patient seen before for current problem	66.0	56.8

[a] Adapted from *Office Visits to Internists: National Ambulatory Medical Care Survey, United States, 1975.* Advance data, no. 16, February 7, 1978; and from *National Ambulatory Medical Care Survey of Visits to General and Family Practioners, January–December, 1975.* Advance data, no. 15, December 14, 1977.
[b] Percentage will not add to 100 because most patient visits required the provision of more than one treatment or service.
[c] Includes prescription and nonprescription drugs.
[d] Signifies time spent in face-to-face encounter between physician and patient.

Table 1.6.
Percentage Distribution of New Problem Office Visits by Time since Onset of Complaint or Symptom, According to Selected Principal Reasons for Visit: United States, January to December 1977[a]

Principal Reason for Visit	Total	Time since Onset of Complaint or Symptom					
		1 Day	1–6 Days	1–3 Wk	1–3 Mo	>3 Mo	Not Applicable
		%					
All new problem visits	100.0	8.2	37.3	15.6	10.3	13.9	14.8
Symptoms of throat	100.0	6.9	77.9	10.6	2.3	1.9	0.4
Cough	100.0	3.3	73.0	18.6	2.9	2.1	0.2
Head cold, upper respiratory tract infection	100.0	6.2	72.5	16.5	3.0	1.1	0.7
Fever	100.0	17.6	76.4	4.7	0.2	1.0	
Headache	100.0	5.1	35.6	19.0	16.5	19.7	3.2
Back symptoms	100.0	6.5	37.6	26.4	11.8	16.2	1.5
Chest pain	100.0	7.6	45.8	22.6	9.3	13.6	1.2
Laceration, upper extemity	100.0	70.4	15.4	7.8	3.0	2.1	1.3

[a] From *National Ambulatory Medical Care Survey, 1977, Summary.* Hyattsville, MD, National Center for Health Statistics, 1979.

Table 1.7.
Profile of 5 Years in the Care of an Elderly Patient (Each Problem *Italicized*)

Feature	1975	1976	1977	1978	1979
ENCOUNTERS	Initial visit, 4 office visits, many phone calls	3 office visits, many phone calls	5 office visits, 2 hospital admissions, 1 home visit, many phone calls	4 office visits, many phone calls	4 office visits, many phone calls
PRINCIPAL MEDICAL PROBLEMS	*Acute myocardial infarction* (mild congestive heart failure; digitalized; home management by patient's choice)	Stable (digoxin)	Stable (digoxin)	Congestive heart failure (diuretic added)	Stable (digoxin, diuretic)
	Degenerative joint disease (knees for years; cervical spine for years)	Waxes and wanes (aspirin, Motrin)	Same (coated aspirin)	Same (coated aspirin)	Same (coated aspirin)
	Temporal headaches for 1 year (erythrocyte sedimentation rate 30)	Rarely	Rarely	Rarely	Rarely
	Hearing loss (ear, nose, and throat examination: senile high frequency deficit, no prescription)	Stable	Stable	Stable	Stable
	Bilateral cataracts	Stable	Stable	Referred (not mature)	Stable
	Leukoplakia, mouth (biopsy: not malignant)	Stable	Stable	Stable	Referred for change in appearance (biopsy: not malignant)
	Hematocrit 35 (guaiac-negative)	Stable	Stable	Stable	Stable
	Constipation (for years)	Waxes and wanes (over-the-counter (OTC) laxative as needed)	Same (OTC laxative as needed)	Same (OTC laxative as needed and stool softener)	Same (OTC laxative as needed and stool softener)
		Leg cramps (quinine at bedtime)	Minimal (quinine at bedtime)	Same (quinine at bedtime)	Same (quinine at bedtime)
		Left cerebral *transient ischemic attack* (TIA)	*Left cerebrovascular accident* (CVA) (hospital, physical therapy)	Stable (right hemiparesis)	Recurrent left CVA (home management)

OVERALL PROFILE				
87-year-old widow living with daughter's family, ambulatory and independent in the home, mentally intact, crochets and cans food; weight 166; multiple medical problems identified at initial visit (above)	88 years old, status the same; weight 160; 2 new problems (above)	89 years old, ambulation with walker assistance after CVA; weight 151; 4 new problems (above), hospitalized twice	90 years old, status the same; weight 140; 3 new problems (above)	91 years old; ambulation more impaired after second CVA; mentally intact, crochets and cans food; weight 139; no new problem
		Dog bite (cellulitis)	*Family temporarily "exhausted"* (Visiting Nurses Association)	No recurrence
		Rectal bleeding (hospital, negative workup)	*Painful toe* *Appetite lost temporarily*	No recurrence
		Dysuria (culture negative)		Family doing well
				Persists (codeine) No recurrence
				No recurrence

cisions in influencing the course of events in ambulatory medicine.

The Temporal Dimension in Ambulatory Medicine

The longitudinal nature of ambulatory care cannot be appreciated in the information from NAMCS contained in Tables 1.1 to 1.6. Table 1.7 shows the 5-year profile of care, mostly ambulatory care, for an elderly woman followed from 1975 through 1979. This patient's story illustrates each of the following important questions for which only the passage of time provides the answers:

1. *What is the significance of a recent symptom?* (e.g., the temporal headache for 1 year reported in 1975, subsequently stable for 5 years.)

2. *What is the advisability of initiating a referral for a problem?* (e.g., cataract problem identified but asymptomatic in 1975, evaluated when more symptomatic in 1978 and classified as not mature.)

3. *How well will the patient (or the patient's family) adhere to recommended care?* (e.g., the digoxin for heart failure, taken reliably for 5 years.)

4. *What is the impact of treatment upon the patient's health?* (e.g., adding a diuretic in 1978; heart failure gradually improved during the month following diuretic.)

5. *What is the impact of intercurrent medical problems upon the patient's usual activities?* (The answer to this question varied over time depending upon intercurrent problems: during the 5 years the patient's ambulation deteriorated greatly; however, other valued activities, such as crocheting and canning, did not.)

GOALS OF AMBULATORY CARE

The Patient's Expectations

The goals of ambulatory care are determined by the fact that the patient is residing at home, not in an institution. Residence at home creates expectations that differ greatly from those created by hospital confinement. They are the same expectations that are held by an individual who has not in fact become a patient: that he will play as active a role as possible in the life of his family and community; that he will be as capable as possible of taking care of basic needs such as nutrition, clothing, hygiene, travel, etc; that on an average day he will be as free as possible of physical and emotional symptoms while engaging in his usual activities; and that he will be generally satisfied with his situation in life. Depending on the severity of his medical problem, an ambulatory patient may be greatly, moderately, or not at all constrained from attaining these expectations. But by virtue of living at home, he will be dealing with these expectations daily, in contrast to hospitalized patients for whom these expectations must await return to home.

In ambulatory medicine, then, the ultimate goals of care can be equated with those goals of any individual who is living at home in his community. These goals contain certain implications for the practice of ambulatory medicine.

Implications for Practice

First, in order to decide how any patient is doing, the physician must know about the individual's particular expectations; this usually involves learning about the make up of the patient's household, about the patient's usual role in the household, about the patient's occupation, about the patient's level of formal education, and about the patient's recreational and religious activities.

Second, the kind of information described above is particularly important in clinical preventive medicine (see Chapter 2), in which the patient's degree of "wellness" rather than his degree of illness is assessed. Assessing wellness means determining how successfully patients are meeting their own expectations and determining what health risks they have. For example, a 40-year-old mother who is happily married, free of chronic disease, has stopped smoking, has had periodic negative Pap smears and breast examinations, and drinks alcohol only socially would be assessed as very well. If everything was the same but she smoked three packs of cigarettes daily she would be assessed as only relatively well because of the major risk posed by heavy tobacco exposure. If she was recently divorced, had stopped seeing friends, and was smoking and drinking heavily, she would be assessed as not very well, even though she might not complain of any particular symptoms or have objective evidence of any disease.

Third, knowledge of how well a patient is meeting his expectations is often critical in managing that patient's medical problems. This is because management of an ambulatory patient should be directed not just at physiological disturbances, but also at social disruptions that accompany an illness. This point can be illustrated by a common example, namely, that of the head of a household who has had an uncomplicated myocardial infarction. After 3 months, the patient might be assessed as "status post myocardial infarction—doing well." If he is back at work, then he is indeed "doing well." If he is not back at work, is financially stressed, and his wife reports that he has become irritable, then he is "not doing well" (even though his cardiovascular status is stable), and he needs additional support from his physician.

KNOWLEDGE AND SKILLS CENTRAL TO AMBULATORY MEDICINE

The picture provided by the National Ambulatory Medical Care Survey and other studies of office practice has clear implications for the knowledge and the skills that are most important in the practice of ambulatory medicine. These are knowledge derived from clinical epidemiology and skills in communication with patients, in record keeping, in coordination of care, and in containing costs.

Clinical Epidemiology

Feinstein has defined clinical epidemiology as follows:

"The territory is the clinicostatistical study of diseased populations. The intellectual activities of this territory include the following: the occurrence rates and geographic distribution of disease; the patterns of natural and post-therapeutic events that constitute varying clinical courses in the diverse spectrum of a disease; and the clinical appraisal of therapeutic agents" (2) and of diagnostic tests (*author's addendum*).

In patient care, the principal uses of clinical epidemiology are (a) making a working diagnosis, (b) understanding the natural history of a condition and the capacity of treatment to alter it, and (c) planning and monitoring treatment.

Making a Working Diagnosis

In ambulatory medicine, the working diagnosis (or assessment) may range from "healthy without any significant risk factors," to "healthy with risk factors A and B for disease X," to "disease X."

In evaluating a patient for the presence of a risk factor or of an established disease, the physician should be aware of the *prevalence* (i.e., proportion of the population affected at one particular time) and the *incidence* (i.e., proportion of the population newly affected during a specified interval of time) of the suspected condition in the general population and in the particular subgroup(s) to which the patient belongs. This information enables a physician to follow a strategy that is particularly important in reaching a working diagnosis in ambulatory medicine: *focusing upon the probable and not upon the possible*. A familiar example of this strategy is the evaluation of a patient for hypertension. The crude prevalence of hypertension is 10 to 20% in adult citizens of the United States. The prevalence of renovascular hypertension is probably less than 0.1% in the population of black hypertensive patients. Based on this information, screening for hypertension is appropriate in all adult patients, but screening for renovascular hypertension is not appropriate in most black hypertensive patients.

Three principal types of clinical data are utilized to reach a working diagnosis:

1. *A single diagnostic test*, for example, a biopsy that shows a malignant neoplasm.

2. *A quantitative deviation* in a single physiological function, for example, a fasting blood gucose which satisfies a criterion for diabetes.

3. *A cluster of criteria*, which includes symptoms, signs, and duration; for example, the DSM-III (*Diagnostic and Statistical Manual-III*) criteria for most psychiatric disorders.

There are a number of qualities by which diagnostic and screening tests can be characterized:

1. The *reliability* of the test, which is a measure of its repeatability on more than one occasion.

2. The *objectivity* of a test, which indicates the repeatibility of results of a test by multiple observers.

3. The *sensitivity* of a test, which means the percentage of affected individuals with a positive test (true positive rate). The sensitivity of a test is determined systematically by utilizing the test on a large group of patients known to have the condition being tested for.

4. The *specificity* of the test, which means the percentage of nonaffected individuals with a negative test (true negative rate). The specificity of a test is determined systematically by utilizing the test on a large group of patients who are known not to have the condition.

5. The *predictive value* of the test, which means the probability that a specific patient has a suspected condition when the test is positive (positive predictive value) or does not have the suspected condition when the test is negative (negative predictive value). The predictive value of a test is dependent upon the prevalence of that condition in the population to which the patient belongs. The predictive value of a positive test is highest when the prevalence of a condition is relatively high (*i.e.*, ≥5%) and the specificity and sensitivity of the test are also relatively high. As shown in Figure 1.1, the predictive value of a test can be calculated when the prevalence of a condition in the population plus the sensitivity and the specificity of the test are known or can be estimated.

In the examples shown at the bottom of Figure 1.1, it can be seen that approximately 10 patients with a positive test from population A (1% prevalence) would have to undergo additional evaluations in order to identify one with condition X, while only two patients with a positive test from population B (10% prevalence) would have to undergo additional evaluations in order to identify one with condition X.

Understanding the Natural History and the Impact of Treatment

This information is derived from longitudinal studies.

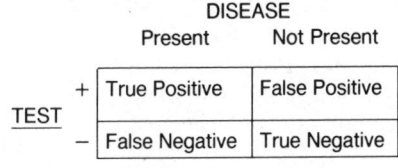

DISEASE

Present   Not Present

TEST

+ | True Positive | False Positive
− | False Negative | True Negative

$$\text{Sensitivity} = \frac{\text{True Positive}}{\text{True Positive} + \text{False Negative}}$$

$$\text{Specificity} = \frac{\text{True Negative}}{\text{False Positive} + \text{True Negative}}$$

Independent of prevalence of the disease in the population to which a specific patient belongs

$$\text{Predictive value of positive test} = \frac{\text{True Positive}}{\text{True Positive} + \text{False Positive}}$$

$$\text{Predictive value of negative test} = \frac{\text{True Negative}}{\text{False Negative} + \text{True Negative}}$$

Dependent on prevalence of the disease in population to which the patient belongs

← EXAMPLES:		Test Characteristics			
Population to Which Patient Belongs	Prevalence of Condition	Sensitivity	Specificity	Predictive Value of a Positive Test	Predictive Value of a Negative Test
A	1%	90%	90%	9%	99.9%
B	10%	90%	90%	50%	98.7%

Figure 1.1. Methods for determining sensitivity, specificity, and predictive values of a test.

In order to *learn the natural history of a condition* (including a risk factor), a group of subjects representative of the universe of patients affected by the condition must be followed longitudinally. Ideally the longitudinal study is conducted prospectively, meaning that the questions to be asked and the data to be collected are chosen before subjects are enrolled. In reality, many of the studies of the natural history of conditions have been performed retrospectively (meaning that the primary data were generated before the study was planned and that the patients selected were those available for review at the time the study was planned). At times, a satisfactory "prospective" study can be reconstructed from events which preceded the planning of the study.

In order *to delineate the impact of treatment*, the study design should assure that treated subjects are compared with untreated subjects who are similar in every important characteristic except treatment. Again, ideally, the study is conducted prospectively; participating subjects are allocated randomly to two groups for concurrent study or the same subjects are allocated randomly to study and comparison treatments for crossover study; the study is double blind, meaning that neither the investigator nor the subjects know who is receiving which treatment; and a simulation of treatment in the form of a placebo is utilized in the comparison group. For many of the conditions seen in ambulatory medicine, longitudinal studies of treatment are either inadequate or have not been conducted at all. One or more of the following flaws are found commonly in existing studies: retrospective methods are used to evaluate treatments; the study group is representative of a narrow subgroup of the universe of patients affected by a condition but the results are generalized to all who are affected; the comparison group differs significantly from the study group; or the impact of therapy (or of a diagnostic test) on the overall health status of study subjects is not measured.

In the absence of definitive information, the physician must base his decisions upon evaluation of existing information. A good example of this approach is Liang and Fries' (5) discussion of a common problem: the management of asymptomatic hyperuricemia.

Planning and Monitoring Treatment

Two questions that occupy much of the physician's time in the care of ambulatory patients are: What treatment shall I recommend? What events related to the treatment should I anticipate after initiating it? The answers to these questions may be found in studies of the effectiveness of a treatment and sources describing the clinical pharmacology of drugs utilized in ambulatory patients.

The *effectiveness* of a treatment is a measure of its impact in patients being cared for in the "real world," meaning representative community and practice settings. This concept is different from the familiar concept of the *efficacy* of a therapy, which is a measure of its impact in cooperating patients who belong to formal study groups (described above). For a number of reasons, there are few available studies of effectiveness. In recent years, patient compliance—a major determinant of the effectiveness of treatment in ambulatory patients—has been studied in "real world" settings for a variety of conditions (see Chapter 4). Such studies have generally demonstrated that adherence to a prescribed regimen in ambulatory patients is highly variable, and that a number of factors related to patient behavior must be considered if treatment is to be effective for the individual patient.

Clinical pharmacology is the source for the many details needed for appropriate administration of drugs. Apart from the impact of a drug upon a patient's condition, the physician should be aware of the following aspects of each drug that he prescribes:

1. *Practical information about initiating the drug*: appropriate starting dose and schedule; modifications in dose and schedule dictated by patient age, by concurrently administered drugs, and by the presence of diseases affecting drug metabolism; time interval for the effect of the drug to be apparent; duration of a course of the drug (when not a maintenance drug); how to assess the impact of the drug; and potential interaction with other drugs the patient is taking. (It is also important to know the approximate cost of a prescription to the patient and to select the least expensive drug, including a generic preparation if available, whenever there are one or more alternatives.)

2. *The major side effects of the drug*: when to anticipate them, and how to detect and manage them. (It should be remembered that the risks associated with new drugs are often not completely delineated until several years after release of the drugs for general use.)

3. *The major reasons for inadequate response to a drug*: nonadherence, insufficient dose of drug, antagonism of the drug by patient behavior or by concurrent drugs, and primary refractoriness to the drug; and how to recognize and manage each of these problems.

Since administering/prescribing drug therapy is the single most common action taken by generalists in ambulatory medicine (see Table 1.5), access to these practical types of information is particularly important.*

---

* A number of sources provide timely and critical reviews of this information, e.g., *The Medical Letter*, The American Medical Association (AMA) Drug Evaluation, and regular reviews such as the "Drugs in Perspective" reports in the *Annals of Internal Medicine* and the "Drug Therapy" reports in the *New England Journal of Medicine*.

Communication and Patient Education

As stated earlier, the goals of care in ambulatory medicine can be equated with the patient's expectations for himself at home and in his community. Attaining these goals is an ongoing process, requiring some measure of continuous care for most patients and recognition that the patient has the major responsibility for carrying out the plan of care. Given these characteristics of ambulatory medicine, skills in interpersonal communication and in providing patient education are fundamental to effective practice, for it is through these skills that the physician motivates the patient for his role in adhering to the plan of care. In recent years, many of the skills in these areas that are important in patient care have been delineated, and a growing number of investigations have confirmed the positive impact of these skills on the outcome of care. This topic is covered in depth in Chapter 3, The Doctor-Patient Relationship: Communication and Patient Education.

Clinical Records

Clinical records are valuable chiefly for reference at some later time. In ambulatory medicine, the interval between visits is usually weeks or months, so that the physician must rely largely upon those facts that he has recorded and not on his memory. The various characteristics of ambulatory medicine that have been discussed earlier point to the essential information that should be available in the patient's office record if it is to provide useful points of reference for subsequent care.

As stated earlier, the goal for the patient in ambulatory medicine is attaining/maintaining his expectations in the community despite his medical conditions. To facilitate the patient's attainment of this goal, the physician should know (therefore, should record) three sets of information about his patient:

1. A *social profile*, including information about family, occupational, educational, and recreational circumstances that determine the patient's expectations (see example, Fig. 1.2).

2. A *problem list*, that is, a list of all medical problems with dates that have been identified in the course of the patient's care (see example, Fig. 1.2).

3. A *preventive care profile* that provides a record of periodic care with the objective of reducing risks of subsequent disease (see example, Chapter 2, Fig. 2.3).

Although the patient is responsible for carrying out the plan of care in ambulatory medicine, the physician is responsible for advising the patient, developing the plan with the patient, and assessing its success at serial visits. Specific recording of clinical evidence, of the interpretation of that evidence, of the specific details of the treatment plan, and of the patient's reported adherence is essential if the record is to provide a reliable reference for serial visits. The writing of *brief problem-oriented notes* (notes which cover separately each problem being addressed) and the use of the S (subjective) O (objective) A (assessment) P (plan) format (6) for progress notes are recording techniques well suited to these needs. To record observations about adherence to medication or about the course of one or more facets of the patient's condition, separate medication records or flow sheets may also be useful in long term care (see example, Chapter 2, Fig. 2.3).

Coordination of Care

The third general skill that is particularly important in ambulatory medicine is skill in coordinating the patient's care. Coordination of care refers to actions that promote appropriate use of services which the patient may need. During the past 20 years, the number of available laboratory services, supportive services, and specialty consultative services grew enormously: there are currently more than 200 health-related professions and occupations; and the ratio of nonphysician health workers to physicians grew from 10:1 in 1960 to more than 20:1 in 1980. The availability of so many services requires the generalist to be prudent in recommending them and in utilizing the information they provide. The physician should always be aware of the cost of a service to his patient, the nature of the experience the patient will undergo, and the likelihood that the service will be of value to the patient.

The services recommended for patients may involve permanent, temporary, or partial transfer of responsibility for the patient's care, or they may be strictly consultative, meaning that they provide information to be utilized directly by the referring generalist (ranging from laboratory test results to specific recommendations by a consultant).

There are two sets of guidelines that define the role of the general physician in the coordination of services that he recommends for a patient:

1. The physician should begin by assuring that the patient understands the reason for services that are recommended; he should arrange to obtain information promptly after a service has been performed; and he should assure that the patient learns, as soon as is appropriate, the meaning of this information for the care of his condition.

2. Whenever a physician requests a service for a patient, he should be sure that proper information is given to the person providing the service. For example, there should be a clear indication of what laboratory test is required or of the facts generally needed by consultants (see Table 1.8).

Patients sometimes obtain services for medical problems without the intercession of their personal physician. These most often include visits to emergency rooms or to specialists such as ophthalmologists. Obtaining information about treatment changes or new diagnoses related to these visits is another way in which the generalist should attempt to coordinate his patient's care.

FRANCIS SCOTT KEY MEDICAL CENTER
Department of Medicine

PRIMARY CARE PROFILE

Mrs. Jane Doe

Date This Form Initiated _Feb. 5, 1985_
Name of Provider _Dr. Jones_

Social Profile

Marital Status _Widow (2/83)_   Highest Education _High School_   Income Source _Social Security_

Work History/Hazard Exposure: _Munitions Plant WWII, salesLady 1950s-1976 (Ret.)_

Children/Immediate Family: _2 daughters, 6 grandchildren - all live in town_

Lives with ? _Alone_   Permanent Impairments: _Hearing Loss (uses aid)_

Persons (relations) to contact in event of emergency _Mrs. James Smith (daughter) 533-0000_

Other (activities, major life events, social support system, etc.): _Bowls weekly, active in church, 2 dogs (walks them daily), several neighbors whom she sees weekly_

Allergic/Drug Reactions (Year)

None _____
Penicillin (hives 1968)

Risk Profile

Smoker	Ⓝ	Y _____	(quit 1977)
Etoh	Ⓝ	Y _____	(_____)
Drugs	Ⓝ	Y _____	(_____)
Exercise	N _____	Y _Bowls_	(_____)

Cholesterol: _3/79 - 186 mg%_
Other:

Operations (Year)

1968 hysterectomy
1982 Ⓡ carpal tunnel

Problem List

Date of Onset / Identification	#	Problem & Comments (Key Tests/Consults)
— / —	1	HM (Health Maintenance)
/1976	2	COPD Fvc/FEV-1 $\frac{1.9}{1.3}$ 1979
1950s/1976	3	Smoker - stopped 1977
/1976	4	Pneumonia
/1976	5	Mitral Valve Prolapse Echo 1976
/198	6	Prolonged Grief p̄ husband ↓
1983/1983	7	Stress incontinence → learned self control technique
/1984	8	Immature cataracts ⇗ Ophth 1983

FSKMC #6037-001   REV. 8/84   28-3357-7773   335-12950

Figure 1.2. Example of form for recording social profile, problem list, and other baseline data in an office record.

Table 1.8.
Information That Subspecialty Consultants
Generally Need from the Referring Physician

The specific reason for the consultation
Relevant current medical problems
Relevant current medications
What the patient has been told about the referral
The patient's attitude about the problem (if relevant)

Containing Costs

This chapter has emphasized that the patient has a dominant role in ambulatory medicine, particularly with regard to carrying out the plan of care recommended by the physician. However, just as in hospital medicine, the office-based physician is largely responsible for deciding what services the patient should purchase. Although the ways in which patients pay for services in ambulatory care vary from prepayment for all services to paying out of pocket for each service when it is rendered, the impetus for purchasing those services almost always comes from the physician. This is similar to many situations in our society in which the consumer entrusts to a professional or expert the decision to purchase a particular service.

Owing to the extraordinary increase in available medical services in the past two decades and because of the parallel increase in the cost and the utilization of these services, the containment of the cost of medical care is generally recognized as a national imperative. The need to contain costs has critical implications for generalist physicians in office practice, for it is they who coordinate most of the medical care provided in our society. Table 1.5 indicates that, in addition to paying for the office visit, the patient, on the recommendation of his physician, purchases one or more discrete services at the majority of office visits (diagnostic testing, office procedures, prescribed medications, consultant opinions, etc). There is little doubt that many of these services are not necessary for the health of these patients.

There are important ways in which the generalist physician can limit the costs of care. Taking a history carefully and allowing some time to pass before embarking on an extensive diagnostic workup of a new symptom is one way. Keeping himself well informed about the *value to the patient's health* of a costly diagnostic procedure is a second way. Devoting sufficient time to educating a patient about his condition (especially about conditions that often lead to inappropriate and costly doctor shopping by the patient) is another way. Prescribing only necessary medications and selecting the least expensive preparations are further ways. Utilizing home health services and other community services to forestall the need for hospital admission is yet another way.

Unhappily, third party reimbursement patterns have promoted excessive utilization of technical services in the United States and have discouraged physicians from engaging in the inquiry and counseling that might obviate much inappropriate purchasing of health services. It would be helpful if, in parallel with their recent efforts to reduce the utilization of hospital beds, the federal government and other third party payors will develop ways to reward physicians for practices such as inquiry and counseling, practices which tend to promote the health of patients and to reduce the unnecessary use of costly technical services.

General References

The National Ambulatory Medical Care Survey (periodic publications issued by the Department of Health and Human Services. Washington, DC).
> Nationwide study of a probability sample of office-based physicians from all medical specialty areas, utilizing physician- and patient-generated information to delineate the ambulatory care activities of physicians and patients, started 1973.

Feinstein AR: Clinical epidemiology. I–III. *Ann Intern Med* 69:807, 1037, 1287, 1968.
> Series of three articles describing lucidly the domain and the uses of clinical epidemiology.

Fletcher RH, Fletcher SW: Clinical research in general medical journals: a 30-year perspective. *N Engl J Med* 301:180, 1979.
> A critical review of the clinical research methods utilized in studies reported in three general medical journals from 1946 to 1976; it is important to note that a decrease in longitudinal studies was found.

Fletcher RH, Fletcher SW, Wagner EH (eds): *Clinical Epidemiology: The Essentials.* Baltimore, Williams & Wilkins, 1982.
> Lucid book written for clinicians. Uses case examples to illustrate all points.

Fries JF, Vickery DM (eds): *Take Care of Yourself: A Consumer's Guide to Medical Care.* Reading, MA, Addison-Wesley, 1976.
> Good book to recommend to interested patients; contains sound advice about self-care for most common symptoms.

Fry J: *Common Diseases: Their Nature, Incidence and Care,* ed. 2. Philadelphia, JB Lippincott, 1979.
> Unique account of the longitudinal course of many common diseases, based upon over 25 years of general practice in a single community.

Fuchs VR (ed): *Who Shall Live? Health, Economics, and Social Choice.* New York, Basic Books, 1974.
> Lucid account of the interrelationship of medical services and the economy.

Griner PF, Mayewski RJ, Mushlin AI, Greenland P: Selection and interpretation of diagnostic tests and procedures. *Ann Intern Med* 94:553, 1981.
> Lucid guidelines for appropriate use of diagnostic tests (special supplementary issue).

Mendenhall RC, Tarlov AR, Girard RA, *et al*: A national study of internal medicine and its specialities. II. Primary care in internal medicine. *Ann Intern Med* 91:275, 1979.
> Nationwide study of a large sample of internists (including subspecialists), utilizing physician-generated information to delineate the primary care activities of internists.

Noble J (ed): *Primary Care and the Practice of Medicine.* Boston, Little, Brown, and Co, 1976.
> A multiauthored book which discusses in detail many of the relationships between primary care and contemporary society.

Specific References

1. Bartlett EE: The contributions of consumer health education to primary care practice: a review. *Med Care* 18:862, 1980.

2. Feinstein AR: Clinical epidemiology. I–III. *Ann Intern Med* 69:809, 1968.
3. Fry J: *Common Diseases: Their Nature, Incidence and Care,* ed 2. Philadelphia, JB Lippincott, 1979, chap 1.
4. Kohn R, White KL: *Health Care.* New York, Oxford University Press, 1976.
5. Liang MH, Fries JF: Asymptomatic hyperuricemia: the case for conservative management. *Ann Intern Med* 88:666, 1978.
6. Weed LL: *Medical Records, Medical Education, and Patient Care.* Chicago, Year Book, 1969.

CHAPTER TWO

Preventive Medicine in Ambulatory Practice

DAVID E. KERN, M.D., AND L. RANDOL BARKER, M.D.

The practicing physician's tasks in preventive medicine consist of disease prevention, early detection and treatment of presymptomatic disease, and promotion of optimal functioning once disease has become clinically manifest. Two characteristics distinguish preventive from curative care:

1. The physician, not the patient, usually initiates preventive care.

2. Preventive care is designed to protect health *prospectively*; this is true even when "health" may mean, for an individual patient, a sedentary exist-ence in his home instead of a hospital admission for a preventable problem.

A number of considerations underlie the importance of incorporating preventive strategies into routine office practice: (a) It has been estimated that 50% of mortality from the 10 leading causes of death in the United States can be traced to alterable behavioral patterns, often termed "life style" (5). (b) Early detection and treatment of several common disorders—such as hypertension, hypercholesterolemia, breast cancer, and cervical carcinoma *in situ*—are effective in reducing the morbidity and mortality caused by these conditions. (c) While infectious diseases have been controlled to a large extent in the industrialized nations by public health measures, including immunization, outbreaks continue to occur, particularly in under- or unprotected individuals and segments of the population. Influenza, for example, remains a major preventable cause of death. (d) The value of a comprehensive approach to prevention is demonstrated by the reduction in maternal and perinatal morbidity and mortality that may be attributable to prenatal care (12). In addition, a comprehensive, preventive approach to care has recently been shown to reduce mortality, acute hospitalizations, and nursing home placement in high risk elderly patients, while improving their functional status and morale (14, 15). (e) Finally, while documentation is difficult to obtain, a significant proportion of iatrogenic illness is probably preventable.

TYPES OF PREVENTIVE CARE

Prevention of disease and disability can be sub-divided conceptually into three types according to where in the course of a disease process the preventive intervention occurs (Fig. 2.1).

Primary prevention is any intervention that prevents a pathological process from occurring. Immunization against infectious diseases, for example, neutralizes infectious agents before disease processes can begin. In a similar fashion, identification and control of risk factors (such as cigarette smoking) in healthy individuals can be considered primary prevention, since control or elimination of the risk factors prevents the development of specific diseases.

Secondary prevention occurs when there is intervention after a pathological process has been initiated but before symptoms occur. Secondary prevention is of value when two important conditions exist: (a) the pathological process is detectable during the presymptomatic stage of disease and (b) treatment initiated before symptoms occur is more beneficial than treatment initiated after sympotms occur. The early detection and treatment of breast and cervical cancers are examples of secondary prevention (a) since the former can be detected presymptomatically by periodic physical examination and mammography and the latter by periodic cytological screening of the uterine cervix, and (b) since early treatment reduces morbity and mortality from these diseases. Behavior modification leading to weight reduction in an obese individual with impaired glucose tolerance would also be considered secondary prevention, since weight loss in such a patient may improve glucose tolerance and forestall or prevent symptomatic diabetes.

Tertiary prevention refers to the prevention of progressive disability or other complications in individuals with chronic symptomatic disease. Physical and occupational therapy designed to prevent flexion contractures and to restore independent functioning in a stroke victim is an example of tertiary prevention. Tertiary prevention has also been termed *prevention in clinical medicine* (17).

While conceptually useful, the distinctions between primary, secondary, and tertiary prevention occasionally become cloudy in practice. The detection and treatment of hypertension, for example, would be considered secondary prevention if one considers hypertension a disease and congestive heart failure, stroke, and renal failure complications of that disease. On the other hand, hypertension is a risk factor for atherosclerotic disease, so detection and treatment of hypertension to prevent myocardial infarction or atherosclerotic cerebral or peripheral vascular disease can be considered primary prevention. Smoking cessation, as another example, represents primary prevention in the healthy individual but tertiary prevention in the patient with established coronary artery or chronic obstructive pulmonary disease.

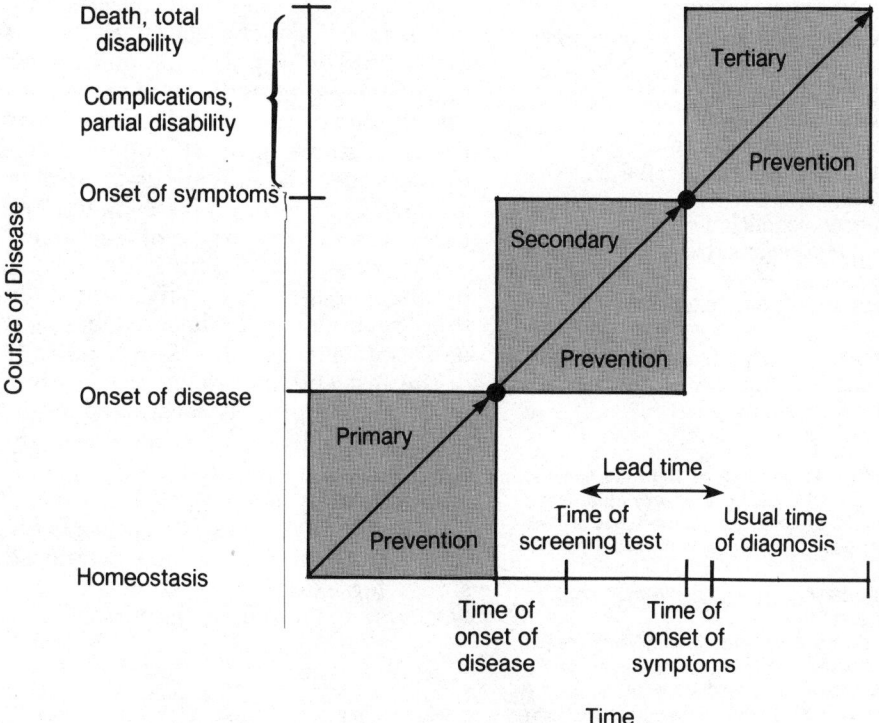

Figure 2.1. Primary, secondary, and tertiary prevention in the spectrum of a disease.

Within the practice of preventive medicine, *screening* is defined as "the process of identifying individuals with one or more remediable asymptomatic diseases or risk factors in a defined population group" (17). When screening tests are applied to large populations, independent of visits to physicians, the process is called *mass screening*. Screening for asymptomatic conditions in office practice is most readily accomplished through a procedure called *case finding*. This is the application of screening tests to patients by their physicians during consultations for unrelated problems.

EVALUATING PREVENTIVE MEASURES FOR USE IN AMBULATORY PRACTICE
(Table 2.1)

The first step in integrating preventive care into office practice is deciding which measures to offer

Table 2.1.
Questions to Ask in Evaluating a Recommended Preventive Measure

IS THE PREVENTABLE CONDITION IMPORTANT?
What is the prevalence and/or incidence?
What is the size of the attributable morbidity?
What is the mortality rate?
IS PREVENTIVE INTERVENTION EFFECTIVE IN RESEARCH SETTINGS?
Is the intervention efficacious[a] in study groups?
Are compliance levels in study situations acceptable?
Are side effects acceptable?
Is intervention in the asymptomatic stage more beneficial than intervention after symptoms?
DO EFFECTIVE SCREENING TESTS EXIST?
Do they have acceptable sensitivity, specificity, and predictive value?[b]
Are they reliable?[b]
Are they practical and reasonably priced?
Are the side effects of screening acceptable?
WOULD USE OF THE MEASURE BE EFFECTIVE IN ROUTINE OFFICE PRACTICE?
Have suitable field trials been conducted?
Is the measure effective in reducing morbidity and mortality in nonstudy situations?[a]
Are the compliance levels in nonstudy situations acceptable?
Are side effects in nonstudy situations acceptable?
What are the reliability, sensitivity, specificity, and predictive value of screening tests in one's own setting?
Is the measure cost effective?

[a] A measure is *efficacious* if it results in more benefit than harm to those who are completely compliant. Efficacy is usually established in clinical trials where participants are selected on the basis of their compliance and where special efforts are made to minimize complications from the intervention.
A measure is *effective* if it results in more benefit than harm to those to whom it is offered in practice.
A measure may be extremely efficacious yet minimally effective in practice if patient compliance is lower and/or complications/costs are substantially higher in practice than in controlled study situations.
[b] See Chapter 1 for a discussion of reliability, sensitivity, specificity, and predictive value.

patients routinely. To make these decisions, it is necessary to consider the importance of each preventable condition, in terms of its prevalence and severity, the efficacy and effectiveness of treatment, the availability of effective screening tests, and the usefulness of each measure in office practice (see Table 2.1). Recommendations which are periodically published by organizations such as the Canadian Task Force on the Periodic Health Examination, the American Cancer Society, the American College of Physicians, the American Medical Association, the Center for Disease Control, and others may also be consulted (see "General References"). The Canadian Task Force's reports, which are firmly grounded in clinical epidemiology, provide the most scientific framework to date for evaluating which preventive health measures should be included in periodic health examinations. In the United States, the Public Health Service has established a Preventive Services Task Force that will serve in a similar function.

In evaluating a given measure, the physician should be aware of certain pitfalls and special considerations. *Lead time* refers to the interval between early detection by a screening test and usual time of diagnosis (Fig. 2.1). In evaluating the efficacy of early detection and treatment, the lead time must be subtracted from the survival times reported for screened patients to avoid *lead time bias*. Otherwise, a preventive measure might be proposed that simply increases the duration of patients' awareness of their disease without reducing morbidity or increasing longevity. *Time-linked biased sampling* or *length bias* occurs when the same disease (e.g., some malignancies, autoimmune diseases, dementia syndromes) is characterized both by less aggressive forms with long presymptomatic stages and more aggressive forms with presymptomatic stages that are significantly shorter than the screening interval. Hence, a greater proportion of screened, as opposed to nonscreened, individuals will have the less aggressive forms of the disease and a better prognosis irrespective of the timing of treatment.

The process of screening itself can cause morbidity, independent of any physical complications from the screening test, by falsely labeling some individuals as ill (*false positives*—related to the specificity of the test and the prevalence of the disease*) (2), while inappropriately reassuring other patients that they are healthy (*false negatives*—related to the sensitivity of the test and prevalence of the disease*). Even correctly labeling patients can be associated with morbidity, a risk which has been documented for a number of common conditions (2, 6–8). In one study, for example, absenteeism rose in screened workers diagnosed as hypertensive, especially if

_____
* See Chapter 1 for a discussion of sensitivity, specificity, and predictive values.

they had previously been unaware of the condition and if they complied poorly with treatment (7). A disadvantage of mass or nonoffice-based screening is that a significant proportion of labeled individuals will not seek recommended follow-up with a physician. The physician who screens for presymptomatic disease in his own patients may prevent much of the morbidity created by labeling (a) by confirming that a problem is present, usually by repeat or additional observations, before presenting a patient with a diagnosis; (b) by taking time to explain the meaning of a problem to a patient and to respond to his questions; (c) by only screening for conditions for which detection is likely to benefit the patient; and (d) by ensuring appropriate follow-up.

Finally, caution must be exercised in adopting recommendations based solely upon proof of effectiveness in highly controlled study situations, especially when the proposed measure is expensive or associated with significant complications. Costs and conditions may be different in office practice. Before recommending yearly mammography to all women age 50 and over, the physicians in a large group practice might wish to negotiate the lowest price with local radiologists and obtain some assurance that the sensitivity and specificity of their readings approach published norms. Before recommending routine sigmoidoscopy to all patients age 45 and over in one's practice (a recommendation based upon less than conclusive evidence in study situations), the costs, availability of diagnostic services, and complication rate in one's own setting must be considered. While colon perforation rates of up to 1 per 1000 examinations have been reported among trained gastroenterologists, the complication rate for trained and untrained generalists remains to be established.

Despite the above precautions, there is sufficiently strong evidence to support the integration of numerous primary and secondary preventive measures into office practice (see below). Failure to do so represents an inadequacy in the provision of primary care.

THE COMPONENTS OF PREVENTIVE CARE

The General Examination and Baseline Data

Most physicians will perform a *baseline general examination* (history, physical, and selected laboratory tests) for some or all of their ambulatory patients. In addition, some physicians will update all or part of this examination on a periodic basis. In many practices patients complete self-administered history forms. As contrasted to the periodic health examination discussed below, there is no firm scientific evidence linking the general examination to reductions in morbidity and mortality. Most clinicians would agree, however, that knowledge of a patient's past hospitalizations and operations, past and present illnesses, medication and allergic his-

tory, diet history, habit history, social history, and family history is indispensable to the provision of effective preventive and curative care for that patient. General examinations may be advantageous in other ways as well. For example:

1. Baseline information may be of value in assessing symptoms which are likely to occur at a later date (e.g., EKG in a patient with a high risk of coronary artery disease or chest X-ray in a patient exposed to asbestos).

2. Occasionally a general approach will detect a treatable asymptomatic condition, such as an abdominal aneurysm, which, because of low prevalence or lack of a highly accurate screening test, cannot justify a directed screening effort.

3. Periodic updates of the medical history may assist the primary care physician in coordinating the patient's care.

4. Comprehensive general examination of individuals, upon whom other lives are dependent (e.g., airline pilots), may be of use.

5. A "normal" general examination can provide reassurance, especially to the patient who expressly wants to know if he is in good health.

The Periodic Health Examination

Periodic health examinations consist of the periodic provision of selected preventive measures to groups of patients, based upon their age, sex, and risk status. Recommended measures are summarized in Table 2.2. For each recommendation, the table provides the following information:

1. The required assessment by the physician.

2. Preventable condition(s) for which the assessment is performed.

3. The patient population to which the measure should be applied (age, sex, risk status).

4. Type of prevention (primary, secondary, tertiary).

5. Nature of the action to be taken by the generalist.

6. Quality of the evidence for improvement in health status through intervention (effectiveness).

7. Location of additional information elsewhere in this book.

These recommendations are based upon a critical review of selected existing evidence and upon recommendations compiled by others (see "General References"). For a number of the health assessments recommended in the tables, the evidence for the effectiveness of intervention is rated as fair or weak. Nevertheless, these are included because the disease consequences related to them are significant and because there is a consensus that preventive intervention is probably effective. For some of these health assessments and for others not yet recommended, future investigations will probably provide more conclusive evidence for the effectiveness of intervention in improving health status. The physi-

Table 2.2.
Recommended Periodic Health Assessment

Health Assessment by Generalist	Preventable Condition	Patient Population (Age, Sex, Risk Status)	Time Interval	Type of Prevention	Nature of Action by Generalist	Evidence for Effectiveness of Intervention	Chapter to See for Details
INFECTION							
Gonococcal culture	*Gonorrhea* and complications	Sexually active high risk F	Discretionary	2°	Antibiotics, report case, counsel regarding prevention	Fair	27, 94
Risk of hepatitis B	*Hepatitis B* and complications	High risk M, F of all ages	Once	1°	Hepatitis B vaccine	Established	32, 42
Risk of influenza	*Influenza* and complications	(a) High risk M, F of all ages	1 year	1°	Influenzal vaccine	(a) Established	32
		(b) Institutionalized M, F of all ages				(b) Established	
		(c) Healthy M, F ≥ 65				(c) Weak	
Risk of pneumococcal pneumonia	*Pneumococcal pneumonia*	(a) High risk M, F of all ages	Once	1°	Pneumococcal vaccine	(a) Good to established	32
		(b) Healthy M, F ≥ 65				(b) Weak	
Rubella antibody titer or documented history of rubella vaccination	(a) *Rubella* (b) Congenital rubella syndrome	F of childbearing age	Once	1°	Rubella vaccine	(a) Established (b) Good	32
Serological test for Syphilis (STS)	*Syphilis* and complications	High risk M, F	Discretionary	2°	Antibiotics, report case, counsel regarding prevention	Good (for early stages)	27, 94
History of tetanus and diphtheria vaccine within last 10 years	*Tetanus, diphtheria*	All M, F	10 years	1°	Tetanus-diphtheria vaccine	Established	32, 33
Travel to developing countries	Hepatitis, malaria, gastroenteritis, cholera, yellow fever, typhoid fever, poliomyelitis, etc	All M, F	Varies	1°	Immunization, prophylactic medication, counseling regarding preventive health practices	Established for most	32, 33
Tuberculin skin test	*Tuberculosis*	High risk M, F	Discretionary	2°	Chemoprophylaxis, immunization—depends on age of patient and clinical circumstances	Established	29
CANCER							
Breast examination by physician	*Breast cancer* morbidity and mortality	(a) All F ≥ 50 (b) All F 40–49 (c) All F 20–40	1 year 1 year 1–3 years	2° 2° 2°	Referral	(a) Established (b) Fair (c) Weak	89
Mammography	*Breast cancer* morbidity and mortality	(a) All F ≥ 50 (b) All F 40–50 (c) High risk < 50	1 year 1 year 1 year	2° 2° 2°	Referral	(a) Established (b) Fair (c) Fair	89
Teach/encourage monthly breast self-examination	*Breast cancer* morbidity and mortality	All F ≥ 20	1 month	2°	Referral	Weak	89

test)	morbidity and mortality	activity or age 18 (whichever comes later) to age 34 (b) F, 35–60	(b) 3 years, after 2 normal cytologies	2°			
Stool for occult blood	Colorectal cancer morbidity and mortality	M, F ≥ 40 High risk < 40	1 year	2°	Referral	Fair	37
Sigmoidoscopy	Colorectal cancer morbidity and mortality	High risk M, F	1 year (×2), then 3–5 years	2°	Referral	Fair	37
Rectal exam	Colorectal cancer morbidity and mortality	M, F ≥ 40	1 year (×2), then 3 years	2°	Referral	Weak	37
Oral inspection, toluidine blue mouth wash (can be done during dental visits)	Oral cancer morbidity and mortality	High risk M, F ≥ 40	Discretionary	2°	Referral	Weak	101
Skin inspection	Skin cancer morbidity and mortality	High risk M, F	Discretionary	1°, 2°	Counseling regarding reduction of risk factors, referral	Weak	100
CHRONIC DISEASE Blood pressure	Stroke, congestive heart failure, chronic renal failure	All M, F	1 year	1°, 2°	Confirm high blood pressure, treat	Established	62
Plasma cholesterol level (or lipid profile)	Atherosclerotic disease	All M, F	Once late adolescence to early adulthood, once early middle age	1°, 2°	Confirm abnormal level, treat	Established	75
Assessment of oral hygiene practices and dental inspection	Dental caries, periodontal disease, premature loss of teeth	All M, F	Discretionary	1°, 2°, 3°	Counsel regarding proper dental hygiene (brush, floss), fluoride, diet, and regular dental visits	Fair to good	101
Comprehensive (medical, psychosocial, accident risk, and functional) evaluation	Premature morbidity and mortality in high risk geriatric populations	High risk M, F ≥ 65	Once	2°, 3°	Management of detected disorders	Established	6
Hearing assessment, assessment of risks for hearing loss	Hearing impairment	All M, F	5 years	1°, 2°, 3°	Noise control, hearing protectors, confirm abnormal assessment, treat when possible, selective referral	Established	96
Weight, height	Morbidity and mortality related to morbid obesity	All M, F	1 year	1°, 2°, 3°	Counseling regarding diet and weight reduction, referral	Weak	76

Table 2.2.—Continued

Health Assessment by Generalist	Preventable Condition	Patient Population (Age, Sex, Risk Status)	Time Interval	Type of Prevention	Nature of Action by Generalist	Evidence for Effectiveness of Intervention	Chapter to See for Details
None	Osteoporosis, hip and other fractures	White F starting at menopause	Not applicable	1°	(a) Estrogen replacement[b] (b) Calcium supplements[b] (c) Exercise[b]	(a) Fair to good (b) Fair (c) Weak	74, 77
History of bothersome visual impairment[c]	Visual impairment	All M, F	Discretionary	3°	Referral for diagnosis and correction of impairment	Good	97, 98
LIFE STYLE-RELATED DISEASE							
Alcohol abuse	Physical and psychosocial complications of alcoholism	All M, F	1–5 years	1°, 2°, 3°	Counseling, referral	Weak to fair	21
Birth control	Unwanted pregnancy	M, F childbearing years	1–5 years	1°	Counseling, prescribing, referral	Established	93
Dietary assessment	Cardiovascular, dental, and other health problems	M, F all ages	1–5 years	1°, 3°	Counseling, diet prescription	Weak to good	62, 75, 76, 101
Drug abuse	Physical and psychosocial complications of drug abuse	All M, F	1–5 years	1°, 2°, 3°	Counseling, referral	Weak	20
Exercise practices	Premature mortality, cardiovascular disease, obesity, osteoporosis, some psychosocial problems, unfavorable plasma lipoprotein levels, lack of physical fitness	M, F all ages	1–5 years	1°, 3°	Counseling, exercise prescription	Good	58, 75, 76
Smoking	Premature morbidity and mortality from cancer, pulmonary, cardiovascular	All M, F	1–5 years	1°, 3°	Smoking cessation counseling	Established (small to moderate increases in cessation rates)	20
PREGNANCY							
Prenatal care	Low birth weight infants and fetal/infant mortality	Pregnancy F	Multiple visits during pregnancy	1°, 2°, 3°	Counseling, monitoring, management of detected problems	Fair	
Alcohol use	Impaired fetal growth, birth defects, mental re-	Pregnant F	Once or more	1°	Alcohol cessation counseling	Fair	21

Amniocentesis	Chromosomal disorders, neural tube defects, *etc*	Pregnant F ≥ 35, other high risk pregnant F	Once	2°	Abortion	Established	
Hematocrit/hemoglobin	Severe *anemia* (and its potential maternal and fetal complications)	Pregnant F	Twice	2°, 1°	Iron and folate therapy	Established	49
Cervical culture for *Chlamydia*	Infection in newborn	Pregnant F	Once	1°	Antibiotic therapy, report cae, counsel regarding prevention, monitor newborn	Weak	
Plasma glucose, history of diabetes	Increased perinatal and maternal morbidity and mortality related to maternal *diabetes*	Pregnant F	Once	2°, 3°	Strict diabetic control	Established	72
Cervical gonococcal culture	Maternal *gonorrhea* and its complications, infection in newborns	Pregnant F	Once	2°, 1°	Antibiotic therapy, report case, counseling regarding prevention, monitor newborn	Established	94
Hepatitis B antigen	Neonatal *hepatitis*	High risk pregnant F	Once	1°	Immunization of infant and household/sexual contacts	Established	32
Blood group Rh incompatibility	Erythroblastosis fetalis	Pregnant F	Once	1°	Rh hyperimmune globulin	Established	
Smoking	Impaired fetal growth, perinatal mortality	Pregnant F	≥ 1	1°	Smoking cessation counseling	Established	20
STS	Maternal *syphilis* and its complications, congenital syphilis	Pregnant F	Once	2°, 1°	Antibiotic therapy, report case, counsel regarding prevention, monitor newborn	Established	20
Toxoplasma gondii titer	*Congenital toxoplasmosis*	High risk pregnant F (raw meat eaters, cat owners)	Every 3 months	1°	Counseling on hygiene, treat, consider abortion if first trimester infection, close monitoring and early treatment of newborn	Weak	
Urine culture	Pyelonephritis, fetal complications	Pregnant F	Once	2°	Antibiotic therapy	Fair	27

[a] Effectiveness of intervention established, required intervals for examination less well established.

[b] Estrogen replacement is particularly indicated in patients with symptoms of estrogen deficiency and in patients who have experienced premature surgical/radiological menopause. Because of established and possible complications from estrogen use, calcium supplementation and exercise counseling are the preferred intervention in most postmenopausal women. The use of cyclical estrogen/progestin therapy will abolish the increased risk of endometrial cancer attributable to estrogen therapy, but will result in the return of menses (for further details see Chapter 77).

[c] Note: Routine tonometry by the generalist is *not* recommended (10).

cian can decide for himself the value of these and other preventive measures by asking the questions listed in Table 2.1.

The preventive measures recommended in Table 2.2 are guidelines for average adults. Factors that may dictate expanded or more limited surveillance for the individual patient may not be included. A characteristic that the physician should always consider when planning preventive care, for example, is the expected longevity of an individual patient. Thus, a 55-year-old patient with inoperable lung cancer should receive influenza and pneumococcal vaccines but should not receive the other preventive care recommended for his age and sex. On the other hand, a 50-year-old patient who has survived an uncomplicated myocardial infarction at the age of 48 has a reasonable life expectancy and should be offered all of the preventive care recommended for an individual in his age group.

Preventive Care for Established Conditions (Tertiary Preventive Care)

Preventive care pertains to the management of a patient's established condition as well as to early detection and treatment for asymptomatic conditions. In an office practice consisting largely of patients with such established conditions as diabetes, congestive heart failure, and degenerative joint disease, the physician may improve the health of his patients as much by preventive care for these conditions as by screening systematically for asymptomatic conditions. Appropriate preventive care for an established disease depends upon the disease, its treatment, and the expectations of the individual patient. This type of care ranges from concrete actions, such as periodic monitoring of the serum potassium in patients taking digitalis and diuretics, to such techniques as short term counseling for a survivor of a myocardial infarction who is showing early symptoms of depression. The strategies for optimal preventive management of specific conditions are emphasized in subsequent chapters of this book.

Extending Prevention to the Family and the Community

The physician should take action to extend preventive care beyond the individual when this is appropriate. In some instances, he should recommend preventive treatment for members of a patient's family and other close contacts. Gamma globulin prophylaxis for the family of a patient with infectious hepatitis and treatment of sexual contacts of patients with sexually transmitted bacterial diseases are classic examples. In other situations, the physician should recommend evaluation of the relatives of patients with certain chronic diseases that show a tendency to occur in families. For example, relatives of patients with familial hypercholesterol-

emia should have plasma lipid levels determined, and routine screening should be encouraged for at risk relatives of patients with breast and colon cancers. Prevention should be extended to the community at large when a notifiable communicable disease is diagnosed in an individual patient (see Table 2.3). Similarly, any suspected occupational disease in an individual worker should be reported to local health authorities. Such reporting may be critical in protecting the health of other workers in that environment (see Chapter 7).

PRACTICING PREVENTIVE CARE

Physician Performance

Despite a sound scientific base that supports the routine provision of selected preventive measures, recent studies have shown that physicians in both academic (9, 13) and community (4) practice often fail to provide them. In the practices studied, roughly 50% of highly indicated measures were offered to patients, with compliance rates highest for Pap smears, breast examinations, and blood pressure measurements (over 75%), lower for stool occult blood (20 to 50%), and lowest for mammography, tetanus, influenzal, and pneumococcal vaccinations

Table 2.3.
Notifiable Diseases, United States[a]

AIDS	Meningococcal infections
Amebiasis	Mumps
Anthrax	Pertussis
Aseptic meningitis	Plague
Botulism	Poliomyelitis
Brucellosis	Psittacosis
Chancroid	Rabies
Chickenpox	Rheumatic fever,
Cholera	acute
Diphtheria	Rubella
Encephalitis	Rubella congenital
Gonorrhea	syndrome
Granuloma inguinale	Salmonellosis
	Shigellosis
Hepatitis A	Syphilis
Hepatitis B	Tetanus
Hepatitis, non-A, non-B	Toxic shock syndrome
Hepatitis unspecified	Trichinosis
	Tuberculosis
Legionellosis	Tularemia
Leprosy	Typhoid fever
Leptospirosis	Typhus fever
Lymphogranuloma venereum	Rocky Mountain spotted fever
Malaria	
Measles	

[a] Adapted from Annual Summary and most recent issue, Morbidity and Mortality Weekly Report (see "General References"). Many individual states require reporting by physicians of additional diseases, including occupational diseases, food poisoning, animal bites, and regionally significant infectious diseases.

(30% or lower). Interestingly, in one study (4) the performance of periodic complete physical examinations correlated with improved provision of preventive measures. Favorable physician attitudes toward the preventive measures were even better predictors of performance.

Implementing a Practice Plan for Prevention

It is generally agreed that preventive care must be planned carefully if it is to be offered routinely and effectively to patients in a busy practice. First, a policy must be developed that outlines which measures are to be offered to which patients (see above). This policy can be posted, in abbreviated form, for quick reference in each examining room (Fig. 2.2). Second, a plan must be developed to implement the policy. Including "health maintenance" as a problem at the top of each patient's problem list and including a risk profile on the front sheet in the chart of each patient are means of cueing the physician to provide indicated preventive care (see Fig. 1.2, Chapter 1). Maintenance of a preventive care flow sheet (Fig. 2.3) is necessary to determine efficiently which measures are due and which have already been done. Otherwise, much time may be spent trying to retrieve relevant information that has become "buried" in the text of the chart. When an office-based computer is availalbe, it can be programmed to generate flow sheets and produce preventive care reminders for each visit, which are then attached to the front of each patient's chart (11). Nurses (3) or midlevel practitioners can be also

FRANCIS SCOTT KEY MEDICAL CLINIC

GUIDELINES FOR ROUTINE HEALTH MAINTENANCE

Baseline

History and Physical Examination (see clinic forms for physical exam and complete self-administered history)		All patients
Alcohol history		All patients
Teaching breast self-exam and giving booklet		All ♀
Cholesterol ×2		♂ & ♀, < 60
EKG		♂ ≥ 40, ♀ ≥ menopause
Osteoporosis prevention		♀, postmenopausal white
PPD (purified protein derivative)		All patients
Rubella titer		♀ childbearing age
Smoking history		All patients
STS (serological test for syphilis)		All patients

Periodic

History update	Every 5 years	All patients
Birth control	Every 1 year	♀, childbearing age
Blood pressure	Every 1 year	All patients
Breast exam	Every 1 year	All ♀ ≥ 40 High risk ♀ ≥ 30
Mammogram	Baseline and every 1–2 years	♀ age ≥ 50 High risk ♀ ≥ 35–40
Dental assessment	Discretionary	All patients
Exercise history	Discretionary	All patients
Gonococcal culture of cervix	Every 1 year	High risk
Hearing assessment	Discretionary	All patients
Hemoccult	Every 1 year	♀ & ♂, ≥ 45
Rectal, prostate	Every 2 years	♀ & ♂, ≥ 45
Influenzal vaccine	Every 1 year	High risk, age ≥ 65
Pap/gyn	Every 1 year until 35, then every 3 years if normal	♀, onset of sexual activity to age 60
PPD	Every 1 year	High risk
STS	Every 1 year	High risk
Tetanus/diphtheria immunization	Every 10 years	All patients
Visual assessment	Discretionary	All patients
Pneumococcal vaccine	Baseline, good at least 8 years	High risk

Health Maintenance Flow Sheet		All patients
Problem List		All patients
Problem-oriented Flow Sheet		Most patients with chronic active problems

Figure 2.2. Sample of abbreviated preventive care standards posted in each examining room of the Francis Scott Key Medical Center, Baltimore.

PREVENTIVE PROFILE / FLOW SHEET

DATE/STATUS	DATE/STATUS	DATE/STATUS
PPD 1979/⊖	Vision/Glaucoma 1980 glasses/⊖	Baseline Hx/PE 1979
STS 1979/⊖	Hearing 1980 nl	
Pneumovax 1979	Dental dentures	
Tetanus/Dipth. 1979	Seatbelts 1979⊖/counseled	

MEASURE\YEAR:	1979	1980	1981	1982	1983	1984				
Stool Occult Blood	⊖x3	⊖x3	⊖x3	⊖x3	⊖x3	⊖X3				
Rectal-Prostate	⊖		⊖		⊖					
Breast/Br.Self Exam	⊖ / ✓	⊖ / ✓	⊖	⊖	⊖	⊖ / ✓				
Mammogram			⊖							
Pap	I	I			I					
Flu Shot	✓	✓	✓	✓	✓	✓				

FLOW SHEET FOR SPECIFIC PROBLEMS

PARAMETER\DATE	7/79	8/79	10/80	10/81	10/82	10/83	10/84								
FEV./FVC	1.25/3.1				1.31/2.9										
RA ABG	7.42/68/40				7.46/70/68										
theophylline	4.2	12.6	14.0	11.6	12.8	13.1	ND								
theo. dose	200 qid	300 qid	—	—	—	—	—								
SMOKING	1PPD	1PPD	⊖	⊖	⊖	⊖	⊖								

Figure 2.3. Sample preventive care flow sheet. (Department of Medicine, Francis Scott Key Medical Center, Baltimore.)

trained to monitor or provide preventive care within the office. Whatever the approach, it is essential that it be an organized one.

While it is desirable to schedule special time for a baseline history and physical examination for patients new to a practice, ongoing preventive care is best incorporated into routine office visits. This is so since few visits to the doctor are purely preventive and since attendance rates are lower for preventive than for problem-based visits (16). The low attendance rates for preventive visits may be explained by low patient motivation and/or by the additional cost and inconvenience of an extra visit for purely preventive care. For otherwise healthy patients who see their physicians infrequently, however, health maintenance visits should be scheduled

and appointment reminders sent to increase attendance rates.

Motivating Patients

Unfortunately, simply recommending a preventive measure to a patient is not sufficient to ensure compliance. When the preventive measure involves an unpleasant procedure (such as sigmoidoscopy or pelvic examination) or requires active participation (such as collection and return of stool samples or the taking of chronic medication), poor compliance is likely. It is most likely to be a problem when the preventive intervention requires change in behavior on the part of the patient (such as smoking cessation).

Motivating patients to comply with recommen-

Health Hazard Appraisal

UNIVERSITY OF CALIFORNIA, SAN FRANCISCO
DEPARTMENT OF EPIDEMIOLOGY AND INTERNATIONAL HEALTH

```
JOHN Q. PATIENT                       123456    CODE  RECOMMENDATIONS               BENEFIT
CHRONOLOGIC AGE          51 YRS                  E     EXERCISE PROGRAM             3.6 YRS
APPRAISAL AGE            60 YRS      (MALE)       Q     QUIT SMOKING                 2.6 YRS
ATTAINABLE AGE          52 YRS                   W     LOSE 60 POUNDS               1.4 YRS
FOR COMPARABLE AGE AND SEX,                      R     YEARLY PROCTOSIG             0.4 YRS
   PATIENT RISK IS 2.1 TIMES AVERAGE             S     WEAR SEAT BELTS 100%         0.0 YRS

                                                       TOTAL RISK REDUCTION          8 YRS
CAUSE              DEATHS/100K    RISK TO PATIENT (AVERAGE RISK = 1)
OF DEATH          AVG.    PAT.    0        1        2        3        4        5
                                  : . . . . . . . . : . . . . . . . . : . . . . . . . . : . . . . . . . . : . . . . . . . . :

HT DIS            5874    18679   :XXXXXXXXXXXXEEEEEEEEEEEQQQQQQWWWW
                                  :XXXXXXXXXXXXEEEEEEEEEEEQQQQQQWWWW
                                  :XXXXXXXXXXXXEEEEEEEEEEEQQQQQQWWWW
                                  :XXXXXXXXXXXXEEEEEEEEEEEQQQQQQWWWW
                                  :XXXXXXXXXXXXEEEEEEEEEEEQQQQQQWWWW

CA LUNGS          1040    2392    :XXXXXXXXXXXXXXXXXXXQQQQQ
                                  :XXXXXXXXXXXXXXXXXXXQQQQQ

STROKE            666     1131    :XXXXXXXXXXXXXXXQQ

CIRRHOSIS         567     113     :XA

M- V ACC          373     216     :XXXXSS

SUICIDE           324     324     :XXXXXXXXXX

EMPHYSEMA         319     734     :XXXXXXXXXXXXXXXXXQQQQQQQQ********************K3*DISCLAIMER***

CA INTEST         303     909     :XXXXXXXXXRRRRRRRRRRRRRRRRRRRRRRR

PNEUMONIA         297     653     :XXXXXXXXXXXXXXXXXXXXXXQQ

RHEUM HT          191     19      :X
                                  : . . . . . . . . : . . . . . . . . : . . . . . . . . : . . . . . . . . : . . . . . . . . :

OTHER             4336    4336
TOTAL             14290   29507
```

*** THESE DATA SHOW ONLY RISKS OF DEVELOPING DISEASES. IF ANY OF THESE DISEASES EXIST, THEIR RISK FACTORS BECOME MEANINGLESS. DISCLAIMER. EVIDENCE OF THIS DISEASE WAS GIVEN IN THE QUESTIONNAIRE. THUS, THE RISK OF DEATH IS GREATER THAN THE APPRAISAL AGE INDICATES.

Figure 2.4. Printout of a health hazard appraisal in a 51-year-old man (17).

dations requires considerable skill on the part of the physician. Important ingredients for success include establishment of a trusting, friendly, and supportive patient-physician relationship (Chapters 3 and 4), effective patient education (Chapters 3 and 4), involvement of the patient in planning and monitoring his own health maintenance plan (Chapters 3 and 4), use of behavioral strategies to enhance compliance (Chapters 4 and 20), and the promotion of more healthy beliefs, attitudes, values, and self-perceptions in one's patients (Chapter 4). A patient's perceived *self-efficacy* or expectations for success may be the best predictor of whether he will initiate and persist in an activity (1, 19). It should always be remembered that a patient's motivation to comply may be different than the physician's motivation in wanting him to comply. Patients tend to be less impressed than physicians with long term and more impressed with short term benefits. Accordingly, the physician should stress the factors that seem to motivate the patient.

One specific and sophisticated motivational strategy, which is designed to prevent long term risks to patients in a very concrete and immediate fashion, is called health hazard appraisal. After completing a questionnaire that explores numerous health risks, the patient receives a computer-based report that (a) provides him with his risk compared to an average patient's risk of dying within a defined period of time and (b) provides him with an estimate of the amount of reduction in risk that could theoretically be accomplished if he complied with specific health-promoting recommendations (18). A sample printout is displayed in Figure 2.4. Prices for such printouts range from $3.00 to $30.00. A list of providers of such services can be obtained from the Society for Prospective Medicine (4405 East-West Highway, Suite 311, Bethesda, 20014). Preliminary studies suggest that health hazard appraisals are modestly effective counseling tools in helping some people reduce their risks. They should be considered adjuncts rather than substitutes for the personalized approach outlined above.

General References

ACS report on the cancer-related health check. Recommendations and rationale. *Ca* 30:194, 1980.

> American Cancer Society recommendations for early detection of breast, cervical, and colorectal cancer. Rationale is discussed and the report is well documented. Updated discussions of mammography appeared in the July/August 1982 issue and of fecal occult blood and sigmoidoscopy screening in the May/June 1984 issue of *Ca–A Cancer Journal for Clinicians*. This journal is available free from the American Cancer Society.

Adult Immunization, Recommendations of the Immunization Practices Advisory Committee (ACIP). Morbidity and Mortality Weekly Report Supplement 133:15, 1984.

> Overview of immunizations for adults and specific immunization recommendations.

Canadian Task Force on the Periodic Health Examination: The periodic health examination. *Can Med Assoc J* 121:1193, 1979.

> Critical evaluation of 78 preventive measures and recommendations regarding their use in periodic health examinations.

Canadian Task Force on the Periodic Health Examination: Cervical cancer screening programs: summary of the 1982 Canadian Task Force Report. *Can Med Assoc J* 127:581, 1982.

> Revised recommendations regarding screening for cervical cancer, which reduces the recommended interval between examinations from 3 years to 1 year for sexually active women between the ages of 18 and 35.

Canadian Task Force on the Periodic Health Examination: 1. Introduction. 2. 1984 update. 3. An evolving concept. *Can Med Assoc J* 130:1276, 1984.

> Re-evaluations of preventive measures for five previously reviewed conditions (chlamydial genital infections, hearing impairment in adults, hypertension, cancer of the skin, scoliosis) and for five conditions reviewed for the first time (coronary artery disease in asymptomatic individuals, carotid bruits in asymptomatic individuals, cancer of the testis, infant feeding technique, hepatitis B).

Council on Scientific Affairs, American Medical Association: Medical evaluations of healthy persons. *JAMA* 249:1626, 1983.

> Summary of recommendations for the periodic health examination from the Canadian Task Force, American Cancer Society, and others.

Guide for Adult Immunization, ed 1. Philadelphia, American College of Physicians, 1985.

> Practical and exhaustive paperback manual. Includes references. Can be ordered from American College of Physicians, P.O. Box 7777-RO325, Philadelphia, PA 19175.

Hamburg DA, Elliott GR, Parron DL (eds): *Health Behavior, Frontiers of Research in the Behavioral Sciences.* Washington, DC, Institute of Medicine, National Academy Press, 1982.

> A 359-page book which comprehensively reviews behavioral risk factors for morbidity and mortality, their effects on health, and their alteration.

Health Information for International Travel. Published yearly by the Center for Disease Control, U.S. Department of Health and Human Services, as a supplement to the Morbidity and Mortality Weekly Report.

> This monograph provides up-to-date and comprehensive information on immunization requirements and health recommendations for international travelers.

Healthy People. The Surgeon General's Report on Health Promotion and Disease Prevention, US Department of Health, Education and Welfare/Public Health Service (publication no. 79-55071), 1979.

> A readable 177-page philosophical and factual account of the present health status of Americans, by age group, and of the broad range of specific preventive care and health-promoting actions recommended for the 1980s.

Medical Practice Committee, American College of Physicians: Periodic health examination: a guide for designing individualized preventive health care in the asymptomatic patient. *Ann Intern Med* 95:729, 1981.

> Summary of recommendations from the Canadian Task Force, American Cancer Society, and others.

Morbidity and Mortality Weekly Report. Atlanta, Center for Disease Control, Department of Health and Human Services. Printed and distributed by the Massachusetts Medical Society, SCPO Box 9120, Waltham, MA 02254-9120.

> A weekly report containing very current information about communicable disease incidence (for example, regional incidence of influenza), updated recommendations of communicable disease prevention, and timely reports on outbreaks of a wide variety of preventable diseases.

Specific References

1. Bandura A: Self-efficacy; toward a unifying theory of behavior change. *Psychol Bull* 84:191, 1977.
2. Bergman AB, Stamm SJ: The morbidity of cardiac non-disease in school children. *N Engl J Med* 276:1008, 1967.

3. Davidson RA, Fletcher SW, Retchin S, Duh S: A nurse-initiated reminder system for the periodic health examination. Implementation and evaluation. *Arch Intern Med* 144:2167, 1984.

4. Dietrich AJ, Goldberg H: Preventive content of adult primary care. Do generalists and subspecialists differ? *Am J Public Health* 74: 223, 1984.

5. Hamburg DA, Elliott GR, Parron DL (eds): The contribution of behavior to the burden of illness. In *Health and Behavior, Frontiers of Research in the Behavior Sciences*. Washington, DC, Institute of Medicine, National Academy Press, 1982, p 33.

6. Hampton ML, Anderson J, Lavizzo BS,, Bergman AB: Sickle-cell "nondisease": a potentially serious public health problem. *Am J Dis Child* 128:58, 1974.

7. Haynes RB, Sackett DL, Taylor DW, *et al*: Increased absenteeism from work after detection and labeling of hypertensive patients. *N Engl J Med* 299:741, 1978.

8. Knibbs S, Jackson JGL: In Keen H, Jarrett J (eds): *Complications of Diabetes*. Chicago, Year Book, 1975, p 265.

9. Kosecoff J, Fink A, Brook RH, *et al*: General medical care and the education of internists in university hospitals: An evaluation of the Teaching Hospital General Medicine Group Practice Plan. *Ann Intern Med* 102:250, 1985.

10. Leske MC, Rosenthal J: Epidemiologic aspects of open angle glaucoma. *Am J Epidemiology* 109:250, 1979.

11. McDonald CJ, Sui LH, Smith DM, *et al*: Reminders to physicians from an introspective computer medical record. A two-year randomized trial. *Ann Intern Med* 100:130, 1984.

12. Milio N: *Primary Care and the Public's Health*. Lexington, MA, DC Heath, 1983, p 34.

13. Romm FJ, Fletcher SW, Hulka BS: The periodic health examination: comparison of recommendations and internist's performance. *South Med J* 74:265, 1981.

14. Rubenstein LZ, Josephson KR, Wieland GD, *et al*: Effectiveness of a geriatric evaluation unit. A randomized clinical trial. *N Engl J Med* 311:1664, 1984.

15. Rubenstein LZ, Rhee L, Kane RL: The role of geriatric assessment units in caring for the elderly: an analytic review. *J Gerontol* 37:513, 1982.

16. Sackett DL, Snow JC: The magnitude of compliance and noncompliance. In Haynes RB, Taylor DW,, Sackett DL (eds): *Compliance in Health Care*. Baltimore, Johns Hopkins University Press, 1979, p 11.

17. Stokes J, Noren J, Shindell S: Definitions of terms and concepts applicable to clinical preventive medicine. *J Community Health* 8:33, 1982.

18. Werra RJ, Petrakis NL: Prospective medicine. In Rakel RE (ed): *Textbook of Family Practice*. Philadelphia, WB Saunders, 1984, p 175.

19. Wilson GT: Cognitive factors in life style changes: a social learning perspective. In Davidson PO, Davidson SM (eds): *Behavioral Medicine: Changing Health Lifestyles*. New York, Brunner/Mazel, 1980.

CHAPTER THREE

The Doctor-Patient Relationship: Communication and Patient Education

ARCHIE GOLDEN, M.D., MARSHA GRAYSON, M.A., EDWARD BARTLETT, PH.D., AND L. RANDOL BARKER, M.D.

After leaving the hospital, a patient who has emphysema was overheard telling her husband, "You know I don't really feel any better. This going into the hospital for a few days and then not feeling better afterwards hardly seems worth it." When her husband asked, "What do you think the problem is?," the patient replied, "I think it's the medication. I told the doctor, but he didn't really seem to pay any attention. But I really think it's the medication. If it isn't any better in a few days, I'm going to see another doctor."

The evolution of American medical practice over the last 50 years has witnessed a movement from office practice mixed with house calls to a pattern of practice characterized by a much more rapid pace, a greatly enlarged armamentarium of diagnostic tests and therapeutic regimens, and virtually no house calls. Because of the elimination of the house call, there is a tendency to know less about the personal, social, and psychological side of the patient and to rely more on test results to assess a patient. This trend was already noted in 1927 by Francis Peabody when he wrote in the *Journal of the American Medical Association*, "The most common criticism made at present by older practitioners is that young graduates have been taught a great deal about the mechanism of disease, but very little about the practice of medicine—or, to put it more bluntly, they are too 'scientific' and do not know how to take care of patients" (14). He went on to say, "One of the essential qualities of the clinican is interest in humanity, for the secret of the care of the patient is in caring for the patient."

THE DOCTOR-PATIENT RELATIONSHIP

Our society's concept of the doctor-patient relationship has evolved through the years. Over three decades ago, Parsons described the patient's role as essentially passive (13). Later Szasz and Hollender (17) outlined the following three types of interactions between physician and patient: the *active-passive* relationship, in which the physician has all authority (similar to Parson's conceptualization); the *guidance-cooperation* relationship where the physician still is somewhat authoritarian and the patient cooperates; *mutual participation*, where there is active collaboration between patient and physician and the patient assumes more responsibility for his care. The consumer movement of the 1960s and 1970s promoted an increase in the mutual participation relationship between doctors and patients (9). This relationship requires the physician to get to know his patient better, restoring to practice a feature which was integral to the house call.

Each doctor-patient relationship is established through a person-to-person interaction. The goals of the doctor-patient interaction are to (a) obtain valid information from patients; (b) provide information and ensure that the patient comprehends it; (c) achieve patient satisfaction; (d) assure patient compliance; and (e) attain optimum outcome for patients. The attainment of these goals depends equally upon the physician's knowledge of medicine and upon his use of effective and efficient communication.

COMMUNICATION

The Importance of Effective Communication

The importance of effective communication has been confirmed in a variety of studies of the doctor-patient relationship.

Gathering of *valid information* and getting the

patient to disclose fully the reasons for a visit are two goals which are achieved better by physicians trained to utilize effective communication skills (7). *Satisfaction* with the physician correlates well with high interactional skills in the physician (8), and *compliance* with medical regimens is related strongly to satisfaction (5). In addition, medication errors occur less frequently when the physician utilizes effective techniques to communicate instructions (6). Finally, there is mounting evidence that the incidence of *malpractice* is related to the communication between the physician and the patient (15).

While information gathering and receiving may appear to be the primary reason for direct communication with patients, the *therapeutic nature* of the interaction is an essential component of the healing power of the physician. If data gathering and giving were the only goals of the interaction, then patients could fill out a questionnaire on their symptoms, and the physician could read the response and provide a treatment plan. This would result in an efficient and cost-effective method of providing medical care but would not produce much satisfaction for the patient or the physician. As summarized by Reiser and Schroder (16):

"Repeatedly, physicians will feel the power of something intangible, yet unmistakable, in the nature of the doctor-patient relationship that helps a sick person to get better. It is hard to overestimate the potency and curative potential of this very unique and special relationship. For all our technical advances, this relationship remains one of medicine's most powerful therapeutic tools."

The Fundamental Communication Skills

Recognizing Patient Expectations

Over the past 20 years, research on the doctor-patient relationship has delineated the communication skills that are effective in interactions with patients. The appropriate use of these skills requires that the physician understand the patient's expectations about an office visit.

It is essential for physicians to understand *what it is like for a patient to be seen by a doctor*. Patients come to the office with anxieties concerning what the doctor may find wrong with them. Patients know that their doctor has a busy schedule, and they are reluctant to ask what the doctor may regard as trivial questions. Some social distance often exists between doctor and patient, and the combination of this and the physician's special knowledge gives the physician a great deal of authority. As a result, patients may be reluctant to contradict or correct their physicians' statements; may block or misrepresent their thoughts or feelings in order to provide answers they think the physician wants to hear; and may not ask

for clarification despite being confused by medical terminology. Finally, during the physical examination, some patients feel embarrassment at being exposed, and this may further inhibit disclosure of important concerns. While a long-standing relationship with a physician will diminish these sources of discomfort, it can be expected that most patients possess some degree of uncertainty during an office visit, and it behooves the physician to ask, "If I were this patient, how would I be feeling during this visit?"

The component of communication that most facilitates disclosure of concerns by the patient is the *development and maintenance of rapport*. Rapport is basically a feeling that one has of being with a "friend." Three basic elements of rapport are trust, respect, and understanding. Rapport develops when a physician demonstrates genuine interest in the patient and when both the doctor and the patient feel they have been heard and understood. These conditions create a safe atmosphere so that the patient feels comfortable talking about matters that he might otherwise feel reluctant to discuss. Essential to the development of rapport is the ability of the physician to *be empathetic* toward the patient's problems. Empathy requires careful listening by the physician and demonstration of understanding of the problem to the patient. The physician can indicate listening by maintaining eye contact and leaning forward. Empathetic statements include both content and feeling, e.g., "I can tell that you're feeling angry because your retirement plans are on hold." Each of the other behaviors and skills described below facilitates the development of rapport.

Planning the Interaction

It is important to review critical information about a patient before actually seeing him. Scanning the record will remind the physician of the reason for this visit, will assure that he is updated on important information from previous visits, and will help him to establish a tentative agenda. This preinteraction planning, accomplished in 1 or 2 minutes, allows the physician to indicate a familiarity with the patient's problems when greeting him and eliminates the need to rummage through the chart in the presence of the patient. With the information the physician has gained from the record review, the message transmitted to the patient is one of familiarity and interest.

Opening the Interaction

Upon first greeting a patient, the physician should shake the patient's hand, use the patient's name, and, if it is a first visit, introduce himself. The first few moments are crucial because the physician and the patient are sizing up one another, and nonverbal behavior will take precedence over what is being said. Both the physician and the patient are paying attention to physical features, type of handshake, voice tone and pitch, age, dress, and overall demeanor. *The seating arrangement* of the office should be conducive to the development of rapport. Where space allows, the patient's and the physician's chairs should be arranged so that the patient and the physician are facing one another without a desk between them. Thus, the patient's chair should be situated on the side of the physician's desk rather than opposite the desk. An attentive posture should be maintained by leaning forward slightly.

The eyes are a primary medium of expression and often tell more about an individual's message than words. *Eye contact* is thus an essential element in establishing and maintaining rapport. Looking at one's watch or at the chart while discussing a patient's problem signals to the patient that the physician is not listening, is not interested, or is too busy to be answering questions that the patient may be reluctant to ask. While eye contact is one of the best methods for conveying interest, staring can be uncomfortable and should be avoided.

Gathering Information

For gathering information about a patient's problems, it is pertinent to *begin with an exploratory approach* and move to a more directive approach as needed. An exploratory approach is usually more efficient, aids the physician in detecting underlying problems, and indicates interest in the patient. The most appropriate method for initiating an inquiry is the *use of open-ended or exploratory questions.* Open-ended questions allow patients to discuss symptoms or express concerns in their own words. Asking the patient "How have you been doing since your last appointment?" is an appropriate open-ended question for a follow-up visit. For a new patient visit, or a visit requested by the patient, the physician will want to explore the reason for the visit by asking "Please tell me what brings you in today?" This type of opening provides an opportunity for the patient to describe his reasons for the visit and does not imply that there is a problem. There is a tendency for physicians to ask "What seems to be the problem?" This question implies that a problem exists when the patient may be there for preventive care. Once the patient defines the reason for the visit, the physician can continue to use open-ended questions.

In response to the physician's opening inquiry, a patient might respond "Well, I haven't been doing so well lately. My shoulder has been giving me a problem." While the physician might go on to explore the shoulder problem, he will find it helpful with most patients to ask if there are any other problems that the patient wants to discuss at the visit. If the physician assumes that the patient wishes to discuss only one problem and goes on to

ask about the shoulder problem, then, as the interview progresses, the physician may find himself frustrated as additional problems are brought up throughout the visit. By having the patient name each of his concerns at the outset, this dilemma can be avoided. If several issues are mentioned by the patient, it is quite appropriate to ask "Which problems seem to be bothering you the most?"

If the patient does not name other problems, the physician should continue with open-ended questions to explore the main problem. For example, "Tell me about the shoulder pain." The patient will then be able to describe the problem in his own words. Open-ended questions should be curtailed with patients who tend to produce extraneous information.

Exploratory questions can be used throughout the interaction. When the physician wants to inquire about the patient's life situation, an appropriate question is "Tell me, how have things been going at home?" When the patient produces information that needs clarifying, additional exploratory questions are helpful to establish a common meaning. For example, if the patient complains for the first time of constipation, the physician will want to explore what this means to the patient, e.g., "What do you mean by constipation?" The physician may discover that the patient moves his bowels every other day and yet believes that this means constipation.

The patient rarely provides all of the information needed to evaluate a problem, and the physician will have to use more direct questions to obtain the additional information. *Direct questions* are those questions that require a specific response. For example: "When did you first notice the pain?" or "What words would you use to describe the pain?" or "Can you show me where the pain is?" When seeking specific information, physicians should *avoid asking leading questions,* i.e., questions that tend to elicit predetermined answers, usually in the form of a simple "yes" or "no." For example: "You don't have the pain every day, do you?" This leading question gives the message to the patient that the physician does not expect the pain to occur every day. If the patient is somewhat passive, he may agree to whatever the physician suggests even if the answer is not accurate. Once the patient has responded inaccurately, he may become distracted and forget to report important information related to his symptoms.

When a patient is unable to provide needed information, it is sometimes necessary to *give the patient a number of choices* from which to select. For example, if the patient reports chest pain but is unable to provide accurate information about whether the pain radiates, the physician might ask "Does the pain seem to go anywhere else, such as to your back, one of your arms, your neck, or your legs?" While the physician may have an idea of the likely response, this will not be obvious to the patient since the patient is given several choices. This is contrasted with a question such as "Does the pain move to your left arm?" which is a leading question giving the patient the distinct impression that this is the correct answer.

A patient will at times give a vague, aggregate description of an episodic symptom, and the physician will find it extremely helpful to have the patient *describe in detail a single episode*. For example, "Let's discuss the last time you felt the nausea and crampy pain . . . ."

When asking questions, it is important to *ask only one question at a time* and to phrase each question so that it refers to one piece of information. Thus, when the patient responds the physician knows what the patient is referring to in his response. For example, to questions such as "Are you having any problems sleeping or eating?" or "Are you constipated or do you have diarrhea?" a positive response may not reveal which is the problem. Conversely, a negative response may only refer to one of these problems, but the physician may incorrectly assume that the patient is not having either problem.

While responding to questions, the *patient may give verbal cues* related to the discussion or concerning other issues that will need exploration. At times, it is appropriate to pursue a verbal cue when it is mentioned, and at other times it will be more appropriate to pursue it later in the interaction. If a verbal cue is pertinent to the present discussion, it is helpful to repeat the patient's words or to ask an open-ended question to explore what the patient means. For example, in response to a question about pain, a patient may respond "Well, it seems to have gotten worse lately, but maybe its just my nerves." Here, an appropriate response would be an open-ended question such as "Your nerves?" or "What do you mean?" An example of a verbal cue the physician would explore at a later time would be a response to a question about sleep disturbance due to pain, such as "Sometimes I wake up in the middle of the night, but it isn't because of the pain." Since the physician is exploring the pain at this time, it would not be appropriate to pursue the patient's sleep problem. However, it would be an important problem to pursue later in the interaction.

A patient's *nonverbal cues* may provide important information. The physician not only needs to pay attention to the content of the message but to the vocal message as well, including the pitch, the tone, and the tempo; each of these may confirm or contradict the content of the patient's verbal message. Nonverbal messages also include what has been called "body language." When interpreting nonverbal messages, the particular situation and person should be taken into account. The physician needs to distinguish between a patient's usual habits of seating, talking, and gesturing and any nonverbal

behavior that is out of character for that patient. For example, although crossing one's legs when seated may be a sign of defensiveness, many people do so out of habit and for comfort. It may be presumptuous to assume such patients are feeling defensive based on seating alone. Elements of body language that can be observed are the patient's seating position (e.g., sitting on the edge of the chair suggests apprehension, facing away from the physician suggests mental discomfort); head position (e.g., held back in defiance, anxiety, or fear; or held down in sadness); facial expression (eyes, eyebrows, and forehead show the greatest range of emotions, including surprise, fear, anger, happiness, disgust, sadness); hands (ringing or rubbing of hands can show anxiety, clenched fists or pounding on the table can show anger); arms and legs (crossing of the arms and legs can signify resistance or defensiveness). An astute physician will routinely notice when there is congruity or incongruity between what the patient says and his body language. At times, incongruity in these factors will be the only indicator of an important problem which the patient is hesitant to disclose.

When gathering data, it is important to ensure that one's *judgments* are not visible to nor imposed upon the patient. Generally, judgmental statements are conveyed by the way in which one speaks rather than by the content of the message. The inflection and tone of voice can convey judgment on the part of the physician.

The data-gathering phase should always include inquiry about the *patient's life situation*. Awareness of the patient's life situation can be instrumental in developing a diagnosis or management plan, and attention to this information makes the patient aware of the physician's interest in him. This includes information about family, household members, work, stress, personal relationships, support systems, finances and daily activities, and other family members.

Organizing the Flow of the Interview

The importance of setting a tentative agenda before greeting the patient and then having the patient disclose his own additions to the agenda has been mentioned above. There are a number of other ways in which a visit can be organized to assure optimal effectiveness and efficiency. They are:

1. Keeping the interview focused upon *one problem at a time.*

2. *Delineating the essential features of each problem,* including the meaning of the problem to the patient. The following checklist is useful to keep in mind when assessing new problems: (a) chronology—onset date and time, duration, frequency and time of day of symptoms, duration of symptoms during a typical episode, course over time, remote history of a similar problem; (b) quality—nature of

a symptom (in the patient's words), location, radiation; (c) quantity—severity of symptoms and of functional impairment; (d) aggravating and alleviating factors; (e) associated factors or symptoms; (f) description of a descrete episode; (g) patient's working diagnosis for the problem and associated fears or concerns related to that working diagnosis.

3. *Utilizing transitional statements* to assure that the patient understands when the focus of the interview is changing. This is especially important when the physician wishes to explore a sensitive topic, such as the patient's personal life (e.g., "Since this is your first visit, I would like to find out more about you.").

4. *Summarizing periodically.* This helps by letting the patient know that the physician has heard what he said and by giving the patient the chance to clarify or expand on important information.

5. *Using vocabulary consistent with the patient's background* and avoiding formulations which may confuse the patient, e.g., telling a patient that his test results are "negative" may convey to the patient that something is wrong.

6. *Taking notes in a fashion that does not diminish rapport* with the patient. It is helpful to point out that one will be making a few notes during the visit; it is equally helpful to suspend the interaction entirely while writing or dictating the complete note for the chart.

7. Communicating appropriately during the *physical examination.* This includes describing what one is doing and avoiding the tendency to give important information (diagnosis and plan) during the physical or when the patient is getting dressed; both are instances when the patient is distracted and cannot be expected to focus upon the physician's message or to formulate his questions as well.

Closing

At the close of a visit, it is important to accomplish a number of rather concrete tasks, i.e. (a) summarize, by problem, the assessment and plan, assuring that the patient comprehends these (see patient education below); (b) ask if there are any further questions; (c) schedule a follow-up visit at an appropriate interval; (d) instruct the patient explicitly to phone back when this is indicated, e.g., when there is a symptom whose status is important to the physician or when the physician will know the results of a diagnostic test of interest to the patient, *etc.* At the end of the visit the physician should use rapport-generating techniques that will re-emphasize interest and concern for the patient. Actions such as shaking the patient's hand or touching the patient on the shoulder, using the patient's name, and encouraging him to call for any interval problems will help to impress upon the patient the physician's interest in him.

Difficult Situations

All physicians have been faced with difficult patients and situations in medical practice. Patients may be difficult for the physician to care for because of their style of communicating, because of the nature of their disease(s), because of their failure to adhere to appropriate treatment or behavior, because they rarely or never respond positively to the physician's efforts, or because they have lifelong maladaptive personalities. Difficult situations occur because of a lack of understanding on the part of the physician, the patient or the patient's family or because of the nature of the illness. A number of these situations are covered in Section 2 of this book (Psychiatric and Behavioral Problems).

It is common for physicians to react negatively in a variety of ways to difficult patients and situations. Table 3.1 summarizes common negative reactions of physicians and strategies for dealing with these reactions.

Here we discuss three difficult situations common in practice (the need to communicate bad news, dealing with angry patients, and dealing with demanding patients) and communication strategies that may be useful in dealing with them.

Communicating Bad News

Physicians frequently must inform patients of the seriousness of their condition. While some patients will be aware of their condition before hearing a specific diagnosis from the physician, other patients will not realize the seriousness of their problem. When the physician is ready to discuss the problem with the patient (and family), he should be direct and use terminology that the patient can understand. Because patients are often incapable of comprehending much information upon first learning of their illness, treatment, and prognosis, it is essential to give patients an opportunity to let the information "sink in" by using silence or an empathetic inquiry. The physician can present the options of care to the patient at this time but will probably have to repeat this information at a later time. For example:

Doctor Jones: Mrs. Smith, How are you today?

Mrs. Smith: I'm okay, but I've been anxious about the results.

Doctor Jones: Well, I'm sorry to tell you Mrs. Smith, but the test showed that the lump is cancer. (Direct and understandable)

Mrs. Smith: I was afraid of that. (Patient looks down and begins to cry)

The physician at this point has several choices: (a) remain seated and silent; (b) go over to the patient, put a hand on the patient's shoulder, and remain silent; (c) encourage the patient to talk about what

Table 3.1.
Common Negative Responses of Physicians to Difficult Patients and Strategies to Cope with These Responses[a]

Physician's Emotional or Behavioral Reaction	Coping Strategies
Avoidance	Analyze why; attempt to understand and master feelings that lead to avoidance; stay with the patient; discuss with colleagues
Identification with patient	Recognize, avoid tendency to deny seriousness of disease or to give way to despair; stay with the patient
Hostility/rejection	Acknowledge and analyze; do not attempt to like the unlikable patient; use behavioral approaches; if situation is intolerable, transfer patient to another physician
Feelings of impotence, inadequacy (e.g., in caring for dying patient)	Discover areas in which help and comfort can be rendered physical and emotional; be realistic about limitations of medicine; give the patient time to go through the stages of bereavement
Feelings of loss of control or threatened authority	Acknowledge and analyze; be realistic about personal limitations and actual range of influence and authority; be aware that patient's need for control over his own body may conflict with physician's urge to control the situation
Frustration, confusion, uncertainty about dealing with the patient; coping strategies not effective	Request psychiatric consultation/referral
Anxiety, guilt, and frustration about meeting patient's recognized emotional needs	Allocate time realistically according to need; request consultation/referral

[a] From Gorlin R, Zucker HD: Physicians' reactions to patients. *N Engl J Med* 308:1059, 1983.

she is thinking by using an empathetic statement such as "This is really frightening to you."

Later, after the patient has calmed down:

Doctor Jones: I know this seems terrible to you, but let's talk for a few minutes about the treatment options and what's going to happen. There does not appear to be any spread of the cancer . . . .

Communicating with Angry Patients

Anger displayed by patients can be appropriate or inappropriate. Anger should be recognized as an appropriate response to serious illness or poor treatment, especially if the anger is displayed by a patient who generally does not display traits of anger. Anger is inappropriate when it is displayed by individuals who are hostile for reasons that are not evident. Such patients usually have underlying psychosocial disorders (see Section 2, Psychiatric and Behavioral Problems).

Most people respond with anger when confronted with someone who is angry. The physician should try always to avoid becoming angry and rather should ask himself why the patient is angry. If the physician does not understand the source of the anger, then it is appropriate to say to the patient, "You seem angry." Approaching the patient with understanding and recognizing the anger and its source will help to reduce the anger. If the source of the anger is the physician, a nurse, a technician, or other office or hospital personnel, then the physician should apologize even if he is not personally respon-

sible. For example, if a patient is upset with something a nurse said, the physician should respond: "I'm sorry this has happened. I will try to find out what the problem is." For example:

A 30-year-old female patient has been complaining of chest pain. Several tests were ordered and the results were negative. The patient, however, is still experiencing the chest pain. At her next visit her husband comes with her.

Doctor Jones: How are you doing, Mrs. Smith?

Mrs. Smith: Well, I'm still having these chest pains.

Doctor Jones: Have they changed any since our last visit?

Mrs. Smith: Well, I'm not sure; I think they may be getting worse, I . . . .

Mr. Smith: You know, doctor, you keep saying that everything is okay, but she's still got the chest pain. They're getting worse. What are you gonna do if something happens to her?

Doctor Jones: You seem angry and quite concerned about your wife. I understand your concern, but I don't understand your anger.

Mr. Smith: You're right, I'm angry. You haven't done a thing to get her better.

The physician has uncovered an initial source of anger, the husband's concern over his wife and the feeling that the physician has not done anything. The physician could ask Mr. Smith, "What do you mean?" but this may sound rather defensive. Another approach would be to review what has occurred thus far in the diagnosis and treatment of the chest pain. After a full discussion, if Mr. Smith still seems uncomfortable with Dr. Jones' care, he should ask if Mrs. Smith would like to see another physician to get a second opinion.

Communicating with Demanding Patients

Physicians often have difficulty with demanding patients. A demanding patient is one who requests certain tests and medications repeatedly, who calls frequently, or who has many visits with multiple complaints. Usually there is an underlying dependency, as well as anger, and this manifests itself when the physician gets angry himself or attempts to avoid the patient's demands. When dealing with a demanding patient, the physician must first recognize the source of his anger and/or avoidance (4); then deal with it. The danger in such a reaction is that real medical problems will be overlooked and/or the patient will move on to another physician following the same demanding pattern.

Patients who are demanding can be dealt with and helped, although one should not expect changes in their basic character. First, the physician must set limits and be firm in maintaining the limits. Phone calls should be limited in number, as should the number of office visits. A common type of demander is one who requests specific medications, e.g., penicillin for a cold. A frequent patient ploy is the threat to go to another physician if the requested medication is not granted. A full explanation and firmness in sticking to the appropriate treatment are essential.

The demanding patient has illnesses that need treatment. The good physician can deal with these if he tries to understand the patient and his own feelings and sticks to the limits that have been set with the patient.

PATIENT EDUCATION

Introduction

The word doctor means "teacher." Most practicing physicians today would not identify their doctoring as teaching, and most would agree that little of their medical education concerned the acquisition of teaching skills. Observational studies have shown that physicians caring for ambulatory patients devote about 25% of their direct patient care time to patient education and counseling (3). This represents a substantial amount of time. It is generally not necessary to devote more time than this to educating and counseling. It is important, however, to assure that these activities are conducted effectively and efficiently.

If a physician has been effective as a teacher, then his student (in this case the patient) should confirm this (a) by demonstrating understanding of his illness; (b) by carrying out actions favorable to his health; and (c) by gaining the health benefits which accrue to these actions. A useful exercise for physicians is to imagine the "tests" a patient's spouse probably administers when the patient returns home from visits to the doctor. The patient's answers to his spouse's questions indicate how effective his teacher (doctor) has been. Questions such as the following are commonly asked:

So what does he think it is?
But how long will you feel this way?
Will it get worse?
Will it ever come back?
Did he tell you whether this could be an early sign of cancer?
Do you think we can still take the hot air balloon ride to Peoria?
How long will you be taking these new pills?
Will the new ones be okay to take with the old pill?
If you don't feel anything wrong why should you have to take the medicine anyway?
What were the three tubes of blood taken for? Sounds like you have something serious!
Does the echo test hurt much?
How long will you have to be in the hospital for the catheterization?
How do we get hold of the doctor if you do black out again?
Do you really think that Dr. Smith is right about all these things?

The previous section of this chapter describes the fundamental communication skills needed to elicit an accurate history. These are the same skills that are essential to effective patient education. The following discussion defines patient education and provides guidelines for integrating it into office practice.

Definition of Patient Education

Patient education is defined as a process whereby a patient learns about his health status and then adopts behavior(s) favorable to his health. All members of the staff of an office practice may contribute to patient education, including physician, nurse, secretary, and others. For example, the office secretary may explain to the patient how the practice works, while a nurse may learn of special concerns that the patient is hesitant to discuss with the physician.

Clinical experience and research have supported the principle that *knowledge is necessary, but not sufficient, to assure behavior change.* Studies of the impact of patient education upon a number of conditions have confirmed this principle (1, 2, 11, 12). More than information is usually needed when the patient is expected to make a life style change, varying from fitting a medication regimen into his daily routine to altering long-standing pleasurable habits, such as overeating and smoking.

Integrating Patient Education into the Visit

Patient education occurs throughout the three phases of a typical office visit—history taking, physical exam, and closure of the visit. The process begins when an *educational diagnosis* is made, i.e., the patient's informational and/or behavioral needs are identified. Some degree of educational diagnosis occurs at every visit. The patient may state his needs in the form of specific questions; the physician may note misinformation or information gaps in what the patient says; or the *physician may infer the patient's needs* (e.g., a patient newly diagnosed with chronic lymphocytic leukemia in its asymptomatic stage, or a regular patient in whom the physician suspects noncompliance as the explanation for poorly controlled hypertension). At times, a patient's informational needs may be the source of significant psychological distress (see "Meeting Informational Needs" in Chapter 11).

When an educational diagnosis has been made, the physician has the task of assuring that the patient learns both the information he needs and the skills (behaviors) he needs to deal with his medical

problem. The case report on page 38 illustrates the process of making an educational diagnosis and designing an effective educational intervention.

Guidelines for Providing Information

In most chapters of this book, the patient education content related to specific problems is described. The following general guidelines are important in providing information to patients.

1. *Assure that rapport has been promoted* in the various ways noted earlier (see page 31) and that the patient is able to give his full attention to you (e.g., not getting dressed, not trying to discuss another subject, *etc*).

2. When explaining a problem, its treatment, and the expected outcome, *summarize using explicit categorization*, as this is the most effective approach. Table 3.2 compares this approach to the usual approach for conveying the same information to a patient with a chest infection.

3. *Have the patient demonstrate comprehension* of the most important information you have just conveyed. Because it has been found that patients

Table 3.2.
The Effect of Explicit Categorization on Recall of Verbal Medical Information Given to a Layperson[a]

Usual Presentation of Information	Explicit Categorization of Information[b]
1. You have a chest infection.	'I am going to tell you: what is wrong with you
2. And your larynx is slightly inflamed.	what tests we are going to carry out;
3. But I think your heart is all right.	what I think will happen to you;
4. We will do some heart tests to make sure.	what treatment you will need; and
5. We will need to take a blood sample.	what you must do to help yourself'.
6. And you will have to have your chest X-rayed.	First, what is wrong with you . . . (statements 1–3)
7. Your cough will disappear in the next 2 days.	Second, what tests we are going to carry out . . . (statements 4–6)
8. You will feel better in a week or so.	Third, what I think will happen to you . . . (statements 7–9)
9. And you will recover completely.	Fourth, what the treatment will be . . . (statements 10–12)
10. We will give you an injection of penicillin.	Finally, what you must do to help yourself . . . (statements 13–15)
11. And some tablets to take	
12. I'll give you an inhaler to use.	
13. You must avoid cold draughts.	
14. You must stay indoors in fog.	
15. And you must take 2 hours' rest each afternoon	

[a]Adapted from Ley P, Bradshaw, PW, Eaves D, Walker CM: A method for increasing patients' recall of information presented by doctors. *Psychol Med* 3:217,1973.
[b] When the information in the left column was explicitly categorized (see right column), recall of information was 50% higher.

tend to recall the diagnosis better than the treatment plan (10), it is especially important to ascertain retention of the essentials of the plan, e.g., for a streptococcal throat infection, that penicillin will be taken for a full 10 days (not the exact dose or schedule, which will be transcribed onto the pill bottle).

4. *Whenever appropriate, provide written information* as an adjunct to what you tell the patient. Since patients retain only about one-half of the essential information communicated at a visit (10), some written information should be given to the patient at the end of most visits. Written information includes *individual instructions* (e.g., modification in the way a current medication is to be taken, instructions to call back on a certain day, *etc*; see example, Fig. 3.1), in addition to *preprinted patient education materials*. When individual instructions are given in writing, consider having the patient sign those instructions, indicating comprehension or agreement with what is written. When a printed item is given to a patient, it is a good idea to personalize it by underlining important points, writing down additional information that you judge important, and writing the day's date on it. A useful collection of printed educational handouts is available in the book by Griffith (see "General References").

Guidelines for Overcoming Obstacles to Behavior Change

There are four steps to overcoming obstacles to behavior change:
1. Assessing the extent of compliance with indicated behavior.
2. Identifying the obstacles to compliance.
3. Using indicated educational intervention(s).
4. Assessing the response to educational interventions.

General strategies for carrying out these four steps are outlined in Chapter 4, Patient Compliance with Medical Advice. Specific strategies are described in chapters covering the many conditions for which behavior change is fundamental to treatment. Table 3.3 lists common problems identified in behavioral diagnosis and educational strategies for addressing them.

Case Illustrating Educational Diagnosis and Intervention

The following case example illustrates the process of making an educational diagnosis and designing specific educational interventions.

A 30-year-old black male actor sought care because "his blood pressure was up again." Severe hypertension was diagnosed in this patient at least 5 years ago and has been treated intermittently since that time. As the patient stated, he had "gotten rid of his high blood pressure several times," only to have it come back again, despite having seen several physicians and having taken "lots of medicine."

Further questioning revealed that, although the patient always tried to do what the doctor said, it was troublesome to remember or to take the time to ingest all 12 pills each day because he worked and had family responsibilities. Moreover, it was hard to keep all of the doctor's appointments and even more difficult to maintain a salt-free diet because he did not do the family cooking. His wife could not understand his illness, since he did not feel or look bad, and thus it was very difficult to ask her to cook separate meals for him. In general, his family found his treatment needs demanding and interfering.

The patient was quite aware of why hypertension needed treatment, and he desired to keep his blood pressure under control. He was willing to come for

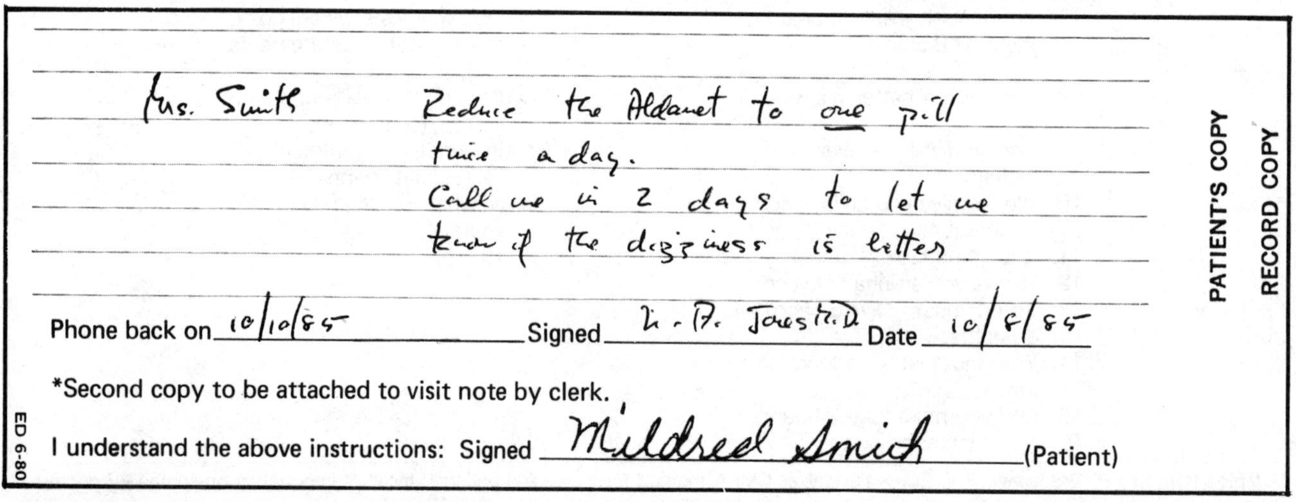

Figure 3.1. Examples of written instructions for a patient (form makes a copy for the patient's folder). (Source: Francis Scott Key Medical Center, Baltimore.)

Table 3.3.
Common Problems Affecting Behavior and Some Strategies for Addressing Them[a]

Finding of Behavioral Diagnosis	Educational-Behavior Strategies
INDIVIDUAL	
1. Lack of awareness or understanding	Teaching, instructional aids, repetition
2. Lack of confidence to control condition	Reassurance, encouragement, attribution, peer group discussions
3. Forgetfulness	Simplifying regimen, cueing pill taking to other activities, providing weekly pill dispenser, involving friend or family member
4. Denial	Supportive exploration of patient's feelings and perceptions, avoiding "sledgehammer" method of sharing diagnosis
5. Inadequate motivation	Pointing out dangers of untreated condition (fear arousal) and benefits of therapy, paradoxical mention, increasing frequency of visits
6. Fear of getting hooked on drugs	Trying nonpharmacological treatment, reassuring patient that drugs will be used as little as possible, explaining known side effects
7. Lack of skills	Demonstration and guided practice
8. Behaviors that are repetitive and unconscious (smoking, diet)	Applying behavior modification techniques (stimulus control, contingency management, recording behavior, contracting, cueing, modeling, etc)
9. Reluctance to accept sick role	Giving patient as much freedom and respect as possible, exploring patient's feelings
10. Psychiatric disturbance	Psychiatric referral, psychotherapy, chemotherapy
11. Skepticism toward provider's statements	Respecting patient's feelings, providing medical textbooks and journals, referring for second opinion
SOCIAL	
12. Lack of support from family, friends, and teachers	Calling significant other on telephone, inviting to accompany patient to next clinic visit, making home visit, asking patient to talk to significant other, using mass media
13. Poor relationships with health provider	Developing provider communication skills, improving accessibility and continuity of care
ENVIRONMENTAL	
14. Inadequate money to purchase medications	Prescribing generic drugs, giving free drug samples, prescribing less expensive drugs, referral to social worker
15. Inadequate money to pay for health care	Providing free care, referral to social worker, community organizing
16. Long clinic waiting time	Using practice management to decrease waiting time, having patient see only nurse at follow-up visit
MEDICAL REGIMEN	
17. Side effects	Taking medications with meals, substituting medications
18. Complex regimen	Simplifying regimen, cueing medication taking with other activities, reducing dosage

[a] From Bartlett EE: Behavioral diagnosis: A practical approach to patient education. *Patient Counseling Health Educ*, 4:29, 1982.

care in order to control his blood pressure but was "getting tired of not getting anywhere." In brief, he simply wanted a safe, effective, and relatively simple way to control his blood pressure.

From an educational perspective, the following problems of the patient were diagnosed:

1. Lack of family understanding and support.
2. Difficulty incorporating the requirements of therapy into his daily life situations.
3. Belief that the problem would "go away."

4. Increasing discouragement regarding his ability to control his high blood pressure.

Thus the approach taken to address these perceived problems included the following educational efforts:

1. Inviting the patient's wife to come to the office to educate her regarding hypertension, the need for dietary and drug therapy, and how she could positively support her husband.
2. Decreasing the number of medications, and

developing with the patient mechanisms by which the drug-taking behavior could be cued to other daily behaviors, e.g., taking pills twice daily, with breakfast and dinner.

3. Educating the patient regarding his belief that hypertension could be cured, with the accompanying frustration and discouragement when it was not.

4. Explicitly describing the specific behaviors that the patient should follow regarding maintenance of diet, appointment keeping, and medication taking.

5. Providing management and support to the patient to follow the regimen.

The effectiveness of the educational efforts was evaluated in the following ways:

1. Self-reports of dietary and medication adherence.

2. Appointment-keeping behavior.

3. Patient's perception of family understanding and support.

4. Patient's reported sense of confidence to control his hypertension.

5. Level of blood pressure.

After 1 year of treatment and educational support, the patient found it much easier to remember to take his pills twice a day, and reported that he took his medication about 80% of the time. He also reported that he added salt to his food very infrequently and that he felt more support and cooperation from his family. He was cautiously optimistic about continuing to control his blood pressure in the future. His blood pressures at his last two visits have averaged 150/94, as contrasted to readings averaging 200/138 1 year ago.

Integrating Patient Education into an Office Practice

It is possible to enhance the overall patient education effort in an office practice by addressing some practical management issues.

1. *Nurses* frequently have considerable interest in patient education, and involving them in this effort can save physician time and can enhance the effectiveness of care. Of course, a nurse engaging in patient education should have the communication skills needed for effective patient education. These have been described earlier in this chapter. Many office practices involve the nurse in educating patients about preventive measures such as breast self-examination, family planning, and the like. In other practices, nurses play a larger role in patient education by working with patients newly diagnosed with such chronic illnesses as diabetes, asthma, or hypertension. In these instances, it is important to delineate in advance which information will be covered by the nurse and which will be covered by the physician.

2. A certain amount of general patient education can be promoted in the waiting room, by setting up a *pamphlet rack* containing 10 to 15 of the most useful printed materials. These might include pamphlets on smoking cessation, weight reduction, low salt diets, exercise, and other topics of interest to patients and their families. Some practices have found it helpful to have a bulletin board with newspaper clippings about current health topics. Finally, removal of ashtrays and a no-smoking policy are important ways in which the waiting room can be a healthful atmosphere that reminds smokers of the possibility of discontinuing their habit.

3. One of the most innovative methods of actively involving patients in their care is the establishment of a *patient advisory group*. This idea has been tried in small and large practices. A patient group can be effective not only in channeling suggestions and complaints but also in helping to promote patient education in the office and to develop community health education programs.

General References

Bartlett EE (Ed): *The Patient Education Newsletter.*
> Twice-monthly newsletter published since 1978, covering new developments, scientific perspectives, controversies, publications related to patient education. (Address for subscription: 720 South Twentieth St., Birmingham, AL 35294.)

Enelow AJ, Swisher SN: *Interviewing and Patient Care.* New York, Oxford University Press, 1978.
> A sound general outline of interviewing with practical applications.

Green LW, Kreuter MW, Deeds SD, Partridge KB: *Health Education Planning, A Diagnostic Approach.* Palo Alto, CA, Mayfield, 1980.
> A valuable book that takes the reader from educational diagnosis to education techniques in patient care.

Griffith HW: *Instructions for Patients,* ed 3. Philadelphia, WB Saunders, 1982.
> Soft-bound collection of one to two page instructions, which can be reproduced for individual patients, on over 200 conditions. Includes anatomical sketches of most organ systems, useful for instructing patients.

Specific References

1. Bartlett EE: The contributions of consumer health education to primary care practice: a review. *Med Care* 18:862, 1980.
2. Cogan R: Effects of childbirth education. *Clin Obstet Gynecol* 23:1, 1980.
3. Flynn B: Completion of referrals for hypertension screening. *Physician's Patient Education Newsletter,* December, 1980.
4. Groves JE: Taking care of the hateful patient. *N Engl J Med* 298:883, 1978.
5. Hulka BS, Kupper LL, Cassell JC, et al: Medication use and disuse: physician-patient discrepancies. *J Chronic Dis* 28:7, 1975.
6. Hulka BS, Kupper LL, Cassel JC, et al: Doctor-patient communication and outcomes among diabetic patients. *J Community Health* 1:15, 1975.
7. Hutler MJ, Dungy CI, Zakus GE, et al: Interviewing skills: a comprehensive approach to teaching and evaluation. *J Med Educ* 52:328, 1977.
8. Korsch B, Negrete V, et al: Doctor-patient communication. *Sci Am* 227:66, 1972.
9. Levin K, Katz AH, Holst E: *Lay Initiatives in Health.* New York, Prodist, 1976.
10. Ley P: Psychological studies of doctor-patient communication. In Rachman S (ed): *Contributions to Medical Psychology,* I. Oxford, Pergamon Press, 1977.

11. Mazzuca SA: Does patient education in chronic disease have therapeutic value. *J Chronic Dis* 35:521, 1982.
12. Morisky DE: Five year blood pressure control and mortality following health education for hypertensive patients. *Am J Public Health* 73:153, 1983.
13. Parsons T: *The Social System.* Glencoe, IL, The Free Press, 1951.
14. Peabody FW: The care of the patient. *JAMA* 89:1127, 1927.
15. Reeder LC: The patient-client as a consumer: some observations on the changing professional-client relationship. *J Health Soc Behav* 13:406, 1972.
16. Reiser DE, Schroder AK: *Patient Interviewing: The Human Dimension.* Baltimore, Williams & Wilkins, 1980.
17. Szasz T, Hollender MH: A contribution to the philosophy of medicine—the basic models of the doctor-patient relationship. *Arch Intern Med* 97:585, 1956.

CHAPTER FOUR

Patient Compliance with Medical Advice

DAVID E. KERN, M.D., AND WALTER F. BAILE, M.D.

The first section of this chapter reviews in detail what is known about patient compliance with medical advice. The short section at the end provides practical guidelines for preventing or managing noncompliance and refers the reader to relevant information contained in the first section.

INTRODUCTION

The following case example is representative of a common problem in office-based practice:

Example: Mr. Y is a 45 year-old black male who feels dizzy at work. A blood pressure check shows a reading of 180/110. He is told that his "pressure is up" and is referred to a physician. Mr. Y has not seen a doctor in 20 years. After an appropriate physical examination and laboratory work the diagnosis of essential hypertension is confirmed. The physician is happy because he knows that there are efficacious medicines which will prevent complications of hypertension such as stroke and congestive heart failure. The patient is given medication, takes it for a couple of weeks, feels better, and then stops taking it.

In the above example, the physician might have been more successful if he had addressed the following questions: What is Mr. Y's understanding of hypertension and its management? What is the source of his information? What are his beliefs about the relationship between symptoms and high blood pressure? (A symptom precipitated its detection.) Why has Mr. Y not seen a doctor in 20 years? How does he view himself (in control of his destiny or controlled by forces beyond himself, at risk of or magically protected from disease, *etc*)? What is his value system, and where do health promotion and disease prevention fit in?

Before consulting a physician, a patient may already have tried a number of remedies for his symptoms, consulted family, friends, or lay practitioners, and developed half-formed or inaccurate models to explain his illness. His age, sex, race, ethnic background, family, social class, education, past experience, and place in history will have affected his view of the problem and the world. While he is likely to be more informed about medical care than patients were in the past, he is also more likely to be skeptical of the medical profession. He may have read about successful malpractice suits and medical mistakes, heard about bad experiences in medical care from friends, or had them himself. He is likely to come from a lower socioeconomic class, be less educated, and have a different value system than the physician. He may have underlying fears and concerns, and certain expectations for the visit, but be reluctant to express them for fear of being thought foolish.

The physician may be well motivated and highly trained in the diagnosis and treatment of physical disease. He is less likely to have developed his interviewing, communication, and teaching skills to an equivalent degree. Although he may make a diagnosis and prescribe effective treatment, he may not detect or allay the patient's underlying concerns or meet the patient's expectations for the visit. It is likely he will assume that the patient's value system is similar to his own. It is even more likely he will fail to uncover the patient's beliefs about and understanding of the illness. If he has failed to establish rapport and to explain things adequately, the patient may not trust him.

Given the difference in perspectives, it is not surprising that patient noncompliance with medical advice is an extremely prevalent condition. Fortunately, our understanding of this common problem has improved during the past two decades, during which over 2000 articles on the subject have been published. While methodological problems still exist in compliance research, a sufficient number of well designed studies and a sufficient amount of concordance in results among studies exist to provide clinically useful guidelines. It is true that most studies of factors associated with compliance are cross-sectional, making inferences of causality subject to error. However, an increasing number are prospective. Most studies of compliance have involved hospital-based ambulatory patients, leaving questions about their general applicability; but when private patients have been studied, results tend to be similar. Numerous studies now exist which evaluate the short term effectiveness of various interventions designed to improve patient compliance. The development and assessment of strategies to maintain such improvements are areas where research is needed.

DEFINITIONS AND CLASSIFICATION

Patient compliance is defined as the extent to which the patient adheres to medical advice. It encompasses taking medications, keeping appointments, undertaking recommended preventive measures, and, with respect to activities such as dieting, exercising, and ceasing to smoke or take alcohol, changing possibly deep seated behavioral patterns. Some clinicians favor the term *patient adherence* to *patient compliance*, but the latter is more widely used.

Noncompliance can be caused by a failure to understand instructions, *noncomprehension*, or can exist in the presence of adequate understanding, *volitional noncompliance*.

Noncompliance in medication taking can be classified as *errors of omission* (a prescribed medicine is not taken), *errors of commission* (a nonprescribed medicine is taken), *dosage errors* (the wrong dose is taken), and *scheduling errors* (the medicine is taken according to the wrong schedule, e.g., once daily instead of twice).

Noncompliance should be viewed as a neutral term with neither negative nor positive connotations. It describes one aspect of patient behavior which may be either appropriate or inappropriate to the patient's best interests. For example, it may be appropriate for a patient with mild chronic obstructive pulmonary disease to be noncompliant in taking a regularly prescribed medicine, such as aminophylline, if it causes more distress (e.g., nausea) than relief. On the other hand, it would be inappropriate for a patient with severe hypertension to stop taking antihypertensive medication because of denial of his medical problem. In view of the not insignificant frequency of documented prescribing errors and unwise prescribing patterns, patients are justified in critically questionning their particular regimen (7, 25, 27, 30, 32, 33). That patients may exercise sound judgment is suggested by higher compliance rates for seemingly more important medications, such as cardiac, diabetic, and antihypertensive agents, than for seemingly less important agents, such as sedatives, antacids, and drugs prescribed for symptomatic relief (2, 14–16). Finally, it should be realized that responsibility for noncompliant behavior often rests with the physician. It is not valid, for example, to blame noncompliant patients for failure to understand instructions or to realize the importance of therapy when there has been ineffective communication by the physician (see Chapter 3 on patient education).

IMPORTANCE OF COMPLIANCE

Problems Caused by Noncompliance

Patient noncompliance is potentially important from at least four perspectives: individual patient care, public health efforts, interpretation of the medical literature, and economic consequences.

First, patient noncompliance with efficacious therapeutic regimens may thwart the goals of both physician and patient in reducing suffering, preventing illness, improving functional status, and increasing longevity. If the physician is unaware of the patient's noncompliance, he may falsely attribute a poor outcome to inadequate dosage, failure of the regimen itself, or incorrect diagnosis. Any of these conclusions could lead to inappropriate action by the physician. Thus medication might be changed or dosage might be increased, and new diagnoses entertained, so that the patient could be subjected to unnecessary procedures and testing.

Second, noncompliance may increase the cost and reduce the effectiveness of screening, immunization, and disease control programs. For example, a screening program which identifies undiagnosed hypertensives will be less effective and will cost more for each hypertensive complication prevented if the dropout rate after screening is high or compliance with medication is low.

Third, noncompliance may influence the outcome of the therapeutic trials upon which important recommendations are based. Dose-response curves (dose plotted on the abscissa and response on the ordinate) may be shifted to the right by noncompliance, resulting in falsely high estimates for toxic and therapeutic doses. A falsely large response range for a given dose may be reported because of variation in subjects' compliance. In therapeutic trials, noncompliance in the treatment group will reduce the power of the study to detect significant differences between treatment and placebo. Furthermore, differences in compliance among different treatment groups may lead to false conclusions regarding their relative efficacy. Most therapeutic trials now include methods to exclude noncompliers at entry and to monitor compliance in participants. However, subjects chosen on the basis of proven compliance may not be representative of the population from which they were drawn. Patients with type A (competitive, driving, and independent) personalities, for example, may be less likely to enroll in a coronary prevention program (26) but more likely to have a myocardial infarction. Their under-representation in prevention programs could decrease the overall risk of myocardial infarction for enrollees compared to controls. In the Coronary Drug Project trial of the usefulness of lipid-lowering therapy (3), those subjects who adhered strictly to their regimen of clofibrate had a substantially lower 5-year mortality than those who did not, but so did those control subjects who adhered strictly to their prescribed placebo.

Fourth, noncompliance with indicated medical regimens has been shown to increase medical costs by increasing hospitalization rates for cardiac and other patients, by causing nursing home placement in the elderly, and by increasing utilization of outpatient services (31).

Prevalence of Noncompliance

The high prevalence of noncompliance underlines the importance of the problem. Reported noncompliance rates must be viewed critically and compared with caution, because of differences in definition from study to study. Nevertheless, the results of extensive reports are almost unanimous in identifying noncompliance, variably defined, as an *extremely prevalent* condition. Rates vary from less than 10% to over 90%, depending on the setting. Owing to previous dropouts, cross-sectional studies of patients taking medication chronically tend to underestimate noncompliance, but even then noncompliance is often in the 20% to 70% range. Among newly diagnosed hypertensives, for example, up to 50% fail to follow through with referral advice; over 50% of those who begin treatment drop out by 1 year; and only about two-thirds of those who stay under care consume enough prescribed medications to achieve adequate blood pressure reduction (13).

A review of the literature leads to the following additional conclusions:

1. Noncompliance rates tend to be higher for preventive care than for treatment of established illness.

2. There is a marked increase in noncompliance with duration of therapy.

3. Noncompliance is highest for regimens that require significant behavioral change, such as smoking cessation or weight loss.

4. Missed appointments are more common for provider-initiated than patient-initiated visits. Asymptomatic patients are more likely to miss appointments than symptomatic patients.

5. Lack of comprehension of a regimen is a common cause of noncompliance. Unfortunately, most studies do not separate noncomprehension from willful noncompliance, but where studied, noncomprehension has been shown to be responsible for 20% to 70% of objectively measured noncompliance.

MEASUREMENT OF COMPLIANCE

General Considerations

Various methods are available for measuring compliance. Unfortunately, there is no gold standard of validity and each method has strengths and weaknesses. Of general concern are the following issues:

First, it should be recognized that compliance is usually defined arbitrarily. Ideally compliance should be defined in terms of its relationship to therapeutic efficacy. For example, 80% compliance may be required to ensure blood pressure reduction (12), while evidence suggests that consumption of only about one-third of prescribed medicines provides some protection from recurrence of rheumatic fever (22).

Second, compliance reported in terms of percentages does not reflect sequential behavior. For example, omitting medications for 1 week could have an impact on therapeutic efficacy quite different from missing a few doses per week over a much longer period; yet the percentage compliance might be identical.

Third, measuring compliance in populations requires additional considerations. The magnitude of the noncompliance problem will depend upon the particular population at risk (*i.e.*, the denominator), which should be clearly stated. Compliance rates will be higher, for example, for a clinic population studied at a single time than for a clinic population studied longitudinally from the inception of therapy, since only the latter approach adequately accounts for patients who completely drop out from care. The compliance distribution (percentage of patients versus percentage of compliance) should also be reported, since its pattern can vary markedly (Fig. 4.1). Reported compliance distribution curves have varied from U-shaped in children given rheumatic fever prophylaxis (10), to skewed bell-shaped for patients taking chronic antacid therapy (28), to relatively uniform for patients taking antituberculous (18), chronic oral hypoglycemia (8), or psychopharmacological (23) therapy. The shape of the curve may influence the choice of strategies designed to improve compliance. For example, in the case of a U-shaped distribution, attempts to improve compli-ance might best be directed toward the most non-compliant group of patients, whereas the entire population might be a better target when compliance is normally distributed.

Methods of Measurement

There are several approaches to assessing compliance behavior in patients. Since each method has some limitations, it is *often necessary for the physician to use more than one method* to arrive at a reasonably valid estimate of compliance in the individual patient.

Asking

The simplest and most practical method of assessing compliance behavior is to ask the patient. Self-reports of noncompliance are generally valid, although the degree of noncompliance tends to be underestimated. There is even some evidence that patients who admit to being noncompliant may be more amenable to intervention than those who do not (19).

Only about 40% to 80% of patients admit their noncompliance, however, so self-reported compliance cannot be relied upon. In studies of various patient populations, reported compliance rates have almost always overestimated true compliance rates.

Since the *manner of asking* influences response, it is generally agreed that patients should be questioned about compliance in an open-ended, facilitative, nonthreatening, nonjudgmental way. For example:

Ineffective Method:

Doctor: Now, Mrs. Smith, are you taking your medications as prescribed? (judgmental; leading question, which allows a "yes/no" and promotes a "yes" answer; confines response to medications)

Patient: Yes, every day.

Result: The doctor raises dose or adds new medication because her blood pressure is still not adequately controlled. The patient becomes frustrated.

Effective Method:

Doctor: Now, Mrs. Smith, can you tell me what you are doing to control your blood pressure? (open-ended; nonjudgmental; focuses responsibility on patient; does not confine response to medications)

Patient: Well, I've stopped adding salt to my food and have pretty much cut out all salted snacks. I do occasionally have a frozen dinner when I'm alone. And, of course, I'm taking the medication.

Doctor: Uh, huh . . . . (facilitative)

Patient: Yes, that blue pill.

Doctor: And how are you taking it? (directive, not leading)

Patient: Twice a day.

Doctor: Any other medications? (directive, not leading)

Patient: No. I stopped the fluid pill when we started the blue one.

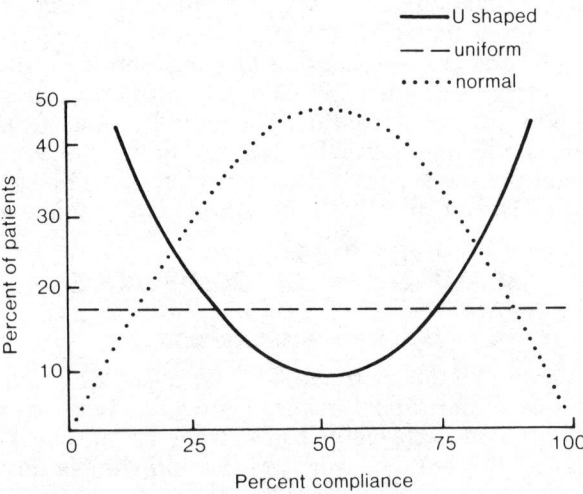

Figure 4.1. Possible compliance distributions.

Doctor: And did you take the blue one this morning? (directive)

Patient: No, I never take my medicine the day I come to the office!

Doctor: What about yesterday? (directive)

Patient: Yes ... at least in the morning. Yesterday afternoon was so hectic! You know how busy my days are!

Doctor: I guess it's hard to take that afternoon dose? (facilitative, nonjudgmental)

Patient: Yes, because my schedule varies so much.

Doctor: What did you decide about starting on an exercise program? (directive, nonjudgmental, shifts responsibility to patient)

Patient: Thought about it, but haven't done anything yet. Do you really think it's important?

Result: The doctor congratulates (positively reinforces) the patient on salt restriction, tailors a medication regimen to the patient's schedule, explains why she should take her medication on the day of an office visit, provides more information on the value of regular exercise, and provides written instructions/contract to which both he and the patient agree. He decides not to restart the diuretic (which he had not planned to discontinue), because of the patient's compliance with salt restriction and the lack of a blood pressure reading on the current medication regimen. If the dietary history had been less convincing or the patient had gained weight, he might have asked her for a 24-hour diet recall (which is more accurate than general questioning) on this and subsequent visits.

Medication Counting

Medication counting provides a more objective measure of compliance than does simply asking patients, and it has been used to demonstrate the lack of reliability of patient-reported compliance. Results are usually expressed in terms of percentages, which facilitate the construction of population distribution curves. The ability to measure sequential behavior depends upon the use of short intervals between counts, which is usually not feasible. While more accurate than reported compliance, medication counts are still not perfect. If the patient is suspicious of being monitored, he can remove medicines from containers without ingesting them. Overestimates of compliance can also occur if other persons are using medicine from the same container. Compliance may be underestimated if the patient is using more than one medication container but only makes one available for counting. Furthermore, many patients do not bring their medication containers with them to the physician's office, despite reminders. Finally, some patients might take offense at having their medications counted, resulting in deterioration of the physician-patient relationship.

The medication count can be approximated by the more practical and less intrusive method of prescribing quantities of medication which should be consumed within a reasonable interval of time, and then observing the *frequency with which prescription renewals are requested.*

Ingenious medication dispensers have been devised which monitor not only the amount but also the regularity with which medicine is removed. They are bulky, however, and are not commercially available.

Assays

Another objective method of estimating compliance behavior involves testing drug levels in blood, urine, breath, or saliva. Drug levels have been shown to correlate with compliance determined by other methods as well as by outcome. Marked variation in drug levels may reflect inconsistencies in medication taking. Monitoring drug levels and relaying results to the patient may also serve as stimuli to improve compliance.

However, there are limitations to the method. Assays can be expensive. For accurate assessment, multiple measurements are required over an extended period. There is the possibility that, if the patient knows he is being monitored, he may take medicine immediately before the collection of specimens but not at other times. More important may be differences in drug absorption, distribution, metabolism, and excretion among individuals, making it impossible in the individual patient to decide whether a low level represents noncompliance or inadequate dosage. The absence of any drug in the specimen suggests noncompliance, assuming the specimen has been collected appropriately. The physician should have a working knowledge of the pharmacokinetics of the medicine being assayed, so that the collection of specimens can be timed correctly. Compliance with short acting drugs, which are rapidly cleared from the blood and excreted, is difficult to monitor by assay techniques because of the difficulty in collecting specimens at appropriate times. Finally, assays are not available for many medications.

Practical information on routinely available assays is presented in Table 4.1.

Outcome

An even more indirect but objective method of estimating compliance is the monitoring of expected therapeutic or physiological outcomes. For example, blood pressure can be followed in a patient taking antihypertensive medication, weight in a patient on a weight reduction diet, and pulse rate in a patient prescribed a β-blocker. Many of the limitations of drug assays also affect assessment of outcome, which can be influenced by variations in drug bioavailability, absorption, distribution, and excretion; multiple measurements are required. Furthermore, other factors can influence outcome. For example, a reduction in stress may lower blood pressure or the presence of concomitant heart disease might be responsible for bradycardia.

Table 4.1.
Drug Assays Routinely Available for Monitoring Patient Compliance with and/or Response to Prescribed Medication[a]

Medication	Half-Life (Hours)[b]	Time to Peak Level (Hours)	Preferred Timing of Specimen[c]	Usual Therapeutic Level in Serum
Anticonvulsants				
Phenytoin (diphenylhydantoin, Dilantin)	22 (range 7–42)	1.5–3 (prompt action) 4–12 (extended release)	Trough	10–20 µg/ml
Phenobarbital	72 (range 50–140)	6–18	Trough	15–40 µg/ml
Primidone (Mysoline)	3–12[d] 72[e]	2–4[d] 6–18[e]	Morning trough[d] Trough[e]	6–12 µg/ml[d] 15–40 µg/ml[e]
Carbamazepine (Tegretol)	10–30	2–18	Trough	4–12 µg/ml
Ethosuximide (Zarontin)	60 (adults) 30 (children)	1–7	Morning trough	40–100 µg/ml
Valproic acid (Depakene)	6–16	1–4	Morning trough	50–150 µg/ml
Clonazepam (Clonopin)	20–40	2–4 (range 1–8)	Morning trough	0.005–0.07 µg/ml
Antiarrhythmics				
Quinidine	5–8[f]	1–2 2–5 (sustained release)	Trough	1–6 µg/ml[g]
Procainamide (Pronestyl)	2–5	0.5–1.5	Trough	3–8 µg/ml
Phenytoin (diphenylhydantoin, Dilantin)	22 (range 7–42)	1.5–3 (prompt action) 4–12 (extended release)	Trough	10–20 µg/ml
Digoxin (Lanoxin)	36–48	1.5–5	Post distribution phase (8–24 hours after last dose)	0.5–2.0 ng/ml
Lithium	Average 24 (range 10–36)[h]	1–4 4–12 (extended release)	12 hours after last dose[h]	Maintenance: 0.7–0.9 mEq/liter Acute treatment: 0.9–1.4 mEq/liter
Salicylate	3–6 (low doses) 15–30 (high doses)	1.5–2	Peak (2–3 hours after last dose)[j]	5–10 mg/dl analgesia 15–30 mg/dl antiarthritic
Theophylline	4 to >24[j]	2–3 3–14 (sustained release)	Trough[k]	10–20 µg/ml
Tricyclic antidepressants				
Amytriptyline (Elavil, Endep)	15–45[l]	2–12	Morning trough (about 10 hours after last dose)	>120 ng/ml[m]
Desipramine (Norpramin, Pertofrane)	10–76[l]	2–8	Morning trough (about 10 hours after last dose)	>125 ng/dl[m]
Doxepin (Sinequan, Adapin)	6–19		Morning trough (about 10 hours after last dose)	>90 ng/ml[m]
Imipramine (Tofranil, SK-Pramine, Presamine)	8–24[l]	1–8	Morning trough (about 10 hours after last dose)	>95 ng/ml[m]
Nortriptyline (Aventyl, Pamelor)	16–90+	4–9	Morning trough (about 10 hours after last dose)	50–140 ng/dl
Protriptyline (Vivactil)	50–200	24–30	Morning trough (about 10 hours after last dose)	70–170 ng/dl

Supervision

An additional approach to assessing compliance is to compare drug levels or outcome of therapy during supervised versus unsupervised periods of medicine consumption. Depending upon the pharmacokinetics of the drug, supervision may be accomplished either in the office or in the hospital.

Physician's Ability to Predict Compliance

The need to measure compliance becomes obvious if one considers that studies have shown that physicians are *poor* at predicting compliance behavior in their patients, sometimes performing no better than would be expected by chance. Whether physicians can improve their performance by making determined efforts or by specific training remains to be evaluated.

FACTORS ASSOCIATED WITH COMPLIANCE

There are multiple determinants of compliance behavior, and no single factor or small group of factors seems to account for all of the noncompliance in any study population. Factors associated with noncompliant behavior can be classified as being related to the patient, the disease, the environment, the treatment, or the physician-patient relationship (Table 4.2). Physicians need to be aware of the most important of these associations in order to improve their ability to predict and manage noncompliance in their own patients.

Patient Characteristics

Surprisingly, such *sociodemographic* variables as age, sex, race, education, occupation, income, and marital status usually do not correlate with compliance behavior. Elderly patients, however, have been shown to have difficulty in opening childproof medication containers, and they may be at increased risk for noncomprehension. *Alcoholism and drug addiction* tend to correlate highly with noncompliance. *Previous compliance or concurrent compliance* with one aspect of treatment usually correlates with adherence to other aspects of the regimen. *Psychological factors*, such as depression, immaturity, impulsivity, paranoia, hostility, fear of dependence, denial, commitment to a bad decision, and type A personality, might be expected to correlate with noncompliance, and in some studies such associations have been demonstrated. Internal locus of control, or the extent to which a patient feels in control of his environment, rather than vice versa, is usually associated with compliant behavior. Factors which affect the patient's ability to comprehend, including a language barrier, dementia or mental retardation, or the presence of a major psychiatric illness, such as schizophrenia, which affects the patient's ability to organize and initiate deliberate behavior, should be expected to affect compliance adversely. More-

---

[a] See also Chapters 15, 59, and 80 and References 1a, 9a, 14a, 19a, 23a, 26a, 33a, and 33b.

[b] Steady state serum concentrations of a drug are reached after approximately four half-lives. It is, therefore, advisable to delay measurement of serum drug level until four to five half-lives after the last dosage change. (Serum level is 94% of steady state at four half-lives, 97% of steady state at five half-lives.)

[c] Recent drug studies of anticonvulsants and antidepressants, on which therapeutic ranges are based, have used morning trough levels. For some well absorbed drugs, peak levels may be nearly twice trough levels. Drugs which are slowly absorbed and have long half-lives, such as phenobarbital and phenytoin, have small daily fluctuations. For such drugs, use of trough levels is less crucial.

[d] For primidone.

[e] For phenobarbital (metabolite of primidone).

[f] Sustained release forms of quinidine prolong its release into the gastrointestinal tract over 8 to 12 hours. The elimination half-life of quinidine is 5 to 8 hours, once absorbed.

[g] Therapeutic levels of quinidine, based on nonspecific assay methodology, are usually 1.5 to 7.0 µg/dl. Quinidine levels are generally lower when specific assays are used, and effective reduction of ventricular premature contractions has been reported with levels <1.0 µg/ml. Physicians should check the methodology and the recommended therapeutic range for their laboratory.

[h] Lithium elimination occurs in two phases. There is an initial steep drop in serum lithium levels for 5 to 6 (up to 12) hours, followed by a slower elimination over the next 24 hours or more. Hence, serum levels should be drawn 12 hours after the last dose.

[i] Timing is not critical when used in high dose because of prolonged half-life.

[j] Theophylline's half-life averages 4 to 5 hours in smokers, 7 to 9 hours in nonsmokers. Older adults with obstructive pulmonary disease and any patients with heart failure or liver disease may have much lower clearance rates, with half-lives over 24 hours. Various preparations are available that prolong the duration of effect by delaying absorption.

[k] Use of trough levels is less important for the sustained than for the regular release preparations.

[l] Half-life is longer in elderly than in younger patients.

[m] Upper limit is not established.

Table 4.2.
Factors Associated with Compliance

Patient characteristics
    Health beliefs and values (+ or −)[a]
    Alcoholism and drug addiction (−)
    Psychological factors (+ or −)
    Patient symptomatic (+)[b]
    Previous noncompliance (−)
Disease features
    Schizophrenia, personality disorders, paranoid disorders,
       and dementia (−)
Environmental factors
    Stable, supportive family and social support system (+)
    Waiting time (−)[b]
    Individual *versus* block appointment system (+ *vs* −)[b]
    Time between referral and appointment (−)[b]
Treatment factors
    Complexity of regimen (−)
    Duration of therapy (−)
    Requirement for behavioral change (−)
    Side effects (−)[c]
    High cost (−)[c]
    Medication class (+ or −)
Features of the physician-patient relationship
    Supervision (+)
    Effective transfer of information (+)
    Justification of regimen (+)
    Provider confidence (+)
    Provider friendliness (+)
    Provider effort to motivate patient (+)
    Negotiation, rather than dictation of regimen (+)
    Meeting of patient expectations (+)
    Patient satisfaction (+)
    Continuity of provider care (+)

[a] +, positively associated with compliance; −, negatively associated with compliance.
[b] Compliance with appointment keeping.
[c] While cost and side effects may be responsible for noncompliance in individual patients, they usually have not been a significant overall determinant of noncompliance in study populations.

over, many patients who come to physicians are experiencing considerable anxiety, which may interfere with cognitive functioning of which comprehension is one element. Understanding may be further hampered by the tendency of many patients, such as blue-collar workers, to ask few questions of their physicians even when they desire information (11).

Other important patient characteristics which are often overlooked are "*health beliefs.*" Patients' beliefs about the severity of an illness, their susceptibility to an illness or its complications, the efficacy of treatment, and barriers to therapy have usually been found to be associated with compliance behavior. As distinguished from disease, which is an objective entity based upon the presence of independently verifiable findings, a patient's experience of illness is a subjective state which is shaped by personal, interpersonal, and cultural factors. It is the patient's perceptions of disease and treatment that correlate with compliance rather than the objective realities. An extreme example occurs in patients who deny illness. Thus, myocardial infarction patients, who answer "no" or "maybe" rather than "yes" when asked if they have experienced a heart attack, are less likely to comply with physicians' instructions for decreased activity and reduced cigarette smoking (4).

Patients often have their own *models of disease* and treatment. If this model conflicts with the regimen prescribed for the patient, noncompliance may follow. For example, the not uncommonly held perception of hypertension as an intermittent, symptomatic, stress-related condition encourages an erratic approach to medication taking. Some patients with clearly diagnosable soft tissue injuries may feel that their evaluation was incomplete without an X-ray and therefore mistrust the physician's diagnosis. Ethnic concepts of disease and treatment can also conflict with the physician's approach to diagnosis and management and result in noncompliance. Such concepts are more prevalent among ethnic group members who experience a language barrier, are generationally close to immigration, live in segregated neighborhoods, are lower in education level and socioeconomic class, and experience barriers to receiving personalized medical care—i.e., these who are least integrated into the mainstream culture. For example, some black patients might change physicians or refuse treatment if they are told they have both "high blood" pressure and a "low blood" count (anemia). According to some folk beliefs these diagnoses are mutually exclusive, so the physician making them may be regarded as ignorant. Among Mexican Americans, lay understanding and management of *caide de la mollera* ("fallen fontenelle") in infants can result in a failure to understand the importance of rehydration therapy in diarrheal disease.

Finally, the patient's *value system* may conflict with that of the physician. An elderly patient, for example, may prefer to accept an increased risk of death rather than endure the inconvenience, impersonalization, and separation from house and family resulting from hospitalization.

Features of the Disease

Unlike severity as perceived by the patient, actual disease severity is usually not associated with compliance behavior. Diagnosis *per se* shows little correlation with compliance, except for patients with schizophrenia and certain personality disorders, especially those with paranoid or antisocial features, who tend to be less compliant.

Environmental Factors

Patients who have stable *support systems* and stable *family situations* tend to be more compliant. A spouse's concern about a patient's illness can encourage compliance with medication taking, appointment keeping, and prescribed behavior changes (such as diets and smoking cessation). On the other hand, adherence to the *cultural norms* of social class, ethnicity, family, age, and sex are likely to supersede adherence to the norms of the medical profession when the two are in conflict. It should be remembered that a patient's previous experience of *similar disease among* his *relatives or friends* can profoundly affect his beliefs about his illness. *Advice from friends, family, and lay practitioners* can also be influential.

Appointment keeping is positively correlated with *appointment scheduling systems* which reduce waiting time, give individual rather than block appointments, minimize the time between scheduling and the actual appointment date, and make referrals to specific doctors rather than to clinics.

Treatment Factors

The *complexity of the medical regimen* usually correlates inversely with compliance. In the studies done to date, the number of medications seems more important than the number of daily doses, although both can be important. Unsynchronized schedules (e.g., one drug every 4 hours and another every 6 hours) should also be expected to affect compliance adversely. *Side effects* of medications are mentioned relatively infrequently in the compliance literature, but clearly may cause noncompliance when they cause significant symptoms or interfere with an important function in the individual's life (e.g., impotence secondary to an antihypertensive drug in a young sexually active man). *Medication class* has already been noted to be related to compliance, with seemingly more important drugs (such as cardiac and diabetic agents—over 70% compliance in cross-sectional studies) resulting in higher compliance rates than seemingly less important medicines (such as antacids and drugs prescribed for symptomatic relief—less than 50% compliance). The reason for these differences is unknown and could conceivably be due either to sound patient judgment or to increased physician emphasis, supervision, and teaching. The relationship between independently audited medication need and compliance remains unexplored.

The *duration* of therapy and the requirement for significant *behavioral change* (e.g., weight reduction or smoking cessation) have been previously mentioned as negatively associated with compliance.

Doctor-Patient Relationship

Close supervision of the patient by the physician (or his assistant) has proved a consistent and significant correlate of compliant behavior. In most studies, *continuity* in provider care has also contributed.

Establishment of a good patient-physician relationship is being increasingly recognized as an important determinant of patient compliance. While *effective communication* is a prerequisite to the establishment of such a relationship, studies show that physicians commony communicate poorly with their patients (6, p 29; 9, 33). However the necessary skills can be learned (see Chapter 3) and are being taught with increasing frequency in medical schools, residencies, and continuing education courses. Among the aspects of the communication process that have a demonstrated relationship to patient compliance are the following:

Effective transfer of information is important, since the patient must first understand a regimen before he can be expected to comply with it. To improve retention, instructions need to be clear, concise, explicit, and categorized by subject matter, with important features emphasized and repeated (21). Since patient factors, such as anxiety and reluctance to ask questions, may interfere with understanding, it has been found useful to test the patient for receipt and retention of instructions and to supplement verbal with written instructions. The use of medical jargon needs to be avoided, while use of language should be geared to the educational and cultural backgrounds of the recipient.

It should be remembered that the physician may be the last resource on a long road of self-medication and lay consultation, and that the patient may already have some ideas and concerns about his problem. The physician must, therefore, *justify* or explain the rationale behind a regimen, and in the process detect and correct or accommodate any misconceptions which might interfere with compliance.

Other features of the communication process which seem to correlate with patient compliance include: fulfillment of patient expectations (requires detection of and attention to the patient's underlying concerns); physician friendliness; a positive, confident approach on the part of the physician; physician response to patient complaints; encouragement of patient questions; a supportive, nonjudgmental method of eliciting and responding to patient admissions of noncompliance; encouragement of patients to become actively involved in their own care; negotiation rather than dictation of a treatment plan; congruence between patient and physician in their understanding of a problem and its management; physician effort to motivate the patient; and patient satisfaction.

Transference, or the subconscious redirection to one person of feelings and attitudes toward others (e.g., toward parents or authority figures), may further influence the patient's relationship to his physician. Depending upon its nature, which is based on previous experience, the transference reaction can promote compliance (e.g., the patient who finds it rewarding to please authority figures) or impede it (e.g., the patient who distrusts authority figures). *Countertransference*, the redirection toward the patient of previously developed physician attitudes and feelings, may also be detrimental or beneficial to the patient-physician relationship.

Many of the above features contribute to the development of *patient-trust in the physician*, and trust is one of the most important factors in any approach to helping people change. Since a key element of trust is self-disclosure and self-disclosure exposes the patient to possible rejection, ridicule, shame, or exploitation, the importance of eliciting and responding to admissions of noncompliance in a nonjudgmental manner, in the context of a positive and supportive relationship, is clear.

Understandably, busy practitioners prefer patients who do not ask too many questions and who simply follow instructions. While this active-passive relationship may be appropriate for some patients, to be effective with most ambulatory patients the physician must enter into a relationship of mutual participation in which he must listen to the patient, educate, and negotiate with him. Such an approach need not be time consuming. It is the quality of the interaction and not the amount of time spent which correlates with compliance and satisfaction (6, p 53).

COMPLIANCE-IMPROVING INTERVENTIONS

The techniques designed to improve patient compliance which have been evaluated include organizational, instructional, and behavioral interventions. Successful intervention has increased compliance rates by less than 10% to almost 70%, averaging between 25 and 30% (percentage change = percentage of compliant patients in the experimental group minus percentage of compliant patients in the control group). When studied, compliance-improving interventions have also been shown to have favorable cost-benefit ratios (31).

Appointment Keeping

A number of factors have been shown to improve appointment keeping by patients.

Telephone and mail reminders, in which the patient receives a message several days before his scheduled visit informing him of the date and time of the appointment or a message inviting the patient to reschedule after a missed appointment, have consistently improved compliance, usually in the range of 10 to 20%. Wording of the message may be influential. In one study of high risk patients (20), postcards with a persuasive educational message resulted in a significantly higher compliance rate for influenzal vaccination than those with a "neutral" message simply announcing the availability of the vaccine.

The introduction of *individual rather than block appointment systems* and the *substitution of a single*

for multiple providers have resulted in *decreased waiting time* and improved appointment keeping. Individual appointment systems give each patient a precise time for his appointment; block systems schedule several or all patients for one time, usually at the beginning of office hours.

If *referral* is required, *educating the patient* about the purpose of referral, *minimizing the elapsed time* between the referral and the referral appointment, secretarial assistance to facilitate scheduling and transportation, and *referral to a specific physician* and not simply to a specialty group or clinic have also been shown to improve appointment keeping for diagnostic studies and/or specialty consultations.

Short Term Therapy

Compliance with short term courses of medication has been increased by the use of verbal and written instructions, the use of long acting parenteral therapy, the use of clearly labeled medication containers, pill calendars (devices on which patients keep track of their medication taking), and special pharmaceutical packaging designed to aid memory.

Although *verbal and written instructions* are clearly important, physicians often communicate poorly both the purpose of a specific regimen and precise directions about how it should be administered (6, p 37; 33). Furthermore, as already noted, psychological factors such as high anxiety levels may interfere with the patient's ability to comprehend initial instructions. Verbal instructions should be brief, clear, explicit, categorized by subject matter, with repetition for emphasis and testing for the effectiveness of the communication (21). Written instructions provide a remedy for forgetfulness and can be reviewed at leisure in the less stressful environment of the patient's home. Interestingly, informing patients of likely drug side effects seems to increase compliance, at least with respect to antidepressant therapy (24).

Long acting parenteral therapy is especially useful in situations where compliance is known to be low. For example, the use of a single intramuscular long acting penicillin rather than 10 days of an oral preparation will improve the effectiveness of therapy.

Chronic Therapy

Behavioral Strategies

Strategies which incorporate various combinations of increased supervision, tailoring of the medical regimen to individual patients' needs or habits, reinforcement, and patient involvement have improved compliance with chronic therapy. Instruction alone tends to be less effective in this setting, probably because most patients have already learned their regimen and have been taught something about their disease. Verbal and written instructions, however, would still be important at the initiation of therapy and whenever the regimen is changed.

Increased supervision includes scheduling of more frequent provider-patient contacts, the use of reminders, the use of drug assays, and the eliciting of family or community support to assist in administering and monitoring treatment. For example, the physician may request more frequent blood pressure values in a hypertensive patient. The blood pressures can be taken either by a nurse at the physician's office, a nurse at work, by a family member, or by the patient himself.

Tailoring refers to a process whereby the therapeutic regimen is fitted to the patient's characteristics and environment. Effective tailoring requires personal knowledge of the patient—his beliefs, life style, social and family support systems, and specifically, any barriers to compliance. Forgetful patients may benefit from linking medication taking or prescribed activities to daily routines, such as eating meals, brushing teeth, getting up in the morning, or going to bed at night. In addition, medication should be kept available where it is taken (e.g., at the breakfast table). If possible, the patient should avoid taking medication during times of the day when his activities are variable or when he is likely to be distracted (e.g., at work). Other examples of tailoring include involving patients who like to be in control in planning and monitoring their own therapy, substituting liquid medication for tablets in patients who have difficulties swallowing pills, increasing supervision and peer support for patients who are having difficulty on their own following a desired regimen (such as a weight reduction diet), and recommending exercise programs that can be incorporated into the schedules of extremely busy, time-pressured individuals that eliminate travel and waiting time and the need for special scheduling. The physician needs specifically to search for barriers which interfere with compliance. When cost is a factor, less expensive regimens can be prescribed or financial assistance sought. When a patient's health beliefs or ethnic model of disease interferes, they can sometimes be accommodated. For example, Mexican American or Puerto Rican patients who ascribe to the hot-cold theory of health and disease avoid the use of "hot" substances during pregnancy and, therefore, may refuse to take "hot" medications such as iron and vitamins. Compliance in this situation may be obtained by encouraging the patient to "neutralize" the hot properties of these medications with cool substances such as fruit juices or herb teas.

Reinforcement consists of behavioral feedbacks which can either promote or discourage compliance. It is the physician's task to identify existing reinforcers, support or initiate those which promote, and attempt to eliminate or diminish those which discourage compliance. For example, through *classical (Pavlovian) conditioning* a patient may have learned the habit of eating whenever he watches television, even when he is not hungry. To eliminate this behavior, the physician might try to reach an agreement whereby the patient eats only at the dining room table with the television off. *Operant*, in contrast to classical, conditioning reinforces behavior through its consequences and is more commonly used in clinical medicine. Feeding back to the patient results of drug level assays and therapeutic outcomes (e.g., decrease in blood pressure or weight) are examples of operant conditioning. Since positive feedback is more effective in changing behavior than negative, measures and outcomes which indicate compliance should be praised, otherwise rewarded, or viewed by the patient as rewards in themselves. When measures or outcomes suggest noncompliance, the problem should be discussed. Education and use of family and friends may be required to optimize reinforcers at home and in the community. Two common examples of such an intervention are: reversal of reinforced psycho-social disability in the physically capable postmyocardial infarction patient and maintenance of abstention in the detoxified alcoholic patient.

When a regimen is particularly complex or difficult, compliance may be improved by "*graduated regimen implementation*" or "*shaping*," whereby the patient is initially rewarded for adhering to only part of the regimen. Once the first part is achieved, additional components of the regimen are added in stepwise fashion with rewards being given only when there is compliance with all of the components that have been implemented.

Mechanisms of *enhancing patient involvement* have included various forms of self-monitoring, such as taking blood pressures at home, and the signing of contracts between patients and physicians. Therapeutic regimens which have been negotiated with rather than dictated by the physician are more likely to result in patient compliance. By taking active responsibility for their own care, patients may become more motivated to comply with therapy.

Combination strategies utilize two or more of the above methods and are generally much more effective than single interventions. Such a combination strategy utilized to improve behavior in noncompliant postmyocardial infarction patients has been described by Baile and Engel (1). Patient involvement was effected by having patients set their own goals and monitor their own behavior. Frequent contact with the physician allowed reinforcement, modification of goals on a negotiated basis, and discussion of problems with the regimen. Involvement of the spouse also increased supervision.

Following is an example of tailoring, negotiating, use of reinforcement, and actively involving the patient in her own care (continuation of example from pages 44 to 45):

Doctor: Well, Mrs. Smith, your blood pressure remains elevated today. It's 150/100, which is better than when we started, but not as low as we'd like it. ("We" implies shared responsibility.)

Patient: Oh . . . .

Doctor: Of course, not taking your medicine this morning could be a factor, as I've already explained. I also think it's very important that we decide on a schedule that you can keep 100% of the time. How about taking that afternoon dose at the same time and place every day? Is dinner a good time for you?

Patient: My meal times are irregular and I don't always eat at home.

Doctor: How about bedtime?

Patient: Sometimes I'm so exhausted, I just fall to sleep while I'm reading, before I've brushed my teeth or anything. Don't you have a pill that can be taken just once a day?

Doctor: As a matter of fact, that's a possibility. When would you take it?

Patient: With my morning coffee. I never miss that!

Doctor: Fine, I'll give you a prescription for which you can take once a day with your morning coffee . . . 100% of the time, *even the mornings you come to my office.* Is that a deal?

Patient: Yes! (solution achieved through tailoring and negotiation)

Doctor: The side effects for this medicine are the same as for the other. Since you experienced none with the other, you should tolerate this one well.

Patient: Good.

Doctor: Together with your diet and exercise program, this medicine alone may be enough to control your blood pressure. Of course, we'll start with a low dose, so we may have to increase it. Can you come back in 2 weeks?

Patient: How about 2 months?

Doctor: Well, I'd really like to see you more frequently until your blood pressure is controlled. Of course, if you monitored your own blood pressure at home, you could call the results into me and there would be less need for frequent office visits. (The doctor prefers not to yield on the follow-up interval and uses the opportunity to motivate the patient to become further involved in her own management and to create a new environmental reinforcer.)

Patient: How can I do that?

(Doctor proceeds (*a*) to explain the process of getting a blood pressure cuff, coming to the office to have it checked, and learning how to use it; (*b*) to test the patient for her understanding of her responsibilities; (*c*) to get her verbal commitment; and (*d*) to write down for her the new management plan it.)

Direct Supervision of Medication Taking

Direct supervision of drug intake is especially helpful for ensuring compliance in patients with impaired intellectual or psychological functioning, such as those with alcoholism, dementia, and schizophrenia. Examples include the use of intermittent supervised oral antituberculosis therapy and the use of long acting parenteral drugs in the ambulatory management of schizophrenia.

Maintenance of Compliance/Motivating Patients

No matter how successful the intervention, compliance tends to decay toward baseline after cessation of the intervention. Hence, there is a need to continue some form of intervention. Unfortunately, there has been little effort to date to study maintenance strategies.

DiMatteo and DiNicola ("General References") point out that compliant behavior is unlikely to be maintained once external supports are removed. Based upon their review of the relevant compliance, sociological, and behavioral literature, they suggest an approach which promotes "*internalization*" of the patient's motivation to comply. Thus, new *beliefs, attitudes, or values* may have to become integrated into the patient's life, and perhaps others may have to be dropped. Since the physician is the major source of health information for most Americans (6, p 37), he can assist in this process. He is more likely to succeed, if he has earned the patient's trust (see "Doctor-Patient Relationship" above).

The first step for the physician in promoting change in health attitudes is to explore the patient's present knowledge, beliefs, attitudes, and values, as well as his social and cultural norms. Education about his disease and regimen can then be tailored to correct misconceptions, fill in gaps in his knowledge base, and motivate him in the context of his value system. Simply taking time for discussion will raise the salience in the patient's mind of the issue being discussed. Threat or fear messages can motivate behavioral change but should not be too strong (can cause patient denial or paralysis) or too weak. Furthermore, they should be combined with a positive message about a feasible (for the patient) and effective therapeutic regimen. Because patients are often more present than future oriented, short term, as well as long term, benefits of any regimen should be stressed. Since behavior can influence attitudes, as well as *vice versa*, the practitioner should point out the patient's own behaviors which support the attitude being promoted. He can help integrate the new attitude into the patient's total system of beliefs by noting how it correlates with other beliefs the patient has. He can also note how it adheres to cultural and social norms.

Actively involving the patient in the reasoning behind the regimen, enhancing the patient's feeling of responsibility for belief change, repeatedly exposing him to the message, and having positive expectations for him all help. Once the patient has adopted a new attitude or belief, it is useful to inoculate him against likely challenges from his environment by rehearsing them with him in role-playing sessions (e.g., to the recovering alcoholic ... "How are you going to handle it, when people try to get you to drink at your niece's wedding this weekend?"; or to the hypertensive patient who is sensitive to being viewed as ill by others ... "How are you going to respond when one of your colleagues at work sees you taking your medication and says 'Oh, you have to take medicine now! What's wrong with you?'"). Of course, new attitudes and beliefs need positive reinforcement as discussed earlier.

Some patients with unhealthy *self-perceptions* may need to be convinced that they can indeed effect a change in their lives. The practitioner can help by emphasizing the patient's past and present behaviors which demonstrated self-control, by pointing out inaccuracies in the patient's negative self-perceptions, and by having and projecting a positive attitude to the patient about her abilities to change (e.g., "On the one hand you say you have no self-control. On the other, you tell me you stopped smoking for the entire period of your second pregnancy. That must have taken tremendous will power! Did you know that persons who have successfully stopped smoking in the past for a month or more are more likely to succeed in quitting altogether than those who have never tried?").

Efforts to help patients adopt beliefs, attitudes, and values consistent with health-promoting behaviors can be integrated into ongoing care and should usually span several office visits. Referral to *supportive groups* which expose patients to others with similar problems (e.g., asthmatic, postmyocardial infarction, ostomy, and mastectomy groups, Alcoholics Anonymous, Weight Watchers, *etc*) is an important adjunct to management.

Education of Physicians as a Compliance-Improving Strategy

That educating physicians about the importance, recognition, and management of noncompliance can result in improved compliance outcomes in their patients has been demonstrated in one carefully executed controlled study of hypertensive patients (17) but not in another (5). Additional research is required to identify the components necessary for effective educational intervention.

Ethical Considerations

It has been suggested that the following three conditions be met before attempting to improve compliance: (a) the diagnosis should be correct, (b) the therapy should be proven efficacious and benefits should outweigh adverse effects, and (c) the patient should be an informed and willing partner in the intervention (29).

While the first two conditions are probably appli-cable to interventions directed toward populations, they may be too rigid for application to individual patients. In some circumstances, it may be reasonable to prescribe an efficacious medicine as a therapeutic trial, when the diagnosis is in question. Furthermore, many medicines have not been unequivocally proven to be efficacious, although some evidence supports their usefulness. The physician is justified in encouraging the use of such medications in an attempt to determine whether they relieve symptoms or improve functional status. How else will the physician know whether a given antiarrhythmic or analgesic, for example, is effective for a given patient?

In individual practice, therefore, the first two conditions might be replaced with the following requirements: (a) that the therapy be rational and based upon sound medical knowledge, and (b) that the potential risks of therapy be small compared to the potential benefits.

The third condition, that of an informed and willing partner in the intervention, is even more difficult to satisfy. In medical practice one may encounter individuals who willfully fail to comply against their own best interest. Is the physician justified in increasing supervision or attempting to elicit familial support in order to improve compliance, without obtaining explicit consent from the patient? On the one hand, the patient has come to the doctor's office and voluntarily entered into the patient-physician relationship, suggesting implicit consent. On the other hand, the patient is willfully noncomplying, suggesting a rejection of this aspect of the relationship. The dilemma may be somewhat artificial since most compliance-improving strategies require participation of the patient and, therefore, implicit consent. Going beyond the patient-physician relationship to enroll family help, however, requires consideration of the patient's feelings with respect to this intervention. The situation becomes more difficult when patients are mentally or psychologically impaired in their ability to make sound decisions. An example might be the symptomatic schizophrenic patient who fails to comply in taking his oral antipsychotic medication, when introduction of long acting parenteral therapy could reduce symptoms, rate of relapse, and rehospitalization. There are no definitive guidelines in these situations, but the following suggestions may be helpful: (a) The physician should attempt to determine the patient's own best interest, considering not only the disease but also the patient's desires, values, psychological makeup, and social environment, and he should use this information as a guide to action. (b) The physician should weigh the relative benefits *versus* risks of intervention (self-monitoring of blood pressure in some individuals, for example, might markedly increase their anxiety). (c) The physician should respect the patient's legal rights. (d) In particularly difficult situations, such as the case of mentally incompetent patients, the physician should consult with others before deciding on a course of action. (See Chapter 10 for determination of mental competence.)

Finally, there is the question of where the patient's responsibilities begin and those of the physician end. Is the physician ethically bound to identify and treat noncompliance when it compromises the health of his patient? Once a patient-physician relationship has been entered, it is certainly the physician's responsibility to improve the health status of the patient to the best of his ability, taking into consideration the severity of the problem, economic constraints, time constraints, and competing obligations to other patients. To achieve this end a physician should use not only the traditional methods of diagnosis, treatment, and instruction of patients, but when appropriate, interventions for improving compliance as well.

PRACTICAL APPROACH TO NONCOMPLIANCE

In practice, the problem of noncompliance should be handled in the same way as are other clinical problems. Whenever possible it should be prevented. When present, it should be diagnosed and treated by accepted diagnostic approaches and treatment modalities.

Noncompliance with Therapeutic Regimens

Prevention (Table 4.3)

It is usually more efficient to use some strategies that will improve compliance with all patients at the inception of treatment, rather than to attempt to

Table 4.3.
Prevention of Noncompliance

Development of rapport and patient trust
Use of simplest possible medical regimen
Tailoring of medical regimen
Verbal and written instructions
Concise
Clear
Explicit
Categorization
Repetition
Testing for comprehension
Targeted education
Correction of misconceptions
Motivation of patient
Discussion of:
Likely side effects
Cost
Alternative therapies
Consequences of nontherapy
Parenteral therapy (when an option)

identify the noncompliers at a later time. Minimal preventive strategies for all patients would include (a) *development of rapport and patient trust* (see pages 49 to 50); (b) the use of the *simplest possible medical regimen* (page 49); and (c) *brief, clear, explicit, categorized instructions*, which include the purpose and duration of therapy, with subsequent repetition and testing for the effectiveness of the communication (pages 49 to 50). *Written instructions* (in addition to what the pharmacist transcribes onto the pill bottle) should be given when the patient is anxious, the regimen complex, or the instructions incompletely retained. *Education targeted to correct misconceptions and motivate the patient*, and *discussion of likely side effects*, what to do in the event of side effects, approximate *cost* of medications, *alternative therapies*, and *consequences of nontherapy* may further enhance compliance. Negative transference and countertransference reactions should be recognized and controlled.

Tailoring of care to the individual needs of the patient from the outset may increase his satisfaction and improve the chances for compliance. This requires that the physician routinely answer some of the following questions about most patients: (a) *Who* is this patient? What are his personality traits? Does he need more or less information about and involvement in his own care? (b) *What* are the patient's explanations for and beliefs about his illness? What are his attitudes about care? What perceived barriers to compliance exist? (c) *Where* does the patient come from? What environmental factors, such as family and work hours, might influence his ability to follow a therapeutic regimen? (d) *Why* is the patient here? What are his expectations, motivations, and concerns in seeking care? What triggered today's visit? (e) Does the patient *understand and accept* the physician's explanation and prescription? These answers may then be utilized as described above (page 51). Familiarity with the beliefs and practices of commonly served ethnic groups can also be of assistance (see pages 48 and 51).

The use of *parenteral therapy* in lieu of more complicated and prolonged oral regimens (e.g., in the treatment of gonococcal urethritis or streptococcal pharyngitis) will reduce noncompliance and thereby increase the effectiveness of therapy.

The use of printed *patient education materials* may be an efficient way to enhance patient understanding of a disease and its management from the outset (see also Chapter 3).

Diagnosis (Table 4.4)

The possibility of noncompliant behavior should be considered in all patients, because of its high prevalence and the inability of physicians to predict it intuitively. The failure to see expected therapeutic or side effects should raise suspicions, as should the presence of other factors known to be associated

Table 4.4.
Diagnosis of Noncompliance

Suspicion
  All patients (special emphasis on patients who fail to achieve expected therapeutic effects or side effects and those with associated risk factors for noncompliance)
Measurement
  Questioning of patient or family (see the text)
  Frequency of patient-requested prescription renewals or medication count
  Inspection of all pill bottles
  Drug assays
  Expected outcomes
  Supervised medication taking (office or hospital)
Cause
  Noncomprehension
  Volitional noncompliance
    Determine cause of volitional noncompliance

with noncompliance (see discussion above, pages 47 to 50 and Table 4.2).

The first step in diagnosing noncompliance is to *ask* patients what they are doing to treat their problem in an open-ended, nonthreatening, nonjudgmental manner (see example, pages 44 to 45). Questioning should continue until the patient has provided information about what medicines he is taking, how frequently he is taking them, how frequently doses are missed, and what nonpharmacological modes of treatment he is using. Patients should be specifically asked about compliance on the day of and the day preceding their visit (some diabetic patients, for example, routinely omit all drugs including insulin at the time of a morning visit; 24-hour recalls are more accurate than general reports, which tend to be idealized). Using such techniques, 50% or more of noncompliers (and all those who do not comply because they do not understand the requirements) will be identified. Sensitivity can be increased by asking family members or housemates.

When the patient appears confused or is unable to provide sufficient information, having him *bring all medication containers to the office* (for both prescribed and over-the-counter medications) may provide invaluable information. For example, it may be discovered that a patient is still taking a discontinued medication or is taking two different preparations of the same drug. Selected patients should be encouraged to bring their medication containers with them at every visit.

If volitional noncompliance is suspected despite denial by the patient, objective measures are required. Medication counts may be instituted but are often impractical as discussed above (page 45). Instead observations of the frequency of actual *versus* expected *prescription renewals* may be substituted for formal pill counts. (A method for keeping track

of prescription renewals should be incorporated into the office record, especially when prescriptions are filled by more than one physician.) Review of the longitudinal relationship between medication and *outcome measures* (greatly assisted by the appropriate use of flow sheets) can provide important clues of noncompliant behavior, such as widely varying blood pressures on a constant regimen. The absence of a *drug* upon *assay* is virtually diagnostic of noncompliance (assuming that the assay is reliable and the samples have been obtained at appropriate times). The failure to achieve therapeutic drug levels or expected outcomes, however, could be secondary either to noncompliance or inadequate therapy. To distinguish between these two alternatives it may sometimes be necessary to observe drug levels or outcome of treatment during a period in which drugs are taken under *direct supervision*. This may require a period of hospitalization. In one common condition, hypertension, hospitalization can be avoided by measuring the patient's blood pressure for several hours after supervised ingestion of medication in the office (for example, see cases in Chapter 62).

Once the presence of noncompliance has been established, its *cause* should be determined. Noncomprehension will be detected by simply asking the patient to describe his regimen. If the patient knows his regimen but does not comply, possible reasons for the noncompliance should be explored (e.g., inappropriate beliefs about the illness or therapy, presence of side effects, cost of medicines, inconvenience of taking medicines, depression, *etc*). The ways in which these factors may affect compliance behavior have been discussed above (pages 47 to 50).

Treatment (Table 4.5)

Once noncompliance has been established and it has been decided to try to treat it (after a review of the ethical considerations previously discussed, pages 53 to 54), several methods are possible. If the problem is *noncomprehension*, the use of further

Table 4.5.
Treatment of Noncompliance

Noncomprehension
  Verbal and written instructions
  Simplification and tailoring of medical regimen
  Supervision of medication taking
Volitional noncompliance
  Targeted education and persuasive communication
  Simplification and tailoring of medical regimen
  Increased supervision
  Patient involvement (self-monitoring, negotiation, contracts)
  Positive reinforcement
  Familial/environmental support
  Supervised medication taking
  Combined interventions
  Maintenance of intervention that helps

verbal and written instructions and/or simplification and tailoring of the medical regimen may be indicated. If the patient is still unable to comprehend, supervision of medication taking by family members or by health personnel, such as visiting nurses, will be required.

When there is *volitional noncompliance*, a strategy designed to improve compliance must be tailored to each individual's needs. Underlying problems, such as depression or alcoholism, should be treated. The use of behavioral methods (see pages 50 to 52) will often be required, including simplification and tailoring of the regimen, use of special pharmaceutical packaging or drug charts to aid memory, patient self-monitoring, negotiation and involvement of the patient in planning his own care, obtainment of patient verbal commitments and written contracts, increased medical and environmental supervision, monitoring and feedback of blood levels or outcome measures, and alteration of environmental reinforcers. Further education and persuasive communication in an attempt to motivate the patient, correct important misconceptions, and introduce or alter certain beliefs, attitudes, or values is usually a necessary concomitant of treatment (see pages 52 to 53). Long acting parenteral therapy is occasionally an option. Since compliance tends to decline after the termination of such interventions, effective strategies may have to be continued indefinitely. Attempts to simplify or to discontinue a successful strategy should be done in stepwise fashion, while continuing to monitor compliance.

Noncompliance with Appointment Keeping (Table 4.6)

Techniques to improve appointment-keeping rates in general have been discussed above (page 50). When follow-up is important, the physician can (a) logically "*bridge*" to the next visit by discussing its purpose with the patient (*e.g.*, monitoring for recurrence, review of test results, decision about therapy, *etc*); (b) *negotiate a visit interval* that is mutually acceptable; (c) *tailor the appointment time* to the patient's needs; (d) *obtain* a verbal *agreement* from the patient to comply; and (e) *schedule the appointment* instead of giving the patient instructions to "call for" one. Components (a) and (e) of this strategy have been tested in one successful clinical

Table 4.6.
Preventing Dropouts and Missed Appointments

Appointment system which minimizes waiting time
Bridging to next visit
Negotiation of interval between visits
Tailoring of appointment time
Contracts
Scheduling of next visit at present visit
Daily review and follow-up of missed appointments
Telephone and mailed reminders

trial (34). Since *missed appointments* could presage dropouts from treatment, the charts and/or names of these patients should be reviewed daily by the physician. When indicated, the patient can be contacted by telephone, letter, or postcard.

General References

Bartlett E (ed): *Physician's Patient Education Newsletter*. Birmingham, University of Alabama.

> Bimonthly newsletter published since 1978. Contains timely accounts and reviews of behavioral approaches to patient compliance. Available by subscription.

Becker MH, Maiman LA: Strategies for enhancing patient compliance. *J Community Health* 6:113–134, 1980.

> Review article. Readable, comprehensive, referenced article on compliance improving interventions.

Bernarde MA, Mayerson EW: Patient-physician negotiation. *JAMA* 239:1417, 1978.

> Practical discussion of the components of patient-provider communication, including negotiation, which can enhance patient compliance.

DiMatteo MR, DiNiola DD: *Achieving Patient Compliance: the Psychology of the Medical Practitioner's Role*. New York, Pergamon Press, 1982.

> Important recent contribution which describes an in-depth social-psychological approach to the understanding and management of noncompliant behavior.

Eraker SA, Kirscht JP, Becker MH: Understanding and improving patient compliance. *Ann Intern Med* 100:258, 1984.

> Recent review. Develops "health decision model," which combines decision analysis, behavioral decision theory, and patient beliefs, as a conceptual aid for understanding and managing patient noncompliance.

Garrity TF: Medical compliance and the clinician-patient relationship: a review. *Soc Sci Med* 15E:215, 1981.

> Critical review of studies from which derive recommendations regarding instructional techniques, meeting patient expectations, increasing patient involvement, and fostering good provider-patient rapport.

Harwood A: *Ethnicity and Medical Care*. Cambridge, MA, Harvard University Press, 1981.

> Useful reference on ethnic health beliefs and practices.

Haynes RB, Taylor DW, Sackett DL (eds): *Compliance in Health Care*. Baltimore, Johns Hopkins University Press, 1979.

> Excellent comprehensive reference with annotated bibliography. Still the single best source of information on compliance.

Schmidt JP: A behavioral approach to patient compliance. *Postgrad Med* 65:219, 1979.

> Practical discussion of some behavioral change techniques designed to improve compliance.

Specific References

1. Baile WF, Engel BT: A behavioral strategy for the treatment of noncompliance following myocardial infarction. *Psychosom Med* 40:413, 1978.
1a. Burrows GD, Norman TR: *Psychotropic Drugs, Plasma Concentration and Clinical Response*. New York, Marcel Dekker, 1981.
2. Closson R, Kikuwago C: Noncompliance with drug class. *Hospitals* 49:89, 1975.
3. Coronary Drug Project Research Group: Influence of adherence to treatment and response of cholesterol on mortality in the Coronary Drug Project. *N Engl J Med* 30:1038, 1980.
4. Croog SH, Shapiro DS, Levine S: Denial among heart patients. *Psychosom Med* 33:385, 1971.
5. Dickinson JC, Warshaw GA, Gehlbach SH, *et al*: Improving hypertension control: impact of computer feedback and physician education. *Med Care* 19:843, 1981.
6. DiMatteo MR, DiNicola DD: Practitioner-patient relation-

ships: the communication of information. In DiMatteo MR, DiNicola DD (eds): *Achieving Patient Compliance, The Psychology of the Medical Practitioner's Role.* New York, Pergamon Press, 1982.

7. Durbin WA, Lapidas B, Goldman DA: Improved antibiotic usage following introduction of a novel prescription. *JAMA* 246:1796, 1981.

8. Eshelman FN: Drug compliance in diabetics. *Br Med J* 1:581, 1978.

9. Fletcher C: Listening and talking to patients. I. The problem. *Br Med J* 281:845, 1980.

9a. Gilman AG, Goodman LS, Gilman A (eds): *The Pharmacologic Basis of Therapeutics.* New York, Macmillan, 1980.

10. Gordis L, Markowitz M, Lillienfeld AM: Studies in the epidemiology and preventability of rheumatic fever. IV. A quantitative determination of compliance in children on oral penicillin prophylaxis. *Pediatrics* 43:173, 1962.

11. Hackett TP, Cassem NH: White-collar and blue-collar responses to heart attack. *J Psychosom Res* 20:85, 1976.

12. Haynes RB: Strategies in improving compliance with referrals, appointments, and prescribed medical regimens. In Haynes RB, Taylor DW, Sackett DL (eds): *Compliance in Health Care.* Baltimore, Johns Hopkins University Press, 1979, p 123.

13. Haynes RB, *et al:* Management of patient compliance in the treatment of hypertension. Report of the NHLBI Working Group. *Hypertension* 4:415, 1982.

14. Hemminki E, Heikkila J: Elderly people's compliance with prescriptions, and quality of medication. *Scand J Soc Med* 3:87, 1975.

14a. Hollister LC: *Clinical Pharmacology of Psychotherapeutic Drugs.* New York, Churchill Livingstone, 1978.

15. Hulka B, Kupper L, Cassel J, *et al:* Medication use and misuse: physician-patient discrepancies. *J Chronic Dis* 28:7, 1975.

16. Inui TS, Carter WB, Pecoraro RE, *et al:* Variations in patient compliance with common long term drugs. *Med Care* 18:986, 1980.

17. Inui TS, Yourtee EL, Williamson JW: Improved outcomes after physician tutorials: a controlled trial. *Ann Intern Med* 84:646, 1976.

18. Ireland HD: Outpatient chemotherapy for tuberculosis. *Am Rev Respir Dis* 82:378, 1960.

19. Johnson AL, Taylor DW, Sackett DL, *et al:* Self-recording of blood pressure in the management of hypertension. *Can Med Assoc J* 119:1034, 1978.

19a. Knobbin JE, Anderson PO: *Handbook of Clinical Drug Data.* Washington, DC, Drug Intelligence Publications, 1983.

20. Larson EB, Bergman J, Heidrich F, *et al:* Do postcard reminders improve influenza vaccination compliance? A prospective trial of different postcard "cues." *Med Care* 20:639, 1982.

21. Ley P: Memory for medical information. *Br J Soc Clin Psychol* 18:245, 1979.

22. Markowitz M: Eradication of rheumatic fever: an unfilled hope. *Circulation* 41:1077, 1970.

23. Mason AS, Forrest IS, Forrest FM, Butler H: Adherence to maintenance therapy and re-hospitalization. *Dis Nerv Syst* 24:103, 1963.

23a. McEvoy GK (ed): *Drug Information 1985.* Washington, DC, American Society of Hospital Pharmacists, 1985.

24. Meyers ED, Calvert EJ: Knowledge of side effects and perseverance with medications. *Br Med J* 1:1577, 1976.

25. Muller C: Medical review of prescribing. *J Chronic Dis* 18:689, 1965.

26. Oldright NB, Wicks JR, Hanley C, *et al:* Noncompliance in an exercise rehabilitation program for men who have suffered myocardial infarction. *Can Med Assoc J* 118:361, 1978.

26a. Pribor HC, Morell G, Scherr GH: *Drug Monitoring and Pharmokinetic Data.* Pathotex Publishers, 1980.

27. Ray WA, Federspiel CF, Shaffner W: A study of antipsychotic drug use in nursing homes: epidemiologic evidence suggesting misuse. *Am J Public Health* 70:485, 1980.

28. Roth HP: Accuracy of doctors' estimates and patients' statements on adherence to a drug regimen. *Clin Pharmacol Ther* 23:361, 1978.

29. Sackett DL: Introduction. In Sackett DL, Haynes RB (eds): *Compliance with Therapeutic Regimens.* Baltimore, Johns Hopkins University Press, 1976, p 1.

30. Sheckler WE, Bennett JV: Antibiotic usage in seven community hospitals. *JAMA* 213:264, 1970.

31. Smith M: The cost of noncompliance and the capacity of improved compliance to reduce health care expenditures. In: *Improving Medication Compliance, Proceedings of a Symposium.* National Pharmaceutical Council, 1985, p 35.

32. Stolley PD, Lasagna L: Prescribing patterns of physicians. *J Chronic Dis* 22:394, 1969.

33. Svarstad BL: Physician-patient communication and patient conformity with medical advice. In Mechanic D (ed): *The Growth of Bureaucratic Medicine.* New York, John Wiley & Sons, 1976, p 243.

33a. Tricyclic antidepressants—blood level measurements and clinical outcome: an APA task force report. *Am J Psychiatry* 142:155, 1985.

33b. Troupin AS: The measurement of anticonvulsant agent levels. *Ann Intern Med* 100:854, 1984.

34. Waggoner DM, Jackson EB, Kern DE: Physical influence on patient compliance: a clinical trial. *Ann Emerg Med* 10:348, 1981.

CHAPTER FIVE

Adolescent Patients: Special Considerations

LARRY N. SCHERZER, M.D.

INTRODUCTION

As indicated in Chapter 1 (Table 1.2), patients in the age group 15 to 24 account for about 9% of visits to internists and 16% of visits to family or general practitioners in the United States.

From a developmental perspective, adolescence is a time of dynamic changes, with tremendous physical, sexual, intellectual, and psychological growth. This chapter describes the normal changes and the major problems associated with each of these four spheres of development; an understanding of these changes is critical to the proper management of adolescent patients. The last section of the chapter recommends a number of special strategies for conducting ambulatory visits by adolescent patients.

ADOLESCENT MORTALITY AND MORBIDITY

Adolescence is the healthiest period of life; morbidity and mortality rates are low compared with other age groups; but the absolute number of adolescents who die or suffer from chronic illnesses is considerable. Since the number of productive years at stake for a teenager with a significant illness is large, adolescent health deserves a special priority.

Accidents are by far the leading cause of death among adolescents and young adults (see Table 5.1). Preventive measures have, by and large, been bypassed by the victims of accidental death; and, in many instances, behavioral problems underlie those deaths. For example, alcohol is implicated in over 50% of automobile accidents, and there may be an element of suicidal intent in many of them.

The second and third leading causes of death in older adolescents (and an important problem in young adolescents) are homicide and suicide, problems that are discussed later in this chapter (page 69).

The fourth leading cause of death among adolescents and young adults is neoplasia. The most frequent diagnoses are acute leukemia (both lymphocytic and myelogenous), lymphomas (including non-Hodgkin's lymphoma and Hodgkin's disease), central nervous system tumors (especially supra- and infratentorial gliomas), bone tumors (especially osteogenic sarcomas and Ewing's sarcomas), and solid organ tumors (especially of genital organs).

As medical treatment improves, conditions that were previously fatal in childhood are being seen more frequently in adolescents and young adults. It is not uncommon that patients with cystic fibrosis, nephritis, congenital heart disease, and leukemia survive into adolescence and young adulthood. The transfer of their care from their pediatrician to an internist may threaten these patients, make it more difficult for them to adapt to their illness, and may even lead to complications requiring hospitalization.

Most visits to a physician by adolescents are for preventive care or are for problems that are relatively minor (Tables 5.2 and 5.3). However, a number of more severe medical problems are either limited chiefly to the adolescent period or are problems of adulthood which begin during adolescence (Table 5.4). The data in the tables do not demonstrate the significant distress that many adolescent patients (and their physicians) experience. This distress is often related to the pressures unique to the several chronological stages of adolescence.

The *young teen* (i.e., 11 to 15 years old) with his special concern over physical development, may have anxieties about mutilation and death. Hostility toward an illness may be expressed in a fantasy of invincibility leading to an uncooperative, noncompliant patient. Other young adolescents become

Table 5.1.
Major Causes of Death Ages 15 to 24: United States 1975[a]

Cause of Death	Annual Rate/10⁵ Individuals
Accidents	60.3
Homicide	13.7
Suicide	11.8
Neoplasms, malignant and benign	7.1
Cardiovascular disease	4.4
Ill defined conditions	3.8
Infectious illnesses[b]	3.0
All other external causes	2.5
Congenital anomalies	1.6
Gastrointestinal diseases	0.8
Anemias	0.4
Diabetes mellitus	0.4
Complications of pregnancy and childbirth	0.4
Respiratory diseases	0.3
Nephritis and nephrosis	0.3
Nutritional deficiencies	0.1
All other disease	8.0
Total	118.9
Estimated number of persons (in millions)	39.98
Number of deaths	47,545

[a] Adapted from data presented in *National Center for Health Statistics Monthly Vital Statistic Reports* (vol 25, no. 10, December 30, 1976 and vol 25, no 11, February 11, 1977).
[b] All infectious illnesses including those related to specific organ systems, *e.g.*, diarrheal diseases, pneumonia, meningitis, and pyelonephritis.

greatly depressed by their illnesses and become annoying, complaining, whiny patients, frequently regressing to a child-like dependence on adult caretakers.

The *middle adolescent* (i.e., 14 to 19 years old) who is ill suffers from the loss of valued contact with friends and schools. Important aspirations may be interrupted (and dreams shattered) through illness. Body image is at a critical developmental stage in midadolescence, and the teen may be more worried about a cosmetic defect resulting from an illness than about the disease or its therapy. Such fears need to be faced early and dealt with honestly.

The *older adolescent* (i.e., 18 to 21 years old) shares many adult concerns. For example, anxiety may be expressed over the cost of an illness and the length of hospitalization, and the burdens these place on the family.

An understanding of adolescent development will help the clinician to recognize and deal with these and other special problems.

PHYSICAL DEVELOPMENT

Normal Patterns and Concerns

Physical maturation is an important feature of the second decade of life. Although the rate and the timing of maturation may vary, they follow the hormonal changes of puberty in a given individual.

There is a notable *growth spurt* occurring during the adolescent years, with a 20 to 25% increase in height over a period of 2 to 3 years. This spurt usually occurs earlier in the female than in the male (as does sexual maturation).

During puberty, there is an average 2-fold increase in both lean and nonlean *body mass*. The ratio of lean to nonlean body mass is greater in males than in females. It has been suggested that the greater proportion of fat in females may be related to reserves needed for the onset of menarche and ovulation. Fat accumulation tends to be greatest at the point that growth ceases and may extend into adulthood.

The *musculoskeletal system* has special characteristics during adolescence. To accommodate growth, the ligaments and tendons become lax and elastic, frequently giving the teen a slouched-over appearance. Similarly, there is an increase in skeletal growth, particularly in long bones; and metaphyseal-epiphyseal junctions remain soft. Thus, the actively

Table 5.2.
Thirty Most Common Reasons for Physician-Patient Contact for Patients 10 to 24 Years Old (Based on 2-Year Experience of 118 Family Physicians)[a]

Medical examination for preventive and pre-symptomatic purposes	11,877
Pharyngitis	8,245
Lacerations, contusions, and abrasions	7,714
Prenatal care	4,872
Strains and sprains	4,560
Vulvitis, vaginitis, and cervicitis	2,753
Coryza	2,725
Bronchitis	2,691
Febrile cold	2,388
Menstrual disorders	1,992
Abdominal pain other than colic	1,630
Otitis media, acute	1,561
Headache	1,342
Cystitis	1,313
Contact dermatitis	1,256
Warts	1,032
Sinusitis	1,001
Anxiety neurosis	986
Allergic rhinitis	909
Otitis externa	894
Depressive neurosis	871
Acne	853
Asthma	849
Gonorrhea	780
Acute gastritis or duodenitis	738
Other local infections of skin	730
Specific allergies	717
Physical disorders presumably of psychogenic origin	587
Hypertension	567
Hypochromic anemia	507

[a] Adapted from Marsland DW, *et al*: Content of family practice. *J Fam Practice* 3:37, 1976.

Table 5.3.
Number of Office Visits Made by Adolescents and Percentage Distribution by the 20 Most Frequent Principal Diagnoses, According to Age: United States, 1980–1981[a]

Age, Principal Diagnosis, and ICD-9-CM Code[b]		No. of Visits in Thousands	Percentage Distribution	Age, Principal Diagnosis, and ICD-9-CM Code[b]		No. of Visits in Thousands	Percentage Distribution
11–14 years				**15–20 years**			
Total		40,269	100.0	Total		87,172	100.0
General medical examination	V70	2,832	7.0	Normal pregnancy	V22	7,926	9.1
Allergic rhinitis	477	1,760	4.4	Diseases of sebaceous glands[c]	706	7,306	8.4
Diseases of sebaceous glands[c]	706	1,629	4.0	General medical examination	V70	5,457	6.3
Acute pharyngitis	462	1,297	3.2	Acute pharyngitis	462	2,439	2.8
Acute upper respiratory infections of multiple or unspecified sites	465	1,296	3.2	Acute upper respiratory infections of multiple or unspecified sites	465	2,242	2.6
Suppurative and unspecified otitis media	382	1,177	2.9	Special investigations and examinations[e]	V72	1,756	2.0
Asthma	493	1,109	2.8	Disorders of refraction and accommodation	367	1,525	1.7
Disorders of refraction and accommodation	367	1,054	2.6	Allergic rhinitis	477	1,482	1.7
Routine infant or child health check	V20.2	930	2.3	Other diseases due to viruses and chlamydiae	078	1,427	1.6
Certain adverse effects not elsewhere classified[d]	995	808	2.0	Follow-up examination	V67	1,345	1.5
Acute tonsillitis	463	791	2.0	Acute tonsillitis	463	1,254	1.4
Other diseases due to viruses and chlamydiae	078	770	1.9	Contact dermatitis and other eczema	692	1,146	1.3
Contact dermatitis and other eczema	692	684	1.7	Suppurative and unspecified otitis media	382	955	1.1
Fracture of radius and ulna	813	551	1.4	Contraceptive management	V25	866	1.0
Disorders of external ear	380	527	1.3	Asthma	493	851	1.0
Curvature of spine	737	460	1.1	Disorders of menstruation and other abnormal bleeding from female genital tract	626	820	0.9
Bronchitis, not specified as acute or chronic	490	*435	1.1	Bronchitis, not specified as acute or chronic	490	78.8	0.9
Observation and evaluation for suspected conditions	V71	*422	1.0	Disorders of external ear	380	731	0.8
Other noninfective gastroenteritis and colitis	558	*413	1.0	Chronic sinusitis	473	722	0.8
Follow-up examination	V67	*405	1.0	Neurotic disorders	300	719	0.8
Residual	...	...	52.1	Residual		...	52.3

[a] From Cypress BK: *Health Care of Adolescents by Office-Based Physicians: National Ambulatory Medical Care Survey, 1980–1981*. Advance Data from Vital and Health Statistics. No. 99, September 28, 1984.
[b] Based on US Public Health Service and Health Care Financing Administration: *International Classification of Diseases, 9th Revision, Clinical Modification* (ICD-9-CM). Department of Health and Human Services, Publ no. (PHS) 80-1260. Public Health Service. Washington, DC, US Government Printing Office, September 1980.
[c] Chiefly 706.1, acne other than varioliformis.
[d] Chiefly 995.3, allergy unspecified.
[e] Chiefly V72.3, gynecological examination.

growing teen, who may not have developed a muscle mass to correspond to his skeletal growth, may be prone to some special injuries, particularly joint dislocations and fractures along epiphyseal plates.

As with all areas of development, the adolescent may have particular concerns about growth and weight. The principal reason for this is that adolescents often base judgment of each other's adequacy and acceptability on size or (for males) on athletic ability; and adult criteria of social status based on other standards (or prejudices) are of less importance.

Children called "squirt" or "runt" are given various types of parental advice; much of it is not

helpful. Some children adapt by engaging in an activity where size is unimportant (e.g., debating, chess, fencing, swimming, body building, etc). Occasionally, normal children, with a familial basis of their short stature will require some psychological counseling to promote effective adaptation to their stature. Some individuals who are very sensitive about height and strength limitations may try radical and potentially harmful solutions such as self-injections of purported growth stimulants.

The concern of the adolescent about height may be generalized to many other aspects of appearance, including body habitus, beauty (or lack of beauty), skin condition, etc. The physician should be pre-

Table 5.4.
Selected Medical Problems Limited to Adolescence or Persisting into Adulthood

Limited Chiefly to Adolescence	Chronic Problems That May Begin in Adolescence
Slipped epiphysis	Obesity
Distortion of body image	Hypertension
Delinquency[a]	Diabetes
Anorexia nervosa	Hypercholesterolemia
Primary amenorrhea	Duodenal ulcer
School or learning problems[b]	Inflammatory bowel disease
	Irritable colon
	Dental caries
	Drug abuse
	Alcoholism
	Personality disorders
	Somatization disorder (hysteria)
	Depressive neurosis

[a] May begin earlier.
[b] Often develops earlier.

pared to recognize when concern about body image is the patient's primary concern and to provide reassurance that he or she is medically and biologically normal. This reassurance can be greatly facilitated at times by suggesting a book in which the adolescent can learn more about normal growth (see page 71).

Common Problems

Short Stature

(See "Short Stature and Delayed Sexual Maturation," page 65.)

Obesity

A practical definition of obesity is a weight of 20% or more over ideal body weight (see also Chapter 76). This can be estimated by determining the weight that corresponds to the growth chart height percentile for the age and sex of the child, and dividing this into the actual weight (see Fig. 5.1). A result of greater than 1.2 would be suspect. This ratio should be compared with the clinical appearance of the child, since the fat distribution changes at puberty in men, when extra weight may be transformed into musculature, and in women, who normally increase their storage of fat. Obesity remains a clinical diagnosis. Adolescent obesity is usually due to overeating. Most estimates place the prevalence between 4 and 10%, with the highest frequency among the lower socioeconomic groups. Frequently, the obesity began in early childhood, but becomes a concern in adolescence because of desires to conform to peer standards.

In order to treat adolescent obesity successfully, the teen himself must be motivated and must accept the physician's assessments and recommendations.

Frequently, the patient has attempted to cope with the problem by himself. Certain fad diets, such as fasting, water diets, *etc*, may yield rapid weight loss, but will deplete the strength of the child. Generally, since no modification of long term eating habits is attempted, the weight is regained upon cessation of the diet. Occasionally, there are serious biological complications to prolonged adherence to highly restrictive diets. Macrobiotic diets have been associated with symptoms of protein and vitamin deficiencies and liquid protein diets have cardiotoxic effects that have resulted in deaths. Severely calorie-restricted diets will lead to a cessation of linear growth and may cause menstrual irregularities.

Medications have been of no value in weight control. Amphetamines and metamphetamines are contraindicated in adolescents because of their potential for abuse.

Surgical treatment (e.g., jejunal-ileal bypass or gastric stapling) of obesity is rarely indicated, particularly in the adolescent years.

One is left with methods of dietary control by modification of behavior together with moderate calorie restriction. These methods, while successful for some, are not successful for all. Frequently, the teen who wants to diet is well motivated, if for personal and emotional reasons rather than for reasons of health. A group meeting of obese teens provides a nucleus of peer support, with an opportunity for mutual discussions of problems of dieting and appetite control that may not be aired in a brief office visit. Such a group may also help to alleviate home pressures. (Parental coercion and control of diet in the context of a normally antagonistic parent-teen relationship may result in an angry, rebellious youngster who is gaining rather than losing weight.)

For overweight young to midadolescents a reasonable goal is to maintain their current body weight, since excess caloric restriction may result in a loss of lean body weight. For the late adolescent, the goal may be weight loss. For all obese patients, one wishes to achieve a change in long term eating patterns.

Some adolescents overeat beacause of unresolved psychological difficulties. If there are expressions of problems in peer, school, or parental relationships, these should be explored further. Obesity alone, however, is not an indication of psychopathology.

Anorexia Nervosa

Anorexia nervosa is an infrequent but serious disorder of growth in adolescents. It is marked by extreme loss of appetite and of weight (at least 25% of the baseline weight) that is not attributable to a medical or psychiatric illness ordinarily associated with weight loss (i.e., inflammatory bowel disease or a major affective disorder). Patients characteristically exhibit an intense fear of becoming obese and, even when very thin, have a distorted body

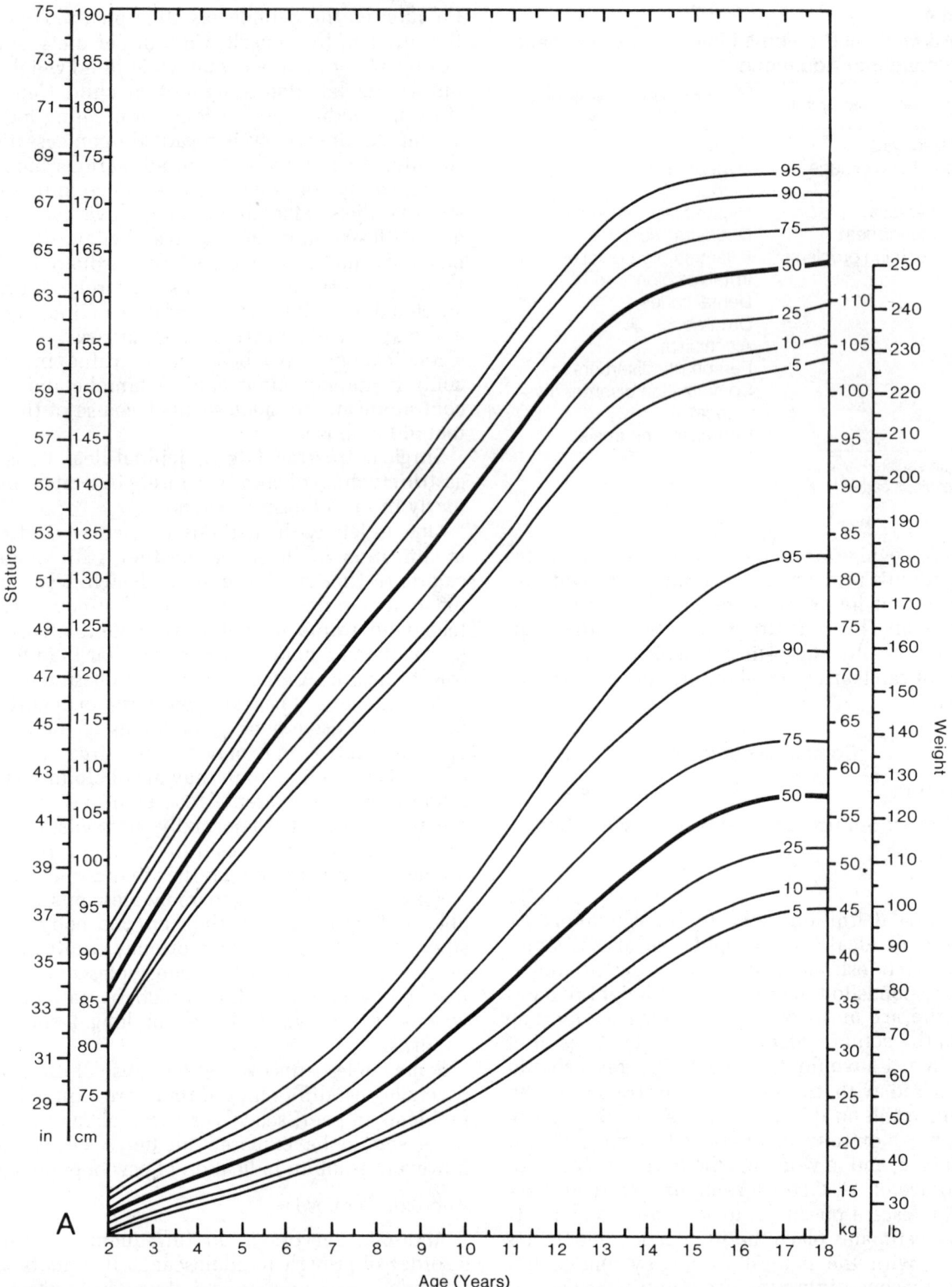

Figure 5.1A.   Physical growth in girls. Plot height and weight against chronological age at each encounter. The curve so obtained should parallel percentile lines within the clear area (growth patterns of 90% of children/adolescents). If the curve deviates from percentile lines, an abnormal growth pattern is likely. The upper series of curves represent the normal range of height at various ages and the lower series of curves, the normal range of weight at various ages. (From National Center for Health Statistics: NCHS Growth Charts, 1976. Monthly Vital Statistics Report. vol 25, no. 3, supp. (HRA) 76-1120. Rockville, MD, Health Resources Administration, June 1976.)

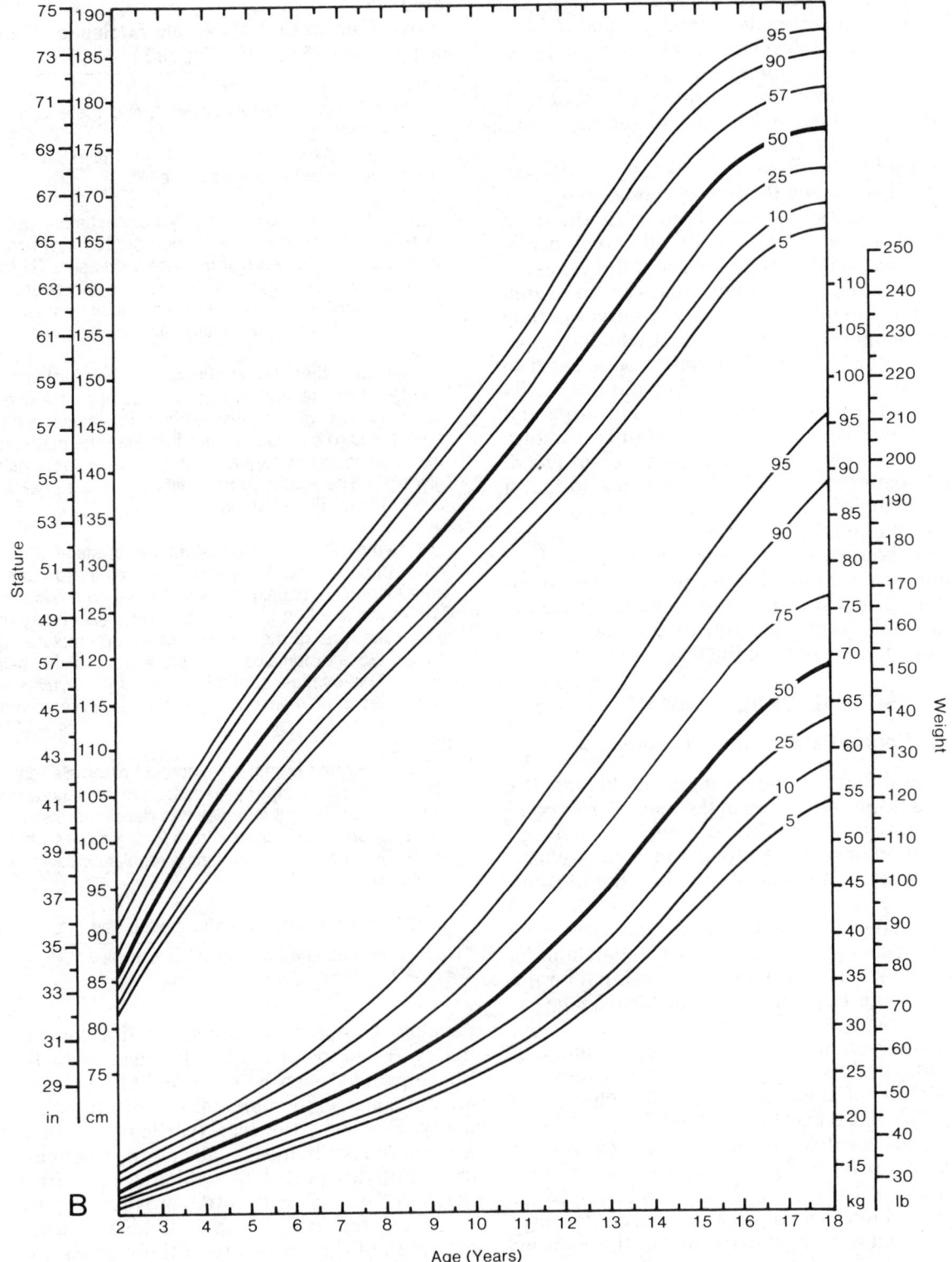

Figure 5.1B. Physical growth in boys.

image so that they still consider themselves over-weight.

Occasionally, a patient will periodically gorge herself, only to follow this by self-induced vomiting and by further self-reprisals through abstinence from food. As the disease progresses, patients may become withdrawn and depressed, leading to further appetite suppression. Amenorrhea is common in these patients, and it may be the presenting complaint.

Anorexia nervosa is most commonly a disease of

young adolescent girls (about 90% of cases); but occasionally it affects males or older females. Most often, the problem develops in children of upper middle class families. Before their illness, the patients typically have been considered "model children," who have done well in school and have been obedient to their parents.

The cause of the disease is unknown. Although there have been many theories proposed to explain it, none is entirely satisfactory. Frequently there has been some stress in the family (divorce, death, change of location) before the onset of the illness.

There is no simple treatment that can be recommended for patients with anorexia nervosa. Help should be sought from a psychiatrist who has experience with the problem. The best results seem to be achieved by involving the patient and her family in an intensive program in which counseling and behavior modification are employed to restructure the patient's eating habits and attitude toward food. Cachectic patients should be hospitalized so that a proper program of nutrition can be instituted.

Complete remission of anorexia nervosa is unusual, but about 75% of patients achieve an acceptable improvement in both their physical and emotional state. The rest remain chronically undernourished and maladapted, and 10% of the total population die of complications of the disease.

SEXUAL DEVELOPMENT

Normal Patterns and Concerns

A major difference between the child and the adolescent is the conversion of the teen into a sexual being. The onset of puberty is associated with an intensification of sexual feelings and desires which lead to sexual exploration. With the liberalization of sexual mores in recent years, the problems of adolescent pregnancy and venereal diseases have grown to epidemic proportions. An understanding of adolescent sexual development is essential for the practitioner interested in counseling his teenage patients in these areas.

The staging of physical sexual development of adolescents established by Tanner is a widely accepted method of following the physical changes of puberty (Tables 5.5 and 5.6 and Fig. 5.2).

As the adolescent enters puberty, he also assumes a role as a sexual being. He must begin to meet expectations of his society, family, and peer group and is pushed into sexual propriety and conformity. These expectations are transmitted to the teen by multiple messages. However, these messages are often conveyed poorly, and many teens remain ignorant and insecure about sexual issues.

Early adolescence is characterized by a bisexual period, in which close friendships are formed with members of the same sex, but heterosexual attitudes

Table 5.5.
Typical Progression of Female Adolescent Sexual Development (See Also Fig. 5.2.)[a]

STAGE 1:
> There is no pubic hair present, and there is no breast enlargement.
> The ovaries have begun to enlarge. The external genitalia are preadolescent or those of a child.

STAGE 2:
> Breast bud formation usually begins before pubic hair growth. A small mound is formed by the elevation of the breast and papilla. Areolar diameter increases. The adolescent height spurt begins, and there is an acceleration in the deposition of total body fat. The adult female habitus emerges as the breasts enlarge and the hips widen.

STAGE 3:
> There is further spread of pubic hair and further enlargement of breasts and areola with no separation of their contours. The vagina enlarges and the vaginal epithelium, responding to estrogen stimulation from the maturing ovaries, increases in thickness, with considerable deposition of glycogen. The height spurt usually reaches a peak early in stage 3, prior to menarche.

STAGE 4:
> If menarche has not occurred late in stage 3 it should occur during stage 4. Axillary hair appears just before or after menarche, usually in early stage 4. There is a projection of the areola and papilla to form a secondary mound above the level of the breast. The areolar mound may be absent (25% of females). The breasts and pubic hair progress. The ovaries continue to enlarge. Ovulation may occur just after menarche, but it is usually delayed until stage 5.

STAGE 5:
> Pubic hair and breast development resemble that of the adult female; the areola has recessed to the general contour of the breast. Height increase has decelerated since menarche; height may increase from 2 to 4 inches after menarche. By 2 years after menarche regular ovulation may be expected.

STAGE 6:
In 10% of females there is a further spread of pubic hair.

[a] From Tanner JM: *Growth at Adolescence*: New York, Appleton-Century-Crofts, 1966.

develop. One sees young teens developing "best buddy" relationships. The closeness of these relationships may even be on a sexual level, but they are not considered characteristic of adult homosexuality. However, the teen (particularly male) may fear that he is a homosexual; and the frequent name calling of this period (in which people are called "gay" or "queer" with little provocation) may be taken too seriously. Such individuals need to be reassured of the normality of these concerns. Masturbation tends to be a frequent practice in this period, and there may be associated guilt which increases as the sex drive stimulates the teen to continue the practice. Again, where appropriate, problems associated with masturbation should be met with reassurance of its normality.

Table 5.6.
Typical Progression of Male Adolescent Sexual Development[a]

STAGE 1:

The male has no pubic hair or increase in size of the penis.

This describes the male as a preadolescent or child. However, the testes are beginning to mature. Usually there is considerable acceleration in height and weight gain along with changes in body composition (especially more body fat).

STAGE 2:

There is early growth of the testes and scrotum before pubic hair appears. The height spurt accelerates; the male physique begins to change as fat and muscle are added; and the areola of the breast increases in size and darkens slightly.

STAGE 3:

There is further enlargement of the testes and scrotum, enlargement of the penis (mainly in length), and spreading and darkening of the pubic hair. Facial hair first appears at the corners of the upper lip. The height spurt accelerates further; there is broadening of the shoulders relative to the hips and generalized increased moulding of the body, with considerable increase in muscle mass relative to fat. Hair appears in the perineum. Facial expression is significantly altered and appears more adult. The cartilage of the larynx enlarges, and the voice may begin to deepen. There is transient gynecomastia with a slight projection of the areola.

STAGE 4:

Axillary hair first appears. There is continued enlargement of the scrotum, testes, and penis (the last, mainly in breadth). The pubic hair begins to appear adult. Facial hair is still limited to the upper lip and chin. The first ejaculation, indicating considerable growth of the prostate gland, occurs early in stage 4. Sebaceous glands are approaching adult size and function. The voice deepens further.

STAGE 5:

Genital size and pubic hair distribution are adult in appearance. Hairs are present on the sides of the face. Gynecomastia has disappeared. The height spurt has decelerated and the physique is that of the mature male.

STAGE 6:

Some adolescents have a further spread of pubic hair up the linea alba, which may be described as stage 6. This later development, often not reached until the early twenties, occurs in 80% of males.

[a] From Tanner JM: *Growth at Adolescence.* New York, Appleton-Century-Crofts, 1966.

In mid- to late adolescence, dating and heterosexual activities begin in earnest. Sorenson (9) found that 52% of all adolescents and 45% of single females have had intercourse by age 19. Frequently, teens rush into sexual activity before they fully understand their own feelings about it. It is often part of the dating relationship—a prerequisite to communication, rather than *vice versa*. It may be part of thrill-seeking behavior for some teens, and others use it to escape from loneliness and depression.

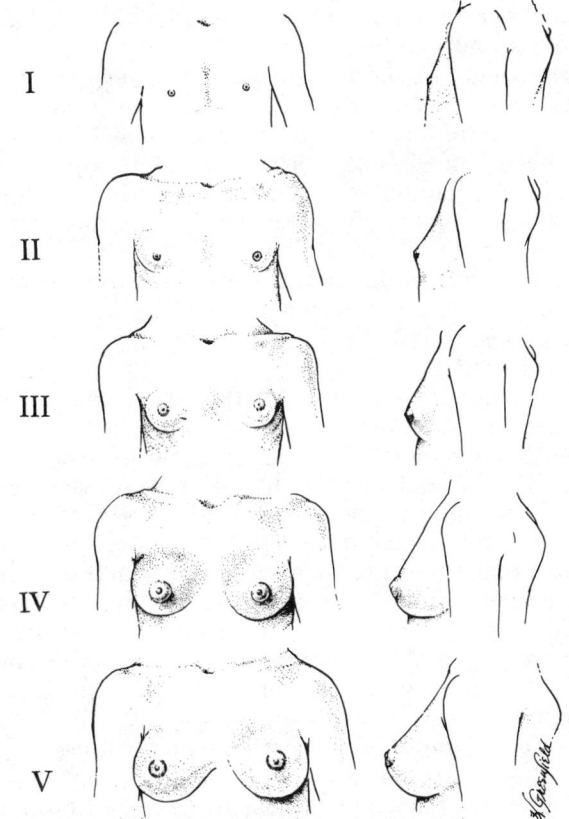

Figure 5.2. Diagrammatic representation of Tanner stages I to V of human breast maturation. (Adapted from Marshall WA, Tanner JM: Variations in pattern of pubertal changes in girls. *Arch Dis Child* 44:291, 1969.)

Sexuality may also be used as reward or punishment in some relationships, emulating parental behavior.

Common Problems

Short Stature and Delayed Sexual Maturation

A frequent problem that comes to the attention of physicians is the teenager with short stature and/or delayed puberty. These two symptoms are often interrelated, and the medical investigation is similar, so they will be discussed together. However, the presence of one does not necessarily indicate a problem with the other.

Most of these patients simply are at one end of the spectrum of normal development (3). Many teenage boys may not appreciate the fact that some individuals fall into the 10th percentile of a normal curve, and therefore will not respond well to a cursory dismissal of their complaints. Some may be helped by looking at normal growth curves which indicate the predicted ultimate height for persons in their percentile (see Fig. 5.1). Detailed discussion may be necessary for patients to comprehend fully and to cope with normal findings.

Assessment of short stature and delayed puberty by the generalist consists of the following steps:

1. A careful history of the onset of puberty and of the height of siblings, parents, and grandparents should be obtained. In particular, it should be noted if there is a history of several short family members (males under 5'6", females under 5'0").

2. Growth records of the patient should be reviewed. Heights and weights should be plotted on an appropriate growth curve (see Fig. 5.1). If a child has followed a single curve throughout life, a significant metabolic reason for this short stature is unlikely. If, however, there is a falling away from a growth line, a metabolic problem is more likely.

3. The medical history should be reviewed, including a prenatal and neonatal history. A history of operations, head injuries, or chronic medical conditions that could predispose the individual to failure to thrive should be noted. If the child had a low birth weight, a review of underlying factors may disclose a possible chromosomal abnormality or toxic exposure (e.g., maternal cigarette smoking) that could produce long term growth delay.

4. A developmental and psychosocial history may indicate possible familial problems and/or emotional neglect that could predispose to constitutional growth delay (so-called psychosocial dwarfism).

5. Inquiries into the teen's general health and daily habits may reveal problems needing investigation, such as poor appetite, frequent infections, chronic abdominal pain, or general fatigue and listlessness.

A physical examination is essential, including an accurate height and weight and Tanner stage assessment (Tables 5.5 and 5.6). If the testes are softening and show enlargement, or if breast budding is present, there usually will be a normal sexual development. Unusual facies or ears, unusual hand creases, clinodactyly (deviation or deflection of the fingers), obesity, or delayed intellectual development may suggest a recognizable hereditary syndrome.

The initial laboratory investigation should include the following: urinalysis; measurement of serum urea nitrogen, creatinine, and electrolytes; hematocrit value and white cell count; as well as X-rays of the hands and wrists to assess skeletal growth (2).

More specific laboratory investigations may be suggested by the history and physical examination. Examples are: (*a*) thyroid enlargement (testing for hypothyroidism); (*b*) normal physical examination and appearance but markedly short stature which is falling away from growth lines (testing for growth hormone deficiency); (*c*) girls with delayed puberty, heights under the 3rd percentile, associated with a short "webbed" neck, a systolic murmur, or widely spaced nipples (buccal smears performed to rule out Turner's syndrome, i.e., X-O chromosomes); (*d*)

striking pubertal delay without a history of similar delay in other family members (testing for gonadal failure: measurement of serum follicle-stimulating and luteinizing hormones, and estradiol and of urinary 17-ketosteroids and 17-hydroxysteroids; vaginal smear for maturation index and buccal smear for chromosome analysis).

Definitive diagnosis and planning for adolescents with suspected endocrine, metabolic, genetic, or psychological reasons for maturation delay require referral to an appropriate specialist. Patients with hereditary disorders may benefit from genetic counseling, particularly those who will be unable to bear children—for example, patients with Turner's syndrome.

Venereal Disease

Venereal diseases are epidemic in 15- to 19-year-olds. This is partially due to more casual attitudes toward sex, with frequent changes of sex partners.

The diagnosis and treatment of various venereal diseases are discussed elsewhere in this book (see Chapters 27 and 94).

Public health professionals find it disheartening to witness the failure of the medical system in combating the spread of venereal disease. Many teens seem to avoid therapy and continue to pass on their disease. Physicians have not uniformly reported cases of venereal disease, and there has been a tendency to delay treatment and not reach out to case contacts.

Sex education programs have had little impact on the problem. Fear of infection apparently does not deter some teens, who seem irresponsible, impulsive, emotionally insecure, and who appear to have little respect for others. Frequently parents have failed to provide basic information about sex and the risks of infection and pregnancy which accompany it.

In most states, adolescents have a right to receive treatment for venereal disease without the parents' knowledge. The practitioner should be receptive to the teen seeking treatment. Visits for treatment should also be utilized to explain the mechanism of acquiring venereal infection and to explain and encourage the use of condoms to prevent reinfection.

Pregnancy

Each year over a million women under the age of 20 become pregnant, half of them out of wedlock. Many of these pregnancies are associated with serious medical risks for the mother and the fetus. Mothers under 14 have particularly high risks of toxemia, anemia, prematurity, infants with low birth weight, prolonged labor, and postpartum complications. Many of these problems can be prevented by good obstetrical care, so that the first goal in adolescent pregnancy should be early diagnosis and entry into a comprehensive treatment program.

There are multiple social and behavioral reasons for the high number of teenage pregnancies. For many adolescents, pregnancy may be part of a maladaptive attempt to solve psychological issues, such as independence from a clinging mother, or manipulation of a boyfriend. Such patients may have previously engaged in other maladaptive activites, such as drug abuse or delinquency. There may also be an underlying ignorance about methods and availability of birth control (see Chapter 93).

The teenager herself may be ambivalent about her pregnancy. Often, the manipulations that led to the pregnancy in the sense of achieving a prolonged relationship, *etc*, have not succeeded and a sense of abandonment is felt. Furthermore, the pregnancy may have resulted in hostility from the family when the teenager is in greatest need of help from her parents.

Clearly the teenager about to make important decisions about herself and her pregnancy requires counseling. It can be provided by the primary physician or by a staff member of a counseling agency such as Planned Parenthood. In either case, the primary physician should be aware of the patient's plan and make himself available for any problems she may wish to discuss. If the teenager decides to continue with the pregnancy, she should be prepared to assume a parenting role. Furthermore, she should be educated about future pregnancies and given medical assistance for the pediatric care needed for her infant. If possible, day care, vocational, and educational services should be available for the mother so that she may continue her education after the birth of her child. As an integral part of counseling, a stable caring person should be identified (a parent, if possible) who can assist the teen emotionally and financially, and who can help her see the future for herself and her baby in a realistic manner.

Rape

Rape is a sexual act, usually intercourse, with a nonconsenting victim. The most frequent type of adolescent rape has been called "acquaintance rape," and it is probable that most instances are never reported. In acquaintance rape, the victim is sexually misused by a boyfriend during a date or by a casual friend, or a trusting teen may accompany her friends to a strange place where she is gang raped.

Teens, in exploring sexuality, may not have set limits to their petting, or, if limits have been set unilaterally, they may afford little protection for the victim, especially when the assailant is an adolescent for whom limit setting has not been successful in other areas. Some teens may also, in their uncertainty, present themselves in provocative, pseudomature ways; for example, by wearing outrageous and provocative clothing which may be viewed as sexually inviting by male acquaintances.

There is a tendency in dealing with adolescent rape victims to imply that the assault may have been invited by the victim. Regardless of this possibility, rape should be treated as a very serious problem for the victim who reports it.

Initial care for the rape victim should be handled by a physician, with follow-up by a rape counseling service if one exists in the community. Often, a physician who is already acquainted with the patient can provide the best care.

There are several important considerations in caring for the rape victim:

1. Rape is a crime of violence, not a sexual act.

2. Above all else, the adolescent reporting rape has usually had a very frightening experience and needs short term counseling (see Chapter 11). She will usually have a number of questions about the physical meaning of her experience, and it is important to provide answers to them.

3. She should be examined carefully for evidence of trauma, both to the pelvic organs and to the rest of her body, and the information should be carefully recorded.

4. She must decide whether she wishes to report the rape to the police. In this instance, it is essential to obtain a wet and fixed smear of the vaginal contents as early as possible to confirm the presence of spermatozoa.

5. Most rape victims will need counseling by their physician and or a counselor for a number of months to discuss persisting anxieties and questions.

PSYCHOSOCIAL DEVELOPMENT

Normal Patterns and Concerns

The major psychosocial developmental task for the adolescent as he approaches adulthood is to increase independence from his parents and to establish a positive identity congruent with social norms.

In early adolescence, the young teen is faced with the dilemma of seeking independence from parents while at the same time relying on them for emotional and physical support. The conflict over independence is evidenced by contradiction and ambivalence. For example, a teen may refuse to listen to parents' suggestions about study habits, but blame mediocre grades on the fact that the parents did not help with homework assignments.

As the teen enters into middle and late adolescence, he demonstrates a remarkable resourcefulness in coping with anxiety over separation and in learning more mature behavior. Much assistance comes through peer relationships. Teens support each other by experimenting with adult roles which mirror societal expectations of behavior; a sense of moral responsibility begins to take shape. In this period, individual identity tends to be blunted by the seeking of independence from the family. Peers tend to look alike, dress alike, date alike, and experiment with drugs and sex alike. Later, as teens address their concerns about careers, a greater differentiation of personalities takes shape and individual identities emerge.

Normal development also requires the example of secure, healthy parents in an environment in which the teen can feel secure. Thus, parents, who are preoccupied with their own psychological problems at work, in their marriage, or with their own families, may have difficulties helping and coping with the development of their adolescent offspring. Often such parents have not previously succeeded at their own adolescent tasks and so are unable to proceed with the task of adulthood—they have not developed the ability for intimacy, for close personal feelings, for the sharing of feelings and thoughts with others, and for adhering to reasonable limits.

One clear fact about adolescent development is that its emotional course is variable, even among "normal" adolescents. The idea that adolescence is usually a time of crisis, in which persistent neurotic behavior is essential for development of a personal identity, has not been borne out by longitudinal research. On the other hand, Kysar et al's study (4) of college freshmen showed that 22% had psychological problems, usually personality disorders of the compulsive, schizoid, or passive-aggressive type expressed as difficulties in academic, social, and psychosexual functioning. Offer et al's longitudinal study of teenage boys (8) points out that achievement of identity is a long term process. His subjects were first studied when they were high school freshmen, and were followed for 7 years. At the end of this interval, most subjects had yet to consolidate their identities to the point where they could develop an intimate relationship, one of the best indicators of progress to adulthood. Despite this, self-satisfaction and parental satisfaction were the norm. For many, adolescence is a crisis but an internalized, noiseless one.

Generally the teen must succeed in the other spheres of development in order to meet tasks in the psychosocial sphere successfully. In retarded, handicapped, or chronically ill children the dependence-independence struggle may persist, impairing the development of self-esteem needed to develop a sense of identity.

Common Problems

Juvenile Delinquency

Juvenile delinquency is a legal term for youthful behavior that violates the law and would be adjudicated and punished if it had been committed by an adult. It is a major social problem, and will, at times, be brought to the attention of the practitioner who is asked whether there is an underlying psychological cause for the delinquent behavior. In order to deal with this issue, it is necessary to distinguish between three broad categories of delinquency, described by Weiner (10) as sociological delinquency, characterological delinquency, and neurotic delinquency.

Sociological delinquency refers to illegal acts organized by a subcultural group, i.e., street gang. The delinquent acts are adaptive in that the teen receives the approval of his peers. The following four features of the clinical history suggest sociological delinquency: first, the delinquent acts are performed with valued companions, rather than alone or with strangers; second, these teens see themselves as accepted and integral members of their peer group and rarely exhibit feelings of alienation or inadequacy; third, sociological delinquents give little evidence of neurotic symptom formation or basic character flaws; and fourth, these delinquents frequently have had supportive family relationships during early childhood, although there may have been more recent problems which have led to their current activities. Frequently, involvement in other positive group activities will change the delinquent orientation of these teens.

Characterological delinquents reflect a basically antisocial attitude toward life. Their acts do not evoke in them any guilt or remorse. Such teens are frequently loners who have not established a strong relationship of basic trust in their life. Their past history suggests a series of problems, with a flurry of destructive acts, such as fighting, fire setting, and cruelty to animals, preceding their more destructive delinquent activity. Such children often require long term psychiatric treatment.

The *neurotic delinquent* commits destructive acts as an atypical (for him) behavior pattern to illustrate and emphasize certain needs. These acts may reflect feelings of being ignored by family or peers, or indicate that the teen is suffering from some form of psychological distress, most frequently depression. The acts are committed in such a way that the teen will be caught in the process or will give himself away soon after. (Generally, if concealment of illegal acts is repetitive and successful, a neurotic basis of the delinquency is unlikely.) There is rarely a history of early behavioral problems, and typically the delinquent has enjoyed a loving relationship with parents and family members. Occasionally, however, some recent family stress may serve as the trigger for the delinquent act. In general, neurotic delinquency may be treated by the interested practitioner through short term counseling (see Chapter 11).

Substance Abuse

Although substance abuse, including tobacco use, is a major problem of adult life, it frequently begins during the adolescent years (see Chapter 20 on tobacco use, Chapter 21 on alcoholism, and Chapter 22 on illicit drugs). Since adolescence is a period of experimentation, it is the rare teen who has not had a drink of alcohol, smoked a cigarette, or tried marijuana. A major concern is to identify the adolescent abuser—one whose life is being disrupted by his aberrant activities. It is this teenager who is most likely to continue to abuse alcohol or drugs in adult life.

The routine examination of a teen should include direct questioning about his use of alcohol and of drugs. If the use of a substance is excessive and hazardous, the physician should explore the factors that might have led to abuse. Drugs and/or alcohol used to excess are generally an escape from some psychological problem, and it is only by identifying the problem that the abuse may be stopped. Lecturing on the dangers of alcohol, drugs, or tobacco seems to have little impact on adolescents.

Occasionally, the serious abuser of hazardous substances will develop physiological symptoms that are dramatic enough to come to the physician's attention. Hospitalization for observation is almost always indicated for the teenager presenting with drug intoxication, even if emergency room evaluation indicates that there are no immediate medical risks. The possibility of attempted suicide may be real and must be explored. Even if this is not a factor, there is still concern about the teen's ability to control his own drug abuse behavior.

How and when to intervene in drug abuse behavior is a difficult question. In part, it is a moral question, where the physician's behavior may be influenced by his own beliefs about the dangers of cigarettes, alcohol, or drugs and about his right to interfere with the actions (albeit dangerous) of an autonomous individual. Furthermore, intervention in this problem is made difficult by the fact that treatment is often ineffective.

Depression and Suicide

A behavioral hallmark of adolescents is mood shifts, from the peaks of elation to the depths of despair. Depressive symptoms are normal parts of psychosocial development. The quest for identity is balanced by a sense of loss once independence is achieved. Similarly, rejections by peers (e.g., first loves) may be felt very deeply. It is not unusual, as part of these depressions, for the adolescent to contemplate suicide.

Mattsson (6) describes five depressive states of adolescence. Normal *depressive mood swings* represent transient reactions to personal disappointments or family difficulties. They rarely affect other life functions. *Acute depressive reactions* are more severe states, often lasting weeks or months. They are normal reactions, similar to states of grief (see Chapter 19), often related to separation or to loss of

a close friend, relative, or teacher. The adolescent who does not successfully work through his grief, and who becomes increasingly depressed and incapacitated by his loss, suffers from a *depressive neurosis*. Such teens withdraw from their normal functioning, are chronically sad, and begin to entertain suicidal ideation. This is a fairly severe level of depression and demands professional intervention. A fourth form of depression, the *masked depressions of adolescence*, can be viewed as a subgroup of the depressive neuroses. Such teens cannot tolerate their painful feelings, and express them through a variety of somatic or behavioral complaints. They may be frequent visitors to the primary care physician, suffering from ill defined, atypical symptoms without a clear organic basis. Their behavior may include overeating, delinquent acts, exhibitionist acts resulting in "accidental" self-destruction, drug and alcohol abuse, etc. *Psychotic depressive disorders* are marked by impaired reality testing, thought disorders, paranoia and suicidal intention, in addition to depressive symptomatology.

The primary care physician is sometimes asked to evaluate the depressed or suicidal adolescent. In taking the history, the physician should try to uncover recent events that may have precipitated the depressive disorder: any long-standing family, school, or peer problems; possibilities of organic brain disease or of drug abuse that may mimic depressive symptoms; symptoms of cognitive or reality disturbances, suggesting a psychosis; and symptoms suggesting a masked depression. The physician should not hesitate to talk about depression with the teen. Indeed, such openness may put the adolescent at ease and let him feel that the physician truly understands what he may be feeling. A physical examination will help the physician rule out physical problems, and communication with the school will give the physician some additional observations about the teen in his daily activities.

Most adolescents with depressive symptoms need some counseling. If the primary care physician feels medication is necessary, and is unfamiliar with the use of psychoactive drugs in adolescents, conjoint treatment with a psychiatric consultant may prove helpful. Patients with long-standing depressive symptoms, which suggest thought disturbances, and possible suicide attempts should be referred for psychiatric intervention. Additional details about the office management of depression are contained in Chapter 15.

INTELLECTUAL DEVELOPMENT

Normal Patterns and Concerns

In adolescence, a major change occurs with respect to education and intellect. Schools differentiate students, placing them into vocational or academic tracks. The emphasis shifts from the learning of tasks (e.g., basic reading, writing, and arithmetic) to the accumulation of facts and the ability to think abstractly. As teens prepare for college, learning becomes a competitive task. Career choices become limited as an individual's abilities and talents become manifest. Upon entering college, a greater amount of independence and responsibility is expected. Symbolically, the university begins to resemble the workplace both in terms of potential rewards and of potential pressures.

Scholastic Failure

Academic achievement is strongly related to parental aspirations, socioeconomic status, and intellectual ability. Occasionally, the child cannot meet parental expectations, and the resultant crisis may lead to a visit to the physician's office. Failure in school may also be a symptom of a physical impairment, mental retardation, specific learning disabilities, or emotional stress. By making an accurate diagnosis of the underlying problem, a caring practitioner may help such children.

First a history is necessary, to determine the nature of the school difficulties. When did they begin; has educational achievement been a problem throughout a school career, as with a global intellectual deficit, or is it specific to certain subjects or tasks, as with learning disorders? Is there a family history of poor school performance, as is seen with familial dyslexics? How does the teen act with his family and peers? Is there evidence of disturbed behavior outside of school as with emotional disorders? Is the family structure stable, or has there been separation, divorce, or death of a parent or grandparent? Is there evidence of substance abuse on the part of the teen or a member of the family? What has the family done to try to work through problems?

Second, a physical examination, with a careful neurological examination, is indicated, with emphasis on looking for signs of minimal cerebral dysfunction, such as "soft" neurological signs, right-left discrimination or orientation difficulties, or overt signs of cerebral palsy (1). (In such patients, there may be suggestions of a neurological problem in the past medical history; the birth may have been abnormal; or the patient may have shown hyperactivity or attention deficits as a child.) Vision testing and office assessment for slight or moderate hearing loss (see Chapter 96) are also particularly important.

Third, some specific intelligence testing is indicated. Children who are mentally retarded will tend to show low I.Q. scores, and achievement tests will show a delay of several grades in math and reading levels. Children with dyslexia will have a normal I.Q. but will show a wide scatter of scores on subtests, indicating a nonglobal deficit. Achievement tests may also show a difference between abilities in reading and mathematics.

Recent research in learning disabilities indicates that some learning problems may appear relatively late in a school career (5). The recent criticism of the ability of some college students to write well has given credence to the notion of expressive language disorders, which may not become manifest until adolescence. Some individuals with fine perceptual problems may not reveal difficulties until geometry or drafting is studied in high school.

The Congress, in 1974, passed Federal Law 94-142, assuring a free, appropriate educational placement for all children up to age 21. Thus, adolescents with specific learning problems, retardation, or emotional difficulties are entitled to be placed in a classroom setting where they will learn. If he suspects an unrecognized problem in one of these spheres, the physician may help by referring the patient and his parents for evaluation, usually available through the child's school or the local education system. Unfortunately, problems remain unrecognized for many children, and, out of frustration, they will drop out of school.

A SUGGESTED APPROACH TO THE ADOLESCENT PATIENT IN THE OFFICE SETTING

The physician who deals even occasionally with teens and young adults must be aware of their perspective. Each adolescent approaches the developmental pressures of this period of life with his own particular skills and emotions. From a health perspective, an adolescent can be a responsible partner in maintaining his well-being and complying with medical care; or he can be infantile, dependent, uncommunicative, aggressive, or irresponsible. The physician who cares for adolescents must have a temperament equal to coping with them and be a patient and perceptive listener and inquirer.

As shown in Table 5.2, although a general examination is the single most frequent reason for office visits by adolescents, the majority of visits are for specific medical problems. In either of these situations, the practitioner should use appropriate strategies in interviewing and examining the patient and should be alert for clues suggesting problems in any of the major spheres of development described in the preceding sections.

Interviewing Strategies

The physician, in obtaining a history, should interview adolescents in private. The adolescent needs to feel that he is the patient and that his problems are being listened to and taken seriously. Then it is often useful to talk to the parents separately as well.

The Patient

Some adolescent patients are difficult to interview. An uncommunicative patient may have been sent to a physician against his will or may lack verbal skills needed for coherence. The physician must be verbally active with such patients and watch for any nonverbal cues as wedges to try to get the patient to speak. Examples of nonverbal cues are: a look of interest or initiation of eye contact when a subject is mentioned which the patient would like to discuss; a clenched fist when an anger-provoking subject is raised; frequent position change and fidgeting when the patient is anxious about a specific subject or about the visit to the physician in general. Because adolescents are often reticent about their major concerns, an open-minded invitation to share information ("Is there anything else you wanted to talk about?") should be included in each office contact. The initial comprehensive interview may require several sessions. At the first visit, warmth and interest in the adolescent may open the way to better communication in future sessions.

Many adolescents continue to go to their pediatrician for medical care until they enter college, take a job, or marry. Because of this long term association, their relationship may be almost like that of a father and child—warm, intense, and comradely. These feelings cannot be transferred easily to a new physician, and it is unwise to attempt to transfer them.

The physician can most effectively surmount such problems by explaining his *modus operandi* in advance, emphasizing that he will be primarily the adolescent's physician, rather than an agent of the patient's parents as had been the case previously. Communications should be adult-to-adult whenever possible.

The internist should encourage the adolescent to initiate patient-doctor contacts, guard against patriarchal advice giving, and avoid showing disapproval or surprise when the adolescent attempts to impress him with tales of sexual exploits, with the use of vulgar language, *etc.*

It is wise to establish other ground rules with adolescents. Patient-doctor confidentiality, for example, can be assured to adolescents only insofar as they do not reveal that they are comtemplating harmful acts, such as running away or committing suicide. However, certain privileged communications should be kept confidential from parents. In particular, adolescent minors have the right to be seen for venereal disease or for sex offense-related examinations without the prior consent of a parent. The teen may also wish to keep some health-related or emotional problems, such as drug experimentation, from a parent's knowledge.

The Parents

How does an adolescent's physician communicate with the parent? It is suggested that, whenever possible, a parent should be involved with and concerned about the health of the teen. A separate interview with a parent, immediately before or after the examination, may prove helpful and can emphasize particular concerns downplayed or denied by the patient. The parents of adolescent patients may be useful in aiding treatment, providing emotional support, and ensuring compliance with therapy; therefore, informing them about the adolescent's problems and needs is important.

Some parents ask physicians to take on the role of health educator or counselor for their adolescent child. Usually, these requests are for anticipatory guidance about birth control or drug usage. At times, the physician is asked to help the child work through an upcoming family crisis, such as divorce, serious illness, or death. Frequently, adolescents welcome the opportunity to discuss these issues in private. Their knowledge in these areas is often found wanting, and the sensitive physician may help the adolescent grasp realities and make intelligent decisions. A number of books are directed to an adolescent audience in these areas, and it may be useful to make these titles available:

R. A. Gardner: *Boys and Girls Book about Divorce (Grades I and Up).* Burtan, New York, 1971.
E. Kay: *Sex and the Young Teenager (Grades 7–12).* Franklin-Watts, New York, 1973.
H. Soethcord: *Sex before Twenty: New Answers for Young People.* E. P. Dutton, New York, 1971.
K. McCoy and C. Wibbelsman: *The Teenage Body Book.* Pocket Books, New York, 1978.

Parents often have questions about specific adolescent behavior. A particular episode or issue may come to the parents' attention, and they may ask the physician whether they should exert control over it. In such instances, the physician should not offer specific advice, but should try to discern any moral or behavioral conflicts between the parents and the adolescent. When the parent's behavior is inconsistent with the parent's own stated values, adolescents will often act in opposition to those values. Miller (7) suggests that parents are not helped in this instance by being told how to behave. Advice either increases the parent's uncertainty when faced with later difficulties or implies that the parent's own opinions are inappropriate. Adolescents probably turn out mentally healthier when presented with models of adult behavior with which their parents are comfortable, whether consistent with societal norms or not. Parents must be prepared, however, to make allowances so that their children have freedom to make their own "mistakes." Family counseling is a technique which the general physician can utilize when several members of a household are involved (see Chapter 11).

Health Assessment

The initial interview(s) should be comprehensive enough to ensure that the adolescent is meeting

Table 5.7.
Disqualifying Conditions for Sports Participation by the Adolescent[a]

Conditions	Collision[b]	Contact[c]	Noncontact[d]	Other[e]
General				
Acute infections:				
Respiratory, genitourinary, infectious mononucleosis, hepatitis, active rheumatic fever, active tuberculosis	X	X	X	X
Obvious physical immaturity in comparison with other competitors	X	X		
Hemorrhagic disease:				
Hemophilia, purpura, and other serious bleeding tendencies	X	X	X	
Diabetes, inadequately controlled	X	X	X	X
Diabetes, controlled	[f]	[f]	[f]	[f]
Jaundice	X	X	X	X
Eyes				
Absence or loss of function of one eye	X	X		
Respiratory				
Tuberculosis (active or symptomatic)	X	X	X	X
Severe pulmonary insufficiency	X	X	X	X
Cardiovascular				
Mitral stenosis, aortic stenosis, aortic insufficiency, coarctation of aorta, cyanotic heart disease, recent carditis of any etiology	X	X	X	X
Hypertension on organic basis	X	X	X	X
Previous heart surgery for congenital or acquired heart disease	[g]	[g]	[g]	[g]
Liver, enlarged	X	X		
Skin				
Boils, impetigo, and herpes simplex gladiatorum	X	X		
Spleen, enlarged	X	X		
Hernia				
Inguinal or femoral hernia	X	X	X	
Musculoskeletal				
Symptomatic abnormalities or inflammations	X	X	X	X
Functional inadequacy of the musculoskeletal system, congenital or acquired, incompatible with the contact or skill demands of the sport	X	X	X	
Neurological				
History or symptoms of previous serious head trauma or repeated concussions	X			
Controlled convulsive disorder	[h]	[h]	[h]	[h]
Convulsive disorder not moderately well controlled by medication	X			
Previous surgery on head	X	X		
Renal				
Absence of one kidney	X	X		
Renal insufficiency	X	X	X	X
Genitalia				
Absence of one testicle	[i]	[i]	[i]	[i]
Undescended testicle	[i]	[i]	[i]	[i]

[a] From Committee on Sports Medicine, American Academy of Pediatrics: *Sports Medicine: Health Care for Young Athletes.* Evanston, IL, American Academy of Pediatrics, 1983.
[b] Football, rugby, hockey, lacrosse, and so forth.
[c] Baseball, soccer, basketball, wrestling, and so forth.

appropriate developmental tasks. Inquiries should be made into the teens' relationships and functioning with their families, at school, and with peers. It is important to determine whether the teens are establishing positive personal identities (Have they hobbies? Do they voice their own opinions? Can they choose their own friends or must friends be approved by the parents? Do they have plans for the future?); whether they are accepting their sexuality and adjusting to adult sexual roles (Do they date? Are they sexually active? Do they have a knowledge of contraception? Is contaception used?); whether they are establishing independence from the family (Do they drive? Do they earn money on their own? What sort of hours do they keep?); whether they are working toward a career (What are their plans after high school? What subjects in school do they like? What are their grades? Do they plan to go to college? Are their goals realistic and are they supported by the family?); whether they have established good health habits (What are their views about nutrition? Have they experimented with alcohol, tobacco, or other recreational drugs? What drugs? Have they ever been drugged or high when driving or when attending school?); and whether affective swings are interfering with functioning (Do they often feel down? What makes them happy? Have sad feelings ever made them consider harming themselves?).

As part of the review of systems before examination, a self-administered medical questionnaire may be useful and timesaving. Such a questionnaire should be brief with language simple enough to be understood by teens with poor reading skills. Positive answers often need to be explored further. A physical examination should be performed in the absence of parents. Teenage girls examined by male physicians may be more comfortable with an adult female in the room with them. Some parts of the physical examination occasionally omitted by physicians but essential for adolescent patients include blood pressure measurement, examination of the entire integument, of the spine (for scoliosis), and of the external genitalia (for signs of venereal disease and for assessment of sexual development using Tanner's staging—see Tables 5.5 and 5.6). All sexually active adolescent girls should have a pelvic examination, including gonorrheal cultures and a Pap smear. If the physician is uncomfortable doing this examination, the teen should be referred to a gynecologist who is used to dealing with adolescents.

There are several useful adjuncts to the physical examination of the healthy adolescent. These include testing for myopia and hyperopia (using a Snellen chart) and screening for deafness (by speaking softly). Adolescence is a period marked by noise pollution, in the form of loud music which can cause permanent damage to the eighth nerve (see Chapter 96). Those adolescents who have difficulty in school should be screened for learning disorders. Having a teenager read a newspaper paragraph out loud or do some simple arithmetic may reveal a previously undetected learning disability.

Laboratory screening tests for healthy adolescents should include a full urinalysis, a complete blood count, and tuberculin testing. Screening for hyperlipidemias (Chapter 75) is indicated in adolescents with family histories of myocardial infarction or of stroke under the age of 50. Blood chemical screens, chest X-rays, and electrocardiograms are not indicated in healthy adolescents. Specific recommendations regarding healthy periodic health assessment in adolescents and young adults are found in Chapter 2 (Table 2.1).

Examining the Adolescent Athlete

As public interest in physical fitness has increased, more adolescents and young adults have turned to competitive sports and vigorous physical activities. Physicians have taken on important new responsibilities in the field of sports medicine, advising and providing health services for athletes of all ages. The examination of adolescent athletes requires an evaluation of the individual's health and a consideration of his functional ability, growth, and maturation. Thus, the physician should help the less fit or physically immature adolescent to choose a sport that may require minimal physical impact or less endurance.

Most principles of sports medicine are a part of general medical knowledge and everyday practice. Special understanding of the physical demands of various sports and the injuries possible in them can

---

[d] Cross country, track, tennis, crew, swimming, and so forth.

[e] Bowling, golf, archery, field events, and so forth.

[f] No exclusions.

[g] Each patient should be judged on an individual basis in conjunction with his cardiologist and surgeon.

[h] Each patient should be judged on an individual basis. All things being equal, it is probably better to encourage a young boy or girl to participate in a noncontact sport rather than a contact sport. However, if a patient has a desire to play a contact sport and this is deemed a major ameliorating factor in his or her adjustment to school, associates, and the seizure disorder, serious consideration should be given to letting him or her participate if the seizures are moderately well controlled or the patient is under good medical management.

[i] The Committee approves the concept of contact sports participation for youths with only one testicle or with an undescended testicle(s), except in specific instances such as an inguinal canal undescended testicle(s), following appropriate medical evaluation to rule out unusual injury risk. However, the athlete, parents, and school authorities should be fully informed that participation in contact sports for youths with only one testicle carries a slight injury risk to the remaining healthy testicle. Fertility may be adversely affected following an injury. But the chances of an injury to a descended testicle are rare, and the injury risk can be further substantially minimized with an athletic supporter and protective device.

be gained from books and journals on sports medicine.

The purpose of the preparticipation health evaluation is to identify medical conditions that might preclude safe and effective athletic participation, including those that might become worse by partic-ipation in sports activities. It is in the examination of the young athlete that these conditions become known. As athletes become more experienced, the most commonly encountered abnormalities are residuals of previous sports injuries.

By and large, the preathletic physical is similar to

Table 5.8.
Screening Preparticipation History for the Adolescent Athlete[a]

NAME _____   DATE _____

PREPARTICIPATION EVALUATION—HISTORY

Completed by ATHLETE or PARENT

	YES	NO
1. Have any members of your family under age 50 had a "heart attack" or "heart problems"?	_____	_____
2. Have you ever been told you have a heart murmur, high blood pressure, extra heart beats, or a heart abnormality?	_____	_____
3. Do you have to stop while running around a (¼ mile) track twice?	_____	_____
4. Are you taking any medications?	_____	_____
5. Have you ever "passed out" or beeen "knocked out" (concussion)?	_____	_____
6. Have you ever had any illness, condition, or injury that:		
a. Required you to go to the hospital either as a patient overnight or in the emergency room or for X-rays?	_____	_____
b. Required an operation?	_____	_____
c. Lasted longer than a week?	_____	_____
d. Caused you to miss a game or practice?	_____	_____
e. Is related to allergies (hayfever, hives, asthma, or medicine)?	_____	_____

[a] Adapted from Committee on Sports Medicine, American Academy of Pediatrics: *Sports Medicine: Health Care for Young Athletes.* Evanston, IL, American Academy of Pediatrics, 1983.

Table 5.9.
Orthopaedic Screening Examination for the Adolescent Athlete[a]

The orthopaedic screening examination[b] requires about 90 seconds. Time studies indicate it is most efficiently done one athlete at a time rather than in small groups. It is designed to reveal previous inadequately rehabilitated injuries or those few previously unrecognized orthopaedic conditions that might be adversely affected by participation in a sports activity. Positive findings require a more extensive examination and/or history. A more detailed examination should not be attempted at the screening examination.

Athletic Activity (Instructions)	Observation
Stand facing examiner	Acromioclavicular joints; general habitus
Look at ceiling, floor, over both shoulders; touch ears to shoulders	Cervical spine motion
Shrug shoulders (examiner resists)	Trapezius strength
Abducts shoulders 90° (examiner resists at 90°)	Deltoid strength
Full external rotation of arms	Shoulder motion
Flex and extend elbows	Elbow motion
Arms at sides, elbows 90° flexed; pronate and supinate wrists	Elbow and wrist motion
Spread fingers; make fist	Hand or finger motion and deformities
Tighten (contract) quadriceps; relax quadriceps	Symmetry and knee effusion; ankle effusion
"Duck walk" four steps (away from examiner with buttocks on heels)	Hip, knee, and ankle motion
Back to examiner	Shoulder symmetry; scoliosis
Knees straight, touch toes	Scoliosis, hip motion, hamstring tightness
Raise up on toes, raise heels	Calf symmetry, leg strength

[a] From Committee on Sports Medicine, American Academy of Pediatrics: *Sports Medicine: Health Care for Young Athletes.* Evanston, IL, American Academy of Pediatrics, 1983.
[b] May require reflex hammer, tape measure, pin, and examination table.

a general physical examination. Most conditions that would disqualify an adolescent from sports participation are obvious and easily determined through a careful history and physical examination (Table 5.7). The examination should be directed toward the more clinically silent conditions that can present a significant risk of health hazard with sports participation. The preparticipation screening history and screening orthopaedic examination recommended by the Committee on Sports Medicine, American Academy of Pediatrics, are shown in Tables 5.8 and 5.9. Those exercise-related orthopaedic injuries which can be managed in the office are described in Chapter 67.

General References

Blos P: *On Adolescence.* New York, The Free Press, 1962.
    A standard treatise on adolescence, with a psychoanalytic perspective.
Committee on Sports Medicine, American Academy of Pediatrics: *Sports Medicine: Health Care for Young Athletes.* American Academy of Pediatrics, Evanston, IL, 1983.
    An updated reference on sports medicine for children and adolescents.
Erickson EH: *Identity, Youth and Crisis.* New York, WW Norton, 1968.
    The most widely used theoretical model of adolescent psychosocial development.
Gallagher JR, Heald FP, Garell DC (eds): *Medical Care of The Adolescent,* ed 3. New York, Appleton-Century-Crofts, 1976.
    An excellent textbook on adolescent medicine. Emphasizes patient-doctor relationship.
Garell DC (ed): Symposium in adolescent medicine. *Pediatr Clin North Am* 20:769, 1973.
    A good series of reviews of clinical problems of adolescents.
Haggerty RJ: Adolescence. In *Ambulatory Pediatrics,* ed 2. Philadelphia, WB Saunders, 1977.
    A brief review of adolescent disorders.

Kenniston K: *Youth, Transition to Adulthood.* Vol II: *American Handbook of Psychiatry,* ed 2. New York, Basic Books, 1974.
    Another standard text; the perspective is sociological.
Litt IF: Symposium on adolescent medicine. *Pediatr Clin North Am* 27:1, 1980.
    Another set of reviews highlighting psychosocial issues of adolescents.
Sorenson RC: *Adolescent Sexuality in Contemporary America.* New York, World, 1973.
    A good overview of sexual problems of adolescents and proposed social policy approaches.
Tanner JM: *Growth at Adolescence,* ed 2. Springfield, IL, Charles C Thomas, 1962.
    A classic system for describing the physiological changes of adolescents.

Specific References

1. Desmond MM, Volderman AL, Fisher ES: Assessment of learning competence during the pediatric examination. *Curr Prob Pediatr* 8:2, 1978.
2. Greulich WW, Pyle SI: *Radiographic Atlas of Skeletal Development of the Hand and Wrist.* Palo Alto, CA, Stanford University Press, 1974.
3. Kogut MD: Growth and development in adolescents. *Pediatr Clin North Am* 20:789, 1973.
4. Kysar JR, Zaks MS, Schuchman HP, *et al*: Range of psychological functioning in "normal" late adolescents. *Arch Gen Psychiatry* 21:515, 1969.
5. Levine MD, Zallen BG: The learning disorders of adolescence: organic and non-organic failure to thrive. *Pediatr Clin North Am* 31:345, 1984.
6. Mattsson A: Adolescent depression and suicide. In Hockelman RA, Blatman S, Bounell PA *et al* (eds): *Principles of Pediatrics.* New York, McGraw-Hill, 1978, pp 665–669.
7. Miller D: Adolescent crisis: challenge for patient, parent, and internist. *Ann Intern Med* 79:435, 1973.
8. Offer D, Marcus D, Offer JL: A longitudinal study of normal adolescent boys. *Am J Psychiatry* 126:917, 1970.
9. Sorenson RC: *Adolescent Sexuality in Contemporary America.* New York, World, 1973.
10. Weiner IB: Delinquent behavior. In *Psychological Disturbance in Adolescence.* New York, John Wiley & Sons, 1970, chap 8.

CHAPTER SIX

Geriatric Medicine: Special Considerations*

JOHN R. BURTON, M.D., AND WILLIAM R. HAZZARD, M.D.

Geriatric medicine permeates all aspects of adult medical practice. Accordingly, information pertinent to the care of the elderly patient is presented in the various sections of this textbook. This chapter contains a discussion of special aspects of geriatric medicine that do not fit as well in other sections, yet are fundamental for the physician to provide appropriate care for the elderly patient.

THE DEMOGRAPHIC IMPERATIVE

The population of elderly individuals has increased dramatically in recent decades (Fig. 6.1). In 1980, 11% of the population (25.5 million people) were over the age of 65 years (4), but they accounted for approximately 30% of the health care expenditures in this country (9). This disproportionate con-

---

* Dr. Edmund G. Beacham contributed to this chapter in the first edition of this book.

sumption of health care resources was applicable to all categories of expenditures: hospital, professional services, nursing homes, and drugs (Fig. 6.2). The office physician, especially, will experience the effects of this demographic trend. Elderly patients visit their physicians almost 50% more often than do middle-aged patients. In 1980, a typical elderly patient visited a physician in his office more than six times (15).

Particularly important is the recent rapid growth of the population of those over 75 which contains most of the *frail elderly* (see below). Fig. 6.3 depicts this remarkable growth, and it is anticipated that increasingly this population will be the major focus of most physicians' practices. In parallel with this heavy utilization of health care services, there is an age-related increase in disability and loss of independence (14). Table 6.1 shows this increasing disability, which affects nearly 35% of people over the age of 85 years. Also, the elderly have multiple health problems with a typical clustering of disorders in several organ systems: cardiovascular, neurological, psychological, and musculoskeletal.

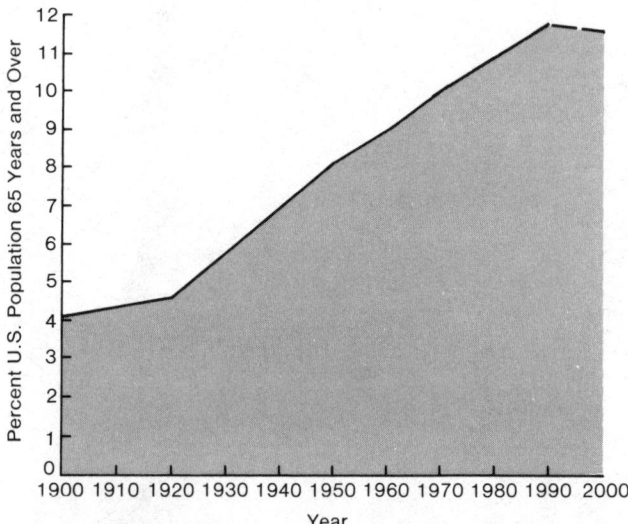

Figure 6.1. Elderly patients in the United States. (Adapted from US Department of Health, Education and Welfare, prepared by the National Institute of Health: *Our Future Selves: A Research Plan toward Understanding Aging.* NIH publ no. 80-1096. Bethesda, MD, National Institute on Aging Information Office, 1980.)

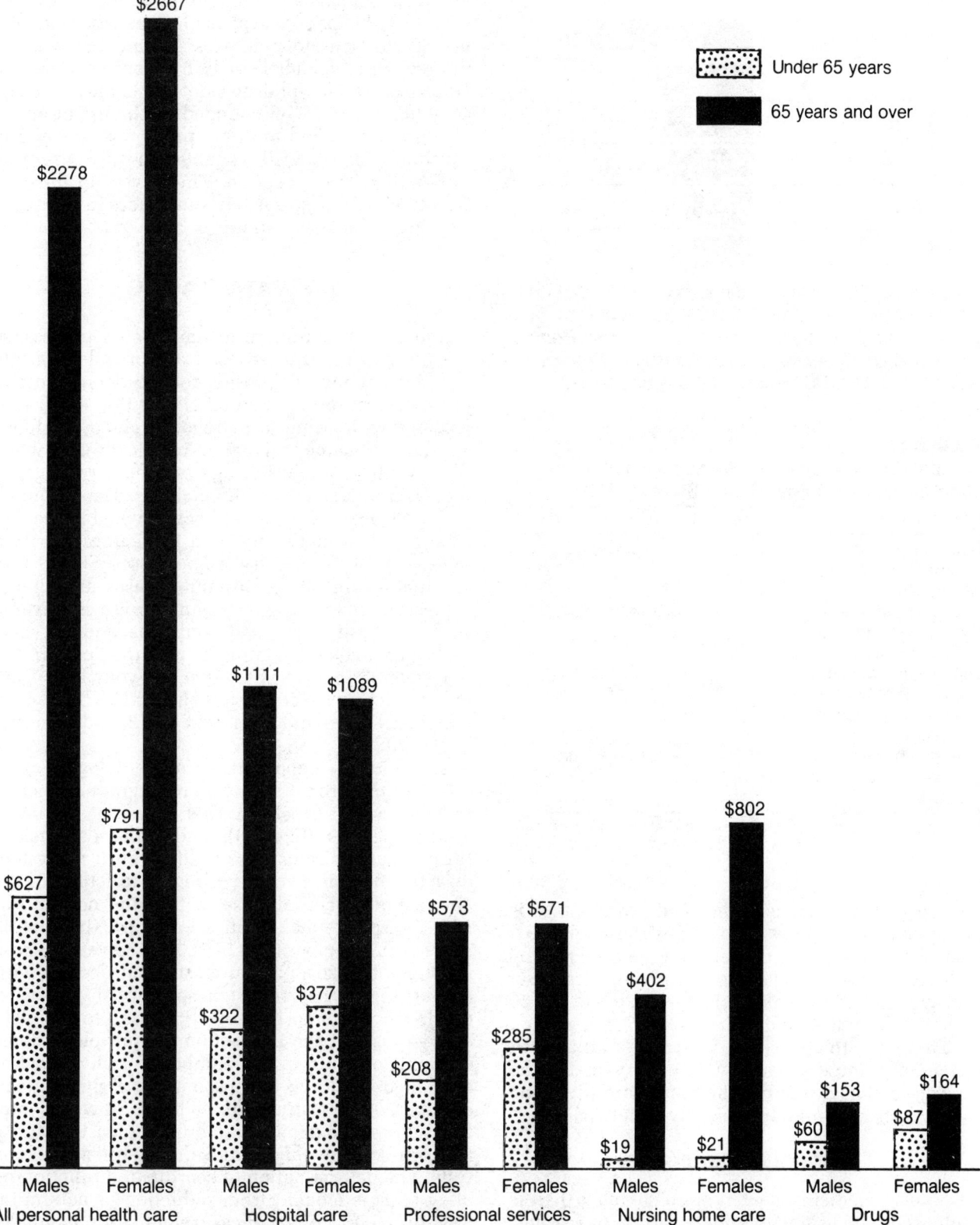

Figure 6.2. *Per capita* personal health care expenditures, according to type of care, age, and sex: United States, 1980. The elderly comprised 11% of the population but consumed disproportionate amounts of health care resources. (Redrawn from Hodgson TA, Kopstein AN: Health care expenditures for major diseases in 1980, National Center for Health Statistics. *Health Care Financing Rev* 5:1, 1984.)

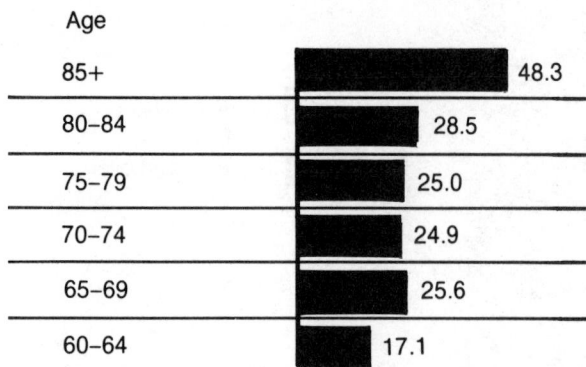

Figure 6.3. Percentage change from 1970 to 1980 in the population of United States residents by age groups. (Adapted from Bureau of Census: General population characteristics. *1980 Census of Population*. Washington, DC, US Department of Commerce.)

Table 6.1.
Percentage of Adults Who Need Assistance, by Type of Need and Age: United States, 1979[a]

Type of Need	65–74 Yr	75–84 Yr	>85 Yr
Needs help in one or more basic physical activities	5.3	11.4	34.8
Needs help in one or more home management activities	5.7	14.1	39.9
Usually stays in bed	1.1	2.6	5.1
Has device to control bowel movement or urination	0.5	1.1	2.9
Needs help of another in one or more of the above	7.0	16.0	43.7

[a] Adapted from National Center for Health Statistics: Advancedata, from *Vital and Health Statistics*, Sept 14, 1983.

Of special importance to the health care system is the predominance of women among those who survive into old age, 3:2 overall and ever increasing with age. There is an even greater preponderance of elderly women living alone. Just over 25% of the 25 million elderly live alone, of which 80% are women (3). Therefore, the physician has to be familiar with systems of community support in order to assure the most optimal health care to the community-dwelling elderly, especially the frail elderly female patient.

SPECIAL ISSUES

Geriatric medicine is even more complex than is adult medicine as a whole for a variety of reasons: new problems are often confused with manifestations of aging itself; the elderly—especially, the frail elderly—may have blunted, nonspecific, or frankly misleading manifestations of acute illness; normal loss of physiological functions in aging often compromises the patient's physiological reserves, and hence, compensatory homeostatic mechanisms are limited; drug metabolism is frequently altered in elderly patients, and drug side effects may be exaggerated as well as compounded by the use of multidrug regimens; and multiple problems—social and psychological as well as physical—are the rule rather than the exception. The physician must be sensitive to these special circumstances in providing care for the elderly patient.

NORMATIVE AGING

Aging is by definition a time-related process; so are the chronic diseases that are prevalent in old age. Also, many of the time-related decrements in physiological reserve and efficiency that occur universally with aging, e.g., relative glucose intolerance, are the same that define specific diseases when they occur at an earlier age or are more flagrant, e.g., symptomatic diabetes mellitus. Hence, much gerontological research has been devoted to the definition of "normal aging" and its segregation from the effects of specific disease processes. Suffice it to say that while many chronic diseases are phenocopies of universal aging, aging *per se* is never a sufficient basis for clinical symptoms, and the stock reply to a given complaint, for example, pain in the left knee, "What do you expect at your age?," not only reflects insensitivity but also invites the sarcastic retort, "My right knee is just as old, and it doesn't hurt a bit!"

The clinically important aspects of biological aging relate to the progressive, generally gradual decline in homeostatic capability that begins at maturity, around age 30 (Fig. 6.4), and proceeds linearly throughout the remainder of life. Yet in no system does this decline critically threaten function, in the absence of specific disease, within the normal human life span, usually defined as approximately 85 years with an upper limit of 110 to 120 years. Those functions that display the most rapid decline with age are ones that reflect a specific physiological challenge, the imposition of a time limit to complete a given task, or the interaction of multiple systems or points of control. An example of a physiological challenge would be the response to a glucose load as opposed to a fasting glucose level. Slower mental function can be demonstrated by decreasing ability to assimilate new information during timed learning tests. The determination of coordinated functioning of systems is evident from reduction of maximum breathing capacity, a measurement, for example, that evaluates the maximum coordination of the function of respiratory nerves, muscles, and the lungs over a given time period. This complete interaction can be contrasted with vital capacity that

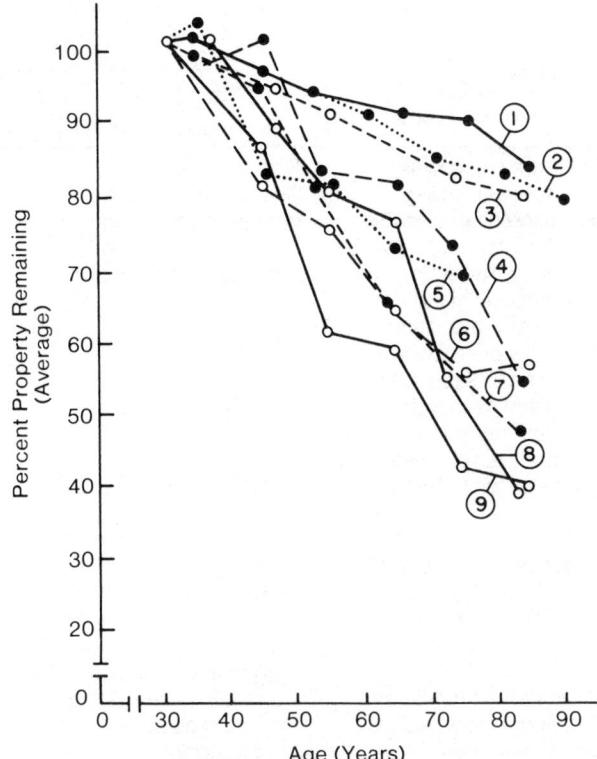

Figure 6.4. Organ system function and aging. *1*, conduction velocity; *2*, basal metabolic rate; *3*, standard cell water; *4*, cardiac index; *5*, standard glomerular filtration rate (inulin); *6*, vital capacity; *7*, standard renal plasma flow (Diodrast); *8*, standard renal plasma flow (para-aminohippurate (PAH)); *9*, maximal breathing capacity. (Adapted from Shock NN: The physiology of aging. *Sci Am* 206:100, 1962.)

involves but a single, maximal respiratory excursion without a time limit.

Two additional features of physiological aging of great clinical significance are less measurable. One is the greater interindividual variability among older persons: old people are less alike than young people. Hence, individualization of physiological assessment is critical, and rules of thumb (e.g., "normal systolic blood pressure is 100 plus your age") are of little use in the practice of geriatric medicine. A second feature is the contribution of potentially reversible or preventable disease processes to age-related physiological decrements, so-called "secondary aging," in contrast to the immutable changes, defined as "primary aging." Examples of the effects of these changes, primary and secondary, are given in Table 6.2. Hence, what is currently accepted as normative aging may in the future be redefined taking into account the effects of reduction in such prevalent risk factors as cigarette smoking and a diet high in animal fat.

These principles of normal *versus* abnormal aging

underlie much of what remains in this chapter, to wit: individualized evaluation of a given elderly patient's status, *geriatric assessment*—physiological, psychological, and socioeconomic—is a key element of successful geriatric practice. Certain challenges to test homeostatic control mechanisms may be introduced in the course of such an assessment to ascertain limited reserves that may become critical in circumstances of disease or social collapse. The interaction of multiple factors produces a final common pathway of dysfunction that may blur conventional organ system or disease-based diagnostic categories. Adjustment of the health care system to meet the needs of frail elderly patients may preserve to the maximum a life of satisfaction and independence; *home care* (see below) is one such adjustment that is a vital part of geriatric practice. Preservation of function and avoidance of trigger phenomena that may initiate a catastrophic cascade of collapse are essential in the elderly. Such care entails an aggressive approach to *preventive medicine*, recognition of the *nutritional* basis of much geriatric decline, especially when disease is superimposed upon a precarious nutritional state, and the special role of drugs and the necessity of careful *pharmacological* management to minimize the common occurrence of *iatrogenic* problems in the elderly. Those iatrogenic problems are most likely to occur in hospital; hence, expertise in ambulatory care is of critical importance to avoid unnecessary, expensive, and dangerous hospitalization of elderly patients.

COMPREHENSIVE ASSESSMENT

The physician will encounter a patient in need of geriatric assessment in several circumstances: a patient age 75 or over (or a disabled, dependent, fragile, younger patient, *i.e.*, a "frail elderly patient") whom the physician is seeing for the first time because of a change in health status, change in locale, death or retirement of a lifelong physician, or on referral by a worried family member or by a physician not comfortable with geriatrics. Also, an established elderly patient will be seen when there has been a major change in health status perceived either by the patient or his family and, very importantly, whenever there is consideration of placement in a long term care facility. The aim of assessment in all of these instances is to detect and treat reversible disease, preserve function, and facilitate the care of the patient by arranging for the service(s) available in the community that most appropriately fit the person's needs, including long term institutional care if necessary. Cure of disease or establishment of a specific diagnosis is not usually as important as stabilization or an improvement of functional status. If the elderly patient is so unstable that his life may be at risk, then the physician should most appropriately hospitalize him for the assessment process.

Table 6.2.
Examples of Age and Age-Related Disease Effects

Organ System	Anatomical and Physiological Phenomena in the Elderly	Primary Age-Related Change	Diseases, Iatrogenic Effects and Secondary Aging Factors
Skin	Wrinkling; Purpura with minor trauma; Susceptibility to pressure sores and slower healing; Dry skin/pruritis; Hair loss; hair graying	Atrophy (especially subcutaneous), decreased elasticity, increased vascular fragility/decreased extravascular tamponade; decreased sweating and sebaceous gland secretions; decreased hair and hair pigment	Sun exposure; Chemical exposure; Iatrogenic (or self-induced changes in hair color or amount)
Eyes	Presbyopia, decreased dark adaptation; ? Cataract; ? Glaucoma; ? Macular degeneration	Altered lens elasticity Altered physiology of vitreous, retina	Diabetes ? Cataract; ? Glaucoma; ? Macular degeneration; Drug effects (miosis)
Ears	Decreased hearing, especially high frequency; Decreased sound discrimination; Diminished position sense—"dizziness"	Diminished function of hair cells Diminished vestibular function	Traumatic hearing loss; Ménière's disease; Drug toxicities; "Benign positional vertigo"
Nose and mouth	Decreased taste and food enjoyment; Dry mouth	Diminished olfaction Diminished number of taste buds and salivation	Zinc deficiency; Periodontal disease; Drug-induced dry mouth, salivation
Gastrointestinal tract	Dysphagia, gastric contents reflux; Hypochlorhydria with bacterial overgrowth; Constipation; Retarded drug metabolism	Diminished esophageal motility and sphincter function; Diminished acid, pepsin, trypsin; Decreased intestinal motility; Altered hepatic enzymes	Hiatus hernia Pernicious anemia; Constipation secondary to a low residue diet; Drug toxicities
Respiratory	Decreased vital capacity, FEV_1,[a] maximum breathing capacity	Diminished lung elasticity Diminished respiratory musculature	Chronic obstructive pulmonary disease secondary to smoking, pollution
Cardiovascular	Diminished cardiac reserve (increased dependence on Frank-Starling mechanism), increased pulse pressure, increased vulnerability to hypotension and syncope	Diminished myocardial cell number, increased left ventricular and arterial resistance, diminished chronotropic response (especially maximum heart rate), diminished vascular baroreceptor (adrenergic) sensitivity;	Atherosclerosis-related ischemia, ventricular dysfunction, arrhythmias, CHF,[a] hypertensive heart disease

Table 6.2.—Continued

Organ System	Anatomical and Physiological Phenomena in the Elderly	Primary Age-Related Change	Diseases, Iatrogenic Effects and Secondary Aging Factors
	Tissue ischemia	? Arteriosclerosis (without cholesterol accumulation)	Atherosclerosis and related phenomena
Renal-urinary system	Decreased glomerular filtration rate, tubular resorption	Diminished number of nephrons; changes in basement membranes and tubular function;	Drug-induced renal disease (aminoglycosides, nonsteroidal anti-inflammatory agents);
	Obstructive uropathy; Incontinence; Vulnerability to urinary infection	Decreased bladder tone, decreased bladder capacity, diminished sphincter tone, prostatic hypertrophy (men), diminished pelvic muscular tone (women)	Renal infections
Endocrine-metabolic system	Menopause (vasomotor symptoms, vaginal atrophy, osteoporosis in old age);	Hypogonadism— Relatively abrupt (women); Relatively slow (men);	Accelerated osteoporosis with low calcium intake, smoking;
	Altered male libido, potency, sexual behavior; Relative glucose intolerance;	Diminished insulin response to glucose load; decreased insulin sensitivity (increased adiposity);	Increasing incidence of diabetes mellitus;
	Diminished thyroid reserve	Diminished thyroid response	Autoimmune thyroiditis and hypothyrodism
Musculoskeletal	Decreased strength	Decreased muscle fiber and diameter;	Disuse atrophy (sedentary life style);
	Increased vulnerability to fracture;	Diminished bone mineral and osteoid;	Diet-, alcohol-, tobacco-, and drug-related osteoporosis
	Joint stiffness and inflammation;	Increased stiffness of tendons, connective tissue	Drug-induced osteoarthritis (fluoride)
		Diminished joint cartilage	
Neural regulation	Hypothermia; Hyperthemia; Dehydration	Diminished tolerance to temperature variation;	Hypothermia from hypothyroidism;
	Postural hypotension, "dizziness," syncope, falls;	Diminished thirst and drinking;	Hyperosmolar, nonketotic diabetes mellitus;
	Increased incidence of Alzheimer's disease;	Diminished postural reflexes and autonomic regulation;	Drug-induced dehydration, autonomic insensitivity
	Slowness of movement;	Neuronal loss; nucleus basalis, decreased cholinergic neurotransmitters and choline acetyltransferase activity;	Drug-induced cognitive dysfunction; Delirium;
	Parkinson's disease		Drug-induced parkinsonism
	Retarded positional correction, falls;	Diminished basal ganglia function;	Drug-induced ataxia, Alcohol toxicity
	Altered sleep patterns	Diminished dorsal column function	Alzheimer's disease Parkinson's disease

Table 6.2.—Continued

Organ System	Anatomical and Physiological Phenomena in the Elderly	Primary Age-Related Change	Diseases, Iatrogenic Effects and Secondary Aging Factors
Immune system	Increased susceptibility to infections, malignancies; Impaired response to immunization; Increased autoantibodies	Diminished cellular immunity (decreased helper cells) Diminished primary antibody response; Increased abnormal immunoglobulin and autoimmunity	Nutritional deficiency, autoimmune diseases (thyroiditis), pernicious anemia

[a] FEV_1, forced expiratory volume during the first second; CHF, congestive heart failure.

Parameters of Assessment

To be effective and in order to plan the care of a frail elderly person properly, it is important that the assessment of the individual include five dimensions: physical health, mental health, social and economic resources, environmental situation, and functional status.

When a new patient is seen, often there are medical records available. A summary of previous hospitalizations is very important for the physician to review. Also, often the elderly patient may have seen several specialists and the general physician will need to sort out the available information and opinions to advise properly the patient and the patient's family. The physician must coordinate all of this information and interpret consultant opinions to guide properly the health care a patient receives. One of the many multidimensional questionnaires that are available may be helpful (10). Probably the most utilized is the Older Americans Resources and Services Group (OARS) instrument, which takes approximately 1 hour to administer. This validated instrument, including instructions on how to use it, may be purchased from the Older Americans Resources and Services Group (Duke University Center for the Study of Aging and Human Development, Durham, NC 27710). A validated and somewhat shorter version of the OARS instrument is the Functional Assessment Inventory (FAI). This useful instrument and directions for its use may be purchased from the Suncoast Gerontology Center (University of South Florida Medical Center, Tampa, FL 33612). However, because of the time and, therefore, expense of administering, multidimensional questionnaires are not often practical for a general physician. For a new patient, a simple questionnaire often helps the patient and family to focus their questions and to record certain specific information that may save time during the actual encounter. Unfortunately a brief questionnaire has not yet been validated, though several are under study. A physician may fabricate a questionnaire that reveals information in five domains and this may help to identify important information and may focus the assessment: physicial health, mental health, social and economic resources, environment, and functional ability. These are the general areas of evaluation of the OARS instrument (see above).

Physical Health

A traditional medical history and physical examination are necessary, though they may need to be modified for the elderly to reserve time for the key issues and to provide a different focus.

The history and physical examination require more time and patience because the elderly individual will frequently have a mobility problem, may easily be confused by questions, often is hard of hearing, and may become fatigued. Usually, in an office situation, this assessment is better accomplished over several visits. By this means more rapport may be established, and visits of short duration help to minimize fatigue or undue stress on the patient.

The focus of the examination requires special emphasis to search for common yet functionally disabling problems: eyes (Chapter 97), ears (Chapter 96), nervous system (Chapter 78), teeth (Chapter 101), skeletal system–osteoporosis (Chapters 74 and 77), and mobility are especially important. Also no assessment is complete without a very careful search for drug toxicity (see below).

Mental Health

Because depressive illness, delirium, and dementia are very common in the elderly, specific focus by the physician on cognitive function and mood is imperative. The usual questions and observations for evaluation of these problems can be augmented, if there is an indication of a problem, by the use of simple scales, such as depression or mental assessment scales. These are described more fully in Chapters 15 and 17, respectively.

Social and Economic Resources

A social assessment is imperative so that the physician will be able to understand the patient's resources and properly guide the patient's caretakers. This assessment should include determination of the care providers available to the patient, and designation of those whose support may be of unlimited duration, such as family members living at home, those whose support is available on short notice to the patient, and those whose support is ancillary, such as church groups or other nonfamily support. In the case of a frail elderly patient, it is mandatory to understand and assist the patient's supporters so that the patient can be maintained in the community rather than in a long term care institution. The dependence on a caregiver increases with the age of the patient, and the sickness or death of this supporter may precipitate institutionalization of the frail elderly patient.

A brief financial appraisal also is necessary in order for the physician to consider realistic care options for a frail elderly patient. Also it is important to know if a patient is eligible for public support of home care services or if he has the means to purchase such services.

Environmental Situation

The physician should understand the environment in which the individual lives: Are there stairs to climb? Is the bathroom available easily to the patient? Is there adequate heating/cooling? Is there access to food and other vital needs? Are there obstacles that create a risk to the patient, such as poorly lighted areas or loose throw rugs, which might endanger the patient, especially when there is a mobility problem?

Functional Status

All care provided to a frail elderly patient must be planned with a sensitivity to the limits of a person's functional ability. This may be a simple quantification of functions that the patient can perform; for example, is the patient able to dress, to feed himself, or to bathe? What is most vital to maintain independence is the ability of the patient to perform these activities of daily living (ADL). There are many elaborate functional scales; however, a well known and easy to administer scale is the Katz Functional Assessment (Table 6.3) (11). This measure scores six functions: bathing, dressing, toileting, transferring, continence, and feeding. Also, scales which assess instrumental activities of daily living (IADL) have been developed (12). These and similar scales evaluate more complex activities than those in the Katz ADL and include such activities as meal preparation, shopping, taking care of finances, housekeeping, public transportation, taking medications, and doing laundry. For each frail elderly

Table 6.3.
Areas and Levels of Assessment in the Katz Index of Independence in Activities of Daily Living [a]

Bathing:	____Receives no assistance ____Receives assistance in bathing only one part ____Receives assistance in bathing more than one part
Dressing:	____Gets clothes and dresses without assistance ____Needs assistance in tying shoes only ____Needs assistance greater than above or stays undressed
Toileting:	____Needs no assistance ____Needs assistance only in getting to toilet room or in cleaning self ____Does not go to toilet room
Transferring:	____Needs no assistance from another person ____Needs assistance with transferring ____Does not get out of bed
Continence:	____Continent ____Occasional accident ____Needs supervision, uses catheter, or is incontinent
Feeding:	____Needs no assistance ____Needs assistance in cutting meat or buttering bread ____Needs more assistance or is tube or intravenously fed

[a] From Katz S, Ford AB, Moskowitz RW, et al: Studies of illness in the aged: The index at ADL; standardized measure of biological and psychosocial function. *JAMA* 185:94, 1963.

patient, the physician will want to have a simple system of following some elemental indicators of function.

Value of Assessment

Preservation of function and independence are the overriding goals.

Often at the time of assessment, the elderly patient is in transition: there may be exacerbations of multiple chronic problems; new disease causing functional loss may be present; there may be apprehension or concern of family members or friends; and questions about independent living are frequent. The physician's task then is to identify the reasons for change (physical, mental, social, or environmental) and to preserve or improve function whenever possible. The physician must understand that small gains in function are far more likely and achievable than is cure. This mind set is unique to geriatric medicine and is the reason that formulation of functional goals is often more important than establishing a precise diagnosis. To accomplish this the physician must define the reversible precipitating factors, *e.g.*, drug toxicity causing delirium or the recent loss of a pet causing depression, and strive to reverse what is possible. If reversible factors are not identified, then the goal is the complete identification of the patient's support needs and the arrangement or the facilitation of the arrangement of community or family resources to maintain function and to preserve independence. This requires that the physician become familiar with community resources (see below).

Careful studies have emphasized that almost 50% of elderly persons have been institutionalized inappropriately (26), and now evidence is accumulating that geriatric assessment in specialized in-patient units (17) or in a community-based program (25) is helpful in improving outcomes in a significant proportion of elderly individuals (Table 6.4).

Even when the physician has not been able to identify any potential for improvement in functional status, the comprehensive assessment will have provided for the physician the necessary data base and rapport to help the family effectively. This may take the form of talking with the family to remove any guilt they may have about institutionalization or to help the family obtain support in the home for the burdens of continued care they are having to provide.

Logistics of Assessment

Geriatric assessment must be multidimensional (see above), is time consuming, and frequently, in an office situation, requires several visits. Often it necessitates obtaining records from other institutions and requires the physician to review the history with the patient's family or friends. Because of the importance for the physician to understand the social, functional, and environmental status of the patient in order to provide good management, achieve the best functional status, and provide the most congruous service available for the patient's need, an *assessment in the patient's home by the physician* is usually the most expeditious way to gain the needed information and insight (5). This is especially important for a physician who does not have a team of professionals, such as social workers, occupational or physical therapists, nurses, or psychiatric resources, to help accomplish the assessment. A home visit permits the physician readily to assess the patient's social and environmental status, which is immediately apparent, while reviewing the history, performing a physical examination, and assessing the mental function. A home visit frequently saves the physician considerable time and provides an understanding of the patient and his support system never realized in an office encounter. Also, it is very much appreciated by the elderly patient and is accordingly extremely helpful in the establishment of rapport necessary to manage the elderly patient.

NONSPECIFIC PRESENTATION OF ILLNESS

Elderly patients frequently respond differently than do younger patients to acute illness (19). It is important, accordingly, for the physician to be familiar with some of these responses if he is to diagnose a frail elderly patient properly. Table 6.5 reviews the prejudices that too often compromise the development of a proper data base by the physician.

In the frail elderly patient, a constellation of nonspecific syndromes frequently signals a change in

Table 6.4.
Results of Careful Assessments Arranged by Site

Situation	Comment	References
Long term care facility	1. Approximately 50% inappropriately placed	Health Care of the Aged, Monroe County (8a)
Inpatient unit—VA hospital	1. Lower 1-year mortality 2. Less nursing home placement 3. Less acute hospital care utilization 4. Approximately 50% of patients placed at a better than expected level of care 5. Significant new diagnosis 6. Decrease in number of drugs prescribed	Rubenstein *et al* (17)
Outpatient clinic	1. Of patients referred for nursing home placement, only one-third required same. 2. One-third referred for rehabilitation and of these >50% improved. 3. 20% of patients required further diagnostic studies and many were identified as having a reversible problem (*e.g.*, drug toxicity)	Williams *et al* (26)

stability or the development of a new problem. The so-called *geriatric quintet* (Fig. 6.5) shows the interaction of these syndromes which are found separately or together in almost every acute or long term problem posed by an older patient (6).

Table 6.6 lists some common problems of the elderly patient that often present atypically from their presentation in younger patients. Symptoms of pain and fever are often not present in a frail elderly patient and pose a particular threat to the diagnostician. Not uncommonly a normal temperature, a slight elevation, or even hypothermia is a manifestation of serious infection. Caution is justified when encountering an elderly patient with a new change in status even when that change is nonspecific. Open-minded, repeated observations and close telephone surveillance by the physician is often the most important diagnostic method. Also, because there are many reasons an elderly patient minimizes a new symptom, the physician should always corroborate the history with the patient's family or friend. Time invested by the physician in doing so

Table 6.5.
Some Common Prejudices or Errors (of Patient and/or Physician) That Compromise the Development of a Proper Data Base for an Ill Elderly Patient

Symptoms attributed to normal aging
New symptoms attributed to chronic problem
Drug toxicity not considered
Fear that symptom, if revealed, might result in hospitalization
Concern of the cost or discomfort of evaluation results in stoicism
Patient too old to undergo evaluation
Classical or typical manifestation of illness not present
Longer time requirement for evaluation not provided

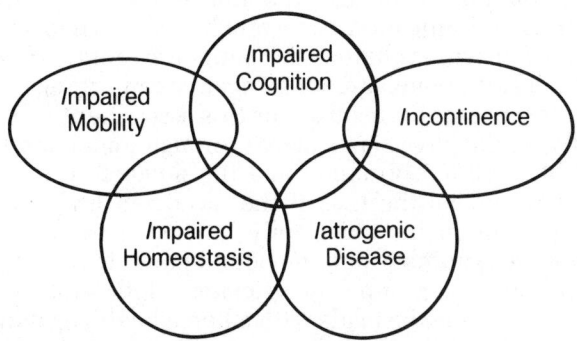

Figure 6.5. The geriatric quintet or "O complex" emphasizes the interaction of problems very commonly seen in the frail elderly patient. It has also been called the five *I*'s of geriatrics and represents the core of geriatric teaching. (Adapted from Cape R: *Aging: Its Complex Management*. Hagerstown, MD, Harper and Row, 1978, p 82.)

Table 6.6.
Some Common Problems of the Elderly that Frequently Present "Atypically"

Intra-abdominal surgical problem (*e.g.*, appendicitis, intestinal ischemia)
Myocardial infarction
Hyperthyroidism
Hypothyroidism
Pyleonephritis
Pneumonia
Vasculitis
Alcoholism
Affective disorder
Drug toxicity

usually will provide direction and order to an evaluation.

PRERETIREMENT COUNSELING AND PLANNING

Many problems of the elderly can be minimized if they are contemplated before people become old. Not only are books available to help the older person in planning (see "General References") but also large corporations, senior citizen centers, and college centers offer courses in preretirement counseling and planning. The American Association of Retired Persons (AARP) has a wide range of materials to assist in such planning in their National Gerontology Resource Center (1901 K Street NW, Washington, DC 20049; (202) 728-4883). Important topics for the older person to consider are: anticipated economic changes, preparation of wills and estate planning, changes in tempo and nature of activities, the importance of developing hobbies and activities for leisure time, health care resources, and systems of health care and social support. A useful publication on the Medicare insurance program, *Your Medicare Handbook* (8), is available to patients and physicians. It may be obtained from the Superintendent of Documents, US Government Printing Office, Washington, DC 20402.) This concise booklet explains services and provides definitions of terms used by Medicare, e.g., skilled nursing facility care. An understanding of the Medicare program is vital to every elderly citizen. However Medicare covers only 44% of total health expenditures for the elderly (1), and therefore the aging patient and his family will need sound advice to plan properly for potential health care needs. The physician should encourage utilization of all of these resources by his "young" elderly patients before they attain the age at which frailty is more common.

COMMUNITY RESOURCES

Physicians working with the elderly should be aware of the resources available to assist in the management of their patients' care. Local or state health departments may have special geriatric divisions. If not, all local or state health departments will have information on availability of nurses, home health care, homemaking services, eating together programs, pet therapy programs, transportation, as well as other activities of special interest to the elderly. Further, there are many senior citizen centers available where the elderly can find friends, recreation, and social stimulation. The physician should be aware of the location of these and the method of referral of his patients to them. The health department or the social work department of a local hospital will usually be able to provide the physician with appropriate information. Finally, when a patient is hospitalized, detailed planning between the patient and the physician for the use of available resources will avert future problems.

HOME CARE

As the population of frail elderly individuals in this country increases, there will be an increased need for physicians to make house calls. Approximately 7% of noninstitutionalized elderly persons are homebound and cannot be transported without specially equipped buses or vans (2). In spite of this, only a small number of patient-physician encounters occur in the home (1.2% with elderly between the ages of 65 and 74 and 2.9% with elderly age 75 and over) (16). To manage the patient properly and assist the patient's family, and to coordinate other home services effectively (see Chapter 9, Selected Special Services: Disability, Vocational Rehabilitation, and Home Health Services) the physician caring for homebound elderly patients should see that individual regularly in his/her home. In addition to the fact that this will obviously provide a needed service to the patient, it develops a deep rapport between the patient and family and the physician and can be immensely rewarding for the physician. The time efficiency of house calls may be minimized by scheduling regular visits at the beginning or at the end of an office session.

To evaluate and follow a frail elderly patient properly, the physician must focus on aspects of care which include, as above, medical, psychiatric/mental, social, functional, and environmental factors. While the psychiatric/mental and medical aspects of a patient's care needs can be readily identified in a physician's office, the social, functional, and environmental assessment and needs estimates are very often much more efficiently and fully understood by the physician evaluating the patient in the home.

There are many home health services available to help support a patient in his/her home and to assist the physician in the provision of care. Home health agencies are rapidly proliferating and are sponsored by proprietary and nonproprietary agencies as well

as by many hospitals. Home health services include provision in the home of skilled nursing services, home health aides and other nursing assistants, social work, physical therapy, occupational therapy, and other supportive and rehabilitative services. These services, if they are to be covered by Medicare insurance, require that the patient be in need of a skilled level of care. The assignment of a level of care is derived from the data supplied by the physician to the home health agency (and reviewed by a Professional Standards Review Organization (PSRO)), usually on a standard form supplied by the agency. A skilled level of care requires that a high level of professional service (nursing, physical therapy, etc) be needed. Examples of this level of care are the provision of a supervisory or monitoring service (blood pressure assessment, drug surveillance) or patient/family education (treatment of an open wound, diabetes instruction, use of a walker or rehabilitative exercise). By design, skilled care is short term and aimed at functional improvement; it is not a service for a stable chronic disability. In addition, many communities have well developed resources that are available to homebound elderly citizens. Examples are home-delivered meals, home building maintenance services, and home assistants for shopping and other chores. These are sponsored by agencies of the city and state government as well as by many private voluntary and church organizations. Each community is unique, and the physician should be aware of what resources exist in the community within which he practices. Most often, sources of information may be gained from the city, county, or state health department or a state office on aging or the department of social work of a hospital.

Communication regarding the coordination of care of a frail elderly person between physician and home health agency is often difficult because there may be little contact and little or no familiarity between physician and the home health agency staff. Communication is so much easier when the physician has evaluated the patient at home; also, often a staff member from an agency can arrange to be present simultaneously for this assessment. This will give the physician a more thorough understanding of the home situation and the home care team than would be the case if the physician had seen the patient in his office only. In instances where there are a number of homebound patients that the physician or a group of physicians is following, arrangements can be made with a home health agency that permit easier communication. For example, the home health agency may provide one nurse to coordinate the care for all of the patients followed by a physician or a physician group, and the agency might be willing to have this nurse meet on a regular basis to improve communication relevant to the coordinated care of the patient(s).

It is only in this way that the physician can fully understand the situation and needs of the patient, properly coordinate the various services that may be available to the patient, and remain the leader of the care provided to the patient by other professionals or lay people.

PREVENTIVE MEDICINE

To be maximally effective, much of the potential benefit of measures to prevent or delay the onset of diseases that occur in the elderly must be instituted long before old age. Hence, preventive gerontology applies to the young and middle-aged as much (and perhaps even more so) as to the aged: avoidance of cigarette smoking, maintenance of an active, challenging life style, and eating a well balanced diet relatively low in cholesterol and saturated fat. No data reject the benefit of such a hygienic life style even in old age, as long as health and vigor permit. Thus, the reduction in atherosclerotic cardiovascular disease mortality that has been so striking in the United States over the past two decades, a reduction generally attributed to population-wide changes in life style, has applied across the entire adult life span (and in both sexes), notably including those over 85 years of age (22).

At a practical level, however, preventive medicine in the elderly focuses upon relatively short term goals, carefully weighing the risks and costs as well as the benefits of any intervention (and their estimated duration). This reinforces the central role of assessment in geriatric practice and the prevention of phenomena that may trigger physiological collapse: immunizations as justified (notably one-time polyvalent pneumococcal vaccination, maintenance of adequate tetanus protection, and annual influenza vaccination, see Chapter 32); elimination of environmental hazards (classically the scatter rug); and preservation of adequate activity, nutrition, and socialization. The content of an annual assessment by a physician from the perspective of prevention becomes heavily weighted toward social, psychological, and functional issues.

NUTRITION AND AGING

Geriatric medicine is notable for its focus upon certain final common pathways of functional decline. One of these is the central role of nutrition in determining health or disease.

Much has been written of nutritional requirements in old age; yet remarkably few data have been gathered that suggest any aspects of nutrition that are unique to old age. Indeed current Recommended Dietary Allowances (RDA) specify essentially equal requirements for all adults (Table 6.7). Moreover, most surveys of free-living, healthy American adults have demonstrated remarkably little evidence of

Table 6.7.
Recommended Daily Dietary Allowances for Adults (Revised 1980)[a]

Nutrient	Men[b]		Women[c]	
	Ages 25–50 Yr	Ages 51+ Yr	Ages 23–50 Yr	Ages 51+ Yr
Protein, g	56	56	44	44
Fat-soluble vitamins				
Vitamin A, g retinol equivalent[d]	1000	1000	800	800
Vitamin D, g[e]	5	5	5	5
Vitamin E, mg tocopherol equivalent[f]	10	10	8	8
Water-soluble vitamins				
Vitamin C, mg	60	60	60	60
Thiamine, mg	1.4	1.2	1.0	1.0
Riboflavin, mg	1.6	1.4	1.2	1.2
Niacin, mg niacin equivalent[g]	18	16	13	13
Vitamin B_6, mg	2.2	2.2	2.0	2.0
Folacin, g	400	400	400	400
Vitamin B, g	3.0	3.0	3.0	3.0
Minerals				
Calcium, mg	800	800	800	800
Phosophorus, mg	800	800	800	800
Magnesium, mg	350	350	300	300
Iron, mg	10	10	18	10
Zinc, mg	15	15	15	15
Iodine, g	150	150	150	150

[a] Recommended Dietary Allowances. From Shank RE: Nutrition principles. In Andres R, Bierman EL, Hazzard WR (eds): *Principles of Geriatric Medicine*. New York, McGraw-Hill, 1985, chap 39.
[b] Relates to reference man weighing 70 kg and 178 cm in height.
[c] Relates to reference woman weighing 55 kg and 163 cm in height.
[d] One retinol equivalent = 1 g of retinol or 6 g of carotene.
[e] As cholecalciferol; 1 g of cholecalciferol = 40 IU.
[f] One tocopherol equivalent = 1 mg of D-tocopherol.
[g] One niacin equivalent = 1 mg of niacin or 60 mg of dietary tryptophan.

clinical nutritional deficiency among the elderly. More prevalent, and more debatable, given the uncertainties of nutritional requirements in the elderly, is marginal or potential nutritional deficiency, a phenomenon of great relevance in ambulatory geriatric medicine. Moreover, such surveys have generally excluded or underrepresented those older persons least likely to seek a physician's care, and it is specifically those elderly in whom malnutrition is most pervasive. On a physiological level it is readily apparent that multiple age-related changes jeopardize nutritional intake: smell and taste perception decline, so enjoyment of food is less; salivation decreases, and mastication is impaired through dental losses and malfunction; swallowing is difficult, choking is more common, esophageal motility is decreased; gastric acid and pepsin secretion are diminished, and gastric motility is impaired (as is that of the small and large intestine); biliary secretion is commonly impaired; perhaps, most important, if activity is diminished, appetite is decreased and intake of micro- as well as macronutrients is diminished. Finally, social and psychological cues to eating are commonly reduced; e.g., the loss of a spouse may not only cause anorexia from the depression of bereavement but remove the incentive to prepare a tasteful and nutritious meal.

Beyond these physiological and social factors are those attributable to the diseases that are so prevalent among the elderly. While the mechanism of the anorexia and weight loss accompanying disease remains largely obscure, the magnitude and impact of these phenomena are obvious, and prevention of malnutrition in the sick and frail elderly is a major thrust of geriatric medicine. Sometimes the cause of weight loss is clear, e.g., carcinoma. More often it is not; the anorexia of depression, tuberculosis, chronic lung disease, heart failure, or digitalis toxicity may be the presenting feature of one of these serious underlying diseases. Nevertheless, the prognostic significance of weight loss is nowwhere more evident than among the elderly, especially since malnutrition is a barrier to recovery and may lead to complications, such as pressure sores, infections, muscle wasting, and weakness that prevent ambulation and self-care.

Nutritional assessment in the elderly is not unlike that in the nonelderly. While some physicians, notably those based in hospitals, may choose to monitor laboratory tests such as serum albumin or transferrin concentrations, or lymphocyte count, these add little to measurement of weight/height or, more valuable, documentation of a change in weight. Skinfold thickness estimates add little to simple weight measurements and, unless performed and interpreted carefully, invite confusion. Calorie counts or dietary intake reviews may be helpful, particularly if extremes of food avoidance are suspected. Other laboratory measurements are of derivative usefulness only, e.g., folate and/or B_{12} levels if the patient has a macrocytic anemia.

Nutritional therapy is frequently attempted in the elderly, though success is not easily attained. Most commonly, multivitamins and mineral supplements are taken to prevent micronutrient deficiency (calcium supplementation at 1500 mg daily is now widely prescribed in women). The risk of such supplementation in the healthy is small, and a placebo or, in the case of calcium, an actual (see Chapter 74) benefit may accrue. The addition of liquid, calorie-rich supplements in the malnourished may be helpful, though their specific role has not been justified in patients without functional barriers to adequate nutrition; i.e., the determinants of disease and recovery play the dominant role, and nutritional supplements only a permissive role in recovery. Where functional impediments exist (e.g., a swallowing disorder following a stroke), a specific nutritional regimen may be critical in promoting recovery, e.g., enteral or parenteral feeding.

Thus, nutritional disorders are epidemic among the sick elderly; weight loss is a cardinal manifestation of disease and nutritional deficiency is a barrier to recovery; the physician must be especially attuned to the role of nutrition in determining the longitudinal course and outcome of disease in this population.

PHARMACOLOGICAL ISSUES

Iatrogenic disease is of special concern in geriatric medicine, and pharmacological misadventures feature prominently in this concern. The elderly characteristically have multiple disorders; consequently, they are likely to be treated with multiple medications, appropriately as well as inappropriately. While much has been written of the special characteristics of the elderly that place them at increased risk of pharmacological toxicity, none is so important as this: Multiple drugs multiply the hazard of complications.

Surveys of ambulatory geriatric populations have indicated that up to 90% may take at least one medication, and the majority take two or more (23). The most commonly prescribed medications are cardiovascular agents, antihypertensives, analgesics, and anti-inflammatory agents. Importantly, over-the-counter medications account for over 40% of the total and must not be overlooked in reviewing drug regimens. Patients in long term care facilities receive even more medications, psychotropics (in up to 75%, as compared with 25% in ambulatory patients) surpassing all others. Adverse drug reactions, often difficult to detect in disabled elderly patients, occur in 6 to 40% of those over 60 years of age in various series and are a common cause of hospitalization. Risk factors for such reactions, in addition to advanced age and multiple drug usage, include female sex, small body size, hepatic or renal insufficiency, and previous drug reactions. Whether age is a factor independent of its association with the other risk factors is not clear; that such reactions are more prevalent among the elderly is, however, all too clear.

Other aspects of drug therapy in the elderly are also germane to ambulatory care. Compliance is one such issue (23). Various studies have disclosed that 25 to 50% of outpatients fail to take their medications as prescribed (18). In one study 59% of ambulatory patients above age 60 made one or more medication errors—26% potentially serious ones and, commonly, multiple errors (especially frequent in patients above 75 years of age) (20). The basis of such errors is complex, including problems in communication and understanding, multiple drugs, and complicated and changing regimens. Whether such problems are actually more common among the elderly as compared with younger, equally vulnerable patients is not certain; however, their greater aggregate risk is clear.

Much has also been made of age-related differences in pharmacokinetics and pharmacodynamics. These are summarized in Table 6.8. However, the similarities between age-related physiological changes and pathological conditions in older *versus* younger patients outweigh the differences. Several key differences are worthy of note, however: (*a*) *Body water and lean body mass are diminished* relative to adipose mass in the elderly. Hence, water-soluble drugs have a lesser space of distribution (and, therefore, a higher concentration) for a given dose in the elderly. Alcohol is a notable water-distributed agent, this accounting at least in part for the greater susceptibility of older patients to a given amount of alcohol. (See Chapter 21 for a discussion of alcoholism.) (*b*) *Renal clearance declines* progressively with age. Hence, drugs excreted by the kidney such as digoxin should be given in lower doses to prevent accumulation and toxicity. (*c*) Lest one be tempted to generalize that all drugs are to be given in lower doses, β-blockers may have to be given in higher quantities, reflecting the *relative insensitivity* of adrenergic receptors in the elderly to both agonists and antagonists. Overall, however, prudence in drug prescription in the elderly is to be exercised both in quantity of agent and number of drugs prescribed, and reduced dosages are commonly employed (Table 6.9).

These principles of physiology and pharmacology converge in the rationale for prescribing drugs depicted in Table 6.10.

URINARY INCONTINENCE

Urinary incontinence affects 15 to 20% of ambulatory elderly people and has profound implications. Frequently it is a stated reason for admission to a long term care facility; it is a major reason for social isolation of elderly individuals; and when severe it can lead to skin maceration and pressure sores. In spite of the high prevalence of urinary incontinence in the elderly, especially in women, the problem is not recognized frequently by their physicians. In part this is because patients fail to report urinary incontinence, assuming it is part of normal aging—"one of the curses of age"—and in part because physicians fail to inquire of their patients about urinary incontinence. General physicians usually have not been involved in the care of the incontinent patient because younger patients with this problem have been managed by urologists and/or gynecologists. In a younger population, most patients are women with urinary incontinence due to sphincter insufficiency (or stress incontinence, see below) and this insufficiency is treated very effectively by urologists or gynecologists. In the elderly, however, the general physician must be involved in the care of

Table 6.8.
Summary of Factors Affecting Drug Disposition in the Geriatric Patient[a]

Pharmacokinetic Parameter	Age-Related Physiological Changes	Pathological Conditions
Absorption	Increased gastric pH Decreased absorptive surface Decreased splanchnic blood flow Decreased gastrointestinal motility	Achlorhydria Diarrhea Gastrectomy Malabsorption syndromes Pancreatitis
Distribution	Decreased cardiac output Decreased total body water Decreased lean body mass Decreased serum albumin Increased body fat	Congestive heart failure Dehydration Edema or ascites Hepatic failure Malnutrition Renal failure
Metabolism	Decreased hepatic mass Decreased enzyme activity Decreased hepatic blood	Congestive heart failure Fever Hepatic insufficiency Malignancy Malnutrition Thyroid disease Viral infection or immunization
Excretion	Decreased renal blood flow Decreased glomerular filtration rate Decreased tubular secretion	Hypovolemia Renal insufficiency

[a] From Vestal R: Clinical pharmacology. In Andres R, Bierman EL, Hazzard WR (eds): *Principles of Geriatric Medicine*. New York, McGraw-Hill, 1985, chap 38.

Table 6.9.
Examples of Drugs[a] Usually Given in Reduced Dosage in the Elderly[b]

Drug (or Drug Class)	Possible Consequences of Standard Dosage Regimen
Aminoglycosides	Ototoxicity and nephrotoxicity
Benzodiazepines	Unwanted CNS depression—more common with larger doses
Carbamazepine	Drowsiness or ataxia may develop
Chlormethiazole	Confusion can occur with larger doses
Digoxin	Digitalis toxicity
Haloperidol	Extrapyramidal reactions
Levodopa	Hypotension common
Meperidine	Respiratory depression
Metoclopramide	Confusion common
Thioridazine	Confusion common
Thyroxine	Myocardial infarction
Vitamin D	Renal toxicity

[a] The drugs listed are examples only.
[b] Source: World Health Organization: Health care in the elderly: report of the technical group on use of medicament by the elderly. *Drugs* 22:279, 1981. From Vestel R: Clinical pharmacology. In Andres R, Bierman EL, Hazzard WR (Eds): *Principles of Geriatric Medicine*. New York, McGraw-Hill, 1985, chap 38.

the incontinent patient for several reasons: There are too many patients for referral; the elderly are often resistant to consultation; they often refuse to have an invasive evaluation; frequently the incontinence is multifaceted; and, in general, surgery is not often as beneficial in frail elderly as it is in young patients.

Physiology of Micturition

In order for the physician properly to evaluate and manage patients with urinary incontinence, an understanding of the basic knowledge of the physiology of voiding is necessary. The bladder functions as a part of an autonomous spinal reflex arc which can be modulated effectively by the cerebral cortex, permitting the patient, under normal circumstances, to evacuate the urinary bladder in a socially acceptable fashion. Sensory fibers from the bladder that sense stretch or fullness connect to the S1-S2 area of the spinal cord where they synapse with motor fibers going *via* pelvic ganglia to the detrusor muscle of the urinary bladder. This spinal reflex may be modulated by a second neural pathway to the cerebral cortex *via* a synapse in the brainstem. It is this higher loop that permits the purposeful supression or augmentation of the bladder reflex so that voiding

Table 6.10.
Principles of Geriatric Prescribing[a]

1. Evaluate the need for drug therapy.
   a. Not all diseases afflicting the elderly require drug treatment.
   b. Avoid drugs if possible, but do not withhold on account of age drugs which might enhance the quality of life.
   c. Strive for a diagnosis prior to treatment.
2. Take a careful history of habits and drug use.
   a. Patients often seek advice and receive prescriptions from several physicians.
   b. Knowledge of existing therapy, both prescribed and nonprescribed, helps one anticipate potential drug interactions.
   c. Smoking, alcohol, and caffeine may affect drug response.
3. Know the pharmacology of the drug prescribed.
   a. Use a few drugs well, rather than many drugs poorly.
   b. Awareness of age-related alterations in drug disposition and drug response is helpful.
4. In general, use smaller doses in the elderly.
   a. Often the standard dose will be too large for the elderly patient.
   b. While the effect of age on hepatic drug metabolism is less predictable, renal excretion of drugs and their active metabolites tends to decline.
   c. The elderly are particularly sensitive to drugs affecting central nervous system function.
5. Titrate drug dosage with patient response.
   a. Establish reasonable therapeutic end points.
   b. Adjust dosage until end points are reached or unwanted side effects prevent further increases.
   c. Use an adequate dose for the patient. This is particularly important in the treatment of pain associated with malignancy.
   d. Sometimes combination therapy is appropriate and effective.
6. Simplify the therapeutic regimen and encourage compliance.
   a. Try to avoid intermittent schedules. Once- or twice-daily dosage is preferred.
   b. Select a dosage form appropriate for the patient.
   c. Label drug containers clearly. When appropriate, specify standard containers.
   d. Give careful written instructions to both patient and a relative or friend.
      Explain why the drug(s) is (are) being prescribed.
   e. Suggest the use of a medication calendar or diary.
   f. Encourage the return or destruction of old medications.

[a] From Vestel R: Clinical pharmacology. In Andres R, Bierman EL, Hazzard WR (eds): *Principles of Geriatric Medicine*. New York, McGraw-Hill, 1985, chap 38.

may be accomplished on desire. A third pathway is a spinal reflex arc with sensory input from the pelvic and perineal tissues that synapse in the lower spinal cord with motor fibers that, *via* the pelvic ganglion, innervate the periurethral muscle fibers. A fourth reflex neural pathway is similar but initiates with sensory fibers in the periurethral musculature and travels *via* the spinal cord synapses to the cortex of the brain. From the motor cortex of the brain, fibers emanate with synapses in route to the motor horn of the S1-S2 spinal segments, and stimulation results in contraction of the skeletal muscle of the perivesical, periurethral, perineal areas as well as of the urethral and anal sphincter. Spontaneous contraction of the detrusor muscle usually occurs when the urinary bladder fills to approximately 150 to 250 ml; however, most individuals under normal circumstances can suppress this urge to void. Also, conditioning by chronic high or low volume voiding can change the bladder capacity considerably, in either direction.

Reasons for Urinary Incontinence

It is simplest to classify disorders of urinary continence into two groups: disorders of storage and disorders of emptying (Table 6.11).

Disorders of Storage

The two disorders of storage are the uninhibited urinary bladder (spastic bladder, urge incontinence) and sphincter insufficiency (stress incontinence). Incontinence from an *uninhibited bladder* occurs when there is an inability by the patient to suppress sensations of bladder fullness; consequently, when a certain bladder volume is achieved, voiding occurs often within moments (the urge to void is very transient and incompletely suppressible). This problem is common in patients with dementia or those who have had a stroke. *Sphincter insufficiency* (stress incontinence) occurs because there is an inability to increase the resistance to the bladder outflow tract necessary whenever there is an increase in muscle tone (stress) transmitted to the urinary bladder. This might occur with increased abdominal tension such as when carrying packages, coughing,

sneezing, or laughing. In all of these instances increased muscle tone (stress) is transmitted to the urinary bladder, the outlet sphincters are unable to resist the increased pressure, and urinary incontinence occurs. This problem is very common in women who have borne children (resulting in perineal trauma) and who are menopausal such that tissue relaxations (from estrogen deficiency) result in malalignment of the bladder and urethra. Also, sphincter insufficiency is frequently present in combination with the uninhibited bladder in elderly women and, occasionally, in men who have had prostatic surgery.

Disorders of Emptying

The two disorders of emptying are overflow incontinence and functional incontinence. *Overflow incontinence* occurs when there is inadequate detrusor function and/or inadequate sensory perception within the bladder wall, or significant outlet obstruction. Overdistension of the bladder results until incontinence occurs at high bladder volumes. This is a typical result of diabetic neuropathy or may occur due to obstructive uropathy, as, for example, from prostatic hypertrophy in males. *Functional incontinence* occurs when under ideal circumstances the voiding mechanism is adequate but because of impaired mobility or an increase in urinary volume (e.g., from diuretics) the reserve is overcome and incontinence results. This pattern is typical in older persons who are in a new environment where they are unable to reach a toilet or when they have been given medications which may interfere with their voiding, either neurologically (e.g., antidepressant or antiparkinsonian drugs) or volumetrically (e.g., diuretics).

Evaluation of a Patient with Urinary Incontinence

The simultaneous combination of several of these four major patterns is very common in elderly patients.

Reversible Causes

When a patient with urinary incontinence is seen, it is important for the physician first to evaluate the patient for the possibility of a functional disorder (see above) and/or an acute reversible cause of urinary incontinence. The most common reversible causes are changes in mental state for any reason, drug effects (especially diuretics, anticholinergics, sedatives, and neuroleptics), urinary tract infections, fecal impactions, and, in women, atrophic vaginitis. In the latter three of these instances, incontinence results from increased bladder sensory stimulation, which may be incompletely suppressed (because of a marginal decrease in suppressor function). In the case of atrophic vaginitis, also there may be relaxation of the tissues of the urinary bladder outlet, resulting in a pattern of sphincter insufficiency.

Table 6.11.
Classification of Disorders or Urinary Continence

Disorders of Storage
    Uninhibited urinary bladder (spastic bladder, urge incontinence)
    Sphincter insufficiency (stress incontinence)
Disorders of Emptying
    Overflow incontinence
    Functional incontinence—normally adequate control but imbalance due to drugs (*e.g.*, anticholinergics or diuretics), diminished mobility (arthritis), or environment change (away from home)

These problems should be considered routinely and, when identified, treated appropriately. Even so, some patients, especially those with infection, often have persistence of incontinence after eradication of the problem.

History

If reversible causes are not present, it is important for the physician to establish the pattern of urinary incontinence by taking a careful history. Usually, after reviewing the symptoms with the patient, it is best to ask the patient to record the episodes of incontinence and to void on a regular schedule. Figure 6.6 provides a sample of a *bladder record*. The physician should fabricate a similar record, provide the patient with 7 to 14 copies, and instruct him to void at timed intervals (usually every 2 hr), record the time, and describe any voiding accidents. The physician can review these data with the patient at a follow-up office visit. Usually, in the patient with an *uninhibited bladder*, there are episodes of urinary incontinence of large volume that are frequently described as occurring when the patient simply was not able to suppress the urge to void or could not get to a lavatory in time (Fig. 6.6A). *Sphincter insufficiency* (stress incontinence) is associated with episodes of small volume loss or of dribbling that occurs in association with increased abdominal pressure, e.g., coughing or sneezing (Fig. 6.6B). The physician should also inquire about symptoms that might relate the incontinence to a *neurological cause* (e.g., paresthesia; gait abnormality), a *structural cause* (e.g., prostatism), or a *metabolic disorder* (e.g., diabetes.)

Examination

The physical examination should include observations that will help in the classification of the incontinence and will rule out reversible causes (see above). The bladder should be *carefully palpated* with the patient in the supine position. A palpable bladder is strongly suggestive of overflow incontinence, but a nonpalpable bladder does not rule out this problem. A *neurological examination* should include an assessment of anal sphincter tone and sensation (using fine touch or pin) in the perineal and perianal area. Also, in men, the bulbocavernosus reflex should be tested (contraction of the bulbous portion of the urethra caused by tapping the penis near the scrotum). Diminished or absent sensation in these areas or lack of sphincter tone suggests a neurological cause of the urinary incontinence. A *rectal examination*, besides assessing sphincter tone, is necessary to evaluate the possibility of fecal impaction and, in men, to assess the prostate for cancer, benign enlargement, or infection. In women, a *pelvic examination* is necessary to evaluate for atrophic vaginitis (see Chapter 94). It is also necessary to test for urinary sphincter ade-

quacy. This may be accomplished by having the patient cough after her bladder is full. If urinary sphincter insufficiency is present, a small urine leak will result. If the patient has a leak following cough, a *Bonney's test* may be performed: Incontinence due to a cough is prevented by lifting the urethra and base of the bladder with the tips of two fingers in the vagina. While the test is more likely to be positive in young women, it should be tried in elderly patients as well. The correction of the incontinence by this maneuver correlates well with a good surgical outcome if sphincter insufficiency is the only mechanism of incontinence.

After the patient has voided, it is important to perform carefully a *straight catherization of the urinary bladder* to assess the postvoiding residual volume. If this volume is greater than 100 ml of urine, overflow incontinence may be present; this is especially a concern with very large residual volumes (>200 ml). Overflow incontinence (also see Chapter 48) is important for the physician to recognize because it requires that the patient be referred to a urologist for further evaluation and treatment (e.g., for relief of obstruction or, in the case of an atonic bladder, for consideration of educating the patient in intermittent self-catheterization if the general physician is not familiar with this technique). The urologist may perform cystometric evaluation and cystoscopy and may consider a trial of urochloline if an atonic bladder is confirmed. The analysis of the urine (microscopically and by dipstick) can be accomplished on the urine specimen obtained by the catheterization and is helpful in evaluating for an infection or in raising concern for another problem (e.g., hematuria may suggest a tumor).

Patient experience. Straight catheterization may be performed simply by obtaining a catheterization kit, which contains all of the materials necessary (cleansing solutions, a catheter, sterile gloves, collection containers, and lubricant). After preparation of the urethral meatus, the sterile catheter is inserted gently into the bladder. In male patients, it is important that the shaft of the penis be extended and lifted in a cephalad direction to align the urethra with the bladder outlet. The urine volume is measured and the catheter removed. When carefully performed, the incidence of infection is less than 1% and only 3 to 4% of patients—usually males—experience mild discomfort, typically a burning sensation. This discomfort may be minimized by careful placement of a well lubricated catheter and by thoroughly explaining the procedure to the patient prior to its performance.

Referral

Younger patients with urinary incontinence should be referred to a urologist or gynecologist for cystoscopy and, often, cystometrographic studies, which are necessary to classify the voiding disorder,

Bladder Record

Name _____   Date_____

Instructions: 1. In the first column, mark the time every time you void.
2. In the second or third column, mark every time you accidentally leaked urine.
3. Write "dry" if no accident occurred in the 2-hour interval.

Time Interval	Urinated in Toilet	Leaking Accident	or	Large Accident	Reason for Accident
6–8 AM	✓				
8–10 AM					
10–12 AM	✓				
12–2 PM					
2–4 PM	✓	✓			Running water
4–6 PM					
6–8 PM				✓	Waited too long
8–10 PM	✓				
10–12 PM				✓	Running water
Overnight					

Number of pads used today: _____

Comments: _____

_____

Exercises: _____

_____

_____

Total: _____

Figure 6.6A.   Bladder record from patient with urinary incontinence: Uninhibited bladder. (Patient data, for *A* and *B*, courtesy of Kathryn L. Burgio, Ph.D., Gerontology Research Center, National Institute on Aging, Baltimore, MD. Bladder record from Whitehead WE, Burgio KL, Engel BT: Behavioral methods in the assessment and treatment of urinary incontinence. In Brocklehurst JC (ed): *Urology in the Elderly*. New York, Churchill Livingstone, 1984, p 81.)

and for consideration for definitive therapy. Frequently, however, this is not possible in frail elderly patients, who generally are very resistant to consultation from a specialist or to the performance of an invasive procedure. Also the value of cystometrographic studies has not been fully validated in elderly patients. Especially when the pattern of incontinence is highly suggestive of the uninhibited urinary bladder (large volume accidents often occurring within moments of the first urge to void), there is no indication for further evaluation by a urologist since at present these patients are not surgical can-

Bladder Record

Name _____ Date _____

Instructions: 1. In the first column, mark the time every time you void.
              2. In the second or third column, mark every time you accidentally leaked urine.
              3. Write "dry" if no accident occurred in the 2-hour interval.

Time Interval	Urinated in Toilet	Leaking Accident	or	Large Accident	Reason for Accident
6–8 AM	✓	✓			Fast walking
8–10 AM	✓				
10–12 AM	✓				
12–2 PM					
2–4 PM	✓				
4–6 PM		✓			Coughed
6–8 PM	✓				
8–10 PM		✓			Sneezed
10–12 PM	✓				
Overnight					

Number of pads used today: 2   _____

Comments: _____

_____

Exercises: _____

_____

_____

Total: _____

Figure 6.6B.   Bladder record from patient with urinary incontinence: Sphincter insufficiency.

didates. Elderly women who have a pure pattern of sphincter insufficiency (stress incontinence) may be surgical candidates. The surgical success in correcting this problem is especially dramatic in younger women; and now with the newer techniques of endoscopic suspension of the bladder neck, a procedure with less operative stress than earlier operations, many elderly women with predominantly sphincter insufficiency may be helped (21).

Therapy

It is most important to recognize that small therapeutic gains often are extremely important to an elderly patient. Cure is not accomplished often, but if incontinent episodes can be minimized, the patient and his/her family may express considerable satisfaction.

The symptom record (see above) may provide an

important clue to the treatment (as well as the cause) of the incontinence. The physician might advise, for example, avoiding situations that increase the urge to void (the patient who comments that incontinence occurs only when drinking warm milk or listening to running water). Also, having the patient void at timed intervals permits the beginning of a *behavioral modification program*. The patient learns to empty the bladder by the clock and therefore before a bladder volume is achieved that results in spontaneous detrusor contraction. Not uncommonly, when asked to void at 2-hourly intervals, a patient with an uninhibited bladder (urge incontinence) will become continent. If that happens, the physician can educate the patient to increase the interval between voidings by 30 to 60 minutes every week or so until incontinence recurs. Then by continuing to void by the clock (at the longest interval without incontinence) acceptable continence often will result and the patient (and caretakers) will be satisfied.

Also, the mechanism of incontinence from sphincter insufficiency should be explained to the patient, if the patient is not severely demented. The patient should learn to avoid increasing abdominal pressure. The pattern of fluid ingestion also may be modulated so that the patient avoids consuming a large volume of fluid 2 to 6 hours prior to his being in a situation in which easy access to a toilet would not be possible.

Kegel exercises may help some women, especially younger individuals with stress incontinence. With the women in a lithotomy position, the physician places two fingers in the vagina and separates them as much as possible. Then the patient is asked to squeeze the introitus around the fingers. The physician will sense when the musculature has been properly contracted and he should instruct the patient to practice repeatedly contracting this muscle group. Once the patient learns how to do this, she should contract these muscles several times every day. At follow-up visits, the examination should be repeated and the patient advised as to the adequacy of her effort.

Drug therapy. While there are many drugs touted as effective in the treatment of urinary incontinence, currently there are only three that have been shown, by controlled trials, to have significant efficacy in the treatment of elderly patients: estrogen, imipramine, and oxybutynin.

Estrogen therapy for female patients with atrophic vaginitis has been beneficial in improving incontinence. Atrophic vaginitis may be diagnosed during the pelvic examination and if there is doubt on inspection, the physician may perform a *maturation index* as described in Chapter 94. If atrophic vaginitis is diagnosed, a course of estrogen therapy should be tried. At first, it is probably simplest to provide the patient with topical estrogen cream such as Premarin vaginal cream (if acceptable) or to administer oral conjugated estrogen (Premarin, 0.625 mg taken one time by mouth each day). A 1-month trial should be adequate; if there is significant improvement, the physician should discuss with the patient the possibility of long term estrogen therapy. It must be recognized that even topical estrogen therapy has a systemic effect, and the physician must be sensitive to the complications (such as uterine cancer) of continuous progestin-unopposed estrogen given in relatively high dose. In general, it is best that the physician treating the patient for atrophic vaginitis use the lowest dose of estrogen possible and cycle it with progestin. Such a regimen is described fully in Chapter 77, and it minimizes or eliminates most risks previously associated with estrogen therapy.

Imipramine (Tofranil, 25 mg) has been shown to be effective in some elderly patients with either sphincter insufficiency or an uninhibited bladder (7). It is the only antidepressant carefully studied for this effect. The drug probably works by increasing bladder capacity and increasing sphincter tone. It should be tried in a regimen of 25 mg orally every night, then increasing every third night to a maximum of 150 mg/night or until side effects occur. The most common side effects are postural hypotension, constipation, dizziness, and mucous membrane dryness. While the drug may be partially effective in 50 to 60% of patients, over half experience some side effects and approximately 20% will discontinue the medication because of intolerance. Nevertheless, when behavior modification (see above) has not been effective and, in women, when atrophic vaginitis has not been identified or found to be responsive to estrogen therapy, a trial of imipramine may be considered.

Oxybutynin (Ditropan, 5 mg) has been shown to be effective when administered in short term studies in patients with either an uninhibited bladder or sphincter insufficiency (13). It probably works by increasing sphincter tone and increasing bladder capacity. Oxybutynin is administered orally as a 5-mg tablet three times a day. It is effective in approximately 50% of patients, but the side effects of dryness of the mouth, blurred vision, abdominal cramps, or constipation are encountered in nearly 50%; also 20% of patients stop the drug because of intolerance. A trial of this drug for 2 to 3 days may be considered if imipramine fails. Long term studies with this agent are not available.

Garments and catheters. Increasingly, there are available comfortable diapers or briefs that may be worn to avoid embarrassing incontinent accidents, e.g., Attends (Proctor and Gamble), Depend (Kimberly-Clarke), Absorb-fil (Sears), or Tranquility (Devilbiss) available from pharmacies, physician supply stores, or large catalogue stores (Sears). For men there are also available relatively comfortable (day and night) drip urinals or supporters with absorbent liners, generally for under $40 to $50. Also, inexpensive condom catheters may be tried. However, if the patient frequently manipulates the external catheter, urosepsis is a frequent complication, and in that instance it is probably wise to use a diaper garment.

Indwelling urinary catheters have no place in the treatment of urinary incontinence, except in instances where there is secondary skin maceration or pressure sore development; and in those instances, the catheter should be used only temporarily until those complications have been resolved. Intermittent self-catheterization is a useful technique for patients with an atonic bladder and overflow incontinence. However, the patient or his/her caretaker must be able and willing to perform the procedure several times a day. When this procedure is considered, usually it is best to refer the patient (and caretaker) to a urologist for education unless the general physician (or his staff) is experienced in educating others in its performance.

Biofeedback techniques are under current investigation, and preliminary studies indicate promise of this being an efficacious way of treating elderly men and women with incontinence from sphincter insufficiency or from an uninhibited bladder (24). Severe dementia is likely to preclude this technique, which requires learning skills.

Surgical techniques of creating artificial urinary bladder sphincters are gaining clinical applicability; a urologist should be consulted, initially by telephone, to help determine which patients might be candidates for artificial sphincter surgery.

OTHER IMPORTANT PROBLEMS OF THE ELDERLY PATIENT

The following problems are discussed in detail elsewhere in this book: constipation (Chapter 38), diverticular disease (Chapter 40), musculoskeletal problems (Section 9), menopause (Chapter 77), osteoporosis (Chapter 77), hearing loss (Chapter 96), skin problems (Chapter 100), dental problems (Chapter 101), disorders of the feet (Chapter 102), hypertension (Chapter 62), cataracts (Chapter 97), psychiatric illnesses of old age such as dementia (Chapter 17), delerium (Chapter 17), depression (Chapter 15), and bereavement (Chapter 19), and urinary problems such as infection (Chapter 27) and retention (Chapter 48).

General References

Action for Independent Maturity: *Looking Ahead: How to Plan Your Successful Retirement*. Washington, DC, American Association of Retired Persons, 1984.
> A 92-page paperback on retirement planning which covers: retirement planning, health and fitness, housing, use of leisure time, and other related topics.

Andres R, Bierman EL, Hazzard WR (eds): *Principles of Geriatric Medicine*. New York, McGraw-Hill, 1985.
> A valuable comprehensive textbook of geriatric medicine.

Bowman FJ: *The Complete Retirement Handbook*. New York, Peregee Books, 1983.
> A 249-page paperback covering various aspects of retirement planning.

Cape RDT, Coe RM, Rossman I (eds): *Fundamentals of Geriatric Medicine*. New York, Raven Press, 1983.

Cassel CK, Walsh JR (eds): *Geriatric Medicine*. New York, Springer-Verlag, 1984.
> A comprehensive two-volume textbook covering all aspects of geriatric medicine.

Downs H: *The Best Years Book*. New York, Delacorte Press, 1981.
> A well known television personality gives his thoughts on retirement.

Kane RL, Ouslander JG, Abrass JB: *Essentials of Clinical Geriatrics*. New York, McGraw-Hill, 1984.
> A short textbook that contains much practical information.

Williams RE: Urinary incontinence in the elderly: physiology, patholophysiology, diagnosis, and treatment. *Ann Intern Med* 97:895, 1982.
> An excellent review article.

Specific References

1. Aiken LH, Bays KD: The Medicare debate—round one, special report. *N Engl J Med* 311:1199, 1984.
2. Brody SJ: Health services: need and utilization. In Brody SJ, Persily NA (eds): *Hospitals and the Aged*. Rockville, MD, Aspen, 1984, p 30.
3. Bureau of Census: Social and economic characteristics of the older population: 1978. Series P-23, No 85. Washington, DC, US Department of Commerce, 1979.
4. Bureau of Census: General population characteristics. *1980 Census of Population*. United States Summary 1–27. Washington DC, US Department of Commerce, 1983.
5. Burton JR: Housecalls: an important service for the frail elderly. *J Am Geriat Soc* 33:291, 1985.
6. Cape R: *Aging: Its Complex Management*. Hagerstown, MD, Harper and Row, 1978, p 82.
7. Castleden CM, George CF, Renwick AG, et al: Imipramine—a possible alternative to current therapy for urinary incontinence in the elderly. *J Urol* 125:318, 1981.
8. Health Care Financing Administration: *Your Medicare Handbook*, Publication no. HCFA 10050, DMHS, January, 1984.
8a. *Health Care of the Aged*. Rochester, NY, Health Council of Monroe County and Department of Preventative Medicine, University of Rochester School of Medicine and Dentistry.
9. Hodgson TA, Kopstein AN: Health care expenditures for major diseases in 1980, National Center for Health Statistics. *Health Care Financing Rev* 5:1, 1984.
10. Kane RA, Kane RL: *Assessing the Elderly: A Practical Guide to Measurement*. Lexington, MA, Lexington Books, DC Health, 1981.
11. Katz S, Ford AB, Moskowitz RW, et al: Studies of illness in the aged: the index at ADL: standardized measure of biological and psychosocial function. *JAMA* 185:94, 1963.
12. Lawton MP: Assessing the competence of older people. In Kent D, Kastenbaum R, Sherwood S (eds): *Research Planning and Action for the Elderly*. New York, Behavioral Publications, 1972.
13. Moisey CU, Stephenson TP, Brendler CB: The urodynamic and subjective results of treatment of detrusor instability with oxybutynin chloride. *Br J Urol* 52:472, 1980.
14. National Center for Health Statistics: Advancedata, from *Vital and Health Statistics*, Table 1, #92, Sept 14, 1983, p 2. From selected data from the Home Care Supplement to the 1979 National Health Interview survey.
15. National Center for Health Statistics: Number of physician visits and number of physician visits per person per year. In *Physician Visits: Volume and Interval Since Last Visit, U.S.*

1980, Table 3. Data from National Health Survey, Series 16, #144. Washington, DC, Department of Health and Human Services.

16. National Center for Health Statistics: Percent distribution of physician visits by place of visit. In *Physician Visits: Volume and Interval Since Last Visit, U.S. 1980.* Table 17. Data from National Health Survey, Series 16, #144. Washington, DC, Department of Health and Human Services.

17. Rubenstein LZ, Josephson KR, Wieland GD, *et al*: Effectiveness of a geriatric evaluation unit: a randomized clinical trial. *N Engl J Med* 311:1664, 1984.

18. Sachett DL, Haynes RB (eds): *Compliance with Therapeutic Regimes.* Baltimore, Johns Hopkins University Press, 1976.

19. Samily AH: Clinical manifestations of disease in the elderly: symposium on clinical geriatric medicine. *Med Clin North Am* 67:333, 1983.

20. Schwartz D, Wang M, Zeitz L, *et al*: Medication errors made by elderly, chronically ill patients. *Am J Public Health* 52:2018, 1962.

21. Stamey TA: Endoscopic suspension of the vesical neck for surgically curable urinary incontinence in the female. *Ann Surg* 192:465, 1980.

22. Stamler J: Lifestyles, major risk factors, proof and public policy. *Circulation* 58:3, 1978.

23. Vestal RE: Clinical pharmacology. In Andres R, Bierman E, Hazzard WR (eds): *Principles of Geriatric Medicine.* New York, McGraw-Hill, 1984, chap 38.

24. Whitehead WE, Burgio KL, Engel BT: Behavioral methods in the assessment and treatment of urinary incontinence. In Brocklehurst JC (ed): *Urology in the Elderly.* New York, Churchill Livingstone, 1984.

25. Williams TF: Comprehensive functional assessment: an overview. *J Am Geriatr Soc* 31:637, 1983.

26. Williams TF, Hill JG, Fairbank, ME, Knox KG: Appropriate placement of the chronically ill and aged: a successful approach by evaluation. *JAMA* 226:1332, 1973.

CHAPTER SEVEN

Occupational and Environmental Disease

JAMES P. KEOGH, M.D.

This is an era characterized by widespread proliferation of new and potentially toxic chemicals which are encountered in homes, schools, the general environment, and especially in the workplace. This proliferation has altered our overall environment in ways that affect the health of many individuals. Contamination of air and water from industrial discharges of hazardous waste is reported nearly every day in newspapers all over the country. The extent to which such exposures may be causing unrecognized health problems is a grave concern. In the future, few communities in the United States will escape public scrutiny of the health hazards of pesticide spraying, asbestos in school buildings, contaminated drinking water, or toxic waste disposal.

This chapter provides an overview of how environmental diseases occur and outlines an approach to enable the physician to recognize and deal with them. Its emphasis on the workplace reflects the fact that clinically diagnosed illness is much more likely to be related to the higher levels of toxic exposure found in such settings. Each year in the United States over 100,000 people die and over 400,000 become ill as a direct result of occupational disease. Every practitioner will see patients with occupational problems, and he must be prepared to recognize these problems and to provide appropriate care to the patients.

THE VITAL ROLE OF THE PRIMARY PRACTITIONER

Primary practitioners have frequently been the first professionals to recognize the hazards of a particular exposure by documenting the link between their patients' illnesses and their patients' work. While the task of following up on such observations involves public health specialists, practitioners should remember that theirs is the most critical role. When patients get sick from a hazardous exposure, they do not call an epidemiologist; they come to see their own doctor.

It is vitally important that primary practitioners take the time to report and follow up suspected occupational diseases. Although theoretically there is a system of surveillance and inspection of workplaces through the Occupational Safety and Health Administration (OSHA), there are, in fact, only enough inspectors to visit every workplace once in about every 200 years. Furthermore, most workers are unaware of their right to request investigation of potential hazards at work, and corporate medical departments and executives usually do not want government inspectors in their plants. Inspectors who do visit workplaces may lack medical training, so that they often focus on safety, rather than on health issues. For these reasons, if a patient has an occupational health problem or is exposed to a dangerous situation at work, the physician and his patient need to initiate action to protect the patient and his co-workers. Table 7.1 illustrates the sequence of events that may follow the recognition of an occupational disease by a primary physician.

THE PATHOGENESIS OF OCCUPATIONAL DISEASE

The pathogenesis of occupational disease is complex and involves not only the interaction between the host and a toxic substance, but a complex set of social interactions as well.

Toxin-Host Interaction

For an occupational disease to occur, there must be a triad consisting of a toxic agent, a host, and an environment in which the host is exposed. The illness that may result depends on the toxic properties of the substance, its route of entry, the dose received by the host, and the susceptibility of the host to the toxin.

Toxic agents can be inhaled, ingested, or absorbed through the skin. With inhalation, the dose received depends on whether the substance is present as a fume or a dust. Deposition of dust in the lungs depends to a great extent on particle size and distribution, since smaller particles can more easily enter the alveoli and become trapped. The concentration of the substance in the air (which is related to room ventilation, temperature, and humidity), the rate at which the worker is exercising and breathing, protective factors such as special clothing or respirator use are other factors that affect the likelihood of illness.

Once the toxic substance is absorbed there may be an instantaneous effect as in the case of carbon monoxide poisoning, a brief latent period, as in the case of occupational asthma, or a latent period of years or decades as in the pneumoconioses. A brief, high dose exposure may cause serious illness and death and be relatively easy to recognize. On the other hand, prolonged exposure to a low dose of a toxin may not cause symptoms at the outset, and yet may produce disease years later.

Economic Factors Affecting Pathogenesis

Thousands of new chemicals are introduced into industrial processes every year; few have had testing to detect their potential toxicity. Even when toxicological screening tests are done on a compound, these may not predict human disease. In all too many cases, the hazardousness of a chemical is recognized only after an outbreak of illness.

Economic factors play a major role in determining how safe a workplace is. Industrial hygiene programs to monitor exposure are common only in the largest plants. Important decisions such as improv-

---

Table 7.1.
Chronology of a Case of Lead Poisoning Diagnosed by a Primary Practitioner

Date	
7/7/81	28-year-old construction worker sees his physician with a history of 3 weeks of arthralgia and malaise. Physical examination is normal.
7/14	At follow-up visit, all initial laboratory tests are normal. Screening occupational history reveals patient began new job 2 months ago, burning off sections of steel on a highway bridge that was covered with red lead paint. Blood for lead level sent to lab.
7/19	Blood lead is 93 μg/dl (nl < 30). Patient told to stop work. Local health department called. Health department provides name of consultant to discuss clinical management.
7/20	Health department takes samples for blood lead level from all co-workers and alerts OSHA.
7/25	Patient and two co-workers admitted to hospital for chelation therapy, as suggested by consultant. OSHA completes preliminary monitoring of lead in air at bridge site and advises use of air-supplied respirators.
8/2	Patients discharged following first course of therapy. Workup reveals mild nerve conduction abnormalities and some abnormalities on psychological testing. One patient has low sperm count.
8/6	Patients apply for worker's compensation benefits by filling out claim at Worker's Compensation Commission office.
8/10	Patients readmitted for second course of chelation.
9/2	OSHA issues citations to employer under general duty clause as lead standard does not cover construction workers. Fines total $800.
9/6	Employer contests worker's compensation claims.
9/7	Demolition phase of project completed.
9/10	Hospital social worker intervenes to prevent eviction of first patient who has been without income since 7/19. Urges all patients to get attorney to represent them.
9/11	Complete medical records requested by worker's compensation insurance carrier. Brief summary and copies of records sent by the physician.
9/30	Company agrees to compromise settlement with OSHA covering future practices on other jobs. Fines dropped to $400.
10/1	Social worker persuades insurance carrier to agree to early hearing after workers' story appears in local newspaper.
10/15	Hearing held, Worker's Compensation Commission orders patients to be given back benefits.
11/3	Primary physician and consultant write to urge state OSHA to extend protections of OSHA lead standard to construction workers.
3/1/82	First hearing held on proposed new rule by state OSHA agency, which promises future study of issue.
4/3	Last of patients returns to work on new job.
1/16/83	Primary physician convinces state legislator to introduce bill mandating coverage of construction workers.
2/3	Patients, social worker, and physician testify before legislature.
4/16	Governor signs bill extending protection to construction workers, mandating monitoring, education, protective equipment, and pay retention if poisoned.

ing ventilation or decreasing exposure to noise may involve significant expense. Therefore management must weigh the benefits of protecting employee health against the cost of doing so. A company that consistently chooses health over profits may find itself at a distinct competitive disadvantage.

The worker may be reluctant to complain about working conditions for fear of losing his job. This is especially likely during periods of high unemployment, when acceptance of unpleasant and potentially unhealthy working conditions may be the price of having a job. The physician who fails to recognize this may be perplexed by his patient's unwillingness to take action to secure better conditions at work.

Even when workers are strongly organized, the desire for a safer workplace may be balanced by a concern that increased production costs may result in a company's decision to relocate its plant to areas where unions are less effective or do not exist.

Despite these factors that tend to make occupational illness more common, progress has been made. Increasingly, American workers and businessmen are both developing the knowledge needed to prevent workplace illness and demonstrating a willingness to place a higher priority on people than on profits. Stringent health and safety regulations with strong enforcement can put competitors on a more equal footing and protect responsible businesses from being undercut by irresponsible ones.

DIAGNOSING WORK-RELATED DISEASE

Although episodes of illness caused or exacerbated by the patient's work are frequently seen in ambulatory practice, they are frequently not recognized as such, and even less often are they appropriately managed. The practitioner who is prepared to recognize the connection between the patient's symptoms and the patient's work can make a big difference for both the individual and the community. The practitioner who fails to think about the patient's occupation may

1. miss the diagnosis entirely and pursue the wrong therapy;
2. permit continuation of poor working conditions which may subsequently injure others or even result in death.

Two cases illustrate these points:

Case: A Teenager with Bronchitis

An 18-year-old woman complained to her physician of a severe cough and some wheezing. He treated her with erythromycin and fluids and advised her to stay in bed for a few days. She recovered and returned to work feeling well. Several days later she had a severe recurrent cough with wheezing

and dyspnea and saw her physician again. He again prescribed erythromycin and rest. She remained off work for a week. She felt better and returned to work. After 2 days she became extremely short of breath and was brought to the emergency room. She had severe bronchospasm and was admitted, improving on bronchodilators and corticosteroids after a few days.

History on admission disclosed that her work involved grinding drill bits made of tungsten carbide, a known pulmonary sensitizer. Having been sensitized, each fresh exposure to the dust caused symptoms after a shorter incubation period. Had the first physician considered the diagnosis of extrinsic asthma and inquired about occupational exposures he could have prevented the patient's subsequent deterioration.

Case: A Grouchy Man with a Headache

A 25-year-old man presented to the emergency room of a community hospital with a chief complaint of headache. When seen by the physician he was hostile and complained bitterly about having waited 45 minutes to be seen. He said he had had increasingly severe headaches for several weeks. He initially refused physical examination, pointing out that the pain was only in his head, and insisted "what I really need is something stronger for the pain." Physical examination was negative and he was given an aspirin-narcotic compound.

Seen some weeks later, a co-worker warned him that his lead level might be high, and a family member contacted the health department. In addition to the persisting headaches, a history of irritability, abdominal pain, insomnia, and constipation was elicited. The patient worked in an automobile assembly plant where he used a grinding wheel to smooth joints filled with a lead-containing solder. He had actually been under surveillance for lead poisoning, with regular measurement of blood lead level, but the plant physician did not inform workers of their results. His blood lead level had been steadily rising and was 3 times normal. After therapy with a chelating agent he became symptom free. Subsequent investigation revealed that most of his co-workers had high blood lead levels; three of them were subsequently treated for lead poisoning. Questioning the patient about his work could have saved him weeks of discomfort and prevented some of his co-workers from being poisoned.

To avoid the pitfalls these cases demonstrate, the primary practitioner needs to remember only three important principles:

1. *Ask every patient about his or her job.*
2. *Consider the possibility that the patient's illness is related to work or home environment.*
3. *Follow up on your suspicions. Others may be in danger.*

Taking an Occupational History

Inquiring about a patient's job will not only help to identify occupational disease, it will provide other information useful in caring for a patient. Clearly the physical demands of the job are important when advising a patient about a health problem, such as coronary artery disease or diabetes. Knowing the patient's work schedule is also important since shift work affects medication schedules, diet, and family life. Medications can dramatically affect the patient's comfort or safety at work (e.g., diuretics in an interstate truck driver or antihistamines in an ironworker). Financial and psychological stress may result from layoffs, whereas regular overtime may bring about chronic fatigue and psychological problems of its own.

The diagnosis of an occupational disease cannot be made unless the physician asks every patient about his job as part of the medical history (Table 7.2). Usually, a brief discussion of the current job, including a brief description of how the patient spends his working day, is sufficient. This rarely takes more than 3 minutes.

When some aspect of the medical or occupational history has raised suspicions of a work-related condition, further questioning will flow naturally. In general the questioner will be looking for a temporal relation between symptoms and possible exposure, for an exposure to an agent known to cause disease, or for a pattern of similar illness among co-workers. Because every patient, every job, and every medical presentation is different, there is no single way of taking a history. Building skill in occupational history taking requires that the physician be interested and be willing to adopt the role of learner. If the

patient uses jargon or job titles that are unfamiliar, he should be asked for an explanation. Once patients get over their surprise that the physician is interested in what they do, they are always happy to describe their work.

The screening history will sometimes reveal the need to take a comprehensive lifelong work history. An account of the previous jobs and exposures is especially important when the patient has a chronic illness or the possibility of work-related neoplasia. In such cases, the following approach is recommended:

1. *Begin with parents' jobs and childhood exposures.*

2. *Review each of the patient's jobs in chronological order.*

3. *Elicit relevant aspects of each period of employment (see Table 7.2).*

Are Some Diseases More Likely to Be Work Related?

The astute clinician is alert to the possibility of an environmental etiology in all situations. Getting in the habit of asking about the patient's work will rapidly build the physician's awareness of local industries and particular problems.

The occupational diseases a physician will encounter depend upon his location in the United States, the industry in the immediate vicinity, and the demographic makeup of the practice. For example, practitioners near retirement communities may see retired workers with previous exposure in all types of industry. Table 7.3 lists selected examples of clinical problems grouped according to the organ system affected.

Dermatitis and *pneumoconiosis* are the most frequently reported occupational illnesses. This probably reflects both true incidence (skin and pulmonary epithelium are most in contact with the outside environment) and the greater likelihood of recognition of these disorders as being occupational in origin.

The number of chemicals that are toxic to the *liver* and *kidney* is so great that a careful exposure history should be taken from all patients with hepatitis and hepatic or renal failure. Many chemicals can affect the gastrointestinal tract and cause functional disturbances that may be misdiagnosed as peptic disease or irritable bowel syndrome.

Low level exposure of the respiratory organs to a variety of substances may result in the production of *nonspecific upper respiratory syndromes* that the patient may describe as an intractable cold or as sinus trouble.

Although occupational diseases periodically present with striking and unusual signs (such as acroosteolysis in vinyl chloride workers or nasal septal perforation in patients exposed to chromates), more

Table 7.2.
Components of an Occupational History

Description of the job:	Physical exertion
	Body mechanics
	Pace of work
	Repetitive tasks
	Job stress
Exposure to hazards:	Risk of trauma
	Dusts, fumes, mists
	Contamination of skin and clothing
	Noise and vibration
	Heat and cold
	Ionizing and nonionizing radiation
Protective measures:	Ventilation and respiratory protection
	Protective clothing
	Medical surveillance
Effects of exposure:	Temporal relation of any symptoms to work, *e.g.*, relation to time of day, day of week, change of symptoms on vacation, weekends
	Similar symptoms in co-workers

Table 7.3.
Selected Occupational Problems

Clinical Problem	Causative Agent[a]	Clinical Problem	Causative Agent[a]
CONSTITUTIONAL		Painful burns	Hydrofluoric acid (deep pain out of proportion to appearance of burn)
Fever	Heat		
	Radiant heated air	Skin cancer	Soots
	Microwaves		Tars
	Metal fumes:		Arsenic
	Zinc		Coke oven emissions
	Copper		Cutting oils
	Magnesium	NERVOUS SYSTEM	
	Cadmium	*Central Effects*	
	Dinitrophenol	Altered conscious-	Hundreds of chemicals have cen-
	Pentachlorophenol	ness	tral nervous system (CNS)-
	Dinitro-*o*-cresol		depressant properties and
	Polymer fume (polytetrafluorethy-		other CNS effects
	lene)	Convulsions	Aldrin
	Cotton dust		2-Aminopyridine
	Bagasse		Camphor
	Moldy hay		Chlordane
SKIN			Crag herbicide
Sweating	Organophosphates		DDT
	Pentachlorophenol		Decaborane
	Dinitro-*o*-cresol		2,4-Dichlorophenoxyacetic acid
Cyanosis	Methemoglobin formers:		Dieldrin
	Aniline		1,1-Dimethylhydrazine
	Anisidine, ortho- and para- iso-		Endrin
	mers		Heptachlor
	Dimethylaniline		Hydrazine
	Dinitrobenzene, all isomers		Lindane
	Dinitrotoluene		Methoxychlor
	Monomethylaniline		Methyl bromide
	p-Nitroaniline		Methyl chloride
	Nitrobenzene		Methyl iodide
	p-Nitrocholorobenzene		Methyl mercaptain
	Nitrogen trifluoride		Monomethylhydrazine
	Nitrotoluene		Nicotine
	Perchloryl fluoride		Nitromethane
	n-Propyl nitrate		Oxalic acid
	Tetranitromethane		Pentaborane
	o-Toluidine		Phenol
	Xylidine		Rotenone
Contact dermatitis	Many chemicals with irritant or		Sodium Fluoroacetate
	sensitizing properties		Strychnine
Chronic eczematous	Solvents		Tetraethyllead
dermatitis	Detergents		Tetramethyllead
Folliculitis	Oil exposure		Tetramethylsuccinoitrile
	Grease exposure		Thallium, soluble compounds
Acne	Polychlorinated biphenyls		Toxaphene
	Chlorinated naphthalenes	Headaches	Carbon monoxide
	Paraffin		Nitrites
	Coal tar		Nitrates
	Dioxin		Alcohols
Photosensitization	Coal tar		Lead
	Pitch		Organic lead compounds
	Asphalt		Methemoglobin formers (see un-
	Anthracene		der cyanosis)
	Creosote	Behavioral change	Mercury
	Fluorescein		Lead
	Phenanthrene		Carbon disulfide
Granulomas	Beryllium		Carbon monoxide
Corns	Asbestos		Methyl chloride
	Fiberglass		Methyl bromide
Punctate ulcers	Chromic acid		

Table 7.3.—Continued

Clinical Problem	Causative Agent[a]	Clinical Problem	Causative Agent[a]
Ataxia, tremor, spasticity	Manganese	Lens deposits and discoloration	Copper
	Organic lead compounds		Iron
	Organic tin compounds		Mercury
Hyperreflexia, micrographia	Compounds		Phenylmercuric salts
	Mercury		Silver
	DDT	Optic neuritis—visual acuity and visual field defects	Carbon dioxide
Peripheral neuropathy	Peripheral neurotoxins:		Carbon monoxide
	Acrylamide		Carbon disulfide
	Arsenic and compounds		Cyanide
	Calcium arsenate		Methanol
	Carbon disulfide		Methyl mercury
	n-Hexane		Naphthalene
	Lead and inorganic lead compounds		Thallium
			Lead
	Lead arsenate		Acetylphenylhydrazine
	Dimethylaminopropionitrile		Benzene
	Lucel-7 (2-t-butylazo-2-hydroxy 5-methyl hexane)		Triethyl tin
			Phosphorus
	Mercury		Ethylene glycol
	Methyl bromide	Nystagmus and extraocular muscle palsy	Carbon disulfide
	Methyl butyl ketone		Dieldrin
	Thallium, soluble compounds		Ethanol
	2,4,6-Trinitrotoluene		Ethylene Glycol
	Tri-o-cresyl phosphate		Lead
EYE			Methyl bromide
Conjunctivitis	Ultraviolet radiation (welder's flash)		Methyl chloride
			Methyl iodide
	Many irritant chemicals		Triethyl tin
Corneal irritation or scarring	Acids	Eye strain—visual fatigue	Visual display terminals
	Alkalies	**HEARING**	
	Dimethyl sulfate	Decreased acuity and tinnitus	Noise exposure especially above 85 decibels
	Formaldehyde		
	Methyl dichloropropionate	Acoustic neuritis	Aniline
	Osmic acid		Arsenic
	Sulfur dioxide		Carbon monoxide
	1-Butanol		Hypoxia
	Xylene		Lead
	Diazomethane		Organic mercury
	Dichlorobutenes		Phosphorus
	Ethylene oxide		Sodium nitrate
	Ethylenimine	Otitis externa	Contamination of earplugs used for noise protection
	Hydrogen sulfide		
Corneal edema producing "haloes" around lights	Allyl alcohol	Ear pain	Acute shifts in pressure
	Amines	**SMELL**	
	Morpholines	Anosmia	Arsenic
	Diethyldigylocolate		Benzine
	Diisopropylamine		Benzol
	3-Dimethylamino propylamine		Cadmium
	Ethylenediamine		Carbon disulfide
	Tetraethylbutanediamine		Chromium
	Triethylenediamine		Ethyl acetate
Scarring and discoloration	Benzoquinone		Formaldehyde
	Aniline		Hydrazine
Corneal discoloration as a manifestation of systemic intoxication	Arsine		Iodine
	Nitrobenzene		Ketone
	Silver		Lead
Cataracts	Radiant heat		Mercury
	Microwave exposure		Nickel
	Dinitro-o-cresol		Osmium tetroxide
	Dinitrophenol		Phosphorus oxychloride
			Phthalic anhydride

Table 7.3.—_Continued_

Clinical Problem	Causative Agent[a]	Clinical Problem	Causative Agent[a]
	Potassium iodide	Maple bark-stripper's disease	_Cryptostroma corticale_
	Selenium		
	Sulfuric acid	Miller's bronchitis	_Aspergillus glaucus_ and _Penicillium glaucum_
TASTE			
Decreased acuity	Bromine	Mill fever	_Corchorus capsularis_ and _chorchorus olitorius_
	Caprolactam		
Alterations in taste	Iodine	Mother of pearl (nacre)	Conchiolin
	Phosgene		
	Antimony	Mushroom-picker's lung	
	Arsenic		
	Bismuth	Paprika-splitter's lung	_Mucor stolinifer_
	Cadmium		
	Copper	Sequoiosis	_Graphium_ sp.
	Gallium	Bronchospasm	Pulmonary sensitizers:
	Lead		Castor bean pomace
	Mercury		Cobalt, metal fume and dust
	Nickel		Enzymatic detergents
	Nitrogen dioxide		Grain dusts
	Selenium		Maleic anhydride
	Tellurium		Methylene bisphenyl isocyanate
	Thallium		Methyl isocyanate
	Vanadium		Nickel, metal
	Zinc oxide		_p_-Phenylenediamine
			Phthalic anhydride
RESPIRATORY			Platinum salts
Nasal septal perforation	Chromic acid and other chromates		Polyvinyl chloride (fume from heated film: meat-wrapper's asthma)
Laryngeal carcinoma	Asbestos		
Laryngitis, bronchitis, tracheitis, pneumonitis	Many irritants including:		Toluene 2,4-diisocyanate
	Ammonia		Tungsten carbide
	Chlorine		Western red cedar dust
	Oxides of nitrogen		Wood pulp dust
	Ozone	Pulmonary fibrosis	Asbestos
	Phosgene		Silica
	Sulfur dioxide		Silicates including diatomaceous earth
	Vanadium pentoxide		
	Mercury		Beryllium
	Manganese		Talc
	Cadmium dust		Coal dust
Bronchiolitis obliterans	Nitrogen dioxide		Cobalt
			Hematite
Allergic alveolitis:			Kaolin
Bagassosis	_Thermoactinomyces vulgaris_ and _Micropolyspora_ sp.		Yttrium
		Benign pneumoconiosis deposits in lung without fibrosis	Aluminum powder
Bird-breeder's lung (pigeon-breeder's disease)	Avian proteins		Barium
			Graphite
			Iron oxide
			Tin
Byssinosis (Cannabosis)	Cotton, flax, and soft fiber hemps		Cerium oxide
			Silver
Cheese-washer's lung	_Penicillium caseil_		Titanium
			Ultramarine
Coffee-worker's lung	Chlorogenic acid	Pleural effusion	Asbestos
			Paraquat
Detergents	_Bacillus subtilis_		Talc
Farmer's lung	_Micropolyspora faeni_ and _Thermoactinomyces vulgaris_	Carcinoma of lung	Arsenic
			Asbestos
Feathers	Feather proteins		Bis(chloromethyl)ether
Furrier's lung	Keratinized particles of hair		Chloromethylmethylether
Kapok	_Ceiba pentandra_ (fruit) and _Eriodendron anfractuosum_ (seed-pod)		Coke oven emissions
			Chromates
		Pleural mesothelioma	Asbestos
Malt-worker's lung	_Aspergillis clavatus_		Zeolite

Table 7.3.—*Continued*

Clinical Problem	Causative Agent[a]	Clinical Problem	Causative Agent[a]
GASTROINTESTINAL		Abdominal pain	Antimony
Gingivitis and gum pigmentation	Mercury		Arsenic
	Lead		Bromine
	Bismuth		Cadmium
Dental erosion	Acetic acid		Lead
	Hydrochloric acid		Mercury
	Lactic acid		Nicotine
	Nitric acid		Organophosphates
	Nitrogen dioxide		Thallium
	Sulfuric acid		Many other chemicals when ingested
Tongue paresthesias	Furfural		
	Rotenone	CARDIOVASCULAR SYSTEM	
	Cresol	*Heart*	
Green discoloration	Vanadium	Myocardial damage	Antimony
Esophagitis	Ingestion of a variety of irritants		Arsine
Esophageal carcinoma	Asbestos		Carbon disulfide
		Ischemic disease	Nitroglycerin
Nausea and vomiting	Many chemicals including:		Nitrogycol
	irritants		Other vasodilating nitrates
	CNS depressants	*Peripheral Vascular Disease*	
	Cholinesterase inhibitors		
	Methemoglobin formers	Hypertension	Noise exposure
Constipation	Lead		Aminopyridine
	Barium sulfate		Arsenic
	Thalium		Barium
	Tellurium		Boron hydride
	Vanadium		Carbon disulfide
	Fluorides		Cobalt
	Nitrous fumes		Diphenyl
Hepatomegaly	Hepatoxins:		Lead
	Acetylene tetrabromide		Mercury
	Carbon disulfide		Thallium
	Carbon tetrachloride	Vasospastic disorders "White finger"	Vibrating tools
	Chlorodiphenyl, 42% chlorine		
	Chlorodiphenyl, 54% chlorine	Raynaud's phenomenon	Vinyl chloride
	Chloroform	GENITOURINARY	
	p-Dichlorobenzene	Renal disease	Nephrotoxins:
	Dimethylacetamide		4-Aminodiphenyl
	Dimethylformamide		Carbon disulfide
	Dioxane		Carbon tetrachloride
	Ethylene chlorohydrin		Chloroform
	Ethylene dibromide		Dioxane
	Ethylene dichloride		Ethylene chlorohydrin
	Hexachloronaphthalene		Ethylene dibromide
	Kepone		Lead
	Nitroethane		Mercury
	Octachloronaphthalene		Oxalic acid
	Pentachloronaphthalene		Picric acid
	Picric acid		Tetrachloroethane
	Tetrachloroethane		2,4,6-Trinitrotoluene
	Tetrachloroethylene		Turpentine
	Tetrachloronaphthalene		Uranium (natural), soluble and insoluble compounds
	Trichloronaphthalene		
	2,4,6-Trinitrotoluene	Renal carcinoma	4-Aminodiphenyl
Jaundice	Hepatoxins (see above)		Auramine
	Hemolytic agents:		Benzidine
	Arsine		*β*-Naphthylamine
	Butyl cellosolve		4-Nitrodiphenyl
	Naphthalene		Magenta
	Phenylhydrazine	Urinary retention	Dimethylaminopropionitrile
	Stibine		
Angiosarcoma of liver	Vinyl chloride		

Table 7.3.—Continued

Clinical Problem	Causative Agent[a]	Clinical Problem	Causative Agent[a]
Urinary frequency	Chloroform		Marrow depressants:
	Fufuryl alcohol		Benzene
	Oxalic acid		Dinitrophenol
REPRODUCTIVE AB-NORMALITIES			Tetryl
			2,4,6-Trinitrotoluene
Female sterility	Arsenic	Leukemia	Benzene
	Lead		Radiation
	Phosphorus		Styrene-butadiene
Male sterility	Arsenic		Ethylene oxide
	Benzene	Splenomegaly	Beryllium
	Cadmium		Methyl chloride
	Carbon disulfide		Naphthalene
	Carbon monoxide		Naphthol
	Chlordecone (Kepone)		Nitrobenzene
	Dibromochloropropane		Phosphorus
	Lead		Resorcinol
	Manganese	MUSCULOSKELETAL	
	Methyl chloride	Muscle cramps	Boron hydrides
	Microwaves to testes (radar workers)		Camphor
			Chlorobenzenes
	Phosphorus		Dinitrophenol
	Stilbestrol		Hydrofluoric acid
	Trichloroethylene		Lead
HEMATOLOGICAL PROBLEMS			Manganese
			Mercury, organic
Anemia	Lead		Nicotine
	Hemolytic agents:		Ricin
	Arsine		Tricresol phosphates
	Butyl cellosolve	Osteonecrosis	Phosphorus
	Naphthalene	Osteomalacia	Cadmium
	Phenylhydrazine	Osteosclerosis	Fluorine
	Stibine	Acro-osteolysis	Vinyl chloride

[a] The types of occupations which most often provide risk of exposures to these agents are most easily identified in Key et al (see "General References").

commonly they present with the vague systemic symptoms typical of early intoxication.

There are a few specific clinical situations that deserve to be highlighted:

Any change in personality or behavior. Poisoning due to mercury, lead, pesticides, and a wide variety of other central nervous system toxins may present this way.

New onset of asthma. Owing to the time lapse when an immunological mechanism is involved, wheezing and dyspnea may not be noted until after the workday is over.

Any case of pulmonary fibrosis. A prolonged latent period between exposure and disease onset means that abnormalities that appear on X-ray must have resulted from a job the patient had decades ago.

Peripheral neuropathy. A toxic neuropathy may be recognizable by an unusual pattern of presentation, but in most cases only careful history taking will reveal the cause.

Hearing loss. Noise-induced hearing loss occurs gradually and usually in older workers, so that it is rarely recognized in time to prevent severe damage.

Inability to conceive. More and more compounds that affect the reproductive system and cause sterility are being identified.

Lung cancer. Exposure to asbestos and cigarette smoke causes synergistic action. Such synergism is likely but less established with the other pulmonary carcinogens.

Other cancers. Specific carcinogens are identified in Table 7.4.

Determining Work Relatedness

The key to identifying occupational disease is to be sure that a toxic/environmental etiology is at least considered. The physician needs to think of possible agents that could cause the patient's symptoms and to consider the temporal relationship to changes at work or in the home environment. In addition, the patient should always be asked, "*Do you think this problem could have anything to do with your work?*" and, "*Does anyone else at work have this same problem?*" Very often if there is a connection, the patient will be able to identify it. The literature of occupational medicine is replete with episodes where workers knew for months or years of an unusually high incidence of a syndrome

Table 7.4.
Cancers Presently Known to Be Caused by Environmental Agents

Site/Cell Type	Toxic Agent	Industry/Occupation
Liver/hemangiosarcoma	Vinyl chloride monomer	Vinyl chloride polymerization industry
	Arsenical pesticides	Vintners
Nose	Hardwood dusts	Woodworkers, cabinet, furniture makers
	Radium	Radium chemists and processors, dial painters
	Chromates	Chromium producers, processors, users
	Nickel	Nickel smelting and refining
	Unknown agent	Boot and shoe industry
Larynx	Asbestos	Asbestos product manufacture, shipbuilding, construction and maintenance work
Lung	Asbestos	Asbestos product manufacture, shipbuilding, construction and maintenance work
	Coke oven emissions	Topside coke oven workers
	Radon daughters	Uranium and fluorspar miners
	Chromates	Chromium producers and processors, users
	Nickel	Nickel smelters, processors, users
	Arsenic	Smelters
	Mustard gas	Mustard gas formulators
	Bis (chloromethyl) ether, chloromethyl methyl ether	Ion exchange resin makers, chemists
Pleura and peritoneum/ mesothelioma	Asbestos	Asbestos product manufacture, shipbuilding, construction and maintenance work
Bone	Radium	Dial painters, radium chemists and processors
Scrotum	Mineral/cutting oils	Automatic lathe operators, metalworkers
	Soots and tars, tar distillates	Coke oven workers, petroleum refiners, tar distillers
Bladder	Benzidine, α- and β-naphthylamine, auramine, magenta, 4-aminobiphenyl, 4-nitrophenyl	Rubber and dye workers
Esophagus	Asbestos	Asbestos product manufacture, shipbuilding, construction and maintenance work
Stomach	Asbestos	Asbestos product manufacture, shipbuilding, construction and maintenance work
Colon	Asbestos	Asbestos product manufacture, shipbuilding, construction and maintenance work
Kidney	Coke oven emissions	Coke oven workers
Hematopoietic/lymphoid leukemia, acute	Unknown	Rubber industry
	Ionizing radiation	Radiologists
Myeloid leukemia, acute	Benzene	Refining, chemical, and manufacturing industries
	Ionizing radiation	Radiologists
Erythroleukemia, acute	Benzene	Refining, chemical, and manufacturing industries

and were unable to get their physicians to listen to them.

If neither the physician nor the patient knows if a syndrome is occupational in origin, there are resources available that identify: (*a*) toxic causes of a given symptom complex, (*b*) toxic exposures of given professions, and (*c*) the effects of exposure to given substances (see Table 7.5).

FOLLOW-UP OF OCCUPATIONAL DISEASE

Follow up on Suspicions: Others May Be in Danger

If there is suspicion that a patient became ill from an occupational exposure, it is the physician's re-

sponsibility to follow up. Not only does diagnosing an occupational disease affect therapy and eligibility for compensation for a patient, but it may indicate that the health of others is also in danger. Often physicians overcome their own uneasiness about a patient's job by advising the patient to change jobs. Then, instead of the potentially hazardous job being made safe, another unsuspecting person is brought in to take the risk.

There are some circumstances where occupational disease is recognized but the original hazard has been eliminated—for example, a patient with asbestosis who worked in a now closed shipyard. Even in these circumstances, former fellow workers

Table 7.5.
How to Determine the Potential Hazards of an Exposure

1. Characterize the exposure to the extent possible, including the chemical identity of substances; type and wavelength of radiation, light, or noise; likely route of entry; concentration of chemical substance or intensity of energy source; available protection
2. Look it up in available references:

If you know:	*Then:*
Only a trade or code name	Call the employer to get the chemical identity or at least the name of the manufacturer, then call the manufacturer of the substance to learn the contents;
	or use:
	Gosselin RE, Smith RP, Hodge HC: *Clinical Toxicology of Commercial Products*, ed 5. Baltimore, Williams & Wilkins, 1984.
Only the general nature of the patient's work	Get an idea of exposures from the patient, the employer or union, or a consultant (see below).
The identity of the chemicals or energy	Call your local poison control center for fast help;
	or look it up in:
	Proctor N, Hughes J: *Chemical Hazards in the Workplace*. Philadelphia, JB Lippincott, 1976;
	or
	Rom WN (ed): *Environmental and Occupational Medicine*. Boston, Little, Brown, and Co, 1983;
	or
	some toxins have separate listings in *Index Medicus*.

3. Call a consultant:
   Your state or local health department may be able to help identify the nature of the problem and even help you get clinical advice. A number of states with "right to know" laws have set up information clearinghouses.
   The National Institute of Occupational Safety and Health has a Clearinghouse for Occupational Safety and Health Information. Staff members welcome physicians' inquiries and have rapid access to information and expertise. Telephone numbers: 513-684-8328 or 513-533-8326.

need to be informed of the risk resulting from previous exposure.

The physician should not wait for absolute proof of etiology before beginning an investigation of a possible workplace hazard. The least severely affected member of a group of workers may be the one who seeks attention. Moreover, for most occupationally induced diseases, proof of a relationship rests on epidemiological data rather than on diagnostic study of the individual patient. Often the most practical way to learn if a patient's problems are caused or exacerbated by his occupation is to find out if fellow workers are similarly affected.

Health Department

In many states, there is a health department unit for investigation of occupational disease. Some states require physicians to report all cases of suspected occupational disease. Such laws should and probably will become more widespread. Reporting any suspected occupational disease problem to the local health department can be the first step in follow-up.

Occupational Safety and Health Administration

While health departments generally have authority to investigate occupational diseases, regulation of workplace conditions is usually the responsibility of a separate state agency or of the local office of the Occupational Safety and Health Administration in the United States Department of Labor (telephone number is listed under US Government, Labor Department, OSHA). Where a state has taken over OSHA enforcement, its regulations are required to be as strict as the federal regulations. In every state, every employer is obligated to report workplace injuries and illness to OSHA.

If other workers may be in imminent danger of being made ill, the physician should communicate this urgently to OSHA to promote an immediate investigation. In most cases OSHA enforcement officers are able to determine relatively easily if regulations are being violated at a workplace, and they will provide a follow-up report to the referring physician. In some cases, the inspection may suggest that the patient's illness was job related, but that at the time of the inspection no specific OSHA regulation was being violated. If a continuing hazard does exist, OSHA can force changes by invoking the employer's "general duty" to maintain a safe workplace. Especially in these situations the physician may need to be patient but persistent to see that appropriate action is taken.

National Institute of Occupational Safety and Health

If there is difficulty in clarifying the potential relationship of illness to environment, or if the concerns raised are not addressed by a specific OSHA regulation, it may be helpful to request assistance from the National Institute of Occupational Safety and Health (NIOSH).* This institute is that part of the US Public Health Service's Centers for Disease Control that conducts research on occupational disease. An employer, union, or any three employees can request a formal Health Hazard Evaluation (HHE) of a workplace. Furthermore, NIOSH now has Educational Resource Centers (where consultants are available to help physicians, employers, and workers) available in each region of the country. These centers can provide literature searches and information on available publications and current areas of research, and can refer a physician to others who are experts in the field. (Access to regional centers can be provided by the central office.)

In addition to its investigatory function, NIOSH can provide assistance directly regarding a physician's concern about a patient's exposure. Its clearinghouse responds to practitioners' inquiries with information about the hazards of particular trades and toxic substances.

WORKER'S COMPENSATION

Every state has a worker's compensation act which provides a system of dispensing funds for medical expenses related to occupational disease and injury and for employee's lost earnings. These laws were passed to provide a "no-fault" system of compensating workers injured on the job, and to provide employers with a statutory protection from being sued for negligence by their employees. In almost all states an injured worker or his family may not sue an employer, but is supposed to be able rapidly to receive compensation for lost earning ability without having to go through a lengthy legal proceeding.

While this system works well in some situations for on-the-job injuries, it does not respond well to the needs of a worker with an occupational disease. Here the burden of proof that the disease is work related falls squarely on the worker, and the process of obtaining compensation is often slow and difficult. Because most small employers insure themselves with an insurance company, the insurer may delay

---

* NIOSH may be contacted at the following address:
NIOSH
Clearinghouse for Occupational Safety and Health Information
ATTN: Information Retrieval and Analysis Section
4676 Columbia Parkway
Cincinnati, OH 45226
Telephone: 513-684-8328 or 513-533-8326

action on a claim even when the employer himself believes the illness was caused by the job. Usually the worker can obtain legal assistance without having to pay an attorney directly, because provision is made for cases to be taken on a contingency basis (*i.e.*, the attorney receives no fee unless the claim is upheld, and then receives a fixed percentage). Because illness claims are usually complex, the worker will often need such expert advice.

If a physician concludes or even strongly suspects that a patient has an illness caused or made worse by his job, the patient should be encouraged to file for worker's compensation (through his employer, the worker's compensation local office, or his lawyer).

There are two reasons for this. First, if a claim is pursued and won (even though it takes time), the patient is usually guaranteed lifetime medical coverage from worker's compensation funds for that illness. Compensation may lift some of the financial burdens from the patient and his family, particularly in cases of chronic or fatal diseases. Second, worker's compensation has the potential to encourage safety and to penalize careless employers.

To a great extent worker's compensation has failed in the area of occupational disease, chiefly because of inadequate physician diagnosis and follow-through. For example, a 1980 Department of Labor survey showed that only 3% of workers disabled by occupational respiratory disease were receiving compensation. The 97% of the disabled workers who were not receiving worker's compensation were living on Social Security or welfare. Their medical bills were being paid by health insurance, Medicare, or state welfare funds. Thus, the economic and social costs of industrial disease are largely borne not by the companies who may have acted irresponsibly but by the victims and the taxpayers, including those businesses who are trying to protect their employees properly.

Physicians are often reticent about involvement with worker's compensation, feeling a claim may tie them up in court. This is an unsubstantiated fear since the medical record usually provides sufficient medical evidence and the physician does not have to appear at the hearing. If the record does not provide adequate information, the attorneys involved will almost always be willing to take a statement from the physician at his convenience.

THE PART TIME PLANT PHYSICIAN

A primary practitioner may become involved in a workplace at the invitation of the employer or the union representing the employees. Many small and medium-sized workplaces need the assistance of part time physicians to conduct effective programs to detect and prevent occupational disease. The practitioner should welcome the chance to do something to prevent illness, but must take special care to meet the ethical obligations such a role requires. Many physicians in occupational medicine regard themselves as responsible to the management of the company that pays them, rather than to the patients they serve. In some instances, physicians have withheld information from patients about work-related diseases. In other cases, physicians modify their therapy for illnesses and injuries to meet the needs of production rather than the needs of the patient. This role of the "company physician" as servant of management rather than of the patient has had tacit acceptance in the past. In the last decade the American Occupational Medical Association, composed principally of industry-employed physicians, has called for adherence to ethical practice, and many abuses have been ended. Any physician today who practices as a plant physician differently from the way he practices in his own office may face professional discipline and malpractice suits. In some plants, workers and management are following the Swedish model of jointly selecting a plant physician. Table 7.6 summarizes the principal ethical responsibilities of a plant physician.

HAZARDS AT HOME AND IN THE COMMUNITY

Exposures at Home

The average American home is a Pandora's box of potentially harmful exposures. Between kitchen, bathroom, garage, and garden, family members may have access to caustics, a variety of aerosols, pesticides, solvents, paint removers, adhesives, and electrical equipment. Practitioners often think of these kinds of exposures when warning about childproofing for toddlers and when evaluating dermatoses

and allergic reactions. Exposures at home may also produce illness in ways that come less readily to mind (see Table 7.7). Case reports have documented poisoning from unwise use of cosmetics and vitamin supplements. Many hobbies can involve exposure to chemicals with fewer protections than workers in industry may enjoy. For example, lead poisoning has been documented from ceramics, stained glasswork, and cosmetics; paint strippers containing methylene chloride can produce carbon monoxide poisoning sufficient to aggravate angina and precipitate infarction; and injudicious combinations of cleaning materials can release hazardous fumes.

Homes themselves may have hazards. For example, lead-containing paints are a risk to both children and do-it-yourselfers, and formaldehyde-urea foam insulation can release sensitizing fumes. In cases of illness caused by such exposures, physicians need to take a careful history to recognize the cause.

Heating and ventilation systems deserve special mention. Even up-to-date heating systems can produce carbon monoxide poisoning if flues are blocked or inadequate air for combustion is provided. Because symptoms of early carbon monoxide poisoning are nonspecific and mimic those of stress and depression, a high level of suspicion is critical, especially early in the heating season. With the current emphasis on increased insulation and barriers to air infiltration, houses are often poorly ventilated by fresh air. The increasing use of wood, coal, and kerosene heaters may make matters worse. Use of scrap lumber treated with chemical preservatives is an additional hazard.

Office and commercial buildings are also increasingly "tight," due to recirculation of heated or cooled air. A large number of epidemics of illness caused by chemical or biological agents circulated through the air are being reported.

Exposures from Sources in the Community

Physicians are increasingly being asked for advice relating to concerns about contamination of drinking water and air and the cleanup of toxic wastes. Many communities dependent on groundwater have had their supplies threatened by illegal dumping of chemicals or by leakage from licensed landfills.

Table 7.6.
Responsibilities of the Plant Physician

The primary responsibility of the physician is to the individual patient, no matter who is paying the bill.

The physician may reveal nothing to others, including management, about the patient without his permission. Reports should be limited to a statement about the patient's fitness to work and any specific limitations of activity.

The physician must acquire all available information about the workplace that may be relevant to a patient's health.

Everything that the physician learns or may deduce about the safety of the workplace must be explained to those whose health may be affected.

The physician should report occupational disease to the local health department or state OSHA.

The physician should not take sides in any dispute between the management, the workers, or the government, but should only provide accurate information and honest opinion to all concerned.

Table 7.7.
Common Hazards at Home

Heating and air conditioning
Insulation and lack of ventilation
Vitamins and health foods
Cleaning chemicals
Electrical appliances
Water supply
Hobbies
Home repair
Neighborhood pollution sources

The discovery of a chronic source of contamination is an experience few American communities will escape. There is no substitute in such situations for enlisting the assistance of appropriate experts, and physicians in a community need to take the lead in getting help from state and local agencies. Often there is a continuing role for practitioners to play in facilitating the resolution of problems. In many cases, the specialists, whose knowledge is so valuable, have difficulty in translating what they have to say into language that the lay public can understand. The doctor who spends his entire day translating medical science into advice for his patients in the office is well suited to serve in this role. At the same time, community members may need someone who can represent their acute personal concerns to the authorities in a reasoned way. The physician may have to serve as the community's advocate and critical reviewer, making sure that the statements and positions of all of those involved are supported by factual evidence and calling on independent expertise when appropriate.

Air Pollution

Patients with respiratory disease are especially concerned about the effects of air pollution. There is little evidence to implicate general community air pollution as the primary cause of individual patient illness, except in unusual circumstances. Patients often do develop symptoms of upper respiratory irritation during periods of severe pollution, and patients with cardiac or respiratory disease may suffer exacerbations. Prudent advice is in order in such situations. Advice to move to less polluted areas is rarely a good idea, and such advice should be given only after a great deal of thought about the impact of a move on the patient's entire life. The lack of convincing data linking air pollution with huge excesses in mortality is not a reason for physicians to be complacent about it in their own communities. Alleviating the immediate discomfort air pollution causes to nearly everyone and freeing patients with pulmonary disease from imprisonment in their homes during pollution alerts ought to be motivation enough for physicians to join in the battle for clean air. Pollution of indoor air in workplaces and in public facilities from cigarette smoking is an equally important challenge to the medical profession.

Hazardous Materials: Accidents and Disposal

Physicians with no special background in toxicology or public health may be pressed into service in cases of accidental emissions of toxic fumes or accidents involving transport of hazardous materials.

In responding to such emergencies, a practitioner should clarify immediately that the hazard is being contained to the extent possible, that individuals not

Table 7.8.
Checklist for Physicians Involved in Hazardous Substances Incidents

1. What toxic and hazardous substances have been identified?
   a. What are the concentrations in air, water, and soil?
   b. What are the known health hazards at these concentrations?
   c. What are the potential hazards of fire, explosion, or chemical interactions?
2. How many persons have been exposed and how many are likely to become exposed in the near future?
   a. What groups in the exposed population are likely to be most susceptible to health effects?
   b. How many exposures are resulting in hospital admissions?
   Outpatient visits?
   c. What clinical findings, if any, are being observed?
3. What technical resources are available on short notice to assist in evaluation and control?
4. Is the community adequately handling the casualties?
   a. What is the capacity of local hospitals, clinics, and physicians to absorb the additional caseload?
   b. Should hospital disaster plans be mobilized?
   c. Are intensive care or specialty services adequate or available to the degree needed?
   d. Are local physicians experienced and knowledgeable about this kind of problem? If not, what is the best way to obtain expert help quickly?
5. Is this community covered by a control data repository (such as a tumor registry or population-based research study) that could be used to follow the exposed population in the future?

needed at the scene are not being allowed to become exposed, and that orderly procedures for the care of casualties are being set up. A checklist is provided in Table 7.8.

General References

Himmelstein JS, Frumkin H: The right to know about toxic exposures. New Engl J Med 312:687, 1985.
   Critical review of facts clinicians should know about the subject.
Key MM, Henschet AF, Butlee J, et al: Occupational Diseases: A Guide to Their Recognition, rev ed. Washington, DC, National Institute for Occupational Safety and Health, 1977.
   An excellent guide to the hazards of a large number of chemicals.
Levy BS, Wegman DH (eds): Occupational Health: Recognizing and Preventing Work-Related Disease. Boston, Little, Brown, and Co, 1982.
   Excellent introductory text for the practitioner.
Morgan WK, Seaton A: Occupational Lung Disease. Philadelphia, WB Saunders, 1975.
   This text covers all the pneumoconioses.
Proctor NH, Hughes JP: Chemical Hazards of the Workplace. Philadelphia, JB Lippincott, 1978.
   A thorough text on chemical hazards. It includes a section on diagnostic principles.
Rom WN (ed): Environmental and Occupational Medicine. Boston, Little, Brown, and Co, 1983.
   An up-to-date text.

CHAPTER EIGHT

Primary Care of the Patient with Cancer

LARRY WATERBURY, M.D.

In recent years there have been significant advances in the treatment of many different cancers. A massive body of medical literature continues to grow; multidisciplinary cancer treatment centers have arisen around the country; and there has been a marked increase in the amount of basic knowledge pertinent to the diagnosis and treatment of cancer. The general physician may feel overwhelmed by the growing body of specialized knowledge in oncology and inadequate to handle the problems of cancer patients. There is a tendency to relegate the care of all cancer patients to specialists. Although appropriate in certain patients and clinical situations, there are other settings where general physicians should remain active in the cancer patient's care. To the patient with a progressive metastatic tumor, unresponsive or poorly responsive to therapy, the continuing involvement of his personal physician is increasingly important, especially if that doctor-patient relationship has been a long-standing one.

The purpose of this chapter is not to discuss specific cancers, but to examine in a more general way the role of the general physician in the care of patients who have cancer. Common cancers are discussed in other chapters (breast, Chapter 89; lung, Chapter 56; gastrointestinal, Chapter 37; prostate, Chapter 48; gynecologic, Chapter 95).

Table 8.1 lists a number of nonoperable cancers in which survival may be prolonged by modern treatment regimens; patients with such cancers should be referred to cancer specialists. These patients frequently benefit from multimodality treatment. Even within this group of cancers, when specialty help is needed, the general physician will continue to play an important role, especially if the

relationship with the patient or the family has been a lengthy one.

INITIAL REFERRAL AND TREATMENT

When possible the general physician should refer patients to specific oncologists whom he trusts and whom he knows to be helpful, considerate clinicians. Multimodality treatment regimens involving the combined efforts of surgical, medical, and radiation oncologists frequently result in a bewildered patient who does not know who the primary responsible physician is. Thus the general physician may need to play a coordinating role or to intercede in order to identify that physician who will be the coordinator for the patient's care and who will be accessible to the patient to answer questions, provide support, improve communications, *etc.* The general physician should expect to receive up-to-date and complete information about the diagnostic and therapeutic plans and about the patient's current status. His continuing interest in the case is especially helpful if he will be involved in follow-up care after the initial treatment. The general physician may be able to assess the overall picture and, as time goes on, to identify when problems resulting from treatment (side effects, expense, family disruption, deteriorating psychological status of patient, *etc*) outweigh the likely benefits of continued therapy.

FOLLOW-UP CARE

Many oncologists welcome participation of the primary physician in the patient's follow-up and continuing care. This is particularly important when treatment has been given in an oncology center in a distant city. Some less toxic ambulatory treatment regimens may even be given by the primary physician under the direction of the specialist.

CARE OF PATIENTS UNRESPONSIVE OR POORLY RESPONSIVE TO TREATMENT

Table 8.2 lists a number of cancers less responsive to therapy, where the impact of therapy on survival is unproven or controversial. Diagnosis and initial therapy usually require surgery, but when metastasis is proven, the effect of chemotherapy or radio-

Table 8.1.
Some Nonoperable Cancers in Which Treatment Prolongs Survival[a]

Acute leukemia
Hodgkin's disease
Lymphoma
Metastatic testicular cancer
Metastatic ovarian cancer
Small cell carcinoma of the lung
Metastatic breast cancer

[a] Patients with these cancers require specialized treatment, frequently in centers where multimodality therapy is available.

Table 8.2.
Some Cancers in Which Treatment Provides Palliation in Some Patients: Effects on Survival Unproven or Controversial

Non-small cell lung cancer (unresectable)
Metastatic large bowel cancer
Metastatic stomach cancer
Metastatic pancreatic cancer
Metastatic malignant melanoma
Hepatoma
Metastatic soft tissue sarcomas
Metastatic cervical cancer
Metastatic endometrial cancer
Metastatic hypernephroma
Metastatic prostate cancer (posthormonal therapy with relapse)

therapy is at most palliative. In such situations, knowledgeable general physicians may be in the best position to evaluate the total picture and to make recommendations.

1. *Should palliative therapy be recommended?* Although difficult to generalize, a number of factors must be considered in attempting to help patients and their families decide whether the patient is likely to benefit from palliative therapy. More than age, the functional status of the patient must be considered in such therapeutic decisions. The infirm, ill, poorly functional patient with widely disseminated and rapidly progressive disease may be more harmed by the side effects and discomforts of palliative treatment than benefited, especially if response rates are small and toxicity of treatment is high. Weight loss prior to therapy correlates remarkably with poor response rates in clinical chemotherapy trials in these less responsive cancers (6). Other patients, even if elderly, in good functional status are much more suitable candidates for attempts at palliation. The patient who feels that any chance of response is worth the price of toxicity, and who cannot feel comfortable unless attempting some therapy, should generally be offered treatment.

2. If some attempt at palliative treatment seems worthwhile, *should it be conventional therapy or experimental protocol therapy?* Every oncology cen-

ter and large cooperative group has a current protocol for the metastatic cancers that are listed in Table 8.2. Clinical protocols designed to attempt to find improved methods of treatment are important for advances in oncology and to improve the outlook and the comfort of future patients. However, experimental therapy may have less than desirable consequences for the individual patient. Frequently, such protocols involve the investigation of treatments with more toxicity than current conventional therapies. They usually require more frequent visits to the physician as well as more frequent diagnostic tests, because of the necessity to document precisely the objective response. They may therefore also involve increased expense to the patient. Obviously patients agreeing to experimental protocol therapy must be well informed about the implications of the therapy, and that requires that they understand what is to be done. Patients need to realize the differences between experimental treatment and conventional treatment in terms of expense, time, and discomfort. In those diseases where the beneficial effects of therapy remain questionable, the responsible general physician must make sure that both he and the patient are informed about the side effects and likely benefits of therapy (19). The physician very much needs an experienced and sensitive practical clinical oncologist to give him counsel, including an honest appraisal of effects of treatment in terms of its benefit and toxicity. The helpful consultant must be able to do more than describe the currently popular treatment for the patient's disease; he should be able to tailor the recommendation to the specific patient. No treatment, conventional low dose palliative chemotherapy or radiotherapy, and experimental therapy are all appropriate choices for individual patients in various different clinical situations. In order to make sensitive and responsible recommendations with regard to treatment of patients with metastatic cancer the physician needs to be able to process and integrate a large amount of data of various kinds (Table 8.3).

Table 8.3.
Factors Affecting Treatment Recommendations in Patients with Cancer

The natural history of the untreated cancer
The proven effect of treatment on the natural history
    Likely effects on survival
    Likelihood of lessening morbidity
Toxicity of treatment
Functional status of the patient
Ability of the patient to comprehend the implications of treatment
Psychological state and philosophical position of the patient
Emotional strength, and attitudes of immediate family
Financial situation, health coverage status

The general physician because of his involvement with the patient and family over a long time may be in the best position to do this.

If he feels therapy is likely to be helpful for the patient, the primary physician must know something about what the patient will experience when he receives radiotherapy or chemotherapy.

RADIOTHERAPY

The patient with cancer frequently has misconceptions about and limited knowledge of radiotherapy. The primary physician, at the time that he discusses with the patient possible referral for radiotherapy, must spend time in explaining the rationale and the hoped for response from the treatment, and he should outline what the patient will experience during treatment. The initial visit usually includes a relevant history and physical examination by the radiotherapist. Further diagnostic tests (X-rays, computerized tomography (CT) scan, *etc*) may be obtained. If the therapist agrees that treatment is appropriate, the radiotherapy ports may actually be determined at the first visit; and the patient may receive his first treatment at that time. The patient should be told that skin markings may be placed in order to facilitate the uniformity of subsequent treatments, and that these markings must not be removed. It is important to explain that the therapy machines are bulky and somewhat overwhelming in appearance. Many patients are likely to be frightened by the experience; and if the referring physician appreciates this, it is useful to contact the radiotherapist and to explain the particular fears of the patient ahead of time. Therapists will often give patients and their families a tour of the radiotherapy treatment rooms before starting therapy and will spend extra time answering questions about the treatment and its benefits and complications. The patient should be aware that the treatment itself is *not* painful. The initial consultation is usually time consuming (several hours), but subsequent treatments are usually scheduled precisely and require only a small amount of time (30 minutes). Treatments are usually given several days a week, and the entire course may take several weeks to complete. The patient usually will not see the radiotherapist at the time of each treatment, but will be seen by a radiotherapy nurse or technician. He therefore needs to know precisely with whom to communicate if he has side effects or questions during radiotherapy. The primary physician should be available for phone consultation in order to intercede for the patient should communication problems arise. Also, the follow-up plans after treatment should be outlined.

In addition to the timing and types of side effects which the patient may experience, it is important for him to know that the response to treatment is frequently delayed and that sometimes the maximal effect is seen a few weeks after the course of radiotherapy is completed. For example, radiotherapy is useful in the palliation of pain secondary to local bony metastases but may require 2 to 3 weeks of treatment before improvement, which may continue after treatment has been discontinued. Some responses are more rapid, occurring after only a few days of therapy (e.g., relief of superior vena caval obstruction and neurological deficits from spinal cord obstruction or CNS metastasis).

Side Effects

Table 8.4 describes important side effects of radiotherapy. The patient will be most concerned by those common side effects which occur during treatment and by those which may remain for a few weeks after treatment is discontinued.

Dermatitis secondary to radiotherapy is less common than it used to be, owing to the use of the modern high energy machines. Severe burning requiring specialized treatment is quite uncommon; however, skin discoloration may occur. The patient should be told that the radiation field should not be exposed to sunlight or extreme cold, and that total, but temporary, hair loss will usually occur in the areas being radiated and that complete return of hair, after high dose radiation, may take many months.

The most troublesome side effects that occur during radiotherapy are *gastrointestinal*. Patients receiving radiation to the chest or upper back frequently experience symptoms of radiation esophagitis (odynophagia and sometimes reflux symptoms which may respond to elevation of the head of the bed and to antacids). Severe esophagitis is more likely to occur when radiotherapy has been used in patients who have had prior chemotherapy with adriamycin. Superinfection of the irritated esophagus with *Candida* is not unusual, especially in patients who are receiving steroids. This usually responds to treatment with oral nystatin (Mycostatin, suspension 100,000 U/ml, 5 ml every 4 hours). Clotrimazole troches (Mycelex troches, one troche dissolved in the mouth five times daily) are also effective and more palatable. Oral ketoconazole (Nizoral) is frequently effective in nystatin failures (200-mg tablets, one daily by mouth). Patients should improve within 1 week of therapy. Occasionally short courses of amphotericin (5 to 12 mg/day for 14 days) are necessary to cure *Candida* esophagitis, but that treatment is best given in the hospital. Abdominal irradiation may cause some troublesome *diarrhea* that may persist to some degree during the entire course of treatment. Other than the importance of replacing fluids and electrolytes, there are some dietary maneuvers which may minimize diarrhea; these are listed in Table 8.5. *Nausea* and *anorexia*

Table 8.4.
Important Side Effects of Radiotherapy (5, 7, 11, 12, 17, 18, 22, 23)

Dermatitis (less common with newer high energy machines; avoid sunlight and extreme cold).

Acute radiation pneumonitis (transient, usually occurring 6–12 weeks after treatment; precipitated by corticosteroid withdrawal, concomitant chemotherapy; clinical manifestations include nonproductive cough, dyspnea, fever, leukocytosis with parenchymal infiltrates on X-ray in the area of the radiation ports; usually responds to steroid treatment) (12).

Pulmonary fibrosis (occurs 6–12 months after treatment, not responsive to steroids) (12).

Esophagitis (usually occurs during treatment; particularly severe when radiotherapy and adriamycin are administered together).

Nausea, vomiting, and diarrhea (occur during treatment with most abdominal radiotherapy, usually self-limited).

Enteritis (rare, more likely with very high dose treatment; small bowel more sensitive than large bowel and stomach; occurs weeks to years after radiotherapy; manifestations include obstruction, bleeding, perforation; pelvic irradiation, *e.g.*, in the treatment of bladder or prostate cancer, may cause acute *proctitis* which occasionally becomes chronic sometimes leading to bleeding or stricture formation) (11, 17).

Pericarditis (occurs months to years after radiation, usually resolves, occasionally progresses to constrictive pericarditis or to tamponade requiring pericardiectomy) (18).

Neurological side effects (transverse myelitis, very rare; side effects from CNS irradiation in adults are infrequent (5); Lhermitte's sign (the sensation of electric shocks passing down the body when the head is flexed) seen in 10% of patients undergoing mantle irradiation for Hodgkin's disease; after radiotherapy herpes zoster is common).

Hypothyroidism (common in patients treated for Hodgkin's disease with mantle field; may develop years after treatment).

Sterility (usually temporary).

Growth retardation in children (occurs both from direct skeletal effects and from hypopituitarism from CNS irradiation).

Dental side effects (severe dental problems are common after head and neck irradiation because of decrease in saliva formation, increased sensitivity to caries, osteonecrosis) (23).

Cystitis (occurs during treatment with pelvic irradiation; clinical manifestations include urgency dysuria and hematuria occurring usually during the third and fourth weeks of treatment; usually self-limited and treated symptomatically with fluids and phenozopyridine (Pyridium), 200 mg four times a day; chronic bladder fibrosis is a rare late complication manifested usually by painless hematuria).

Table 8.5.
Dietary Maneuvers for Therapy-Induced Diarrhea (22)

Clear liquids (warm or at room temperature)
Avoid fiber (roughage) in the diet
Take smaller amounts of food more often
Avoid fatty foods
Avoid highly spiced foods
Avoid carbonated drinks, beans, cabbage, broccoli, cauliflower, and corn

---

are the most troublesome side effects of abdominal irradiation and are discussed separately below.

Patients who receive radiotherapy to the head or neck are subject to special *dental complications.* Before treatment all patients should have a complete dental examination by a dentist experienced in the treatment of patients who have undergone radiotherapy. Damage to the teeth, gums, and bone, plus the xerostomia that results from high dose radiotherapy to the oral mucous membranes and salivary glands may result in severe problems. Many of these can be prevented by appropriate prophylaxis (aggressive treatment of periodontal disease and of infected teeth before radiation) and an ongoing program during and after radiotherapy, which should be strictly followed. The use of artificial saliva (Saliva Substitute, Roxane Laboratories) may be helpful for patients with xerostomia.

The patient's personal physician may sometimes be involved with the *early treatment of CNS metastases* or spinal cord compression, using corticosteroids. Multiple regimens are used. A common regimen consists of dexamethasone (Decadron), 4 to 25 mg four times a day, continued until the patient has received several courses of radiotherapy and then rapidly tapered off over several days. Steroids decrease the local edema which occurs in these situations and help to protect against radiation-induced edema during the first few days of therapy.

An excellent monograph is available free from the National Institutes of Health, to patients undergoing radiotherapy (22). Unfortunately not all radiotherapists make this monograph available to their patients. Primary physicians who refer patients for radiotherapy should have this monograph available in their offices and should make sure all patients have access to it before their radiotherapy consultation.

CHEMOTHERAPY

The chemotherapy experience for the patient is so varied (depending on the disease being treated) that it is hard to give a general description. The medical oncologist giving therapy can best explain to the patient the specifics of treatment, including how it is administered, the frequency of treatment, the hoped for response, and the side effects. The most frequent troublesome side effects for the patient are hair loss and nausea and vomiting. The frequency and degree of hair loss vary with the treatment regimen, but it is helpful for the patient to know that hair will regrow once the treatment is discontinued. The treatment of nausea and vomiting is discussed below.

There is an excellent free monograph on chemotherapy written for patients which is available through the National Institutes of Health (4). Primary physicians who refer patients for chemotherapy should have this monograph available for patients, preferably before their first visit with the medical oncologist.

Table 8.6 lists other acute and chronic side effects of various chemotherapeutic agents. Knowledge of the long term side effects of various agents is particularly important for the primary physician who may be responsible for follow-up care of patients with good prognoses following chemotherapy.

NAUSEA, VOMITING, AND ANOREXIA

Nausea and vomiting are by far the most troublesome and common side effects of both radiotherapy and chemotherapy. Unfortunately the symptomatic treatment of nausea is only moderately effective. However, there are a number of maneuvers which may help to limit the degree of nausea following chemotherapy or radiotherapy. For example, it is frequently helpful for the nauseated patient to be extremely still, lying down in a quiet room without external stimuli. Antiemetics may help, but unfortunately may not eliminate the nausea completely, especially that associated with intense chemotherapy regimens. However, for more mild regimens the use of conventional antiemetics by tablet or by rectal

suppository (e.g., prochloperazine, 10 mg orally every 6 hours) may be helpful. Patients receiving intensive chemotherapy programs, especially with regimens including cis-platinum, are benefited by treatment with high doses of metoclopramide (60 mg/m^2 intravenously every 2 hours during cis-platinum infusion) and corticosteroids (1, 2, 16).

There are a number of dietary maneuvers which may be helpful to the patient experiencing nausea and vomiting after therapy (Table 8.7). The patient who experiences severe nausea and vomiting after therapy should probably only drink clear liquids until the symptoms are decreased. In general it is more helpful to take smaller portions of food frequently than to take larger meals less often, to take foods that are low in fat, and to avoid overly sweet foods. Mild nausea, especially that experienced before therapy or in anticipation of therapy, may be helped by taking dry toast or crackers in small quantities. It is recommended that patients do not lie down just after eating. Some patients find also that it is helpful not to drink liquids with their food which may increase their feeling of bloating and subsequent nausea. Many patients become nauseated at the smell of food cooking, and it may be helpful for them to go to another part of the house or to stay out of the house when food is being prepared. Greasy and fried foods seem to be the worst offenders in this regard and are best avoided.

One of the major problems with intensive cancer therapy is the general *anorexia* which may result in considerable nutritional problems and weight loss. Consultation with a dietitian may be extremely helpful in such a situation. There is an excellent monograph available through the National Institutes of Health which contains all sorts of dietary advice for cancer patients including many recipes (9). It is available free of charge to physicians for their patients and is strongly recommended.

TERMINAL CARE

The primary physician who has participated in various phases of the cancer patient's care and who has an ongoing relationship with him and his family is frequently in the best position to help during a patient's terminal illness. The physician who develops some expertise in this regard can find enormous

Table 8.6.
Common Side Effects of Chemotherapy (4, 20)[a]

Hair loss—alkylating agents, vincristine, vinblastine, adriamycin, mithramycin, daunomycin (8).
Hypercalcemia—estrogens, antiestrogens (tamoxifen).
Fluid retention—estrogens, androgens, steroids.
Skin darkening—adriamycin (nails), 5-FU, bleomycin, busulfan (8).
Dermatitis—methotrexate, 6-MP, 6-thioguanine (8).
Marrow depression—alkylating agents, vinblastine, nitrosoureas, methotrexate, adriamycin, cytosine arabinoside, daunomycin, 5-FU, mithramycin, mitomycin C, cis-platinum, procarbazine, hydroxyurea, 6-MP (13).
Neurological—cis-platinum (deafness), vincristine, vinblastine, methotrexate, hexamethylmelamine, 5-FU, procarbazine (14).
Gastrointestinal ulcerations—methotrexate, 5-FU, bleomycin (mucocutaneous), adriamycin.
Cardiomyopathy—adriamycin, daunorubicin (25).
Pulmonary fibrosis—bleomycin, alkylating agents, mitomycin-C (10).
Renal damage—cis-platinum, methotrexate, streptozotocin, nitrosoureas (24).
Red urine—adriamycin, daunomycin.
Hepatic toxicity—mithramycin, methotrexate, nitrosoureas, cytosine arabinoside, 6-MP (21).
Sexual and gonadal dysfunction—(3).
Secondary neoplasm—alkylating agents, combination chemotherapy (15).

[a] 5-FU, 5-fluorouracil; 6-MP, 6-mercaptopurine.

Table 8.7.
Dietary Maneuvers for Therapy-Induced Nausea (4, 9, 22)

Smaller portions eaten more slowly
Avoid foods high in fat, and greasy and fried foods
Clear, cool liquids between meals
Crackers or toast
Rest (sitting, not lying) after eating
Avoid food odors (during preparation)

gratification from this role. Chapter 19 deals with many of the issues important to consider in caring for terminal patients including the very important issue of pain control.

In the last several years the *hospice concept* has received much support in this country. Central to the concept is the premise that dying patients have specific unique needs which are different from other patients. Although initially hospices were conceived as free standing units separate from acute hospitals, the concept has grown considerably as a general way of caring for terminal patients, rather than as a specific place for their care. One of the primary goals is to provide support for the family so that the patient may be able to spend a large amount of time at home. Many community hospitals are developing hospice programs with coordinated home support services utilizing visiting nurses, volunteers, physical and occupational therapists, home health aids, *etc.* Such programs can help the primary physician provide physical and emotional support for the patient and his family. An excellent publication entitled *Coping with Cancer: A Resource for the Health Professional* is available free of charge from the National Institutes of Health (see "General References"). In addition to other useful information, it lists organizations and agencies that provide useful services which may aid the physician in his attempt to provide home support for the dying cancer patient.

General References

Cancer chemotherapy. *The Medical Letter* 27:13, 1985.
> Useful review of drugs, toxicities, and indications.

Coping with Cancer: A Resource for the Health Professional. National Institutes of Health publ no. 80-2080. Bethesda, MD, National Cancer Institute, Office of Cancer Communications, Sept, 1980.
> An excellent general review of many aspects of the care of the patient with cancer. Free copies are available by writing to the Office of Cancer Communications, Department of Health and Human Services, NIH, Bethesda, MD 20205. Telephone (301) 496-4070.

Portlock CS, Goffinet DR (eds): *Manual of Clinical Problems in Oncology.* Boston, Little, Brown, and Co, 1980.
> Excellent, brief, clinically oriented oncology manual.

Rubin P (ed): *Clinical Oncology: A Multidisciplinary Approach,* ed 6. New York, American Cancer Society, 1983.
> Provided free of charge by the American Cancer Society. Excellent condensed data about all cancers and their treatment.

Specific References

1. Aapro MS, *et al*: Double-blind crossover study of the antiemetic efficacy of high-dose dexamethasone *versus* high-dose metoclopramide. *J Clin Oncol* 2:466, 1984.
2. Cassileth PA, *et al*: Antiemetic efficacy of dexamethasone therapy in patients receiving cancer chemotherapy. *Arch Intern Med* 143:1347, 1983.
3. Chapman RM: Effect of cytotoxic therapy on sexuality and gonadal function. *Semin Oncol* 9:84, 1982.
4. *Chemotherapy and You: A Guide to Self-help during Treatment.* National Institutes of Health no. 80-1136. Bethesda, MD, Office of Cancer Communications, Aug 1980.
5. Deutsch M, Parsons JA, Mercado R: Radiotherapy for intracranial metastases. *Cancer* 34:1607, 1974.
6. Dewys WD: Prognostic effect of weight loss prior to chemotherapy in cancer patients. *Am J Med* 69:491, 1980.
7. Donaldson SS, Lenon RA: Alterations of nutritional status: impact of chemotherapy and radiation therapy. *Cancer* 43:2036, 1979.
8. Dunagin WG: Clinical toxicity of chemotherapeutic agents: dermatologic toxicity. *Semin Oncol* 9:14, 1982.
9. *Eating Hints: Recipes and Tips for Better Nutrition during Cancer Treatment.* National Institutes of Health publ no. 80-2079. Bethesda, MD, Office of Cancer Communications, 1980.
10. Ginsberg SJ, Comis RL: The pulmonary toxicity of antineoplastic agents. *Semin Oncol* 9:34, 1982.
11. Goffinet D, *et al*: Bladder cancer—results of radiation therapy in 384 patients. *Radiology* 117:149, 1975.
12. Gross NJ: Pulmonary effects of radiation therapy. *Ann Intern Med* 86:81, 1977.
13. Hoagland HC: Hematologic complications of cancer chemotherapy. *Semin Oncol* 9:95, 1982.
14. Kaplan RS, Wiernik PH: Neurotoxicity of antineoplastic drugs. *Semin Oncol* 9:103, 1982.
15. Kyle RA: Second malignancies associated with chemotherapeutic agents. *Semin Oncol* 9:131, 1982.
16. Meyer BR, *et al*: Optimizing metoclopramide control of cisplatin-induced emesis. *Ann Intern Med* 100:393, 1984.
17. Morgenstern L, Thompson R, Friedman NB: Radiation enteritis. *Am J Surg* 134:166, 1971.
18. Muggia EA, Cassileth PA: Constrictive pericarditis following radiation therapy. *Am J Med* 44:116, 1968.
19. Penman DT: Informed consent for investigational chemotherapy: patients' and physicians' perceptions. *J Clin Oncol* 2:849, 1984.
20. Perry MC: Chemotherapy, toxicity and the clinician. *Semin Oncol* 9:1, 1982.
21. Perry MC: Hepatotoxicity of chemotherapeutic agents. *Semin Oncol* 9:65, 1982.
22. *Radiation Therapy and You: A Guide to Self-Help during Treatment.* National Institutes of Health publ no. 80-2227. Bethesda, MD, Office of Cancer Communications, 1980.
23. Regeyi JA, Courtney RM, Kerr DA: Dental management of patients irradiated for oral cancer. *Cancer* 38:994, 1976.
24. Schilsky RL: Renal and metabolic toxicities of cancer chemotherapy. *Semin Oncol* 9:75, 1982.
25. Van Hoff DD, Rozencwieg M, Piccart M: The cardiotoxicity of anticancer agents. *Semin Oncol* 9:23, 1982.

CHAPTER NINE

Selected Special Services: Disability Insurance, Vocational Rehabilitation, and Home Health Services

L. RANDOL BARKER, M.D.

INTRODUCTION

Maintenance of a patient's overall health often requires efforts beyond those of the physician and the patient. Frequently assistance comes from community-based agencies to which physicians may refer their patients. Many of these agencies provide services for patients with specific types of illness; the roles of such "categorical" community services are described in the appropriate chapters in this book. Other services are designed to assist sick persons regardless of their type of illness. This chapter describes two fundamental services of this kind: (a) Social Security income support programs for disabled persons and (b) home health services. The purposes of the chapter are to explain eligibility for these services, the nature of the benefits, and the role of the physician in enabling his patients to receive these services. Chapter 7 provides similar information about another "noncategorical" program, workmen's compensation, which is designed to provide income support to persons with work-related diseases.

SOCIAL SECURITY PROGRAMS FOR DISABLED PERSONS

Loss or decrease of a person's ability to earn his living accompanies many illnesses. Beginning with 1954 amendments to the Social Security Act, income support for medically disabled persons has been available in the United States. Further modifications since 1954 have led to the program that exists today.

Five fundamental benefits are present available: Disability Insurance (DI), Supplemental Security Income (SSI), Vocational Rehabilitation (VR), Medicare (for DI recipients), and Medicaid (for SSI recipients). Detailed information about each of these services is available from any local Social Security Office.

Definition of Medical Disability

Under Social Security, disability is defined as "inability to engage in any substantial gainful activity by reason of a medically determinable physical or mental impairment which can be expected to result in death or has lasted or can be expected to last for a continuous period of not less than 12 months...."

Disability Insurance (DI—Title II)

Eligibility

To be eligible for disability insurance payments, a *disabled worker* must have paid into the Social Security program for a minimum period of time before becoming disabled; in addition there is a requirement for coverage during 5 of the 10 years before the onset of disability. Today, 9 of 10 workers pay Social Security. For younger workers (up to age 31) there are modified requirements to meet insured status.

The *dependents* of a fully insured worker who is retired, disabled, or deceased may be eligible for disability insurance payments in two situations: (a) a child who became disabled before age 22 (eligible for disability insurance payments at the time that his parent retires, becomes disabled, or dies; payments continue as long as the child's disability lasts); and (b) a widow or widower who is between 50 and 59 years of age and who did not work under Social Security but who become medically disabled before or within 7 years of the death of a fully insured spouse.

Benefits

Disability insurance payments go to disabled workers before the age of 65 (after 65, Social Security Retirement Income replaces disability payments) and to eligible children, widows, or widowers as long as they remain disabled. The first monthly disability insurance check is not paid for the first 5 months after the onset of the worker's disability (for example, if a patient is certified as disabled 6 calendar months after he actually became disabled, he immediately becomes eligible for a check covering the 1 month in excess of the required 5-month wait). Supplemental Security Income (see below) is often awarded to persons who qualify for disability benefits, effective the date they apply for benefits. There is no waiting period. Income from DI for a disabled worker is the same amount as the retirement income the worker would receive if he were 65. The average monthly payment to a disabled worker in 1983 was $441, and to a worker with a wife and dependent children, $841. In that year, 2,591,000 workers were receiving DI benefits; 3,893,000 workers and dependents were receiving DI benefits; and 944,000 children were receiving DI benefits.

In addition to income support, disabled persons under 65 receive Medicare (Social Security Health Insurance) after they have been eligible for disability benefits for 24 months.

The Process of Disability Determination

There are three basic steps in the process of determining medical disability.

First step. The patient completes a detailed application at a local Social Security Office. The patient must not be gainfully employed at the time of application. Most patients will initiate disability claims by themselves, but at times the physician may be helpful in suggesting early application to a patient who may not be aware that his medical condition qualifies him for medical disability.

Second step. The patient's physician receives a request for medical information and returns his report to the state Disability Determination Office. The report sent by the patient's physician should be succinct and precise; and it should provide objective data regarding the condition for which disability is being claimed. It should be divided into the following subheadings: history, physical, laboratory reports, diagnosis, treatment, and response. The information provided should permit the claims reviewers to determine both the severity and the duration of the patient's condition. If malingering is suspected, the report should describe the circumstances that raise doubts rather than recording this assessment without supporting information. In this report the physician is not expected to rate the work disability of the patient. The most helpful guide for completing these medical reports is the booklet entitled *Disability Evaluation under Social Security: A Handbook for Physicians* (available free from any Social Security Office or the State Disability Determination Office). This manual, which was most recently published in 1979, contains the criteria for medical disability for most common conditions. These criteria are the basis for most allowances made by disability claims reviewers. Tables 9.1 through 9.6 contain excerpts

from this manual (and from modifications to be published in 1985) illustrating the criteria for several common conditions that may cause medical disability: symptomatic ischemic heart disease, chronic obstructive airways disease, cerebrovascular accident, epilepsy due to major motor seizures, arthritis of a major weight-bearing joint, and rheumatoid arthritis. Since 1980, the Social Security Administration has paid a small fee to physicians for medical reports for the DI program; a small reporting fee has also been paid for SSI reports of evidence of record since the inception of that program in 1974. Previously patients were expected to pay for these reports. In some states, doctors also have access to a free teledictation service for dictating their reports.

Third step. The information provided by the patient and the physician (the disability claim) is reviewed at the State Disability Determination Office by a team consisting of a disability claims examiner and a physician. If deemed necessary, an independent medical examination is purchased by the Disability Determination Office. In keeping with the 1974 Freedom of Information Act, patients may have access to their disability claims files. If an insured worker has an impairment that does not meet the standard criteria for disability but that nevertheless prevents the individual from doing his usual job, other factors (limitations of age, education, training, work experience) may also be considered by the Disability Determination team. Most findings of disability are, however, based on the standard Social Security criteria.

Appeal Process

If the initial claim of disability has been denied, the claimant may file for reconsideration within 60 days of receiving a denial notice. The case will then be re-evaluated by a different claims examining team. If the claim is denied at this reconsideration, the claimant then has 60 days to file a request for a hearing. Hearings are conducted by administrative law judges. If the claim is again denied, the claimant may make an additional appeal for review by the Appeals Council. After that the case may be taken to the United States District Court.

The patient's personal physician can be instrumental in assuring that his patient gets the fullest consideration throughout the Disability Determination process. If the physician feels that there are aspects of the patient's illness that make it more severe than the criteria indicate, he should communicate this information in writing, together with support for his opinon, to the Disability Determination Office.

Return to Work

All claims are reviewed for referral to Vocational Rehabilitation (see below) at the time the disability decision is made. In addition, every person with a

Table 9.1.
Impairments Qualifying a Person with *Ischemic Heart Disease* for Medical Disability under Social Security[a]

Ischemic heart disease with chest pain of cardiac origin as described in 4.00E. With:

A. Treadmill exercise test (see 4.00F and G) demonstrating one of the following at an exercise level of 5 METs[b] or less:
  1. Horizontal or downsloping ischemic depression (from the standing control) of the ST segment to 1.0 mm or greater, lasting for at least 0.08 second after the J junction, and clearly discernible in at least two consecutive complexes which are on a level baseline in any lead; *or*
  2. Junctional depression occurring during exercise, remaining depressed (from the standing control) to 2.0 mm or greater for at least 0.08 second after the junction (the so-called slow upsloping ST segment), and clearly discernible in at least two consecutive complexes which are on a level baseline in any lead; *or*
  3. Premature ventricular systoles which are multiform or bidirectional or are sequentially inscribed (3 or more); *or*
  4. ST segment elevation (from the standing control) to 1 mm or greater; *or*
  5. Development of second or third degree heart block; *or*
B. In the absence of a report of an acceptable treadmill exercise test (see 4.00G), one of the following:
  1. Transmural myocardial infarction exhibiting a QS pattern or a Q wave with amplitude at least one-third of R wave and with a duration of 0.04 second or more. (If these are present in leads III and aVF only, the requisite Q wave findings must be shown, by labeled tracing, to persist on deep inspiration); *or*
  2. Resting ECG findings showing ischemic type (see 4.00F1) depression of ST segment to more than 0.5 mm in either (a) leads I and aVL and V$_6$ or (b) leads II and III and aVF or (c) leads V$_3$ through V$_6$; *or*
  3. Resting ECG findings showing an ischemic configuration or current of injury (see 4.00F1) with ST segment elevation to 2 mm or more in either (a) leads I and aVL

and V$_6$ or (b) leads II and III and aVF or (c) leads V$_3$ through V$_6$; *or*
  4. Resting ECG findings showing symmetrical inversion of T waves to 5.0 mm or more in any two leads except leads III or aVR or V$_1$ or V$_2$; *or*
  5. Inversion of T wave to 1.0 mm or more in any of leads I, II, aVL, V$_2$ to V$_6$ and R wave of 5.0 mm or more in lead aVL and R wave greater than S wave in lead aVF; *or*
  6. "Double" Master Two-Step test demonstrating one of the following:
    a. Ischemic depression of ST segment to more than 0.5 mm lasting for at least 0.08 second beyond the J junction and clearly discernible in at least two consecutive complexes which are on a level baseline in any lead; *or*
    b. Development of a second or third degree heart block; *or*
  7. Angiographic evidence (see 4.00H) (obtained independent of Social Security disability evaluation) showing one of the following:
    a. 50% or more narrowing of the left main coronary artery; *or*
    b. 70% or more narrowing of a proximal coronary artery (see 4.00H3) (excluding the left main coronary artery); *or*
    c. 50% or more narrowing involving a long (greater than 1 cm) segment of a proximal coronary artery or multiple proximal coronary arteries; *or*
  8. Akinetic or hypokinetic myocardial wall or septal motion with left ventricular ejection fraction of 30% or less measured by contrast or radioisotopic ventriculographic methods; *or*
C. Resting ECG findings showing left bundle branch block as evidence by QRS duration of 0.12 second or more in leads I, II, or II and R peak duration of 0.06 second or more in leads I, aVL, V$_5$, or V$_6$, unless there is a coronary angiogram of record which is negative (see criteria in 4.04B7).

---

[a] From *Disability Evaluation under Social Security: A Handbook for Physicians, 1979.* (Revised criteria due to be implemented in 1985).
[b] MET, metabolic equivalent.

permanent impairment is re-evaluated every 7 years; and all other persons (*i.e.,* those with impairments that may not be permanent) are re-evaluated at least every 3 years to determine whether they are still disabled. Even if the original impairment, on review, is judged not to be severe, payments are continued if there has been no improvement. These two processes and the following conditions are designed to encourage disabled persons to return to work: (a) Disabled beneficiaries may test their ability to work for 9 months while continuing to receive benefits. After this trial work period, a determination is made as to whether the work constitutes substantial gainful activity (defined as an activity which yields a monthly income of $300 or greater); if it does, benefits are suspended after an additional

3-month adjustment period. (b) If a person who still has a disabling impairment stops work again within 15 months after Social Security payments have been suspended because of substantial gainful activity, the monthly DI benefits can be resumed, usually without a new application. (c) Medicare coverage generally can continue for 3 years after a person's DI benefits stop because of return to substantial gainful activity. If a worker starts receiving DI benefits again within 5 years after the DI was stopped, and if the patient was previously entitled to Medicare, that protection will resume immediately. (d) Work expenses related to the impairment that are paid for by a disabled person may be deducted from the patient's earnings in determining whether these constitute substantial gainful activity. This is true

Table 9.2.

Impairments Qualifying a Person with *Chronic Obstructive Pulmonary Disease* for Medical Disability under Social Security[a]

Chronic obstructive pulmonary disease (due to any cause). With: Both FEV_1[b] and MVV equal to or less than the values specified in table (below) corresponding to the person's height without shoes.

Height without Shoes (Inches)	FEV_1 Equal to or Less Than (liters, BTPS)	and	MVV (MBC) Equal to or Less Than (liters/min, BTPS)
60 or less	1.0		40
61–63	1.1		44
64–65	1.2		48
66–67	1.3		52
68–69	1.4		56
70–71	1.5		60
72 or more	1.6		64

[a] From *Disability Evaluation under Social Security: A Handbook for Physicians*, 1979. (Revised criteria due to be implemented in 1985).
[b] FEV_1, forced expiratory volume in 1 second; MVV, maximum voluntary ventilation; MBC, maximum breathing capacity.

Table 9.3.

Impairments Qualifying a Person with *Cerebrovascular Accident* for Medical Disability under Social Security[a]

Central nervous system vascular accident. With one of the following more than 3 months postvascular accident:
A. Sensory or motor aphasia resulting in defective speech or communication; *or*
B. Significant and persistent disorganization of motor function in two extremities, resulting in sustained disturbance of gross and dexterous movements, or gait and station.[b]

[a] From *Disability Evaluation under Social Security: A Handbook for Physicians*, 1979.
[b] See Handbook for additional important details.

even if these expenses also apply to needs for daily living (such a wheelchair). (e) In addition to disabled workers, persons diasabled before the age of 22 and disabled widows and widowers can also have a trial work period.

Supplemental Security Income

Supplemental Security Income is a federal program which was introduced in 1974. It is paid for out of general funds rather than Social Security funds, but it is administered by the same state agencies which administer the Disability Determination program. The application process is similar to that described above for Social Security Disability Insurance. The same criteria are used to evaluate SSI disability claims as are used for DI claims.

The basic differences between SSI and Social Security benefits are as follows: (a) *Eligibity*: SSI is available for two groups of persons when they are not insured by Social Security: persons under 65

Table 9.4.

Impairments Qualifying a Person with *Epilepsy Due to Major Motor Seizures* for Medical Disability under Social Security[a, b]

Major motor seizures (grand mal or psychomotor), documented by EEG and by detailed description of a typical seizure pattern, including all associated phenomena: occurring more frequently than once a month, in spite of at least 3 months of prescribed treatment.[c] With:
A. Diurnal episodes (loss of consciousness and convulsive seizures); *or*
B. Nocturnal episodes manifesting residuals which interfere significantly with activity during the day.

[a] From *Disability Evaluation under Social Security: A Handbook for Physicians*, 1979.
[b] See Handbook for additional important details.
[c] Adherence to therapy must be objectively confirmed by measurements of drug levels that are in the therapeutic range.

Table 9.5.

Impairments Qualifying a Person with *Arthritis of a Major Weight-Bearing Joint* for Medical Disability under Social Security[a]

Arthritis of a major weight-bearing joint (due to any cause): With history of persistent joint pain and stiffness with signs of limitation of motion or abnormal motion of the affected joint on current physical examination. With:
A. Gross anatomical deformity of hip or knee (*e.g.*, subluxation, contracture, bony or fibrous ankylosis, instability) supported by X-ray evidence of either joint space narrowing or bony destruction *and* markedly limiting ability to walk and stand; *or*
B. Reconstructive surgery or surgical arthrodesis of a major weight-bearing joint and return to full weight-bearing status did not occur, or is not expected to occur, within 12 months of onset.

[a] From *Disability Evaluation under Social Security: A Handbook for Physicians, 1979.* (Revised criteria due to be implemented in 1985).

Table 9.6.

Impairments Qualifying a Person with *Rheumatoid Arthritis* for Medical Disability under Social Security[a]

Active Rheumatoid Arthritis and Other Inflammatory Arthritis. With both A and B:
A. History of persistent joint pain, swelling, and tenderness involving multiple major joints (see 1.00D) *and* with signs of joint inflammation (swelling and tenderness) on current physical examination despite prescribed therapy for at least 3 months, resulting in significant restriction of function of the affected joints, and clinical activity expected to last at least 12 months; *and*
B. Corroboration of diagnosis at some point in time by either:
  1. Positive serological test for rheumatoid factor; *or*
  2. Antinuclear antibodies; *or*
  3. Elevated sedimentation rate; *or*
  4. Characteristic histological changes in biopsy of synovial membrane or subcutaneous nodule (obtained independent of Social Security disability evaluation).

[a] From *Disability Evaluation under Social Security: A Handbook for Physicians, 1979.* (Revised criteria due to be implemented in 1985).

who are medically disabled and all uninsured persons over the age of 65.* In addition to these two groups, persons who have "presumptive disability" (claim for total disability being processed) and disabled persons who are in the 5-month waiting period for their DI payments to begin may be eligible. Eligibility in all of these groups is based on need (total resources below a certain defined level) and the absence of gainful employment (defined as earned monthly income of $300 or more for disability claims). (b) There is *no waiting period*: a person becomes eligible for the first SSI payment in the month when he files his disability claim. (c) In most states, persons who are approved for SSI are *also eligible for Medicaid* and other social services provided by their state. (d) All persons receiving SSI are *reviewed once each year* to determine whether their income and other resources still make them eligible to receive SSI.

The maximum monthly income from SSI in 1984 was $314 for an individual and $472 for a couple. In 1984, there were 4.8 million recipients of SSI, on the basis of disability, blindness, and age (over 65 and without Social Security).

The patient's personal physician plays the same pivotal role in SSI application that he plays in DI application (see above). Until his report is received, no income support can be initiated for his patient.

Vocational Rehabilitation

State Vocational Rehabilitation agencies existed before the federal Disability Determination program was created in 1954. In many states, these agencies administer the Disability Determination program in addition to providing vocational rehabilitation services.

Eligibility

To be eligible for Vocational Rehabilitation, a person must have a disability that interferes with his capacity to obtain suitable employment or that is a threat to his present career; this does not mean that the person has to meet the criteria for medical disability discussed above. The individual must have a reasonable chance of being able to engage in a suitable occupation after Vocational Rehabilitation services are provided. A "suitable occupation" would include assistance provided by being a housewife provided that Vocational Rehabilitation would enable her to remain in her own home instead of requiring institutional care.

Services

The services provided by Vocational Rehabilitation agencies vary from state to state. However, they

usually include the following: (a) A *medical examination*. A complete medical examination is provided to determine the extent of a person's disability. (b) *Counseling and guidance*. A trained rehabilitation counselor is assigned to guide each client through the rehabilitation process. (c) *Physical aids*. Items such as artificial limbs, braces, hearing aids, eyeglasses, and wheelchairs may be provided if needed. (d) *Job training*. Training for the proper job is provided when necessary. This may be given in a vocational school, college or university, rehabilitation facility, or in the home. (e) *Help with living expenses*. Board, room, transportation expenses, and other necessary expenses may be provided if needed. (f) *Equipment and licenses*. Tools, equipment and licenses necessary for getting started in the right job may be provided. (g) *Job placement*. Placement in the right job is an important part of the rehabilitation process. The abilities of each handicapped individual are carefully matched to job requirements. (h) *Follow-up*. The counselor follows up on each placement to make sure that the client's job is suitable.

The Physician's Role

As noted above, all persons applying for Social Security disability benefits are screened for referral to Vocational Rehabilitation. For those persons, the report of the patient's physician (see above) may be utilized by the Vocational Rehabilitation agency. For persons who are not applying for medical disability, the physician will often be asked to provide a general medical report for the Vocational Rehabilitation agency. Perhaps the most important role of the general physician in this regard is to provide encouragement to the patient to apply for Vocational Rehabilitation and to maintain continued interest in the patient's progress. It has been estimated that every $1,000 spent for Vocational Rehabilitation increases by $35,000 the lifetime earnings of those who are rehabilitated. This economic consequence for society, in addition to the benefit to the individual, makes support of Vocational Rehabilitation a particularly important role for the physician.

HOME HEALTH SERVICES

A consequence of illness as distressing to the patient as the loss of the ability to earn an income is the temporary or permanent loss of the ability to remain at home. Most people will require acute hospital care one or more times in their adult life, and a small proportion will also require long term institutional care. The principal objectives of home health services are to minimize the need for admission to either acute or long term care facilities and to decrease the length of stay in these facilities. Numerous studies have shown that these objectives are attained when home health services are utilized appropriately; but studies have also shown that

---

* SSI for persons over 65 is similar to Social Security retirement. These claims are not handled by Disability Determination services.

home health services are underutilized and that much institutional care could be prevented by broader and more frequent utilization of these services.

Evolution of Home Health Services

The provision of home care services is a long established concept, beginning in this country with a home care program offered by the Boston Dispensary in 1796. A resurgence of interest in home care began in 1947, with the establishment of the Coordinated Home Care Program at Montefiore Hospital in New York City. The provision of a broad array of home health services to a growing number of chronically ill patients caught the imagination of those who recognized the disadvantages and high cost of institutionalization. Home health agencies throughout the country have used Montefiore as a model in developing or expanding home care services. The inclusion of home health services in the coverage provided by Medicare, Medicaid, and other third party insurers has enabled home health agencies to expand greatly in the past two decades.

Range of Services

Health care provided to sick persons at home includes (a) basic care provided by nonprofessional family members and friends (at times with the help of Red Cross or similar training in basic care technique); (b) home food services available at a nominal cost to the patient ("Meals on Wheels"); (c) care provided by physicians or their associates who make home visits; and (d) services provided by the personnel of certified home health agencies, under the supervision of the patient's physician. Even when professional help is involved, most of the responsibility for carrying out care is given to the patient or to a member of the patient's family; as noted in Chapter 1, it is this assumption of responsibility by the patient and his family that most clearly distinguishes ambulatory medicine from hospital-based medicine.

Today there are approximately 3500 home health agencies in the United States. Agencies may be part of state and local health departments, nonprofit voluntary agencies, or for-profit proprietary agencies. The home care provided by voluntary agencies is coordinated by a visiting nurse. A substantial proportion of the care is often carried out by home health aides, analogous to nursing aides on hospital wards, under the supervision of the nurse. In recent years, nurse practitioners have been added to the staffs of many home health agencies, so that more sophisticated care can be provided. In addition to nursing, the services may include physical, occupational, and speech therapy, dietary and social work counseling, and homemaker services. Home health agencies also provide the nursing component

of hospice programs (see Chapter 19) in many communities.

Recently, numerous companies have begun to supply and administer *in-home intravenous therapies*, ranging from short term normal saline and electrolyte infusions to courses of antibiotics, cancer chemotherapy, and total parenteral nutrition. These initiatives have emerged in response (a) to efforts to reduce the length of hospitalization and (b) to patients who prefer home care to hospital care for parenteral therapy that may have to be administered during 1 or more weeks. These sophisticated home therapies require careful supervision by the referring physician. Adequate day-to-day supervision of the overall care of patients receiving in-home parenteral therapy is usually *not* provided by the company that supplies the equipment; therefore, this responsibility should be delegated to a visiting nurse who knows the physician's comprehensive plan for the patient and is in close contact with the supplier.

The types of clinical problems most frequently referred to home health agencies are listed in Table 9.7.

Third Party Coverage

Any patient (or patient's family) may purchase services from a home health agency. During the past 20 years, patients meeting certain criteria have been eligible for coverage of much of the cost of home care by Medicare, Medicaid, and other third party payors (Table 9.8). The minimal criteria are that (a) the patient is under the care of a physician and (b) the patient has an active medical problem that requires skilled nursing or other skilled professional service such as physical or occupational therapy.

Table 9.7.
Problems Most Commonly Referred for Home Health Services

Postsurgical wound care (teach and/or provide dressing changes)

Rehabilitation after hospitalization for orthopaedic problems

Congestive heart failure (provide dietary counseling, assess medication compliance)

Diabetes (supervise insulin technique, provide dietary counseling, teach urine testing, care of the lower extremities, *etc*)

Hypertension (supervise and reinforce compliance with medication, check blood pressure response in patient's home)

Incurable cancer (provide dietary counseling, psychological support, and other aspects of hospice care)

Stroke and other incapacitating neurological problems (provide physical and occupational therapy)

Decubitus and stasis ulcers (teach and/or provide debridement and dressing changes)

Dementia and older person living alone (assess environment for health hazards)

Chronic obstructive pulmonary disease (assess home for oxygen therapy)

Table 9.8.
Criteria for Third Party Reimbursement for Home Health Services, Current 1981

Part A[a] or Part B Medicare
Part A pays for all covered services (skilled nursing, home health aide, social work, physical, occupational, and speech therapy). Care must be provided by a certified Home Health Agency and must be medically necessary. There is no limit to the number of visits, as long as the patient's condition meets criteria for services. The following conditions must be met to qualify for reimbursement:

1. Patient is confined to his home.
2. Need for intermittent skilled nursing, physical therapy, or speech therapy. (One of these three services must be needed to qualify for reimbursement for the other services provided by home health agencies, *i.e.*, social work, occupational therapy, nurses aid, and nutrition services.)
3. Physician must sign renewal of certification every 60 days.

Medicaid
Coverage for home health services varies by state.
Blue Cross and other private health insurance.
Coverage for home health services varies by plan.

---

[a] Note that effective July 1, 1981, Part A Medicare, like part B, covers patients even if they have not been recently discharged from a hospital.

Because of the criterion that the patient must have an active medical problem requiring skilled care, payment for the services of a home health aide is often denied after the active problem becomes stable, even when the home health aide's services are important in maintaining the patient's health.

The Physician's Role

All physicians should be well acquainted with the home health services available in their community and with the third party coverage that their patients may have for the services. Although anyone (the patient's family, a nurse, a social worker, *etc*) can refer a patient for home health services, orders written by the patient's physician are always needed for third party reimbursement.

The quality of the communication between a patient's physician and the visiting nurse often determines how much the patient will benefit from home health services. When the physician provides clear and thorough initial information, when the physician is accessible to the nurse when needed, and *vice versa*, patients who would otherwise require in-hospital care can receive excellent care in their homes. Some problems are best managed at home, such as adjustment of insulin and diet in a diabetic patient with an intercurrent illness, adjustment of diuretics and diet in a patient with worsening congestive heart failure, assessment of compliance and the response to medication in a patient whose high blood pressure seems refractory to treatment at office visits, and debridement, dressing, and monitoring of a sacral pressure sore.

General References

Brickner PW: *Home Health Care for the Aged.* New York, Appleton-Century-Crofts, 1979.
    Extensively referenced resources covering all aspects of home care services for elderly persons.
Davidson RC: The future of home health agencies. *J Community Health* 4:55, 1978.
    Excellent review of the present and future place of home health agencies in patient care.
Disability Evaluation under Social Security: A Handbook for Physicians. Department of Health, Education and Welfare publ no. (SSA) 79-10089. August, 1979.
    Gives criteria for impairments that qualify a person for medical disability under Social Security (available free from local Social Security Office and State Disability Determination Service). A number of criteria were updated in 1985 (published in the *Federal Register*).
Family Health and Home Nursing. Garden City, NY, Doubleday, 1979.
    Inexpensive Red Cross publication for the lay person explaining in detail all aspects of caring for sick persons at home. Available in most bookstores.

SECTION 2

Psychiatric and Behavioral Problems

CHAPTER TEN

Evaluation of Psychosocial Problems

L. RANDOL BARKER, M.D., AND CHESTER W. SCHMIDT, JR., M.D.

INTRODUCTION

Patients with psychological and social problems often consult their general physicians, usually complaining of not feeling well in some physical sense. The problems these patients present range from temporary distress to rather enduring and disabling conditions.

The *temporary disturbances* which are most often seen by the generalist are anxiety regarding the meaning of a new symptom (*e.g.*, cancer fear), frustrations attending an illness which interrupts valued activities (*e.g.*, recovery phase following myocardial infarction), or dysphoric mood related to recent social stress (*e.g.*, anxiety in the mother of a teenager who has run away from home). Such problems occur frequently in persons with excellent previous mental health. These disturbances usually resolve when the interviewing and counseling skills discussed in Chapters 3 and 11 are utilized in conjunction with management of the patient's medical problem.

Those patients with *more persistent psychosocial problems* are difficult to care for unless one has a knowledge of common psychosocial syndromes and utilizes a systematic approach to the patient. This chapter and the following chapter provide general approaches for the evaluation and management of such patients. Subsequent chapters cover the specific psychosocial syndromes seen by generalists. The chronic psychosocial syndromes that occur most frequently in American communities are listed in Table 10.1, in rank order for major age-sex groups. It is of interest that the household interviews utilized to obtain these data disclosed a high prevalence of two chronic problems—phobia and antisocial personality—that are not diagnosed commonly in medical practice. It is likely that these two problems, and alcoholism—the most prevalent disorder in males under 65 years of age—account for a great deal of illness that is attributed to other causes by physicians and laypeople.

SYNDROMAL DIAGNOSIS

Accurate diagnosis of a psychosocial problem is essential for prognosis and management. The *Diagnostic and Statistical Manual-III* (DSM-III), issued in 1980 by the American Psychiatric Association, is a particularly useful resource, as it provides diagnostic criteria, epidemiological information, and prognostic profiles for most of the psychosocial syndromes encountered in office practice. DSM-III criteria are stated wherever relevant in the chapters which follow.

Despite the availability of diagnostic criteria, reaching an accurate psychosocial diagnosis in the generalist's office can be difficult. There are several reasons for this: (*a*) When the presenting symptoms are somatic, physical illness must always be considered, even when the patient's presentation suggests a psychosocial problem. (*b*) Psychosocial symptoms or findings are not often specific for one syndrome. (*c*) The necessary information is different from that needed to evaluate a physical symptom. The most salient information is obtained by inquiring about or observing thoughts, feelings, behaviors, events, and relationships.

After initial information gathering, it is usually possible to decide which general phenomenon is the dominant problem, *e.g.*, anxiety, depression, somatization, cognitive impairment, maladaptive behavior, *etc.* To refine the diagnosis, additional information is needed. For example:

The patient has a depressed mood. With a systematic approach, the diagnosis of "depression" may be more accurately formulated as one of the following:
1. adjustment disorder with depressed mood;
2. major depression;
3. dysthymic disorder (depressive neurosis);
4. depression related to a recently prescribed drug;
5. alcoholism presenting as depression.

Table 10.1.
Four Most Frequent DIS:DSM-III Psychiatric Disorders by Sex and Age Based on 6-Month Prevalence Rates[a,b]

Rank	18–24 Yr	25–44 Yr	45–64 Yr	65+ Yr	Total
Men					
1	Alcohol abuse/ dependence	Alcohol abuse/ dependence	Alcohol abuse/ dependence	Severe cognitive impairment	Alcohol abuse/ dependence
2	Drug abuse/ dependence	Phobia	Phobia	Phobia	Phobia
3	Phobia	Drug abuse/ dependence	Dysthymia	Alcohol abuse/ dependence	Drug abuse/ dependence
4	Antisocial personality	Antisocial personality	Major depressive episode without grief	Dysthymia	Dysthymia
Women					
1	Phobia	Phobia	Phobia	Phobia	Phobia
2	Drug abuse/ dependence	Major depressive episode without grief	Dysthymia	Severe cognitive impairment	Major depressive episode without grief
3	Major depressive episode without grief	Dysthymia	Major depressive episode without grief	Dysthymia	Dysthymia
4	Alcohol abuse/ dependence	Obsessive-compulsive disorder	Obsessive-compulsive disorder	Major depressive episode without grief	Obsessive-compulsive disorder

[a] From Myers JK, Weissman MM, Tischler GL, et al: Six-month prevalence of psychiatric disorders in three communities. *Arch Gen Psychiatry* 41:959, 1984.
[b] Dysthmia included. The basis for ranking was the mean 6-month prevalence rates for New Haven, Baltimore, and St. Louis combined. DIS indicates Diagnostic Interview Schedule.

INFORMATION GATHERING

The order in which information is gathered and the particular information gathered will vary depending upon the style which one has developed with previous patients and the diagnosis being considered. With a minimum amount of prompting, many patients will volunteer information that would otherwise require systematic questioning. Both the efficiency and the accuracy of the interview are probably enhanced when this occurs. Other interviewing skills useful in eliciting a psychosocial history are described in Chapter 3.

Building upon the patient's initial account, one should assess relevant aspects of the social history, the patient's mental status, the patient's personality and coping styles, the chronology of the patient's problem, and the family history of psychosocial problems. With the patient's permission, additional information should be obtained from family members, other physicians, and previous medical records whenever possible. Current medications should be identified, as psychological disturbances can be caused or worsened by a large number of drugs (see "General References" and Table 12.2, Chapter 12).

Social and Developmental History

This should always include a profile of the patient's current life situation (e.g., marital status, family structure, household makeup, educational level, occupation, recreational activities, and substance use). At times, it is also helpful to know the principal patterns and events that have characterized his development from childhood until the present (e.g., family makeup, interactions, losses; relationships in school, the armed services, jobs; and the patient's depiction of the type of person he is and has been). Some of this information will be known already to the patient's personal physician, making the assessment of a new psychosocial problem simpler at times. When a psychosocial problem seems likely, the presenting symptom should be re-explored in the context of social interactions (e.g., "Tell me just where you were and who was there the last time you noted the nausea and quivering in your stomach"), and the patient should be asked to describe any recent changes in his life situation and to discuss the nature of critical relationships (e.g., with spouse, children, and work associates). If substance abuse is suspected, skillful inquiry will be needed to make a diagnosis (see Chapter 21 on alcoholism and Chapter 22 on illicit drugs).

Much psychosocial illness is related to stresses and maladjustments which will be disclosed by the patient during this inquiry. McWhinney has summarized the social factors most commonly related to psychosocial distress (see Table 10.2). The significance of a report of one of these factors becomes clear when it is integrated into the rest of the history (e.g., an interpersonal conflict may be the *stressor*

Table 10.2.
Common Social Factors Related to Psychological Symptoms[a]

1. *Loss*: (*a*) Personal loss—loss of a loved one through death or desertion. (*b*) Loss of things—imposed loss of home, cherished possession, or job.
2. *Conflict*: (*a*) Interpersonal—conflict within family, with neighbors, or at work, where hostility is recognized. (*b*) Intrapersonal—role conflict or conflicting demands on the patient (as in a working mother).
3. *Change*: (*a*) Development—where time of life is the major problem (as in adolescence, menopause, or senescence). (*b*) Geographic—where a move to an unfamiliar environment is the major problem (as in immigration).
4. *Maladjustment*: (*a*) Interpersonal—problems between people with no overt conflict (as in failure to achieve a satisfactory sexual relation without hostility between partners). (*b*) Personal—failure to adjust to the environment (home or job) in the absence of the above-mentioned loss, conflict, or change.
5. *Stress*: (*a*) Acute—unexpected event not covered under loss, conflict, or change (for example, the sudden illness of self or of a family member or friend). (*b*) Chronic—long term situation not included in loss, conflict, or change (for instance, the presence of a handicapped child in the family).
6. *Isolation*—not due to any recent loss, change, or conflict (as in an elderly widow).
7. *Failure or frustrated expectations*—when the patient's goals in life are not fulfilled and when there is no evidence of an intervening event covered by loss, conflict, or change (*e.g.*, failure at school or failure to achieve occupational promotion).

[a] From McWhinney IR: Beyond diagnosis, an approach to the integration of behavioral science and clinical medicine. *N Engl J Med* 287:384, 1972.

causing an adjustment disorder or it may be *a symptom of* alcoholism, depression, or sexual dysfunction).

In addition to providing clues to the diagnosis, the social history will usually disclose important assets and liabilities in the patient's life. This information is always useful in planning management for a psychosocial problem.

Mental Status

In those instances when the patient's behavior is the principal problem and/or when psychological symptoms are causing a great deal of subjective distress (e.g., marked anxiety or depression) or suggest a major psychiatric disorder (e.g., dementia, schizophrenia, or manic-depressive illness), a brief mental status examination should be performed.

The mental status examination is a systematic assessment of the patient's current mental functioning. The elements of the mental status examination most useful for the general physician include:

Appearance: Grooming, motor activity (quiet versus agitated).

General level of consciousness: Alert, sleepy, stuporous, obtunded.

Orientation: The patient knows who he is, where he is, and the date (day, month, and year).

Speech: Ability to use customary syntax. Note slurring, inability to find the right word, pressured speech, flight of ideas, looseness of association, muteness.

Memory: Recent memory—knowledge of recent events, capacity to remember names of current treating physicians. Remote memory—ability to give history and present illness in proper historical sequence.

Attention and concentration: Ability to understand and follow questions or instructions.

Intelligence: Can be estimated from level of schooling achieved, vocational history, use of language.

Mood: A pervasive, sustained emotion (depressed, euphoric, neutral).

Affect: An observable and immediately expressed emotion (anger, anxiety, sadness, fear, humor, lability, *etc*). Note whether display of affect is consistent with the content of speech, thoughts, and behavior.

Perceptions: Presence of hallucinations (i.e., visual, auditory, or somatic perception occurring in the absence of appropriate external stimuli), delusions, (i.e., fixed beliefs, which are false), paranoid ideas, or persistent phobias (i.e., fears directed toward specific objects or situations).

Suicidal thoughts. Statement or actions that indicate the patient wishes to harm or kill himself.

Homicidal or violent thoughts: Statements or actions that indicate patient wishes to harm or kill others.

Judgment: Capacity to understand the situation in which the patient finds himself and demonstrate appropriate compliance with instructions for care.

Most of the data needed for a brief mental status examination are observable while the patient gives his history. Depending upon the cues the patient provides, he should be questioned more about his mental status and other features of the syndrome(s) suggested by his history. For patients whose mental status suggests dementia, a more formal cognitive examination can be administered in a few minutes (see Mini-Mental Status Exam, Table 17.1, Chapter 17).

Personality and Coping Responses

Personality refers to the relatively enduring attitudes and patterns of behavior which typify an individual. Generally a physician becomes acquainted with a patient's personality, particularly the patient's behavior pattern in the face of illness, through caring for that patient during months or years. Some patients will exhibit the features of a maladaptive personality, and recognition of this may be very helpful in planning the patient's care, as discussed in more detail in Chapter 14.

Coping responses are behaviors which people assume in adapting to life's stresses. There are several common coping responses which should be recognized since patients may use them to avoid confronting a problem for which help is needed. When maladaptive coping is recognized, the patient can often be assisted to disclose the primary problem and to reach a healthier adaption to it.

Denial is a common response by which a distressing problem is avoided. Denial may be relatively silent (i.e., a patient with blood in his stools may keep this information to himself to avoid confronting his fear of cancer) or it may be voiced openly (e.g., a patient who greatly fears sudden death during convalescence from a myocardial infarction may boast of robust health and deny angina or other symptoms he may be experiencing).

Rationalization serves the same function as denial. It is a process in which a patient gives plausible explanations for behavior designed to avoid unpleasant realities (e.g., a relapsing alcoholic explains that his work load increased so much lately that it was impossible to continue to go to Alcoholics Anonymous meetings).

Regression is reversion to dependent behavior typical of childhood. Regressive behavior is a common response to major illness or other circumstances which threaten a person's autonomy (e.g., a man who is recovering slowly from a hip fracture complains excessively about small problems at home, gets upset when his son cannot continue to visit daily, and expects his wife to order for him when they go out to a restaurant on the weekend).

Projection is a process in which an unpleasant aspect of one's self is ascribed to another person (e.g., a teenager who is very angry about limits set by her mother criticizes her older sister for being hostile to their mother).

Displacement is a process in which feelings toward one individual are directed toward another (i.e., a researcher who is furious at a colleague who has beaten him to an important finding becomes very irritable toward his wife for no apparent reason).

Chronology

Accurate information about the chronology of a psychosocial problem is important for diagnosis, prognosis, and management. Therefore, as the interview is closing, one should assure that the patient has provided the following essential information: (*a*) duration of the present episode; (*b*) the time(s) and circumstances during which the current symptoms have either improved or worsened (if temporal relationships are unclear, it is helpful to have the patient *keep a log* of symptoms and events for one or more weeks); (*c*) the patient's optimal level of functioning during the past year (when was it and how long did it last?); (*d*) the time and circumstances of any previous episode of similar symptoms or of previous mental illness.

Family History

In the family of a patient with a chronic psychosocial disorder, occurrence of the same disorder or other psychiatric problems is common. Information about psychiatric illness in the family may strengthen one's diagnostic hunches and may help the patient to recognize the nature of his own problem.

Table 10.3.
Severity of Current Psychosocial Stressors[a]

Code[b]	Term	Adult Examples	Child or Adolescent Examples
1	None	No apparent psychosocial stressor	No apparent psychosocial stressor
2	Minimal	Minor violation of the law; small bank loan	Vacation with family
3	Mild	Argument with neighbor; change in work hours	Change in school teacher; new school year
4	Moderate	New career; death of close friend; pregnancy	Chronic parental fighting; change to new school; illness of close relative; birth of sibling
5	Severe	Serious illness in self or family; major financial loss; marital separation; birth of child	Death of peer; divorce of parents; arrest; hospitalization; persistent and harsh parental discipline
6	Extreme	Death of close relative; divorce	Death of parent or sibling; repeated physical or sexual abuse
7	Catastrophic	Concentration camp experience; devastating natural disaster	Multiple family deaths
0	Unspecified	No information, or not applicable	No information, or not applicable

[a] Adapted from *Diagnostic and Statistical Manual of Mental Disorders*, ed 3. Washington, DC, American Psychiatric Association, 1980.
[b] Code numbers used in DSM-III.

OVERALL FORMULATION OF THE PROBLEM

When the essentials of a patient's psychosocial history have been collected, a useful way to formulate the problem is the five-axis approach recommended by the American Psychiatric Association. The five axes refer to the different classes of information which are relevant in caring for a patient.

Axis I—Psychosocial syndrome(s), plus conditions not attributable to a mental disorder that are a focus of attention (e.g., malingering, uncomplicated bereavement, noncompliance with medical treatment, academic or occupational problems, *etc*).

Axis II—Personality disorders or styles and specific developmental disorders.

Axis III—Physical disorders and conditions.

Axis IV—Severity of current psychosocial stressors (see Table 10.3).

Axis V—Highest level of adaptive functioning in past year (see Table 10.4).

Case example. Mr. J., a 60-year-old married security guard, underwent coronary bypass graft surgery (CABG) in January 1984. His postoperative hospital course was uneventful. Shortly after discharge, he came twice in the same day to the emergency department complaining of severe chest pain and also of cold upper extremities. Evaluation revealed mild tenderness at the location of his sternotomy scar. The next day he returned, this time describing inability to sleep in addition to the previous symptoms. A thorough evaluation, including an exercise

Table 10.4.
Highest Level of Adaptive Functioning in Past Year[a]

Code[b]	Levels	Adult Examples	Child or Adolescent Examples
1	*Superior*—Unusually effective functioning in social relations, occupational functioning, and use of leisure time.	Single parent living in deteriorating neighborhood takes excellent care of children and home, has warm relations with friends, and finds time for pursuit of hobby.	A 12-year-old girl gets superior grades in school, is extremely popular among her peers, and excels in many sports. She does all of this with apparent ease and comfort.
2	*Very good*—Better than average functioning in social relations, occupational functioning, and use of leisure time.	A 65-year-old retired widower does some volunteer work, often sees old friends, and pursues hobbies.	An adolescent boy gets excellent grades, works part time, has several close friends, and plays banjo in the jazz band. He admits to some distress in "keeping up with everything."
3	*Good*—No more than slight impairment in either social or occupational functioning.	A woman with many friends functions extremely well at a difficult job, but says "the strain is too much."	An 8-year-old boy does well in school, has several friends, but bullies younger children.
4	*Fair*—Moderate impairment in either social relations or occupational functioning, or some impairment in both.	A lawyer has trouble carrying through on assignments, has several acquaintances, but hardly any close friends.	A 10-year-old girl does poorly in school, but has adequate peer and family relations.
5	*Poor*—Marked impairment in either social relations or occupational functioning, or moderate impairment in both.	A man with one or two friends has trouble keeping a job for more than a few weeks.	A 14-year-old boy almost fails in school and has trouble getting along with his peers.
6	*Very poor*—Marked impairment in both social relations and occupational functioning.	A woman is unable to do any of her housework and has violent outbursts toward family and neighbors.	A 6-year-old girl needs special help in all subjects and has virtually no peer relationships.
7	*Grossly impaired*—Gross impairment in virtually all areas of functioning.	An elderly man needs supervision to maintain minimal personal hygiene and is usually incoherent.	A 4-year-old boy needs constant restraint to avoid hurting himself and is almost totally lacking in language skills.
0	*Unspecified*	No information.	No information.

[a] Adapted from *Diagnostic and Statistical Manual of Mental Disorders*, ed 3. Washington, DC, American Psychiatric Association, 1980.
[b] Code numbers used in DSM-III.

stress test, did not disclose a physical basis for his symptoms.

The patient's wife described regressive behavior since the patient returned home (e.g., he wanted her to bring his meals to him in bed, asked her to pick his clothes for him each day, was having occasional urinary incontinence, and had put her in charge of dispensing all of his medicines). He was not sleeping well and awakened his wife whenever he could not sleep. Additional inquiry and observation revealed a somewhat diminished sense of self-worth and some doubts regarding his future. He was worried specifically that he would not return to work, as he had expected to preoperatively, and his calculations suggested that his income would be significantly lower if he applied for Social Security.

The patient eventually disclosed that he was sure that he had been "on the pump too long" and that he feared that his incision would break down (this had happened to a friend following CABG).

Mr. J had always seemed to be a self-reliant man. He had worked as a security guard, on medical therapy for his angina, for several years. The CABG was recommended when his angina worsened in November 1983, making it difficult for him to walk the distances required at his job. He had never developed markedly regressive behavior in the past, although he had depended on his wife to make decisions about almost all purchases they made, had never been separated from her for a full day during their long and tranquil marriage, and often referred to her as "Mother." There was no history of significant psychiatric illness in his family.

Based upon this story and additional inquiry, the formulation of Mr. J's illness was:

Axis I—Adjustment disorder, with depressed mood and somatization.

Axis II—No personality disorder; history of dependency which made him vulnerable to the behavior he exhibited following CABG.

Axis III—(a) Coronary artery disease. (b) Status post-coronary artery bypass graft, with good technical result.

Axis IV—Current stressors moderate to severe, i.e., (a) temporary disability due to major surgery; (b) uncertainty regarding his future financial security.

Axis V—Highest level of adaptive functioning in past year good, i.e., no more than slight impairment in either social or occupational functioning.

CO-MORBIDITY IN THE PATIENT'S FAMILY

Psychosocial problems create substantial stress for spouses, children, or other persons with close ties to the affected patient. This is particularly true of chronic problems such as alcoholism, affective disorders, anxiety disorders, and the somatoform disorders. The impact of the patient's illness on others should always be considered in the evaluation of psychosocial problems. As pointed out in other chapters in this section, there are important ways in which the co-morbidity of the family can be alleviated as part of the overall approach to these trying problems.

ASSESSMENT OF MENTAL COMPETENCE

Occasionally, the general physician will be expected to assess the mental competence of a patient. Common civil issues of mental competence include competence to accept or refuse medical care, commitment to hospitals, contesting of wills, and guardianship decisions.

The usual test of the patient's competence in selecting medical care is the determination of whether the patient understands the nature, benefits, and risks of that care and the consequences of not selecting it. This determination can usually be made by the primary care physician for patients with mental retardation or dementia and for patients with psychological problems short of frank psychosis. Similarly, the primary care physician can evaluate a patient's competence in the office, utilizing a standard test such as the Mini-Mental Status Exam outlined in Table 17.1, in order to assist a lawyer in planning the management of the patient's routine financial affairs (e.g., Social Security checks and monthly bills).

In the ambulatory setting, perhaps the commonest problem presented by marginally competent patients is unreliable self-care; here, the assistance of a competent household member or of a visiting nurse is essential.

Although commitment laws in most states require examination by a physician and do not specify psychiatric examination, the primary care physician will rarely be required to make commitment determinations. In those instances when a psychiatrist is not available, a complete psychiatric evaluation, including a complete mental status examination, is necessary to determine whether the patient is dangerous to himself or to others, which is the usual test for commitment.

It is even less likely that the primary care physician will be called upon to examine and provide expert testimony in contesting of wills or in determining the need for guardianship for a patient. The ultimate decision in such cases is made by an administrative law judge. These legal proceedings are often adversary in nature, and familiarity with principles of forensic psychiatry and experience as an expert witness are required of the physician participating. Most psychiatrists hesitate to become involved in these proceedings unless they have had special training and experience. Therefore, it is unlikely that the primary care physician will or should be involved unless he, too, has had the necessary training and experience.

General References

American Psychiatric Association: *Diagnostic and Statistical Manual of Mental Disorders*, ed 3. Washington, DC, American Psychiatric Association, 1980.

    Recently updated diagnostic criteria and epidemiological information for all recognized psychiatric disorders.

Cadoret RJ: Gathering data. In Cadoret RJ, King LJ (eds): *Psychiatry in Primary Care*. St Louis, CV Mosby, 1983, chap 2, pp 9–41.

    Chapter which covers in greater depth the approaches to evaluation by the generalist which are described in this chapter.

Drugs that cause psychiatric symptoms. *Med Lett* 26:75, August 17, 1984.

    Entire issue consists of a table listing psychiatric symptoms or syndromes that have been reported as effects of use or withdrawal of more than 80 currently used drugs. Includes references for every drug.

CHAPTER ELEVEN

Psychotherapy in Ambulatory Practice

CHESTER W. SCHMIDT, Jr., M.D., AND L. RANDOL BARKER, M.D.

Psychotherapy consists of a number of verbal and behavioral processes which are used in the management of psychosocial problems for the purpose of relieving symptoms and resolving intra- and inter-personal conflicts. Although many different techniques have been described, there are fundamental principles which are common to all. Since general physicians have many opportunities to use psychotherapy effectively, either formally or informally, it is important that they have a working knowledge of these principles and of the techniques most useful in ambulatory practice.

GENERAL PRINCIPLES

Transference

Patients come to physicians for the relief of pain, suffering, and fear associated with illness and disease. They recognize and accept the expertise of the physician and are hopeful and trusting that the physician will relieve their distress. The basic attitudes of hopefulness and trust are positive attributes of the relationship between patient and doctor. There are potent psychosocial roots to the generally positive initial expectations of the patient as he enters into the relationship with the physician. Each patient brings with him a history of psychosocial development in which pain, fear, and other forms of distress have been repeatedly responded to by parents or by parent surrogates. Through these experiences, individuals both consciously and unconsciously come to expect that new people in their lives will behave with them in ways similar to the ways their parents behaved. These expectations are what are known as *transference phenomena*. Patients will project onto the patient-physician relationship these conscious and unconscious expectations. In fact, at times patients may react to the physician as if the physician were an important parental figure. To the degree that the transference is *positive*, the physician can exercise powerful supportive and healing psychological forces over the patient. Positive transference may explain placebo responses, and its effect must always be kept in mind when evaluating any therapeutic intervention.

Not all transference reactions are positive. Virtually no one comes through their childhood and adolescence without some psychological scars from disappointments, frustrations, and anger that are the results of unmet expectations and other deprivations experienced during the process of growing up. These psychological scars are the historical-developmental roots of maladaptive and negative personality traits such as dependency, passivity, hostility, obsessive-compulsivity, and sociopathy (see Chapter 14). The conscious and unconscious conflicts associated with these traits can also be projected onto the physician-patient relationship. These *negative* transference reactions often cause troubled physician-patient relationships. The more seriously the patient is deprived of parental affection and support during his childhood, the more likely it is that he will manifest these negative traits as an adult, and therefore the more likely it is that negative transference reactions will develop within the patient-physician relationship.

The significance of the transference phenomenon to psychotherapeutic techniques is that it is a basic tool for bringing about positive attitudinal and behavioral change in the patient. For most ambulatory patients psychological distress results from problems within their current relationships with family, friends, and associates. The transference will recreate, within a controlled setting, modified but reasonably accurate representations of the patient's current and past relationships. As the patient begins to disclose conflicts and to react to the physician as if he were one of the individuals with whom he (the patient) is having difficulty, difficult relationships can be clarified and changes in the patient's attitudes and behavior to improve the relationship can then be considered.

The more intense the therapeutic relationship between patient and physician, the more likely it is that both positive and negative transference reactions will appear and become part of the therapeutic effort. Techniques like short term counseling (see below) do not produce intense therapeutic relationships and therefore tend to involve chiefly positive transference.

Countertransference

Physicians, like their patients, must go through the trials and tribulations of childhood, adolescence, the maturation, and therefore are not immune to the development of negative personality traits. However, society and the medical profession assume that physicians will not allow these traits to affect the physician-patient relationship. The physician is expected to maintain an objectivity in his relationship with his patients, and to be supportive and empathetic.

When practicing psychotherapy, the physician must be aware of his own idiosyncracies and must keep them under control and out of the therapeutic relationship; i.e., he must avoid countertransference. Chapter 3, "The Doctor-Patient Relationship," describes a number of interviewing skills that are helpful in avoiding countertransference.

The Therapeutic Contract

In mental health care settings, whenever a therapist and a patient agree to engage in counseling, the details of the treatment are spelled out and agreed to by both parties. A similar process may be helpful in general practice settings when formal counseling is undertaken. The details of the "therapeutic contract" usually include the frequency of visits, the length of the visits, the fee for the visit, the place in which the treatment is to be conducted, and the approximate length of the treatment program. These details form the boundaries within which the treatment, regardless of specific technique, will take place. The boundaries, although they seem obvious, can become extraordinarily significant during the course of treatment. Patients often react to the boundaries as part of the transference phenomenon by objecting to them, or by attempting to change or violate them. Although there are exceptions, the boundaries should not be modified because of a change in the relationship between the patient and the physician that arises as a result of transference. The contractual agreements are important boundaries and should remain stable throughout the course of the treatment.

Treatment Process

Psychotherapeutic techniques are like all human relationships: they have a beginning, a middle, and an end. The *initial phase* involves continued collection of data about the patient, sharpening of the formulation of the case, and, in collaboration with the patient, development of treatment goals. The initial phase of treatment is like a honeymoon during which the patient's expectations and hopes are expressed by positive transference toward the physician. The *middle phase* of treatment consists of the work of accomplishing the treatment goals agreed to by the patient and the therapist. Efforts to achieve those goals are met with by resistance from the patient as he attempts to avoid making the attitudinal and behavioral changes that are necessary to attain the goals. As the patient's avoidance of doing the work is pointed out or interpreted by the therapist, the patient becomes frustrated and annoyed and may develop negative transference toward the therapist. Recognition of the negative transference reactions and the resolution of them are important parts of the middle phase of treatment.

The *last phase* of treatment is a review of the work accomplished and a preparation for separating the patient from the treatment and the therapist. Separation is an extremely important part of the treatment process. It forces the patient to give up any residual dependency on the therapist. The experience of separating in a constructive fashion strengthens the ego functions of the patient. It is not unusual for the patient to experience a recurrence of the symptoms that originally brought him to treatment. However, in order to allow the patient to benefit fully from the separation experience it is important to complete the treatment on schedule as agreed. Inasmuch as general physicians will continue to have a relationship with their patients, separation may not be complete. However, shifting from the psychotherapeutic mode back to the primary care mode (see "Supportive Therapy" below) is a form of separation and contains within it some of the same benefits that would result from a formal psychotherapeutic situation.

PSYCHOSOCIAL TREATMENT TECHNIQUES

Since disclosure of delicate information and feelings may in itself be beneficial to the patient, it is artificial to separate evaluation from therapy for psychosocial problems (general aspects of evaluation for psychosocial problems are described in Chapter 10). This section describes the principal techniques utilized in counseling, and the following section describes those forms of counseling useful in office practice.

Establishing a Therapeutic Relationship

As noted earlier (see "Transference"), the therapeutic relationship recapitulates to some extent the parent-child relationship. Several elements are generic to an effective therapeutic relationship. Above all, the patient must trust his physician. Trust is promoted by being consistent in show of interest, by accepting sensitive information without being judgmental, by taking the patient's concerns seriously, and by controlling inappropriate reactions to difficult patients (see Table 3.1, Chapter 3). In addition to establishing trust, a physician should ensure that the patient understands ways in which there will be access to him (the physician) during ongoing treatment. When embarking on counseling, it is a good idea to reflect on whether these trust-promoting and condition-setting actions have been accomplished at the outset.

Chapter 3 contains a detailed description of the communication skills which foster an effective doctor-patient relationship.

Example: A physician listened empathically to a bereaved woman; in closing, he summarized what she had expressed to him, assured her of his willingness to talk with her about any additional problems, and asked her to telephone him twice a week for the next few weeks.

Identifying and Addressing Informational Needs

Much psychosocial distress or harmful behavior is related to misinformation or lack of information. Fear of dread illness, misunderstanding of an established condition, or conviction that one's symptoms must be due to physical illness are common forms of misinformation which patients bring to office visits. Through skillful interviewing, the physician can usually have a patient identify and clarify his informational needs. Providing information, tailored to the patient's needs, and assuring that the patient has received that information is the next step. Clear explanation of normal physiology, disease processes, treatment regimens, *etc* is often overlooked as a powerful aid in counseling. Besides imparting knowledge, this effort draws the patient into a collaborative relationship with the physician. Depending upon the problem, other counseling techniques may be as important or more important than this first step, particularly when somatic complaints are due to a psychosocial problem.

Commonly encountered informational needs are the following:

1. *Identification/clarification regarding feared or existing physical disorder.* For example:

The son of a recently deceased diabetic patient, who thinks he also has diabetes, receives reassurance and advice following a negative workup for diabetes.

A woman with mitral valve prolapse who has adopted inappropriate activity limitations receives reassurance regarding the relatively benign course of her condition and assurance that she can resume valued activities which she had curtailed. The American Heart Association booklet entitled *Mitral Valve Prolapse* is given to her; it reinforces what her physician has said.

2. *Identification/clarification regarding a psychophysiological basis for somatic symptoms.* For example:

A man with panic disorder obtains partial relief from an explanation of how hyperventilation leads to central nervous system symptoms.

3. *Identification/clarification of the role of a psychosocial stressor in producing symptoms.* For example:

A man with an adjustment disorder, with anxious mood, recognizes the role of his impending job layoff in precipitating his symptoms, and his and his family's fear that he is "going crazy" is alleviated.

4. *Identification of a working diagnosis, the plan, and the likely prognosis.* For example:

A woman with the syndrome of major depression develops some hopefulness when she is told the diagnosis, the plan to utilize gradually increasing doses of antidepressants, and the likelihood of significant improvement after a few weeks.

A man with the syndrome of hypochondriasis is *not* given the name of his syndrome, but he reaches a truce with his physician after being informed that he will probably continue to have some symptoms but that he can engage in valued activities which he has curtailed.

Eliciting Feelings

The discomfort of psychosocial illness is often due to the feelings the patient is experiencing. The fundamental ways in which the physician can help the patient to deal with feelings are (a) through empathic listening and (b) having the patient "ventilate" in the office.

Empathic Listening

It is very supportive and reassuring to the patient for the physician to indicate that he is listening and paying close attention to what the patient is saying. Remembering details of the history, responding with appropriate affect to situations described by the patient, and indicating to the patient that his feelings have been observed are actions that demonstrate to the patient that the physician is concerned and that increase the patient's self-esteem. For example:

A man with generalized anxiety disorder feels better after a visit to his physician at which the physician listens attentively, summarizes what the patient has told him, and tells him that he understands how distressing it must be to have tension headaches and difficulty concentrating on his work when he is plagued by worries.

Ventilation of Feelings

Patients who keep to themselves strong feelings about past or current experiences usually feel better after releasing their pent-up emotions. An outpouring of emotion can be elicited sometimes by stating that the patient looks tense, angry, or depressed or by commenting that the experience which the patient has just described must have made the patient feel upset. Encouraging the patient to express feelings may loosen his defenses just enough to allow the ventilation to take place. For example:

A middle-aged woman with chronic depressive neurosis (dysthymic disorder) always feels better temporarily when her physician encourages her to ventilate to him, and to cry in the office, about her feelings of guilt due to the anger she develops toward members of her family in her week-to-week life.

Problem Solving

In general, the physician who engages in counseling should be an observer-participant and should avoid acting as a powerful, all-knowing figure. His strategy is to help the patient recognize assets (e.g., supportive people, activities he enjoys) and to make choices that favor resolution of current problems. There are times, however, when the physician may have to be somewhat directive in helping a patient work out plans.

Contingency Planning

The life situations that create stress for patients are often manageable even after slight changes. Distressed patients often cannot see a means of making these changes. Once the physician has a clear understanding of the situation, he and the patient can engage in creative plans for dealing with specific problems that may arise in the days or weeks ahead. In making contingency plans, it is useful to present hypothetical situations and to have the patient decide how he will try to handle them. For example:

A woman who lives alone is distraught because her only child, a grown daughter who recently moved to another city, has hinted that she may not be able to get home for Christmas. The woman's physician encourages her to make another plan for Christmas rather than face the prospect of being alone. She phones later in the week to say that she still does not know if her daughter will be able to come for Christmas; she has, however, invited several friends to have Christmas dinner with her and feels much better.

Advice (Persuasion)

The physician is considered by the patient to be an expert and should judiciously exercise that expertise. Concrete recommendations may be very helpful for patients who are upset and temporarily unable to use their own coping skills. The physician's advice provides the patient with something to hang on to until he can make decisions himself. For example:

A middle-aged man with major depression who is beginning to improve is tactfully dissuaded from entering a doctoral program which is known to be particularly demanding. (This example makes the point that stressful life changes should be discouraged during recovery from a major depressive illness.)

Advice may also be used in a confrontational manner, forcing the patient to face up to the fact that he is engaging in dangerous or destructive behavior. The shock value of the confrontation may pierce the complacence and defensiveness of the patient, thereby allowing the physician to persuade the patient to change behavior.

Managing Illness Behavior

Illness behavior is present when the patient's symptoms/impairments are disproportionate to detectable disease. Patients with somatoform disorders (see Chapter 12) express their distress mainly in terms of somatic complaints and/or dreaded conditions; patients with other psychosocial problems also do so at times. The following general strategies are useful in patients whose psychosocial problems present mainly as illness behavior:

1. *Do not facilitate/reinforce illness behavior.*
   a. Avoid unnecessary testing.
   b. Avoid unnecessary prescribing.
   c. Avoid unnecessary referral to specialists.
   d. Schedule regular visits (*i.e.,* do not make visits contingent on a new or worsening symptom) and stay within a time frame agreed upon for visits.
2. *Permit the patient to have some symptoms (do not view elimination of symptoms as an essential goal).*
3. *Encourage the patient to talk about his life situation instead of about somatic symptoms.*

Example: A patient with somatization disorder and an unremarkable recent urinalysis states that she plans "to see the urologist who took care of my friend's bladder problem" and is persuaded to come for brief weekly visits to her primary physician instead. At the weekly visits, the physician focuses chiefly on the patient's efforts to keep her teenage daughter in school, and he commends her for any success that she reports in handling these and other domestic problems.

Involving Family, Friends, and Environment

Two fundamental psychosocial influences external to the patient are family/close friends and the patient's environment. The physician can facilitate optimal involvement of family and the patient's environment in several ways.

1. *Meeting the family's informational needs.* The family and close friends of a patient with a psychosocial syndrome frequently suffer much because of the patient's illness. They often have the same informational needs as the patient (see above). If they are to understand the patient's feelings/behavior and to handle appropriately their own feelings toward the patient, these needs must be addressed. For example:

The grown son of a man with the recent onset of a major depression telephones the patient's physician and says that he is very concerned. He reports that his father has been angrily criticizing his young grandchildren for all kinds of petty reasons and that this is not the way he used to treat the children. Furthermore, the son is worried that his father must have an ulcer because he leaves the table rubbing his stomach and shaking his head after eating a few bites of each meal. The physician empathizes with the patient's son and explains that the behavior change is very typical for a depressed man, that the antidepressant medication which has just been started should lead to some improvement within 1 to 2 weeks, that a thorough physical exam did not reveal evidence for anything like an ulcer, and that it is very likely that his father will recover entirely within 2 to 4 months.

2. *Enlisting the family's help.* For some conditions in which the patient demonstrates a failure to make choices favoring improvement, the family may be instrumental in promoting such choices. For example:

The family of an alcoholic patient agrees to participate in a family intervention (see Chapter 21) in order to get the patient to accept treatment.

3. *Facilitating healthy choices regarding the patient's environment.* For example:

A woman with a long-standing depressive neurosis (dysthymic disorder) is encouraged to take a job as a companion and housekeeper for an elderly lady with a stroke, and her chronic depressive symptoms improve.

Knowing and Utilizing Community Resources

Support groups, recreational opportunities, vocational opportunities, and home health services are among the community resources that may greatly alter the status of patients with psychosocial problems. The physician's awareness of and enthusiasm about a community resource can be instrumental in determining its impact on the patient. For example:

The depressed and anxious wife of an alcoholic man experiences marked improvement in the symptoms from this common adjustment disorder after she has been active in Al-Anon, an idea suggested by her physician.

An elderly woman joins a geriatric day center, which provides supervision and activity for her 5 days/week. This idea, which was suggested by her physician, enables the patient's family to continue to have her live with them and alleviates the patient's own negativism and a feeling of guilt toward family members who felt compelled to check on her frequently during the day.

FORMS OF COUNSELING

Short Term Counseling

This form of intervention is especially useful in a patient who accepts a psychological formulation for symptoms and who wants professional help in resolving a crisis related to those symptoms. It is a *suppressive* form of psychotherapy, meaning that the

goals of treatment are to strengthen the defenses of
the patient and to relieve symptoms without uncovering, in depth, long-standing intrapsychic conflicts
underlying the current problem. Any or all of the
techniques discussed above may be utilized. Key
elements in all short term counseling are the following:

1. *Agreement on the problem area and the goal,* in
specific terms related to feelings and behavior.

2. *A timetable,* usually 4 to 10 weekly or twice
monthly visits 15 to 30 minutes in length.

3. *Contingency planning* (see above).

4. *Weekly plans* which are essential steps toward
the stated goal; this requires the counselor and the
patient to explore and mobilize existing resources.

Supportive Therapy

Supportive therapy utilizes the techniques of
counseling and, similarly, does not attempt to uncover or resolve psychodynamic issues. Unlike short
term counseling, the duration of supportive therapy
is open ended; and it is often incorporated into the
routine management of a chronic disease. Patients
should participate in the decision about the frequency of visits, and in so doing make a contribution
at least to that portion of the treatment contract.
This form of psychotherapy is useful, for example,
in the long term management of a diabetic patient
with a history of poor compliance and multiple
family problems. Such a patient is seen once a month
for 15 to 30 minutes. The strategies for the sessions
are the following:

1. To monitor the patient's diabetic condition.

2. To enhance compliance.

3. To review family problems.

The verbal exchange between the physician and
the patient during the visit consists of a review of
the therapeutic regimen, an assessment of symptoms, a brief review of what has occurred in the
patient's life since the last visit, and a discussion of
ways to cope with existing family problems. In this
manner, a significant supportive service is provided
in the context of management of the patient's organic disease.

Crisis Intervention

Crisis intervention is a form of short term counseling in which the acuteness of the crisis and the
severity of the symptoms demand somewhat more
vigorous and frequent initial treatment.

Faced with an acute crisis, patients experience a
rise in emotional tension that initiates their usual
problem-solving responses. If the crisis is not resolved, there is a further rise in tension, accompanied by a state of partial or complete ineffectiveness.
If the stress continues with no resolution, further
tension is followed by mobilization of internal resources in a final attempt to cope. If all efforts fail, a
breaking point is reached and psychic disorganiza-

tion results. If feelings of anxiety, depression, hopelessness, and helplessness continue, the patient may
engage in self-destructive acts (e.g., drug overdose)
or may develop regressive behavior such as uncontrolled crying, muteness, and inability to perform
basic self-care.

The theoretic basis of crisis intervention includes
a focus on the immediate event (stressor) accompanied by a recognition that the stressor is both a
threat to the patient and an opportunity for personal
growth if the problem can be overcome. During the
initial contact with the patient, the physician's task
is to identify the details of the event that has precipitated the crisis. Next, the physician assesses the
physiological effects of the stress on the patient,
identifies the patient's psychological strengths and
social resources, and develops a strategy for reducing
the stress. During this phase of intervention, medications may be prescribed to alleviate specific symptoms such as anxiety or sleep loss (see Chapters 13
and 85, respectively). When symptoms are partially
controlled, discussion of a way of resolving the problem begins. Contingency planning is especially important at this point. If during this phase of treatment
the patient experiences strong feelings of rage, anger,
or guilt the patient is allowed to ventilate these
feelings. However, through his physical presence, a
physician helps the patient control the level of affects so that the feelings do not generate destructive
behavior. The next phase of treatment is the implementation of the specific interventions, mutually
agreed upon by the physician and the patient, that
are expected to resolve the effects of the crisis. The
final step of treatment is a review of the entire
process to help the patient consolidate the gains
made in achieving a resolution to crisis. For example:

The patient is a 32-year-old mother of two young children. Her husband died 2 weeks ago following an industrial accident. She has managed to handle the funeral of
her husband with the help and support of several friends.
Her own family lives in another part of the country and
is not readily available during the crisis. She has been
encouraged by friends to come for the evaluation because
of severe headaches and insomnia.

Initial evaluation reveals that the patient is in good
physical health but she feels abandoned, overwhelmed,
and grief stricken. Her headaches and insomnia are adding
to the obvious stress of the situation and further sapping
her emotional and physical resources. She is judged to be
nonsuicidal, but even so the analgesics and sedatives
prescribed are given in small amounts.

The physician schedules a follow-up visit for *the next
day,* which is devoted to a review of her perception of her
social and financial situation. The patient gives a reasonable summary of the steps she must take to stabilize her
situation but suggests that she might not be up to the task.
The physician reviews the effectiveness of the prescribed

medicine, makes adjustments as necessary, asks the patient to prepare a list of specific tasks she must accomplish over the next 2 weeks and gives her an appointment *in 2 days.*

During the next visit the patient is asked to review her list. She indicates a need to make contact with insurance companies, the personnel office of her husband's employer, Social Security, lawyer, bank, *etc.* The physician goes over the list with her, encouraging her efforts and calling to her attention that she omitted from the list time to be spent in the company of close friends who might help her with her grief and sense of abandonment.

Subsequent sessions, spaced according to the judgment of the physician and preferences of the patient, are reviews of the patient's progress in accomplishing the outlined tasks. During one visit the patient becomes very angry, expressing frustration over her inability to contact an insurance agent: "Nobody really gives a damn about me." The physician allows the patient to ventilate, is empathic by indicating that people are not always as helpful as they could be, but then continues with the review of the tasks.

Following two or three additional visits the physician judges the patient to be handling her situation competently. The headaches and insomnia have disappeared. He suggests a final visit during which he reviews the process of their meetings and enumerates the steps the patient has taken in order to gain control of her situation. He does not schedule another meeting but offers her future availability if needed.

Family Counseling

The goals of this form of counseling are (a) to create effective communications among the family members, (b) to bring to their awareness maladaptive patterns of behavior that may be destructive to one or more members of the family, and (c) to change those maladaptive patterns to constructive patterns of behavior. The specific techniques are similar to those used in individual counseling.

Example of family counseling. A couple asked their family physician for help in dealing with their adolescent daughter who was continually misbehaving at school and at home. Evaluation of the problem revealed that the parents had not been consistent in limit setting for their daughter and the family considered the girl to be "the black sheep" of the family. Counseling for the whole family was recommended. During the first session the family members (parents and children) attacked the daughter, blaming her for all of the family's troubles. The physician interrupted the attack by focusing the discussion on the development of a contract between the parents and their daughter designed to define the rules they expected her to follow and the consequences of violating the rules. The next session was a review of the parents' and daughter's adherence to the contract. The parents reported that the daughter broke the contract by misbehaving, but one of the older siblings pointed out the parents were inconsistent in their application of the agreed-upon limit-setting rules. This revelation confronted the family with the fact that the girl's behavior was a shared responsibility within the family. Over the remaining sessions, the physician continued to encourage the family to establish fair rules to which all could adhere consistently. By focusing on the behavior of the entire family, the pressure on the "bad member" was relieved, destructive patterns of interacting were interrupted, and new, constructive patterns were introduced.

General References

Dubovsky SL, Weissberg MP (eds): *Clinical Psychiatry in Primary Care*, ed 2. Baltimore, Williams & Wilkins, 1982.
> A practical book which gives excellent examples of good and poor techniques for management of psychosocial problems by the primary care practitioner.

Frank J: *Persuasion and Healing*, revised ed. Baltimore, Johns Hopkins University Press, 1974.
> Presents model of the patient in distress and of the components of practical psychotherapy.

Frank JD: The influence of patients' and therapists' expectations on the outcome of psychotherapy. *Br J Med Psychol* 41:349, 1968.
> A classic paper on the subject of expectations and treatment outcome.

Imboden JB, Urbaitis JC: *Practical Psychiatry in Medicine.* New York, Appleton-Century-Crofts, 1978.
> Two books containing useful sections on therapeutic techniques appropriate for use in office practice.

Jacobson GF: Programs and techniques of crisis intervention. In Arieti S (ed): *American Handbook of Psychiatry*, ed 2. New York, Basic Books, 1974, vol 2, pp 811–825.
> A concise review of the subject of crisis theory and technique.

Mann J: The specific limitation of time on psychotherapy. *Semin Psychiatry* 1:375, 1969.
> A paper which describes how best to structure short term psychotherapy.

CHAPTER TWELVE

Minor Mood Disturbances and Psychosomatic Conditions

WALTER F. BAILE, M.D., AND L. RANDOL BARKER, M.D.

INTRODUCTION

This chapter describes those emotional and behavioral disturbances which are most often expressed as somatic complaints, with or without associated psychological symptoms. Aside from their effects on patients, such disturbances present problems for the physician since patients often present with symptoms that *mimic* those associated with organic disease, *coexist* with organic disease, or serve as "*triggers*" for visits to the physician.

Illness Behavior

The response of a particular individual to a perceived change for the worse in his physiological state is called *illness behavior*. Illness behavior incorporates two independent but complementary concepts: the notion of "illness" (in contradistinction to "disease," *i.e.*, a biological lesion or dysfunction that can be observed objectively), and the notion of an action taken by an individual to deal with his illness.

Illness

It is generally acknowledged that the task of the clinician is not only to treat disease but to alleviate distress (14); this is as it should be, because it is distress which usually brings the patient to the physician in the first place. The patient may be distressed by worry over a painless breast lump or by the pathophysiological changes of a disease process. Moreover, there may be much disease and little illness (e.g., as in a silent myocardial infarction or asymptomatic coin lesion) or much illness and little disease (e.g., as in severe low back pain for which no anatomical cause can be detected). Thus, illness is a *subjective* experience of distress. It is unique to each individual, affects the whole person, is expressed as "symptoms," and may be experienced in the absence of disease. It involves a complex interaction among perceptual, attitudinal, emotional, evaluative, cultural, and physical factors. This is illustrated by the fact that while certain individuals have a tendency to amplify, focus on, and worry about relatively minor changes in their bodily processes (see Barsky, "General References"), others will rationalize and attempt to ignore such alarming bodily changes as the pain associated with a myocardial infarction.

The distinction between treating disease and treating illness is not new. Long before scientific principles were applied to the understanding and treatment of disease, ritual and reassurance, empathy and encouragement were the mainstays of healing. Rarely was the course of disease changed. However, if success is measured in terms of relief of distress, the results were often impressive.

Since physicians in ambulatory practice tend to see many patients in distress, the ability to distinguish between illness and disease is crucial. Although the distress may be a response to the pathophysiology of disease, distress often seems out of proportion to the amount of disease, or it may be present even when no disease process can be detected. This often presents a diagnostic dilemma for the clinician. Much of this chapter focuses upon the role that emotional distress plays in the symptoms of many of these patients.

The Decision to Seek Care

The patient's decision to seek care is the action by which he brings his illness to the attention of a professional. Studies have shown that the relationship between the presence of symptoms and care-seeking behavior is far from linear. White and his colleagues (15) reviewed English and American studies and calculated that during an average month in a population of 1000 adults 16 years of age and older, 750 experience what they recognize as an injury or illness on at least one occasion. Among this population, 250 consult a physician, 9 are hospitalized, 5 are referred to another physician, and 1 is referred to a university medical center. In terms of actual disease, there may be little which distinguishes those who come under treatment from those who do not. Thus, in an annual report on health problems in the United States, it was found that about 13% of deaths in 1976 would have been preventable with medical intervention (7), suggesting that many patients with obvious signs and symptoms of disease failed to pay attention to their problem. On the other hand, in this report it was also noted that the largest proportion of ambulatory visits were for problems rated as "not serious" by the physician; similar findings have been reported in general practice in England (13).

Many factors determine whether a particular individual seeks medical care at a given time. The simplest assumption is that pain, malaise, and other symptoms cause discomfort and distresss that interfere with normal functioning or may exceed the individual's threshold for tolerance. Nevertheless many persons avoid medical care despite obvious signs and symptoms of disease, while others appear to overreact to minor problems. Clearly, nonphysiological factors may serve as important "triggers" for utilization of medical care. The importance of these factors is illustrated by the study of Zola (17), who surveyed patients at the time of their first visit to a university medical outpatient clinic to determine why they decided to visit the clinic at that particular time. Extensive interviews and follow-up of the patients indicated the following: First, the physical complaints of the patients were often of long duration, and many had tolerated considerable disability before initiating the visit. Second, in most cases the symptom, although it may have caused distress, was influenced by the person's psychosocial environment. Zola distinguished in his patient population several nonphysiological "triggers" for the decision to seek medical help:

1. The occurrence of an interpersonal crisis (e.g., a young lady who is fighting with her mother over her dating behavior complains of symptoms related to her chronic ear infection).

2. The perceived interference of the symptom with interpersonal or social relationships (e.g., a teenager complains about his acne at a time when his classmates are making dates for the upcoming prom).

3. "Sanctioning"—seeking medical attention because a family member or friend insists (e.g., a woman finally sees a doctor for a painless breast mass after weeks of badgering by her husband).

4. The idea that the symptom will interfere with vocational or physical activity (e.g., a middle-aged man with a long-standing hernia becomes concerned that it will interfere with his sexual performance, soon after he has begun "dating" a year after his wife's death).

5. Providing a time limit for symptoms to abate (e.g., the setting of external time criteria—"if it isn't better in a week, I'll take care of it").

Clearly the interplay between symptoms and care-seeking behavior is complex. In examples 2 through 4 above, the decision to seek care was prompted by *distress* associated with the symptoms rather than by physical discomfort, and there was a direct relationship between the symptoms and the social problem. In example 1, on the other hand, the symptoms were not directly related to the social problem, but the problem exacerbated existing symptoms of an unrelated illness. Thus visits to physicians may be prompted by psychosocial factors that are related in various ways to concomitant disease.

Somatic symptoms may be the principal symptoms of an acute or chronic psychiatric disorder. *Acute disorders* are often precipitated by discrete environmental stressors, tend to occur in adulthood, and present with symptoms that for the most part are somatic expressions of anxiety and mood disturbance. In many cases the patient has functioned fairly well in job, family, and interpersonal spheres, but a specific event will be associated with the onset of symptoms. The onset of *chronic disorders* may often be traced to adolescence or early adulthood. By the time the patient is seen in later life there is often global disturbance of functioning. These patients are more likely to have severe personality disturbances that are associated with the unconscious use of symptoms and of the sick role to establish some level of functioning, albeit an unsatisfactory one (see chapter 14, Maladaptive Personalities).

Prevention of Iatrogenic Illness Behavior

Given the powerful reinforcers existing in the medical system (e.g., ordering tests, prescribing drugs, inquiring about physical symptoms), the physician who is aware of the role psychosocial problems may play in generating physical complaints and medical visits may be instrumental in preventing some abnormal illness behavior. Although it is sometimes difficult to avoid certain tests for fear of missing a diagnosis, the decision for further workup, of a patient whose history and physical examination are unrevealing, should always be balanced against the knowledge that this may promote excessive physician utilization and prolong the sick role. Questioning the patient briefly about his ability to function in personal, family, and occupational spheres and allowing some time to elapse after the patient has presented his symptoms are the most efficient ways to determine whether psychosocial factors are involved, and thus to avoid actions which may reinforce illness behavior.

The place of this general preventive approach is pointed out in more detail in the description of each of the specific problems discussed below.

MINOR MOOD DISTURBANCE AND ADJUSTMENT DISORDER

Description

Psychiatric morbidity in office practice most often presents as a minor mood disturbance, related to a stressor in the patient's life. When certain criteria are met, the American Psychiatric Association's Diagnostic and Statistical Manual of Mental Disorders (DSM-III) diagnosis for a minor mood disturbance is adjustment disorder (see Table 12.1). Table 10.2 (page 129) lists the usual categories of stressors that cause adjustment disorders. These illnesses are called "minor" because they do not cause the overwhelming symptoms of major depression (Chapter 15) or of chronic anxiety neuroses (Chapter 13) and somatoform disorders (below) and because the prognosis is usually favorable. However, patients with adjustment disorders, and their families, may suffer much anguish while the problem is active.

Minor mood disturbances usually result from "life crises" reflecting problems in adjusting to demands of the environment (11). In these situations, environmental stressors (physical, interpersonal, economic, etc) temporarily impair the individual's ability to cope and result in increased tension, worry, demor-

alization, and irritability. Often, the patient with an adjustment disorder expresses his distress in somatic terms, both because somatic complaints "legitimate" a visit to the doctor and because anxiety and depression cause well known somatic symptoms, such as light-headedness, fatigue, gastrointestinal problems, cold intolerance, increased frequency of micturition, palpitations, precordial pain, breathlessness, and flushing. These are often the presenting symptoms of the patient, as seen in the following case.

Example: A 26-year-old, usually shy, parochial school teacher was evaluated for symptoms of dizziness, abdominal cramps, nausea, excessive urination, and a sensation of fullness in the bladder. When physical examination and laboratory tests revealed no physiological disturbance, a more detailed history was taken. It showed that his symptoms began shortly after a confrontation with his school principal over his attempt to organize a teacher's union and his criticism of several school policies. In his ensuing anger he applied for a job that he did not really want. His symptoms prevented him from taking the scheduled examination for the position. (Diagnosis: adjustment disorder with anxious mood.)

Individuals such as this patient are often unaware (or only partially aware) of the relationship between their psychological disturbance and somatic symptoms. Symptoms brought on by anxiety and depression can mimic almost any disease entity. As illustrated in the following example, diagnosis may be particularly difficult when the symptoms of psychosocial distress mimic those of a patient's established disease process.

Table 12.1.
Diagnostic Criteria for Adjustment Disorder[a]

A. A maladaptive reaction to an identifiable psychosocial stressor (including a recent illness), that occurs within 3 months of the onset of the stressor.
B. The maladaptive nature of the reaction is indicated by either of the following:
    1. Impairment in social or occupational functioning
    2. Symptoms that are in excess of a normal and expected reaction to the stressor
C. The disturbance is not merely one instance of a pattern of overreaction to stress or an exacerbation of one of the mental disorders previously described (in DSM-III).
D. It is assumed that the disturbance will eventually remit after the stressor ceases or, if the stressor persists, when a new level of adaptation is achieved.
E. The disturbance does not meet the criteria for any of the specific disorders listed (in DSM-III) previously or for uncomplicated bereavement.

Note: DSM-III subgroups adjustment disorders into the following categories, based on the manifestations that predominate:
1. *With depressed mood* (e.g., depressed mood, tearfulness, hopelessness).
2. *With anxious mood* (e.g, worrying, jitteryness, insomnia).
3. *With mixed emotional feelings* (includes more than one emotional pattern, e.g., sadness, anger, anxiety, ambivalence).
4. *With disturbance of conduct* (e.g., truancy, vandalism, reckless driving, fighting, defaulting on legal responsibilities).
5. *With mixed disturbance of emotion and conduct* (see 3 and 4 above)
6. *With work (or academic) inhibition* (e.g., inability to write papers or reports).

[a] From American Psychiatric Association: *Diagnostic and Statistical Manual of Mental Disorders*, ed 3. Washington, DC, American Psychiatric Association, 1980.

Example: A 54-year-old widowed white woman recovering from a recent myocardial infarction complained to her physician on several occasions of fatigue, breathlessness, and pleuritic-like chest pain unrelated to exertion. Her physical examination and ECG were unchanged from when she left the hospital. Questioning revealed that she was forced to leave her job after her heart attack and was barely able to afford the $40/month needed for medication. She tearfully revealed that although her son had offered to help pay for her medication, her daughter-in-law hinted they could really not afford to help out. This proud and, until recently, self-sufficient woman who was initially reluctant to accept any help was now made to feel like a "charity case" by her son's wife; and yes, she reported that the periodic symptoms in her chest invariably occurred while she was thinking about her plight. (Diagnosis: adjustment disorder, with mixed emotional features.)

In this case anxiety and mild depression produced symptoms, some of which suggested cardiac decompensation. The correct diagnosis was made when psychiatric consultation was eventually requested to rule out a functional disorder and the appropriate history was elicited.

Distress which is provoked by life crisis is usually *self-limited.* Often the complaints will seem trivial to the physician. The frequency with which episodes of dysphoria occur depends upon the stability of the individual's environment and upon his own internal coping resources. The assumption of the "sick role" on the part of the patient may allow him to relinquish responsibilities temporarily, regroup his forces, and mobilize new resources for coping. A visit to the physician is an attempt to obtain help and it is also legitimizes the "sick role."

Evaluation

Two strategies are important in evaluating patients who seem to have minor mood disturbances:

1. *Eliciting the relevant history.* Asking the patient open-ended questions such as "How are things at home (or at work)?" will generally provide some clue about whether there are psychosocial disturbances. If so, diagnosis may be confirmed by a history of sleep and/or appetite disturbance, increased irritability, difficulty in concentrating, excess worry, increased tension, or loss of interest in social activities or sexual relations. It is important to allow the patient to expand on his personal history. Most patients are grateful for a physician's interest in their personal problem, will respect time limits, and with a little advice, reassurance, and encouragement will go on to solve the precipitating problem themselves. Even before the physician has taken a psychosocial history, there may be indicators of a psychosocial problem, such as verbal and nonverbal cues suggesting distress (e.g., the comment "things aren't the way they used to be" or hand wringing and looking

away when describing a new somatic symptom), a bizarre description of the symptoms, or failure to respond to previous treatment known to work specifically for a somatic disorder (5).

In some instances, patients may be defensive and reluctant to admit psychosocial problems even when these problems are clearly present. In such cases the physician should try to build a trusting relationship, in the expectation that the patient will eventually disclose the problems underlying his distress.

2. *Tempering the workup.* Obviously the patient should be examined and laboratory tests needed to evaluate a symptom should be ordered. However, extensive workups to exclude possible diagnoses may prolong the sick role and increase the risk that the patient will develop chronic illness behavior. This may occur especially when factors such as compensation claims or other gains are involved or when the stressor is prolonged and beyond the patient's capability to remove, influence, or change it. In these instances unproductive workups and doctor shopping tend to imbed the patient in the sick role.

Management

Management of patients with minor mood disturbance or adjustment disorder is based upon several considerations:

1. Patients who are not coping well often feel at once that they have failed and that they are powerless to overcome the stressors that have produced their dilemma. When the physician, in taking the history, explores the possible role of a psychosocial stressor as an etiological factor in the patient's symptoms, he allows the patient to relinquish his embarrassment and guilt at this perceived failure.

2. The fundamental processes of office psychotherapy, described in Chapter 11—e.g., transference, meeting informational needs, catharsis (achieved by ventilation), and problem solving—facilitate the resolution of most adjustment disorders.

3. Explaining the role of psychosocial stressors provides a rationale to the patient for his symptoms.

4. There are often concrete ways in which the patient can be helped to modify, or adapt to, the stressor(s) that underlies his symptoms. Examples are (a) encouraging a socially isolated person to begin a regular activity such as bowling, volunteer work, or an "eating together" program; (b) referring a patient to a self-help group which specifically addresses the patient's needs—e.g., group therapy for families of Alzheimer patients (see Chapter 17) or Al-Anon for the spouse of an alcoholic (see Chapter 21); (c) persuading a patient to agree to family counseling, when it is clear that there are serious interpersonal conflicts in the patient's household.

5. Short term prescription of anxiolytic or hypnotic medication (see Chapter 13, The Anxious Patient, and Chapter 85, Sleep Disorders) may be help-

ful. Such prescribing is not likely to lead to abuse when it is agreed upon for a short interval, especially with a patient whose distress is likely to be limited in duration, such as a patient who has recently suffered an important loss.

6. A number of drugs can exacerbate dysphoric symptoms and should be avoided in patients with minor mood disturbances (see next section).

The identification of a psychosocial basis for a patient's somatic complaints is often sufficient to allow him to begin to marshall his own resources for coping (8). However, when this information and the other measures listed above fail to help, the patient may need goal-focused short term counseling (described in Chapter 11) to facilitate problem solving.

Outcome of management. There have been only a few reports of the outcome of minor mood disturbances managed by generalists (2, 3, 8, 13). From these studies, the following tentative conclusions can be stated:

1. A large proportion of patients get better *after just one office visit.* Most often, this visit includes empathic listening, a partial physical examination, and reassurance that the patient does not have a serious physical problem.

2. Short term prescribing of drugs for anxiety or insomnia may not increase the proportion of patients who show significant improvement—about two-thirds of patients—when they are re-evaluated after 1 month (2). This conclusion derives from a single careful study of this important issue, in which patients with minor mood disturbances were allocated at random to receive brief counseling plus a benzodiazepine drug or just brief counseling.

Several practical considerations regarding longitudinal management are suggested by these outcome findings:

1. It is generally prudent to determine the impact of an initial visit upon a patient's distress—by brief telephone or office follow-up within a week—before prescribing a psychotropic drug for a minor mood disorder.

2. Psychotropic drugs may have their biggest impact when they are prescribed for just 1 to 2 weeks to the patient whose symptoms have not improved within a week of the initial visit.

3. Some patients (approximately one-third) who seem to have an adjustment disorder do not respond to the above management strategies. At follow-up visits, such patients should be interviewed more systematically to look for evidence of other syndromes, in particular panic disorder or generalized anxiety disorder (see Chapter 13), a major affective disorder (see Chapter 15), alcoholism or another chemical dependency (see Chapters 21 and 22), or one of the somatoform disorders (see below). For all of these problems, specific treatment in addition to office psychotherapy is indicated.

DRUG-INDUCED DYSPHORIA

In evaluating patients with mood disturbances, it is important to identify all drugs that they are taking, for medical or recreational reasons, since a number of drugs may either cause or exacerbate dysphoria (see Table 12.2). As noted above, such drugs should be avoided in the patient with a stressor-induced mood disturbance. Whenever use of a drug or withdrawal of a drug appears to be the primary cause of the patient's dysphoria, this should be explained to the patient; management consists of discontinuing the offending drug or, for drugs of abuse, getting the patient to agree to treatment (see Chapter 21 on alcoholism, and Chapter 22 on illicit drugs).

Common examples of drug-provoked mood disturbances are (a) symptoms of depression following the initiation of a central acting antihypertensive (*i.e.*, beta β-blockers, clonidine, gunabenz, methyldopa, reserpine); (b) physical symptoms of anxiety (tremulousness, palpitations, *etc*) associated with overuse of multiple over-the-counter cold remedies containing sympathomimetic decongestants; or excessive use of caffeine, and withdrawal from caffeine or nicotine after habitual use; (c) symptoms of depression or anxiety associated with abuse of or withdrawal from alcohol and sedative-hypnotic drugs.

Table 12.2.
Drugs and Other Substances That May Exacerbate (or Produce) Symptoms of Dysphoria

SYMPTOMS OF DEPRESSION
   Antihypertensives
      Clonidine
      Methyldopa
      Reserpine
      β-Blockers
   Antidepressants
   Antihistamines
   Anxiolytic drugs
   Cimetidine
   Neuroleptic drugs
   Sedative-hypnotic drugs
   Alcoholic beverages
SYMPTOMS OF ANXIETY
   Anticholinergic drugs
   Stimulant drugs of abuse (see Chapter 22)
   Sympathomimetic drugs:
      Decongestants (found in most over-the-counter cold remedies)
      β-2 bronchodilators
      Weight reduction agents
   Xanthine-containing drugs, foods, and beverages:
      Bronchodilators with theophylline
      Many over-the-counter cold and arthritis remedies
      Use and discontinuation of caffeine
   Thyroid hormone
   Discontinuation of alcohol, sedative-hypnotic drugs, and tobacco

SOMATOFORM DISORDERS

Grouped together in the DSM-III classification are three serious and often chronic disorders whose essential feature is the presentation by the patient of physical symptoms (a) for which there are no demonstrable findings of organic disease and no known physiological mechanisms to explain the symptoms and (b) for which there is positive evidence, or a strong presumption, that they are related to psychological factors or conflicts. These disorders are hypochondriasis, somatization disorder, and conversion disorder. Table 12.3 summarizes the salient features of these three disorders. Because most patients are seen by internists and family physicians and do not often come under extended psychiatric observation, our understanding of the etiology and natural history of the disorders is incomplete.

Unlike factitious disorder and malingering (see below), symptom production is not under voluntary control in patients with the somatoform disorders.

Hypochondriasis

Description

Hypochondriasis (see Table 12.4) is a disorder commonly seen in medical practice, the cardinal manifestation of which is an unrealistic interpretation by a patient of normal physical signs or sensa-

Table 12.3.
Major Features of the Principal Somatoform Disorders

Characteristics	Hypochondriasis (Hypochondriacal Neurosis)	Somatization Disorder (Briquet's Syndrome, Hysteria)	Conversion Disorder (Hysterical Neurosis, Conversion Type)
Essential features	Fear of or belief in presence of serious disease in absence of objective findings; misinterpretation of normal physical symptoms or signs	Multiple somatic complaints without organic pathology; long history of questionable medical treatment, procedures, and surgeries; vague, tangential verbal style	Loss or alteration of sensory or voluntary motor functioning not explained by pathophysiology; usually involves one organ or system
Associated features	May be component of somatization disorder or other disorders; history of doctor shopping, anxiety, depression	Interpersonal difficulties; history of depression or suicide attempts or anxiety; lack of insight	May be component of somatization disorder or other disorders; symptoms often suggest neurological disease
Prevalence	Probably common; equal in men and women	May affect as many as 1% of all women; rare in men	Prevalence in ambulatory practice unknown
Age at onset	Adolescence, thirties, or forties	Adolescence or young adulthood	Adolescence, early adulthood
Course	Chronic, fluctuating	Chronic, fluctuating	Generally unknown; 50% may recover in 1 year
Impairment and complications	Variable; strained doctor-patient relations	Related to substance abuse, doctor shopping, medical, surgical procedures; serious depression may lead to suicide attempt	Marked effect on life style; disuse may lead to atrophy; 10–30% of patients develop organic disease related to symptom
Predisposing factors	Psychosocial stressors; (?) previous organic disease	Unknown	Presence of "model," life stress (usually unrecognized by patient)
Familial pattern	Unknown	Occurs with greater than chance frequency in female family members; history of alcoholism and sociopathy in first degree male relative	Unknown
Differential diagnosis	Physical disorder; major psychiatric disorders (especially depression)	Physical disorders (*e.g.*, hyperparathyroidism, multiple sclerosis (MS), systemic lupus erythematosus (SLE); schizophrenia with multiple somatic delusions; major depression; conversion disorder)	Physical disorders (*e.g.*, MS, SLE), somatization disorder, hypochondriasis

Table 12.4.
Diagnostic Criteria for Hypochondriasis[a]

A. The predominant disturbance is an unrealistic interpretation of physical signs or sensations as abnormal, leading to preoccupation with the fear or belief of having a serious disease.

B. Thorough physical evaluation does not support the diagnosis of any physical disorder that can account for the physical signs or sensations or for the individual's unrealistic interpretation of them.

C. The unrealistic fear or belief of having a disease persists despite medical reassurance and causes impairment in social or occupational functioning.

D. Not due to any other mental disorder such as schizophrenia, affective disorder, or somatization disorder.

[a] From American Psychiatric Association: *Diagnostic and Statistical Manual of Mental Disorders*, ed 3. Washington, DC, American Psychiatric Association, 1980.

tions leading him to believe that he suffers from a serious disease. This misbelief is usually refractory to energetic efforts to reassure the patient to the contrary.

Hypochondriasis most commonly has its onset in midlife. It is equally frequent in both sexes and tends to affect all social classes. It usually runs a chronic, fluctuating course. Symptoms and impairment may be severe or mild. Patients often have obsessive compulsive personality traits, are egocentric and unduly sensitive to criticism, and have difficulty expressing feelings.

In some cases hypochondriasis will dominate the person's entire personality and govern his lifestyle. In others it may exist in milder forms, especially as part of obsessive compulsive personality disorders, and not significantly disturb the individual's functioning. An example of the milder form follows.

Example: A 30-year-old accountant had always been preoccupied about his physical appearance. He attempted to allay this concern by weight lifting and by constantly comparing himself to other individuals. After his father died of a heart attack he became concerned that he might have heart disease and was fearful about the implication of any insignificant chest pain. He also worried about his blood pressure, which was transiently elevated at the time of his yearly physical examinations. His most recent examination revealed insignificantly elevated activity of liver enzymes, which he fretted over for weeks. Despite these concerns he rarely missed a day's work. He was not sure that he did not have a serious disease but thought he had best trust his physician. He was a minor annoyance to his physician because of the difficulty in reassuring him.

While the physician will see patients such as this young man, it is the chronic, older hypochondriac who presents the most difficult management problem. Often he will "doctor shop" because of preoc-

cupation with a single dreaded illness or with a single organ system or several systems. Two striking features of this illness are the amount of worry or concern invested in even a minor symptom such as a scratchy throat or a cough, and the amount of time invested in seeking a diagnosis. In severe cases there may be interference with work, and the individual may develop the life style of an invalid, creating constant or periodic stress for his family and friends. When there is increased psychosocial stress in the patient's life, his hypochondriacal behavior will predictably increase.

The etiology of this disorder is unknown. Personality traits and psychosocial stressors predispose to its onset, as does previous disease in the patient or in a family member who may serve as a "model."

The DSM-III criteria for the diagnosis of hypochondriasis are listed in Table 12.4. Additional features that may be part of hypochondriasis are (a) a history of past illnesses that cannot be confirmed in medical records and that may, in fact, be the patient's own diagnostic formulations for past symptoms (e.g., "I had scarlet fever lasting almost 2 years" or "Almost once a year I have a couple of weeks of back pain due to kidney stones"); and (b) the patient's report that he knows a lot about his illnesses because he reads about them in his "doctor book." The fact that the patient's symptoms are usually limited to one or two organ systems, the degree of conviction that the patient expresses in having a disease, the *cognitive* nature of the patient's distress, and pre-existing obsessive compulsive personality traits distinguish it from somatization disorder (see description below).

Management

Treatment of the hypochondriac is difficult and frustrating, especially when the disorder is chronic and severe. Patients are taxing, demanding, and generally refuse to consider the possibility that they may have an emotional problem.

The viewpoint of Aldrich (1) and the strategy for management he suggests may be useful for both chronic hypochondriasis and for the other somatoform disorders mentioned in this chapter. Management of the patient is based upon the following considerations:

1. The symptoms serve a purpose, by means of which a person who is not coping can save face. The sick role exonerates people from normal responsibility.

2. Early learning probably plays a part in the process; persons with chronic hypochondriasis probably were put to bed for minor ailments and had parents who worried excessively about their health.

3. Adults cannot ask for reassurances or nurture unless they are helpless. The health care system is a way to get this support; medicines, examinations, and procedures serve to provide attention.

4. New symptoms are ways of assuring attention;

intermittent reinforcement by physician, family, *etc* strengthen symptom reporting.

5. The motivating forces behind the patient's behavior are beyond his level of awareness.

It follows that: (*a*) Attempting to reassure the patient of absence of disease will not be effective and will be seen as a rejection (*b*) Administration of medicines (especially placebos), tests, and procedures just to "see if there's something we missed" or to prove that the patient is not really sick will reinforce symptoms (this is difficult to avoid in the "age of malpractice"). (*c*) Referring the patient to a psychiatrist will probably be unsuccessful since it threatens the face-saving purpose of the symptoms. (*d*) Positive medical diagnoses and specific treatments will not satisfy the patient, and new symptoms will emerge.

Treatment of the hypochondriac, therefore, is based upon the understanding that the patient has learned to cope with everyday problems by avoiding them; this is in part a learned response and has been reinforced by the medical system and the environment. Only by reduction of "illness behavior" and removal of the reinforcers will the patient be able to deal better with everyday stresses. Treatment must be undertaken by the patient's general physician; the chronic hypochondriac will not see a psychiatrist since it merely will be interpreted by the patient that "it's all in your head." Once the diagnosis of hypochondriasis is made, the following strategy should be utilized:

1. Schedule regular visits (e.g., 15 minutes every 2 to 4 weeks) so that the patient does not need a new symptom to initiate a visit "only when necessary."

2. Tell the patient that his problems are partially due to tension and stress and that visits will focus on these.

3. Do not attempt to "take away" the patient's somatic symptoms; rather, the patient is encouraged to carry on despite the presence of symptoms.

4. Stay within the time framework decided even if the patient attempts to prolong the session.

5. Encourage the patient to talk about his or her life situations; clarify alternatives, but remind the patient that the choice among them is his (i.e., avoid giving advice).

6. Likewise resist the patient's plea for numerous tests or for referrals to specialists.

7. Be tolerant of being tested by the patient. At first the patient may telephone between visits with new symptoms; treat new symptoms professionally and detachedly; manage contacts between sessions pleasantly and as quickly as possible; treat frequent between-visit telephone calls with *increased* contact.

Although not always effective, this strategy enables one to gain some control in a difficult situation. The greatest danger to its success will be the physi-cians' impatience. One should be prepared for improvement to take a long time consistent with the treatment of any chronic physical or psychiatric disorder.

Somatization Disorder (Briquet's Syndrome, Hysteria)

Description (9a)

This clinical entity was previously known as "Briquet's syndrome" after the French physician Paul Briquet who first described and categorized the symptoms of more than 400 patients with this disorder. The etiology is unknown; however, it runs in families, affects 1 to 2% of adult women, and the frequency of sociopathy and alcoholism is increased in first degree male relatives of the patient. It is important for the generalist to recognize this entity because it is not uncommon, is often associated with substance abuse, and frequently results in the patient having unnecessary medical and surgical procedures.

The DSM-III criteria for the diagnosis of somatization disorder are listed in Table 12.5. The main clinical characteristics of the disorder are: (*a*) The patient presents with multiple vague somatic complaints (more than 10), which involve several different organ symptoms. When seen early in the course, when the patient is usually in her early twenties the most frequent mode of presentation is with complaints referable to the reproductive tract: painful menstruation, menstrual irregularity, excessive bleeding, severe vomiting throughout pregnancy. Later on there is a shift of symptomatology: headaches, fainting spells, nausea, vomiting, abdominal pains, bowel difficulties, and fatigue predominate. (*b*) The presenting symptoms have little or no organic basis. One or more symptoms may have the characteristics of a conversion disorder (see below). (*c*) The patient's medical history will usually include: treatment by a multiplicity of physicians, multiple surgical and medical procedures (laparotomy, removal of "adhesions," and multiple cystoscopies are common) for which there is no organic basis; and possible substance abuse. (*d*) The mode of presentation of the symptoms is often circumstantial and somewhat incoherent. The physician may feel particularly frustrated and perplexed not only by the variety of somatic complaints, but also because the patient may be unable to give any coherent history of the problems, often interjecting descriptions of how they have affected life style and relationships, relating irrelevant details about treatment, yet being unable to describe crisply the nature, character, location, onset, and duration of the symptoms. (*e*) Patients often show manifestations of the histrionic personality or the borderline personality (see Chapter 14). (*f*) Typically the patient's attitude is that she has been sick most of her life

Table 12.5.
Diagnostic Criteria for Somatization Disorder[a]

A. A history of physical symptoms of several years' duration beginning before the age of 30.
B. Complaints of at least 14 symptoms for women and 12 for men, from the 37 symptoms listed below. To count a symptom as present the individual must report that the symptom caused him or her to take medicine (other than aspirin), alter his or her life pattern, or see a physician. The symptoms, in the judgment of the clinician, are not adequately explained by physical disorder or physical injury, and are not side effects of medication, drugs, or alcohol. The clinician need not be convinced that the symptom was actually present, *e.g.*, that the individual actually vomited throughout her entire pregnancy; report of the symptom by the individual is sufficient.

Sickly: Believes that he or she has been sickly for a good part of his or her life.

Conversion or pseudoneurological symptoms: Difficulty swallowing, loss of voice, deafness, double vision, blurred vision, blindness, fainting or loss of consciousness, memory loss, seizures or convulsions, trouble walking, paralysis or muscle weakness, urinary retention or difficulty urinating.

Gastrointestinal symptoms: Abdominal pain, nausea, vomiting spells (other than during pregnancy), bloating (gassy), intolerance (*e.g.*, gets sick) of a variety of foods, diarrhea.

Female reproductive symptoms: Judged by the individual as occuring more frequently or severely than in most women: painful menstruation, menstrual irregularity, excessive bleeding, severe vomiting throughout pregnancy or causing hospitalization during pregnancy.

Psychosexual symptoms: For the major part of the individual's life after opportunities for sexual activity: sexual indifference, lack of pleasure during intercourse, pain during intercourse.

Pain: Pain in back, joints, extremities, genital area (other than during intercourse); pain on urination; other pain (other than headaches).

Cardiopulmonary symptoms: Shortness of breath, palpitations, chest pain, dizziness.

[a] From American Psychiatric Association: *Diagnostic and Statistical Manual of Mental Disorders*, ed 3. Washington, DC, American Psychiatric Association, 1980.

and that she has no insight into the true nature of her disorder. (g) There may be a history of a suicide attempt or overt depressive symptoms. (h) The patient often has a history of psychosexual problems—sexual indifference, lack of pleasure during intercourse, painful intercourse.

The following case illustrates several of the features of this disorder:

The patient was a 43-year-old married white woman who was referred for psychiatric evaluation by her internist who, noting her presentation with, "ill defined symptoms" was requesting information about management. She had presented with complaints of generalized muscle aching, and periodic sensations throughout her body described as "what one has when hearing someone scratch his fingers on a blackboard." She also complained of skin lesions on her back and stated that she was hypothyroid and suffered from a chronic urinary tract infection. Her past history included tonsillectomy, groin lymph node biopsy (twice), hysterectomy, bladder suspension (twice), rectocele repair, removal of adhesions, multiple cystoscopies, appendectomy, and removal of a tongue papilloma. The patient stated she suffered from Ménière's disease and episodes of hyperventilation. She also carried a diagnosis of "fibrositis" for which she had taken steroids in the past and "restless leg syndrome." She had stopped having sexual intercourse with her husband because of pain that "10 gynecologists could not cure." Her current medicines were Clinoril, Valium, and Bellergal. She mentioned that she had "always been ill" and that she "hated men." Her psychosocial history included marriage to an alcoholic who abused her, and a positive family history of suicide. In presenting her symptoms, the patient was extremely vague and interjected facts about her emotional life with an inappropriate laugh. She had little insight into the nature of her problem, believing her symptoms were due to "food allergy." She had stopped eating everything and at the time of her initial visit to her internist had ingested only distilled water for 4 days. Physical examination and laboratory tests were normal.

Somatization disorder tends to run a chronic but fluctuating course characterized by episodes of aggressive doctor shopping and interludes in which the patient remains "stably symptomatic." This disorder is not difficult to recognize since the history suggests that it has been present for a number of years. The diffuseness and vagueness of the multiplicity of symptoms, the mode of presentation of complaints, and a past history of doctor shopping in the context of a mostly negative physical examination and laboratory tests are the essential criteria for making the diagnosis. The features that distinguish somatization disorder from hypochondriasis are (a) the fact that the patient's symptoms involve many systems; (b) the drama and dysphoria attached to symptoms, in contrast to the cognitive distress which typifies hypochondriasis; (c) the onset is usually in late teens or early twenties (thirties and forties for hypochondriasis); and (d) somatization disorder occurs almost exclusively in women (about 1% of women) while hypochondriasis occurs equally in both sexes. Since these patients, like hypochondriacs, may indeed experience organic disease, new symptoms need to be evaluated carefully.

Management

Treatment of these patients is difficult because of their lack of insight. To tell the patient "I can't find anything wrong with you" is inviting doctor shopping. Since many of these patients lead chaotic lives with marital and domestic turmoil, psychosocial crises may precipitate or maintain complaining behavior. The physician, in taking the patient's history, can invite her to talk about her social problems, which may succeed in shifting the focus away from the bodily complaints. An approach similar to that outlined above for the treatment of the chronic hypochondriac may succeed in settling the patient down and in stabilizing an emotional crisis. The patient should be prevented from undergoing multiple unnecessary diagnostic procedures and surgery. When the family structure is fairly stable, an attempt may be made to work with family members to achieve limited therapeutic goals for the patient.

Family members are usually frustrated and may insist that the physician do more to diagnose and treat the patient. In this situation, Murphy (9a) recommends having concerned family members recount what has already transpired; this helps them to recognize the fundamental facts about the patient's problem, i.e., that no serious disease has ever been found and that the patient seems to be wedded to a life of multiple symptoms. The physician's strategy of giving attention without embarking on complicated evaluations may then be appreciated and supported by the patient's family. It is not necessary, and it may be counterproductive, to tell the family the name of the patient's disorder.

Prognosis for lasting improvement in this disorder is poor. Some patients may improve with intensive, expert psychotherapy, but for most management consists of careful handling of new complaints as they arise and attempts to help the patients stabilize their living situation.

Conversion Disorder

Description

Conversion disorder or hysterical neurosis, conversion type, is a disorder in which the patient complains of loss or alteration in physical functioning, most often loss of a voluntary motor function or another neurological symptom. The symptom suggests an organic problem, but is instead an expression of an unconscious psychological conflict or need. The symptom can mimic any organic problem. The most obvious and classic symptoms are paralysis, aphonia, and seizures.

Example: A 15-year-old girl abruptly lost her voice and developed an unremitting cough for which there was no organic pathology. The symptoms had their onset shortly after her brother had been transferred to the school that she attended. Family counseling by a psychiatrist revealed that the girl's brother had been experiencing emotional problems with which the family had failed to deal, and which recently had been worsening to the point of incip-

ient psychosis. With her brother in the same school, the patient felt even more intensely the burden of keeping the family "secret." By becoming the patient herself she was able to avoid the stressful situation. Her aphonia allowed her to deal with the conflict between her brother's deterioration and the family mores. Family therapy allowed the identification of the real problem and permitted the patient to relinquish her symptom.

Often, as in the above case, the symptom has symbolic value in that it may serve to solve an internal conflict created by a feeling, impulse, or wish that the individual may find morally or ethically unacceptable (primary gain). The conversion may also allow the individual to gain certain support from the environment (secondary gain). A conversion disorder is likely to involve a single symptom during a single episode. Sometimes the symptom mimics those of a previous illness or illnesses of others significant to the patient ("modeling"). The expression of the symptom, however, will often follow the *patient's* notion of an anatomical distribution or function that will be reflected in the sensory or motor loss.

Conversion symptoms usually have their onset in adolescence or childhood. Their prevalence in ambulatory settings is unknown. Their significance for the generalist is that not only do they mimic organic disease, but also several follow-up studies of hospitalized patients diagnosed as having conversion disorders showed that from 13% to 30% subsequently developed organic disorders, most of them neurological, related to their "conversion" symptoms (9). The physician must thus be cautious in his approach to these patients.

The DSM-III criteria for the diagnosis of conversion disorder are listed in Table 12.6. Additional features that may be present in patients with conversion symptoms are the following: (a) the pathological process follows the patient's notion of bodily functions; (b) a history of previous conversion reactions or undiagnosable physical symptoms; (c) a symptom "model" (i.e., a significant person who has or did have a similar loss of function, often a person remembered from childhood); and (d) associated psychopathology, especially somatization disorder, depression, schizophrenia, or a personality disorder.

The course of the illness is quite variable. The effect on life style may be severe, and atrophy from disuse may cause further impairment. Moreover, there is a significant incidence of later organic illness, a high incidence of subsequent major depression or other incapacitating mental illness, and a greatly increased suicide rate.

Conversion disorder may be distinguished from other somatoform disorders by the "nonphysiological" nature of the symptom, the fact that there is actual "loss" of function, and the symbolic significance of the symptom.

Table 12.6.
Diagnostic Criteria for Conversion Disorder[a]

A. The predominant disturbance is a loss of or alteration in physical functioning suggesting a physical disorder.
B. Psychological factors are judged to be etiologically involved in the symptom, as evidenced by one of the following:
  (1) there is a temporal relationship between an environmental stimulus that is apparently related to a psychological conflict or need and the initiation or exacerbation of the symptom;
  (2) the symptom enables the individual to avoid some activity that is noxious to him or her;
  (3) the symptom enables the individual to get support from the environment that otherwise might not be forthcoming.
C. It has been determined that the symptom is *not* under voluntary control.
D. The symptom cannot, after appropriate investigation, be explained by a known physical disorder or pathophysiological mechanism.
E. The symptom is not limited to pain or to a disturbance in sexual functioning.
F. Not due to somatization disorder or schizophrenia.

[a] From American Psychiatric Association: *Diagnostic and Statistical Manual of Mental Disorders*, ed 3. Washington, DC, American Psychiatric Association, 1980.

Management

In general, treatment of conversion symptoms is most likely to succeed in those patients with good premorbid adjustment; where the symptoms are recent in onset and obviously precipitated by a life stress; where the patient is able to express feelings and to experience distress over the symptoms; and where there is not a coexisting major psychiatric or organic illness. A psychiatric consultation may be useful in helping make the diagnosis and in providing suggestions for management, but few patients will comply with long term psychotherapy.

When the diagnosis is made, the physician should avoid confronting the patient about the possible psychological basis for the symptom, but should explain to the patient that he is interested in investigating all possible etiological factors, including the relationship of the disorder to stress. This may allow the patient gradually to accept the role of psychosocial factors, to articulate the feelings against which the symptom defends, and to give up the symptom. The solicitation of the aid of the family and practical interventions to reduce stresses that underlie the conversion symptom are often important. The physician should be aware, however, that conversion symptoms often mask serious psychiatric disorders such as depression. Furthermore, since a significant number of patients do develop organic disease, any changes in symptoms or the development of new symptoms should be taken seriously.

PSYCHOGENIC PAIN

Spectrum of Disorders

Patients whose complaints of pain have little or no organic basis may have one of several psychiatric and/or behavioral syndromes. These are: (*a*) minor mood disturbance (adjustment disorder, see above); (*b*) major depressive disorder (Chapter 15); (*c*) one of the somatoform disorders (conversion disorder, somatization disorder, or hypochondriasis, see above); (*d*) schizophrenic disorder (Chapter 16); (*e*) malingering (see below); (*f*) factitious disorder (see below); and (*g*) chronic benign intractable pain syndrome.

In *minor mood disturbances*, the dysphoric mood lowers the threshold for both pain tolerance and pain perception; as a result there are complaints about insignificant problems that may be newly developed, such as a pulled muscle, or that may be long-standing but stable, such as arthritis. Most of these disorders are acute; there is usually a detectable stressor in the environment; and the stress is temporally related to the onset of the symptom. These patients have been described as temporarily dependent (13), which means that they are looking to the medical system for support in a time of stress or crisis. Their pain can thus be viewed as a "ticket" to the doctor. Evaluation and management of these patients is described above.

Not uncommonly patients with *major depressive disorder* (see Chapter 15) present with symptoms of pain. Somatic complaints in fact are frequent in seriously depressed patients (16) and are considered as primary manifestations of a disturbed, vegetative state along with anhedonia, fatigue, and sleep disturbance. Treatment of the depression often relieves the pain complaints.

Some patients with *acute or chronic schizophrenia* (see Chapter 16) may present with unusual sensations of pain as an expression of somatic hallucination or delusional thinking. Complaints such as "electricity shooting through my head" or "snakes biting out my intestines" should suggest questioning the patient about other symptoms of schizophrenia. In some patients, the complaint of pain may be the only manifestation of an incipient psychosis (4). In contrast to overtly psychotic patients who express their pain with an unusually flat affect, in this case complaints often have a desperate quality and may be accompanied by suicidal ideation. Careful psychiatric examination may reveal an underlying delusion, excessive suspiciousness, or subtle thought disturbance.

Chronic Benign Intractable Pain Syndrome

Sometimes what began as acute pain (*i.e.*, pain lasting 2 months or less) evolves into a chronic pain state that fails to respond to medical or surgical therapies and results in global interference with patient functioning. In recent years the dynamics of this disorder has been clarified, and it has been called the "chronic benign intractable pain syndrome." Some believe that this syndrome has reached almost epidemic proportions in the United States, with an estimated prevalence of 7 million cases and a cost in health care, unemployment benefits, and lost productivity of $5 billion/year (10). Patients typically have pain that has lasted anywhere from 6 months to several years and has failed to respond to multiple interventions. This disorder, which affects men more than women, usually has its onset after an injury that is job related.

Origins

Some years ago Engel (6) pointed out that in many of the patients he saw with chronic pain there were often developmental histories marked by physical or sexual abuse, parental deprivation, or loss of parents in childhood. He felt that these experiences predisposed individuals to several unresolved conflicts and needs that were expressed later in chronic pain. Common features in the patients history were (*a*) an unconscious yearning to be cared for in a passive-dependent way; this striving was often defended against with a pseudoindependent facade; (*b*) a tendency to use pain in place of other feelings to communicate emotional needs (such as a need for love); (*c*) a tendency toward depression, which most patients attribute to their pain but which may, in fact, have preceded it; (*d*) life stressors represented by job or family problems that the patient was not coping with but could not admit to.

Because of these characteristics Engel coined the term "pain prone" to indicate that developmental factors play a significant part in the syndrome, which is seen today as a "systems disorder" with important social, psychological, physical, and other inputs. A proposed schema for the evolution of the intractable pain syndrome is seen in Figure 12.1. Through chronic pain the patient with this disorder is able to avoid problems he feels he cannot cope with and to have his unconscious passive-dependent needs satisfied. However, this occurs at a great price and causes much ambivalence in the patient, who on one level is gratified by his dependency but on the other is angered and frustrated by it.

Manifestations and Diagnosis

The working diagnosis of chronic benign intractable pain syndrome can be made when a patient presents with a history that includes a number of typical features. It is, of course, important to verify the evidence that a *bona fide* cause of persistent pain has been excluded when making this working diagnosis.

In patients with this disorder, the most common

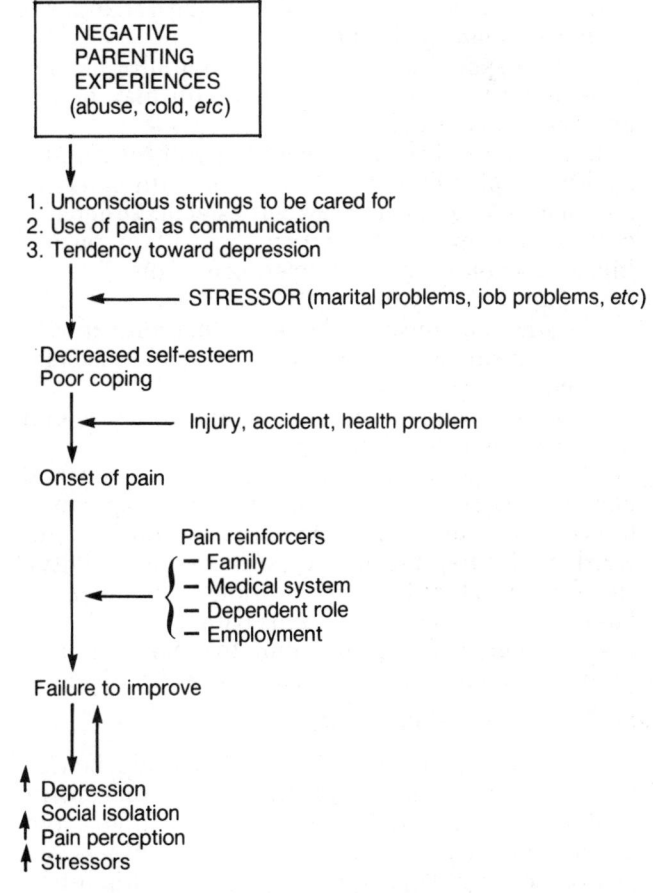

Figure 12.1. A proposed schema for development of the chronic benign intractable pain syndrome. (Adapted from Violon A: The process involved in becoming a pain patient. In Roy R, Tunks E (eds): *Chronic Pain*. Baltimore, Williams & Wilkins, 1982, pp 20–35.)

location of pain is the lower back, and usually the original injury that led to the pain was diagnosed as a sprain. Headache, facial pain, and neck pain are also common. Following the onset of pain the patient may have seen his local doctor and attempted to go back to his usual work or other activities that he had temporarily discontinued. The history reveals that soon after his return to work the patient's pain recurred (sometimes following apparent reinjury) or he was unable to perform the tasks required of his job. After this, the patient will usually have consulted a series of specialists (e.g., orthopaedic surgeons, neurosurgeons, or neurologists); conservative treatment, such as physical therapy, will have been tried and will not have helped; there may have been an attempt at surgical relief, followed by transient improvement; then recurrence of a pain described as "worse than ever." By 6 to 12 months after the onset of symptoms, some of the following patterns will have developed in the patient's life style:

1. He is out of work and experiencing a significant decrease in family income.

2. He is spending a significant amount of his day in sedentary activity, and weight gain may be exacerbating his discomfort.

3. His family has taken over many of his responsibilities. This unwittingly reinforces pain behavior and inactivity and decreases self-esteem. Other secondary gain may occur when the patient pushes himself beyond his "pain tolerance," complains of pain, and is told by his family to rest.

4. He has significantly decreased his contact with persons outside of the home and has become socially isolated.

5. He is dependent on narcotic analgesics, which he takes whenever he has pain.

6. He easily becomes angry and frustrated and usually has some symptoms of major depression (especially guilt, anhedonia, negative outlook toward the future, loss of interest in sexual activity). He often feels that health professionals and even his family may not be regarding his pain as "real."

7. He is enmeshed in litigation to obtain compensation for the injury that preceded the chronic pain.

Management and Prognosis

When the working diagnosis of chronic benign intractable pain syndrome is made, the management strategies that are most likely to help are (a) to avoid actions that will reinforce the patient's illness behavior (see page 00) and (b) to refer the patient to a center specializing in the treatment of chronic pain. The overall goal of treatment is not to relieve pain totally but to return the patient to as functional a state as possible, focusing upon increased autonomy, vocational rehabilitation, and self-management of stress and pain. The family plays a crucial role in helping to motivate the patient and to maintain healthier behavior. In general, the prognosis for improvement is best when appropriate management is started before more than 2 years of chronic pain behavior have elapsed.

Centers for Treatment of Chronic Pain

Multidisciplinary centers for treatment of chronic pain have become widely available in recent years. They utilize both inpatient and outpatient treatment programs. Good results (up to 60% of patients showing improvement in functioning 1 year after treatment) have been reported in patients admitted for 4 to 6 weeks to an inpatient pain treatment unit (12).

Initially, it is often difficult to engage these patients in psychological treatment, since they are very nonpsychologically minded and ambivalent about wanting to get better. Treatment focuses upon modifying maladaptive behavior, extinguishing reinforcers in the patient's environment that propagate pain complaints, treating depression, detoxifying the

patient from narcotics or other drugs, and providing individual, family, and group psychotherapy.

By assuring that all who are involved in treating the patient agree on the strategy and goals, these programs attempt to break the pattern of multiple approaches by multiple providers that has previously fostered the patient's pain as a way of life.

In many ways, the management of the chronic pain patient is analogous to that for another problem whose management has been clarified in recent years, chronic alcoholism: improvement depends both upon consistency in the approach to modifying behavior and upon eliminating reinforcement of that behavior by physicians, family members, and others in the patient's environment. Recognizing the patient's problem and motivating him to obtain appropriate treatment are perhaps the most important roles which the patient's personal physician plays in dealing with both of these vexing problems.

OTHER PSYCHOSOMATIC CONDITIONS

Psychological Factors Affecting Physical Condition

Description

In many patients, emotional factors or psychological stressors may initiate or exacerbate somatic symptoms due to a physical disorder. The resulting symptoms, which are called "psychophysiological," are usually not accompanied by significant tissue damage. In the presence of underlying disease, however, the potential for irreversible injury is present. For example, myocardial infarction may occur when strong emotion leads to increased heart rate or coronary vasoconstriction in the presence of underlying atherosclerotic heart disease. A listing of the most common conditions in which psychophysiological symptoms may occur is found in Table 12.7.

The reason that certain individuals react to a stressor with such bodily changes is unknown. Heredity, learning, and personality factors probably all play a part. However, it is clear that the rich connections between the cerebral centers of emotion and arousal, on one hand, and the autonomic nervous system and the hypothalamic-pituitary neuraxis, on the other, permit excitation to be transmitted virtually anywhere in the body. Moreover, stimuli that evoke excitation may be a threat to one person or a pleasure to another (for example, the thought of dangling from a cliff at the end of a tether would terrify most people, but might delight a mountain climber). Thus, a key determinant of the emotional arousal and physical responses caused by a particular stimulus is its meaning to the individual.

Most of the conditions listed in Table 12.7 may occur either as psychophysiological disorders or as disorders without a predominantly psychological basis. Diagnostic criteria for most of these conditions

Table 12.7.
Common Conditions in Which Psychophysiological Symptoms Are Important

Physiological System	Symptomatic Condition	For Further Information, See Chapter
Cardiovascular	Migraine headache	79
	Vasovagal syndrome (fainting)	81
	Hypertension (usually asymptomatic)	62
	Supraventricular tachycardia	59
	Angina	57
Gastrointestinal	Irritable bowel syndrome	39
	The following symptoms may occur singly or together: anorexia, nausea, vomiting, abdominal cramps, diarrhea, constipation, aerophagia, acid-peptic symptoms	35, 36, 38
Genitourinary	Menstrual disturbances	77
	Difficulties in micturition: frequency (in both sexes); retention (females); hesitancy (in males)	
	Sexual disorders	18
	Dyspareunia	
	Anorgasmia	
	Inhibited sexual excitement; (impotence, frigidity)	
	Delayed ejaculation; premature ejaculation	
Musculoskeletal	Pain secondary to increased muscle tension: occipital or bitemporal headaches, backaches, myalgia in various muscle groups	65, 79
	Fatigue	
	Tremor	82
	Rheumatoid arthritis	70
Respiratory	Hyperventilation syndrome	13
	Bronchospasm	55
	Dyspnea	53
Skin	Hyperhidrosis	100
	Pruritis	100

are found elsewhere in this book, as indicated in the table. For a patient's symptoms to be labeled as chiefly psychophysiological, stressful life situations should be present and should have a temporal relationship to the onset of symptoms; and symptoms should subside when the stressful situation abates. Most of the conditions listed in Table 12.7 tend to occur intermittently over a long period of time, without evidence of significant progression in severity.

Conversion symptoms are differentiated from psychophysiological symptoms by the lack of physical changes (except for disuse atrophy), and by the fact that the symptom protects the patient from anxiety while in psychophysiological disorders there is often overt anxiety. Psychophysiological problems are closely related to adjustment disorders, but are distinguished from them by the fact that physical symptoms dominate the picture rather than mood disturbance and by the fact that symptoms may occur in the absence of psychosocial stressors as well as in response to them.

Management

When initiation or exacerbation of a physical condition is related to environmental stressors, management is the same as that described for adjustment disorder (page 143).

Factitious Illness

Description

Factitious illness is characterized by deliberate simulation of physical or psychological symptoms, with the singular objective of assuming the role of "patient." When this behavior is chronic and leads to multiple hospitalizations, it is known either as chronic factitious disorder with physical symptoms (Munchausen's syndrome) or factitious disorder with psychological symptoms (see DSM-III criteria, Table 12.8). Although fully expressed factitious disorders are probably quite rare, minor forms of factitious behavior are probably relatively common, i.e., symptoms that enable an individual to achieve the patient role but are not severe enough to warrant hospitalization, such as dermatitis caused by excoriation or voluntary shoulder dislocation. Factitious illness differs from malingering in that for the malingerer the hospitalization or the patient role always

Table 12.8.
Diagnostic Criteria for Factitious Disorders[a]

Chronic Factitious Disorders with Physical Symptoms
A. Plausible presentation of physical symptoms that are apparently under the individual's voluntary control to such a degree that there are multiple hospitalizations.
B. The individual's goal is apparently to assume the "patient" role and is not otherwise understandable in light of the individual's environmental circumstances (as is the case in malingering).

Factitious Disorder with Psychological Symptoms
A. The production of psychological symptoms is apparently under the individual's voluntary control.
B. The symptoms produced are not explained by any other mental disorder (although they may be superimposed on one).
C. The individual's goal is apparently to assume the "patient" role and is not otherwise understandable in light of the individual's environmental circumstances (as is the case in malingering).

[a] From American Psychiatric Association: *Diagnostic and Statistical Manual of Mental Disorders*, ed 3. Washington, DC, American Psychiatric Association, 1980.

has a readily identified ulterior motive attached to it (e.g., avoidance of jail, debtors, etc) while the patient with a factitious disorder has no other apparent goal than to assume the patient role.

Chronic factitious disorder usually begins in early adult life, often shortly after hospitalization for a *bona fide* physical illness. It is more common in males, while minor factitious illness is more common in females. Because of the recurrent hospitalizations, this disorder is usually incompatible with stable work, family life, or other social relationships. The etiology is unknown, but in many patients there is a strong history of parental abuse and/or deprivation.

Patients with the Munchausen syndrome may simulate almost any physical illness. The illness may be feigned through reporting invented symptoms or by deliberate production of physical signs by injecting noxious substances to cause abscesses or by using drugs such as anticoagulants or insulin. Common presenting symptoms in these patients are severe right lower abdominal pain with nausea and vomiting, dizziness and blacking out, massive hemoptysis, generalized rashes, abscesses, and unexplained protracted fever. The time interval between discharge from one hospital to presentation at another hospital varies from less than a day to several months.

In taking the history, the physician may note that it is presented with a dramatic flair and that on careful questioning the information given by the patient becomes vague and inconsistent. In its most exaggerated form, the patient will tell fantastic stories about prior medical treatment in hospitals located in many cities, may attempt to impersonate famous individuals, and will have an extensive knowledge of medical history and hospital routines. Often the patient has been a health professional or has been well acquainted with one.

Management and Prognosis

Successful treatment has virtually never been reported for a patient who is fully enmeshed in a chronic factitious disorder. Management consists chiefly of keeping the patient out of hospitals and avoiding risk-laden procedures. When the syndrome is suspected strongly, consultation with a psychiatrist early after admission may help in deciding on management. Management in the hospital focuses mainly on physician-staff relations, on tactfully confronting the patient with his diagnosis, and on persuading the patient to accept psychiatric hospitalization.

Patients with minor factitious illness behavior, who do not have hospitalization as their singular objective, may, in fact, have underlying depressions or other problems that are amenable to treatment. Therefore, tactful confrontation of these patients with the evidence for factitious illness—in which

one acknowledges that the patient must need to emphasize his distress—may clarify the patient's problem and lead to acceptance of psychiatric evaluation.

Malingering

Description

Malingering is the deliberate simulation of physical (or psychological) symptoms in order to achieve a specific benefit. It occurs in trivial forms in most households from time to time. It occurs as an important and relatively common problem in settings where sickness is rewarded with certain benefits—e.g., avoidance of military service or court appearances, monetary reward for injuries or disability. Ford (see "General References") divides malingering into three broad categories:

1. Pure malingering, in which there is a deliberate deception by the description and/or production of nonexistent symptoms and signs (rare).

2. Partial malingering, which involves the conscious and voluntary exaggeration of symptoms of a real disease.

3. The deliberate attribution of an actual disability to an injury or accident that did not cause it.

The diagnosis of malingering should be suspected whenever there is the combination of (a) symptoms or impairments that greatly exceed associated objective evidence; and (b) an obvious benefit contingent upon having those symptoms. Important observations suggesting the diagnosis are inconsistency of the patient's impairment (e.g., a blind person who is detected reading or a back pain sufferer who is observed playing touch football with his friends) and presentation of symptoms in a vague way, with exaggeration, or with defensiveness when challenged.

It may be difficult to differentiate malingering, in which the patient is strictly trying to deceive others, from conversion disorder (see above), in which the patient is deceiving both himself and others. The features that favor malingering are the inconstancy of symptoms, the clear linkage of symptoms to benefit, and, usually, the lack of symbolic meaning or modeling in the patient's environment. Careful inquiry and observation are needed to establish that malingering is the fundamental problem.

Management

A number of treatment strategies have been successful in having malingerers give up their symptoms/impairments:

1. Responding minimally to the patient's report of symptoms and responding with interest to reports of healthy behavior.

2. Gradually and tactfully making the patient aware that malingering is suspected.

3. "Treating" the patient with environmental

changes that diminish his gratifications in the sick role—e.g., reducing access to television and to valued social interactions in a jail setting.

Because serious psychiatric illness may underlie suspected malingering, it is helpful to persuade a patient to accept psychiatric evaluation when malingering persists despite measures such as those outlined above.

General References

American Psychiatric Association: *Diagnostic and Statistical Manual of Mental Disorders*, ed 3. Washington, DC, American Psychiatric Association, 1980.
> Recently updated diagnostic criteria and epidemiological information for all recognized psychiatric disorders.

Barsky AJ III: Patients who amplify bodily sensations. *Ann Intern Med* 91:63, 1979.
> Excellent review focusing on the underlying mechanisms leading to somatization as it presents in the generalist's practice.

Cadoret RJ, King LJ: *Psychiatry in Primary Care*. St Louis, CV Mosby, 1983.
> Excellent account of common problems, emphasizing epidemiology, treatment, and outcome; extensively referenced.

Ford CV: *The Somatizing Disorders: Illness as a Way of Life*. New York, Elsevier Biomedical, 1983.
> Practical, well referenced monograph covering all disorders in which somatization is the principal feature.

Reiser MF (ed): Vol 4: *Organic Disorders and Psychosomatic Medicine*. In Arieti S (ed): *American Handbook of Psychiatry*. New York, Basic Books, 1975.
> Contains excellent reviews of most psychophysiological conditions.

Specific References

1. Aldrich CK: The severe chronic hypochondriac. *Postgrad Med* 69:140, 1981.
2. Catalan J, Gath D, Edmonds G, Ennis J: The effects of nonprescribing of anxiolytics in general practice. I. Controlled evaluation of psychiatric and social outcome. *Br J Psychiatry* 144:593, 1984.
3. Catalan J, Bath D, Bond A, Martin P: The effects of nonprescribing of anxiolytics in general practice. II. Factors associated with outcome. *Br J Psychiatry* 144:603, 1984.
4. Delaney JF; Atypical facial pain as a defense against psychosis. *Am J Psychiatry* 133:1151, 1976.
5. Drossman DA: The problem patient: evaluation and care of medical patients with psychosocial disturbances. *Ann Intern Med* 88:366, 1978.
6. Engel GL: "Psychogenic" pain and the pain-prone patient. *Am J Med* 36:899, 1959.
7. *Health—United States*. US Department of Health, Education and Welfare publ no. (PHS) 78-1237, December, 1978.
8. Johnstone A, Goldberg D: Psychiatric screening in general practice. *Lancet* 1:605, 1976.
9. Lazare A: Conversion symptoms. *New Engl J Med* 305:745, 1983.
9a. Murphy GE: The clinical management of hysteria. *JAMA* 247:2559, 1982.
10. National Institute on Drug Abuse: *New Approaches to Treatment of Chronic Pain: A Review of Multidisciplinary Pain Clinics and Pain Centers*, Research Monograph 36. Rockville, MD, Department of Health and Human Services, DHHS publ no. (ADM) 81-1089, May, 1981. (Available from National Institute on Drug Abuse, Division of Research, 5600 Fishers Lane, Rockville, MD, 20857.)
11. Stoeckle J, Zola IK, Davison GE: The quantity and significance of psychological distress in medical patients. *J Chronic Dis* 17:959, 1964.
12. Swanson DW, Maruta T, Swenson WM: Results of behavior modification in the treatment of chronic pain. *Psychosom Med* 41:55, 1979.
13. Thomas KB: Temporarily dependent patient in general practice. *Br Med J* 1:625, 1974.
14. Tumulty PA: What is a clinician and what does he do? *N Engl J Med* 28:20, 1970.
15. White KL, Williams TF, Greenberg BG: The ecology of medical care. *N Engl J Med* 265:885, 1961.
16. Wittenborn J, Buhler R: Somatic complaints among depressed women. *Arch Gen Psychiatry* 36:465, 1979.
17. Zola IK: Pathways to the doctor—from person to patient. In Albrecht GI, Higgens PC (eds): *Health, Illness and Medicine, A Reader in Medical Sociology*. Chicago, Rand McNally, 1979.

CHAPTER THIRTEEN

The Anxious Patient

WALTER F. BAILE, M.D.

INTRODUCTION

Anxiety is a general term given to a group of signs, symptoms, and sensations (Table 13.1) which may be present in a number of psychiatric and nonpsychiatric disturbances (see Table 13.2). Anxiety disorders are a group of psychiatric syndromes in which anxiety is the primary manifestation. Whether primary or secondary, anxiety manifests itself in one or more of the following ways: (a) as a *cognitive experience*, e.g., apprehension, worry, or anticipation of danger or threat; (b) as *motor tension* manifesting itself in jumpiness, trembling, inability to relax, and autonomic signs and symptoms such as palpitations, breathlessness, giddiness, and gastrointestinal disturbances; (c) as *behavioral disturbances*

such as irritability, poor concentration, insomnia and sometimes panic. All three manifestations of anxiety are closely associated.

Anxiety is encountered commonly in office or hospital practice. Anxiety disorders may be present in as many as 10 to 15% of patients seen in these settings. Recognition of these patients is important because patients with primary anxiety disorders are over utilizers of medical services. Often underlying anxiety goes unrecognized because of the patient's undue preoccupation with disease (hypochondriasis, see Chapter 12), fear that he may have a medical disorder (medical phobia, see below), or the concurrent presence of a physical disorder. The difficulty of recognizing anxiety and other psychiatric disturbances in the medical patient is illustrated by a study of general practice patients (14a) which found that 15% of patients had somatic symptoms related to ongoing psychiatric problems and another 10% had physical disease with associated psychiatric disorder. This and other studies (19, 38) indicate that a generalist is as likely as a mental health practitioner to be consulted by patients with anxiety as the primary disorder.

Before discussing the clinical entities associated with pathological anxiety, it is important to note that in older classification systems some disorders in which anxiety was not a presenting symptom (e.g., conversion disorder, dissociative disorder) were classified together with the anxiety disorders under the category of "neuroses." This system of classification for the most part reflected psychoanalytic thinking that postulates that anxiety results when unconscious wishes, impulses, drives, and thoughts, which have been repressed because they are unacceptable, threaten to emerge into consciousness as a result of internal or external stressors. Anxiety acts as a "signal" to the self that this "unrepression" is occurring. When the ego is strong enough, other defense mechanisms, such as conversion, may come into play. When they do not, the anxiety continues to be felt and is called "free floating." In the third edition of the American Psychiatric Association's *Diagnostic and Statistical Manual of Mental Disorders* (DSM-III) this more intrapsychic and mechanistic approach has been abandoned in favor of a more descriptive one. While this also has its disadvantages, it allows a more expanded view of anxiety that takes into account other etiological

Table 13.1.
Symptoms and Signs of Anxiety[a]

Symptoms	Signs
NERVOUS SYSTEM	**NERVOUS SYSTEM**
Tense, unable to relax	Strained facial expression
Difficulty concentrating, difficulty with memory, loss of interest in usual activities	Stereotypic behavior, *e.g.*, facial tic, nail biting, chain smoking
Lightheadedness,[b] dizziness,[b] syncope[b]	Cold, clammy handshake
"Bad mood," general irritability, unable to tolerate even mild frustration	Pacing, restlessness
Sleep disturbances: nightmares, difficulty going to sleep[b]	Irritability during physical examination
Ill defined fear of the unknown, terrifying sense of dread	Postural tremor
Fatigue, weakness[b]	Proptosis and stare
Headaches,[b] poor coordination	Dilated pupils
Trembling, numbness and tingling of fingers, toes, and face[b]	Positive Chvostek's sign[b]
Piloerection ("goosebumps")	Carpal-pedal spasm[b]
	Hyperreflexia
CARDIOVASCULAR	**CARDIOVASCULAR**
Palpitations[b]	Sinus tachycardia[b]
Substernal pressure, precordial pain unrelated to exertion[b]	Transient elevated systolic blood pressure
Flushing of face	Functional systolic ejection murmur
PULMONARY	**PULMONARY**
Difficulty breathing adequately[b]	Hyperventilation[b]
Sense of suffocation[b]	Increased frequency of sighing respiration[b]
GASTROINTESTINAL	
Epigastric distress: fullness,[b] belching,[b] heartburn, dyspepsia	
Diarrhea, constipation	
Anorexia, compulsive eating	
GENITOURINARY	
Increased frequency of micturition	
Amenorrhea, excessive menstrual cramps and flow	
Impotence, premature ejaculation	

[a] Adapted from Favazza AR, Royer JA: Anxiety, acute and chronic. In Rakell RS, Conn HS (eds): *Family Practice*, ed. 2. Philadelphia, WB Saunders, 1978.
[b] Denotes symptoms and signs which may be due to hyperventilation.

theories (including behavioral and metabolic theories) which have led to significant advances in the treatment of anxiety disorders (13). These theories are discussed under "Treatment of Anxiety."

PHOBIC DISORDERS

The term *phobia* derives from the Greek word "phobes" which means fear, flight, or terror. The essential feature of a phobia is thus a persistent, irrational fear of an object, activity, or situation which compels an individual to avoid the feared stimulus. Over time, a phobic stimulus may induce the symptoms of anxiety. The affected person realizes that his reaction is out of proportion to the actual dangerousness of the stimulus, but he is unable to overcome it with logical reason. Nor is the reassurance of others helpful as a remedy. Related to phobia are the phenomena of *avoidance*, which is the behavior undertaken to remain distant from the phobic stimulus in order to avoid unpleasant anxiety, and *counterphobic behavior*, which is an attempt to master the phobia sometimes by forcing oneself into contact with it. *Extinction* refers to the process by which phobias remit either spontaneously or with therapy.

DSM-III divides the phobic disorders into agoraphobia, social phobia, and simple phobia. Agoraphobia is discussed after the entity "panic disorder" (page 160) as there is evidence that agoraphobia most often results from a conditioned response to repeated anxiety attacks. In all phobias *anticipatory anxiety* may result if an individual is forced into contact with the phobic stimulus. For example, the prospect of a business trip for an individual phobic for flying may trigger significant anticipatory anxiety. Symptoms of anticipatory anxiety resemble those of generalized anxiety disorder (see below).

An important property of phobic stimuli is their tendency to *generalize* to previously neutral stimuli. Thus the same person who is afraid of flying may eventually stay away from airports altogether or even roads leading to airports. Phobic generalization is most common in agoraphobia. When there is generalization to multiple stimuli, chronic anxiety may result and make the distinction between specific phobic disorders and generalized anxiety disorder difficult.

Table 13.2.
Anxiety-Related Syndromes

Acute psychosis
Adjustment disorder with anxious mood
Anxiety disorders (DSM-III)
  Generalized anxiety disorder
  Obsessive compulsive disorder
  Panic disorder
  Phobic disorders
  Post-traumatic stress disorder
Dementia and delirium
Depression
Drug toxicity or withdrawal
  Alcohol
  Anxiolytics
  Cocaine
  Phenothiazines
  Quinidine
  Sympathomimetics
  Xanthines (including caffeine)
Hypercalcemia
Hyperthyroidism
Hypoglycemia
Pheochromocytoma
Schizophrenia
Temporal lobe epilepsy

Prevalence

Phobic symptoms are extremely common in the general population. Depending on the setting, anywhere from 2 to 23% of the general population will meet the criteria for phobic disorder (2, 29). In only a small percentage, however, is it significantly disabling. Phobias may be minor complaints, as well, in such other psychiatric disorders as depressive illness. Phobic disorders make up only a small percentage (2 to 3%) of the problems seen in psychiatric office practice, and among these agoraphobia represents 60% of all patients treated. The prevalence of phobias in the general medical setting is unknown, but they are probably not uncommon. Medical phobia (see below) may be a particularly underrecognized problem, which may lead to noncompliance when avoidance or counterphobic behavior exists.

Simple Phobia

DSM-III criteria for simple phobia (also called single phobia) include:

A. A persistent, irrational fear of, and compelling desire to avoid, an object or a situation other than being alone, or in public places away from home (agoraphobia, see below), or of humiliation or embarrassment in certain social situations (social phobia, see below).
B. Significant distress from the disturbance and recognition by the individual that his or her fear is excessive or unreasonable.
C. The problem is not due to another mental disorder,

such as schizophrenia or obsessive compulsive disorder.

The true incidence and prevalence of simple phobia have not been established. From existing data (2, 10), the following generalizations can be made, however:

1. Simple phobias are most common in early childhood, often involve fear of animals, cause little impairment, and tend to extinguish themselves spontaneously by the midteens.
2. The patients with simple phobia who come for psychiatric treatment are primarily adults whose childhood phobias failed to be extinguished or have worsened and are interfering with functioning. Patients with simple phobias represent about 20% of all patients with phobias who are treated in psychiatric settings.
3. Most adult cases of simple phobia show a female-male ratio of at least 3 to 1. Many more women than men appear to seek treatment.
4. The most commonly feared objects/situations are animals, storms, heights, and enclosures. These follow the pattern of acquisition early in life, with early extinction in most cases. Less common phobias, such as of darkness and strangers, seem to be acquired until late childhood but also gradually extinguish over time.
5. Most simple phobias are not disabling. Community surveys have found that only 0.2% of patients had severely incapacitating simple phobias (2, 10).

Medical phobias—that is, fear of death, injury, illness, and medical procedures—deserve special mention because of their impact on the delivery of medical care. These phobias are very common: in one study they represented 42% of all phobias in a population surveyed (2). They are important because they are acquired throughout life and are particularly common in middle age and old age, when physical illness is also common. Patients with apparent medical phobia must be distinguished from those with the somatoform disorder hypochondriasis (see Chapter 12). It would seem plausible to diagnose medical phobias in individuals who acquire fears of medical situations by becoming sensitized to them through experience. Where fear of disease is not based in reality, it is more likely that the patient has hypochondriasis. For example, a simple medical phobia could explain why a person avoids a hospital where the untimely death of his spouse occurred, but hypochondriasis would be more likely in someone who has never had sexual intercourse but has a persistent fear of having syphilis.

Medical phobias may have a significant impact, as when a diabetic fearful of needles is unable to administer insulin or when a patient with kidney failure is unable to utilize a dialysis machine. More dramatic is the case when individuals who are recovering from an acute illness like a myocardial infarction develop counterphobic behavior, such as doing pushups, in order to challenge their fear. In addition to counterphobic behavior many patients with myocardial infarction demonstrate phobic avoidance by delaying unnecessarily return to work and normal activities, presumably because of fears related to the consequences of activity. Fortunately, exercise programs, which provide a way of extinguishing these fears, have contributed greatly to the rehabilitation of the cardiac patient. However, many equally harmful medical phobias and the behaviors related to them probably go unrecognized and untreated.

Special mention should be made of *cancer phobia*. The publicity given to cancer in general and to the negative experiences occurring with cancer, especially pain, the perception of a progressively downhill course, and the large number of individuals in the population with a relative or acquaintance who has suffered from cancer, make it a prime concern for many individuals who encounter a new symptom or lesion. Cancer phobia is especially common in depressed patients, and in such individuals there is sometimes a delusional belief of having cancer rather than a fear of it. The overly concerned patient should always be asked whether he has been preoccupied about having some serious illness such as cancer and whether he has been depressed. In this context, then, specific evaluation and reassurance can be undertaken.

The symptoms occurring in patients with simple phobias are those of anxiety. They occur when the phobic stimulus is approached or contact is foreseen. Phobic avoidance is common. Occasionally a patient may have associated depression or multiple phobias. Systematic desensitization or flooding is the treatment of choice, and response to treatment is usually good (see discussion of treatment below).

Social Phobia

The DSM-III criteria for social phobia are:

A. A persistent, irrational fear of, and compelling desire to avoid, a situation in which the individual is exposed to possible scrutiny by others and fears that he or she may act in a way that will be humiliating or embarrassing.

B. Significant distress because of the disturbance and recognition by the individual that his or her fear is excessive or unreasonable.

C. The problem is not due to another mental disorder, such as major depression or avoidant personality disorder.

The individual affected by a social phobia worries about how he appears to other persons, is extremely self-conscious, and fears that he will do something to attract the attention of others and make him feel more uncomfortable. Sweating, trembling, clumsiness, stuttering, or simply appearing conspicuous are constant preoccupations. In a recent study of social phobia (3), 87 patients rated the following situations as giving rise to severe anxiety: (a) meeting people one does not know; (b) meeting people in authority; (c) being observed by others; (d) being in situations where one may be criticized. Because they have already experienced anxiety in a variety of social situations, social phobics become very aware that their manifestations of anxiety might also be noticed by others.

Social phobias are fairly common. They occur almost equally in men and women. The usual age of onset is the midteens, but they may occur in predisposed individuals whenever new social obligations are encountered. In a series of phobic patients seen in a psychiatric outpatient setting, social phobics comprised approximately 8% (25) of all cases of phobia. Nearly half had some history of depression. Moderately severe generalized anxiety was present in 13% and alcohol abuse in 18%. Fifty per cent of patients had a history of excessive timidity in childhood and adolescence. Many came from broken homes.

There has been some discussion as to whether social phobia is a syndrome truly distinct from agoraphobia (see below) since both groups avoid social situations, public transport, and enclosed spaces. However, the agoraphobic avoids these situations because of his fear of being away from home or because he cannot escape from crowded surroundings if he has an anxiety attack. The social phobic avoids situations because he is overly aware of being observed. Moreover, agoraphobia occurs more often in women, has its onset later in life with more rapid occurrence of symptoms, and patients often have multiple other phobias. Social phobics, on the other hand, show more use of alcohol to treat symptoms, have often recently been upwardly socially mobile (necessitating new social obligations), and in one study 14% had suicide gestures (3).

Strategies and techniques for the treatment of social phobias are described below.

ANXIETY NEUROSES

Anxiety neuroses are divided into generalized anxiety disorder, panic disorder, and post-traumatic stress disorder. Obsessive compulsive disorder, classified as an anxiety neuroses in DSM-III, is discussed in Chapter 14, Maladaptive Personalities.

Generalized Anxiety Disorder

The DSM-III criteria of this disorder are:

A. Generalized, persistent anxiety is manifested by symptoms from three of the following four categories:

(1) *motor tension*: shakiness, jitteriness, jumpiness, trembling, tension, muscle aches, fatigability, inability to relax, eyelid twitch, furrowed brow, strained face, fidgeting, restlessness, easy startle

(2) *autonomic hyperactivity*: sweating, heart pounding or racing, cold, clammy hands, dry mouth, dizziness, lightheadedness, paresthesias (tingling in hands or feet), upset stomach, hot or cold spells, frequent urination, diarrhea, discomfort in the pit of the stomach, lump in the throat, flushing, pallor, high resting pulse and respiration rate

(3) *apprehensive expectation*: anxiety, worry, fear, rumination, and anticipation of misfortune to self or others

(4) *vigilance and scanning*: hyperattentiveness resulting in distractibility, difficulty in concentrating, insomnia, feeling "on edge," irritability, impatience

B. The anxious mood has been continuous for at least *1 month*.

C. The problem is not due to another mental disorder, such as a depressive disorder or schizophrenia.

D. The person affected is at least 18 years of age.

This disorder is commonly encountered by generalists. Patients often present with somatic complaints or "bad nerves." Origins of the problem can usually be traced to childhood. There is often a history of a poor home environment or of overly anxious parents. Parents who worry excessively often overreact to childhood illnesses, setting up a preoccupation with physical functioning in the child. Excessive timidity, insecurity, and shyness are accompanying problems. Childhood anxiety symptoms may have been present and include enuresis, nail biting, somnambulism, temper tantrums, and separation anxiety when entering school. As the anxious child develops, anxiety often increases with developmental challenges. These include puberty, which brings on concerns about competition and later dating; marriage, which brings concerns about separation from family of origin and obligation to spouse and children; and occupational stresses. During adolescence one or more social phobias may develop, causing further impairment. At times when stress is increased, such as in the sickness of children or conflict with an employer, baseline anxiety will increase. Excessive worrying, sleep disturbance, inability to concentrate on normal tasks, and somatic sensations reflecting the physical symptoms of anxiety will occur. In order to deal with anxiety, compulsive rituals, phobic avoidance, alcohol abuse, and, in situations of acute stress, secondary symptoms such as conversion or dissociation disorders may occur. These behaviors are sometimes sufficient to allow coping, and when the stress resolves itself the patient will return to baseline functioning. Persons with chronic anxiety also often have dependent personality characteristics, further reducing self-reliance and increasing the tendency to look toward outside sources such as the family or the medical system for help. When stress persists, however, the patient may develop depressive symptoms or have acute anxiety attacks. For example:

A 42-year-old divorced woman had a history of excessive worrying over small details, a generalized inability to relax, and episodes of hyperventilation (acute anxiety attacks) as an adolescent. Her son had recently left for a tour in Germany with the military, and this had increased her worrying. One day while working at her job as a cashier in a supermarket she observed a customer stuffing a carton of cigarettes into his coat. This male customer was unusually tall and menacing to the patient and the thought of confronting him caused the patient to experience intense acute anxiety and she rushed into the bathroom and hyperventilated.

Anxiety attacks such as those occurring in this patient illuminate the predisposition of such patients to respond to cognitive anxiety with autonomic hyperactivity. In this regard, some patients with generalized anxiety disorders resemble those with panic disorder (see below); if stress continues they may develop that condition. In most cases, however, patients with generalized anxiety experience symptoms of muscle tension and overconcern, and it is these symptoms that bring them to the physician. Correct diagnosis depends upon eliciting a history of (a) "chronic worrying," especially when under stress; (b) a childhood history of parental separation, divorce, abuse, or poor home environment; (c) symptoms of anxiety in childhood; (d) dependent personality characteristics; and (e) a recent stressful event. This latter feature is not always easy to detect without persistence, and at times one may have to see family members to obtain further information. When depressive affect is present, generalized anxiety may resemble a depressive disorder, but most individuals with depression will not have symptoms of severe chronic anxiety or developmental problems.

Strategies and techniques for the treatment of generalized anxiety disorder are described below.

Panic Disorder

Panic disorder or "anxiety state" is manifested by recurrent episodes of somatic and psychic anxiety which may range from palpitations and diarrhea to immobilizing panic. The DSM-III criteria for panic disorder include:

A. At least *three* panic attacks within a *3-week* period in circumstances other than during marked physical exertion or in a life-threatening situation. The attacks are not precipitated only by exposure to a circumscribed phobic stimulus.

B. Panic attacks are manifested by discrete periods of apprehension or fear, and at least *four* of the following

symptoms appear during each attack:
  (1) dyspnea
  (2) palpitations
  (3) chest pain or discomfort
  (4) choking or smothering sensations
  (5) dizziness, vertigo, or unsteady feelings
  (6) feelings of unreality
  (7) paresthesias (tingling in hands or feet)
  (8) hot and cold flashes
  (9) sweating
  (10) faintness
  (11) trembling or shaking
  (12) fear of dying, going crazy, or doing something uncontrolled during an attack.

Three characteristics distinguish this disorder from other anxiety disorders: (*a*) The anxiety which is experienced appears to come "out of the clear blue sky" and is not directly precipitated by a stressful event; (*b*) anxiety usually reaches "panic" proportions with patients usually describing the anxiety in terms such as fear of dying, fear of suffocating, or "going crazy"; (*c*) panic attacks are accompanied by intensely uncomfortable autonomic symptoms, especially palpitations.

There is some overlap between this and other anxiety disorders, and some patients with generalized anxiety do experience primarily autonomic symptoms at times of stress. Furthermore, generalized "anticipatory" anxiety may result from repeated panic attacks.

Before the recognition of the primary role of anxiety in panic disorder, it was known under a variety of names, such as DaCosta's syndrome, effort syndrome, neurocirculatory asthenia, cardiac neurosis, and irritable heart (11, 32, 42, 43). These names evolved from wartime studies of the disorder when it disabled large numbers of soldiers. Although the central role of anxiety was not well recognized and its relationship to cardiac findings still remains to be clarified, many important observations were made then which are still valid. These include observations about premorbid personality characteristics, the tendency of the disorder to run in families, exercise intolerance, and biochemical abnormalities. The prevalence of the disorder today in the general population is estimated to be from 2 to 5% (14). Patients with this and related acute anxiety syndromes frequently seek help from the generalist because of the predominance of somatic signs and symptoms (36). In surveys of general medical practice, as many as 14% of patients with cardiovascular symptoms have been identified as having the disorder. Recently, symptoms of this disorder have been identified in a large proportion of patients undergoing cardiac catheterization and having insignificant findings (4).

Panic disorder is primarily a problem of young adults, although it may begin in childhood. It is much more common in women than in men. As in generalized anxiety disorder, a history of neurotic symptoms in childhood, parental divorce, separation anxiety, and excessive shyness may be found as predisposing factors. This disorder tends to run in families and there may be a genetic predisposition, as is suggested by a higher rate of concordance among monozygotic than dizygotic twins. Patients with panic disorder may show higher rates of major depression than usual, and their first degree relatives may be affected at a higher than usual rate with alcoholism and major depressive disorders.

Many of the secondary symptoms of panic disorder result from repeated exposure to panic attacks. After an anxiety attack a patient never quite feels well and often may be left with a nagging precordial ache, extreme fatigue, or occasional breathlessness. Several panic attacks can lead to serious anticipatory anxiety and avoidance of the situation in which the panic occurred. For example, several panic attacks occurring while driving will produce anticipatory anxiety when a patient arises on a workday, phobic anxiety as he approaches his car, and avoidance behavior when he takes a bus to work. Panic attacks that occur in many different situations over time may lead to several phobias, and the patient will avoid many situations in which she or he does not feel secure. The most extreme form of this phobic avoidance is seen in agoraphobia (see below) where the patient does not feel secure even venturing from the house. As disability continues, depression may occur as a secondary phenomenon. In addition, the patient may become very somatically preoccupied and focused on his body. At times a vicious cycle occurs wherein his own perception of palpitations or other somatic symptoms can lead to anticipatory anxiety of a full blown panic attack; if anxiety increases enough an attack may indeed occur (39).

Patients with panic disorder may also develop *chronic hyperventilation* and acquire a habit of breathing which maintains an abnormally low arterial pCO_2 (23). Chronic alkalosis then places an individual at or near the threshold for hypocapneic symptoms, such as paresthesias and lightheadedness. The symptoms themselves (and perhaps what the patient has been told about them) then also become a source of anxiety for the patient and contribute to the vicious circle. In its chronic form, the hyperventilation syndrome is frequently overlooked because the patient is hyperpneic (deep, at times sighing respiration), which he may not notice, instead of tachypneic which most patients notice and report (30). Therefore, complaints of dizziness, paresthesias, breathlessness, and other symptoms for which there are no obvious explanation should be investigated as possible manifestations of chronic anxiety. Sometimes having the patient hyperventilate by breathing rapidly for about a minute can reproduce symptoms. Chronic hyperventilation can also produce transient T wave inversion and ST segment depression on electrocardiogram. Because of this, it is sometimes necessary to exclude coronary artery disease or pulmonary embolism before ascribing a patient's presentation to anxiety-induced hyperventilation.

A syndrome also related to panic disorder is the *syndrome of mitral valve prolapse* (MVP; see Chapter 60). This syndrome is of interest because symptoms associated with it resemble those associated with anxiety—dyspnea, faintness, chest pain, palpitations, and fatigue. True panic attacks rarely occur, however. Moreover, patients with panic disorder are not more likely to have MVP than controls. It is not clear at this time whether anxiety and MVP are both manifestations of an underlying disturbance or whether symptoms occurring in MVP serve to trigger anxiety in patients who are biologically predisposed to panic attacks.

Strategies and techniques for treating panic disorder are described below.

AGORAPHOBIA

Often the occurrence of severe anxiety or panic attacks will result in intense fear of recurrence of attack and especially of fear of finding oneself in situations where escape might not be possible. With recurrent panic attacks occurring over a period of several months, an individual might initially begin to avoid tunnels, elevators, crowded areas, *etc* that he feels he might not be able to "escape" from when an anxiety attack occurs. Later, with more and more frequent attacks, the person may fear to leave the house altogether. This state of markedly constricted activity is termed agoraphobia. Although the name means "fear of open spaces," this is a misnomer since it actually is the fear of having a panic attack away from a protecting person (24). Chronic anticipatory anxiety, somatic preoccupations, and depression may become superimposed upon the agoraphobia as an individual becomes more and more immobilized.

Agoraphobia is the commonest of all serious phobias in adults. Among a sample of members of a British organization for phobia suffers, 80.6% of 569 persons reported having agoraphobia (6). Agoraphobia represents over half of all those phobias that cause impairment in living. Its true prevalence is unknown, but it may affect almost 1% of the population. Age of onset is in the twenties and thirties and parallels that of panic disorder. A large majority of sufferers are female. Although some of these patients see psychiatrists for treatment, the majority consult their personal physicians. Mostly this is for treatment of somatic symptoms related to panic or generalized anxiety. Agoraphobia can be an extremely disabling problem. Strain in marriages, reduction of employment opportunities, restriction of social activities, and decrease in self-esteem, often leading to significant depression, are common. Once

Table 13.3.
Frequency of Strategies Adopted by Patients with Agoraphobia to Reduce Anticipatory Anxiety[a]

Strategy	Percentage of Patients
When out, having a way open for a quick return home	91
Being accompanied by husband/wife	85
Sitting near a door in hall, restaurant, *etc*	76
Focusing my mind on something else	63
When out for a walk, taking dog, perambulator, *etc*	62
Talking problem over with a friend	62
Talking problems over with my doctor	62
Being accompanied by a friend	60
Talking "sense to myself" (reassuring myself)	52
Wearing sunglasses	36

[a] From Burns LE, Thorpe GL: Epidemiology of fears and phobias. *J Int Med Res* 5:1, 1977.

agoraphobia has been initiated, phobic avoidance will be generalized to a variety of situations as mentioned above and the individual will adapt a variety of strategies to allow himself to feel better. Table 13.3 lists the 10 most common strategies adopted by agoraphobic patients to decrease anticipatory anxiety.

Strategies and techniques for treating agoraphobia are described below.

POST-TRAUMATIC STRESS DISORDER

When an individual undergoes a psychologically traumatic event which is outside the range of everyday stressful human experiences (e.g., severe automobile accident, destructive house fire, *etc*), disturbances of mood, autonomic hyperactivity, and impaired cognition may be associated with mental recapitulation of the traumatic event. The trauma may have caused physical harm to the individual (e.g., an assault), or it may not have caused harm but still have been recognized as physically threatening (e.g., an automobile crash). Symptoms may have their onset immediately after the event, or they may be delayed for as long as a year. In general, the shorter the time between onset of symptoms and the traumatic event the better the prognosis.

The main characteristic of the disorder is the recapitulation by the individual of the traumatic event. This may occur in nightmares, intrusive thoughts, or dissociative states in which the person behaves as if he is in the midst of the trauma. Associated with the experience of the stressor, there is usually emotional blunting, apathy, autonomic hyperarousal and difficulty in sleeping, irritability, explosions of aggressive behavior, impulsiveness, and inability to concentrate; typical symptoms of anxiety and depression may also occur. Symptoms may last for periods of 6 months or more and may be exacerbated by situations which resemble circumstances of the original trauma. In general, the longer the disorder persists, the worse is the prognosis for remission.

In its severe form, this disorder may impair functioning considerably. The individual may avoid circumstances that evoke memories of the event. The ability to experience warm and interpersonal relationships may be impaired. Suicidal behavior and substance abuse are serious complications. Because of these problems, patients with post-traumatic stress disorder should be referred to a psychiatrist for expert help.

DIFFERENTIAL DIAGNOSIS OF ANXIETY

It may be difficult to distinguish anxiety disorders from one another (see Table 13.4) and from other

Table 13.4.
Principal Differences among DSM-III Anxiety Disorders

Feature	Generalized Anxiety	Panic Disorder	Phobia	Post-Traumatic Stress Disorder
Onset	Teens or early adulthood	Usually adulthood	Anytime; medical phobias later	Anytime
Antecedents	Unstable home life; neurotic symptoms (school phobia, nail biting, shyness, insecurity)	Occurs in families; neurotic symptoms in childhood	May occur in families	Unknown
Precipitants	Worsened by environmental stressors and challenges to coping	Often environmental stressors, especially separations	Unknown; agoraphobia likely to be conditioned by panic attacks; social phobics show neurotic histories	Calamatous experience
Symptoms	Usually motor tension, apprehension, dependency, somatic complaints	Autonomic signs and symptoms; episodic, spontaneous panic	Specific fears with anticipatory anxiety (autonomic or motor)	Mood changes, nightmares, flashbacks
Treatment	Benzodiazepines and other anxiolytics; psychotherapy; self-regulation strategies; problem solving	Antidepressants, alprazolam, behavior therapy	Desensitization, flooding	Antidepressants, anxiolytics, psychotherapy
Prognosis	Chronic with acute exacerbations	Acute episodes may be successfully treated; recurrences are frequent	Good to variable	Unknown
Differential diagnosis	In adjustment disorders with anxious features anxiety is usually not chronic; in panic disorder episodic anxiety is present; in phobias avoidance is present	In organic disease symptoms are usually not episodic and the physical exam is positive; in generalized anxiety disorder there is no history of recurrent panic attacks; in phobic disorder there are specific feared stimuli	In generalized anxiety disorders there are no phobic stimuli; in panic disorder attacks come out of "clear blue sky"	In major depression, other anxiety disorders there are not calamatous incidents
Major complications	Excessive use of medical system; dependency on medication, especially tranquilizers	Agoraphobia; excessive use of medical system; major depression; substance abuse; generalized anxiety	Phobic avoidance; alcohol abuse (especially in social phobia)	Depression Substance abuse

conditions for which the treatment and prognosis are different. Depending upon the symptoms described by the individual patient, the differential diagnosis may include the medical conditions, drug toxicities, and drug withdrawal syndromes listed in Table 13.2. In a recent review of a number of patients presenting with somatic symptoms and later diagnosed as having anxiety disorders, only 11% of patients initially related their problems to psychosocial difficulties (20). The three most common presenting complaints of these patients were cardiac, gastrointestinal, and neurological symptoms. In most instances an adequate history and physical examination would have directed the physician away from a medical disorder.

Transient anxiety, at times combined with symptoms of depression, occurs frequently in patients who are being followed for long-standing but stable medical conditions. Usually these minor mood disturbances (adjustment disorders) occur as a reaction to situational stress in patients who are coping well; and the symptoms of anxiety respond well to brief counseling and appropriate use of psychotropic drugs (7, 8). Patients with adjustment disorders often present their anxiety symptoms as somatic complaints (see additional information in Chapter 12).

It is sometimes difficult to distinguish generalized anxiety disorder from other anxiety disorders because patients with specific phobias, agoraphobia, and panic disorder often report chronically high levels of anxiety that result from anticipating an episode of severe anxiety. Moreover, as mentioned previously, some patients with chronic generalized anxiety do have classic panic attacks when stressors in their lives increase. Some of these patients may respond to the treatments that are relatively specific for panic disorder (see below). In differentiating generalized anxiety disorder from panic disorder, it should be established that the chronic anxiety is not simply anticipatory anxiety. This is best done by looking for a simple phobia or agoraphobia or panic attack as the primary cause of anxiety.

In some patients, anxiety may be associated with office visits for medical conditions. This *"normal" anxiety* occurs as a response to threats to one's health and may be heightened by the following factors: (*a*) situational factors such as unfamiliarity with a new physician or a scheduled visit for a potentially painful procedure; (*b*) individual factors such as a patient's interpretation of the gravity of his problem, expectations of disability, and his capacity to assume a dependent and trusting relationship with the physician; (*c*) certain cultural factors which color the meaning of disease and the role of the medical care system in general; and (*d*) preexisting psychopathology in the form of anxiety disorders which may be exacerbated by the stress of disease or a concurrent stress in the patient's life. While not reaching the intensity of an anxiety dis-

order, heightened anxiety may interfere with a patient's ability to remember details relevant to his medical history, to tolerate pain, and to comprehend the physician's message. This is illustrated by Figure 13.1 which shows the relationship between anxiety and performance. At low levels, anxiety may actually increase alertness, attentiveness, learning, and comprehension. Beyond a certain point, however, anxiety is no longer adaptive and interferes with normal function. Clinically, this has been illustrated pointedly by Mayou *et al* (28), who found that survivors of myocardial infarction and their spouses recollected little of the information and explanations given to them during in-hospital recovery from the heart attack. Thus, not only is it important to detect significant anxiety in a patient but also to treat it skillfully by reassuring the patient, anticipating his concerns, providing an opportunity to ventilate, and, wherever possible, giving essential information in a written form.

Finally, although anxiety may occur periodically in many psychiatric disorders, *schizophrenia* and *dementia* (or delirium) may initially present with it as the most striking feature. The manifestations of these two disorders are described in Chapters 16 and 17, respectively.

GENERAL PRINCIPLES FOR THE TREATMENT OF ANXIETY

The treatment of anxiety requires a combination of pharmacological and other approaches. The identification of anxiety, problem solving related to concurrent stressors, and pharmacological and nonpharmacological management are three essential steps. A number of behavioral techniques, briefly described below, are best applied by mental health professionals with experience dealing with the more complicated anxiety disorders. Stepwise practical

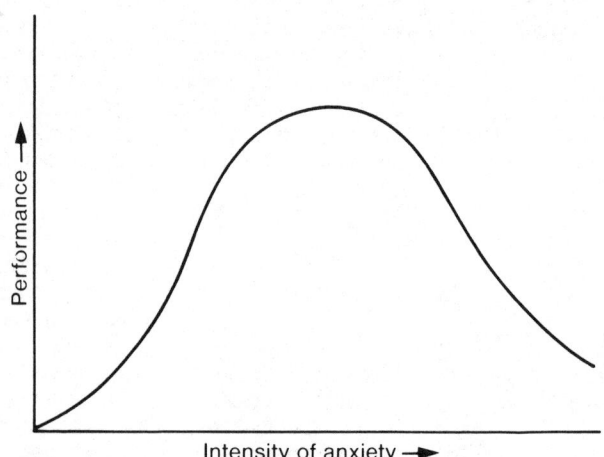

Figure 13.1. Schematic representation of the effect of anxiety on performance.

approaches for office management of the commonest anxiety syndromes are described below (page 171).

Theoretical Basis for Treatment

Current management of anxiety is based upon efforts to delineate better the specific anxiety disorders. The specificity reflected in the classification system of DSM-III was prompted by a series of observations beginning with Klein's finding (21) that imipramine but not benzodiazepines blocked spontaneous anxiety attacks in patients with panic disorder. He suggested that the noradrenergic system was important in the production of symptoms of panic attacks. Later, experimental evidence for a specific benzodiazepine receptor emerged. This receptor was associated with the neurotransmitter γ-aminobutyric acid (GABA). Currently two psychopharmacological models of anxiety are postulated: one located in the pons, mediated by noradrenergic activation and corresponding to "alarm" (having as its principal clinical manifestation the panic attack); another located in the telencephalon, mediated by the GABA-benzodiazepine system and corresponding to "fear" (having as its principal manifestation generalized anxiety disorder) (9, 18). Future research will probably yield a better understanding of the psychopharmacology of anxiety and to the development of more specific antianxiety drugs with fewer side effects.

Behavioral techniques for managing anxiety are based upon well established models of conditioning. In classical conditioning, it is postulated that phobic disorders and generalized anxiety are acquired when an unconditioned stimulus is paired with a conditioned stimulus. For example while a panic attack may occur as a result of some internal defect in the modulation of stress and anxiety, stimuli (places, events, *etc*) associated with the anxiety attack will be avoided. Thus an individual having an anxiety attack in a supermarket will begin to avoid supermarkets. This theory provides the conceptual basis for such treatments as flooding and systematic desensitization (see below). In operant conditioning, behaviors are seen to have rewards or punishments that serve to reinforce or extinguish those behaviors. Those behaviors which are reinforced regularly often become the most difficult habits to break. Anxiety that elicits admonitions to rest or attention from the doctor is an example of this. Extinction of such behaviors is often accomplished by putting the patient on a program that encourages active coping with anxiety, as described below.

Nonpharmacological Techniques

Explanation-Education

Patients with chronic anxiety which suddenly flares up, those who are phobic of situations, places, and people, or those who are fearful of leaving the house usually suffer from feelings of loss of control. Often they have no explanation for their symptoms, which appear confusing to them. Moreover, patients are often unaware of environmental factors that may be increasing their anxiety. Sometimes merely providing a name for a particular disorder and information about it gives the patient confidence that he has a recognized entity for which there is treatment. In some places, there are self-help organizations that provide education and mutual support.

Self-Regulation Techniques

The self-regulation techniques useful in treating anxiety include muscle relaxation, biofeedback, meditation, and self-hypnosis. They are targeted at the motor tension and autonomic hyperactivity that accompany anxiety. They are called "self-regulation" because patients are taught to apply the techniques themselves. This often restores a sense of control to the patient. The techniques are useful (a) in patients with generalized anxiety disorder; (b) as an adjunct to other therapies, such as flooding, in which relaxation techniques allow the subject more easily to tolerate contact with a phobic stimulus; (c) together with imagery in systematic desensitization therapy for phobias; (d) in decreasing arousal that may be playing a role in initiating or exacerbating medical problems such as asthma attacks or hypertension. These techniques are briefly described. Their role in managing anxiety is critically reviewed in a recent paper by Goldberg (see "General References").

In *progressive muscle relaxation*, which is widely used, patients are taught to contract then relax individual muscle groups in sequence (see Table 13.5). The objectives are to teach the patient to identify tension and to facilitate relaxation. The theory underlying this technique is that muscle relaxation is incompatible with anxiety and that as one learns to relax muscles, anxiety will be mastered. Of course the patient must also be helped to identify anxiety-producing stimuli in the environment so that he will know when to use the technique. Home practice is important for mastery. There are many commercially available audio tapes to guide the patient through the procedure (see General References). Often therapists make their own tapes for patients. Benson *et al*'s article (5) entitled "The Relaxation Response" is written for the lay person and may be helpful.

In *biofeedback* (13) the patient receives visual or auditory signals about the tension in one or more muscle groups. Electrodes register electromyographic activity that is not normally available to the patient. He is then in a position to alter this activity to receive immediate feedback on the results of his effort, and to learn how to achieve desirable results (in this instance, muscle relaxation). For example,

Table 13.5.
Essential Steps in (A) Progressive Muscle Relaxation and (B) Rapid Muscle Relaxation Techniques[a]

Muscle	Exercise
	(A) PROGRESSIVE MUSCLE RELAXATION[b]
Forehead/scalp	Raise the eyebrows high; hold; feel strain; relax.
Forehead	Scowl or frown; bunch eyebrows with nose upward; relax.
Eyes	Squeeze eyes shut; hold; feel strain in temples; relax.
Mouth	Smile broadly until mouth quivers slightly; relax; press lips tightly inward; hold; relax.
Jaw	Grit teeth gently but firmly; hold, relax; part lips slightly.
Neck/arm/shoulder	Press head back against right hand; relax; repeat exercise with left hand.
Neck/arm/shoulder	Press head forward against right hand placed on forehead; relax; repeat with left hand.
Back/legs/abdomen	Sitting, grip chair sides firmly; raise legs slightly; lift buttocks 1 inch from chair; point toes forward, then backward; relax.
Hands/arm	Make fist; clench tightly; relax.
	(B) RAPID RELAXATION[c]
Step 1:	Sit or lie down. The quieter the place, the better.
Step 2:	Take a deep breath through your mouth, hold it for 10 seconds, and exhale slowly.
Step 3:	Mentally repeat the word "relax" 4 times in a calm manner.
Step 4:	Gradually space out repeating "relax" until each repetition takes about 7 seconds.
Step 5:	Keep practicing until you achieve the level of relaxation you desire.

[a] Reproduced with the permission of Dr. Richard Waranch.
[b] Subject instructed to practice this seated comfortably or reclining.
[c] For immediate relaxation in everyday stressful situation.

successful frontalis muscle relaxation may be accompanied by a decrease in the amplitude of a tone which is transmitted to the patient *via* earphones.

In teaching *self-hypnosis* therapists often induce deep states of muscle relaxation in addition to facilitating increased reception to suggestion. One technique is to use a standardized hypnotic induction technique and then ask the patient to focus on the toes and feet and notice the warm, tingling feeling. The therapist guides the movement of this feeling throughout the body. He sometimes uses the suggestion of pleasant, relaxing scenes. The patient is taught how to self-induce hypnosis and repeat the sequence and is given home practice, with repetitions in the office several weeks apart to provide reinforcement. Tapes of the therapist's voice may also be made. Hypnosis is a skill which can be easily learned by attending seminars given by professional organizations such as the Society for Clinical and Experimental Hypnosis.

Meditation techniques such as Zen, yoga, and transcendental meditation have been practiced for centuries but have recently become more fashionable because they induce physiological effects opposite to those which accompany anxiety. These beneficial effects include decreased respiratory rate and oxygen consumption and decrease in galvanic skin response, a measure of autonomic activity. Benson et al (5), who studied the physiological states induced by various meditation techniques, believe that the following factors are necessary to induce what they call the "relaxation response." (a) *A mental device.* There should be a constant stimulus such as a sound, word, or phrase repeated silently or audibly, or fixed gazing at an object. The purpose of these procedures is to shift attention away from logical, externally oriented thoughts. (b) *Passive attitude.* If distracting thoughts occur during the repetition or gazing, they should be disregarded and attention should be redirected to the technique. The patient should not worry about the quality of his performance. (c) *Decreased muscle tonus.* The patient should be in a comfortable position so that minimal muscular work is required. (d) *Quiet environment.* An environment with decreased environmental stimuli should be chosen. Most techniques instruct the subject to close his eyes.

Studies designed to demonstrate the efficacy of meditation in inducing a hypometabolic state and decreased autonomic activity have yielded inconsistent results. Moreover, although the technique is easy to understand it is not so easy to learn, especially for anxious patients who cannot control unwanted thought intrusions and restlessness. Therefore, only patients who are highly motivated to overcome these initial difficulties are likely to benefit.

Scrignar (37) explains a technique that he calls "encephalic reconditioning," which is known more commonly in the US as "*cognitive restructuring.*" In one modification of this technique the patient is taught to monitor thoughts associated with anxiety such as "what will happen if. . . ." The patient helps to create scenes from fantasy or past memory of happy events. After they are practiced daily and well rehearsed, he is instructed to substitute them when an anxiety-related thought comes into mind. Patients who are likely to misinterpret somatic stimuli, whether normal or related to somatic anxiety, are first educated about the significance of these stimuli and then are taught to use positive reinforcing statements when they experience these sensations. For example:

1. I feel comfortable.
2. I am experiencing pathological anxiety.
3. I have had these feelings before and they have passed.
4. They are not related to a physical problem.

This cognitive form of therapy is often used together with relaxation techniques or self-hypnosis.

The interested generalist can develop skill in teaching his patients one or more of the techniques described above.

Specialized Techniques for Phobic Disorders

The treatment of phobias has benefited greatly from behavioral therapies aimed at fear extinction through a variety of methods. Three commonly used techniques are desensitization, participant modeling, and social skills training.

Systematic desensitization is a counterconditioning technique in which the patient's own imagery is used to expose the phobic stimuli gradually. The anxiety-provoking properties of the stimuli are eliminated by having the patient exercise a response incompatible with anxiety—that of relaxation—when images associated with anxiety are presented visually or in fantasy to the patient. This treatment occurs over a series of sessions until the patient is comfortable enough to encounter the stimulus *in vivo*. Related to systematic desensitization is *flooding* or implosion in which the imagery is not presented in a gradual way but instead the patient is helped to confront it quickly through imagery.

In vivo desensitization usually combines several approaches such as systematic desensitization, relaxation training, and education. The central element, however, is gradual exposure of the patient to the feared stimulus in real life in a stepwise manner and in repeated fashion. The patient is often accompanied by the therapist but gradually this support withdraws. For example, a severe agoraphobic may go through a series of more anxiety-producing tasks such as taking excursions a certain distance from the house, riding the bus, shopping, *etc.* Progress from less to more anxiety-producing tasks is accomplished by mastering anxiety at each level. The basis for the techniques is that repeated exposure produces extinction.

Participant modeling is a form of *in vivo* desensitization in which the therapist models the desired interaction with the feared object. Taylor and his colleagues (40) describe the use of this procedure with severe needle phobics whose refusal of procedures was potentially life threatening. The particular therapy involved the following steps:

1. education aimed at providing realistic information about the feared object;
2. response modeling in which the therapist handles the feared object;
3. joint performance which exposes the patient to the feared object together with the therapist;
4. self-directed practice. (In the case of a needle phobic, the first step was inserting the needle into an orange.)

Social skills training is used especially with social phobias. It is also called assertiveness training. Its object is to promote the development of comfortable social interactions using techniques such as modeling and role playing that aim to reduce specific social fears such as speaking in public, attending meetings, *etc.* Treatment usually occurs over 12 to 15 sessions.

Behavioral techniques like these have been used successfully for phobias related to such situations as hemodialysis, needles, and return to work after medical illness. They have several advantages: (*a*) They are time limited and when successful can be carried out within 15 sessions; (*b*) they have clear outcome measures related to reduction of fear and avoidance of phobic stimulus; (*c*) they may be administered by paramedical personnel, such as nurses; (*d*) they appear to be cost effective. Marks (24, 26) has reported that difficult-to-treat fear, hypochondriacal symptoms, and work adjustment improve within 6 months. More impressive in his series of patients, visits to general practitioners decreased by 60% and to specialists by 43%, and the net reduction in nonhospital health care resource usage was 61%.

The results of desensitization are particularly impressive with agoraphobics, who are usually markedly impaired. The most frequently reported improvements are reduction in fear of leaving the house, decrease in other phobic symptoms, a decrease in generalized anxiety, decreased depression, improvement in social relationships, and enhanced ability to return to work (31). It is important to note that, although most patients report global improvement, for many residual distress remains that is tolerated and affects life style minimally. Several studies have shown clearly that *in vivo* desensitization alone and desensitization plus antidepressant therapy produce results which have been maintained for as long as 5 years of follow-up (35). Interestingly, predictors of outcome are for the most part unrelated to severity or duration of phobia but rather to social support measures, such as level of marital satisfaction, and to degree of generalization of phobia (1).

Psychotherapy is also important in the treatment of phobias. Its efficacy for the most part appears to lie in promoting confidence in the patient to encounter feared stimuli and thus facilitate extinction. In addition, exploration of such issues as separation, which sometimes triggers anxiety, can be helpful in providing a rationale to the patient for his symptoms and promoting anxiety reduction. Psychotherapy techniques useful in office practice are described in Chapter 11.

Pharmacological Treatment

Benzodiazepines

In the late 1960s and early 1970s there was a dramatic increase in the use of benzodiazepines in the United States so that diazepam quickly became the most frequently prescribed drug in the country (17). Since then usage has dropped amid adverse publicity that caused public concern over problems such as inappropriate use, addiction, and "national tranquilization." In part these concerns are valid since studies have shown that in some communities up to 20% of adults in the general population have used these or related drugs in a single year, and they have been used daily for at least 1 week by approximately 10% of adults (41). On the other hand, recent epidemiological surveys indicate that not only has the prevalence of psychopathology in the general population been significantly underestimated but that those patients with the most serious disorders are still receiving inadequate therapy (38). Recently the discovery of (a) specific brain receptors for benzodiazepines and (b) benzodiazepine antagonists that induce behavioral symptoms similar to anxiety suggests that biochemical abnormality may underlie many anxiety disorders.

Pharmacological properties of benzodiazepines. Benzodiazepines have anxiolytic, sedative-hypnotic, and anticonvulsant properties. "Anxiolytic" refers to their capacity to decrease apprehension, uncomfortable sensations associated with arousal, and avoidance behavior.

After intravenous injection, all benzodiazepines rapidly cross the blood-brain barrier, producing onset of effect in less than 1 minute. Intramuscularly only lorazepam has been shown to have rapid and complete absorption consistently. In cases of acute, severe anxiety, if diazepam is the only drug available it should be injected into the deltoid muscle area where higher blood flow will increase absorption (15). There are differences among the benzodiazepines in *onset of action* following oral administration (Table 13.6). Drugs with rapid absorption from the gastrointestinal tract have a prompt clinical effect, but sedation is more likely to occur. Those absorbed slowly may cause less drowsiness. Chlorazepate, a long acting benzodiazepine, is hydrolyzed into its active metabolite in the stomach. Patients with low gastric acidity and those taking antacid medication will absorb only minimal amounts of

this drug. *Duration of action* of benzodiazepines depends upon differences in distribution. Those drugs with high affinity for fat tissue are distributed rapidly into peripheral tissues, chiefly adipose tissue, thus diminishing their concentration and effect in the brain after a single dose and prolonging their presence in the patient (elimination half-life) (16). Because duration of anxiolytic action following a single dose depends more upon drug distribution than elimination half-life, more lipophilic agents (i.e., agents with a long half-life, such as diazepam) may have a shorter duration of anxiolytic action than those with a short half-life (e.g., lorazepam) following a single oral dose.

For multiple dosing on a maintenance schedule, unwanted side effects such as drowsiness and sedation are more likely to occur with the drugs that have high *indices of accumulation* (i.e., longer elimination half-life). Long term users of benzodiazepines appear to adjust to the sedating property of the long acting benzodiazepines because of *tolerance.* Another aspect of accumulation revolves around *withdrawal.* Withdrawal symptoms are more likely to occur in patients taking drugs with high rates of accumulation such as diazepam. Unpleasant reactions such as agitation and even seizures can occur upon abrupt withdrawal, especially in patients taking large doses for long periods of time (12). Finally there are two principal *routes of clearance* for benzodiazepines—oxidation and conjugation by the liver. Factors that influence hepatic oxidation, such as hepatitis, cirrhosis, or drug therapy, may lead to excessive accumulation.

The most commonly encountered *side effects* of benzodiazepines are related to central nervous system depression. This may result in drowsiness, poor motor coordination, ataxia, and decreased cognitive abilities, such as impaired concentration and memory. Benzodiazepines with more rapid onset of action (Table 13.6) are more likely to cause these effects. Patients may be sensitive to even small doses of medication and should be warned ahead of time that sedation may occur. On the other hand, tolerance to side effects (but usually not to anxiolytic effects) commonly occurs after 1 or 2 weeks.

Prolonged use of benzodiazepines in recommended doses usually does not result in physiological dependence. Termination of drug therapy, however, may result in re-emergence of symptoms of anxiety. This usually occurs over a period of a week or two after discontinuation and should be distinguished from withdrawal, which tends to occur more rapidly and to decrease over time. Withdrawal symptoms occur more frequently with abrupt discontinuation of short acting drugs. Typically, there is autonomic nervous system hyperactivity signified by tremulousness, sweating, photosensitivity, abdominal discomfort, and systolic hypertension. Readministering the drug on a slowly tapering

Table 13.6.
Usual Dose and Pharmacokinetics of Anxiolytic Benzodiazepines

Drug (Trade Name) Year Introduced	Onset of Effect after Oral Dose[a]	Available Strengths	Oral Daily DoseRange Divided Two or Three Times a Day	Active Metabolites Present	Elimination Half-life
		mg	mg		hr
Alprazolam (Xanax) 1981	Intermediate	0.25, 0.5, 1 (scored tablets)	0.25–8	No	8–16
Chlordiazepoxide[b] (Librium) (Libritabs) 1960	Intermediate	5, 10, 25 (capsules) 5, 10, 25 (tablets)	15–150	Yes	5–30
Clorazepate dipotassium (Tranxene)	Rapid	3.75, 7.5, 15 (capsules)	15–60	Yes	36–200
(Tranxene SD) 1972		11.25, 22.5 (tablets)	22.5 (single doses are intended for patients stabilized on 3.75 or 7.5 mg three times a day)	Yes	36–200
Diazepam[b] (Valium) 1961	Rapid	2, 5, 10 (tablets)	4–40	Yes	20–50
Diazepam (Valrelease) 1982	Slow	15 (capsules)	15–30 (single dose is equivalent to 5 mg of Valium three times a day)	Yes	20–50
Halezepam (Paxipam) 1981	Slow to intermediate	20, 40 (tablets)	80–160	Yes	50–100
Lorazepam[b] (Ativan) 1977	Intermediate	0.5, 1, 2 (tablets)	1–6	No	10–20
Oxazepam (Serax) 1963	Slow to intermediate	10, 15, 30 (capsules) 15 (tablets)	30–120 30–120	No	5–10
Prazepam (Centrax) 1977	Rapid	5, 10 (capsules)	20–60	Yes	36–200

[a] Drugs with more rapid onset of action are those more rapidly absorbed. Elimination half-life reflects degree of lipophilic activity.
[b] Generic available.

schedule over a period of a week is the treatment of choice for this withdrawal syndrome.

Benzodiazepines are not frequently abused by "hard core" drug abusers. However, their extensive availability results in significant misuse. They are sometimes used to "boost" the effects of methadone, and when other drugs are not available benzodiazepines may be ingested in quantities up to the equivalent of several hundred milligrams a day of diazepam. However, harmful overdosages with benzodiazepines alone are rare due to their very high index of safety; fatal overdoses may, however, occur when benzodiazepines are used with alcohol or other substances that depress the nervous system. For further details, see Chapters 21 (alcoholism) and 22 (illicit drugs).

In prescribing benzodiazepines, one should be aware of several important influences on drug metabolism. These include: (a) the effect of antacids in reducing the amount of the active metabolite of clorazepate available for absorption from the gastrointestinal tract; (b) the effect of disulfiram in decreasing the plasma clearance of diazepam and chlordiazepoxide; and (c) the reduced clearance found for most benzodiazepines in the elderly and in the presence of liver disease.

Practical use of benzodiazepines. In placebo trials all benzodiazepines have been found to be effective in the management of anxiety. Selection of a particular drug will be determined by the intended use, characteristics of the patient, and such other factors as drug cost. In this regard, chlordiazepoxide is now produced in a generic form. For the extremely agitated patient, where rapid sedation is desirable, intramuscular lorazepam or diazepam given in the deltoid muscle is probably the agent of choice. Where rapid initial effect is not a concern and when drug accumulation is undesirable, a short acting benzodiazepine such as lorazepam may be selected. This may be particularly important in elderly or chronically ill patients, who seem especially prone to undesirable side effects; these patients should be given low starting doses and be followed up soon to assess the effect (16). Compared to previously used anxiolytics, such as barbiturates, the benzodiazepines are less sedating at equivalent doses, rarely associated with fatalities when used alone in overdoses, and have relatively low abuse potential.

Benzodiazepines are for the most part indicated for the treatment of patients with generalized anxiety, either acute or chronic. Patients with a low baseline level of anxiety who become symptomatic during a time of acute stress are likely to go into remission more promptly with a short course of benzodiazepine treatment, although several studies indicate that counseling alone may suffice for a majority of these patients (7, 8).

Other patients whose anxiety is always near an intense level may benefit from *periods of long term treatment.* It does not appear that such patients develop tolerance to the anxiety-reducing effect. Discontinuation of benzodiazepine administration after several months in patients with chronic generalized anxiety is associated with the return of symptoms in the majority of patients (34). Patients most likely to benefit from prolonged (e.g., several months) benzodiazepine treatment are those with relatively severe anxiety and without significant depression, those who have responded previously to anxiolytics, those with stable relationships, and those with realistic treatment goals (33). Physicians who are perceived as warm, empathetic, and having a positive attitude toward drugs are more likely to be successful in helping such patients.

With the exception of alprazolam, benzodiazepines do not block panic attacks, and they are not indicated in patients with specific phobias. As noted elsewhere in this chapter (page 172), there are other therapies available for these disorders and there is potential for benzodiazepine abuse. Benzodiazepines are useful, however, as an adjunct in patients with agoraphobia and generalized anxiety.

The decision to treat with benzodiazepines must be a clinical judgment. The physician should always attempt to elicit a history of recent stress. Often this allows the patient to ventilate and to be reassured that support is available, and often minor tranquilizers may not be necessary. This is often the case when anxiety is mixed with depression as part of an adjustment disorder (see Chapter 12). If anxiety is the prominent feature, if it is interfering with functioning, or if the patient has a pre-existing anxiety disorder, a trial of benzodiazepines is worthwhile. The benzodiazepine should be intergrated into an overall practical approach to managing anxiety (see below).

Barbiturates

These substances are rarely used for treatment of anxiety today. In addition to the fact that doses that relieve anxiety also produce sedation, these drugs have more side effects, more potential for abuse, and are more lethal when taken in overdose than benzodiazepines.

β-Adrenergic Blockers

Propranolol and other β-blockers may be more effective than benzodiazepines in reducing the marked autonomic symptoms—such as palpitations, tachycardia, and breathlessness—that occur in some anxious individuals (22). β-Blockers may be particularly helpful prophylactically in acute stress situations that elicit autonomic anxiety, such as public speaking, giving musical performances, and taking examinations. In these situations the cognitive impairment which may be produced by benzodiazepines is undesirable. β-Blockers do not appear to be very useful in blocking panic attacks; however, they may be tried in a patient who does not tolerate the drugs of choice for this disorder (alprazolam or tricyclic antidepressants, see below). They also do not appear to be particularly effective in eliminating the subjective distress of an anxious person unless it is connected with disturbing autonomic sensations. Details regarding the use of β-blocking drugs are found in Chapter 62.

Antihistamines

Antihistamines are used to control anxiety as alternatives to benzodiazepines. They appear to be safer for patients with chronic obstructive pulmonary disease in whom benzodiazepines may suppress respiration, and they are useful in patients in whom benzodiazepines may represent potential agents of abuse. Their major disadvantage is that they sedate the patient significantly. Hydroxyzine (Atarax, Vistaril) is most frequently prescribed and is preferable to diphenhydramine, which sometimes increases muscle tone and affects the peripheral autonomic nervous system. Hydroxyzine is prescribed in doses ranging from 10 to 25 mg three times a day.

Antidepressants

Both tricyclic antidepressants and monamine oxidase inhibitors have been shown to be effective in blocking panic attacks that occur spontaneously or that are induced experimentally by lactate infusion or a variety of other methods. The two most frequently used drugs are imipramine and phenelzine. Patients usually require dosages similar to those indicated for depressive disorders, imipramine between 100 and 250 mg/day and phenelzine 60 to 90 mg/day. The latter drug is not used much in the United States because of its interaction with dietary tyramine (see Table 15.5) and sympathomimetic drugs. Details regarding the use of antidepressant drugs are found in Chapter 15.

Antidepressants alone do not appear to help symptoms due to agoraphobia (27, 39). Although they block panic attacks, phobic avoidance usually remains a problem and usually desensitization is needed (see above). Many patients in Britain are treated successfully for agoraphobia without drugs and have remittance of panic attacks. Therefore, whether panic attacks are secondary to the anxiety which invariably accompanies agoraphobia or represent the primary problem leading to agoraphobia is unclear. There is some suggestion that agoraphobics with severe depression respond better to antidepressants.

Antidepressants are not indicated for generalized anxiety but may play a role in adjustment disorder with depressed and anxious mood (see Chapter 12).

GUIDELINES FOR TREATING SPECIFIC ANXIETY SYNDROMES

Practical steps in assessing and managing patients with discrete anxiety syndromes are outlined here.

Prevention and Management of Anxiety Associated with Any Illness

The generalist's role in the *prevention* of unnecessary anxiety is important. As mentioned previously, patients often have illness fears which are worsened by a variety of factors. The following approaches are helpful:

1. Assume that patients with new symptoms often have concerns about serious illness. Asking the patient if he or she has thought of what the problem might be due to can be very helpful. Frequently, a relative or friend will have had a similar symptom related to a serious disease.

2. Avoid comments or jargon that might sensitize or frighten patients (e.g., commenting, while examining a skin lesion, "It's been a long time since I've seen one like that").

3. Take the opportunity to reassure the patient routinely, even if prognosis is guarded. The physician can find a way to communicate some hope and optimism to the patient in many adverse situations.

4. Prepare the patient for painful procedures with explanations. Assume that any procedure may be potentially frightening to a patient.

5. Assume that any patient recovering from serious illness will be anxious about the future; determine if any unnecessary disability is due to fear or inadequate education. Hospitalized patients often get incomplete explanations of their illnesses at the time of their discharge.

6. Show a warm and personal manner that will inspire trust and will encourage the patient to disclose what is on his mind.

Generalized Anxiety Disorder

By following a number of practical steps, one can usually help a patient with generalized anxiety disorder (see diagnostic criteria, page 159) to reach lower levels of anxiety and of functional impairment.

1. Elicit a history of situational stressors which may be amenable to problem solving, and encourage the patient to ventilate and to explore ways to reduce stress in his life. (See Chapter 11, Psychotherapy in Ambulatory Practice.)

2. Determine the necessity for medication. Agitation, poor sleep and concentration, and unremitting worry are indications for medication. In less severe anxiety, periodic visits at which the patient ventilates may be sufficient treatment.

3. Involve the patient in the decision to use medication. Tailor the medication to the patient's needs. Drugs with slow onset of action (see Table 13.6) may minimize the risk of sedation in those needing to drive or to operate machinery. Advise the patient of possible side effects. Patients will often know through experience which medication has helped them in the past.

4. Advise the patient that medication is an adjunct to therapy. Agree upon the length of drug treatment.

5. Begin treatment with a dose suited to the level of anxiety. For severe problems consider starting at a relatively high dose. Troublesome side effects can be dealt with by instructing the patient to titrate the dose down if they occur.

6. Schedule a return visit or a return phone call in a week or so. Improvement can be gauged by reports of decreased subjective distress and somatization, increased sleep, and diminished preoccupation with specific worries.

7. Continue to explore issues exacerbating anxiety. In motivated patients use relaxation or meditation as adjunctive therapies (see pages 165–166).

8. Obtain additional psychosocial history. This may help to determine a need for chronic therapy.

9. After 4 to 6 weeks, a trial off medication is indicated. This should be done by gradual tapering over a week's time.

A number of difficulties may occur in the management for generalized anxiety:

1. Some patients will be so somatically focused that they will frustrate one's attempt to elicit a psychosocial history. These patients are often psychologically unsophisticated, and one needs time to form an alliance with them. In this case one should rely on significant others for some of the history.

2. Some patients will experience a return of anxiety after a trial off medication. This usually occurs within 1 to 4 weeks after medication is terminated. When symptoms are related to withdrawal they typically occur in the first few days after the drug is stopped. If marked symptoms recur, one should consider extending the trial to 4 months (34) or look for persisting psychosocial stressors that are amenable to change. Referral to a mental health facility for adjunctive therapies, such as family counseling, may be helpful.

3. Some depressive affect may emerge during history taking, especially in a patient whose anxiety is accompanied by agitated behavior. Further exploration for symptoms of depression is important in such a patient, since he may in fact have a major depression (possibly "atypical") in which benzodiazepines can exacerbate the illness (see Chapter 15, Affective Disorders).

Panic Disorder

In new onset of panic disorder (see diagnostic criteria, pages 160–161)—before phobic avoidance, dependence, and persistent generalized anxiety have evolved—the following practical steps should be followed:

1. Educate the patient about the nature of anxiety as the source of his problem. If there is a history of the disorder in a family member, this fact can be cited to persuade the patient that this is a real illness and that the course is predictable.

2. Elicit a history of current stressors, especially recent separations. Discuss the impact of this with the patient.

3. Suggest to the patient a trial of alprazolam (39). Begin at 0.5 mg three times a day and increase slowly over the next 2 to 4 weeks until attacks have abated. A total daily dose of 3 to 8 mg is usually required to achieve satisfactory control of attacks.

4. If the frequency of panic attacks does not dramatically decrease after a 3-week trial of alprazolam, consider tapering this drug and adding a tricyclic antidepressant (imipramine is most commonly used). Very small doses (begin with 25 mg/day) may be adequate in some patients but doses in the range of usual treatment for depressive disorders (e.g., 100 to 250 mg of imipramine) may be required.

5. After a satisfactory response has been achieved, the patient should remain on medication until he is symptom free for 6 to 12 months. During this time,

the daily dose can sometimes be reduced. After 6 to 12 months, medication can be tapered *slowly* (over 2 to 3 months). Relapse occurs in a majority of patients after medication is discontinued. If relapse occurs, medication should be reinstituted and maintained indefinitely.

The most common problems that occur are drug side effects and lack of response to therapy. The former should be monitored carefully, including regular checking for orthostatic hypotension when an antidepressant is used. Failure of response on a trial of two different medications should be cause for specialty referral.

Post-traumatic Stress Disorder

Because this disorder is relatively new in psychiatric classification (see diagnostic criteria, page 162), treatment trials have not been reported. Antidepressants appear to be helpful in improving mood, nightmares, and flashbacks. Because of the lack of precise treatment guidelines, however, patients who are significantly disturbed by this disorder should be referred for psychiatric treatment.

Phobias

The techniques used in the treatment of phobic disorders (see diagnostic criteria, page 157) are best administered by those with the expertise to tailor them to the patient's individual situations. While some phobias can be rapidly extinguished using systematic desensitization over one to five sessions, some patients require as many as 24 sessions to accomplish treatment. This is especially true for agoraphobia (35). For this reason patients with this and other phobic disorders should be referred to professionals with expertise in managing these problems. The various behavioral techniques used in the management of phobias are described above under "Specialized Techniques for Phobic Disorders."

CASE EXAMPLES

Because anxiety is such a pervasive symptom in office practice, its evaluation represents a significant challenge to the physician. The following cases illustrate the possible modes of presentation of anxiety and provide guidelines for evaluation and management.

The Patient with "Bad Nerves"

A 42-year-old married woman is seen by a physician for the first time. She states: "Doctor, I've been so nervous for so long. Can't you refill my prescription?" She presents the physician with a prescription bottle containing a few minor tranquilizer tablets which she received at a local emergency room. She is about to run out of the medicine. The patient appears apprehensive, mildly tremulous, fidgity, and distressed as she sits toward the edge of her chair.

Typically this is the presentation of a patient with chronic "free-floating" anxiety and general anxiety disorder. The following points are helpful.

Evaluation

In eliciting a history from the patient, the physician needs to focus on the following psychological elements:

1. How long has the patient felt nervous? Even in patients with generalized anxiety disorder, the onset of symptom exacerbation may be related to recent life stresses. Most common among these are separations (divorce, loss of job, relatives, and children by death or other circumstances, marital strife, employment difficulties).

2. Has the patient ever had this problem before or been treated for it? Patients with chronic anxiety are high utilizers of medical care and psychiatric services. Many patients depend upon minor tranquilizers chronically, but others seek out physicians when external and sometimes internal stresses push their anxiety above the threshold of tolerability. Precipitants of previous episodes of anxiety are helpful to know.

3. In differentiating among the various causes of anxiety, are any of the following syndromes present?

a. *Panic attacks.* Patients with a history of episodic severe autonomic anxiety with or without agoraphobia often develop generalized anxiety. Separations will sometimes precipitate the onset of panic disorders in predisposed individuals. In generalized anxiety disorder, however, most often anxiety is experienced as motor tension, does not occur in acute, sudden episodic fashion, and is not associated with avoidance or agoraphobia.

b. *Phobias.* The anxiety associated with phobia is usually specific to the phobic stimulus and is not generalized. Anticipating necessary contact with the feared object may lead to anticipatory anxiety.

c. *Post-traumatic stress.* This is usually initiated by a calamity of unusual proportions.

d. *Depression.* Depressed mood, low self-esteem, and sleep disturbances are often mixed with symptoms of anxiety, especially in patients with adjustment disorders.

e. *Medically related.* A review of the symptoms will reveal other symptoms such as nausea and vomiting, recent increase in irritation, new drugs, or alcohol abuse as a precipitant.

4. Does the patient's past history reveal information that would be helpful in supporting any of the above diagnoses? Developmental histories are often easily elicited during the physical examination and may serve to distract the patient's attention from uncomfortable maneuvers. The physician can casually inquire about:

a. The patient's early home environment.

b. The presence of "bad nerves" or othe psychiatric problems in the family.

c. A history of childhood neurotic symptoms—late thumb sucking, nightmares, fingernail biting, school phobia, shyness, timidity, social anxiety that would predispose one to generalized anxiety.

d. Is the patient a chronic worrier who frets about minor problems?

5. What current stressors is the patient experiencing? This may be elicited by asking the patient how things are at home, on the job, and with the family and about specific worries the patient may be having. How the patient has dealt with anxiety in the past is important information.

The doctor finishes his physical examination, which reveals no evidence of such conditions as mitral valve prolapse, hyperthyroidism, medication or alcohol withdrawal. The patient denies full blown panic attacks but does state that when she gets very anxious she gets palpitations. She has always been a worrier just like her mother. Her father was an alcoholic, and one time she hyperventilated when she saw him threaten her mother. She had been doing well up until a month ago when her current husband, who had been going to Alcoholics Anonymous, went on a drinking binge. This has happened before and usually makes her nerves worse, and she gets some medicine from her family doctor. Also, last year her family doctor passed away and she had to go to the emergency room to get a prescription. Finally, her daughter moved to another state several weeks ago. In addition to the above symptoms, she mentions that she has trouble getting to sleep because of her problem.

Assessment, Using DSM-III Formulation

Axis I: Generalized anxiety disorder.

Axis II: Dependent personality traits.

Axis III: No physical disorder or condition.

Axis IV: Psychosocial stressors—exacerbation of husband's drinking problem; daughter's moving out of town; loss of family physician.

Axis V: Highest level of adaptive functioning past year—fair to good.

Management

The following techniques are likely to be helpful in following the patient's anxiety and promoting functioning.

1. Empathetic listening (see Chapter 11). A neutral but understanding approach will reduce the patient's sense of isolation in handling the problem and provide emotional support. In the past her daughter was in town to give her this kind of support.

2. Empathize with the patient's current difficulty, but avoid probing into the patient's long-standing difficulties with self-esteem. Stick to working on the source of the current anxiety.

3. Consider prescribing anxiolytics, especially if they have been helpful to the patient previously. Ask the patient what previously prescribed medicine has helped her. Advise the patient that you will re-evaluate the need for medication on a regular basis. Prescribe medication in doses sufficient to produce anxiolytic effects. Allowing the patient to participate in the selection of medication and the dosage will decrease her sense of helplessness.

4. Advise the patient to seek outside sources of support (Al-Anon, family, *etc*). If the patient is being physically abused, consider referral to a social work agency. Inquire about other modes she successfully used to cope previously and encourage reliance on them. Determine the patient's insight into the current cause of her anxiety. Agreement on the causes of the problem will facilitate agreement on the treatment strategy.

5. Follow-up. In a week's time reassess the patient's anxiety and her actions to follow through with recommendations. When the patient's situation is stabilized, consider referral for specialized services to deal with chronic anxiety (relaxation procedures, assertiveness training) and family problems (family therapy).

Adjustment Disorder with Anxious Mood

A 55-year-old married man suffered a heart attack 3 months ago. Today he appears in the office with a history of chest pain, dizziness, and breathlessness. His ECG is unchanged. A recent submaximal stress test showed no signs of coronary insufficiency or serious arrhythmia. The patient appears mildly depressed, and his wife is very anxious.

Evaluation

1. Is an anxiety disorder present? Some patients may feel it is not "manly" to admit they are not coping. Confirmation of psychiatric disturbance may come from information from the spouse, from associated symptoms of sleep disturbance or increased irritability, or from frequent sighing observed during the evaluation.

2. Has there been avoidance behavior and counterphobic behavior (e.g., shoveling snow)? This could be elicited by asking the patient to describe a typical day. Inactivity or inappropriate activity may be a response to fear or poor education and advice. Determine the patient's understanding of his disease. Many patients fail to understand the relationship.

3. What fear(s) does the patient have about activity? Fears of another heart attack and of sudden death are common in such patients.

4. Have there been similar problems in friends or family that have sensitized him to negative experiences (e.g., has a friend who had a heart attack died suddenly?). Elicit the patient's other fears, such as

not returning to work or giving up being provider for the family.

5. Are his spouse's fears also contributing to the patient's disability?

6. Is the patient demoralized?

The physical examination and laboratory information show no evidence of changes in the patient's condition. His wife reports that the patient has not been himself since he left the hospital and that any little thing gets on his nerves. She says he is afraid to go any place and is taking a lot of nitroglycerin without much help. She says he is tense all of the time and yesterday she had to stop him from shoveling snow. She complains that she is at her wits end and has not slept well in weeks. She claims that before his heart attack he was on the go all of the time and worked two jobs.

Assessment, Using DSM-III Formulation

Axis I: Adjustment disorder with anxious mood.
Axis II: Possible type A personality.
Axis III: Physical disorder—recent myocardial infarction, stable.
Axis IV: Psychosocial stressors—spouse's anxiety; inactivity.
Axis V: Previous level of functioning—good.

Management

1. Educate. Provide exact information about the nature of the illness to the patient and his spouse and determine their comprehension of the information. Elucidate the relationship of chest pain to anxiety and hyperventilation. Consider hyperventilating the patient for a minute to determine the reproducibility of symptoms (this may occur in only 30% of patients).

2. Provide information about prognosis based on medical information.

3. Encourage independence and provide mastery over the fear by having the patient plan his own activity program. Have him make a list of things he would like to do so you can give specific guidance.

4. Prescribe specific activities in a graded fashion. Use relaxation techniques to assist in this. Pulse rate monitoring by the patient after each activity demonstrates ease of tolerance. Consider referring the patient to a cardiac rehabilitation program to assist him in return to physical activities.

5. Involve the patient's partner in treatment.

6. Respect the patient's possible fear of dependency. Give as much control to the patient as possible by counseling in terms of advice and not commands.

7. Allow the patient to depend upon you without encouraging dependency. Establish regular visits until you feel progress has been made.

General References

American Psychiatric Association: *Diagnostic and Statistical Manual of Mental Disorders*, ed 3. Washington, DC, American Psychiatric Association, 1980.

Recently updated diagnostic criteria and epidemiologic information for all recognized psychiatric disorders.

Benson H: *The Relaxation Response.* New York, William Morrow, 1975.

The popular best seller that introduced the "relaxation response" to the public. Emphasizes transcendental meditation but is a bit overenthusiastic. Easy to read and use.

Brown JT, Mulrow CD, Stoudemire GA: The anxiety disorders. *Ann Intern Med* 100:558, 1984.

Extensively referenced and up-to-date review.

Cadoret RJ and King LJ *Psychiatry in Primary Care.* C. V. Mosby, St. Louis, 1983.

Excellent account of common problems, emphasizing epidemiology, treatment, and outcome; extensively referenced.

Goldberg RJ: Anxiety, Biobehavioral Diagnosis and Therapy. New Hyde Park, NY, Medical Examination Publishing Co, 1982.

A comprehensive practical text emphasizing practical management of anxiety disorders; well referenced.

Goldberg RJ: Anxiety reduction by self-regulation: theory, practice, and evaluation. *Ann Intern Med* 96:483, 1982.

Readable, critical review of hypothesized mechanisms and impact of muscle relaxation, biofeedback, and meditation in anxiety disorders and in other psychosocial and medical conditions.

Greenblatt DJ, Shader RI, Abernethy DR: Current status of benzodiazepines. *N Engl J Med* 309:354, 1983.

Exhaustive review of characteristics and uses of benzodiazepines.

Relaxation Cassettes: A variety of cassette programs which provide self-introduction in relaxation techniques are available from the following publishers: Guilford Publications, Inc., 200 Park Avenue South, New York, NY 10003; and New Harbinger Publications, 2200 Adeline, Suite 305, Oakland, CA 94607.

Specific References

1. Agras WS, Chapin HN, Jackson M, Oliveau DC: The natural history of phobia. *Arch Gen Psychiatry* 26:315, 1972.
2. Agras WS, Sylvester D, Oliveau D: The epidemiology of common fears and phobias. *Comp Psychol* 10:151, 1969.
3. Amies PL, Shaw PM: Social phobia: a comparative clinical study. *Br J Psychiatry* 142:174, 1983.
4. Bass C, Wade C, Gardner WN, *et al*: Unexplained breathlessness and psychiatric morbidity in patients with normal and abnormal coronary arteries. *Lancet* 1:605, 1983.
5. Benson H, Beary JF, Carol MP: The relaxation response. *Psychiatry* 37:37, 1974.
6. Burns LE, Thorpe GL: The epidemiology of fears and phobias. *J Int Med Res* 5(Suppl 5):1, 1977.
7. Catalan J, Gath D, Bond A, Martin P: The effects of non-prescribing of anxiolytics in general practice. II. Factors associated with outcome. *Br J Psychiatry* 144:603, 1984.
8. Catalan J, Gath D, Edmonds G, Ennis J: The effects of non-prescribing of anxiolytics in general practice. I. Controlled evaluation of psychiatric and social outcome. *Br J Psychiatry* 144:593, 1984.
9. Charney DS, Heninger GR, Brever A: Noradrenergic function in panic anxiety. *Arch Gen Psychiatry* 41:751, 1984.
10. Costello CG: Fears and phobias in women: a community study. *J Abnorm Psychol* 91:280, 1982.
11. Craig H, White PD: Etiology and symptoms of neurocirculatory asthenia. *Arch Intern Med* 53:633, 1934.
12. De la Fuente JR, Rosenbaum AH, Martin HR, Niven RG: Lorazepam-related withdrawal seizures. *Mayo Clinic Proc* 55:190, 1980.
13. Gaarder KR, Montgomery PS: *Clinical Biofeedback: A Procedural Manual for Behavioral Medicine,* ed 2. Baltimore, Williams & Wilkins, 1981.
14. Goldberg R: Anxiety, A Guide to Biobehavioral Diagnosis and *Therapy for Physicians and Mental Health Clinicians.* New Hyde Park, NY, Medical Examination Publishing Co, 1982.
14a. Goldberg D, Blackwell B: Psychiatric illness in general practice: a detailed study using a new method of case identification. *Br Med J* 2:439, 1970.
15. Greenblatt DJ, Shader RI, Abernethy DR: Current status of benzodiazepines. *N Engl J Med* 309:354, 1983.
16. Greenblatt DJ, Shader RI, Abernethy DR: Current status of benzodiazepines. *N Engl J Med* 309:410, 1983.
17. Hollister L: Benzodiazepines 1980: current update: a look at the issues. *Psychosomatics* 21:4, 1980.
18. Isel TR, Ninan PT, Aloi J, et al: A benzodiazepine receptor-mediated model of anxiety. *Arch Gen Psychiatry* 41:741, 1984.
19. Johnstone A, Goldberg D: Psychiatric screening in general practice. *Lancet* 1:605, 1976.
20. Katon W: Panic disorder and somatization. Review of 55 cases. *Am J Med* 77:101, 1984.
21. Klein DF: Delineation of two drug-responsive anxiety syndromes. *Psychopharmacologia* 5:397, 1964.
22. Lead article: Beta-adrenergic blockade and anxiety. *Lancet* 2:611, 1976.
23. Lum LD: The syndrome of habitual chronic hyperventilation. In Hill O (ed): *Modern Trends in Psychosomatic Medicine.* Woburn, MA, Butterworths, 1976.
24. Marks I: *Fears and Phobias.* London, Heinemann, 1969.
25. Marks I: The classification of phobic disorders. *Br J Psychiatry* 116:377, 1970.
26. Marks I: Recent results of behavioral treatments and phobias and obsessions. *J Int Med Res* 5(Suppl 5):15, 1977.
27. Mavissakalian M, Michelson L, Dealy RS: Pharmacological treatment of agoraphobia: imipramine *versus* imipramine with programmed practice. *Br J Psychiatry* 143:348, 1983.
28. Mayou R, Williamson B, Foster A: Attitudes and advice after myocardial infarction. *Br J Med J* 1:1577, 1976.
29. Meyers JK, Weissman MM, Tischler GL, *et al*: Six-month prevalence of psychiatric disorders in three communities 1980 to 1982. *Arch Gen Psychiatry* 41:959, 1984.
30. Missiri JC, Alexander S: Hyperventilation syndrome: a brief review. *JAMA* 240:2093, 1978.
31. Munby M, Johnston DW: Agoraphobia: the long-term clinical follow-up of behavioral treatment. *Br J Psychiatry* 137:418, 1980.
32. Noyes R, Clancy J: Anxiety neurosis: a 5 year follow-up. *J Nerv Ment Dis* 162:200, 1976.
33. Rickels K: Psychopharmacologicl approach to treatment of anxiety. In Fann WW, Katacan I, Porkorny AD, Williams RL (eds): Phenomenology and Treatment of Anxiety. New York, SP Medical and Scientific Books, 1979.
34. Rickles KR, Case G, Downing RW, Winokur A: Long-term diazepam therapy and clinical outcome. *JAMA* 250:767, 1983.
35. Rohs RG, Noyes R: Agoraphobia: newer treatment approaches. *J Nerv Ment Dis* 166:701, 1978.
36. Salkind MR: Anxiety neurosis in general practice. *Postgrad Med J*, 34, 1972.
37. Scrignar CB: *Stress Strategies.* Kargar Biobehavioral Medicine, Series 1. New York, Karger, 1983.
38. Shapiro S, Skinner EA, Kessler LG, *et al*: Utilization of health and mental health services. Three epidemiologic catchment area sites. *Arch Gen Psychiatry* 41:971, 1984.
39. Sheehan DV: Current perspectives in the treatment of panic and phobic disorders. *Drug Ther*, 179–190, 1982.
40. Taylor CB, Ferguson JM, Wermuth BM: Simple techniques to treat medical phobias. *Postgrad Med J* 53:28, 1977.
41. Uhlenhuth EH, Balter MB, Mellenger GD, *et al*: Symptom checklist syndromes in the general population. *Arch Gen Psychiatry* 40:1167, 1983.
42. Wheeler EO, White PD, Reed EW, Cohen ME: Neurocirculatory asthenia: a 20-year follow-up of 173 patients. *JAMA* 142:878, 1950.
43. Wood P: Da Costa's syndrome (or effort syndrome). *Br Med J* 1:767, 1941.

CHAPTER FOURTEEN

Maladaptive Personalities

WALTER F. BAILE, M.D.

INTRODUCTION

Because of the uniqueness of each individual and the dynamic interaction of the person with his environment, any attempt to classify personality in a systematic way may seem too ambitious. However, as the physician gets to know a patient he will usually detect certain "themes"; these themes comprise relatively consistent attitudes and patterns of behavior, and as such they make up the patient's personality. This chapter describes a number of personality styles which are associated with inflexible or maladaptive behavior. The ability to recognize patients with these personality styles is important, for effective management of medical problems in these patients often requires strategies adapted to their personality.

OBSESSIVE COMPULSIVE PATIENT

Definition and Recognition

Obsessive compulsive individuals lead lives characterized by extreme orderliness, adherence to convention, perfectionism, and conscientiousness. On the job they dress very neatly, are always on time, and have a meticulously clean and orderly desk. An over-restrictive conscience provides a strong sense of duty, so that they are blindly loyal and hardworking; they are extremely responsive to the praise of superiors, which inspires in them renewed energy and enthusiasm to tackle new assignments. On the other hand, colleagues or fellow workers will see an obsessive compulsive person as stiff, formal, inhibited, and dogmatic; they may admire his ability for logical thinking and working with details, but they will be annoyed and frustrated by his rules and regulations. Above average intelligence and a liking for working with factual information, when present, will often bring success to the obsessive compulsive individual in jobs such as accounting; but his dogmatic approach to problem solving and the tendency to be uncomfortable in situations that are unstructured prevents ascendency to positions of greater responsibility. At home there may be a rigid insistence on following a fixed routine; at times this may provoke anger in the rest of the family who become tired of always going to the same places to eat, for vacations, *etc.* Excessive frugality may also be a source of friction, and the children may use terms such as "tightwad." A spouse may complain that there is a lack of feeling, an inflexible and uncomprising approach to decisions, and a paucity of imagination. Typically, the obsessive compulsive person will have disdain for others, for no one can do a job as thoroughly as he can.

For the general physician the obsessive compulsive personality is important for several reasons. First, this personality type has often been found to be associated with classical psychosomatic disorders such as peptic ulcer and ulcerative colitis. Second, because of their conscientiousness, their high standards for performance, and their need to be in control, these individuals may encounter situations at home or at work where their performance needs are frustrated, and they may develop partially decompensated states manifested as somatic symptoms (see Chapter 12). Third, they cooperate well with the management of whatever medical problem they may have if their personality needs are met.

Origins

It is hypothesized that such a rigid, overly controlled personality structure results from premature parental insistence on obedience in the child—that is, before the child's intellectual and motor development is up to the task. Thus, as a child the patient may have been expected to be neat at the table, to have been toilet trained early, and to have controlled his emotions. In submitting to these parental pressures the child must repress strong aggressive and defiant drives that are characteristic of all children. The price paid is an overly strict conscience wherein the traits of obedience and conformity on the one hand, and obstinacy and stubbornness on the other, coexist and mirror the original parental struggle.

Management Strategies

If this personality style is recognized, these individuals can be managed quite easily when medical care is required. Identification with the orderliness and methodical approach of the physician is a source of comfort. Since reliance on factual information and logic are cornerstones of the obsessive compulsive individual's approach to reality, informing him in detail about his illness and about the rationale for required tests and treatment, etc will be helpful. Such patients also respond to being included in the decision-making process. Because of the need to "do something" to get approval, the patient will often feel better about participating in any treatment plan, such as home blood pressure monitoring. However, this must be balanced against his tendency to become overly attentive to detail. He will also respond well to reinforcement and praise.

OVERLY EMOTIONAL HISTRIONIC PATIENT

Definition and Recognition

This personality type is seen mostly in women. Typically, the physician is struck by the patient's excessive preoccupation with her physical attractiveness, even when she is in the hospital. This is an attempt to draw attention to herself. Although superficially charming and appealing there will be a lack of emotional balance; thus, behavior is overreactive and often coquettish. Initial warmth and intensity of emotional expression may mask a tendency toward premature intimacy in relationships, and although at first this may appear charming, the expectation for others to respond in the same eager, warm, and personal way transforms the charm into demanding, egocentric, and inconsiderate actions. Men with this disorder may feel the need to show their manliness, courage, and attractiveness to female doctors and nurses.

These patients are often attractive and seductive. In relationships with the opposite sex there is often an attempt to control or to enter into a dependent relationship. Thus their histrionic behavior may be seen as a way to take care of unmet dependency needs or to counter feelings of helplessness, inadequacy, and anxiety prompted by an interpersonal relationship. Such feelings may also lead to an overly trusting attitude and an initially positive response to the authority of someone whom they believe will provide a magical answer to their problems. Often when these individuals are disappointed, there will be dramatic acting out (including suicide gestures or threats). It is common for patients with this disorder to complain of poor health, such as weakness or headaches. These personality characteristics may be seen in some patients who exhibit conversion disorders and very frequently in patients with somatization disorder (see Chapter 12).

Origins

The principal traits of this personality type are said to be derived from the period of development when the child is between the ages of 3 and 6. During this period, the foundation for sexual identity is laid down when an initially strong attachment to the parent of the opposite sex is relinquished and patterns of identification with the parent of the same sex are strengthened. The superficial warmth, charm, exaggerated emotionality, and sexual provocativeness of the histrionic patient are hypothesized to be derived from impulses stemming from the early affection for the parent of the opposite sex.

Management Strategies

In dealing with this type of patient, the physician should begin by attempting to answer two important questions: Is this personality part of another entity such as a somatization disorder? Do the physical complaints reflect organic disease?

As mentioned above, these patients may be very seductive and may make the physician uncomfortable. Their overly warm and friendly approach on the other hand may make the physician feel charmed and challenged. However, it is important to remember that underneath this behavior are strong feelings of dependency and of a desire to control. The physician should therefore avoid getting trapped into an overly familiar relationship with the patient (e.g., by avoiding the use of first names, by assuring a professional posture during office visits, and by having a nurse present when he examines the patient). When these patients do become seriously ill, they may feel that they are unattractive and unsuccessful. During these periods they may become particularly depressed and overemotional or make extra demands on the physician. When the patient is vulnerable and feeling more helpless, reassurance and explanations about the illness will help the patient distinguish realities from fantasies. At these times it may also be important for the physician to be more supportive, since dependency needs aroused by the illness make the patient more vulnerable to anxiety and depression.

OVERLY SUSPICIOUS QUERULOUS (PARANOID) PATIENT

Definition and Recognition

The characteristic features of this personality type are suspiciousness, hypersensitivity to criticism, and restriction of emotional expansiveness. Thus these individuals tend to be suspicious not only of other people and their motives, but also may show a general cynicism about institutions, about the motives of organizations such as charitable groups whom they may accuse of "ripping off the public," and about legitimate competitions, which they will claim are "fixed." Their overall posture toward life is defensive. Such persons question the loyalty of others, exaggerate the need to be self-sufficient, and may be seen by others as guarded and secretive. They may harbor considerable hostility that, together with their querulousness, leads them to be argumentative and litigious and to overplay small difficulties with others. Sometimes hypervigilance associated with their defensive attitude toward life will be expressed in tenseness of expression and inability to relax. The individual with a paranoid personality has great difficulty in admitting the possibility that he has made a mistake; thus he will be overly sensitive to criticism and quick to defend himself. Often he will attribute his own failures to the faults of others (projection). At times this need to defend himself from any hint of failure will result in a certain unrealistic self-importance and a disdain for people who are considered as weak, soft, sickly, or defective. Thus, there will be a denial of any passive, soft, or tender feelings in himself; and he will often be seen by others as cold, unemotional, and humorless.

Origins

It is hypothesized that individuals with this personality type have been subjected to excessive parental anger. The features of the personality may be conceptualized as the persistence of childhood defenses against parental anger and rage. The hypervigilance, suspiciousness, and feelings of being taken advantage of are a result of feeling that others will treat him the same way as his parents treated him.

Management Strategies

Two problems confront the physician who manages such patients when they become ill. The first is the meaning of the illness. Because the patient denies being vulnerable and disdains this trait in others, physical disease in himself may arouse strong threats. This can be seen very clearly in illnesses such as myocardial infarction. In this situation, the physician may see "counterphobic" behavior in which the patient struggles to protect himself against the threat of perceived weakness by prematurely engaging in physical activity or avoiding the disclosure of symptoms to the physician. The second difficulty lies in forming a therapeutic alliance. Because of his oversuspiciousness the patient may struggle to stay in charge of his treatment, questioning the physician's diagnosis, reasoning, and the appropriateness of the treatment plan. This may arouse strong competitive urges in the physician, leading to anger toward the patient or refusal to treat the patient. These responses only serve to confirm the patient's view of the world as hostile.

The best approach to management is to provide routinely the fullest possible explanation of the illness and any related procedures. Allowing the patient to share in the treatment plan by exercising options wherever possible will also be helpful. This will help to develp some sense of mastery over a situation in which he feels weak and vulnerable. When symptoms are withheld, or behavior is inappropriate, the physician may sometimes have to confront the patient and to define reality, which may allow the patient to identify with the strength and authority of the physician at a time when he is feeling out of control. A pleading, solicitous approach by the physician, however, will only be seen by the patient as a sign of weakness. A trusting relationship will be developed only with time and patience.

PASSIVE-DEPENDENT PATIENT

Definition and Recognition

Individuals of this type are often unable to make their own decisions, deferring almost all choices to spouses or relatives; they assume passive roles and are convinced that they have very few assets or characteristics that others find admirable. For example, this sense of unworthiness may often result in a man's continually taking jobs that are below his true potential or a woman's willingness to tolerate a husband's abuse rather than leave him. In some cases the individual will attempt to compensate for low self-esteem by investing most of his or her energy in caring for others. As a consequence, the individual with a dependent personality who has invested a strong interest in another person or activity may become anxious or depressed if the situation alters, i.e., if the person leaves or the job changes. In these instances the patient may develop the psychological or somatic symptoms of minor or major mood disturbances (see Chapters 12 and 15) and present symptomatically to the generalist.

In addition these patients may develop various degrees of dependency on the physician. Generally their relationship with him will be "idealized." That is, the physician, in showing warmth, concern, and interest, may elicit emotions related to similar feelings the patient desired in the parent. It is not uncommon in these instances to see affectionate feelings develop in these patients toward physicians of the opposite sex. Sometimes these become overly sexual, but for most patients they remain on an idealized, platonic level.

On some occasions the physician will meet persons whose anxiety about coping with even the most minimal demands makes them into desperate, clinging, dependent individuals. Such persons are overwhelmed with social problems, which exacerbate dependency and increase anxiety. These patients may become overdependent on their doctors, behaving like young children who turn to their parents when they are frightened or overwhelmed. They may learn that somatic complaints get attention and medicine and that being sick allows them to avoid feeling that they are not coping (illness behavior, see Chapter 12). These patients may badger their physician with phone calls at the most inopportune times with their worries about nausea or arthritis that is "acting up again."

Origins

An individual's self-esteem is a reflection of his ability to feel competent in roles defined by society and to "feel good" about himself. In general this is a function of the warmth and degree of support a person received from his environment, especially parental figures, as he tackled the developmental tasks which lay on the road to adulthood. A parent overly critical of a child's accomplishments in school and in other spheres because they did not meet his high standards will have seriously undermined the child's morale. This and similar childhood experiences may produce an adult with a predominantly dependent personality style.

Management Strategies

The patient with a very dependent personality who is unable to make his own decisions but whose dependency needs are being met in a reasonable way is unlikely to change; here, in decisions regarding treatment the physician will usually have to include the person responsible for care. This will be especially important in a situation where there is serious illness, in which case the patient may experience further threats to security.

For the dependent patient who still has some capacity for interpersonal growth and is able to develop warm relationships, insight-oriented psychotherapy may be helpful. When the patient's positive feelings toward the physician become an issue

in such work, the physician may interpret them by telling the patient that it is not unusual for people to feel warm toward those who take an interest.

The exceedingly clinging individual needs a different management strategy. These persons use their symptoms to get intermittent reinforcement, the most potent kind of reward in operant conditioning. At times they seem to be holding all of the cards, since there always lurks the possibilty that a new complaint may represent a real change in physical status. The physician is most likely to succeed with these patients when he understands the nature of the process. The patient will not give up his behavior or symptoms until he is sure he does not need them to get attention. Thus an approach such as the one described in the section on hypochondriasis in Chapter 12 will be helpful. Unfortunately, since these individual do get sick, the physician must stay attentive for new signs and complaints.

PASSIVE-AGGRESSIVE PATIENT AND SELF-SACRIFICING PATIENT

Defintion and Recognition

Two other styles of functioning may be seen in patients who, like the passive-dependent patient, have difficulty with the responsibilities of adulthood.

The first of these is the *passive-aggressive personality*, in which the maturational block is associated with resistance to demands for adequate performance in both social and occupational spheres. Typically, individuals with this style will demonstrate passive-resistant behavior when required to increase their performance level. Thus they may continually "forget" important tasks such as doctors' appointments, medication administration, *etc.* They may procrastinate in decision making until an opportunity has been allowed to slip by, or they may sabotage arrangements made by others to provide them with an opportunity for advancement. Although such a patient rarely expresses anger directly, the physician eventually recognizes that the patient, through forgetfulness, dawdling, stubbornness, and deliberate inefficiency, is actually saying "see if you can get me to do anything—I'm staying right where I am." It is important to recognize that the tendency toward passive-resistant behavior can be pervasive and persistent, in which case it is the hallmark of the passive-aggressive personality, or it can be an isolated regressive phenomenon in an individual who is attempting to cope with an overwhelming stress. Thus it may be seen not infrequently in adolescents who have major illnesses that increase dependency; yet the adolescent will not wish to express his needs, because he is at a stage when increased independence is an important issue.

A similar desire to be taken care of can be seen in

the *long suffering, self-sacrificing* patient. These persons seem always to be subject to some misfortune and disappointment. If examined more carefully, this can usually be shown to be due to an error in judgment made by the patient himself. Furthermore these patients often wear their misfortune as a "badge of courage" and sigh that no matter how much they try, things never seem to work out. Some hint of the problems of these patients may be seen when anger is expressed in statements such as "when things go wrong no one ever seems to be around to help me." Their tendency often to disregard their own comfort and be of service to other people exacerbates the situation.

Management Strategies

It is helpful for the physician to think of both passive-resistant and self-sacrificing behavior as indirect ways of demanding to be taken care of. The physician should avoid getting into a "parent-child" struggle with the patient. For the resistant patient the physician may gently explain the resistant behavior, acknowledge that it is difficult to weather illness alone, and thus acknowledge the patient's dependency needs. With the adolescent patient the approach can be the same; but since the behavior is a reaction to a catastrophic event, the patient can be encouraged to acknowledge his feelings about being ill, which can then be explained by the physician.

The self-sacrificing patient may increase his "martyred" behavior when struck by illness. Helpful suggestions and comfort with this patient are usually met with increased complaints, dismissal of evidence of recovery, and accentuation of negative feelings. It is as if the patient is telling those around him that they have to love him because he suffers so much. This often leads to feelings of irritation and anger on the part of the doctor. With such patients the physician may try to explain that improvement in symptoms is an additional benefit for others—emphasizing the patient's important role in assisting others, so that becoming well becomes a route back to his habitual style of coping.

PATIENT WITH EXAGGERATED SELF-IMPORTANCE

Definition and Recognition

Individuals with this personality problem are self-centered, vain, and in need of constant attention and admiration. Their behavior is thus focused on doing the "right things" or being with the "right people" in order to create an "image." An excessive focus on themselves creates a lack of awareness of the feelings of others and in fact often leads to an exploitation of others in order to satisfy needs of self-aggrandizement. As a result relations with others tend to be superficial. Their fantasy life also reflects a grandiose sense of self-importance or uniqueness. Thus an overestimation of abilities may lead to fantasies of achieving more power, wealth, brilliance, beauty, or ideal love.

Behind the exaggerated sense of self-importance and the attempt to maintain such an image is a very fragile ego. Thus there is continuous preoccupation with performance, acceptance, and admiration by others. This is revealed best by rage or humiliation in response to even constructive criticism. Normal setbacks are experienced as failures, criticism is poorly tolerated, and unrealistic expectations, exploitativeness, and a sense of entitlement often lead to disappointment. Thus periods of depressed mood and feelings of isolation often result; during severe stress transient psychotic symptoms (e.g., hallucinations or delusion) may be seen.

This personality type is important to the general physician for several reasons. First, because of the inappropriate preoccupation with self, individuals with these characteristics are prone to worry excessively over minor physical symptoms and at times may be refractory to reassurance to the point of hypochondriasis. Second, there may be unrealistic expectations of special consideration from the physician, which often lead to disappointment when these are not met. This is complicated by the fact that the patient's own grandiosity leads him to choose a physician whom he considers to be an eminent expert.

Origins

It is hypothesized that this personality style may reflect an attempt to compensate for loss of self-esteem that occurred early in childhood; for example, the loss of self-esteem in a child who experiences abrupt loss in parental attention because of the birth of a sibling or because of remarriage of a single parent.

Management Strategies

The physician's approach to the patient should be realistic. He must avoid getting into a competitive situation if his competence is challenged, which is especially likely to occur if immediate results are not forthcoming. If the physician is able to acknowledge his own limitations to the patient, the situation may be defused. Furthermore, the physician should try to establish the idea that an illness often does not interfere with achieving goals in life and with being appreciated by others. If the illness is short-lived, reassuring the patient that he will soon return to his usual functional status will be helpful in the overall management.

THE ANTISOCIAL PERSONALTIY

Definition and Recognition

The problems of individuals affected with this disorder usually begin to manifest themselves by adolescence. Delinquent behavior, persistent lying, frequent fights with peers, alcohol and drug abuse, truancy, and running away from home are characteristic behaviors.

In adulthood, the antisocial traits are reflected in an inability to assume responsibility for mature, goal-directed behavior and to follow accepted norms for conduct. Inability to hold a job, superficial, exploitative relationships, and failure to meet financial obligations are characteristic. As a parent, the individual with an antisocial personality is likely to be neglectful, abusive, and unreliable. He may travel often from place to place, surviving by "conning" others or by illegal behavior. This impulsive and wandering behavior is oriented toward pleasure seeking and appears to ward off boredom or depression. Although not all sociopathic individuals are criminals, thievery, drunk-driving offenses, and disorderly conduct are common.

Many sociopaths adopt a slovenly appearance and associate with groups who flaunt their nonconformity, such as motorcycle gangs. Higher functioning sociopaths may instead manifest an ingratiating, glib, or colorful style in their interactions with people. Diagnosis in this latter group is supported by a history of disturbed childhood, delinquency, and poor socialization.

Origins

It is hypothesized that the acting out in the adolescent sociopath represents an attempt to avoid anxiety and depression that emanate from a home environment characterized by the absence of nurturing emotional ties. There may be a history of childhood neurotic problems, such as persistent enuresis and sleep walking, which is also related to lack of nurturing. Hereditary factors are also felt to contribute to the development of antisocial personality. Studies of twins reared apart suggest that parental sociopathy, especially in the father, increases the likelihood of this disorder in offspring. This disorder is more common in males. It is felt to be underdiagnosed in women, who are more likely to be classified as borderline personalities when they have this disorder.

Management Strategies

The sociopathic individual's contact with the medical system is most likely to be engendered by legal difficulties, or drug seeking. There are some reports also that suggest that as some of these individuals get older sociopathic behavior decreases but hypochondriasis and somatic concerns increase.

Particular problems result when the antisocial individual needs to be hospitalized because he will often quarrel with staff, manipulate staff in order to obtain special treatment, such as narcotic analgesics, and threaten to sign out against medical advice if he does not get what he wants. A physician who is acquainted with such a patient can render invaluable service by telling the hospital staff about the patient's style and helping to set limits from the outset of the hospital stay.

BORDERLINE PERSONALITY

Definition and Recognition

This personality type has recently received considerable attention in the psychiatric literature as its characteristics have become more clearly defined. It is called "borderline" because it refers to patients whose behavior and sense of reality approach those seen in patients with schizophrenic disorders (see Chapter 15). At one time this disorder was known as "pseudoneurotic schizophrenia" because of the presence of neurotic phenomena such as phobias and anxiety in these marginally functioning patients. This disorder is more common in women than in men, and it may be found in as many as 1 to 2% of the population.

Because his personality organization is impulsive and infantile, the borderline patient will always demonstrate some psychological impairment. When not in the midst of a crisis he may complain of intense emptiness and moods of anger and depression. During a crisis this anger often intensifies and the patient may become argumentative, demanding, and self-destructive. At times conversion symptoms and hypochondriacal complaints may be present (see Chapter 12). In addition, there may be transient psychotic episodes (e.g., paranoid ideation) when the patient becomes frustrated in an interpersonal relationship. Although anger is often a salient feature in these patients, clinging dependency is also prominent. When they feel dependent, a psychological phenomenon called "splitting" may occur, in which people in their environment are categorized either as good persons, who are seen as protective and nurturing, or as bad persons, who are seen as cruel and unsupportive. The borderline patient often turns to alcohol or drug use to control chronic tension and anxiety.

Because these patients may present with neurotic symptoms, such as conversion or anxiety, their primary problem may not be recognized unless their overall history is reviewed. A history which includes suicide gestures, pervasive anxiety, mood swings, identity disturbance, and inappropriate anger should suggest borderline personality and should prompt a psychiatric referral.

Origins

It is hypothesized that the borderline personality results from difficulties in the separation phase of human development (which occurs at 16 to 25 months of age) that leave the individual vulnerable to emotional crisis when separation is experienced as an adult.

Management Strategies

In managing the medical problems of a patient with borderline personality, it is important for the physician to realize that he is dealing with an individual who suffers greatly because of his chronic feelings of emptiness, of his fear of being alone, and of the chaos in his interpersonal relationships. Thus, he deserves empathy and understanding. Since this may be difficult when the patient is being demanding, hostile, or manipulative, such a patient is best managed in conjunction with a psychiatrist.

When these patients become seriously ill, their dependency may increase, and the crisis of disease may be enough to trigger transient breaks with reality. At such times, it is particularly important for the general physician to enlist the help of the patient's psychiatrist, especially if the patient requires hospitalization. This is because these patients can present serious management problems in the hospital, characterized by "splitting" the staff into all good and all bad, by exhibiting demanding, infantile, and at times hostile behavior, and by threatening self-destructive acts. Ideally the psychiatrist should not wait for a crisis to develop but should see the patient as soon as possible after admission. In this way, he can work with the staff to explain the dynamics and behavior of the borderline personal-ity. Strategies can thus be developed to deal with staff splitting, acting out, and other disruptive behavior. The occurrence of behavior suggestive of a partial break with reality may necessitate the use of a neuroleptic drug (see Chapter 16).

General References

American Psychiatric Association; *Diagnostic and Statistical Manual of Mental Disorders*, ed 3. Washington, DC, American Psychiatric Association, 1980.
> Recently updated diagnostic criteria and epidemiological information for all recognized psychiatric disorders.

Bowden CL, Burstein AG: *Psychosocial Basis of Health Care*, ed 3. Baltimore, Williams & Wilkins, 1983.
> An introduction to human behavior in the clinical setting, with excellent accounts of a number of difficult personality types.

Kahana RG, Bibring G: Personality types in medical management. In Zinberg NE (ed): *Psychiatry and Medical Practice in a General Hospital*. New York, International Universities Press. 1964, pp 108–123.
> Clear definition of a number of common maladaptive patterns and their management.

Neill JR, Sandifer MG: *Practical Manual of Psychiatric Consultation*. Baltimore, Williams & Wilkins, 1980.
> A short, practical text of general hospital psychiatry, particularly useful for managing patients with difficult personalities when they are hospitalized.

Sharpiro D: *Neurotic Styles*. New York, Basic Books, 1965.
> Describes in fine detail the cognitive experiences and behavioral manifestations of the paranoid, hysterical, and impulsive personalities.

CHAPTER FIFTEEN

Affective Disorders

J. RAYMOND DePAULO, M.D.

INTRODUCTION

The most common psychological disturbance in the general population is a disturbance of mood characterized by depression with or without anxiety. The prevalence of this type of disturbance ranges from 10 to 20% for general populations, to 20 to 50% for patients seen in general practice settings, to 30 to 60% for general hospital inpatients (3, 4).

Implicit in these figures are two powerful arguments for the diagnosis and treatment of many of these patients by general physicians rather than by psychiatrists. First, there are too many patients for psychiatrists alone to provide the primary care, and second, there is a clear association between these mood disturbances and medical illnesses.

There are five factors which tend to hinder the generalist in helping these patients: (a) inadequate detection of a mood disturbance, (b) difficulty in classifying a mood disturbance when it has been detected, (c) difficulty in treating the correctly classified patient because of insufficient knowledge of antidepressant medications or inadequate time to allocate to the counseling of such patients, (d) inadequate knowledge of the prognosis of and the impact of treatment on the various mood disorders, and (e) difficulty in persuading patients with refrac-

tory affective disorders to accept referral to a psychiatrist.

The principal mood disturbances are the following:

1. major affective syndromes (major depression, atypical depression, and mania);
2. organic affective syndromes (mania or depression secondary to medication (see Chapter 12) or brain disorders (i.e., dementia, Chapter 17; stroke, Chapter 83);
3. dysthymic disorder (synonyms: depressive neurosis, characterological depression, minor depression);
4. adjustment disorder with depressed mood (see Chapter 12);
5. uncomplicated bereavement (depression related to recent loss; see Chapter 19).

DETECTION OF PATIENTS WITH AFFECTIVE SYMPTOMS

Complaints of loss of energy, poor sleep, poor appetite, weight loss, decreased libido, etc (i.e., vegetative symptoms) should alert physicians to the possibility of depression. However, depressed patients may not complain of those symptoms initially. Studies (14) have shown that these patients, in fact, usually present to generalists with three types of more vague complaints: ill defined somatic symptoms, pains of undetermined etiology in a wide variety of anatomical sites, and nervous complaints such as increased tension and feelings of anxiety. Primary complaints about marital distress or job difficulty are also common.

When the physician specifically asks about mood changes and associated symptoms, most depressed patients will acknowledge them. The presence of a mood disturbance should not be taken to explain or to invalidate all physical complaints since coexistence of psychiatric and medical disorders is the rule rather than the exception. Conversely, it is a mistake to conclude that depression (or any other psychiatric illness) is present simply because no objective signs of organic disease can be found in a patient with somatic symptoms. If the patient does suffer from a mood disturbance and if appropriate inquiries are made, it is likely that at least some of the classic features of an affective disorder will be detected.

It is appropriate to ask patients about their mood,

their sense of self-esteem and general physical and mental well-being, their sleep, appetite, libido, and their feeling about their future. The diagnostic significance of each of these factors is pointed out in the sections on the principal mood disorders below.

Family members, if available, should be asked to confirm and augment the information obtained from the patient. With the patient's agreement, the physician should share with the family his assessment and plans for treatment.

Manic symptoms are usually detected by family members or co-workers. They most commonly include rapid, sometimes incoherent speech, insomnia or refusal to sleep, hyperactivity, hypersexuality (often recognized as inappropriate for the particular patient), and hostile aggressive behavior. Manic patients usually feel there is nothing wrong with them and often resist medical attention. If they do ask for medical attention, it is because they recognize something wrong in their sleep or level of activity, because they feel that others want to hurt them, or because they want the doctor to reassure their "nagging" family that there is nothing wrong with them.

DYSTHYMIC DISORDER (DEPRESSIVE NEUROSIS, CHARACTEROLOGICAL DEPRESSION, MINOR DEPRESSION)

Dysthymic disorder is the current name given by the American Psychiatric Association to depressions which lack the severity of major depression (described below) and which are sustained over a 2-year period.

This category, which is related to earlier constructs of "depressive neurosis" and "characterological depression" is a heterogeneous grouping for those patients, many with primary personality disorders, who are chronically troubled people. One important subgroup consists of alcoholic patients who have chronically low moods which would improve with sobriety. It is also apparent that a fraction (perhaps 10 to 20%) of patients in this grouping have mild but persistent forms of an endogenous depressive disorder. These patients are often revealed by strong family histories for major affective disorders and often respond well to antidepressant medications (1). Dysthymic disorder is separated from adjustment disorder with depressed mood (the other form of minor depression) by the duration of the depressed mood, which is long-standing in dysthymic disorder. Diagnostic criteria and clinical aspects of adjustment disorder are found in Chapter 12.

Patients with minor depressions outnumber those with major depressive syndromes by approximately 10 to 1. For reasons that are not clear, neurotic depression is far more common among women than among men. Onset usually occurs around 18 to 30 years, and recurrence during periods of increased stress may characterize the patient's entire adult life. Serious medical illness is likely to precipitate a recurrence.

Diagnosis

The minor depressive disorders are only quantitatively distinct from normal mood responses. The patient's own sense of what is a normal response will often determine why one patient goes to the doctor while another attempts to deal with the perceived problem by other means. However, there is no absolute level of severity which distinguishes normal mood from dysthymic disorder or depressive neurosis.

Minor depression is a disturbance that arises from personality traits which make the patient more susceptible to particular stessful events or environmental demands. Although there is a strong association between certain personality traits (see Chapter 14) and depressive symptoms, different environmental stresses lead to depressive responses in people with different personality traits. For example, a dependent person may be more likely to become depressed when a source of security is threatened than would a relatively independent person. The depressive symptoms in such a patient should concern the general physician when the patient asks for help or when the mood change affects the patient's ability to function effectively.

Presenting or complicating problems associated with depressed mood in these patients include: (a) suicide attempts or self-injurious behavior—usually nonfatal but often requiring heroic medical interventions to prevent a fatal outcome, (b) multiple medical complaints and excessive medical care-seeking behavior or "illness behavior" (see Chapter 12 for additional detail), (c) alcohol and drug abuse (see Chapters 21 and 22), (d) family and marital discord, and (e) job difficulties.

These patients do not usually have the characteristic sustained changes in self-attitude and vital sense (i.e., unwarranted feelings of hopelessness and worthlessness and of bodily deterioration), the psychomotor retardation (i.e., slowed speech and movements), or the characteristic early morning awakening with diurnal mood variation (worse in the morning), which are seen in patients with major depression (see below). However, difficulty in getting to sleep, lack of appetite, mild weight loss, and loss of energy, and libido are common, as are anxiety symptoms (subjective tenseness, tremulousness, and shortness of breath).

Table 15.1 shows the specific criteria of the American Psychiatric Association (APA) for making the diagnosis of dysthymic disorder.

Management

Detection of the depressed mood and further interviewing to help delineate the external and per-

Table 15.1.
American Psychiatric Association Diagnostic Criteria for Dysthymic Disorder (Depressive Neurosis)[a]

A. During the past 2 years (or 1 year for children and adolescents) the individual has been bothered most or all of the time by symptoms characteristic of the depressive syndrome but they have not been of sufficient severity and duration to meet the criteria for a major depressive episode (see Table 15.2).

B. The manifestations of the depression syndrome may be relatively persistent or separated by periods of normal mood lasting a few days to a few weeks, but no more than a few months at a time.

C. During the depressive periods there is either prominent depressed mood (e.g., sad, blue, down in the dumps, low) or marked loss of interest or pleasure in all, or almost all, usual activities and pastimes.

D. During the depressive periods at least three of the following symptoms are present:
Insomnia or hypersomnia
Low energy level or chronic tiredness
Feelings of inadequacy, loss of self-esteem, or self-depreciation
Decreased effectiveness or productivity at school, work, or home
Decreased attention, concentration, or ability to think clearly
Social withdrawal
Loss of interest in or enjoyment of pleasurable activities
Irritability or excessive anger (in children, expressed toward parents or caretakers)
Inability to respond with apparent pleasure to praise or rewards
Less active or talkative than usual, or feels slowed down or restless
Pessimistic attitude toward the future, brooding about past events, or feeling sorry for self
Tearfulness or crying
Recurrent thoughts of death or suicide

E. Absence of psychotic features, such as delusions, hallucinations, or incoherence, or loosening of associations.

F. If the disturbance is superimposed on a pre-existing mental disorder, such as obsessive compulsive disorder or alcohol dependence, the depressed mood, by virtue of its intensity or effect on functioning, can be clearly distinguished from the individual's usual mood.

[a] From American Psychiatric Association: *Diagnostic and Statistical Manual of Mental Disorders.* ed 3. Washington, DC, American Psychiatric Association, 1980. Some of the criteria for children have been omitted from this table.

sonal antecedents of the depression are often therapeutic; the interest shown in the patient's story can help to restore lost self-esteem. Whereas occasionally some specific guidance and reassurance will help, more often empathic listening and encouraging the patient to outline his own synthesis of the problem and his approach to solving it provide more durable improvement. Weekly or biweekly visits for brief supportive psychotherapy for 3 to 6 weeks will often help during an episode of increased depressive

symptoms. Useful psychotherapeutic techniques for the generalist are described in more detail in Chapter 11. Ocassionally, adjunctive medication may be helpful in more severely affected patients. If generalized anxiety symptoms and/or insomnia predominate, a nighttime dose of a benzodiazepine sedative-hypnotic may be helpful (see Chapter 85).

If the depressed mood persists, despite several weeks of initial therapy, or if the patient has panic attacks (see Chapter 13), an antidepressant may be tried. A detailed account of antidepressant drugs is found below in the discussion of the treatment of major depression. It is important to explain to the patient that these are adjunctive treatments so that he does not fear that he is being treated for a major mental disorder. Treatment should be simple, with avoidance of combination preparations and polypharmacy, and relatively brief, i.e., 1 to 6 months. Use of neuroleptics and lithium should not be considered in these patients due to their potentially irreversible side effects. With minor depressive disorders it is equally important to explain and treat concurrent medical conditions and to avoid drugs which may produce or exacerbate depression (see Table 12.1 Chapter 12). If the depression worsens despite treatment, referral to a psychiatrist is indicated.

Prognosis

In contrast to the major effective syndromes, prognosis in dysthymic disorders cannot be estimated with much confidence. Some general features of outcome have been gleaned from large epidemiological studies. It is probably safe to conclude that *episodes of depressive neurosis* usually have a limited course even if untreated; the best available data suggest an average duration between 1 and 2 years after diagnosis (11). Although short term beneficial effects have been shown with the use of benzodiazepines and tricyclic antidepressants, they are modest at best. Various forms of psychotherapy as well as no treatment have been associated with positive outcomes. Poor outcomes are most common in patients with chronic medical disorders, severe social maladjustments, and coexistent personality disorders (see Chapter 14).

Recurrence of minor depression commonly occurs in the setting of later social stress or of medical illness. This is particularly true during the years of peak risk (i.e., 18 to 30 years).

MAJOR AFFECTIVE SYNDROMES

Mania and major depression are the two syndromes that give the traditional name *manic depressive disorder* to this group of disorders. These disorders are characteristically episodic with complete remissions between episodes. Most patients suffer only recurrent depressive episodes (the unipolar group), few suffer only manic episodes (they are grouped with bipolar patients), and the remainder suffer both manic and depressive episodes (the bipolar group). In its *Diagnostic and Statistical Manual of Mental Disorders* (see "General References), the APA estimates that 18 to 23% of women and 8 to 11% of men experience at least one major depressive episode during their adult life; it may occur at any age. Only 0.4 to 1.2% of adults develop a bipolar disorder; it is equally common in men and women; the first manic episode usually occurs before age 30.

Major Depression

Diagnosis

It is important to differentiate major depression from other major disorders, *i.e.*, schiozophrenia and dementia (see Chapters 16 and 17), from depressive neurosis (see above) and anxiety neurosis (see Chapter 13), and from adjustment disorder with depressed mood (see Chapter 12).

The concept of the "endogenous" depression, although flawed, has provided a durable, usable account of major depressive illness. The fully developed syndrome is characterized by a sustained alteration in mood, self-attitude, and vital sense. The *sustained lowering of mood* is relatively impervious to environmental influence when depression is severe. A major life stress frequently occurs at the onset of symptoms, and, thus, is not useful for making or excluding the diagnosis. The *change in self-attitude* is usually manifested in the development of feelings of guilt, inferiority, uselessness, and hopelessness regarding the future as the mood descends. The *changes in vital sense* (*i.e.*, the subjective assessment of one's physical and mental functioning) usually include feelings of confusion or poor memory with the inability to concentrate, a lack of energy and easy fatigability, and occasionally fears of delusions of dying of cancer, losing one's mind, *etc.*

Marked psychomotor retardation (*i.e.*, slowed speech and movements), delusions with depressive content, and diurnal mood variation (worst mood in the morning) occur in a minority of patients but are diagnostically useful when present since they are fairly specific to this disorder.

A patient presenting with a history of an episodic disorder and a fully developed symptom cluster as described is not difficult to diagnose. However, many patients with major depressions present either with few of these characteristic "endogenous" symptoms, with a dominant somatic symptom, or with a clear reason to be depressed, guilty, or hopeless. In such patients, recognition of major depression may be delayed, and either the patient may be insufficiently treated or may receive no treatment for this eminently treatable disorder. If the diagnosis is uncertain, the facts should be examined for the specific criteria of the APA for major depressive episode (see

Table 15.2). These criteria state that patients with 2 weeks of markedly depressed mood and without characteristic symptoms of schizophrenia who have four of eight symptoms of vegetation and depression should be considered to have a major depressive disorder and treated accordingly. Obviously these criteria will result in misclassification of some patients, even though they would be easily classified

Table 15.2.
American Psychiatric Association Diagnostic Criteria for Major Depressive Episode[a]

A. Dysphoric mood or loss of interest or pleasure in all or almost all usual activities and pastimes. The dysphoric mood is characterized by symptoms such as the following: depressed, sad, blue, hopeless, low, down in the dumps, irritable. The mood disturbance must be prominent and relatively persistent, but not necessarily the most dominant symptom, and does not include momentary shifts from one dysphoric mood to another dysphoric mood, *e.g.*, anxiety to depression to anger, such as are seen in states of acute psychotic turmoil.

B. At least four of the following symptoms have each been present nearly every day for a period of at least 2 weeks:
Poor appetite or significant weight loss (when not dieting) or increased appetite or significant weight gain
Insomnia or hypersomnia (see Chapter 85)
Psychomotor agitation or retardation (but not merely subjective feelings of restlessness or being slowed down)
Loss of interest or pleasure in usual activities, or decrease in sexual drive not limited to a period when delusional or hallucinating
Loss of energy; fatigue
Feelings of worthlessness, self-reproach, or excessive or inappropriate guilt (either may be delusional).
Complaints or evidence of diminished ability to think or concentrate, such as slowed thinking, or indecisiveness not associated with marked loosening of associations or incoherence
Recurrent thoughts of death, suicidal ideation, wishes to be dead, or suicide attempt

C. Neither of the following dominate the clinical picture when an affective syndrome is present (*i.e.*, symptoms in criteria A and B above):
Preoccupation with a mood-incongruent delusion or hallucination (*i.e.*, mood-incongruent psychotic features). Delusions or hallucinations whose content does not involve themes of either personal inadequacy, guilt, disease, death, nihilism, or deserved punishment. Included here are such symptoms as persecutory delusions, thought insertion, thought broadcasting, and delusions of control, whose content has no apparent relationship to any of the themes noted above.
Bizarre behavior

D. Not superimposed on either schizophrenia, schizophreniform disorder, or a paranoid disorder (see Chapter 16).

E. Not due to any organic mental disorder or uncomplicated bereavement (see Chapters 17 and 19).

[a] From American Psychiatric Association: *Diagnostic and Statistical Manual of Mental Disorders*, ed 3. Washington, DC, American Psychiatric Association, 1980. Special criteria for children have been omitted from this table.

with more traditional diagnostic concepts. However, these criteria are useful in supporting the working diagnosis of major depression in order to begin therapy. Recent work suggests that the dexamethasone suppression test may be useful in differentiating a major depressive episode (plasma cortisol not suppressed by dexamethasone) from a minor affective disturbance. However, a sizeable number of medical conditions interfere with its interpretation. This and other problems make it more useful in an inpatient psychiatric population than in an ambulatory medical population (5).

So-called *atypical depressions* are those major depressions in which symptoms such as hypersomnia, overeating, and agitation or anxiety are seen more frequently than the usual insomnia, anorexia, and psychomotor retardation (12). Such patients usually show the characteristic depressive changes in self-attitude and vital sense, but may describe their mood changes more in terms of fatigue than sadness.

Management

Drugs

For the patient who is maintaining good nutrition and hydration, who is cooperative with treatment, and who is neither overwhelmed with depressive delusions nor suicidal, antidepressant medication is the appropriate initial treatment. Although very useful, the antidepressant drugs—tricyclic antidepressants (TCA) and monoamine oxidase inhibitors (MAOI)—are not always effective in eradicating depressive symptoms. Probably only 65% of patients will have a complete remission of symptoms with any one particular medication. For most patients, TCAs are more effective than MAOIs and are, therefore, regarded as the drugs of first choice, although MAOIs may be equally useful for patients with atypical depression with prominent anxiety and panic attacks. The tricyclics derived from amitriptyline (*i.e.*, amitriptyline and nortriptyline) and imipramine (*i.e.*, imipramine and desipramine) are the best studied and most frequently prescribed. Among patients with the syndrome of depression, those with delusions, hallucinations, and profound psychomotor retardation tend to be less responsive to drugs than those without these stigmata; referral for psychiatric consultation and consideration for electroconvulsive therapy are appropriate for such patients. Among patients with suicidal intent (see "Suicide Prevention") the tricyclics should be dispensed in small amounts since even a 10-day supply provides enough drug for a lethal overdose.

The mechanism of therapeutic action of antidepressant drugs is unknown. Although much indirect evidence suggests that they exert their therapeutic effects by enhancing catecholaminergic and serotonergic neurotransmission, their clinical use remains empirical. The TCAs can be divided into two groups

(see part A of Table 15.3): the *secondary amines* (e.g., desipramine and nortriptyline) and the *tertiary amines* (e.g., amitriptyline, doxepin, and imipramine), which have been more widely used but which have more anticholinergic activity and cause more orthostatic hypotension than the secondary amines. At a recent consensus development conference at the National Institute of Mental Health, the secondary amine TCAs were selected as drugs that should be recommended to nonpsychiatrists as effective antidepressants with acceptable toxicity. This approach would suggest beginning with a secondary amine such as nortriptyline or desipramine. The average effective doses would be nortriptyline 100 mg/day or desipramine 200 mg/day. Nortriptyline has been shown to have its therapeutic effect linked to a steady state blood level of 50 to 140 ng/ml of the drug.

Four novel drugs have recently been approved by the Food and Drug Adminisration for use in depressed patients: alprazolam (Xanax), the only benzodiazepine approved for depression; amoxapine (Ascendin), a compound with neuroleptic and antidepressant properties; maprotiline (Ludiomil), a tetracyclic drug; and tradazone (Desyrel), a novelly structured antidepressant (10). All have been promoted as drugs which are as effective as and less toxic than tricyclic antidepressants. None of them represents a major advance in the treatment of major endogenous depressive disorders, however, and amoxapine and tradazone have potential toxicity which exceeds that of several established tricyclic agents (see part C, Table 15.3). The new antidepressants are also more costly than the standard TCAs. Alprazolam lacks the potential of TCAs for cardiotoxicity and thus may be useful in patients with unstable cardiac conditions; however, its efficacy in endogenous depression is less well established than the efficacy of TCAs. Both alprazolam and trazadone are practically devoid of anticholinergic effects and so may be tried in patients who cannot tolerate these effects in tricyclics. However, maprotiline, which, of the four, is most like a traditional tricyclic preparation, also has very modest anticholinergic effects, is not as sedating as either of the aforementioned drugs, and is well established as being equally effective as tricyclics in treating depression.

In general, treatment with TCAs should begin at 25 to 75 mg/day (exceptions: 5 to 15 mg for protriptyline and 25 to 50 mg for nortriptyline) and be increased in 25-mg increments as tolerated to 150 mg/day, the average effective dose for most of these drugs (exceptions: 40 mg for protriptyline and 100 mg for nortriptyline) (see Table 15.3). Starting doses should be reduced by about 50% in older patients (especially those with medical illnesses). TCA dosage may be increased every 2 to 4 days in young physically healthy patients, but weekly increases are safer for older or infirm individuals. Giving the

Table 15.3.
Selected Characteristics of Antidepressant Drugs

A. TRICYCLICS

Amine Group	Generic Name	Proprietary Name(s)	Strengths of Oral Preparations (mg)	Usual Effective Total Daily Dose in mg (Range)	Therapeutic Plasma Level (ng/ml)	Side Effects		
						Antihistamine (Sedation)	Anti-α-adrenergic (Hypotention)	Anticholinergic[a]
Secondary amines	Desipramine	Norpramin, Pertofrane	25, 50	200 (50–300)	—	+	++	+
	Nortriptyline	Aventyl, Pamelor	10, 25	100 (50–150)	50–140	+	++	++
	Protriptyline	Vivactil	5, 10	40 (15–60)	70–170	+	++	++
Tertiary amines	Amitriptyline	Elavil, Endep	10, 25, 50, 75, 100	150 (50–300)	>120[b]	+++	+++	+++
	Doxepin	Sinequan, Adapin	10, 25, 50, 100	150 (50–300)	>90[b]	+++	++	++
	Imipramine	Tofranil, SK-Pramine, Presamine	10, 25, 50	150 (50–300)	>95[b]	++	+++	++

B. MONOAMINE OXIDASE INHIBITORS

Generic Name	Proprietary Name	Strengths of Oral Preparations (mg)	Usual Effective Total Daily Dose in mg (Range)	Side Effects	
				Risk of Hypertensive Crisis	Orthostatic Hypotension
Tranylcypromine	Parnate	10	30 (20–60)	++	++
Phenelzine	Nardil	15	45 (30–90)	+	++
Isocarboxazide	Marplan	10	30 (20–60)	+	++

C. NEW ANTIDEPRESSANTS

Generic Name	Proprietary Name	Strengths of Oral Preparations (mg)	Usual Effective Total Daily Dose in mg (Range)	Major Advantage Over Tricyclics	Major Disadvantage Compared to Tricyclics
Maprotiline	Ludiomil	25, 50, 75	200 (100–300)	Few anticholinergic effects. Not sedating	May have greater CNS toxicity after overdoses (seizures, myoclonus)
Trazadone	Desyrel	50, 100	300 (200–600)	Almost no anticholinergic effects	Very sedating (like amitriptyline). Appears to have greater direct cardiotoxicity than TCAs. Priapism requiring surgery reported.
Amoxapine	Ascendin	25, 50, 100, 150	150 (100–300)	Few anticholinergic effects	Neuroleptic activity of metabolites may result in extrapyramidal syndromes, possible tardive dyskinesia after long term use. Three times a day schedule initially.
Alprazolam	Xanax	0.25, 0.5, 1	0.75–4	A benzodiazepine without anticholinergic or other tricyclic side effects	Not established as fully effective in depression. Some addictive potential. Fairly sedative. Three times a day schedule.

[a] Dry mouth, blurred vision, decreased intestinal motility, decreased bladder tone, tachycardia.
[b] Upper limited not established.

total daily dose at bedtime is desirable for most patients. Since TCAs may interact with a number of commonly prescribed drugs (Table 15.4), simultaneous prescribing of other drugs with TCAs should be avoided; if this is not possible, close monitoring is very important (for example, when a patient is taking antihypertensive drugs and a TCA).

Dosage with MAOIs should begin at 15 mg two times a day for phenelzine or 10 mg two times a day for tranylcypromine or isocarboxazide, be increased by 10–15 mg per week to the maximum dose unless therapeutic response or toxicity dictates otherwise (see Table 15.3). The use of MAOIs, particularly tranylcypromine, requires caution with respect to

Table 15.4.
Drugs Which May Interact with Tricyclic Antidepressants (TCAs)[a]

Drug	Interaction
Anticholinergic antispasmodics	Enhanced anticholinergic side effects
Antihypertensive drugs	Enhanced orthostatic hypotension
Exception: clonidine and guanethidine	TCA may interfere with antihypertensive effectiveness
Antiparkinsonian drugs (L-dopa and anticholinergic drugs)	Enhanced anticholinergic side effects (also decreased L-dopa effect)
Dilantin	May block TCA effectiveness
Cimetidine	Increased imipramine effect
Methylphenidate (Ritalin)	May increase TCA plasma levels
Monoamine oxidase inhibitors (MOAIs)	Levels of both TCA and MAOI may be increased, enhanced risk of hypertensive crisis
Sedating drugs (alcohol, antihistamines, anxiolytics, hypnotics, neuroleptics)	Enhanced sedation
Sympathomimetics (decongestants, weight reduction agents, stimulants)	TCA may potentiate blood pressure-raising effects of these drugs

[a] From Richelson E: *Psychiatr Ann* 9:16, 1979.

Table 15.5.
Restrictions Needed to Avoid Hypertensive Crisis in Patients Taking Monoamine Oxidase Inhibitors[a]

Items To Be Avoided[b]	Comments
FOODS	
Chicken liver	Tyramine content varies from little to 113 mg/g
Pickled herring	Tyramine content reported at 3.03 mg/g
Cheese	Tyramine content may increase with aging. Sharp cheeses, especially cooked and uncooked cheddar, are highly implicated, but no problem with cream and cottage cheese
Yogurt	
Sour cream	
Beer	
Wine	Not all wines are implicated equally; the problem is noteworthy with Chianti and sherry in small amounts
Broad beans (fava beans *Vicia faba*)	Several reported hypertensive crises; these beans are an ingredient in pasta fasula
Canned figs	
Bananas	
Avocados	
Active yeast preparations	No problem with bread
Soy sauce	
Excessive caffeine	
Raisins	
Chocolate	
DRUGS	
Any sympathomimetic drug (decongestants in cold remedies, weight reduction agents, stimulants)	Can lead to hypertensive crisis
Stop monoamine oxidase inhibitors 2 weeks before planned surgery	Hypertensive crisis can occur if sympathomimetic given for vasoconstriction during surgery

[a] From Lipman AG: *Modern Med* 48:133, 1980.
[b] As little as 6 mg of tyramine may produce a hypertensive reaction in a patient taking a monoamine oxidase inhibitor.

diet and the effects of coadministered drugs, in order to avoid a hypertensive crisis (see Table 15.5).

The newer antidepressants vary in recommended dosing schedules. Average effective daily doses are listed in Table 15.3. Maprotiline can be given once a day like the TCAs, starting at 75 mg and increasing by increments of 25 mg every 2 weeks. Trazadone is initiated at 150 mg, given in a once or twice daily schedule, and it may be increased by 50 mg every 3 to 7 days. Amoxapine is started at 50 mg three times daily and may be increased every 3 to 7 days. When an effective daily dose is found, the entire dose can be taken at one time. Alprazolan is started at 0.25 mg three times daily and may be increased every 3 to 7 days.

Improvement usually occurs after 2 weeks of administration of a therapeutic dose of any antidepressant; maximum benefit usually occurs after 4 to 8 weeks at this dose. Obtaining TCA blood levels may be helpful if after 2 weeks at a stable dose the patient has shown no response to treatment; either noncompliance or rapid metabolism of the drug can be responsible for drug levels below the therapeutic range (Table 15.3). Nortriptyline levels above the upper limit of the therapeutic range may be associated with a loss of therapeutic response (Table 15.3 shows therapeutic ranges). Combination pills containing TCAs and phenothiazines should be not used in the treatment of depressive disorders, since they carry the risk of side effects from both drugs and they provide no demonstrated advantage over carefully selected TCAs in nondelusional patients.

Drug Side Effects

The antidepressants cause *side effects*, many of which can be grouped according to probable physiological mechanism (see Table 15.3). The physician and the patient must decide which side effects are worth tolerating. Since depressed patients tolerate even mild side effects poorly, the patients should be reassured that the treatment is safe and potentially very helpful. Apart from the specific warnings contained in Tables 15.4 and 15.5, there are no known measures that are clinically useful in preventing or alleviating the side effects of antidepressant drugs. In addition to the side effects named in Table 15.3, TCAs may produce mild paresthesias, increased appetite with weight gain, granulocytopenia (rarely), anticholinergic delirium (rarely), hypomania, slowed cardiac conduction, and cardiac arrhythmias. Because of the cardiac effects, these drugs should be given cautiously to those patients who have pre-existing conduction abnormalities and to those with unstable cardiac conditions, such as a recent myocardial infarction. However, tricyclics are quite safe even in patients with pre-existing stable heart disease (13). The major problem associated with the use of MAOIs is acute hypertension caused by foods containing the sympathomimetic agent, tyramine. Thus, patients taking MAOIs must eliminate certain foods from their diet (Table 15.5).

Duration of Drug Treatment

After recovery from a first or infrequently recurrent depressive syndrome the medication that induced the remission should be continued usually for 3 to 6 months (a period of high risk for relapse); during this interval, dosage should remain at the level which relieved the depression. Occasionally, a lowering of the dose to reduce side effects will be justified. The patient should be told that withdrawal symptoms (nausea, dizziness, headache, increased perspiration, and increased salivation) may occur when tricyclics are discontinued abruptly. For this reason tricylics which have been given for 2 months or more should be tapered in 25- to 50-mg increments/week prior to discontinuation. After electroconvulsive therapy (see below), maintenance treatment with tricyclic antidepressants also reduces the risk of relapse. Exceptions to these guidelines include the occurrence of drug toxicity, the appearance of manic symptoms (which can be induced by the antidepressants), and a history of such regular relapses that indefinite maintenance therapy with a tricyclic or lithium is needed (see section on long term management).

Office Psychotherapy

For the first 6 to 8 weeks, the patient with major depression should be seen at least weekly both for adjustment of medication and for brief supportive psychotherapy by the techniques described in Chapter 11. Major life decisions and major shifts in personal relationships should be gently discouraged until the patient returns to his or her premorbid

condition. Frank discussion of suicidal feelings, plans, intentions, risk, and alternatives should be a routine part of each visit (see "Suicide Prevention" below). The patient should be checked routinely for side effects of drugs by being asked about dry mouth, tremor, blurred vision, orthostasis, tachycardia, and constipation, and by examining heart rate and rhythm and blood pressure (sitting and standing). The more depressed the patient is, the less tolerant he will be of minor adverse drug effects. The support of the doctor in encouraging persistence with drug therapy can be crucial.

Discussion of prognosis with the patient and his family is extremely important in the management of depression (see page 185, "Prognosis" and page 194, "Counseling the Distressed Family").

Referral for Management

The general physician may choose to manage those patients in whom he diagnoses major depression or he may refer them to a psychiatrist. There are four types of patients who should always be referred for the expertise of a psychiatrist: those who have shown no improvement after 2 to 4 weeks of treatment with therapeutic doses of antidepressant drugs (about one in three patients); those who cannot or will not take antidepressant medications; those who are overtly suicidal; and those who show delusions, hallucinations, or depressive stupor (the patient becomes mute and unresponsive). In these patients, either hospitalization, intensive psychotherapy, more aggressive drug therapy, or electroconvulsive therapy will usually be suggested by the psychiatric consultant. Some patients will be resistant to the idea of seeing a psychiatrist. A physician with whom a patient has good rapport can be very persuasive if he explains that additional drug treatments are available, but that their use requires the expert experience of the psychiatrist, and that there is an excellent chance of improvement.

Electroconvulsive Therapy

Electroconvulsive therapy (ECT) is an effective and rapid treatment for major depressive disorder. The decision to use ECT should be made by the psychiatrist with the concurrence of the patient and/or the patient's family. This treatment is given only to hospitalized patients; during ECT the patient is anesthetized with a short acting barbiturate anesthetic. There is general agreement that this treatment is not useful for patients with "neurotic" depression (dysthymic disorder). There is even some evidence that among patients with clear-cut major depression those with the more severe symptoms will have a better therapeutic response. In a recent double blind, controlled study (in which the control group were treated by sham ECT) of a large number of patients with endogenous depressions, only a modest, but statistically significant advantage accrued to the ECT-treated patients. Failure of drug therapy, the need for a rapid response (as in the starving or suicidal patient), and overwhelming severity of the depression are the principal indications for trying ECT.

The mechanism of action of ECT is unknown, but it appears that the electrical seizure discharge is required for benefit, which comes in an all-or-none fashion after the application of current. There is usually transient memory loss, related to the passage of current through cerebral hemispheres, but therapeutic benefit is not linked to the memory disturbance. Although there are other methods of inducing seizures, electric current is easiest to control and, therefore, safest. The usual risk of general anesthesia is the major hazard associated with ECT.

The *adverse effects* which follow ECT primarily involve memory. Commonly, retention of new and occasionally old memories is mildly defective for weeks to months following a series of ECT treatments. This defect is usually "spotty"—that is, it will be apparent for specific domains of memory, but will not affect many others. Typically, the patient in whom this effect becomes clinically apparent (perhaps 40% of treated patients) will have trouble recalling names of recent acquaintances including doctors, nurses, and other patients. Clinically, apparent memory defects typically resolve within a month. More detailed formal testing reveals mild defects up to 3 months, but none at 6 months after treatment.

Depressed patients with brain tumors ordinarily should not receive ECT. Patients with dementias from neuropathological causes treated with ECT may have temporary worsening of their cognitive impairments, but not infrequently the removal of depression actually helps overall social functioning. ECT should be avoided, if possible, within 3 months of myocardial infarction, cerebrovascular accident, or perforated viscus repair. Neither anticoagulation therapy nor the presence of a cardiac pacemaker is a contraindication for ECT.

Mania

Diagnosis

The manic syndrome, like major depression, is defined by a sustained change in mood with parallel changes in self-attitude and vital sense. The manic patient's *mood* may be euphoric or irritable and angry or may alternate between the two. *Self-attitude* becomes one of overconfidence and of an inflated sense of power, position, and importance. *Vital sense* reflects a subjective sense of quickened, acutely accurate thinking, unusual ease in decision making, a sense of heightened perception of sounds, colors, tastes, *etc.* In addition there is usually a sense of increased energy and a decreased need for sleep.

This central triad is often accompanied by parallel psychomotor symptoms. Delusions and hallucinations which are either persecutory or consistent with mood are not uncommon. Occasionally even characteristic symptoms of schizophrenia (see chapter 16) occur in manic patients, leading to the clinical rule of thumb that so-called "schizophrenic" symptoms are not in themselves diagnostic but should be judged by the company they keep. In the presence of the characteristic manic syndrome and first rank symptoms of schizophrenia some would diagnose "schizoaffective disorder—manic type." Whether or not this is a useful practice, acute treatment and projected outcomes are similar to those for typical mania. The specific criteria of the American Psychiatric Association for mania are shown in Table 15.6.

Management

Because the disruptive and bizarre symptoms of mania are not seen frequently by the generalist and because it is treated with a drug, lithium, which requires supervision by someone familiar with its use, mania is a problem which should be referred to a psychiatrist. The generalist may play a crucial role in persuading a severely manic patient to accept referral and in following the patient with the psychiatrist if the patient also has a chronic medical problem. Knowledge of lithium treatment and of management techniques for severe mania is therefore important for the generalist.

Lithium

In its milder form (called hypomania), the manic syndrome may be successfully treated with a neuroleptic (see Chapter 16 for details on neuroleptics) or lithium alone. Since the neuroleptics reduce manic behavior more rapidly, they are often used in combination with lithium in the early phases of treatment. This combined treatment involves greater risk of adverse effects and should be carried out by a psychiatrist. For both short and long term treatment, lithium carbonate is the most useful drug in the manic patient.

Lithium is given in divided doses. Beginning with 300 to 600 mg on the first day and increasing the dose in small increments every 3 to 4 days to the desired level minimizes nausea (as does taking the dose on a full stomach). The usual maintenance dose is 600 to 1800 mg given in divided doses (three or four times daily with standard preparations and once or twice daily with slow release preparations). Blood levels, which should be measured 12 hours after a dose, should be monitored once or twice/ week at first. Even when thoroughly stabilized in a compliant patient, lithium levels should be checked at least six times/year. In addition, because of the possibility of long term renal effects, maintenance dosage should be aimed at maintaining the lowest therapeutic level (probably 0.7 to 0.9 mEq/liter) and

Table 15.6.
American Psychiatric Association Diagnostic Criteria for a Manic Episode[a]

A. One or more distinct periods with a predominantly elevated, expansive, or irritable mood. The elevated or irritable mood must be a prominent part of the illness and relatively persistent, although it may alternate or intermingle with depressive mood.

B. Duration of at least 1 week (or any duration if hospitalization is necessary), during which, for most of the time, at least three of the following symptoms have persisted (four if the mood is only irritable) and have been present to a significant degree:

Increase in activity (either socially, at work, or sexually) or physical restlessness

More talkative than usual or pressure to keep talking

Flight of ideas or subjective experience that thoughts are racing

Inflated self-esteem (grandiosity, which may be delusional)

Decreased need for sleep

Distractibility, *i.e.*, attention is too easily drawn to unimportant or irrelevant external stimuli

Excessive involvement in activities that have a high potential for painful consequences which is not recognized, *e.g.*, buying sprees, sexual indiscretions, foolish business investments, reckless driving

C. Neither of the following dominates the clinical picture when an affective syndrome is present (*i.e.*, symptoms in criteria A and B above):

Preoccupation with a mood-incongruent delusion or hallucination (*i.e.*, mood-incongruent psychotic features). Delusions or hallucinations whose content does not involve themes of either personal inadequacy, guilt, disease, death, nihilism, or deserved punishment. Included here are such symptoms as persecutory delusions, thought insertion, thought broadcasting, and delusions of control, whose content has no apparent relationship to any of the themes noted above.

Bizarre behavior

D. Not superimposed on either schizophrenia, schizophreniform disorder, or a paranoid disorder (see Chapter 16).

E. Not due to any organic mental disorder, such as substance intoxication (see Chapters 17 and 22).

---

[a] From American Psychiatric Association: *Diagnostic and Statistical Manual of Mental Disorders*. ed 3. Washington, DC, American Psychiatric Association, 1980. *Note:* A hypomanic episode is a pathological disturbance similar to, but not as severe as, a manic episode.

Table 15.7.
Important Drug Interactions with Lithium

Drugs that may enhance lithium toxicity:
Amiloride[a]
Ethacrynic acid[a]
Furosemide[a]
Indomethacin (and probably other nonsteroidal anti-inflammatory drugs (NSAIDs))[a]
Methyldopa[b]
Phenytoin[b]
Carbamazepine[b]
Spectinamycin[a]
Spironolactone[a]
Tetracycline[a]
Thiazide diuretics[a]
Thiramterene[a]
Drugs that may diminish lithium effect:
Theophylline[c]
Acetazolamide[c]
Drugs that may aggravate lithium tremor:
Neuroleptics[b]
Tricyclic antidepressants[b]

---

[a] Decreased renal excretion.
[b] Mechanism not established.
[c] Increased renal excretion.

The number of possible side effects from the *maintenance dose* is large enough to warrant a medical review of systems to detect them. The three most important ones are hand tremor, thyroid disturbances, and renal toxicity.

1. An accentuated physiological tremor (see Chapter 82) appears in a large percentage of patients (perhaps 60%) but is rarely severe. A family history of benign essential tremor and of concomitant use of other psychotropic drugs is often associated with more severe tremor.

2. In about 3% of patients, lithium therapy causes nontoxic goiter and mild alterations of thyroid function tests (*i.e.*, borderline low thyroxine levels or elevated thyroid-stimulating hormone values). Less frequently, frank hypothyroidism may occur, usually in patients who had subclinical hypothyroidism before receiving lithium. For these reasons thyroid function should be assessed before lithium treatment is begun.

3. Finally, and of greatest concern, long term lithium therapy is associated with renal abnormalities: a renal concentrating defect (partial nephrogenic diabetes insipidus) and mild defects in glomerular filtration rate (GFR). These abnormalities may cause symptoms of diabetes insipidus (polyuria, hypernatremia) in about 10% of patients. The concentrating defect predisposes the patient to dehydration and, therefore, to frank lithium intoxication. Patients must be counseled to maintain good hydration even under circumstances which might inhibit their interest in adequate water intake (including depression) or which would increase water loss (e.g., hot weather). They should also be instructed to report

not necessarily the level required for acute antimanic activity (0.9 to 1.4 mEq/liter). Lithium should be used cautiously with other medications since there are a number of important drug interactions associated with its use (see Table 15.7).

The *adverse effects of lithium* can be divided into three groups: early (associated with rapidly rising blood levels), maintenance (associated with stable levels within the therapeutic range), and toxic (usually associated with high lithium levels).

The *early* side effects include nausea and vomiting, diarrhea, mild lassitude, and drowsiness. These effects typically resolve as the serum level stabilizes in the therapeutic range.

the onset of polyuria at any time in the course of lithium treatment. The GFR should be assessed (see Chapter 47) before lithium is started and reassessed yearly thereafter.

The *toxic* effects of lithium occur uncommonly at normal serum levels, but increase in frequency as serum levels rise past 1.5 mEq/liter. Premonitory signs are the recurrence of gastrointestinal side effects and worsening of polyuria and hand tremor, lethargy, and clumsiness. Obvious changes in the level of consciousness are reflected in confusion, delirium, stupor, and finally coma. Focal as well as nonlocalizing neurological signs are often present. Peak levels near or above 4.0 mEq/liter are potentially fatal; death in coma or due to aspiration pneumonitis can occur. The toxic syndrome is not usually relieved rapidly, even though blood levels can be reduced rapidly. A rather prolonged 10- to 14-day resolution of the mental state is usual. Management of suspected lithium intoxication begins with an emergency measurement of serum lithium level and the discontinuation of lithium when the early signs of the disorder appear. If the clinical or laboratory evaluations suggest the likelihood of the toxic syndrome, hospitalization is mandatory.

The most important lesson to be learned about lithium intoxication is to prevent it. Overingestion and inadequate renal excretion (at times, related to one of the drugs listed in Table 15.7) are the only causes of the disorder.

Treatment of Severe Mania

Severe acute mania requires treatment with both lithium and neuroleptics, which is usually carried out in the hospital. The generalist's role with such patients may include initial diagnosis and then assessment of the acute manic state, persuasion of the manic patient to accept hospitalization voluntarily if needed, assessment of the patient for possible civil commitment, and the management of the acutely manic patient at home or in the office. These last three steps are outlined below.

Relating to the acutely manic patient can be very difficult. The euphoric or irritable manic patient often will not be able to accept the notion that his or her behavior is disturbed and requires inpatient therapy. A rationale for treatment which does not call attention to the obviously disordered behavior is usually more palatable to the patient. Consultation with the family about the plan of treatment should be arranged before, not after, confrontation with the patient. The family should be willing to accept responsibility if they refuse to follow the physician's recommendation.

Although laws on commitment vary from state to state, all states currently have legal provisions to allow the involuntary hospitalization of patients with mental disorders who are clearly dangerous to themselves or others and for whom no less restrictive alternative is appropriate.

For acute manic agitation the use of parenteral haloperidol (Haldol) is usually quite effective. Modest doses (5 to 10 mg intramuscularly) will calm most patients with little or no depression of blood pressure and little sedation. The sedating phenothiazines such as chlorpromazine (Thorazine) are more apt to produce severe orthostatic hypotension, and repeated doses are often necessary to break the agitated manic state. Within 15 to 20 minutes, intramuscular haloperidol usually brings about a calming trend which lasts for several hours. This period can be used to get the patient admitted to hospital. Even in this short period, however, patients may develop extrapyramidal side effects from haloperidol, most frequently acute dystonic reactions. This condition will be alleviated by 50 mg of intramuscular diphenhydramine (Benadryl).

Prognosis and Long Term Management of Major Affective Disorders

Because of the fundamental similarities, the prognoses of major depression and mania are discussed together. Before modern treatment, patients with these disorders usually recovered spontaneously within 6 to 18 months. With antidepressants, lithium, and ECT, remissions usually can be achieved much more quickly. However, even with modern treatment, about 20% of patients with severe major depressions may not recover fully in a 2-year period after entering treatment (7). Predictors of poor outcome include severity sufficient to require hospitalization and long duration of major symptoms (1 year) before treatment. It is also noted that many nonrecovering patients have not been aggressively treated after failure to respond to a trial of antidepressant medications. Although some patients will fail to respond to all treatments, clinical experience teaches that most correctly diagnosed patients who are initially treatment failures will eventually respond to a second, third, or fourth treatment effort.

A hallmark of the course of major affective syndromes is the tendency to relapse. The frequency of relapse is quite variable. However, fewer than 20% of major affective syndromes resolve without relapsing at some point. There is a tendency for relapses to become more frequent later in the life of the patient (or later in the course of the illness). There is some evidence that depressions in later life are more severe and treatment resistant as well. Formerly, this was part of the justification for the now discarded term "involutional melancholia."

The use of lithium and antidepressants has been shown to be beneficial in preventing recurrent affective episodes (9). Depressive relapses which occur in patients taking lithium or tricyclics are usually less severe and of shorter duration. Lithium is the only treatment demonstrated to reduce the frequency of manic relapses.

The foundations of long term care of patients within bipolar or unipolar affective disorders are the following: a trusting doctor-patient relationship; education and counseling of the patient and his family regarding the course of the illness, the early signs of relapse, and the benefits and hazards of treatment; and maintenance on lithium carbonate or tricyclic antidepressant. Maintenance treatment is usually continued indefinitely for a clearly relapsing disorder. The patient's personal physician can often provide the basic treatment, particularly if he is following the patient for chronic medical problems. Brief visits every 2 to 3 months are sufficient when the patient is well. The objectives of these visits are to monitor the mood state, the drug therapy, and the social progress of the patient. If the patient has a well established trusting and predictable relationship with the doctor, even patients with the most grandiose manic or pessimistic depressive states will be more amenable to accepting necessary additional treatment.

The patient and his family should be educated with respect to the relapsing and remitting course of the illness, which is greatly modified but not usually eradicated by drug therapy. Individual aspects of the illness need to be obseved and remembered by the patient, the family members, and the doctor, in particular, (a) the early symptoms of relapse (which differ from patient to patient); (b) certain signs or symptoms which specifically point to the affective syndrome in contrast to other reasons for changed feelings or behavior; and (c) recognized signs for suicidal or other dangerous behavior, as well as ways to relieve the danger.

Counseling the Distressed Family

Family members of patients with serious affective disorders often experience feelings of confusion, hopelessness, guilt, and recrimination toward the patient. These are not only painful feelings—they positively impede the family's attempts to support or care for their ill relative. Physicians need to address the family's needs directly through educational meetings with them. Above all, the family must recognize major affective disorders as diseases and realize that these disorders are not caused by the family, by the patient, or by social predicaments affecting the patient. The family also should know that, although the pathophysiology of affective disorders is unknown, empirical treatments are quite effective and the prognosis for complete recovery from an episode is generally good, although relapses occur frequently. These points will usually require some repetition and are best repeated in response to questions which the family should be encouraged to raise in such a meeting or consultation. The recently published book by Greist and Jefferson (see "General References") can also be recommended to patients and families.

It is equally important to reassure families and patients with dysthymic and transiently demoralized mood states that the patients are not suffering from major mental illness.

Evidence from studies of concordance in identical as compared to nonidentical twins suggests a substantial genetic contribution to the etiology of major affective disorders. Since no single pattern of inheritance has been discerned, the evidence for a genetic contribution has been interpreted in several ways: (a) not all cases are genetically transmitted, (b) there is genetic heretogeneity in familial cases, and (c) the condition may be polygenic. Overall, it appears that a sibling or offspring of a patient with a major affective disorder has a 10% chance of developing the disorder. However, in a family in which there is no evidence for a genetic contribution, the risk would not be greater than that in the general population, while in some families this risk may be as high as 50%. Counseling patients and their families about the genetic risk needs to be tailored to the needs and relevant past history in each family. The major themes of counseling should be that most, but not all, cases are genetically influenced, that effective treatment is available, and that treatment is much enhanced by early detection of the disorder.

CYCLOTHYMIC DISORDER

A bipolar affective disorder that is sufficiently mild or so brief that the episodes fail to meet the APA criteria for major depression or mania (Tables 15.2 and 15.5) is categorized as a cyclothymic disorder. These patients must be distinguished from patients with the personality traits of emotional lability and self-dramatization, who will often report rapid but unsustained mood changes. The family histories of cyclothymic patients are similar to those of patients with a bipolar affective disorder, as is their response to medication. The prognosis is also similar to that of bipolar disorder, as 35% of such patients were found to suffer full blown manic, hypomanic, or depressive episodes in a 2- to 3-year period (2).

SUICIDE PREVENTION

The rate of suicide in most countries is low enough (11 per 100,000 in the United States) that successful prediction of an individual suicide at a given point in time is very unlikely.

Practical strategies in this area are to protect those with relatively high risk in the short term and to reduce the risk in these patients over a longer term. *Risk factors* for successful suicide include older age, male sex, depressive disorder, alcoholism, living alone, previous suicide attempt, and refusal to accept referral for psychiatric treatment. Retrospective studies of patient groups with major affective disorders in the era before effective drugs were available suggest that about 15% of the deaths were due to suicide. In addition, clinical observations suggest that the risk of suicide increases when improvement begins (or just after a depressed patient is discharged from the hospital) or when the depressive's ruminations become frankly delusional convictions. Retrospective studies also suggest that there are fewer suicides in patients treated with ECT or long term lithium.

The most crucial activities of physicians in preventing suicides are the recognition, treatment, and prophylaxis of major depressive episodes. When evaluating any patient with depressed mood, direct and open inquiry should be made regarding suicidal ideas, specific plans, and available means which the patient might be inclined to use. This information as well as information about the capability and availability of constant family supervision are essential in determining whether treatment may be attempted safely on an outpatient basis. This evaluation should also be guided by the knowledge that delusionally depressed patients have a significantly increased risk of suicide and that patients with prior suicide attempts are more likely than others to attempt it again when depressed. When treating depressed outpatients it should be recalled that a majority of people who commit suicide with pills have obtained the lethal dose in a single prescription at a recent visit to a physician (8). This could represent as little as a 1- to 2-week supply of antidepressant medication. Thus, small prescriptions and, at times, family supervision of medications, will be needed. Finally, short term protection of patients with suicidal intent *via* hospitization, including involuntary commitment, is often required.

The majority of patients who present to emergency facilities after overdose of pills do not suffer from major depression, but from adjustment disorders and personality disorders, and they usually do not die by suicide. However, they should be methodically evaluated in the same manner as noted above since many such patients are prone to take overdoses again when stressed. These patients may benefit from very brief hospital admissions when social support for them is lacking and suicidal feelings are intense. All should have some outpatient counseling.

General References

American Psychiatric Association: *Diagnostic and Statistical Manual of Mental Disorders*, ed 3. Washington, DC, American Psychiatric Association, 1980.
Recently updated diagnostic criteria and epidemiological information for all recognized psychiatric disorders.
Baldessarini RJ, Lipinski JF: Lithium salts: 1970–1975. *Ann Intern Med* 83:527, 1975.
Excellent review of the history of practical aspects of lithium use for manic-depressive illness.
Crowe RR: Electroconvulsive therapy—a current perspective. *N Engl J Med* 311:163, 1984.
An up-to-date review of ECT.
Greist JH, Jefferson JW: *Depression and Its Treatment*. Washington, DC, American Psychiatric Press, 1984.
A brief book written for patients and families.
Hollister LE: Tricyclic antidepressants. *N Engl J Med* 299:1106, 1978.
Good review of the most useful antidepressant drugs.
Lake CR (ed): Clinical psychopharmacology I. *Psychiatr Clin North Am* 7, 1984.
An up-to-date review of the major drugs used to treat affective disorders.
Mood Disorders: Pharmacologic Prevention of Recurrences. Consensus Development Conference, Consensus Statement, vol 5, no. 4, US Department of Health and Human Services, National Institutes of Health.
The distilled wisdom of a committee of experts on maintenance treatment for major affective disorders. (Available by request from the National Institutes of Health.)

Specific References

1. Akiskal HS: Dysthymic disorder: psychopathology of proposed chronic depressive subtypes. *Am J Psychiatry* 140:11, 1983.
2. Akiskal HS, Djenderedjian AH, Rosenthal RH, Khani MK: Cyclothymic disorder: validating criteria for inclusion in the bipolar affective group. *Am J Psychiatry* 134:1227, 177.
3. DePaulo JR, Folstein MF: Psychiatric disturbance in neurological patients: detection, recognition and hospital course. *Ann Neurol* 4:225, 1978.
4. Goldberg DP, Day C, Thompson L: Psychiatric morbidity in general practice and the community. *Psychol Med* 6:565, 1976.
5. Health and Public Policy Committee, American College of Physicians: The dexamethasone suppression test for the detection, diagnosis, and management of depression. *Ann Intern Med* 100:307, 1984.
6. Johnstone EC, Deakin JFW, Lawler P, et al: The Northwick Park electroconvulsive therapy trial. *Lancet* 1:1317, 1980.
7. Keller MB, Klerman GL, Lavori PW, et al: Long-term outcome of episodes of major depression. *JAMA* 252:788, 1984.
8. Murphy GE: The physcian's responsibility for suicide. I. An error of commission. II. Errors of omission. *Ann Interm Med* 82:301, 305, 1975.
9. Prien RF, Klett CJ, Caffey EM Jr: Lithium carbonate and imipramine in prevention of affective episodes: a comparison in recurrent affective illness. *Arch Gen Psychiatry* 29:240, 1973.
10. Settle EC: Recently introduced antidepressants: their place in clinical practice. *Postgrad Med* 72:87, 1982.
11. Shepherd M, Gruenberg EM: The age for neuroses. *Milbank Mem Fund Q* 35:258, 1957.
12. Sovner RD: The clinical characteristics and treatment of atypical depression. *J Clin Psychiatry* 42:285, 1981.
13. Veith RC, Raskind MA, Caldwell JH, et al: Cardiovascular effects of tricyclic antidepressants in depressed patients with chronic heart disease. *N Engl J Med* 306:954, 1982.
14. Widmer RB, Cadoret RJ, North CS: Depression in primary care—changes in pattern of patients visits and complaints during subsequent developing depressions. *J Fam Pract* 9:1017, 1979.

CHAPTER SIXTEEN

Schizophrenia

CHESTER W. SCHMIDT, Jr., M.D.

Schizophrenia is a mental disorder or group of disorders of unknown etiology. The American Psychiatric Association lists the essential features of the disorder as the presence of certain psychotic features during the active phase of the disease, characteristic chronic symptoms involving multiple psychological processes, deterioration from a previous level of functioning, onset before the age of 45, and duration of at least 6 months. As noted below, none of these symptoms is pathognomonic for schizophrenia and each is seen in other psychotic states associated with both functional and organic mental disorders.

Familiarity with schizophrenia is important to the generalist for two principal reasons: (a) in the prodromal stage, the patient frequently presents first to a general physician, and (b) the generalist can provide most of the care for a patient with this lifelong disorder.

EPIDEMIOLOGY

Schizophrenia has been found in all societies throughout the world. The distribution is assumed to be similar through all populations. Epidemiological studies in Western societies have found the incidence of schizophrenia to range from 50 to 250 cases/100,000 population/year. Lifetime incidence rates have been reported to range from 0.75 to 2.75%. Studies of incidence and prevalence in Europe using strict and somewhat narrow criteria of schizophrenia have produced case numbers and rates lower than similar studies done in the United States using broader criteria. Currently it is estimated there are 200,000 patients hospitalized in the United States with a diagnosis of schizophrenia. These patients occupy one-half of all the psychiatric beds in the country. In 1943, Lemkau et al (3) determined that 15 to 25% of patients with schizophenia never enter the hospital. Developments in psychopharmacology which occurred in the 1950s and the wide availability of ambulatory treatment resources have expanded that number and have greatly reduced the duration of confinement for those schizophrenics who require hospitalization.

Schizophrenia is found with equal frequency in males and females. Onset is usually during young adulthood, with the first hospitalization generally occurring between the ages of 25 and 34 years. Most schizophrenics are single and are found in lower socioeconomic groups. The proposed reason for the clustering of patients in the lower socioeconomic groups is a downward social drift resulting from deterioration of social and vocational function.

ETIOLOGY

The cause or causes of schizophrenia remain unknown. Numerous theories have been offered: constitutional, genetic, neurological, anatomical, biochemical, nutritional, psychosocial, and psychoanalytical. It is known that people related to schizophrenics are at higher risk for the disorder. The increased risk ranges from 3% for second degree relatives, to 7 to 15% for siblings and children of one schizophrenic parent, to 40% for children of two schizophrenic patients. Concordance rates in dizygotic twins are 10 to 15%, and in monozygotic twins 45%. This evidence indicates there is a genetic factor, but such a factor has yet to be defined. A more recent clue to the etiology of schizophrenia has emerged from studies of the pharmacological effects of neuroleptic antipsychotic agents on schizophrenia. These antipsychotic agents have been found to antagonize dopamine-mediated neurotransmission, leading to the speculation that excessive activity of the dopamine systems may be part of a biochemical defect in schizophrenics (4).

NATURAL HISTORY OF SCHIZOPHRENIA

Although the first episode of acute psychosis usually occurs in late adolescence or early adulthood, prodromal manifestations of the disease are often present for years before the acute episode. During the *prodromal phase*, individuals gradually withdraw from social relationships into their own inner psychological world. They become indifferent to their grooming, develop suspicious attitudes about others, and ignore social graces and social rituals. They appear different, peculiar, and sometimes bizarre. Withdrawal often results in a gradual deterioration of scholastic and vocational abilities although some patients who have achieved substantial social skills (including marriage and family), educational skills (college and/or graduate level work), and vocational skills (stable and productive work) show little deterioration of their baseline function. The development of these skills may be a function of the age at onset of the disorder: the older the patient is, the more likely it is that he or she will have developed social, educational, and vocational talents. In other patients the deterioration of social and vocational skills may be so striking that the patient seems to have a changed personality. In many cases of early onset schizophrenia, the patients will have developed only marginal social and vocational skills so that their deterioration appears more insidious.

In one study of the prodromal stage of schizophrenia (6), the majority of patients demonstrated some dysphoria (anxiety or depression) in association with social deterioration; and it is significant that over half of them developed vague somatic complaints for which they sought help from a general practitioner.

Acute psychotic episodes are marked by the presence of a variety of symptoms: delusions (content of thought); hallucinations (perception); blunted, flattened, or inappropriate affect; illogical thinking and loosening of associations (form of thought); preoccupation with fantasies and an inner psychological world (autism); inability to carry out goal-directed behavior because of preoccupation with consequences of alternatives (ambivalence); and stereotyped, bizarre, and sometimes rigid posturing. These episodes are often associated with stressful life events. Before neuroleptics were available, these episodes could last from weeks to years. Currently most episodes are brought under pharmacological control within several weeks to 2 months. After treatment, full blown psychotic symptoms subside and in some cases seem to have disappeared completely. Most patients then resume the withdrawn, distant, odd social manner they manifested before the psychotic episode. Scholastic and vocational ability may slip further. With each subsequent psychotic episode the patients slip further and further into a dependent, regressed state in which they are unable to function and become entirely dependent on family or society. Less than 20% work full time;

the majority are financially supported by welfare programs or by federal disability programs. Institutionalization is required in some cases because the patients lose all ability to care for themselves.

Thus, schizophrenia is a lifelong disease consisting of (*a*) psychotic symptoms which periodically become intense, and (*b*) an arrest or deterioration of social and vocational functioning probably caused by massive withdrawal of interest in the outside world.

DIAGNOSIS

The diagnosis of schizophrenia, especially during the initial episodes of acute psychosis, is based on clinical judgment and diagnostic criteria which, until recently, were unreliable. There are no pathognomonic symptoms, signs, or laboratory findings which point to the diagnosis. The medical history of the patient does not contribute to the diagnosis and, as discussed above, family history of the disease provides only partial information.

The diagnostic criteria for schizophrenia described in the American Psychiatric Association's *Diagnostic and Statistical Manual of Mental Disorders* (DSM-III) are an excellent synthesis of several recognized diagnostic schemas (see Table 16.1). Diagnosis rests upon the findings of the symptoms of psychosis elicited by a mental status examination (see Chapter 10) and a history which documents the prodromal phase.

DIFFERENTIAL DIAGNOSIS

Any kind of psychotic state may resemble acute schizophrenia. However, differences in symptomatology permit differentiation and diagnosis. *Organic mental disorders* (see Chapter 17) are marked by disturbances in consciousness (delirium), by disorientation with respect to time, place, and person, and by impairment in intellectual functions (memory, calculations, *etc*). In addition, especially in persons under 50, there is usually evidence from the history, physical examination, and laboratory tests of specific organic findings which are etiologically related to the mental condition. *Illicit drugs*, especially amphetamine and phencyclidine (see Chapter 22), may mimic the acute phase of schizophrenia. In addition, a number of *prescription drugs* may occasionally produce hallucinations and other manifestations suggesting psychosis (see Table 16.2). History of drug usage and absence of the prodromal phase help to differentiate these conditions from schizophrenia.

The psychotic symptoms of *major affective episodes* (both mania and depression, see Chapter 15) can also be similar to those seen during acute episodes in the course of schizophrenia. Affective disorders differ from schizophrenia in that psychotic

Table 16.1.
Diagnostic Criteria for Schizophrenic Disorders[a]

A. At least one of the following during a phase of the illness
Bizarre delusions (content is patently absurd and has no possible basis in fact), such as delusions of being controlled, thought broadcasting, thought insertion, or thought withdrawal
Somatic, grandiose, religious, nihilistic, or other delusions with persecutory or jealous content
Delusions with persecutory or jealous content if accompanied by hallucinations of any type
Auditory hallucinations in which either a voice keeps up a running commentary on the individual's behavior or thoughts, or two or more voices converse with each other
Auditory hallucinations on several occasions with content of more than one or two words, having no apparent relation to depression or elation
Incoherence, marked loosening of associations, markedly illogical thinking, or marked poverty of content of speech is associated with at least one of the following:
    Blunted, flat, or inappropriate affect
    Delusions or hallucinations
    Catatonic or other grossly disorganized behavior
B. Deterioration from a previous level of functioing in such areas as work, social relations, and self-care.
C. Duration: Continuous signs of the illness for at least 6 months at some time during the person's life, with some signs of the illness at present. The 6-month period must include an active phase during which there were symptoms from A, with or without a prodromal or residual phase, as defined below.
    Prodromal phase: A clear deterioration in functioning before the active phase of the illness not due to a disturbance in mood or to a substance use disorder and involving at least two of the symptoms noted below
    Residual phase: Persistence, following the active phase of the illness, of at least two of the symptoms noted below, not due to a disturbance in mood or to a substance use disorder
    Prodromal or residual symptoms:
    Social isolation or withdrawal
    Marked impairment in role functioning as wage earner, student, or homemaker
    Markedly peculiar behavior (*e.g.*, collecting garbage, talking to self in public, or hoarding food)
    Marked impairment in personal hygiene and grooming
    Blunted, flat, or inappropriate affect
    Digressive, vague, overelaborate, circumstantial, or metaphorical speech
    Odd or bizarre ideation, or magical thinking, *e.g,* superstitiousness, clairvoyance, telepathy, "sixth sense," "others can feel my feelings," overvalued ideas, ideas of reference
    Unusual perceptual experiences, *e.g.*, recurrent illusions, sensing the presence of a force or person not actually present
        Examples: Six months of prodromal symptoms with 1 week of symptoms from A; no prodromal symptoms with 6 months of symptoms from A; no prodromal symtoms with 2 weeks of symptoms from A and 6 months of residual symptoms; 6 months of symptoms from A, apparently followed by several years of complete remission, with 1 week of symptoms from A in current episode.
D. The full depressive or manic syndrome (criteria A and B of major depressive or manic episode)[b] if present, developed after any psychotic symptoms, or was brief in duration relative to the duration of the psychotic symptoms in A.
E. Onset of prodromal or active phase of the illness before age 45.
F. Not due to any organic mental disorder or mental retardation.

[a] Adapted from American Psychiatric Association: *Diagnostic and Statistical Manual of Mental Disorders*, ed 3. Washington, DC, American Psychiatric Association, 1980.
[b] See Chapter 15, Tables 15.2 and 15.6.

symptoms (delusions, hallucinations, *etc*) appear after the development of the affective disturbance (depression or mania). In schizophrenia, marked depression or mania may appear, but the affective disturbance occurs after the onset of the psychotic symptoms. These principles of differential diagnosis are far from perfect, and patients with both types of disorder have been mislabeled. Because of the often poor prognosis associated with schizophrenia, mislabeling is not without significant consequence in terms of the physician's attitudes toward the patient and the actual treatment provided.

There are several *other functional psychotic conditions* that have symptoms similar to the acute psychotic phase of schizophrenia. However, these psychoses do not include a prodromal phase of withdrawal and deterioration, and patients return to their baseline level of function after recovery from the psychotic episode and do not experience progressive deterioration of function or recurrence of psychotic episodes.

TREATMENT AND PROGNOSIS

Neuroleptic Antipsychotic Drugs

The primary treatment of the acute and chronic psychotic manifestations of schizophrenia in ambulatory or hospitalized patients is with the "neuroleptic" antipsychotic agents (agents that may produce unwanted symptoms which resemble neurological disease). There are several classes of neuroleptics, with numerous drugs in each class. The common

Table 16.2.
Prescription Drugs Which Have Been Reported Occasionally to Cause Hallucinations or Other Manifestations of Psychosis[a]

Amandatine (Symmetrel)
Anticonvulsants
Antihistamines
Atropine and anticholinergics
Chloroquine (Aralen)
Cimetidine (Tagamet)
Corticosteroids (prednisone, cortisone, ACTH, others)
Dextroamphetamine
Diazepam (Valium)
Digitalis glycosides
Disopyramide (Norpace)
Disulfiram (Antabuse)
Ethchlorvynol (Placidyl)
Indomethacin (Indocin)
Isoniazid (INH, others)
Levodopa (Dopar, others)
Methyldopa (Aldomet)
Methylphenidate (Ritalin)
Nalidixic acid (NegGram)
Pantazocine (Talwin)
Phenelzine (Nardii)
Phenobarbital
Phenylephrine (Neo-Synephrine)
Procainamide (Pronestyl)
Procaine Penicillin G
Propoxyphene (Darvon)
Propranolol (Inderal)
Quinacrine (Atabrine)

[a] Adapted from Drugs that cause psychiatric symptoms. *Med Lett* 23:9, 1981.

drugs are listed in Table 16.3, together with available strengths and potency equivalents to chlorpromazine.

Although the structures of the various antipsychotics are well known, the pharmacology is not. Dose-response relationships have not yet been worked out for humans. The drugs produce effects within 1 hour after oral administration and within 10 to 15 minutes after intramuscular injection. They are lipid soluble with a high affinity for cell membranes. The drugs and their metabolites are distributed generally throughout the central nervous system with no local or regional accumulation. Metabolites are partially excreted each day with significant portions retained in lipid-rich tissues and connective tissues. As these tissues become saturated, the drugs undergo slow turnover. The drugs are detoxified and inactivated mainly through oxidation by hepatic microsomal enzymes, and excreted through both the bile and the urine.

There is no evidence that these agents are addicting, although tolerance to some of the side effects (sedation, hypotension, anticholinergic effects and parkinsonian symptoms) has been reported. The drugs are relatively safe; massive amounts must be taken acutely to produce symptoms of stupor or coma.

The mechanisms of action of the antipsychotics are not fully understood. Although it has been speculated that specific antipsychotic activity may be due to the dopamine-antagonist action of these agents, the drugs have a variety of effects on many metabolic processes.

Treatment of Acute Psychotic Episodes

All of the neuroleptic antipsychotics are equally efficacious for controlling psychotic symptoms associated with schizophrenia. The choice of one drug over another depends upon predicted differences in side effects, history of a particular patient's response, and the clinician's familiarity with the agent. The treatment of acute psychotic episodes should begin with the equivalent of 300 to 400 mg of chlorpromazine (Thorazine) a day, in divided doses (usually three times daily). Only one antipsychotic should be given at a time because administration of more than one agent increases the probability of side effects.

Combativeness, hyperactivity, and agitation are usually controlled within 24 to 48 hours after beginning treatment. If these symptoms are not modified within that period of time, the dosage should be increased 100 to 200 mg a day, up to the equivalent of 800 to 1000 mg of chlorpromazine. It may be necessary to administer the drugs intramuscularly during the acute phase of agitation if the patient is unable to take oral medication. The butyrophenone, haloperidol (Haldol), 2 to 5 mg, is a good choice for intramuscular injection because of its minimal effects upon circulatory regulation; an equivalent intramuscular dose of chlorpromazine (25 mg) can also be used, but the likelihood of orthostatic hypotension (occasionally leading to syncope) is greater.

Delusions, hallucinations, associational defects, negativism, and withdrawal begin to subside within 1 to 2 weeks after treatment begins. Continued improvement of these symptoms may take place over an additional 4- to 8-week period. If very high doses of antipsychotic agents were initially required, the dosage should be reduced to the equivalent of 400 to 600 mg of chlorpromazine as soon as possible. This adjustment in dosage can usually be made 1 to 2 weeks after reaching the peak dose.

Early Side Effects

Antipsychotic drugs with lower potency per milligram, such as chlorpromazine (see Table 16.3) produce *sedation*, which may be a useful side effect in treating hyperactive or combative patients but a disadvantage in regressed, withdrawn patients. The *anticholinergic* property of all antipsychotics produces annoying symptoms of dry mouth, stuffy nose, blurred vision, and occasional urinary retention in older patients. These side effects often disappear within 2 to 4 weeks. The most worrisome side effect

Table 16.3.
Available Strengths and Equivalent Doses of Commonly Used Neuroleptic Antipsychotic Agents[a]

Generic Name	Trade Name	Available Strengths of Oral Preparations	Approximate Equivalent Dose
		mg	*mg*
Phenothiazines			
Aliphatic			
Chlorpromazine	Thorazine (also generic)	10, 25, 50, 100, 200	100
Triflupromazine	Vesprin	10, 25	30
Piperidines			
Mesoridazine	Serentil	10, 25, 100	50
Piperacetazine	Quide	10, 15	12
Thioridazine	Mellaril	10, 15, 25, 50, 100, 150, 200	95
Piperazines			
Fluphenazine[b]	Prolixin, Permitil	1, 2.5, 5, 10	2
Perphenazine	Trilafon	2, 4, 8, 16	10
Trifluoperazine	Stelazine	1, 2, 5, 10	5
Thioxanthene			
Aliphatic			
Chloroprothixene	Taractan	10, 25, 50, 100	65
Piperazine			
Thiothixene	Navane	1, 2, 5, 10, 25	5
Dibenzazepine			
Loxapine	Loxitane, Daxolin	10, 25, 50	15
Butyrophenone			
Haloperidol[c]	Haldol	0.5, 1, 2, 5, 10	2
Indolone			
Molindone	Moban	5, 10, 25	10

[a] Adapted from Baldessarini RJ: The neuroleptic antipsychotic drugs. *Postgrad Med 65:*108, 1979.
[b] Long acting fluphenazine decanoate or enanthate, for injection once weekly, comes in a concentration of 25 mg/ml.
[c] Haloperidol for injection comes in a concentration of 2 mg/ml.

is *drug-induced Parkinson's syndrome*. It occurs with greatest frequency in association with drugs of higher potency per milligram, such as haloperidol (see Table 16.3). The syndrome usually appears within 5 to 30 days of the beginning of treatment and includes tremor, rigidity, bradykinesia, fixed facies, drooling, and stooped posture. Because this problem commonly causes patients to discontinue antipsychotic treatment, it should be managed properly (5). Management consists of: (*a*) reduction of dosage, if possible; (*b*) change to another drug; or (*c*) antiparkinsonism medication (for details, see Chapter 82). In most cases reduction of dosage and/ or addition of small amounts of an antiparkinsonism agent will control these side effects. The parkinsonian effects of neuroleptic drugs tend to decrease after 1 or 2 months. Therefore withdrawal of antiparkinsonism drugs should be attempted after 6 to 12 weeks. Prophylactic treatment of all patients with antiparkinsonism drugs is generally not a good idea because of the additional anticholinergic effects of these drugs.

Acute dystonias occur in occasional patients, within 1 to 5 days of initiating neuroleptic treatment. The symptoms are the sudden onset of severe, tonic contractions of the musculature of the neck (torticollis), of the neck, back, and heels (opisthotonos), of extraocular muscles (oculogyric crises) of the mouth, and of the tongue. These symptoms remit promptly after parenteral injection of either diphenhydramine (Benedryl, 25 to 50 mg intramuscularly) or benztropine (Cogentin, 2 mg intravenously). Neuroleptic treatment can be continued in these patients; an antiparkinsonism agent should be added for about 1 month to protect against recurrent dystonia. *Akathisia* may also occur early in treatment. This side effect is marked by motor restlessness with pacing, fidgeting, and "restless legs." Treatment is the same as that prescribed for drug-induced parkinsonism. Diazepam (Valium), 5 mg two or three times daily, may also help to control this side effect.

A number of non-neurological side effects can result from administration of the antipsychotics. *Cardiovascular toxicity* is usually limited to orthostatic hypotension; frank syncope rarely occurs after intramuscular administration of low potency antipsychotics. Ventricular tachycardia is a very rare side effect; there are no baseline characteristics that help one to recognize persons at risk for this problem. Reversible *cholestatic jaundice* may occur as an allergic response. *Agranulocytosis* is an exceedingly rare side effect.

Since older schizophrenics are more prone to the development of the common side effects, dose levels should be lower by the equivalent of 100 to 200 mg of chlorpromazine. The very high dose range described for treatment of combativeness and hyperactivity should be avoided in elderly patients.

Long Term Drug Treatment of Schizophrenia

The responsibility for the long term care of schizophrenics can be assumed by generalists or by nonmedical mental health professionals under the supervision of a physician.

Pharmacotherapy is the principal mode of long term treatment. Many studies have shown that 60 to 70% of schizophrenics relapse within 1 year if they do not receive medication (2). Most patients require antipsychotics indefinitely, but all patients should be treated for at least 2 years following an acute episode.

The goal of long term pharmacotherapy is to minimize psychotic symptoms with the lowest dose of antipsychotic possible. For most patients this dose is the equivalent of 100 to 200 mg of chlorpromazine daily. Patients on this dose often continue to have psychotic symptoms but do not seem to be disturbed by them (e.g., "I still hear the voices but they don't seem to bother me").

Some patients temporarily have difficulty maintaining a regular medication schedule because of psychotic disorganization, negativism, or fear of medication (5). Inability to comply with the medication regimen may signal the onset of an acute episode. With the first indication of a disruption in medication schedule, the patient should be evaluated, frequency of visits increased to at least once a week, and medication increased if warranted. If the patient remains unable to comply, a long acting intramuscular agent, fluphenazine (Prolixin), 1 to 2 ml once a week, should be used. The patient can be returned to an oral medication when symptom control is re-established. Long acting intramuscular agents are also useful for new patients for whom no information is available on compliance in aftercare or ambulatory programs.

Late Side Effects

Side effects are rarely a problem for patients on maintenance doses of antipsychotics. When an increase in medication is necessary, drug-induced *parkinsonism* may appear. Patients who experience symptoms of parkinsonism over a long period of time should try other antipsychotic medications until one is found that does not produce the side effect. As noted above, long term use of antiparkinsonism medication is to be avoided if possible (see Chapter 82 for further discussion of drug-induced parkinsonism).

Tardive dyskinesia is an extrapyramidal syndrome which occurs in about 10 to 15% (only 3 to 5% according to some reports) of patients following prolonged (months to years) moderate to high dose antipsychotic chemotherapy. The incidence of this disorder increases with age (3 times more common over the age of 40 years), and it is more common in women. The disorder has been reported in association with long term treatment with anticonvulsants. Up to 25% of neuroleptic treated patients who are evaluated for drug-induced tardive dyskinesia are found to have another disorder causing their dyskinesia. The syndrome consists of involuntary or semivoluntary movements of choreiform, ticlike nature, sometimes associated with a dystonic component which classically involves the tongue, facial, and neck muscles. Early manifestations include fine worm-like movements of the tongue at rest, facial tics, and jaw movements. Later symptoms are buccolingual-masticatory movements, chewing motions, lip smacking, puffing of cheeks, blinking of eyes, and choreoathetoid movements of the extremities. Younger patients often have significant involvement of the extremities and trunk. Although the syndrome is painless, it can be socially embarrassing and can interfere with the patient's ability to feed and care for himself. In general, the prognosis is poor, regardless of treatment, and symptoms last for years if not indefinitely. In an occasional patient, the symptoms slowly subside after several years.

There is no satisfactory treatment for tardive dyskinesia. Antiparkinsonism medications usually worsen the symptoms. One short term effective treatment is the use of more potent antipsychotics to suppress the symptoms, but this usually requires increasing doses of the suppressing agent, and subsequent withdrawal of antipsychotics often leads to worsening of the symptoms for a period of time. The emphasis of treatment should be on prevention of tardive dyskinesia. At the first sign of the disorder, neuroleptics should be gradually lowered and discontinued it possible. Symptoms will gradually disappear over several months in about one-third of patients who can be taken off of drugs early. Benzodiazepines, pure lecithin, lithium, and sodium valproate have been reported to be useful in a limited number of cases.

Overall Management of the Patient

The schizophrenic patient is sensitive to change or instability in any aspect of his life. Therefore one practicioner should provide continuity and consistency in his relationship with each of these patients so that the clinician becomes a predictable resource for assisting the patient to develop and maintain his social role in the community. Although few schizophrenics work full time (≤20%), the clinician should refer patients for vocational rehabilitation (see Chapter 9) or sheltered workshops when requested. Most patients determine their own level of social activity, and it is fruitless to push them into unwanted activities. The clinician should be available to the patient's family or to foster care providers for periodic review of the patient's progress and expectations. The recently published book *Surviving Schizophrenia* should be recommended to the patient's family (see General References).

Recreational or social activities are enjoyed by some patients, but many do not care for them. Ideally, residential facilities are available when there is no family for the patient to live with or when the family has a harmful influence. However, in many communities such facilities do not exist. For some patients the clinician and the ambulatory center itself become the source of the few social contacts which the patient has outside of his home and his inner psychological world.

Office visits should be scheduled on a regular basis, as frequently as once a month, or as infrequently as twice a year. Frequency of visits should be determined on the basis of the current status of the patient, history of the course of the patient's illness, reliability of the patient in taking medication, and the patient's ability to recognize early signs of onset of acute episodes. Office visits need last only 15 to 20 minutes and should include an interim history, a brief mental status examination, a review of the effectiveness of medications and of significant side effects, and provision of support or advice regarding the ways in which the patient is dealing with day-to-day matters. In other words these office visits may be defined as supportive therapy, which is described in Chapter 11.

In addition to individual office visits a family management approach may be useful for patients who are having difficulties with their families (1). The method involves a two-step process:

Step 1—sessions devoted to educating the patient and family about the nature, course, and treatment of schizophrenia.

Step 2—family sessions aimed at reducing existing family tensions and improving problem-solving skills of the family in coping with causes of stress. (See chapter 11 - "Family counseling").

Management is enhanced if the clinician has ready access to social services, emergency mental health services, and psychiatric day care and inpatient services. Social services, especially for financial support (welfare, food stamps, disability payments, *etc*) are very important in the management of schizophrenics, because of the usual dependent status of these patients (many acute episodes of psychosis are precipitated by threatened or actual withdrawal of welfare and disability payments).

The generalist caring for a schizophrenic patient may need psychiatric consultation for confirmation of initial diagnosis, for decisions regarding hospitalization, or for treatment recommendations when symptoms respond poorly to antipsychotics or when side effects are intolerable.

Prognosis of the Treated Patient

Schizophrenia is a lifelong disease requiring an open-ended commitment by the clinician. The patient's life is disrupted by periodic psychosis, sometimes necessitating hospitalization, and by an arrest or deterioration of social function. Some patients are able to work and maintain fair levels of interpersonal relationships. Many lead lonely, withdrawn, socially marginal existences. Psychopharmacological treatment is very effective for controlling the symptoms of acute psychosis and for suppressing the intensity of psychotic symptomatology over long periods of time. Suppression of psychosis may permit the patient to use his intellectual and social talents more effectively in developing and maintaining some role in the community; however, the antipsychotics have no direct effect on the deterioration of social function which is so characteristic of schizophrenia.

General References

American Psychiatric Association: *Diagnostic and Statistical Manual of Mental Disorders*, ed 3. Washington, DC, American Psychiatric Association, 1980.
> Recently updated diagnostic criteria and epidemiological information for all recognized psychiatric disorders.

Baldessarini RJ: Antipsychotic agents. In *Chemotherapy in Psychiatry*. Cambridge, MA, Harvard University Press, 1977.
> A well referenced primer on the pharmacology and actions of antipsychotic agents.

Bleuler E: *Dementia Praecox or the Group of Schizophrenias*. New York, International Universities Press, 1950.
> A classical work on schizophrenia.

Torrey EF: *Surviving Schizophrenia: A Family Manual*. New York, Harper and Row, Publishers, 1983.
> A thorough book which contains invaluable information for families of schizophrenia patients and for generalist practitioners.

Tune LE, McHugh PR, Coyle JT: Management of extrapyramidal side effects induced by neuroleptics. *Johns Hopkins Med J* 148:149, 1981.
> Brief, helpful review of current information.

Specific References

1. Falloon IR, Boyd JL, McGill CW, *et al*: Family management in the prevention of exacerbation of schizophrenia. *N Engl J Med* 306:1437, 1982.
2. Hogarty GE, Goldberg SC, Schooler NR, Ulrich RF: Drug and sociotherapy in the aftercare of schizophrenic patients: two year relapse rates. *Arch Gen Psychiatry* 31:603, 1974.
3. Lemkau PU, Tietze C, Cooper M: Survey of statistical studies on prevalence and incidence of mental disorder in sample population. *Public Health Rep* 58:1909, 1943.
4. Snyder SH: The dopamine hypothesis of schizophrenia: focus on the dopamine receptor. *Am J Psychitry* 133:197, 1976.
5. Van Putten T: Why do schizophrenic patients refuse to take their drugs? *Arch Gen Psychitry* 31:67, 1974.
6. Varsamis J, Adamson JD: Early schizophrenia. *Can Psychiatr Assoc J* 16:487, 1971.

CHAPTER SEVENTEEN

Psychiatric Problems of Old Age

JOHN C. BREITNER, M.D., AND PETER V. RABINS, M.D.

At any one time at least 25% of individuals aged 65 and over have a significant mental disorder. Their disorders comprise many different diagnostic entities requiring various approaches to treatment. This chapter summarizes a number of general principles important in geriatric psychiatry, provides recommendations regarding specialty referral for psychiatric disorders in the elderly, and discusses specifically three categories of psychogeriatric disorder that are encountered commonly by the general physician in ambulatory practice: depression, dementia, and delirium.

GENERAL PRINCIPLES

Importance of Diagnosis

Age *per se* does not cause major changes in mental functioning. Instead, the elderly become prone to the development of a host of *specific disorders*. These disorders frequently occur in complex combinations affecting both mind and body, and the reduction of the composite picture to specific diagnostic entities may be challenging. The British geriatrician Sir W. Ferguson Anderson said, "The greatest gift that a physician can give his elderly patient is a diagnosis ... provided, of course, that it is the right diagnosis." This statement applies emphatically to the care of elderly individuals who are mentally ill. Because of the interactions of their multiple disorders, elderly patients frequently present a perplexing array of signs and symptoms, often including mental confusion. The clinician must avoid the temptation to group these patients under such non-informative terms as "senile" and must instead evaluate each patient systematically; the goal of this evaluation is a comprehensive and concise diagnostic formulation of the patient's behavioral or mental disorder. Fulfillment of this goal is frequently difficult, and the generalist should not hesitate to seek specialty psychogeriatric or neurological consultation in complicated cases.

Epidemiology and Presentation

Although the psychiatric disorders seen in older patients are the same as the disorders seen in younger adults, important differences exist. New onset of most common psychiatric disorders is unlikely in the elderly (see discussions of the epidemiology in other chapters in this section), except for in those few conditions seen particularly in older people, especially dementia.

Unusual presentation is common in psychogeriatric disorders, as in many other diseases among the elderly (see Chapter 6). For example, depressive illness in old age may present initially not with depressed mood but instead with agitation, confusion, or hypochondriasis.

Interrelationships between Physical Illness and Mental State

These interrelationships are of particular importance in both geriatric psychiatry and geriatric medicine. The following types of problems illustrate this principle:

1. *Idiosyncratic psychological reactions of the elderly to physical disorder.* The elderly suffer high rates of physical illness at a time in life when many possess only modest social and financial resources to deal with illness. It is not surprising, therefore, that many physically ill old people show despondency, anxiety, frustration, irritability, dependency, or other maladaptive responses to their problems. Such responses become an important part of the patient's total problem, since they often exaggerate severity of dysfunction or complicate clinical management.

2. *Specific psychiatric complications of neurological disease.* Patients with a variety of organic brain diseases have a marked vulnerability to major depressive syndromes. These "organic" depressions re-

spond to pharmacotherapy with tricyclic antidepressants (see below), but poorly to counseling and psychotherapy.

3. *Iatrogenic psychosyndromes.* There is a risk of producing or exacerbating psychiatric symptoms—especially cognitive impairment and mood disturbance—by the administration of many commonly used medicines (e.g., β-blockers, anticholinergics, clonidine, digitalis, methyldopa, reserpine, ibuprofen, cimetidine). Although variable in intensity, such symptoms may reach the proportions of a major affective disorder or delirium, and suicides have been reported. A list of these and other drugs that may cause psychiatric disturbance is found in Table 12.2, Chapter 12.

4. *Dementia and delirium secondary to primary medical problems.* As discussed below, cognitive impairment may be a complication, at times reversible, of a variety of primary medical problems.

5. *Alcoholism in the elderly.* This important mental health problem, which may be the basis for a variety of physical problems in older persons, is discussed in Chapter 21.

Principles of Psychotropic Drug Use in the Elderly

Drug treatments for specific psychosocial disorders are discussed below and in other chapters. Several general principles of psychotropic drug use in the elderly are enumerated here:

1. Use lower doses and increase doses slowly. Changes in drug distribution, metabolism, and excretion occur with aging, and these changes are compounded by diseases common in the elderly which affect drug metabolism. Furthermore, the elderly are more prone to develop cognitive side effects of drugs, suggesting that the brain may also be more sensitive to toxic effects. In general, then, it is wise to start at 50% of the dosage used in younger persons and to increase dosages slowly.

2. Use particular caution when prescribing psychotropic drugs to patients with dementia since they are at high risk of developing cognitive deterioration. Thus starting at very low doses and choosing drugs with less effect on cognition (e.g., thioridazine 25 mg or haloperidol 0.5 μg; nortriptyline 10 to 25 mg or desipramine 25 to 50 mg) can minimize the likelihood of adding drug-induced cognitive impairment.

Elderly and demented patients are also particularly prone to developing cognitive deterioration with nonpsychotropic drugs. Specific compounds and classes of compounds likely to impair cognition are discussed below under delirium. The concomitant use of several different drugs which can adversely affect cognition should be minimized.

3. Remember that drug half-lives may be very prolonged in the elderly. For example, diazepam may have a 5-day half-life in an older patient. Using the rule of thumb that steady state blood levels are reached in five half-lives, one should expect that steady state blood levels may not be reached until 1 month after diazepam is initiated and that toxic side effects from this drug may appear long after it has been started. In elderly patients, the benzodiazepines with intermediate or short half-lives (e.g., lorazepam for anxiety, triazolam for sleep) are the most logical choice.

4. Consider side effect profiles when choosing a psychotropic drug for an individual patient. When initiating a neuroleptic, one might choose a drug which minimizes extrapyramidal symptoms (e.g., thioridazine), which minimizes hypotension and sedation (e.g., haloperidol, thiothixene), or which maximizes sedation (e.g., thioridazine). When initiating an antidepressant, one might choose a drug with the least effect on blood pressure (nortriptyline) or a drug with more sedative properties (imipramine or trazodone).

Importance of the Patient's Social Network

Of special importance when dealing with elderly patients who are ill is awareness of the patient's milieu and social supports. The elderly often suffer financial impoverishment, social isolation, and personal losses, as well as physical illnesses. The ongoing support needed by many elderly individuals in dealing with these problems is provided by family and by other informal sources; the physician must be especially sensitive to the needs of these other caregivers in such cases, as well as to the needs of the patient himself. For patients lacking this informal support system, the physician can make an important impact by referring the patient for help to an effective social worker or to a community agency for the elderly.

SPECIFIC PSYCHOGERIATRIC DISORDERS

Many common psychiatric disorders (e.g., personality disorders, substance abuse) present only subtle differences in diagnosis and treatment in elderly *versus* young patients. Other specific syndromes (e.g., late onset schizophrenia and the dementia syndrome of depression) take special forms in the elderly and should be referred for specialty care. Late onset schizophrenia is characterized by delusions and hallucinations and an absence of both mood symptoms and cognitive impairment. The dementia syndrome of depression presents with symptoms of major depression (see below) and cognitive decline. Beyond these, three types of mental disorders—depression, delirium, and dementia—are especially common or important in old age. They are discussed here since each of these presents practical problems in diagnosis, management, or referral for the general physician.

Depression

Depressed mood is the most common psychiatric symptom in old age. A major reason for its frequency is the fact that it may result from many predisposing conditions, such as stroke, that are themselves common in the elderly.

Forms of Depression

The types of depression as classified by the American Psychiatric Association's *Diagnostic and Statistical Manual of Mental Disorders* (DSM-III) are: adjustment disorders with depressed mood; dysthymic disorder (depressive neurosis), major affective disorders (major depression and manic-depressive illness), and the organic affective syndromes.

An *adjustment disorder* with depression is differentiated from dysthymic disorder by its relatively acute onset, by the presence of a recent well defined precipitating circumstance (often death or separation, see Chapter 19), and by the expectation of a fairly rapid and spontaneous recovery. *Dysthymic disorder* implies chronicity, a less well defined or more distant precipitant, and underlying personality difficulty as a predisposing condition. Both adjustment and dysthymic disorders are appropriately understood as reactions of a particular individual to psychosocial threat or loss. All but the most severe cases of adjustment disorder are best treated by a general physician who, because of an established relationship with the patient, may be more effective than a psychiatrist. The techniques of short term and supportive counseling (see Chapters 11 and 12) may be applied with good results in such cases. Among individuals with dysthymic disorder a careful history often reveals evidence of lifelong personal maladjustment or of previous depressive episodes; management of this disorder, described in Chapter 15, may require specialty referral.

The multiple forms and diagnostic criteria of the *major affective* disorders are described in Chapter 15. Not only do new cases appear quite commonly in late life, but the frequency of recurrence in established cases tends to increase with age, while in bipolar patients the proportion of depressed (as opposed to manic) episodes increases steadily with aging. The description of this disorder and its treatment, given in Chapter 15, is generally applicable to the elderly, although older victims show agitation more often than retardation, and they almost always show hypochondriacal features. Suspiciousness (paranoia) may be seen as well. The syndrome is often severe and may account for the high rate of completed suicides among old people. Treatment relies mainly on drugs (tricyclic antidepressants) and/or electroconvulsive therapy. The most useful of the tricyclics for the elderly appear to be nortriptyline (Aventyl, Pamelor), desipramine (Norpramin, Pertofrane), and doxepin (Sinequan, Adapin). These drugs are given in preference to other agents such as amitriptyline (Elavil, Endep) because of their fewer side effects, particularly anticholinergic effects. These drugs are not without risk (hypotension with dizziness or falling, arrhythmia, urinary retention, delirium), and conservative practice dictates a reduced initial daily dosage in older patients (e.g., 25 mg for nortriptyline, 50 mg for desipramine) and a gradual increase in dosage to the level of therapeutic efficacy or plasma levels in the "therapeutic range." Practical details about the use of tricyclics are found in Chapter 15.

"Organic" depressions are similar in appearance to major depressions in patients without organic pathology. The diagnosis is made in the presence of significant symptoms of major depression as well as of evidence or organic neurological disease—*e.g.,* stroke (see Chapter 83), tumor, trauma—judged to be etiologically related to the disturbance. Because such organic conditions are common in the elderly, organic depressions are relatively common. Treatment with the tricyclic antidepressants recommended in the preceding paragraph is generally successful (8), but these drugs must be used particularly cautiously in brain-damaged patients because of the increased possibility of provoking delirium.

Dementia Syndrome of Depression (3)

The dementia syndrome (see below) may occur as a manifestation or complication of a depressive illness. Severe depressions can cause reduced mental acumen and performance in any age group, but depressed elderly individuals in particular may show a significant decline in intellectual performance. The term pseudodementia has been applied to this condition, implying both that it is not a "true" dementia (e.g., based on organic pathology) and that its clinical features differ somewhat from those of dementia syndromes provoked by structural brain pathology. We prefer the label "dementia syndrome of depression," since the term dementia strictly signifies a clinical syndrome of mental life without implications for etiology or mechanism (see below). The dementia syndrome of depression is usually of relatively acute onset, similar to the course of development of depressive illness; this differs from the more gradual and insidious onset of many dementias caused by structural brain disease. A history of previous depressive episodes is often obtained. In addition, the patient often complains about his cognitive defect, whereas those with other types of dementias, such as Alzheimer's or multi-infarct disease, show a greater tendency to mask or hide their difficulties. Most important, the patient will show the characteristic signs and symptoms of depression, usually major depression, in both the history and examination of the mental state (see Chapter 15 for details). The importance of diagnosis in this type of dementia syndrome cannot be overemphasized. The disorder is generally reversible and resolves with successful treatment of the underlying affective illness; as such it is probably the most common type of reversible dementia syndrome.

Dementia

Definition and Epidemiology

Dementia is the clinical syndrome of global deterioration in intellectual function(s). It occurs in clear consciousness and is of sufficient severity to interfere with social or occupational functioning. The global nature of the defect differentiates dementia from amnestic syndromes (isolated short and/or long term memory loss), focal aphasic syndromes, or other focal defect states. The term deterioration implies a documented reduction in ability from some previously established level, (contrasted with mental retardation). Its occurrence in clear consciousness differentiates dementia from delirium (see below). Like delirium, dementia is a clinical syndrome which may have many different etiologies, pathologies, or mechanisms, some of them treatable. It is commonly but by no means invariably chronic. With the notable exception of its occurrence as a part of depressive illness (and possibly other major psychiatric illnesses), dementia is generally due to an organic disease affecting the brain.

Dementia has become a major public health problem. About 5% of the population over 65 is demented. Most dementia occurs, however, among the "very old" or "frail elderly" aged 75 and up. The prevalence of dementia is 20% in persons aged 80 and over; and it is present in approximately one in three persons over age 90. These rates have not decreased in recent years while larger portions of the population have reached advanced age (5). If anything, the age-specific prevalence of dementia (determined by both incidence and duration of illness) has increased as patients now survive longer. Since even larger portions of the population are now reaching late old age, the overall prevalence of dementia is increasing at an alarming rate. As a result, dementing illnesses and their complications have become a leading cause of death, perhaps the fourth or fifth most common cause of mortality in the United States (6).

Diagnosis and Evaluation of Dementia

The diagnosis of dementia is often delayed by two factors: the tendency for demented patients to attempt to hide their embarrassing problem by rationalization for memory lapses and other defects; and the fact that the earliest changes are often more apparent in the patient's environment than in a physician's office (for example, leaving a stove burning all night, writing checks inappropriately, forget-ting appointments, neglecting personal hygiene or appearance, taking the wrong bus home from shopping). When the possibility of dementia is present, the physician should evaluate the cognitive domain of the patient's mental status. As noted in Chapter 10, this part of the mental status examination is often accomplished through observations made while taking a general medical history or performing a physical examination. The "mini mental status examination," which systematically tests the cognitive domain, is summarized in Table 17.1; this test is useful not only to confirm the presence of significant dementia but to quantify the initial severity of dementia and the changes in severity over time. Equally important, information should be sought at frequent intervals from the patient's spouse, children, or other close friends.

There are numerous etiologies of the dementia syndrome. Table 17.2 subdivides them into four groups—conditions in which dementia is (a) the only manifestation of disease, (b) associated with other neurological signs and symptoms but not with other medical disease, (c) secondary to a medical disease, (d) secondary to another major psychiatric syndrome (pseudodementia). The frequency of these etiologies is not known; it is likely, however, that idiopathic cerebral degenerative disease explains a sizeable proportion of the cases for which an etiology is not apparent. (Formerly most of these cases were attributed to atherosclerosis.) Recent studies (1) indicate that a large proportion of these cases may be due to the familial form of Alzheimer's disease. This entity, which may be transmitted as an autosomal dominant trait, is identified clinically by prominent aphasic or apractic symptoms accompanying a gradually progressive decline in memory. The diagnosis of Alzheimer's disease is strictly clinical, i.e. other causes of dementia are excluded in a patient with typical features; there is no laboratory test that confirms the diagnosis of this disease.

In evaluating the patient with dementia, the general physician should first determine whether there are manifestations that suggest a specific etiology for the patient's dementia. This evaluation always includes a careful history and physical examination. Laboratory tests should be based chiefly upon the information obtained by history and physical examination.

In some patients the cause of dementia will be suggested by the history and physical examination alone. Examples include (a) the patient with long-standing hypertension or diabetes who has had a stair-step deterioration (sudden worsenings followed by stability or slight improvement) and focal neurological signs, findings suggesting multi-infarct dementia; and (b) the patient who has dementia following severe anoxia or hypoglycemia. In other patients, certain clues suggesting a primary medical or psy-

Table 17.1.
Mini-Mental Status Examination: Instructions for Administration and Scoring[a]

The test takes 5 to 10 minutes to administer.

ORIENTATION

1. Ask for year, season, date, day, month. Then ask specifically for parts omitted. One point for each correct. (0–5)

2. Ask in turn for name of state, county, town, hospital or place, floor or street. One point for each correct. (0–5)

REGISTRATION

Ask the patient if you may test his memory. Then say the names of three unrelated objects, clearly and slowly, about 1 second for each. After you have said all three, ask him to repeat them. This first repetition determines his score (0–3) but keep saying them until he can repeat all three up to six trials. If he does not eventually learn all three, recall cannot be meaningfully tested.

ATTENTION AND CALCULATION

Ask the patient to begin with 100 and count backward by 7. Stop after five subtractions (93, 86, 79, 72, 65). Score total number of correct answers, one point for each. (0–5)

If the patient cannot or will not perform this task, ask him to spell the word "world" backward. The score is the number of letters in correct order, e.g., dlrow = 5, dlrwo = 3. (0–5)

RECALL

Ask the patient if he can recall the three words you previously asked him to remember. Score 0–3.

LANGUAGE

Naming: Show the patient a wrist watch and ask him what it is. Repeat for pencil. Score 0–2.

Repetition: Ask the patient to repeat this phrase after you: "No ifs, ands, or buts." Allow only one trial. Score 0 or 1.

Three-stage command: "Take a piece of paper in your right hand, fold it in half, and put it on the floor." Give the patient a piece of blank paper and repeat the command. Score 1 point for each part correctly executed. (0–3).

Reading: On a blank piece of paper print the sentence "Close your eyes," in letters large enough for the patient to see clearly. Ask him to read it and do what it says. Score 1 point only if he actualy closes his eyes. (0–1)

Writing: Give the patient a blank piece of paper and ask him to write a sentence for you. Do not dictate a sentence; it is to be written spontaneously. It must contain a subject and verb and be sensible. Correct grammer and punctuation are not necessary. (0–1)

Copying: On a clean piece of paper, draw intersecting pentagons, each side about 1 inch, and ask him to copy it exactly as it is. All 10 angles must be present and 2 must intersect to score 1 point. Tremor and rotation are ignored. (0–1)

Estimate the patient's level of sensorium along a continuum, from alert on the left to coma on the right.

[a] From Folstein MF, Folstein SE, McHugh PR: "Mini-mental state": a practical method for grading the cognitive state of patients for the clinician. *J Psychiatr Res* 12:189, 1975. Total possible score is 30 points. Patients with totals of 20 points or less usually have either dementia, delirium, schizophrenia, or a major affective disorder (pseudodementia).

Table 17.2.
Etiological Classification of Dementia[a]

DEMENTIA THE ONLY MANIFESTATION OF ILLNESS
  Idiopathic degeneration of the cerebral cortex (Alzheimer's or Pick's disease, called primary degenerative dementia in DSM-III)
DEMENTIA ASSOCIATED WITH OTHER NEUROLOGICAL CONDITIONS:
  Invariably associated with other neurological signs:
    Huntington's disease (choreoathetosis)
    A large variety of rare degenerative syndromes—most of them of unknown etiology
    Dementia with Parkinson's disease
  Often associated with other neurological signs:
    Cerebral arteriosclerosis
    Brain tumor[b]
    Brain trauma, such as cerebral contusion, midbrain hemorrhage, chronic subdural hematoma[b]
    Normal pressure hydrocephalus (always with ataxia of gait and often with sphincteric incontinence)[b]
DEMENTIA DUE TO SPECIFIC MEDICAL CONDITIONS:
  Arteritis (e.g. systemic lupus erythematosis)[b]
  Hypothyroidism[b]
  Cushing's disease[b]
  Nutritional deficiency states such as pellagra, the Wernicke-Korsakoff syndrome, and subacute combined degeneration of spinal cord and brain (vitamin B_{12} deficiency)[b]
  Neurosyphilis: general paresis and meningovascular syphilis[b]
  Hepatolenticular degeneration, familial and acquired
  Bromidism, chronic barbiturate intoxication[b]
DEMENTIA SECONDARY TO MAJOR PSYCHIATRIC DISTURBANCE
  The dementia syndrome of depression (pseudodementia)[b]

[a] Adapted from Adams RD: Derangements of intellect, mood, and behavior. In Isselbacher KJ et al (eds): *Harrison's Principles of Internal Medicine*, ed 9. New York, McGraw-Hill, 1980.
[b] Potentially reversible dementia.

chological basis for the dementia will enable the general physician to reach a working diagnosis based upon a selective evaluation and to initiate management. Examples are the patient with signs, symptoms, and laboratory confirmation of hypothyroidism (see Chapter 73), vitamin B_{12} deficiency (see Chapter 49), or neurosyphilis (see Chapter 30); or the patient with a prior history of major depression who develops dementia in association with typical symptoms of recurrent depression (see description of the dementia syndrome of depression above).

For a number of patients the probable explanation for dementia cannot be determined by a simple office evaluation. For these patients, radiological or neurological evaluation should be considered, especially in the following situations:

1. *The patient in whom the evidence suggests a treatable cause.* Common examples are the patient with findings suggesting brain tumor (relatively rapid progression of symptoms, focal signs—partic-

ularly frontal lobe signs, known primary extracranial malignancy such as carcinoma of the lung or breast); the patient with possible subdural hematoma (history of falls and head trauma, anticoagulation therapy); the patient with the syndrome typical of normal pressure hydrocephalus (relatively rapid onset, apathy progressing to dementia, bladder and bowel incontinence, gait apraxia—particularly if there is a history of subarachnoid hemorrhage, head trauma, or chronic meningitis).

2. *The patient for whom objective diagnosis is important in order to provide prognostic information to the family*, even though there is nothing to suggest a treatable cause. Common examples are the patient who has responsibility for others and who may need to have a legal guardian named or the elderly person who is not yet institutionalized or totally dependent at home.

3. *The patient in whom dementia appears to be part of a clinical neurological syndrome*, such as Parkinson's disease or Huntington's disease, for which a neurologist may provide both diagnostic confirmation and recommendations about prognosis and management.

While many practitioners feel it is unnecessary to undertake the etiological evaluation of patients with many years' history of dementia or with coexisting debilitating disease, this practice carries some risks of ignoring a treatable condition. It is reasonable, therefore, to obtain a small number of screening tests as part of the initial evaluation of most patients. These tests are simple, inexpensive, noninvasive, and they may identify reversible causes of dementia which are not apparent in the history and physical

examination. They include a hemogram (if the hematocrit is low and the mean corpuscular volume is high, the vitamin B_{12} level should be measured), serum thyroxine, and serological test for syphilis. These, and other tests utilized in the evaluation of dementia that should not be regarded as screening tests, are summarized in Table 17.3.

Management

The management of the irreversibly demented patient can be divided into five aspects:

1. *The assessment process* itself is the first step. The diagnosis has often been suspected by the family or patient, but at times abnormal behavior has been misinterpreted as purposefully irritating. As specific a diagnosis as possible should be made and conveyed to the family. The family may ask about long term prognosis. The average patient with dementia lives 7 to 10 years after early symptoms but life span ranges from 3 to 20 years. In general a dementia which has progressed slowly will continue to do so while a more rapid progression by history presages future rapid decline. While the patient has the right to know his diagnosis, many lack the ability to realize they have a deficit. In our experience patients who, when asked, deny they have any problems with their memory usually do not accept that there is a memory problem when directly told.

The evaluation process should also elicit specific problems in behavior caused by the dementia (see commonly-cited problems, Table 17.4). Difficulty in speaking, dressing, and such potentially dangerous activities as driving, smoking, and cooking should be inquired about. When present, these problems

Table 17.3.
Laboratory Tests Useful in the Etiological Evaluation of Dementia

Test	Etiology
Blood tests:	
Hematocrit and mean corpuscular volume (MCV)[a]	Vitamin B_{12} deficiency
(If hematocrit is low and MCV high, measure vitamin B_{12} level)	
Thyroid function tests[a]	Hypothyroidism
Serum creatinine[a]	Uremia
Serological test for syphilis[a]	Neurosyphilis
Liver function tests	Hepatolenticular degeneration
Electroencephalogram	Helps confirm cerebral disturbance (if normal, suggests nonorganic diagnosis, *i.e.*, depression)
Computerized axial tomograpy	Identifies abscess, tumors, subdural hematoma, or hydrocephalus. May show atrophy.
Lumbar puncture	Confirms neurosyphilis, identifies other chronic meningoencephalitis.

[a] Reasonable to obtain as screening test for treatable etiology in all patients.

Table 17.4.
Behavior Problems of Patients and Problematic Activities of Daily Living Cited by Families of Demented Patients[a]

Behavior	No. of Families Responding[b]	Families Reporting Occurrence, No. (%)	Families Reporting Behavior to Be a Problem, No. (%)
Memory disturbance[d]	55	55 (100)	51 (93)
Catastrophic reactions[c,d]	52	45 (87)	40 (89)
Demanding/critical behavior	52	37 (71)	27 (73)
Night waking	54	37 (69)	22 (59)
Hiding things	51	35 (69)	25 (71)
Communication difficulties	50	34 (68)	25 (74)
Suspiciousness[d]	52	33 (63)	26 (79)
Making accusations[d]	53	32 (60)	26 (82)
Meals	55	33 (60)	18 (55)
Daytime wandering	51	30 (59)	21 (70)
Bathing	51	27 (53)	20 (74)
Hallucinations	49	24 (49)	16 (42)
Delusions	49	23 (47)	19 (83)
Physical violence[d]	51	24 (47)	22 (94)
Incontinence[d]	53	21 (40)	18 (86)
Cooking	54	18 (33)	8 (44)
Hitting[d]	50	16 (32)	13 (81)
Driving	55	11 (20)	8 (73)
Smoking	53	6 (11)	4 (67)
Inappropriate sexual behavior	51	1 (2)	0 (0)

[a] Based on an open-ended interview with the primary care-givers of 55 patients with irreversible dementia. Adapted from Rabins PV, Mace NL, Lucas MJ: The impact of dementia on the family. *JAMA* 248: 333, 1982.
[b] "Don't know" answers excluded.
[c] See example in text.
[d] Cited as *most* serious problem.

should be explained as the result of the illness. The family or other caregivers should then try to adapt the environment to the disordered behaviors and take steps to eliminate dangerous behaviors. Helping the caregivers specifically to identify each problem can enable them to institute common sense solutions they have not otherwise tried. Families needing legal and financial advice should be advised to seek this out early and not wait for a crisis. Guidelines for assessing competence or for obtaining legal guardianship are described in Chapter 10.

2. *Good general medical care* (7). Congestive heart failure, urinary tract infection, and other seemingly minor medical abnormalities can lead to marked deterioration of the demented patient's functioning. Likewise, drugs which can affect cognition (e.g., cimetidine, β-blockers, clonidine, methyldopa, digoxin anticholinergics) should be carefully monitored since they may worsen the already poor memory. A search for superimposed medical illness should be instituted if there is a sudden deterioration in behavior or cognition.

3. *Behavioral management and treatment of depression.* Not sleeping at night, suspiciousness, and easy irritability (so-called catastrophic reactions) can be more problematic than cognitive impairment. Nonpharmacological management approaches should be tried first. For sleep disorder these might include keeping the person more active in the day-

time (day care centers are a significant help in this regard) and not letting the patient nap during the day. Irritability, suspiciousness, and frustration are often best managed by avoiding tasks which the patient can no longer do or situations which frustrate the patient. If pharmacological therapy is necessary, very low doses should be tried first and increases should be made slowly. When both irritability and sleep disorder are serious enough to necessitate drug treatment, useful drugs are thioridazine (Mellaril), 25 to 50 mg, or haloperidol (Haldol), 1 to 2 mg/hour before bedtime. A regular dosage schedule rather than as occasion requires is favored. Patients taking these drugs must be monitored for two common side effects—orthostatic hypotension and extrapyramidal symptoms (see details in Chapter 16). If only sleep disorder is a problem, chloral hydrate, 500 to 1500 mg, causes the least paradoxical agitation and daytime drowsiness. When daytime irritability is being treated, low doses of thioridazine or haloperidol two or three times daily should be tried. These drugs can worsen cognition and this should be watched for. Suspiciousness sometimes decreases with neuroleptic drugs, but we favor non-drug therapy for this symptom unless it is causing severe problems.

Depression is present in 20% of patients with dementia. When it has the characteristics of an *adjustment disorder* or demoralized state (see above) it is best managed with supportive therapy (see Chapters 11 and 12). However, *major depressions* with symptoms of early waking, anorexia, notions of guilt, self-blame, or worthlessness, nihilistic attitudes, or morbid hypochondriasis also occur. Their treatment is discussed above under "organic" depression.

Demented patients with at least partial insight into their disability may become profoundly distressed when brought into a situation where they are forced to confront their failing abilities. There often ensues an overwhelming sense of frustration, fear, anger, or anxiety. These poorly controlled emotions further impair the patient's already limited functional ability, and a "positive feedback" effect is created which results in total decompensation of a previously coping individual.

Example: A 72-year-old woman with a history of several small strokes suffered from moderate forgetfulness and confusion but was generally calm and pleasant. Keeping track of the date with a calendar and making copious notes to herself, she managed to maintain an independent existence at home. At the supermarket check-out counter she could not find her wallet but insisted she had money to pay for her food. The clerk grew impatient, and the patient became increasingly agitated, tearful, and accusatory. When the store manager was called, she picked up grocery items and began throwing them.

These *catastrophic reactions* may have an extremely important impact on both the patient and his caregivers. The explanation of their cause and their prevention through avoidance of provoking circumstances can forestall the need for institutionalization. The use of small doses of the neuroleptic drugs haloperidol (Haldol) or thioridazine (Mellaril) may be beneficial in preventing recurrence of these reactions.

4. *Family support.* Family distress is common. Treating it starts with the assessment and problem-solving approach outlined above. The latter gives families a sense of control and hope that problems can be better managed in spite of the irreversibility and probable progression of the underlying disorder. Feelings of guilt, anger, discouragement, and demoralization are common. Other common types of distress are concern about loss of friends, hobbies and leisure time; family conflicts; and worry that the caregiver will become ill. Allowing families time to ventilate these feelings and concerns and acknowledging that they are common can be helpful. Referral to one of the support groups which are emerging in the United States is sometimes invaluable. The Alzheimer's Disease and Related Disorders Association can provide information about nearby resources and has a free "800" phone number (1-800-621-0379). It is also helpful to recommend *The 36-Hour Day* (see "General References"), a book which explains dementia and provides practical advice for dealing with all of the vexing problems created by a demented family member.

5. *Longitudinal care.* Because the dementing illnesses are progressive (new symptoms appear while old symptoms worsen), changes should be explicitly pointed out to families. Also it is prudent to discuss the possibility of eventual nursing home placement soon after the diagnosis is made. While the majority of families report that they do not want to place their loved one in a nursing home, we urge them not to promise this unconditionally since medical issues or behavioral problems may develop to the point where placement is necessary. The family's emotional needs may change over time. Here again, a nonjudgmental, listening approach helps family members feel supported.

Drugs for Dementia

Although statistically significant improvement in mental status and in behavior has been reported in institutionalized demented patients who were treated with an ergot derviative (Hydergine) (4), neither this nor any other drug for dementia has been shown to improve the quality of life for demented persons living in the community. Therefore, there is no basis for recommending such drugs for demented patients followed in ambulatory settings.

Delirium (Acute Organic Brain Syndrome)

Definition and Diagnosis

The hallmark of delirium is clouding of consciousness, with secondary changes in behavior, cognition, or perception. The delirious patient often seems strangely inaccessible or unable to concentrate on his environment or on the task at hand. Bizarre, dream-like hallucinations may occur. The patient commonly suffers illusions, misinterprets his environment, and may fail to recognize persons well known to him. Because of the bizarre, threatening quality of his perceptions, the delirious patient may become wildly agitated. On the other hand, psychomotor underactivity may also dominate the picture. The onset of delirium is acute or subacute, developing over hours or days rather than over weeks or months. The intensity of the disturbance often waxes and wanes through the day and night.

Table 17.5 summarizes the criteria of the American Psychiatric Association for the diagnosis of delirium. When the manifestations are not florid, the diagnosis of delirium is easily missed (2). This error can lead to two catastrophes for the patient—failure of the physician to identify and treat a reversible cause of delirium and, at times, inappropriate referral to a mental hospital for custodial care. The most helpful data in diagnosing delirium in the patient with less florid symptoms are the duration of behavioral change (obtained from a reliable observer), a

Table 17.5.
Diagnostic Criteria for Delirium[a]

Clouding of consciousness (reduced clarity of awareness of the environment), with reduced capacity to shift, focus, and sustain attention to environmental stimuli
At least two of the following:
Perceptual disturbance: misinterpretations, illusions, or hallucinations
Speech that is at times incoherent
Disturbance of sleep-wakefulness cycle, with insomnia or daytime drowsiness
Increased or decreased psychomotor activity
Disorientation and memory impairment (if testable)
Clinical features that develop over a short period of time (usually hours to days) and tend to fluctuate over the course of a day
Evidence, from the history, physical examination, or laboratory tests, of a specific organic factor judged to be etiologically related to the disturbance

[a] From American Psychiatric Association: *Diagnostic and Statistical Manual of Mental Disorders*, ed 3. Washington, DC, American Psychiatric Association, 1980.

Table 17.6.
Etiological Classification of Delirium[a]

IN A MEDICAL OR SURGICAL ILLNESS (NO FOCAL OR LATERALIZING NEUROLOGICAL SIGNS; CEREBROSPINAL FLUID USUALLY CLEAR):
Metabolic disorders: hepatic stupor, uremia, hypoxia, hypercapnea, hypoglycemia, porphyria, hyponatremia
Congestive heart failure
Typhoid fever
Pneumonia
Septicemia
Rheumatic fever
Thyrotoxicosis
Postoperative and post-traumatic states
IN NEUROLOGICAL DISEASE THAT CAUSES FOCAL OR LATERALIZING SIGNS OR CHANGES IN THE CEREBRO-SPINAL FLUID:
Cerebrovascular disease
Subarachnoid hemorrhage
Hypertensive encephalopathy
Cerebral contusion
Subdural hematoma
Tumor
Abscess
Meningitis
Encephalitis
Status epilepticus (by EEG)
Postconvulsive delirium
THE ABSTINENCE STATES AND EXOGENOUS INTOXICATIONS (SIGNS OF OTHER MEDICAL, SURGICAL, AND NEUROLOGICAL ILLNESSES ABSENT OR COINCIDENTAL):
Withdrawal of alcohol (delirium tremens), barbiturates, and nonbarbiturate sedative drugs, following chronic intoxication
Drug intoxicaitons due to sedatives, opiates, psychotropic agents, anticholinergics, digitalis, illicit drugs (see Chapter 22), *etc*
BECLOUDED DEMENTIA:
Senile or other brain disease in combination with infective fevers, drug reactions, heart failure, or other medical or surgical disease.

[a] Adapted from Adams RD: Delirium and other acute confusional states. In Isselbacher KJ, *et al* (eds): *Harrison's Principles of Internal Medicine*, ed 9. New York, McGraw-Hill, 1980.

careful history of all current drugs or exposure to toxins, new symptoms or signs of physical illness, and the patient's performance in a mental status examination (particularly orientation and recall of events during the past few hours).

Elderly individuals are particularly prone to delirium, probably because (a) the frequency of many of the conditions causing delirium is higher in the elderly, and (b) the aging brain seems particularly susceptible to the development of delirium. In the patient with known dementia, rapid development of clouded consciousness (the feature which distinguishes delirium from dementia) should always invite prompt evaluation for an intercurrent medical problem. Catastrophic reactions (see above) in the demented patient may resemble delirium; however, catastrophic reactions generally occur abruptly and in response to an easily identified stressful circumstance.

Etiological Evaluation

Like dementia, delirium usually has an identifiable cause, a point stressed in the criteria in Table 17.5. Unlike dementia, most causes of delirium are treatable or are self-limited, and the prognosis for return to baseline mental function is good. Table 17.6 subdivides the etiologies of delirium into medical conditions, neurological conditions, drug/toxin excess or withdrawal, and beclouded dementia (the occurrence of delirium superimposed on an irreversible dementia syndrome).

Management

When delirium is diagnosed in the office setting, it is usually necessary to hospitalize the patient for management. However, in some patients, the delir-

ium may be due to a known cause which is transient or which can be readily reversed in the office setting. Examples are the mild delirium which may follow the initial dose of a benzodiazepine or of a potent analgesic such as pentazocine (Talwin); or the delirium accompanying insulin-induced hypoglycemia.

The treatment of delirium begins with diagnosis and *specific treatment* of the underlying disorder. If appropriate treatment is initiated, delirium generally resolves within a period of 24 hours. In a substantial portion of cases, however, exhaustive efforts fail to reveal the etiology. In these instances one can only offer supportive management while awaiting spontaneous resolution of the syndrome.

Delirious patients require *supportive management* in addition to specific treatment. The room should be well lit and stimuli maintained at a moderate level. Frequent reality orientation and reassurance help the patient to remain calm during his frightening ordeal. Extremely disruptive patients may require restraints, but these are rarely required in older patients. Sedation should be given with caution, except in those patients whose delirium is attributable to withdrawal of sedating drugs (e.g., alcohol, sedative-hypnotics). Some agitated elderly delirious patients may respond positively to small doses of haloperidol (Haldol); trial doses of 1 or 2 mg every hour may safely be given for a few hours.

General References

Birren JG, Sloane RB (eds): *Handbook of Mental Health and Aging*. Englewood Cliffs, NJ, Prentice-Hall, 1980.

Encylopedic, thorough, and up-to-date.

Busse E, Blazer X: *Handbook of Geriatric Psychiatry*. Princeton, NJ, Van Nostrand Reinhold, 1980.

An up-to-date, authoritative source of information.

Isaacs AD, Post F (eds): *Studies in Geriatric Psychiatry*. New York, John Wiley & Sons, 1978.

A concise, authoritative work with British orientation.

Mace NL, Rabins PV: *The 36-Hour Day*. New York, Warner Brooks, 1981.

An invaluable book, for the family/caretakers of a demented person, containing detailed practical information. Available at most bookstores.

Thompson TL, Moran MG, Nies AS: Psychotropic drug use in the elderly. *N Engl J Med* 308:134, 194, 1983.

Two-part, exhaustive review article.

Specific References

1. Breitner JCS, Folstein MF: Familial Alzheimer dementia: a prevalent disorder with specific clinical features. *Psychol Med* 14:63, 1984.
2. Engel GL, Romano J: A syndrome of cerebral insufficiency. *J Chronic Dis* 9:260, 1959.
3. Folstein MF, McHugh PR: Dementia syndrome of depression. In Katzman R, Terry RD, Bick KL (eds): *Alzheimer's Disease, Senile Dementia and Related Disorders*. New York, Raven Press, 1978.
4. Gaitz CM, Varner RV, Overall JE: Pharmacotherapy for organic brain syndrome in late life: evaluation of an ergot derivative vs. placebo. *Arch Gen Psychiatry* 34:839, 1977.
5. Gruenberg EM: Epidemiology of senile dementia. *Adv Neurol* 19:437, 1978.
6. Katzman R: The prevalence and malignancy of Alzheimer disease: a major killer. *Arch Neurol* 33:217, 1976.
7. Larson EB, Reifler BV, Featherstone HJ, English DR: Dementia in elderly outpatients: a prospective study. *Ann Intern Med* 100:417, 1984.
8. Lipsey JR, Robinson RG, Pearlson GD, *et al*: Nortriptyline treatment of post-stroke depression: a double blind study. *Lancet* 1:297, 1984.

CHAPTER EIGHTEEN

Sexual Disorders

CHESTER W. SCHMIDT, JR., M.D.

The sexual difficulties described by patients to their physicians are evenly divided into sexual problems that accompany physical illness, those that are secondary to side effects of medication or abuse of drugs, and those that are unrelated to physical problems and are purely psychological in origin. Typically the psychologically based sexual problems are related to both psychosocial antecedents and to current stressful life situations which are often self-limited. Those physically related and stress-related problems which are minor and are reversible lend themselves to treatment by counseling techniques that rely heavily on catharsis, reassurance, and education. Although there are limited data to document results of treatment for these types of problems in the ambulatory setting, clinical experience suggests that the outcome for reversible sexual problems is usually good, with improvement rates approaching 75%.

THE NORMAL SEXUAL RESPONSE CYCLE

In order to assess these disorders rapidly and accurately it is helpful for the clinician to be familiar with the normal sexual response cycle and the major physiological factors mediating each phase of the cycle. The human sexual response cycle is divided into four phases.

The first phase is one of *desire* and consists of fantasies and wishes to engage in sexual activity. This response is psychic in origin, but the psychic stimulation is mediated by circulating androgens.

The second phase is the *excitement* phase and consists of a number of physiological changes plus the subjective sense of sexual pleasure. In both sexes there is an increase in heart rate, an increase in breathing rate, and development of muscular tension throughout the body, most pronounced in the pelvic area and thighs. For both sexes the major physiological change is the development of vascular congestion in the genital area. For females the manifestations of vasocongestion are vaginal lubrication and swelling of the external genitalia. In males, vasocongestion leads to erection. Vasocongestion may occur via either of two neurological pathways: (a) a *local reflex pathway* initiated by tactile stimulation of the penis or clitoris and mediated by sensory fibers entering the dorsal root ganglia at S_2 through S_4 and by parasympathetic fibers from these ganglia to the perivesicular, prostatic, and cavernous plexuses; postganglionic fibers from these plexuses go to the blood vessels of the corpora cavernosa. (b) A *cortical pathway* initiated by psychic stimuli and mediated by parasympathetic and sympathetic fibers which originate at the T_{12}–L_1 level of the spinal cord. Each of these pathways promotes rapid inflow and retention of blood in the penis and the vulva.

The presence of these two spinal centers governing erection has important clinical implications. Patients with complete cord transections above the sacral center but below the thoracic center may still be capable of psychogenic erections mediated by impulses descending from higher centers and exiting the cord at T_{12}-L_1. With a cord lesion above both spinal centers, psychogenically produced erections are blocked, but the patient may still be capable of reflexogenic erections from direct tactile stimulation of the penis or clitoris even though he or she is unable to experience the sensation.

In addition to neurological pathways, erection in the male depends upon intact arterial blood flow from the right and left internal pudendal arteries.

The third phase is *orgasm*. Subjectively for both sexes orgasm is a peaking of sexual pleasure accompanied by a sense of release from sexual tension. Physiologically in the male, the most obvious manifestation of orgasm is ejaculation. Ejaculation is mediated by the sympathetic nervous system and consists of two processes: emission, resulting from contraction of the vas deferens, prostate, and seminal vesicles; and actual ejaculation, resulting from rhythmic contraction of the muscles of the pelvic floor and from closure of the internal sphincters of the bladder (preventing retrograde ejaculation). In the female, the rhythmic contractions take place within the musculature of the outer third of the vagina and in the perineal muscles. The subjective component of orgasm is a cortical sensory phenomenon, purely psychic in origin; it can occur without ejaculation or bladder neck closure.

The fourth phase is called *resolution*, which subjectively is accompanied by a sense of pleasure, warmth, well-being, and relaxation. Physiologically there is a gradual return of heart rate, breathing rate, and muscle tension to the baseline state. Most males are refractory to entering another cycle of sexual activity for some period of time (minutes in younger men and an hour or longer in middle-aged and older men). Women are not subject to this refractory period and may have multiple orgasms following continued or additional stimulation.

COMMON SEXUAL DISORDERS

The nomenclature and criteria used to classify sexual disorders in this chapter are based upon the 1980 edition of the American Psychiatric Association's *Diagnostic and Statistical Manual of Mental Disorders* (DSM-III). The assessment and management of the following common sexual disorders are discussed below: inhibited sexual desire (loss of libido); inhibited sexual excitement (impotence); inhibited orgasm; dyspareunia; vaginismus; and premature ejaculation.

Organic Etiologies

As is pointed out below in the criteria for each of these disorders, a physical basis must be excluded before the disorder can be attributed to psychologi-

cal factors. Since sexual functioning involves neural, vascular, and endocrine physiological mechanisms, there are many physical conditions and drugs which can interrupt normal function. To make matters more complicated these pathological conditions can adversely affect one or more phases of the sexual response cycle (see Tables 18.1 to 18.4).

General Characteristics

Incidence

The exact incidence of sexual disorders is not known. Estimates of lifetime incidence have ranged from a high of 75% in marriages and other long term relationships to a low of 25%. In all likelihood, the higher estimates include these disorders in their milder and more transient forms. Each type of sexual dysfunction can be found in both hetero- and homosexual couples. The sex ratio varies for the particular dysfunction. For example, inhibited orgasm is more common in females. By definition, premature ejaculation is confined to men and vaginismus is restricted to women.

Age of Onset of Common Sexual Disorders

Psychological and behavioral antecedents of these disorders can sometimes be found in both adolescent and childhood sexual behaviors and fantasies; however, the common age of onset is early adulthood. Onset can occur at any time during adult life, especially for those dysfunctions which are associated with physical conditions or drugs and for those which are situational or transient.

Predisposing Personality Factors

In general, competent and satisfying sexual function is considered to be associated with a healthy and adaptive personality development. Therefore, defects in personality structure accompanied by maladaptive personality traits or psychopathology may affect sexual function. *Compulsive* traits in men and women may be associated with inhibited sexual desire and inhibited sexual excitement. *Passive-aggressive* traits appear to be associated with premature ejaculation. *Histrionic* traits in both men and women may be associated with inhibited sexual excitement and inhibited orgasm. *Negative attitudes toward sexuality* due to particular experience, internal psychic conflicts, or adherence to rigid cultural values can predispose individuals to the development of these dysfunctions.

Course and Severity

The course of sexual dysfunctions is variable. They may develop after a period of normal functioning or they may be lifelong. They may be generalized, occurring with all partners, or situational, limited to certain partners. There are differing degrees of impairment from partial to total. Usually, early

Table 18.1.
Organic Factors Which May Affect Sexual Response in Both Sexes

Organic Factor	Sexual Disorders
Alcoholic neuropathy	Inhibited excitement, inhibited orgasm
Angina pectoris	Inhibited desire
Any chronic systemic disease	Decreased desire, inhibited excitement
Chronic pain	Decreased desire
Degenerative arthritis and disc disease of lumbo-sacral spine	Inhibited desire, inhibited excitement
Diabetes mellitus	Inhibited excitement; retrograde ejaculation (men) Inhibited orgasm (women)
Endocrine disorders (thyroid deficiency states, Addison's disease, Cushing's disease, hypopituitarism, hyperprolactinemia)	Decreased desire, variable effect on excitement
Multiple sclerosis	Decreased desire, inhibited excitement, inhibited orgasm
Cord lesions:	
Low lesion	Inhibited reflex excitement (psychogenic excitement, and reflex ejaculation may be preserved)
High lesion	Inhibited psychogenic excitement (reflex excitement, and ejaculation may be preserved)
Radical pelvic surgery	Inhibited excitement, inhibited orgasm
Temporal lobe lesions	Decreased or increased desire
Vascular disease:	
Large vessel (Leriche syndrome)	Inhibited excitement
Small vessel (pelvic vascular insufficiency)	Inhibited excitement

Table 18.2.
Organic Factors Which May Affect Sexual Response: Men Only

Organic Factor	Sexual Disorders
Dyspareunia (genital pain during intercourse):	Inhibited desire, inhibited excitement, and inhibited orgasm are disorders which may occur with any of the organic factors listed at the left.
Disturbed penile anatomy (chordee, Peyrone's disease, traumatic fracture, traumatic amputation)	
Penile skin infections	
Prostatic infections	
Testicular disease (orchitis, epididymitis, tumor, trauma)	
Urethral infections (gonorrhea, nonspecific urethral infections)	
Hypogonadal androgen-deficient states (Klinefelter's syndrome, testicular agenesis, Kallman's syndrome, testicular tumors, orchitis, hyperprolactinemia, castration)	Inhibited desire, inhibited excitement, inhibited orgasm
Mechanical problems (inguinal hernia, hydrocele)	Inhibited excitement
Surgical procdedures:	
Abdominoperineal bowel resection	Inhibited excitement
Lumbar sympathectomy	Inhibited orgasm
Radical perineal prostatectomy	Inhibited excitement

Table 18.3.
Organic Factors Which May Affect Sexual Response: Women Only

Organic Factor	Sexual Disorders
Complications of surgery:	Inhibited desire, inhibited excitement, inhibited orgasm, and vaginismus are disorders which may occur with any of the organic factors listed at the left.
Ovarian approximation to vagina	
Posthysterectomy scarring	
Shortened vagina	
Dyspareunia (painful intercourse):	
Agenesis of the vagina	
Clitoral phymosis	
Imperforate hymen, rigid hymen, tender hymenal tags	
Infections of external genitalia: herpes genitalis, labial cysts, furuncles, Bartholin cyst infections	
Infections of the vagina: herpes genitalis, *Candida albicans*, *Trichomonas*	
Injuries due to birth trauma: episiotomy scars, tears, uterine prolapse	
Irritations of the vagina: chemical dermatitis (douches), atrophic vaginitis, intercourse with insufficient lubrication	
Miscellaneous pelvic problems	
Cystitis, urethritis, urethral prolapse	
Endometriosis, ectopic pregnancy, pelvic inflammatory disease, ovarian cysts and tumors, pelvic tumors	
Intrauterine device complications	

age of onset and total impairment indicate chronicity and a poor treatment outcome. Conversely, a history of prior adequate sexual function, situational symptoms, and partial impairment indicate a self-limited course and a favorable treatment outcome.

Complications

The major complications are disrupted marital or sexual relationships. In addition, presence of the dysfunction may give rise to a variety of symptoms such as depression, anxiety, guilt, shame, frustration, and anger. These symptoms affect not only the individual but may intrude into most of his or her relationships.

General Approach to the Patient

Since patients often have difficulty discussing sexual problems, the presentation of the chief complaint and history of the present problem may be imprecise. Thus it is important to set aside sufficient time with the patient to achieve a clear statement of the problem. Occasionally, more than one scheduled session may be necessary. The setting for the dis-

cussion of the sexual problem should be private. For those patients whose difficulties involve a partner or a spouse, it is important to have the partner's view of the problem. Sometimes the more functional partner will seek help in order to gain support for bringing the less functional partner into the evaluation.

The evaluation should be organized to obtain information about the onset and duration of the problem, about factors that make the problem better or worse, about concurrent events, such as birth of children, changes in relationships or vocation, onset of physical or emotional illness, and about use of new medications. It is always important to elicit from patients their ideas about the etiology of sexual problems and their expectations of treatment.

Table 18.4.
Drugs Which May Affect Sexual Response[a]

Drugs	Sexual Disorders
Alcohol and sedatives (high dose)	Decreased desire, inhibited excitement, delayed orgasm
Androgens	Increased desire (women)
Antidepressants	Decreased or increased desire, inhibited excitement
Antihypertensives:	
Centrally acting (β-blockers, clonidine, guanabenz, methyldopa, reserpine)	Decreased desire, inhibited excitement, (?) inhibited orgasm
Peripherally acting (guanethidine, guanadrel)	Retrograde ejaculation
Antipsychotics	Decreased or increased desire, inhibited excitement, retrograde ejaculation (Mellaril)
Cimetidine	Decreased desire
	Inhibited excitement
Digoxin	Decreased desire
	Inhibited excitement
Disopyramide	Inhibited excitement
Disulfiram	Inhibited excitement, delayed ejaculation
Diuretics	Inhibited excitement
Estrogens, progesterone	
Men	Decreased desire, inhibited excitement, inhibited orgasm
Women	Decreased desire
L-Dopa	Increased desire (elderly men)
Lithium	Decreased desire
	Inhibited excitement
Marijuana (high dose)	Inhibited excitement (low dose may produce increased desire in men)
Narcotics	Decreased desire, inhibited excitement, inhibited orgasm
Stimulants (high dose) (cocaine, amphetamines)	Decreased desire, inhibited excitement, inhibited orgasm (low dose may produce increased desire)

[a] See also: Drugs that cause sexual dysfunction. *Med Lett* 25:73, 1983, for an exhaustive list, with references.

Inhibited Sexual Desire (Loss of Libido)

DSM-III Diagnostic Criteria

Persistent and pervasive inhibition of sexual desire. The judgment of inhibition is made by the clinician's taking into account factors that affect sexual desire such as age, sex, health, intensity, frequency of sexual desire, and the context of the individual's life.

Assessment

As can be seen from Tables 18.1 to 18.4 there are many pathological conditions and drugs that have the potential for inhibiting sexual desire. In practice, most of these conditions will be known or easily diagnosed by the physician. Only a few conditions may present with the initial complaint of inhibited desire.

Congenital or acquired *hypogonadism* may be associated with inhibited sexual interest in men (10). Since the testosterone level needed to maintain libido is usually lower than that needed for full stimulation of the prostate and seminal vesicles, the patient should also complain of a decrease or absence of emission when loss of sexual desire is due to hypogonadism. Hypogonadism which occurs before puberty results in eunuchoidism (lack of development of secondary sex characteristics). Similar striking physical findings are not present in patients who acquire hypogonadism after puberty; however, subtle physical changes do occur; decrease in beard growth, tendency to female body habitus, and decreased size of testes. An evaluation for hypogonadism should be undertaken in any male with persistent loss of libido (see details in Chapter 77).

In both sexes *prolactin-secreting microadenomas* of the pituitary can cause loss of sexual interest. In men this is partly due to a prolactin-mediated decrease in gonadotropin output, and the testosterone level is low. Hyperprolactinemia causes amenorrhea and galactorrhea in females, but galactorrhea is rare in affected men. Diagnosis can be made in both sexes by measuring serum prolactin levels (normal less than 15 mg/ml). (See additional details in Chapter 77.)

In both sexes *alcohol or other substance abuse* can cause inhibited sexual desire. Patients who abuse drugs are usually guarded or untruthful about their habits; therefore, persistence and use of collateral interviews are often necessary in diagnosing the primary problem.

Depression is a common cause of inhibited sexual desire. Even mild depressive states may result in loss of sexual desire, but in patients suffering from severe depressions this loss is universally observed. The relationship between inhibited sexual desire and the presence of depression may be recognized by noting the patient's mood as well as by obtaining a history of depressive symptoms (see Chapter 15).

Life stresses (loss of a job, death of a family member or of a friend, birth of a new family member, recent illness such as myocardial infarction, *etc*) are common sources of libido loss related to depression or anxiety.

In married couples inhibited sexual desire in one or both partners is often the result of *marital strife*. The differences that arise between the partners create anger which eventually interferes with their sexual relationship. Although spouses may be aware of their anger toward each other, they may fail to draw a connection between loss of sexual interest and their mutual problems, if such problems are not sexual in nature. Assessment requires taking a history from the couple together and from the partners separately. Review of their current life situation will usually elicit the precipitating stresses and highlight the conflicts. The uncovering of extramarital relationships during the assessment requires careful handling by the physician. If both partners are aware of the relationship, then it can be discussed openly. If the extramarital relationship is revealed to the physician during the individual interviews, the physician should ask what the partner intends to do about the relationship, and with the "secret" information now shared with the physician. The responsibility for telling the other partner should be left with the patient. In some cases the extramarital relationship is a peripheral issue, and airing it could be destructive to an otherwise salvageable relationship.

Finally, inhibited sexual desire can be caused by the anxiety and frustration of repeated sexual failure associated with one of the other sexual disorders discussed beow.

Treatment

Depending upon the etiology, *hypogonadism* in men may be treated by surgery, radiotherapy, hormone replacement, or hormone suppression (in the case of hyperprolactinemia). These treatment modalities are discussed in Chapter 77.

In both sexes, if a *drug* (see Table 18.4) is suspected of interfering with sexual desire, it should be discontinued, if possible, as a diagnostic-therapeutic test. If loss of sexual drive is secondary to alcohol or substance abuse, then treatment should be aimed at controlling the abuse (see Chapters 21 and 22).

Patients with *coronary artery disease*, especially postmyocardial infarction, have particular problems associated with sexual function. The management of these patients is discussed as part of the overall approach to rehabilitation after infarction in Chapter 58.

For transient loss of sexual desire secondary to *psychological factors* such as stress, anger, or other interpersonal problems, short term counseling is effective in most instances. When alcoholism, depression, or another psychosocial disorder is the primary problem, specific treatment for that disorder should of course accompany the counseling (see chapters on these disorders). The design of a counseling program should include an agreement between the patient or couple and the physician to meet for a specific number of sessions (usually two to five) for approximately 30 minutes/session.

Example. A couple in their midtwenties presents with a history of recent loss of sexual desire on the husband's part, and a decrease in the frequency of their sexual relationships. Assessment reveals a past history of mutually satisfying sexual experiences until 1 month ago when the husband was threatened with a job layoff. Although the husband still has his job, the layoff is still a possibility. The wife reports the husband has become quiet, sullen, and has increased drinking of alcohol. They report fighting frequently over small issues. The assessment is that the husband has an *adjustment disorder* with depressive features (see Chapter 12). During the initial counseling session the physician suggests that a relationship exists between changes in the husband's behavior and the threatened layoff. The wife indicates that the husband has refused to discuss his concerns because "it is unmanly." During the next counseling session the physician assists the couple in developing contingency plans to cope with the potential layoff. As they are drawn into the discussions of planning, the couple's anger with each other subsides and a collaborative relationship is re-established. The third session is utilized to review what contingency plans they have made. As an aside, they report that they have resumed their sexual relationship. During the final session the physician (*a*) reviews the relationship between stress, anger, and the change in sexual functioning; (*b*) points out that anger subsided when they worked together and that good sex is difficult to experience when they are angry with each other; and (*c*) encourages them to use what they have learned when stresses arise in the future.

Patients and their physicians often attempt to treat inhibited sexual desire with drugs such as testosterone, alcohol, antianxiety compounds, or stimulants. There is no scientific basis for prescribing drugs for sexual disorders, except testosterone for the treatment of confirmed hypogonadism and bromocriptine for treatment of hyperprolactinemia (8), as discussed in Chapter 77.

Inhibited Sexual Excitement (Impotence)

DSM-III Diagnostic Criteria

A. Recurrent and persistent inhibition of sexual excitement during sexual activity manifested by partial or complete failure to attain or maintain erection until completion of the sexual act in males, or partial or complete failure to attain or maintain the lubrication and swelling response of sexual excitement until completion of the sexual act in females.
B. A clinical judgment that the individual engages in sexual activity that is adequate in focus, intensity, and duration.

Assessment

An initial history (including psychosocial evaluation—see Chapter 10) and physical examination will usually lead to a formulation that the problem is probably organic (*i.e.*, one of the causes in Tables 18.1 to 18.4) or probably psychogenic. The general features in the patient's history listed in Table 18.5 are helpful in making this important distinction.

Organic basis. In both sexes, partial or complete failure to begin and maintain genital vasocongestion can be caused by a large number of pathological conditions and drugs. In male medical patients, drugs are the commonest organic causes of impotence (Table 18.4). The other conditions that may cause inhibited sexual excitement (Tables 18.1–18.3) usually present with other manifestations before the patient complains of this problem.

In patients with *diabetes mellitus* it is estimated that impotence will eventually affect 25 to 60% of males (3). Because some patients present with impotence as the initial symptom of diabetes, a fasting blood glucose is indicated for any male patient who presents with a chief complaint of impotence that is not due to an obvious psychosocial stressor or a

Table 18.5.
Clinical Features Differentiating Predominantly "Psychogenic" from Predominantly "Organic" Erectile Dysfunction[a]

	Psychogenic	Organic
Onset	Usually abrupt, with temporal relationship to specific stress (marital difficulties, loss of job, bereavement, fatigue, *etc*)	Usually insidious decline from previous competency (90–95% of cases)
Course	Selective, intermittent, episodic, transient	Usually persistent, with progressive deterioration
Degree of impairment	Evidence of potential to respond to erotic stimuli and fantasies, with masturbation, alternate partner	Unable to obtain erection with masturbation, erotic stimuli, other partner
Nocturnal or morning erection	Generally present	Generally absent or reduced in frequency and intensity

[a] From Vliet LW, Meyer JK: Erectile dysfunction: progress in evaluation and treatment. *Johns Hopkins Med J* 151:246, 1982.

recently started drug. There is no definitive information at this time about the effect of diabetes on the excitement phase in women; clearly, it can inhibit orgasm in women (7).

There are two conditions in women that may contribute to inhibition of sexual excitement: *vaginitis* and *atrophic vaginal changes* secondary to estrogen deficiency (see Chapter 94). Surprisingly, some women do not associate the presence of vaginitis or atrophic changes with the discomfort or pain these conditions can cause when intercourse is attempted. The history should therefore include questions that determine whether there is pain during intercourse, and the physical examination should include a pelvic examination and collection of a specimen for determining maturation index if there is doubt about the presence of atrophy (see Chapter 94).

Occlusive vascular disease causing diminished blood flow to the internal pudendal arteries is more likely to affect men than women. Inhibited sexual excitement has been described with large vessel disease (Leriche's syndrome) as well as with medium and small vessel disease. If it is suspected that there is a vascular basis for impotence, the patient should be referred to a vascular surgeon for evaluation. The diagnostic techniques which may be employed included angiography of the medium size vessels of the corpus cavernosa, comparison of penile systolic pressures to limb systolic pressures, Doppler measurement of penile blood flow, and nocturnal penile tumescence studies (NPT) (5).

The *hypogonadal states* which cause inhibited desire (see above) can also cause inhibited excitement (10), and the approach to diagnosis is the same (see Chapter 77).

Psychogenic basis. If the assessment for an organic etiology, which will often include a trial off of a potentially offending drug, does not yield a convincing diagnosis, a *psychogenic basis* should be assumed and further inquiry followed by appropriate brief counseling (see below) should be utilized as a diagnostic-therapeutic trial.

Inability to attain and maintain levels of excitement that permit a smooth and trouble-free progression from the beginning of a sexual experience to its completion can be caused by any external event or internal psychological event that interferes with the patient's ability to focus on the stimuli which are creating the sexual excitement. A dramatic example of an external event is the ringing of a telephone during the midst of the sexual experience. An internal psychological event might be a recurring thought. The history and assessment should be structured to uncover the presence of external events and the specific content of the psychological events when present. A common finding is a *persistent preoccupation and anxiety about performing successfully.* This problem may be primary or may occur as a secondary response to the frustration associated with organic dysfunction. Worry about a successful performance becomes more and more absorbing during the course of the sexual experience so that the psychological activity crowds out the patient's capacity to focus on the sexual stimuli which create the excitement response. When such patients realize they are losing their level of excitement, they try all the harder, shutting off completely their ability to respond to sexual stimuli. Masters and Johnson have called this process "*spectatoring*" (see "General References"). The term describes a process whereby the patient, through observation of his performance, psychologically takes himself out of the experience. The mental process is guaranteed to result in loss of sexual excitement. Typically this process may begin after one or two failed performances secondary to external events or stresses. Once the process begins, it becomes internally reinforcing, leading to further worry and further failure. When this process is suspected, the history should focus on the patient's mental experiences during sexual intercourse. Such information is difficult for most patients to describe, and more than a single interview will be required to obtain it.

Other common causes of psychologically inhibited sexual excitement are *stressful life situations.* Patients who have recently lost a job, have lost a relative, are concerned about retirement, have developed an illness, *etc* may not be able to clear their minds of their worries during a sexual experience and therefore cannot respond. Similarly, feelings of anger or resentment directed toward the sexual partner can interfere with the ability to become sexually excited.

If the patient with suspected psychogenic impotence does not respond to brief counseling (see below), then he should be offered *referral to a sleep laboratory for NPT studies (5).* The diagnostic usefulness of NPT monitoring is based on the assumption that during sleep, the psychological factors impeding erectile function during wakefulness are no longer operative, allowing a demonstration of the integrity of one's physiological capacity. Organic deficits, however, would persist during sleep, and therefore inhibit the number and duration of erectile episodes. Research has tended to confirm this assumption, with two exceptions: first, in certain psychiatric disorders (*e.g.*, endogenous depression) in which REM sleep patterns are also disrupted; and second, in a few men with organically proven erectile failure who occasionally have an episode of full erection during sleep, such as in patients with lower body spasms due to spinal cord injury, patients with a vascular "steal" syndrome, and in a previously unrecognized syndrome of impaired penile tumescence in the presence of sleep apnea, hypoventilation with decreased oxygen saturation, myoclonic jerks, and bradycardia.

Patient experience. This is similar to the experience for evaluation of sleep disorders (see Chapter 85). The patient will usually be scheduled to sleep on 3 consecutive nights in the sleep laboratory. Paramaters monitored include electroencephalography, eye movements (to document the presence of REM sleep), heart rate, blood pressure, changes in penile circumference at the tip (just proximal to the glans) and base using two mecury-filled strain gauges, and an assessment of the degree of penile rigidity during at least one of the erectile episodes. Rigidity is assessed using a specifically designed tonometer which measures the amount of force required to "buckle" the erect penis. The patient is also briefly awakened to observe his erection, and asked to evaluate the quality of this erection, and to estimate its sufficiency for intromission. The technician records his estimate of the degree and rigidity of the erection. A photograph of the erect penis is taken, and later reviewed with the patient. This photograph provides visual evidence of normal erectile capacity to the patient with psychogenic dysfunction; it aids in the interpretation of numerical data obtained; and it reveals or confirms the presence of an anatomical deformity interfering with normal erection and/or intromission.

A do-it-yourself device (the Dacomed Snap-Gauge) for assessing nocturnal erections has been promoted in recent years. Because the role of this potentially cost-saving device has not been validated in careful studies, its place in the evaluation of impotence is not yet clear.

If NPT study indicates an organic disorder (*i.e.*, no or only partial erections occur during sleep), additional evaluation for vascular or neurological disorders should be carried out. If NPT study supports psychogenic impotence, psychiatric referral is warranted.

Treatment

Treatment of *organically based inhibited sexual excitement in men* will depend on whether the physiological impairment is reversible.

If the disease process (usually an infection or another condition that has caused dyspareunia) has not caused irreversible anatomical or physiological changes, treatment of the disease is dictated. Similarly, side effects of drugs can be reversed by reduction of dosage or, ideally, discontinuation of the drug. An adequate trial off of a drug would be 1 or more weeks. Testosterone replacement for hypogonadism produces improvement in sexual excitement within a few weeks (see Chapter 77 for details). Whenever one is managing a patient with a probably reversible organic cause, the treatment should be accompanied by encouragement and practical advice such as that discussed below.

When a disease process has caused permanent impairment of neural, vascular, or anatomical function in males, surgical measures can be considered. Currently there are two types of penile prosthetic devices which allow the impotent male to engage in intercourse. The Small-Carrion (9) prosthesis is a set of semirigid Silastic rods which are placed in the penis, creating a permanent modest erection. The second prosthesis is a hydraulic device (4) which, when implanted, permits voluntary stiffening of the penis. The commonest indication for penile prosthetic devices has been in impotent diabetics who are otherwise healthy. Counseling of the patient and his spouse or partner is an essential element of a rehabilitative program before and after surgery.

Little is known about the response to treatment in *women* with disease processes which impair the physiological capacity for sexual excitement. As in men, side effects of drugs can be eliminated by adjustment of dosage or discontinuation of the drug, and dyspareunia due to vulvovaginal conditions and atrophic vaginitis can usually be eliminated (see Chapter 94).

The strategy for management of *psychologically based* inhibited sexual excitement in both sexes depends on whether the patient has had the dysfunction for a sustained period of time or whether the dysfunction has appeared recently and there is a prior history of competent sexual functioning. As discussed earlier, transient inhibition of sexual excitement is often secondary to stressful life situations and/or marital discord (adjustment disorders). These clinical situations often respond to brief counseling. The elements of counseling are similar to those desribed in the above example of the couple with inhibited sexual desire (see page 218). The role of the physician is to help the couple recognize the effect of the stress on their relationship as well as the effect of their feelings (often anger) on their ability to relate sexually. Encouragement of collaborative contingency planning for resolving problems reduces anxiety and anger, often helping the couple to return to their baseline level of sexual function. The same principles and steps are applicable to an individual patient.

When spectatoring is the major problem and this problem does not remit after open discussion, referral to a professional skilled in sex therapy usually brings excellent results. The treatment is that developed by Masters and Johnson; it combines cognitive as well as behavioral techniques to replace spectatoring with appropriate sexual focus and behavior.

The following factors favor a good prognosis following treatment for psychogenic impotence: history of adequate prior sexual functioning, acute *versus* insidious onset, short duration of sexual impairment, heterosexual orientation, stable social situation, motivation for treatment, presence of sexual desire, willingness of partner to participate in treatment, absence of severe marital conflicts, and absence of significant concurrent psychopathy.

Even in patients for whom excellent function can

be expected, the return to normal sexual excitation can be impaired by worry and hesitation. This is especially true when the impaired excitation has been present for more than a few weeks, which is often the case. Such patients should be invited to discuss this situation freely and should be given permission and encouragement to experiment in one or more ways (e.g., masturbation, erotic pictures or movies, new techniques) in order to test or promote their sexual functions. Such advice should, of course, be consistent with the patient's moral and ethical beliefs.

Patients who have suffered with inhibited sexual excitement over a long period of time or have never functioned competently may be given a trial of short term counseling (Chapter 11). If the counseling does not result in reasonable improvement, referral for more expert help should be considered.

Inhibited Orgasm (Anorgasmia)

DSM-III Diagnostic Criteria for Women

Recurrent and persistent inhibition of the female orgasm is manifested by delay in or absence of orgasm following a normal sexual excitement phase during sexual activity that is judged by the clinician to be adequate in focus, intensity, and duration. Some women are able to experience orgasm during noncoital clitoral stimulation, but are unable to experience it during coitus in the absence of manual clitoral stimulation. There is evidence to suggest that in some instances this represents a normal variation of the female sexual response. The judgment to assign the diagnosis is assisted by a thorough sexual evaluation which may even require a trial of treatment (see below).

DSM-III Diagnostic Criteria for Men

Recurrent and persistent inhibition of the male orgasm is manifested by delay in or absence of ejaculation following an adequate phase of sexual excitement.

Assessment

The orgasmic response is physiologically governed by the autonomic nervous system in both sexes. The organic conditions which inhibit orgasm are for the most part neurological disorders, drugs which affect the autonomic system, and surgical or traumatic interruption of the involved neural pathways (see Tables 18.1 to 18.4) History-taking and physical examination should focus on these possibilities. In women, diabetic autonomic neuropathy is probably the most common organic cause of inhibited orgasm (7). Men who are experiencing retrograde ejaculation often state they have lost their ability to have orgasms. If history reveals the patient has the subjective sensations of orgasm but has no ejaculate (and the patient is not taking a drug which can cause

retrograde ejaculation, see Table 18.4), then the patient should have a urological evaluation of the function of the internal sphincter of the bladder.

Isolated *psychogenic* anorgasmia in *men* is a rare disorder and is associated with severe personality disturbances. Cases can be divided roughly into two personality types: severe obsessive compulsive character disorder and severe sadomasochistic character disorder.

Psychologically caused inhibited orgasm is a common problem in *women*. Numerous studies estimate that 10% of the female population is anorgasmic to any stimuli and 30 to 50% of all married women are occasionally anorgasmic with intercourse. Assessment should focus on the duration of the problem, a past history of sexual functioning, the status of the relationship with the spouse or partner, and the presence of a stressful situation. A history of recent onset, competent past functioning, and identifiable precipitating stresses predicts a good response to treatment. Patients who have been anorgasmic for many years and are seeking help because of a change in their relationship or life situations are more difficult to treat.

Some women will present with a complaint of anorgasmia but evaluation will reveal the patient is actually experiencing inhibited sexual excitement. Since treatment may differ for these disorders, clarification of the phase in which the dysfunction is operating may be important.

Treatment (Men)

It is unusual for men to experience loss of orgasmic capacity due to organic factors while retaining the capacity for erection. In fact it is more usual for men to lose their potency while retaining the capacity for emission and some of the subjective sensations associated with orgasm. Most of the physical conditions, diseases and drugs listed in Tables 18.1, 18.2, and 18.4 will affect the capacity for erection before orgasmic function is impaired. There may be isolated instances of side effects of drugs in which males report loss of ability to experience orgasm, but retain the capacity for erection. In these instances, it is important to distinguish *retrograde ejaculation* from inhibited orgasm. Retrograde ejaculation can occur with some drugs, including thioridazine (Mellaril) and guanethidine (Ismelin) while the other components of orgasm remain intact.

Men who suffer from inhibited orgasm on a psychogenic basis usually have long-standing personality disorders requiring expert psychotherapy to effect improvement.

Treatment (Women)

Apart from managing local vaginal conditions and discontinuing possible causal drugs, there are no organic therapies for this dysfunction in women. Therefore, in female patients with known neuronal damage, including diabetic neuropathy, the goal of therapy should be to help the patients adjust to the permanent loss of their sexual responsiveness.

Transient forms of anorgasmia caused by psychogenic factors are amenable to treatment with counseling. A history of previous orgasmic response is a good prognostic indicator. The block in orgasmic response is often due to the process of "spectatoring" described above. The interfering process is usually secondary to stressful life situations and/or marital discord. Counseling for married women and women who have a regular sexual partner should include the partner provided that it is agreeable to the patient. Counseling should be aimed primarily at resolving the dominant problems which are usually life stresses or interpersonal strife. With the single patient, counseling should be directed at helping the patient suppress or remove the psychological events (i.e., spectatoring) which are occurring at a critical time, when the patient has reached a high plateau level of excitement and is prepared for orgasmic release. The interfering psychological events may be removed by having the patient focus to the best of her ability on the physical stimuli that she is experiencing during the excitement phase.

Women with anorgasmia of long duration can be given a trial of counseling. If counseling does not result in substantial improvement, referral for additional evaluation and treatment should be made.

Dyspareunia

DSM-III Diagnostic Criteria

Coitus is associated with recurrent and persistent genital pain in either sex.

Assessment

The common causes of genital pain during intercourse (dyspareunia) are presented in Tables 18.2 and 18.3. In both sexes the complaint of discomfort or pain during intercourse requires a careful history, physical examination, and laboratory testing. The commonest causes are infectious or atrophic vaginitis in women, and urethral or prostatic infection in men. Psychogenic dyspareunia is uncommon, and this diagnosis should be made only after organic causes have been excluded.

Treatment

The treatment of dyspareunia caused by organic conditions in both men and women is directed at the condition causing the pain (see Chapters 27 and 94). Patients with psychogenic dyspareunia will have many of the features described for those with psychogenic inhibited sexual excitement or inhibited orgasm; that is, the patients will report a prior history of competent sexual function without pain and will have current life stress and/or marital

discord. Therefore, the counseling techniques used in the treatment should be very similar to those described for the other two disorders. An important strategy in counseling is to allow the patient a face-saving way of giving up the pain without directly confronting him with the idea that the pain is of psychogenic origin.

A few patients have psychogenic dyspareunia over a sustained period of time. Such patients usually have severe underlying psychiatric conditions and require referral for expert evaluation and treatment.

Vaginismus

DSM-III Diagnostic Criteria

Vaginismus is diagnosed by a history of recurrent and persistent involuntary spasm of the musculature of the outer third of the vagina that interferes with coitus.

Assessment

By definition this is a disorder of women. There are relatively few causes of organic vaginismus, and they are usually secondary to dyspareunia. Diagnosis of functional vaginismus may be made when pelvic examination is attempted and the physician finds it impossible to pass a finger or speculum into the vagina because of contraction of the musculature around the vaginal outlet.

Treatment

The treatment of organic vaginismus is the same as the treatment of the organic causes of dyspareunia.

The treatment of functional vaginismus is based upon *desensitizing* the patient to the experience of penetration. Couples are provided with a series of exercises to be performed in the privacy of their home. Following a relaxing bath, the couple engages in general body touching, excluding the genitals. Next, they repeat general touching but include the genitals, avoiding any touching that is frankly stimulating. At following sessions, they repeat the touching but add the passage of graded sized dilators, still avoiding stimulating, touching, or efforts to attain orgasm. When dilators have reached the size approximating the size of the penis, then the penis can be substituted as a dilator. The same process can be applied by having the individual woman dilate herself. One problem with the single patient is the possibility that the experience during the sessions at home will not generally apply to a sexual experience with a partner. Should this occur, treatment may have to be delayed until the patient has a regular partner with whom she has a reasonably good relationship and who can participate in the outlined program.

Premature Ejaculation

DSM-III Diagnostic Criteria

Ejaculation occurs before the individual wishes it, because of recurrent and persistent absence of reasonable voluntary control of ejaculation and orgasm during sexual activity. The judgment of "reasonable control" is made by the clinician, taking into account factors that affect duration of the excitement phase, such as age, novelty of the sexual partner, and frequency and duration of coitus.

Assessment

There are no known organic causes for premature ejaculation; therefore, the assessment of this dysfunction should focus on psychological issues. Whereas some men recognize that orgasm regularly occurs too soon for their partner to enjoy intercourse fully, others do not; therefore it is necessary to interview both partners in order to make the diagnosis. Typically the couple will report that the male experiences orgasm as he is attempting to penetrate, just as he has penetrated, or within several thrusts after penetration.

Patients usually have had the dysfunction since they became sexually active. Although occasionally patients may report the recent onset of premature ejaculation, these men have invariably experienced this disorder for a sustained period in the past. Another variation is the patient who reports good control with a girlfriend but premature ejaculation with his spouse.

The personality structure of the premature ejaculator is often passive-aggressive. Evaluation of the relationship usually reveals an ongoing struggle between the couple. The woman is openly angry about some issue (not necessarily the sexual problem), and the man is complacent, content, and puzzled that his partner is upset. Transient episodes of premature ejaculation may be precipitated by marital conflict. Some men who are sufficiently frustrated by the disorder may develop inhibited sexual excitement (impotence) secondarily.

Treatment

There are several behavioral methods of treatment which may be adaptable to the ambulatory setting. The key to helping the premature ejaculator is to teach him to become aware of his progression through the sexual response cycle and then, with his partner, to practice one of two control techniques. Patients without regular partners cannot readily use this behavioral method. The techniques are "squeeze technique" and "stop and go." The squeeze technique requires the female partner to place her thumb and first two fingers around the coronal ridge of the penis and press firmly for 10 seconds. The pressure will result in a 10 to 25% loss of erection and a decrease in the subjective sense of arousal. The technique teaches the couple a method of control that can be practiced well before the patient reaches high levels of sexual arousal. The stop and go method accomplishes the same thing by discontinuing all forms of stimulation. The patient and his partner alternately stimulate and practice control with these techniques until they are confident of their ability to exercise control. At this point they progress to coitus, interrupting the experience as necessary with the squeeze or stop and go technique. Additional details can be found in Masters and Johnson's *Human Sexual Inadequacy* (see "General References").

HOMOSEXUALITY

General Characteristics

Although homosexuality is no longer classified as a sexual disorder, it is the most common sexual deviation that will be seen by the generalist. Thirty years ago Kinsey *et al* (6) estimated that 10% of white American men and 5% of white women were predominantly homosexual. Estimates of the prevalence of homosexuality in blacks have not been published. The only disorder including homosexual behavior listed in the DSM-III is "ego dystonic homosexuality." The principal feature of this diagnostic classification is a pattern of overt homosexual arousal which is experienced by the individual as unwanted and a source of distress. Further, the diagnosis is reserved for those homosexuals for whom changing sexual orientation is a persistent concern.

Predisposing Factors

Various attempts to relate homosexuality to abnormal pituitary and sex hormone function have been unsuccessful. There is no evidence to support the contention that homosexuality is genetically determined. Many theories about the etiology of homosexuality involving psychosocial predisposition have been proposed. However, no studies have clearly demonstrated psychosocial etiological precipitants.

Course

Most individuals who make a choice of a homosexual orientation continue that orientation as a lifelong pattern. Some homosexuals are socially open about their life style; others are covert.

Complications

In the past, but to a lesser degree at the present time, the principal complication was the social stigma. Bias against homosexuals leads to occupational and other social problems for some, as summarized in Table 18.6. Recently, criminal penalties

Table 18.6.
Influence of Homosexuality on Vocation and Social Life (Results of a Study of 143 Subjects)[a]

	Male Homosexuals N = 86	Female Homosexuals N = 57
	%	%
SOCIAL:		
No negative influence[b]	51	72
Deprived of family life	35	9
Social contacts limited to other homosexuals	14	19
AMBITIONS:		
No negative influence	68	88
Imposed restrictions on choice of work or advancement	32	12
JOB:		
No negative influence	84	88
Reprimanded, fired, or asked to resign because of homosexuality	16	12

[a] From Saghir M, Robins E: *Male and Female Homosexuality—A Developmental, Psychiatric, and Sociological Investigation.* Baltimore, Williams & Wilkins, 1973.
[b] All negative influences listed are those that subjects felt were specifically a result of being identified as a homosexual.

for homosexuality have been eliminated for consenting adults. The only legal difficulty currently is for those individuals who are promiscuous and who use public facilities for their sexual activities. Homosexuality *per se* is no contraindication for developing sustained, affectionate, long term relationships. There is little evidence to support the contention that homosexual individuals are subject to or manifest greater levels of psychopathology than heterosexual individuals.

Assessment and Management

Assessment of patients who express concerns about homosexual fantasies or experiences should focus on the frequency of the experiences, on the patients' decisions to continue with homosexual experiences, and on whether they feel comfortable with those decisions. Patients who ultimately choose a homosexual orientation and are comfortable with that choice do not present problems. However, patients who are anxious or depressed about their homosexual inclinations may need therapy. Adolescents or adults who anxiously report isolated episodes of homosexual experiences or fantasies may need brief supportive counseling (see Chapter 11).

Most homosexuals prefer their personal physician to know of their homosexuality and indicate that they are more satisfied with the care they obtain when their physician is so aware (2).

Homosexuals require special considerations in their *routine medical care.* Those who have multiple partners should always be asked about the presence of symptoms that might be caused by venereal dis-

ease, including the acquired immune deficiency syndrome (AIDS—see Chapter 52) and the "gay bowel syndrome" (see Chapter 26); and they should be screened periodically for type B hepatitis (Chapter 42), syphilis (Chapter 30), and gonorrhea (Chapter 27). Physical examination should include inspection for oral or pharyngeal gonorrhea in addition to a genital and rectal examination.

SPECIAL CONSIDERATIONS FOR SELECTED AGE GROUPS

Elderly Patients

Aging individuals do not lose their capacity for sexual function on the basis of the aging processs alone. Elderly patients who have any of the sexual disorders discussed above should be evaluated in the same manner as a younger patient. The changes associated with aging are slower excitement phase, increased ability to stay at plateau levels of excitement, and, in men, a longer refractory period.

Children

It is unusual for children to complain of sexual difficulties. However, parents will occasionally ask their own physician questions about the developing sexuality of their children. Parents may express concern about the appearance of sexual behavior in children such as mutual exploration of playmates' genitalia or masturbation. The parents can be assured that the behavior is normal and that the behavior should be discouraged in a nonpunitive fashion. Failure to control the behavior may require further evaluation of both the child and the family.

Occasionally the physician may recognize the presence of *sexual abuse* within a family. If the abuse has been committed by someone outside the family, both the child and parents may require supportive counseling to help them vent their fear and anger about the experience. Discovery of sexual abuse within a family needs to be fully evaluated. This should be initiated by reporting the problem to the local department of social services; in each state, this department has a division of protective services to investigate suspected sexual abuse.

Adolescents

Adolescent sexual difficulties (see Chapter 5) may be brought to the attention of the physician either by the adolescent or by the adolescent's parents. Adolescents who are sexually active may have questions about their sexual function, birth control, venereal disease, or abortion. In most states, the physician may provide service for sex-related problems to the adolescent with or without the parental consent.

Adolescents may request consultation about isolated homosexual experiences and/or homosexual fantasies. In most cases, the physician's role is to reassure the adolescent that these experiences are normal and are not indicative of the development of lifelong homosexuality. Adolescents who have decided on a homosexual orientation or who are in the process of doing so may be brought to the physician by parents disturbed at the discovery of homosexual activities. In these instances, counseling should be given to the parents in order to help them accept the decision of the adolescent. Older adolescents (above 17 years) are unlikely to change their orientation. Younger adolescents (16 years and below) have not consolidated their personality development and should be referred for psychiatric evaluation and possible treatment.

GENDER IDENTITY DISORDERS

Gender identity disorders are divided into (a) transsexualism and (b) gender identity disorders of childhood. The essential feature of both disorders is the incongruence between anatomical sex and gender identity.

Predisposing Factors

No known genetic or biochemical predisposing factors have as yet been elucidated. There is some evidence that these disorders may stem from faulty parent-child relationships in situations where parents have confused sexual identity, or have a need to raise a child of one sex in the role of the opposite sex.

Prevalence

These disorders are apparently rare. Male cases are more common than female, the reported ratio varying from 8 to 1 to as low as 2 to 1.

Age of Onset

For children the initial expression of the wish to be in the cross-gender role may take place as early as the fourth birthday. For adults, the manifestations of this disorder usually become apparent in early adulthood, although the adults usually state that they had been aware of wishes to be in the cross-gender role since childhood or adolescence.

Course

The course of the disorder for children is as yet unknown. An undetermined number of affected boys and girls may adopt a homosexual orientation during adolescence or as adults. The course in adults is variable. For some it is chronic and unremitting, with a persistent drive toward attaining surgical reassignment. For others, the intensity of the desire for living and functioning in the cross-gender role waxes and wanes, often associated with current life stress and the appearance of psychiatric symptoms, principally depression. Females who are interested in sexual reassignment are a more homogeneous group than the males, in that they are more likely to have a history of homosexuality and by and large have a more stable course with or without treatment.

Complications

The principal complications are those associated with the desire and attempt to live and function socially and occupationally in the cross-gender role. In addition, there is a moderate degree of associated psychopathology, including episodes of depression and of suicide attempts. In rare instances, affected males may attempt to mutilate their genitals.

Assessment

The assessment of these disorders in adults is relatively simple in that most individuals will identify themselves as being unhappy with their anatomical sex and interested in a surgical reassignment. No endocrinological studies are indicated, and physical findings show that the individuals seeking surgical reassignment are genetically normal men or women. However, the generalist may see rare cases of patients who have a congenital intersexed condition and who are confused about their sexual identification.

Treatment

Patients with gender identity disorders should be referred to psychiatrists or to special programs which have the expertise to treat these problems. Transsexuals who are in a cross-gender program and who need continuous administration of cross-gender hormones may be transferred to the generalist. Some physicians may not agree with such treatment, and these patients should select physicians who are comfortable working with these types of problems.

THE PARAPHILIAS

This is a group of disorders in which sexual interests are directed primarily toward objects other than other human beings, toward sexual acts not usually associated with coitus, or toward coitus performed under bizarre conditions.

Fetishism

Fetishism is the relatively exclusive displacement of erotic interest in sexual satisfaction to an object, or to a body part other than those usually associated with genital sexuality. Common fetish objects are female undergarments (particularly worn or soiled ones), feet, and shoes. Orgasmic release may be achieved by any of the behavior used by adults in sexual activities.

Zoophilia

Zoophilia is the use of animals as a preferred or exclusive method of achieving sexual excitement. The animal may be the object of intercourse or may be trained to excite the human partner sexually by licking or rubbing. The animal is preferred no matter what other forms of sexual outlet are available.

Pedophilia

Pedophilia is a condition in which adults compulsively involve children in their sexual activities. The sexual behavior that results in orgasmic release may be heterosexual or homosexual, and include any behavior utilized by adults in their sexual activities. In the majority of cases, however, the pedophile is concerned with mutual masturbation or fondling rather than coitus.

Exhibitionism

Exhibitionism is the displaying of the genital organs for the purpose of sexual gratification. This perversion is predominantly a male activity. Orgasmic release is usually achieved through masturbation.

Voyeurism

Voyeurism is a deviation in which sexual stimulation and gratification are obtained from looking at the sexual organs of others or from observing their sexual activities. Orgasmic release is usually achieved by masturbating during, or just following, the period of observation.

Sadism and Masochism

Sadism and masochism are deviations in which sexual arousal and gratification are dependent either upon inflicting pain (sadism) or experiencing it (masochism). There is a broad spectrum of behavior ranging from the dim awareness of cruelty or suffering as part of the sexual experience to overt behavior, including extreme physical injury and murder. Aspects of sadism and masochism are usually found in the same individual, even though one or the other behavior appears dominant.

General Characteristics of the Paraphilias

Predisposing Factors

The etiology is unknown. However, history of physical and/or sexual abuse during childhood appears in a modest number of the cases.

Prevalence

The disorders are rare. The sex ratio is predominantly in favor of males, with the exception of sexual sadism and masochism.

Course

The course of these disorders is usually chronic. Peaks of deviant activity may accompany current life stress or be associated with psychiatric symptomatology, principally depressive episodes. If the deviant behavior brings the individual into conflict with society, the outcome can often include arrest and incarceration. Treatment is difficult because of the ego-syntonic nature of the behavior. Anxiety and depression may be associated with the fear of being discovered, arrested, or punished; however, once these dangers have passed, the uncomfortable affect disappears, and the individual has little motivation for treatment.

Complications

Inasmuch as these disorders are often associated with other defects in personality development the capacity for developing long term, affectionate relationships may be impaired. The possibility of being involved in criminal violations has already been mentioned. In some instances the behavior may bring the individual into extremely dangerous situations, resulting in severe injury or death.

Assessment

It is not difficult to diagnose a specific paraphilia once the history is obtained. No specific laboratory tests are indicated. The physical examination will usually be normal. Sadistic or masochistic behavior may produce physical injuries. Hypersexuality, including some deviant behavior, has been reported to be associated with temporal lobe epilepsy (1). Thus, in cases in which there is suggestion of a seizure disorder, an electroencephalogram is indicated. Psychiatric disorders, principally depression secondary to loss, may precipitate bursts of deviant behavior in paraphiliacs. Abuse of alcohol or of other substances may also increase the behavior.

Stress, anxiety, organic brain syndrome, and mental retardation may lead to episodic deviant behavior, but these episodes are not diagnosed as paraphilia.

Treatment

Psychotherapy or other psychological treatment designed to control or eliminate paraphiliac behavior is best provided by a psychiatrist. The general physician's role in the care of these patients is in the management of concurrent medical problems. Of major concern are recognition and treatment of venereal disease in those patients whose sexual behavior is promiscuous, and the possibility of child abuse in families which have paraphiliac members. Many individuals who engage in paraphilias were subjected to physical or sexual abuse as children. The pattern is often passed on from generation to generation.

General References

American Psychiatric Association: *Diagnostic and Statistical Manual of Mental Disorders*, ed. 3. Washington, DC, American Psychiatric Association, 1980
  Recently updated diagnostic criteria and epidemiological information for all recognized psychiatric disorders.
Masters WH, Johsnon VE: *Human Sexual Inadequacy*. Boston, Little, Brown, and Co, 1970.
  The original and still used descriptive work on the behavioral treatment of common sexual disorders.
Meyer JK, Schmidt CW, Wise TN (eds): *Clinical Management of*

Sexual Disorders. Baltimore, Williams & Wilkins, 1983.
A current textbook which addresses the evaluation, diagnosis, and treatment of a wide variety of sexual disorders.

The Medical Letter. *Drugs That Cause Sexual Dysfunction,* vol 25 (issue 641), August 5, 1983.
Review article listing drugs that cause sexual dysfunction with excellent reference list.

The Psychiatric Clinics of North America: Sexuality. Philadelphia, WB Saunders, 1980.
A current, concise review.

Vliet LW, Meyer JK: Erectile dysfunction: progress in evaluation and treatment. *Johns Hopkins Med J* 151:246, 1982.
An in-depth review article which focuses on impotence but which provides a methodology of evaluation for the practitioner which can be applied to any sexual dysfunction.

Specific References

1. Blumer D: Changes of sexual behavior related to temporal lobe disorders in man. *J Sex Res* 6:173, 1970.
2. Dardick L, Grady KE: Openness between gay persons and health professionals. *Ann Intern Med* 93:115, 1980.
3. Ellenberg M: Impotence in diabetes: the neurologic factor. *Ann Intern Med* 75:213, 1971.
4. Furlow WL: Surgical treatment of erectile impotence using the inflatable penile prosthesis. *Sex Disabil* 1:299, 1978.
5. Karacan I: Diagnosis of impotence in diabetes mellitus: an objective and specific method. *Ann Intern Med* 92:334, 1980.
6. Kinsey AC, Pomeroy WB, Martin CE: *Sexual Behavior in the Human Male.* Philadelphia, WB Saunders, 1948, pp 610–666.
7. Kolodny RC: Sexual dysfunction in diabetic females. *Diabetes* 20:557, 1971.
8. Schmidt CW: Biochemical treatment of sexual disorders. *Psychiatr Clin North Am* 3:89, 1980.
9. Small MP: The Small-Carrion penile prosthesis: surgical implant for the management of impotence. *Sex Disabil* 1:282, 1978.
10. Spark RF, White RA, Connolly PB: Impotence is not always psychogenic: newer insights into hypothalamic-pituitary-gonadal dysfunction. *JAMA* 243:750, 1980.

CHAPTER NINETEEN

Dying, Death, and Bereavement

KRIPA S. KASHYAP, M.D., AND L. RANDOL BARKER, M.D.

The family physician traditionally took care of his patients from cradle to death, and when they died, he managed the grief and bereavement of the survivors. This situation has changed dramatically in the last 40 to 50 years, in part because of the mobility of the society, in part because of the increased specialization of physicians. Now 80% of people come to hospitals to receive terminal care, which cannot be given at home either because of the specialized nature of the care or because of lack of family resources. Up until 40 or 50 years ago a dying patient stayed at home or returned home from the hospital to be with his family when death was imminent. Death was not a taboo and was openly discussed with the patients and their families. The physician had a major role in managing the moment of death. The role of the primary physician has become somewhat limited as the responsibility of this care has shifted to hospitals.

During the second half of the 20th century interest in the care of dying patients has steadily grown, stimulated in the last decade by the growth of the hospice movement. It is likely that, because of this interest, the general physician again will be able to manage many dying patients in their own homes.

SOCIOPSYCHOLOGICAL ISSUES

Fear of Death

Man is the only creature known who buries his dead; this he has done since the very dawn of human culture, possibly as far back as 50,000 B.C. Before the 11th century A.D., life after death was seen as a kind of sleep for an indeterminate period. Death was calmly accepted, without fear. Then the concept of the Last Judgment began to be taken seriously. An awe and fear of death became manifest in art and culture. The image of purgatory, heaven, and hell which preoccupied the mind of medieval man continues to exert its influence on a significant sector of society today.

Although aware that death is his ultimate fate, contemporary man is often incapable of facing his own death. In the unconscious, death is always the death of the other. The fear of death is intricately linked with the facing of the finality of one's being and the separation from one's loved ones. Therefore, it is unusual for a person to reflect upon death unless his own life is threatened or unless a close friend or relative is dying.

Fear of Dying

Fear of dying should not be confused with fear of death. Death is the ultimate moment of the cessation of life, and dying is the process whereby that moment is approached. Fear of dying is actually a combination of fear of death and fear of living in dread of death. Whether a man is dying at home or in a hospital, he cannot escape the agony of dying. Writings of doctors who attended many death beds give vivid descriptions of patients ravaged by pain and disease to such a point that they were either beyond caring or were a foul-smelling embarrassment to their family and friends. On the other hand, dying in a hospital's impersonal environment surrounded by machines and by unfamiliar staff cannot be glamorized either. The technology which has given us the knowledge and equipment to prolong life is greatly responsible for "the medicalization of death" which we see today. Death is no longer synonymous with the irreversible loss of consciousness. It is a technical phenomenon obtained by cessation of care based upon the decision of the doctor and the family. The management of a dying patient ends with the onset of irreversible coma—and what is left afterward is management of death. Death has been dissected and seen as a phenomenon of several steps—cessation of consciousness, cessation of breathing, and cessation of brain activity, manifested by a flat electroencephalogram. The fear of dying also involves the dread of protracted death.

The fear of dying is further compounded by the following factors: (a) helplessness over the hopelessness of the treatment; (b) self-blame and guilt feelings; (c) fear of physical injury, multilation, and crippled existence; and (d) fear of being abandoned.

A dying person continues to hope for a miraculous recovery; but when the hopelessness of the treatment becomes quite evident, a strange sense of helplessness comes over the patient. He starts blaming himself for not having taken good care of himself. He may also feel guilty over his conduct and may see the terminal illness as some kind of punishment. The fear of physical injury and multilation from a drastic investigative procedure, chemo-, radio-, and/or surgical therapy is not to be discounted. Finally, the fear of a crippled existence and of being left alone to die in isolation away from family, friends, and children is present in the back of the mind of every terminal patient.

Emotional Reactions in the Face of Death

Terminally ill patients often go through a series of five stages in accepting the reality of their impending death (4). The duration of these stages and the intensity and sequence with which they are experienced are highly variable from one individual to the next. The stages are:
1. Shock and denial;
2. Anger;
3. Bargaining;
4. Depression;
5. Acceptance.

During the *first stage*, when the patient is informed of his diagnosis and poor prognosis, he is usually unable to "hear" it. Some patients may be shocked and surprised temporarily, but a profound sense of disbelief in the physician's pronouncements keeps them calm. They may go from physician to physician to find someone to tell them what they would like to hear—that their condition is not serious. This denial of illness can be best summed up in a phrase—"No, not me." Eventually, all such attempts are deemed to be futile and the patient has to face reality.

During the *stage of anger* it is often difficult to deal with the patient. He complains about his care and, as a result, he is often avoided by his family, friends, and physicians. This rejection further increases his rage. He is likely to ask "Why me?" He often feels cheated and envious of others. If a person does not feel guilty and lose his self-esteem, he is likely, after this period of anger, to move on to the stage of bargaining. On the other hand, if he feels that he deserves punishment for his past doings as an explanation of his illness, he is likely to become very depressed. From being very "mad" he moves to being very "sad."

During the *stage of bargaining* the dominant theme is—"Yes, it is me, but. . ." With the realization of an impending death the patient, in exchange for the prolongation of his life, offers to do things which he did not do before or to live his life differently. A number of patients go thruogh a religious experience, and some of them believe that they are "born again." Often at this stage the patient will look comfortable and peaceful, but that sense of well-being is short lived. As the illness advances and suffering is compounded, the patient becomes depressed.

During the *stage of depression* the reality of death sinks even deeper. The patient may have already gone through many real (and imagined) losses by this time; e.g., he may have lost a body organ, or he may have missed important events in the life of his family, or he may have lost his job or his savings. Depression at this stage is not so much compounded by anger as it is colored with resignation. The patient begins to separate himself from everyone and everything he loved before. At this time he does not want any false hopes. It is a very private and personal time in his life. He may not want any visitors and may not even say much to his own immediate family members. He wants his family's love, affection, and respect but may not be able to give them anything in return. He may exhaust his caregivers by developing regressive behavior patterns, such as failing to accomplish activities of daily living of which he is capable, making many small demands, and becoming incontinent. This stage is very difficult for the family.

Finally, when the patient has finished his business—experienced anger and experienced grief—he moves to the *stage of acceptance*. If the patient has the strong support of his family, he will go through all stages to arrive at his final stage of equanimity characterized by tranquility—where the patient is neither happy nor sad. He may simply say "My time is coming close," "It is all right," or "I am ready," etc.

CARE OF A DYING PERSON

The vast majority of patients who experience prolonged but predictable dying are patients with terminal cancer. This discussion focuses on terminal care, much or all of which can be provided out of hospital. Chapter 8 covers the care of the cancer patient before the terminal stage.

Patients are often quite realistically concerned about the impact of their terminal illness and its expensive treatment on their family. The dying person needs to know that he is loved and will always be loved and missed, but at this stage he should not be told how much he is needed for the survival of the family.

Clearly a general physician may see a terminal patient at any moment in the course of the illness, e.g., he may himself diagnose the patient and inform him of the poor prognosis; or he may become involved in the care after the diagnosis has been made at a hospital and the patient has been sent home (or to a hospice) to receive terminal care. In order to provide excellent care for a terminally ill patient, the physician should know his patient as a person. The physician should make a determination not only of the stage of the terminal illness, but also of the patient's psychological stage of accepting impending death (see above). Terminally ill patients' needs differ widely, and every effort should be made to provide care which is adapted to these unique needs.

Often terminally ill patients receive attention during the early stages of their illness, when the diagnosis is first made, but unfortunately attention wanes as their disease progresses. The stages of denial, anger, and depression often cause a withdrawal of family, friends, and physicians which establishes a vicious cycle; i.e., the more the patients are ignored, the more unmanageable and inaccessible they become. For these reasons, the most important principle of the care of a terminal patient is to maintain a *consistency* of involvement. The physician should plan regular contacts with the patient, either by scheduling office visits or making visits to the home. The patient must be reassured that he will continue to get adequate medication to relieve his pain and suffering. However, the most important thing about the continued and consistent involvement in the care of a dying person is that the physician's continued presence gives dignity to the dying person. The patient continues to feel like a *person* till the very end.

Communication

Communication of Diagnosis, Treatment Plan, and Prognosis

People have different opinions about the need and importance of communication of the diagnosis, treatment plan, and prognosis of terminal patients. A common practice in the past has been to maintain a conspiracy of silence where the physician in collusion with the family members actively has covered up the diagnosis of a terminal illness in order to "protect" the dying man from emotional shock. This practice is now recognized usually to be wrong. Honesty and sincerity in dealing with terminally ill patients make effective management possible. Although patients may get temporarily upset in the beginning, they appreciate the truth in the long run. Moreover, it is then easier for their families to relate to them in an open and honest manner. Families participating in a conspiracy of silence have greater emotional difficulties than do families in situations where truth has prevailed. Occasionally, a patient will indicate that he does not want to know the unpleasant truth; in that case, the physician should respect the patient's wish. However, invariably these patients come to know the nature of their illness even if it has not been expressed to them.

When the physician is ready to discuss the diagnosis and expected course of the illness with his terminally ill patient, he should sit down with the patient and his family in a private place. He should avoid lengthy introductions. He should be precise and concise and should not be hurried. It is important that he pay attention to the emotional reactions of the patient and of the family members; silent pauses, followed by verbal acknowledgement of the patient's emotional reactions, are usually much more helpful than details about the patient's disease. He should also pledge that he will do whatever can be done to reduce suffering as much as possible, and should affirm that he will be involved and supportive to the very end. A majority of patients "do not hear" the bad news when it is first delivered and must be told the truth in small doses in the course of several interviews.

Communication of Positive Attitudes of Caregivers

More important than all the kind words of the physician is the nonverbal message the dying person gets from his caregivers. It is extremely important that the physician and his staff continue to maintain positive and consistent attitudes toward the patient. Genuine *concern* should be visible in both words and deeds as well as *equanimity* on the part of the caregivers, which is often the most reassuring element in the care of the terminally ill. It not only reduces the patient's anxiety, but also makes it easier for him to express his feelings and to ask questions without worrying about the physician's emotional state. It makes honest communication possible.

Management of Pain, Anxiety, Depression, Delirium

Pain

Over 50% of patients with cancer have significant pain during the terminal stage of their illness. Therefore, a very basic principle in the care of these patients is to provide adequate relief of pain. This often requires the administration of narcotics. Narcotics do not always eliminate the perception of pain but by diminishing the patient's affective response to pain, they reduce his distress. Because of the physician's fear of inducing addiction, patients may receive doses of narcotics that are too small or too infrequent to relieve pain adequately. Physicians should be aware that the risk of addiction, in this setting, is slight and that narcotics should be given on schedule (not "as occasion requires"), including at night, when it is preferable to disturb the patient for his medication than to wait for pain to waken him.

Important considerations in selecting medication for pain are effectiveness, route of administration (e.g., the cachectic patient may have few sites for injections), available forms for oral administration (e.g., some patients may be able to take only liquids easily; liquid morphine is especially useful for such patients), and duration of pain relief. Table 19.1 summarizes practical information about a number of narcotics which are used in controlling pain. All narcotic analgesics may cause the following *side effects*: sedation, respiratory depression, emesis, suppression of cough, constipation, bladder spasm, or urinary retention. Because of the likelihood of constipation, a bulk laxative such as Metamucil should be started when regular narcotics are prescribed. The synthetic narcotics may cause less nausea and constipation than does morphine; however, they may also produce less euphoria than morphine at equivalent analgesic doses.

In order to determine the appropriate dose of a narcotic, pain control should be assessed approximately 1 hour after a dose is given. If the patient reports that he is not getting good relief from pain, the next dose should be higher. In order to determine the appropriate interval between doses, pain control should be assessed at the end of an interval. If the patient reports that pain control regularly abates before the next dose of narcotic, the dosing interval should be reduced.

Because of the problem of oversedation and respiratory suppression, it is unwise to use multiple narcotics simultaneously. If one agent is not providing adequate relief, another drug should be substituted for, not added to, that agent. Table 19.1 gives the approximate equianalgesic doses of commonly used doses of narcotics.

Phenothiazines such as fluphenazine 2 to 10 mg daily (see Chapter 16), and tricyclic antidepressants, such as a amitriptyline 25 to 100 mg daily (see Chapter 15), used alone or in combination, may provide significant relief from the anxiety and depression accompanying intractable pain; and at times these drugs may diminish the patient's need for narcotic analgesics. Antihistamines such as hydroxyzine (Atarax, Vistaril) may be useful in this situation also, as noted below.

Anxiety

The physician's concern and accessibility may be all that are necessary to relieve the anxiety of the dying patient. *Tranquilizers* also can be of some help in the management of these patients. Commonly prescribed tranquilizers belong to the benzodiazapine group; their use for the control of anxiety is described in detail in Chapter 13. When insomnia is also a major problem, a benzodiazepine hypnotic can be used to induce sleep (see Table 85.6). Hydroxyzine (Atarax, Vistaril), another important minor tranquilizer, has a number of properties which may make it more beneficial than one of the benzodiazepines (1). It has not only sedative but has antispasmodic, antiemetic, and (when given intramuscularly) analgesic effects. In this regard, hydroxyzine has advantages over phenothiazines, which are not analgesic and which may produce hypotension. Hydroxyzine, 25 to 50 mg by mouth, three times daily is often prescribed to patients who have anxiety as the result of prolonged pain.

Table 19.1.
Selected Drugs for Treating Pain

Constituents	Trade Name	Available Preparations	Usual Dose Range[a]	Approximate Equivalent Intramuscular Dose of Morphine	Peak Effect (Hr)	Duration (Hr)	Federal Narcotic Schedule
MODERATELY POTENT							
Codeine phosphate		Tablets 30,60 mg; Injectable 10 mg/5 ml	30–120 mg	2–10 mg	2	3–4	II
Codeine-acetaminophen[b]	Tylenol #3; Tylenol #4	Tablets (30 mg codeine); Tablets (60 mg codeine); Elixir (12 mg codeine/5 ml)	1–2 tablets; 1 tablet; 15–30 ml	2 mg	2; 2	3–4; 3–4	III
Oxycodone[c]-aspirin-phenacetin-caffeine	Percodan	Tablets (5 mg oxycodone)	1–3 tablets	2–4 mg	1	3–4	II
Oxycodone[c]-acetaminophen	Tylox[d]; Percocet[b]	Capsules (5 mg oxycodone); Tablets (5 mg ocycodone)	1–3 capsules; 1–3 tablets	2–4 mg; 2–4 mg	1	3–4	II
MOST POTENT							
Morphine sulfate[a]		Liquid; Injectable 10 mg/ml; Tablets 5,10 mg	20–60 mg; 10–15 mg; 2.5–20 mg	4–10 mg	1/2; 1; 2	2–3; 3–4; 4–5	II; II; II
Methadone[c,f]	Dolophine	Injectable 10 mg/ml		4–10 mg; 10 mg	2	3–4	II
Meperidine[c]	Demerol	Tablets 50,100 mg; Syrup 50 mg/5 ml; Injectable 25 mg/ml, 50 mg/ml, 75 mg/ml, 100 mg/ml	50–300 mg	2–10 mg	2	3–4	II
Hydromorphone[c]	Dilaudid	Tablets 1,2,3,4 mg; Suppository 3 mg; Injectable 1 mg/ml, 2 mg/ml, 3 mg/ml, 4 mg/ml	2–8 mg; 1–2 mg	4–10 mg	1; 1/2	3–4; 3	II
Levorphanol[c,f]	Levo-Dromoran	Tablets 2 mg; Injectable 2 mg/ml; Tablets 50 mg	2–4 mg; 2 mg; 50–150 mg	5–10 mg; 10 mg; 2–10 mg	2; 1; 1	4–5; 4–5	II
Pentazocine[e]	Talwin	Injectable 30 mg/2 ml, 45 mg/2 ml, 60 mg/2 ml	60 mg	4–10 mg	1	3–4	IV

[a] Higher doses needed in patients who develop tolerance.
[b] Each tablet contains 300 mg of acetaminophen.
[c] Synthetic.
[d] Each capsule contains 500 mg of acetaminophen.
[e] A weak narcotic antagonist, may block analgesic effect of simultaneously administered narcotic and may cause abstinence reaction in patient dependent on narcotics.
[f] The plasma half-life of methadone and levorphanol is long (≥ 15 hours) and cumulative effects may occur with continual use of these drugs.

Depression

Most patients go through the depressive stage without requiring antidepressant medications, although periodically some may require antianxiety medications. The family's and the physician's support is most therapeutic for this kind of depression. Some patients develop severe depression, particularly after a brief stage of anger when they conclude that they are being punished for their sins. Loss of self-esteem, guilt feelings, psychomotor retardation, early morning awakening with a diurnal variation in mood, even suicidal thoughts, may appear in this setting. When five of the eight diagnostic criteria for depression are present (see Table 15.2), tricyclic antidepressants may bring relief. There is a detailed discussion of depression and its treatment in Chapter 15.

Delirium

Periodic or persistent delirium (inattentiveness, inaccessibility, nonrecognition of loved ones, gross confusion, *etc*) is very common in the final days or weeks of terminal disease (5). The cause is almost always an identifiable metabolic derangement, excess analgesic or psychotropic medication, tumor metastasis to the brain, or a combination of these factors. Loss of clear communication due to delirium is very distressing to the patient's family. Management of easily reversible causes is therefore very important except in the patient whose death is imminent. A list of the principal causes of delirium is found in Chapter 17.

Special Concerns for the Family

Gratification of Small Needs

Removing restrictions from food, alcohol, and cigarettes is not only humane but sensible.

Access to the Children

A dying person has a great need to have access to his children. Likewise, children have a great need to be close to their dying parent. The physician should encourage these necessary contacts.

Emotional Support for the Family

The emotional problems of the family of a dying person need attention from the physician. Family members often go through stages of emotional adjustment and have difficulties in accepting the diagnosis and projected course of a terminal illness, just as the patient does. By encouraging honest communication between the patient and his family, the physician can make an important contribution in the care of the dying person. Family members will react differently to the impending death of a person, depending on his age, personality, role, and the status of his relationship with the rest of the family members. To be effective, the physician must be sensitive to these variations and to the needs of individual family members.

An excellent booklet for families, *Taking Time*, is available from the National Cancer Institute (Bethesda, MD 20205). It was prepared by terminal cancer patients and their families to help others deal with many draining and awkward experiences they will face.

Often, there is time for a dying patient or the patient and his family to decide whether cardiopulmonary resuscitation or other extraordinary life supports are wanted in the event of a sudden change in status. With skill, the personal physician can help both patient and family to express their preference. As this preference is frequently not to have "heroic" intervention, the patient will be spared inappropriate care in the event that a physician who is unfamiliar with him may render care in a crisis.

Hospice Care

In many communities, patients and their families can be cared for by their physician in cooperation with a hospice, a program devised to provide terminal care, including relief of pain, to the dying patient and to provide support to his family. Services are delivered either in the patient's home or in a hospital by a multidisciplinary team under the direction of the physician (see *The Management of Terminal Disease* in the "General References" list).

In hospice care the primary focus of the physician changes from curing to caring, and the overall goal changes from prolongation of life to the enhancement of the quality of life during the patient's final days. Since the introduction of the hospice movement in the United States and founding of the first hospice here in 1974, more than 1000 hospices have become operational. This mushrooming of programs may create an erroneous impression that hospice type care can only be provided in hospices. Comprehensive humanistic treatment for the dying patient and his family can be offered by any physician right in the patient's home. Home health agencies can play a pivotal role in this care (see Chapter 9). The essential ingredients of the delivery of hospice type care at home are (a) the physician's knowledge and skill in prescribing for symptom relief; (b) his willingness and ability to work with a multidisciplinary team; and (c) his willingness to spend extra time and effort to foresee and alleviate the many problems faced by the dying patient and his family. Recent surveys have shown that dying patients and their families report particular satisfaction when the place of care is changed at appropriate moments from acute medical services to hospice services or to home.

A clearing house for information on hospice care in the United States is provided by the National Hospice Organization, 1750 Old Meadow Road, McLean, VA 22102.

THE MANAGEMENT OF GRIEF

If death of a loved one has been unexpected, grief usually begins with an initial stage of shock and disbelief accompanied by a general numbing of all affect. If death has been anticipated, however, this stage is less prominent. There is often a feeling of relief that the dead person's suffering has ended. Soon afterward (within hours to a few days) there is a more demonstrative phase characterized by protest and anguish, often accompanied by tears. These feelings come in waves and may be precipitated by even an indirect reference to the lost person; ordinarily, they do not persist for more than 1 or 2 months. Mourning, however, normally with a slow recovery over a period of a year, is virtually universal. As time passes there often is a preoccupation with memories of the lost person. Guilt feelings for not having done enough for the deceased are very common. In some cases, this guilt may be expressed as hostility toward the physician. Bereaved people often have experiences of "seeing" the dead person in a crowd or in some other individual, fleetingly seen, which is then followed by the reality of permanent loss. The bereaved is likely to visit the grave during the first year of loss more frequently than in later years. Sometimes, there is a dramatic change in personality, and the manners and the terminal symptoms of the dying individual are assumed by the bereaved person. This is another way of resolving grief, by attempting to make the lost person a part of the survivor.

Approximately 80% of bereaved people are depressed and have disturbed sleep; 40% have a poor appetite, weight loss, difficulty in concentrating, and general loss of interest in daily life (2). Depression is especially common in spouses in the middle or later years of their lives. In fact, one-third of this latter group have symptoms which meet the criteria of a diagnosis of a probable affective disorder (Chapter 15) (3). While depression usually lasts for many months, 80% of individuals do show some improvement within 10 weeks (3). However, two-thirds of bereaved spouses at the end of the first year of bereavement continue to have some symptoms of apathy, aimlessness, and a disinclination to look to the future. Only a small fraction of these survivors develop complicated and/or atypical mourning.

The *management of normal grief* during the first year of bereavement should be individualized, depending on the patient's personal, family, and social background. Some bereaved persons may need short term medication for the relief of insomnia and anxiety. A benzodiazepine hypnotic (Chapter 85) at bedtime if needed for sleep, or one of the benzodiazapines with a shorter half-life (Chapter 13) two or three times a day as needed for anxiety, should be considered for 1 to 2 weeks in the management of normal grief. On the other hand, many patients may feel quite satisfied with an empathetic, supportive,

and concerned physician. These patients need to be reminded that their grief and its psychophysiological concomitants are normal. This has to be done with special care, acknowledging the irreparable loss while, at the same time, encouraging the bereaved person to pull his life together. The survivors need to be encouraged to lead a full life without feeling guilty. When severe emotional reactions become prolonged, pastoral counseling or psychotherapy may be necessary. Patients with physical symptoms without any clear-cut organic etiology should not be referred to a psychiatrist at first; but they should be seen frequently, examined carefully, and reassured of their physical health. Extensive diagnostic work-ups should be avoided as much as possible as they reinforce illness behavior. Furthermore, supportive therapy (see Chapter 11) is more likely to be helpful than is more extensive and complicated psychotherapy. In time, with the completion of their grieving reaction, they will give up their physical symptoms and again become actively engaged in a new life.

During the first year of bereavement special attention should be paid to the patient during holidays, anniversaries, or on other important dates. Some symptoms of acute grief are likely to resurface around these times. Supportive therapy at such times will usually control the symptoms.

The physician is in a good position to detect the early signs of *pathological mourning* when a person either shows no signs of grieving or shows the exaggerated features of grieving characterized by excessive and/or prolonged (longer than a year) social isolation, unmoderated guilt or anger, panic attacks, and physical symptoms without any clear-cut organic etiology. In such cases, consultation with a psychiatrist is appropriate to help remove obstacles which have inhibited the mourner from undergoing a normal grief reaction (6).

General References

Bowlby J: *Separation.* New York, Basic Books, 1973.
> This is the second volume of Bowlby's classic work on attachment and loss, and deals with the issues of anxiety and anger generated in the anticipation of and in the event of separation from a loved one.

Bowlby J: *Loss.* New York, Basic Books, 1980.
> This is the third and final volume of Bowlby's work on attachment and loss. This is probably the best book ever written on the subject of bereavement.

It's Your Choice, the Practical Guide to Planning a Funeral. Glenview, IL, Scott Foresman, 1982.
> A practical paperback on making funeral plans in the face of impending death.

Kübler-Ross E: *On Death and Dying.* New York, Macmillan, 1969.
> A classic work on the subject of death and dying.

Reuler JB, Girard DA, Nardone DA: The chronic pain syndrome: misconceptions and management. *Ann Intern Med* 93:588, 1980.
> Excellent review by general internists, that covers both psychogenic and organic aspects of chronic pain, physiology of placebo effect, drug treatment of terminal cancer pain, nondrug modalities (transcutaneous nerve stimulation, acupuncture, neurological block/ablation biofeedback, hypnosis, behavior modification).

Saunders C (ed): *The Management of Terminal Disease.* Chicago, Year Book, 1978.

This book is an excellent guide to any professional involved in the care of a dying patient; it includes a complete discussion of the hospice concept.

Specific References

1. Beaver WT, Fleise G: Comparison of the anaglesic effects of morphine, hdyroxyzine, and their combination in patients with postoperative pain. In Bonica JJ, Albe-Fessard D (eds): *Advances in Pain Research and Therapy.* New York, Raven Press, 1976, vol 1, p 553.
2. Clayton PJ, Halikas JA, Maurice WL: The bereavement of the widowed. *Dis Nerv Syst* 32:597, 1971.
3. Clayton PJ, Halikas JA, Maurice WL: The depression of widowhood. *Br J Psychiatry* 120:71, 1972.
4. Kübler-Ross E: *On Death and Dying.* New York, Macmillan, 1969, chap 3–7.
5. Massie MJ, Holland J, Glass E: Delirium in terminally ill cancer patients. *Am J Psychiatry* 140:1048, 1983.
6. Melges FT, DeMaso DR: Grief-resolution therapy: relieving, revising, and revisiting. *Am J Psychother* 34:51, 1980.

CHAPTER TWENTY

Tobacco Use and Dependence

GEORGE E. BIGELOW, Ph.D., CAROL S. HAINES, M.D. M.P.H., AND MAXINE L. STITZER, Ph.D.

Chronic tobacco use, primarily in the form of cigarette smoking, is the most pernicious of the substance abuse disorders and represents the greatest single cause of chronic illness, disability, and death in the United States. The perniciousness of the habit relates largely to smoking's long history of broad social acceptability, and to the reluctance by society and by many health professionals to recognize smoking as a health-damaging behavior deserving professional medical attention.

Physicians must deal with patients' tobacco dependency primarily in two contexts: (*a*) occasional self-motivated patients who request aid or advice in quitting smoking or in managing the tobacco abstinence syndrome, and most commonly (*b*) relatively unmotivated patients whose smoking either contributes to their illness or increases their risk of illness.

The purpose of this chapter is 2-fold: (*a*) to provide an overview of current scientific information concerning tobacco use and dependence, and (*b*) to provide specific recommendations concerning how the practicing physician should respond to patients' tobacco use.

ETIOLOGY

The determinants of tobacco dependence are uncertain. The smoking habit is so widespread that it defies substantial correlation with discrete environmental, physiological, or psychological factors. Smoking typically begins in the teenage years or in early adulthood. It appears that social influences (e.g., peer pressures, efforts to display independence and to appear mature and self-confident) are major factors in promoting and sustaining initial smoking experiences (4). The aversive properties of those initial experiences (e.g., coughing, nausea, dysphoria) are described even by individuals who subsequently develop into chronic dependent smokers. Nicotine is generally presumed to be the active pharmacological agent responsible for maintaining the habit. Whatever the factors that sustain smoking through the period of initial exposure, those individuals who do persist in the exposure are highly likely to become chronic dependent smokers.

Risk Factors

Despite our inability to identify causal factors, it is possible to identify certain risk factors associated with increased likelihood of becoming a chronic cigarette smoker. Chief among these is *family history*. Cigarette smoking runs in families, and this is generally thought to be due to a social modeling process. An individual with parents and siblings who smoke is 4 times as likely to become a smoker as is an individual from a nonsmoking family. This familial relationship can sometimes be used persuasively to motivate parents with young children to stop smoking in an effort to reduce the likelihood that their children will adopt the habit. The possibility of genetic or physiological predisposing factors accounting for this familial aggregation has received little study, but data from twin studies suggest some genetic contribution (9).

Since smokers almost universally begin the habit during *adolescence or early adulthood*, age is a significant risk factor for initiation of smoking; it is the rare smoker who acquires the habit at an age beyond the early twenties. In the past males were more likely to smoke than females, but this is no longer the case. There is a modest inverse relationship between smoking prevalence and both educational level and socioeconomic status. There is no personality type which is characteristic of smokers, but on the average they tend to be somewhat more extroverted than nonsmokers, to be more adventuresome or risk taking, and to be more likely to deviate from social norms or rules. These latter characteristics may, in adolescence, increase the probability of experimenting with smoking—with a consequent increased risk of chronic dependence.

PRIMARY PREVENTION

Because of the relatively narrow age window during which individuals are at risk for becoming smokers, it is necessary that primary prevention efforts be directed to adolescents and preadolescents. Unfortunately, the age of greatest risk is also the age of greatest resistance to the influence of parents and other authorities. It is thought that the optimal timing of formal preventive interventions is at the fourth, fifth, and sixth grade levels in school. Some progress is being made in developing effective preventive interventions for this age group (14). These interventions focus upon teaching specific behavioral skills for resisting social pressure and include explicit instruction and rehearsal with peers in vignettes about resisting cigarettes. Teaching about the health risks of smoking is appropriate and necessary, but has weak preventive effects in the absence of behavioral skill training. Due to the nature of preventive interventions it is unlikely that physicians will play a major role in this area. However, physicians should advocate and support the implementation of preventive programs, and should support restrictions on tobacco advertising directed toward or glamourizing smoking for youth.

RECOGNITION AND DIAGNOSIS

The greatest impediment to effective professional response to smoking is the widespread failure of health professionals to recognize and diagnose tobacco dependence and to treat it as an active problem when it is identified. The determination of smoking status should be a regular part of the examination and should not be treated as an item in the history to be recorded only at initial contact.

Only infrequently will patients present with the primary complaint of tobacco dependence, although certainly a small number of patients will initiate requests to their physician for advice on smoking cessation. In such cases the physician can generally rely upon the patient's reports of the extent and nature of the tobacco habit. Far more common is the smoker whose visit is not motivated by a concern about smoking. In these less motivated patients it is wise not to rely completely upon a negative response to the question "Do you smoke?"; some patients, especially those who recognize the ill effects of smoking, will "quit" a few hours or perhaps a day before their appointments. A more accurate depiction of current smoking status is revealed by such questions as "Have you ever been a smoker?" and "When did you last have a cigarette?"

Diagnostic Criteria

Tobacco dependence is now recognized as a substance abuse disorder in the third edition of the American Psychiatric Association's *Diagnostic and Statistical Manual of Mental Disorders* (DSM-III). Diagnostic criteria include regular smoking of at least 1 month's duration, and at least one of the following: (*a*) tobacco withdrawal syndrome; (*b*) failure to quit smoking in serious prior attempts; or (*c*) continuing to smoke despite a severe tobacco-related illness. In practice, there is rarely a need to rely upon these formal diagnostic criteria.

Objective Assessment

In virtually all patients the assessment of smoking status will be based solely upon patient self-report. However, under some conditions it may be desirable to assess smoking status with an objective biological assay. Three primary indices can be used: (a) thiocyanate, a product of the cyanide compounds in tobacco, can be measured in blood, saliva, or urine; (b) cotinine, the major metabolite of nicotine, can be measured in blood, saliva, or urine; or (c) carbon monoxide, a combustion product, can be measured in blood (as carboxyhemoglobin) or in expired breath. While none of these is in routine clinical use, all are widely used in clinical research. Assessment of carbon monoxide (CO) concentrations in expired breath is the least intrusive and least expensive procedure and is widely used in smoking cessation programs (7). Devices for measuring breath CO that would be suitable for routine office use are currently marketed for about $1000. Some smoking experts have suggested that office assessment of expired breath CO should become as routine as the recording of blood pressure. The value of objective assessment of smoking status is indicated by the fact that up to 20 to 30% of self-reported quitters may show biological evidence of continuing to smoke.

COURSE OF THE HABIT

Until recently, the typical course of the habit was one of relatively unabated chronic smoking from the time of initiation throughout the remainder of the smoker's life. In more recent years, as the health hazards of smoking have become more widely recognized and as the social acceptability of smoking has declined, there has been a growing tendency for smokers to discontinue the habit. Now, in the United States there are nearly as many former smokers (approximately 30 million) as there are current smokers (approximately 50 million).

Most continuing smokers feel considerable ambivalence about their habit. Over one-half of current smokers report having made at least one serious attempt to stop smoking, and about 90% of smokers say they would like to quit if there were an easy method to do so. About 30% of smokers report that they have made an active attempt to stop smoking within the preceding year. As described below, advice from physicians can be a potent force in promoting increased cessation efforts by patients.

Patterns of Quitting and Relapse

Approximately 60 to 80% of smokers who attempt to quit achieve at least a minimal period of abstinence. However, the relapse rate is high, and approximately two-thirds of quitters resume smoking within 3 to 6 months, often within only a few days. Only 15 to 20% of quitters remain cigarette free for 6 months or more.

A cessation attempt should not be considered successful until at least 6 months of abstinence have been sustained. The probability of relapse following 6 months of abstinence is relatively small. About 1% of smokers permanently quit each year, yielding about one-half million new ex-smokers annually.

Smokers express interest in a wide variety of aids for cessation. Most popular are instructional and self-help aids that smokers can use at their own convenience. A substantial proportion of smokers express interest in formal cessation treatment programs; but when such services are offered, even at optimal cost and convenience, fewer than 10% of those expressing interest will actually attend.

Approximately 95% of smoking cessation occurs as the result of smokers' self-directed personal efforts, without formal treatment. Abrupt (so-called "cold turkey") cessation is more likely to be successful than are approaches involving gradual reduction. Most quitters require more than one attempt before becoming successful ex-smokers. The probability of success actually increases with successive attempts.

The physician should recognize that cyclic quitting and relapse are characteristic of the normal, successful cessation process. Smokers are vulnerable to interpreting initial relapse as proof of an inability to quit. When relapse occurs the physician should offer nonjudgmental understanding coupled with encouragement to plan another cessation attempt.

The risk of relapse to smoking is increased (a) when patients are under emotional stress (e.g., anger, frustration, anxiety, depression); (b) when ex-smokers are exposed to cues associated with prior smoking (e.g., after meals, when consuming alcoholic beverage); and (c) in individuals whose spouse or friends continue to smoke (19).

HEALTH CONSEQUENCES

Risk of Disease

Although smoking dramatically increases overall population morbidity and mortality, its effects on individual smokers are unpredictable, and some smokers will escape major health consequences. The overall mortality rate for smokers is 70% greater than that for nonsmokers; the mortality rate for the two-pack-a-day smoker is twice that of an age-matched nonsmoker. Life expectancy is significantly shortened by smoking, being 8.1 years less for the 30-year-old, two-pack-a-day smoker than for a comparable nonsmoker. Risk is dose related, in that it increases with increasing number of cigarettes smoked, with increasing number of years smoking, with depth of inhalation, and with increasing yield of tar and nicotine of the cigarettes smoked.

Smoking is associated with increased risk of cancer (especially of the respiratory tract), cardiovascular disease, chronic obstructive pulmonary disease, and gastric ulcer. Smoking by pregnant women reduces fetal growth, and therefore birth weight, and increases the risk of fetal death; smoking interacts with the use of oral contraceptives by women and increases their risk of myocardial infarction, subarachnoid hemorrhage, and thromboembolic disease.

The risks of cancer and of chronic pulmonary disease in smokers are 10-fold the risks in nonsmokers. The risk of atherosclerotic cardiovascular disease is approximately doubled in smokers. Because of the much greater population prevalence of cardiovascular disease, it is in this area that the greatest overall health benefits of smoking cessation occur.

While it is important that patients understand the risks associated with smoking and be motivated to discontinue the habit, it is not generally necessary for the physician to emphasize this global risk information. Surveys indicate high public awareness that smoking is a health risk. Simple knowledge of risk or fear of adverse health consequences is not an effective motivator for changing complex, ingrained habits such as smoking. Advice to patients should be brief, highly personal, and not laden with threatening or terrifying images. It is better to stress positive outcomes to be gained rather than traumas to be avoided (see details under "Treatment" below).

Benefits of Cessation

The greatest immediate benefit of smoking cessation is the reduction of cardiovascular risk. Within hours of smoking cessation both carbon monoxide and nicotine, the two cigarette products thought to be primarily responsible for cardiovascular disease, are dissipated from the body, with a consequent reduction in cardiac work requirement concurrent with an increase in oxygenation. There is also prompt reduction in the risk for upper respiratory infection. Slower to accrue is a reduction in the rate of pulmonary decline and a reduction in cancer risk; benefits of cessation are measureable in these domains within 3 to 5 years after smoking cessation.

Health benefits of smoking cessation are greater for those smokers who quit prior to the development of symptoms; however, the benefits of cessation can extend to those individuals who have already experienced symptoms of smoking-related disease. For example, individuals who stop smoking after myocardial infarction have improved survival rates compared to those who continue smoking (2).

Abstinence Syndrome and Craving

Upon cessation of smoking, an abstinence syndrome may occur. The physiological correlates of the tobacco abstinence syndrome are generally in-consequential, consisting of a slight and gradual decline in heart rate and blood pressure. However, the subjective aspects of the syndrome can be very distressing to patients. Symptoms can include irritability, restlessness, sleep disturbances, difficulty in concentrating, anxiety, gastrointestinal disturbances, hunger, weight gain, and most important, craving for cigarettes. Relatively little is known about the course of the tobacco abstinence syndrome, but most patients feel normal again within approximately 2 weeks of abstinence, except that craving for tobacco may persist for months or years (5, 20).

In an effort to reduce the intensity of withdrawal discomfort some practitioners recommend that patients preparing for cessation should reduce their level of dependence by reducing their number of cigarettes per day or by smoking a brand of lower nicotine and tar yield for 2 to 3 weeks prior to the quit date. It is not clear whether this strategy has any merit.

Recently nicotine chewing gum has been approved as a prescription drug in the United States (see details below). Its primary purpose is to facilitate tobacco abstinence by suppressing the abstinence syndrome. Prior to the availability of nicotine gum there was no specific treatment available for the tobacco abstinence syndrome.

Craving for tobacco is an extraordinarily persistent obstacle to sustained abstinence. More than an occasional ex-smoker reports craving 5 or even 10 years after cessation. The duration of craving is highly variable, but it should be expected to persist for at least 3 to 6 months, with its frequency and urgency diminishing over that interval.

Low Yield Cigarettes

Because the risks of smoking are dose related, it is reasonable to advise patients that, even in the absence of total cessation, risks are decreased by reducing the amount of smoke intake. This might be achieved by any of a variety of techniques—reducing the number of cigarettes smoked, taking fewer or smaller puffs per cigarette, inhaling less, or switching to a cigarette with lower tar and nicotine yield. Epidemiological data generally indicate that the overall risks are lower among individuals smoking lower yield cigarettes. However, as a cautionary note, it should be mentioned that these epidemiological data were generally collected at a time when the average tar and nicotine yield of marketed cigarettes was considerably higher than it is today. In the mid-1950s the average yield was 2 to 3 times the level of cigarettes in the 1980s; the extent to which the earlier data can be extrapolated to the present era is not clear. Several reports have appeared in recent years suggesting that variations in current tobacco yields may have relatively little health impact (11, 21).

When patients switch to lower yield cigarettes they should be cautioned not to change the pattern of their smoking in a compensatory fashion that could maintain the same biological intake of smoke—e.g., by smoking more cigarettes or inhaling more smoke. Extensive research has documented that such compensatory behavioral changes are common when cigarette yields are changed (8, 23). Cross-sectional studies of smokers have found negligible correlations between the stated yield of the brand smoked and blood levels of nicotine and its major metabolite, cotinine (1). Thus, it appears that biological yield may differ substantially from the yield values published by the Federal Trade Commission.

Physicians and patients should understand that the published cigarette yields are not the "dosages" delivered to the smoker; the yield figures represent the delivery during standardized machine puffing assays. They do not represent either the content of the cigarette or the amount delivered to a human smoker. The delivery to the smoker depends upon how the individual smokes. The primary manufacturing technique for producing current low yield cigarettes is to place ventilation holes in the sides of the filter to dilute the smokestream with air. With these low yield brands it is especially likely that biological delivery will significantly exceed assay delivery since the smoker's fingers will tend partially to block these ventilation holes (12).

Passive Smoking

The long term effects of passive smoking—exposure of nonsmokers to air contaminated by the smoking of others—are not clear, although such exposure is certainly an irritant to many nonsmokers. In addition, data indicate that measurable amounts of smoke products are absorbed by those passively exposed, suggesting that passive exposure may have health effects. Although smoke products are detected in the blood and urine of passively exposed nonsmokers, the levels are quite low relative to those of smokers.

The strongest evidence for deleterious health effects of passive smoking comes from studies of nonsmokers in families with smokers. Nicotine metabolites are detected in the urine of infants of smoking mothers, indicating their uptake of the parent's smoke (6). Nonsmokers married to smokers have been found to have reduced forced midexpiratory flow rates (10). Children of smokers have been found to have increased rates of respiratory infections (16) and to have a slowed rate of increase in forced expiratory volume in 1 second (22).

The effects of maternal smoking on the developing fetus can also be considered an example of the adverse effects of passive smoke exposure. It is clear that maternal smoking contributes to reduced birth weight and that smokers who stop the habit during pregnancy have significantly heavier babies than those who continue smoking (18).

The adverse effects of smoking upon other family members—and especially on young children—might be effectively used in persuading smokers to attempt cessation. Also, as a general practice, physicians should try to protect nonsmokers from cigarette smoke. Smoking (including employee smoking) should be considerately but emphatically prohibited at the physician's practice site, and physicians should support similar efforts in all public settings, but especially in health care facilities.

TREATMENT

Role of the Physician

The primary role for the physician in the treatment of tobacco dependence is to encourage patients to stop smoking. Most smokers who quit the habit do so by their own self-directed efforts rather than by formal treatment. Therefore, interventions which motivate these self-directed efforts can have greater overall impact than formally organized treatment programs.

Physicians are in a uniquely effective position to encourage and motivate smoking cessation. A major reason that patients stop smoking is concern about their health, and smokers cite physicians as the individuals most able to influence their decisions to attempt to stop smoking. The appearance of specific smoking-related symptoms often serves as a stimulus for patients' efforts to break the smoking habit, although many patients continue smoking despite obvious disease.

The most prevalent error in physician management of the smoking patient is to do nothing. Despite the overwhelming adverse consequences of smoking, usually the smoking patient receives no communication from the physician. Only 25% of smokers report ever having any physician talk with them about their smoking.

Research indicates that brief physician advice giving can significantly increase rates of smoking cessation (13). The levels of cessation achieved will, however, vary considerably depending upon the patient population and the setting for contact. Studies have demonstrated a 3-fold increase in smoking cessation rates (from 1% to 3%) when physicians simply cautioned each smoker to quit during routine office visits for other problems. Additional efforts beyond the cautionary advice yield even higher quit rates. Physicians who also provide a take-home pamphlet with how-to-quit suggestions have generated quit rates of 7 to 12% in general practice. Investing a few more moments to negotiate a "quit date" in addition to delivering the cessation message increases the quit rate to 15%. Even higher cessation rates are reported in certain settings—prenatal care and coronary care settings, in particular. For example, reports indicate that the smoking cessation rate following a first myocardial infarction is approximately 50% for patients given directive smoking cessation advice by their physician, compared to about 35% for patients receiving usual care (2). Similarly high rates of cessation are seen in prenatal care settings—where up to 20 to 30% of smokers may quit during a pregnancy (18).

It is important to recognize at the outset that the achieved rates of cessation are likely always to be frustratingly low. In an individual practice small changes in smoking cessation rate will be unnoticed. However, in terms of overall health benefit to a patient population, routine smoking cessation advice from the physician can be very worthwhile; even the lowest figures cited above—a change from 1% to 3% cessation rates—would yield an additional 1 million ex-smokers per year in the United States.

It is important that the physician not allow the frustrations of the nonresponders to deter him from delivering beneficial health advice to those who would respond. There is a small minority of smokers who are so dramatically frustrating that physicians might overestimate the resistance of all smokers to cessation advice. The most extreme cases are those patients who smoke through tracheostomies or while in critical care units where oxygen is used. Overinvolvement with these highly resistant patients should be avoided, since it can drain the physician of enthusiasm and desire to assist more responsive and cessation-receptive patients.

Professional Communication

The physician is in a uniquely persuasive position as an authority figure, but has little in the way of medically specific skills, techniques, or remedies to offer the smoker. Rather, one must rely largely upon the patient's willingness to comply with medical advice. Therefore, it is the physician's responsibility to provide persuasive and motivating advice which will maximize the likelihood of patient compliance. A frequent failing in physician communication is excessive reliance upon fear as a motivator; fear is at best a weak motivator of complex behavior change, and at its worst may stimulate denial and resistance ·which will actually inhibit behavior change. Patient commitment and confidence are strengthened by enumerating the nonhealth benefits of smoking cessation—its importance to significant others, the financial savings, the increased self-esteem and sense of self-control which result.

The smoking advice to patients should be personally relevant, should describe in a positive way the benefits to be gained, and should directively prescribe a particular course of action. The communication can be made personally relevant (a) by pointing out the association between smoking and the specific symptoms, illnesses, or health risks of the individual patient; (b) by pointing out that smoking cessation can prevent, reverse, or stop the progression of disease (whichever is appropriate); and (c) by stating clearly, simply, and directively the course of action to be taken—to stop smoking. A general statement that "Smoking is bad for your health and you can kill yourself if you continue" fails on all three of these points. It is not specifically personal; it describes no benefit; and it is not sufficiently directive. Many patients will not perceive this as an instruction to stop smoking. A more personalized and directive statement can be more persuasive; for example: "I strongly advise you to stop smoking; especially for people like you who use oral contraceptives the risk of heart disease or stroke is very substantially increased as long as you continue to smoke"; or "Both your coughing and your recurring colds and flus are caused in part by your smoking; I want you to try to quit smoking, and then we should see some improvement."

Recommended Office Procedure

Described below is a three-step procedure for delivering brief, persuasive smoking cessation advice in office practice. The procedure requires less than 5 minutes and follows a structured format which ensures effective content to the message; without this structure it is easy to lose control both of time and of the content of the message. Use of the procedure is facilitated if the smoker completes a brief questionnaire, such as that shown in Figure 20.1, prior to the examination. The questionnaire provides cues to guide the physician through the structured procedure and makes it possible to tailor smoking cessation advice to the individual patient. Although the description below is based upon use of the questionnaire, this same three-step procedure can be readily adapted for use without the questionnaire.

Step 1: Focus on smoking. The opening sentence must specify the physician's intent, and preferably will begin with "I"; for example: "I am concerned that you are still smoking cigarettes and I want you to quit." A punctuating silence is effective here in gaining the smoker's attention. Then it is necessary to speak very specifically about the patient's personal status; items 1 to 4 from the questionnaire facilitate this. Example: "You have smoked two packs a day for 15 years; that is too much." An additional brief comment about the patient's health status, especially if it relates smoking to a complaint prompting the current visit, is advisable here. Next, repeat the smoker's aspirations as reflected in items 5 and 6. Example: "You must feel the same way, for I see you have tried to quit before and your desire to quit is quite high."

Step 2: Build confidence. "Quitting is extremely difficult, one of the most challenging things you can ask of yourself." This statement builds the smoker's

Francis Scott Key Medical Center
Medical Clinic
Smoker's Questionnaire

1. How many cigarettes a day do you smoke? _____ Cigarettes each day
   How many years have you been a smoker? _____ Years as a smoker

2. Have you ever had a job for 6 months or longer that exposed you to (circle one or more answers)
       Asbestos   Coal   Cotton Fiber   None of these

3. Has smoking harmed your health?   Yes   No

4. Have you ever tried to quit smoking?   Yes   No
   Were you ever successful in quitting for a full month?   Yes   No

5. How strong is your desire to quit smoking?   Let 0 = no desire and 10 = great desire. Give a number from 0 to 10 that rates your desire to quit: _____

6. Rate your chances of quitting smoking in the next 6 months:
   ____ Very sure that I will quit
   ____ Fairly sure that I will quit
   ____ Fairly sure that I won't quit
   ____ Very sure that I won't quit

People have different reasons for wanting to quit smoking. Are the following reasons for quitting *Not*, *Somewhat*, or *Very* important to you?

	How important to you?		
7. Food tastes better	Not	Somewhat	Very
8. Save money	Not	Somewhat	Very
9. Breath and clothes smell better	Not	Somewhat	Very
10. No more nagging from family and friends	Not	Somewhat	Very
11. More in control of myself	Not	Somewhat	Very
12. Set a good example for my kids	Not	Somewhat	Very
13. Get sick less often	Not	Somewhat	Very
14. Not so short of breath on stairs	Not	Somewhat	Very
15. Fewer colds and sinus problems	Not	Somewhat	Very

(6/84)

Figure 20.1.   Example of questionnaire useful in office smoking cessation counseling.

confidence in his physician; the physician establishes expertise—for this is one truth about smoking of which all smokers are certain—and compassion—because smokers and significant others are quick to berate their inability to quit. Next, the physician and smoker must agree that to quit is indeed beneficial. Items 7 to 15 will assist the physician in quickly reviewing patient-perceived benefits. The physician then adds firmly "I am confident your [specific health status] will improve also, and that you will find more energy and vitality." A final general confidence builder is to offer encouragement if a prior quit attempt has occurred. "You have quit before, and you can do it again. Almost all ex-smokers tried more than once."

Step 3: Contract for behavior change. Next it is mandatory that the physician obtain a commitment from the smoker. A contract, signed by both the physician and the patient, is useful. The example shown in Figure 20.2 provides a practical stepwise plan for the patient to follow. The physician describes each item in succession, pauses for emphasis, then inquires "Can you do that?" Every smoker should be approached with the first two requests—agreement to read the smoking cessation brochure, and agreement to tell important others that the doctor has told him or her to stop smoking; the other preparatory steps are discretionary. A *specific quit date* is very important. It should be within 3 weeks; beyond that time the likelihood that cessation will be attempted diminishes dramatically. Every effort should be made to have the patient phone the physician on the quit date. From one-third to one-half of smokers seen in ambulatory settings will agree on a quit date when this stepwise procedure is recommended.

Dr. John A. Smith, M.D.

For _____

Address _____ Date _____

℞

I AGREE TO:
___ Read *Quit for Good*
___ Tell people at home and work that Dr. Smith
wants me to stop smoking.
THESE ARE THE STEPS I'M READY TO TAKE:
___ Buy only by the pack
___ Switch brands every pack
___ Wait until ___ A.M. to have my first smoke
___ Write down every cigarette I smoke
I'M QUITTING. MY QUIT DATE IS: _____

Dr. Smith and I will permit ____ pounds weight gain
in the first 60 smoke-free days.

_____
Smoker's Signature
Refill 0-1-2-3-4 _____ M.D.

Figure 20.2. Example of a contract for specific steps
leading to smoking cessation.

Brochures for Office Use

Self-help brochures concerning smoking cessation
increase the efficacy of cessation advice by expanding the patient's understanding of cessation techniques. To be effective, though, provision of these
materials must be accompanied by directive physician advice to stop smoking; simply making smoking
brochures available within the office has minimal
effect.

Various smoking cessation brochures are available
and can generally be obtained by contacting local
offices of the American Lung Association, American
Heart Association, or American Cancer Society. One
superb office aid is the *Quit for Good* series (see
contents, Fig. 20.3). This series is produced by the
National Cancer Institute and is available to physicians without charge through its Office of Cancer
Communications (Room 10-A-18, National Cancer
Institute, Bethesda, MD 20205; phone (800)-4-CAN-
CER). An additional useful source of information
and materials about smoking and smoking cessation
is the US Public Health Service's Office on Smoking
and Health (Room 110 Park Building, 5600 Fishers
Lane, Rockville, MD 20857; phone (301)-443-5287 or
(301)-443-1690).

Nicotine Chewing Gum

Nicotine chewing gum, which has been available
for a number of years in Europe and Canada, was
approved in 1984 for marketing as a prescription
drug in the United States. The gum—a nicotine resin
complex—is to be used by individuals who have
stopped smoking, with the intent that the nicotine
substitution should reduce the likelihood of craving,
withdrawal discomfort, and smoking relapse. The
gum has documented therapeutic value when used
in this way. *It is important to understand, however,
that the gum is not intended for use by continuing
smokers who hope that the nicotine substitution will
induce either a cessation attempt or a reduction in
smoking*; rather, it is to be used as an aid for maintaining smoking cessation once the patient has made
the cessation decision and committed himself to that
decision. Thus, the physician must still engage in
persuasion and motivation and in the selection/
prescription of a quit date.

Available data indicate that use of nicotine chewing gum may approximately double the long term
smoking cessation rates which are achieved. The
absolute rates of cessation depend, of course, upon
the context. In organized cessation programs use of
the gum has led to cessation success rates of about
45% compared to about 20% in program participants
receiving placebo gum (17). In general office practice
prescription of nicotine gum in combination with
brief directive cessation advice from the physician
led to successful cessation in 9% of patients, compared to 4% in control patients receiving the advice
without the gum (15).

Nicotine gum is commercially available as Nicorette, in packages of 96 pieces. In 1984 the cost to
pharmacists was approximately $15 per package.
Each piece of gum contains 2 mg of nicotine—approximately equivalent to the nicotine yield of two
cigarettes. The manufacturer's basic instructions for
use are reproduced in Figure 20.4. Similar information is contained in the package insert for the patient. Investigators who have worked with nicotine
gum emphasize that patients tend to use too little of
the gum and to use it for too short a period. Therefore, it is important to emphasize to patients that
they should use the gum regularly for about 3
months and should use it repeatedly through the
day. It is also important to emphasize that the gum
is a medication and must be chewed differently than
popular sweet chewing gums; a common problem is
too vigorous chewing, resulting in the unpleasant
side effects of nicotine toxicity (see Fig. 20.4).

Weight Gain

Weight gain is a frequent, distressing consequence
of cessation for smokers and may contribute to relapse. The magnitude of likely weight gain is medically insignificant relative to the health benefits of
smoking cessation. However, the social, cosmetic,
and economic (e.g., wardrobe cost) consequences of
weight gain may be sufficient to deter some smokers
from quitting and to lead others to relapse. There-

A   TABLE OF CONTENTS ("Quit It")

INTRODUCTION
1. **STRIKE UP A MASTER PLAN TO QUIT**
   When thinking about quitting
   Involve someone else
   Switch brands
   Cut down on the number of cigarettes you smoke
   Just before quitting
2. **THE DAY YOU PACK IT IN**
   On the day you quit
3. **HOW TO GET RID OF AN OLD FLAME FOR GOOD**
   Immediately after quitting
   Avoid temptation
   Find new habits
   When you get the "crazies"
4. **ON BECOMING AN "EX"**
   Marking progress
   One popular four-step program
   About gaining weight
   When you have called it quits
   Other sources of information on quitting

B   TABLE OF CONTENTS ("For Good")

1. **CONGRATULATIONS! YOU'VE KICKED THE HABIT.**
2. **NO BUTS ABOUT IT, YOU WILL BE TEMPTED.**
3. **HOW TO PUT OUT THE FIRE BEFORE IT STARTS.**
   Review your reasons for quitting.
   Know when you're rationalizing.
   Anticipate triggers and prepare in advance how to avoid them.
   Reward yourself for not smoking.
   Use positive thoughts.
   Use relaxation techniques.
   Seek social support.
4. **GAMES NONSMOKERS CAN PLAY.**
   Stress: Pressure from the boss.
   Frustration: Dealing with daily hassles.
   Anxiety: Being in an unfamiliar setting.
   Craving: Fighting withdrawal symptoms.
   Depression: Feeling bad.
   Partying: Stopping off at a bar.
   Celebrating: Going to a restaurant.
   Relaxing: An evening at home.
5. **NOT SMOKING IS HABIT FORMING.**
   Recognize that you've had a slip.
   Don't blame yourself.
   Identify the trigger.
   Know and use various skills.
   Sign a contract to remain a nonsmoker.

Figure 20.3.   Table of contents from (A) *"Quit It, A Guide to Help You Stop Smoking"* and (B) *"For Good,* *A Guide to Living as a Non-Smoker."* Both are available from the National Cancer Institute.

fore, it may be advisable to provide anticipatory guidance concerning weight control to patients for whom this risk is a concern. Such anticipatory guidance includes advice on attending to weight early—preferably even prior to the quit date—*via* a schedule of frequent weighings; in addition, keeping only low calorie snacks on hand and initiating a moderate, pleasurable exercise program can be helpful. Snacking is a common substitute for smoking even among successful abstainers (3). Explicit *a priori* specification of a "ceiling" weight gain which will be tolerated during the cessation attempt can be useful and is included in the treatment contract illustrated in Figure 20.2.

Organized Treatment

Physicians often state that they would like to have information concerning formal cessation programs to which they might refer patients. However, only a small minority of patients will utilize such programs even when they are available. Therefore, the physician's time is more effectively utilized providing personal, directive cessation advice than in persuading smokers to enroll in organized programs. Information concerning available smoking cessation services can generally be obtained through the local offices of the Lung Association or Heart Association.

For those patients who desire them, organized programs at little or no cost are often available through local voluntary service associations. Commercial programs may be somewhat more comprehensive, but are also more costly and require greater investment of time by the patient. There is little difference in outcome among organized treatment programs. Most such programs have now incorporated the behavioral principles which have been characteristic of the most successful treatments (self-

1. Starting now you must give up smoking completely. Gradually cutting down your tobacco consumption will not work.
2. Your physician has prescribed Nicorette as part of a program to help you stop smoking.
3. Whenever you feel that you want to smoke, put *one* piece of gum into your mouth.
4. When you chew the gum, nicotine is slowly released and is absorbed through the lining of your mouth.
5. Chew the gum *very slowly* until you taste it or feel a slight tingling in your mouth. (This is *usually* after about 15 chews—the number of chews is not the same for all people.) Because of its nicotine content, the gum does not taste like an ordinary chewing gum.
6. As soon as you get the taste of the gum, stop chewing.
7. After the taste or tingling is almost gone (about 1 minute), chew *slowly* again until you taste the gum. Then stop chewing again.
8. The gum should be chewed slowly and intermittently for about 30 minutes to release most of the nicotine.
9. Most people find that 10 to 12 pieces per day of 2 mg Nicorette are enough to control their urge to smoke. Depending on your needs, you can adjust the rate of chewing and the time between pieces.
10. WARNING: If you chew the gum too fast, you may get effects like people get when they inhale a cigarette for the first time, or when they smoke too fast. These effects include light-headedness, nausea and vomiting, throat and mouth irritation, hiccups, and stomach upset. Most of these side effects are controlled by chewing more slowly. See instructions above. Some other effects sometimes seen—particularly during the first few days of using the gum—include mouth ulcers, jaw muscle ache, headaches, heart palpitations, and more than the usual amount of saliva in the mouth. In addition, the mechanical effects of gum chewing (any gum) include traumatic injury to oral mucosa or teeth, jaw ache, and belching from swallowing air. These side effects may be minimized by proper chewing technique (see steps 5 through 8 above). *There are other side effects which have been infrequently reported with the use of Nicorette. Your physician can answer any questions you may have as to possible side effects. Report any disturbing symptoms to your doctor.*
11. *Not more than 30 pieces of 2 mg gum should be chewed in any one day.*
12. If you accidentally swallow a piece of gum you should not experience adverse effects. If you do experience adverse effects, call your doctor. Overdosage could occur if many pieces are chewed simultaneously or in rapid succession. IN CASE OF ACCIDENTAL OVERDOSE OR IF A CHILD CHEWS OR SWALLOWS ONE OR MORE PIECES OF THE GUM, YOU SHOULD CONTACT YOUR PHYSICIAN OR LOCAL POISON CONTROL CENTER IMMEDIATELY.
13. As your urge to smoke fades, gradually reduce the number of pieces of gum you chew each day. This may be possible within 2 to 3 months. Unless your physician tells you otherwise, do not attempt to stop using the gum until your craving is satisfied with one or two pieces a day, but do not use the gum for more than 6 months.
14. Remember to carry the gum with you at all times in case you feel the sudden urge to smoke again. DO NOT FORGET THAT ONE CIGARETTE IS ENOUGH TO START YOU ON THE SMOKING HABIT AGAIN.

Figure 20.4. Manufacturer's basic instructions for the use of nicotine chewing gum (Nicorette). (From Merrell Dow Pharmaceutical Company.)

monitoring, analysis of environmental stimulus factors, and scheduling of rewards).

Patients seeking to stop smoking are often tempted by one of the many fads that advertise effective treatment. In the absence of any established and clearly effective technique one should not denigrate innovations which at least sustain the motivation of some smokers to attempt cessation. Smokers should, however, be cautioned against excessively costly involvements and against the expectation of any "magic cure" requiring no personal motivation and effort.

Relapse

It is unknown what preventive role physicians might play regarding relapse. It is likely that support, advice, and encouragement—especially regarding craving and weight gain—in the first weeks and months are of value.

Smoking cessation is a remarkably difficult process. It is to be expected that many attempts will end in relapse (see page 236). This should not frustrate or discourage either the physician or the patient, but should be recognized as a predictable part of the quitting process. Unsuccessful attempts often precede successful cessation; it is important and worthwhile to try again. The relapsed patient will often be disappointed in himself or herself and fearful of a nagging or humiliating response from the physician. Therefore, it is important that the physician's response to relapse be understanding and nonjudgmental.

OTHER FORMS OF TOBACCO USE

The above discussion has focused upon cigarette smoking because it is the most prevalent form of tobacco use and has the greatest health impact. Other forms of tobacco use—cigars, pipes, snuff, chewing tobacco—also have deleterious health effects. The mortality rates associated with these other forms of tobacco use are intermediate between those of cigarette smokers and nonusers of tobacco. While the total mortality of cigarette smokers is increased by about 70%, the total mortality of cigar or pipe smokers is about 15 to 20% higher than that of nonsmokers.

Cigar and pipe smoking is usually associated with reduced exposure to carbon monoxide and with reduced exposure of lung tissue to smoke; some cigar and pipe smokers do, however, continue to inhale. Use of snuff or chewing tobacco eliminates both of these exposures. However, with all of these noncigarette products nicotine is absorbed through the mucous membranes, and there is topical exposure to tobacco or smoke in the oral-nasal cavity and throat. Site-specific cancer rates in these areas are 5 times as great as in nonusers of tobacco. In addition, there is a slight elevation in cardiovascular disease risk.

Treatment approaches for these other varieties of tobacco dependence are the same as those described above for cigarette smoking.

Acknowledgment. Preparation of this chapter was supported in part by research grants HL 28401, CA 37736, and DA 03893, training grant T32 HL 07180, and Research Scientist Development Award DA 00050 from the U.S. Public Health Service.

General References

Darby TD, McNamee JE, van Rossum JM: Cigarette smoking pharmacokinetics and its relationship to smoking behavior. *Clin Pharmacokinetics* 9:435, 1984.
> Review article discussing the pharmacokinetics of nicotine and smoke absorption.

Gritz ER: Smoking behavior and tobacco use. In Mello NK (ed): *Advances in Substance Abuse.* Greenwich, CT, JAI Press, 1980, vol 1, pp 91–158.
> Review of behavioral and pharmacological research on tobacco dependence.

US Public Health Service: *Smoking and Health: A Report of the Surgeon General.* DHEW publ no. (PHS) 79-50066. Washington, DC, US Government Printing Office, 1979.
> The most comprehensive compilation and review of biomedical and behavioral data available. Subsequent annual volumes for the years 1980 to 1984, respectively, have focused on the special topics of Women, The Changing Cigarette, Cancer, Cardiovascular Disease, and Chronic Obstructive Lung Disease; all are excellent.

Specific References

1. Benowitz NL, Jacob P: Nicotine and carbon monoxide intake from high- and low-yield cigarettes. *Clin Pharmacol Ther* 36:265, 1984.
2. Burling TA, Singleton EG, Bigelow GE, et al: Smoking following myocardial infarction: a critical review of the literature. *Health Psychol* 3:83, 1984.
3. Burling TA, Stitzer ML, Bigelow GE, Russ NW: Techniques used by smokers during contingency motivated smoking reduction. *Addict Behav* 7:397, 1982.
4. Eckert P: Beyond the statistics of adolescent smoking. *Am J Public Health* 73:439, 1983.
5. Gilbert RM, Pope MA: Early effects of quitting smoking. *Psychopharmacology* 78:121, 1982.
6. Greenberg RA, Haley NJ, Etzel RA, Loda FA: Measuring the exposure of infants to tobacco smoke. *N Engl J Med* 310:1075, 1984.
7. Henningfield JE, Stitzer ML, Griffiths RR: Expired air carbon monoxide accumulation and elimination as a function of number of cigarettes smoked. *Addict Behav* 5:265, 1980.
8. Hill P, Haley NJ, Wynder EL: Cigarette smoking: carboxyhemoglobin, plasma nicotine and thiocyanate vs self-reported smoking data and cardiovascular disease. *J Chronic Dis* 36:439, 1983.
9. Kaprio J, Hammar N, Koskenvuo M, et al: Cigarette smoking and alcohol use in Finland and Sweden: a cross-national twin study. *Int J Epidemiol* 11:378, 1982.
10. Kauffmann F, Tessier JF, Oriol P: Adult passive smoking in the home environment: a risk factor for chronic airflow limitation. *Am J Epidemiol* 117:269, 1983.
11. Kaufman DW, Helmrich SP, Rosenberg L, et al: Nicotine and carbon monoxide content of cigarette smoke and the risk of myocardial infarction in young men. *N Engl J Med* 308:409, 1983.
12. Kozlowski LT, Frecker RC, Khouw V, Pope MA: The misuse of "less-hazardous" cigarettes and its detection: hole-blocking of ventilated filters. *Am J Public Health* 70:1202, 1980.
13. Pederson LL: Compliance with physician advice to quit smoking: a review of the literature. *Prev Med* 11:71, 1982.
14. Perry C, Killen J, Telch M, et al: Modifying smoking behavior of teenagers: a school-based intervention. *Am J Public Health* 70:722, 1980.
15. Russell MAH, Merriman R, Stapleton J, Taylor W: Effect of nicotine chewing gum as an adjunct to general practitioners' advice against smoking. *Br Med J* 287:1782, 1983.
16. Schenker MB, Samet JM, Speizer FE: Risk factors for childhood respiratory disease. The effect of host factors and home environmental exposures. *Am Rev Respir Dis* 128:1038, 1983.
17. Schneider NG, Jarvik ME, Forsythe AB, et al: Nicotine gum in smoking cessation: a placebo-controlled, double-blind trial. *Addict Behav* 8:253, 1983.
18. Sexton M, Hebel JR: A clinical trial of change in maternal smoking and its effect on birth weight. *JAMA* 251:911, 1984.
19. Shiffman S: Relapse following smoking cessation: a situational analysis. *J Consult Clin Psychol* 50:71, 1982.
20. Shiffman SM, Jarvik ME: Smoking withdrawal symptoms in two weeks of abstinence. *Psychopharmacology* 50:35, 1976.
21. Sparrow D, Stefos T, Bosse R, Weiss ST: The relationship of tar content to decline in pulmonary function in cigarette smokers. *Am Rev Respir Dis* 127:56, 1983.
22. Tager IB, Weiss ST, Munoz A, et al: Longitudinal study of the effects of maternal smoking on pulmonary function in children. *N Engl J Med* 309:699, 1983.
23. Wald NJ, Idle M, Boreham J, Bailey A: Inhaling habits among smokers of different types of cigarette. *Thorax* 35:925, 1980.

CHAPTER TWENTY-ONE

Alcoholism

CHARLES L. WHITFIELD, M.D., JOHN E. DAVIS, PH.D., AND
L. RANDOL BARKER, M.D.

The medical consequences of alcoholism range across a spectrum from the relative mildness of a hangover, to death due to trauma, bleeding, or infection. Along with cardiovascular disease and cancer, alcoholism ranks among the top three causes of death and disability in the United States. Its estimated cost to society in 1984 approached $150 billion, with an untold additional cost in the suffering of those people who are close to alcoholics. It is also estimated that over three-fourths of the alcoholics in the United States do not receive treatment for their alcoholism.

Until recently, the average physician or lay person has viewed alcoholism as a hopeless condition due to underlying psychological problems, with a poor prognosis for recovery. Yet alcoholism is one of the most treatable of all medical and psychiatric conditions, with about a 70% long term success rate when appropriate modern treatment methods are employed.

DEFINITIONS

While there are several accurate definitions of alcoholism available (Table 21.1), perhaps the most useful is *recurring trouble associated with drinking*. The trouble may occur in one or more of several

Table 21.1.
Some Definitions of Alcoholism

Definition	Reference
"... use of any amount of alcohol to such an extent that it interferes recurringly in the functional life of the person, manifest by resulting difficulties in any one or more of the following life areas: family or other close relationships, educational, legal, health, or job (commonly progressing in that order). Interference in financial and spiritual life is usually affected progressively.	Whitfield and Williams (43)
"... an illness that is a reciprocal relationship between the individual and the social environment. It is characterized in the individual by the developing dependency on alcohol resulting in alienation, dependency, loss of self-esteem, role dysfunction, and an apparent irreversible inability to safely ingest alcohol ... characterized in the community by responses and practices that actively reinforce individual alienation and dependency ... further characterized by denial of the problem by the individual and/or community, unless and until visible dysfunction results in recognition."	Zuska and Pursch (47)
"... a disease characterized by the repetitive and compulsive ingestion of any sedative drug, ethanol representing but one of this group, in such a way as to result in interference with some aspect of the patient's life, be it health, marital status, career, interpersonal relationships, or other required societal adaptations."	Gitlow and Peyser (see 47)
"... an illness characterized by preoccupation with alcohol and loss of control over its consumption which usually leads to intoxication if drinking is begun; by chronicity; by progression; and by the tendency toward relapse. Typically associated with physical disability and impaired emotional, occupational, and/or social adjustments as a direct consequence."	American Medical Association, Handout on Alcoholism, Chicago.
"... a chronic, progressive and potentially fatal disease. It is characterized by tolerance, psychologic and physical dependence, pathologic organ changes, or both, all of which are the direct or indirect consequences of the alcohol ingested."	National Council on Alcoholism (7)

domains, including *interpersonal* (e.g., valued relationships, especially within the family), *educational*, *legal*, *financial*, *medical*, or *occupational*. While there are many exceptions, trouble due to alcoholism usually occurs in that order of progression, so that one's health and job are the last areas to be overtly affected. The definitions in Table 21.1 emphasize these fundamental features of alcoholism.

The American Psychiatric Association's definitions of alcohol abuse and alcohol dependence (Table 21.2) in the *Diagnostic and Statistical Manual of Mental Disorders* (DSM-III) have several drawbacks: (a) the definition of *alcohol abuse* is in reality a description of alcoholism at an early to middle stage; and (b) the definition of *alcohol dependence*, which DSM-III notes may also be called alcoholism, actually represents middle stage to advanced alcoholism. We believe that there is no purpose in disguising the diagnosis of alcoholism with another term such as "alcohol abuse" or "alcohol dependence." By doing so, the diagnosis of alcoholism is delayed, and thus the initiation of treatment is delayed. Finally, DSM-III states that "When abuse or dependence develops, it is usually within the first five years after

regular drinking is established." There is no convincing evidence for this statement in the medical or psychiatric literature. Indeed, there is strong evidence that alcoholism can develop at *any time* after drinking begins.

Alcoholism often occurs concomitantly with other drug problems, so that one now uses the term *chemical dependence* (CD) to describe the overall condition, whether it be due to alcohol, other drugs, or both. The above definitions of alcoholism also apply to drug or chemical dependence, and *most of the diagnostic and treatment principles for alcoholism also apply for other forms of chemical dependence.* Chapter 22 describes patterns of abuse and dependence for a number of substances other than alcohol.

Alcoholism is characterized as being *insidious, progressive, chronic, malignant, primary, family centered, and treatable.* These cardinal features are described throughout this chapter.

ETIOLOGY

The etiology of alcoholism is multifactorial and poorly understood. A predisposition to alcoholism

Table 21.2.
DSM-III Criteria for Alcohol Abuse and Alcohol Dependence[a,b]

Diagnostic Criteria for Alcohol Abuse

A. *Pattern of pathological alcohol use*: need for daily use of alcohol for adequate functioning; inability to cut down or stop drinking; repeated efforts to control or reduce excess drinking by "going on the wagon" (periods of temporary abstinence) or restricting drinking to certain times of the day; binges (remaining intoxicated throughout the day for at least 2 days); occasional consumption of a fifth of spirits (or its equivalent in the wine or beer); amnesic periods for events occurring while intoxicated (blackouts); continuation of drinking despite a serious physical disorder that the individual knows is exacerbated by alcohol use; drinking of nonbeverage alcohol.

B. *Impairment in social or occupational functioning due to alcohol use*: e.g., violence while intoxicated, absence from work, loss of job, legal difficulties (*e.g.*, arrest for intoxicated behavior, traffic accidents while intoxicated), arguments or difficulties with family or friends because of excessive alcohol use.

C. Duration of disturbance for at least 1 month.

Alcohol Dependence (or Alcoholism)

A. Either a pattern of pathological alcohol use (A above) or impairment in social or occupational functioning (B above).

B. Either tolerance or withdrawal:

  Tolerance: need for markedly increased amounts of alcohol to achieve the desired effect, or markedly diminished effect with regular use of the same amount.

  Withdrawal: development of Alcohol Withdrawal (*e.g.*, morning "shakes" and malaise relieved by drinking) after cessation of or reduction in drinking.

[a] See comments in the text.
[b] From American Psychiatric Association: *Diagnostic and Statistical Manual of Mental Disorders*, ed 3. Washington, DC, American Psychiatric Association, 1980.

---

appears to be inherited by at least half of all alcoholic patients (12). Social conditioning, enabling behavior by others close to the individual (see "Co-Alcoholism" below) and, for about 10%, a concomitant major psychiatric condition also probably play etiological roles in this disease. None of these factors accounts for all alcoholism. They only add credence to the concept that alcoholism is a disease entity that is complex and not the result of moral turpitude. For a particularly helpful discussion of the etiology of alcoholism, the reader is referred to Vaillant's monograph (see "General References") and the 1980 Rand Corporation report (21).

ALCOHOLIC BEVERAGES: CONTENT AND METABOLISM

Alcoholic beverages can be divided into nondistilled (wine and beer) and distilled varieties. The concentration of alcohol (ethanol) in wine ranges from 10 to 22% by volume and is 12 to 14% in most wines. Beer usually contains 4 to 5% alcohol by volume. The distilled alcoholic beverages are whiskey, brandy, rum, gin, and vodka. Alcoholic fermentation ceases when the concentration of alcohol exceeds 15% by volume, and, therefore, to manufacture more potent beverages distillation is necessary. In the United States, the word "proof" is preceded by a number that is double the percentage of alcohol by volume: thus 90 proof whiskey contains 45% alcohol by volume. In a 154-pound or 70-kg person on an empty stomach, one drink of distilled alcohol (usually 1 fluid ounce or 30 ml), which normally contains about 15 ml of absolute ethyl alcohol, produces a blood alcohol level (BAL) of about 25 mg/dl. The metabolism of alcohol follows zero-order pharmacokinetics: about 15 mg/dl (or approximately 10 ml)/hour are metabolized, no matter how high the BAL. The alcohol in about 120 ml of whiskey (*i.e.*, four drinks each containing about 15 ml of alcohol) or in about 1.2 liters of beer would take about 5 to 6 hours to be metabolized. The rate of metabolism is higher—even in the range of from 20 to 25 mg/dl/hour—in the alcoholic who drinks heavily each day for many months. To reach a BAL of 300 mg/dl, which is diagnostic of alcoholism, a 70-kg person generally has to consume between 14 to 20 drinks because of the body's metabolism of alcohol.

EPIDEMIOLOGY

Prevalence

In a recent national survey, alcoholism was found to be the commonest psychosocial disorder in American men between the ages of 18 and 65 and the fourth most common in American women in the age range 18 to 24 years (19). The exact prevalence of alcoholism is unknown, but the most conservative estimate is that it involves 10 million Americans and perhaps as many as 15 million (21). Another 10 million are heavy users of alcohol, but have not yet developed alcoholism. The apparent annual national consumption of alcohol is 2.7 gallons of pure alcohol or the equivalent of 2.6 drinks a day for every person over the age of 15. Since about one-third of the adult population is abstinent, the consumption of alcohol is concentrated in the approximately 94 million drinking Americans. About one-third of that number (30 million) consume approximately 70% of all the alcohol produced. It is this group that uses the health system more frequently, is most at risk of trauma, and has the recurring problems that constitute the disease alcoholism (46). In spite of these data, alcoholism is frequently overlooked and remains largely untreated.

Alcoholism is common in medical and psychiatric patients. Among general hospital inpatients, alcoholism has been documented in 15 to 42% of men and in 4 to 35% of women (16). Similar percentages have been reported from emergency departments, clinics, and office practices. A conservative estimation would be that *at least* 1 in 10 ambulatory patients has alcoholism or another form of chemical dependence and that at least another 10 or 20% are suffering from a concomitant condition seen in family members that is now called "co-alcoholism" (see below, page 269). Alcoholism afflicts all ethnic, cultural, and socioeconomic groups, and no single group is immune.

Morbidity and Mortality

In a prospective study of 899 alcoholics matched against 921 controls for age, sex, socioeconomic class, and geographical location, the 5-year mortality rate for alcoholics was 12%, compared with 3.7% for the controls (20), substantiating the general impression that alcoholism is a treacherous disease. The most common causes of early death in alcoholics were cirrhosis of the liver, cancers of the respiratory and gastrointestinal tracts, accidents, suicide, and ischemic heart disease. Many other prospective studies of alcoholism and mortality have shown similar results, with alcoholics having a 2 to 4 times higher death rate than matched controls. Overall, 1 in 10 deaths in the United States is alcohol related (37).

In the prospective study cited above, even alcoholics who reported that they stopped drinking retained considerable excess morbidity and mortality. This may be because certain diseases initiated during active drinking may be irreversible or because personal habits adversely affecting health may have persisted, including surreptitious continued use of alcohol. The authors concluded that the excess sickness and death may have been due to toxic effects of the alcohol itself, cigarette smoking, use of other drugs, poor diet, and emotional disturbances.

Alcoholics who are untreated for their alcoholism tend to be high users of medical care. Overall, it is estimated that 20% of spending for hospital care and 12% of the total expenditure for adult health care is for problems caused by alcoholism (37). In a study of 2238 medical records selected at random from six contrasting hospital populations, it was found that alcoholics constituted a major proportion of the high cost 13% of patients who consumed as many resources as the low cost 87% (46). The high cost group was further characterized by having repeated hospitalizations for the same disease and having a 5 times higher incidence of unexpected complications of their illnesses than the low cost group. In a related study, 161 alcoholic patients, while they were drinking actively, used the health care system at a rate 3 times that of the general population. When they were successfully treated for alcoholism, their use of the health care system decreased to that of the general population (5).

MANIFESTATIONS OF ALCOHOLISM

Alcoholism is a protean disease, and it is probably the most common "great masquerader" today. It should be looked for in every patient, and should be searched for in more detail in any patient with high risk complaints, such as depression, repeated trauma (29), or sexual dysfunction. Table 21.3 lists medical, psychiatric, legal, and other manifestations that are often associated with alcoholism. Manifestations are ranked in the table according to their strength as diagnostic features, ranging from those which are diagnostic of alcoholism to those which should make one at least consider alcoholism. A number of the most important manifestations of alcoholism are discussed here.

Legal Problems

A driving-while-intoxicated (DWI) history or record is highly suggestive of alcoholism. In one study of about 21,000 consecutive people with DWIs, about 75% of first time offenders were found to be alcoholic. Of those with two DWI arrests, over 90% were alcoholic, and of those with three, essentially 100% were alcoholic (11). A prison record is also strongly suggestive. Reports indicate that about 65% of prison inmates are alcoholic and another 15% are dependent upon other drugs, making a total of about 80% of prison inmates who have a history of chemical dependence. Child and spouse/partner abuse are additional sociolegal problems highly associated with alcoholism.

Behavioral and Psychiatric Problems

Miscellaneous

Accidents and trauma are frequently associated with alcoholism; in more than half of patients with severe trauma, alcohol or other recreational drug use can be detected (29). Among patients with symptoms of chronic mental illness, especially symptoms of depression and anxiety, alcoholism is very common (19). Usually alcoholism is the primary problem, and treatment of mental symptoms is not successful until the alcoholism is treated.

Alcohol Intoxication

The best known acute consequence of alcoholism is alcohol intoxication, which should usually pre-

Table 21.3.
Medical, Psychiatric, Legal, and Other Findings Suggestive (0 to *) to Highly Suggestive (to ***) or Diagnostic (****) of Alcoholism and Other Chemical Dependence**

Presenting Complaint and History

**** Drinking or drug-related problem, recurring	* Night sweats
*** Blackouts with drinking	* Depression
*** Spouse/other complains of patient's drinking	* Suicide attempt
*** Driving-while-intoxicated (DWI) record	* Sexual dysfunction
*** Prison record	* Legal problem
*** Change in alcohol/drug tolerance	* Noncompliance in treatment
*** Frequent requests for mood-changing drugs	* School learning problem
** Gastrointestinal bleeding, especially upper	* Hypertension
** Automobile accident	Heart trouble
** Traumatic injuries, fracture	Palpitations
** Parent, grandparent, or relative alcoholic	Abdominal pain
** Friends alcoholic or other chemical dependence	Amenorrhea
** Family or other violence	Weight loss
** Child abuse or neglect	Vagus complaints
** First seizure in an adult	Seizure
** Job performance problem	Insomnia
* Multiple gastrointestinal complaints	Anxiety or panic attacks
* Untoward responses to a number of medications (see page 262)	Marital discord
* Unexplained syncope	Financial problem
* Frequent infections	Behavior problem

Alcohol or Other Drug Use History

**** Alcohol use recurringly interfering with health, job, or social functioning	*** Word "drinker" said in rounds or report
*** Patient says, "I can stop drinking anytime," or the equivalent; or patient gets evasive or angry, or talks glibly during taking of drinking history	** Heavy alcohol use (more than 3 drinks/day or more than 5 drinks at an occasion for a 154-lb person)
	** Other drug misuse or dependence
*** Patient states that he has consciously stopped drinking completely for any length of time	* Cigarette smoker

Physical Examination

*** Odor of beverage alcohol on breath	* Unexplained arrhythmias, especially chronic borderline tachycardia
*** Parotid gland enlargement, bilateral	* Thin extremities in proportion to trunk
*** Spider nevi or angioma	* Splenomegaly
*** Edematous, "puffy face" (may be subtle); unexplained edema	* Hypertension
*** Tremulousness, hallucinosis, and/or 1 or 2 seizures	Diaphoresis, day or night
** Cigarette stains on fingers	Very neat and clean
** Breath mints odor	Depression
** Many scars or tattoos	Alopecia
** Hepatomegaly	Corneal arcus
** Gynecomastia	Abdominal tenderness
** Small testicles	Cerebellar signs (e.g., nystagmus)
** Unexplained bruises, abrasions, or cuts	Any depressed alteration in consciousness
	Anxiety

Laboratory Abnormalities

**** Blood alcohol level greater than 300 mg/100 ml	** Abnormal liver function tests
*** Blood alcohol level greater than 100 mg/100 ml	** Anemia, macrocytic or megaloblastic
*** High serum osmolality	** Hyperlipoproteinemia-type 4 or 5
*** High serum ammonia	* Positive blood or urine for mood-changing drugs
*** SGOT elevated on admission, and normal by discharge	* Hyperuricemia (7 to 12 mg/100 ml most often; may be transient)
*** GGT elevation	* Small intestinal absorption test abnormalities
*** Negative workups for hyperthyroidism	* Hypophosphatemia or hypomagnesemia
* Creatinine phosphokinase elevation	Electrolyte imbalance
** Blood alcohol level positive, any amount	Elevated or low blood glucose
** High amylase	Low white blood cell or platelet count

Table 21.3.—Continued

X-ray Film Findings

*** Pancreatic calcification	* Hepatomegaly
*** Multiple rib fractures	* Splenomegaly
** "Aspiration pneumonia"	* Nonfilling gallbladder

Diagnosis

**** Hepatitis, alcoholic	** Attempted suicide
*** Pancreatitis, acute or chronic (40 to 95%)	** Gastritis
*** Cirrhosis (85%)	** Refractory hypertension
*** Portal hypertension	** Cerebellar degeneration
*** Wernicke-Korsakoff syndrome	** Peripheral neuropathy
*** Frequent automobile or other accidents	** Aspiration pneumonia
*** Cold injury	* Cerebral
*** Nose and throat cancer	* Cardiomyopathy
** Hepatitis, non-A or B	** Anxiety
** Other chemical dependence	** Any symptom or sign, cause not found, or unknown
** Drownings	* Depression
** Burns, especially third degree	* Marital discord or family problem
** Leaves hospital against medical advice (40 to 80%)	* Fatty liver

sent no diagnostic problem. But just because this condition is so common, diagnostic errors are made when the physician forgets that "drunken behavior"—often with evidence of recent alcohol use—may be caused by a host of conditions, such as infection, metabolic disturbance, neurological disease, or other drug toxicity. Because the alcoholic is especially prone to many disorders that may be manifested as deranged behavior, he should be examined systematically before a diagnosis of simple drunkenness is made.

Alcohol intoxication may be characterized by one or more of the following: relaxation and sedation, euphoria, impaired coordination, loudness, lowered inhibitions, poor memory and judgment, labile mood, slurred speech, nausea, vomiting, and obtundation (see Table 21.4). An initial period of excite-

ment and euphoria is often followed by depression and sleep, or possibly coma. The duration and magnitude of the intoxication depend on dose, the rapidity with which the alcohol was drunk, and on whether the patient drank on an empty stomach (enhancing the rate of absorption). Tolerance is also a significant factor. As noted above, normal persons metabolize ethanol at a rate of about 15 mg/dl (or 10 ml)/hour, no matter how much is ingested, but an alcoholic may acquire the (reversible) capacity to increase his rate of alcohol metabolism. Moreover, alcoholics characteristically develop substantial central tolerance, so that they appear fairly sober at blood alcohol levels of 150 mg/dl or more. Most nonalcoholic individuals become intoxicated at levels between 100 and 200 mg/dl, and some, at levels as low as 30 mg/dl. Levels over 400 mg/dl

Table 21.4.
Expected Effects According to Blood Alcohol Level for a Person without Tolerance to Alcohol

Blood Alcohol Level Rising mg/dl	Expected Effect	Approximate Location of Physiological Disturbance
to 50	Relaxation, sedation	
to 100	Coordination impaired; euphoric; loud conversation; apparent reduction of social inhibitions	Cerebral cortex
to 200	Ataxia; depressed fine motor ability, decreased mentation, attention span and memory; poor judgment; labile mood; beginning of slurred speech	Limbic system and cerebellum
to 300	Marked ataxia and slurred speech, nausea and vomiting, tremor, irritable	Reticular activating system
to 400	Stage 1 anesthesia (unconsciousness) memory lapse	Reticular activating system
above 400	Respiratory failure, coma, death	Medulla oblongata

may be lethal, death usually resulting from depressed respiration or aspiration of vomitus.

Blackouts

"Blackouts," amnesia for events that occurred during a period of intoxication, are common. However, from 10 to 25% of alcoholics do not have memory blackouts, and some normal drinkers have experienced one or two blackouts. If they recur more than two times, blackouts are usually an indication of alcoholism.

Alcohol Idiosyncratic Intoxication

Alcohol idiosyncratic intoxication (pathological intoxication) is an uncommon syndrome characterized by an extreme, often aggressive reaction to drinking alcohol, which is frequently followed by amnesia for the episode. The behavior is atypical of the person when not drinking. The duration of this condition is brief (hours), and the person returns to his normal state as the blood alcohol level falls. Temporal lobe epilepsy, sedative-hypnotic use, and malingering should be ruled out (2).

Alcohol Amnestic Disorder (Korsakoff's Psychosis)

Alcohol amnestic disorder is characterized chiefly by short term memory impairment, associated with some loss of long term memory, in the absence of clouded consciousness (delirium) or general loss of intellectual abilities (dementia). (For definitions and detailed discussions of delirium and dementia, see Chapter 17.) Patients with less advanced forms of this disorder may be substantially impaired, but they may appear superficially to be normal, particularly as they frequently attempt to minimize their impairment and to confabulate in order to fill in memory gaps.

The amnestic disorder frequently follows an episode of *Wernicke's encephalopathy* (a syndrome of global confusion, ataxia, and impaired eye movement, due to thiamine deficiency, which may occur suddenly or gradually over several days). Parenteral thiamine given during an acute episode of Wernicke's encephalopathy may prevent the amnestic syndrome. Some of these patients recover entirely from the alcohol amnestic syndrome. Many remain grossly impaired and require institutional care; of these about 20% improve modestly with good long term institutional support (22a).

An amnestic syndrome resembling alcohol amnestic disorder may be caused by bilateral damage to certain diencephalic and medial temporal structures due to head trauma, surgery, hypoxia, or infarction in the territory of the posterior cerebral arteries.

Dementia Associated with Alcoholism

When more generalized intellectual impairment develops after years of heavy drinking, the diagnosis of dementia (chronic organic brain syndrome) associated with alcoholism is appropriate. An estimated 70% of actively drinking chronic alcoholics will have some damage, as measured by psychological testing. Perhaps 10% of these will have dementia that is sufficiently apparent so that it can be noticed without psychological testing. Since even detoxified alcoholics are likely to show some cognitive impairment for a period of time after cessation of drinking (1), this diagnosis should not be made unless dementia persists for at least 3 weeks after drinking has stopped. Other causes of dementia must be excluded (see Chapter 17).

All alcoholics with any signs of dementia should be treated with high dose thiamine (i.e., 100 mg daily) and multivitamins long term. Some will improve.

Other Medical Complications

Miscellaneous

The various deficiency states involved in a diet composed largely of nutritionally empty alcoholic calories (7 calories/g), as well as the direct toxic actions of alcohol itself, have been implicated in the pathogenesis of the medical consequences of alcoholism. These disorders are legion, spare no body system, and most are related to the quantity and duration of alcohol consumed (8). Among the commoner medical complications of alcoholism are gastritis; fatty liver, hepatitis, or cirrhosis; pancreatitis; cerebellar ataxia; peripheral neuropathy; unexplained elevation of serum creatinine phosphokinase with or without muscle pain and weakness; pulmonary infections suggesting aspiration or impaired defenses (tuberculosis and pneumonia); cancers of the liver and gastroinestinal tract; unexplained cardiomyopathy; and hypertension.

Hypertension is becoming a more frequently recognized manifestation of alcoholism. It is found in about one-third of actively drinking alcoholics. Since it frequently remits within 1 week of discontinuing alcohol, and since the patient usually remains normotensive for the duration of abstinence (24), it may be the most common reversible cause of hypertension.

Fetal Alcohol Syndrome (17)

Because it appears to be both serious and preventable, the fetal alcohol syndrome deserves special mention. It is manifested by morphological abnormalities, low birth weight, and developmental and cognitive impairment. This syndrome is a consequence of alcohol ingestion by the mother during pregnancy. The risk of minor abnormalities (e.g., low birth weight) begins with the consumption of one drink per day; this risk increases with increasingly larger amounts of alcohol consumption. Because of this, it is prudent to advise women not to drink during pregnancy.

Medical Consequences: A Summary View

Nearly all of the medical consequences of alcoholism tend to have certain common characteristics:

1. Excessive drinking causes them.

2. A poor diet generally makes most of them worse and makes them occur earlier.

3. Harmful habits—such as cigarette smoking, the misuse of other drugs, and "overdoing it" in many life areas—also tend to compound the medical consequences.

4. If the patient continues to consume alcohol, damage involving major organs progresses slowly, but relentlessly, over the course of a few years, often ending in organ failure.

This progression of organic damage will occur no matter what medical or psychological intervention the patient may receive, as long as drinking continues. If the patient stops drinking, many of the pathophysiological processes due to alcohol will reverse rapidly, such as those in the blood and bone marrow (cytopenias), those in the small intestine (malabsorption), hypertension, and fluid and electrolyte imbalance. Other processes do not reverse rapidly with sobriety, but they usually do not progress and often improve over weeks and months. Alcoholic hepatitis, chronic pancreatitis, and organic brain syndrome are conditions that tend to improve more gradually. When providing treatment and follow-up of the medical consequences of alcoholism, after acute conditions have been stabilized, the physician caring for an alcoholic should devote most of his energy to the patient's alcoholism rather than the medical consequences. As discussed below, this task begins by getting the patient to accept the fact that he has the disease alcoholism or, at least, that he should begin specific treatment for his drinking problem.

Alcoholism in the Elderly (37)

Alcoholism is an important problem in older persons. Almost half of older alcoholics develop the disease well after middle age; the rest are long term survivors of lifelong alcoholism. Older alcoholics are subject to the entire array of complications of alcoholism, and there is evidence suggesting that they actually have an increased sensitivity to the toxic effects of alcohol, although their metabolic clearance of alcohol is identical to that of younger alcoholics.

For a variety of reasons, the manifestations of alcoholism may be missed in a substantial proportion of older persons with the disease, even those who are being seen regularly by a physician. Elderly alcoholics are more likely to be single, divorced, or widowed and to be spending much of their time alone. Because of reduced involvement in family life, retirement from the work setting, and decreased social interactions in general, they are less likely to have the recurring troubles in these spheres that bring younger alcoholics to medical attention. Mis-

management of their financial affairs, recurring minor injuries, such as cigarette burns and falls without fractures, or mental/physical deterioration leading to nursing home admission are typical ways in which advanced alcoholism may be manifest in older persons. Often, these alcoholics are "protected" from the troubles attending alcoholism by embarrassed, frustrated or well meaning children and friends.

DIAGNOSING ALCOHOLISM

Taking the History

Except when a patient presents with overt behavioral or medical complications of alcoholism, skillful inquiry is needed to make the diagnosis of alcoholism. In taking the alcohol use history from any patient, the following guidelines are useful:

1. Begin with an open-ended approach, asking the patient: *How do you use alcohol?* If the patient manifests any avoidance, anger, or glibness; or if he gives a history of heavy alcohol use; or if you know of *any other indication* that alcohol might be a problem, including nonspecific but important clues among the manifestations listed in Table 21.3, then ask the following questions.

2. *Have you ever been concerned about your drinking?* You may wish to add: What does your wife (or other significant partner, parent) think about your drinking? If these probes suggest a possible problem, try getting the patient to talk about alcoholism in the following ways.

3. *Do you think you are an alcoholic?*

4. *What is an alcoholic? How would you recognize an alcoholic?* (Here you tell the patient the definition noted at the beginning of this chapter, *i.e.*, recurring trouble in previous life areas associated with drinking, after he has told you his definition).

5. *How do you fit this definition?*

If questions such as these are asked in a nonjudgmental manner, most patients will give valid answers. The trust that develops during an ongoing doctor-patient relationship is very helpful in getting an alcoholic to acknowledge his problem. Thus, in patients who appear to be denying their problem initially, the information needed to make the diagnosis of alcoholism may be more effectively obtained at subsequent visits.

Two cardinal features will eventually emerge in the interview of most patients who have alcoholism: (a) evidence of inability to control the use of alcohol, and (b) denial that a significant problem exists.

Loss of Control

Continuous inability to control the use of alcohol is not always present in alcoholics. Indeed, many can go for periods of a few hours (*e.g.*, at a social gathering) to a few months of apparently "normal" drinking. Therefore, the absence of overt loss of control for a period of time does not rule out alcoholism. In such patients, the loss of control returns eventually. Inability to control one's drinking may be manifested acutely, where the person drinks more than he intended to or is unable to stop drinking and becomes intoxicated, or it may follow a chronic pattern, where the patient drinks heavily for a few days or most days of the week and cannot seem to stop. Normal persons do not drink in these ways, and it is a sign of a serious problem. Control of alcohol consumption is always an issue for the alcoholic.

Denial

Denial is present in nearly all actively drinking alcoholics. What at first appears to be simple "denial" is actually a response that is due to one or more of the following mechanisms: (a) conscious lying (one of the least common mechanisms); (b) classic denial (an adaptive coping response to avoid a distressing problem); (c) a memory blackout; (d) euphoric recall (the patient remembers only the good times when drinking); (e) the fact that no one points out problems related to drinking; (f) wishful thinking; (g) denial on the part of the family and other close people, including helping professionals; (h) ignorance of what an alcoholic is; (i) toxic effects on information processing and memory; (j) stigma related to the term "alcoholic"; (k) fear of the unknown; and (l) a complex thinking quandary (4, 34, 39). This last mechanism consists of genuine confusion on the part of the patient; he knows that something is wrong in his life but somehow cannot connect it with drinking alcohol (34). *The clinician who knows how to recognize and appropriately manage denial will be able to reach a successful outcome in the treatment of many or even most alcoholic patients (see below, page 255).*

Screening Tests

Several screening questionnaires have been developed to assist physicians and others in diagnosing alcoholism. If the interviewing approach above does not clarify whether a person has alcoholism, or if one wishes to characterize an alcoholic's condition fully, these tests are extremely helpful.

Michigan Alcoholism Screening Test (MAST)

The MAST is a screening test that has the advantages that it can be given by nonprofessional persons without extensive training, it is simple, and it is reliable as a diagnostic screening test (22, 28). It was standardized in several populations of men and was further standardized and refined in women and in adolescents. It can also be modified for use with persons with possible drug problems other than alcohol.

The test consists of 24 "yes" or "no" questions pertaining to the effects of drinking on a person's ability to function. It usually takes about 5 minutes to administer and score. If alcoholism is defined as drinking interfering repeatedly with relationships, health, job, or legal status, then this test measures three or more parameters in *each* of these major areas. The MAST is shown in Table 21.5. If the patient scores 10 or more points, he is definitely alcoholic. If he scores between 5 and 9 points on the MAST, the probability appears to be about 80% that he is alcoholic. With a score of 3 points or less, he is probably a normal drinker. A score of 4 points is considered borderline.

It is often worthwhile to show the patient his test, explaining it to him and discussing the meaning of the questions on which he scored points. In this way, the MAST can be helpful in confronting the alcoholic with objective evidence ("a test designed by experts") that he is an alcoholic. It is also of value in treating and following up a patient (43).

It may be helpful to give the MAST to family members of a patient, to answer for the patient as though he were answering honestly, and to compare their answers to those of the patient. This approach has been shown to detect alcoholism with nearly the same validity as when the patient takes the test (18). It may also be a way to learn how much the alcoholic patient is denying. The MAST may also be used with teenagers by modifying key words, e.g., "education" for "job" or "work," and "parents" for "spouse" (43).

Since the development of the MAST in about 1970, investigators have found that several additional questions can be helpful in screening for alcoholism. These are included in Table 21.6. While these seven questions have not been rigorously validated, they have been especially helpful in confirming the diagnosis in patients with scores of less than 10 points on the standard MAST. These questions, plus three additional ones (8 to 10 in Table 21.6) related to observations by the clinician, are called the MAST Addendum.

CAGE Questionnaire

Another validated alcoholism screening instrument, the CAGE questionnaire has the advantage of being perhaps less incriminating than the MAST, while being easier to administer and score (9). The four CAGE questions are: (a) "Have you ever felt you should *Cut* down on your drinking?" (b) "Have people *Annoyed* you by criticizing your drinking?" (c) "Have you ever felt bad or *Guilty* about your drinking?" (d) "Have you ever had a drink first thing in the morning to steady your nerves or get rid of a hang-over (*Eye-Opener*)?" Two positive responses are suggestive of alcoholism, and three of four positives are diagnostic. Other screening tests are available for use, although they are not as well standardized as the MAST and the CAGE.

Table 21.5.
Michigan Alcoholism Screening Test (MAST)[a]

	YES	NO
0. Do you enjoy having a drink now and then?	0	
1. Do you feel you are a normal drinker? (By normal we mean you drink less than or as much as most other people and you have not gotten into any recurring trouble while drinking.)		2
2. Have you ever awakened the morning after some drinking the night before and found that you could not remember a part of the evening?	2	
3. Does either of your parents, or any other near relative, or your spouse, or any girlfriend or boyfriend ever worry or complain about your drinking?	1	
4. Can you stop drinking without a struggle after one or two drinks?		2
5. Do you feel guilty about your drinking?	1	
6. Do friends or relatives think you are a normal drinker?		2
7. Are you able to stop drinking when you want to?		2
8. Have you ever attended a meeting of Alcoholics Anonymous (AA)?	5	
9. Have you gotten into physical fights when you have been drinking?	1	
10. Has your drinking ever created problems between you and either of your parents, or another relative, your spouse, or any girlfriend or boyfriend?	2	
11. Has any family member of yours ever gone to anyone for help about your drinking?	2	
12. Have you ever lost friends because of your drinking?	2	
13. Have you ever gotten into trouble at work or at school because of drinking?	2	
14. Have you ever lost a job because of drinking?	2	
15. Have you ever neglected your obligations, your school work, your family, or your job for 2 or more days in a row because you were drinking?	2	
16. Do you drink before noon fairly often?	1	
17. Have you ever been told you have liver trouble? Cirrhosis?	2	
18. After heavy drinking have you ever had severe shaking, or heard voices or seen things that really weren't there?	2(5 DTs)	
19. Have you ever gone to anyone for help about your drinking?	5	
20. Have you ever been in a hospital because of drinking?	5	
21. Have you ever been a patient in a psychiatric hospital or on a psychiatric ward of a general hospital where drinking was part of the problem that resulted in hospitalization?	2	
22. Have you ever been seen at a psychiatric or mental health clinic or gone to any doctor, social worker, or clergy for help with any emotional problem, where drinking was a part of the problem?	2	
23. Have you ever been arrested for drunk driving, driving while intoxicated, or driving under the influence of alcoholic beverages or any other drug? (IF YES, How many times? ____)	2 each	
24. Have you ever been arrested, or taken into custody, even for a few hours, because of other drunk behavior, whether due to alcohol or another drug? (IF YES, How any times? ____)	2 each	

[a] Interpretation: *Standard MAST*—0 to 3 points = probable normal drinker; 4 points = borderline score; 5 to 9 points = 80% associated with alcoholism/chemical dependence; 10 or more = 100% associated with alcoholism.

Summary of Diagnostic Approach

One or all of the diagnostic approaches outlined in the preceding text and tables may be needed to help establish the diagnosis of alcoholism. These approaches, which include direct questioning, inductive reasoning, and diagnostic testing, are summarized in the algorithm in Figure 21.1.

Under inductive reasoning the following question is included: "Are any NCA (National Council on Alcoholism) major criteria present?" Recognizing a need to establish a helpful set of criteria for diagnosing alcoholism, the NCA and the American Medical Society on Alcoholism selected an expert committee whose goals were to provide uniform nomenclature and to promote early detection of alcoholism. The product of this committee's deliberation, an article entitled "Criteria for the Diagnosis of Alcoholism" (7), is helpful because it uses objective criteria obtained from the patient or those closest to him. These criteria are similar to those in Table 21.3. The NCA criteria are divided into *major* (any one of which is considered diagnostic) and *minor* (strongly suspicious, or possible or incidental). Similar to the criteria of DSM-III, a problem with some of the major criteria is that they may be *late* manifestations of alcoholism. The NCA is currently testing these diagnostic criteria.

Table 21.6.
Addendum[a] to the MAST

In patients in whom a drinking problem is suspected, yet who score 9 points or less and especially those who score 4 points or less, one may ask seven additional Yes-No questions:[b]

1. Have you ever consciously stopped drinking for a period of time?
2. Can you or could you at any time in your life drink more than other people without showing it?
3. Did either of your parents ever have a problem with drinking, or were you ever concerned about either of their drinking?
4. Have you ever been stopped while driving or apprehended by a law officer for any reason while you were drinking, yet you did not get arrested or receive a citation, but probably should have?
5. Have you ever gone to a doctor for a medical problem, other than liver disease or cirrhosis, that you or he suspected was caused by drinking?
6. Have you ever been dependent upon or ever had recurring problems with using a drug other than alcohol?[c]

A "Yes" answer to any of these questions should be scored two points. For question 2, if the answer is "Yes" for both parents, score 4 points.

7. Did you *often* have hangovers (feeling bad or sick after drinking) during the first few years of your heavy drinking?

A "No" answer to question 7 should be scored 2 points.

Three additional observations can be helpful, and these are to be answered by the clinician.

8. Does the patient display any "red flags" during the taking of the drinking history? (*e.g.*, glibness, avoiding, anger, defensiveness) ("Yes" answer = 3 points)
9. At any time during the interview did the patient say anything like "I can quit anytime", "I don't need it", "I can take it or leave it", or the like? ("Yes" answer = 3 points)
10. If there is a blood alcohol level available, does it fulfill any of the following criteria?
    a. 100 mg/100 ml at an office visit
    b. 150 mg/100 ml without gross evidence of intoxication
    c. 300 mg/100 ml at anytime
    ("Yes" answer to any one of a, b, or c = 5 points)

Although these ten questions are not a part of the standardized MAST, one of us (CW) finds them to be of value in patients with doubtful or negative MAST scores. They can provide up to 27 additional points.

Rarely, patients who are alcoholic will score 3 points or less on the standard MAST. In these patients, the clinician can usually find other information that indicates that the patient may be or is alcoholic. It may also be helpful to give the MAST and the Addendum to a family member, such as the spouse, to answer for the patient, as though the patient were answering truthfully. In such a case the MAST score will be as accurate as if the patient answered it honestly. In recording the patient's score, the MAST score should be listed first, followed by the sum of both the MAST and the Addendum, *e.g.*, 15/22 (MAST/MAST and Addendum).

Explanation for MAST Addendum

Answers by the Patient/Client

Question 1. Normal drinkers normally do not *consciously* stop drinking. Any person who consciously stops drinking is giving evidence that he has found drinking to be a negative experience. Alcoholics usually stop drinking periodically toward the middle and advanced stages of their alcoholism. Consciously stopping drinking usually indicates that the person has some form of struggle with drinking.

2. This demonstrates tolerance to alcohol, either or both of an acquired or congenital tolerance. Alcoholics commonly manifest one or both of these.

3. About two-thirds of alcoholics have a family history of a drinking problem in a parent. If you are now seeing a person for suspicion of an alcohol problem who discloses that his/her parent was an "alcohol abuser" or was concerned about the parent's drinking, or the parent was a heavy drinker, this is further evidence of either risk or an actual problem. For those people with both parents having had a drinking problem, there is probably an even higher risk of being or becoming alcoholic. If the person has some doubt about a parent's alcoholism, taking the MAST for the parent as though the parent were answering honestly is usually helpful and can help remove the doubt.

4. This can be called a "near arrest." It commonly occurs in women and VIP drunk drivers, where the law officer often does not issue a citation because, for example, the woman cries or the VIP uses other influence.

5. This questions a medical consequence of alcoholism other than liver disease or cirrhosis. Any person who has such should be suspected of having alcoholism.

6. People with drug dependence to one type of drug tend to develop dependence to other types of psychoactive drugs. Alcoholism is the most common drug dependence. Thus, having another type of drug dependence places a person at a higher risk of becoming or being alcoholic.

7. In a pilot survey by one of us (CW), from 25 to 65% of 400 people who identified themselves as recovering alcoholics said that they rarely, if ever, experienced a hangover after heavy drinking during the first few years of their alcoholism, contrasted to less than 5% of a smaller nonalcoholic population so surveyed.

Observations by the Clinician

8. These responses indicate struggle, similar to question 1.
9. These statements or the like also indicate struggle. Normal drinkers do not make this type of statement. Some alcoholism experts consider this to be almost diagnostic of alcoholism.
10. These blood alcohol levels are those set forth by the National Council on Alcoholism's expert committee on the diagnosis of alcoholism. Any one of these is considered to be a major diagnostic criterion and therefore is diagnostic of alcoholism.

[a] The authors have developed these additional questions to facilitate diagnosis in patients with low MAST scores. While we have found them to be helpful over about 5 years of experience with hundreds of patients, these questions have not been standardized.

[b] These questions may also be asked of those who score above 9 points on the MAST to provide additional data.

[c] If the patient answers "No" to this question, yet the clinician knows that the patient has or had a drug problem, 2 points should be scored. This principle also applies to other questions on the MAST and this addendum as well.

PRINCIPLES OF TREATMENT

Definition of Successful Treatment

Alcoholism is a highly treatable disease. Successful treatment depends largely on a positively motivated health professional who has effective diagnostic and treatment skills, many of which are outlined here. Treatment success can be defined as *the achievement of abstinence for progressively longer periods of time from alcohol (and other drugs), with*

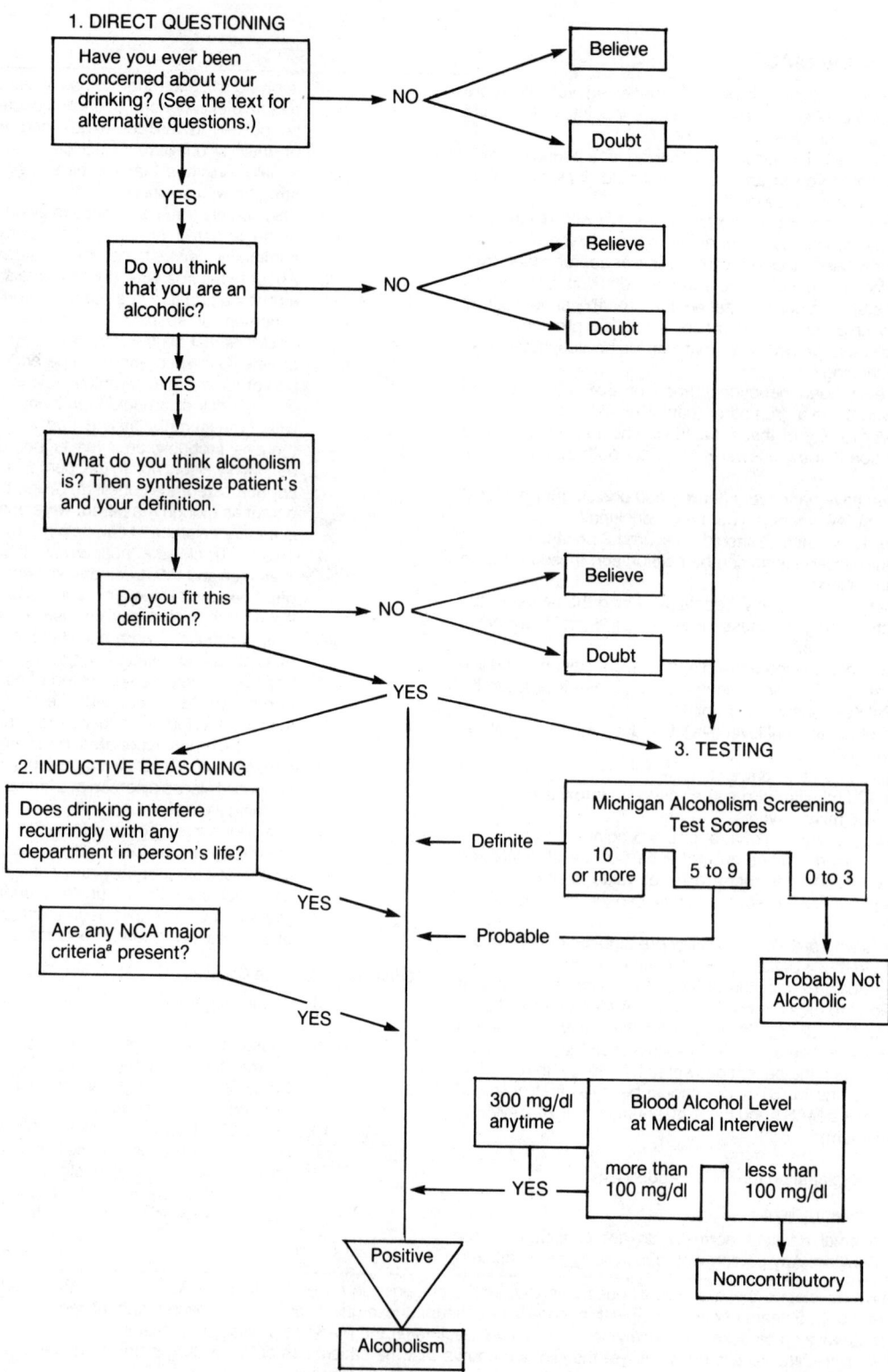

Figure 21.1. An algorithmic approach to diagnosing alcoholism. (From Whitfield CL, Liepman MR (eds): *The Patient with Alcoholism and Other Drug Problems.* Baltimore, University of Maryland, 1980.)

[a] NCA (National Council on Alcoholism) major criteria: Evidence of dependence or tolerance (see Table 21.2); or either of the following major alcohol-associated illnesses: alcoholic hepatitis, alcoholic cerebellar degeneration; or drinking despite strong medical or social (*e.g.,* job loss, threatened marriage) contraindication known to the patient; or blood alcohol level >300 mg/100ml.

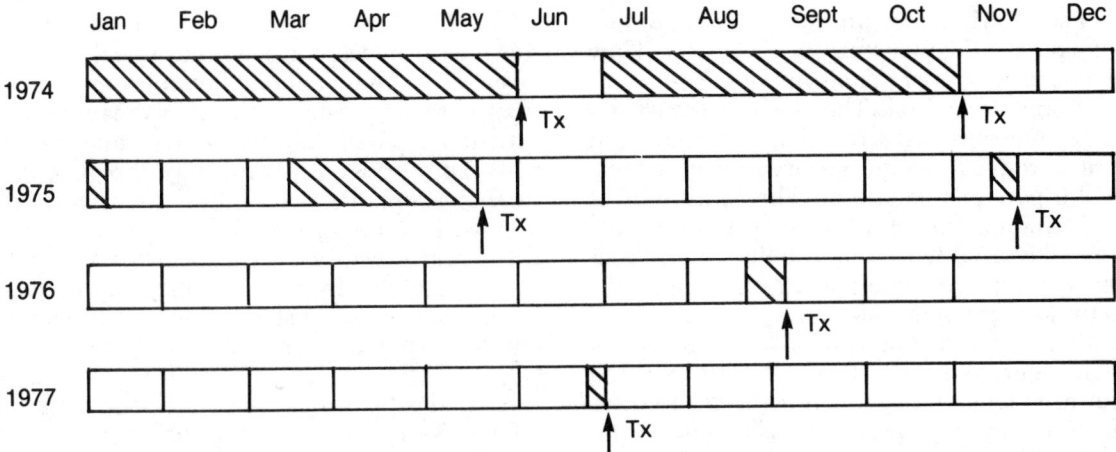

Figure 21.2. Drinking-sober profile of a 53-year-old factory supervisor who had been alcoholic for 15 years. The achievement of longer and longer periods of abstinence is typical of the process of recovery from alco-holism. *Hatched areas* = drinking; *clear areas* = absti-nence; *Tx* = came in for treatment, after having dropped out of treatment.

improved life functioning for the patient and his family. (A case example is shown in Fig. 21.2.) Using this definition, when treatment is initiated and maintained for about 3 years, 70% of alcoholic patients will successfully recover from alcoholism (6, 15, 21, 39). This rate of recovery compares favorably with reported rates of spontaneous recovery from alcoholism, which range from 4 to 26%. Factors associated with good and poor outcomes after treatment are summarized below (see "Prognosis with Treatment" below).

The appropriate terms for describing an alcoholic in recovery are "recovered" alcoholic (a public or polite term) or "recovering" alcoholic (a personal or clinical term). The terms "ex-," "reformed," "former," or "cured" alcoholic are misnomers and are inappropriate.

Despite initial reports that some alcoholics can learn "controlled drinking" (30), this goal of treatment has been shown in careful studies to be totally unrealistic (37).

Avoiding a Psychoanalytic Approach

It has been repeatedly shown that treating alcoholics as though their abnormal drinking behavior were secondary to underlying psychopathology is usually unsuccessful and often countertherapeutic. Insight-oriented or in-depth psychotherapy early in the treatment of alcoholism is, therefore, contraindicated. By contrast, supportive and directive psychotherapy, using the treatment methods outlined below and focused on the alcoholism as a primary disease, is usually effective in helping the alcoholic patient reach a successful recovery.

Outpatient Treatment: Overview

A trial of outpatient treatment is appropriate initially for most alcoholics. It is more economical, allows the patient to continue working and to continue daily activities, and promotes recovery in the more realistic environment of the patient's unique day-to-day life. However, to be successful, outpatient treatment must be *intensive, thorough, and monitored consistently and regularly* over a long period of time. Even with optimal outpatient treatment, up to half of all alcoholics also require inpatient treatment (discussed below, page 267). Treatment consists of motivating the patient, initiating a treatment plan, and providing regular follow-up, as described below.

Motivating the Patient into Treatment

Breaking down denial is the most difficult part of treatment and is an ongoing process. By persistently and patiently using motivational techniques, denial can be broken. And, surprisingly, it can be enjoyable for the therapist.

There are three common, effective techniques to break down denial in patients—and in their family members if necessary: *confrontation, empathy, and offering hope.* Confrontation is telling the person what you observe, including that you have diagnosed the disease alcoholism. This may be the most difficult of the three actions; for the motivation to be effective, however, it must be accomplished. The patient will usually deny the diagnosis and may even get angry. However, with persistent and nonjudgmental confrontation, the patient will eventually admit that he has a problem with alcohol.

Empathy and offering hope are supportive and help to allay the person's denial, anxiety, and anger. They should be used with every confrontation.

Offering hope is crucial. The therapist must deliver a clear message that there is a "way out" and that there is relief from the misery and bewilderment of the patient's condition. The "way out" is through abstinence from alcohol and other sedative drugs—one day at a time—and the liberal and regular use of group treatment, which includes self-help groups and group therapy.

Motivation is an ongoing process. In follow-up, denial will recur, and it can be dealt with by using the same three techniques. It can be useful to refer to the facts recorded at previous visits and to the patient's Michigan Alcoholism Screening Test results, if available, to help break down the recurring denial.

A Formal Intervention

All too frequently, an alcoholic with a concerned family does not respond to efforts to motivate him to accept treatment. In this situation, the physician should offer the family the option of using a powerful method known as the "intervention." The intervention consists of a meeting at which persons closest to the alcoholic (immediate family members, concerned friends, or employer) create a crisis which motivates the alcoholic to accept treatment. An individual with expertise in coordinating formal interventions can usually be identified through the local office of the National Council on Alcoholism. An available film illustrates this technique well (see "General References").

The intervention team is composed of as many persons as possible (up to a dozen) who are emotionally important to the alcoholic. Before the actual intervention this team meets several times to talk about the alcoholism, to come together in their thinking, and to break down their own denial that this intervention is necessary.

The focus of this process is to show the patient in unmistakable terms that there is a problem and that he needs treatment. This is done by having each participant put in writing specific dramatic instances of drinking-related incidents which led to anger, fear, disappointment, sadness, embarrassment, or other distress for the team member. The team rehearses confronting the alcoholic with care and concern and in as nonjudgmental a fashion as possible. Each person begins with an expression of caring and concern for the alcoholic, then describes the disturbing event and how it made that person feel. In the meantime arrangements are made to have the person admitted for alcoholism treatment. Alcoholism treatment centers are familiar with this technique and cooperate. Details of financing of treatment, packing clothes, arranging for absence from work, *etc* must all be worked out by the team ahead of time.

Team members must decide upon the severity of the measures they are willing to take in order to ensure that the alcoholic gets into and sticks with treatment. For instance, a spouse may be willing to threaten separation; an employer may be ready to threaten job loss; a parent may threaten to cut off financial support; a child may threaten to refuse to play with the alcoholic parent. The person making the threat must be prepared to carry it out if the "bluff is called" by an alcoholic who refuses treatment. The team must be prepared to support one another to make it possible to carry out their threats (42).

After the team has rehearsed, the consequences for not going into treatment are agreed upon, and the details of treatment are worked out, the patient is told that the family wants to meet to talk about some family concerns. The patient is asked to hear the family out and is told that he will be given an opportunity to express his concerns. It is hoped that the intervention will conclude with the patient accepting treatment.

If properly constructed and properly prepared, such an intervention can have enormous power with even an unmotivated alcoholic. Faced with the crisis created by the intervention, the alcoholic will find that there is nowhere left to turn should the entire team pull out its support if treatment is refused. Although an alcoholic may respond angrily to the coercion that drives him into treatment, he will usually eventually be grateful for the help.

Motivating through Employee Assistance Programs

Increasingly employers have recognized the economic and human costs of alcoholism and have developed employee assistance programs to motivate and assist alcoholics into treatment. Employers threaten to terminate employees who have deteriorating job performance due to alcoholism unless they get treatment and remain in treatment. Such programs have demonstrated recovery rates as high as 90% for alcoholics. Cost savings have been estimated to be in the range of $4 to $7 saved for every dollar invested in an employee assistance program. Physicians asked to write work excuses can often work with employee assistance programs to coerce the denying alcoholic to get appropriate treatment for alcoholism. This approach uses the strong motivation to keep a job as leverage for getting treatment and following through to recovery—leverage the physician alone may not have on the patient.

The problem of the impaired professional and the use of measures similar to employee assistance programs are discussed below (page 272).

Initiating a Treatment Plan: Eight Basic Actions

The steps which have proved most effective in getting alcoholics into treatment can be described as *eight basic actions*:

1. Tell the patient his diagnosis: Alcoholism.

2. Tell him it is a disease.

3. Tell him it is not his fault for having it.

4. Tell him it is treatable, that with treatment recovery is likely, and that you or someone else will tell him how it is treated.

5. Tell him it is his responsibility to accept treatment for his disease.

6. Offer him a specific treatment "menu" or treatment alternatives, and initiate a specific treatment plan (or utilize referral to a program; see page 267).

7. Interview the spouse or closest family member.

8. Provide strong and regular follow-up (39).

Whether or not the patient admits to having a drinking problem, the initiation of treatment is most effective if the term *alcoholism* is used. The term "drinking problem" may be used early in the discussion, before the patient's feelings regarding alcoholism are known. Even in the most denying and uncooperative patient, naming the diagnosis is useful, because it "plants a seed" that is likely to grow, given time and motivation.

Telling the patient that *he has a disease*, and that it is not his fault for having it, is a powerful motivator for patient cooperation. This information relieves guilt, a powerful and painful emotion in most alcoholics. If the patient tries to avoid responsibility for further drinking because he "has a disease," one should tell him it is his responsibility to seek treatment (action 5 above).

The first goal of treatment is *abstinence from alcohol.* However, it is never sufficient simply to tell the patient to stop drinking. Early in treatment, the physician must tell the patient *how* to get help in this difficult undertaking. This *help is multidimensional.* Among the most important elements are a concerned, supportive physician who believes the patient can recover, a plan for detoxification (see below, page 264), disulfiram (Antabuse, see page 261), family involvement, Alcoholics Anonymous (AA), and group therapy that provides the patient with successful role models. Inpatient treatment in a specialized alcoholism treatment facility will often be needed (see below, page 267). Most facilities can provide detoxification, but more important are the education, counseling, and positive orientation to the treatment process that these programs offer patients. It is important to explain each of the possible treatment options to the patient and his family. If the physician is not familiar with these, he can ask an alcoholism specialist or counselor to see the patient to explain them. If the patient is in a crisis and not enough time is available during the first visit, a return appointment should be scheduled within a few days, or the patient should be immediately referred to a reliable treatment specialist or program.

Alcoholics Anonymous and Group Therapy

Alcoholics and other chemical-dependent people seem to recover best in group therapy settings. Groups effectively break down the denial process and heal the associated guilt and shame through a combination of identification, confrontation, and support. Every alcoholic should be strongly encouraged to attend AA regularly. Many physicians who are specialists in alcoholism consider it the single most important aspect of treatment, and studies have shown that regular AA attendance is strongly correlated with long term recovery and improved functioning (3, 32). Formal alcoholism group therapy is also successful. The method of referral and the selection of a group are crucial. The referral should be made with enthusiasm and clarity. Many patients will be reluctant to attent AA or a therapy group. Therefore, the clinician should be familiar enough with these treatments and know how to obtain them so that he can be persuasive, and he should be ready to act immediately when a patient agrees to try treatment (44). Immediate action, taken while the patient is in the office, may consist of (a) telephoning the local AA office and letting the patient request a contact to take him to a convenient AA meeting, ideally on the same evening or within a day, or (b) telephoning an alcoholism treatment program and arranging an intake appointment for the patient.

The best way for physicians to learn about these programs is to attend one or more AA and open group therapy meetings. To locate such meetings, one should call the local AA office or the local National Council on Alcoholism (to find an open group therapy meeting). The AA process is summarized in Table 21.7.

Psychotherapy

It is commonly thought that all alcoholic patients have a primary and causative underlying psychological problem. If treatment of this condition is successful, the alcoholism is expected to resolve, since it is considered to be chiefly a manifestation of the underlying psychological problem. While this approach may seem theoretically valid, experts in treating alcoholism agree that this therapeutic strategy rarely works unless there happens to be a coexisting psychosis. Even in the latter case, the alcoholism must also be treated (44). After establishing rapport, therefore, the initial effort in psychotherapy should be to work with the patient toward *abstinence* and toward *regular participation in group treatment.*

For most nonalcoholics in psychotherapy it is best for the patient to arrive at his own "diagnosis," in order to reinforce insight. This technique works well for patients with emotional problems who are not chemical dependent, do not have an organic brain syndrome, or are not psychotic. However, active alcoholics are, by definition, chemical dependent, with a strong denial system, and they often have some degree of cognitive impairment, sometimes severe. Therefore, achieving insight is difficult and often impossible. To circumvent this problem, it is suggested that the therapist utilize confrontive, sup-

Table 21.7.
The Process of Alcoholics Anonymous

AA was founded in 1935 by two chronic alcoholics, one a stockbroker and one a physician.

Meetings

AA meetings are held frequently in all communities in the United States and in most other countries. Meetings are either open or closed (most are open and most welcome nonalcoholics interested in treating alcoholism). A published directory of meetings, places, times, and information by telephone are available from each local chapter of AA. By contacting AA, an alcoholic can almost always arrange to be taken to a meeting in his community, often on the day he makes the request. Many AA members attend meetings several times a week. Some attend at least one meeting per day. Lifelong activity in AA is the basis for maintaining health for many recovering alcoholics.

Meetings are usually 1 hour in length. Most are held in the evening, although there are many daytime meetings as well. Meetings begin with a recitation by one member of the Twelve Steps and the Twelve Traditions and are devoted to examination and interpretation of these—as illustrated in personal experiences described by a number of members. One member of the group chairs the meeting and calls on speakers. Speakers introduce themselves by their first names (*e.g.*, "I'm Joe—I'm an alcoholic . . . ."). Meetings end with a recitation of the Lord's Prayer by the entire group.

AA on the surface can sometimes look insubstantial and unsophisticated, often turning off newcomers. Frequently the spiritual overtones of the program are rejected. The program however is *profound and life changing*. Without an administrative structure, owning no property, and having no dues or fees, it continues to grow because it works and meets human need.

Publications

AA provides printed educational aids in the form of pamphlets (available at meetings) and "the Big Book" (*Alcoholics Anonymous*, a collection of personal stories that illustrate vividly the ways that lives are damaged by alcoholism and the AA path to recovery). One can obtain this book or other literature at meetings, at the local AA office, or by writing AA World Services, Box 459, Grand Central Station, New York, NY 10017.

The 12 Steps and the 12 Traditions

The 12 Steps

1. We admitted we were powerless over alcohol, that our lives had become unmanageable.
2. Came to believe that a Power greater than ourselves could restore us to sanity.
3. Made a decision to turn over will and our lives over to the care of God *as we understood Him*.
4. Made a searching and fearless moral inventory of ourselves.
5. Admitted to God, to ourselves and to another human being the exact nature of our wrongs.
6. Were entirely ready to have God remove all these defects of character.
7. Humbly asked Him to remove our shortcomings.
8. Made a list of all persons we had harmed, and became willing to make amends to them all.
9. Made direct amends to such people wherever possible, except when to do so would injure them or others.
10. Continued to take personal inventory, and when we were wrong promptly admitted it.
11. Sought through prayer and meditation to improve our conscious contact with God, *as we understood Him*, praying only for knowledge of His will for us and the power to carry that out.
12. Having had a spiritual awakening as the result of these Steps, we tried to carry this message to alcoholics, and to practice these principles in all our affairs.
    Boiled down, these steps mean, simply:
    a. Admission of alcoholism.
    b. Personality analysis and catharsis.
    c. Adjustment of personal relations.
    d. Dependence upon some Higher Power.
    e. Working with other alcoholics.

The 12 Traditions of AA

1. Our common welfare should come first; personal recovery depends upon AA unity.
2. For our group purpose there is but one ultimate authority—a loving God as He may express Himself in our group conscience. Our leaders are but trusted servants; they do not govern.
3. The only requirement for AA membership is a desire to stop drinking.
4. Each group should be autonomous except in matters affecting other groups or AA as a whole.
5. Each group has but one primary purpose—to carry out its message to the alcoholic who still suffers.
6. An AA group ought never endorse, finance, or lend the AA name to any related facility or outside enterprise, lest problems of money, property, and prestige divert us from our primary purpose.
7. Every AA group ought to be fully self-supporting, declining outside contributions
8. Alcoholics Anonymous should remain forever nonprofessional, but our service centers may employ special workers.
9. AA, as such, ought never be organized; but we may create service boards or committees directly responsible to those they serve.
10. Alcoholics Anonymous has no opinion on outside issues; hence the AA name ought never be drawn into public controversy.
11. Our public relations policy is based on attraction rather than promotion; we need always maintain personal anonymity at the level of press, radio, and films.
12. Anonymity is the spiritual foundation of our Traditions, ever reminding us to place principles before personalities.

portive and directive approaches, such as the eight basic actions listed above. Using this approach, the process of admission and acceptance of having a problem is initiated.

Individual supportive psychotherapy, which all physicians can provide, is useful to continue the patient's education about the disease of alcoholism and about the recovery process; to monitor the patient's functioning in important life areas, such as family, job, and interpersonal relations; to evaluate the patient's ego strength and psychopathology; and to assist the patient in change and growth (44).

Interview with the Spouse or Closest Family Member(s)

An interview with the spouse or person closest to the patient is helpful; it should, of course, be conducted without breaking the patient's confidentiality. Through this interview, one can (a) gather additional information to establish the diagnosis; (b) ensure that the family agrees with the goal of abstinence; (c) explore the drinking pattern of the spouse; (d) discern any special problems occurring in any of the close family members, including the children; (e) educate the spouse about the enabling process; (f) refer the spouse to Al-Anon, teenage children to Alateen, or some other available family resource; and (g) schedule a follow-up visit after the spouse has attended several Al-Anon meetings (44). *If the family does not change and grow, usually through regular attendance at Al-Anon meetings, it will be more difficult for the patient to recover.* Family treatment is discussed further below under "Co-Alcoholism" (the Al-Anon process is summarized in Table 21.16).

Disulfiram (Antabuse)

Consideration should be given to the use of disulfiram (Antabuse) for every alcoholic patient. Experience with this drug now approaches 40 years and includes hundreds of thousands of patients. Although physicians with the most experience in prescribing disulfiram consider it safe, many who have never prescribed it are fearful of using it (44). The dangers have probably been overemphasized. Very few deaths attributed to its interaction with alcohol have been recorded in the medical literature. Most of these occurred early in the drug's history and usually at daily doses exceeding 1000 mg (more than 4 times the present recommended daily dose of 250 mg). Disulfiram is available, as Antabuse, in the form of scored tables containing 250 mg or 500 mg. The dose range is 125 to 500 mg/day (47). Disulfiram should be prescribed with the patient's full knowledge and consent and when the patient is alcohol free (usually between 12 and 24 hours after the last drink). To assist the physician in this process, Ayerst Laboratories has published a helpful patient education booklet entitled *Guidelines for Antabuse Users.* The major points from this booklet are summarized in Table 21.8.

The Disulfiram-Alcohol Interaction

Alcohol is initially oxidized by the hepatic enzyme alcohol dehydrogenase to acetaldehyde; the acetaldehyde is immediately oxidized by the enzyme aldehyde dehydrogenase. Disulfiram works by inhibiting acetaldehyde oxidation by interfering with aldehyde dehydrogenase. Resulting elevated levels of blood acetaldehyde produce the symptoms of the alcohol-disulfiram reaction. These symptoms

---

Table 21.8.
Important Information for the Patient Who Takes Disulfiram (Antabuse)

1. Antabuse helps you remain sober by giving you time to get over the temptation of the moment to drink. The desire to drink will pass if you do not drink.
2. Antabuse is not a cure for alcoholism. Recovery requires growth in many areas of your life. Antabuse is an aid to remaining alcohol free and is best used in combination with AA, group therapy, and other treatment that helps you develop recovery strengths and skills.
3. Beware of hidden alcohol. Read labels and where there is alcohol content do not use. Many products contain alcohol. Beware of these:

Mouthwash	Paint solvents
Cough syrups	Salads prepared with wine dressings
Liquid medicines	Desserts prepared with liqueurs
Nebulizer sprays	Foods prepared with alcohol

4. At parties where alcohol is served never leave your nonalcoholic drink unattended. By accident alcohol could be added to it or you could pick up someone else's drink. If you're not sure, be safe—get a fresh drink.
5. If you should drink on Antabuse and feel frightened, contact your doctor immediately or go to an emergency room.
6. It is a good idea to carry the Antabuse identification card found in the booklet *Guidelines for Antabuse Users*. It tells helpers you are on Antabuse should you be unable to give them that information.
7. Tell your family and friends you are on Antabuse and about the reaction that will occur if you should have alcohol. Some people not knowing the dangers might want to experiment, but would not do so if they had all of the facts.

Table 21.9.
Drug Interactions with Disulfiram

Disulfiram may potentiate the effect of:
  Anesthetics
  Sedatives and hypnotics
  Anticonvulsants (particularly phenytoin, requires careful monitoring)
  Oral anticoagulants
Disulfiram with isoniazid:
  Can occasionally cause confusion, changes in mental status and unsteady gait
Disulfiram with metronidazole (Flagyl):
  May produce a psychotic reaction

are proportional to the amounts of disulfiram and alcohol ingested. Some people will have typical symptoms after drinking as little as 7 ml of alcohol. Disulfiram also interferes with other hepatic microsomal enzymes, sometimes resulting in a potentiation of the therapeutic effects of certain other drugs (see Table 21.9).

The alcohol-disulfiram reaction is described by patients as decidedly unpleasant, though a very small percentage of patients seem to be able to drink on disulfiram with no significant symptoms. In these latter patients the dosage can be increased up to 500 mg once daily, but only if the patient seems motivated to sobriety rather than to drinking.

The most commonly reported symptoms of the alcohol-disulfiram reaction usually begin within 10 minutes of drinking and include flushing, throbbing in head and neck, headaches, anxiety, general discomfort, sweating, and respiratory difficulty. The reaction typically lasts between 30 minutes and several hours. Less frequently nausea, vomiting, hypotension, thirst, chest pain, palpitation, dyspnea, hyperventilation, tachycardia, syncope, weakness, blurred vision, and confusion can occur. Very rarely, disulfiram may cause an acute exacerbation of a coexisting problem—e.g., respiratory depression, congestive heart failure, convulsions, arrhythmias, angina, or myocardial infarction. These very rare risks must be weighed against the certain risks of continued alcohol drinking.

Treatment for the alcohol-disulfiram reaction is usually supportive to restore blood pressure and treat shock. These measures should be instituted in an emergency department. A massive dose of the antioxidant vitamin C (1 g) may reduce the production of acetaldehyde by allowing alcohol to be excreted unchanged.

Disulfiram at recommended doses is tolerated well by most patients. Some patients complain of drowsiness, fatigability, headaches, a garlic-like or metallic aftertaste and breath odor and acneform eruptions. These symptoms usually subside within a few days or weeks with continued therapy or reduced dosage. More rarely confusion (particularly in the elderly), optic neuritis, polyneuritis, and peripheral neuritis may occur.

There are several advantages to disulfiram: (a)

Since the drug is taken daily, it is a constant reminder that the person cannot safely drink; (b) it provides evidence of compliance in the treatment program; (c) it is compatible with other forms of treatment of alcoholism; and (d) it can also provide family and employer with reassurance that, as long as it is taken daily, the alcoholic cannot get drunk (44). There are four additional advantages for the patient to consider. These are (a) while he takes it he cannot drink alcohol without getting sick; (b) because of this, he tends not to worry about whether he can drink or not; (c) not worrying or thinking about drinking saves him considerable energy; and (d) this makes his recovery easier.

Compliance and Duration

Assessment of compliance with the prescribed regimen is done mostly by patient report and observation. About 20% of patients who report that they are taking their disulfiram will not actually be doing so. However, many of these patients will not be drinking. Urine and breath tests to measure disulfiram metabolites have been developed, although they are not presently commercially available. A decision to stop the drug is best made jointly by the therapist, the spouse, or other close person, the AA sponsor, and the patient. It should be based on the strength of the person's recovery. Important guidelines in this decision are active AA and/or group therapy participation, coping with crises without recourse to drinking, improved family relationships, dissolution of denial, social ease (diminution in social anxiety), growth in self-esteem, and over 1 to 2 years of abstinence (47).

Alcohol-Drug Interactions (14, 27)

Because of their erratic behavior, alcoholics frequently fail to take prescribed drugs regularly or correctly. In this sense, alcoholism, like other forms of chronic mental illness, adds greatly to the difficulty of treating coexisting medical conditions. There are a number of hazards and drug interactions that must be considered when prescribing to alcoholics. Some of the interactions between alcohol and other drugs may, in fact, provide initial clues to the existence of alcoholism.

Alcohol-drug interactions may involve (a) antagonism, (b) additive and supra-additive (synergistic) effects, and (c) cross-tolerance or synergism.

Antagonism between drugs and alcohol, such as occurs with disulfiram, can cause specific, deleterious reactions. Some common drugs in this category are:

Drug	Effect
Chloral hydrate	Generalized vasodilatation
Chlorpropamide and other sulfonylureas	Disulfiram-like reaction
Some antimicrobials: chloramphenicol, griseofulvin, isoniazid, metronidazole, and quinacrine	Disulfiram-like reaction

The *additive* and *synergistic* category of drugs includes agents whose effects may be aggravated by alcohol; for example, in the presence of alcohol, salicylates might be more likely to induce bleeding or antihypertensive drugs to lower blood pressure. Common drugs in this category are:

Drug	Effect
Tolbutamide and other sulfonylureas	Hypoglycemia
Salicylates	Gastrointestinal bleeding
Antihypertensives, nitroglycerine, tricyclics	Hypotension
Warfarin	Hemorrhage (prothrombin time increased)
Sedative-hypnotics	Central nervous system (CNS) depression
Anxiolytic drugs	CNS depression
Antidepressant drugs	CNS depression
Neuroleptic drugs	CNS depression, hypotension, respiratory depression, impaired hepatic function
Antihistamines	CNS depression
Opiates	CNS depression
Metoclopramide	CNS depression

Either *cross-tolerance or synergism* can occur with some drug-alcohol combinations, depending on the time of drug administration. For example, chronic alcoholics may require an unusually large dose of anesthetic because of cross-tolerance, but at the same time would be susceptible to CNS depression with a low dose of anesthetic when alcohol has been ingested shortly before the need for emergency surgery and anesthesia (e.g., following major trauma). Examples of these drugs include: tolbutamide and other sulfonylureas, phenytoin, anesthetics, warfarin, CNS depressants, and tricyclic antidepressants.

Finally, *cimetidine* may inhibit hepatic metabolism of alcohol and/or increase gastrointestinal absorption of alcohol; patients placed on cimetidine may thus become intoxicated with less consumption and should be forewarned.

Psychoactive Drug Prescribing

Although many alcoholics present with symptoms that might be helped by sedatives, such as anxiety, insomnia, and tremors, in actuality *these drugs usually interfere with successful recovery.* Sedative drugs may have a role in acute detoxification (see below, page 266) and major tranquilizers, antidepressants, and lithium have usefulness in treating, respectively, the schizophrenic, the severe protracted depressive, and the manic-depressive alcoholic (as long as these patients are being treated concomitantly for alcoholism). Psychoactive drugs should be avoided in the postdetoxification treatment of alcoholics because (a) all of the sedatives are cross-tolerant with alcohol, and thus have a "built-in" escalation factor; (b) combining sedatives with alcohol is often dangerously synergistic; (c) inability to control consumption, a cardinal feature of alcoholism, occurs with prescribed sedative drugs; (d) memory blackouts may also occur with other sedatives and minor tranquilizers; (e) patients may alter the prescription in order to obtain excess quantities of these drugs; (f) prescribing these drugs reinforces sedative ingestion as a coping mechanism; alcoholics already have difficulty in using another sedative—alcohol—in this way; (g) they prevent development of the patient's coping mechanism; (h) they interfere with learning to relate to others in a healthy manner; and (i) using the drugs may alienate the patient from perhaps the best treatment he could receive, i.e., Alcoholics Anonymous (39, 44). Bissell (4) has said "I do think we need to give our patients a substitute for alcohol, but I don't think that substitute can be another sedative. I think it has to be our concern, our time, our caring, and ourselves."

Urine Monitoring in the Alcoholic with Chemical Dependence

For the patient with chemical dependence to one or more drugs other than alcohol, urine monitoring is indicated. This is in part because it can be difficult to recognize that a person is using drugs, especially early in the course of a relapse. Urine monitoring is also therapeutic, in that it gives the patient another type of structure through which to recover. Finally, it is often to the patient's advantage (e.g., to protect his job or to meet court-ordered conditions) to have negative urines documented for a substantial period of time. Low priced urine screens that check for from 30 to 40 different psychoactive drugs are available in most large communities. For communities that lack these services, specimens can be mailed to a regional laboratory. This should be done by a reliable person other than the patient. The sample should be collected at random and witnessed by a reliable observer. In patients being treated for multidrug dependence, weekly urine monitoring should continue for a minimum of 1 year.

Follow-up Treatment

Next to dealing with denial and motivating the patient, follow-up is the most difficult part of treatment. One reason is that when an alcoholic recovers there may be an early "honeymoon period" during which the patient feels and looks so good that the therapist is lulled into believing that regular follow-up is not necessary. However, because it takes about *2 to 3 years of appropriate treatment* before recovery can be secure, regular follow-up is indicated.

During the first 6 weeks after stopping drinking, the patient is most likely to relapse. Therefore, at least weekly visits are indicated for this time, with a gradually decreasing frequency thereafter. During this early period many patients are fragile and need much support and direction. Therefore, the treating clinician should try to spend at least 30 minutes with them at each of these early visits. High risk times for potential relapse may include special days and occasions, such as vacations, holidays, business trips, birthdays, anniversaries; or crises such as separation, divorce, death of a close person, or illness in the family. Other relapse danger times are when a patient stops taking disulfiram or stops going to AA or group therapy meetings.

The "dry drunk" is also a danger time. A dry drunk is a flare-up of negative emotions and behavior reminiscent of that when the patient was drinking. It may be an anxiety or panic attack; or the patient may be depressed, angry, feeling a wish to drink and not accepting the disease, or simply having a bad day. Dry drunks may last from a few hours to several weeks or even months, and they are frequently part of the natural history of recovery. Treatment is by recognition, education, and alteration of the diet and other current life habits. Dry drunks are often associated with eating "junk food." A nutritious diet should be prescribed. Caffeine intake, including coffee, tea, colas, and chocolate, should be markedly decreased or discontinued. Sweets and sugar should be avoided, and a substantial breakfast is helpful. Increased attendance at AA and/or group therapy meetings at this time is also important. Moderation in the patient's work, and recreational activities and rest should be advised.

The "dry drunk" is a part of the relapse *process* or dynamic, which generally begins long before the person drinks. This relapse process often progresses in the following sequence: (*a*) reactivation of denial; (*b*) progressive isolation and defensiveness; (*c*) building a crisis to justify symptom progression; (*d*) immobilization; (*e*) confusion and overreaction; (*f*) depression; (*g*) loss of control over behavior; (*h*) recognition of loss of control; (*i*) option reduction; and (*j*) debilitation—which ends in drinking, using other drugs, or in some other debilitating condition (13).

Although it should not be telegraphed to the patient, relapse is part of the natural history of successful recovery (see Fig. 21.1 illustrating the long term course of a typical recovering alcoholic), and the therapist should not become discouraged if it happens. Instead, he should *immediately* recruit the patient back into treatment. *Relapse is a time for both the patient and the therapist to learn about their mistakes* and to correct them by strengthening treatment.

DETOXIFICATION

It has been shown that about 90% of alcoholics can be detoxified from alcohol by outpatient procedures (10, 38, 39, 44, 45), leaving about 10% that require hospitalization for detoxification. While many alcoholics can be detoxified at home, many will also benefit from a community "social setting" detoxification center, described below.

Alcohol Withdrawal Symptoms

A history of a recent bout of drinking lasting at least a week—although the duration is usually longer—and the absence of other conditions which could cause symptoms mimicking withdrawal, usually confirm the diagnosis of alcohol withdrawal. The four major manifestations of alcohol withdrawal in alcohol-dependent patients are tremors, hallucinosis, seizures ("rum fits"), and delirium tremens. These occur also in other conditions, ranging from meningitis to withdrawal from other sedative-hypnotic drugs (see list of causes of delirium, Chapter 17, Table 17.6).

The *alcohol hallucination* is almost never the mythical "pink elephant." Rather, it is usually one of moving insects, small animals, or threatening voices. In a series of 50 consecutive patients, 58% of their hallucinations were purely visual, 16% were purely auditory, and 26% were mixed (33). In certain patients these hallucinations may not be all negative, *i.e.*, the patient becomes used to them and is no longer frightened. Hallucinations may begin up to several days after the patient stops or markedly reduces alcohol (usually in the first 48 hours). Typically, alcoholic hallucinosis lasts from minutes to days (usually less than 1 week) but in a very small percentage of patients hallucinosis may continue for weeks or months and, rarely, as a continuous symptom.

At least half of ambulatory alcoholic patients who stop drinking have *none* of the four major manifestations of withdrawal. Additional minor symptoms are common. Anorexia, nausea, and sometimes vomiting are present in varying degrees. Generalized weakness may be prominent, and tinnitus, hyperacusis, itching, muscle cramps, mood and sleep disorders are sometimes experienced. The patient is often hyperalert, becomes startled easily, and usually craves alcohol or other drugs to quiet his symptoms. The patient usually experiences varying degrees of disorientation and difficulty concentrating.

Nondrug Detoxification

This technique of detoxification is used in many settings, including home and social settings and in some inpatient treatment programs and hospitals. It is sometimes erroneously called "nonmedical" detoxification. However, medical and nursing input and supervision are integral features of this approach.

Candidates for nondrug detoxification should be *ambulatory* or semiambulatory and, except for their chronic alcoholism and acute withdrawal, should be *otherwise free from serious illness*. As described below, nondrug detoxification can be utilized for both "social setting" and home detoxification. These settings are appropriate if they are available and if the patient does not have one of the indications for being taken to an emergency room for treatment (see Table 21.10).

The primary aim in nondrug detoxification is to provide a nonthreatening, positive environment for the patient (Table 21.11). The patient should be kept ambulatory when possible and given a regular diet. Except when asleep or resting comfortably, he should be encouraged to perform purposeful activities, such as carrying out small duties or attending introductory group education and therapy sessions. If the patient becomes unduly agitated, someone he trusts should provide the "three R's"—Reassurance, Reality orientation, and Respect.

The patient will nearly always benefit from positive attitudes and benign persistence on the part of physician, staff, or family. It is now clear that nondrug therapy can be just as effective and usually is

Table 21.10.
Some Indications for Taking a Withdrawing Alcoholic to an Emergency Department

1. Vomiting blood
2. A fever greater than 100.5°F (38.1°C)
3. Shortness of breath or respiratory rate >20
4. Sudden onset of chest pain
5. Heart rate >120 in absence of tremulousness or hallucinosis, or as part of withdrawal that does not improve with a talk down
6. A seizure that occurs more than once, or from which the patient does not awaken within 15 minutes, or a localized seizure
7. Shaking chills
8. Severe abdominal pain
9. Protracted vomiting
10. Any trauma other than minor trauma
11. Depression of consciousness where the patient is not arousable
12. History of a recent head injury (within 3 days)
13. Recurring hallucinations
14. Marked agitation that does not respond to talk down
15. Delirium
16. Delirium tremens
17. Uncontrolled violence

Table 21.11.
Environmental Modification in Treating Alcohol and Other Sedative Withdrawal[a]

Sense	Therapeutic	Countertherapeutic
Visual	Lights on, not bright Familiar people, pictures, clock, clothes	Lights off Marked shadows
Sound	Soft music Soft conversation Reassurance and reality Orientation by staff	Loud or abrupt noises
Touch	Reassuring touch by staff (*e.g.*, taking pulse, hand on shoulder) Comfortable chair Low bed Regular clothes	Bed clothes High bed Restraints IVs and tubes
General	Respect Positivity, optimism	Hostility, even if subtle Negativity or pessimism

[a] Modified from Baum R, Iber FL: Initial treatment of the alcoholic patient. In Gitlow SE, Peyser HS (eds): *Alcoholism: A Practical Treatment Guide*. New York, Grune and Stratton, 1980, chap 4, pp 73–87.

less hazardous than drug therapy in the detoxification of ambulatory and otherwise uncomplicated patients (10, 38, 45).

The advantages of nondrug detoxification, as compared with traditional detoxification with drugs, include:

1. It is shorter in duration.
2. It can be done by nonmedical personnel.
3. It is less expensive.
4. It permits earlier diagnosis of psychiatric conditions.
5. It decreases dependence on other drugs.
6. The patient is more alert and, therefore, better able to participate in treatment.
7. The patient remembers the withdrawal experience and is thus more likely to realize the damaging consequences of his or her drinking behavior.

The use of all psychoactive drugs should be avoided, and routine medications should not be given unless they are clearly indicated for an ongoing condition. Antimicrobials and antidiabetic and cardiac medications usually should be continued. Antihypertensive drugs should be discontinued during the patient's withdrawal from alcohol. The only routine medication should be vitamins, i.e., 50 to 100 mg of thiamine daily, 1 mg of folate a day, and a potent multivitamin daily. Some centers give the first dose of these vitamins intramuscularly. These vitamins should be continued for the first month or more of recovery.

For patients with a history of withdrawal seizures, phenytoin in a dose of 300 mg daily for 5 days can prevent most withdrawal seizures, even though therapeutic levels are not reached initially (23). Should a withdrawal seizure occur, the nurses and aides should monitor the patient carefully. If the patient does not recover fairly rapidly following a seizure, he should, of course, be checked by a physician.

Social Setting Detoxification (See Table 21.12)

In the past 10 years, many communities have established alcoholism facilities that provide a sheltered, supportive environment to care for alcoholics using a social model for detoxification. Patients are screened and evaluated to detect any obvious medical problems before or shortly after being admitted. Should complications arise, backup hospital/medical support is available.

The detoxification is carried out without use of medications by substituting for drugs the involvement of staff and other patients in support, encouragement, and caring for the acutely detoxifying patient. The atmosphere is usually home-like, and the facility is typically free standing rather than being located in a hospital.

The length of stay varies in each program from 3 days to more than 30 days. Most social setting programs use AA extensively, and many of the larger programs use all of the techniques used in other alcoholism treatment centers. These centers can be either day treatment or inpatient facilities.

Table 21.12.
Suggested Procedure for Nondrug Detoxification in a Social Setting Treatment Unit

1. Diet and fluids as desired (regular diet).
2. Juices as needed between meals.
3. Decaffeinated coffee or tea only.
4. No smoking in bed or during acute withdrawal symptoms.
5. Vital signs (temperature, blood pressure, pulse) every 4 hours.
6. History and physical examination by the physician or designee within 8 hours of admission to the center.
7. Thiamine 100 mg, folate 1 mg on admission, then same amount by mouth daily thereafter.
8. Multiple vitamin by mouth daily.
9. Acetaminophen (Tylenol), antacid as needed.
10. No psychoactive drugs or physical restraints.
11. Provide a nonthreatening, positive environment (Table 21.11).
12. Bed rest as desired.
13. For withdrawal signs keep patient active, as tolerated.
14. Reality orientation, reassurance, and respect in abundance.
15. Call physician or take patient to emergency department as indicated (see Table 21.10).

Home Detoxification

For detoxification at home without the use of drugs, there should be a trusted family member or other person to observe the patient for 2 full days. The physician should have training and experience in supervising such detoxification and should be in touch with the patient or the family member daily during the 2 days required for detoxification. The following is a checklist for home detoxification:

1. The patient should be motivated to do it at home.
2. A reliable person should be with the patient or frequently check on him.
3. There should be access to a phone to call the physician or counselor twice or more daily for reassurance and to monitor withdrawal.
4. No active medical problems requiring aggressive treatment, and no high dose chemical dependence to drugs other than alcohol.
5. Ability to see physician, nurse, or counselor each day for 2 days.
6. Use no drugs, preferably.
7. If sedatives are required, use antihistamines (e.g., Vistaril 50 mg orally every 3 to 4 hours).
8. Keep the patient as active as he can tolerate.
9. Attend AA if patient can tolerate.
10. Food and fluid as desired.
11. Multivitamins daily.
12. No caffeinated beverages.
13. Strong outpatient program started upon detoxification.

Using Psychoactive Drugs in Detoxification

Psychoactive drugs are clearly beneficial in selected patients who are withdrawing from alcohol. Characteristics of such patients include the following: (*a*) those hospitalized in intensive care and coronary care units (usually nonambulatory); (*b*) those hospitalized with an ongoing *acute* medical problem (also usually nonambulatory); (*c*) those in situations where the physicians and staff are not trained in and committed to using a nondrug detoxification approach; (*d*) those for whom nondrug detoxification techniques are delivered by trained staff and do not work (probably less than 1% of ambulatory, relatively uncomplicated alcoholics); and (*e*) as a reserve, for those persons undergoing detoxification at home or in a social setting detoxification center.

Detoxification using psychoactive drugs appears to be most effective when combined with the nondrug techniques described above, when treatment is given early, and when low doses of the drugs are used. The safest and most effective drugs for this purpose are the benzodiazepine sedative-hypnotics. It seems to matter somewhat less *which* sedative-hypnotic drug is used than *how* it is used. (An exception is that oxazepam, Serax, is probably safer in patients with overt liver disease, as it is not metabolized by the liver.) What is important is *early recognition* of withdrawal, *early treatment*, *frequent monitoring*, and *continual treatment*. Given the decision to use sedative drugs to help the detoxification process, one can choose low or high doses (see Table 21.13).

Low doses of sedative-hypnotic drugs may be tried first for most patients who are not already in active delirium tremens. The advantage of low dose treatment is that it allows a clearer sensorium in the patient, thereby preserving some of the advantages of using nondrug detoxification techniques listed above. Low dose drug treatment should be used in *combination with the nondrug techniques* described and should be started early in the course of withdrawal, preferably at its first sign.

High doses of these drugs may be indicated (*a*) where the low dose approach is not effective and (*b*) in patients where a high degree of sedation seems necessary, such as a patient already in active delirium tremens, or a patient with an obvious acute medical or surgical problem. Nondrug techniques will also help with these patients. The acute medical condition should be appropriately and vigorously treated.

The aim of drug treatment is to alleviate the bothersome symptoms and signs of withdrawal, when nondrug techniques alone are not indicated or feasible, and to prevent their future progression. The drug should be given such that withdrawal symptoms are improved but without oversedating the patient. The total single dose, daily dose, and frequency of administration will vary with the patient's and the staff's needs. Thus the schedule of the drug will usually be between every 2 to 12 hours "as needed." The route of administration of benzodiazepines should be by mouth, or if this is not possible, by slow intravenous push (diazepam or chlordiazepoxide). (Hydroxyzine, diphenhydramine, and barbiturates can be given intramuscu-

larly, but not the benzodiazepines, which are inconsistently absorbed.)

For the 70-kg patient *actively* in delirium tremens (DTs), a slow intravenous push of diazepam 10 mg may be the most effective initial treatment, to be repeated every 30 to 60 minutes as needed to lessen the agitation. At times it may be needed more frequently. After diagnosis and initial therapy, patients with DTs should be admitted to the hospital.

REFERRAL

The clinician who initially motivates an alcoholic to accept treatment may elect not to treat him but to refer him elsewhere. It is far better to refer than to become involved with alcoholics in a partial or countertherapeutic manner. If the decision is made to refer the patient, the referring physician's major responsibilities are recognition of the disease alcoholism, selection of an effective source of help, and avoidance of placing problems in the path of the recovering patient such as prescribing sedative medication or advising to cut down on drinking (44).

For this important referral, one should select a specialist or a program with demonstrated expertise in helping alcoholics to recover. The simplest ways to find such expert help are to call the local National Council on Alcoholism (listed in the yellow pages of the phone book under alcohol), to ask a colleague who has had experience in referring or treating alcoholics, or to refer the patient to an existing community alcoholism treatment program. In selecting skilled help, one should look for several characteristics. The effective alcoholism specialist or program tends to (*a*) be abstinence oriented; (*b*) use AA and/or group therapy as a mainstay of treatment; (*c*) offer disulfiram to patients; (*d*) avoid the use of psychoactive drugs in long term treatment, especially the sedative-hypnotics; (*e*) refer the spouse to Al-Anon or family therapy; (*f*) provide close follow-up; and (*g*) avoid insight-oriented psychotherapy, unless indicated later in the course of recovery. The physician who makes the referral, if he is the patient's personal physician, should reinforce participation in the treatment program, as well as any agreed-upon treatment aid, whenever he sees the patient in follow-up.

The responsibility of physicians to be competent in handling alcoholism has been highlighted in legal decisions in recent years. There are accumulating cases in which physicians have lost suits brought by families and patients for (*a*) failure to diagnose alcoholism; (*b*) failure to refer alcoholics for treatment; or (*c*) failure to provide treatment for alcoholism.

INPATIENT TREATMENT

Inpatient treatment for 2 to 6 weeks is a powerful aid for breaking down denial and motivating the

Table 21.13.
Selected Sedative-Hypnotic Drugs in Low and High Oral Doses as Treatment Aids in Detoxification

Drug	Low Dose[a]	High Dose[a]
	mg	*mg*
Benzodiazepines		
Chlordiazepoxide (Librium)	25	100
Diazepam (Valium)	2–5	10
Oxazepam (Serax)	10	30
Antihistamine-Antianxiety		
Hydroxyzine (Vistaril, Atarax)	25–50	100
Diphenhydramine (Benadryl)	25–50	100
Barbiturates		
Phenobarbital	30	100

[a] Every 2 to 12 hours.

patient to remain in a long term outpatient treatment program. There are situations where it is especially appropriate and should be used in concert with outpatient treatment. Indications for inpatient treatment are (a) strong denial, especially if it persists in outpatient treatment; (b) unsuccessful or too slow recovery despite adequate outpatient treatment; (c) weak or unavailable support systems; (d) danger to self or others; (e) severe medical, psychiatric, or other problems or consequences; and (f) patient's desire for inpatient treatment.

Perhaps 50% of alcoholic patients will require at least one admission to an inpatient treatment facility during the long course of their alcoholism treatment. Such treatment should be given in a facility that specializes in treating alcoholism and chemical dependence.

While treatment goals among inpatient treatment programs vary, some of the major goals include (a) breaking down denial; (b) educating about alcoholism/chemical dependence; (c) providing an introduction to group treatment: self-help and group therapy; (d) becoming aware of feelings and learning to handle them; (e) learning how to ask for help; (f) learning how to communicate directly and honestly; (g) learning how to enjoy life while abstinent; (h) beginning family restoration; and (i) developing a specific, appropriate, and structured long term recovery program.

PROGNOSIS WITH TREATMENT

With appropriate and continued treatment for at least 2 years, the prognosis for a successful recovery in alcoholism is about 70% (6, 15, 21, 25, 26, 32, 39). However, this figure does not apply to every alcoholic. For example, even with appropriate treatment, it is rare to see a "skid row" alcoholic (homeless, jobless, and derelict for 2 years or more) make a successful recovery. By contrast, the alcoholic patient with a home, a family, a job, and a strong incentive or coercive mechanism to continue appropriate treatment will have a high chance for success, usually in the range of from 80 to 90%.

Table 21.14 lists factors that are associated with a high chance of success and factors that are associated with a low chance of success.

Factors Associated with a Good Prognosis

The first of these factors is *clinician and patient motivation*. Most patients are only marginally motivated to get well. They can be characterized as having a strong ambivalence: a part of them wants to get well, and another part of them wants to continue drinking and stay sick (the patient usually does not know what is wrong with him because no one has told him of the diagnosis in an effective way). If the patient's personal physician is not motivated, the patient will almost never attain a pro-

Table 21.14.
Some Factors That Positively and Negatively Influence the Quality and Duration of Recovery in Alcoholism

Factors Associated with an Increased Likelihood of Recovery

1. Clinician and patient motivation
2. Crisis situation (*e.g.*, job, driving while intoxicated, family)
3. Appropriate treatment—minimum 2 years
4. Continued threatened loss for stopping treatment (therapeutic coercion)
5. Job, health, and intelligence intact (early diagnosis)
6. Family intact, with treatment for alcoholism
7. Prompt and strengthened treatment at relapse
8. Caring, nonjudgmental clinician—uses disease view
9. Constructive clinician: learns from relapses and mistakes
10. Three-fold recovery model used—physical, mental, and spiritual

Factors Associated with a Decreased Likelihood of Recovery

1. No threatened loss from continued drinking
2. Inappropriate or short treatment
3. Continued self-destructive bent
4. Cognitive impairment or psychosis
5. Acceptance of derelict subculture status
6. Powerful enablers (see "Co-Alcoholism")
7. Relapse treatment delayed or not strengthened
8. Avoiding, negative, or rejecting clinician—does not use disease view
9. One-dimensional recovery model
10. Patient uses other psychoactive drugs (lithium and major tranquilizers are exceptions in highly selected patients)

longed recovery. It is therefore up to the clinician to help motivate the patient into treatment, by using the skills described earlier in this chapter.

The presence of a crisis situation is also a positive prognostic factor *if the clinician uses the crisis as a motivational tool*. The crisis may be the threat of a job loss, family separation or divorce, a driving-while-intoxicated charge, a health-related crisis, an organized formal intervention (see page 258), or some other dramatic event. To be most effective, it is important to capitalize on the presence of this crisis within about 10 days of its onset. Such action will mean getting the person started in treatment that is specific for the alcoholism. Probably the most effective way to do so is either to have the patient see a trained alcoholism counselor or to have the patient admitted to an inpatient alcoholism treatment facility. The physician can also precipitate a "mini-crisis" in the office, hospital, or emergency room by emphasizing to the patient that he or she has a *serious* problem, and then taking the eight basic actions listed earlier (see page 258). If exploitation of this crisis does not work, at least a seed has been planted that may eventually yield results.

The third factor associated with a good prognosis is *appropriate treatment for at least 2 years*. Those people whose alcoholism began before age 25 usually require at least 3 years of treatment. Many alcoholics who begin treatment will either believe they can "do it on their own" or they will return to drinking and drop out of treatment. They frequently offer other "reasons" or excuses for stopping treatment. However, nearly always patients *cannot remain abstinent from alcohol (and other drugs) continuously and substantially improve their lives "on their own."* A major barrier to recovery is the isolation that alcoholism breeds. To recover effectively, most alcoholics need to be with people who are themselves recovering successfully. This favorable environment is found most easily in self-help groups such as Alcoholics Anonymous and in group therapy (see above, page 259). Thus, when the patient shows any indication of dropping out of treatment, the effective clinician immediately motivates him back into treatment.

It is very helpful, in keeping the patient motivated to stay in treatment, for him to have a *continued threatened loss for stopping treatment*. However, most clinicians are not trained to use such a therapeutic coercion, and some, especially those trained in the mental health fields, find doing so especially difficult. If the alcoholic patient knows that his physician genuinely cares, he will be more likely to cooperate in treatment that is somewhat coercive. In this regard, the following are helpful ways to obtain participation in treatment: (*a*) using a therapeutic contract between physician and patient, or (*b*) a patient-employer contract making job security contingent upon continued sobriety (see "Motivating through Employee Assistance Programs", page 258), or (*c*) assuring that the family continues to threaten the actions named in a formal intervention (see page 258).

The prognosis also tends to be better if *job, health, and intelligence are intact*. These are often not completely intact early in treatment, but they are usually salvable, and will improve with abstinent time and continued treatment. Job, health, and intelligence, plus family support, are factors that usually correlate with how far along the alcoholism has advanced. Thus, making a diagnosis early in the course of the alcoholism generally portends a better prognosis, since these factors tend to be more intact early in the illness. Also, in early illness the patient's and family members' denial system and other defense systems tend not to be as strong.

If the patient's *family is intact* and one or more of them are receiving treatment for their co-alcoholism (discussed below, page 269), the patient generally has a better prognosis.

If *relapse occurs, it should be treated immediately.*

At this time the treatment should be strengthened. The clinician can exert much positive influence if he is *open to learning from his mistakes*, either during diagnosis, treatment, or at relapse. Finally, if a 3-fold recovery model is used, emphasizing that alcoholism is a *physical, mental, and spiritual illness* (40), the patient is more likely to make a successful recovery.

Generally, the more of the above factors that are present and maintained, the better the chance for reaching a successful recovery.

Factors Associated with a Poor Prognosis

If the patient has *no perceived threatened loss* from continued drinking, the prognosis for recovery is generally worse.

A second factor which may worsen the prognosis is *one of the following forms of inappropriate treatment*: (*a*) disulfiram (Antabuse) alone; (*b*) psychoanalytically oriented psychotherapy in the first year of alcoholism treatment; (*c*) "controlled drinking" treatment; (*d*) inpatient or outpatient treatment that does not treat alcoholism as a primary process; and (*e*) treatment that is too short in duration.

While many patients who have a *continued self-destructive bent* do not tend to recover, some do. Often, intensive inpatient alcoholism treatment for 2 months or longer can be helpful in such patients.

Cognitive impairment or psychosis often makes treatment difficult. However, the presence of these factors alone does not preclude a full attempt at treatment. With abstinence there is often surprising improvement over time.

Acceptance of a derelict subculture status by the patient makes the prognosis virtually hopeless. However, it can be helpful to screen for a potentially reversible derelict status by looking at prior career and duration of dereliction. For example, a person who up until 2 years ago was in a productive profession or trade, and is now on skid row, has potential for recovery. By contrast, a skid row person who has had no constructive activities for many years generally has little chance for reaching a successful long term recovery.

If the patient has *powerful enablers* (see "Co-Alcoholism") to deny, cover up, and protect him from the consequences of his drinking or drug using, it is less likely that he will make a successful recovery. Treatment for the family and other people close to the patient may eliminate this enabling process.

Additional factors associated with a poor response to treatment are listed in Table 21.14.

CO-ALCOHOLISM

Co-alcoholism can be defined as *ill health or maladaptive, problematic, or dysfunctional behavior that is associated with living, working with, treating, or otherwise being close to a person with alcoholism.*

Co-alcoholism affects not only individuals, but families, communities, businesses, and other institutions, and even whole societies. Its "signs and symptoms" range from passive acceptance and absence of symptoms to (a) behaviors that protect or "enable" the alcoholic, (b) chronic somatic or psychiatric symptoms, and (c) a myriad of other manifestations as shown in the following lists of examples.

In Individuals Close to an Alcoholic (Children, Spouses, Friends)

1. Behavioral or psychological symptoms, such as anxiety, depression, insomnia, hyperactivity, aggression, anorexia nervosa, bulimia, and suicidal gestures.
2. Functional or psychosomatic illness.
3. Family violence or neglect.
4. Alcoholism or another chemical dependence or a "drug problem."

In Helping Professionals

1. Failure to diagnose alcoholism.
2. Failure to treat alcoholism as a primary illness.
3. Treating the alcoholic with long term sedatives or minor tranquilizers.
4. Treating the co-alcoholic with sedatives or minor tranquilizers.

(As noted earlier, some of these co-alcoholic behaviors have been the basis for a number of successful suits against physicians in recent years.)

In Society at Large

1. Not confronting relatives, friends, and colleagues who are inappropriately intoxicated or who are misusing alcohol or drugs.
2. Placing a positive social value upon those who drink.
3. Stigmatizing those who are alcoholics or those who do not drink.

Co-Alcoholism in the Individual

The following is a typical case history of co-alcoholism in an individual.

A 38-year-old white, married woman presented with recurring episodes of upper abdominal pain of about 4 years' duration. During that time she had been worked up by two internists and had been hospitalized once. After extensive evaluations, the working diagnosis was functional abdominal pain. She was treated with antispasmotics and sedatives but there was no substantial improvement. The pain occurred almost every day. On a follow-up visit 6 months later, the patient said that a friend had suggested that she attend the self-help group Al-Anon because her husband's drinking had been bothering her for at least 5 years. The patient reported that after attending 12 Al-Anon meetings over 3 months, her abdominal pain gradually abated. On follow-up 2 years later, she had continued to attend Al-Anon and the symptoms had not recurred. In the meantime, the patient's husband had continued to drink.

This patient illustrates a common manifestation of co-alcoholism, *i.e.*, a functional or psychosomatic illness that resolved after recognizing an alcohol problem in the family and attending Al-Anon regularly. The diagnosis and treatment of co-alcoholic patients is often more complex. The diagnostic and treatment principles described here can be applied to the family that has a member suffering from chemical dependence due to other drugs, in which the analogous condition can be called "co-chemical dependence," often abbreviated as "co-dependence" (35, 36).

Diagnosis and Management of the Co-Alcoholic Individual

When a patient presents with unexplained somatic or psychological symptoms, it is helpful to ask if the patient has ever been concerned about the drinking (or drug use) of anyone close to him or her. If the answer is yes, the patient should be asked to describe the problem. If the patient is vague or doubtful, one can administer the Family Drinking Survey shown in Table 21.15. One can also ask the possible co-alcoholic to answer the questions on the Michigan Alcoholism Screening Test (Table 21.4) as though the questions were addressed to, and answered honestly by, the potentially alcoholic person to whom he or she is close. A positive score on either test is a strong indication of co-alcoholism.

Initially, the psychological and behavioral adjustments of the co-alcoholic are normal responses to an abnormal situation. However, these adaptive responses eventually lead to the individual becoming dysfunctional. Co-alcoholism, like alcoholism, is chronic, progressive, and characterized by denial, ill health, or maladaptive behavior and by a lack of knowledge about alcoholism. While there is little in the literature about co-alcoholism, there appear to be effective aproaches to its treatment.

The family member with co-alcoholism often meets the DSM-III criteria for *adjustment disorder*, *i.e.*, a maladaptive reaction to a stressor (in this instance, alcoholism) leading to social or occupational impairment or to symptoms in excess of a normal or expected reaction to the stressor; and expected to improve when the stressor ceases or, if the stressor persists, when a new level of adaptation is achieved (2). It should be emphasized that improvement for the co-alcoholic may occur even if the alcoholic (stressor) does not get treatment, as illustrated in the case example above. The co-alcoholic may also meet the DSM-III criteria for *posttraumatic stress disorder*: (a) a recognizable stressor;

Table 21.15.
Family Drinking Survey

	YES	NO
1. Does someone in your family undergo personality changes when he or she drinks to excess?	——	——
2. Do you feel that drinking is more important to this person than you are?	——	——
3. Do you feel sorry for yourself and frequently indulge in self-pity because of what you feel alcohol is doing to your family?	——	——
4. Has some family member's excessive drinking ruined special occasions?	——	——
5. Do you find yourself covering up for the consequences of someone else's drinking?	——	——
6. Have you ever felt guilty, apologetic, or responsible for the drinking of a member of your family?	——	——
7. Does one of your family member's use of alcohol cause fights and arguments?	——	——
8. Have you ever tried to fight the drinker by joining in the drinking?	——	——
9. Do the drinking habits of some family members make you feel depressed or angry?	——	——
10. Is your family having financial difficulties because of drinking?	——	——
11. Did you ever feel like you had an unhappy home life because of the drinking of some members of your family?	——	——
12. Have you ever tried to control the drinker's behavior by hiding the car keys, pouring liquor down the drain, *etc*?	——	——
13. Do you find yourself distracted from your responsibilities because of this person's drinking?	——	——
14. Do you often worry about a family member's drinking?	——	——
15. Are holidays more of a nightmare than a celebration because of a family member's drinking behavior?	——	——
16. Are most of your drinking family member's friends heavy drinkers?	——	——
17. Do you find it necessary to lie to employers, relatives, or friends in order to hide your spouse's drinking?	——	——
18. Do you find yourself responding differently to members of your family when they are using alcohol?	——	——
19. Have you ever been embarrassed or felt the need to apologize for the drinker's actions?	——	——
20. Does some family member's use of alcohol make you fear for your own safety or the safety of other members of your family?	——	——
21. Have you ever thought that one of your family members had a drinking problem?	——	——
22. Have you ever lost sleep because of a family member's drinking?	——	——
23. Have you ever encouraged one of your family members to stop or cut down on his or her drinking?	——	——
24. Have you ever threatened to leave home or to leave a family member because of his or her drinking?	——	——
25. Did a family member ever make promises that he or she did not keep because of drinking?	——	——
26. Did you ever wish that you could talk to someone who could understand and help the alcohol-related problems of a family member?	——	——
27. Have you ever felt sick, cried, or had a "knot" in your stomach after worrying about a family member's drinking?	——	——
28. Has a family member ever failed to remember what occurred during a drinking period?	——	——
29. Does your family member avoid social situations where alcoholic beverages will *not* be served?	——	——
30. Does your family member have periods of remorse after drinking occasions and apologize for his or her behavior?	——	——
31. Please write any symptoms or medical or nervous problems that you have experienced since you have known your heavy drinker? (Write on back if more space needed).		

If you answer "YES" to any 2 of the above questions, there is a good possibility that someone in your family may have a drinking problem.

If you answer "YES" to 4 or more of the above questions, there is a definite indication that someone in your family *does* have a drinking problem.

(These survey questions are modified or adapted from the Children of Alcoholics Screening Test (CAST), the Howard Family Questionnaire, and the Family Alcohol Quiz from Al-Anon.)

(b) symptoms of re-experiencing the trauma; (c) symptoms or signs of psychological numbing; and (d) other manifestations, such as hyperalertness or survival guilt (2). This disorder is discussed in Chapter 13.

The major strategies in treating an individual with co-alcoholism are remarkably similar to those for treating the alcoholic:

1. Have the patient accept the fact that he or she is a co-alcoholic.

2. Motivate the patient to get help (occasionally by using a coercive intervention, such as the family intervention described on page 258).

3. Refer the patient to Al-Anon or Alateen (as is true of AA referrals, enthusiasm for and a good understanding of the Al-Anon process on the part of the referring physician are critical to successful referral. The Al-Anon process is described in Table 21.16).

4. Provide supportive psychotherapy at follow-up visits (see description of techniques, Chapter 11) and refer the patient or the family for additional therapy, especially group therapy for spouses and other family members.

5. Assist in the process of getting the alcoholic(s) who is the source of the problem into treatment (this is *not* the responsibility of the co-alcoholic, however).

Co-Alcoholism in the Helping Professions

Co-alcoholism includes behavior on the part of professionals that "enables" alcoholics to remain enmeshed in their disease, as noted above. Enabling behavior often coexists with otherwise excellent clinical skills. The Professional Enablers Screening Test (Table 21.17) is useful for identifying the various ways in which enabling may occur in the context of medical practice. Societal norms (including one's own approach to the use of alcohol) plus unawareness of modern approaches to diagnosis, motivation, and management of the alcoholic—usually due to a lack of appropriate training in medical or other professional school—are probably the major reasons for the co-alcoholism in helping professionals. Several steps are recommended for the professional who wishes to cease being an enabler:

1. Update one's knowledge of alcoholism.

2. Attend a number of AA and Al-Anon meetings.

3. In one's own practice, try using skills such as those described in this chapter. The best "cure" for co-alcoholism in the physician is success in getting a number of alcoholics and their families into the recovery process.

A Summary View of Co-Alcoholism

It is estimated that for each of the 10 to 15 million alcoholics in the United States there are three to five people who are seriously affected by their association with the alcoholic. Focusing on this enormous segment of the population that, in addition to family members, includes many helping professionals, law enforcement workers, politicians, employers, and others could result in a cultural change that would force the alcoholic or other chemical dependent into earlier treatment. In other words, education of this co-alcoholic group could stop the enabling, cover-up, and seductive promotion of alcohol to those afflicted with or destined to be afflicted with the disease alcoholism.

THE IMPAIRED PHYSICIAN OR OTHER PROFESSIONAL

Each year the United States loses an estimated 400 or more physicians and countless persons from other helping professions to chemical dependence and suicide. Conservatively, at least 8% of physicians become chronically impaired because of alcohol or other substance abuse at some time in their careers. Most of these individuals could be successfully treated with early recognition and follow-up. Since the mid-1970s, the American Medical Association and each state medical society have developed helpful programs for troubled or impaired physicians. Because of this, each year several hundred dysfunctional physicians are now being rehabilitated and returned to productive practices and better lives. In recent years, numerous other professional organizations have implemented such programs, including organizations of nurses, dentists, pharmacists, psychologists, social workers, lawyers, and others.

Definitions

A physician or other professional can be considered to be impaired when one or more problems cause him to be dysfunctional, recurringly, in the quality of patient or client care, other professional activities, education, or private life. The impaired professional may be further defined as a person who is troubled by personal difficulties to the extent that (a) he cannot offer reasonable patient care, effectively help others through interpersonal skills, or maintain skills by continuing education; or (b) he demonstrates a definite decline from his prior level of functioning, even if he is currently performing adequately. Impairment may be further characterized by denial and ambivalence on the part of the physician, the family, and the community, all of whom may ignore the problem until it is too late. Intervention with appropriate treatment as soon as it is recognized is a major goal of the impaired physician movement.

Impairment may be either transient or chronic and varies along a spectrum of severity of degree and causes. One problem is that presently there is no way to monitor *transient impairment*. For example, any physician who has been intoxicated has

Table 21.16.
The Al-Anon Process

Al-Anon began in the 1940s as an AA auxiliary and initially called itself AA Family Groups. In 1952, the wives of the two founders of AA established Al-Anon.

Al-Anon is a fellowship of family members of alcoholics who meet together to share their experience, strengths, and hopes so that they can achieve health and serenity. The organization is modeled after AA and uses the 12 Steps of AA as its principles for individual recovery. Its focus is not on the alcoholic but on the family members, and by so doing it powerfully frees families from their dependence on the alcoholic.

Al-Anon meetings are all open to the public and frequently meet at the same time and location as AA meetings. In most communities, Al-Anon has a telephone listing where meeting information, help, and literature can be obtained. Where there is no local Al-Anon office, the AA office can provide Al-Anon information.

Al-Anon meetings generally last 1 hour and follow the format of AA meetings (see Table 21.7), but they are usually smaller and discussion of topics is often freer than in AA.

Al-Anon is the sponsor of Ala-Teen and Ala-Tots, which are organizations for teenage and young children of alcoholics, respectively. These groups follow the Al-Anon discussion format and in general are not open to the nonalcoholic public, but helping professionals are usually welcome if they request to attend. In the last several years in some areas, Al-Anon members have begun groups for adult children of alcoholics. These groups offer help to adults who may no longer live with an alcoholic family member, but whose life continues to be adversely affected by the legacy of growing up in an alcoholic home. These are especially powerful, and many patients with this background can be profoundly helped.

Al-Anon publishes a number of pamphlets for families that are available at meetings. *Al-Anon Faces Alcoholism*, Al-Anon's "Big Book," describes the family's plight with alcoholism through a variety of stories that graphically describe how families become sick in response to the alcoholic. Its other major book, *Living with an Alcoholic*, offers practical suggestions for recovery.

More information can be had by writing Al-Anon Family Group Headquarters, Box 182, Madison Square Station, New York, NY 10010.

The Al-Anon 12 Steps

Al-Anon uses the same 12 Steps as AA. It can be helpful to clarify these steps for Al-Anon members or prospective members. Because there are many co-dependents who will not be familiar with 12-Step programs, Wegsheider-Cruse (36) has paraphrased the steps for co-dependents:

1. We acknowledge and accept that we are powerless in controlling the lives of others, and that trying to control others makes our lives unmanageable.
2. We have come to believe that a power greater than ourselves can restore enough order and hope in our lives to move us to a growth framework.
3. We make a decision to turn our lives over to this power to the best of our ability, and honestly accept that taking responsibility for ourselves is the only way growth is possible.
4. We make an inventory of ourselves, looking for our mental, emotional, spiritual, physical, volitional, and social assets and liabilities. We look at what we have, how we use it, and how we can acquire what we need.
5. Using this inventory as a guide, we admit to ourselves, to God as we understand Him, and to other caring persons, the exact nature of what is within that is causing ourselves pain.
6. We give to God as we know Him, all former pain, hurt and mistakes, resentments and bitterness, anger and guilt. We trust that we can let go of the hurt we cause and receive.
7. We can ask for help, support, and guidance and be willing to take responsibility for ourselves and to others.
8. We begin a program of living responsibly for ourselves, for our own feelings, mistakes, and successes. We become responsible for our part in relationship to others.
9. We make a list of persons to whom we want to make amends and commence to do so, except where doing so would cause further pain for others.
10. We continue to work our program, each day checking out our progress and asking for feedback from others in our attempt to recover and grow. We do this through support groups.
11. We see through our own power and a Higher Power, awareness of our inner selves. We do this through reading, listening, meditation, sharing, and other ways of centering and getting in touch with our inner selves.
12. Having experienced the power of growing toward wholeness, we find our bodies, minds, and spirits awakened to a new sense of physical and emotional relief which leaves us open to a new awareness of spirituality. We seek to explore our meaning in life by honest sharing with others, remembering that BECOMING WHO WE ARE is a lifetime task which must be done one day at a time.

Wegsheider-Cruse (36) sees these 12 Steps for co-dependents as useful guidelines and reminders of their tasks in recovery. They are not meant to imply affiliation with AA, Al-Anon, or any other self-help group structured around a 12-Step format.

Al-Anon 12 Traditions

1. Our common welfare should come first; personal progress for the greatest number depends upon unity.
2. For our group purpose there is but one authority—a loving God as He may express Himself in our group's conscience. Our leaders are but trusted servants—they do not govern.
3. The relatives of alcoholics, when gathered together for mutual aid, may call themselves an Al-Anon Family Group, provided that, as a group, they have no other affiliations. The only requirement for membership is that there be a problem of alcoholism in a relative or friend.

Table 21.16.—Continued

4. Each group should be autonomous, except in matters affecting another group or Al-Anon or AA as a whole.
5. Each Al-Anon Family Group has but one purpose: to help families of alcoholics. We do this by practicing the 12 Steps of AA *ourselves*, by encouraging and understanding our alcoholic relatives, and by welcoming and giving comfort to families of alcoholics.
6. Our Family Groups ought never endorse, finance, or lend our name to any outside enterprise, lest problems of money, property, and prestige divert us from our primary spiritual aim. Although a separate entity, we should always cooperate with Alcoholics Anonymous.
7. Every group ought to be fully self-supporting, declining outside contributions.
8. Al-Anon Twelfth Step work should remain forever nonprofessional, but our service centers may employ special workers.
9. Our groups, as such, ought never be organized; but we may create service centers or committees directly responsible to those they serve.
10. The Al-Anon Family Groups have no opinion on outside issues; hence our name ought never be drawn into public controversy.
11. Our public relations policy is based on attraction rather than promotion; we need always maintain personal anonymity at the level of press, radio, TV, and films. We need guard with special care the anonymity of all AA members.
12. Anonymity is the spiritual foundation of all our Traditions, ever reminding us to place principles above personalities.

Table 21.17.
Professional Enablers Screening Test[a]

Please check your answer to each question. For medically oriented questions, please check the space to which you would subscribe, even though you may not be a physician.

	Yes	No
1. Do you sometimes avoid raising sensitive issues related to drinking because it might offend your patient, or make him or her angry or feel bad?	(2)	
2. Do you generally treat the heavy drinking person's problems without focusing most of the treatment on the drinking behavior?	(5)	
3. Do you avoid confronting your heavy drinking patient when there is good evidence that he or she has misinformed you about his or her drinking?	(2)	
4. Do you generally suggest to your alcoholic patients that they cut down on their drinking?	(3)	
5. Do you believe what your heavy drinking patient tells you about his or her drinking without using other sources such as a spouse, employer, a screening test, blood alcohol level, or other laboratory test?	(5)	
6. Do you generally prescribe a sedative or minor tranquilizer for the nervous conditions or sleep problems of your alcoholic patients?	(5)	
7. Do you refer most of your alcoholic patients to attend Alcoholics Anonymous meetings regularly?		(5)
8. Do you refer many of your alcoholic patients to an alcoholism therapy group?		(3)
9. Do you prescribe disulfiram (Antabuse) to many of your alcoholic patients?		(3)
10. When your alcoholic patient has a minor crisis requiring hospitalization, do you routinely hospitalize him or her in a community hospital general ward?	(5)	
11. Do you refer most of the spouses or family members of your alcoholic patients to attend Al-Anon meetings regularly?		(5)
12. Do you subscribe to the theory that most alcoholics have an underlying psychological disorder that is the major cause of their alcoholism?	(5)	
13. Do you believe that most alcoholics will not respond positively to treatment for their alcoholism?	(5)	

[a] A score of 0 to 3 points indicates a probable nonenabler; 4 to 6 points may indicate a possible enabler; 7 points or more indicates a probable enabler. We can change our enabling behavior.

been transiently impaired, since during the period of intoxication he would have provided suboptimal care. Also, physicians can be episodically exposed to extreme personal stresses, i.e., their own or family members' change or loss of important relationships or financial disruptions which render them temporarily impaired. How long impairment should be present to indicate *chronic impairment* is difficult to specify; 6 months might be a reasonable minimum (41).

Troubled physicians have been described in three major categories—those who are:
1. Incompetent, due to lack of skill or knowledge.
2. Unethical, malicious, or uncaring.
3. Ill, either physically or mentally.
The ill physician is by far the most common. The illness may be alcoholism, other chemical dependence, emotional illness, senility, or another condition. Programs for impaired physicians are analogous to "broad brush" employee assistance pro-

grams, in that they must sort out the source of the problem and arrange appropriate intervention and follow-up.

Recognition, Diagnosis, and Management

The manifestations, symptoms, or signs of impairment from alcoholism and other chemical dependence among professionals are the same as those seen in nonprofessionals (see Table 21.3). A checklist of particular clues to assist in the recognition of impairment in helping professionals is shown in Table 21.18. Note that many of these manifestations are late indicators of impairment, especially those listed under "Manifestation at Hospital." Early signs are indicated with an *asterisk*.

Once impairment is recognized, an evaluation should be made to determine the cause of the impairment. Two approaches may be used. First, the director of the impaired professional program or the identified person's supervisor can discreetly call two close associates to substantiate that impairment is present. At that time the likely cause of the impairment can be explored. Alternatively, the director or supervisor can order an evaluation by a professional with expertise in the area of chemical dependence and other causes of job impairment. Alcoholism or another chemical dependence will be the cause of the impairment in from 40 to 85% of those evaluated, with the remainder being due to psychiatric illness such as major affective disorder, schizophrenia, se-

---

Table 21.18.
Clues to Impairment in the Physician, Nurse, or Other Helping Professional[a,b]

Home and Family	*Physical Status*
* Medicinal use of alcohol or drugs	* Insomnia
* Mood swings or inconsistency	* Personality and behavior changes
* Behavior excused by family and friends	* Amnesias
Drinking or substance-using activities more important than other activities	Multiple physical complaints and illnesses
Children neglected, abused, or in trouble, often with drugs	Many prescriptions for self and family
Extreme temper	Frequent emergency room visits and hospitalizations
Fights, arguments, and violent outbursts	Inappropriate tremulousness or sweating
Sexual problems	Poor hygiene and appearance
Withdrawal, isolation, and fragmentation of social and family life	Long sleeves in warm weather
Family isolating itself from social supports	*Manifestations at Hospital*
Financial problems	* Heavy drinking at staff functions
Spouse in psychotherapy or taking psychoactive medication	Often late, absent, or ill
Lack of problem resolution	Decreased work/chart performance
Separation or divorce	Inappropriate orders
	"Hospital gossip"
Manifestations at Office	Unavailability
* Overwork	Alcohol on breath while in hospital
Disorganized schedule	Drunk when on call, even at home
Spasmodic work pace	
Unreasonable behavior	*Friends and Community*
Inaccessible to patients and staff	* Neglected social commitments
Excessive drug use, prescriptions, and supply	* Embarrassing behavior
Liberal in prescribing psychoactive drugs to patients	Personal isolation
Medical errors	Overreaction to criticism
Patient complaints	Exaggerates work accomplishments and finances
Frequent absences	Drunk driving arrests
Decreased work load and tolerance	Legal problems
Frequent days off for vague reasons	Neglected social commitments
Taking sexual advantage of patients or co-workers	Lessening of ethical values
	Unpredictability or unreliability
Employment Applications	
Frequent job changes or relocations	
Unusual medical history	
Vague letters of reference	
Inappropriate qualifications	
Time lapse unexplained in work	
Inappropriate job now	
Refusal of physical examination or spouse interview	

[a] Modified from Talbott GD, Benson E: Impaired physicians: the dilemma of identification. *Postgrad Med* 68:56, 1980; and Whitfield CL, Bissell L, Wesson DW: Treatment of the professional or "VIP" alcoholic. In Whitfield CL, Liepman MR (eds): *The Patient with Alcoholism and Other Drug Problems.* Baltimore, University of Maryland, 1980. See also Table 21.3.
[b] An *asterisk* indicates early signs.

nility, or severe neurosis or character disorder and severe chronic problems, sometimes due to compulsive gambling, and occasionally miscellaneous other causes, including co-alcoholism (see above). Rarely, more than one cause will be present.

Alternatively, direct, private, individual approaches to the impaired person and/or family are often appropriate and effective. However, one must assure that the helping professional(s) involved are skilled in the successful treatment of chemical dependence.

The family members of the troubled physician or other professional are often suffering in varying degrees from co-alcoholism or co-dependence or an equivalent debilitating condition. They should be evaluated and appropriately treated.

General References

Alcoholics Anonymous: The Story of How Many Thousands of Men and Women Have Recovered from Alcoholism ("The Big Book"), ed 3. New York, Alcoholics Anonymous World Services, 1976.

> The nature of alcoholism and the recovery process using AA are illustrated in a large number of personal stories.

Bean M: Alcoholics Anonymous. I. Principles and methods. *Psychiatr. Ann* 5:5, 1975.

> A psychiatrist's lucid account of the AA process, based on her personal visits to 40 different AA groups.

Drews T: *Getting Them Sober: A Guide for Those Who Live with an Alcoholic*, Plainfield, NJ, Haven Books, 1980.

> Widely available paperback, for families of alcoholics. Quick reading. Advice regarding numerous practical issues ("hide the car keys?"; "don't beg him to stay"; "don't pour out the booze," etc).

Health and Public Policy Committe, American College of Physicians: Chemical dependence. *Ann Intern Med* 102:405, 1985.

> Consensus paper defining the responsibilities of practicing physicians to recognize alcoholism and other forms of chemical dependence and to assure that affected patients get appropriate treatment.

Kwentus J, Major LF: Disulfiram in the treatment of alcoholism. *J Stud Alcohol* 40:428, 1979.

> Reviews biochemistry, history of therapeutic uses, current indications and contraindications.

"The Enablers" and "The Intervention." Minneapolis, Johnson Institute, 1978.

> Two of the best films ever made on alcoholism. Must viewing for all helping professionals. Technique of formal intervention shown.

Vaillant G: *The Natural History of Alcoholism*. Cambridge, MA, Harvard University Press, 1983.

> Detailed monograph, much of it based on the author's longitudinal studies.

West LJ: Alcoholism. *Ann Intern Med* 100:405, 1984.

> Recent review covering biomedical consequences, alcoholism in older persons, and controversies regarding treatment.

Specific References

1. Allen RP, Faillace LA, Wagman A: Recovery time for alcoholics after prolonged alcohol intoxication. *Johns Hopkins Med J* 128:158, 1971.
2. American Psychiatric Association: *Diagnostic and Statistical Manual of Mental Disorders*, ed 3. Washington, DC, American Psychiatric Association, 1980.
3. Bill C: Probability of continuation of sobriety. *Q J Studies Alcohol* 26:283, 1965.
4. Bissell L: The treatment of alcoholism: what do we do about long-term sedatives? *Ann NY Acad Sci* 252:396, 1975.
5. Buckey SF, Edwards D, Berz NH: *Hospitalizations and Discharge Rates of Men Treated at the Navy's Alcohol Centers.* Report No. 75-41. San Diego, Naval Health Research Center, May, 1975.
6. Cahalan D: *Problem Drinkers: A National Survey.* San Francisco, Jossey-Bass, 1970.
7. Criteria for the diagnosis of alcoholism. Criteria Committee, National Council on Alcoholism, New York, New York. *Ann Intern Med* 77:249, 1972.
8. Eckardt MJ, Harford TC, Kaelber CT, et al.: Health hazards associated with alcohol consumption. *JAMA* 246:648, 1981.
9. Ewing JA: Detecting alcoholism: the CAGE questionairre. *JAMA* 252:1905, 1984.
10. Feldman DJ, Pattison EM, Sobell LC, et al: Outpatient alcohol detoxification: initial findings on 564 patients. *Am J Psychiatry* 132:407, 1975.
11. Fine E, et al: Philadelphia DWI Study. *US J Alcohol Drug Abuse*, 19, March, 1983.
12. Goodwin DW: *Is Alcoholism Hereditary?* New York, Oxford University Press, 1976.
13. Gorski TT, Miller M: *Counseling for Relapse Prevention.* Independence, MO, Independence Press, 1982.
14. Hansten PD: *Drug Interactions: Clinical Significance of Drug-Drug Interactions*, ed 5. Philadelphia, Lea and Febiger, 1985.
15. Kissin B: Theory and practice in the treatment of alcoholism. In Kissin B, Begleiter H (eds): *The Biology of Alcoholism.* Vol 5: *Treatment and Rehabilitation of the Chronic Alcoholic.* New York, Plenum Press, 1977, pp 1–51.
16. Lewis DC, Gordon AJ: Alcoholism and the general hospital: the Roger Williams Intervention Program. *Bull NY Acad Med* 59:181, 1983.
17. Mills JL, Graubard BI, Harley EE, et al: Maternal alcohol consumption and birth weight: how much drinking during pregnancy is safe? *JAMA* 252:1875, 1984.
18. Morse RM, Swanson WM: Spouse response to a self administered alcoholism screening test. *J Stud Alcohol* 36:400, 1975.
19. Myers JK, Weissman MM, Tischler GL, et al: Six-month prevalence of psychiatric disorders in three communities. *Arch Gen Psychiatry* 4:959, 1984.
20. Pell S, D'Alonzo CA: A five-year morbidity study of alcoholics. *J Occup Med* 15:120, 1973.
21. Polich JM, Armor DJ, Braiker HB: *The Course of Alcoholism: Four Years after Treatment.* Santa Monica, Rand Corporation, R-2433, NIAAA, 1980.
22. Powers JS, Spickard A: Michigan Alcoholism Screening Test to diagnose early alcoholism in a general practice. *South Med J* 77:852, 1984.
22a. Reuler JB, Girard DE, Coomes TG: Wernicke's encephalopathy. *N Engl J Med* 312:1035, 1985.
23. Sampliner R, Iber F: Diphenylhydantoin control of alcohol withdrawal seizures. *JAMA* 230:1430, 1974.
24. Saunders JB, Beevers DG, Paton A: Alcohol-induced hypertension. *Lancet* 1:163, 1981.
25. Schuckit MA: *Drug and Alcohol Abuse.* New York, Plenum Medical Book Co, 1979, pp 59–62, 180.
26. Schuckit MA: Treatment of alcoholism in office and outpatient settings. In Mendelson JH, Mello NK (eds): *The Diagnosis and Treatment of Alcoholism.* New York, McGraw-Hill, 1979, pp 229–255.
27. Seixas FA: Alcohol and its drug interactions. *Ann Intern Med* 83:86, 1975.
28. Selzer M: The Michigan Alcoholism Screening Test (M.A.S.T.): the quest for a new diagnostic instrument. *Am J Psychiatry* 127:1653, 1971.
29. Skinner HA, Holt S, Schuller R, et al: Identification of alcohol abuse using laboratory tests and a history of trauma. *Ann Intern Med* 101:847, 1984.
30. Sobell MB, Sobell LC: Individualized behavior therapy for alcoholics. *Behav Ther* 4:49, 1973.
31. Talbott GD, Benson E: Impaired physicians: the dilemma of identification. *Postgrad Med* 68:56, 1980.
32. Vaillant G, Clark W, Cyrus C, et al: Prospective study of alcoholism treatment. *Am J Med* 75:455, 1983.

33. Victor M, Hope JM: The phenomenon of auditory hallucinations in chronic alcoholism. *J Nerv Ment Dis* 126:451, 1958.

34. Wallace J: Alcoholism from the inside out: a phenomenological analysis. In Estes NJ, and Heinemann ME (eds): *Alcoholism: Development, Consequences, and Interventions.* St Louis, CV Mosby, 1977.

35. Wegsheider S: *Another Chance: Hope and Health for the Alcoholic Family.* Palo Alto, CA, Science and Behavior Books, 1981.

36. Wegsheider-Cruse S: *Choice-Making.* Pompano Beach, FL, Health Communications, 1985.

37. West LJ: Alcoholism. *Ann Intern Med* 100:405, 1984.

38. Whitfield CL: Treatment of alcohol withdrawal without drugs. In Masserman J (ed): *Current Psychiatric Therapies.* New York, Grune and Stratton, 1980.

39. Whitfield CL: Outpatient management of alcoholism. *Psychiatr Ann* 12:447, 1982.

40. Whitfield CL: *Alcoholism, Other Drug Problems and Spirituality: Stress Management and Serenity during Recovery.* Baltimore, MD, The Resource Group, 1984.

41. Whitfield CL, Bissell L, Wesson DW: Treatment of the professional or "VIP" alcoholic. In Whitfield CL, Liepman MR (eds): *The Patient with Alcoholism and Other Drug Problems.* Baltimore, University of Maryland, 1980.

42. Whitfield CL, Liepman MR: Motivating the alcoholic patient into treatment. In Whitfield CL, Liepman MR (eds): *The Patient with Alcoholism and Other Drug Problems.* Baltimore, University of Maryland, 1980.

43. Whitfield CL, Williams KH: Diagnosis of alcoholism. In Whitfield CL, Liepman MR (eds): *The Patient with Alcoholism and Other Drug Problems.* Baltimore, University of Maryland, 1980. (Can be obtained by writing The Resource Group, 7402 York Road, Suite 101, Baltimore, MD, 21204.)

44. Whitfield CL, Williams KH: Treatment of the alcoholic patient. In Whitfield CL, Liepman MR (eds): *The Patient with Alcoholism and Other Drug Problems.* Baltimore, University of Maryland, 1980.

45. Whitfield CL, et al: Detoxification of 1,024 alcoholics without psychoactive drugs. *JAMA* 239:1409, 1978; and letter response 241:2597, 1979.

46. Zook CJ, Moore FD: High-cost users of medical care. *N Engl J Med* 302:996, 1980.

47. Zuska JJ, Pursch JA: Long-term management. In Gitlow SE, Peyser HS (eds): *Alcoholism: A Practical Treatment Guide.* New York, Grune and Stratton, 1980, pp 131–163.

CHAPTER TWENTY-TWO

Use and Abuse of Illicit Drugs and Substances

BURTON D'LUGOFF, M.D., AND JAMES HAWTHORNE, PH.D.

DEFINITIONS

Illicit drugs are substances which are taken for nonmedical reasons, to modify mood or behavior. The use and abuse of such substances dates back thousands of years. Plant alkaloids, alcohol, and an ever increasing array of newly synthesized chemicals have been used in these endeavors. Patterns of use and the social acceptance of use of these agents have differed from time to time and from place to place. Successive generations of the same society have held discordant views about which substance to use, at what age, in what amount, and under which circumstances (e.g., attitudes regarding alcohol use in the pre- and postprohibition eras in the United States). Also, in a single historical epoch, neighboring cultures have differed about the sanctioned use of psychoactive substances. Currently, in 20th-century Western society the use of illicit substances is expressed in two ways:

1. *Experimental.* The experimental use of illicit substances is sporadic; the initial trial and experience usually are associated with youthful rites of passage. These experiments usually have little impact on mental health. Medically they are dangerous only to the extent that possible dosage errors and bizarre or unsterile methods of exposure may occur. Incorrect labeling of such drugs (a common problem) increases the risk of an untoward effect. Experimentation is commonplace. A 1983 national high school survey (11) revealed that 57% of all respondents had engaged in an experimental trial of an illicit drug (primarily marijuana) and 93% had tried alcohol on at least one occasion.

2. *Social-recreational.* The social and recreational use of illicit substances suggests that they have been used repetitively but that control has been exerted over the dose and the time of use. The risks due to unintended overdosage, improper exposure, and mislabeling are increased by the frequency of use. To the extent that control is effectively exerted to maintain a high degree of social and behavioral function, recreational use also is not psychologically disabling. Most American use of alcohol and marijuana conforms to this pattern of social-recreational use.

Abuse refers to the combination of three characteristics (1):

1. *There is a pattern of pathological use* of a particular substance. Depending upon the substance, this may be manifested by intoxication throughout the day, inability to cut down or stop use, repeated efforts to control use, continuation of use despite a serious physical disorder that is exacerbated by the substance, need for daily use for adequate functioning, and episodes of a medical complication of substance intoxication.

2. *Impairment in social or occupational functioning* is caused by the use of an illicit substance. This refers to failure to meet important obligations to friends and family, to erratic and impulsive behavior, and to behavior leading to legal difficulties or problems with employment.

3. *Duration is of at least 1 month.* Signs of the drug-abusing pattern do not have to be present continuously throughout the month, but should be sufficiently frequent that a pattern of pathological use causing interference with social or occupational functioning is apparent.

Succeeding sections of this chapter describe the manifestations and the principles of management for the forms of substance abuse most common in the United States today. A cursory listing of all drugs extant today which have abuse potential would be extremely long. It is possible, however, to group the various substances into broad classes, the members of which share common characteristics and are readily distinguishable from other classes (Table 22.1). Psychoactive substances may thus be classified as (a) depressants, (b) stimulants, and (c) drugs which alter perception (including hallucinogens).

PREVALENCE

Survey data indicate that with the exception of cocaine and other stimulants, the prevalence of drug abuse has declined slightly between 1978 and 1983.

Table 22.1.
Categories of Psychoactive Drugs

DEPRESSANTS
  Narcotics:
    Morphine, hydromorphone (Dilaudid), heroin, meperidine (Demerol), codeine, methadone
  Sedative-hypnotics:
    Alcohol, barbiturates, glutethimide (Doriden), methaqualone (Quaalude)
  Minor tranquilizers:
    Diazepam (Valium), chlordiazepoxide (Librium), meprobamate (Equanil or Miltown)
  Inhalants:
    Nitrous oxide, toluene, volatile hydrocarbons
STIMULANTS
  Cocaine, amphetamine methylphenidate (Ritalin), phenmetrazine (Preludin)
DRUGS WHICH ALTER PERCEPTION (INCLUDING HALLUCINOGENS)
  Marijuana, lysergic acid diethlamide (LSD), dimethylamine tryptamine (DMT), psylocybin, phencyclidine (PCP), belladonna alkaloids (atropine, scopolamine)

This is a welcome departure from the consistent pattern of year by year increases which marked the mid and early 1970s. The percentage of high school students who have ever used marijuana, for example, has fallen from a peak of 60% in the years 1979 through 1981 to 57% in 1983. The number of seniors reporting daily marijuana use has declined from 10.7% in 1978 to 5.5% in 1983 (11).

Recent estimates of the prevalence of drug use by young Americans are available from the 1982 *National Survey on Drug Abuse* (15) (see Table 22.2). These data were obtained in household interviews, omitting subsets of the population in which drug abuse is probably even more common (*i.e.*, transients, military base personnel, college dormitory residents, and prisoners). A major trend during the early 1980s has been the emergence of cocaine as a drug of abuse and its use by Americans in both the middle and upper social classes. Twenty-eight per cent of young adults in the 1982 sample had used cocaine at least once and 7% had used it within the last year (see Table 22.2).

ECONOMIC COST OF DRUG ABUSE

A study commissioned by the National Institute on Drug Abuse placed the economic cost of drug abuse in the US during fiscal year 1980 at approximately $47 billion (9). This figure includes both direct expenditures of funds and economic losses attributable to drug abuse. Comparable cost estimates for alcoholism and mental illness were $90 billion and $54 billion, respectively. Major expenditures related to drug abuse were for law enforcement, treatment of drug abuse and its medical consequences, and drug abuse prevention. The largest economic losses to society occurred in the form of

Table 22.2.
Percentage of People Ages 12 through 25 Who Report Nonmedical Use of Drugs[a]

	Youth (12–17 Years)								Young Adults (18–25 Years)							
	Ever Used				Current Use[b]				Ever Used				Current Use[b]			
	1972	1977	1979	1982	1972	1977	1979	1982	1972	1977	1979	1982	1972	1977	1979	1982
Marjuana and hashish	14	28	31	27	7	17	17	12	48	60	68	64	28	27	35	27
Hallucinogens	5	5	7	5	1	2	2	1	+	20	25	21	+	2	4	2
Cocaine	2	4	5	7	1	1	1	2	9	19	28	28	+	4	9	7
Heroin	1	1	1	*	*	*	*	*	5	4	4	1	*	*	*	*
Stimulants	4	5	3	7	x	1	1	3	12	21	18	18	x	3	4	5
Sedatives	3	3	3	6	x	1	1	1	10	18	17	19	x	3	5	3
Tranquilizers	3	4	4	5	x	1	1	1	7	13	16	15	x	2	2	2
Analgesics	x	x	3	4	x	x	2	1	x	x	12	12	x	x	1	1
Alcohol	x	53	70	65	x	31	37	27	x	84	95	95	x	70	76	68
Cigarettes	x	47	54	50	x	22	—	15	x	68	83	77	x	47	—	40

[a] Adapted from Miller JD, Cisin IH, Gardner-Keating H, *et al: National Survey on Drug Abuse: Main Findings 1982.* Washington, DC, US Government Printing Office, 1983.
[b] Used at least once in last 30 days.
Symbols: +, not tabulated; x, not asked; *, less than 0.5%; —, alternate definition.

worker absenteeism and lost productivity due to underemployment, hospitalization, or incarceration. As of 1980, the authors of the study estimated that the cost of drug abuse in 1983 would be approximately $60 billion.

The connection between property crime and heroin addiction has been well established. One recently published study (3) reported that heroin addicts commit 4 times as many crimes while addicted than when abstinent. The addicts interviewed in this study reported committing an average of over 250 crimes a year during the 9-year period under investigation. It is important to note that the cost estimates given earlier did not include the cost of stolen property because economists think of theft as an "involuntary transfer" of goods. From an economic standpoint, goods are considered to be lost only when they are destroyed.

THE GENERAL PHYSICIAN'S ROLE: DIAGNOSIS AND REFERRAL

The care of the drug-abusing patient by the generalist should consist basically of diagnosis and referral. Diagnosis is often difficult since patients generally take great pains to deny and conceal their use of drugs. Techniques which are especially helpful in getting a patient to disclose his substance abuse and to agree to treatment are described in Chapter 21 (Alcoholism). Information obtained from the patient's spouse, parent(s), or other closely associated person(s) is often important.

It is important to remember that people from all walks of life can abuse drugs. The stereotype of the drug abuser is of a young, antisocial male of unkempt appearance who uses drugs for their euphoric effect. However, the abuse of illicit drugs such as marijuana and cocaine is now commonplace among middle and upper class Americans, and the misuse and abuse of prescription analgesics and anxiolytics by individuals who are in the mainstream of American society have been recognized for many years. Patients with chronic anxiety, insomnia, or pain are at high risk of abusing medications used to treat those conditions. In most instances, abuse develops not because the patient is seeking drug-induced euphoria or intoxication but because the tolerance that develops during continued use leads the patient to increase the dosage to inappropriate levels. Elderly patients are at particular risk because they are more likely to be given medications and more likely to be receiving multiple prescriptions. Changes in the pharmacokinetics of drugs secondary to the aging process also make the elderly more vulnerable to normally prescribed doses (24) (see also Chapter 6). Furthermore, they often have less recourse to nonpharmacological alternatives in coping with pain, psychological distress, or insomnia.

All forms of drug abuse require both acute and long term intervention. Acute intervention includes the management of overdose, toxicity, and withdrawal, which requires medical treatment and is concerned primarily with the physical effects of drug ingestion. It is important to recognize, however, that when the immediate physical consequences of drug abuse have been successfully treated, there remains a critical need to identify and treat the underlying conditions that motivated drug misuse in the first place. Most drug abusers will be found to have significant problems of psychological and social adjustment and will require counseling and rehabilitation over extended periods of time before they are capable of sustained abstinence. If the underlying problems are not addressed, detoxification of the patient, regardless of how it is carried out, is unlikely to result in meaningful periods of abstinence.

Insight-oriented psychotherapy has not proven particularly successful in the treatment of drug abusers, particularly those with extensive problems of social adjustment. Effective approaches stress basic rehabilitation, the development of practical social and vocational skills, and the avoidance of social environments conducive to drug use. In recent years, there has been an increasing recognition that families may actually "enable" drug abuse by one or more members. Family therapy has been used successfully with narcotic addicts (21) and would appear to be the treatment of choice with teenage drug abuse patients who are still living with their parents.

Since many drug abusers have important deficits in education and vocational preparation, lack basic social and recreational skills, and are handicapped by problems of poor impulse control and low self-esteem, the process of rehabilitation will often take considerable time. As with alcoholics, relapse is commonplace and recurrent treatment episodes will frequently be required.

There is evidence that existing treatment modalities shorten the course of substance abuse disorders and reduce the amount of injury to both the individual and the community. An economic assessment of the effects of drug abuse treatment (20) has yielded evidence that treatment reduces the economic costs that result from drug abuse and that these cost reductions substantially exceed the actual cost of providing care. However, while treatment appears to be cost effective, it must also be acknowledged that definitive treatment methods that result in lasting abstinence from drugs in a significant proportion of patient do not presently exist. The modalities currently available, while beneficial, generally require time, patience, and the recognition that recurrent episodes of treatment will often be required.

Specialized treatment facilities, inpatient, ambulatory, and residential, are now widely available and can be located through state and local health departments.

Self-help groups have also proved to be beneficial to many patients with drug and alcohol problems. A trusted physician can be instrumental in persuading a patient to try self-help groups. Alcoholics Anonymous, Al-Anon, and Ala-Teen groups (see descriptions in Chapter 21) are primarily oriented to alcoholics and their families, but most groups welcome participation by individuals and family members where any type of drug abuse is the primary problem. Even when a patient refuses treatment, the physician should recommend Al-Anon to the spouse and Ala-Teen to the children if this is possible. These groups help family members deal with the shame and guilt that family members often experience and help them to regain their own confidence and self-esteem. They also stress the importance of discontinuing "enabling" behavior—actions which are intended to "help" but in fact only shield the substance abuser from the consequences of his or her abuse and serve therefore to delay serious efforts at recovery. Narcotics Anonymous and Nar-Anon are groups specifically designed for narcotic abusers that are based on the Alcoholics Anonymous and Al-Anon models. They are a relatively recent development and are not as widely available as the latter groups, but both organizations are growing. All of these groups can be located by consulting the local telephone directory.

DEPRESSANT DRUGS

Tolerance and Addiction

Central nervous system (CNS) depressants all share the capacity to induce *psychoactive tolerance*. Psychoactive tolerance is habituation of the CNS to repetitive drug dosages given in a schedule so that there is at all times a measurable level of the drug in the blood. Tolerance results in a diminution or absence of the expected biological effect of a given dose of the drug. Markedly increased amounts of drug are required to achieve the initially desired effect. Psychoactive tolerance is distinguishable from "*pharmacological*" *tolerance*, which reflects the induction of catabolic enzymes that metabolize a drug more rapidly on repeated use. Psychoactive tolerance depends upon a change in the neuronal membrane receptors, independent of the rate of metabolism of the drug. Barbiturates induce both pharmacological and psychoactive tolerance. Narcotics produce only psychoactive tolerance.

The time required for the induction of psychoactive tolerance varies from a matter of days following repeated intravenous or intramuscular administration of narcotics, to weeks or months following repeated oral administration of narcotics, barbiturates, alcohol, and other sedatives.

Physiological addiction (dependence) is defined as the point in the induction of tolerance where abrupt cessation of a drug results in withdrawal symptoms (the abstinence state). Withdrawal symptoms are often the mirror image of the biological effects exerted by the drug in question (Table 22.3). As can be seen in the table, narcotic withdrawal, while uncomfortable, is not life threatening. Sedative withdrawal has both a minor and relatively innocuous symptom complex that occurs initially in all sedative-tolerant individuals and the possibility of a major symptom complex, in a smaller fraction of tolerant individuals, which includes seizures and death. This sequence is the same as that referred to as delirium tremens in alcohol withdrawal (see Chapter 21). Alcohol- and sedative-tolerant individuals should have a tapering detoxification in a hos-

Table 22.3
Characteristics of Dependence on Depressant Drugs

Drug	Physiological Effect	Withdrawal Symptoms (from 1 to 7 Days after Last Dose)	
Narcotics	Pupillary constriction Analgesia Constipation Respiratory depression	Pupillary dilation Myalgia Diarrhea Stimulation of respiratory centers ("yawning")	
Barbiturate, alcohol, sedative, tranquilizers	Induction of sleep (hypnosis) Sedation Alcohol increases seizure activity All other sedatives decrease seizure activity Depression of seizure threshold	Insomnia Tremulousness Irritability Hyperpyrexia	Minor symptoms Onset 24–72 hr after last dose Duration 72–96 hr after last dose
		Delirium Seizures Death	Major symptoms Onset 72 hr to 1 week after last dose Duration up to 2 weeks after last dose

pital under medical supervision and an absolute prohibition of sudden abstinence or "cold turkey" withdrawal. The inhalants, which also are CNS depressants, do not usually induce tolerance because their volatility and short term use never lead to high blood levels long enough to habituate the neuronal membranes.

Prescribing Patterns

It has been widely observed that the fear of causing addiction has led physicians to undermedicate in the management of acute pain (2). Conversely, there has been a tendency in managing chronic pain patients to continue the use of analgesics when the development of tolerance has rendered them ineffective or even countertherapeutic. Patients who have been on narcotic analgesics for long periods may experience little pain relief and may, in fact, confuse incipient withdrawal toward the end of a dosing interval with the onset of pain (18). An understanding of the induction of tolerance and of physiological addiction can assure more rational prescribing patterns. Narcotic analgesics should be given in adequate doses for short term intense pain, and sedatives and tranquilizers should be used for emotional crises, with a recognition of the need to limit and taper these drugs when the period of intense symptoms is over. Chronic pain, insomnia, anxiety, and emotional distress cannot be treated with a prescribed daily depressant drug without inducing tolerance and physiological addiction. *Intermittent* use is required to avoid addiction. Other modalities, *i.e.*, psychotherapy, relaxation techniques, biofeedback, physiotherapy, and exercise regimens, should therefore be utilized also, in order to increase the interval between doses and/or permit intermittent use of depressant drugs. Additional details on prescription of depressant type drugs for medical conditions are found elsewhere (anxiety—Chapter 13; pain control—Chapter 19; insomnia—Chapter 85).

A recent change in prescribing patterns de-emphasizing barbiturates and other potent sedatives in favor of the benzodiazepine tranquilizers is to be welcomed for reducing the potential of serious overdosage. The benzodiazepines do, however, induce tolerance and physiological addiction (the shorter acting benzodiazepines are associated occasionally with major withdrawal symptoms). Benzodiazepines are also potentiated by alcohol and other psychoactive substances and must be treated with caution in prescription and use, with adherence to intermittent short term regimens.

Sedative-Hypnotics

Usual Effects

Intoxication with sedatives is similar to intoxication with alcohol. Sufficient amounts are taken to produce a depression of cortical function and to relax social and personal inhibitions. This disinhibition is called "a high," a state of euphoria in which mood is elevated and anxiety is reduced. Depending on dose, route of administration, rate of metabolism, and body size, exact effects of the sedative may vary widely from time to time and from individual to individual.

Acute Adverse Effects

Overshooting the mark may lead to more profound intoxication: slurred speech, impaired judgment, and unsteady gait. Even greater overdose may lead to stupor, coma, respiratory depression, vasomotor collapse, and death. Intoxication from sedatives, as with alcohol intoxication, impairs motor coordination and the ability to make intellectual judgments.

Chronic Adverse Effects

A different population of abusers of sedatives is characterized not by the intent to reach disinhibition (a "high") but by the intent to calm anxiety or induce sleep. Physicians frequently prescribe sedatives (including tranquilizers) without instructions that they should be used only for short term intermittent treatment. Patients will then use the medications on a regular basis, induce tolerance, and increase the dose (sometimes obtaining prescriptions from multiple physicians) in a misguided effort to control anxiety. The escalating drug use may go undetected until the confusion, irritability, slurred speech, and ataxia together are recognized as sedative intoxication. Often the only distinguishing physical features are ecchymoses which result from the patient being uncoordinated during an intoxicated state. Prescribing and use of individual new sedatives vary widely, almost in a fad-like pattern. Despite assertions to the contrary, all induce tolerance, are dangerous when consumed with alcohol or other CNS depressants, and produce dependency. None should be used in a chronic dosage schedule without serious regard for the possible consequences.

Treatment

Sedative overdose is a life-threatening emergency which should be treated in an emergency room.

Because of physiological dependence, patients who use excessive doses of sedative drugs are at risk of serious withdrawal reactions (including life-threatening seizures). Detoxification of these patients should only be attempted in hospital under close medical supervision. There are clinical reports (5, 19, 27) suggesting that dangerous withdrawal symptoms can occur also in patients who have taken therapeutic doses of benzodiazepines continuously for periods in excess of 1 year.

Patients who have used therapeutic doses of diazepam (Valium) for less than 6 months should be able to discontinue by gradually reducing their dosage. The use of phenobarbital as a detoxification agent may be helpful to those who are unable to do so. Detoxification using phenobarbital may be done on an outpatient basis provided that daily diazepam intake has not exceeded 40 mg. Fifteen milligrams of phenobarbital should be substituted for every 5 mg of diazepam, and the total daily intake should be divided and administered in three separate doses. After 2 or 3 days, the dosage may be reduced at the rate of 15 mg/day. The phenobarbital should be dispensed in the smallest available dosage units in order to maximize the number of tablets taken by the patient, and the patient should report on a daily basis. Daily reporting is important because these patients often require considerable support and close monitoring of their progress.

Heroin and Other Narcotics

The heroin addict will not generally be seen in office practice seeking treatment of his addiction, although a review of medical histories given by patients entering a large methadone maintenance program indicates that these patients do receive treatment for a range of other medical problems. Addicts may also appear in office practice settings attempting to obtain prescription drugs when they experience difficulty in obtaining heroin (diacetylmorphine). Morphine, hydromorphone (Dilaudid), and meperidine (Demerol) are the narcotics most preferred by addicts, but they will readily use the whole range of less potent narcotic and non-narcotic analgesics if preferred drugs are unavailable. If analgesics are difficult to obtain, addicts will temporarily use virtually any depressant drug, but will prefer the barbiturates and other potent sedatives such as methaqualone (Quaalude), glutethimide (Doriden), and ethchlorvynol (Placidyl). Alcohol, the benzodiazepines, and promethazine hydrochloride (Phenergan) are often abused by patients maintained on methadone because of their tendency to potentiate the effects of methadone.

Usual Effects

The acetyl groups on the heroin molecule allow it to penetrate the blood-brain barrier more rapidly than do other narcotics. In the CNS the acetyl moieties are removed, yielding the active compound, morphine. Heroin is usually injected intravenously but can also be injected intramuscularly (skin-popping) or sniffed (snorting). The effects following intravenous injections consist of a brief and intense period of euphoria followed by several hours of a pleasant dreamy state in which the user may slowly nod as if he is falling off to sleep. He may also experience itching of the skin which leads to characteristic scratching movements.

Acute Adverse Effects

Narcotic overdose is characterized by depressed consciousness and depressed respiration. Pulmonary edema, a common complication of narcotic overdose, contributes to hypoxia and may cause death, even while the needle is still in the vein. Experimental evidence suggests that a massive sympathetic discharge is responsible for this effect.

Chronic Adverse Effects

The adverse effects of chronic heroin use result from use of dirty needles, the adulterants mixed with the heroin, and the associated life style (poor nutrition and health care) rather than from the drug itself. Heroin generally constitutes only 2 to 5% of the content of a street dose and is usually mixed with milk sugar (lactose) and quinine under nonsterile conditions in which other, more dangerous, adulterants may also be included to mask the dilution of the heroin. Chronic heroin abusers will have needle marks or scars, usually in the antecubital fossae of both arms, on the forearms and wrists, or on the backs of the hands. The presence of abscesses or old abscess scars and of bluish phlebitis scars from past injections also indicates chronic use. Long time users are usually forced to seek out new injection sites as old sites become unusable owing to scarring, and may exhibit fresh needle marks on the legs and neck. In addition to abscesses, chronic intravenous drug use will result in an increased incidence of hepatitis B antigenemia, viral hepatitis, chronic liver disease, cellulitis, endocarditis, and pulmonary hypertension due to microembolization. It has been estimated that at least one-half of all heroin addicts develop chronic liver disease.

Tolerance to heroin develops quickly and can be demonstrated to some degree after only a few days of administration of the drug. The degree of tolerance and the consequent severity of withdrawal symptoms will depend primarily on dosage levels, and the frequency and duration of use. However, the severity of a patient's addiction to heroin cannot be defined purely in terms of tolerance or withdrawal symptoms since heroin addiction is as much a function of psychological and social factors as it is a simple consequence of physical tolerance or of withdrawal symptoms.

Narcotic withdrawal is characterized by anxiety, nausea, yawning, diarrhea, sweating, rhinorrhea, dilated pupils, and piloerection ("goose flesh"). In the advanced stages of withdrawal the patient experiences vomiting and muscle spasms which often appear as jerky "kicking" movements of the legs. Acute narcotic withdrawal may be inadvertently induced when a narcotic-tolerant individual is given pentazocine (Talwin) or nalbuphine hydrochloride (Nubain), analgesics which combine agonist and antagonist properties. While the untreated addict will experience significant anxiety and discomfort during withdrawal, the process itself presents no serious medical risks. Narcotic addicts tend to confuse anxiety with the early symptoms of withdrawal, so that the diagnosis of withdrawal should be made on the basis of observable symptoms rather than on subjective reports of anxiety and nausea.

Treatment

Narcotic overdose must be treated in an emergency room. Emergency treatment requires cardiorespiratory monitoring and support. A narcotic antagonist (nalorphine, Narcan) is extremely safe and effective in countering the central nervous system depression caused by narcotic overdose.

As a practical matter, any patient who has been abusing heroin or other narcotics and is willing to accept help should be referred for treatment. The physician should realize, however, that few addicts voluntarily seek treatment until the destructive effects of their drug use have made continued use intolerable. The most widely used methods of treatment for narcotic addiction are methadone maintenance and methadone detoxification, both of which are normally administered on an ambulatory basis by specially licensed drug treatment programs. The Food and Drug Administration has recently approved naltrexone, an orally administered, long acting narcotic antagonist for the treatment of narcotic addiction. When taken three times a week, naltrexone effectively blocks the effects of narcotics. While naltrexone is highly effective in preventing narcotic use in patients who take the drug faithfully, patient compliance has been a problem and its utility may be limited to highly motivated patients. Therapeutic communities offer drug-free residential treatment to highly motivated patients who are able to withdraw from narcotics before entry.

Inhalants: Solvent Abuse

The inhalation of solvents is a form of substance abuse that is most commonly found among young people. Since solvents are easily obtainable and inexpensive, they are likely to be preferred by individuals who lack the money or other resources needed to obtain more desirable drugs. A far from exhaustive list of specific substances subject to this type of abuse includes gasoline, ignition spray, airplane glue, paint thinner, spray paint, lighter fluid, nail polish remover, cleaning fluid, and shoe polish. Inhalation is typically accomplished by saturating a rag with the substance and holding it directly over the face or placing it in a bag that is then placed over the nose and the mouth.

Usual Effects

The effects of solvents are immediate and of short duration, usually dissipating in an hour or less. Acute intoxication is similar to alcohol intoxication except for a shorter duration.

Acute Adverse Effects

A hangover, with symptoms of headache and nausea similar but perhaps milder than the hangover produced by alcohol, has been observed. Some users will experience apparent delirium characterized by tactile hallucinations, spatial distortions, and macropsia or micropsia (body image distortions). Sudden sniffing deaths have been described where inhalants were used during strenuous activity or under conditions where blood oxygen is reduced. Such deaths apparently occur as a result of cardiac arrhythmias. Other deaths have been caused by suffocation when the user loses consciousness while his nose and mouth are covered by the bag containing the solvent.

Chronic Adverse Effects

While current information does not permit clearcut conclusions concerning the extent of organ damage caused by inhalant abuse, there is cause for concern. The effects of solvents on the central nervous system, liver, kidneys, and bone marrow are not known. Numerous studies have demonstrated organ damage from long term exposure to relatively low concentrations of industrial solvents, but it is not clear to what extent these findings can be generalized to the short term, high concentration exposures experienced by inhalant abusers. Furthermore, in studies contrasting solvent abusers with control subjects, adverse effects were found in solvent abusers, but the possibility that these were due to factors other than inhalant abuse was not ruled out.

There is evidence that tolerance develops with chronic solvent abuse, but no withdrawal syndrome has been reported, probably because the concentration of the substance in neurons is not sustained.

Treatment

Because the acute effects of solvents are usually of short duration, abusers rarely present for medical treatment. On rare occasions a patient may be brought in for treatment of a solvent-induced delirium. Chronic solvent abuse requires the same type of intense counseling and rehabilitative intervention indicated for other forms of self-destructive substance abuse (see below).

STIMULANT DRUGS: COCAINE AND AMPHETAMINES

Cocaine and the amphetamines are the most commonly abused stimulant drugs.

Cocaine

At this time there is a major epidemic of cocaine use in the United States. Current trafficking has spread cocaine use to millions of persons in middle income segments of the population. The affluence of the middle income population is such that this expensive drug, heretofore reserved for the super-rich, is now in daily repetitive use in quite common-place settings, including business offices and sales-rooms, as well as social and recreational settings. Cocaine is generally available as a white powder that is sniffed ("snorted") so that it is absorbed directly into the bloodstream through the mucosa of the nose. This method of ingestion, which leaves no telltale needle marks and which gives short lived effects because only a modest amount of drugs is absorbed by this route, accounts for the popularity of the drug in so-called "straight" circles. Cocaine may occasionally be injected, swallowed, or smoked as well; when taken by these routes, the duration of action and the unwanted dysphoric effects are enhanced.

Amphetamines and Other Stimulants

Amphetamines are swallowed or injected intravenously. Two nonamphetamine stimulants, methylphenidate (Ritalin) and phenmetrazine (Preludin), which can mimic the effects of naturally occurring stimulants such as cocaine, are taken orally or intravenously.

Usual Effects

Central nervous system stimulants produce euphoria, increased confidence and energy, increased heart rate and blood pressure, dilated pupils, constriction of peripheral blood vessels, and increased body temperature and metabolic rate. All of these effects are caused by a massive sympathetic discharge induced by these drugs. Single doses of amphetamines produce effects lasting 2 to 4 hours. The effects of cocaine are similar but of much shorter duration. When the acute effects of stimulants subside, users often experience lethargy or depression, somnolence, and a voracious appetite. The preference for cocaine over amphetamines and other stimulants is related to its greater potency. Cocaine absorbed in small quantities yields euphoria disproportionate to the dysphoric sympathetic side effects (increased heart rate, increased blood pressure, increased temperature, and sensations of irritability and anxiety). These side effects are more commonly associated with higher dosages of cocaine and with the longer acting amphetamines. As cocaine use becomes more widespread and intravenous injection and smoking ("free-basing") become more common, the adverse effects associated with higher doses will also become more commonplace. The minimal dysphoria induced and the lack of impairment of function (as opposed to the sedation associated with alcohol and the narcotics) make cocaine at "snorted" doses the exemplar of an ideal pure euphoriant.

Acute Adverse Effects

Extremely large doses of all stimulants may cause hyperpyrexia, hypertension, convulsions, cardiovascular collapse, and death (26). Large amounts of cocaine, in addition, cause depression of the medullary centers, and death may result from respiratory arrest as well. Death from overdose of CNS stimulants is still unusual; however, this is probably due to the relatively low doses used until lately.

Chronic Adverse Effects

Long acting stimulants. The chronic abuser of *amphetamines and other long acting stimulants* is typically hyperactive, jittery, and irritable. There is a history of insomnia and anorexia and weight loss. The patient may be emotionally labile, and his periods of irritability may alternate with periods of elation and enthusiasm ("mania"). Physical examination may reveal needle marks, teeth worn from bruxism (grinding of teeth), ulcers on the lips and tongue, tremor, flushing, cardiac arrhythmias, and excessive sweating. Heavy users may exhibit rapid, repetitious, and ritualistic body movements, or such movements may be described by companions.

Chronic abusers of these stimulants rapidly develop *pharmacological tolerance* so that markedly increased doses are required to experience effects previously obtained with lower doses. This is clearly true of amphetamine use and is probably true of cocaine as well.

Repeated exposure to high doses of long lasting stimulants exhausts the supply of preformed noradrenaline. It has been proposed that the resultant excess of other neurotransmitters in the CNS, notably dopamine and serotonin, explains the development of a *reversible organic delusional disorder* that resembles paranoid schizophrenia (25). This syndrome may occur in normal subjects with no previous psychiatric history (8). Subjects who have taken higher doses of a stimulant (e.g., 10 mg of dextroamphetamine every hour) have developed the disorder within 24 hours. The more typical pattern is that of gradual onset over a period of days or weeks as the user gradually increases his intake. Initially, the onset of a delusional disorder may be signaled by increased suspiciousness and distrustfulness. In the final stages the subject becomes markedly paranoid, with delusions of persecution, ideas of reference, and, in many cases, visual or auditory hallucinations. Displays of aggressiveness, hostility, anxiety, and psychomotor agitation are also commonly observed.

While a stimulant-induced delusional disorder is difficult to distinguish from paranoid schizophrenia, it may be inferred from (a) a history of recent stimulant use; (b) intravenous injection sites, malnourishment, bruxism, or other physical symptoms suggestive of amphetamine abuse; or (c) laboratory studies indicating the presence of stimulants. A stimulant-induced delusional disorder differs from phencyclidine (PCP)- or lysergic acid diethylamide (LSD)-induced psychosis (see below) in that it begins much more insidiously. Also the LSD or PCP user may be cognizant of the fact that he is hallucinating, whereas the stimulant abuser is typically unable to distinguish his hallucinations from reality. Delirium, a common feature of PCP abuse, is a rare consequence of stimulant abuse.

Stimulant abusers who abruptly terminate their use of the drug experience a withdrawal reaction (a "crash") characterized by fatigue, depression, and irritability. Patients who develop a high level of pharmacological tolerance for stimulants may experience severe depression and, therefore, may be suicide risks.

Cocaine. People who sniff cocaine no more than two or three times a week are not likely to experience serious side effects, although they do, of course, run the risk of developing psychological dependence leading to repetitive and increasing dosage. Repetitive use of substantial doses of cocaine will interfere with normal sleeping and eating patterns and produce irritability, impaired concentration, and weight loss, undifferentiated from that of the chronic amphetamine abuser, and manic, paranoid, or delusional thinking.

The extent to which chronic use of cocaine produces *physiological tolerance* in humans is unclear. However, cocaine users seem to experience a milder form of the symptoms associated with stimulant withdrawal, probably as a result of the shorter exposure of the neurons to the drug due to the extreme difficulty of achieving the duration and dosage equivalence of the other stimulants, in the usual manner of ingestion.

In the current cocaine epidemic, in which massive amounts are being used by some people, syndromes indistinguishable from those associated with chronic use of longer acting stimulants have been observed.

Treatment

Its capacity to produce a "high" without dysphoria, without impairment of function, and without significant expenditure of mental, emotional, or physical energy makes cocaine a particularly destructive drug for otherwise gainfully involved members of society. The press is replete with items describing heavy cocaine use among highly performing members of society. Athletes, business executives, salesmen, and housewives have now joined heretofore exotic celebrities in abusing cocaine. Cocaine abuse may be masked by intercurrent use of alcohol, sedatives, and other depressants to relieve the anxiety, insomnia, and irritability of chronic abuse. Recognition of the disorder is quite difficult under these circumstances of widespread use, masked effects, and less than obvious impairment of function. Recognition often occurs only as the result of unexplained financial distress due to the high costs of chronic use.

Treatment is difficult. Because intermittent use produces so little dysphoria, there is often little incentive for the patient to seek help. Chronic abuse, debilitating physically and financially, may decrease the patient's reluctance to seek help, but the reinforcing psychological dependence on the cocaine "high" makes outpatient treatment relatively ineffective. Most therapists insist on inpatient treatment to effect a temporary cessation of use and a determined use of "contracting for aversive consequences" (loss of job, loss of spouse, *etc*) upon resumption of use to maintain a drug-free state. No longitudinal studies exist to evaluate the efficacy of this or any other treatment studies. Unlike the experience gained in alcohol and depressant drug treatment, where deficits in educational and vocational preparation and social function underlie much of the abuse and point to a method of successful rehabilitation, cocaine abuse often occurs in highly functional and creative members of society. The insidiousness of a drug that predictably mimics the pure euphoria heretofore reserved as reward for great achievement, great honor, or great love explains both its explosive spread in populations previously immune to other forms of drug abuse and the difficulty it poses in treatment.

In summary, the generalist should have a high index of suspicion in ostensibly productive persons who experience unusual financial problems or who come for unexplained tranquilizers or sedative prescriptions to help mask the chronic effects of stimulant use. When a patient accepts the fact that he is abusing stimulant drugs, referral to a specialized treatment center is imperative since, as stated above, ambulatory treatment is almost invariably a failure.

DRUGS WHICH ALTER PERCEPTION

This category encompasses substances which may be CNS stimulants or depressants, but which in their commonly used dose and *via* their usual route of administration produce exaggerated imaginings, visual hallucinations, altered time perceptions, and subjective feelings of enhancement of sensation.

Marijuana/Hashish

Marijuana consists of the dried leaves of the marijuana (*Cannabis sativa*) plant, which are usually smoked in pipes or cigarettes ("joints"). *Hashish* is a concentrated resin of cannabis and contains approximately 5 to 10 times as much of the psychoactive ingredient, tetrahydrocannabinol (THC) as does marijuana. The discussion that follows applies to both marijuana and hashish, although the effects associated with higher doses are more likely to occur with hashish than with marijuana.

Usual Effects

The effects of marijuana usually last from 3 to 6 hours. The more common effects are elation, relaxation, an increased tendency to laughter and silliness, a sense of sharpened perception and increased insight, increased vividness and appreciation in all sensory modalities, decreased concentration, loosened associations, increased appetite, tachycardia, mild feelings of paranoia, and a sense of detachment or depersonalization. Lower doses tend to produce relaxation and euphoria, while higher doses tend to result in increasing visual and auditory perceptual distortions. Doses 3 to 5 times higher than those producing relaxation and mild euphoria can result in psychotomimetic effects (depersonalization, auditory and visual hallucinations). Thus, some of the usual effects of marijuana which might be enjoyable to the experienced user can be frightening to the inexperienced user. The setting is also very important in determining the effects of the drug. Marijuana, when smoked in a pleasant and familiar setting, is less likely to produce a negative response than when used in an unfamiliar or threatening setting.

There is substantial evidence that marijuana in dose levels associated with common social usage interferes with intellectual and psychomotor performance. A number of studies indicate that marijuana use will significantly impair driving skills. In the dosage commonly used (10 mg/cigarette), marijuana impairs recent memory, thus interfering with cognition and learning (14).

Acute Adverse Effects

Considering the large number of regular users in the United States it is clear that adverse reactions to marijuana requiring medical treatment are rare. The most frequent adverse response is an *acute anxiety* reaction which is similar to the panic attacks described in Chapter 13. The acute anxiety reaction that is induced by marijuana is different in that it frequently includes paranoid ideation, which is not typically a feature of panic attacks. Acute panic reactions are most likely to occur in novice users or in users who unexpectedly receive a much higher than usual dose. This reaction is characterized by the appearance of many of the usual effects of the drug in an exaggerated form and by mounting anxiety which often stems from a sense of losing control and which is often expressed as a fear of "going crazy" or, less frequently, of dying. Acute panic reactions can vary in intensity and duration, but most last only the few hours it takes for the effects of the drug to wear off. Some patients experience

persistent anxiety for several days after the initial panic subsides. It has been estimated that three intense panic reactions occur per 100,000 exposures (22).

There have also been reports of *delirium*, in the form of an organic delusional disorder induced by marijuana. A *dysphoric reaction* characterized by disorientation, catatonia-like immobility, acute panic, and heavy sedation has also been reported. As with the anxiety/panic reaction, these conditions tend to remit within 2 to 4 hours as the effects of the marijuana diminish.

Reports of *enduring psychotic reactions* following heavy marijuana use have appeared largely in countries where marijuana is used in much higher doses than in the United States. Reports of confirmed psychotic reactions to marijuana in this country have been rare.

Chronic Adverse Effects

It is clear that smoking marijuana, even a few cigarettes daily for only a few weeks, adversely affects pulmonary function (23). It has also been reported that marijuana smoke contains 70% more carcinogens, such as benzopyrene, than does tobacco smoke (16). While there is reason for concern regarding the carcinogenic potential of marijuana smoke, there are no data yet that demonstrate an association of neoplasia with marijuana. There have been conflicting findings concerning possible adverse effects of marijuana on the *immune system*. Some studies have reported changes in immunological responsiveness, but the clinical implications of these changes are not currently known. There is evidence that marijuana reduces testosterone levels in men, although the average level for users remains within normal limits (12). The clinical implications are unclear, but concern has been expressed over possible effects of even small changes in testosterone levels in adolescent males.

Animal studies involving very high doses of THC have yielded evidence of teratogenicity. However, while there is widespread use of marijuana among women of reproductive age, there have not been reports of a higher level of birth defects among children born to mothers who were regular users of marijuana during pregnancy. Several studies (6, 7, 10) suggest that more subtle effects, such as neurological abnormalities and reductions in birth weight and height, may be associated with maternal use of marijuana.

It should be noted that all reviews of the literature on marijuana include the admonition that the available data simply are not adequate to draw clear conclusions about the effects of chronic use. The current status of marijuana research is quite analogous to the status of research on the effects of smoking some 30 years ago.

Tolerance and withdrawal. Marijuana is clearly a CNS depressant. It is cross-tolerant with the barbiturate sedatives; high doses induce psychoactive tolerance and physiological dependence (see page 281), and it is additive with all other depressants (narcotics, sedatives, alcohol) in depressing the function of the central nervous system. Heretofore, because of the low potency of the marijuana used in the United States (1 to 10 mg/cigarette) these effects were not generally appreciated. With greater potency (new plants yielding 20 mg/cigarette) and greater concentration of the active ingredient in hashish or oil of hashish, users ingesting doses as high as 30 to 100 mg report more adverse reactions, greater frequency of hallucinations, and more pronounced CNS depression. In one study (17) volunteers who smoked an average of five marijuana cigarettes a day for 64 days exhibited restlessness, sleep disturbance, loss of appetite, and irritability when they stopped using marijuana.

Treatment of Acute Reactions

Since they must be closely observed and may take several hours to recover, patients suffering from panic reactions are best managed in a setting such as a drug abuse program, mental health center, or emergency room where continuing observation and supportive contact can be provided. Generally, these patients require simple reassurance and an explanation that they are experiencing a drug reaction which will dissipate as the drug is eliminated from their bodies. A critical or moralizing attitude will only undermine rapport with the patient, thereby compromising a critical element in management.

Delusional or delirious patients should be seen in an emergency room since they present more complicated management problems and may require sedation or hospitalization. Furthermore, other causes of a delirium or an organic delusional disorder such as trauma or infection should be ruled out. Restraints should only be used when absolutely necessary for the safety of the patient or of others. Drugs should also not be used unless the patient is extremely agitated and difficult to control. In such cases, diazepam (Valium) is preferred in an initial dose of 20 mg intramuscularly with subsequent doses of 10 mg each hour to a maximum of 60 mg.

Phencyclidine (PCP)

Phencyclidine, a derivative of ketamine, a known barbiturate-like anesthetic, is quite clearly a CNS depressant, capable of inducing psychoactive tolerance (see page 281). However, PCP exhibits selective action as an anesthetic, appearing to depress sensory tracts, including proprioception, pain, touch, and temperature, to a greater degree than it depresses cortical function. The resultant state of sensory deprivation and relative cortical wakefulness makes for a peculiar sense of detachment, disembodiment, and weightlessness. These sensations are intensely pleasurable for some, while for others they induce intense anxiety and even panic. Prolonged sensory deprivation, whether chemically induced or provoked mechanically by shielding out visual, auditory, and tactile stimuli, will predictably induce delusions and hallucinations even in normal subjects.

PCP was developed as an anesthetic, but was abandoned for this purpose when it was found to cause disturbing side effects. It continues to be used by veterinarians as an animal tranquilizer or immobilizing agent. Pure PCP is a white powder which dissolves in water. It is usually sprinkled on marijuana, dried parsley flakes, or other organic material and smoked. Less frequently, it is obtained in powder or tablet form and ingested or sniffed ("snorting"). Street names for the drug vary considerably from region to region, but it is most commonly known as angel dust, flakes, crystal, hog, or sheets. An excellent summary of the literature on PCP has been prepared by Luisada (13).

Usual Effects

The effects of PCP tend to be dose related, although there can be marked differences in the response of different individuals to a given dose or in the response of an individual to the same dose at different times. Individuals who take PCP in the relatively low doses normally associated with street use may experience exhilaration, euphoria, a sense of great strength and power, inebriation, tranquilization, and perceptual disturbances. Some unpleasant effects commonly reported include disorientation, hallucinations, anxiety, paranoia, hyperexcitability, and irritability. At usual street dosages, most users reach peak intoxication in 5 to 30 minutes and remain "high" for 4 to 6 hours. It may take 24 hours before the user feels completely normal again.

Acute Adverse Effects

Even in relatively low doses, PCP is capable of occasionally causing severe reactions which may precipitate extreme agitation and *acts of violence* toward oneself and others. With higher doses users are more likely to exhibit *delirium.* The delirious patient can present a bewildering array of symptoms, which can fluctuate markedly over relatively short periods of time. He may be hypervigilant or drowsy, anxious or aggressive, fearful or dauntless. His behavior may fluctuate during the day, alert at times and stuporous at other times.

A cardinal symptom of delirium is clouding of consciousness, defined as a reduction in the clarity of awareness of the environment (1). While obvious in the stuporous or comatose patient, clouding of consciousness will appear in other patients in the form of impairments in concentration, memory, arithmetical ability, orientation, and complex motor functions, such as in writing a sentence or drawing an abstract design. Thinking may appear fragmented and disorganized or it may be unusually accelerated or slowed. Delirious patients may also experience hallucinations, illusions, and delusions. They frequently show a blank stare, and in some instances they may appear almost catatonic.

Luisada distinguishes between the delirium that is seen in acute PCP toxicity and what he refers to as a *PCP psychosis*, a disorder closely resembling schizophrenia that develops following acute intoxication and persists for 24 hours or more. Such psychoses may develop out of the original intoxication or may occur days after the intoxication has cleared. Approximately one-fourth of the patients who experience a PCP psychosis will go on to develop a schizophrenic psychosis within 2 years, despite abstinence from PCP. Luisada reports that in his experience, at least half of the patients treated for PCP psychosis use the drug again within 2 weeks of discharge (13).

Ataxia, nystagmus, and ptosis are common features of acute PCP toxicity. Very high doses of PCP, which are normally the result of oral ingestion rather than of smoking, can result in coma, severe respiratory depression, seizures, and death.

Chronic Adverse Effects

Chronic use of PCP may produce persistent changes in personal habits (hygiene or dress), problems with memory or speech, sleep disturbances, mood changes (depression, irritability), paranoid or frankly delusional thinking, and unusual excitability or lethargy. Little is known about long term physical effects.

Treatment of Acute Reactions

Burns and Lerner (4) reported consistent correlation between the patient's initial level of consciousness and the time course of improvement. Patients who presented with delirium cleared in 3 to 8 hours; patients who remained stuporous or comatose for 1 to 4 hours cleared in 5 to 62 hours; and patients whose stupor or coma lasted 6 or more hours cleared in 75 to 288 hours. Therefore, patients who are delirious at presentation can be treated in an emergency room and do not require hospitalization. Repeated mental status examinations should be performed to insure that the patient is in a state of clear consciousness for at least 4 hours prior to discharge. Members of the family should be cautioned that the patient should stay in the company of family members or reliable friends for several days. Patients can have the onset of severe depression or a PCP psychosis for several days after the acute effects of the drug have subsided.

Patients who remain comatose or stuporous for more than 2 hours or who develop a PCP psychosis require hospitalization.

Lysergic Acid Diethylamide (LSD)

Lysergic acid diethylamide is the prototype of a number of alkaloid substances of such great potency that small doses predictably cause hallucinations. These hallucinogens, including psylocybin, dimethyltryptamine (DMT), and mescaline, are all CNS depressants in higher doses. LSD ("acid") is sold illicitly in the form of powder, tablets, or capsules. Sugar cubes, small squares of gelatin ("window pane"), or paper ("blotter acid") that have been impregnated with the drug are also available. LSD is usually ingested orally and its effects appear within 15 minutes, reaching a peak at about 90 minutes, and lasting for approximately 8 to 10 hours.

Usual Effects

LSD usually produces some combination of the following subjective effects: depersonalization, altered time perception, labile mood, profound perceptual distortions (usually visual), body image distortion, and feelings of profound insight. Objective effects include tachycardia, palpitations, anorexia, elevated blood pressure, fever, lack of coordination, and dilated pupils.

Acute Adverse Effects

Inexperienced users may experience an acute panic reaction that occurs because the normal effects of the drug are unfamiliar or unexpected. In more severe reactions, users of LSD may experience hallucinations (usually visual) and delusions that may persist beyond the time during which the drug is circulating in the blood.

Flashbacks, spontaneous recurrences of the original LSD experience, have been estimated to occur in 1 of every 20 users (from days to years later). They are more likely to occur in chronic users. There have also been reports of prolonged psychotic reactions following the use of LSD, although these are rare.

LSD toxicity differs from PCP toxicity and from schizophrenia in several ways. LSD causes dilation of the pupils, which is absent in PCP toxicity and in schizophrenia. PCP toxicity usually is characterized by clouding of consciousness, and the patient will often exhibit ataxia, nystagmus, and ptosis, which are not features of LSD toxicity or of schizophrenia.

Chronic Adverse Effects

Some degree of tolerance develops with repeated use of LSD, but no withdrawal syndrome has been observed.

Treatment

Adverse reactions to LSD usually remit in 8 to 24 hours, and hospitalization is usually not necessary. However, the patient should be observed until symptoms clear. Referral to an emergency room or to a drug abuse program that can provide this type of support will usually be necessary. The same supportive measures described earlier for the treatment of adverse reactions to marijuana are appropriate. Extremely agitated patients should be given diazepam (Valium), 20 mg intramuscularly, before being sent to a treatment center.

Belladonna Alkaloids

Belladonna derivatives such as atropine (the active ingredient in jimsonweed) and scopolamine are acetylcholine inhibitors that in high doses will also regularly produce hallucinations, delirium, and varying states of excitement, insomnia, and/or amnesia. These effects may be followed by CNS depression and coma. The side effects of these drugs—dryness of the mouth, blurred vision, anhidrosis, and tachycardia—limit their appeal as psychoactive agents. Thus, the rare instances of abuse are mostly by youngsters experimenting with jimsonweed in rural areas or, in the past, by use of over-the-counter soporifics which contained scopolamine until banned by the Food and Drug Administration some years ago. Treatment of toxic overdose is a medical emergency requiring gastric lavage and ingestion of activated charcoal to limit intestinal absorption. Physostigmine, 1 to 4 mg, injected intravenously, intramuscularly, or subcutaneously is a specific antidote that abolishes both the peripheral and CNS effects of these alkaloids. Repeated injection at 1 to 2 hours may be necessary.

General References

Bourne PC (ed): *Acute Drug Abuse Emergencies*. New York, Academic Press, 1976.
> Covers the treatment of overdose and toxic reactions to commonly abused drugs.

Brecher EM (ed): *Licit and Illicit Drugs*. Boston, Little, Brown, and Co, 1972.
> While somewhat dated, still an excellent overview of the history of drug abuse in the United States.

Lowinson JH, Ruiz P: *Substance Abuse: Clinical Problems and Perspectives*. Baltimore, Williams & Wilkins, 1981.
> An excellent general reference for the field of drug abuse.

National Academy of Sciences Institute of Medicine: *Marijuana and Health*. Washington, DC, National Academy Press, 1982.
> A comprehensive review of physical and psychological effects of marijuana.

Specific References

1. American Psychiatric Association: *Diagnostic and Statistical Manual of Mental Disorders*, ed 3. Washington, DC, American Psychiatric Association, 1980.
2. Angell M: The quality of mercy. *N Engl J Med* 306:98, 1982.
3. Ball JC, Nurco DN: Criminality during the life course of heroin addiction. In *Problems of Drug Dependence 1983*. Rockville, MD, Department of Health and Human Services, 1984.
4. Burns RS, Lerner SE: Perspectives: Acute phencyclidine intoxication. *Clin Toxicol* 9:477, 1976.
5. Dysken MW, Chan CH: Diazepam withdrawal psychosis: a case report. *Am J Psychiatry* 134:573, 1977.
6. Finnegan LP: Pulmonary problems encountered by the infant of the drug-dependent mother. *Clin Chest Med* 1:311, 1980.
7. Fried PA; Marihuana use by pregnant women: neurobehavioral effects in neonates. *Drug Alcohol Dependence* 6:415, 1980.
8. Griffith JD, Cavanaugh JH, Oates JA: Psychosis induced by the administration of d-amphetamine to human volunteers. In Efron DH (ed): *Psychotomimetic Drugs*. New York, Raven Press, 1970.
9. Harwood HS, Napolitano D, Kristiansen P, Collins J: *Economic Cost to Society of Alcoholism and Drug Abuse and Mental Illness: 1980*. Washington, DC, US Government Printing Office, 1984.
10. Hingson R, Alpert JJ, Day N, et al: Effects of maternal drinking and marijuana use on fetal growth and development. *J Pediatr* 70:539, 1982.
11. National Institute on Drug Abuse: *Drugs and American High School Students, 1975–1983*. Rockville, MD, US Department of Health and Human Services, 1983.
12. Kolodny RC, Lessin PJ, Toro G, et al: Depression of plasma testosterone with acute marijuana administration. In Braude MC, Szara S (eds): *Pharmacology of Marijuana*. New York, Raven Press, 1976.
13. Luisada PV: Phencyclidine. In Lowinson JH, Ruiz P (eds): *Substance Abuse: Clinical Problems and Perspectives*. Baltimore, Williams & Wilkins, 1981.
14. Melges FT, Tinklenberg JR, Hollister LE, Gillespie HK: Temporal disintegration and depersonalization during marijuana intoxication. *Arch Gen Psychiatry* 23:204, 1970.
15. Miller JD, Cisin IH, Gardner-Keating H, et al: *National Survey on Drug Abuse: Main Findings 1982*. Washington, DC, US Government Printing Office, 1983.
16. Novotny M, Lee ML, Bartle KD: A possible chemical basis for the higher mutagenicity of marijuana smoke as compared to tobacco smoke. *Experientia* 32:280, 1976.
17. Nowlan R, Cohen S: Tolerance to marijuana: heart rate and subjective "high." *Clin Pharmacol Ther* 22:550, 1977.
18. O'Brien CP, Weisbrot MM: Behavioral and psychological components of pain management. In Brown RM, Pinkert TM, Ludford JP (eds): *Contemporary Research in Pain and Analgesia, 1983*. Washington, DC, US Government Printing Office, 1983.
19. Prevnick JS, Jasinski DR, Haertzen CA: Abrupt withdrawal from therapeutically administered diazepam. *Arch Gen Psychiatry* 35:995, 1978.
20. Rufener BL, Rachal JV, Cruze AM: *Management Effectiveness Measures for NIDA Drug Abuse Treatment Programs*. Rockville, MD, US Department of Health, Education and Welfare, 1984, vol 1.
21. Stanton MD, Todd TC: *The Family Therapy of Drug Abuse and Addiction*. New York, Guilford Press, 1982.
22. Talbott JA; Emergency management of marijuana psychosis. In Bourne PC (ed): *Acute Drug Abuse Emergencies*. New York, Academic Press, 1976.
23. Tashkin DP, Sharpiro BJ, Lee YE, Harper CE: Subacute effects of heavy marijuana smoking on pulmonary function in healthy men. *N Engl J Med* 294:125, 1976.
24. Thompson TL, Moran ML, Nies AS: Psychotropic drug use in the elderly. *N Engl J Med* 308:134, 1983.
25. Van Kammen DP: The dopamine hypothesis of schizophrenia revisited. *Psychoneuroendocrinology* 4:37, 1979.
26. Wetli CV, Wright RK: Death caused by recreational cocaine use. *JAMA* 241:2519, 1979.
27. Winokur A, Rickels K, Greenblatt DJ, et al: Withdrawal reaction from long-term, low-dosage administration of diazepam. *Arch Gen Psychiatry* 35:101, 1980.

Allergy and Infectious Diseases

CHAPTER TWENTY-THREE

Allergy and Related Conditions

MARTIN D. VALENTINE, M.D.

INTRODUCTION

Allergy is a state of increased immunological reactivity resulting from the synthesis of immunoglobulin E (IgE) antibodies after man is exposed to foreign immunogenic protein. Subsequent allergen-IgE antibody interaction causes release of chemical mediators which cause the symptoms of allergy. Although allergy symptoms are undesirable, the allergen-antibody-mediator sequence may have originally evolved as a host defense mechanism.

It is estimated that 17% of Americans suffer from acute and chronic conditions generally considered to be allergic in origin (see Table 23.1); approximately 9% of all office visits to physicians are for one of these conditions (1). The majority of visits are for conditions which are known to be mediated by antibodies of the IgE class or for conditions which resemble IgE-mediated allergy. Since the symptoms in these patients result from the release or formation of a limited number of chemical mediators, effective pharmacological treatment may be similar whether or not allergy in the true sense is involved.

It is believed that the ability to synthesize relatively large amounts of IgE with specificity for certain antigens may be inherited. The risk of developing an allergy for a child if one parent is allergic is one chance in three, increasing to two in three if both parents are allergic.

This chapter is concerned with IgE-mediated allergy and similar conditions (with the exception of asthma which is discussed in Chapter 55). Other immunopathological conditions which are not IgE mediated (drug-induced hepatitis, autoimmune hemolytic anemia) are discussed elsewhere in this book.

PATHOPHYSIOLOGY

Antibody

Acute allergic reactions are mediated by IgE, which was the fifth class of antibody to be discovered in humans. Never present in large amounts, its level in serum is greatest between puberty and young adulthood. As indicated in Figure 23.1, IgE binds to surface receptors on tissue mast cells and blood basophils. The release of histamine and other chemical mediators from these cells is initiated by the bridging of a pair of IgE molecules on the surface of the cells by an antigen molecule of appropriate specificity.

Allergens

Allergens which have clinical relevance are usually proteins with a molecular weight between 10,000 and 40,000. Low molecular weight substances are generally not allergens unless they, like penicillin for example, are capable of combining as a hapten with a protein.

Mediators

The release or formation of biologically significant chemical mediators is a prerequisite to the devel-

Table 23.1.
Estimated Prevalence of Common Allergic Conditions in the General Population[a]

Condition	Prevalence (%)
Allergic rhinitis alone	7
Miscellaneous conditions (eczema, urticaria/ angioedema, food/drug/insect allergy)	6
Asthma	4

[a] From *Asthma and the Other Allergic Diseases*, NIAID Task Force Report. NIH publ no. 79-387, May 1979.

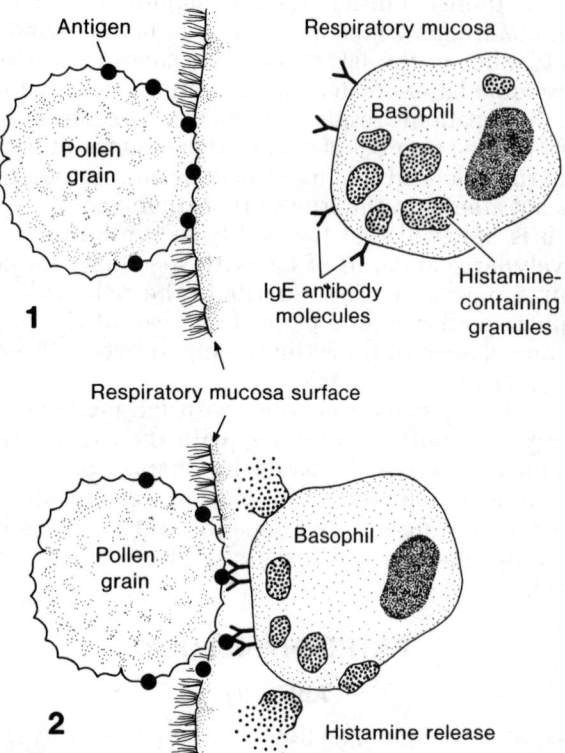

Figure 23.1. Steps in the IgE-mediated response of respiratory mucosa to pollen antigen. *Step 1*, pollen grains containing antigen reach nasal mucosa containing mast cells and basophils with IgE antibodies to antigen. *Step 2*, antigen bridges adjacent IgE molecules, initiating histamine release.

opment of allergic symptoms. In general, mediators affect smooth muscle contractility and vascular tone and permeability. *Histamine*, released from mast cells and basophils, causes pruritus, flushing, nasal stuffiness, conjunctival injection, bronchoconstriction, uterine contraction, increased permeability of venules, and hypotension. *Anaphylatoxin*, a substance formed during complement activation, induces histamine release. *Bradykinin* and similar polypeptides with potent vasodepressor activity may be responsible in part for the shock of anaphylaxis. Members of the leukotriene family have been identified as the slow reacting substances of anaphylaxis

(SRS-A), arachidonic acid metabolites with bronchoconstrictor and vasodilator activities. These and prostaglandin D_2 (PGD_2) have recently been found in the nasal secretions of allergic rhinitis patients challenged intranasally with allergen.

PHYSIOLOGICAL BASIS FOR TREATMENT
Pharmacological

Drugs can favorably influence the outcome of an allergic condition by acting at various sites in the sequence of the allergic reaction (see Table 23.2). Although no drug prevents antigen-antibody interaction, *disodium cromoglycate* (cromolyn, Intal) prevents mediator release after this interaction has occurred. The formation or release of some mediators is modulated by variation in cellular and tissue levels of cyclic adenosine monophosphate (cAMP), which acts as a "second messenger" for certain energy-requiring metabolic steps. β-Adrenergic agonists appear to inhibit mediator release and relax bronchial smooth muscle by increasing cAMP. The *methylxanthines*, such as theophylline, produce similar effects by preventing enzymatic breakdown of cAMP. Conventional (H-1) *antihistamines* inhibit histamine effects by competing with histamine for H-1 receptor sites. The usefulness of antihistamines is limited by their inability to compete successfully with relatively high tissue concentrations of histamine adjacent to its cellular sites of origin, and also because nearly all antihistamines are central nervous system (CNS) depressants. Corticosteroids have

Table 23.2.
Sites of Action of "Antiallergic" Drugs

Drug	Action Site	Mode of Action
Cromolyn	Mast cell	Inhibits mediator release
Adrenergics		
α	Postcapillary venules, arterioles	Vasoconstriction
β_2	Mast cell, basophil	Inhibits mediator release (increases cyclic AMP)
	Bronchial muscle	Relaxes bronchial muscle
Methylxanthines	Mast cell, basophil	Inhibits mediator release (increases cyclic AMP)
	Bronchial muscle	Relaxes bronchial muscle
Antihistamines	Histamine receptors	Competitive inhibition
Corticosteroids	Basophil	Inhibits histamine release

a topical vasoconstrictor effect and inhibit histamine release from basophils, but not mast cells.

Immunological

Immunization of humans with extracts of pollens has been shown to result in the appearance in serum of "blocking" antibody (immunoglobulin G), suppression of specific IgE production, and a reduction in the sensitivity of mediator-containing cells to antigen challenge.

ALLERGIC RHINITIS AND SIMILAR NASAL CONDITIONS

Epidemiology and Natural History

The prevalence of allergic rhinitis in the United States varies from region to region, depending upon the amount and type of airborne allergens present. Onset of symptoms is most common between the ages of 10 and 20. The prevalence is approximately 10% in the age group 16 to 64 and may be as high as 20 to 25% in young adults (1).

During the 10 years after onset, about one-third of young adults get better, and almost one-half get worse (1). Some have a permanent remission of symptoms; in the longitudinal study of the Tecumseh population, typical allergic rhinitis remitted entirely in 8% of subjects during a 4-year interval (2). The severity of symptoms tends to decrease in most subjects after the age of 40. Therefore, it is important to consider other causes for apparent allergic rhinitis which begins after age 40. While it is generally thought that asthma develops in many people with allergic rhinitis, in fact only about 10% develop this condition (1).

Differential Diagnosis of Noninfectious Rhinitis

Noninfectious rhinitis refers to those conditions in which there is no purulent discharge from the nose; purulent discharge is typical of nasal and paranasal infections such as viral upper respiratory infection and acute and chronic sinusitis (see Chapter 28). Occasionally grossly purulent secretions occur in noninfectious rhinitis; microscopically, large numbers of eosinophils are seen. Subjects with noninfectious rhinitis may belong to one of three categories: typical seasonal allergy, perennial (year-round) allergy, and miscellaneous nonallergic causes for nasal symptoms (see Table 23.3). The classification of an individual patient depends chiefly upon information obtained in the history. Some patients may have elements of more than one of these conditions.

History

Symptoms of noninfectious rhinitis. The symptoms which trouble patients most are obstruction of nasal airflow, dry mouth (from mouth breathing) nasal

Table 23.3.
Miscellaneous Nonallergic Causes of Noninfectious Rhinitis

RHINITIS MEDICAMENTOSA
Antihypertensive medication:
β-Blockers
Guanethidine
Methyldopa
Reserpine
Aspirin sensitivity
Topical decongestant abuse (rebound rhinitis)
ENDOCRINE
Hypothyroidism
Pregnancy
Oral contraceptives
ANATOMICAL
Nasal polyp
Deviated nasal septum
Nasal tumor
VASOMOTOR RHINITIS

discharge (usually clear), itching of the nose and the soft palate, and sneezing. In addition, discharge, itching, and puffiness of the eyes may occur, and there may be periodic loss of smell and taste. Occasionally acute sinusitis (see Chapter 28) or serous otitis media (see Chapter 96) may occur as complications. While these symptoms are not incapacitating, they may interfere significantly with an individual's usual activities and may lead to minor mood disturbance (see Chapter 12) in susceptible individuals. As shown in Figure 23.2, there is considerable day-to-day variability in the severity of symptoms in patients with typical seasonal allergy. Furthermore, the symptoms may vary substantially from year to year.

In nasal allergy due to seasonally prevalent allergens, symptoms will recur each year at approximately the same time. Pollen counts are higher in the morning, and outdoor symptoms are apt to be worse at that time. In nonseasonal allergy, symptoms may be induced by exposure to allergens (such as animal dander) any time during the day. In vasomotor rhinitis (see below), obstructive symptoms are prominent and, in contrast to allergic rhinitis, irritative symptoms (sneezing, itching, and discharge) are usually not pronounced.

Environmental exposures. In seasonal allergy ("hay fever"), the specific source of the patient's trouble can often be identified by careful history taking. Skin testing and *in vitro* immunological tests can be utilized to provide definitive evidence; these measures are appropriate when the incrimination of a specific allergen, such as dog dander, will assist in environmental treatment or when immunotherapy is being considered (see below). In patients with year-round allergic symptoms, differentiation from nonallergic rhinitis may be more difficult. Indirect evidence for an allergic etiology for nasal symptoms

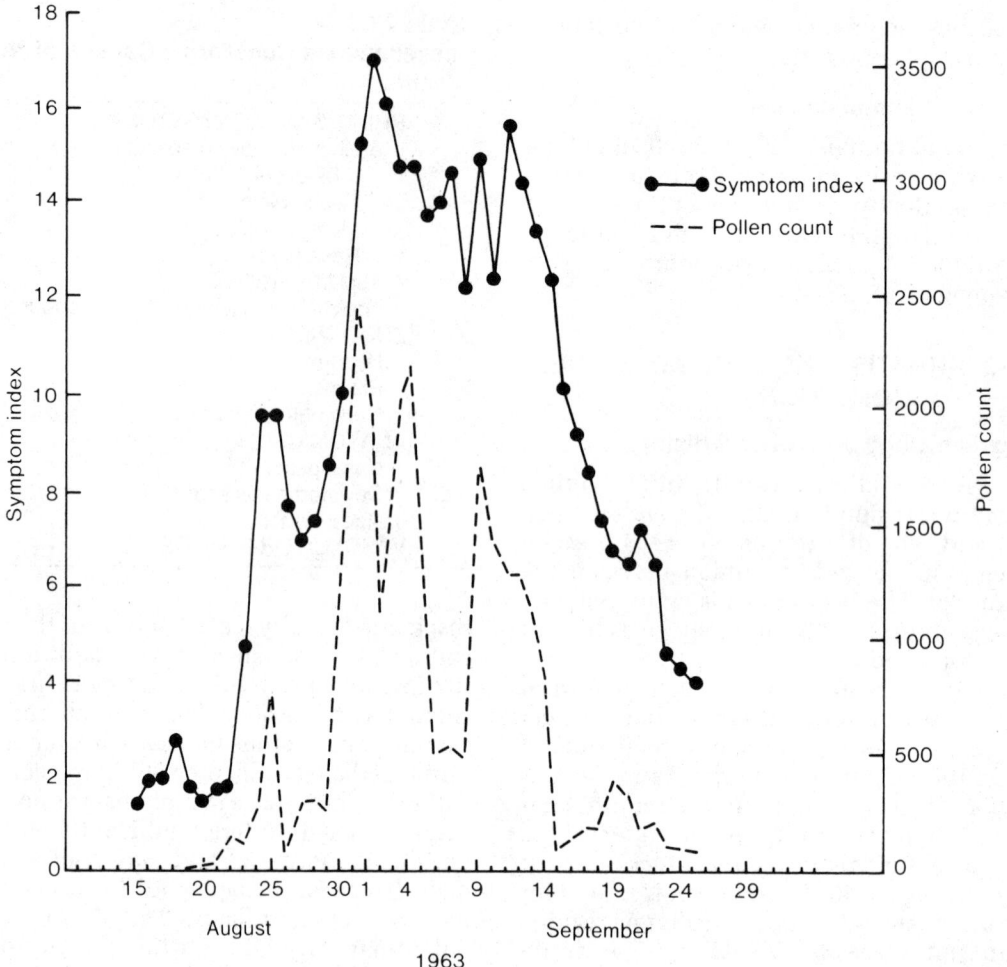

Figure 23.2.   Day-to-day variation in self-reported symptoms during the pollen season, in an untreated patient with allergy to ragweed pollen.

includes other manifestations of atopy (see Table 23.1) and a history of typical allergic rhinitis in one or both parents. The absence of blood or nasal eosinophilia (<25% eosinophils in Giemsa-stained nasal smear) mitigates against an allergic etiology.

To a certain extent, even a limited knowledge of local flora will assist the physician in history taking. The general rule is that plants capable of causing nasal allergy produce copious quantities of pollen in inconspicuous, unattractive flowers which depend on wind for pollination. Therefore, pollen from attractive, pleasantly scented flowers, such as roses, is not allergenic, since these flowers depend on insects for pollination. So-called "rose fever" is usually due to allergy to grass pollen, which is prevalent during that period of time when roses are in bloom; the pleasant scent of the rose simply aggravates the patient already irritated by the allergic reaction initiated by grass pollen. In those sections of the country where the seasons are well demarcated, tree pollens are found in early spring, followed in late spring by grass pollen (Fig. 23.3). Late summer pro-

duces ragweed pollen in the east and midwest and cedar pollen in other sections. Mold spores are also prevalent in the fall, but snow during the winter usually prevents further dissemination of spores.

House dust, a mongrel material of uncertain heritage, can be more of a problem during the heating season in northern climes, since all heating systems, but particularly forced air systems, tend to disperse dust particles. Among important components of urban dust are the following; fragments of cockroach exoskeleton and excreta; the house dust mite, a nonparasitic organism which exists on human skin scales after they are shed; and aerosolized fragments of the saliva and skin of mammalian pets. Animal hair *per se*, comprising primarily insoluble collagen, is allergenic only by virtue of its burden of dander (shed skin). Symptoms due to animal allergens may be more pronounced in pollen seasons in pollen-sensitive patients and in circumstances when the patient and his pet spend more time indoors, e.g., during the winter months.

Miscellaneous causes of nasal symptoms. As noted

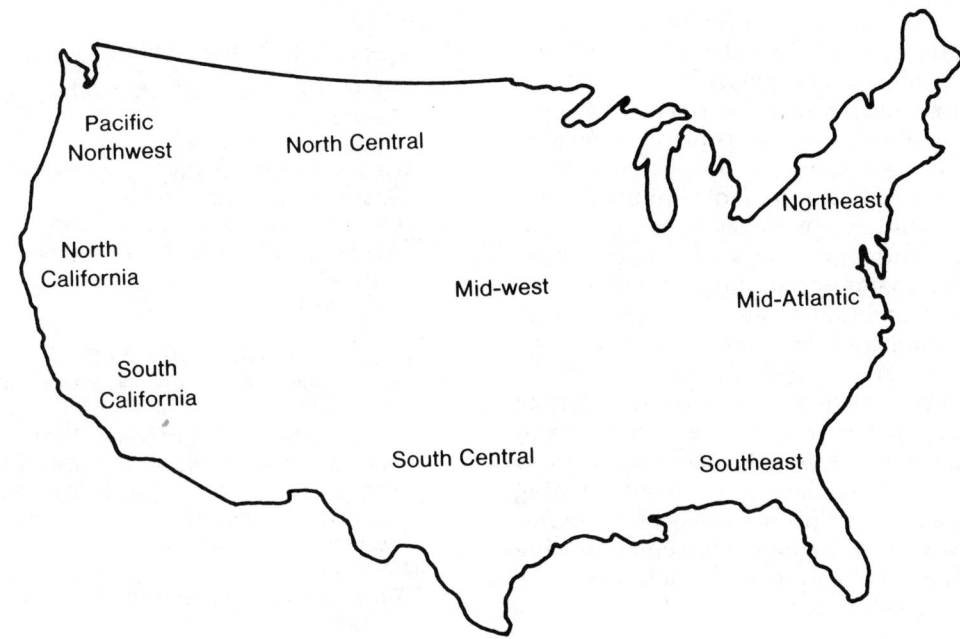

Figure 23.3.   Seasonal occurrence of pollens, selected regions:

Pacific Northwest
Trees: Apr–May
Grasses: Apr–Oct
Weeds: June–Sept
North California
Trees: Feb–May
Grasses: Apr–Sept
Sagebrush: July–Oct
Other weeds: Mar–Oct
South California
Trees: Feb–June
Grasses: Apr–Oct
Sagebrush: July–Oct
Other weeds: June–Oct

North Central
Trees: Mar–May
Grasses: May–Aug
Ragweed: Aug–Sept
Other weeds: June–Sept
MidWest
Trees: Mar–May
Grasses: May–July
Ragweed: Aug–Oct
Other weeds: July–Oct
South Central
Mountain Cedar: Dec–Feb
Other trees: Feb–Apr
Grasses: Feb–Aug
Ragweed: Aug–Oct
Other weeds: June–Oct

Northeast
Trees: Apr–May
Grasses: May–July
Ragweed: Mid-Aug–Sept
Other weeds: May–Sept
Mid-Atlantic
Trees: Mar–May
Grasses: May–June
Ragweed: Mid-Aug–Sept
Other weeds: May–Sept
Southeast
Trees: Feb–May
Grasses: May–Oct
Ragweed: Aug–Oct
Other weeds: May–Oct

above, there are a number of other conditions which may cause symptoms of chronic nasal obstruction. Most of these can be diagnosed or excluded on the basis of the history and physical examination.

Rhinitis medicamentosa refers to symptoms produced by the administration of several sympatholytic drugs (see Table 23.3) or of aspirin, and to symptoms associated with abuse of topical decongestant sprays (abuse refers to frequent use which leads, after 1 to 2 weeks, to tolerance and then to rebound engorgement of submucosal blood vessels as the vasoconstrictive effect of the medication fades). The diagnosis of rhinitis medicamentosa can be made most efficiently by discontinuing the suspected drug. In the case of topical decongestants, the persistence of symptoms after the drug has been stopped suggests allergic or vasomotor rhinitis.

The nasal symptoms, chiefly obstructive, which

may accompany *pregnancy, oral contraceptive use, and hypothyroidism*, are most readily recognized because of their temporal association with one of these conditions and their remission when the inciting condition is no longer present.

The recognition of *anatomical causes* for chronic nasal symptoms depends chiefly upon the physical examination (see below). An uncommon problem such as a tumor may be suspected if there are new and progressive symptoms, especially in older individuals. Polyps or deviated nasal septum may produce chronic obstructive symptoms which are difficult to separate from perennial allergy or vasomotor rhinitis. In patients with the combination of aspirin-induced bronchospasm and nasal symptoms (see below, page 309), polyps are common. Whenever one of these anatomical causes is suspected, the patient should be referred to an otolaryngologist.

In over half of the patients with chronic, nonseasonal nasal symptoms, the clinical evidence will not support the diagnosis of perennial allergy or one of the miscellaneous causes just described. These patients are thought to have the poorly understood condition known as *vasomotor rhinitis* (10). As is true of allergic rhinitis, symptoms of vasomotor rhinitis are also thought to be provoked by environmental stimuli. The pathophysiology of this condition seems to involve inappropriate heightened reactivity of the nasal membranes to a variety of stimuli. Typically the patient awakes in the morning without symptoms but develops nasal congestion, with or without discharge and sneezing, shortly after getting out of bed; moreover, exposure to a cold bedroom or bathroom, particularly to cold bathroom tiles, is frequently identified by the patient as an inciting stimulus. Pleasant scents (in perfumes or in household products such as soaps and detergents), cooking odors, products of combustion, and emotional stress may all precipitate symptoms.

Physical Examination

Allergic and vasomotor rhinitis, with or without conjunctivitis, usually presents with swollen nasal membranes and enlarged turbinates which are often described as "pale" or "blue." The usual healthy pink appearance is absent. It may be difficult to differentiate edematous membranes or turbinates from nasal polyps; the appearance of pearly glistening globules, resembling peeled green grapes, in the nasal cavity suggests polyps and requires the opinion of an otolaryngologist. Polyps usually arise from stalks originating in the ethmoid sinuses. They are usually visible on speculum examination; at times, they may fill the nasal cavity.

Management of Allergic Rhinitis

The management of the patient with seasonal or perennial allergic rhinitis is outlined in Table 23.4.

Avoidance and Environmental Control

The treatment of choice is removal of a suspected allergen from the environment. It this is not possible, other environmental manipulations may be carried out. Since the allergic patient is rarely affected by only one allergen, general control of the environment with respect to removal of as many irritants as possible is often beneficial, even though the irritants play only a contributory role. Thus, the allergic patient will benefit from avoiding smoke in the environment, although smoke is not usually regarded as an antigen-containing substance. Clearly *animal-sensitive* patients will benefit by removing the animal from the home or attempting to reduce direct contact with it. Improvement of symptoms thereafter is gradual owing to the tendency of microscopic fragments of dander to persist in the environment, even for several months; thorough vac-

Table 23.4.
Management of Allergic Rhinitis

AVOIDANCE AND ENVIRONMENTAL CONTROL
  Control dust
  Isolate furred animals
  Obtain machine-washable polyester pillows
  Seal mattress in zippered cover
  Close windows, use air-conditioning
  Adjust humidity to 30–40% in winter
  Filter air
    Electrostatic
    HEPA
PHARMACOLOGICAL TREATMENT
  Antihistamine alone (for discharge, sneezing, itchy eyes)
  Decongestant alone (for obstruction)
  Antihistamine-decongestant combination
  Topical disodium cromoglycate (cromolyn)
  Topical corticosteroid
  Systemic corticosteroid
IMMUNOTHERAPY
  Rational choice of allergens
    History
    Skin testing
  Adequate dosage essential

uum cleaning and washing, if feasible, of all fabrics and surfaces are indicated. If it is questionable whether a pet is actually producing allergic symptoms, it is appropriate to send the patient, not the pet, for a short stay away from home. If the symptoms improve outside the home, but recur on return to home, this is presumptive evidence of the presence of allergen(s) in the home, usually from an animal or an unsuspected source of mold or related fungal growth, such as a contaminated humidifier reservoir.

The *quality of the air* in closed environments can have a significant impact on symptoms. Regulation of the relative humidity is useful; it should be maintained between 35 and 40% during the winter. Humidifier reservoirs must be kept clean. Reduction of humidity in warm, humid summer weather may also be beneficial, although this is less critical unless the degree of humidity is such that it supports visible mold growth. Air conditioning and dehumidifiers are thus often necessary where the relative humidity is always high. Any heating, humidifying, or air-cooling device which depends upon the delivery of forced air must have an effective air filter. Two types of air filtration devices may be used. One depends on electrostatic precipitation of particulate matter as it is drawn through a charged field by a blower. The second type depends on the trapping of particulate matter in a specially treated cellulose filter (the so-called HEPA type). Maintenance of the electrostatic filtration devices merely requires cleaning (usually by washing) of the particle-trapping device. With a HEPA type of filter, accessory filters may need to be replaced on a regular basis. These prefilters are necessary for trapping larger particles which would otherwise impair the efficiency of the unit. In addition to air-filtering devices, the following are desirable: floors which are bare or carpeted with washable rugs; windows that are curtained with washable curtains rather than dust-catching venetian blinds; bedrooms furnished with washable materials and containing a minimum of dust-catching books and bric-a-brac; and use of pillows of washable polyester and mattresses encased in zippered plastic covers.

Drug Therapy

Symptomatic drug treatment of allergic rhinitis is empiric and usually involves striking a satisfactory balance between the beneficial effects of the drug and the undesirable side effects. The goal of therapy is reduction of symptoms to a level which enables the patient to function normally, since complete elimination of symptoms is usually not possible (see Fig 23.4). Antihistamines are the mainstays of em-

piric therapy. Sympathomimetic decongestants, cromolyn, topical or systemic corticosteroids, and topical ophthalmic agents may be added to antihistamines depending upon the individual patient's needs.

In many patients, an *antihistamine alone* may provide adequate relief most of the time. This is particularly true when irritative symptoms (sneezing, itching, discharge) are the major problems. Many antihistamines are available. Nearly all produce some sedation and drying of the mucous membranes. Efficacy in suppressing nasal symptoms generally parallels the degree of these two side effects. As indicated in Table 23.5, there are several chemical classes of antihistamines from which to choose in the treatment of allergic rhinitis. Individual patients may respond more readily to a given class, but within classes, differences in efficacy tend to be slight. Once an effective class has been found for a patient, preference within the class will be determined by relative absence of side effects. There is

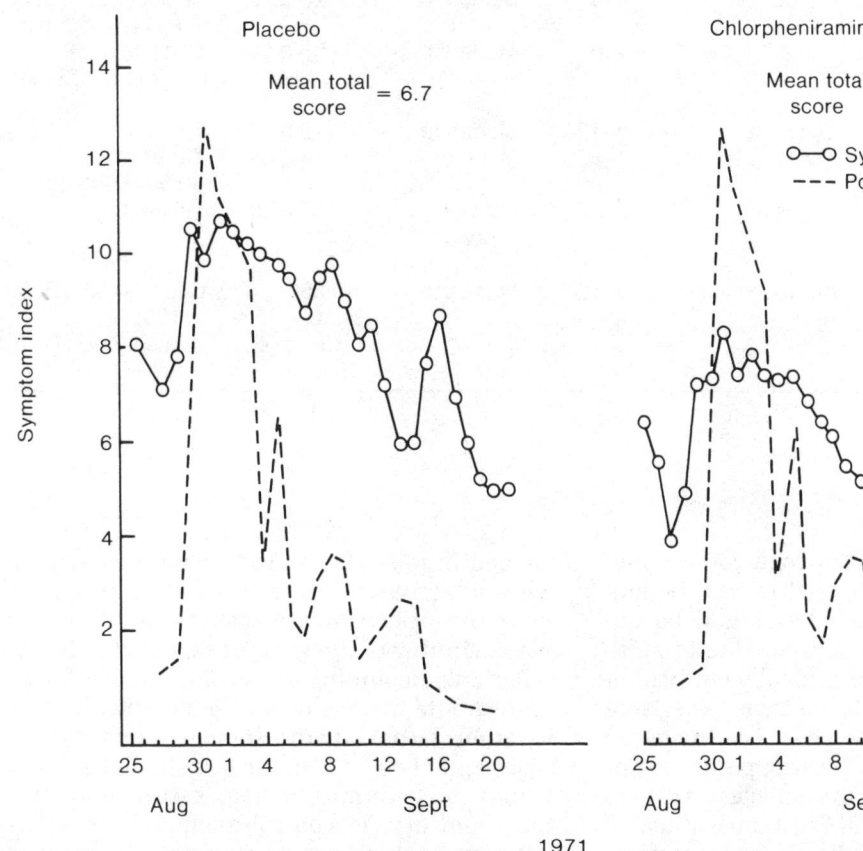
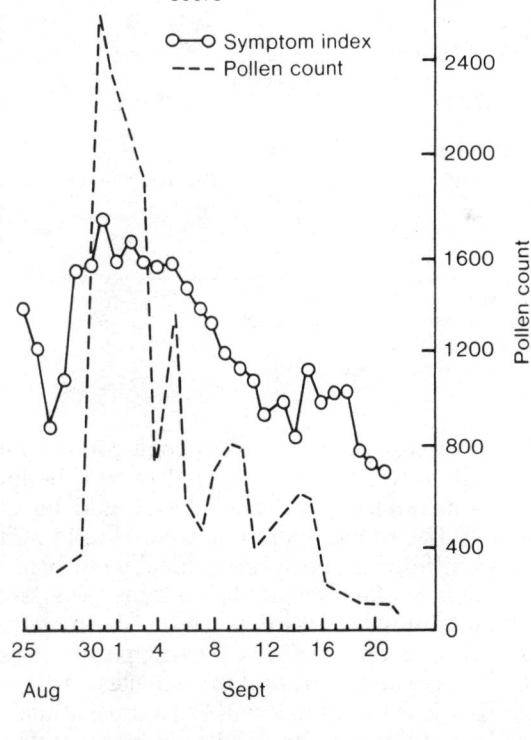

Figure 23.4. Symptom level in patients with allergic rhinitis taking antihistamines. These two sets of data compare the response of carefully matched groups of ragweed-allergic patients either to placebo or to an antihistamine (chlorpheniramine) during the ragweed pollen season. It can be seen that the antihistamine reduces but does not eliminate symptoms (the symp-

toms recorded by patients were: sneezing, stuffy nose, running nose, red itchy eyes, and cough). (Adapted from Valentine MD, Norman PS, Lichtenstein LM: Evaluation of an antihistamine in ragweed hay fever. In McMahon FG (ed): *Evaluation of Gastrointestinal, Pulmonary, Anti-Inflammatory, and Immunological Agents.* Mount Kisco, NY, Futura, 1974.)

Table 23.5.
Representative Antihistamines Useful in Treatment of Allergic Rhinitis

Generic Name	Trade Name	Duration of Action	Sedation	Recommended Adult Dose	Available Preparations
		hr		mg	mg
ETHANOLAMINES					
Diphenhydramine[a, c]	Benadryl	4–6	Marked	25–50 q.i.d.	Capsule (25, 50), elixir (12.5/5 ml)
Carbinoxamine[b]	Clistin	3–4	Moderate	4 q.i.d.	Tablet, elixir
Doxylamine	Decapryn	4–6	Moderate	12.5–25 q.i.d.	Tablet, syrup
ETHYLENEDIAMINES					
Tripelennamine[a, b]	Pyribenzamine	4–6	Moderate	50 q.i.d.	Tablet (25, 50), elixir (37.5/5 ml)
ALKYLAMINES					
Chlorpheniramine[a, b, c]	Chlor-Trimeton	4–6	Mild	4 q.i.d.	Tablet (4), syrup (2/5 ml)
Dexchlorpheniramine[b]	Polaramine	4–6	Mild	2 q.i.d.	Tablet (2), syrup (2/5 ml)
Brompheniramine[a, b, c]	Dimetane	4–6	Mild	4 q.i.d.	Tablet (4), elixir (2/5 ml)
Triprolidine[a, c]	Actidil	8–12	Mild	2.5 b.i.d.	Tablet (2.5), syrup (1.25/5 ml)
PHENOTHIAZINES					
Promethazine[a]	Phenergan	4–6	Moderate	12.5–25 q.i.d.	Tablet (12.5, 25, 50), syrup (2.5/5 ml)
Trimeprazine[a, b]	Temaril	4–6	Moderate	2.5–7.5 q.i.d.	Capsule (2.5), syrup (2.5/5 ml)
PIPERIDINES					
Azatadine	Optimine	8–12	Moderate	1–2 b.i.d.	Tablet
Cyproheptadine[d]	Periactin	4–6	Marked	4 q.i.d.	Tablet (4), syrup (2/5 ml)
Terfenadine	Seldane	8–12	Little or none	60 b.i.d.	Tablet (60)
PIPERAZINE					
Hydroxyzine[a, d]	Atarax, Vistaril	6–12	Moderate	10–25 b.i.d., t.i.d.	Capsule (10, 25, 50, 100), suspension (10/5 ml)

[a] Generic available.
[b] Sustained-release preparation available.
[c] Over-the-counter drug.
[d] More useful in urticaria and pruritus.

an enormous cost differential between generic and brand name antihistamines, so that once a patient has found an effective product, he should be encouraged to try an equivalent generic. Subtle manufacturing differences between clinically equivalent products may make a particular one more suitable for a given patient. A useful procedure is to choose one drug from each class as a starting point, beginning with the drug names first in each class in Table 23.5. At first it is better to avoid "sustained-release" preparations; they may be used later as a convenience once the right drug is found.

As shown in Table 23.5, antihistamines are available in a variety of strengths and in liquid, tablet, and sustained-released preparations; some are available without prescription. All have their onset of action in 10 to 30 minutes. Sustained-released preparations must be taken at least every 6 to 8 hours

for continuous effect. Antihistamines appear to be more effective if dosing is begun in anticipation of symptoms, i.e., before exposure to animals, or before the beginning of the grass or ragweed pollen season.

Patients beginning antihistamine use for the first time should always be advised about the hazard of sedation. To obviate this some patients omit daytime doses and choose to utilize a sustained-release preparation at bedtime, to help assure a good night's sleep and also to control adequately the irritative symptoms which are so common upon awakening in the morning. Terfenadine (Seldane), which lacks CNS depression, has recently been approved by the Food and Drug Administration (FDA). Astemizole, also nonsedating, is awaiting approval.

Sympathomimetic decongestants may add significantly to the beneficial effects of antihistamines. They may be particularly effective in patients who have pronounced obstructive symptoms due to nasal mucosal edema; presumably decongestants work by vasoconstriction which decreases the blood flow to nasal mucosa. A second beneficial property of these agents is that they have a stimulatory effect on the central nervous system, which may counteract antihistamine-induced sedation. Table 23.6 summarizes practical information about a number of commonly prescribed antihistamine-decongestant combinations (all require written prescription). Extendryl and Histaspan-D incorporate the anticholinergic agent methscopolamine for additional drying effects.

Sympathomimetic decongestants are also available alone in oral preparations and in topical drops and sprays. These forms may be useful in patients with allergic rhinitis whose most troublesome symptom is nasal obstruction or in those who cannot tolerate antihistamines. Decongestant treatment without antihistamine is the treatment of choice in patients with acute sinusitis and serous otitis media, two conditions which may complicate any allergic or nonallergic process producing congestion of the nasal mucosa. Details regarding available decongestant preparations are found in the discussion of serous otitis, Chapter 96.

In therapeutic doses, sympathomimetic decongestants may cause tachycardia and blood pressure elevation (6). Therefore, it is important to determine the individual patient's blood pressure response before prescribing a sympathomimetic for prolonged use; this can be done within 1 to 3 hours of administration of the drug. Patients with allergic rhinitis should be strongly warned against the routine use of nasal decongestant sprays or drops, as this may lead to rhinitis medicamentosa (see above). Perhaps the best advice for the patient who cannot part with a decongestant spray is that he utilize it only at times when symptom relief is crucial—for example, at bedtime if nasal obstruction makes it difficult to get to sleep (and when the stimulatory effects of oral sympathomimetic decongestants may interfere with sleeping).

For patients whose nasal symptoms are not controlled adequately by antihistamines or decongestants, *topical corticosteroids* may provide excellent relief, at times enabling an almost incapacitated individual to return to normal function. Steroids have a major impact upon obstructive nasal symptoms; simultaneous antihistamine use may, however, be needed to suppress irritative symptoms.

Table 23.6.
Representative Antihistamine-Sympathomimetic Combinations Useful in Treating Allergic Rhinitis

Trade Name	Ingredients	Mg. per Tablet or Capsule	Recommended Adult Dosage	Available Preparations[a]
Pyribenzamine with ephedrine	Tripelennamine	25	1 or 2 tablets q.i.d.	Tablet
	Ephedrine	12		
Co-Pyronil	Thenylpyramine	25	1 capsule t.i.d.	Capsule
	Pyrrobutanine	15		Suspension
	Cyclopentamine	12.5		
Omade	Chlorpheniramine	12	1 Spansule b.i.d.	Timed-release spansule
	Phenylpropanolamine	75		
Naldecon	Chlorpheniramine	5	1 tablet t.i.d.	Sustained-action tablet
	Phenyltoloxamine	15		Syrup
	Phenylpropanolamine	40		
	Phenylephrine	10		
Extendryl or Histaspan-D	Chlorpheniramine	8	1 capsule b.i.d.	Timed-action capsule
	Phenylephrine	20		Syrup
	Methscopolamine	2.5		
Isoclor[a]	Chlorpheniramine	4	1 tablet q.i.d.	Tablets
	d-Isoephedrine	25		Syrup
				Sustained-release capsule
Dimetapp[a]	Brompheniramine	12	1 Extentab b.i.d.	Extended-release tablet
	Phenylpropanolamine	75		Elixir
Actifed[a, b]	Triprolidine	2.5	1 tablet t.i.d.	Tablet
	d-Isoephedrine	60		Syrup
Disophrol	Dexbrompheniramine	6	1 tablet b.i.d.	Chronotab
Drixoral[b]	d-Isoephedrine	120		Extended-release sustained-action tablet
Rondec	Carbinoxamine	2.5	1 tablet q.i.d.	Tablet, syrup
	Pseudoephedrine	60		
Trinalin	Azatadine	1	1 tablet b.i.d.	Extended-action tablet
	Pseudoepinephrine	120		

[a] Generic available.
[b] Over-the-counter drug.

Two agents, beclomethasone (Vancenase, Beconase) and flunisolide (Nasalide), have been extensively tested and shown to be effective when administered intranasally as aerosols. One or two puffs of beclomethasone may be used two to three times daily to both nostrils; a similar regimen may be used with flunisolide, although the fact that flunisolide is a liquid solution as opposed to the micronized powder of beclomethasone makes it more difficult for a small nasal passage to retain the liquid flunisolide if administered more than one spray at a time. Thus, if it is desired to use more than one spray of flunisolide per dosing, the patient is advised to wait several minutes between sprays. In the use of both beclomethasone and flunisolide, the patient should be instructed to sniff more or less synchronously with the administration of the spray so that distribution of the agent within the nasal cavity will be enhanced. Each of these agents may cause mild burning; rare side effects include localized *Candida*, epistaxis, mucosal ulceration, and nasal septal perforation. Patients must be told to expect gradual improvement, over the course of days, in contrast to the immediate response to be expected from a topical vasoconstrictor. The pump spray device used with flunisolide may be difficult for patients with muscle weakness or poor coordination; for such individuals the freon-propelled device used for administering beclomethasone may be preferable. Dexamethasone as a nasal aerosol has also been available for some time, but is rarely indicated because of the increased risk of adrenal gland suppression which is present with this preparation, when used in maximum dosage. Both flunisolide and beclomethasone can be used safely for prolonged periods. All nasal aerosols occasionally cause transient, mild local irritation.

Patients who are using intranasal corticosteroids occasionally report symptoms suggesting a new, infectious rhinitis. Although the manufacturers have advised patients to notify their physician in this instance, there is no evidence for a need to discontinue the topical spray.

Systemic steroids are occasionally justified in treating seasonal allergy. For example, in a patient who usually requires topical steroids for obstructive symptoms, a 3- or 4-day course of prednisone (20 mg/day) may be needed to relieve nasal obstruction sufficiently so that the aerosol can effectively reach the nasal mucosa. Only rarely should a longer course of steroids (2 to 3 weeks) be utilized to treat allergic rhinitis. The prednisone can usually be tapered rapidly during the last few days of treatment (see further discussion of steroid use in Chapter 74). Although parenteral, "depot" steroid injections are convenient, they are generally contraindicated because they entail greater risk of adrenal suppression.

A nasal aerosol of cromolyn sodium (Nasalcrom) was introduced in the United States in 1983 (5). As indicated in Table 23.2, this agent inhibits mediator release in the mast cells of the nasal mucosa. Aerosolized cromolyn must be administered approximately every 4 hours by metered dose to each nostril in order to prevent symptoms. Mild side effects (chiefly nasal irritation) are common, but they are transient and well tolerated. The disadvantages of this drug are high cost to the patient and the frequent dose schedule. However, for selected patients with unequivocal seasonal allergic symptoms, a trial of cromolyn may be worthwhile because of the absence both of antihistamine sedation and risk of steroid-induced adrenal suppression.

Management of Eye Symptoms

Frequently the nasal symptoms of allergic rhinitis are controlled by one of the above drugs, but the eye symptoms persist. In this situation any of the number of topical preparations containing α-adrenergic agents such as Vasocon, Prefrin, Albalon, and Opcon, may be effective; 2 drops should be instilled three to four times daily. The latter two agents include "artificial tears" in their formulas. Of these agents, Prefrin can be obtained without prescription. Several are available in the "A" form, denoting inclusion of antihistamine. For the patient who is seriously impaired by conjunctival symptoms despite topical vasoconstrictors, either of two relatively weak topical steroids (HMS Liquifilm or FML Liquifilm) may be tried for brief periods; however, an ophthalmologist should be consulted, at least by telephone, first. Prolonged use of ophthalmic steroids should be avoided unless the patient has periodic slit-lamp examinations by an ophthalmologist, because of the danger of herpetic keratitis. Ophthalmic cromolyn (available as Opticrom) recently received FDA approval; trials in the US and abroad show that it is a promising alternative with less risk of side effects than ophthalmic steroids. The dose is 1 drop in each eye every 4 hours. This preparation is not compatible with "soft" contact lenses; any contact lens wearer should consult an ophthalmologist before using any eye drop.

Referral to an Allergist

If the patient fails to respond to the measures outlined above he should be referred to an allergist for evaluation, to confirm the diagnosis of allergic rhinitis or to disclose any other cause for nasal symptoms, and to determine whether the patient may be a candidate for immunization treatment.

The *immunological tests* done by an allergist are primarily scratch or intracutaneous tests using solutions of suspected offending allergens. These skin tests are more sensitive, although no more specific, than *in vitro* RAST (RadioAllergoSorbent Test) in which the patient's level of allergen-specific IgE antibody is measured. Moreover, the skin test is far less expensive than the RAST; therefore, the latter should be reserved for instances where either the skin is not suitable for testing (such as in patients with dermatographism or generalized atopic dermatitis) or where skin reactivity seems to be equivocal when compared to negative and positive controls.

Immunization with sufficient doses of appropriate allergens has been shown to reduce symptoms in 95% of patients with seasonal allergic rhinitis due to ragweed or grass pollens (see Fig. 23.5): however, nearly one-third of patients seem to benefit from a placebo (7). Although there are few controlled studies of animal dander immunotherapy, some allergists try this mode of therapy in selected animal-hypersensitive patients when manipulation of the environment and pharmacological control are ineffective. The house dust mite (*Dermatophagoides* species), a commensal occupant of human habitats, is an important source of airborne allergen in some areas. Control is difficult and no practical miticide

is available at present. Mite extract is also available for diagnosis and immunotherapy.

Because allergic rhinitis is often present in multiple family members, parents may question their physicians about the value of immunotherapy for their affected children. Immunotherapy is rarely indicated in early childhood. Although it may yield apparently good results in the prepubertal child, it should be borne in mind that puberty may also be accompanied by a diminution in symptoms of allergic rhinitis. Therefore, immunotherapy is indicated chiefly in the postpubertal patient.

Immunotherapy is often arbitrarily recommended for a period of 2 to 3 years. Initially, the patient is given frequent injections of the selected allergen extract in progressively higher doses until a maintenance dose is selected, after which maintenance injections are given approximately once or twice per month for the duration of immunotherapy. After 2 or 3 years, a decision must be made whether to

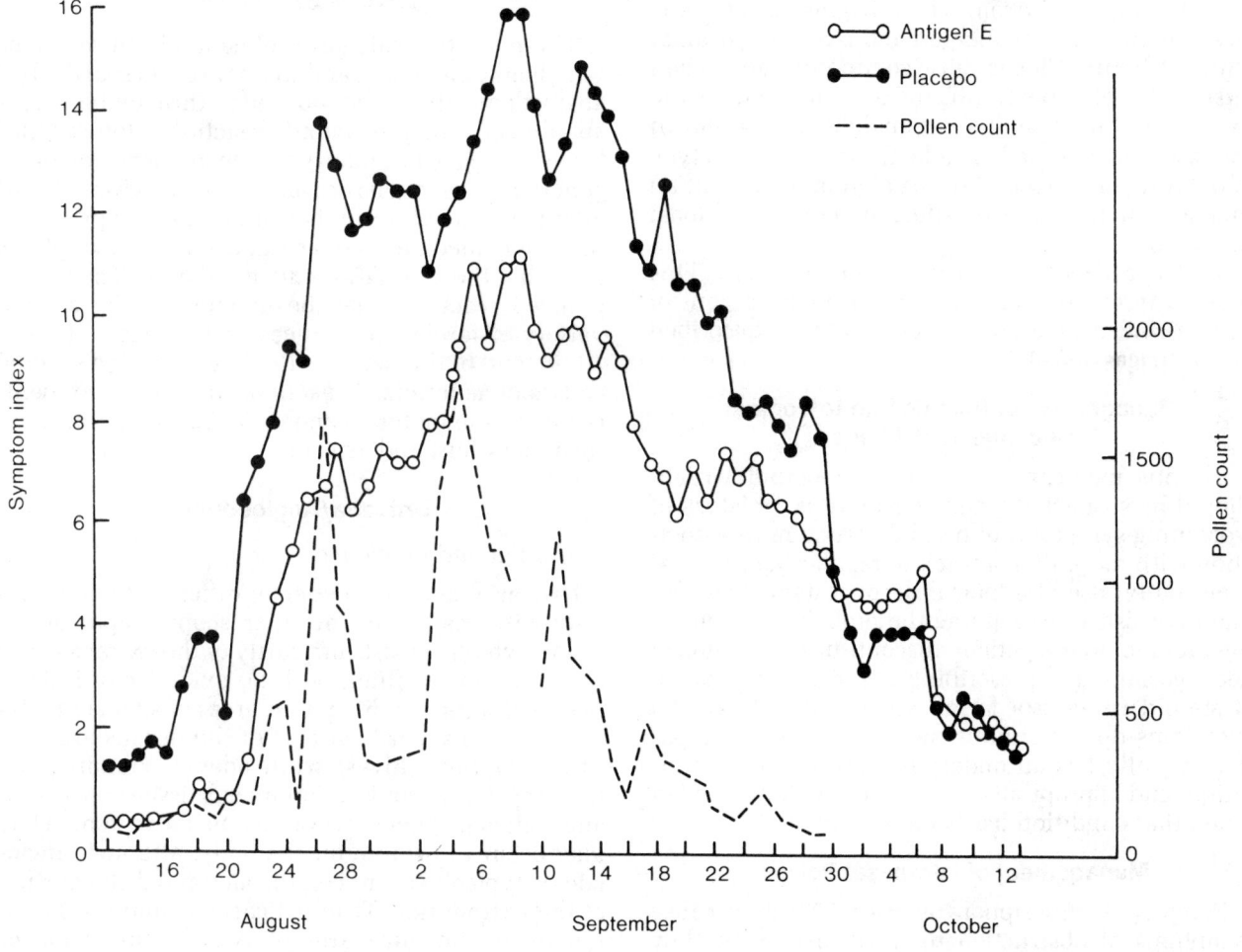

Figure 23.5. Daily symptom scores of patients immunized with a ragweed antigen (Antigen E), compared with matched patients "immunized" with a placebo. (From Lichtenstein LM, Norman PS, Winkenwerder WL: A single year of immunotherapy for ragweed hay fever: immunologic and clinical studies. *Ann Intern Med* 75:663, 1971.)

continue treatment or to stop it and watch for recurrence of symptoms. Some patients who respond well to several years of immunotherapy may continue to enjoy reduced symptoms even after immunotherapy is stopped. Allergen preparations modified with formalin ("allergoid") or glutaraldehyde are awaiting FDA approval; this sort of chemical modification allows less frequent dosing and a somewhat reduced risk of systemic reactions to therapy.

The patient's general physician may at times be asked to administer maintenance subcutaneous allergen injections. There are three types of *untoward reactions* which may occur following allergen injections:

1. *An immediate reaction*, characterized by formation of a wheal and flare at the site of injection. An eruption which is as large as a half dollar is an indication not to increase the dosage of allergen in the subsequent injection. This type of reaction may result from inadvertent administration of the dose too superficially.

2. *A delayed reaction*, which begins 2 to 4 hours after the injection of allergen and reaches a peak at 18 to 24 hours. This is most commonly seen when dust and mold spore antigens are included in the extract, and may be due to nonallergens present in the raw material used to make the extract. This type of delayed, large local skin reaction may prevent an increase in the dose of allergen because of local discomfort.

3. *Generalized or constitutional reaction.* This may be immediate or delayed; the management of generalized urticaria and anaphylaxis is described below (pages 306–307).

Management of Rhinitis Due to Topical Decongestant Abuse

Rhinitis medicamentosa of the rebound variety should be suspected whenever there is a history of worsening symptoms of nasal obstruction in association with more than a week of regular (*i.e.,* several times daily) use of a topical decongestant. Management consists of explaining the probable reason for the problem to the patient, discontinuing the topical decongestant, and prescribing a 1- to 2-week course of steroid in aerosol form, which will relieve the symptoms due to rhinitis medicamentosa. The patient usually has an underlying chronic nasal condition, and appropriate management will be needed when that condition has been identified.

Management of Intranasal Polyps

Polyps (see description on page 298) may cause symptoms of obstruction to nasal airflow or they may be asymptomatic. They may be seen in association with asthma precipitated by aspirin (see below, page 309), and there is often associated chronic or acute sinusitis. The treatment of symptomatic polyps consists of topical steroids or polypectomy.

When polyps are suspected, the patient should be referred to an otolaryngologist to confirm the diagnosis and to plan appropriate management.

Management of Vasomotor Rhinitis (10)

This nonallergic condition shows little or no response to antihistamines, but symptoms may diminish when the patient is treated with oral decongestants alone (see Chapter 96 for details regarding these preparations). Symptoms may respond to intranasal steroids (see above), which can be prescribed for use during troublesome exacerbations. The most important consideration in management for patients with vasomotor rhinitis is assuring that the patient understands the chronicity of his condition, the limited symptomatic treatment available, and the importance of avoiding irritants in his environment and of not abusing topical decongestants.

GENERALIZED ALLERGIC AND ALLERGIC-LIKE REACTIONS

There are two categories of generalized reactions which may be seen in ambulatory settings: urticaria/angioedema (usually not life threatening) and anaphylaxis/anaphylactoid reactions (often life-threatening). The underlying mechanisms for these generalized reactions are either classic IgE-mediated allergy or one of a number of nonallergic processes in which mediator release and clinical symptoms resemble those in IgE-mediated allergy. These generalized reactions may be precipitated by a wide variety of foreign substances and physical stimuli. At the end of this section, the following five specific causes of generalized reactions are discussed: penicillin, Hymenoptera venom, foods, iodinated contrast materials, and aspirin.

Urticaria/Angioedema

Definition and Incidence

Urticaria and angioedema differ pathologically only with respect to the microscopic depth of the lesion, which consists primarily of the extravascular accumulation of fluid, with no evidence of inflammation. Raised erythematous areas of edema involving only the superficial part of the dermis are urticarial eruptions (hives), while edema extending into the deep dermis and subcutaneous tissue constitutes angioedema. These eruptions usually itch. They may occur anywhere on the body, although angioedema typically occurs on the face and distal portion of the extremities. True urticarial eruptions do not remain in the same area of skin for much longer than 24 hours; persistence of lesions for 72 hours or longer in the same area of skin suggests the possible presence of cutaneous vasculitis as an underlying cause. During a typical episode of acute urticaria, evanescent eruptions may arise in different areas for 1 or more days. Urticaria ceases being acute and becomes chronic after eruptions have continued to appear, recur, or persist for 6 weeks or longer.

Urticaria is particularly common in prepubertal females but occurs at some time in approximately one-fifth of the population.

Etiology and Evaluation

A number of etiologies are recognized for urticaria/angioedema. These etiologies are summarized in Table 23.7. Both urticaria and angioedema may occur alone or together in each of the conditions listed in the table; the exception to this rule is the rare syndrome *hereditary angioedema* (HAE) in which angioedema alone occurs.

The definite (or most likely) cause of *acute* urticaria can often be determined by a history of an exposure preceding the onset of symptoms. The onset of acute urticaria/angioedema may occur from minutes to hours after the exposure to an *inciting substance* (additional discussion of reactions to selected common substances is found in a later section of this chapter). There are a number of urticaria/angioedema states initiated by *physical stimuli.* The most common is dermatographism, a linear wheal with flare which occurs at the site of brisk stroking with a firm object; the eruption fades within 30 minutes. There are several less common conditions induced by physical stimuli: (*a*) pressure urticaria/angioedema, which is characterized by local swelling, sometimes painful, which occurs immediately

Table 23.7.
Etiology of Urticaria/Angioedema

ACUTE (Episode Lasting 6 Weeks or Less)
  Allergy (IgE-mediated):
    Foods, drugs, insect stings
  Infection:
    Virus (mononucleosis, hepatitis)
    Bacterial (β-hemolytic streptococcus)
  Idiosyncrasy:
    Nonsteroid anti-inflammatory drugs (NSAID)
    Iodinated contrast material
  Physical agents:
    Dermatographism
    Heat:
      Generalized ("cholinergic")
      Localized
    Cold
    Solar
    Pressure
  Idiopathic
CHRONIC OR RECURRING
  Hereditary angioneurotic edema (HAE)
  Hepatitis
  Parasitic infestation
  Neoplasm (especially Hodgkin's lymphoma)
  Collagen-vascular disease:
    Systemic lupus erythematosus (SLE)
    Polyarteritis
    Idiopathic

---

or within 4 to 6 hours after constant pressure has been applied (for example by tight garments); (*b*) exposure to low temperatures (cold urticaria); (*c*) exposure to sunlight or intense artificial light (solar urticaria); (*d*) so-called "cholinergic" urticaria (because it can be reproduced locally in affected subjects by the injection of cholinergic agents) which develops after an increase in core body temperature due to a hot bath, exercise, fever, *etc*: and (*e*) urticaria developing shortly after the local application of heat (heat urticaria).

It is particularly important to consider the rare but potentially life-threatening condition, HAE, in any patient with isolated episodes of angioedema, particularly if there is a history of other family members with angioedema. Onset of symptoms usually occurs before age 20. Typically, the patient does not describe itching. Local trauma may precipitate peripheral attacks. Visceral attacks may occur spontaneously, characterized by abdominal pain. Life-threatening oral or laryngeal edema may occur during any attack. HAE is a nonimmunological problem, due to deficiency of the inhibitor of the first component of complement. The diagnosis is suggested by a low level of serum C4 and a normal C3 level. Patients with these findings should be referred to an allergist for definitive evaluation, which involves a functional assay for the inhibitor. An acquired form of C1 inhibitor deficiency has recently been recognized in which the pathophysiology involves consumption of the inhibitor through chronic activation of C1 by circulating immune complexes, the entire syndrome being secondary to lymphoproliferative or other malignant disorders. In both the inherited and the acquired forms, the diagnosis must be confirmed immunologically. Specific therapy with impeded androgens, such as danazol or stanozolol is indicated in these syndromes but *not* in other forms of angioedema. Another cause of low C4 values in urticaria is cutaneous vasculitis; this is usually accompanied by an elevated erythrocyte sedimentation rate.

It is often difficult to determine the etiology for *chronic* urticaria. The diagnostic workup may include complete blood counts with differential, sedimentation rate, urinalysis, stool examination for ova and parasites and tests for hepatitis antigen (see Chapter 42), cytomegalovirus antibody, heterophile antibody (Mono-spot test, see Chapter 52), cold agglutins, cryoglobulins, C3, C4, or antinuclear antibody. Despite screening tests for underlying conditions, in over 70% of patients with chronic urticaria no etiology is found (so-called idiopathic urticaria).

Management

Many patients with minor episodes of urticaria/angioedema simply tolerate it or learn by trial and error how to eliminate the causative factor(s). Others will seek help from their physician.

The intense *itching* of acute urticaria usually responds promptly to the subcutaneous administration of epinephrine (for adults: 0.2 to 0.5 ml of a 1:1000 solution of aqueous epinephrine, repeated after 15 minutes if necessary). An antihistamine such as dyphenhydramine (50 mg) or chlorpheniramine (4 mg) orally should be given at the same time. If the parenteral route is used, the initial dose should be reduced 50% to avoid marked sedation.

Additional antihistamines are helpful in preventing prolonged symptoms from urticaria. Hydroxyzine (Vistaril or Atarax) appears to be the most effective for controlling itching (8), particularly in chronic urticaria. A low dose (10 mg every 8 hours) should be tried initially, as the usual dose (25 mg every 8 hours) is much more likely to cause significant sedation. If hydroxyzine is ineffective, cyproheptadine (Periactin) may be tried, beginning with 2 mg every 8 hours and increasing to a maximum of 4 mg four times daily. The addition of an H2 antagonist (cimetidine or ranitidine) may enhance the effectiveness of conventional (H1) antihistamines in the management of urticaria. Ephedrine, 25 mg every 4 to 6 hours, may be added to H1 plus H2 regimens with some additional beneficial effect resulting from the α-, β_1-, and β_2-adrenergic effect of this compound.

These measures are useful in most of the allergic and nonallergic urticaria/angioedema states. There are exceptions, however. Cold urticaria seems to respond best to cyproheptadine (Periactin), 4 mg every 8 hours. Pressure urticaria, when severe enough to require treatment, usually does not respond to antihistamines and may require a short course of corticosteroids. Solar urticaria should be managed with a combination of topical sunscreens and hydroxyzine. As noted above, specific therapy for HAE involves preventive treatment with a nonvirilizing androgen derivative (3). If C4 levels are less than 50% of normal, any surgical procedure proposed for such patients should not be attempted because of the risk of precipitating local attacks through trauma. Two units of fresh frozen plasma may be administered prophylactically to such patients provided that an attack is not in progress; when an attack is in progress, such therapy may aggravate edema formation and is contraindicated. Life-threatening attacks require admission for observation in an intensive care unit.

Where there is a clear indication that certain conditions promote urticaria, it is important to avoid re-exposure, since more severe reactions may result. Acute generalized urticaria/angioedema following exposure to a foreign substance signifies that there is a risk of a life-threatening reaction (see below) on re-exposure. In addition, in patients with a history of solar, cold, or cholinergic urticaria, there is a small risk of vascular collapse on subsequent exposure. These disquieting facts should be made known to affected subjects and their families in order to emphasize the importance of avoiding exposure, of obtaining immediate medical attention if recurrent exposure occurs, and of administering emergency treatment if there is a severe reaction (anaphylaxis, see next section).

Anaphylaxis/Anaphylactoid Reactions

Definition

Life-threatening acute generalized reactions are not uncommon in ambulatory practice. Table 23.8 lists selected therapeutic and diagnostic substances which have been documented as causes of such reactions; other important causes are insect stings and ingested foods (see below, pages 308–309).

Anaphylaxis is an immune response to an agent to which an individual has become hypersensitive by prior exposure. A variety of symptoms may occur. Initially, there may be a diffuse erythema of the skin followed by a sense of warmth and then generalized urticaria. Severe and rapidly progressive respiratory distress due to bronchospasm and/or angioedema involving the larynx may follow. Gastrointestinal symptoms may include vomiting, abdominal cramps, and diarrhea (occasionally bloody). Vascular collapse, with or without other symptoms, can occur (anaphylactic shock). Reactions clinically indistinguishable from anaphylaxis can also occur when no allergic basis can be established for the reaction (anaphylactoid reactions).

Table 23.8.
Selected Therapeutic and Diagnostic Substances Reported to Have Caused Anaphylaxis or Anaphylactoid Reactions[a]

Adriamycin
Antisera (produced in animals)
Aspirin (and other nonsteroidal anti-inflammatory agents)
Barbiturates
Blood and blood products
Bromsulfophthalein (BSP)
Cephalosporins
Cyclophosphamide
Dehydrocholate (Decholin)
Diazepam (and other benzodiazepines)
Insulin
Iodinated radiopaque contrast agents
Local anesthetics (procaine, lidocaine)
Penicillins
Phenytoin (and other antiepileptics)
Protamine
Streptomycin
Sulfonamides
Tetanus toxoid
Tetracyclines
Various peptide hormones

[a] Modified from *Asthma and the Other Allergic Diseases*, NIAID Task Force Report. NIH publ no. 79-387, May 1979.

Management

The recommendations of the National Institutes of Health Task Force on Allergy for the initial management of anaphylaxis and anaphylactoid reactions are summarized in Table 23.9. Because bronchospasm, hypotension, and other hazardous manifestations can recur over a number of hours, the patient should either be hospitalized or kept in an emergency department for observation during the 12 to 24 hours following anaphylaxis.

Avoidance of the offending substance is, of course, critical in patients with a history of anaphylaxis. The self-treatment kit described below under Hymenoptera sting reaction should be prescribed for subjects who are at risk of recurrent accidental exposures.

Selected Causes of Generalized Reactions

Penicillin

Penicillin allergy is a common concern in ambulatory practice, where short courses of penicillin or one of the semisynthetic penicillins are frequently prescribed. The physician may be confronted with either of two problems.

The commonest problem is the patient who needs penicillin and gives a *history of penicillin "allergy."* For the infections treated in ambulatory practice, there is almost always a suitable alternative to a penicillin (throughout this volume, the appropriate alternative is named wherever a penicillin is recommended). The most prudent strategy is to select an alternative drug whenever there is a possibility of prior penicillin allergy, even though this will lead to some unnecessary substitution, as almost half of patients giving a history of penicillin allergy do not in fact show allergic reactions when rechallenged with penicillin (11). In an ambulatory patient who has been labeled "allergic to penicillin" on the basis of an atypical "allergic" reaction, genuine penicillin allergy can be confirmed or excluded by skin testing, ideally utilizing both major and minor determinant penicillin antigens (11); this may be particularly desirable in a young adult who may be denied access to penicillin throughout his life on the basis of unsubstantiated "penicillin allergy." When such a patient is seen in ambulatory practice, the best plan is to select alternatives to penicillin when antibiotics are needed and to refer the patient to an allergist for administration and interpretation of these critical skin tests.

Approximately half of patients with confirmed penicillin allergy also have positive skin tests to cephalosporin antigens (11). Therefore, cephalosporin antibiotics should not be given to persons allergic to penicillin, and *vice versa.*

Less commonly, the physician in ambulatory practice will have to manage a *first reaction to penicillin.* Table 23.10 shows the approximate incidence of each of three types of allergic reactions (immediate,

Table 23.9.
Treatment of Anaphylaxis[a]

1. When applicable, place tourniquet above site of injection or sting to obstruct venous return or stop the administration of the causative agent. Remove tourniquet temporarily every 10–15 minutes.
2. Place patient in recumbent position and elevate lower extremities.
3. Administer aqueous epinephrine 1:1000, 0.3–0.5 ml subcutaneously or intramuscularly (or if necessary 0.1 ml in 10 ml of saline solution given intravenously over several minutes) and repeat as necessary.
4. Inject aqueous epinephrine 1:1000, 0.1–0.3 ml at the site of the injection.
5. Establish and maintain airway, first with oral airway. If necessary, use endotracheal tube.
6. Give oxygen as needed.
7. Monitor vital signs frequently.
8. If patient is not responding, give diphenhydramine hydrochloride (Benadryl), 60–80 mg intravenously over 3 minutes (maximum, 5 mg/kg in 24 hours).
9. If blood pressure cannot be obtained, give normal saline intravenously and maintain blood pressure with levarterenol bitartrate (Levophed), 1 or 2 ampules (8 to 16 mg) in 500 ml of 5% glucose in water. Titrate to maintain blood pressure.
10. If severe asthma without shock give aminophylline, 500 mg intravenously over 10–20 minutes.
11. While corticosteroids will not be helpful for the acute anaphylaxis, they may prevent protracted anaphylaxis.

[a] Modified from *Asthma and the Other Allergic Diseases*, NIAID Task Force Report. NIH publ no. 79-387, May 1979.

Table 23.10.
Estimated Incidence of Allergic Reactions to Penicillin[a]

Type of Reaction	Manifestations	Time of Occurrence after First Dose of Penicillin	Percentage of Treated Patients Showing Reaction
Late reactions	Skin rash	≥72 hr	1.4
Accelerated reactions	Urticaria	1–72 hr	0.3
Immediate reactions	Generalized urticaria	2–30 min	0.3
	Anaphylaxis	2–30 min	0.04
	Anaphylactic deaths[b]		0.001

[a] Modified from *Asthma and the Other Allergic Diseases*, NIAID Task Force Report. NIH publ no. 79-387, May 1979. Results are based upon 70 to 80 million therapeutic courses of penicillin or semisynthetic penicillin or cephalosporin given per annum in the United States.
[b] From 400 to 800 deaths per year in the United States.

accelerated, late) following either parenteral or oral administration of penicillin. The management of the more common late reactions (usually nonurticarial morbilliform rashes) is reassurance and a short course of an antihistamine if itching is a problem. The acute management of accelerated and immediate reactions is described in the preceding sections on urticaria and anaphylaxis. Long term management requires assuring that the patient and his immediate family know that all forms of penicillin and the related cephalosporin antibiotics should be avoided.

Ampicillin Rash

Ampicillin commonly causes a nonallergic maculopapular rash which is not pruritic. It occurs in approximately 9% of all patients given ampicillin and as high as 50% of patients with mononucleosis (1). The risk of developing this type of rash is also higher in patients with lymphatic leukemia, hyperuricemia, and those taking allopurinol. Rechallenge with ampicillin at a later time often causes no recurrence of the rash or other adverse reactions; therefore, a well documented history of this kind of ampicillin rash is not a contraindication to subsequent ampicillin (or other penicillin) treatment.

Hymenoptera Venom

Stings by yellow jackets, hornets, honeybees, and wasps result in generalized allergic reactions of varying severity in approximately 0.4% of the population (1).

IgE-mediated hypersensitivity to these insect venoms may be confirmed by skin testing with suitable dilutions of available venoms; this is most appropriately done by an allergist. Since victims, unless already familiar with the distinguishing features of the various Hymenoptera, are often unable to tell bees from yellow jackets, hornets, or wasps, skin testing with individual venoms is particularly important. After a generalized allergic reaction to an insect sting has been treated (see above) the general physician should immediately initiate a plan to protect the patient's future health. Avoidance of recurrent exposure is critical. In particular, wearing shoes at all times is the single most important safeguard to the patient. However, because of the possibility of unavoidable re-exposure, despite the patient's best efforts, the patient (and ideally a companion whenever the patient is out of doors) should know both the early signs of a generalized reaction and how to administer emergency treatment. An *emergency self-treatment* kit containing syringes preloaded with epinephrine should be prescribed. An example is the Ana-Kit (Hollister) which contains a two-dose syringe which allows administration of two measured doses (0.3 ml each) of epinephrine; two 4-mg tablets of chlorpheniramine; two sterile

swabs; tourniquet; and instructions. The Epi-Pen and Epi-Pen, Jr. (Center Laboratories) provide a single 0.3- or 0.15-mg dose of epinephrine, respectively, in an automatic injector which some patients may prefer. The general physician should familiarize himself with one of these kits, keep one in his office, and review its use with any susceptible patient.

Any adult patient with sensitivity to one of these venoms confirmed by skin test who has had a past history of a potentially life-threatening reaction has a greater than 50% chance of a similar reaction if stung again and should therefore be offered *immunization* with those venoms to which he is reactive. Such treatment is analogous to that described above (page 298) for seasonal allergy; it reduces the likelihood of a future severe reaction to less than 5%. Once immunotherapy is instituted for insect venom hypersensitivity, it must be maintained through the use of booster injections at 4- to 6-weekly intervals indefinitely. Children through age 16 whose systemic reactions have been confined to the skin (urticaria or angioedema) have a 10 to 20% risk of future systemic reactions of similar or milder type, and a minuscule risk of a more severe reaction. Therefore in this group of patients, immunotherapy may be offered but may be of relatively small benefit.

Even patients who do not have life-threatening reactions (i.e., those who have urticaria/angioedema or other cutaneous symptoms) may be at increased risk of a more severe reaction on re-exposure; therefore, such patients also should be referred to an allergist for skin testing and for a careful explanation of the available methods of protection (immunization or an emergency self-treatment kit). Patients whose reactions have been local (confined to an area contiguous to the site of the sting) are not considered candidates for immunotherapy, even if the reaction is large.

Food

The gastrointestinal tract is sufficiently permeable to antigens found in food that some individuals experience one or more manifestations of allergy after the ingestion of a food to which they have become sensitive. Clinically apparent food allergy is much more common in young children than in adolescents or adults. In adults food allergy usually manifests as urticaria/angioedema or anaphylaxis. In children (particularly those sensitive to cow's milk), rhinitis, eczema, asthma, and colic may also occur. The most common causes of food allergy are listed in Table 23.11. Allergy to shellfish has nothing to do with susceptibility to the nonimmunological reactions to iodinated contrast materials seen after administration of these materials (see below).

Evidence of sensitization to food antigens can be confirmed by skin testing. It has been established, however, that many subjects exhibit positive skin

Table 23.11.
Foods Which Most Often Cause Allergic Reactions

MOST COMMON:
  Seafood
  Eggs
  Nuts
  Seeds
OTHERS:
  Milk
  Chocolate
  Grains (barley, rice, wheat)
  Fruits (citrus, melons, bananas, strawberries)
  Vegetables (tomatoes, celery, spinach, corn, potatoes, soy bean)

tests to certain foods but have no clinically relevant symptoms; because of these "false positives," skin tests are not useful in the routine evaluation of food allergy. At present, the only ways of *establishing* that a certain food is a cause of allergic manifestations are by elimination diets or by blind challenge and objective evaluation of the results. A blind challenge should not be carried out when an anaphylactic reaction is thought to be due to a particular food, because of the potential danger of the reaction.

There is no good evidence for nonantibody-mediated food hypersensitivity, although many practitioners claim to be able to use various techniques to substantiate food sensitivity. Various symptoms, including hyperactivity, depression, difficulty in concentration, and memory loss, have been blamed on food "allergy." Evidence to support such notions consists of uncontrolled observations by physicians who strongly believe in the existence of such entities.

The management of food allergy is avoidance and, in selected instances, prescription of and education about self-treatment kits (see above). No evidence exists that food sensitivity can be "neutralized" by injections of food extracts or by the administration of food extract drops sublingually.

Iodinated Contrast Materials

Patients receiving intravenous iodinated contrast materials may develop one of three reactions which resemble allergic reactions. Neither IgE-mediated allergy nor other immunological mechanisms have been found to explain these reactions, although complement activation may be shown *in vitro*. The three types of reaction are:

1. *Rash.* Onset of urticaria/angioedema, usually accompanied by generalized itching.
2. *Anaphylactoid.* Cough, dyspnea, wheezing, syncope, with or without urticaria/angioedema.
3. *Vasomotor.* An exaggerated response to dye injection, with more than the usual amount of flushing and nausea, frequently accompanied by a sen-

sation of numbness and tingling of the extremities and transient hypotension of a mild degree.

It is estimated that there is a 1 to 2% risk of developing one of these reactions in the general population and an approximately 35% risk in patients with a prior history of a reaction (1). At the present time, there is no method such as a skin test or a small trial dose to identify prospectively the patient at risk.

Management of the acute reaction is similar to that described for generalized allergic reactions above. The patient should be carefully educated about the risk of recurrence; and repeat studies with iodinated contrast materials should be avoided whenever possible. In the event that a patient with a history of a reaction (either urticaria/angioedema or anaphylactoid) must undergo a later study, the following regimen should be followed: prednisone, 50 mg, is given 13, 7, and 1 hour before the procedure; diphenhydramine, 50 mg, and ephedrine, 25 mg, are given orally 1 hour before the procedure. This regimen reduces but does not entirely eliminate the risk of a subsequent reaction (4).

Aspirin

Aspirin (acetylsalicylic acid) can produce urticaria/angioedema, an anaphylactoid reaction, or severe asthma in susceptible subjects. These reactions usually occur in patients with a prior history of some type of allergy. It is estimated that this type of aspirin sensitivity may develop in up to 10% of asthmatics (1); the problem is particularly common in patients with both bronchial asthma and nasal polyps.

IgE-mediated allergy to aspirin has not been demonstrated. Further evidence against an allergic basis is the fact that affected individuals may show similar reactions to other nonsteroidal anti-inflammatory drugs (NSAIDs) (see Chapter 70) not related antigenically to aspirin. The yellow food-coloring dye, tartrazine (utilized in some foods, beverages, and medications), may also elicit urticaria in NSAID-sensitive patients.

The first generalized reaction to aspirin usually occurs in adulthood, most typically a number of years after the onset of asthma (9). Symptoms may occur immediately after aspirin ingestion or a number of hours later. Because of this delay, the role of aspirin may be overlooked by the patient; therefore, it is important to question any patient with an unexplained generalized reaction about the use of aspirin or one of the other agents known to produce these reactions.

The management of the generalized reactions in these patients is the same as that described earlier for urticaria/angioedema and for anaphylaxis. Avoidance of products containing aspirin (see Table 23.12) and the other agents which may induce these symptoms is essential after the diagnosis has been

Table 23.12.
Aspirin Preparations and Aspirin-Containing Products

Alka-Seltzer[a]
Anacin[a]
Anahist
Arthritis Pain Formula[a]
Ascodeen-30
Ascriptin[a]
Aspergum[a]
Bayer Aspirin[a]
Bufferin[a]
Cama Inlay-Tabs[a]
Cirin
Congespirin[a]
Cope
Coricidin[a]
Darvon Compound
Dristan[a]
Duradyne DHC Tablets
Duragesic Tablets
Easprin
Ecotrin[a]
Empirin
Emprazil
Equagesic
Excedrin
Fiorinal
Goody's Headache Powders[a]
Measurin
Midol[a]
Momentum Muscular Backache Formula
Pabirin
Panalgesic[a]
Percodan
Persistin
Phenaphen
Quiet World Analgesic/Sleeping Aid[a]
Rhinex
St. Joseph Cold Tablets for Children[a]
Sine-off Tablets-Aspirin Formula[a]
Stanback[a]
Stero-Darvon
Supac
Synalgos
Triaminicin[a]
Vanquish[a]
Viro-Med[a]
4-Way Cold Tablets

[a] Over-the-counter.

established. Affected patients should be instructed explicitly to use only acetaminophen (Tylenol or a noncoated generic) when they need a mild analgesic or antipyretic. An oral "desensitization" regimen using aspirin has been reported to result in lessening of chronic nasal and sinus symptoms in some aspirin-sensitive patients. This procedure should be regarded as experimental and should not be undertaken in the ambulatory patient or in the hospitalized patient without expert consultation.

General References

Lichtenstein LM, Fauci AS: *Current Therapy in Allergy, Immunology, and Rheumatology. 1985–1986.* St Louis, CV Mosby, 1985.
Middleton E, Reed CE, Ellis EF (eds): *Allergy: Principles and Practice.* St Louis, CV Mosby, 1983.

> A two-volume compendium with chapters by many recognized authorities on various topics. It is worthwhile to read about a subject in both this and in Samter (see below), since the discussions are often complementary, and at times contradictory.

Mygind N: *Nasal Allergy.* Oxford, Blackwell Scientific Publications, 1978.

> Recommended for the physician who has more than a superficial interest in nasal problems. One author, one style, clearly written, and reasonably concise.

Samter MD (ed): *Immunological Diseases,* ed 3. Boston, Little, Brown and Co, 1978.

> Two-volume work containing more detail on treatment of general problems in immunology than in Middleton *et al.*

Specific References

1. *Asthma and the Other Allergic Diseases,* NIAID Task Force Report. NIH publ no. 79-387, May 1979.
2. Broder I, Higgins MW, Mathews KP, Keller JB; Epidemiology of asthma and allergic rhinitis in a total community, Tecumseh, Michigan. *J Allergy Clin Immunol* 54:100, 1974.
3. Gelfand JA, Sherins RJ, Alling DW, Frank MM: Treatment of hereditary angioedema with danazol: reversal of clinical and biochemical abnormalities. *N Engl J Med* 295:1444, 1976.
4. Greenberger PA, Patterson R, Radin RC: Two pretreatment regimens for high-risk patients receiving radiographic contrast media. *J Allergy Clin Immunol* 74:540, 1984.
5. Handelman NI, Friday GA, Schwartz HJ, et al: Cromolyn sodium nasal solution in the prophylactic treatment of pollen-induced seasonal allergic rhinitis. *J Allergy Clin Immunol* 59:237, 1977.
6. Horowitz JD, Howes LG, Christophidis N, et al: Hypertensive responses induced by phenylpropanolamine in anorectic and decongestant preparations. *Lancet* 1:60, 1980.
7. Norman PS: Specific therapy in allergy. *Med Clin North Am* 58:111, 1974.
8. Rhoades RB, Leifer KN, Cohan R, Wittig HJ: Suppression of histamine-induced pruritis by three antihistamine drugs. *J Allergy Clin Immunol* 55:180, 1975.
9. Samter M, Beers RF Jr: Intolerance to aspirin. Clinical studies and consideration of its pathogenesis. *Ann Intern Med* 68:975, 1968.
10. Stewart TW Jr: Vasomotor rhinitis: neglected cause of nasal congestion. *Postgrad Med* 67:171, 1980.
11. Sullivan TJ, Wedner HJ, Shatz GS, et al: *Skin Testing to Detect Penicillin Allergy.* St Louis, CV Mosby, 1981.
12. Tarlo SM, Cockcroft DW, Dolovich J, Hargreave FE: Beclomethasone dipropionate aerosol in perennial rhinitis. *J Allergy Clin Immunol* 59:232, 1977.

CHAPTER TWENTY-FOUR

Undifferentiated Acute Febrile Illness

NATHANIEL F. PIERCE, M.D.

INTRODUCTION

Acute febrile illnesses are encountered frequently in medical practice. Such episodes have many possible causes, which range in significance from trivial to life threatening. For those which require treatment, accurate diagnosis is obviously needed to guide the choice of therapy. In most instances, fever is accompanied by localizing complaints or physical findings that suggest specific diagnoses and guide the selection of diagnostic laboratory studies. Such episodes can usually be diagnosed promptly and appropriate management can be readily instituted. Thus, for example, fever plus dysuria suggests the diagnosis of urinary tract infection, indicates the need for a urinalysis and urine culture, and is likely to require antibiotic therapy.

A more difficult problem may be posed, however, when fever occurs as an isolated complaint or is accompanied only by nonspecific constitutional symptoms, such as chills, malaise, anorexia, or modest weight loss. Although such episodes of acute undifferentiated febrile illness may raise the fear of serious illness in the minds of both patient and physician, most are benign and resolve spontaneously in 2 weeks or less, without a specific diagnosis being made. In only a very few instances do undifferentiated febrile illnesses persist and remain unexplained despite continued careful observation of the patient and the performance of routine diagnostic laboratory tests. Only when fever has lasted at least 3 weeks in such patients should it be designated "fever of unknown origin" (FUO). Patients with FUO usually require hospitalization for more extensive diagnostic evaluation, whereas unexplained febrile illnesses of shorter duration are usually managed on an ambulatory basis.

The aim of this chapter is to describe a rational approach to the diagnosis and management of acute undifferentiated febrile episodes, emphasizing a careful balance between cautious observation and active investigation.

Normal Temperature Range

In most healthy persons, the normal oral temperature varies between 96.5°F (35.8°C) and 99°F (37.2°C), the lowest value occurring between 2 A.M. and 4 A.M., and the highest between 6 P.M., and 10 P.M. In very hot weather, an individual's temperature may be 0.5°F to 1°F (0.3–0.6°C) higher than normal. Very vigorous exercise, such as marathon running, will also cause the temperature to rise temporarily.

ETIOLOGICAL CONSIDERATIONS

Infections

Infection is undoubtedly the most common cause of acute undifferentiated fever. An abrupt onset of fever is especially suggestive of infection; however, other causes are possible. The majority of episodes of undifferentiated fever due to infection are self-limited, eventuate in complete recovery without treatment, and are likely to be of viral etiology. The viral agents which cause these episodes are rarely identified and attempts to identify causative viruses by cultural or serological methods are not usually warranted.

For certain infections which begin as undifferentiated fever diagnostic signs or symptoms develop after 1 or several days. These account for only a small portion of the episodes of acute undifferentiated fever, but include serious infections which require prompt diagnosis and treatment. Most common among these are viral infections, such as infectious mononucleosis (see Chapter 52), viral hepatitis (see Chapter 42), varicella (chickenpox), rubeola (measles), and rubella (German measles); rickettsial infections, such as Rocky Mountain spotted fever and Q fever; a variety of localized bacterial infections, such as those involving the pleura, biliary tract, retroperitoneum, kidney, liver, and spleen;

Table 24.1.
Some Acute Nonbacterial Infections for Which Undifferentiated Fever May Be the First Manifestation

Infection	Transmission	Incubation Period	Clinical Features
		days	
Chickenpox (varicella)	Person-to-person *via* respiratory secretions and direct contact; highly contagious	10–21	Malaise and fever precede or occur simultaneously with rash. Rash develops in crops as pruritic maculopapules evolving in hours to vesicles and in days to dried scabs. All stages of rash are seen in the same skin area.
German measles (rubella)	Person-to-person, *via* respiratory secretions and direct contact; highly contagious	14–21	1–7-day prodrome of malaise, headache, fever, mild conjuctivitis followed by maculopapular (occasionally confluent) rash which begins on forehead and spreads to trunk and extremities.
Measles (rubeola)	Person-to-person, *via* respiratory secretions	9–11	3–4-day prodrome with fever, malaise, hacking cough, rhinitis, subsiding 1–2 days following onset of maculopapular rash spreading from face to neck to trunk, to feet (by third day)
Q Fever (*Rickettsia burnetti*)	Spread by airborne rickettsiae in dust contaminated by infected animals (cattle, sheep, goats) or by direct contact with infected animals or their tissue	14–26	Headache, chills, fever, anorexia, myalgias lasting 3 days to 2 weeks. Cough with rales after a few days, persisting after fever remits. Treated with tetracycline or chloramphenicol.
Rocky Mountain spotted fever (*Ricksettsia rickettsiae*)	Bite of infected tick or contamination with tick tissues or feces	3–14	Abrupt onset of severe headache, chills, myalgia, fever. Rash (second to fourth day of fever)—initially *macules* on wrists, ankles, palms, soles, extending in 6–12 hours to buttocks, trunk, face; becomes *maculopapular* by day 2–3 and *petechial* by about day 4, progressing to ecchymoses. Rash may be missed on dark skin. Early treatment with chloramphenicol or tetracycline is lifesaving.

and several bacteremic infections, especially acute bacterial endocarditis and *Salmonella* bacteremia. If there has been recent travel to appropriate developing countries (see Chapter 33), the list of etiological considerations should include malaria, dengue fever, scrub typhus, and leptospirosis, and the possibility of viral hepatitis and *Salmonella* bacteremia is increased. Table 24.1 summarizes salient features of important nonbacterial infections that may present with acute undifferentiated fever and that are not discussed elsewhere in this book.

Drugs

A small portion of acute undifferentiated febrile episodes in ambulatory patients is caused by drugs. Almost any drug can cause fever but digitalis preparations, chloramphenicol, insulins, and tetracyclines almost never do. Those most frequently responsible are listed in Table 24.2. Fever may begin promptly after starting the drug or may be delayed by several weeks; however, a drug taken regularly for 3 months or longer is not likely to cause fever. Drug fever may be low grade, or may exceed 104°F (40°C). Chills are uncommon with drug fever, but their presence does not exclude this diagnosis. A maculopapular skin rash or eosinophilia occurs in a minor proportion of cases. Removal of the offending drug is usually followed by defervescence in 1 to 2 days; however, fever may last several days, or up to 2 to 3 weeks, if the drug is eliminated slowly, e.g., iodides. Readministration of the suspected drug usually causes fever within a few hours, thus confirming its causative role. This approach should only be considered if the drug is important for future therapy and the original febrile episode was not associated with organ damage.

Other Causes

Other acute processes that may cause undifferentiated fever include vascular occlusive and/or inflammatory events such as deep vein thrombophlebitis, minor pulmonary emboli, and asymptomatic myocardial infarction. Similarly, fever may be the only manifestation of acute hemolytic episodes, such as occur in acute autoimmune hemolytic anemia or hemolytic anemia due to glucose 6-phosphate dehydrogenase (G6PD) deficiency. Recent immunization with certain vaccines (see Chapter 32) may also cause fever.

Table 24.2.
Important Causes of Drug Fever

Amphotericin B	Isoniazid
Antihistamines	Methyldopa
Atropine	Nitrofurantoin
Barbiturates	Penicillins
Bleomycin	Phenolphthalein[b]
Cephalosporins	Procainamide
Diphenylhydantoin	Quinidine
Ethambutol	Salicylates[c]
Hydralazine	Sulfonamides
Iodides[a]	Thiouracils

[a] Including intravenous contrast media.
[b] Found in many nonprescription laxatives.
[c] When toxic levels occur.

Special Risk Patients

In patients with certain pre-existing conditions, serious infections play an increased role in causing acute undifferentiated fever. Patients with lymphomas, especially Hodgkin's disease, or those receiving therapeutic doses of corticosteroids (more than 20 mg daily of hydrocortisone or an equivalent dose of another corticosteroid), especially if combined with other immunosuppressive agents, are at increased risk of developing primary or reactivation tuberculosis, acquiring or reactivating certain fungal infections (e.g., cryptococcosis, histoplasmosis, and coccidioidomycosis), reactivating certain viral infections (e.g., herpes zoster or cytomegalovirus infections), or developing infections due to *Pneumocystis carinii* or *Toxoplasma*; many of these infections also occur in patients with the acquired immune deficiency syndrome (AIDS—see Chapter 52). Patients with established rheumatic valvular disease, certain types of congenital heart disease (e.g., ventricular septal defect, patent ductus arteriosus, or coarctation of the aorta), or prosthetic heart valves or vascular grafts are at increased risk of bacterial endocarditis (acute or subacute) or other endovascular infection. Patients with multiple myeloma, or surgical splenectomy or autosplenectomy due to sickle cell disease, are at increased risk of serious spontaneous bacteremia, due especially to *Streptococcus pneumoniae*, *Haemophilus influenzae*, or salmonellae. Persons with advanced hepatic cirrhosis, especially when it is accompanied by ascites, may develop spontaneous bacterial peritonitis, often without localizing signs or symptoms. And persons who administer illicit drugs to themselves intravenously are at risk of developing bacterial sepsis due to nonsterile technique.

In other patients, especially elderly people and chronic alcoholics, the usual signs and symptoms of some acute bacterial infections may be diminished or absent. Fever may be the only manifestation of pneumonia, empyema, or localized intra-abdominal infection in such persons; and the febrile response to these infections may be less than usually seen in younger or nonalcoholic patients.

Chronic Fever

The major causes of unexplained fever lasting more than 3 weeks (FUO) differ appreciably from those described above. The most common causes are (a) chronic infections, especially tuberculosis, subacute bacterial endocarditis, chronic osteomyelitis, cytomegalovirus infections, occult intra-abdominal abscesses, and urinary tract infections; (b) collagen-vascular or rheumatic diseases, especially systemic lupus erythematosus, temporal arteritis, rheumatic fever, and rheumatoid arthritis; (c) certain neoplasms, especially lymphoma, acute leukemia, reticulum cell sarcoma, hypernephroma, hepatoma, pancreatic carcinoma, carcinoma of the lung, and malignancies involving bone; and (d) miscellaneous disorders such as granulomatous hepatitis, hyperthyroidism, drug fever, inflammatory bowel disease, sarcoidosis, thyroiditis, and recurrent pulmonary emboli.

Early diagnosis of these chronic disorders is sometimes possible, especially when localizing symptoms or signs are present. Othewise, these diagnoses are usually considered only when fever has been unexplained for at least 3 weeks despite preliminary diagnostic studies.

DIAGNOSTIC APPROACH

General Objectives

There are two general objectives in managing patients with acute undifferentiated fever; first, early diagnosis in those few instances of serious illness which require specific treatment, and second, the avoidance of unnecessary and expensive diagnostic studies and of "blind therapy" for the majority of patients whose course will prove benign and self-limited. The key to achievement of these objectives is careful, repeated evaluation of the patient's history and physical findings and judicious use of diagnostic tests. A sequential evaluation process, which emphasizes frequent re-evaluation combined with increasing diagnostic studies, is summarized in Table 24.3 and described below.

Initial Evaluation

The initial evaluation of most patients with an acute undifferentiated febrile illness requires about 15 minutes. A febrile illness is present if an oral temperature exceeding 99.5°F (37.6°C) is found on examination or by history. The evaluation of such patients should aim to detect the signs, symptoms, or historical background which localizes the cause of fever, as indicated in Table 24.4. A history of similar symptoms among others at home or at work suggests an infectious process. Fever with no other signs or symptoms in a patient recently started on a new drug suggests drug fever. If no localizing signs or symptoms are found and the patients does not seem seriously ill, no further evaluation is needed. The patient should be reassured and instructed to keep a record of morning and evening temperatures at home if the fever persists. A telephone call should be scheduled after 1 or 2 days as a simple means of following the course of the illness, detecting new complaints, and providing reassurance. If undifferentiated fever persists for 7 to 10 days, the patient should return for a thorough re-evaluation.

Exceptions to this pattern of management are patients whose constitutional symptoms are severe, who have those underlying conditions which predispose to serious infections or mask their manifestations (see above), who have been recently hospitalized or have undergone invasive diagnostic studies, or who describe fever of at least 2 weeks' duration when first seen. The initial evaluation of such patients should be expanded to include a thorough history and physical examination, as described below under "Re-evaluation," and the following laboratory studies: chest X-ray with posteroanterior (PA) and lateral views, complete blood count with differential, erythrocyte sedimentation rate, liver function tests, blood cultures (aerobic and anaerobic) from at least two sites, urinalysis, and quantitative urine culture, if the urinalysis reveals pyuria or bacteriuria. Positive findings should be used to guide further studies or treatment. Patients with severe constitutional symptoms may require hospitalization and prompt antimicrobial therapy for possible bacteremia, especially if underlying conditions predisposing to bacteremia are present and/or hematological findings suggestive of bacteremia are found (e.g., Döhle bodies or vacuoles in polymorphonuclear neutrophilic leukocytes (PMNs), or in-

Table 24.3.
Acute Undifferentiated Febrile Illness: Summary of Sequential Evaluation Process

Evaluation Process	Comment
INITIAL EVALUATION	
1. History, physical examination; if negative and not seriously ill, observe 7–10 days; frequent phone contact	Spontaneous defervescence common, benign illness common
2. More thorough evaluation of "special risk" patients, including laboratory studies	Increased risk that fever is caused by serious illness, usually infection
3. If seriously ill: more extensive laboratory studies; may need hospitalization and treatment	
REPEAT EVALUATIONS (AT WEEKLY INTERVALS)	
1. Carefully repeated history and physical examination, expanded laboratory evaluation	Thorough re-evaluation often detects cause of fever
2. Discontinue recent drugs, document fever	
AFTER 3 WEEKS	
1. Begin evaluation for true FUO, usually requires hospitalization	Spontaneous defervescence uncommon, fever usually due to serious illness with substantial risk of mortality

Table 24.4.
Signs or Symptoms to Be Sought during the Initial Evaluation of Patients with Acute Undifferentiated Fever

Anatomical Site	Symptoms	Sign
Ear, nose, throat	Ear pain	Red eardrum
	Nasal discharge	Inflamed nasal passages
	Sinus pain	Sinus tenderness
	Sore throat	Injected pharynx
	Toothache	Tooth tenderness
Eyes	Visual impairment	
Lower respiratory tract	Dyspnea	Abnormal breath sounds
	Pleuritic pain	Pleural friction rub
	Cough	
	Shortness of breath	
Cardiac	Anterior chest pain	New or changing murmur
		Pericardial friction rub
Gastrointestinal	Abdominal pain	Abdominal tenderness
	Nausea, vomiting	Hepatic enlargement, tenderness
	Diarrhea	Jaundice
Genitourinary	Hematuria	Costovertebral angle tenderness
	Dysuria	
	Flank pain	Suprapubic tenderness
	Urethral or vaginal discharge	Urethral discharge
		Tender prostate
		Cervical tenderness
Muscle, bone, joint	Myalgias	Arthritis
	Arthralgias	Focal bone tenderness
Skin		Rash (including petechiae)
		Boils, furuncles, pustules
		Venipuncture marks
Neurological	Severe headache	Meningismus
	Neck pain	Lethargy, delirium
	Seizures	
Lymphoid		Splenomegaly
		Tender, enlarged lymph node(s)

creased numbers of band-forms with an elevated or depressed total white count). If not hospitalized, such patients should be re-evaluated daily by telephone or at an office visit until severe symptoms subside or the cause of fever is determined.

Re-evaluation

Patients with unexplained fever that has lasted 1 week or more after the initial evaluation should be thoroughly re-evaluated. The *history* should be carefully reviewed, including: recent travel (especially to areas of poor sanitation), contact with persons with infectious or febrile illnesses (especially hepatitis or mononucleosis), drug use (including recently prescribed drugs, over-the-counter medications, and illicit drugs), alcohol abuse, homosexual activity, and familial disorders associated with fever or infection. The past medical and surgical history should be thoroughly explored. The review of systems should be repeated to detect any new complaints or subtle complaints missed at the initial evaluation. Trivial symptoms, such as vague abdominal discomfort, may prove of great value in localizing the cause of fever.

The *physical examination* should be meticulously reperformed. As with the history, subtle findings may prove invaluable. Essential procedures sometimes ignored, but which must be included, are funduscopic examination of the eyes (after dilating the pupils, if necessary), examination for a tender or enlarged temporal artery, search for a new or changing heart murmur, detection of enlargement or tenderness of the thyroid gland, search for pericardial, pleural, or hepatic friction rubs, search for hepatomegaly or splenomegaly, detection of subtle abdominal or hepatic tenderness, examination of the rectum and prostate, pelvic examination, thorough search for lymphadenopathy including epitrochlear nodes, and examination of skin and mucus membranes (including conjunctivae) for petechiae, and of nail beds for splinter hemorrhages.

Laboratory studies should also be initiated. A complete blood count, differential white blood cell count, and urinalysis should be performed. Additional studies should include a chest X-ray (PA and lateral views), erythrocyte sedimentation rate, serum alkaline phosphatase, SGOT, SGPT, and a test for occult fecal blood. At least two blood cultures (each cultured aerobically and anaerobically) should be obtained. The urine should be cultured if pyuria or bacteriuria is observed. An intermediate strength purified protein derivative (PPD) skin test should be applied unless there is a documented history of a positive PPD or history of tuberculosis. If there has been travel within 6 months to an area where malaria is endemic, appropriate blood smears should be examined. Any medications started during the previous 2 months should be discontinued or, if that is not possible, replaced by substitutes. This is especially important for those drugs listed in Table 24.2.

Patients should then chart their temperature at least twice daily for another full week. If unexplained fever persists, the history and physical examination should again be reviewed with great care. Additional laboratory studies should include skin tests for cutaneous anergy (if intermediate PPD was negative), an electrocardiogram, serum calcium determination, serum titers of antistreptolysin O, rheumatoid factor and antinuclear antibody, and a monospot test. The complete blood count, differential white blood cell count, and urinalysis should be repeated.

If fever is still unexplained, temperature should be charted again for a full week. Documentation of temperature recordings by an independent observer is important to rule out factitious fever. Patients remaining febrile for at least 3 weeks and lacking a recognized cause or provisional diagnosis despite the evaluations described above should be hospitalized for more extensive studies.

MANAGEMENT OF FEVER

Fever is not usually harmful and antipyretic therapy is not often needed. Moreover, such treatment may confuse the clinical picture by altering the temperature pattern. In certain circumstances, however control of fever is desirable. These include (a) persons with severely compromised cardiac function in whom fever-associated tachycardia further stresses the heart, and (b) persons such as alcoholics or those with senile dementia who develop increasing confusion or delirium when febrile.

Aspirin is usually effective as an antipyretic, but may cause an uncomfortable diaphoresis or actually precipitate shaking chills. These side effects can be minimized by giving the dose of 0.3 to 0.6 g regularly at 3- to 4-hour intervals. Acetaminophen, in similar dosage, may be used in patients allergic to aspirin, in patients with hemorrhagic diatheses, or in patients with a history of gastrointestinal bleeding or with poor tolerance of aspirin.

Antimicrobial drugs have no place in the treatment of patients with acute undifferentiated fever, except in those who appear dangerously ill or who have seriously compromised defenses against infection. The premature use of antibiotics serves only to confuse interpretation of the patient's clinical course, add unnecessary expense, and risk the addition of drug toxicity to the patient's complaints. In most instances, antibiotics should be withheld until a diagnosis for which they are indicated is made.

The daily activities of febrile patients need not be severely restricted, but should be moderated to provide additional rest, light meals, and the avoidance of strenuous or tiring tasks.

General References

Benenson AS (ed): *Control of Communicable Diseases in Man*, ed 13. Washington, DC, American Public Health Association, 1985.
> A concise summary of epidemiological features, management, and prevention of communicable diseases; updated periodically.

Esposito AL, Gleckman RA: A diagnostic approach to the adult with fever of unknown origin. *Arch Intern Med* 139:575, 1979.
> This article includes initial evaluation of patients with acute undifferentiated fever as well as those with true fever of unknown origin.

Larson EB, Featherstone HJ, Petersdorf RG: Fever of undetermined origin: diagnosis and follow-up of 105 cases, 1970–1980. *Medicine* 61:269, 1982.
> A recent follow-up of Petersdorf's original study on fever of unknown origin documenting the changing diagnostic composition of this syndrome.

Lipsky BA, Hirschmann JV: Drug fever. *JAMA* 245:851, 1981.
> A concise review of the problem of drug fever with typical clinical examples and guidelines for management.

Petersdorf RG, Beeson PB: Fever of unexplained origin: report on 100 cases. *Medicine* 40:1, 1961.
> A classic description of true fever of unknown origin.

Vickery DM, Quinnell RK: Fever of unknown origin: an algorithmic approach. *JAMA* 238:2183, 1977.
> A useful example of a systematic approach to evaluation of fever.

CHAPTER TWENTY-FIVE

Bacterial Infections of the Skin

NATHANIEL F. PIERCE, M.D.

INTRODUCTION

Skin infections are extremely common. Although most are trivial and are managed at home without medical assistance, each year about 5% of the population develops skin infections which require medical attention; these are usually caused by *Streptococcus pyogenes* or *Staphylococcus aureus*. The seriousness of these infections depends upon the nature of the infecting organism, especially its array of virulence factors, such as proteolytic enzymes and toxins, and upon the condition of normal host defense mechanisms. Thus, cutaneous infections due to *S. pyogenes* or *S. aureus* in otherwise healthy persons usually cause only modest morbidity and respond rapidly to appropriate treatment. However, the same organisms can cause serious infections in diabetics, in persons with impaired blood supply to, or impaired lymphatic or venous drainage of, the infected site, or in patients with defects in leukocytic or immunological defense mechanisms. Serious infection is also more likely when other bacteria, or combinations of bacteria, are involved such as occurs in bites, or in wounds contaminated with fecal material, animal products, or soil.

This chapter has two aims: first, to aid recognition and guide treatment of those skin infections which can be readily managed on an ambulatory basis, and second, to describe those infections which require more intensive management, either in hospital or by specialists.

SUPERFICIAL INFECTIONS CAUSED PREDOMINANTLY BY *STREPTOCOCCUS PYOGENES*

Impetigo, ecthyma, and erysipelas are due largely to group A β-hemolytic streptococci (*S. pyogenes*), although *S. aureus* may play a causative role in some instances. These infections are all superficial, arising from breaks in the skin which are often so minor that they are unnoticed.

Impetigo

Impetigo occurs mostly among preschool children, especially in warm humid climates and when personal hygiene is poor. Under these conditions, the disease is highly contagious and distinct outbreaks may occur. Older children and adults are only occasionally affected. Although *S. pyogenes* is usually the causative agent, *S. aureus* is often present and sometimes appears to play a pathogenic role.

Impetigo begins as a pruritic, focal, superficial eruption of small 1- to 2-mm vesicles, often on the face near the nares, or on the chin. There is usually no history of preceding trauma. In several days the vesicles change to pustules which break, become crusted, and have an erythematous base. Regional lymphadenopathy is common, but there are no constitutional symptoms. The process may spread due to scratching, or remain localized. Healing occurs without scarring. Streptococcal impetigo may recur if personal hygiene is not improved.

A bullous form of impetigo is caused by S. aureus. It can cause epidemics among newborns, but occurs only sporadically among children; adult cases are uncommon. The process begins as a macular erythematous rash. The characteristic thin-walled, fluid-filled, superficial bullae appear within 1 to 3 days, range from 1 to several centimeters in diameter, and usually involve exposed areas of the body. These rupture, desquamation occurs, and healing without scarring follows in about 7 days. In its most dramatic form, this process causes the "scalded skin" syndrome, a disease of small children in which there is extensive superficial desquamation.

Ecthyma

Ecthyma occurs under the same conditions of poor hygiene that promote streptococcal impetigo. It is characterized by discrete ulcerating lesions (3 to 10 mm diameter) with an adherent necrotic crust and surrounding erythema; a small amount of pus often underlies the crust. The ulcer is sufficiently deep to cause permanent scarring. Lesions are most common on the anterior tibial surface at sites of minor trauma or insect bites. Untreated, the lesions tend to spread distally and there may be associated lymphadenopathy; systemic symptoms, however, are lacking. Cultures of pus may yield both S. pyogenes and S. aureus, but the former appear to play the major pathogenic role.

Erysipelas

Erysipelas involves progressive, often rapid, spread of infection through superficial layers of skin and lymphatics. It may occur after a minor wound in normal skin, but is more likely when prior injury or disease has impaired the lymphatic or venous drainage of the skin or left extensive scarring, as for example in a patient with chronic venous insufficiency of the lower extremities or with a radical mastectomy.

The infection is characterized by a rapidly spreading area of marked erythema with warmth, local pain, an elevated sharp margin between involved and uninvolved skin, and firm edema which gives the skin a typical "orange peel" appearance. Fluctuation and dermal necrosis are lacking, although there may be seropurulent drainage at the inoculation site. Erythema frequently extends centrally along superficial draining lymphatics; regional lymph nodes are often enlarged and tender. Systemic toxicity, chills, and fever are common. If untreated, metastatic infection may occur, and there is appreciable mortality. Facial infections are dangerous because of possible intracranial spread via draining lymphatics or veins. Extensive involvement of the trunk causes increased morbidity and a risk of mortality.

Almost all episodes of erysipelas are due to S.

pyogenes, although a very few are due to S. aureus and these cannot always be distinguished clinically. Infections resembling erysipelas may also be caused by Pasteurella multocida or Erysipelothrix rhusiopathiae (see Table 25.4).

Management

Bacterial cultures of the lesions of impetigo, bullous impetigo, and ecthyma are not usually helpful. Impetigo and ecthyma may reveal mixed cultures of S. pyogenes and S. aureus, whereas lesions of bullous impetigo are frequently sterile. Similarly, cultures of early and mild erysipelas are unnecessary. In contrast, blood cultures should be obtained when erysipelas is extensive or associated with marked systemic toxicity (e.g., temperature greater than 102°F (39°C), shaking chills, severe malaise. Should there be seropurulent drainage at the site of inoculation, this should be cultured as well. Placing the culture swab in a transport medium, such as Carey-Blair medium, preserves the specimen until it reaches the diagnostic laboratory. Attempts to isolate the organism by culturing sterile saline injected and withdrawn at the edge of the lesion are usually unsuccessful.

Systemic antibiotic therapy is required for all streptococcal and related skin infections (Table 25.1 and 25.2). In general, an oral penicillin is adequate except in persons with disease likely to be due to S. aureus (e.g., bullous impetigo), with extensive infection associated with systemic toxicity, or with suspected penicillin allergy. Erythromycin is an ac-

Table 25.1.
Antibiotic Selection for Skin Infections Due to _Streptococcus pyogenes_ or _Staphylococcus aureus_

Infection	Antibiotic[a]	
STREPTOCOCCAL INFECTIONS		
Impetigo	Benzathine pencillin	(i.m.)
	Penicillin V	(oral)
	Erythromycin	(oral)
Ecthyma	As for impetigo	
Erysipelas—mild	Penicillin V	(oral)
	Erythromycin	(oral)
Erysipelas—severe	Penicillin G	(i.m. or i.v.)
STAPHYLOCOCCAL INFECTIONS		
Folliculitis	None	
Furunculosis, boils	Dicloxacillin	(oral)
	Erythromycin	(oral)
Bullous impetigo	As for furunculosis	
Carbuncle	Dicloxacillin	(oral)
	Nafcillin	(i.v.)
	Vancomycin	(i.v.)
Cellulitis	As for carbuncle	

[a] A single antibiotic is given. Choices are in order of preference and include an alternate choice for patients allergic to penicillin. See the text for duration of therapy and adjunctive treatment. Dosage recommendations are in Table 25.2.

Table 25.2.
Antibiotic Dosage and Schedule for Skin Infections Due to *Streptococcus pyogenes* and *Staphylococcus aureus* in Adults[a]

Antibiotic	Dosage
AMBULATORY TREATMENT: MILD INFECTION	
Benzathine penicillin	1,200,000 units i.m., once
Penicillin V	500 mg p.o. 3 times/day
Erythromycin	250–500 mg p.o. 3 times/day
Dicloxacillin	250 mg p.o. 3 times/day
PARENTERAL TREATMENT: SEVERE INFECTION	
Penicillin G	600,000–2,000,000 units i.v. every 6 hours
Nafcillin	1.0–1.5 g i.v. every 4 hours
Vancomycin	0.25–0.5 g i.v. every 6 hours

[a] Choice of antibiotics for specific infections is described in the text and summarized in Table 25.1. The duration of therapy is described in the text.

ceptable substitute in patients who can not receive penicillin. Tetracycline should not be substituted as many strains of *S. pyogenes* are resistant to it. To eradicate group A streptococci, antibiotic treatment should routinely be given for 10 days, even though marked improvement may occur earlier.

Streptococcal impetigo and ecthyma are treated similarly. Penicillin V given orally is adequate. A single parenteral injection of benzathine penicillin is also effective and assures adequate duration of therapy. Oral erythromycin is a satisfactory alternative. Adjunctive therapy includes careful daily soaking of lesions to remove crusted debris using warm water with an iodophor (a *soap* which releases iodine in a nontoxic, nonstaining form, e.g., Betadine skin cleanser) or with a soap which contains hexachlorophene (e.g., pHisoHex). Topically applied antibiotics are of little value and should not be used. Prevention depends primarily upon improved personal hygiene; the most important preventive measure is careful frequent skin cleansing with soap and water.

Treatment of *bullous impetigo* is directed at penicillin-resistant staphylococci. The same treatment should be used for the small portion of patients with impetigo that does not respond to treatment with penicillin V; in such patients *S. aureus* appears to play a pathogenic role and antistaphylococcal therapy is usually effective. Oral dicloxacillin is suitable, with erythromycin as an effective alternative.

Minor episodes of *erysipelas* may be treated with oral penicillin V or erythromycin. Careful local application of moist heat to the affected area appears to hasten clearing of the infection. Serious episodes are those with marked systemic toxicity, extensive lesions, facial lesions, or those occurring in compromised hosts, e.g., diabetics. Such patients usually require hospitalization and more intensive antibiotic treatment (Tables 25.1 and 25.2). Special attention should also be paid to patients with atherosclerotic peripheral vascular disease who have infections of their lower extremities. In such patients, the affected leg should be rested and elevated; sustained pressure on any part of the leg or foot should be avoided.

Persons with pre-existing damage to the veins or lymphatics of an extremity may experience repeated episodes of erysipelas which cause further damage. Patients who have numerous recurrent infections should receive continuous antibiotic prophylaxis with penicillin V (250 mg twice daily), benzathine penicillin (600,000 units intramuscularly monthly), or erythromycin (250 mg twice daily). Reduction of chronic edema by fitted pressure stockings or by diuretics helps to reduce susceptibility to this infection.

Superficial skin infections respond rapidly to appropriate therapy. Systemic toxicity and erythema associated with erysipelas usually abate within 3 or 4 days, and discrete skin lesions show marked healing within 10 days. During this period, activity should be restricted in accord with the extent of morbidity. Minor lesions require no restrictions. Persons with any form of impetigo should avoid contact with infants and small children until lesions heal.

Complications

Group A streptococcal skin infections do not cause rheumatic fever but may cause acute glomerulonephritis, if the streptococcal strain is nephritogenic. Nephritis is not prevented by antibiotic therapy. The average latency period between initial symptoms of a streptococcal skin infection and the onset of glomerulonephritis is 2 weeks. Therefore, if a nephritogenic strain is known to be present in the community, initial and 14-day follow-up evaluation should include a urinalysis. The majority of patients who develop post-streptococcal glomerulonephritis are asymptomatic; but in some, glomerulonephritis will first be suggested by gross hematuria, acute hypertension, or signs of salt and water retention, such as dependent edema or congestive heart failure.

Bacteremia with metastatic infection may complicate neglected or severe episodes of erysipelas. Metastatic infection should be considered in patients with severe disease who respond poorly to treatment or develop findings suggestive of distant localized infection. Possible metastatic infections include meningitis, endocarditis, septic arthritis, infection of pre-existing pleural effusions or ascites, or solid organ abscesses, e.g., in the liver or spleen.

PUSTULAR INFECTIONS CAUSED BY *STAPHYLOCOCCUS AUREUS*

These infections include folliculitis, furunculosis, hydradenitis suppurativa, and carbuncles. They represent increasingly severe effects of the infection of hair follicles, sebaceous glands, or sweat glands by *S. aureus*, the end result being inflammation and abscess formation.

Folliculitis

Folliculitis involves minor inflammation of individual hair follicles, often with formation of small superficial pustules. There is little pain or surrounding erythema. In some persons, lesions may recur for months or even years. A common area of involvement is the bearded part of the face in which minor trauma from shaving may be a contributing factor.

Furunculosis

Deeper infection of follicles or cutaneous glands leads to formation of pustular furuncles (boils are large furuncles). These lesions range in diameter from about 5 mm to 2 to 3 cm and occur most commonly on hairy areas exposed to friction, trauma, or maceration, e.g., the buttocks, neck, face, axillae, groin, forearms, thighs, and upper back. Furunculosis may also complicate the acne of adolescence. Furuncles begin with pruritus, local tenderness, and erythema, followed by swelling and marked local pain. As pus forms in the center of the lesion, the overlying skin becomes thin, the lesion becomes elevated, pain increases, and spontaneous drainage of pus ultimately occurs, usually with prompt relief of pain and rapid healing. Furunculosis may be a recurrent problem in some persons, especially diabetics and persons who are chronic nasal carriers of *S. aureus*.

Hydradenitis Suppurativa

This is a particular form of furunculosis due to obstruction of apocrine sweat glands, usually in the axilla, perineum, or groin. The process is chronic, perpetuated in part by the scars, abscesses, and sinus tracts which develop in the involved skin.

Carbuncles

A carbuncle is a coalescent mass of deeply infected follicles or sebaceous glands with multiple interconnecting sinus tracts and cutaneous openings that drain pus ineffectively. Carbuncles usually occur in the thick skin on the back of the neck or the upper back. Once formed, the lesions steadily worsen, with increasing pain, erythema, swelling, purulent drainage, and lateral enlargement; they vary in diameter from 3 to 10 cm or larger. Fever and systemic toxicity are common. Carbuncles occur with increased frequency in diabetics. Once established, they may recur in the damaged area of skin.

Management

Bacterial cultures of typical lesions are usually unnecessary since virtually all are caused by *S. aureus* and most isolates will prove resistant to penicillin G.

Minimal lesions, such as *folliculitis*, require little therapy. Careful, twice daily cleansing with a mild soap, preferably one containing hexachlorophene, and avoidance of minor trauma and irritants, such as cosmetics or abrasive soaps, are usually sufficient.

Furuncles should be managed initially by application of warm moist heat (either as moist compresses or baths) for about 30 minutes four times a day. Small lesions, i.e., those less than 1 cm in diameter, will often drain spontaneously after 1 to 3 days and require no further treatment. Larger lesions, painful lesions, or lesions that do not drain spontaneously should be drained surgically when they feel fluctuant or contain visible pus. This can be done in the office by making a single incision into the abscess with a scalpel, after the skin has been anesthetized with a topical spray such as ethyl chloride. Antimicrobial therapy is not required except for more extensive lesions such as multiple furuncles, carbuncles, or lesions associated with marked surrounding inflammation. In such cases oral dicloxacillin or erythromycin (Tables 25.1 and 25.2) should be given until signs of inflammation completely subside, which may take 2 weeks or longer. *Carbuncles* may require extensive surgical drainage, which is best done in a hospital. Patients with severe systemic toxicity, such as diabetics with carbuncles, require parenteral therapy with a penicillinase-resistant penicillin; vancomycin is an effective alternative for those allergic to penicillin.

Recurrent furunculosis may prove a frustrating problem. Management of individual episodes is as described above, but other steps should also be taken. The anterior nares should be cultured to determine whether they are the likely source of the reinfecting staphylococci. Patients with positive nasal cultures should be treated by application of bacitracin ointment to the anterior nares three or four times daily for 14 days. Prolonged therapy with bacitracin ointment may be needed if cultures become positive upon cessation of treatment. Bacterial contamination of skin should be meticulously controlled by having the patient bathe and shampoo three times daily with hexachlorophene soaps, and by daily changes of bed and bath linens.

Recurrent furunculosis may occur in certain disorders which impair host defenses. Tests for diabetes mellitus should be made; if positive, strict control of blood glucose may prove beneficial (see Chapter 72). Defects in polymorphonuclear leukocyte function are a rare cause of recurrent furunculosis, but should be considered in patients who show an increased incidence or severity of infections due to staphylococci, Gram-negative bacteria, and fungi (referred to a medical center where there is special expertise with such problems would then be indicated).

Hydradenitis suppurativa is an extremely difficult problem that requires prolonged, often lifelong, treatment by multiple methods. These include selective surgical drainage of abscesses; elimination of irritants, such as tight clothing, antiperspirants, and shaving of the axillae; careful frequent cleansing of skin with antiseptic agents; local application of heat; intermittent or chronic systemic antibiotic therapy; and in some cases local irradiation or excisional surgery. Management of such patients is best done by physicians especially skilled in the treatment of skin disorders. (See additional discussion in Chapter 100, Common Problems of the Skin.)

Complications

Staphylococcal skin infections may disseminate to other sites. This is especially true in patients with extensive inflammation and systemic toxicity, such as those with carbuncles, in whom bacteremia is common. However, even an innocent appearing furuncle may cause metastatic infection, especially in patients with a focus of increased susceptibility, such as a ventricular septal defect, valvular heart disease, or an arthritic joint. Patients with demonstrated bacteremia who have such pre-existing susceptible foci, or whose systemic complaints (fever, focal pain) persist despite antibiotic treatment, should be carefully examined for metastatic infection.

CELLULITIS AND OTHER WOUND INFECTIONS

Any break in the skin may become infected. This includes not only obvious trauma, such as lacerations, burns, abrasions, and animal or human bites, but also minor defects such as scratches and insect bites. The features of the resultant infection vary widely; they depend upon the nature of the wound, the type of infecting organism(s), and the defensive responses of the infected person. In many instances, early appropriate management given on an ambulatory basis is sufficient. In others, recognition of serious infection and prompt hospitalization for vigorous medical and/or surgical treatment are of prime importance. Table 25.3 describes findings which require hospitalization and/or surgical intervention. Table 25.4 lists organisms which may cause life-threatening forms of cellulitis.

Cellulitis Due to S. *Pyogenes* and S. *Aureus*

Acute cellulitis is a spreading infection of skin and subcutaneous tissues. The involved area, which enlarges steadily, is painful, tender, and intensely erythematous. Chills and fever are common and bacteremia may occur. The lesion differs from erysipelas in that its margin is not as sharply demarcated

Table 25.3.
Wound Infections: Findings That Necessitate Hospitalization and/or Surgical Intervention

Finding	Comment
Extensive cellulitis or erysipelas with systemic toxicity	Needs parenteral antibiotics, close observation
Diminished arterial pulse in cool, swollen, pale, infected extremity	Possible fasciitis, a surgical emergency
Cellulitis with cutaneous necrosis and/or subcutaneous gas	Needs parenteral antibiotics and possible surgical drainage/debridement
Closed space infections of the hand	Needs surgical drainage

Table 25.4.
Causes of Life-Threatening Bacterial Cellulitis

Cause	Important Features
Gram-negative enteric bacilli, especially *Escherichia coli*	Occur in fecally contaminated wounds; gas may be present; surgical drainage required for gas or pus
Mixed anaerobic and enteric aerobic bacteria	Occur in fecally contaminated wounds; gas may be present; symptoms may progress rapidly and may include exquisite pain; surgical drainage required
Bacillus anthracis	Causes anthrax when minor wound is inoculated by spore-contaminated animal products (animal hides and hair, especially from goats); local chancre-like lesion develops followed by systemic toxicity
Erysipelothrix rhusiopathiae	Erysipelas-like lesion with central clearing; due to wound contamination with fish or meat products; treated with penicillin V or tetracycline
Pasteurella multocida	Erysipelas-like lesion which follows a dog or cat scratch or bite; treated with penicillin V or tetracycline
Marine vibrios	Necrotizing cellulitis after minor wound is contaminated by sea water or contact with shellfish
Aeromonas hydrophilia	Wound contaminated by fresh water swimming

nor is it elevated. There may be purulent or serous drainage at the inoculation site; in severe cases, patches of involved skin may become necrotic.

The most common causes of acute cellulitis are S. *pyogenes* and S. *aureus*. Presence of Gram-positive cocci in drainage from the wound is presumptive evidence that they are causative. Infection due to these agents may progress rapidly, especially when it involves an area of chronic edema. Lower extremity infection in persons with peripheral arterial insufficiency may precipitate tissue necrosis and secondary infection.

Management of cellulitis should include culture of any wound drainage (as described for erysipelas) and prompt antibiotic therapy. In mild cases, treatment may be given on an ambulatory basis. The treatment selected should be effective for infections due to penicillin-resistant staphylococci, as well as penicillin-sensitive streptococci. Oral dicloxacillin is adequate for infections due to either type of organism; erythromycin is a suitable choice for patients allergic to penicillin and for those who cannot afford the rather high cost of dicloxacillin (Tables 25.1 and 25.2). Local application of moist heat is a useful adjunct to antibiotic treatment; care should be taken, however, to avoid burns, especially in persons with impaired sensitivity to pain. Improvement is usually apparent in 3 or 4 days; during this period, patients should rest the involved area (with elevation when the cellulitis involves an extremity) and be told to report promptly any worsening of the infection or of constitutional symptoms. Severe infections require hospitalization and parenteral treatment with a penicillinase-resistant penicillin or vancomycin. This includes patients with extensive lesions, lesions of the face, or serious toxicity.

Secondarily Infected Ulcers

Cutaneous ulcers are caused by a wide variety of conditions including peripheral vascular disease, arterial insufficiency, pressure sores, neurological disorders, *etc.* Management of the ulcer is generally aimed at the underlying cause and seeks to improve blood flow, reduce edema, and avoid pressure and trauma (see Chapter 88). Control of secondary infection is also of considerable importance. Superficial colonization with a variety of bacteria is unavoidable and without consequence; however, infection which is deeper or laterally invasive prevents healing and may interfere with other treatments, such as skin grafting. Infection is best controlled by repeated careful cleaning and local debridement. Systemic antibiotics should be used only when all other methods fail to control surrounding infection. The choice of antibiotic should be based on cultures of the wound or its purulent drainage. Local antibacterials are sometimes helpful. Those effective against a broad spectrum of bacterial agents include polymyxin-bacitracin-neomycin ointment and topical furacin; these should be applied three times daily until healing occurs or until it is apparent they are ineffective. Soaking with 3% acetic acid three to four times daily is helpful in controlling bacterial growth in ulcers colonized with *Pseudomonas aeruginosa.*

Cutaneous Diphtheria

Cutaneous ulcers or other skin lesions may become secondarily infected with *Corynebacterium diphtheriae*, causing cutaneous diphtheria. Although the cutaneous lesion may appear benign, myocarditis or neuropathy develops in about 3% of cases. Outbreaks have occurred in the northwest and southwest parts of the United States, primarily among Native Americans or urban indigents. The presence of cutaneous diphtheria in a community should increase suspicion that skin wounds may harbor this agent. The diagnosis should be suspected when existing wounds develop a gray-yellow or gray-brown covering membrane and surrounding erythema (1). Typically, the membrane can be easily removed to reveal a clean base. Other minor skin lesions may also become infected. Typical organisms can be seen in methylene blue stains of smears from the wound and confirmed by culture on Loeffler's or tellurite agar. Presumptive cases should be reported to public health officials and treated with equine diphtheria antitoxin (20,000 to 40,000 units intramuscularly or intravenously after testing for hypersensitivity to horse serum) and either erythromycin (1.5 g/day, orally) or procaine penicillin (1.2 million units/day, intramuscularly) for 7 to 10 days.

Bites

Bite wounds become infected with the oral, salivary, or dental flora of the biting person or animal and may cause serious local or systemic infections. Initial management before signs of infection appear is of primary importance in preventing certain infections. Appropriate prophylaxis for tetanus is required for all bite wounds (see Chapter 32).

Human bites are contaminated with a complex variety of aerobic and anaerobic oral bacteria. Without treatment, a severe necrotizing cellulitis frequently results. Minor lesions that break the skin should be washed thoroughly and treated with a combination of dicloxacillin (250 mg three times/day) and ampicillin (500 mg three times/day) given orally; oral clindamycin (150 to 300 mg three times/day) is appropriate for patients allergic to penicillin. Antibiotics should be continued for 7 to 10 days. More severe wounds, including wounds of the hands and knuckles, require meticulous debridement and possible tendon repairs. These shoud be referred for surgical management.

Dog bites carry the risk of local soft tissue infection and raise concern about rabies. Minor abrasions, shallow punctures, or superficial lacerations require no therapy for local infection other than thorough cleansing with soap and water. More extensive or deeper bites require surgical management for debridement and, in some cases, primary closure; ampicillin (500 mg by mouth three times/day for 7 days) should also be given. Rabies precautions should be taken with all dog bites, no matter how minor, including bites by domestic pets, even though the risk of rabies among them is very small. The dog should be quarantined for 10 days; if it is a pet, it may be observed at its home. If it remains well, there is no risk of rabies. If the dog develops suspicious symptoms or dies, its brain should be examined immediately; prophylaxis is required if evidence of rabies is found. If the dog escapes after biting, and especially if the bite was unprovoked, rabies prophylaxis with rabies immune globulin and human diploid cell rabies vaccine is usually indicated (see Chapter 32).

Bites by *other domestic animals*, e.g., cats, should be managed in the same way as dog bites are managed. Bites by *wild animals* carry a greater risk of rabies and are treated similarly, except that rabies prophylaxis is usually required (unless the animal's brain can be examined). Wild animals with the greatest risk of carrying rabies include raccoons, skunks, foxes, coyotes, and bats.

Guidance on the use of rabies prophylaxis, management of the biting animal, and the risk of rabies among various animal species should be sought from local or state health authorities.

Puncture Wounds

Most puncture wounds involve the feet or hands and carry the risk of introduction of infecting bacteria which cannot be removed by washing or debridement. In all instances, patients should receive appropriate prophylaxis for tetanus (see Chapter 32). Low risk wounds, i.e., those not likely to be contaminated by soil or fecal material and in which the wound site is healthy, well vascularized tissue, need only be thoroughly washed and observed for several days for signs of developing infection. Should infection develop, any wound drainage should be cultured and treatment begun with dicloxacillin (250 mg, three times daily) or erythromycin (250 to 500 mg three times daily) for presumptive staphylococcal or streptococcal infection; the wound site should also be soaked in warm soapy water for 30 minutes at least four times a day. Higher risk wounds, i.e., those likely to be contaminated with fecal material, soil, or foreign debris, or occurring in a diabetic or in an extremity with an inadequate blood supply, should be treated with one of the above antibiotics from the outset, and the wound site should be rested and treated with warm soaks as above. The patient should promptly report any evidence of inflammation, swelling, or persisting pain. If purulent drainage develops, this should be cultured. Antibiotic management may need to be altered if Gram-negative bacilli are isolated. If pus develops, surgical drainage is probably required.

Felon

A felon is an infection of the pulp of the distal phalanx of a finger; it usually follows a recognized local wound. Abscess formation and tissue necrosis are common, and bony or articular involvement may occur. If neglected or inadequately treated, severe damage, including loss of function, may occur. The most common causative agents are S. aureus and S. pyogenes, although Gram-negative bacilli may occasionally be recovered. Treatment involves surgical drainage, and this should be done by an experienced surgeon. Concurrent antibiotic therapy should be guided by Gram stain and culture of infected material.

Paronychia

A paronychia is an infection, often chronic or recurrent, which involves tissue immediately adjacent to a fingernail. The affected tissue is warm, tensely swollen, erythematous, and painful. When infection is chronic, the nail may become ridged or discolored and may be lost. Paronychia occur most frequently in persons who bite their nails excessively and in persons whose hands are frequently in water, for example, in mothers of infants or in dishwashers. Diabetics also have an increased risk of this infection. *Candida* species appear to play an etiological role, although a variety of bacteria are also usually present. Management involves keeping hands as dry as possible (e.g., using waterproof gloves for dishwashing) and applying amphotericin B ointment or cream (Fungizone) two to four times a day for several weeks. When localized swelling does not respond to these measures, surgical drainage may be helpful.

Erythrasma

Erythrasma is a superficial infection of moist intertriginous areas (toe webs, axilla, genitocrural area), probably due to *Corynebacterium minitissimum*. Adolescents, diabetics, and persons living in hot, humid climates are most often affected. The management of erythrasma is discussed in Chapter 100.

General References

Koblenzer PJ: Common bacterial infections of the skin in children. *Pediatr Clin North Am* 25:321, 1978.

A useful review of the subject with excellent pictures of typical lesions.

Musher DM, McKenzie SO: Infections due to *Staphylococcus aureus*. *Medicine* 56:383, 1977.

Review article with a section on staphylococcal skin infections, including those which resemble erysipelas.

Peter G, Smith AL: Group A streptococcal infections of the skin and pharynx. *N Engl J Med* 297:311, 1977.

An excellent, thorough review of basic and clinical features of streptococcal skin infections.

Wannamaker LW: Differences between streptococcal infections of the throat and of the skin. *N Engl J Med* 282:23, 1970.

A scholarly discussion by an expert on the subject.

Witkowski JA, Parish LL: Bacterial skin infections. Management of common streptococcal and staphylococcal lesions. *Postgrad Med* 72:166, 1982.

A practical review of the features and treatment of these infections with excellent photographs of typical infections.

Specific Reference

1. Belsey MA, Sinclair M, Roder MR, LeBlanc DR: *Corynebacterium diphtheriae* skin infections in Alabama and Louisiana: a factor in the epidemiology of diphtheria. *N Engl J Med* 280:135, 1969.

CHAPTER TWENTY-SIX

Acute Gastroenteritis and Associated Conditions

R. BRADLEY SACK, M.D., AND L. RANDOL BARKER, M.D.

INTRODUCTION

Acute symptoms of gastroenteritis may follow the ingestion of a wide variety of infectious and chemical agents. Ingestion may occur because of direct person-to-person contact or, more commonly, *via* food or water. With several important exceptions, the acute illnesses caused by these agents are characterized by diarrhea, with or without other gastrointestinal symptoms (nausea, vomiting, abdominal pain) or systemic symptoms (anorexia, fever, malaise, orthostatic hypotension, neurological symptoms).

Diarrhea is defined as an increase in frequency and/or amount of fecal evacuations, which are usually fluid (see Chapter 38). The diarrhea of gastroenteritis usually begins abruptly, sometimes preceded by systemic symptoms, and the hour of onset can usually be documented by the patient. With few exceptions, the illness is self-limited and will terminate within 1 to 5 days.

Table 26.1 (infectious agents) and Table 26.2 (chemical agents) summarize the etiological agents, pathophysiology, clinical and epidemiological features, principles of treatment for those conditions which may occur in the United States.

EPIDEMIOLOGY

The *incidence* of the conditions listed in Tables 26.1 and 26.2 varies from year to year; and the true incidence is never known since a large proportion of cases are not reported to physicians or health authorities. Even when outbreaks of gastroenteritis involving multiple persons are fully investigated, the *etiology* can be established with relative certainty only 50 to 75% of the time. Based upon annual surveillance by the United States Centers for Disease Control (CDC), it is known that the majority of reported outbreaks (and therefore probably the majority of cases) are due to *Staphylococcus aureus*, followed by *Salmonella* species, and *Clostridium perfringens*. Physicians and patients frequently call an illness "viral gastroenteritis," although viral agents probably account for only a modest proportion of acute gastrointestinal illness in adults (14, 23). Studies of outbreaks of viral gastroenteritis in adults have shown that the symptoms it produces overlap with the symptoms produced by several common bacterial pathogens (see Table 26.3). A viral etiology is more likely when secondary cases develop in a household, a pattern which suggests person-to-person spread rather than one-time exposure to a common food.

The *sources and modes of transmission* of the etiological agents causing foodborne illness are summarized in Tables 26.1 and 26.2. These features of the three most common etiological agents illustrate the diverse ways that foodborne disease is acquired (7):

1. Humans whose skin or nasal mucosa is colonized are almost always the source of *Staphylococcus aureus*. Contamination of food with small numbers of staphylococci is undoubtedly very common. Staphylococcal food poisoning occurs when contaminated foods are allowed to stand long enough for organisms to multiply and produce enterotoxin. The principal foods in which this occurs are those high in protein (ham, pork, beef, poultry, either cooked or in salads, and cream-filled cakes and pastries) and those with a relatively high salt or sugar content (ham, salads, and custards).

2. Animals are the source of the *Salmonella* serotypes causing most human disease; only *Salmonella*

typhi and *Salmonella paratyphi* are carried by humans. Transmission from animal to man occurs chiefly by fecal contamination of equipment and personnel involved in the packaging and preparing of foods—most commonly poultry, red meats, and eggs or their by-products.

3. *Clostridium perfringens* is a ubiquitous organism found in human and animal feces and in soil. Meats are the most frequently contaminated foods; transmission of enough organisms to produce illness occurs typically with inadequately heated or reheated meats (spores may survive at normal cooking temperatures and then germinate and multiply while foods are being held at warm temperatures or being rewarmed at temperatures that do not inhibit bacterial growth).

The vast majority of episodes of foodborne illness follow the ingestion of *normally safe foods* which have been rendered unsafe owing to one or more of the following factors (6): failure to refrigerate foods properly or to heat foods thoroughly, preparing foods a day or more before they are served, allowing foods to remain at warm temperatures, failure to reheat or cook foods at temperature that kill vegetative bacteria, incorporating raw (contaminated) ingredients into foods that receive no further cooking, failure to clean and disinfect kitchen or processing plant equipment, and contamination by infected food handlers who practice poor personal hygiene.

A small minority of foodborne illnesses is due to the ingestion of *foods which are always unsafe* owing to the presence of toxins which cannot be rendered innocuous by cooking or other means, i.e., ciguatoxin, scombratoxin, amanita toxins, paralytic shellfish toxin, mushroom toxin, and heavy metals (11, 13).

The *place of ingestion* of the etiological agent is usually the patient's home or a restaurant, and, less commonly, a social gathering or an institutional eating place.

For many of the conditions listed in Tables 26.1 and 26.2, *individuals are at risk at all ages*, and a single episode may not confer protective immunity against a later episode. However, the vast majority of acute diarrheal episodes occur in childen. A particularly high rate of diarrheal illness occurs in people of all ages who travel to developing countries (see Chapter 33).

In the past decade, a wide spectrum of intestinal infections (the *gay bowel syndromes*) has been recognized in homosexual and bisexual men. Several factors favor the acquisition and spread of enteric infections in this population: (a) oral-genital and genital-anal contact between subjects; (b) exposure to multiple sexual partners; and (c) asymptomatic carriage of enteric pathogens, often more than one. The pathogens transmitted to the gastrointestinal tract by homosexual men include common and un-

common enteric pathogens and also a number of genital pathogens (Table 26.4). The syndromes produced by these infections range from oral ulcerations to gastroenteritis to proctitis. Homosexual individuals with one infectious gastrointestinal syndrome often have multiple infections.

PATHOGENESIS

As indicated in Tables 26.1 and 26.2, the majority of the etiological agents produce symptoms due either to inflammation of the gastrointestinal tract or to physiological events related to one or more toxins.

In recent years, the common bacterial diarrheal syndromes have been separated into invasive and enterotoxigenic syndromes (see Table 26.5) (18, 20), an important advance because of the implications for antibiotic treatment. In *invasive disease*, the etiological agent enters the intestinal mucosal cells, often destroying them, and the diarrhea is a result of this destructive process with its accompanying inflammatory response. This usually occurs in the large bowel and produces systemic symptoms (particularly fever), local symptoms (tenesmus, abdominal discomfort), and frequent small amounts of stool which contain pus cells and often blood. Shigellosis is the prototype of this syndrome (15). In *enterotoxigenic diarrhea*, the organisms do not invade tissue, but colonize and multiply on the small bowel mucosal surface; during this process they produce enterotoxins which act as chemical mediators and cause hypersecretion of fluid and electrolytes by the small bowel. Little tissue damage is produced, and inflammation of the mucosa is minimal. Symptoms consist of simple watery diarrhea (which may be voluminous), accompanied by minimal systemic signs, unless dehydration becomes significant. The prototypes of this syndrome are diarrheas caused by *Vibrio cholerae* and by enterotoxigenic *Escherichia coli* (17, 22).

More recently, strains of *E. coli* have been characterized that neither invade mucosal cells nor produce enterotoxins, but rather only tightly adhere to the mucosal surface, and produce diarrhea presumably by interfering with normal absorptive processes. These strains seem to produce diarrhea primarily in small children, and many belong to the classical "enteropathogenic" serotypes (9).

PATIENT EVALUATION

Historical Information

In addition to a history of the specific symptoms the most useful information will be:

1. A history of *food eaten* within the past 48 hours, particularly noting any deviation from the patient's usual pattern, such as eating an unusual food (e.g.,

Table 26.1.
Characteristics of Acute Illness Due to Ingestion of Infectious Agents

Agent	Pathogenesis	Usual Clinical Features	Epidemiological Features					Diagnosis	Specific Therapy
			Frequency in USA	Usual pattern[a]	Source (reservoir)	Transmission to Man	Incubation Period		
BACTERIA									
Bacillus cereus	Enterotoxin produced in food or in intestine	Vomiting if preformed toxin in food, diarrhea	Not common	CSO	Soil	Foodborne	2–16 hr	Culture suspected food	None
Campylobacter jejuni	Invasion of large and small intestine	Fever, abdominal pain, diarrhea	Relatively common	S or CSO	Animal feces	Foodborne or water-borne[b]	? (probably 24–48 hr)	Culture stool, blood	Erythromycin (see text)
Clostridium botulinum	Neurotoxin produced in food	Vomiting, diarrhea, symmetric motor paralysis: cranial nerves, respiratory paralysis, death	Uncommon	CSO	Animal feces, soil	Foodborne (canned, low pH, anaerobic)	12–36 hr	Culture food, identify toxin in food, blood, stool	Polyvalent antitoxin
Clostridium difficile	Cytotoxic enterotoxin produced in large intestine secondary to overgrowth	Fever, abdominal pain, diarrhea (often bloody) in a patient currently or recently on antibiotics	Uncommon	S	Humans (normal intestinal flora)	Probably not necessary but may occur[b]	After several days of antibiotics	Culture stool, identify enterotoxin in stool	Vancomycin (see text)
Clostridium perfringens	Enterotoxin released during sporulation in large intestine	Diarrhea, occasionally vomiting	Relatively common	CSO	Human feces, animal feces, soil	Foodborne (meats)	12–24 hr	Culture suspected food	None
Escherichia coli Enterotoxigenic	Enterotoxin produced in small intestine	Voluminous watery diarrhea without fever (traveler's diarrhea)	Relatively common (travelers)	CSO, S	Human feces	Foodborne	24–48 hr	Culture stool, identify enterotoxin production by bacteria	None
Invasive	Invasion of large intestinal mucosa	Fever, diarrhea (often bloody)	Rare	CSO, S	Human feces	Foodborne (cheeses)	24–48 hr	Culture stool	Same as Shigella (see text)
Adherent	Adheres tightly to small bowel mucosa	Diarrhea, which may be prolonged	Unknown, probably uncommon	S	Human feces	Probably foodborne	?(probably 24–48 hrs)	Culture stool, small bowel	Antibiotics to which organism is sensitive
Salmonella (many species)	Invasion of small and large intestine	Fever and diarrhea (see Table 26.3)	Relatively common	CSO	Animal feces	Foodborne (many foods, see text) person-to-person[b]	12–48 hr	Culture stool	Selected cases only (see text)
Salmonella typhi	Invasion of small intestine mucosa, systemic dissemination	Protracted illness: fever, malaise, headache, constipation more often than diarrhea, splenomegaly, occasionally intestinal perforation	Uncommon	S	Human feces	Person-to-person, food-borne[b]	4 days–3 weeks	Culture blood, stool, antibacterial antibodies	Chloramphenicol
Shigella species	Invasion of large intestine	Fever, diarrhea (often bloody) (see Table 26.3)	Relatively common	S	Human feces	Person-to-person[b]	12–48 hr	Culture stool	Ampicillin (see text)
Staphylococcus	Enterotoxin pro-	Vomiting dominates,	Very com-	CSO	Human skin,	Foodborne	2–8 hr	Culture food, and	None

Organism	Mechanism	Clinical syndrome	Epidemiology (by this mode of transmission)	CSO, S	Source	Mode of transmission	Incubation period	Diagnosis	Treatment
group A	respiratory tract	...gitis syndrome (see Chapter 28)			skin lesions			...sions of food handlers	
Vibrio cholerae	Enterotoxin produced in small intestine	Voluminous watery diarrhea without fever	Rare	CSO, S	Human feces	Waterborne and food borne	12 hr–5 days	Culture stool, antibacterial and antitoxic antibody	Tetracycline
Vibrio parahaemolyticus	Probably both invasion and enterotoxin production; exact mechanism unknown	Diarrhea, abdominal cramps	Uncommon	CSO, S	Seawater	Foodborne (various types of seafood from estuary and seawater)	15–24 hr	Culture stool	None
Yersinia enterocolitica	Invasion of small and large intestine	Fever, abdominal pain, may suggest appendicitis, diarrhea	Uncommon	CSO, S	Animal feces	Foodborne, person-to-person	Probably 3–7 days	Culture stool	Probably tetracycline or trimethoprim-sulfamethoxazole
VIRUS									
Parvovirus-like agents (Norwalk agent)	Invasion of small intestine	Vomiting and diarrhea (see Table 26.3)	? (may be relatively common)	CSO	Human feces	Waterborne, person-to-person (secondary cases)	1–3 days	Rise in antiviral antibody (not generally available)	None
Rotavirus	Invasion of small intestine	Severe gastroenteritis in young children, mild in adults	Relatively common	S	Human feces	Person-to-person (secondary cases)	1–3 days	Virus antigen in stool; Rise in antiviral antibody	None
PROTOZOA AND HELMINTHS									
Entamoeba histolytica	Invasion of large intestine	Diarrhea, often chronic and bloody	Uncommon (travelers)	CSO, S	Human feces	Waterborne, person-to-person[b]	Few days to months	Examine stool for trophozoites	Quinacrine (see text)
Giardia lamblia	Colonization and occasional invasion of small intestine	Diarrhea, flatulence with foul-smelling stools	Uncommon (travelers)	CSO, S	Human feces	Waterborne, person-to-person[b]	1–4 weeks	Examine stool for trophozoites	Metronidazole (see text)
Trichinella spiralis	(a) Encysted trichinae mature, mate, reproduce in small intestine; (b) larvae penetrate intestine, migrate to muscles where they cause inflammation and become encysted	Diarrhea, puffy eyes, muscle aching, fever, occasionally severe heart failure; eosinophilia typical	Uncommon	CSO, S	Animal muscle (swine, many wild animals)	Foodborne	2–28 days	Skin tests, antibody, muscle biopsy	Thiabendazole, occasionally steroids (see text)
Cryptosporidia	Colonization	Diarrhea, acute in children	Chronic in patients with AIDS	S	Human and animal feces	? Probably animal to person	? 2–7 days	Examine stool for trophozoites	None known

[a] CSO, common source outbreak; S, sporadic.
[b] Anal-oral transmission may occur in homosexual men.

Table 26.2.
Characteristics of Acute Illness Due to Ingestion of Chemical Agents

Agent	Pathogenesis	Clinical Features	Frequency in USA	Epidemiological Features				Diagnosis	Specific Therapy
				Pattern[a]	Source	Transmission to Man	Incubation period		
SEAFOOD									
Ciguatoxin	Toxin with character of cholinesterase inhibitor	Vomiting and diarrhea, paresthesia (warmth, extremities), metallic taste, blurred vision, sharp pains in extremities, respiratory paralysis	Uncommon (Florida)	CSO, S	Food chain of bottom-dwelling fish caught in Florida, Hawaii (red snapper, barracuda)	Foodborne	1–6 hr	Clinical and epidmiological features	None (sensory symptoms may last days to months)
Scombrotoxin	Toxin with properties of histamine	Histamine reaction (flushing, headache, dizziness, burning of mouth and throat; urticaria, pruritus, and bronchospasm)	Uncommon (Florida, California)	CSO, S	Bacteria acting on fish flesh (tuna, mackerel, bonito, skipjack)	Foodborne	Minutes to 1 hr	Clinical and epidemiological features	None (lasts few hours—few days)
Paralytic shellfish toxin	Neurotoxin causing motor paralysis	Paresthesia (warmth, extremities), floating sensation, dysphonia, dysphagia, weakness, and respiratory paralysis	Uncommon	CSO, S	Toxic dinoflagellates concentrated in filter feeding bivalves (mussels, clams, oysters, scallops)	Foodborne	<30 min	Clinical and epidemiological features	None (lasts few hours—few days)
MUSHROOMS									
Muscarine	Muscarinic cholinergic response	Colicky abdominal pain, nausea, vomiting, diarrhea, salivation, miosis, blurred vision, bradycardia, hypotension	Uncommon	CSO, S	*Amanita muscaria*	Foodborne	Few minutes-few hours	Clinical and epidemiological features	Atropine 0.1–0.5 mg s.c. or i.v.
Phalloidin (and other toxins)	Diverse cytotoxic effects, multisystemic	*Stage 1:* nausea, abdominal pain, vomiting, bloody diarrhea, marked weakness, hypotension (shock) *Stage 2:* Clinical improvement (day 2 or 3) *Stage 3:* Severe hepatic failure, delirim frequent fatal outcome		CSO, S	*Amanita phalloides* and other *Amanita* species	Foodborne	6–15 hr	Clinical and epidemiological features	None
MISCELLANEOUS									
Heavy metals (antimony, cadmium, copper, iron, tin, zinc)	Upper gastrointestinal irritation	Metallic taste to food, nausea, vomiting, or diarrhea	Uncommon	CSO, S	Containers made of alloy which includes a heavy metal	Foodborne (food prepared in, stored in, or eaten from a container from which heavy metal leached)	5 min—8 hr	Clinical and epidemiological features	None
Monosodium glutamate (MSG)	Idiopathic reaction	Burning sensation in chest, neck, abdomen, extremities	Relatively common	S	Foods prepared with large amounts of MSG	Foodborne (Chinese restaurant foods)	3 min–2 hr	Clinical and epidemiological features	None

[a] CSO, common source outbreak; S, sporadic.

a special fish), eating at a restaurant, attending a picnic or pot-luck dinner, or preparing food in an unconventional container (*e.g.*, in a copper pot).

2. A history of a *similar illness in others* (family members or members of a group who ate with the patient). This will be helpful in suggesting a common source outbreak.

3. The probable *incubation period*. This may be helpful in suggesting the most likely etiology for a patient's illness (see Tables 26.1 and 26.2). For example, the onset of symptoms immediately after ingestion always indicates chemical food poisoning; onset of symptoms within a few hours of eating strongly suggests staphylococcal food poisoning; and onset of symptoms after 1 or more weeks of exposure suggests uncommon problems such as giardiasis.

4. A history of taking antimicrobials (particularly clindamycin), either currently or within the last 2 weeks. This could suggest the possibility of antibiotic-associated diarrhea which, when severe, is most commonly due to *Clostridium difficile* (4).

5. A history of *neurological symptoms* following ingestion of canned foods should always suggest botulism or one of the other sources of neurotoxins (all rare) listed in Table 26.2.

6. A history suggestive of the *acquired immodeficiency syndrome* (see Chapter 52) and chronic diarrhea should suggest the possibility of cryptosporidia (10).

7. A history of *homosexuality* in the male should suggest the possibility of the more unusual agents of diarrheal disease (21).

Physical Examination

The physical examination is usually of minimal help in establishing an etiological agent. Probably

Table 26.3.
Comparison of Symptoms of Viral and Bacterial Gastroenteritis in Adults

Symptom	Percentage with Symptom				
	Viral gastroenteritis		Bacterial gastroenteritis		
	Rotavirus[a]	Norwalk agent[b]	Salmonella[b]	Shigella[b]	Staphylococcus aureus[b]
Nausea	2	85	50	45	62
Vomiting	9	84	23	39	86
Abdominal cramps	26	62	78	60	86
Diarrhea	33	44	73	100	67
Fever	5	32	49	72	10
Headache	NR[c]	37	33	6	8

[a] From Wenman WM, Hinde D, Feltham S, Gurwith M: Rotavirus infection in adults. Results of a prospective family study. *N Engl J Med* 301:303, 1979.
[b] From Adler JL, Zickl R: Winter vomiting disease. *J Infect Dis* 119:668, 1969.

Table 26.4.
Sexually Transmissible Pathogens Resulting in Enteric Infections

Bacteria	Protozoa
Calymmatobacterium granulomatis	*Cryptosporidium* species[a]
Campylobacter species	*Dientamoeba fragilis*
Chlamydia trachomatis	*Entamoeba histolytica*
Haemophilus ducreyi	*Giardia lamblia*
(?) *Mycoplasma hominis*	*Isospora belli*[b]
Neisseria gonorrhoeae	"Nonpathogenic" protozoans
Neisseria meningitidis	
Salmonella species	**Viruses**
Shigella species	Condyloma acuminatum
Treponema pallidum	Cytomegalovirus
(?) *Ureaplasma urealyticum*	Hepatitis A and B
	Herpes simplex
Helminths	
Enterobius vermicularis	
Strongyloides stercoralis	

[a] From Quinn TC: Gay bowel syndrome. *Postgrad Med* 76:197, 1984.
[b] Have been shown to cause enteric disease in homosexual men with acquired immune deficiency syndrome (AIDS), but sexual transmission has not been reported.

Table 26.5.
Characteristics Distinguishing Invasive and Enterotoxigenic Diarrhea

Feature	Invasive Diarrhea	Enterotoxigenic Diarrhea
History	Fever, abdominal pain, tenesmus, may have blood in stool	Watery diarrhea with little or no fever or other systemic symptoms
Physical examination	Fever, abdominal tenderness; proctoscopy may be indicated	May be signs of salt and water depletion
Laboratory studies	Stool culture (may be diagnostic) Fecal leukocytes in large number[a] White count may be elevated	Stool culture usually negative unless special culture techniques available White count usually normal, but may be elevated
Therapy	Oral fluids and electrolytes (usually only small quantities needed) Antimicrobials often indicated[b]	Oral fluids and electrolytes (substantial quantities may be needed) Antimicrobials not indicated
Course	Improvement in 1–2 days, particularly if appropriate antimicrobials used	Duration of 1–2 days usually; may last up to 5 days

[a] Use a drop of methylene blue stain with liquid stool.
[b] See text for recommendations for specific bacterial pathogens.

the most important observation is the temperature: fever or significant abdominal tenderness in association with diarrhea suggests an invasive organism. Poor skin turgor and postural hypotension suggest significant salt and water deficits (relatively uncommon in adults with diarrhea in the United States). Infrequently occurring conditions in which the physical findings may be very helpful are botulism and other neurotoxic forms of food poisoning, and trichinosis (see Tables 26.1 and 26.2).

Laboratory Studies

In the majority of patients with acute gastrointestinal illness, no laboratory studies are indicated. If there is a suggestion of a common source outbreak, however, special cultures and tests for toxins in stools and in food, primarily for epidemiological purposes, should be obtained.

In patients with a combination of diarrhea for more than 24 hours, fever, and blood in the stool or significant dehydration, a minimum number of laboratory studies is indicated (16), i.e., (a) stool culture for *Salmonella, Shigella, Campylobacter* (8), and *Yersinia* (5) (unfortunately enterotoxigenic *E. coli*, invasive *E. coli*, vibrios, and viral agents cannot be identified in routine laboratories because of the special techniques required). (b) Stool examination for fecal leukocytes (more than 10 leukocytes per high power field is indicative of an invasive pathogen). The test is done by mixing a small bit of stool with methylene blue stain on a microscope slide, and placing a coverslip over the mixture. After 2 or 3 minutes, the preparation is examined under the "high dry" objective for the presence of leukocytes. (c) A white blood cell count (an elevated count and/or shift to younger polymorphonuclear forms supports the diagnosis of invasive diarrheal disease).

In suspected cases, the laboratory should be asked to examine the stool for *Giardia lambia, Entamoeba histolytica*, or *Cryptosporidium* (Table 26.1). For optimal identification of trophozoites of these organisms, fresh stools should be examined immediately by an experienced observer. For the diagnosis of giardiasis, stools may need to be examined repeatedly. *E. histolytica* trophozoites are best identified from the mucus taken from the base of ulcerations seen at proctoscopy.

Additional laboratory tests should be ordered for certain conditions (see Tables 26.1 and 26.2). (Also see Chapter 38 for a discussion of the evaluation of patients with chronic diarrhea.)

MANAGEMENT

In all patients with acute diarrhea, symptomatic treatment is of primary importance. In addition, some patients may require specific therapy (i.e., antibiotics), usually indicated on the basis of the history and physical examination. Most episodes of

acute diarrhea are self-limited, lasting 1 to 2 days, or occasionally as long as 5 to 10 days. Resolution of illness is thought to be due to the local secretory immune response of the gastrointestinal tract.

Symptomatic Treatment

Fluid Therapy

With the exception of giardiasis, amebiasis, and the more severe cases of shigellosis and salmonellosis, practically all acute diarrheal disease seen in the United States can be treated with only symptomatic therapy, the mainstay of which is the replacement of fluids and electrolytes lost in the stool. Since in most patients the disease is mild, and the amount of stool is small, replacement is relatively simple. Patients should be encouraged to drink lots of fluids, to avoid spicy foods, and otherwise to eat what they like.

In patients who have a *very large loss of stool* and who experience weakness and a feeling of being "washed out" with or without signs of dehydration, replacement should consist of fluids containing electrolytes and glucose. In many parts of the world, an oral glucose-electrolyte replacement solution is available commercially for this purpose (19). In the US similar commercial glucose-electrolyte solutions are now available. All have been developed primarily for treating children but are perfectly adequate for adults as well. Most have sodium concentrations of 50 to 75 mEq/liter and substitute citrate for bicarbonate (Infalyte, Resol, Pedialyte RS).

Patients experiencing *severe diarrhea or vomiting* which precludes easy ingestion of oral replacement fluids and those who have evidence of moderate to severe salt and water depletion should be hospitalized for initial intravenous fluid replacement with Ringer's lactate or its equivalent.

Other Symptomatic Measures

Two medications are commonly used to treat the diarrhea of gastroenteritis. *Diphenoxylate with atropine* (Lomotil) causes a decrease in intestinal motility and stool frequency; it may be very useful to the patient at times when frequent defecation would be embarrassing. Since this drug does not alter the natural course of the disease, however, and is potentially harmful if invasive pathogens such as *Shigella* are causing the diarrhea, it should only be used infrequently. The dose is 1 to 2 tablets every 6 hours. *Kaolin and pectin mixtures* (e.g., Kaopectate) have primarily a placebo effect. They add to the bulk of the stool, and thus the stools appear to be less watery; actual fluid loss, however, is not affected by these agents.

In patients with *severe vomiting*, commonly seen in staphylococcal food poisoning, the antiemetic drug prochlorperazine (Compazine) may be very helpful, given as a 25-mg rectal suppository two or three times daily.

Specific Treatment

In patients in whom *shigellosis* is strongly suspected, or from whom the organism has been cultured in the stool, appropriate antibiotic treatment should be given as this will shorten the illness from 3 to 7 days to 1 to 2 days (12). Ampicillin, 500 mg four times a day for 5 days, is adequate therapy. For patients allergic to penicillin, or those in whom an ampicillin-resistant organism is isolated, trimethoprim-sulfamethoxazole is a suitable alternative. The dose is 2 tablets every 12 hours for 5 days.

If *Salmonella* is isolated from diarrheal stool, patients should *not* be given antibiotics unless there is evidence of systemic disease, such as high fever or other signs of toxicity, lasting more than 1 day. It has been found that routine treatment of *Salmonella* gastroenteritis with antibiotics leads to a prolongation of the carrier state in some individuals (1). Even without antibiotic treatment, patients may excrete *Salmonella* in the stool for several weeks to months after their acute illness has terminated. If there is systemic disease, ampicillin (as for shigellosis) or chloramphenicol, 500 mg four times daily for 1 week, is adequate.

Patients infected with *Campylobacter* (8) may benefit from antibiotic therapy, but there are no controlled studies to confirm this. Erythromycin, 500 mg four times a day for 7 days, seems to be the drug of choice; most strains are also sensitive to similar doses of tetracyclines.

In patients who develop significant *diarrhea related to antibiotics*, the antibiotic should be stopped and another substituted if antibiotic therapy must be continued. In the majority of cases, however, which are usually due to *C. difficile*, oral vancomycin 500 mg four times a day for 5 days, will usually shorten the illness (4). An alternative effective drug is metronidazole (Flagyl), 250 mg four times a day for 5 days.

Patients with *giardiasis* and *amebiasis* definitely require appropriate therapy. For giardiasis, the drug of choice is quinacrine hydrochloride, 100 mg three times a day, for 5 days. Metronidazole (Flagyl), 750 mg three times a day for 5 to 10 days, is also effective. For moderate to severe amebic dysentery, metronidazole should be administered, 750 mg three times a day for 5 to 10 days, plus diiodohydroxyquin (Diodoquin), 600 mg three times a day for 3 weeks, to prevent the carrier state.

Trichinosis is treated with thiabendazole, 25 mg/ kg twice a day for 5 to 7 days. High doses of prednisone (e.g., 30 to 50 mg daily) should be given simultaneously if symptoms are pronounced (see Table 26.1).

Patients with *suspected botulism* should be hospitalized in an intensive care unit immediately and should be given polyvalent antitoxin, which must be obtained through the local health department.

Patients with mushroom poisoning due to *Amanita muscaria* should be treated with atropine (see Table 26.2).

In patients who are thought to have one or more of the *gay bowel syndromes*, the management for typical enteric infections (e.g., *Salmonella*, *Shigella*, *Entamoeba histolytica*, etc) is identical to that for nonsexually transmitted infections. Patients with proctitis or perianal disease (symptoms include constipation, anorectal discomfort, tenesmus, and mucopurulent discharge) should receive empiric treatment for *N. gonorrhoeae* and *C. trachomatis* (i.e., 4.8 million units of procaine penicillin intramuscularly plus 1 g of probenicid, followed by 500 mg of tetracycline orally four times a day for 7 days). For all patients with a gay bowel syndrome, a serological test for syphilis should be sent.

The Patient's Role in Therapy

Acute gastroenteritis, like the common cold, is an illness which is often diagnosed and handled by the patient without contacting a physician. In some instances, the patient will contact the physician by telephone, and a working diagnosis and plan of therapy can be established without an office visit. This is particularly true for healthy patients with typical symptoms of staphylococcal food poisoning. In all situations, whether the patient is examined by the physician or not, it should be stressed to the patient that care of gastroenteritis requires the regular taking of fluids, at times supplemented by an oral electrolyte solution (see above) and by oral antibiotics if prescribed. The patient will be expected to estimate the severity of his diarrhea in order to plan fluid replacement. He should be advised to notify his physician if his diarrhea becomes worse or if he feels increasingly ill with systemic symptoms such as fever, nausea, and vomiting. He need not return for a follow-up visit unless his symptoms persist beyond 2 to 3 days, or unless stool cultures have been taken and reveal that antibiotic therapy is indicated. Limitation of activity should be dictated entirely by how the patient feels and by his proximity to toilet facilities.

Course of Illness

The dehydrated patient will feel almost immediate improvement when adequate oral replacement fluids are given. When the patient is given antimicrobial therapy for an invasive pathogen, there should be a noticeable decrease in diarrhea and fever within 24 to 36 hours.

An *atypical course* will occasionally occur after initial diagnosis and treatment. Any patient may develop an increase in diarrhea after being initially seen, which could result in unanticipated significant dehydration. An increase in severity of symptoms could also occur if the patient were developing antibiotic-associated enterocolitis. An initial episode of ulcerative colitis could be misdiagnosed as shigellosis, in which case antibiotic therapy would not result in improvement; and the occasional patient with antibiotic-resistant *Shigella* may not respond to initial therapy, indicating the need for an alternative drug.

Rarely, a patient's diarrheal symptoms may not resolve within a few days. In this case, he should return for further evaluation, particularly repeat stool exams, which may be necessary to confirm the diagnosis of protozoal infections.

PREVENTION

Primary Prevention

Primary prevention of the diseases discussed above can theoretically be accomplished by these measures: (*a*) reducing the agent's presence in the environment, (*b*) increasing resistance of the host (by immunization or prophylactic antibiotics), and (*c*) utilizing environmental measures which block the transmission of the agent (2). Regulations governing sewage treatment, water purification, and food processing, packing, and preparation provide the principal protective barriers to foodborne disease *outside the home*. *In the home*, almost all forms of foodborne disease can be prevented if several measures are followed routinely (see Table 26.6). Many people do not realize that some of the food they prepare each day is contaminated before cooking, and that proper cooking and storing, not absence of contamination, is the way in which most food is rendered safe to eat. Whenever food known to be contaminated is eaten raw, the risk of foodborne disease is present; this is particularly important with respect to shellfish, which concentrate microbial organisms from the waters in which they are grown; routine surveillance of these waters by public health authorities is the major mode of protecting persons who eat raw shellfish (13).

Secondary Prevention

After an outbreak of an acute enteric illness, appropriate measures should be taken to prevent additional cases.

In the household, any foods suspected of transmitting illness should be thrown away (in the event that an epidemiological investigation is warranted, a sample should be submitted to the local health department). An error in storage or cooking of the suspected food will often be evident; the patient's physician should point out this error and, most important, review the standard precautions as listed in Table 26.5 to prevent repeated episodes of foodborne illness. When a member of a household has an enteric infection which is transmissible from person

Table 26.6.
Measures to Prevent Foodborne Disease in the Home

1. Refrigerate all foods which are capable of supporting microbial growth (perishable foods)
2. Avoid keeping perishable foods for long periods even in refrigerator
3. Cook all foods at sufficiently high temperatures before serving (212°F (100°C) or higher for all oven-cooked meats and at least 15 minutes boiling time for all boiled foods. Same procedure when foods are reheated)
4. Avoid preparing perishable foods a day or more before they are to be served
5. Avoid allowing foods to stand at warm temperatures for several hours before being served
6. Avoid incorporating raw (contaminated) ingredients into foods that receive no further cooking
7. Thoroughly clean kitchen equipment after it has been in contact with perishable foods
8. Avoid using utensils that may contain toxic metals
9. Avoid foods which are unsafe no matter how they are processed (see text, page 325)

to person (see Table 26.1), this individual should be instructed to wash his/her hands frequently, *especially* before preparing food for others. When shigellosis or salmonellosis occurs in a person involved in food handling, it is critical to obtain three negative stool cultures, assuring eradication of the carrier state, before the individual returns to food handling.

When exposure *outside the home* is suspected by the physician, the problem should be reported immediately to the local health department; it is the health department's responsibility to undertake an epidemiological investigation in order to protect others. Each year, investigations of 400 to 500 outbreaks of foodborne illness are reported to the Centers for Disease Control, and many lead to measures that interrupt potentially widespread outbreaks of diseases, some of them particularly hazardous, such as botulism (3).

Prophylaxis for Travelers to the Developing World

The problem of diarrheal illness and the other problems related to travel are discussed in Chapter 33.

General References

Benenson AS (ed): *Control of Communicable Diseases in Man*, ed 12. Washington, DC, American Public Health Association, 1975.
    A concise summary of epidemiology, management, and prevention of communicable diseases.
Blacklow NR, Cutzor G: Viral gastroenteritis. *N Engl J Med* 304: 397, 1981.
    Excellent review of the role of viruses in gastroenteritis.
Centers for Disease Control: *Foodborne Disease Outbreaks*. Annual Summary, Atlanta.
    This report, published annually, provides the most current overview of foodborne disease epidemiology; it includes detailed reports on important new problems each year.

Hughes JM, Horwitz MA, Merson MH, *et al*: Foodborne disease outbreaks of chemical etiology in the United States, 1970–1974. *Am J Epidemiol* 105:233, 1977.

Excellent review of epidemiological and clinical features of foodborne illness due to toxic and chemical agents.

Specific References

1. Aserkoff B, Bennett JV: Effect of antibiotic therapy in acute salmonellosis on the fecal excretion of salmonellae. *N Engl J Med* 281:636, 1969.
2. Barker WH: Perspectives on acute enteric disease epidemiology and control. *Bull Pan Am Health Org* 9:148, 1975.
3. Barker WH, Weissman JB, Dowell VR Jr, *et al*: Type B botulism outbreak caused by a commercial food product. *JAMA* 237:456, 1977.
4. Bartlett JG: Antibiotic-associated pseudomembranous colitis. *Rev Infect Dis* 1:530, 1979.
5. Black RE, Jackson RJ, Tsai T, *et al*: Epidemic *Yersinia enterocolitica* infection due to contaminated chocolate milk. *N Engl J Med* 298:76, 1977.
6. Bryan FL: Emerging foodborne diseases. II. Factors that contribute to outbreaks and their control. *J Milk Food Technol* 35:632, 1972.
7. Bryan FL: Emerging foodborne diseases. I. Their surveillance and epidemiology. *J Milk Food Technol* 35:618, 1972.
8. Butzler JP, Skirrow MB: *Campylobacter* enteritis. *Clin Gastroenterol* 8:737, 1979.
9. Clausen CR, Christie DL: Chronic diarrhea in infants caused by adherent enteropathic *Escherichia coli*. *J Pediatr* 100:358, 1982.
10. Current WL, Reese NC, Ernst JV, *et al*: Human cryptosporidiosis in immunocompetent and immunodeficient persons. *N Engl J Med* 308:1252, 1983.
11. Gosselin RE, Hodge HC, Smith RP, Gleason MN: *Clinical Toxicology of Commercial Products*, ed 4. Baltimore, Williams & Wilkins, 1976.
12. Haltalin KC, Kusmiesz HT, Hinton LV, Nelson JD: Treatment of acute diarrhea in outpatients. *Am J Dis Child* 124:554, 1972.
13. Hughes JM, Merson MH: Current concepts: fish and shellfish poisoning. *N Engl J Med* 295:1117, 1976.
14. Kapikian AZ, Yolken RH, Wyatt RG, *et al*: Viral diarrhea: etiology and control. *Am J Clin Nutr* 31:2219, 1978.
15. Keusch GT: Shigella infections. *Clin Gastroenterol* 8:645, 1979.
16. Koplan JF, Ferraro MJ, Fineberg HV, Rosenberg ML: Value of stool cultures. *Lancet* 2:413, 1980.
17. Ouchterlony O, Holmgren J (eds): *Cholera and Related Diarrheas*, 43rd Nobel Symposium. Basel, S. Karger, 1980.
18. Pierce NF: Infections of the gastrointestinal tract. In Harvey AM, Johns RJ, McKusick VA, *et al* (eds): *Principles and Practice of Medicine*, ed 20. New York, Appleton-Century-Crofts, 1980.
19. Pierce NF, Hirschhorn N: Oral fluid—a simple weapon against dehydration in diarrhoea: how it works and how to use it. *WHO Chronicle* 31:87, 1977.
20. Plotkin GR, Kluge RM, Waldman RH: Gastroenteritis: etiology, pathophysiology and clinical manifestations. *Medicine* 58:95, 1979.
21. Quinn TC, Stamm WE, Goodell SE, *et al*: The polymicrobial origin of intestinal infections in homosexual men. *N Engl J Med* 309:576, 1983.
22. Sack RB: Enterotoxigenic *Escherichia coli*: identification and characterization. *J Infect Dis* 142:279, 1980.
23. Wenman WM, Hinde D, Feltham S, Gurwith M: Rotovirus infection in adults. Results of a prospective family study. *N Engl J Med* 301:303, 1979.

CHAPTER TWENTY-SEVEN

Genitourinary Infections

JOHN R. BURTON, M.D., AND JAMES K. SMOLEV, M.D.

INTRODUCTION

Urinary tract infection (UTI) is one of the commonest disorders seen by the primary care physician. Although most of these infections are uncomplicated and easily treated, some of them pose a threat to the kidneys and, sometimes, to life itself. This chapter provides a practical approach to the diagnosis, classification, evaluation, management, and follow-up of patients who have urinary tract infections. Sexually transmitted disease and vulvovaginal infections are discussed also in Chapters 30 and 94, respectively.

PATHOGENESIS—GENERAL CONDITIONS

Gram-negative bacteria, particularly *Escherichia coli* account for approximately 80% of UTIs. There are over 100 serotypes of *E. coli*, differentiated by the character of the "O" antigen (a component of the cell wall), but only eight of these commonly cause infection. Other Gram-negative bacteria, such as *Enterobacter*, *Klebsiella*, *Proteus* species, and *Pseudomonas*, and Gram-positive bacteria, especially *Staphylococcus sapophyticus*, also cause UTIs, although less commonly than *E. coli*. Viruses, mycobacteria, fungi, and parasites cause UTIs very rarely.

In women, it is clear that the major cause of UTI is invasion of the urinary tract by bacteria which have ascended the urethra from contamination of the introitus. Women who are prone to infection have colonization of the vaginal introitus with the same serotypes of *E. coli* found in the fecal flora. There is evidence that this colonization is favored by a pH of the introitus greater than 4.4, by the absence of the production of cervicovaginal antibody (a surface antibody produced by the local tissues) to the colonizing bacteria, and by urethral trauma (e.g., during intercourse).

Infection of the bladder and kidneys *in men* is unlikely in an anatomically normal tract (as opposed to its common occurrence in women). The much lower incidence of urinary tract infection in men has been attributed to the long male urethra, to the absence of colonization of bacteria near the meatus, and to an antibacterial factor—*prostatic antibacterial factor* (PAF)—which is present in prostatic fluid (and is markedly diminished in some men with recurrent prostatic infection).

The bladder has unique *intrinsic defenses* against infection. The washout of bacteria by periodic voiding is probably one important defense mechanism. The bladder mucosa also removes surface organisms (perhaps by phagocytosis, the secretion of mucus, surface antibody production, or all of these); this defense mechanism is severely limited if residual urine is present.

Urinary tract infections occur more regularly and persistently in both men and women who have structural abnormalities of the urinary tract (such as an obstruction) or who have been catheterized or instrumented. Vesicoureteral reflux (the retrograde flow of urine from the bladder to the ureters) may be associated with, but is not necessarily a cause of, ascending infection. Infection in women also occurs more frequently in pregnancy (4 to 6% incidence), especially if they also have sickle cell trait (10 to 15% incidence). Diabetes mellitus does not increase the risk of developing a UTI unless there is an associated disorder of bladder emptying or unless the patient has been instrumented. However, once a UTI has developed in a diabetic patient, it may be more virulent. Sobel and Kaye have provided a comprehensive review of host factors in the pathogenesis of UTIs (19). The pathogenesis of other genitourinary infections (vulvovaginitis and sexually transmitted disease) are discussed in Chapters 30 (Syphilis) and 94 (Benign Vulvovaginal Disorders).

GENERAL DIAGNOSTIC CONSIDERATIONS

The diagnosis of urinary tract infection is suggested by the history and physical examination and confirmed by examination of the urine. Sometimes, X-rays and instrumentation of the urinary tract are necessary ancillary procedures. The symptoms and signs of UTI are discussed below, but the process of obtaining and evaluating a urine specimen and the radiological assessment of the urinary tract are the same, regardless of the pattern of infection (see below).

Urine Examination

There are two reasons why the urinalysis is the most important study in the evaluation of the patient suspected of having UTI:
1. A negative urinalysis makes a UTI unlikely.
2. Urinalysis may aid in the localization of an infection within the urinary tract (see below).

Collection

Collection of the urine specimen requires special attention since bacteria and cells on the skin near the urethra may contaminate the urine. However, a carefully instructed patient can usually obtain a *clean caught midstream specimen.*

Men can easily obtain an uncontaminated specimen by cleansing the gland of the penis using one or two 4 × 4-inch gauze wipes containing liquid detergent followed by rinsing with gauze soaked in tap water. In uncircumcised males the foreskin must be retracted. After initially voiding a small amount of urine into the toilet (except when a segmental collection is obtained, page 337) a midstream specimen is collected into a sterile container.

In *women*, the procedure is more difficult and careful instructions are necessary: while sitting on the toilet with one leg swung fully to the side, the labia are separated and the area around the urethra is cleansed two or three times with a 4 × 4-inch gauze soaked with liquid detergent and rinsed with two or three gauzes soaked with tap water. The initial portion of urine is voided into the toilet and a midstream specimen is then collected in a sterile container. Commercial urine collection kits are available but often are expensive and sometimes contain small cotton balls which may be hard for many patients to use. The "clean caught" procedure

may be impossible in women who are very obese or who have other disabilities. The finding of more than an occasional vaginal squamous cell in the urine specimen indicates that contamination has occurred. In this instance, urine must be obtained by either bladder catheterization or by suprapubic tap:

Catheterization of the urinary bladder is accomplished by using a no. 14 catheter, inserted through the urethra into the bladder and removed when the specimen has been obtained. This requires careful preparation and cleansing of the urethra (with an aseptic solution such as Betadine) to minimize the risk of introducing an infection. Alternatively, a *suprapubic tap* may be done if certain precautions are taken. The patient must have a full bladder—uncomfortable to the patient, with palpable suprapubic tenderness on examination, although often in women the bladder is not felt—and the lower abdomen should not have surgical scars. Two to 5 hours after the ingestion of 200 to 300 ml of fluid to the point of having a full bladder, the patient should lie supine for the procedure. The skin is cleansed with a sterilizing solution and the skin above the symphysis pubis is anesthetized with 1% Xylocaine. Then a 21- to 22-gauge 3½-inch spinal needle is gently inserted into the bladder, and a urine specimen is aspirated with a syringe. This procedure is, within the limits described above, preferable to bladder catheterization which has 1 to 2% risk of introducing infection. With experience, and when the patient comes to the office well hydrated, this procedure takes actually less time than catheterization, and is tolerated as well, if not better, by the patient.

Urinalysis

If the urine specimen cannot be processed by the laboratory within 10 to 15 minutes of obtaining it, it must be refrigerated (and transported to a laboratory in this manner) or placed on a dip agar transport device (see below). The *uncentrifuged* specimen can be examined microscopically under a coverslip with use of the oil immersion lens. The finding of bacteria by this method has a 90% correlation with the subsequent culture of over 1 million bacteria/ml of urine. The number of white cells in the uncentrifuged urine can be roughly quantitated microscopically in a counting chamber by the use of the low powered lens. In women the finding of more than seven white cells/mm³ is abnormal (although not specific for infection). The finding of seven or less white cells/mm³ suggests that infection is not present (21). In men the finding of any number of white cells should be considered abnormal.

The urine is more easily analyzed, however, after it is *centrifuged*: a drop of the sediment is examined by use of the high dry lens of the microscope. If bacteria are seen, infection is likely. Quantitation of white blood cells after centrifugation is not very reliable; however, it has been estimated that two to five leukocytes/high power field corresponds to > seven/ml in uncentrifuged urine (11); also, the identification of *white cell casts* is diagnostic of pylonephritis. Red blood cells also are often present in the urine in association with infection but may reflect a number of other processes as well (see Chapter 44).

The urine may also be analyzed by a multiple reagent *dipstick*. There may be a nonspecific positive test for blood and/or protein, but the most important measurement is the urinary pH. In an infected patient, a pH greater than 7.0 (if the patient is not a vegetarian) suggests the presence of infection by a urea-splitting organism, usually a *Proteus* species. The recent addition of the nitrite test to the multiple reagent dipstick should not lead the physician to use it as a reliable method to rule in or out bacteriuria in a symptomatic patient or in a random urine specimen. The use of the nitrite test for the purpose of detecting infection is most valuable when used in mass screening. Bacteria in the bladder reduce nitrate to nitrite and the latter can be measured colorimetrically using a dipstick. Because the generation of nitrite from nitrate by bacteria requires time, the test, when it is used for mass screening, is best performed on the first voided morning specimen and is most sensitive when repeated on three different morning specimens.

Culture

When UTI is suspected and before therapy is given, a culture should always be obtained except, for cost/benefit reasons, in certain circumstances: *women* with first, occasional, or uncomplicated infection (see page 338) or with the urethral syndrome (see page 340)—and in these instances very careful follow-up must be assured. Culture of the urine must be performed within a few minutes after it is collected. Bacteria multiply logarithmically if urine is incubated at room temperature; and, for this reason, the urine should be plated on a dip agar transport device (Uricult, bacteriuria screening test, or Bacturcult—available from commercial laboratories) or it should be refrigerated until it reaches the laboratory. (A refrigerator should be in the vehicle transporting the specimen to the laboratory.) The physician should not process cultures or perform sensitivity testing in his office unless a single individual can be dedicated to this task and quality control measures can be maintained.

Traditionally, 10^5 colonies of bacteria/ml have been considered indicative of significant infection; most patients with UTIs have bacterial counts above this level. However, *any number of bacteria colonies may be significant* if they are present in association with symptoms suggesting an infection. The vast majority of patients with bacterial UTIs have cultured a single species, but occasionally there may be a mixed infection (22).

When urine specimens are contaminated by surface bacteria, cultures may yield bacterial counts of less than 10^5 organisms/ml, or they may yield multiple species. When contamination is suspected, a carefully obtained clean caught urine specimen should be obtained or, if this is difficult, a specimen should be obtained by catheterization or by suprapubic aspiration of the bladder (see above). Not infrequently, a presumptive diagnosis of UTI has been made and antimicrobials have been prescribed by the time the laboratory reports that multiple organisms have been cultured. In this instance, the patient should be contacted by telephone to inquire about symptoms. If improvement has occurred, the antimicrobial course should be completed if it has not been and a repeat culture obtained at follow-up (see below, page 339). If there has not been a significant response to the prescribed therapy, another urine specimen should be obtained for urinalysis and culture, either by a very careful repeated clean caught collection or preferably by a suprapubic aspiration or catheterization.

The culture techniques for sexually transmitted diseases are discussed in Chapters 30 and 94.

Localizing the Site of Infection

There are several techniques which may localize infection in selected cases (15). Three of these are widely available.

The antibody-coated bacteria test takes advantage of the host immune response to invasion by bacteria of tissue, such as kidney, bladder wall, or prostate. The bacteria may be identified in the urine by the use of flourescent antibodies against the immune globulins (generated by the host) which coat the bacteria. This test, while helpful in differentiating bladder bacteriuria from pyelonephritis, is not yet widely reliable when done by commercial laboratories. Furthermore, because it reflects tissue invasion anywhere in the urinary tract, it is not specific pyelonephritis (17). Currently, its use is limited to the evaluation of patients with frequently recurrent UTIs or of pregnant patients with bacteriuria (see below).

Urinary tract infection may also be localized by the *catheterization of the ureters* by a urologist. In this manner infected urine in the upper tracts can be demonstrated. This technique, however, is rarely done except when it is necessary to demonstrate that infection is localized to one kidney (e.g., for consideration of removal of a chronically infected nonfunctioning kidney).

A third method of localization, the *bladder washout technique* (6), is too cumbersome for routine office practice.

In the *male patient*, infection of the prostate and/or bladder can be confirmed by comparison of quantitative bacterial counts on the first 10 ml of voided urine (urethral specimen—voided bladder specimen

1, VB₁), the midstream urine specimen (bladder specimen—voided bladder specimen 2, VB₂), a drop of expressed prostatic secretion (EPS), and the first 5 to 10 ml of urine voided after prostatic massage (prostatic specimen—voided bladder specimen 3, VB₃) (Fig. 27.1). Prostatic massage is accomplished by firm rolling pressure and working from the superior and lateral margin toward the midline and inferior margin. The seminal vesicles should be stripped also. If no secretions result, stripping the bulbar portion of the urethra may provide several drops of prostatic fluid.

In the performance of this *segmented collection technique*, it is important that the patient have some urine in the bladder at the time of the prostatic massage. Occasionally the prostate gland is too tender to massage, in which case a specimen may be obtained by having the patient masturbate and by culturing the ejaculate. The interpretation of the results of this segmented collection is as follows: VB₁ only positive—likely contamination or urethritis alone; VB₂ only positive—UTI; VB₃ or EPS only positive—epididymitis or prostatitis. The VB₁ specimen may be positive in association with a positive VB₂, EPS, or VB₃.

Radiography

The intravenous pyelogram (IVP) is not necessary in the vast majority of patients with uncomplicated UTI. It may help, however, in the evaluation of certain patients (Table 27.1) who are suspected of having structural abnormalities, the correction of which may prevent recurrence or may even be lifesaving. In addition to identifying problems which predispose to infection (such as reflux, a stone, or obstruction), an IVP will help to identify changes in the upper tract, such as scarring or caliectasis, which represent loss of renal parenchyma as well as abnormalities in the lower tract, such as bladder diverticula.

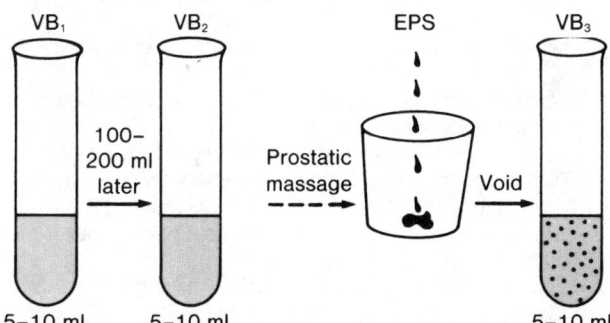

Figure 27.1. Segmented culture of the lower urinary tract in the male patient. VB₁, first voided urine; VB₂, midstream urine; EPS, expressed prostatic secretions; VB₃, first voided urine after massage. (After Stamey TA: *Pathogenesis and Treatment of Urinary Tract Infections.* Baltimore, Williams & Wilkins, 1980.)

Table 27.1.
Indications for Obtaining an Intravenous Pyelogram (IVP) in Patients with Urinary Tract Infection

Acute pyelonephritis in male patients
Acute pyelonephritis in women when symptoms worsen or fail to improve after 2 or 3 days of antimicrobial treatment
Renal colic (see Chapter 47)
Palpable bladder or renal mass
Evidence of a neurogenic bladder (suprapubic mass)
Urea-splitting organism—usually *Proteus* species
Frequently recurrent urinary tract infections in women (more than three or four per year)
Failure to eradicate infection with appropriate therapy
Patients with newly recognized renal failure (an infusion IVP should be performed in the presence of renal failure)

The voiding cystourethrogram may show abnormalities of the bladder outlet and urethra and may demonstrate urethral reflux. In adult patients this procedure is rarely necessary and it is not recommended without a urological consultation.

INFECTIONS IN WOMEN

The Patient with Irritative Symptoms: Diagnostic Approach

Several patterns (see below) of UTI have similar symptoms; therefore, a comprehensive approach to women with these symptoms is important to classify and manage them properly. UTI is characterized by symptoms of bladder irritation (frequency, urgency, and dysuria) and occasionally by hematuria. Chills and fever almost always indicate pyelonephritis, but the absence of these symptoms does not eliminate that diagnosis (7). Also because vaginal infection may mimic UTIs (11) it is important, in the initial evaluation of sexually active women, to ask them if they have a vaginal discharge. If so, a pelvic examination and an examination of the vaginal discharge should be done because vulvovaginitis from candidiasis, trichomoniasis, or other infections may be present and account for the bladder irritative symptoms (see Chapter 94). Also in sexually active women, chlamydial or gonococcal urethritis should be considered (see Chapter 94). *Chlamydia* infection is suggested if the patient has had a sexual partner with recent urethritis, a new sexual partner, or the gradual onset of symptoms (onset over days), or if hematuria is absent. Also cervicitis characterized by mucopurulent cervical discharge with exocervical edema is often present. Gonococcal infection should be suspected in patients with a history of gonorrhea or those whose sexual partners have a urethral discharge. A purulent discharge from the cervical os should be Gram stained (and cultured on Transgrow).

In most practices, several women with urinary infections will be seen weekly. The patients can be classified into several subgroups.

First Infection, Occasional Infection, or Uncomplicated Infection

Women with this very common problem account for the vast majority of patients who have a UTI. The diagnosis of a UTI is confirmed by urinalysis and urine culture, as discussed above (page 335). The infection will often clear spontaneously in time, but treatment dramatically shortens the symptomatic period and should be given.

Treatment

Usually uncomplicated UTIs are sensitive to multiple antimicrobials. Traditionally a 7- to 10-day course of antimicrobials has been given; but, recently, a single dose of a parenteral antimocribial (8, 16) or a single dose or a 3-day course of an oral antimicrobial (1, 5) has been shown to eradicate approximately 90 to 95% of cases of uncomplicated cystitis in young women. There have been several complementary studies which have indicated that the *single oral dose now can be recommended* in preference to the traditional 7- to 10-day course. The single dose is associated with significantly fewer side effects; the flora of the vagina, periurethral area, and rectum are less likely to be altered; the treatment is less expensive; and compliance is more likely (12, 18).

One of the following *single dose oral regimens* is acceptable: amoxicillin, (Amoxil, Polymox, or generic) 3 g (available as 500-mg tablets), sulfisoxazole (Gantrisin or generic) 2 g (available as 500-mg tablets); trimethoprim 160 mg with sulfamethoxazole 800 mg (available in tablets, Bactrim DS or Septra DS). Bactrim DS or Septra DS is preferred because of somewhat better results (2a, 9a). The patient should understand that symptoms may persist for 1 to 2 days, but she should telephone the physician if symptoms persist beyond this time since reassessment is then necessary.

When this regimen is initiated the patient should return in approximately 2 to 7 days so that a repeat urinalysis may be obtained (and if the urinalysis is abnormal, a urine culture and sensitivity testing should be done). By this method the few patients who experience a relapse, because of a renal infection, can be recognized early and can be given a more prolonged course of therapy (4 to 6 weeks of antimicrobial specific therapy, see below). Also this follow-up visit will provide the opportunity for the physician to educate the patient about UTIs (see below, "Follow-up").

However, single dose oral therapy should not be used (and instead a traditional 7- to 10-day course should be used) (*a*) when renal parenchymal infection is suspected (e.g., if fever, chills, or white blood cell casts are present), (*b*) when more than three or four previous episodes have occurred, (*c*) if symptoms have been present >2 days, (*d*) if the patient is older than 65 years of age, (*e*) during pregnancy, (*f*)

if follow-up is uncertain, or (*g*) if there is any suggestion of an underlying systemic problem (such as diabetes mellitus) or urological problem (such as a history of stones, reflux, or renal failure).

If the single dose regimen is not used, the well proven traditional 7- to 10-day course of antimicrobial is a reasonable option. The 3-day or the single parenteral dose regimens do not sufficiently improve upon the single or the 7- to 10-day oral regimens and are therefore not recommended. There is no evidence that treatment beyond 7 to 10 days is beneficial except when tissue infection is present (see below, "Recurrent Infection—Relapse Type in Men and Women"). The selection of an antimicrobial for a 7- to 10-day course should be based on cost and avoidance of any drug to which the patient is allergic. The results of culture sensitivity testing will ultimately guide the choice of therapy for patients with infections with more resistent organisms, but these results often are not available for 48 to 72 hours.

Prompt initiation of therapy is appropriate, before the culture report, to control the patient's symptoms (Table 27.2) Sulfonamides are prescribed more often

Table 27.2.
Antimicrobial Agents Which May Be Used in Uncomplicated Urinary Tract Infection

Agent	Dose
WHEN SINGLE DOSE THERAPY IS USED	
Amoxicillin	6, 500-mg capsules at once
Sulfisoxazole	4, 500-mg tablets at once
Trimethoprim 160 mg and sulfamethoxazole 800 mg (Bactrim DS or Septra DS)	1 double strength tablet at once
WHEN A TRADITIONAL 7–10-DAY COURSE OF THERAPY IS USED	
First Choice	
Ampicillin	250–500 mg 4 times a day
Amoxicillin	250–500 mg every 8 hours
Nitrofurantoin (Furadantin or Macrodantin)	100 mg 4 times a day
Sulfonamides (Gantrisin)[a,b]	500 mg 4 times a day
Trimethoprim[c] and sulfamethoxazole[b] (Bactrim or Septra)	2 tablets twice a day or 1 double strength (DS) tablet twice a day
Second Choice	
Cephalosporins[d] (cephalexin)	250–500 mg 4 times a day
Tetracycline[c]	250–500 mg 4 times a day

[a] Resistance may occur after frequent episodes of urinary tract infection.
[b] Avoid in women who are breast-feeding.
[c] Avoid in pregnancy.
[d] Often more costly.

than are other agents and are recommended except when prior resistance has been noted, in which case trimethoprim/sulfamethoxazole, ampicillin, nitrofurantoin, or tetracycline is a reasonable alternative. The urinary analgesic phenazopyridine (Pyridium) is not required when antimicrobials are prescribed.

A useful way to spare patients given the 7- to 10-day course of treatment the expense of purchasing additional medication if a change in medication is indicated is to provide the patient with a 3-day supply of antimicrobial from the office stock. The patient is instructed to telephone the office after 3 days, to obtain a prescription to complete the 7- to 10-day course. This practice also provides an efficient follow-up at which time a patient with uncomplicated infection should be nearly symptom free. If the symptoms have not significantly diminished, persistent bacteria may be present, and the patient should be re-evaluated (see below, "Persistent Infection in Men and Women"). Recurrences after the eradication of bacteria and after the patient is no longer taking an antimicrobial are common, however, and follow-up is necessary.

Follow-up

It is usual that the first office visit is taken up in establishing the diagnosis and initiating therapy. As cited above, phone follow-up will occasionally identify the need for prompt re-evaluation. If the symptoms have cleared, re-evaluation of the patient in the office in 2 to 7 days if single dose therapy was utilized or in 3 to 4 weeks if a 7- to 10-day course was utilized is recommended, in order to *educate* the patient about UTI (Table 27.3) and to reassess

Table 27.3.
Points to Consider in Educating Women Who Have Had an Uncomplicated Infection

Infections are often recurrent. However, the following measures may decrease the recurrence rate:

Avoid a full bladder. This is an especially important reminder during travel.

High fluid intake (1 liter in 2–3 hours) may eradicate an infection that has just become symptomatic.

Many infections result from the presence of bacteria (identical to bacteria in the feces) near the opening of the urethra. Therefore, after a bowel movement the anus should be wiped in the direction of anterior to posterior.

Irritation to the urethra, as occurs with sexual intercourse, is associated with the movement of bacteria into the bladder. Voiding after intercourse, therefore, may help to prevent recurrent infection.

Infections in the absence of structural urological disorder are rarely, if ever associated with the development of chronic renal failure.

Prompt recognition and treatment will help to control symptoms.

Even if recurrent infections are frequent, there is much that can be done to control symptoms (see discussion of prophylaxis under "Recurrent Infection—Reinfection Type")

the urine. Many patients who have a persisting nidus of infection and who have received only a single dose regimen of a 7- to 10-day course of antimicrobials will have evidence of a *relapse* (see page 344) at follow-up (bacteruria and pyuria), although it is frequently asymptomatic.

Recurrent Infection—Reinfection Type

The vast majority of women with recurrent urinary tract infections have reinfection (rather than an exacerbation of a smoldering quiescent infection). While the infections are symptomatic and occasionally may be associated with pyelonephritis, recurrent reinfection in women with structurally normal urinary tracts rarely, if ever, leads to the development of chronic renal failure.

Treatment

The approach to women with anatomically normal urinary tracts and the syndrome of reinfection has been vastly improved by the understanding of the pathogenesis of UTI in women. In the past, the women were often treated with a variety of painful manipulations, such as urethral dilatation, urethral incision, transurethral resection of the bladder neck, installation of a variety of intravesicle agents, and other inappropriate and ineffective maneuvers. Instead each episode of bacterial infection should be treated as outlined above in the section on first infections (page 338). If there are frequent recurrences, such as three or four or more in a year, prophylactic antimicrobials should be used.

Prophylactic Antimicrobials

After eradicating a recurrent infection, a prophylactic antimicrobial may be initiated.

A number of studies have confirmed the efficacy of prophylaxis in reducing the number of urinary tract infections in women (20, 23). The agents which have been used are effective when given as a single small dose at bedtime. A dose taken after sexual intercourse is also effective, patient acceptance is good, and side effects are uncommon.

Many agents have been shown to be effective prophylactically, but nitrofurantoin (Furadantin) 50 mg at bedtime, trimethoprim-sulfamethoxazole 40/200 mg, half tablet of regular strength Bactrim or Septra at bedtime, and cephalexin (Keflex or generic) 250 mg, half tablet at bedtime, are used most commonly and are recommended. Even with low doses of nitrofurantoin there has been some evidence of serious adverse effects (26) especially in older women; this agent is therefore best avoided in women over age 35. Prophylactic therapy should be continued for 6 months. During prophylaxis, the patient should have a urinalysis performed every 3 to 4 months to ensure that there is no pyuria or bacteriuria. If after the cessation of prophylaxis there are still frequent recurrences, prophylaxis for a longer period (such as a year) should be tried (after a course of appropriate eradicative therapy). Prophylactic therapy has improved dramatically the lives of many women with distressingly frequent UTIs.

In addition to the established efficacy of prophylactic therapy for preventing recurrent urinary tract infections in women, a recent study has shown that patient-initiated single-dose antimicrobial therapy may be just as effective and economically comparable (28). Nevertheless, the method of prophylaxis using a small dose of an antimicrobial every night is recommended until more information can be developed regarding the selection of women for the patient-initiated single-dose method.

Asymptomatic Bacteriuria

Associated with Pregnancy

Asymptomatic bacteriuria in pregnancy is relatively common, affecting up to 4 to 6% of women in the first trimester. Recognition of this fact is important, since eradication of this bacteriuria reduces the high incidence of symptomatic UTI that subsequently occurs during pregnancy and may reduce the risk of immature and premature birth which occurs in women with antibody-coated bacteria in the urine.

Unassociated with Pregnancy

When asymptomatic bacteriuria is identified in women who are not pregnant, the management is uncertain even though asymptomatic bacteriuria may be associated (although not necessarily causally) with increased mortality (3, 4). While a few women will eventually develop symptomatic infection, the likelihood is very much less than it is in pregnant women; in most the bacteriuria will clear spontaneously. Since, if asymptomatic bacteriuria is treated repeatedly, recolonization with another species may occur, asymptomatic bacteriuria in nonpregnant women should be treated only with a single course of therapy; if it recurs, a structural problem should be sought. If found, persistent infection may be present (see page 344). If, on the other hand, no structural problem is found, the bacteriuria is best left untreated unless symptoms develop. Screening for asymptomatic bacteriuria in nonpregnant adult women is not recommended.

Clinical Syndromes That Mimic "Classical" Urinary Tract Infection

Two clinical syndromes in women that mimic "classical" UTI (*i.e.*, $> 10^5$ bacteria/ml of urine) are analogous to prostatodynia in men (see page 343) and because of their high prevalence deserve special attention. They are the urethral syndrome and interstitial cystitis.

Urethral Syndrome (Dysuria-Pyuria Syndrome)

This syndrome is characterized by bladder irritation, frequency, urgency, and dysuria without "sig-

nificant" (greater than 10^5) bacterial colonies/ml on culture. With the increased ability to identify bacteria and other infectious agents in the urinary tract (see above), a new understanding of the syndrome has evolved.

Etiology. Dysuria-pyuria syndrome may be the better term since dysuria is invariable and pyuria (greater than 8 white blood cells/mm^3 of clean uncentrifuged urine) has important etiological implications (21). Studies have shown that many women with the syndrome have bacterial infection (21, 22). Patients may have cultures that show fewer than 10^5 colonies of bacteria (especially of *Escherichia coli*, but occasionally of other bacteria) and yet respond to appropriate antimicrobial eradicative therapy. Also in many women urine cultured by the usual bacteriological techniques appears sterile, but when the urine is cultured by use of special methods, it will grow infectious agents such as herpes simplex virus, *Chlamydia trachomatis*, and other agents (2). Also, this syndrome may be mimicked by vaginitis or gonococcal urethritis.

When *Chlamydia* infection is suspected (see above, page 337), treatment should be empiric because a culture is relatively expensive; however, commercial laboratories increasingly have available diagnostic methods of detecting *Chlamydia trachomatis* in urogenital swab specimens: a fluorescent antibody staining technique and an enzyme immunoassay are the two methods currently available; both are quite accurate and relatively inexpensive. The laboratory should be consulted regarding the method of specimen collection and handling. Satisfactory treatment is achieved with doxycycline (Vibramycin or generic), 100 mg twice a day, or tetracycline, 500 mg four times a day for 10 days. Cervicovaginal gonococcal infection may also be eradicated with this regimen, although penicillin is more effective; therefore, if gonococcus bacteria are identified on Gram stain (or cultured) then procaine penicillin, 4.8 million units intramuscularly plus 1 g of probenecid orally 30 minutes before injection, or ampicillin, 3.5 g orally or amoxicillin, 3 g either following 1 g of oral probenecid may be used. Spectinomycin, 2.0 g intramuscularly is recommended for patients allergic to penicillin or for whom penicillin failed to eradicate the gonococcus. Newer cephalosporins may be used to treat penicillin-resistant gonococci also—as discussed in Chapter 94. Even when gonorrhea is diagnosed, concomitant therapy to eradicate *Chlamydia* is recommended (see above) since these organisms are present commonly (9).

If a sexually transmitted disease is not suspected and if the urinalysis shows pyuria with some bacteria, then the physician should prescribe treatment as outlined above for first, occasional, or uncomplicated UTI in women (see above).

Five to 10% of women who have the urethral syndrome do not have a demonstrable infectious agent even if special cultural methods are used; most often these patients do not have pyuria. The cause of the syndrome in these instances is not known. In this group, treatment with reassurance, sitz baths, and the urinary analgesic phenazopyridine (Pyridium), 200 mg three times a day for 5 to 10 days, will provide some relief. The patient should be informed that the medication often causes the urine to appear orange. If symptoms persist, referral to a urologist is indicated.

Follow-up for patients with this syndrome should be identical to that outlined above (page 339) or, if there is vaginitis or a sexually transmitted disease present, as outlined in Chapter 94.

Interstitial Cystitis

Interstitial cystitis is an occasionally seen disorder affecting middle-aged women which early in its course may be confused with the urethral syndrome. Interstitial cystitis causes symptoms of suprapubic discomfort, especially when the bladder is full, and symptoms are relieved by voiding. The patient may experience progressive urinary frequency and eventually patients may have to void four to six times/ hour, often throughout the night. The urinalysis is often normal but hematuria may be present. The urine is sterile. This disease is difficult to diagnose, and therapy is often unsatisfactory. If suspected on the basis of the history, referral to a urologist is indicated. The urologist will perform a cystoscopy in order to establish the diagnosis (usually a normal appearing mucosa with a very small vesicle capacity is identified; mucosal hemorrhage may appear with bladder filling). Also, a cystoscopic evaluation will permit the urologist to exclude other causes of the symptoms (bladder tumor, for example). No definitive therapy has yet been developed for treatment of this condition.

Vaginitis and Cervicitis

For discussion, see Chapter 94.

INFECTIONS IN MEN

Bacterial Cystitis

This infection is similar in presentation to that in a female patient and is diagnosed by the same method but a urine culture should always be obtained. It suggests the presence, however, of an underlying structural problem, such as prostatic hypertrophy, and a diagnostic workup including a prostatic examination, assessment of renal function by a determination of serum creatinine or creatinine clearance, and an intravenous pyelogram (IVP) and a urological consultation for consideration of cystoscopy are appropriate.

The treatment of bacterial cystitis should be similar to the traditional 7- to 10-day course described above (page 338) and in Table 27.2. The treatment course may need to be prolonged further, however,

if the workup reveals a structural problem (see below, "Persistent Infection in Men and Women" and "Recurrent Infection—Relapse Type in Men and Women"). A single dose or a 3-day regimen of an antimicrobial as described for use in female patients with uncomplicated infection should never be used in men.

Men with bacterial cystitis should be followed carefully even if the initial evaluation was unrevealing, as many will be found to have recurrent infection—relapse type (see below). Many men with relapse infection have bacterial prostatitis; therefore, a follow-up visit in 4 to 6 weeks after the initial infection should include a segmented urine collection.

Prostatitis

Prostatitis is classified as bacterial prostatitis, nonbacterial prostatitis (prostatosis), or the much less common prostatic infections due to a virus, a parasite, tuberculosis, a fungus, or nonspecific granulomatous changes (14).

Acute Bacterial Prostatitis

Acute bacterial prostatitis is characterized often by an abrupt onset of fever, chills, low back pain, and perineal pain with irritative urinary tract symptoms, although on some occasions systemic symptoms are not pronounced. Perineal discomfort may be worsened by defecation. In addition, the patient may have initial, terminal, or occasionally, total hematuria (see Chapter 44). Rectal examination usually discloses a tender, swollen, and boggy prostate. The urinalysis, as well as expressed prostatic secretions (see above, page 336), contain leukocytes, and culture will often grow the responsible bacterial pathogen. The prostate may be too tender to massage and an EPS or VB_3 (see above, page 337) specimen cannot be obtained. Almost always in this situation the urethral (VB_1) or bladder urine (VB_2) specimen will contain bacteria; and sensitivity testing can be performed on bacteria grown from these specimens. If bacteria are not seen in the urine, material for culture may be obtained by having the patient masturbate as discussed above (page 337).

When the diagnosis is made, the patient may occasionally require hospitalization, although if systemic symptoms are minimal, ambulatory therapy is appropriate. Trimethoprim (Proloprim or Trimpex), 100 mg twice a day, trimethoprim-sulfamethoxazole (Bactrim or Septra), 2 tablets twice a day, carbenicillin (Geocillin) 2 tablets four times a day, clindamycin (Cleocin), 150 to 300 mg every 6 hours, or erythromycin, 250 to 500 mg twice a day, achieves a high level of tissue concentration in the prostatic fluid and can be prescribed to an ambulatory patient. Trimethoprim-sulfamethoxazole (Bactrim or Septra) is suggested as initial therapy until culture sensitivity tests are available, and then an adjustment in antimicrobial selection is made if necessary (trimethoprim holds promise as the agent of first choice but further clinical trials are necessary). Therapy with antimicrobials should be continued for 2 weeks.

Bed rest and sitz baths for 20 to 30 minutes two or three times a day may provide comfort. Occasionally, prostatitis results in acute urinary retention, which requires hospitalization and urgent urological consultation. The palpable irregularity of the prostate gland following acute infection may persist for several months. The acute infection is readily controlled, but recurrences may occur, especially in older individuals.

Men below 50, the age where benign prostatic hyperplasia (BPH) occurs, do not need a urological evaluation if the acute prostatitis responds within several days. Men older than 50 should be referred routinely to a urologist because of the likelihood of associated BPH and the high recurrence rate.

Chronic Bacterial Prostatitis

The organisms that cause chronic bacterial prostatitis most often are Gram-negative bacilli, *E. coli* being the most common organism, followed by *Enterococcus*, *Proteus*, and *Klebsiella*. Most patients with chronic bacterial prostatitis present with mild irritative symptoms (frequency, urgency, and dysuria), and occasionally there is a urethral discharge. Fever is absent. Patients may also have painful ejaculation with hematospermia (see Chapter 44). On rectal examination the prostate gland feels somewhat irregular and may be mildly tender, although the examination is often unremarkable.

The diagnosis is confirmed by the presence of greater than 10 to 20 white blood cells/high power field in the prostatic fluid or by the isolation of bacteria from expressed prostatic secretions or from the urine voided after prostatic massage (VB$_3$); at the same time the bladder urine (VB$_2$) is sterile or contains only a few colonies of bacteria and often a small number in the urethral specimen (VB$_1$) (see page 337). Obstructive symptoms are rare. Most often the patients have intermittent symptomatic episodes that have been controlled with a 10- to 14-day course of antibiotics. Unfortunately, however, recurrent infection is frequent because of persistence of bacteria within the urinary tract (see page 344). Chronic prostatitis may also be a reservoir for acute symptomatic cystitis or pyelonephritis.

If the infectious organism is sensitive to trimethoprim-sulfamethoxazole (Bactrim or Septra), a 12-week course consisting of 2 tablets twice a day in patients with chronic prostatitis does offer a 30 to 70% chance of a long term cure (14). For any chance of such a cure, a repeat culture of the expressed prostatic secretions and of the urine voided after prostatic massage should be sterile after 4 weeks of treatment. If the culture at 4 weeks is not sterile, continued therapy will fail and should be stopped.

Some patients in whom oral therapy has failed may be cured by the administration of an aminoglycoside antibiotic parenterally for 7 days, but this requires hospitalization and careful monitoring of renal function to avoid renal injury.

If all efforts to eradicate infection fail, symptoms usually can be controlled with very low dose trimethoprim-sulfamethoxazole, one-half tablet of regular strength Bactrim or Septra nightly indefinitely. The only way to effect a cure is by radical prostatectomy, but the morbidity of this procedure precludes its use for benign disease. Repeated prostatic massage has not been shown to be effective. It is important that patients with refractory chronic bacterial prostatitis be evaluated for the presence of *prostatic stones* by an X-ray of the kidney, ureters, and bladder; if stones are seen, the patient should be referred to a urologist. Patients with prostatic stones are often infected with a *Pseudomonas* species. On the other hand, patients who are not infected and incidentally are found to have prostatic calculi do not need to be referred to a urologist as the stones are frequently of no significance.

Nonbacterial Prostatitis (Prostatosis)

A certain group of patients have all the symptoms of chronic bacterial infection of the prostate, but no organism can be demonstrated; *i.e.*, they have nonbacterial prostatitis (prostatosis). This is the most common form of prostatic inflammation. These patients have mild perineal pain and irritative symptoms on urination, as well as white cells in the smear of the expressed prostatic secretions, or in the third voided urine (VB$_3$); yet, no organisms are cultured. Culture of the secretions and urine by special techniques occasionally reveals infectious agents such as mycoplasma, *Gardernella vaginali*, *Ureaplasma urealyticum*, or *Chlamydia* species; however, the significance of these findings is unknown. It is very difficult to cure patients with this syndrome but they should be given an antimicrobial such as erythromycin, 250 mg four times a day, minocycline (Minocin), 100 mg twice daily, trimethoprim-sulfamethoxazole (Bactrim or Septra), 2 tablets twice a day, or trimethoprim (Proloprim or Trimpex), 100 mg twice a day for a 2-week course; if there is no response to the therapy or if the syndrome recurs, no subsequent antibiotics should be prescribed. Instead, an antispasmodic agent such as oxybutynin (Ditropan), 5 mg two to three times a day, should be tried. Therapeutic prostatic massage has not been shown to be of value.

Interstitial cystitis and *in situ* bladder cancer may mimic symptoms of nonbacterial prostatitis; both conditions require cystoscopic examination for confirmation. Therefore, if the symptoms of nonbacterial prostatitis recur after a single course of treatment, a urological consultation should be requested to exclude these conditions and to educate the patient about the benign nature of prostatosis.

Prostatodynia

Patients with a syndrome called prostatodynia have symptoms suggesting prostatic inflammation, but have no evidence of inflammation on physical examination, have no white blood cells in the urine or expressed prostatic secretions, and have sterile segmented urine cultures. There is some evidence that the syndrome may be due to a neurological disorder and that muscle relaxants or α-sympathetic blocking agents such as phenoxbenzamine (Dibenzyline) are effective in treating it. If this syndrome is suspected, urological consultation is suggested to confirm the diagnoisis, to rule out interstitial cystitis and bladder cancer, and to initiate therapy.

Epididymitis

Epididymitis is a common intrascrotal infection which affects adult male patients. Organisms are thought to reach the epididymis through the lumen of the vas deferens from infected urine, posterior urethra, or seminal vesicles. Epididymitis is manifest as an abrupt swelling of the epididymis which rapidly spreads, presenting often as a generalized inflammation of the entire hemiscrotum and making the differentiation from an acute orchitis impossible. Frequently, fever, chills, and irritative bladder symptoms are also present. The differential diagnosis includes torsion of the testicle, acute orchitis, and tumor of the testicle with hemorrhage or hydrocele. Several observations help to differentiate torsion from epididymitis: torsion occurs in young boys and epididymitis occurs after puberty; the urinalysis is normal in torsion but usually shows pyuria and may show a urethral discharge in epididymitis; elevation of the scrotum often relieves the pain of epididymitis but intensifies the discomfort in torsion. Occasionally, however, it is not possible to distinguish torsion from epididymitis, in which case the patient should be referred to a urologist for emergency evaluation.

Epididymitis may be distinguished from orchitis only in its early stages. However, the presence of a urethral discharge or pyuria suggests epididymitis. A tumor of the testis is usually identified by its hardness and insensitivity to pressure. A hydrocele is usually easy to identify as it is painless and transluminates light. While the gonococcus causes some episodes of urethritis, *Chlamydia* has been found to be a common cause of epididymitis in men less than 50 years; while in older men who have benign prostatic hypertrophy, the coliform organisms are more common. Mumps, although uncommon in adults, may be associated with the development of epididymitis. In some instances no infectious agent can be identified. Once the diagnosis of epididymitis is made on clinical grounds, it should be confirmed by culture of the urine and expressed prostatic secretions, which usually demonstrate an infectious agent.

Treatment with ampicillin, 500 mg four times a day, or tetracycline, 500 mg four times a day, in addition to scrotal support, bed rest, and sitz baths will usually control infection within several days. Treatment should be continued for 14 days, and the patients should be informed that induration and edema in the region of the epididymis may persist for as long as 6 to 8 weeks. In the older patient with acute epididymitis, a search for obstruction at the bladder outlet (see Chapter 48) should be done as soon as the acute symptoms are controlled. On rare occasions, continued pain from chronic epididymitis may occur; if it does, a urologist should be consulted since some of the patients so affected may require an epididymectomy.

Urethritis

Urethritis is an acute inflammation of the urethra which may be classified as gonococcal or nongonococcal (10). Nongonococcal urethritis is more common and the most common cause for it is *Chlamydia trachomatis*. Symptoms of urethritis in the male patient include a discharge from the urethra, dysuria, and a sensation of itching at the distal end of the penis. There is no associated fever. Nearly 25% of men with a *Chlamydia* infection also have no manifestations (24). Culture for *C. trachomatis* is quite expensive and is not recommended for routine clinical use; however commercial laboratories increasingly have available relatively low cost, rapid, and accurate methods of detecting *Chlamydia* in urogenital swab specimens (see above, page 340). The detection methods as they become more widely available will help the clinician accurately diagnose *Chlamydia* urethritis. Diagnosis of gonococcal urethritis depends on the examination and culture of the urethral discharge. Material from the male urethra is best obtained using a sterile calcium alginate swab (Caligiswab, Type 1), available from physician supply stores. The Caligiswab is much smaller than the usual cotton swab and, for this reason, it is much less distressing to the patient.

A culture of the urethra for gonococci using a calcium alginate swab or a culture of the discharge should always be done by plating the swab on Transgrow, which must be at room temperature. (Because of its low cost, culture for gonococci is recommended whereas the high cost of *Chlamydia* culture precludes its routine use.) Approximately 10% of men with gonorrhea are asymptomatic and swabbing the urethra for a culture of *Neisseria gonorrhea* is appropriate whenever there is a history of exposure.

Swartz and co-workers (25) have pointed out the usefulness of counting the white blood cells after staining the discharge with Gram stain. A Caligiswab is passed into the urethra, then rolled over a 1

× 2-cm area on a slide, which is stained by Gram stain. Gonococcal urethritis is almost always associated with greater than 50 white blood cells/high power field compared with less than 2 in normal men and a count of between 4 and 50/high power field in patients with nongonococcal urethritis.

Gonococcal urethritis is diagnosed by the presence on Gram stain of many white blood cells and of extra- or intracellular Gram-negative diplococci; the treatment is either with parenteral penicillin, oral ampicillin, or amoxicillin (all following oral probenecid) or parenteral spectinomycin (Table 27.4).

In *nongonococcal urethritis* the discharge continues for a longer period and is more mucoid, and the smear has fewer white blood cells and no stainable bacteria. Treatment of nongonococcal urethritis is with tetracycline or erythromycin (Table 27.4). The treatment is usually effective but recurrences develop commonly.

Since all the forms of urethritis must be assumed to be sexually transmitted, the patient's partner or partners should be treated with a regimen appropriate for the urethritis and the patient should use a condom until the infection has been controlled.

When patients continue to have recurrences of nongonococcal urethritis or have persistent symptoms unresponsive to antimicrobial agents, they should have bacteriological studies to evaluate the possibility of a chronic bacterial prostatitis (see above), and they should also undergo urological investigation for evaluation of possible urethral stricture, foreign bodies, or other intraurethral lesions.

Gonorrhea in women is discussed in Chapter 94.

PERSISTENT INFECTION IN MEN AND WOMEN

As noted above, treatment in the male or female patient of infection in a normal urinary tract with an appropriate antimicrobial should result in the sterilization of the urine within 72 hours. By this time, symptoms should have abated or, at least, markedly diminished. If symptoms continue, a persistent infection may be present, and it should be established by a repeat urine culture. If any growth of the bacterial species present in the urine before treatment occurs, further evaluation is necessary. Several causes (Table 27.5) should be considered. A test of renal function (determination of a serum creatinine level or of creatinine clearance) and an IVP are suggested if infection persists in a patient who has taken the appropriate antimicrobial therapy. Urinary obstruction is discussed in Chapter 48.

RECURRENT INFECTION—RELAPSE TYPE IN MEN AND WOMEN

Recurrent infection with the same organism is called relapse infection and implies the persistence of bacteria in tissue within the urinary tract. Relapse infection is, in fact, very similar to persistent infection except that in relapse bacterial sterility has been demonstrated either while the patient is on or has completed antimicrobial therapy, whereas sterility is never demonstrated with persistent infection. Relapse occurs most often within 6 weeks of completion of a course of antimicrobial therapy. An underlying structural problem is often present in both men and women with this problem. In women it is very much less common than reinfection (see above, page 339), but it is quite difficult to document because most infections are a result of *E. coli*, which has many serotypes that cannot be differentiated by routine bacteriological laboratory techniques. Therefore, recurrent UTI due to *E. coli* may be either relapse (same serotype) or reinfection (different serotype). On the other hand, relapse of infection with organisms other than *E. coli* may be diagnosed by routine bacteriological culture. In women, if *recurrent* infection with *E. coli* occurs three times in a 12-month period, or if *relapse* infection with other species occurs, evaluation as outlined under "Persistent Infection in Men and Women" to exclude the possibility of structural abnormality is appropriate. If a structural abnormality is identified, it should be corrected if possible; if relapse infection is documented and there is no structural abnormality, a

Table 27.4.
Management of Urethritis in Men

Gonococcal urethritis (one of the following treatments):
  Procaine penicillin, 4.8 million units intramuscularly plus 1.0 probenecid iorally 30 minutes before injection
  Ampicillin, 3.5 g orally in a single dose plus 1.0 g of probenecid orally
  Amoxicillin 3.0 g orally in a single dose plus 1.0 g of probenecid orally
  Spectinomycin, 2.0 g intramuscularly for penicillin-resistant gonococci or for patients allergic to penicillin or intolerant of tetracycline
Nongonococcal urethritis (one of the following treatments):
  Tetracycline, 500 mg orally 4 times a day for 7 days
  Erythromycin, 500 mg orally 4 times a day for 14 days
Treat partner(s) appropriately
Follow-up for recurrence, complications (stricture, prostatitis, epididymitis), or especially in gonococcal urethritis, infection elsewhere (oropharyngeal, arthritis)
Report to local health department as required

Table 27.5.
Differential Diagnostic Possibilities When Urinary Tract Infection Is Not Eradicated by Therapy

Use of an antimicrobial to which the infectious agent lacks sensitity
Failure of the patient to take the antimicrobial
Presence of an underlying structural problem, such as an obstruction, diverticulum, or stone
Renal failure (inadequate urinary concentration of antimicrobial)

more prolonged course (6 weeks) of an appropriate antimicrobial agent should be prescribed.

If a women or man has a structural abnormality of the urinary tract that cannot be corrected, sterilization of the urinary tract usually is not possible. However, *suppressive therapy* may decrease the frequency of symptomatic exacerbations or of episodes of sepsis. Suppressive therapy (as opposed to eradicative or prophylactic therapy) is accomplished for sensitive organisms by the use of sulfisoxazole (Gantrisin), 500 mg twice a day, or trimethoprim-sulfamethoxazole (Bactrim or Septra), 1 tablet twice a day. An alternative to these agents is methenamine hippurate (Hiprex or Urex), 1 g twice a day, or methenamine mandelate (such as Mendelamine or Thiacide), 1 g four times a day. However, for these latter agents to be active the urine pH must be below 6.5, so that acidifying agents such as ammonium chloride, 300 mg three to four times a day must be used and the patient must test the urine regularly and adjust the dose of ammonium chloride accordingly (often several grams/day are required) to assure the acidification of the urine. Thus these agents are unacceptable for most patients.

ACUTE PYELONEPHRITIS IN MEN AND WOMEN

Pyelonephritis is a bacterial infection of the kidney that most often results from an ascending infection. It is suggested by the presence of bladder irritative symptoms, in addition to flank pain, fever, and, frequently, abdominal pain. Bacterial infection of the kidney may also be present without any of these signs of symptoms or with only bladder irritation (7). The urinalysis will show changes as outlined above (page 335), but only the presence of white blood cell casts is diagnostic of pyelonephritis. "Glitter cells" (white blood cells that glitter upon microscopic evaluation because of granules in the cytoplasm) are often touted as diagnostic, but they are not specific (13).

Clinically apparent acute pyelonephritis in men suggests the presence of a structural problem predisposing to infection and is an indication for immediate hospitalization, parenteral antimicrobial therapy, and an urgent IVP. In women, an underlying structural problem is much less likely to be present. Therefore, the decision for hospitalization and evaluation requires careful consideration. The patient can be managed at home if she does not appear severely ill or exhibit sepsis, is reliable, is able to take oral antimicrobials, and if access to the physician is guaranteed should symptoms worsen. If a patient is managed at home, follow-up by the physician in 24–48 hours by phone is necessary. If there has not been significant improvement during that time, the physician should consider the possibility of an undrained infection (due to obstruction or abscess, for example) and arrange for prompt hospitalization for parenteral antibiotics, IVP, and emergency urological consultation.

The initial antimicrobial for the patient who is managed at home can be any of the agents listed in Table 27.2 (except the single dose regimens *should not* be used) with an appropriate adjustment based on the results of the urine culture and on sensitivity testing (see above). Forcing fluid (once an antimicrobial has been started) is not necessary and may theoretically be detrimental, as the concentration of antimicrobials in the urine and in the renal tissue may be diluted (27). However, intake should be adequate to replace fluid losses, including the additional fluid lost by fever or by vomiting.

If the acute episode of pyelonephritis promptly resolves, then follow-up in 3 to 4 weeks is appropriate (see above, page 339). An IVP, unless indicated for evaluation of a nonresponsive patient, should not be done until that time. An IVP performed during the acute state sometimes shows a nonspecific diffuse or segmented decrease in the concentration of dye, a delay in the nephrogram on the effected side, distortion of the collection system, and mild urethral reflux. Also, the kidneys may be enlarged. These changes will reverse in several weeks as the infection subsides. Therefore, to avoid being misled by these transient changes and thus to avoid repeating studies, an elective IVP should be postponed until several weeks after the acute episode has abated.

General References

Earle DP: *Manual of Clinical Nephrology.* Philadelphia, WB Saunders, 1982.
  A practical guide to renal problems with a thorough description of urine collection techniques and urine microbiology.
Kunin CM: Urinary tract infections. In Glassock RJ (ed): *Current Therapy in Nephrology and Hypertensions 1984–1985.* St Louis, CV Mosby, 1984.
  A concise chapter written by a recognized authority.
Stamm WE, Turch M: Urinary tract infection. In Stollerman GH (ed): *Advances in Internal Medicine.* Chicago, Year Book, 1983, vol 28.
  Brief and well referenced.
Stamey TA: *Pathogenesis and Treatment of Urinary Tract Infections.* Baltimore, Williams & Wilkins, 1980.
  A comprehensive, well referenced monograph.

Specific References

1. Bailey RR, Abbott GD: Treatment of urinary tract infection with a single dose of trimethoprim-sulfamethoxazole. *Can Med Assoc J* 118:551, 1978.
2. Berg AC, Heidrich FE, Fihn SD, et al: Establishing the cause of genitourinary symptoms in women in a family practice. *JAMA* 251:620, 1984.
2a. Carlson KJ, Mulley AG: Management of acute dysuria. *Ann Intern Med* 102:244, 1985.
3. Dontas AS, Kasviki-Charvati P, Chem L: Bacteriuria and survival in old age. *N Engl J Med* 304:839, 1981.
4. Evans DA, Kass EH, Hinnekens CH, et al: Bacteriuria and subsequent mortality in women. *Lancet* 1:156, 1982.
5. Fair WR, Crane DB, Peterson LJ, et al: Three-day treatment of urinary tract infections. *J Urol* 123:77, 1980.
6. Fairley KF, Bond AG, Brown RB, et al: Simple test to determine the site of urinary tract infections. *Lancet* 2:7513, 1967.

7. Fairley KF, Carson NE, Gutch RC, *et al*: Site of infection in acute urinary tract infection in general practice. *Lancet* 2:615, 1971.

8. Fang LST, Tolkoff-Rubin NE, Rubin RH: Efficacy of single dose and conventional amoxicillin therapy in urinary tract infection localized by the antibody-coated bacterial technique. *N Engl J Med* 298:413, 1978.

9. Hook EW, III, Holmes KK: Gonococcal infections. *Ann Intern Med* 102:229, 1985.

9a. Hooton TM, Running K, Stamm WE: Single-dose therapy for cystitis in woman. *JAMA* 253:387, 1985.

10. Jacobs NF, Kraus SJ: Gonococcal and nongonococcal urethritis in men. *Ann Intern Med* 82:7, 1975.

11. Komaroff AL: Acute dysuria in women. *N Engl J Med* 310:368, 1984.

12. Kunin CM: Duration of treatment of urinary tract infections. *Am J Med* 71:841, 1981.

13. McGuckin M, Cohen L, McGregor RR: Significance of pyuria in urinary sediment. *J Urol* 120:452, 1978.

14. Mears EM Jr: Prostatitis. *Kidney Int* 20:289, 1981.

15. Pollock HM: Laboratory techniques for detection of urinary tract infection and assessment of value. *Am J Med* 75:79, 1983.

16. Ronald AR, Boutros P, Mourtada H: Bacteriuria localization and response to single-dose therapy in women. *JAMA* 235:1854, 1976.

17. Rumans LW, Vosti KL: The relationship of antibody-coated bacteria to clinical syndromes. *Arch Intern Med* 138:1077, 1978.

18. Sheehan G, Harding GKM, Roland AR: Advances in the treatment of urinary tract infection. *Am J Med* 76:141, 1984.

19. Sobel JD, Kaye D: Host factors in the pathogenesis of urinary tract infection. *Am J Med* 75:122, 1984.

20. Stamey TA, Cindy M, Mihara G: Prophylactic efficacy of nitrofurantoin macrocrystals and trimethoprim-sulfamethoxazole in urinary tract infections. *N Engl J Med* 296:780, 1977.

21. Stamm WE, Wagner KF, Ansel RL, *et al*: Causes of the acute urethral syndrome in women. *N Engl J Med* 303:409, 1980.

22. Stamm WE, Counts GW, Running KR, *et al*: Diagnosis of coliform infection in acutely dysuric women. *N Engl J Med* 307:463, 1982.

23. Stamm WE, Counts GW, Wagner KF, *et al*: Antimicrobial prophylaxis of recurrent tract infections. *Ann Intern Med* 92:770, 1980.

24. Stamm WE, Koutsky LA, Benedett JK, *et al*: *Chlamydia trachomatis* urethral infection in men. *Ann Intern Med* 100:47, 1984.

25. Swartz SL, Kraus SJ, Hermann KL, *et al*: Diagnosis,and etiology of nongonorrhea urethritis. *J Infect Dis* 138:445, 1978.

26. Treatment of urinary tract infections *Med Lett* 23:69, 1981.

27. Whelton A, Walker WG: An approach to the interpretation of drug concentrations in the kidney. *Johns Hopkins Med J* 142:8, 1978.

28. Wong ES, McKevitt M, Running K, *et al*: Management of recurrent urinary tract infections with patient-administered single-dose therapy. *Ann Intern Med* 102:302; 1985.

CHAPTER TWENTY-EIGHT

Respiratory Infections

FREDERICK KOSTER, M.D.

UPPER RESPIRATORY INFECTIONS

Magnitude of the Problem

Upper respiratory infections (URI) are the most common acute illnesses in the United States and the industrialized world. Although these infections are the most common causes of absences from school or work, the vast majority are self-diagnosed and self-treated and do not come to the attention of a physician (Americans spend $500 to $700 million annually for over-the-counter medications for the relief of upper respiratory symptoms). However, 6% of visits to office-based internists are for URI complaints (cough, sore throat, or cold—see Chapter 1 Table 1.2).

Principal Syndromes

The Common Cold

The common cold is a mild, self-limited syndrome caused by viral infection of the upper respiratory tract mucosa and characterized by one or more of the following symptoms: nasal discharge and obstruction, sneezing, sore throat, cough, and hoarseness.

Epidemiology and Transmission

The common cold syndrome is caused by a variety of viruses that are clinically indistinguishable from each other, yet have distinct seasonal peaks for unknown reasons. Rhinoviruses constitute the etiological agent in 25 to 30% of colds, with seasonal peaks in early fall and mid to late spring. Coronaviruses account for another 10 to 15% of annual colds, with a seasonal peak in midwinter. Influenza, parainfluenza, respiratory syncytial viruses, and adenovirus are etiological agents for another 10 to 15%, although this group more commonly presents with the typical influenza syndrome as discussed below.

The incidence of the common cold syndrome decreases with age. On the average, adults have two to four colds per year; children have six to eight (14). Since person-to-person spread of colds occurs mainly in the home and at school, school children usually serve as carriers for introducing colds into the family. Thus mothers tend to have higher secondary attack rates than do fathers. Transmission of rhinovirus is most efficient by direct physical contact (15). Frequent, unconscious touching of virus-contaminated nasal mucosa contaminates the subject's hands. Infectious material can survive on the hand for as long as 4 hours, during which time hand-to-hand contact with susceptible subjects serves to transmit the virus. Exposure to susceptible subjects across even short distances of air is an inefficient method of transmission of rhinoviruses, although aerosol transmission of particles effectively transmits some viruses (e.g., Coxsackie, influenza, and adenovirus). Thus transmission of colds may be low even in congested offices, theaters, buses, etc if hand-to-hand contact is avoided.

Clinical Characteristics

The correct diagnosis of the common cold is readily made by the patient. After an incubation period of 48 to 72 hours, the syndrome begins with mild malaise, rhinorrhea, sneezing, scratchy throat, and variable loss of taste and smell. These symptoms increase to maximum severity on the second to fourth day. Viral excretion and communicability are maximal during the period of severest symptoms. Fever is usually not present but, if present, rarely exceeds 1°F (0.5°C) elevation. Cough and hoarseness may begin later, and their severity and duration are increased in cigarette smokers. Conversely, neither cigarette smoking nor exposure to cold appears to increase the attack rate of colds. Rhinovirus colds usually last 1 week but in one-quarter of cases last up to 2 weeks.

Identification of the causative virus by clinical observation is not possible, nor is it necessary for management. The primary challenge for the physician is to identify the cases with complicating secondary bacterial sinusitis (see below) and otitis media (see Chapter 96), for whom antimicrobials will be beneficial. The physical examination should therefore include the pharynx, nasal cavity, ears, and sinuses. The value of sinus transillumination and radiography, pneumatic otoscopy, and throat culture is discussed in sections on sinusitis (page 353), otitis (Chapter 96), and pharyngitis (page 351), respectively.

Treatment

Most patients with typical URI syndromes can be assessed and managed on the basis of a telephone contact. In view of the absence of specific antiviral therapy for the uncomplicated common cold, symptomatic treatment is the only treatment available. Aspirin is the best drug for relief of fever and myalgias, but it may increase viral excretion, a finding of unknown epidemiological significance (25). Bed rest is not necessary to facilitate recovery. Steam or cool mist helps to liquefy secretions. Sipping hot chicken soup (the only soup studied) increases the clearance of nasal mucus, although it is not clear whether the benefit of this timeless remedy is mediated exclusively through inhaling water vapor or through an additional effect of an aromatic compound (24). There is no symptomatic remedy for hoarseness, which is due to inflammation and edema of the vocal cords; the patient should, however, be advised to rest his voice as this may shorten recovery time.

Nasal congestion is best relieved by *topical decongestants*; sprays rather than drops are preferred for ease of administration. Most over-the-counter short acting (3 to 4 hours) sprays contain 0.5% phenylephrine; some patients prefer the milder effect of 0.25% phenylephrine (sold as Neo-Synephrine). Longer acting topical decongestants (8 to 10 hours) are 0.1% xylometazoline (Otrivin) or 0.05% oxymetazoline (Afrin); they may occasionally produce a stinging sensation when first used. Patients should be cautioned against using drops or sprays for more than 5 days to avoid the rebound effect, defined as an increase in nasal congestion when decongestant medication is discontinued. In contrast to orally administered decongestants, there has not been a blood pressure-elevating effect reported with topical decongestants. (See additional discussion of topical decongestants in Chapter 23).

Oral Decongestants

Phenylpropanolamine (contained in a large number of over-the-counter products) and pseudoephedrine (Sudafed, 30 mg over-the-counter or 60 mg by prescription; also available as Sudafed S.A., a sustained-action preparation containing 120 mg of pseudoephedrine, taken every 12 hours) are somewhat helpful but must be used judiciously because they may cause elevation of blood pressure.

Antihistamines have a marginal effect in attenuating cold symptoms (18). The combination of decongestant and antihistamine, while often helpful in allergic rhinitis (see Chapter 23), is a more expensive, less effective alternative to topical decongestants; this is also true of the many cold remedies containing antihistamines, decongestants, analgesics, caffeine, and a variety of other ingredients (21).

A large number of over-the-counter *cough* remedies are available. These contain various combination of cough suppressants, expectorants, decongestants, analgesics, and alcohol (22). There is no evidence that any expectorant is effective in URIs and it is more rational and far less expensive to utilize the other ingredients individually in appropriate doses (see additional discussion of cough suppressants below, page 357).

Antimicrobials are useless in the uncomplicated cold.

Patient Education

Since transmission of colds occurs chiefly by physical contact, it is reasonable to counsel patients and those around them that transmission can be minimized by handwashing, reduced finger-to-nose contact, and reduced exposure to the cold sufferer. Physicians should be particularly vigilant to avoid contact with the patient's secretions and should wash their hands carefully after examining the infected patient. Although physicians with common colds may examine patients if they wash their hands and avoid sneezing on the patient, physicians with the flu syndrome should avoid patient contact (see below).

Viral upper respiratory infections may be complicated by superimposed bacterial sinusitis, otitis media, or pneumonitis. Therefore, patients should be advised to notify their physician of any symptoms suggesting one of these syndromes, each of which requires antimicrobial treatment (see details below).

Prevention

Prophylactic and therapeutic properties of large doses of *vitamin C* have been examined in a number of trials, and no consistent beneficial effect has been found (4). In those studies suggesting a benefit, the placebo effect could not be excluded since subjects could identify the vitamin C capsule by taste. In doses above 4 g/day, vitamin C may cause diarrhea and has the potential of precipitating urate, oxalate, and cystine stones in susceptible individuals. Other uncommon effects include diminishing the anticoagulant effect of warfarin, and confusing urine glucose tests, causing a false negative glucose oxidase (Dextrostix, Tes-Tape) or a false positive copper reduction test (Clinitest tablets).

It is unlikely that vaccines will ever play a role in preventing the common cold, especially since at least 89 different serotypes of rhinoviruses have been confirmed and since infection occurs despite the presence of specific serum antibody.

Flu Syndrome

Although there is considerable overlap in the two syndromes, the flu syndrome is sufficiently distinct from the common cold syndrome, especially in terms of potential complications, that the two are discussed separately. Flu presents as the abrupt onset of malaise, myalgia, headache, and fever, and substantial morbidity (including prostration in severe cases) persists for 1 to 2 weeks. As many as 85% of cases of flu syndrome may be due to the influenza virus during an epidemic (13). Other viruses, especially parainfluenza, respiratory syncytial, and adenovirus, are agents that produce the same clinical syndrome.

Epidemiology

Epidemic spread of the influenza virus is a function of the appearance of new antigenic variations of the virus in nonimmune populations. Antigenic variations occur almost annually in influenza serotype A, whereas variation occurs much less frequently in influenza B. Major variation is called antigenic shift and results in *pandemic spread* of a new strain, almost always type A, throughout regions of the world where there is little natural immunity. The most recent pandemics were in the winters of 1957–1958, 1968–1969, and 1977–1978, and they varied considerably in severity. In between pandemics, minor antigenic variations occur frequently, resulting in nearly annual epidemics during the winter months. Such *interpandemic spread*, although less dramatic, occurs frequently and therefore accounts for greater cumulative morbidity and mortality than pandemic spread. In some years there are no influenza epidemics, for example in the winters of 1976–1977 and 1978–1979, as measured by excess mortality due to pneumonia or influenza reported to the Centers for Disease Control (Fig. 28.1). Although it is often not possible clinically to separate infections due to type A or B, influenza A is responsible for greater excess mortality than type B.

Influenza virus appears to be transmitted by virus-containing small particle aerosols dispersed by sneezing, coughing, or talking. The incubation period is 18 to 72 hours. Viral shedding persists for 5 to 10 days, but virus is present in high titer in secretions for only 48 hours after the onset of clinical illness. In the community, person-to-person transmission is rapid, with spread initially among children, then adults. In local epidemics the incidence of cases reaches a peak in 2 to 3 weeks and persists for only 5 to 6 weeks.

Clinical Characteristics

Uncomplicated influenza, type A or type B, has an abrupt onset of systemic symptoms including fever, chills, headache, myalgias, and malaise. The fever, which may rise to 106°F (41°C) in some cases, typically lasts 3 days, although frequently it persists

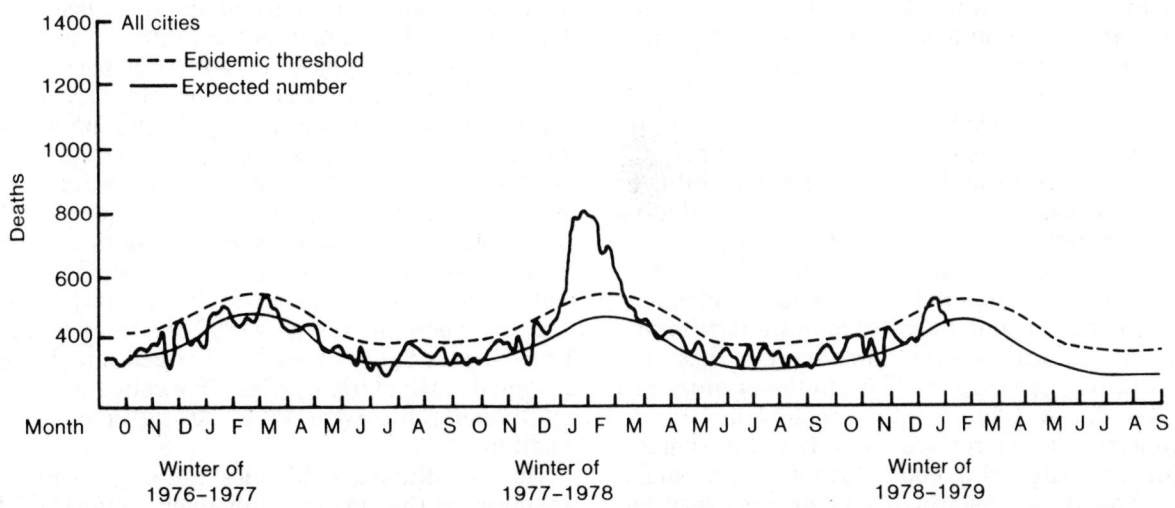

Figure 28.1. Reported pneumonia-influenza deaths in 121 US cities, September 1976 to August 1979. (From *Morbidity and Mortality Weekly Report*, vol 28, no. 54, September 1980.)

for 5 to 7 days. Headache and myalgias, involving the back, arms, legs, and, occasionally, the eyes, are the predominant symptoms, persisting as long as the fever. Respiratory symptoms, such as cough, nasal discharge, hoarseness, and sore throat, appear as systemic symptoms wane. Cough and weakness may persist for 2 or more weeks.

Physical findings include general toxicity, flushed face, hot skin, watery red eyes, clear nasal discharge, tender cervical lymph nodes, and, occasionally, localized rales in the chest. The white cell count and differential count usually demonstrate mild neutropenia and relative lymphocytosis, due to absolute granulocytopenia.

Treatment

One antiviral agent, *amantadine* (Symmetrel), is approved for treatment of type A influenza infections. Amantadine attenuates clinical disease in all patients with influenza A by reducing the fever by 50% and by shortening the duration of illness by 1 or 2 days; these benefits are seen only if the drug is administered within 24 to 48 hours of onset of illness. Side effects, which include insomnia, nervousness, dizziness, and difficulty in concentrating, occur in about 7% of adults, appear a few hours after the first dose, tend to diminish after repeated doses, and disappear upon discontinuation of the drug. The cost of a therapeutic course (200-mg loading dose followed by 100 mg twice a day for 5 days) is approximately $5, in contrast to the more costly prophylactic course (7) discussed in Chapter 32. Treatment with amantadine should be seriously considered for patients at high risk of morbidity and mortality who develop an influenza-like illness in a community where the state or local health department has reported influenza A. Groups at high risk include

1. Unvaccinated children and adults with chronic diseases including pulmonary, cardiovascular, metabolic neuromuscular, or immunodeficiency diseases;

2. Adults whose activities are vital to community function, including selected hospital personnel;

3. Patients with life-threatening primary influenzal pneumonia, although the efficacy of amantadine in such patients has not been demonstrated.

Because of the side effects, only partial effectiveness, difficulty of identifying influenza A infections in the individual, and difficulty in initiating therapy early in clinical illness, amantadine has not achieved widespread use. The physician must balance benefits and side effects in each case.

Supportive measures are important for symptomatic relief. Bed rest and adequate fluid intake should be advised. Aspirin, 600 to 900 mg every 3 to 4 hours, or acetaminophen if aspirin is contraindicated, reduces headache, fever, and myalgia. Sponging with tepid water is effective in lowering high fever, whereas sponging with isopropyl alcohol only

increases the patient's discomfort. Relief of nasal discharge may be obtained by agents discussed in the section on the common cold (page 348). Relief of cough with cough suppressants is discussed in the section on acute bronchitis (page 357).

Complications

Patients should be advised that dyspnea, hemoptysis, wheezing, purulent sputum, fever persisting more than 7 days, and rarely, dark urine, severe muscle pain and tenderness, herald complications that demand prompt medical attention and usually hospitalization.

Pulmonary complications exhibit a continuous spectrum of severity, from mild airway hyperreactivity without pulmonary infiltrates, to segmental influenza pneumonia or secondary bacterial pneumonia, to fulminant bilateral influenza pneumonia with the adult respiratory distress syndrome (ARDS).

Airway hyperreactivity is most common after influenza, but may occur in less severe form following many viral upper respiratory infections (16). It appears to be caused by destruction of epithelial cells secondary to viral invasion and may result from heightened sensitization of afferent cholinergic irritant receptors in the respiratory mucosa. Exposure to inhaled irritants induces a vagally mediated increase in airway resistance, manifested clinically by bronchospasm, coughing, or both; cough may also be due to direct stimulation of cholinergic irritant receptors as these are the receptors which mediate the cough reflex (for additional details, see Chapter 53). Patients with asthma or chronic bronchitis have even greater bronchoconstrictor responses because of their underlying bronchial smooth muscle hyperreactivity. Airway hyperreactivity can be demonstrated for 3 to 8 weeks after influenza and other viral infections, and occasionally it may last for 4 to 6 months even in nonatopic patients.

The relationship between airway hyperreactivity and *persistent symptoms following influenza* is not entirely clear; however, it is likely that nonproductive cough, wheezing, and dyspnea on exertion are related to airway hyperreactivity. These postflu symptoms seem to be particularly common in urban areas during periods of high air pollution. Chest roentgenograms are clear. Both cough and wheezing, following an otherwise uncomplicated flu-like infection, may be treated with a trial of a bronchodilator (see Chapter 55) as needed and at bedtime. Patients troubled particularly by nighttime cough will obtain additional relief with 15 to 30 mg of codeine at bedtime.

During influenza epidemics, there is a 2- to 3-fold increase in the incidence of *pneumonia* (12). The incidence of postinfluenzal bronchitis and pneumonia varies with age: low (5%) below age 50 and very high (60 to 70%) over age 70. Mortality from pneumonia during influenza epidemics clearly increases for those with chronic pulmonary disease and congestive heart failure.

Primary influenza viral pneumonia is a rare complication occurring predominantly among persons with cardiovascular disease, but occasionally in healthy young adults. After several days of typical influenzal symptoms, fever, cough, and dyspnea rapidly progress to cyanosis and delirium, often developing into adult respiratory distress syndrome. Immediate hospitalization and intensive care are required, but mortality remains high.

Milder influenza pneumonia may be restricted to a single lobe. Patients present with persistent fever, cough and dyspnea, localized rales, normal white blood cell count, and subsequently experience a benign course.

Secondary bacterial pneumonia and bronchitis complicate up to 10% of influenza A illness, depending on age group and chronic pulmonary or cardiac disease. Pneumonia complications of influenza B are less common but are becoming increasingly recognized (1). The presentation is typically biphasic: the initial influenzal illness is followed by several days of clinical improvement, and then there is an exacerbation of fever with production of purulent or bloody sputum. The predominant bacterial pathogen is *Streptococcus pneumoniae*, but *Haemophilus influenzae* and *Staphylococcus aureus* are also common; the last mentioned has a mortality rate of approximately 50% in this setting. The diagnosis and management of pneumonia are discussed below (pages 359–362).

Nonpulmonary complications of influenza are unusual. Myositis, with thigh pain and inability to walk, occurs occasionally in children and adolescents. Severe myositis with myoglobinuria and acute renal failure has been observed in adults after both influenza A and B. Guillain-Barré syndrome, encephalitis, and transverse myelitis are neurological complications associated with influenza A, and rarely B, infection, but no firm causal relationship has been established. Reye's syndrome, on the other hand, is a rare but severe complication of influenza, usually type B, presenting as a change in mental status and progressing to coma and hepatic failure. Although the mean age of attack is 6 years, occasional cases of Reye's syndrome have occurred in adolescents. With the exception of mild myositis, all of the nonpulmonary complications of influenza require hospitalization for differential diagnosis and management.

Prevention

The use of influenza vaccine and amantadine prophylaxis in ambulatory practice are discussed in Chapter 32.

Pharyngitis

Sore throat is the fourth most common symptom seen in medical practice (5). The physician's most important task in the evaluation of pharyngitis is to identify and treat group A streptococcal infections in adults, especially those with a history of prior rheumatic fever, and to recognize less common causes of pharyngitis associated with more serious systemic illness.

Nonexudative pharyngitis is usually due to rhinovirus, coronavirus, and respiratory syncytical, parainfluenza, and influenza viruses. In addition, serological evidence for infection with *Chlamydia trachomatis* and *Mycoplasma pneumoniae* has been found in 20% and 10%, respectively, of adults with pharyngitis (20). *Exudative pharyngitis* is seen in some or most patients with infection due to group A β-hemolytic streptococcus, mixed anaerobic infections, *Neisseria gonorrheae*, adenovirus, herpes simplex, and Epstein-Barr virus (infectious mononucleosis). In addition, diphtheria may present early as a simple exudative pharyngitis before pseudomembrane formation, but sore throat is usually not the presenting complaint. Pharyngeal gonorrhea, usually asymptomatic but occasionally exudative and associated with cervical adenitis, is common in partners practicing orogenital sex and may be particularly common in pregnant women. Infectious mononucleosis (see Chapter 52) is characterized by the clinical triad of sore throat, fever, and lymphadenopathy with or without mild tenderness; it can be distinguished with certainty from streptococcal infection on clinical grounds only when hepatosplenomegaly and a maculopapular skin rash (similar to a drug eruption or rubella) are present. Palatal petechiae may be seen in mononucleosis but may also occur with rubella and streptococcal pharyngitis. Pharyngoconjunctival fever is usually accompanied by influenza-like symptoms and can be distinguished by concurrent conjunctivitis in one-third of cases and a history of swimming pool exposure 1 week prior to onset. Herpes simplex, Coxsachie virus A, herpangina and aphthous stomatitis are distinguished by the presence of mucosal vesicles or ulcers (see additional details in Chapter 101).

Diagnosis, Management, and Course

1. GROUP A STREPTOCOCCAL PHARYNGITIS. The incubation period is 2 to 4 days, followed by the abrupt onset of sore throat, malaise, fever, and headache. The "classic syndrome," including tender tonsillar lymph nodes (at angle of jaw), grayish-white exudate on the tonsils, and red soft palate with petechiae, occurs in a minority of cases of streptococcal pharyngitis and may occur in other types of pharyngitis as well. In fact the only clinical feature distinctive of group A streptococcal infection is a rare scarlatiniform rash (*scarlet fever*), characterized by a diffuse red blush appearing on the trunk early in the disease, spreading centrifugally, blanching with pressure, and acquiring a "sandpaper" texture. One week later the skin desquamates in large sheets, particularly over the palms and soles.

Because clinical findings are not specific, the diagnosis of streptococcal pharyngitis requires a throat culture. Office throat culture kits are inexpensive and offer rapid diagnosis and high sensitivity (approximately 95%). Although the technique may appear simple, some physicians use inadequate plating technique, leading to false negatives. The correct procedures are simple. The tonsillar tissue and posterior pharynx are swabbed; the swab is then rubbed on about one-sixth of a blood agar plate and subsequently streaked with a sterile wire loop. The agar is stabbed several times with the loop to enable recognition of subsurface hemolysis. A bacitracin disc is applied and the plate incubated at 37°C for 18 to 24 hours. With a little practice, the physician can readily recognize β-hemolytic colonies, estimate the number, and recognize the inhibition of their growth by the bacitracin disc if they belong to group A. Many physicians prefer to send throat swabs or transport media to state or regional laboratories. Rapid diagnosis using Gram stain of pharyngeal swab material yields variable results even with skilled observers and is thus not recommended.

The standard approach is to make culture studies of all febrile patients with pharyngitis and to treat subsequently only those patients found to be positive for group A streptococcus. If cultures are made from only febrile patients, less than 10% of cases with streptococcal infection will be missed and only 30% of all patients with sore throats will be cultured (10). All patients with a history of rheumatic fever must be tested by culture whether or not fever is present. Although some positive cultures will represent asymptomatic carriage, it is best to assume that all positive cultures are significant in these patients and to treat accordingly.

In three situations in which group A streptococcus is suspected, antibiotic treatment should be started before throat culture results are known: (a) patients with a past history of rheumatic fever not currently on prophylaxis, (b) young patients with a strong family history of rheumatic fever, and (c) all cases of pharyngitis in an explosive epidemic in semi-closed populations. Local health authorities should be notified immediately in this situation.

Symptomatic *family contacts* of patients with streptococcal pharyngitis as well as asymptomatic contacts in families with a history of rheumatic fever or in poor families living in crowded conditions should have cultures made and should be treated if the cultures are positive. It is not clear whether asymptomatic contacts in families living in uncrowded conditions should be tested by culture.

In adults over the age of 15 without a prior history of acute rheumatic fever (ARF), first attacks of ARF are extremely rare. Therefore the principal goals of treatment for streptococcal pharyngitis in such adults are the amelioration of symptoms, the prevention of local suppurative complications, and the prevention of spread. Since early therapy (in the first 2 days) is required for symptomatic relief, most physicians do not wait for culture results in patients with severe pharyngitis. In untreated patients, fever, malaise and sore throat are self-limited, abating in 3 to 5 days; early treatment may reduce modestly the duration and severity of these symptoms. In patients being treated to prevent recurrence of ARF, therapy within 7 days of onset of pharyngitis is sufficient. The mean latent period of ARF is 19 days, with a range of 1 to 5 weeks.

The preferred therapy for streptococcal pharyngitis is parenteral benzathine penicillin, 1.2 million units given once, because it obviates noncompliance. If oral therapy is given, the recommended regimen is penicillin V, 250 mg three times a day for 10 days. For patients allergic to penicillin, erythromycin, 250 mg every 6 hours for 10 days, is recommended (see practical information about antimicrobials, Table 28.3, page 362).

2. GONOCOCCAL PHARYNGITIS. Gonococcal pharyngitis is diagnosed by throat culture. Special culture techniques should be used to detect gonorrhea in specimens from patients practicing orogenital sex. Gram stain of direct pharyngeal smear is insensitive and nonspecific. Calcium alginate swabs should be used, as ordinary cotton swabs contain inhibitory fatty acids. The swab should be immediately plated on a modified Thayer-Martin medium that is incorporated in a number of inexpensive kits for office culture. For throat cultures, however, N. gonorrhoeae must be distinguished from *Neisseria meningitidis* and *Neisseria lactamicus* by carbohydrate fermentation and serology; therefore, cultures should be sent to state or regional laboratories. Effective treatment is either procaine penicillin G, 4.8 million units, divided between two intramuscular sites, plus 1.0 g of oral probenecid, or tetracycline in a 1.5-g loading dose followed by 0.5 g four times daily for 4 days. Ampicillin and spectinomycin are associated with unacceptable failure rates in the treatment of pharyngeal gonorrhea. A follow-up culture 7 days after completion of therapy should be done as a test of cure.

Chapters 27 and 94 discuss in detail sexually transmitted infections, in men and women, respectively.

3. DIPHTHERIA. This diagnosis should be suspected when there is a grayish membrane in the anterior nares, or on the tonsils, uvula, or larynx (infectious mononucleosis and "strep throat" display a creamy white exudate and do not involve the uvula). Treatment must begin before bacteriological confirmation and requires hospitalization for bed rest, close observation, antitoxin, and penicillin. Management of contacts is discussed in Chapter 32.

4. OTHER BACTERIA. Throat cultures often grow pneumococci, staphylococci, groups B, C, and G streptococci, and various Gram-negative enterobacteria. These species colonizing the pharynx have only rarely been shown to be etiological agents in

pharyngitis, and patients who harbor them should not be treated with antimicrobial agents.

5. VINCENTS' ANGINA. This is an anaerobic infection of the pharynx characterized by fever, tender lymphadenitis, a large grayish-brown pseudomembrane in the pharynx and very foul odor. It is a complication of acute necrotizing ulcerative gingivitis, which is described in Chapter 101. Hospitalization for antimicrobial treatment with penicillin or tetracycline is the appropriate managment plan.

Chronic or Relapsing Sore Throat

Some patients will describe a sore throat of several week's duration at their first visit. Others will have either a prolonged course following an illness which began as a typical acute pharyngitis syndrome or frequent recurrence of sore throats. The conditions which may cause prolonged and/or recurrent pharyngitis are listed in Table 28.1. Most are discussed in more detail elsewhere in the book as indicated in the table. One problem, "*chronic tonsillitis*," often related to recurrent streptococcal pharyngitis, may be alleviated best by tonsillectomy. The clinical diagnosis of chronic tonsillitis is made in patients with recurrent sore throats (several in the same year), very large tonsils, and chronically enlarged, periodically tender lymph nodes (6).

Acute Sinusitis

This is a bacterial infection of one or more paranasal sinuses which complicates about 0.5% of viral upper respiratory infections. Sinusitis may also be a complication of noninfectious rhinitis, polyps, foreign bodies, or anatomical nasal obstruction of sinus drainage. Up to 10% of cases of acute sinusitis are an extension of dental abscess. Nursing home or homebound patients with nasogastric tubes occasionally have occult sinusitis as a cause of persistent fever.

Diagnosis

Acute sinusitis in the autumn, winter, and spring usually develops during the course of a viral upper respiratory infection. Sinusitis in the summer often is associated with swimming and diving or with allergic rhinitis (see Chapter 23).

The *pain* of sinusitis is due to periosteal reaction secondary to an expanding purulent inflammation behind an outlet obstruction. The pain is dull in the early stages, but becomes throbbing in later stages. Coughing, dependency, and percussion over the involved sinus exacerbate the pain. Percussion of the teeth is often painful in maxillary sinusitis. The facial pain associated with the noninfectious causes of nasal congestion (see Chapter 23) may resemble the early pain of acute sinusitis, but it is less localized and does not become progressively worse. Other causes of facial pain to be distinguished from sinusitis are dental abscess (Chapter 101), migraine, cluster headache, and trigeminal neuralgia (Chapter 79) (27).

Nontender edema of the eyelids, seen predominantly in children, may occur with uncomplicated ethmoid and maxillary sinusitis. Acute sinusitis may present without pain as in subacute sinusitis (see below), usually in the guise of a cold persisting for more than 2 weeks and accompanied by cough due to postnasal drip, purulent nasal discharge, and headache.

Examination should include the pharynx, nose, ears, and teeth. Transillumination can be a helpful office procedure. In a completely darkened room a small strong light (an ordinary flashlight is not sufficient) is placed under the supraorbital ridges to illuminate the frontal sinuses and through the patient's pursed lips to illuminate the maxillary sinuses. Complete opacification is strong evidence for infection. Complete light transmission rules out active infection. Usually, diminished light transmission is seen; one-quarter of this group of patients will have active infection. Proper interpretation of transillumination findings requires training, preferably in cooperation with an otolaryngologist.

Radiological examination of the sinuses, comprising four views to visualize all paranasal sinuses, is the most sensitive diagnostic test in acute sinusitis. Figure 28.2 shows the typical radiological changes seen in acute maxillary sinusitis. X-rays are not

Table 28.1.
Causes of Chronic or Relapsing Sore Throat

Primary Site of Pain	Condition	See for Details
Pharynx	Chronic tonsillitis	
	Smoking (especially marijuana)	Chapters 20, 22
	Postnasal drip	Chapter 53
	Infectious mononucleosis	Chapter 52
	Agranulocytosis	
	Acute leukemia	
	Pemphigus	
Not the Pharynx	Subacute thyroiditis	Chapter 73
	Angina (radiating to neck)	Chapter 57
	Psychogenic	Chapter 12

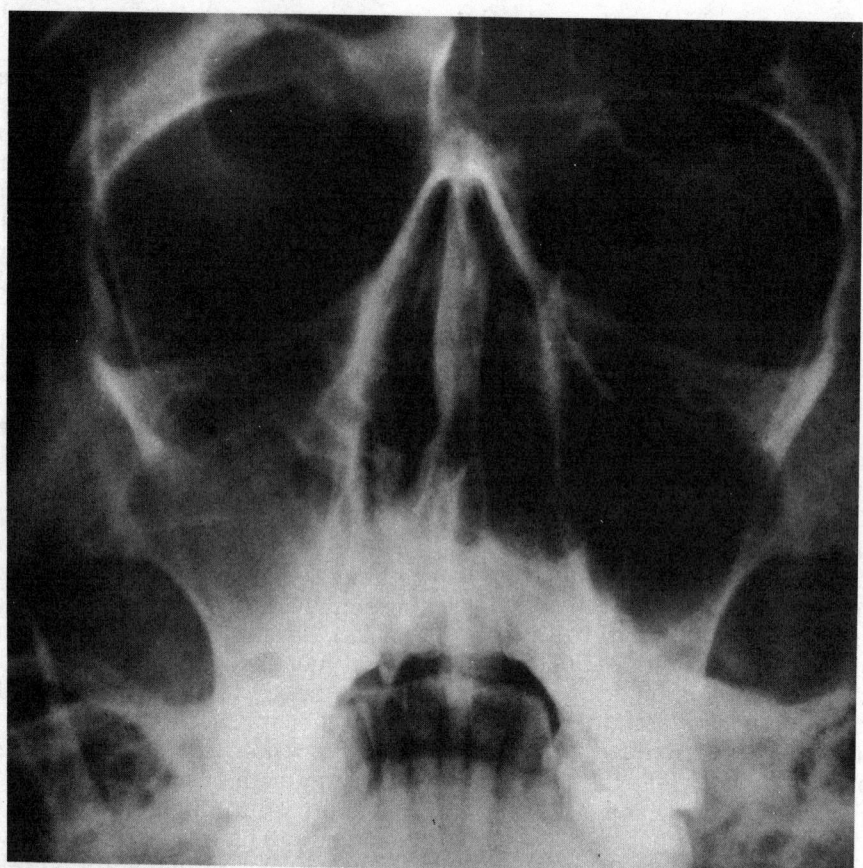

Figure 28.2. Acute infectious maxillary sinusitis. Waters' view shows complete opacity of the right maxillary sinus caused by thickening of the lining mucosa and/or fluid accumulation. The mucoperiosteal line is preserved. The left maxillary sinus is normal in appearance.

necessary in patients with typical signs and symptoms. It is most helpful in the diagnostic workup of headache and in those patients who do not respond to therapy or who are toxic and require accurate diagnosis early.

Most cases of acute sinusitis can be treated without culture. Nasopharyngeal swabs are usually contaminated with normal flora and are of no use. Studies employing antral puncture (9) indicate that *S. pneumoniae* and unencapsulated *H. influenzae* are the bacterial agents in 60% of acute infections and probably in most acute exacerbations of chronic sinusitis. Anaerobes, *Streptococcus pyogenes, Neisseria catarrhalis,* α-hemolytic streptococci, and Gram-negative aerobes each cause a small percentage of infections. *S. aureus* causes less than 5% and tends to be associated with pansinusitis and general toxicity.

Management and Course

ANTIMICROBIALS. Ampicillin or amoxicillin provides the best coverage of the most common bacterial pathogens, in a dose of 250 to 500 mg, four times daily for 10 days. In penicillin-allergic patients, trimethoprim-sulfamethoxazole, 2 tablets twice a day for 10 days, or erythromycin, 500 mg four times a day for 10 days, is a good alternative (see practical information about antimicrobials, Table 28.3, page 362).

Symptomatic therapy to improve sinus drainage is important. A decongestant spray, such as Neo-Synephrine 0.25 or 0.5%, is most convenient, administered as an initial squirt to decrease congestion in the membranes of the anterior nares, followed 5 to 10 minutes later by a second squirt delivered deeper to the middle meatus. This is repeated every 4 hours for 2 to 4 days and followed by oral decongestants (see details on the common cold, page 348) for an additional 2 weeks. Steam inhalation is often helpful. Pain relief is important, and codeine may be required. Patients who plan to fly, especially in nonpressurized aircraft, should take an oral decongestant before takeoff, supplemented with topical decongestant spray every 4 hours.

Resolution of facial pain, headache, and fever is expected within several days. If no response occurs by this time, referral to an otolaryngologist for radiography, antral puncture, or surgical drainage is advisable. Toxic patients, especially those with frontoethmoid sinusitis, should be referred at initial presentation for hospitalization, drainage, and definitive parenteral antibiotics. Patients whose symptoms worsen during the first 48 hours of vigorous ambulatory therapy should be referred. Many patients with severe facial pain are benefited by early antral puncture for pain relief.

Complications of acute sinusitis are unusual, but present as medical emergencies and consist of direct extension of infection to adjacent orbits, bone, blood vessels, and central nervous system. Nontender periorbital edema represents restriction of orbital venous outflow through congested ethmoid veins, is not associated with decreased visual acuity, and is appropriately managed with vigorous medical therapy. However, tender periorbital swelling, associated with proptosis and chemosis, represents orbital cellulitis and requires immediate referral to an otolaryngologist. Subsequent progression of cellulitis to subperiosteal or orbital abscess, associated with ophthalmoplegia and loss of vision, requires emergency surgical drainage. Osteomyelitis is most often a complication of frontal sinusitis. Cavernous sinus thrombosis should be suspected in the patient with signs of orbital complications plus extreme toxicity. Intracranial extension is rare but life threatening, presenting most commonly as meningitis. Abscesses in the brain and epidural and subdural spaces present more insidiously. Frontal lobe abscess may present as mild headache, low grade fever, malaise, and personality change. In poorly controlled diabetics and immunocompromised hosts rhinocerebral mucormycosis begins in the nose and maxillary sinuses and may be recognized by a black eschar on the nasal turbinates.

Subacute and Chronic Sinusitis

When the symptoms of acute sinusitis, especially pain and fever, subside with therapy, but purulent nasal discharge continues, this stage is called *subacute sinusitis*. Despite persistence of radiological changes, this stage usually resolves after an additional 2 to 3 weeks of conservative management, including antibiotics and oral decongestants.

Chronic sinusitis resists accurate definition, but appears to result from episodes of prolonged, repeated, or inadequately treated acute sinusitis. This results in the loss of normal ciliated epithelial lining of the sinus cavity, which becomes populated by anaerobic and Gram-negative bacteria. Acute exacerbations occur, due primarily to the common organisms of acute sinusitis (*H. influenzae* and *S. pneumoniae*). Chronic sinusitis commonly complicates certain systemic diseases, such as sarcoidosis. Wegener's granulomatosis, and allergic rhinitis with asthma. In allergic rhinitis, control of asthma is often facilitated by treatment of the sinusitis.

Diagnosis and Management

Persistent purulent nasal discharge despite adequate medical therapy is the primary feature of chronic sinusitis. Facial pain and tenderness are minimal or absent. The sinuses transilluminate light poorly. Radiological examination usually reveals clouding of the cavities in some patients, thickening (greater than 5 mm) of the mucosal lining, and bony sclerosis (see Fig. 28.3). For this reason sinus films are of limited value in acute exacerbations superimposed on chronic sinusitis.

Referral to an otolaryngologist for appropriate surgical drainage is recommended. Oral penicillin V or ampicillin is the most appropriate antimicrobial, and clindamycin is a successful alternate.

Pharyngeal Abscess

Occasionally, after several days of symptoms due to an upper respiratory tract infection, the patient will develop a complicating infection of one of the closed compartments adjacent to the pharynx. The most common of these pharyngeal abscesses are peritonsillar abscess and retropharyngeal abscess. When one of these conditions is suspected, the patient should be referred immediately for evaluation and management by an otolaryngologist.

PERITONSILLAR ABSCESS. Patients with this condition develop severe odynophagia; they are not only unable to take liquids, but they may be unable to swallow their own saliva, resulting in early dehydration. The voice acquires a muffled quality, and trismus may be present. Fever, malaise, and systemic toxicity are typical. Dramatic relief may occur if the abscess drains spontaneously before the patient seeks medical attention. On physical examination, there is a swelling of the anterior tonsillar pillar at its superior pole. The involved tonsil itself may or may not be enlarged, but it is displaced medially. This condition is almost always unilateral.

RETROPHARYNGEAL ABSCESS. The symptoms of this condition are similar to those of peritonsillar abscess. In addition, there may be respiratory embarrassment if the process extends inferiorly toward the larynx. Trismus is not common. On examination, a swelling in the posterior oropharynx is readily seen. Lateral soft tissue X-rays of the neck may disclose expansion of the soft tissue density in the posterior pharyngeal space.

MANAGEMENT. Incision and drainage, either using an 18-gauge needle or a surgical blade, is the treatment of choice for both of these conditions. This should be performed by an otolaryngologist or an oral surgeon. Antibiotics and warm saline gargles should follow drainage.

Epiglottitis

Acute epiglottitis is a fulminant, life-threatening, but curable condition. The epiglottis serves as a valve which closes over the proximal portion of the trachea during swallowing, to prevent aspiration. When the epiglottis becomes inflamed, the resultant edema causes it to curl posteriorly and inferiorly, thereby reducing the glottic aperture. Inspiration, which draws it down, further reduces the effective airway.

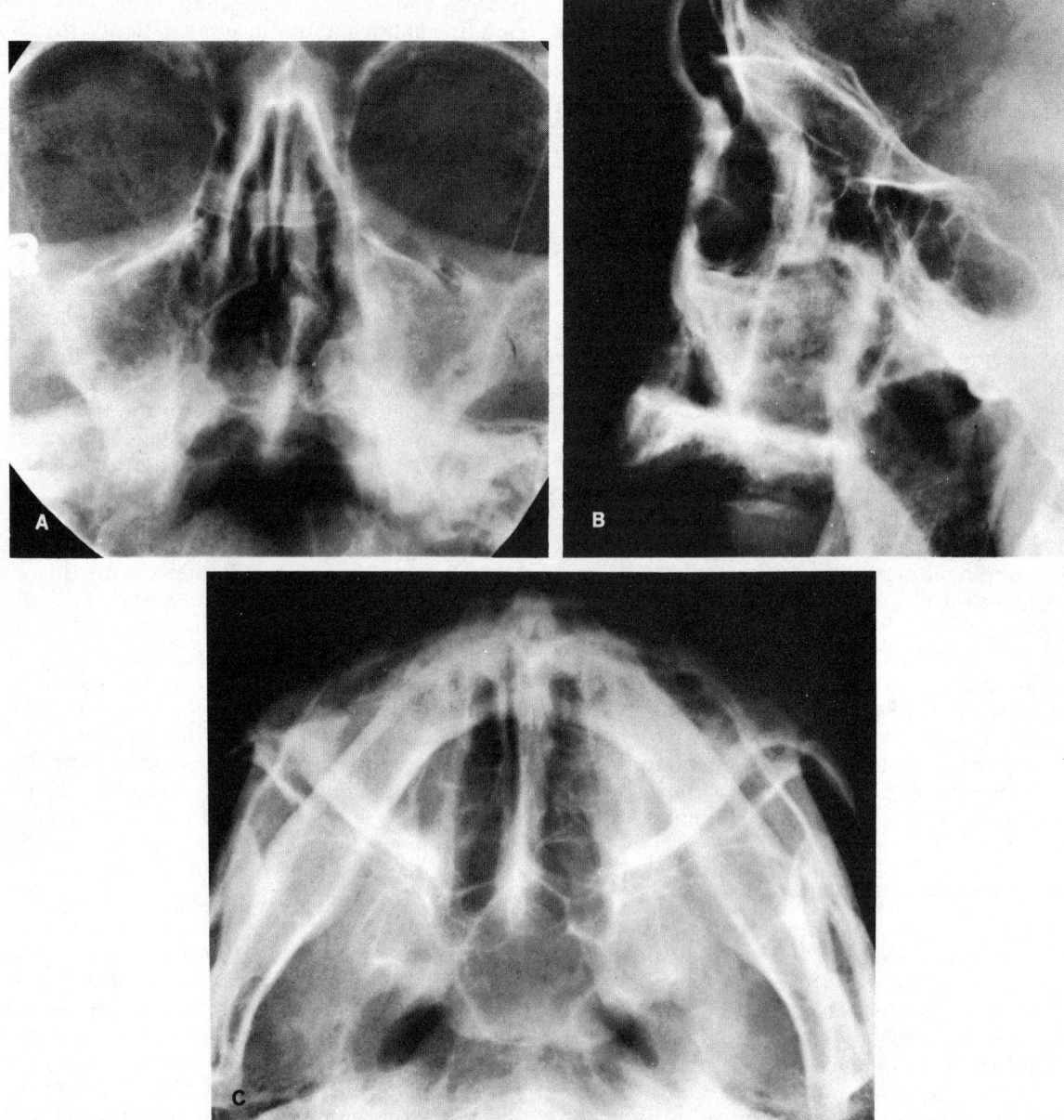

Figure 28.3. Chronic infectious maxillary sinusitis. *A.* Waters' view: marked opacity of the left maxillary sinus and, to a lesser degree, of the right maxillary sinus, with disappearance of mucoperiosteal lines and scle- rosis of the bony walls. *B.* Lateral view: marked bony sclerosis of all of the walls of the maxillary sinuses. *C.* Submentovertical view: marked sclerosis of posterolat- eral walls of the maxillary sinuses.

Epiglottitis is an extremely rare complication of upper respiratory infections. Most cases occur in children, although the condition may occur in adults.

The diagnosis of epiglottitis should be suspected in patients presenting with a sore throat, dysphagia, and progressive respiratory distress, all of short du- ration. On physical examination, stridor may be noted in inspiration. The patients are usually febrile. The oropharynx may be erythematous, but an im- portant clue to the diagnosis is the relatively unin- volved appearance of the oropharynx found in some patients. Soft tissue X-rays of the neck may show edema of the epiglottis and narrowing of the aper- ture. The diagnosis is confirmed by indirect laryn- goscopy which reveals marked edema of the epi- glottis; this procedure must be performed cautiously as it may induce additional obstruction.

Management requires immediate admission to an intensive care unit, where close observation is es- sential since a number of patients with acute epi- glottitis will require emergency tracheotomy.

Telephone Assessment and Self-Care for Upper Respiratory Infection

Most physicians welcome the opportunity to assess URI symptoms initially by phone. The phone assessment should accomplish the following:

1. Differentiate between infectious and allergic problems.

2. Among the patients with acute infections, distinguish those with possible bacterial infections or superinfections who should be examined to decide whether antibiotics should be prescribed.

3. Identify those who may be suffering from complications of a URI that require office evaluation. The following symptoms and signs should be sought: (a) symptoms lasting more than 3 weeks; (b) fever lasting more than 1 week, or associated with delirium; (c) purulent nasal discharge with sinus pain; (d) purulent sputum, chest pain, dyspnea, or hemoptysis; (e) ear pain or discharge; (f) sore throat and a history fo rheumatic fever; (g) the combination of cough and fever over 102°F (39°C) or fever for more than 4 days; (h) hoarseness more than 1 month; (i) pleuritic chest pain; (j) marked odynophagia; (k) the combination of dysphagia, stridor, and difficulty in breathing.

4. For those patients not needing a visit, provide simple instructions for self-care based upon the measures described earlier (see page 348).

Increasing numbers of patients will be consulting self-care algorithms (31). The book *Take Care of Yourself* by Vickery and Fries (see "General References") is one of the most widely distributed collections of algorithms. In one evaluation (3), strict adherence to the algorithms for colds, influenza, cough, and sore throat would have increased the number of patient visits to a physician. Thus, this standard set of instructions exhibited sensitivity, missing few people who need to be examined, yet lacked specificity and led to unnecessary visits. This study points to the need to search for symptom complexes which identify patients likely to be helped by a visit to a physician.

LOWER RESPIRATORY INFECTIONS

Acute Bronchitis

Clinical Characteristics

Acute bronchitis is an inflammatory condition of the tracheobronchial tree that results from respiratory infections with common cold virsuses, influenza, adenovirus, *Mycoplasma pneumoniae*, and rarely *Bordetella pertussis*. The role of secondary bacterial invasion is not clear. The illness is characterized by cough, with or without sputum production, persisting longer than expected (usually 1 to 2 weeks) after the onset of an acute URI.

Rhinovirus and coronavirus, by virtue of their high prevalence, are common etiological agents for mild bronchitis of short duration and without fever. Influenza, adenovirus, and *M. pneumoniae* cause a more severe bronchitis associated with fever and burning substernal pain. Mucoid sputum production develops in half of all cases and is not helpful in distinguishing etiological agents. Frequency and duration of cough are increased in cigarette smokers.

The patient presenting with a cough as the predominant or only respiratory symptom may have pneumonia, bronchitis, or one of a variety of noninfectious conditions associated with persistent cough. Diagnostic efforts should be directed at identifying those patients with pneumonia and with noninfectious causes of cough, leaving acute bronchitis as a diagnosis of exclusion.

The diagnosis of pneumonia is discussed below (page 360). Approaching the patient who has a persistent cough without apparent infectious etiology, the physician should consider the anatomy and physiology of the cough reflex (Chapter 53). Airborne irritants, especially smog containing sulfur dioxide, and allergens cause bronchitic symptoms. Repeated small aspiration of oral and upper airway secretions, especially in the elderly and the alcoholic with incompetent glottic function, is associated with nighttime cough.

Identification of the agent in most episodes of acute bronchitis is not possible. Bacterial cultures of sputum are useless, since the contribution of bacteria to acute bronchitis is unclear and sputum is readily contaminated by nasopharyngeal flora. Culture facilities for viral agents and *M. pneumoniae* are not widely available. *M. pneumoniae* may be implicated if bullous myringitis is observed, or suggested if (a) the patient is a young adult, (b) similar cases are occurring in the family or in the close contacts, and (c) the case occurs in the summer or early fall season. The diagnosis can be confirmed by a 4-fold or greater rise in complement fixation titer in convalescent serum.

Pertussis, rare in adults, is characterized by initial nonspecific symptoms of malaise and rhinorrhea followed by 1 to 4 weeks of severe paroxysms of repetitive coughs without inspiration. The paroxysm is terminated by an inspiratory whoop. The clinical symptoms are attenuated in previously immunized adults and children, who act as reservoirs of infection for nonimmune infants. *B. pertussis* is identified by culture of nasopharyngeal swab on special media, or more rapidly by direct immune fluorescent staining of organisms on smear of nasopharyngeal secretions.

Treatment

It is standard practice to prescribe an antimicrobial such as ampicillin if persistent purulent sputum is associated with acute bronchitis. Only one properly controlled trial has evaluated the efficacy of antibiotic therapy in acute bronchitis in patients without asthma or chronic bronchitis; no difference in time to resolution of symptoms was found between the antibiotic and placebo groups (26). Therefore, more studies must be performed before firm recommendations can be offered. If epidemiological evidence for infection with M. pneumoniae exists (see page 359), a 2-week course of erythromycin, 250 to 500 mg four times a day, or tetracycline, 500 mg four times a day, is indicated. B. pertussis infection is treated with erythromycin (see practical information about antimicrobials, Table 28.3).

Treatment is usually symptomatic. Many patients will have tried an over-the-counter cough suppressant containing dextromethorphan without relief. Cough suppression, primarily to get a good night's sleep, is best obtained with preparations containing codeine, although in titrating up to an effective dose, patients should be warned of problems with drowsiness and constipation (see Chapter 53 for a list of narcotic and non-narcotic cough suppresants and additional details). Except in allergic rhinitis with postnasal drip, antihistamines, present in many combination cough remedies, should be avoided because they dry out secretions. There is no consistent evidence that expectorants or glyceryl guaiacolate alter the course of bronchitis. Maintaining hydration with oral fluids is a reasonable approach to preventing mucous plugs. Inhaled steam and cool mist provide symptomatic relief but fail to deliver water droplets into the smaller airways. Some physicians fear that use of cool mist may contaminate airways with Gram-negative aerobic bacteria that inhabit some home humidifiers and that improperly used steam may cause burns.

Smokers with acute bronchitis should be strongly encouraged to stop smoking at least for the duration of the acute illness. Those smokers with a history of chronic cough before their bronchitis may be more motivated to discontinue smoking permanently in the face of the acute illness. In 50% of those who discontinue smoking, the chronic cough will resolve completely within 1 month. Behavioral approaches to smoking-cessation are described in Chapter 20.

Acute Exacerbations of Chronic Bronchitis

Clinical Characteristics

Respiratory infections contribute to the episodic worsening of cough and increased sputum production in the patient with chronic bronchitis, and they are the most common identifiable causes of death in these patients. Evidence that infections in adulthood play an independent role in the deterioration of pulmonary function is lacking, however (28).

The most important indicator of intercurrent infection is the patient's report of a change in color, consistency, and amount of sputum. Patients who consistently produce purulent sputum most of the time may notice increasing cough, dyspnea, and fatigue. Systemic toxicity with fever and chills is generally absent unless pneumonia is present.

The role of bacteria in acute exacerbations of chronic bronchitis is difficult to assess. The bronchial secretions of patients with chronic bronchitis contain pneumococci, unencapsulated Haemophilus species, and normal pharyngeal flora, which persist through asymptomatic intervals. The development of purulent sputum is not correlated with the presence of one or more specific bacterial species. These bacteria appear de novo during acute exacerbations in only a small percentage of uncolonized patients. Similarly, the acquisition of a new serotype of either pneumococci or encapsulated Haemophilus species is usually not followed by a clinical exacerbation. In summary, a primary role for these bacteria in the pathogenesis of clinical exacerbations remains unclear, and performing Gram stain and a culture of the sputum during acute exacerbations will not provide useful information.

Viruses (influenza, parainfluenza, respiratory syncytial, rhinovirus, and coronavirus) may cause up to 50% of acute infectious exacerbations. M. pneumoniae may be the agent in up to 10% of episodes.

Treatment

Acute exacerbations of chronic bronchitis should always be managed with more vigorous applications of routine therapy for chronic symptoms. Clearance of secretions should be promoted with postural drainage and therapeutic doses of bronchodilators, (see Chapter 55). Cough suppressants and sedatives should be avoided. Smokers should be strongly counseled to discontinue cigarettes at least until their acute symptoms have resolved. As noted above, chronic cough will resolve completely within 1 month in half of those patients who are motivated by an acute illness to discontinue cigarettes permanently.

Antimicrobial prophylaxis is commonly used in the management of chronic bronchitis, but the efficacy of this practice has not been demonstrated convincingly (28). Many studies have suggested that continuous prophylaxis with tetracycline in low doses reduces the frequency of exacerbations during the winter months. The conclusions of most studies, however, do not stand up to rigorous analysis. In addition, there is considerable concern that such widespread use of prophylactic antibiotics without clear effectiveness may promote emergence and dissemination of antibiotic-resistant strains in the community.

Efficacy of *short term antibiotic therapy* given for acute exacerbations is unclear due to the difficulty in assessing therapeutic benefits. For the individual patient, efficacy appears to be based primarily on the patient's reported response to antibiotics during previous exacerbations. A reasonable approach is to provide reliable patients who have three or more acute exacerbations per year with a prescription for tetracycline, 250 mg four times daily for 7 to 14 days. Ampicillin, 250 to 500 mg four times daily, trimethoprim-sulfamethoxazole, 2 tablets twice daily, are alternatives. The patient is instructed to begin the antibiotic within 24 hours of the first sign of a "chest cold," since earlier onset of therapy may be more effective in alleviating symptoms and preventing lost time from work (28). Oral penicillin V and chloramphenicol are not appropriate alternatives, since penicillin is not effective against the *Haemophilus* species; and there are many safer alternatives to chloramphenicol.

Some patients managed at home for acute exacerbations will not improve by any criteria or will deteriorate after self-initiated therapy. The patient should be asked to keep in touch by phone during the acute episode so that symptoms indicating pneumonia will be detected earlier.

Pneumonia

There are over 3,000,000 episodes of pneumonia annually in the United States, responsible for over 30 million days of disability requiring bed rest. With influenza, pneumonia ranks fifth among all diseases as a cause of death and first among infectious diseases (5).

Definition

Bronchitis and pneumonia represent a continuum of lower respiratory infection. Aspirated pathogens including bacteria, mycoplasma, and viruses invade the bronchial epithelium. The extent of involvement of adjacent lung parenchyma determines whether there is an infiltrate on chest roentgenogram. The alveolar inflammation spreads like a grass fire, and the advancing edge of edema and leukocyte infiltration are not radiologically apparent. Patients seen early and those with emphysema and reduced parenchyma may fail to show any infiltrate or may show a patchy infiltrate on their chest film despite the presence of considerable inflammation. Thus the clinical distinction between acute bronchitis and acute pneumonia is often an arbitrary radiological distinction. Early management and the decision for hospitalization must focus on the overall condition of the patient in terms of signs and symptoms of systemic toxicity as well as of localized pulmonary infection.

The clinical presentation of pneumonia can be divided into two categories: "bacterial pneumonias" and "atypical pneumonias." "Atypical" historically referred to cold hemagglutinin-positive pneumonias, which have more recently been identified as being due to *M. pneumoniae*. Atypical pneumonias due to a variety of other viral, bacterial, and chlamydial agents may be clinically indistinguishable from mycoplasmal pneumonia until definitive diagnostic studies are done. The usefulness in separating "bacterial" from "atypical" pneumonia lies in predicting outcome and need for hospitalization, at the time of initial presentation in the office. Thus only a small proportion of patients with mycoplas-

mal and viral pneumonia require hospitalization, whereas probably 80 to 90% of patients with pneumococcal and other bacterial pneumonias require hospitalization. The following discussion is restricted to the recognition of patients requiring hospitalization for pneumonia and to the ambulatory management of patients with pneumonia who do not require hospitalization. Chapter 31 describes the posthospital management of lung abscess, a complication of pneumonia which may require prolonged antimicrobial treatment.

Pneumonia Syndromes

Bacterial Pneumonia

Bacterial pneumonias comprise half of all adult pneumonias, and 60 to 90% of these are due to *S. pneumoniae*. Pneumococcal pneumonia may occur in a previously healthy adult, or following an upper respiratory infection, usually with the abrupt onset of shaking chills, fever, pleuritic chest pain, and cough productive of purulent or rusty sputum. In the setting of compromised pulmonary clearance of secretions (depressed consciousness, morbid obesity, abdominal surgery, chronic bronchitis, congestive heart failure, and alcoholism) that predisposes to pneumococcal and other bacterial pneumonias, onset of clinical symptoms may be more insidious. Other types of bacterial pneumonias are more common in different clinical settings: staphylococcal and *H. influenzae* following influenza A or B; *Haemophilus*, *Klebsiella*, and anaerobic pneumonias in alcoholics; anaerobic and Gram-negative pneumonias in recently hospitalized patients. In the elderly, particularly those in nursing homes, *S. pneumoniae* continues to be the most common cause of pneumonia, but Gram-negative aerobes, nontypable strains of *Haemophilus influenzae*, and mixed pneumococcal-Gram-negative anaerobes are common etiologies. Group B streptococcus, *Branhamella catarrhalis*, and *Legionella pneumophilia* are also occasional etiologies of pneumonia in the elderly (30).

Atypical Pneumonia

The atypical pneumonia syndrome comprises the majority of pneumonias in persons under 40. *M. pneumoniae* is the agent in 60 to 90% of pneumonias in this age group (11). A number of viruses (influenza A and B, respiratory syncytial virus, parainfluenza, adenovirus), *Chlamydia* (psittacosis), rickettsia (Q fever), and bacteria (tularemia and Legionnaires' disease) present as a pneumonitis which clinically is indistinguishable from mycoplasmal pneumonia. The onset is a flu-like illness, with fever, headache, myalgias, and malaise. At onset or several days later a nonproductive hacking cough and substernal chest pain appear, accompanied by dyspnea and respiratory distress in more severe cases. Pleuritic chest pain and hemoptysis are unusual.

Complications of M. pneumoniae are more common in severely ill patients, who probably require hospitalization, but may appear in patients initially managed at home. These complications include sinusitis, otitis media, myringitis (diagnostic of bullae are seen), erythema multiforme or erythema nodosum, intravascular hemolysis, meningoencephalitis, toxic psychosis, myocarditis, and pericarditis. Persistent hacking cough, lasting as long as 6 weeks despite therapy, is common and requires symptomatic relief with codeine (see Chapter 53). Relapse of the primary disease occurs in up to 10% of cases, usually 2 to 3 weeks after the initial illness, and is probably related to the fact that mycoplasma persists in bronchial epithelium for up to 14 weeks.

Diarrhea, relative bradycardia, abdominal pain, liver enzyme elevations, and hematuria may occur in *Legionnaires' disease* but can accompany pneumonia due to viruses or mycoplasma (17). Signs of encephalopathy (confusion, delirium, stupor) are clearly more common in Legionnaires' disease.

Important clues for the etiological diagnosis may be obtained from a knowledge of seasonal, environmental, and occupational predilections of the different agents that cause atypical pneumonias (see Table 28.2).

Physical Examination

The physical examination does not usually distinguish between bacterial and atypical pneumonia syndromes. Crepitant rales that do not clear with cough are suggestive of pneumonia of either type. Signs of consolidation (bronchial breath sounds,

dullness to percussion, and egophony) are more common in bacterial pneumonia. In early stages of pneumonia the examination may be normal, despite an infiltrate on X-ray. On the other hand, rales and rhonchi may indicate pneumonia before the appearance of an infiltrate.

Laboratory Examination

Every patient suspected of having pneumonia should have a chest X-ray, peripheral blood white cell count and differential count, and two blood cultures when possible. A white cell count over 15,000 is usually associated with bacterial pneumonia. Although the X-ray is essential for the firm diagnosis of pneumonia, a normal X-ray does not necessarily rule out pneumonia and X-ray patterns are not specific in terms of the etiology. For example, in one study (29) in which diagnosis was attempted by six radiologists from the chest film alone, mycoplasmal pneumonia was incorrectly identified as bacterial in a significant proportion of patients.

If the chest X-ray or clinical findings indicate pneumonia, a *sputum Gram stain* is often instrumental in directing initial therapy; and cultures of sputum and blood should be obtained. The rapid Gram stain technique requires only 1 to 2 minutes: (*a*) heat fixation; (*b*) 5 seconds crystal violet, water rinse; (*c*) 5 seconds Gram's iodine, water rinse; (*d*) decolorization of the thin part of the smear with 4.5 drops of 95% alcohol, water rinse; (*e*) 5 seconds safranine, water rinse; (*f*) blotting dry. The sputum

Table 28.2.
Epidemiological Clues to the Presumptive Diagnosis of Atypical Pneumonia

Organism or Disease	Peak Seasonal Incidence	Incubation Period *days*	Epidemiological Setting
Mycoplasma pneumoniae	Summer, early fall	14–28	Family—3 weeks between onset among individuals
Respiratory syncytial virus	Late winter and spring	2–8	Bronchiolitis in children <5 years. Mild upper respiratory infection in adult contacts, with mean symptomatic period 9 days. More severe in elderly
Influenza A and B	Winter epidemics	1–3	Adult cases follow school absenteeism
Parainfluenza 1 + 2	Fall	3–8	Croup in children, unusual in adults
Parinfluenza 3	All year	3–8	Family—mild upper respiratory infection in adults, more severe in elderly
Adenovirus (type 4, 7)	Winter	4–5	Military recruits
Psittacosis	All year	6–15	Occupational or household exposure to birds, especially parrots, turkeys, and pigeons (20% have no bird exposure)
Tularemia (pulmonary)	All year	2–4	Handling infected rodents and rabbits
Q fever	All year	14–28	Contact with sheep, goats, cattle
Legionnaires'	Outbreaks in summer, sporadic through year	2–10 (epidemic cases)	Contact with construction sites and stagnant water in air-cooling apparatus (some reports)

sample is probably of lower respiratory tract origin if there are fewer than 10 squamous epithelial cells and more than 25 polymorphonuclear leukocytes/high dry (100×) field, except in leukopenic patients. The appearance of columnar ciliated epithelial cells assures lower tract origin. Sputum smears positive for pneumococci (Gram-positive, lancet-shaped diplococci) are helpful in directing therapy (23). Sputum, often foul smelling, containing mixed flora with pleomorphic Gram-negative bacilli and tiny or pleomorphic Gram-positive cocci, is consistent with anaerobic aspiration pneumonia. Pneumonia due to *Staphylococcus* or *Haemophilus* organisms usually is accompanied by sputum containing abundant large Gram-positive cocci, or small Gram-negative coccobacilli, respectively.

Sputum samples from patients with atypical pneumonia presenting as a flu-like illness characteristically contain few bacteria and only modest numbers of leukocytes. On the other hand, sputum from some mycoplasmal and viral pneumonias contains abundant leukocytes but few bacteria. Many patients produce no sputum, including one-half of patients with *legionella pneumophila*. If such patients are toxic they may require hospitalization for more invasive diagnostic studies such as transtracheal aspiration.

Unlike sputum Gram stains, *sputum cultures* have limited utility in the management of ambulatory pneumonias, since sputum samples are often contaminated by oral pneumococci. Moreover, pneumococci fail to grow in 45% of cultures from cases of pneumococcal pneumonia (2). In view of the confusing data, routine sputum cultures are not recommended, with the following important exceptions: patients, such as nursing home residents or those recently discharged from a general hospital, who are at greater risk for nonpneumococcal pneumonia, and patients with sputum Gram stains demonstrating a predominance of a nonpneumococcal bacterial pathogen.

The majority of pneumonias cannot be diagnosed by blood or sputum culture and do not require definitive diagnosis by *serology*. If, however, the patient fails to respond to 3 to 5 days of therapy and has been ill less than 14 days, an acute serum sample should be obtained and stored. After 3 weeks of illness, a convalescent serum sample should be obtained and both samples submitted to a state or regional health laboratory for diagnostic serology. Guided by epidemiological clues (Table 28.2), complement fixation titers for *M. pneumoniae*, Q fever, psittacosis, influenza, respiratory syncytial and parainfluenza viruses, and adenovirus may be requested. An indirect immunofluorescent assay on paired sera is available to diagnose Legionnaires' disease. Tularemia is usually diagnosed by an agglutination assay.

The presence of serum *cold agglutinins* is often used as a rapid diagnostic test for mycoplasmal pneumonia. This test, however, has several drawbacks. The sample must be maintained at close to 37°C for delivery to the laboratory. In addition, the test is not very sensitive; (only about three-quarters of patients with mycoplasmal infection are positive), and not very specific (half of all positive tests are due to other diseases, including pneumococcal and adenovirus pneumonia).

Management: Hospitalization

The need for hospitalization must be individually determined for each patient, but in general is based on how sick the patient is and what underlying diseases are present. Patients who are toxic, diaphoretic, dyspneic, cyanotic, fatigued from respiratory effort, have hemoptysis, have difficulty clearing secretions, or cannot be expected to follow a course of oral therapy due either to vomiting or to characteristics predictive of poor compliance (see Chapter 4) should be hospitalized.

Other associated features which should prompt hospital admission and the following:

1. Age over 50 years, obstructive or bronchospastic lung disease, congestive heart failure, diabetes, renal insufficiency, malignancy, postsplenectomy, sickle cell anemia, alcoholism, drug abuse, or concomitant tuberculosis.

2. Peripheral white cell count <5000, ileus, or abdominal distention.

3. Suspicion of recent major aspiration due to history of head trauma, sedative use, acute alcoholism, seizures, dental anesthesia, loss of consciousness, or esophageal motility disorder.

4. Extrapulmonary complications (large pleural effusion, meningitis, septic arthritis, peritonitis, metastatic abscesses, *etc*).

5. Hospitalization within the last 4 weeks or residence in nursing home, two situations which increase the chance of having a Gram-negative or a resistant nosocomial pathogen.

6. Sputum smears showing a predominance of Gram-negative bacteria.

7. Inability to care for self if living alone.

8. Failure to respond to initial therapy.

Management: Ambulatory

Antimicrobial Therapy (Table 28.3)

If the clinical presentation supports the diagnosis of pneumococcal pneumonia, the antibiotic of choice is penicillin, 300,000 units of procaine penicillin administered intramuscularly in the office, followed by oral penicillin V, 250 mg every 6 hours for 10 days. If the patient is allergic to penicillin, erythromycin, 250 mg four times daily, is appropriate.

If the clinical presentation is that of the atypical pneumonia syndrome and an adequate sputum smear is nondiagnostic, erythromycin, 250 to 500 mg four times daily for 14 days, is recommended. Patients receiving erythromycin should be advised

Table 28.3.
Oral Antimicrobial Drugs Used in Ambulatory Treatment of Respiratory Infections

Drug	Available Strengths	Usual Adult Dose and Schedule	Common Side Effects	Drug (and Food) Interactions
	mg			
Penicillin V	250, 500	250–500 mg 3 or 4 times daily	Diarrhea, nausea, vomiting, vaginitis, skin rash, urticaria	Rash with infectious mononucleosis or concomitant allopurinol, false positive Clinitest (use Clinistix or Testape)
Ampicillin	250, 500	250–500 mg 3 or 4 times daily		
Amoxicillin	250, 500	250–500 mg 3 or 4 times daily		
Erythromycin	250, 500	250–500 mg 3 or 4 times daily	Nausea, vomiting, abdominal pain, diarrhea	False elevation of aminotransferase, raises serum theophylline levels, potentiates warfarin and glucocorticoids
Tetracycline	250, 500	250–500 mg 3 or 4 times daily	Skin photosensitivity, nausea, vomiting, heartburn, diarrhea, mucosal candidiasis	Food, milk, antacids, iron interfere with absorption
Trimethoprim (T) plus Sulfamethoxazole (S)	400 T/80 S (single strength) 800 T/160 S (double strength)	2 single strength or 1 double strength twice daily	Skin rash, gastrointestinal upset, elevates serum creatinine	Prolongs half-life of warfarin, phenytoin, and oral hypoglycemics

that crampy abdominal pain is a frequent benign side effect which often can be ameliorated by taking the medication with meals (without impairing its absorption) or by lowering the dose. Erythromycin can raise blood theophylline levels, occasionally into the toxic range, and doses of the latter drug should be monitored and adjusted.

Many physicians treat *all* ambulatory patients with pneumonia with erythromycin. The advantage is coverage for pneumococcal and mycoplasmal infections, as well as Legionnaires' and many milder anaerobic infections. Since up to 10% of pneumococcal isolates are resistant to tetracycline, this drug is reserved for the occasional patient who fails to respond to erythromycin or in whom tularemia or Q fever is suspected epidemiologically. In these situations, a 2- to 3-week course of tetracycline, 500 mg four times daily, is appropriate.

Follow-up

The patient should be advised to keep in close contact by phone, maintain good hydration with oral fluids, use aspirin or acetaminophen to control fever and headache, and avoid cough suppressants and cigarettes. A phone call to the patient 24 hours after the initial visit provides a check on antibiotic compliance and side effects and on the status of symptoms; also it reassures the acutely ill patient that he has access to the physician should his condition worsen or fail to improve.

A follow-up visit to the office 3 to 4 days later will help to assess response to therapy. Symptoms of pneumococcal pneumonia in the uncompromised host abate dramatically within 48 to 72 hours of initiation of penicillin therapy. If substantial clinical response to penicillin has not occurred, either switching to erythromycin or hospitalizing the patient for further diagnostic studies should be contemplated.

Erythromycin will substantially reduce fever and systemic symptoms in most patients with mycoplasmal pneumonia by 3 to 6 days.

Early follow-up chest X-rays are mandatory in patients who fail to show clinical improvement by 5 to 7 days of therapy or who have a later relapse. Since 3% of patients who have a bronchogenic carcinoma initially present with a typical pneumonitis with or without consolidation (8), all patients over 40 and all smokers should have a chest X-ray at 4 to 6 weeks, the interval in which radiological clearing is expected for uncomplicated cases of pneumococcal and mycoplasmal pneumonia (19). Old age, chronic obstructive lung disease, and alcoholism may delay radiological clearing for an additional 2 to 6 weeks (19).

Prevention

Polyvalent pneumococcal vaccine and influenza vaccines are discussed in detail in Chapter 32. No special precautions to isolate the ambulatory pneumonia patient need to be taken. Household contacts of pneumonia patients need no special surveillance, with the exceptions of pneumonic disease due to tuberculosis (see Chapter 29), tularemia, plague, and meningococci.

General References

Benenson AS (ed): *Control of Communicable Diseases in Man*, ed 12. Washington, DC, American Public Health Association, 1985.

A concise summary of epidemiology and management of communicable diseases.

Mandell GL, Douglas RG Jr, Bernett JE (eds): *Principles and Practice of Infectious Diseases*. New York, John Wiley & Sons, 1985.

The standard textbook of infectious diseases.

Vickery DM, Fries JF: *Take Care of Yourself: A Consumer's Guide to Medical Care*. Reading, MA, Addison-Wesley, 1976.

Simple algorithms for self-care of common medical problems.

Specific References

1. Baine WB, Luby JP, Martin SW: Severe illness with influenza B. *Am J Med* 68:181, 1980.
2. Barrett-Connor E: The nonvalue of sputum culture in the diagnosis of pneumococcal pneumonia. *Am Rev Respir Dis* 103:845, 1971.
3. Berg AO, LoGerfo JP: Potential effect of self-care algorithms on the number of physician visits. *N Engl J Med* 300:535, 1979.
4. Chalmers TC: Effects of ascorbic acid on the common cold. An evaluation of the evidence. *Am J Med* 58:532, 1975.
5. Current estimates from the Health Interview Survey: United States—1976. Vital and Health Statistics, series 10, no. 119, DHEW pub no. (PHS) 78-1547, 1977.
6. Davidson TM, Calloway CA: Tonsillectomy and adenoidectomy. Its indications and its problems. *West J Med* 133:451, 1980.
7. Delker LL, Moser RH, Nelson JD, *et al*: Amantadine: does it have a role in the prevention and treatment of influenza? A National Institutes of Health Consensus Development Conference. *Ann Intern Med* 92:256, 1980.
8. Drevvatne T, Frimann-Dahl J: Peripheral bronchial carcinomas: a radiological and pathological study. *Br J Radiol* 34:180, 1961.
9. Evans FO Jr, Sydnor JB, Moore WEC, *et al*: Sinusitis of the maxillary antrum. *N Engl J Med* 293:735, 1975.
10. Feinstein AR, Spagnuolo M, Wood HF, *et al*: Rheumatic fever in children and adolescents. *Ann Intern Med* 60:68, 1964.
11. Foy HM, Kenny GE, McMahan R, *et al*: Mycoplasma pneumoniae pneumonia in an urban area. *JAMA* 214:1666, 1970.
12. Foy HM, Cooney MK, Allan I, Kenney GE: Rates of pneumonia during influenza epidemics in Seattle, 1964 to 1975. *JAMA* 241:253, 1979.
13. Fry J: Influenza A cases in 1957: clinical and epidemiological features in a general practice. *Br Med J* 1:250, 1958.
14. Gwaltney JM Jr, Hendley JO, Simon G, Jordon WS Jr: Rhinovirus infections in an industrial population. 1. The occurrence of illness. *N Engl J Med* 275:1261, 1966.
15. Gwaltney JM Jr, Moskalski PB, Hindley JO: Hand to hand transmission of rhinovirus colds. *Ann Intern Med* 88:463, 1978.
16. Hall WJ, Douglas RG, Jr: Pulmonary function during and after common respiratory infections. *Annu Rev Med* 31:233, 1980.
17. Helms CM, Viner JP, Sturm RH, *et al*: Comparative features of pneumococcal, mycoplasmal, and Legionnaires' disease pneumonias. *Ann Intern Med* 90:543, 1979.
18. Howard JC, Kantner TR, Lilienfield LS, *et al*: Effectiveness of antihistamines in the symptomatic management of the common cold. *JAMA* 242:2414, 1979.
19. Jay SJ, Johanson WG Jr, Pierce AK: The radiographic resolution of *Streptococcus pneumoniae* pneumonia. *N Engl J Med* 293:798, 1975.
20. Komaroff AL, Aronson MD, Pass TM, *et al*: Serologic evidence of chlamydial and mycoplasmal pharyngitis in adults. *Science* 222:927, 1983.
21. Oral cold remedies: *Med Lett* 17:89, 1975.
22. Over-the-counter cough remedies: *Med Lett* 21:103, 1979.
23. Rein MF, Gwaltney JM, O'Brien WM, *et al*: Accuracy of Gram's stain in identifying pneumococci in sputum. *JAMA* 239:2671, 1978.
24. Sakethoo K, Januszkiewicz A, Sackner MA: Effects of drinking hot water and chicken soup on nasal mucus velocity and nasal airflow resistance. *Chest* 74:408, 1978.
25. Stanley ED Jackson GG, *et al*: Virus shedding with aspirin treatment of rhinovirus infection. *JAMA* 231:1248, 1975.
26. Stott W: Randomized controlled trial of antibiotics in patients with cough and purulent sputum. *Br Med J* 2:556, 1976.
27. Strome M: Rhino-sinusitis and midfacial pain in adolescents. *Practitioner* 217:914, 1976.
28. Tager I, Spiezer FE: Role of infection in chronic bronchitis. *N Engl J Med* 292:563, 1975.
29. Tew J, Colenoff L, Berlin BS: Bacterial or nonbacterial pneumonia: accuracy of radiographic diagnosis. *Radiology* 124:607, 1977.
30. Verghese A, Berk SL: Bacterial pneumonia in the elderly. *Medicine (Baltimore)* 62:271, 1983.
31. Wood RW, Tompkins RK, Wolcott BW: An efficient strategy for managing acute respiratory illness in adults. *Ann Intern Med* 93:757, 1980.

Acknowledgment. Figures 28.2 and 28.3 are reprinted with permission from Dodd GD, Jing B-S: *Radiology of the Nose, Paranasal Sinuses and Nasopharynx.* Baltimore, Williams & Wilkins, 1977.

CHAPTER TWENTY-NINE

Tuberculosis in the Ambulatory Patient

R. BRADLEY SACK, M.D., Sc.D., AND FREDERICK KOSTER, M.D.

DEFINITION OF THE PROBLEM

Epidemiology

Tuberculosis, though steadily decreasing in frequency in the United States, is still a disease with which all practitioners need to be familiar because of its diverse clinical presentations, most of which are first seen in an ambulatory setting. Approximately 25,500 new cases of tuberculosis, mostly in adults, were diagnosed in the United States in 1982; many of these were in subpopulations (blacks and Indians) and geographic areas (large urban centers) with case rates considerably higher than that of the rest of the population. Table 29.1 summarizes recent national statistics on tuberculosis and the important trends in incidence and mortality from tuberculosis during the past 40 years.

The drop in incidence of tuberculosis is due entirely to decreases in cases of *pulmonary* tuberculosis; new extrapulmonary tuberculosis continues to appear at a rate of about 4000 cases/year.

Reactivation and Primary Tuberculosis

The majority of the sporadic new cases of tuberculosis are due to *reactivation* of a remote primary infection; patients in this situation are those who have had untreated or inadequately treated active tuberculosis and those with positive tuberculin reactions who have neither a past history of active tuberculosis nor documented conversion from tuberculin negativity during an interval of 1 year or less (11). *Primary* tuberculosis means evidence for newly acquired infection (either recent conversion to tuberculin positivity or the onset of active disease shortly after exposure to a patient with known active disease). Persons at highest risk of developing primary tuberculosis are those living with, or having close contact with, a person who has undetected and therefore untreated active disease.

Most patients with tuberculosis are minimally symptomatic or are asymptomatic, which is why public health screening programs are critical for case detection. General physicians, although usually not involved in mass screening efforts, will see patients for routine examinations who have positive skin tests or patients who have specific signs or symptoms suggestive of tuberculosis. This chapter is concerned largely with the detection of the disease in such patients and with the treatment of tuberculosis in the ambulatory setting.

Etiology

The etiology of tuberculosis in the United States is almost always *Mycobacterium tuberculosis*. In some parts of the world, or in immunosuppressed patients, other strains (such as bovine and avian strains) may also be important in human disease. Atypical mycobacteria, such as *Mycobacterium kansasii* and *Mycobacterium intracellulare*, and certain fungi, such as *Cryptococcus neoformans* and *Histoplasma capsulatum*, may produce disease indistinguishable from tuberculosis and should be considered in the differential diagnosis.

DIAGNOSIS

History

Tuberclosis, when symptomatic, almost always presents with signs and symptoms of weeks' to months' duration. Almost the only time it presents as acute disease is in rare cases of acute meningitis or tuberculous pneumonia. The history should be directed toward both defining the symptom complex

Table 29.1.
Summary of National Tuberculosis Statistics, Showing Long Term Trends and Recent Statistics[a]

	INCIDENCE AND MORTALITY TRENDS, 1949–1982					
	1949	1959	1969	1974	1978	1982
Reported new cases	134,865	57,535	39,120	30,122	28,521	25520[c]
Reported mortality	NA[b]	NA	5,567	3,513	2,914	NA

	DISTRIBUTION OF NEW CASES BY AGE, 1979				
Age range	0–4	5–14	15–24	25 and over	Total
Reported new cases	989	631	2,158	23,848	27,669

DISTRIBUTION OF NEW CASES BY REGION AND STATE, 1979

New England	835	Missouri	500	*Western South Central*	3,471
Maine	56	North Dakota	22	Arkansas	382
New Hampshire	25	South Dakota	55	Louisiana	647
Vermont	29	Nebraska	30	Oklahoma	352
Massachusetts	476	Kansas	104	Texas	2,090
Rhode Island	80	*South Atlantic*	6,033	*Mountain*	919
Connecticut	169	Delaware	63	Montana	39
Mid-Atlantic	4,238	Maryland	648	Idaho	21
New York (excl. NYC)	699	Washington, DC	324	Wyoming	19
New York City	1,530	Virginia	747	Colorado	170
New Jersey	933	West Virginia	221	New Mexico	153
Pennsylvania	1,076	North Carolina	990	Arizona	417
Eastern North Central	4,075	South Carolina	483	Utah	46
Ohio	764	Georgia	929	Nevada	54
Indiana	509	Florida	1,628	*Pacific*	4,543
Illinois	1,540	*Eastern South Central*	2,580	Washington	321
Michigan	1,052	Kentucky	635	Oregon	179
Wisconsin	210	Tennessee	748	California	3,642
Western North Central	975	Alabama	644	Alaska	90
Minnesota	190	Mississippi	553	Hawaii	311
Iowa	74				

[a] From *Morbidity and Mortality Weekly Report*, vol 28, no. 54, September 1980.
[b] NA, not available.
[c] *Morbidity and Mortality Weekly Report,* Annual Summary 1982.

and determining possible exposure to known sources of disease.

Since tuberculosis has multiple presentations (12), the physician should be suspicious about anyone with chronic unexplained symptoms. Weight loss (documented over a defined period of time), fever (particularly in the late evenings), night sweats (to be differentiated from environmentally induced sweats), decreased appetite, and the loss of a sense of well-being are the most important nonspecific symptoms. Persistent cough (usually with sputum production), hemoptysis, and pleuritic chest pain are more specific findings suggestive of pulmonary involvement.

It is important to know if the patient has previously had tuberculosis, if the patient has previously been skin tested for tuberculosis (and if so, when he was tested and what the results were), and when the patient has had previous chest films (and where they can be obtained).

Possibly significant history also includes any family member or close friend with known tuberculosis, any person in school or at work with known disease,

and any recent history of travel to the developing world, where tuberculosis is common.

Since *extrapulmonary tuberculosis* may occur in any organ (in particular, pleura, lymph nodes, endometrium, kidneys, ureters, bones and joints, skin, meninges, small intestine, and peritoneum) or as a disseminated (miliary) form, localized symptoms and signs in any organ must raise the possibility of tuberculosis.

Physical Examination

The physical examination often may be entirely negative, even with obvious evidence of pulmonary disease on the chest film. The following positive findings, when present, may be of considerable help in suggesting the diagnosis: auscultatory evidence of pulmonary cavitation (bronchovesicular breathing and whispered pectoriloquy); evidence of pleural effusion; supra- and infraclavicular retraction; lymphdenopathy; evidence of weight loss; and fever. Although rare in the United States, large, matted, nontender cervical lymph nodes (at times with draining sinuses) are almost diagnostic of *scrofula*, a form of tuberculous adenitis (which may also be due to atypical mycobacteria) seen primarily in children.

Tuberculin Skin Tests

If the patient has previously had a negative skin test or has not had a skin test at all, a test with intermediate strength PPD (purified protein derivative), 5 tuberculin units, Tween-stabilized, should be applied intradermally on the volar skin of the forearm. Ideally, a control test should be placed on the opposite arm, containing a ubiquitous antigen, such as *Candida* or mumps. The reactions should be read at 48 hours. A practical method for determining the diameter of the indurated area is the ballpoint pen method (10): a line is drawn from a point 1 to 2 cm away from the margin of a positive reaction; when the pen tip reaches the margin of the indurated area, definite resistance is felt; this is repeated on the opposite side, and the diameter of the indurated reaction is measured. The interpretation and significance of tuberculin tests are summarized in Table 29.2.

A person with a known positive tuberculin skin test does not need to have one repeated; if the test is repeated, there is a small risk of producing a very *strong positive reaction* characterized by tender induration, axillary adenopathy, temperature elevation (as high as 102°F (38.5°C)), and slough of the epidermis after a week. This problem is best treated with a sterile gauze dressing impregnated with a topical steroid, such as 0.1% triamcinolone.

First strength and second strength tuberculin tests are rarely if ever useful in the diagnosis of tuberculosis. Tine tests are used as screening tests, and positive tests should be confirmed by an intermediate PPD.

M. tuberculosis shares antigens with related mycobacteria, and therefore a positive skin test is not completely specific. However, most cross-reactions will be less than 10 mm in diameter. Skin testing with specific atypical mycobacterial antigens is not possible, since the antigens are not available for general use.

It should be remembered that a negative tuberculin skin test does not rule out the diagnosis of tuberculosis; intercurrent febrile illnesses, skin testing within 30 days of vaccination with a live virus, underlying disease or immunosuppressive drugs that may suppress delayed hypersensitivity reactions, and errors in administration of the test material may explain false negative reactions.

The *booster phenomenon* may interfere with the interpretation of the tuberculin test (13). Persons with a remote tuberculous or atypical mycobacterial infection who have become skin test negative may, upon repeat skin testing, develop a positive response because of the *boosting effect* of the repeat test. This boosting effect can be detected by administering a second tuberculin test 1 week after the first test in

Table 29.2.
Evaluation of Tuberculin Skin Tests (5 Tuberculin Units)

Reaction[a]	Associated Features	Significance	Therapy[b]
Positive	Unknown duration:		
	Chest film negative	Probably old infection unless recently acquired disease	Consider INH treatment for 1 yr, if under age 35 yr
	Chest film positive (calcified nodes, apical scarring)	Old tuberculous disease, at increased risk for developing reactivation	Consider INH treatment for 1 yr
	Close contact of patients with tuberculosis	May represent recent disease	Consider INH treatment for 1 yr
Positive	Recent development (<1 yr)	Recent acquisition of tuberculosis	INH treatment for 1 yr
Positive	In patient beginning long term course of corticosteroids	Patient at increased risk of developing clnical tuberculosis	Consider INH treatment for duration of steroid course or for 1 yr
Negative	In patient also negative to ubiquitous antigens	Anergic, noninterpretable	Repeat PPD; follow with chest X-ray if necessary
Negative	In patient with recent close contact with tuberculosis patient	Does not rule out early tuberculous infection	Treat with INH; retest in 3 months. If positive continue for 1 yr. If still negative may stop INH
Negative	In patients taking high dose corticosteroids or immunosuppressives	Uninterpretable	Follow with chest X-rays; treat with INH if disease proved or highly suspected

[a] Interpretation of readings:
Negative: 5 mm induration or less. (See the text for a discussion of factors causing false negative test and of booster phenomenon.)
Intermediate: 5–10 mm induration (needs to be repeated; consider atypical mycobacterial disease).
Positive: 10 mm induration or more.
[b] INH, isoniazid; PPD, purified protein derivative.

persons who initially have a negative response. If the second response is positive, these persons can be said to have had past infection, but are not considered to have a recently acquired infection. The booster phenomemon is important in elderly persons, in whom it is common, and in persons such as hospital employees who may be skin tested frequently.

Laboratory Examination

Chest X-Ray

Both posteroanterior (PA) and lateral views should be obtained. In the patient with strongly suggestive clinical evidence for tuberculosis, an apical lordotic view should also be obtained when the PA and lateral views appear to be normal. The radiological findings typical of tuberculosis (apical scarring, hilar adenopathy with peripheral infiltrate, upper lobe cavitation, miliary infiltrate, *etc*) are not specific; however, a negative chest film rules out pulmonary tuberculosis (with the rare exception of early miliary disease), making the chest film a very sensitive test.

Cultures and Smears

Sputum, for smear (acid-fast stain) and culture, should be obtained at least three times. A positive sputum smear is highly suggestive of tuberculosis (not absolutely diagnostic because of the possibility of atypical infection or of contamination); and a positive culture is diagnostic. If sputum is difficult to obtain, one can obtain morning gastric aspirates, which contain the swallowed sputum (6). Gastric samples should not be examined by acid-fast stain but should be sent for culture only, since smears of gastric contents frequently show commensal acid-fast organisms and are not useful for diagnosis.

In a patient with a positive PPD and persistent pyuria without bacteriuria, three urine samples should be obtained for tuberculosis culture (again a positive acid-fast urine smear is only suggestive, since there are commensal acid-fast organisms such as *Mycobacterium smegmatis*, that inhabit the urinary tract; therefore, only cultures are of diagnostic value).

Tuberculosis cultures become positive within 3 to 4 weeks of plating the specimens. The initial positive cultures from any source should be tested for sensitivity to drugs used to treat tuberculosis since resistant organisms may necessitate a change in treatment.

Miscellaneous Laboratory Tests

Complete blood count. The hematocrit value may be normal or low; the anemia due to tuberculosis is normochromic and normocytic, the so-called anemia of chronic disease (see Chapter 49). The white blood cell count and differential count are usually normal; occasionally a monocytosis is seen in persons with severe disease.

Urinalysis. This should be obtained routinely; if sterile pyuria is found it is suggestive of renal tuberculosis and cultures should be sent as described above.

Liver function tests. Tests of serum aminotransferases, alkaline phosphatase, and bilirubin may be helpful if disseminated disease or liver involvement is suspected.

Other procedures. Other procedures, such as thoracentesis, lumbar puncture, and liver biopsy, are indicated only when specific organ involvement is suspected. These are best done in hospitalized patients.

Presumptive Diagnosis

The *presumptive diagnosis of active tuberculosis* can be made when any of the following is found:
1. A typical chest X-ray;
2. A positive sputum smear;
3. A biopsy showing caseating granulomas with or without acid-fast organisms;
4. A recent change (within 1 year) of the tuberculin skin test from negative to positive, associated with other characteristic systemic symptoms/signs.

The diagnosis of active tuberculosis is *confirmed* by a positive culture from any body fluid or biopsy specimen.

All patients with a presumptive or confirmed diagnosis of tuberculosis must be reported promptly to the appropriate state health authority.

COURSE AND MANAGEMENT

Overview

Most persons infected with *M. tuberculosis* are unaware that they have it; only 5 to 10% of infected persons become ill, and a positive PPD or calcified nodes on chest film may be the only indicators of the past disease. Individuals in the latter group are at continual risk of reactivating their disease, however, since it is known that live *M. tuberculosis* may persist in the tissues of an infected individual for a lifetime. Such individuals have a much higher rate of development of clinical disease than do people not previously infected.

When tuberculosis is diagnosed in association with systemic signs or symptoms, there is no question that the patient should be treated. Persons with positive tuberculin reactions as the only manifestation of disease constitute a more difficult problem (see Table 29.2 and "Isoniazid Prophylaxis" below).

Once the diagnosis is strongly suspected or made, the question arises of how best to initiate therapy. Since it may take 4 weeks before cultures of *M. tuberculosis* become positive, therapy must usually be initiated on the basis of the chest film, sputum-smears, and/or a strong clinical suspicion. If at 3 months all cultures are negative, therapy may be stopped.

If the patient is well enough to care for himself, can take oral medications regularly, and has no extrapulmonary disease, he can be successfully treated without hospitalization.

Treatment

Chemotherapy (Table 29.3)

To treat active pulmonary tuberculosis, *only two oral drugs* are necessary unless the organisms are drug resistant, as shown by *in vitro* testing; a single drug should never be used, because this increases the risk of the emergence of resistant organisms during therapy.

In 1983, The American Thoracic Society issued the following recommendations for the *standard treatment of active pulmonary tuberculosis* (1):

The simplest regimen is based on the administration of isoniazid (INH) and rifampin for *9 months*. In most reported studies, either ethambutol or streptomycin has been added for an initial 2 to 8 weeks. Good results have also been reported using twice weekly administration of the isoniazid and rifampin after an initial 1 month of daily treatment. With these regimens, relapse rates of less than 3% have been reported. Recommended doses for the drugs, all of which can be taken on a once-a-day schedule, are shown in Table 29.3. In those few patients whose sputum is still culture-positive after 3 months of treatment with rifampin and INH, the duration of total treatment

Table 29.3.
Drugs for the Treatment of Mycobacterial Disease in Adults and Children[a]

| Commonly Used Agents | Available Strengths of Oral Tablets or Capsules | Dosage | | Most Common Side Effects | Tests for Side Effects | Drug Interactions[b] |
		Total Once Daily Dose	Twice Weekly Dosage			
	(mg)					
Isoniazid	100, 300	5 to 10 mg/kg up to 300 mg PO or IM	15 mg/kg PO or IM	Peripheral neuritis, hepatitis, hypersensitivity	Aminotransferases (not as a routine)	Carbamazepine— increased toxicity both drugs Disulfiram— psychosis, ataxia Phenytoin— toxicity increased
Rifampin	600	10 mg/kg up to 600 mg PO	10 mg/kg up to 600 mg PO	Hepatitis, febrile reaction, purpura (rare)	Aminotransferases (not as a routine)	May reduce the effect of the following drugs due to increased hepatic metabolism: oral contraceptives, quinidine, corticosteroids, anticoagulants, disopyramide, diazepam, barbiturates, methadone, digitoxin, digoxin, oral hypoglycemics; *p*-aminosalicylic acid may interfere with absorption of rifampin
Streptomycin		15 to 20 mg/kg up to 1 g IM	25 to 30 mg/kg	Eighth nerve damage, nephrotoxicity	Vestibular function, audiograms[b]; blood urea nitrogen and creatinine	Neuromuscular blocking agents— may be potentiated to cause prolonged paralysis
Pyrazinamide	500	15 to 30 mg/kg up to 2 g PO	50 to 70 mg/kg	Hyperuricemia, hepatotoxicity	Uric acid, aminotransferases	
Ethambutol	100, 400	15 to 25 mg/kg	50 mg/kg PO	Optic neuritis (reversible with discontinuation of drug; very rare at 15 mg/kg), skin rash	Red-green color discrimination and visual acuity[c], difficult to test in a child under 3 years	

[a] Adapted from American Thoracic Society: Treatment of tuberculosis and other mycobacterial diseases. *Am Rev Resp Dis* 127:790, 1983.
[b] Reference should be made to current literature, particularly on rifampin, because it induces hepatic microenzymes and therefore interacts with many drugs.
[c] Initial examination should be done at start of treatment.

should be extended to at least 6 months beyond the time of conversion. The combination of isoniazid and rifampin for 9 months is generally considered the present treatment of choice. In patients with drug-sensitive organisms it has been shown that treatment for less than 9 months with isoniazid and rifampin is followed by a higher relapse rate.

If rifampin cannot be used because of drug resistance or intolerance, the duration of treatment must be increased. Regimens shown to be effective when rifampin cannot be used are (a) isoniazid and ethambutol for a total of 18 months, with the addition of streptomycin for an initial period of 1 to 2 months where the initial bacterial population is believed to be high; and (b) isoniazid and streptomycin for a total of 18 months. These regimens have been shown to be effective when given on either a daily or twice weekly basis in appropriate doses. Twice weekly treatment is appropriate in patients requiring directly supervised drug administration.

If isoniazid cannot be used, rifampin and ethambutol can be given for a total of 18 months.

If neither isoniazid nor rifampin can be used, the patient must be given at least two and preferably three drugs to which his organisms are known to be susceptible. These drugs must be given for at least 18 months.

Regimens containing *second line drugs* need to be considered only in patients who have developed adverse reactions to the standard drugs, which is uncommon, or in patients with drug-resistant tuberculosis. This latter group is usually composed of people who have been treated previously for tuberculosis, or who have acquired tuberculosis in Southeast Asia or in Mexico.

Pregnant women can receive isoniazid and rifampin or isoniazid and ethambutol, since both regimens are safe for the fetus.

Patients with *impaired renal function* should be treated with isoniazid and rifampin, since ethambutol is excreted mainly by the kidneys, and its dosage would have to be adjusted.

Because there is not sufficient information regarding 9-month regimens, patients with *extrapulmonary tuberculosis* should be treated with an 18-month course of isoniazid and rifampin, or isoniazid and ethambutol.

Symptomatic Therapy

Usually no symptomatic therapy is required, except that patients should be encouraged to eat an adequate diet. If a patient has symptoms that require special management (such as high fever and toxicity for which steroids may be helpful, or a pleural effusion that needs draining), hospitalization is necessary.

If the patient is eating poorly, pyridoxine (5 mg/day) should be taken with isoniazid to prevent peripheral neuropathy. Pyridoxine should also be taken with isoniazid routinely by pregnant patients and by patients with other diseases that may cause peripheral neuropathy (e.g., alcoholism, diabetes, end-stage renal disease).

Course in Treated Patient

Follow-up Schedule

After treatment has been initiated, the patient should be seen or contacted at least once per month, chiefly to assure drug compliance (see below) and to monitor for drug side effects (see below). Sputum cultures should be obtained monthly for the first 3 months; and at 3 months and 6 months to 1 year a chest X-ray should be obtained. Sputum culture should be negative after 3 months of therapy, although occasionally nonculturable acid-fast organisms will be seen on smear for longer periods. A test-of-cure culture should be done on all patients at 5 or 6 months. Resolution of pulmonary infiltrates is often slow; the former practice of monthly chest films is therefore not warranted. Chest films are most helpful in excluding progression of disease and in documenting the patient's status when the tuberculosis is cured.

At the cessation of traditional chemotherapy regimens (18 months) prolonged follow-up is not necessary. After short course i.e., 9-month, chemotherapy, it is recommended that close follow-up be continued for another 12 months to detect relapses by symptoms and sputum cultures.

Usual Response

Patients diagnosed as having tuberculosis who comply with therapy have an excellent prognosis. The only exceptions are the rare patients with organisms resistant to the usual antituberculous drugs or patients who develop adverse effects from the antituberculous therapy. These problems are discussed in more detail below.

The patient should show some symptomatic improvement within 1 week of being started on antituberculous therapy. Improvement is usually indicated by an increased sense of well-being, an increase in appetite, and a decrease in cough, fever, and night sweats; temperature should be normal within 10 days of initiating treatment. The patient is usually back to his usual state of health in 1 to 2 months.

The improvement is secondary to the antibacterial effects of the drugs, which lead to a decrease in the inflammatory response of the host. After 1 week of therapy, the patient can be considered noninfectious.

Possible Complications

Drug resistance. A number of problems may complicate the management of tuberculosis. The patient may have disease due to *drug-resistant M. tuberculosis* (7). This may occur in 5% of newly diagnosed cases in the United States (4% for isoniazid; 1% for ethambutol or rifampin). The frequency of drug resistance is higher if the disease was acquired abroad, particularly in Southeast Asia (15%) and Mexico. In this case, the patient may show a delayed clinical response during the first few weeks of therapy. Since the laboratory may take 8 to 10 weeks to provide sensitivity data on the original isolates, it may be difficult to detect this problem early. If resistance is strongly suspected (as in a patient with previously treated tuberculosis) or documented, the drug regimen should consist of two antituberculous drugs that the patient has not taken before; ideally these drugs should be selected on the basis of the sensitivity pattern of the organism. It is suggested that consultation be obtained before embarking on a course of therapy with second line, less effective drugs, however.

Drug toxicity. Patients may develop a number of toxicities from antituberculous medications (Table 29.3).

ISONIAZID. Hepatic toxicity is the most common adverse reaction; it occurs at a biochemical level in approximately 20% of persons who take the drug (3); the incidence of toxicity increases with age and with excessive alcohol intake (5, 8). Laboratory evidence of mild injury to the liver is not in itself a reason to stop the drug, however, since in most subjects the aminotransferase level returns to normal while the drug is being continued. If the patient develops clinical jaundice or develops fever and elevated liver enzymes, the drug should, of course, be stopped. The liver injury is usually reversible and will correct itself without further therapy. In some persons, however (elderly men and particularly those with chronic alcohol-related liver disease) the liver injury may be severe and sometimes fatal. Isoniazid liver toxicity most often occurs early in therapy, so that the first 2 to 3 months are the most critical in the detection of adverse drug reactions. Specific guidelines for monitoring for isoniazid hepatitis are contained in the section on prevention (below, page 371). Peripheral neuropathy is an uncommon complication of isoniazid therapy that occurs only in persons on an inadequate diet; it can be prevented by taking 5 mg of pyridoxine every day.

ETHAMBUTOL. The most serious side effect of ethambutol is optic neuritis, resulting in decrease of visual acuity and in inability to distinguish the color green. This problem was seen frequently when the drug was given in a dose of 25 mg/kg. It is extremely uncommon at the recommended daily dose of 15 mg/kg.

RIFAMPIN. Serious allergic complications of rifampin therapy, including thrombocytopenia manifested by purpura, petechiae, and hematuria, acute renal failure, and a "flu syndrome," occur in approximately 1% of patients and necessitate cessation of therapy. There is a modest increase in hepatic toxicity which may be additive to isoniazid toxicity so

that patients taking both drugs should be closely supervised. Patients should be warned that rifampin may result in an orange-red color in secretions such as urine, saliva, *etc.* Rifampin accelerates the metabolism of other drugs (Table 29.3) and may necessitate an increase in the dose of these drugs.

Problems requiring hospitalization. Ambulatory patients started on treatment should not require hospitalization. The few possible exceptions are (*a*) the development of progressive and debilitating disease, due either to resistant organisms or to poor compliance by the patient, and (*b*) severe toxic reactions to drugs, particularly isoniazid.

The Patient's Role in Therapy

The patient's role is of the utmost importance to the successful treatment of tuberculosis, since he must faithfully administer the drugs daily for a period of 9 or 18 months and return for regular follow-up visits.

Because noncompliance accounts for most therapeutic failures, the most important function of monthly visits is the documentation and reinforcement of compliance (see Chapter 4). When therapy is begun, the patient shoud be thoroughly educated about the course and therapy of his disease, so that the illusion of health when symptoms disappear will not cause premature cessation of therapy. The physician should help the patient design a strategy to avoid missing daily medication due to forgetfulness. Pill counts at follow-up visits may be helpful. In noncompliant patients, the twice weekly regimens summarized above may be particularly useful. If there are problems with compliance that cannot be solved by the physician, the patient should be referred to public health authorities for supervision of long term care. Such authorities will provide home visits if necessary and will ensure that the patient is not lost to follow-up.

The patient should be advised about the communicable nature of his disease, which is particularly important until he has been on therapy for at least a week. During that first week, he should minimize his contact with others, and be advised simply to cough into tissue which then should be incinerated. After 1 week, he should be considered not contagious, and his activities can be dictated solely by his sense of well-being. Patients taking isoniazid should be given specific advice and monitored for hepatitis as outlined in the following section.

PREVENTION OF TUBERCULOSIS
Case Detection among Known Contacts

An integral part of initiation of care in any patient with active tuberculosis is case reporting to the local health authority and investigation of contacts. This entails tuberculin testing of all household and intimate "nonhousehold" contacts and retesting of non-reactors in 2 to 3 months. Reactors are examined by chest X-ray and if free of active disease are given chemoprophylaxis with isoniazid for 1 year. With the exception of evaluating family members this type of investigation is usually impossible for a physician to carry out alone and should be done by the local city or county health department. Such departments have trained personnel who are available to visit homes and workplaces in order to detect cases in contacts. In many states, it is required by law that persons with newly diagnosed tuberculosis (or with a strongly suspected diagnosis) be reported to the public health authorities.

Tuberculin Testing in Prevention

(See method, page 366 above, and interpretation, Table 29.2.)

Ideally the tuberculin skin test status of all individuals should be determined at some time in their early adult life. In almost all school age children, screening for tuberculin positivity is coordinated with school health programs. In adult populations, a number of factors such as urban residence, the presence of chronic disease, a history of residence in underdeveloped countries, and health care occupation increase the importance of periodic tuberculin testing. This is particularly true for those individuals for whom isoniazid is recommended if the PPD is positive (see the next section).

Because of the increased risk of contact with unrecognized cases of tuberculosis, physicians and hospital personnel have an increased chance of acquiring infection (twice the risk of the general population). Both for personal protection and because of the risk of transmitting tuberculosis to patients, physicians and other health workers should have annual tuberculin testing and should take isoniazid chemoprophylaxis if they convert from negative to positive.

Isoniazid Prophylaxis

Isoniazid prophylaxis (300 mg daily for 1 year) has been shown to be very effective in preventing new cases of active tuberculosis among special groups of persons at high risk. Because of the recognition of isoniazid-induced hepatitis, however, the indications for the use of isoniazid have narrowed somewhat in recent years. At the present time, isoniazid prophylaxis is recommended for persons in the following groups (2, 4, 9): (a) close contacts of active infectious cases; (b) persons with recent skin test conversion (not those with booster responses, see above, page 366); (c) persons with positive skin tests and an abnormal chest X-ray suggestive of old tuberculosis; (d) persons with a known history of old tuberculosis who have never been given antibacterial treatment; (e) persons with positive skin tests who will be given corticosteroid or immunosuppressive therapy, who have silicosis, who have a history

of a gastrectomy, or who have a malignancy, such as Hodgkin's disease, which reduces T cell activity; and (f) persons with a positive skin test only, who are under the age of 35 years.

The guidelines recommended by the American Thoracic Society for monitoring patients taking isoniazid are the following (2):

Individuals receiving preventive therapy or a responsible adult in a household with children on preventive therapy should be questioned carefully at monthly intervals for (a) symptoms consistent with those of liver damage or of other toxic effects; that is, unexplained anorexia, nausea, or vomiting of greater than 3 days' duration, fatigue or weakness of greater than 3 days' duration, new and persistent paresthesias of the hands and feet; and (b) signs consistent with those of liver damage or of other toxic effects; that is, persistent dark urine, icterus, rash, elevated temperature of greater than 3 days' duration without explanation.

Monitoring by routine laboratory tests (e.g., aminotransferases, serum bilirubin, and alkaline phosphatase) is not always useful in predicting hepatic disease in isoniazid recipients and therefore is controversial. However, in evaluating signs and symptoms such tests are mandatory. Preventive therapy should be reinstituted only if biochemical studies are normal and signs and symptoms are absent.

Because it has been recognized that this monitoring plan may fail to detect an occasional patient with severe hepatitis (3), monthly measurement of aminotransferase levels is recommended by some authorities. This would detect the transient aminotransferase elevation which occurs in approximately 20% of subjects taking isoniazid; a cut-off level, such as a level 3 or 5 times normal, is recommended as the criterion for discontinuing isoniazid. Glassroth (see "General References") suggests monthly measurement of aminotransferase levels in those patients who are in the groups at the highest risk of developing isoniazid hepatitis— i.e., those over 35 years of age, daily "drinkers," patients concomitantly taking other potentially hepatotoxic drugs, and patients with a history of liver disease.

General References

Byrd RB, Horn BR, Solomon DA, et al: Treatment of tuberculosis by the nonpulmonary physician. Ann Intern Med 86:799, 1977.
  Useful summary of the most common mistakes made by general physicians treating patients for tuberculosis.
Glassroth MD, Robins AG, Snider DE Jr: Tuberculosis in the 1980s. N Engl J Med 302:1441, 1980.
  Extensively referenced and up to date review.

Specific References

1. American Thoracic Society: Treatment of tuberculosis and other mycobacterial diseases. Am Rev Respir Dis 127:790, 1983.
2. American Thoracic Society, Medical Section of the American Lung Association: Preventive therapy of tuberculous infection. Am Rev Respir Dis 110:371, 1974.

3. Byrd RG, Horn BR, Solomon DA, Griggs GA: Toxic effects of isoniazid in tuberculosis chemoprophylaxis. *JAMA* 241:1239, 1979.

4. Comstock GW, Edwards PQ: The competing risks of tuberculosis and hepatitis for adult tuberculin reactors. *Am Rev Respir Dis* 111:573, 1975.

5. Garibaldi RA, Drusin RE, Ferebee SH, Gregg MD: Isoniazid-associated hepatitis: report of an outbreak. *Am Rev Respir Dis* 106:357, 1972.

6. Houk VH, Kent DC, Baker JH, *et al*: In-depth analysis of a micro-outbreak of tuberculosis in a closed environment. *Arch Environ Health* 16:4, 1968.

7. Kopanoff DE, Kilburn JO, Glassroth JL, *et al*: A continuing survey of tuberculosis primary drug resistance in the United States: March 1975 to November 1977. A United States Public Health Service cooperative study. *Am Rev Respir Dis* 118:835, 1978.

8. Maddrey WC, Boitnott JK: Isoniazid hepatitis. *Ann Intern Med* 79:1, 1973.

9. Moulding T: Chemoprophylaxis of tuberculosis: when is the benefit worth the risk and cost? *Ann Intern Med* 74:761, 1971.

10. Sokal JE: Measurement of delayed skin-test responses. *N Engl J Med* 293:501, 1975.

11. Stead WW: Pathogenesis of the sporadic case of tuberculosis. *N Engl J Med* 277:1008, 1967.

12. Stead WW, Kerby GR, Schlueter DP, Jordahl CW: The clinical spectrum of primary tuberculosis in adults: confusion with reinfection in the pathogenesis of chronic tuberculosis. *Ann Intern Med* 68:731, 1968.

13. Thompson NJ, Glassroth JL, Snider DE Jr, Farer LS: The booster phenomenon in serial tuberculin testing. *Am Rev Respir Dis* 119:587, 1979.

CHAPTER THIRTY

Syphilis

PETER E. DANS, M.D.

EPIDEMIOLOGY

Syphilis (also known as lues or "bad blood") became a major public health menace when a virulent form of the disease swept through Europe in the late 15th and early 16th centuries. It flourished in settings of sexual promiscuity and of heightened mobility, especially during wars. The combination of effective penicillin therapy and contact tracing brought the incidence of new infections to a low point in the 1950s (Table 30.1). Since the so-called "sexual revolution" of the 1960s, the frequency of early cases has increased somewhat; despite this, the prevalence of late and late latent syphilis has continued to decline.

New cases of infectious syphilis occur more often in large urban centers. Rates per hundred thousand population in 1983 varied from 158.5 in San Francisco and 106.4 in Atlanta and New Orleans to 0.8 in Omaha and 1.7 and 1.9 in Pittsburgh and Des Moines, respectively. The male/female ratio among new cases was 2.6 to 1. Increasingly, syphilis is being

Table 30.1.
Annual Reported Cases of Syphilis in the United States for Selected Years[a]

Stage	1943	1956	1965	1980	1983
Infectious (primary and secondary) syphilis	82,204	6,392	23,338	27,204	32,698
Early latent <1 year duration	149,390	19,783	17,458	20,297	23,738
Late and late latent	251,958	95,097	67,317	20,979	17,896
Total	483,552	121,272	108,113	68,480	94,332

[a] From Blount J, Centers for Disease Control, Department of Health and Human Services, Atlanta, Georgia (personal communication).

traced to male homosexuals or bisexuals. In 1969, approximately 25% of the males acquiring the disease were homosexuals or bisexuals; currently this percentage is about 40%, whereas the proportion of men in the population estimated to be homosexual is approximately 10%. Recent data, however, suggest that homosexuals are altering their sexual practices, avoiding transient anonymous liaisons, and limiting their number of partners because of their fear of the acquired immune deficiency syndrome (AIDS, see Chapter 52). As a result, there may be a decline in their acquisition of syphilis.

STAGES OF THE DISEASE (Table 30.2)

The acquired form of the disease has different stages: primary, secondary, early and late latent, and tertiary or late syphilis. The primary and secondary stages may not be clinically apparent and only a third of untreated patients develop tertiary manifestations.

Primary Syphilis

Primary syphilis is characterized by the development of a "chancre" at the site of intimate sexual contact (genitals, anus, mouth, breast, and occasionally elsewhere). Syphilis infections have been documented in about one-third of the contacts occurring during the past month with patients diagnosed as having infectious syphilis (i.e., primary or secondary) (16). It appears 10 to 90 days (average 21 days) following infection by *Treponema pallidum*, the etiological organism. It usually starts as a single painless papule which varies in size from a few millimeters to a few centimeters in diameter and progresses to an ulcer with indurated edges containing a highly infectious exudate. Multiple lesions occur in about 30% of cases. There is associated painless regional and generalized lymphadenopathy. If secondary infection occurs, the lesions may become painful. Major considerations in the differential diagnosis are summarized in Table 30.3. Definitive diagnosis is made by microscopic examination of the fluid overlying the ulcer (see "Dark-Field Microscopy"). Serological tests for syphilis (STS) are usually positive (see "Diagnosis").

Secondary Syphilis

If untreated during the primary stage, most patients develop secondary syphilis 6 weeks to 6 months after initial contact. When the secondary stage begins, the chancre may still be present. The most characteristic finding is a nonpruritic rash which is usually maculopapular, but not vesicular or bullous. It can involve all areas of the skin, especially the trunk, the palms, and the soles. Scalp and eyelash involvement may lead to alopecia. Mucous patches (gray oral patches on an erythematous base) and lesions in warm, moist areas such as the axillary and genital regions are particularly infectious. Condyloma latum, a flat, wart-like lesion usually found in the genital or anal area, is also highly infectious; it must be distinguished from the more common pointy, fleshy, genital wart (condyloma acuminatum, see Chapter 94). Dark-field examination of moist skin lesions or the condyloma latum should be positive. In as many as one-half of the patients, skin lesions may not occur or may not be detected.

Constitutional symptoms—such as fever, headache, malaise, and generalized lymphadenopathy—are common. Other systemic manifestations occur in 1 to 2% of cases and include hepatitis, immune complex nephropathy, and frank meningitis. The latter is characterized by headache, stiff neck, seizures, and cranial nerve signs including papilledema and involvement of the 3rd, 6th, 7th, and 8th nerves. Associated with involvement of the latter, there is tinnitus, followed by deafness which can be reversed by treatment (1). The diagnosis of *syphilitic meningitis* is made by finding in the cerebrospinal fluid (CSF), mononuclear cells, elevated protein, an abnormal CSF-VDRL, and spirochetes on dark-field examination.

Serological tests for syphilis are positive in virtually 100% of patients at this stage (Table 30.4). The major considerations in differential diagnosis are drug reactions, psoriasis, and pityriasis rosea. The latter occurs in the spring and fall and characteristically begins as a single large initial lesion on the trunk, the "herald patch." This is followed by a pruritic, erythematous, maculopapular rash which develops along the lines of skin cleavage, especially

Table 30.2.
Outline of Clinical Stages of Syphilis[a]

Stage	Characteristic findings	Usual onset after exposure	Duration of stage in untreated patients	Dark field
Primary	Chancre—may be absent or not visible (*e.g*, in vagina or mouth)	10–90 days (average 21 days)	2–6 weeks	+ (Chancre, lymph nodes)
Secondary	Rash, condyloma latum, lymphadenopathy	6 weeks to 6 months	2–6 weeks; recurrences in 25% over 2-year period	+ (Especially moist lesions)
Acute syphilitic meningitis	Headache, cranial nerve lesions, papilledema	6 weeks to 2 years	Not applicable	+ CSF
Latent			May be lifelong since only ⅓ of untreated patients develop tertiary syphilis	–
Early	None	<1 year after infection		
Late	None	>1 year after infection		
Late (tertiary)				
Benign	Gumma	2–10 years	Indolent	–
Cardiovascular	Aortic aneurysm Aortic insufficiency Coronary artery disease especially of the ostia	10–30 years	Progressive; may be fatal	Aorta may be +
Neurosyphilis		2–35 years	Progressive; may be fatal	Brain may be +
Asymptomatic	None			
Meningovascular	Signs of infection depend on area involved	2–10 years		
Paresis	Minor personality change to frank psychosis	15–35 years		
Tabes dorsalis	Signs of posterior column degeneration	5–30 years		

[a] See details in the text.

on the trunk (see Chapter 100). It is not accompanied by systemic symptoms.

Untreated, secondary syphilis lasts 2 to 6 weeks and may relapse in about 25% at some time during the first 4 years after infection; 90% of all relapses occur within a year. Although relapses are usually identical to initial episodes, condyloma latum may be more common.

Latent Syphilis

Latent syphilis is, as the name implies, the period after infection with T. *pallidum* when there are no clinical manifestations. Latent syphilis was formerly divided into an early and late stage at 4 years because the Oslo study of the course of untreated syphilis did not demonstrate relapses after 4 years.

The division has now been set at 1 year because epidemiologists following up contacts of patients with syphilis of more than 1 year's duration rarely turn up infectious cases; so this becomes a useful demarcation for reporting purposes.

The major way that patients with latent disease come to diagnosis is through routine serological testing (see "Diagnosis"). Detection early in this stage is important not only for epidemiological purposes but also to prevent further complications in the one-third of untreated patients who go on to develop late manifestations of syphilis.

Tertiary Syphilis

Tertiary or late disease is divided into three principal forms: late benign syphilis, cardiovascular syphilis, and neurosyphilis. Since the advent of penicillin therapy, all forms of tertiary syphilis have become uncommon (Table 30.1). In addition, the late manifestations have become milder and more subtle (8).

Late benign syphilis, which is rare today, is characterized by the development of a gumma, a lesion which may grow to several centimeters in size. The gumma is a hypersensitivity reaction and rarely contains viable organisms. It usually occurs within

Table 30.3.
Differential Diagnosis of a Genital Sore

Primary syphilis (chancre)
    Incubation period 10–90 days (average, 21 days)
    Usually painless (in absence of secondary infection)
    Not vesicular
    Usually single indurated ulcer but multiple lesions are seen
        in 30% of cases
    Spirochete on dark field examination
    Nontender inguinal adenopathy
Herpes simplex
    Incubation period 24–48 hours
    Usually painful
    Vesicular
    Usually multiple ulcers
    Multinucleated giant cells on Giemsa stain plus virus on
        culture
    Tender inguinal adenopathy
Chancroid
    Multiple soft superficial erosions
    Nontender adenopathy. *Haemophilus ducreyi* on Gram
        stain of dried smear (small Gram-negative bacillus)
Granuloma inguinale
    Soft, occasionally raised, granulating lesions in inguinal
        area: Donovan bodies on smear (histiocytes with intra-
        cytoplasmic encapsulated Gram-negative bacilli)
Other considerations
    Trauma, carcinoma, scabies, lichen planus, psoriasis, fixed
        drug eruption ((especially phenolphthalein), fungus infec-
        tion, folliculitis

2 to 10 years of infection, most commonly on the skin (ulcerative or nodular-ulcerative), in bone, or in the liver. It is especially destructive when it occurs in the brain, liver, or heart. Diagnosis is made on the basis of typical pathological findings and dramatic healing of visible gummas following treatment.

Cardiovascular syphilis, which is very common today, was reported in 13.6% of untreated men and 7.6% of untreated women from 5 to 30 years after acquisition of the disease. Aortitis is the commonest cardiovascular manifestation. The organism destroys the elastic tissue of the media of the aorta and produces an endarteritis of the vasa vasorum. Clinical manifestations include aneurysm of the ascending aorta and progressive dilatation of the aortic ring, resulting in aortic insufficiency and heart failure. When the coronary ostia are involved, angina pectoris may result. Linear calcification of the ascending aorta is a common radiological finding in syphilitic aortitis; it may precede clinical symptoms and signs of aortic involvement.

Asymptomatic neurosyphilis is defined by the occurrence of a positive serological test for syphilis in the spinal fluid of a patient who has no neurological or psychiatric signs or symptoms. A pleocytosis and an elevated protein may be present in the fluid. Asymptomatic neurosyphilis occurred in 10% of all untreated patients in the preantibiotic era. The current prevalence is probably much lower. Exact estimates are hampered by limitations in the diagnostic tests (see below).

Symptomatic neurosyphilis, which is also uncommon, occurred in 9.4% of men and 5% of women with untreated syphilis in the Oslo study. The risk of developing symptomatic neurosyphilis after a primary infection is greater in whites than in blacks. Symptomatic neurosyphilis is divided into various types depending upon the site of major involvement.

1. *Meningovascular syphilis* usually occurs

Table 30.4.
Sensitivity and Specificity of Serological Tests for Syphilis[a] at Different Stages

Stage of syphilis	Percent sensitivity (Sens.) and specificity (Spec.)							
	VDRL[b]		RPR[b]		FTA-ABS[b]		MHA-TP[b]	
	Sens.	Spec.	Sens.	Spec.	Sens.	Spec.	Sens.	Spec.
Primary	80 (59–87)	98 (80–99)	86 (81–100)	98 (80–99)	98 (93–100)	98 (84–99)	82 (64–90)	99 (98–100)
Secondary	100 (99–100)	98	100 (99–100)	98	100 (99–100)	98	100 (96–100)	99
Latent	96 (73–100)	98	99	98	100 (96–100)	98	100 (96–100)	99
Late	71	98	73	98	96	98	94	99

[a] The consensus figures for the sensitivity and specificity are for tests done in the Centers for Disease Control Reference Laboratory (10) on samples derived from a well run STD clinic. The figures in parentheses demonstrate the variability in published reports. Responsible factors include (a) study of populations with different prevalences of syphilis and other confounding illnesses, (b) variable performance by the laboratory and (c) different clinical criteria for the diagnosis of syphilis (see the text).
[b] See text for fuller discussion of these tests.

within 2 to 10 years after untreated primary infection. Common manifestations include headache, irritability, and personality changes. Vasculitis involving small end arteries results in focal neurological signs. The severity of the patient's disability depends upon the extent and location of the accompanying cerebrovascular inflammation and occlusion.

2. *Tabes dorsalis* usually occurs 5 to 30 years after infection. It is characterized by symptoms and signs of posterior column degeneration (ataxia, areflexia, broad-based gait, incontinence, impotence, abdominal pain crises, and paresthesias or "lightning" pains in the extremities). Characteristic findings also include trophic joint changes (Charcot's joints), the Argyll Robertson pupil (small, irregular pupil which accommodates but does not react to light), and optic atrophy (in about 10% of patients).

3. The syndrome of *general paresis* usually occurs 15 to 35 years after infection. It is due to destruction of the parenchyma of the cerebral cortex. It consists of personality changes, irritability, poor judgment, insomnia, and memory loss. The progressive dementia in these patients may be characterized by periodic euphoria and delusions of grandeur.

A definitive diagnosis of neurosyphilis is based upon spinal fluid findings: elevated protein and mononuclear cells, as well as a positive serological test for syphilis (see "Diagnosis").

DIAGNOSIS

Dark-Field Microscopy

As syphilis has decreased in prevalence, both the availability of dark-field microscopy and the competence of those performing it have declined. Large medical centers with special sexually transmitted disease (STD) clinics and larger health departments ordinarily provide reliable testing. One should call ahead to assure availability before obtaining any material. In order to obtain material, one should (*a*) abrade the lesion gently with gauze so as to produce a nonbloody, serous exudate; (*b*) after wiping the surface, squeeze the lesion between gloved thumb and forefinger; (*c*) collect the exudate in a capillary pipette; and (*d*) finally, give it to someone who knows how to do the test. Dark-field microscopy should be performed on 3 consecutive days in highly suspect patients before being called definitively negative. This is especially so if antibiotic ointments have been used. Dark-field examination should not be done on material obtained from oral lesions because of the potential for confusion with *T. microdentium*, a common mouth inhabitant.

Serological Tests in Diagnosis

Serological tests are of *two basic types*; nontreponemal and treponemal. Nontreponemal tests detect reagin, a nonspecific antibody to cardiolipin, a nor-

mal component of many tissues. Wassermann in 1906 was the first to use this reaction to detect patients with syphilis. Since then about 100 different forms of the original Wassermann test have been developed. Those in common use today are the Venereal Disease Research Laboratory (VDRL) and the rapid plasma reagin (RPR) tests which are flocculation tests and, less commonly, the Kolmer complement fixation test.

The treponemal tests include the fluorescent treponemal antibody-absorption test (FTA-ABS) and the microhemagglutination test for *T. pallidum* (MHATP). Both tests detect specific antibodies to *T. pallidum*. Figure 30.1 shows the pattern of reactivity of various serological tests during the course of untreated syphilis. The *Treponema pallidum* Immobilization (TPI) test, once the treponemal test of choice, is now available only on a research basis.

The sensitivity (the percentage of syphilitic patients with a reactive test) varies at each stage of the disease and for different tests (see Table 30.4). The RPR is slightly more sensitive than the VDRL; the FTA-ABS and MHATP are more sensitive than either. The range of values for sensitivity is accounted for by differences in case definition in different studies. Where case definition is more rigorous as, e.g., using a positive dark-field to assure the diagnosis of primary syphilis rather than simply clinical criteria, the sensitivity is higher.

STS *specificity* (the percentage of nonsyphilitic patients with a negative test) is also shown in Table 30.4. Since the FTA-ABS and MHATP measure specific antibody, their specificities are higher than those of the VDRL and RPR. There are two major reasons for the variance in specificity given for each test. First, study populations have differed in the proportion of patients with conditions which cause false positive test results. For example, studies of the

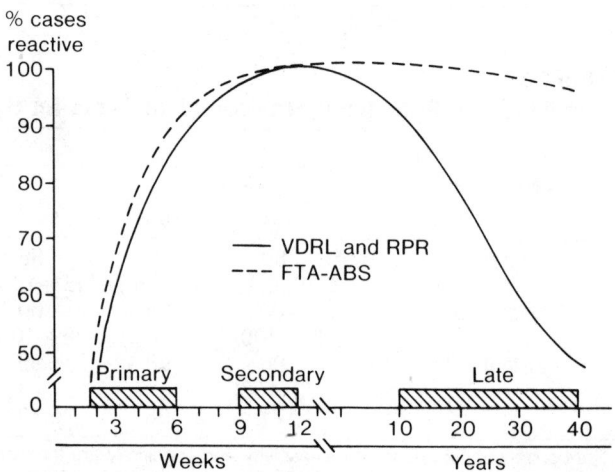

Figure 30.1. Serology of untreated syphilis. (Adapted from Wallace AL, Norins LC: Syphilis serology today. *Prog Clin Pathol* 2:198, 1969.)

specificity of the VDRL or the FTA-ABS in a group of nuns or other healthy volunteer populations have revealed very few false positives. On the other hand, studies in sexually transmitted disease clinic populations, facilities serving drug addicts, or arthritis clinic populations with many patients with systemic lupus have yielded higher rates of false positives and consequently lower estimates of specificity. Second, test performance can vary in different laboratories with devastating effects on both the specificity and sensitivity of such vulnerable tests as the FTA-ABS (2). Table 30.4 gives consensus sensitivity and specificity figures for serological tests done on serum from patients in an STD clinic population and performed at the Centers for Disease Control (CDC) reference laboratory (13). As with any other test, you must determine how applicable they are to tests done in your population and at your laboratory. Most of the discussion of treponemal tests will be confined to the FTA-ABS test which is used more extensively. However, some laboratories are substituting the MHATP as the treponemal test of choice because it is cheaper and less subject to technical error (Table 30.4).

When either the VDRL or RPR is positive and the FTA-ABS or the MHATP is consistently negative, the patient is considered to have a biological false positive test result. "Acute" biological false positive VDRL and RPR tests are defined as those lasting less than 6 months. They have been reported in patients with viral and bacterial pneumonia, hepatitis, pregnancy, mononucleosis, measles, malaria, and following smallpox vaccination. "Chronic" false positive nontreponemal test reactions (those lasting more than 6 months) occur in diseases of disordered immunity, such as systemic lupus erythematosus, rheumatoid arthritis, and Waldenström's macroglobulinemia, as well as in chronic liver disease, heroin addicts, elderly persons (approximately 1% of persons over 70 and 10% of persons over 80), and in a few patients on a hereditary basis. Biologic false positive VDRL or RPR titers are usually 1:8 or lower but occasionally can be higher, especially in hereditary cases. A false positive VDRL or RPR should not be dismissed but should be used as a clue to the diagnosis of the conditions listed above. However, in as many as 50% of cases, no explanation can be found and the patient remains symptom free. Whatever the case, a patient should be informed of his or her test status in order to prevent inappropriate labeling and treatment for syphilis.

When properly performed, the FTA-ABS has a specificity of 98%. False positive reactions do occur, however, in patients with lupus erythematosus, rheumatoid arthritis, chronic liver disease, some infections, and in other patients for unexplained reasons. Since small errors in laboratory technique can affect the results of the FTA-ABS test more than the results of the nontreponemal tests, the FTA-ABS

should be utilized selectively (2), i.e., only when nontreponemal tests are positive. Exception should be made when either primary or tertiary syphilis is highly suspect. This might occur, for example, when the patient has a very suspicious lesion resembling a chancre and dark-field microscopy is negative, when there are neurological or psychiatric signs suggestive of tabes or paresis, or if signs of aortic insufficiency and aneurysm of the ascending aorta are present. In these situations, the treponemal test may occasionally be the only positive test (Table 30.4).

In diagnosing *latent syphilis*, a single positive nontreponemal test, even if confirmed by an FTA-ABS or MHATP test, should not be relied upon as the only datum, especially if there is no other reason to suspect it. The test should be repeated to assure that there was not a mix-up of blood specimens. The implications of this diagnosis are too serious to rely on a single datum.

The sensitivity *of the CSF VDRL* for the detection of neurosyphilis ranges from 10 to 89%. It is highest for meningitis, meningovascular and paretic forms and lowest for asymptomatic neurosyphilis and tabes dorsalis. While virtually 100% specific for neurosyphilis, case reports of false positive CSF-VDRL have been reported after traumatic lumbar puncture and in a case of meningeal tumor. Recent evidence suggests that the CSF FTA-ABS has an excellent sensitivity and specificity when performed at the CDC reference laboratory. However, because of vulnerability to performance error, its use should be restricted to the CDC and only in highly suspect cases. Thus, the CSF VDRL, with all of its limitations, remains the test of choice in the workup for neurosyphilis in selected patients (2a, 11).

Serological Tests in Screening (1a)

A nontreponemal serological test for syphilis should be used as a screening test in patients who are sexually active with multiple partners and who are thereby at increased risk for acquisition of syphilis. This is true for both heterosexuals and homosexuals; however, since the proportion of homosexuals among patients with infectious syphilis is disproportionately high, particular attention should be given to case detection and education in this group. Patients found to have another STD, such as gonorrhea, should also have a screening STS. This is because their pattern of sexual activity puts them at higher risk for having acquired syphilis in the past. The occasional patient who acquires syphilis and gonorrhea simultaneously will have a negative serology when the gonorrhea becomes manifest since the latent periods for the development of both diseases differ so widely. This is of concern only for contact tracing, since penicillin treatment for gonorrhea during the incubation period aborts the development of syphilis (16). In most office settings, an

STS should be done routinely on a sexually active patient's first visit. In subsequent visits, a repeat STS should be done only in those patients deemed to have been at risk for acquiring a new infection during the interval.

Pattern of Serological Tests after Treatment (1a) (Fig. 30.2)

The VDRL reverts to negative in more than 90% of patients adequately treated for primary or secondary syphilis, but the FTA-ABS rarely does so. The FTA-ABS should be repeated once 6–12 months after syphilis is diagnosed and treated. If it remains positive, it should not be repeated. In later serological testing of patients who have had syphilis, the nontreponemal test titer becomes the most useful tool (see "Follow-up") (15). In patients treated for early latent syphilis the VDRL becomes negative within 5 years of treatment in approximatley 75%, while only about 25% of patients with treated late latent syphilis will be seronegative in 5 years (4). Many middle-aged and older persons with a VDRL or RPR of 1:4 or lower reactivity in the nontreponemal test will fall into the category of adequately treated serofast syphilis, but differentiation from late latent syphilis should be made through careful history.

TREATMENT (17)

Regimens

The treatment of choice for *primary, secondary, and early latent syphilis,* as well as for known contacts of a patient with infectious syphilis, is 2.4 million units of benzathine penicillin G (LA Bicillin) intramuscularly (17). Some advocate administering a second injection 1 week later (4). Alternatives for persons allergic to penicillin are total doses of 30 g

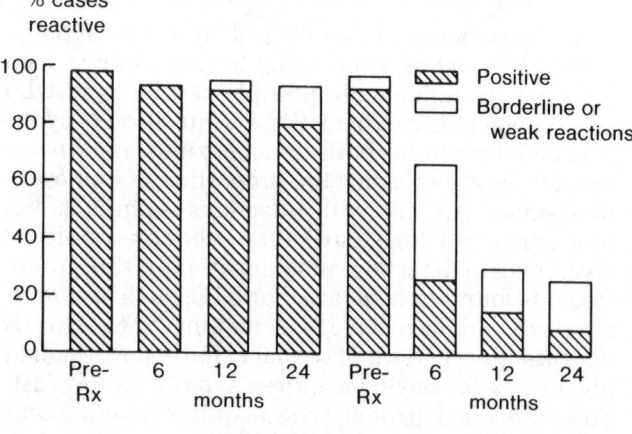

Figure 30.2. Serological reactivity of 80 patients treated for dark-field positive primary or secondary syphilis and observed for 2 years, with use of FTA-ABS and VDRL tests. (Adapted from Schroeter AL, *et al.*: Treatment for early syphilis and reactivity of serologic tests. *JAMA* 221:471, 1972.)

of oral tetracycline or erythromycin (2 g a day for 15 days). As noted above, the usual antimicrobial regimens for gonorrhea are also effective against incubating syphilis, acquired simultaneously (16).

The treatment of choice for late *latent syphilis,* when a spinal fluid examination has not been done to exclude asymptomatic neurosyphilis, is 2.4 million units of benzathine penicillin G (LA Bicillin) weekly for 3 weeks or in patients allergic to penicillin, 60 g total dose of tetracycline or erythromycin (2 g a day for 30 days).

In patients who have *confirmed neurosyphilis,* recommended therapy consists of either

a. Twelve to 24 million units of intravenous aqueous crystalline penicillin G daily for 10 days *followed* by benzathine penicillin G: 2.4 million units, intramuscularly, weekly for three doses or

b. Procaine penicillin G: 2.4 million units, intramuscularly, once daily plus probenecid 500 mg by mouth, four times a day, for 10 days, *followed* by benzathine penicillin G, 2.4 million units, intramuscularly, weekly for three doses.

Benzathine penicillin G (2.4 million units, intramuscularly weekly for three doses), alone is still an option for the treatment of symptomatic neurosyphilis. However, more intensive courses of penicillin are currently recommended because of recent case reports of the failure of benzathine penicillin G alone to eradicate the organism and to arrest the disease (5, 8). Because alternatives to penicillin are less effective for the treatment of neurosyphilis, patients giving a history of penicillin allergy should be evaluated by skin testing (Chapter 23). If negative, a penicillin regimen should be used. In the occasional case where it is positive, consultation with an infectious disease expert is desirable to select the best alternative treatment.

Effectiveness

The effectiveness of treatment varies depending on the stage of syphilis treated. In one study of patients with primary and secondary syphilis, retreatment was required in 5% of patients after the usual doses of benzathine penicillin G, and in 10% of patients after the usual doses of tetracycline and erythromycin (15). The criteria for retreatment in this study were recurrence or persistence of clinical manifestations or failure of the VDRL titer to decrease 4-fold within 1 year.

The effectiveness of treatment in patients with latent syphilis is difficult to assess because of the absence of any markers to follow. However, in one follow-up study, all 469 patients with late latent syphilis treated at various centers with the recommended doses of penicillin were symptom free 12 years later (9).

The effectiveness of treatment of cardiovascular syphilis has been debated (3). Most investigators believe that treatment may arrest the disease, but not reverse it. Because of the weakening of the media of the aorta, aneurysms may continue to enlarge even after adequate treatment.

The results of treatment for neurosyphilis vary directly with the extent of the disease and inversely with its duration. Thus, treatment often reverses the signs and symptoms of acute meningovascular syphilis and stabilizes tabes dorsalis, but is less effective in reversing the signs of general paresis, especially if given late in its course (19).

Jarisch-Herxheimer Reaction (12, 14, 18)

The Jarisch-Herxheimer reaction is characterized by a mild temperature elevation within 6 to 8 hours of administration of the first injection of penicillin. It appears to be caused by microbial lysis and the release of endotoxin. It resolves after several hours and does not occur after subsequent injections. The reaction is estimated to occur in 50% of patients with primary syphilis, 75 to 90% of patients with secondary syphilis, and 30% of patients with late disease. When it occurs during treatment of secondary syphilis, skin lesions become more prominent. Because the Jarisch-Herxheimer reaction is common, patients should be told that the reaction usually is mild and lasts only a few hours and that it can be treated with mild analgesics. Uncommonly the reaction may be quite severe and consist of high fever, chills, headache, muscle and joint pains, sore throat, and transient hypotension. It may produce significant exacerbation of neurological signs in a few percent of patients treated for neurosyphilis. Steroid therapy has been used both before and after the reaction, but its efficacy is not established (18).

PRACTICAL APPROACH TO THE PATIENT

Sexually active patients in whom syphilis is a consideration usually present to their physicians because of (a) a "sore" or rash, (b) referral as a known contact of a patient with syphilis, (c) worry about a recent sexual liaison, or (d) a positive serological test in routine premarital, blood donor, or health screening. The diagnosis of syphilis must be made carefully, as it can have a major impact on the relationships of patients with their contacts and on how they view themselves. A systematic approach to diagnosis and management is outlined here.

Evaluation

The history should include a description of any sore or rash; determination of a previous history of STD especially syphilis; review of previous STS as far back as the last negative one; an inquiry into the patient's type of sexual practices to guide the physical examination; and information about recent partners and their disease status.

The physical examination should include a careful search for typical lesions in all areas of sexual con-tact. Special care should be taken in examining the anogenital area and the mouth. Other features to look for include regional and generalized lymphadenopathy, enlarged liver, and neurological, psychiatric, and cardiovascular signs when late disease is a concern.

Laboratory data should include dark-field microscopy (if available) of suspicious lesions and serological testing for syphilis (see "Diagnosis"). Cerebrospinal fluid (CSF) examination is mandatory in patients with psychiatric or neurological signs or symptoms. In asymptomatic patients who have had syphilis for more than 1 year, the CDC recommends a lumbar puncture to exclude asymptomatic neurosyphilis. However, the CSF examination is virtually always negative in such patients. Furthermore, in the most comprehensive study of the subject, only 1 of 765 patients with asymptomatic neurosyphilis treated with penicillin in doses equivalent to the 3 weekly benzathine penicillin G injections developed clinical neurosyphilis (6). Thus, for patients who are asymptomatic and who have low serum nontreponemal test titers, it is reasonable to administer the recommended regimen for late latent syphilis without performing a lumbar puncture (2a, 18a). An intermediate approach between this and the CDC recommendations has been suggested by Jaffe who lists the following contraindications to lumbar puncture: (a) rapidly fatal underlying disease, (b) initial infection known to have occurred 30 or more years before, (c) unstable angina or coagulation disorder, (d) age greater than 70, and (e) where successful lumbar puncture requires multiple attempts (10).

In patients who were treated for syphilis with heavy metals before the penicillin era, the question arises as to the need for further treatment. Most experts do not recommend retreating such patients whose syphilis acquisition dates back 35 years or more in the absence of signs or symptoms or exposure to infectious syphilis in the interim.

Special difficulty is presented by patients who are pregnant and who are found to have an abnormal serology when a routine STS is performed either at their initial visit or during the third trimester. Although pregnancy has been reported to be a cause of a biological false positive nontreponemal test, the burden of proof is on the person who says that this is not syphilis. Therefore, the FTA-ABS or the MHATP is an essential confirmatory test. If the treponemal test is negative and there is no clinical evidence of syphilis, nontreponemal and treponemal tests should be repeated monthly for 3 months. If the treponemal tests remain negative, this can be considered to be a biological false positive reaction. If there is clinical or serological confirmation of syphilis, the staging is similar to that for nonpregnant patients. The only difference in therapy is that in penicillin-allergic patients, tetracycline is not recommended and erythromycin is the drug of choice. Nontreponemal tests should be performed at monthly intervals to determine therapeutic response and to detect any reinfection. Infants born even to adequately treated mothers will be seropositive at birth because of passive transfer of IgG across the placenta. If the baby appears healthy, no further treatment is indicated but the baby should be followed carefully over the next 6 to 12 months to assure that no signs develop and that the serological reactivity disappears.

Management

The management plan is contingent upon making the appropriate diagnosis. The diagnosis rests on positive dark-field microscopy or on the combination of a positive nontreponemal and treponemal test. When the diagnosis is made, the disease should be staged appropriately, as outlined above.

The most common errors in the diagnosis of syphilis are: (a) failing to take proper note of an abnormal serology and missing the diagnosis entirely; or (b) noting the serological change but inadequately staging the disease or, at the extreme, formulating the assessment and plan as follows: "positive VDRL, treat with penicillin." Treatment of syphilis at a given stage is indicated; not treatment of a positive VDRL. Appropriate antibiotic regimens are listed above for each stage of syphilis.

Follow-up

In following up the patient, the nontreponemal test titer remains the most useful index of the effectiveness of treatment. A high titer is more likely to occur in early syphilis or in active late disease. Where a 1:4 titer or greater is present, a VDRL or RPR should be obtained every 3 months for a year to see if the patient has a 4-fold or greater fall in titer (for example, a 1:32 titer which falls to 1:2). If the expected fall in titer does not occur within 9 to 12 months, the patient should be retreated. It is important to use the same nontreponemal test on all serial specimens because of the differences in their sensitivity, i.e., the RPR titer will often be at least one dilution higher than a VDRL done on the same specimen.

Patients with persistently high titers after 1 year (1:8 or higher) may represent either treatment failures or undetected reinfections and should be retreated. A spinal fluid examination to rule out neurosyphilis is indicated in such patients. Patients who have a 4-fold or greater rise in titer during follow-up should be considered to be reinfected and staged and treated accordingly. In patients with very low titers, as is usually the case in the late latent stage, there is no practical way of assessing the adequacy of therapy.

Contact Tracing

In most jurisdictions, the physician is obligated by law to report the patient's name and the stage of the disease to the health department for both statistical purposes and contact tracing by specially trained investigators. Because of rapport with the patient, the physician may choose to coordinate contact tracing. In this era of freer discussion of human sexuality, this poses less of a problem; however, the physician may encounter a situation where the patient does not wish to be straightforward with partners about outside liaisons. This presents a conflict between patient confidentiality and the binding legal requirement to report the patient. Health department investigators make every effort to keep the patient's name from being divulged; however, where there is a spouse involved, this may be impossible without resorting to deception, which is not recommended. Where the patient balks at informing a spouse or steady partner, it must be impressed upon the patient that the relationship may well benefit from frank and honest discussion of the situation. In any case, not to do so would put the partner at risk and this cannot be condoned. Situations such as this require great sensitivity and ingenuity on the physician's part to be able to keep faith with the patient and the partner, and yet not unduly harm either.

All identified contacts of patients with infectious syphilis should be thoroughly evaluated for signs of syphilis. When the contact has signs of syphilis, the disease should be staged and treated accordingly and *their* contacts should be located. Even if there are no signs or serological evidence of active disease, contacts of patients with syphilis should receive prompt treatment for primary syphilis without waiting for clinical manifestations or a positive serology (7).

Education

Education should focus on prevention. If patients have sexual relations with multiple partners, they should be counseled about the risk this entails for contracting syphilis and other STDs. At the time that a patient is treated for infectious syphilis, he should be told to abstain from sex until the sore or rash disappears or for at least 1 week, whichever is longer. If he plans to continue to be promiscuous, he should be cautioned to use a condom as a protection against venereal disease transmission and acquisition. To be effective, condoms must be used during foreplay, properly worn, and intact. Cutler (1b) and others have shown that contraceptive vaginal creams and jellies may provide some prophylaxis as well. Nonetheless, patients who continue to be promiscuous should have checkups for gonorrhea and syphilis anytime they suspect they may have acquired one of these diseases or on a 6-month or yearly basis.

General References

Clark EG, Danbolt N: The Oslo study of the natural course of untreated syphilis. *Med Clin North Am* 48:613, 1964.
> Long term study of the natural history of syphilis in 1404 subjects.

Fiumara NJ, Shinberg JD, Byrne EM, Fountaine J: An outbreak of gonorrhea and early syphilis in Massachusetts. *N Engl J Med* 256:982, 1957.
> Detailed account of the spread of syphilis and of contact-tracing in a local outbreak.

Holmes KK, Märdh PA, Sparling PF, Weisner PJ (eds): *Sexually Transmitted Diseases.* New York, McGraw-Hill, 1984.
> Detailed accounts of syphilis and other STDs by leading experts.

Jones JH: *Badblood.* New York, Free Press, 1981.
> A popular account of the Tuskegee study.

Rosebury T: *Microbes and Morals.* New York, Vebany Press, 1971.
> Fascinating account of the history of sexually transmitted disease.

Symposium on venereal disease and gay men. *Sex Transm Dis* 4:41, 1977.
> Useful summary of the problem of syphilis in homosexuals.

Specific References

1. Balkany TJ, Dans PE: Reversible sudden deafness in early acquired syphilis. *Arch Otolaryngol* 104:66, 1978.
1a. Brown ST, Zaidi A, Larsen SA, Reynolds GH: Serological response to syphilis treatment. *JAMA* 253:1296, 1985.
1b. Cutler JC: Prophylaxis in the venereal diseases. *Med Clin North Am* 56:1211, 1972.
2. Dans PE, Judson FN, Larsen SA, Lantz MA: The FTA-ABS test. A diagnostic help or hindrance? *South Med J* 70:312, 1977.
2a. Dans PE, Cafferty L, Otter SE, Johnson RJ: The CSF VDRL: a case study of an inappropriately used test. *Ann Intern Med*, in press.
3. Dunlop EMC: Penicillin and the control of syphilis. *Am Heart J* 88:395, 1974.
4. Fiumara NJ: Serologic responses to treatment of 128 patients with late latent syphilis. *J Am Vener Dis Assoc* 6:243, 1979.
5. Greene BM, Miller NR, Bynum TE: Failure of penicillin G benzathine in the treatment of neurosyphilis. *Arch Intern Med* 140:1117, 1980.
6. Hahn RD, Cutler JC, Curtis AC, et al: Penicillin treatment of asymptomatic central nervous system syphilis. I. Probability of progression to symptomatic neurosyphilis. *Arch Dermatol* 74:355, 1956.
7. Hart G: Epidemiologic treatment for syphilis and gonorrhea. *Sex Transm Dis* 7:149, 1980.
8. Hooshmand H, Escobar MR, Kopf SW: Neurosyphilis, a study of 241 patients. *JAMA* 219:726, 1972.
9. Idsoe O, Guthe T, Willcox RR: Penicillin in the treatment of syphilis. The experience of three decades. *Bull WHO* 474:[Suppl] 1972.
10. Jaffe HW, Kabins SA: Examination of cerebrospinal fluid in patients with syphilis. *Rev Infect Dis* 4:[Suppl]S842, 1982.
11. Jaffe HW, Larsen SA, Peters M, et al: Tests for treponemal antibody in CSF. *Arch Intern Med* 138:252, 1978.
12. Jarisch Herxheimer reaction: Editorial. *Br Med J* 1:384, 1967.
13. Larsen SA, Hunter EF, McGrew BE: Syphilis. In Wentworth B, Judson FN (eds): *Laboratory Methods for the Diagnosis of Sexually Transmitted Diseases.* Washington, DC, American Public Health Association, 1984.
14. Putkonen T, Salo OP, Mustarallio KK: Febrile Herxheimer reaction in different phases of primary and secondary syphilis. *Br J Vener Dis* 42:181, 1966.
15. Schroeter AL, Lucas JB, Price EV, Falcone VH: Treatment for early syphilis and reactivity of serologic tests. *JAMA* 221:471, 1972.
16. Schroeter AL, Turner RH, Lucas JB, Brown WJ: Therapy for incubating syphilis. Effectiveness of gonorrhea treatment. *JAMA* 218:711, 1971.
17. Sexually Transmitted Diseases, Treatment Guidelines. *Morbidity and Mortality Weekly Report* 31:50S, 1982.
18. The Jarisch-Herxheimer reaction: *Lancet* 1:340, 1977.
18a. Wiesel J, Rose DN, Silver AL, et al: Lumbar puncture in asymptomatic late syphilis. An analysis of the benefits and risks. *Arch Intern Med* 145:465, 1985.
19. Wilner G, Brody JA: Prognosis of general paresis after treatment. *Lancet* 2:1370, 1968.

CHAPTER THIRTY-ONE

Ambulatory Care for Selected Subacute Infections: Osteomyelitis, Lung Abscess, and Endocarditis

JOHN G. BARTLETT, M.D.

INTRODUCTION

The three types of infections reviewed in this chapter are initially managed with intravenous antibiotics administered in the hospital. They are included here because these patients are often seen first in an office setting and because relatively long courses of antibiotics may be given after hospital discharge. These infections involve diverse bacteria and different anatomical sites but share the propensity for relapse due to persistent bacteria at the infected site. This explains the requirement for prolonged courses of antimicrobial agents. Antibiotics may be administered by two different routes out of hospital: the oral route, to complete a course initiated parenterally during hospitalization, and the intravenous route, utilizing the same regimen provided for inpatients. This latter form of treatment is gaining popularity due to concerns regarding hospital costs, and it is also attractive to patients who would often prefer to receive their antibiotics at home, particularly when other hospital resources are not required. Details about the use of home health services are found in Chapter 9.

OSTEOMYELITIS

Definition

Osteomyelitis is an infection of bone. There are three major categories: osteomyelitis following hematogenous spread of infection, osteomyelitis secondary to a contiguous focus of infection, and osteomyelitis associated with vascular insufficiency. There are major differences between these three categories according to age of occurrence, bones involved, predisposing conditions, usual bacterial pathogens, and presentation (Table 31.1).

Clinical Presentation and Bacteriology

Hematogenous

Hematogenous osteomyelitis is classically described as a disease of children, usually under 16 years of age and usually due to *Staphylococcus aureus*. The tendency for this infection to occur during active growth reflects the enhanced susceptibility of the vascular network of the metaphysis, especially of the femur or tibia. About one-third of patients have a history of preceding nonpenetrating trauma in the area that is subsequently involved. The infection begins in the metaphyseal sinusoidal veins; it is contained by the epiphyseal growth plate and tends to spread laterally with perforation of the cortex and lifting of the loose periosteum. Hematogenous osteomyelitis of the long bones in adults is rare, different in presentation and bacteriologically distinct. In these individuals, the growth cartilage has been resorbed so the subarticular space is more vulnerable and the periosteum is firmly attached so that subperiosteal abscess formation is uncommon. The most frequent form of hematogenous osteomyelitis in adults involves the vertebrae (see Fig. 31.1) and the most common pathogens are Gram-negative bacilli as well as *S. aureus*. The initial site of infection is the richly vascularized bone adjacent to cartilage; there is subsequent involvement of adjacent bone plates and of the intervertebral disc. The infection may extend longitudinally to involve adjacent vertebrae, anteriorly to produce a paraspinal abscess, or posteriorly to form an epidural abscess.

Table 31.1.
Types of Osteomyelitis

	Hematogenous	Secondary to Contiguous Infection	Complication of Vascular Insufficiency
Approximate proportion of all cases	20%	50%	30%
Commonest age group(s)	1–16 years >50 years	Any age	>50 years
Bones involved	Long bones (children) Vertebrae (adults)	Hip, femur, tibia, digits	Feet
Predisposing causes	Trauma Bacteremia	Surgery Soft tissue infection	Diabetes mellitus Vascular insufficiency
Usual bacteria	*S. aureus* Gram-negative bacilli	Often polymicrobial: Gram-negative bacilli, *S. aureus*	Usually polymicrobial: Gram-negative bacilli, anaerobes, streptococci, *S. aureus*
Presentation: Initial episode	Fever, local pain swelling, tenderness, limited movement	Fever, local pain swelling, tenderness, limited movement	Ulceration drainage ± pain
Recurrent eposode	Sinus drainage ± pain	Sinus drainage ± pain	Drainage ± pain

Acute hematogenous osteomyelitis usually presents with precipitous onset of pain, swelling, chills, and fever. With vertebral osteomyelitis there is fever with back pain, stiffness, and often point tenderness over the infected vertebra. Many patients have a more subacute presentation, with vague symptoms of 1 to 2 months' duration prior to presentation with few constitutional complaints. One well described variant is "Brodie's abscess" (also referred to as a "cold abscess")—subacute staphylococcal osteomyelitis located in the metaphysis of a long bone, which presents with local pain and fever. Patients with recurrent or chronic osteomyelitis often simply note increased or persistent drainage and pain following a prior episode involving the same anatomical location.

Contiguous Infection

Osteomyelitis secondary to contiguous foci of infection accounts for at least half of all cases. The most frequent precipitating factor is previous surgery, usually involving the lower extremities, such as open reduction of fractures of the femur or tibia. Next in frequency is a soft tissue infection involving the digits of the hand or feet. These infections usually become apparent within 1 month of a precipitating event, although many patients have chronic or recurrent infections that occur intermittently for years or decades. A variant in this category that is being seen with increasing frequency is infection associated with prosthetic devices. This complication is noted in 0.5–2% of patients with total hip replacement. Infections in the early postoperative period usually result from contamination at the time of surgery. Late infections presumably reflect either persistent perioperative sepsis, hematogenous spread from another infection, or seeding from transient bacteremia in a fashion analogous to the situation in endocarditis. The major pathogens are *S. aureus* and *S. epidermidis*, although multiple different bacteria, including many relatively nonpathogenic organisms, may be involved.

Vascular Insufficiency

Osteomyelitis associated with vascular insufficiency is most frequent in patients with diabetes mellitus and/or severe atherosclerosis. The most common sites of infection are the toes or small bones of the feet, usually with overlying soft tissue infections (see Fig. 31.2). These infections are often detected with the routine X-rays performed to evaluate chronic draining sinuses or skin ulcers that are so common in the patients at risk. Both the adjacent soft tissue infection and the osteomyelitis usually involve a polymicrobial flora that may include anaerobic bacteria, coliforms, pseudomonads, streptococci, and *S. aureus*.

Laboratory Evaluation

Diagnostic studies include X-rays or radionucleotide studies to demonstrate typical bone changes and cultures to identify the etiological organism.

The earliest changes on *plain X-rays* are lytic lesions; other findings may include soft tissue swell-

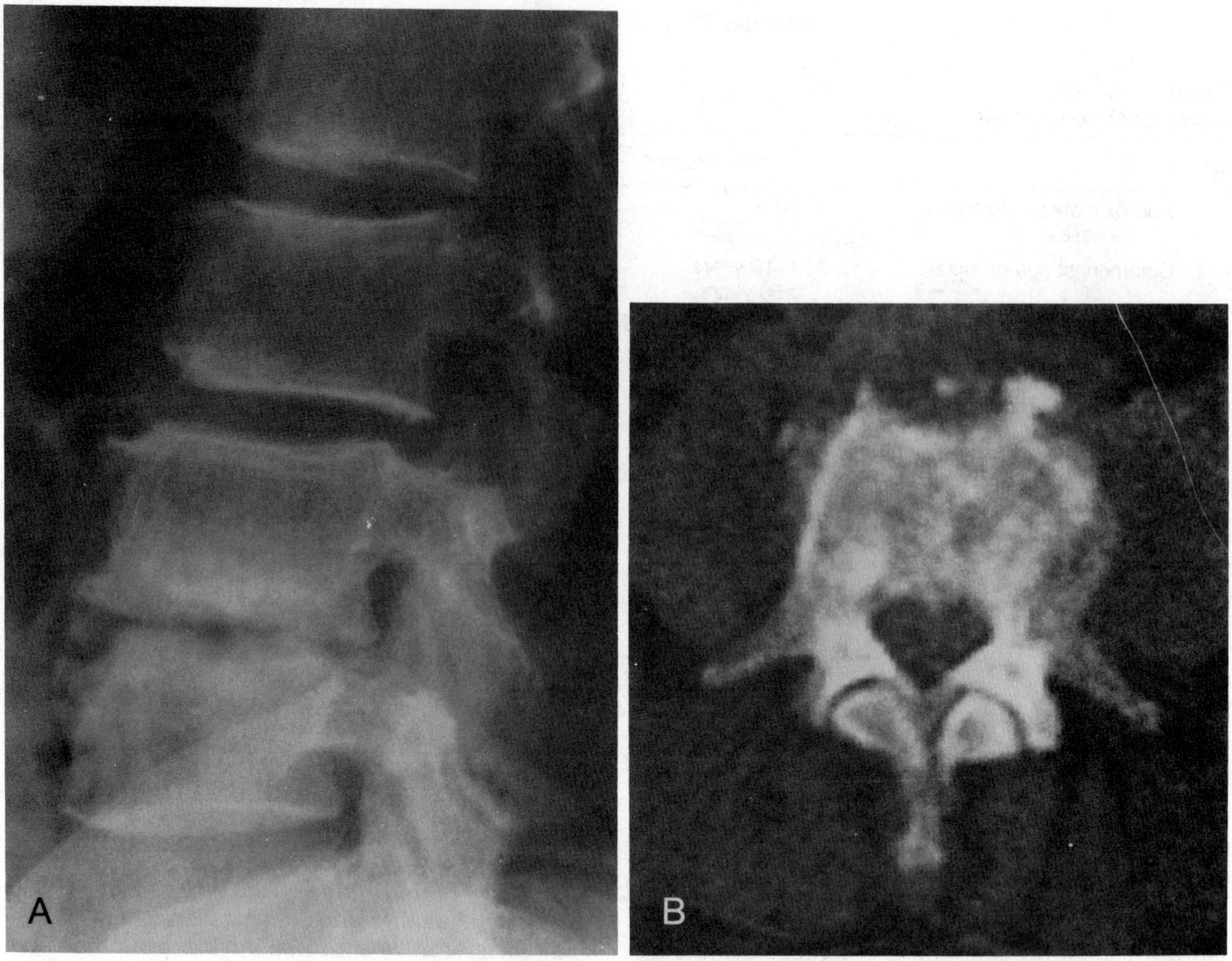

Figure 31.1. *A.* L3-4 staphylococcal osteomyelitis of 3 months' duration with disc narrowing and sclerosis seen on plain film. **B.** Computed tomographic scan in same patient showing small soft tissue abscess and minimal bone destruction. Hazy bone outline. (From Post MJD (ed): *Computed Tomography of the Spine.* Baltimore, Williams & Wilkins, 1984, p 740.)

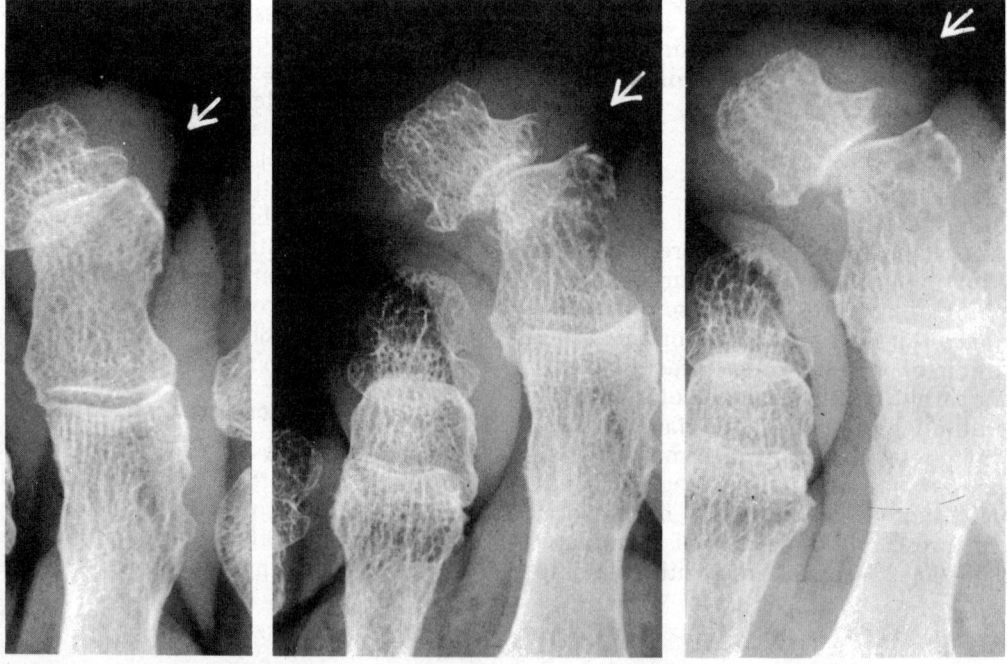

Figure 31.2. Infected soft corn, sinus tract, and osteomyelitis distal interphalangeal joint. As destruction increases, the joint becomes dislocated (From Gamble, FO, Yale I: *Clinical Foot Roentgenology.* Baltimore, Williams & Wilkins, 1966.)

ing, periosteal reaction, cortical irregularity, demineralization, and sequestrum formation. However, typical changes are not visible on plain films until 30 to 50% of the bone has been resorbed, and this usually requires 10 to 14 days. Therefore, in a patient with a normal plain film but suspected osteomyelitis, a *bone scan* should be obtained. The bone scan is a radionuclide examination which employs Tc99 as a marker bound to polyphosphate that concentrates in bone due to incorporation at sites of osteoblastic activity. This scan is positive in nearly all patients with osteomyelitis within 1 to 3 days after the onset of symptoms. Problems with this test are (a) that a "positive" scan may reflect increased blood flow associated with soft tissue infections or with osteoblastic activity due to other processes, such as degenerative joint disease, and (b) that it may show increased uptake for extended periods after eradication of infection due to continuing osteoblastic activity. Thus, the bone scan is sensitive but is nonspecific in detecting osteomyelitis and is not particularly useful for following the course of infection. These problems may be partially overcome with three phase imaging that increases specificity (12). Gallium uptake is not as dependent on bone blood flow and more accurately reflects inflammation than it does osteoblastic activity. Thus, a Ga-67 citrate scan may complement a positive bone scan and is more useful in following the course of an infection.

Since antimicrobial treatment, often prolonged, is the mainstay of management, accurate bacteriological data are imperative for making the diagnosis and for planning treatment. The list of possible organisms is legion, and sensitivity patterns for these organisms show considerable variation, making empiric selection of antimicrobials hazardous. These considerations justify an aggressive attempt to identify the responsible organism. Conclusive bacteriological studies require isolation of the pathogen from either the bone or blood cultures.

When osteomyelitis is suspected, an orthopaedist should perform a needle aspiration over the involved bone, either in an ambulatory setting (when the presentation is not acute) or in the hospital. If subperiosteal pus is obtained, surgical drainage is mandatory. If no pus is obtained, the needle is inserted into bone to obtain a specimen. The diagnostic yield with a needle aspirate of bone is approximately 60%, and for a surgical biopsy it is about 90% (4). Cultures from draining sinus tracts tend to show a poor correlation with cultures obtained directly from bone (11); this experience supports the need for bone biopsy or possibly deep aspiration in patients with chronic osteomyelitis. Care must be exercised in the interpretation of culture results, even of bone aspirates since these are often contaminated, especially if the specimen is obtained by traversing soft tissue infections (15). Organisms recovered in relatively small concentrations, especially those growing only in the broth culture, must be viewed with skepticism. Common skin contaminants include *S. epidermidis*, diphtheroids, and proprionibacteria. These organisms tend to cause osteomyelitis only in the presence of prosthetic devices. Gram stain of exudate or tissue aspirate should verify the culture results and represents an important correlate in deciding upon the etiological organism.

Treatment

General Principles

Immobilization was commonly advocated in the treatment of osteomyelitis in the preantibiotic era. However, this appears to be less important at the present time, and most authorities conclude that strict immobilization is not necessary. The duration of antimicrobial treatment is arbitrary as noted below, although some advocate a sedimentation rate of less than 20 mm/hour as one objective end point.

Antimicrobial Treatment: Acute Osteomyelitis

For newly diagnosed or acute osteomyelitis, optimal management is a 3- to 6-week course of parenteral antibiotics. This recommendation is based on several studies, but particularly the work of Dich and colleagues, who noted that 19% of patients developed recurrent or chronic disease when treatment was less than 21 days compared to only 2% in those who received more prolonged courses (4). The preferred regimen for acute staphylococcal osteomyelitis is a pencillinase-resistant penicillin such as nafcillin given intravenously in a dose of 1.5 to 2 g every 6 hours for adults, 200 mg/kg/day in four divided doses in children. Alternative parenteral regimens are cephalothin (2 g every 6 hours), or clindamycin (600 mg every 8 hours for adults or 30 mg/kg/day for children). In stable patients, these regimens can be initiated in the hospital and completed at home.

To decrease cost, length of hospitalization, and patient discomfort, a modified regimen, consisting of a short course of parenteral antibiotics followed by a prolonged course of oral agents, has been developed (7). The intravenous antibiotic is given for at least 3 days, or until the patient is afebrile, or for an arbitrarily defined period such as 1 to 2 weeks. The same agent is then taken by mouth, usually at home, to complete a total 3- to 6-week course, usually 4 weeks. The drugs recommended for oral administration are clindamycin (300 mg every 6 hours for adults) or an oral antistaphylococcal penicillin such as dicloxacillin or cephalexin (500 mg every 6 hours for adults or 75 to 100 mg/kg/day in four doses for children). It should be noted that this therapeutic approach has been tested successfully in children but that comparable studies have not been done to establish efficacy in adults.

Antimicrobial choice for osteomyelitis involving *Enterobacteriaceae* or *Pseudomonas aeruginosa* should be based on *in vitro* sensitivity tests. The importance of bactericidal activity and the relative merits of drugs for bone penetration as factors in drug selection are debated issues that remain unresolved.

Antimicrobial Treatment: Chronic Osteomyelitis

Therapeutic guidelines are less precise for chronic osteomyelitis. Since necrotic bone may serve as a nidus for sequestered bacteria, surgical excision of dead tissue and adequate debridement are often essential components of treatment. Antibiotic selection should be based on bacteriological diagnosis using deep aspirates or, preferably, cultures obtained from bone. The route of administration and duration of treatment are arbitrary, but most authorities recommend prolonged courses. The initial treatment may be parenteral antibiotics for 1 to 2 months in hospital or in the home, followed by oral agents for several months. An alternative approach is the use of oral agents exclusively for extended periods, such as 6 months or longer (2). In view of the difficulty of obtaining adequate antibiotic levels in avascular bone, there has been an attempt to deliver higher concentrations locally using regional perfusion of the wound following surgery with antibacterial solutions (8). There are no controlled trials to document superiority of this approach, and there is a potential problem of selection for antimicrobial-resistant bacteria.

Late Complications

The major complication of osteomyelitis is recurrence that may occur months, years, or decades after the initial event. The patient should be warned of this potential complication. The clinical features of recurrences are fever, draining sinuses, local pain, elevated sedimentation rate, and the typical changes noted on X-rays or scans as summarized above. Chronic osteomyelitis may be complicated by secondary amyloidosis, although this has become extremely rare since the advent of antibiotics. Another complication is epidermoid carcinoma arising in a draining sinus of osteomyelitis that occurs in 0.2 to 1.5% of cases, with a mean delay of 34 years (17). *Patients with prosthetic joints* are at risk for infections following transient bacteremia and should receive prophylactic antibiotics during procedures, following the recommendations for endocarditis prophylaxis (see below).

LUNG ABSCESS

Definition

Lung abscess refers to pulmonary suppuration with parenchymal necrosis caused by bacterial infection. The lesions are traditionally classified on the basis of clinical and bacteriological observations. Lung abscesses are considered acute or chronic depending on the duration of symptoms at the time of initial presentation, with the usual dividing line being 4 to 6 weeks. Clinically, lung abscesses are often grouped as (a) "putrid lung abscess," in reference to the foul odor of sputum that is regarded as diagnostic of anaerobic infection, or (b) "nonspecific lung abscess," indicating aerobic sputum cultures that do not grow out a pathogen. Anaerobic bacteria are the presumed pathogens in these cases also. Lung abscesses may also be classified clinically as "primary" or "secondary" depending on predisposing conditions. Primary lung abscesses are those which occur in patients who are prone to aspiration or in previously healthy individuals. Secondary abscesses represent complications of a local lesion such as a pulmonary malignancy or of a systemic disease that compromises immunological defenses. Approximately 80% of lung abscesses are primary. Sixty per cent are putrid, and 40% are nonspecific (probably mostly anerobic). Patients with lung abscess frequently present in the ambulatory care setting due to the chronicity of these infections. Most patients are hospitalized for diagnostic studies and initial treatment with intravenous antibiotics. The hospital course is usually followed by prolonged courses of antibiotics and follow-up chest X-rays.

Clinical Presentation and Bacteriology

Many bacteria are potential pulmonary pathogens, but the number of organisms likely to cause parenchymal necrosis is relatively modest. The most common pathogens are anaerobic bacteria that comprise the normal flora of the gingival crevice and are aspirated during periods of altered consciousness. The usual pathogens in such cases are *Bacteroides melaninogenicus*, anaerobic streptococci, and *Fusobacterium nucleatum* (1). The most frequent aerobic bacteria that cause suppurative pulmonary infections are *Staphylococcus aureus* and *Klebsiella pneumoniae*; less frequent causal pathogens are *Streptococcus pyogenes*, *Streptococcus pneumoniae*, *Haemophilus influenzae*, *Pseudomonas aeruginosa*, and enteric Gram-negative bacilli other than *K. pneumoniae*.

Patients with *anaerobic lung abscesses* usually present with indolent complaints that date for weeks or even months. Common symptoms include fever, malaise, cough, and sputum production. Pleuritic pain and hemoptysis are relatively common and may be the factors that persuade a chronically ill patient to seek medical attention. Chills are occasionally noted, but true rigors are rare. The frequent observation of anemia and weight loss reflects the chronicity of many of these infections. The sputum is usually purulent, and putrid odor is noted in about 60% of bacteriologically confirmed anaerobic lung abscesses. The usual sites of involvement are the anatomical segments of the lung where passive aspiration is most likely to occur in the recumbent position. These are the superior segments of the lower lobes and the posterior segments of the upper lobes. Less frequent abscess sites are the basilar segments of the lower lobes, which are dependent in the upright or semiupright position.

Lung *abscesses due to aerobic bacteria* are usually found in specific clinical settings. Staphylococcal pulmonary infections with abscess formation are particularly common in young children and in adults with influenza or with hospital-acquired pneumonia. *Klebsiella* is often suspected as a cause of lung abscess in alcoholic patients, but even in these patients anaerobic organisms are the commonest pathogens. The immunologically compromised patient may have pulmonary suppuration due to a variety of both bacterial and nonbacterial organisms, but anaerobes appear to be distinctly unusual in this population.

Laboratory Examination

The initial evaluations in patients with the symptoms of lung abscess are those recommended for patients with suspected pulmonary infections in general. These include a chest X-ray, a complete blood count, blood cultures, and an examination of expectorated sputum. The lung abscess is generally readily apparent with the chest X-ray (see Fig. 31.3), although other causes of a pulmonary cavity must be considered in the differential diagnosis. Alternative considerations include a cavitating neoplasm, cavitating pulmonary infarction, tuberculosis, fungal infection, an infected pulmonary cyst or bulla, a loculated empyema (*i.e.*, pleural space infection) with an air-fluid level due to a bronchopleural fistula, gas-producing organisms, or Wegener's granulomatosis.

When a cavitary lesion appears to be due to bacterial infection, there is controversy about the approach to identifying the likely pathogen. Sputum should be examined using Gram stain and Ziehl-Neelson stain in order to determine from the outset whether an anaerobic pathogen or *Mycobacterium tuberculosis* is the likely cause of the abscess.

Expectorated sputum is easily obtained from most patients, and standard cultures will usually show a predominance of an aerobic organism when it is the etiological pathogen. The problem with these specimens is that they are not appropriate for anaerobic culture, and the results with aerobic cultures are frequently misleading due to contamination by bacteria that reside in the upper airway. To confirm by sputum culture the presence of anaerobic bacteria, the ideal specimen for patients without an empyema is a transtracheal aspirate. However, this procedure is not necessary in most patients who have a typical presentation. This particularly applies to patients with an associated condition that predisposes to aspiration, to infection involving a typical pulmonary segment, and to patients with putrid sputum. Such individuals may be treated with antibiotics selected empirically.

Bronchoscopy is generally not useful for microbiological studies except for mycobacterial and nonbacterial pathogens; a possible exception is when specimens are obtained with a specialized double catheter and are cultured quantitatively (18).

Antimicrobial Treatment (Table 31.2)

Antimicrobials are the mainstay of treatment for lung abscess. The best studied regimens are those for anaerobic lung abscesses since these account for the majority of cases. Nevertheless, there is considerable controversy regarding the selection of agents and the duration of treatment.

Anaerobic Infections

With regard to drug selection, the initial antimicrobial recommended by most authorities for anaerobic lung abscess is penicillin G, 5 to 10 million units daily, given intravenously until fever resolves and there is definite clinical improvement. Successful treatment has been reported, however, using oral penicillin G from the start, in relatively high doses (750 mg four times daily) (16). The argument favoring high dose parenteral penicillin initially is that this provides a definitive conclusion regarding response to penicillin, thus obviating subsequent changes to a higher dose of penicillin if the patient fails to respond.

The major alternative drug for anaerobic lung abscesses is clindamycin. This drug is more active *in vitro* against the likely pathogens in anaerobic pulmonary infections. In approximately 25% of patients anaerobic organisms resistant to penicillin are present, and nearly all of these organisms are highly sensitive to clindamycin. Not surprisingly, a comparative trial showed that clindamycin was superior to penicillin in terms of the primary response rates and the duration of fever following the institution of treatment (10), two factors which may allow earlier hospital discharge. The advantage of penicillin for initial treatment is that this makes one more confident in prescribing oral penicillin for posthospital treatment. This is desirable because the high cost of clindamycin may lead some patients to discontinue treatment or "spread out" their supply of pills following discharge.

With either penicillin or clindamycin, initial treatment is usually given parenterally until the patient is afebrile and there is subjective improvement. This generally requires 3 to 7 days, but may be considerably longer in patients with very large lung abscesses, patients with prolonged symptoms prior to treatment, and patients with pleural complications (primary empyema).

Aerobic Infections

Guidelines for antimicrobial selection are less precise for lung abscesses involving other organisms. In these cases, the antibiotic is selected on the basis of *in vitro* sensitivity tests. Abscesses involving *S. aureus* or Gram-negative bacilli are regarded as more

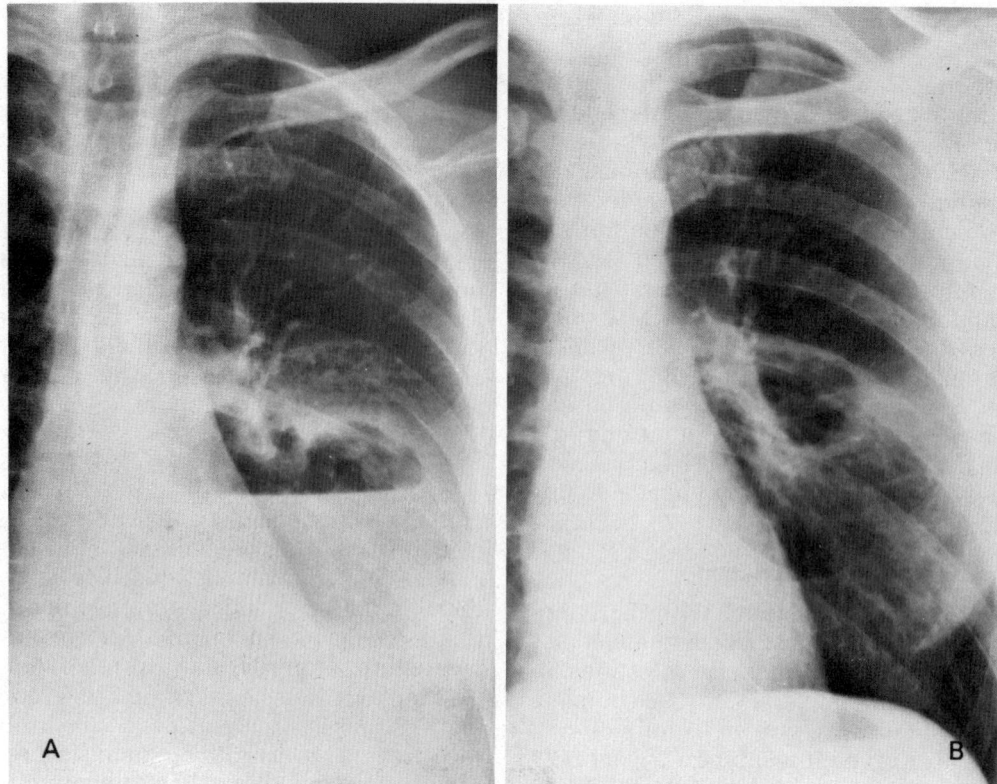

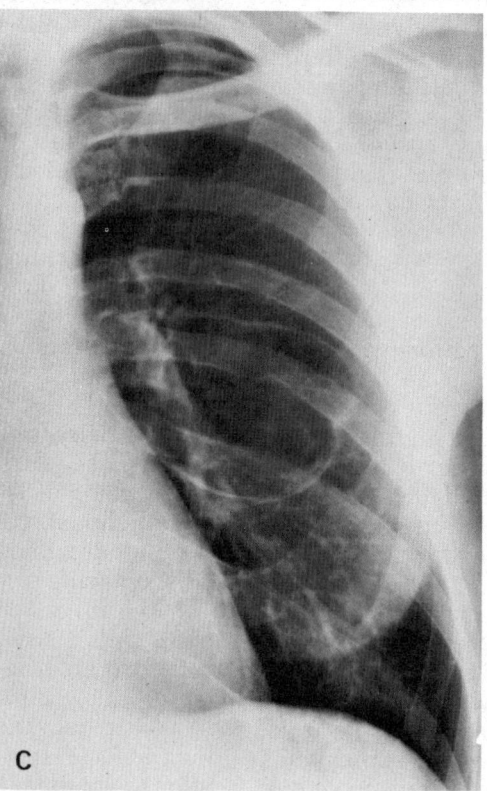

Figure 31.3. Putrid lung abscess. *A.* July 6, 1976. The patient developed fever and coughed up foul sputum after an epileptic attack. The huge cavity with an air-fluid level in the left lower lobe suggests a pyopneumothorax. However, the irregularity of the cavity wall indicates that it lies within the lung rather than in the pleura. *B.* August 3, 1976. On antibiotic therapy, the cavity has become much smaller and there is no longer an air-fluid level. *C.* September 20, 1976. Although the patient was clinically well, the cavity has increased in size. Its wall is thin and smooth and there are no infiltrations in the lung around the cavity. The ballooning of the cavity was noted after an attack of asthma. The increase in size was due entirely to air trapping because of the bronchospasm and does not indicate reactivation of the infection. (From Rabin CB, Baron MG: *Radiology of the Chest*, ed 2. Baltimore, Williams & Wilkins, 1980, p 340.)

Table 31.2.
Antimicrobial Regimens for Primary Lung Abscess

Intravenous[a]	Oral[a]	Commonest
Aqueous penicillin G 5–10 million units/day	Penicillin G or V 500–750 mg four times a day *or* Ampicillin or amoxicillin 500 mg four times a day	Regarded as standard *Advantages:* inexpensive and well tolerated *Disadvantage:* About 20% fail to respond and additional patients have delayed response
Clindamycin 600 mg every 6–8 hours	Clindamycin 300 mg four times a day	*Advantages:* Optimal response rates *Disadvantages:* Expensive; side effects include 10–20% with diarrhea and occasional patients with pseudomembranous colitis

[a] Intravenous treatment until patient is afebrile and clinically improved; oral treatment is given either to complete an arbitrary total course of 3 to 6 weeks of treatment or until chest X-rays show clearance or a small stable residual lesion.

serious infections, and intravenous antibiotics should be given for a more prolonged period; in selected stable patients, the intravenous regimen can be completed at home.

Duration of Treatment

Rigorous studies to determine the optimal duration of antimicrobial treatment for lung abscesses have not been done. Most authorities recommend at least 3 to 6 weeks. It is reasonable to base the duration of treatment also upon observations on serial chest X-rays (weekly or less frequently). Antibiotics are given until the chest X-ray either is clear or shows only a small stable residual lesion (see Fig. 31.3). These recommendations are based on experiences in which patients have had relapses despite treatment for at least 1 month; in these patients the infiltrate was still resolving when drugs were discontinued, and the patients were subsequently readmitted for recurrent abscesses in the same pulmonary segment.

For abscesses due to anaerobes, one of the following oral regimens should be used: penicillin G or penicillin V (500 to 750 mg four times daily), ampicillin or amoxicillin (500 mg four times daily), or clindamycin (300 mg four times daily).

Regardless of the total duration of treatment, adequate follow-up is necessary to assure resolution with serial X-rays. These should be obtained at 2- to 3-week intervals, or earlier if there is clinical deterioration. Most patients with lung abscess treated with antibiotics improve clinically before there is demonstrable improvement in the chest X-ray; cavities gradually close, but 20 to 30% persist beyond 6 weeks, and the roentgenographic criteria

for cure as defined above may require several months (9).

Inadequate Response to Treatment

If the patient is taking oral penicillin at home and does not show continued improvement, a change to clindamycin is appropriate. An alternative regimen, which has been used in Europe with considerable success, is the combination of oral metronidazole (Flagyl), 500 mg four times daily, combined with a penicillin in the doses noted above. It is necessary to use penicillin with metronidazole due to the frequent presence of microaerophilic and aerobic streptococci that are resistant to metronidazole. The anticipated outcome is either a clear X-ray, a small stable residual scar, or a thin-walled cyst. Failure to show progressive improvement, especially if accompanied by clinical symptoms, necessitates a change in therapy, bronchoscopy, or, on rare occasions, surgery. The major indications for surgery are an abscess that is totally refractory to antibiotic treatment, life-threatening or persistent hemorrhage, and abscesses occurring in association with an obstructed bronchus (6).

ENDOCARDITIS

Definition

Endocarditis refers to infections involving heart valves, usually due to bacteria, but occasionally due to other microbes such as *Rickettsia* or fungi. There is a spectrum of clinical findings, but patients with the subacute form of the disease may present with symptoms that are notably vague and nonspecific. The principal criteria for making the diagnosis are documented fever, heart murmur, and positive blood cultures. A unique feature of the disease is that most patients have continuous bacteremia so that blood cultures are positive in 90% of patients, regardless of the temporal relationship between blood samplings and temperature profile. All patients with endocarditis should be hospitalized for complete diagnostic evaluation, supportive care, and initiation of treatment with antibiotics given intravenously. This discussion addresses the management of these patients in the ambulatory care setting following hospitalization.

Treatment

Antimicrobial Treatment Out of Hospital

Antibiotics are selected for patients with endocarditis according to *in vitro* sensitivity tests, with emphasis on bactericidal activity. Most patients are treated with specific regimens according to guidelines from authoritative sources. The duration of treatment is usually 4 weeks of intravenous antibiotics. Exceptions are that some authorities now endorse a 2-week regimen for infections involving penicillin-sensitive strains of viridans streptococci and *Streptococcus bovis* (3), some prefer a 6-week course for straphylococcal endocarditis, and many recommend prolonged courses for patients with prosthetic valve endocarditis (14).

When intravenous antibiotics are planned for several weeks, part of the parenteral course can be administered at home, to expedite hospital discharge. British authorities have even recommended that intravenous antibiotics for 10 to 14 days be followed by an oral regimen, with the proviso that the patient has improved clinically and is afebrile (5). These approaches should be considered only for patients who have been fully evaluated on an inpatient basis, are hemodynamically stable and free of serious complications, and have satisfactory arrangements for home care, with appropriate clinical and microbiological monitoring.

There are two special situations in which out of hospital completion of antimicrobial regimen can be considered:

1. Abbreviated courses of intravenous antibiotics have been suggested for *staphylococcal endocarditis as a complication of intravenous drug abuse* (13). The advantage of this plan is that it limits the period during which an intravenous access is available for the patient to use, surreptitiously, to continue his habit. This occurs frequently and adds the risk of superinfection involving antibiotic-resistant organisms, such as Gram-negative bacilli and *Candida* species. Furthermore, these patients often leave against medical advice, before an intravenous course has been completed. An alternative to the usual 4 to 6 weeks of intravenous treatment is to restrict the intravenous route to 2 weeks or less and then continue oral treatment on an outpatient basis using cephalexin or dicloxicillin (2 to 8 g/day, usually 1 g every 6 hours) to complete a 6-week course of treatment. This approach can be endorsed only in patients who are clinically stable at the time intravenous therapy is discontinued, and when the blood culture isolate is highly sensitive to the drug used orally. Preferably, the shift to an oral agent should be made during hospitalization. After the change the patient should be carefully monitored for 2 to 3 days to ensure that the blood cultures remain negative, there is no fever, and he or she remains clinically stable. Additionally, a serum sample obtained 1 hour after oral dosing should show a bactericidal activity against the patient's blood isolate at a dilution of 1:8 or more.

2. Patients with *prosthetic valve endocarditis* have infections that have proven particularly difficult to cure without intervening surgery. Nevertheless, intravenous antibiotocs are given in the hopes of avoiding reoperation; this is a realistic goal with antibiotic-sensitive organisms. The most common pathogen in these cases is *S. epidermidis*, which is treated for at least 6 weeks with intravenous drugs selected on the basis of *in vitro* sensitivity tests. The

usual regimen is a betalactam (penicillin, a cephalosporin, or nafcillin) or vancomycin for 6 weeks combined with an aminoglycoside for at least 1 week and a prolonged course of rifampin. Many authorities recommend prolonged courses of oral antibiotics, following the initial intravenous regimen, such as dicloxacillin or cephalexin in a dose of 2 g. Because these patients are often stable, it is reasonable to complete a course of dicloxacillin or cephalexin combined with rifampin, 600 mg daily, out of hospital. This oral regimen is continued for arbitrarily defined periods that range from several weeks to 6 months or longer (14).

Long Term Follow-up and Prognosis

Patients with endocarditis treated medically or surgically should be followed carefully after discontinuation of antibiotics. Major complications during this recovery phase include congestive heart failure, relapse, mycotic aneurysms, and recurrences involving new organisms.

Blood cultures are commonly recommended after discontinuation of antibiotic treatment, usually 2 to 3 days later. Patients who have had an inadequate course of therapy will usually relapse within this time frame. Patients most likely to relapse are those with prosthetic valve endocarditis and endocarditis involving organisms resistant to antibiotics. The presence of positive blood cultures without a clearly identifiable portal of entry in the recovery phase is presumptive evidence of relapse. The usual recommendation is another course of antibiotics or surgery for a refractory infection. The choice between these two approaches is made on the basis of the extent of the initial treatment course, underlying valve disease, and the *in vitro* sensitivity of the organism, with particular attention to bactericidal activity. The patient should also be forewarned of the possibility of relapse and should be instructed to monitor temperature with attention to measurements in the evening when elevations are most likely to be noted.

The status of cardiac function should be followed carefully. In recent years, valve replacement has become a rather common practice during active infection and has been performed on the 6 to 20% of patients who satisfy certain, often somewhat arbitrary, criteria. It should be noted, however, that the mortality rate of surgery performed during active infection is substantially higher than surgery performed on an elective basis. When possible, it is preferred that valve replacement be conducted 6 weeks or longer after antibiotics have been discontinued. The major indication is congestive heart failure that proves difficult to control with medical management.

Mycotic aneurysms may become apparent at any time during the course of endocarditis, but most become clinically apparent several months or even years after treatment. These lesions usually occur at arterial bifurcations and have been reported in up

PROPHYLACTIC ANTIBIOTICS TO PREVENT ENDOCARDITIS FOR ADULTS

Dental and Upper Respiratory Procedures

Oral (not recommended for patients with prosthetic valves)

Penicillin V	2 g 1 hour before procedure and 1 g 6 hours later
Erythromycin (penicillin-allergic patients)	1 g 1 hour before procedure and 500 mg 6 hours later
Parenteral regimen Ampicillin	(for patients with prosthetic valves) 1 g IM or IV 30–60 minutes before procedure and repeat once 8 hours later[a]
or Aqueous penicillin G	2 million units IM or IV 30–60 minutes before procedure and repeat once 8 hours later[a]
plus Gentamicin	1.5 mg/kg IM or IV 30–60 minutes before procedure and repeat once 8 hours later[a]
Vancomycin (penicillin-allergic patients)	1 g IV infused over 1 hour beginning 1 hour before procedure

Gastrointestinal and Genitourinary Procedures

Parenteral regimen

Ampicillin	2 g IM or IV 30–60 minutes before procedure and repeat once 8 hours later
plus Gentamicin	1.5 mg/kg IM or IV 30–60 minutes before procedure and repeat once 8 hours later
Penicillin allergy: Vancomycin	1 g IV infused over 1 hour beginning 1 hour before procedure and repeat once 8 hours later
plus Gentamicin	1.5 mg/kg IM or IV 30–60 minutes before procedure and repeat once 8 hours later

Oral (not recommended for patients with prosthetic valves)

Amoxicillin	3 g 1 hour before procedure and 1.5 g 6 hours later

[a] One gram of oral penicillin 6 hours after the first dose of antibiotics may be substituted for the postprocedure parenteral regimen.

Figure 31.4. Contents of wallet-sized card containing recommendations for antimicrobial prophylaxis of bacterial endocarditis (both sides of card are shown). Cards such as this are available from the American Heart Association.

to 15% of cases. The most frequent vessels involved are intracranial; next in frequency are chest and abdominal arteries. The diagnostic evaluation usually consists of computerized tomography, when the central nervous system is involved, and arteriography for lesions suspected there or in other locations. Surgical correction is almost always indicated.

Anticoagulation is usually avoided during active endocarditis due to the danger of bleeding from unrecognized aneurysms or emboli. However, patients who are receiving anticoagulants for prosthetic valves should have anticoagulation continued in the absence of a bleeding complication.

It must be remembered that any patient with endocarditis is at risk for another infection. These patients should be warned about this potential complication with endoscopy, surgery, and dental procedures. It is good practice to supply all patients who are at risk for endocarditis with a wallet-sized card that contains the current antibiotic recommendations for prophylaxis with various procedures (see Fig. 31.4). This serves the dual role of emphasizing the importance of prophylaxis to the patient and assuring that specific guidelines will be available to those health professionals who may be performing procedures on the patient that can cause bacteremia.

General References

Osteomyelitis

Waldvogel FA, Medoff G, Swartz M: Osteomyelitis: a review of clinical features, therapeutic considerations and unusual aspects. I, II, and III. *N Engl J Med* 282:198, 260, 316, 1970.
    A thorough, well referenced review.
Waldvogel FA, Vasey H: Osteomyelitis: the past decade. *N Engl J Med* 303:360, 1980.
    An update of the 1970 review by the same author.

Lung Abscess

Bartlett JG: Lung abscess. *Johns Hopkins Med J.* 150:141, 1982.
Bartlett JG, Gorbach SL: Penicillin or clindamycin for primary lung abscess? *Ann Intern Med* 98:546, 1983.
Gopalakrishna KV, Lerner PI: Primary lung abscess. *Clev Clin Q* 42:3, 1975.
Perlman LV, Lerner E, D'sops N: Classification and analysis of 97 cases of lung abscess. *Am Rev Respir Dis* 99:390, 1969.

Endocarditis

Bayliss R, Clark C, Oakley CM, *et al*: The teeth and infective endocarditis. *Br Heart J* 50:506, 1983.
Bayliss R, Clark C, Oakley CM, *et al*: The microbiology and pathogenesis of infective endocarditis. *Br Heart J* 50:513, 1983.

Specific References

1. Bartlett JG, Gorbach SL, Tally FP, Finegold SM: Bacteriology and treament of primary lung abscess. *Am Rev Respir Dis* 109:510, 1974.
2. Bell S: Further observations on the value of oral penicillins in chronic staphylococcal osteomyelitis. *Med J Aust* 2:591, 1976.
3. Bisno AL, Dismukes WE, Durak DT, *et al*: Treatment of infective endocarditis due to viridans streptococci. American Heart Association Committee on Treatment of Bacterial Endocarditis of the American Heart Association Council on Cardiovascular Disease in the Young. *Circulation* 63:730A, 1981.
4. Dich V, Nelson J, Haltalin K: Osteomyelitis in infants and children. *Am J Dis Child* 129:1273, 1975.
5. Editorial. Infective endocarditis. *Lancet* 1:603, 1984.
6. Hagan JL, Hardy JD: Lung abscess revisited. A survey of 184 cases. *Am Surg* 197:755, 1983.
7. Kaplan SL, Mason EO, Feigin RD: Clindamycin versus nafcillin or methicillin in the treatment of *Staphylococcus aureus* osteomyelitis in children. *South Med J* 75:138, 1975.
8. Kelly P, Wilkowske C, Washington J II: Comparison of Gram-negative bacillary and staphylococcal osteomyelitis of femur and tibia. *Clin Ortho* 96:70, 1973.
9. Landay MJ, Christensen EE, Bynum LJ, Goodman C: Anaerobic pleural and pulmonary infection. *AJR* 134:233, 1980.
10. Levison ME, Mangura CT, Lorber B, *et al*: Clindamycin compared with penicillin for the treatment of anaerobic lung abscess. *Ann Intern Med* 98:466, 1983.

11. Mackowiak POA, Jones SR, Smith JW: Diagnostic value of sinus-tract cultures in chronic osteomyelitis. *JAMA* 239:2772, 1978.
12. Maurer AH, Chen DCP, Camargo EE,, et al: Utility of three-phase skeletal scintigraphy in suspected osteomyelitis: concise communication. *J Nucl Med* 22:941, 1981.
13. Parker RH, Fossieck BE: Intravenous followed by oral antimicrobial therapy for staphylococcal endocarditis. *Ann Intern Med* 93:832, 1980.
14. Sande MA, Scheld WM: Combination antibiotic therapy of bacterial endocarditis. *Ann Intern Med* 92:390, 1980.
15. Sugarman B, Hawes S, Musher DM, et al: Osteomyelitis beneath pressure sores. *Arch Intern Med* 143:683, 1983.
16. Weiss W, Cherniack NS: Acute nonspecific lung abscess: a controlled study comparing orally and parenterally administered penicillin G. *Chest* 66:349, 1980.
17. West WF, Kelly PJ, Martin WJ: Chronic osteomyelitis. I. Factors affecting the results of treatment in 186 patients. *JAMA* 213:1837, 1970.
18. Winberly N, Faling J, Bartlett JG: A fiberoptic bronchoscopy technique to obtain uncontaminated lower airway secretions for bacterial culture. *Am Rev Respir Dis* 110:337, 1979.

CHAPTER THIRTY-TWO

Immunization to Prevent Infectious Disease

R. BRADLEY SACK, M.D., Sc.D., AND L. RANDOL BARKER, M.D.

Protection against infectious diseases can be conferred by *active immunization* with vaccines, and by *passive immunization* with immune globulin preparations. As newly purified antigens become available, and as the mechanisms of the immune response become better understood, there will continue to be new vaccines available for protection against important infectious diseases. This chapter describes available vaccines and immune globulin preparations utilized in the United States, focusing upon the two critical questions commonly considered in practice: (a) Who should receive immunization? and (b) When should they receive it? Chapter 33 provides similar information on immunization for travelers to developing countries.

PATIENT ASSESSMENT

History

There are a number of questions that should be asked whenever immunization is contemplated.

The *history of previous immunizations* should be determined. In young adults, this may be readily known; in older persons, this information is often obscure. Patients may or may not keep personal records which can be of use. For example, persons who have served in the military will have received a large number of immunizations. They and persons who frequently travel abroad may have this information recorded on their International Vaccination Card. Immunization history is particularly important in determining (a) whether to give tetanus toxoid or antitoxin following an injury, (b) whether diphtheria should be seriously considered in the diagnosis of acute pharyngitis (see Chapter 28), and

(c) what immunizations to give to patients traveling outside the United States (see Chapter 33).

A *history of prior allergic reactions* or of other untoward reactions to vaccines or their components should always be excluded before giving an immunization. Most vaccines are now highly purified, and allergic reactions following their use are rare. However, persons allergic to eggs, for instance, should not receive vaccines made in eggs. Some persons experience unusually severe reactions to bacterial vaccines such as typhoid and cholera vaccines. A history of a previous severe response to a vaccine is a contraindication to its use. Some antiviral vaccines contain trace amounts of antibiotics (used often in tissue culture preparations) to which the patient may be hypersensitive; this information should be determined from the package insert before administration of vaccine to susceptible patients.

The following conditions are those for which use of a live virus is contraindicated: patients with either a known *immunodeficiency disease* or recent treatment with an immunosuppressive drug, and *pregnant* women, in whom the live virus vaccine might pose a possible risk to the developing fetus.

A *recent injection of γ-globulin* (within 3 months) requires that use of live virus vaccines be postponed, since there may be interference with the antibody response. For the same reason, γ-globulin should not be administered earlier than 2 weeks following live virus vaccine.

Finally, a patient with an *acute febrile illness* should generally not be immunized until after the illness has resolved, because any side effects might add to the patient's morbidity, and because the effectiveness of the vaccination may be diminished. However, a minor illness is not a contraindication to give a necessary immunization.

Physical Examination

When immunization is contemplated, the physical examination usually adds little to the assessment of the patient. Pregnancy or an active infection (see above) may be confirmed on examination. In one instance, smallpox vaccination, the finding of significant eczema is a contraindication to vaccination because of the risk of dissemination. However, since smallpox has been eradicated, this precaution is only relevant to laboratory workers who are studying the smallpox virus and who should therefore be vaccinated.

Immunological Testing

Immunological tests may be useful in deciding about immunization in two situations: (a) in considering the use of hyperimmune globulin preparations or hepatitis B vaccine for protection against hepatitis B; if the exposed person already has antibody to hepatitis B surface antigen, additional protection is unnecessary; and (b) when considering the use of rubella vaccine for a woman of childbearing age; if she already has antibodies to rubella, further immunization is unnecessary.

IMMUNIZATION PROCEDURES

The physician should always be familiar with the information contained in the *package insert* when giving a vaccine. This information includes dose, route of administration, common and uncommon side effects, contraindications, whether there is contamination with antibiotics, interval between immunizations, and additional detail.

Many of the widely used vaccines can be *given simultaneously*. The Centers for Disease Control list the following guidelines for simultaneous vaccine administration: (a) Inactivated vaccines can be administered simultaneously at separate sites (at the same site in the case of widely used combination vaccines such as tetanus and diphtheria toxoids). However, when vaccines commonly associated with side effects are given together (e.g., cholera, typhoid, plague) the side effects may be accentuated; and consideration should be given to vaccinating on separate occasions (see also Chapter 33); (b) an inactivated vaccine and a live, attenuated virus vaccine can be administered simultaneously at separate sites.

Patients should be told at the time of immunization that they may experience some local soreness and possibly fever and malaise during the following 24 to 48 hours. They can be instructed to take aspirin or acetaminophen if these symptoms are bothersome. Because of the rare possibility of anaphylactic reactions, persons receiving any immunization should wait in the office where they can be observed for about 15 minutes. Finally, patients should be clearly informed of the name of the immunizations they have received and be encouraged to keep a written record of them.

SPECIFIC VACCINES AND IMMUNE GLOBULIN PREPARATIONS

Table 32.1 summarizes information on the major available vaccines and immune globulin preparations. The following sections provide practical information on problems for which immune protection is most likely to be given in ambulatory practice.

Hepatitis (5, 11a, 12)

At present, only passive immunization with preparations of gamma globulin is used widely in the prevention of hepatitis. A vaccine which stimulates active immunity to hepatitis B is now also available. Because of its high cost, it is recommended chiefly for persons at increased risk (see below).

Table 32.1.
Identity, Characteristics, and Administration of Available Vaccines and Immune Globulin Preparations

Vaccine or Immune Globulin (References)	Type Preparation	Population to Be Immunized	Age at Which Immunization Usually Done	Immunization Schedule	Possible Adverse Reactions
Diphtheria vaccine (7, 11)	Killed bacteria and toxoid	All	Child or adult	Series of three primary injections with boosters every 10 yr if known risk exists[a]	Local pain and swelling
Tetanus toxoid (11)	Toxoid	All	Child or adult	Series of three injections with boosters every 10 yr as necessary following injury[a]	Local pain and swelling
Tetanus immune globulin	Human antiserum	Unimmunized person with dirty wound		Single injection for prophylaxis	Not significant
Pertussis vaccine	Killed bacteria	All children	Child only	Series of three injections with boosters to age 6	Fever, occasionally severe neurological reactions
Polio vaccine (6) Oral	Live attenuated virus	All	Child	Primary series of three oral preparations	Not significant, rare clinical disease
Parenteral	Killed virus	All	Child	Primary series of four injections	Not significant
Measles vaccine (9)	Live attenuated virus	All children	Child (>12 months of age)	Single injection	Fever
Rubella vaccine	Live attenuated virus	All children 12 months old and unimmunized adolescents	Child and adolescent females	Single injection	Arthralgias, fever in young women
Mumps vaccine	Live attenuated virus	All children and young adults without history of mumps	Child	Single injection	Not significant
Influenza vaccine (4, 8, 13, 15)	Killed virus (whole virus and "split virus" preparations) preparations of virus change yearly	Persons at risk, chronic illness	Child or adult	Adults: Single injection (whole virus) repeated yearly. Children under 13: split virus preparation, two doses	Mild fever, allergic reactions, Guillan-Barré syndrome rarely
Hepatitis B vaccine[b]	Inactivated viral constituents from infected humans	Health workers and others at increased risk	Usually adults	Three injections (0 time, 1 month, 6 months)	Not significant
Hepatitis globulin (5, 12) Pooled (ISG)	Pooled human γ-globulin	Persons exposed to hepatitis A (and B)	Usually adults	Hepatitis A: 0.02 ml/kg, once Hepatitis B: 0.06 ml/kg, twice	Not significant
High titred (HBIG)	Hepatitis B immune globulin	Persons exposed to hepatitis B only	Usually adults	0.06 ml/kg at time of exposure and again 1 month later	Not significant
Meningococcal vaccine (11a, 14)	Purified polysaccharide (serogroups A and C)	Only during epidemic disease. Persons at high risks (military)	All ages; young adult military	Single injection	Erythema at injection site; not significant
Rabies vaccine (1, 3)	Killed virus (human diploid vaccine)	Persons bitten by possible rabid animal	All ages—postexposure	Multiple injection of vaccine (five) plus rabies immune globulin	Pain, rare neurologic reactions
Pneumococcal vaccine (2)	Polyvalent purified polysaccharides	Persons with asplenia or splenic dysfunction; persons with chronic illness	Any age (over 2 yr)	Single injection, not repeated	Erythema at injection site
Bacillus Calmette and Guérin (BCG) vaccine (10)	Live attenuated bacteria	Used to immunize newborns in developing countries and persons with excessively high risk of developing tuberculosis		Single injection, intradermal	Prolonged granuloma or ulcer at injection site, lymphadenitis

[a] Boosters of diphtheria and tetanus are particularly important for those traveling to underdeveloped countries.
[b] Licensed 1981. Duration of immunity not known.

Hepatitis A

Pooled human γ-globulin (immune serum globulin, ISG) is 80 to 90% effective in preventing hepatitis A in exposed persons. It should be given to the following: (a) Close contacts of persons with known hepatitis A (family members or intimate friends, but not schoolmates or fellow workers unless some unusually high possibility of fecal-oral transmission is suspected). ISG should be given as soon as possible after the known exposure, certainly within 1 week. The usual adult dose is 0.02 ml/kg intramuscularly. (b) Persons traveling to the developing world for more than a few weeks and planning to live in the community rather than in tourist facilities (see Chapter 33 for doses).

Hepatitis B

Pooled γ-globulin (ISG) in relatively large doses (0.06 ml/kg intramuscularly in two doses 4 weeks apart) may also be useful in preventing *hepatitis B*. However, a costly (more than $150/dose in 1984) globulin preparation of high titer (hepatitis B immune globulin, HBIG) is available and is approximately 75% effective in preventing hepatitis in those persons known to have direct exposure to hepatitis B virus. When HBIG is given at the same time as hepatitis B vaccine, this protection is considerably higher. Exposed persons who are known to have antibody to the surface antigen (HBsAg) do not need postexposure prophylaxis.

Table 32.2 summarizes the 1984 recommendations of the Centers for Disease Control (CDC) for *postexposure HBIG and vaccine prophylaxis for persons in the following groups: (a) newborns with perinatal exposure to a mother who has acute hepatitis B or is HBsAg positive (see Table 32.3 for women in whom prenatal HBsAg screening is recommended); (b) sexual contacts of persons who have active hepatitis B or are HBsAg carriers; (c) persons who have had percutaneous, ocular, or mucous membrane exposure to blood from patients who have active hepatitis B or are HBsAg carriers; (d) persons who receive a human bite that penetrates the skin from a patient who has active hepatitis B or is a carrier of HBsAg. (Table 32.4 summarizes strategies for managing persons with similar exposures to patients whose HBsAg status is unknown.)*

Hepatitis B vaccine has an efficacy of about 90% in the primary prevention of hepatitis B in persons who are at high risk of exposure. The immunizing schedule for adults is as follows: 1.0 ml (20 μg of HBsAg protein) intramuscularly followed by the same dose at 1 and 6 months after initial administration. The arm should be used as the hepatitis vaccination site for adults since suboptimal responses to the vaccine have occurred when the vaccine was injected into the buttock (12a). The only side effect of the vaccine is occasional soreness and redness at the injection site. The protection after the completed immunization schedule is about 80 to 95% for at least 2 years. The duration of protection and the need for boosters are not yet known. The vaccine, which is very expensive, is recommended particularly for individuals in the following high risk groups: (a) health care professionals exposed

Table 32.2.
Summary of Postexposure Management of Acute Exposure to Patients Known to Have Active Hepatitis B or to Be HBsAg Positive[a]

Exposure	HBIG		Vaccine	
	Dose	Recommended Timing	Dose	Recommended Timing
Perinatal	0.5 ml IM	Within 12 hours of birth	0.5 ml (10 μg) IM	Within 7 days[b]; repeat at 1 and 6 months
Percutaneous	0.06 ml/kg IM or 5 ml for adults	Single dose within 24 hours	1.0 ml (20 μg) IM[c]	Within 7 days[b]; repeat at 1 and 6 months
		or[d]		
	0.06 ml/kg IM or 5 ml for adults	Within 24 hours; repeat at 1 month		
Sexual[e]	0.06 ml/kg IM or 5 ml for adults	Within 14 days of sexual contact		

[a] From *Morbidity and Mortality Weekly Report*, vol 33, no. 21, p 286, 1984.
[b] The first dose can be given the same times as the HBIG dose but at a separate site.
[c] For persons under 10 years of age, use 0.5 ml (10 μg).
[d] For those who choose not to receive HB vaccine.
[e] Vaccine is recommended for homosexually active males and for regular sexual contacts of chronic hepatitis B virus carriers.

Table 32.3.
Women for Whom Prenatal HBsAg Screening Is Recommended[a]

1. Women of Asian, Pacific Island, or Alaskan Eskimo descent, whether immigrant or US born.
2. Women born in Haiti or Sub-Saharan Africa.

and

Women with histories of:

3. Acute or chronic liver disease.
4. Work or treatment in a hemodialysis unit.
5. Work or residence in an institution for the mentally retarded.
6. Rejection as a blood donor.
7. Blood transfusion on repeated occasions.
8. Frequent occupational exposure to blood in medicodental settings.
9. Household contact with an hepatitis B virus carrier or hemodialysis patient.
10. Multiple episode of venereal disease.
11. Percutaneous use of illicit drugs.

[a] From *Morbidity and Mortality Weekly Report*, vol 33, no. 21, p 287, 1984.

Table 32.4.
Summary of Postexposure Management of Acute Exposures to Patients Whose HBsAg Status is Unknown[a]

Exposure	HBsAg[b] Testing of Source	Recommended Prophylaxis
HBsAg status unknown:		
High risk[c]	Yes	ISG[d] (0.06 ml/kg) immediately, and (a) if source is HBsAg positive, HBIG[e] (0.06 ml/kg) immediately and 1 month later or (b) if source is HBsAg negative, nothing
Low risk[f]	No	Nothing or ISG (0.06 ml/kg)
HBsAg status unknown, source unknown	No	Nothing or ISG (0.06 ml/kg)

[a] Adapted from *Morbidity and Mortality Weekly Report*, vol 30, no. 34, p 433, 1981.
[b] Hepatitis B surface antigen.
[c] Exposure to patient with acute, unconfirmed viral hepatitis; patients institutionalized with Down's syndrome; patients on hemodialysis; persons of Asian origin; male homosexuals; users of illicit intravenous drugs.
[d] Immune serum globulin.
[e] Hepatitis B immune globulin.
[f] Exposure to the average patient.

frequently to blood or blood products (*e.g.*, laboratory and blood bank personnel, operating room staff, surgeons, dentists, endoscopists, pathologists, and the staff in oncology, dialysis, and emergency room units); (*b*) homosexually active men, (*c*) family partners, in particular sexual partners, of chronic HBsAg

carriers; (*d*) patients who frequently receive transfusions of blood or blood products; (*e*) patients in hemodialysis units; (*f*) inmates and staff of institutions for the mentally retarded; (*g*) users of illicit injectable drugs; (*h*) selected international travelers (see Chapter 33). The vaccine is not routinely recommended for individuals who come in contact with HBsAg carriers at work or in school. Screening for antibodies to hepatitis B virus prior to immunization is only cost effective for groups with a very high likelihood of prior infection, particularly homosexuals. Individuals with antibody do not need to be vaccinated. For screening, either anti-HBs or anti-HBc can be tested. However, determination of anti-HBc is preferred. On occasion anti-HBs is nonprotective either because it is a nonspecific reactant or protective only to one subtype of HBsAg. Vaccination of individuals who have anti-HBs from previous infection does not cause adverse effects. (The patterns of appearance of antigens and antibodies in hepatitis B infection are illustrated in Figure 42.1, page 498.)

Non-A, Non-B Hepatitis

There is no immune globulin preparation known to be protective against *non-A, non-B hepatitis*, which is now the most frequent cause of post-transfusion hepatitis.

Hepatitis in ambulatory patients is discussed in Chapter 42.

Tetanus (11)

Currently, 80 to 100 cases of tetanus are reported each year in the United States. There is no known subclinical "natural" immunity to tetanus, so that every person is susceptible unless he has been actively immunized. The majority of cases in the United States occur in persons over 60 years old, a population containing many persons who have never been immunized. Tetanus usually follows penetrating wounds due to accidents and animal bites (see Chapter 25). The incubation period is 4 to 21 days, average 10 days. In persons who have been actively immunized at any time in their life, injection of toxoid once every 10 years is necessary to boost their antitoxin titers to protective levels. If a person at risk of developing tetanus from a wound has received a toxoid booster in the last 10 years, no additional toxoid is required; if such a person has never received toxoid immunization, has not received a toxoid booster within the past 10 years, or is unsure about it, passive immunization with tetanus antitoxin (250 units) should be given. This preparation is made from human serum, and therefore hypersensitivity reactions are not a problem, in contrast to the time when horse serum preparations were used. Persons who require tetanus antitoxin should at the same time (but at a different site) be given their first dose of toxoid, followed by repeat doses of toxoid 1 month and 8 to 12 months later. If these persons have never been immunized against diphtheria, they should be given tetanus and diphtheria toxoids, adult type (Td), as discussed in the next section.

Diphtheria (7, 11)

Currently, 5 to 10 cases of diphtheria are reported each year in the United States. Although subclinical infection may occur and confer immunity in unimmunized persons, it is recommended that persons who have never been given diphtheria toxoid should receive it if their occupation places them at increased risk of exposure to diphtheria (i.e., physicians, nurses, other hospital personnel, teachers, and staff and patients of institutions for the mentally handicapped) or if they plan travel in developing countries (see Chapter 33). For unimmunized school age children and adults, tetanus and diphtheria toxoids, adult type (Td) are used. This preparation contains only about 25% of the diphtheria toxoid contained in the DPT (diphtheria-pertussis-tetanus) combined vaccine utilized in infants; this minimizes the risk of severe reactions in adults, previously a significant problem. Primary immunization consists of an initial dose, a 1-month dose, and a third dose at the 6th to 12th month; a booster is recommended every 10 years to assure protection. In adults, there is a high incidence (25 to 50%) of local soreness, swelling, and itching following Td injections; fever occurs in less than 10% and urticaria in approximately 2% of individuals. Serious reactions (massive swelling of the whole arm, abscess, or anaphylaxis) occur rarely (11).

For asymptomatic unimmunized contacts of patients with diphtheria, management includes: (a) prophylactic antibiotics (600,000 units of benzathine penicillin intramuscularly or a 7-day course of erythromycin, 250 mg four times daily); (b) primary vaccination as outlined above; and (c) daily surveillance for 7 days for clinical evidence of diphtheria (see Chapter 28).

Influenza (4, 8, 13, 15)

Killed virus vaccines have been available for the prevention of influenza for many years. Earlier preparations contained nonspecific protein which frequently led to fever and malaise after the vaccine had been administered. Preparations now available are highly purified, and reaction rates are very low. Each year's vaccine is polyvalent, containing antigenic material from the type A and type B strains which are expected to prevail in a given year.

Influenza vaccine is recommended annually for those persons in whom influenza causes the highest morbidity and mortality: individuals over 60 years old and individuals of all ages with significant heart, lung, or chronic debilitating disease. The vaccine is also recommended for those involved in critical jobs where their absence may be highly detrimental (e.g., firemen, policemen, selected hospital personnel).

Influenza vaccine is about 70% protective, as determined in a number of experimental trials involving healthy adults and in retrospective studies involving young and elderly individuals. The antigens in the vaccine must, of course, be appropriate for the prevailing influenza virus strain. The vaccine should be given in the fall, before the influenza season, which usually occurs between December and April.

During confirmed local outbreaks of influenza A, the antiviral drug *amantadine* (Symmetrel) can be utilized prophylactically as well as therapeutically (see Chapter 28 for a discussion of therapeutic use). Amantadine prevents clinical disease due to influenza A viruses in approximately 70% of subjects. The prophylactic use of this drug has been recommended (13) for the following groups of subjects:

1. Unvaccinated children and adults at high risk of serious morbidity and mortality because of underlying diseases, which include pulmonary, cardiovascular, metabolic, neuromuscular, or immunodeficiency diseases.

2. Adults whose activities are vital to community function and who have not been vaccinated with an appropriate contemporary influenza vaccine—for example, policemen, firemen, selected hospital personnel. Such persons are in frequent contact with others who may have influenza and should be considered at higher risk of contracting influenza than the general population.

3. Persons in semiclosed institutional environments, especially older persons, who have not received the current influenza vaccine.

The drug should be taken once daily (200 mg) during the local outbreak (usually a period of 2 to 3 months). Subjects should be warned of the following transient central nervous system side effects, which may occur during the first few days in 5 to 10% of subjects: insomnia, light-headedness, nervousness, drowsiness, difficulty in concentrating.

Influenza in ambulatory patients is discussed in Chapter 28.

Pneumococcal Disease (2)

A purified polyvalent polysaccharide vaccine is available for the prevention of pneumococcal disease in persons at high risk, including persons who have had a splenectomy, those with sickle cell anemia, and adults with chronic lung disease. The vaccine is about 80% protective against the pneumococcal serotypes which it contains (23 serotypes which are responsible for approximately 90% of pneumococcal disease in the United States). The vaccine produces very few untoward effects and can be given as a single injection. Because of a high incidence of adverse reactions to reinjection of pneumococcal vaccine, second or "booster" doses should not be given.

Pneumococcal pneumonia in ambulatory practice is discussed in Chapter 28.

Rubella

In the interval 1970 to 1982, the number of cases of rubella reported annually in the United States fell from approximately 55,000 to approximately 2,000. The number of reported cases of congenital rubella syndrome remained unchanged during the decade 1970 to 1980 (50 to 60 cases) but fell dramatically in 1982 (11 cases reported) and 1983 (6 cases reported).

Since about 1970, immunization against rubella has been administered routinely to children between ages 1 and 2. The major rationale for this vaccine is to prevent the spread of rubella to pregnant women and thereby to reduce the incidence of the congenital rubella syndrome.

Adolescent females and women in the childbearing age group should be offered immunization also. However, they should first have their rubella antibody titer checked to determine whether they are already immune as a result of prior infection or immunization. Any detectable titer is considered protective. In women with no history of vaccination, vaccine can be given without prior serological testing to decrease costs. Before the vaccine is given, a woman should be cautioned against becoming pregnant (see Chapter 93, Birth Control) for the 3 months immediately following the immunization since there is the possibility of fetal damage by the live virus. However, such an occurrence has not actually been documented and the risk is estimated to be extremely low.

Mumps

In the decade 1972 to 1982, the number of cases of mumps reported annually in the United States fell from approximately 70,000 to approximately 5,000. This decline is probably in part due to the use of mumps vaccine during this interval.

Live attenuated virus mumps vaccine is now recommended routinely for children and for those young adults with no history of mumps; most people over the age of 25, however, can be considered immune. Since in susceptible adults the mumps virus can cause severe symptoms (orchitis, meningitis, or pancreatitis), there is good reason to provide this protection. Unimmunized persons may have had an immunizing subclinical infection, since only one of every three cases of mumps in childhood is symptomatic. Unlike rubella, there is not a reliable test for prior immunity to mumps. However, there are no serious side effects from the vaccine, making prior determinations of immunity less important.

Rabies (1, 3)

In the past 10 years, one to four cases of human rabies have been reported each year in the United

States. Theoretically all of these cases are preventable if protective treatment is given promptly following exposure. The incubation period is usually 2 to 8 weeks, but it may be as short as 10 days or as long as a year or more.

In June 1980, killed virus rabies vaccine produced in human diploid cells was licensed for use in the United States. This vaccine has two major advantages over the previously used duck embryo vaccine: (a) higher levels of antibody are stimulated with fewer doses; and (b) fewer adverse reactions occur. For individuals who are at risk of developing rabies (see Chapter 25), the recommended treatment schedule is as follows: on day 1, simultaneous administration of antirabies globulin (as human rabies immune globulin, HRIG, if available; otherwise as heterologous antiglobulin) and the first dose of rabies vaccine, given intramuscularly, not subcutaneously; vaccine is repeated on days 3, 7, 14, and 30. The effectiveness of this vaccine in stimulating antibody and in protecting patients from rabies has been well established (3). Adverse reactions (urticaria, anaphylaxis, transient headache, and fever) occur in less than 0.5% of persons receiving this vaccine (1). The vaccine and antiglobulin are available from local health departments.

Measles (9)

Measles is a moderately severe illness in most persons and has a case fatality rate of 1:1,000. Since 1963, measles vaccines have been available (initially, killed virus vaccines, and since 1968, attenuated live virus vaccines). In the interval 1960 to 1980, during which measles vaccination of children was introduced generally in the United States, the number of cases reported annually fell from over 400,000 to less than 15,000; in 1982 there were only 1,714 cases reported.

In 1978, the Secretary of Health, Education and Welfare announced the eradication of measles as the goal of the national measles immunization effort. The principal strategy for accomplishing this goal is immunization of all children at approximately 15 months of age. Since the introduction of immunization of this age group, the largest proportion of measles cases has occurred in adolescents and young adults, the subgroups most likely to have missed both live virus immunization and exposure to natural measles. Because neither serological testing nor history of childhood measles is a reliable method to assess immunity to measles, it is difficult to provide a general recommendation for measles protection of this age group. Diminishing the risk of exposure of nonimmune adults by thorough immunization of children is the most practical approach.

Tuberculosis (10)

Efforts to control tuberculosis in the United States are based upon early identification of active disease and upon isoniazid prophylaxis of the contacts of tuberculous patients and other groups at increased risk (see Chapter 29). Because the incidence of new tuberculosis is low in this country (approximately 25,000 cases/year) and because most new cases are due to reactivation of disease in older individuals who acquired their infection in an era when the risk of infection was much higher, the indications for immunization with BCG (bacillus of Calmette and Guérin) vaccine are very limited. The 1975 recommendations of the US Public Health Service (10) are as follows:

1. BCG vaccination should be seriously considered for persons who are tuberculin skin test negative and who have repeated exposure to persistently untreated or ineffectively treated, sputum-positive pulmonary tuberculosis.

2. BCG vaccination should be considered for well defined communities or groups if an excessive rate of new infections can be demonstrated and the usual surveillance and treatment programs have failed or have been shown not to be applicable. Such groups might exist among the socially disaffiliated and those without a regular source of health care, possibly including some alcoholics, drug addicts, and migrants. Groups such as health workers who may be at particular risk of exposure to unrecognized pulmonary tuberculosis should, where possible, be kept under surveillance for evidence of newly acquired tuberculous infection. It must be recognized that only the occurrence of new infections reflects whether transmission is actually occurring.

The recommended route of administration for the BCG strain utilized in this country is intradermal or subcutaneous. If after 2 or 3 months the patient's tuberculin skin test remains negative, vaccination should be repeated. Contraindications to BCG vaccine are compromised immunity due to malignancy or immunosuppressive therapy and pregnancy. After BCG immunization, it is not possible to distinguish between a positive tuberculin skin test resulting from infection with virulent *M. tuberculosis* and one resulting from the BCG vaccine. Because the protective efficacy of BCG vaccine is not absolute, tuberculosis should be included in the differential diagnosis of any tuberculosis-like illness occurring in vaccinated individuals.

General References

Adult immunization: recommendations of the Immunization Practices Advisory Committees. *Morbidity and Mortality Weekly Report*, vol 33, suppl, September 28, 1984.

Summary recommendations, updated periodically.

Benenson AS (ed): *Control of Communicable Diseases in Man*, ed 12. Washington, DC, American Public Health Association, 1985.

A concise summary of epidemiology, management, and prevention of communicable diseases, updated periodically.

Health Information for International Travel: US Department of Health and Human Services, Centers for Disease Control (CDC), Atlanta, Georgia.

This booklet, which is updated yearly, contains recommendations for vaccination and prophylaxis against communicable diseases throughout the world. Available free.

Hilleman MR: Whiter immunization against viral infections? *Ann Intern Med* 101:852, 1984.

An overview of the past, present, and future, with respect to technological possibilities and practical considerations related to vaccine control of viral diseases.

The Immunization Practices Advisory Committee: Recommendations appear periodically in the *Morbidity and Mortality Weekly Report*, published by US Department of Health and Human Services, Centers for Disease Control and available for a modest subscription charge.

These recommendations are also published periodically in the *Annals of Internal Medicine* and *The Medical Letter*.

Morbidity and Mortality Weekly Report, Annual Summary. US Department of Health and Human Services, Centers for Disease Control.

This annual report summarizes the incidence of reportable diseases for the current year and for previous years and decades (beginning with 1940).

Specific References

1. Adverse reactions to human diploid cell rabies vaccine. *Morbidity and Mortality Weekly Report*, vol 29, p 609, December 19, 1980.
2. Austrian R, Douglas RM, Schiffman G, et al: Prevention of pneumococcal pneumonia by vaccination. *Trans Assoc Am Phys* 89:184, 1976.
3. Bahmanyar M, Fayaz A, Nour-Salehi S, et al: Successful protection of humans exposed to rabies infection: postexposure treatment with the new human diploid cell rabies vaccine and antirabies serum. *JAMA* 236:2751, 1976.
4. Barker WH, Mullooly JP: Influenza immunization of elderly persons: reduction in pneumonia and influenza hospitalizations and deaths. *JAMA* 244:2547, 1980.
5. Grady GF, Lee VA, Prince AM, et al: Hepatitis B immune globulin for accidental exposures among medical personnel: final report of a multicenter controlled trial. *J. Infect Dis* 138:625, 1979.
6. Horstmann DM: Viral vaccines and their ways. *Rev Infect Dis* 1:502, 1979.
7. Middaugh JP: Side effects of diphtheria-tetanus toxoid in adults. *Am J Public Health* 69:246, 1979.
8. Parkman PD, Galasso GH, Top FH, Noble GR: Summary of clinical trials of influenza vaccines. *J Infect Dis* 134:100, 1976.
9. Rand KH, Reuman PD: Measles: ready for eradication? *Ann Intern Med* 90:978, 1979.
10. Recommendation of the Public Health Service Advisory Committee on Immunization Practices: BCG vaccines. Centers for Disease Control, Morbidity and Mortality (US DHEW), February 22, 1975.
11. Recommendation of the Immunization Practices Advisory Committee (ACIP): Diphtheria, tetanus, and pertussis: guidelines for vaccine prophylaxis and other preventive measures. *Morbidity and Mortality Weekly Report*, vol 26, p 401, 1977.
11a. Recommendation of the Immunization Practices Advisory Committee: Recommendations for protecting against viral hepatitis. *Morbidity and Mortality Weekly Report*, vol 34, p 313, 1985.
12. Seeff LB, Hoofnagle JH: Immunoprophylaxis of viral hepatitis. *Gastroenterology* 77:161, 1979.
12a. Suboptimal response to hepatitis B vaccine given by injection into the buttock. *Morbidity and Mortality Weekly Report*, vol 34, p 105, 1985.
13. Symposium: amantadine: does it have a role in the prevention and treatment of influenza? A National Institutes of Health and Consensus Development Conference. *Ann Intern Med* 92:256, 1980.
14. Wahdan MH, Rizk F, El-Akkad AM, et al: A controlled field trial of a serogroup A meningococcal polysaccharide vaccine. *Bull WHO* 48:667, 1973.
15. Wright PF, Dolin R, LaMontagne JR: Summary of clinical trials of influenza vaccine II. *J Infect Dis* 134:633, 1976.

CHAPTER THIRTY-THREE

Medical Advice for the International Traveler

STEPHEN D. SEARS, M.D., M.P.H., AND R. BRADLEY SACK, M.D., Sc.D.

INTRODUCTION

Approximately 25 million Americans travel by air to foreign countries each year. This does not include the many who take boats, cruises, or go by car to Canada and Mexico. Of these 25 million, it is estimated that between 3 and 5 million journey to developing areas of the world where infectious diseases are commonly encountered. Malaria, schisto-somiasis, yellow fever, polio, typhoid fever, and amebiasis are just a few of the diseases that are more prevalent in tropical developing countries. Most travelers make little, if any, provision for the prevention of illness while traveling. This is both fool-hardy as well as unfortunate because the overall attack rate for several infectious diseases is much higher in international travelers than it is in comparable populations that remain at home. This fact is well illustrated by the results of a recent study of Swiss travelers that found that three quarters had at least one symptom of infectious illness while traveling; and of the 16,500 travelers surveyed in this study, greater than 30% had at least one episode of a diarrheal illness (9). Another study of 2,000 travelers returning to the United Kingdom found that 43% became ill during or shortly after their journeys (6).

The two previously cited studies offer a small glimpse into the medical problems of travelers. Even so, we do not have any reliable measurement of the amount or severity of disease encountered by the traveler. Only a portion of the most dramatic cases of illness in travelers such as malaria, lassa fever, or African trypanosomiasis are ever reported to public health authorities. At present, there is no mechanism for obtaining accurate surveillance data on either the incidence or prevalence of illness in American travelers, nor are there data on significant risk factors for acquiring infectious diseases. This lack of data hampers scientific investigation of interventional strategies in travelers. Even so, significant progress has been made in the prevention of malaria, travelers's diarrhea, and diseases for which immunizations exist.

One of the major concerns of both public health officials and practicing clinicians is the likelihood of infectious disease becoming manifest in nonendemic areas. Inexpensive air travel has increased the possibility that individuals who have contracted diseases in the tropics will present to their family physicians: A college student on a safari in Kenya can be bitten by an *Anopheles* mosquito carrying sporozoites of *Plasmodium falciparum* and 2 weeks later be back at college when the fever and chills begin.

To prevent unnecessary illness, it is imperative that travelers obtain appropriate pretrip health planning. The developing world offers a wealth of education and experience to the traveler, but unfortunately, most Americans are unthinkingly accustomed to safe drinking water, safe food, and unrestricted access to swimming. Travelers who do not take adequate precautions before and during their trips, are at risk of acquiring serious diseases and of suffering from chronic sequelae.

Because international travel is increasing, it is likely that primary care physicians will be called upon to answer questions concerning the risks of travel. This means that physicians should be prepared to provide adequate pretrip advice as well as post-trip disease surveillance. Physicians also need ready access to a travelers clinic to which complicated problems may be referred or for use as a source of information.

When approached by a person about to embark upon an international journey, the physician needs to ascertain several key aspects of the proposed trip. "Where are you going," "Where will you stay," "What is the purpose of your trip?," "Where will you be eating? In restaurants or in private homes?," are all questions that need to be asked. After the traveler has answered these questions, the physician can categorize the traveler as either high or low risk. The low risk traveler is the businessman staying for a short period of time in a first class hotel in a large city in a developed country. This traveler is rarely if ever at any greater risk than that associated with traveling in the United States. At the other end of the spectrum is the high risk traveler, the college student who will be living at the village level in multiple developing countries. This traveler is at significant risk and should receive complete pretrip health planning. Most travelers fit somewhere between these two extremes. In addition to the risks associated with his itinerary, the traveler's present health status, history of chronic diseases, use of medications, allergies, and immunization record are important in planning for a safe trip.

Immunizations, malaria prevention, food and water safety, diarrhea, schistosomiasis and a number of general health hazards, are topics that may need to be discussed with the traveler. Two useful resources which are updated yearly provide practical information on these issues: "Health Information for International Travel" published by the United States Public Health Service (available from the Centers for Disease Control, Atlanta, GA 30333) and "Vaccination Certificate Requirements for International Travel and Health Advice to Travelers" published by the World Health Organization (available from WHO Publication Center, USA, 49 Sheridan Avenue, Albany, NY 12210).

IMMUNIZATIONS

Vaccines are now available against a number of the major viral and bacterial diseases encountered in developing areas (see Table 33.1). Immunizations can be broadly separated into those that are legally required and those that are recommended. Legally required vaccinations are public health measures that certain countries demand prior to entry, to

Table 33.1.
Vaccines and Immune Globulins for Travelers to Developing Countries[a]

Vaccine	Patient (age, weight)	Route	Dose	Booster
Cholera	6 mo–4 yr	SC	0.2 ml	0.2 ml q 6 mo
	5–10 yr	or	0.3 ml	0.3 ml q 6 mo
	>10 yr	IM	0.5 ml	0.5 ml q 6 mo
Yellow fever	>1 yr	SC	0.5 ml	0.5 ml q 10 yr
Typhoid	<10 yr	SC	1 and 2–0.25 ml	0.25 ml q 3 yr
	>10 yr		1 and 2–0.50 ml	0.50 ml q 3 yr
Poliomyelitis (OPV)	All ages	Oral	3 doses[b]	1 dose[b,c]
(IPV)	All ages	IM	4 doses[b]	1 dose q 5 yr[b]
Tetanus-diphtheria	>7 yr	IM	3 doses	1 dose q 10 yr[b]
Immune globulin (hepatitis prophylaxis)				
Long term prophylaxis	<23 kg	IM	1.0 ml	1.0 ml q 4–6 mo
	23–45 kg		2.5 ml	2.5 ml q 4–6 mo
	>45 kg		5.0 ml	5.0 ml q 4–6 mo
Short term travel (<2 mo)	<23 kg		0.5 ml	
	23–45 kg		1.0 ml	
	>45 kg		2.0 ml	

[a] From Wolfe M: Diseases of travelers. *CIBA Clin. Symp.* 32:4, 1984. (IM, intramuscular; SC, subcutaneous.)
[b] See manufacturer's recommended dose.
[c] The need for further supplemental OPV doses has not been established.

benefit the country as a whole, whereas recommended immunizations are designed only to benefit the individual. In order to enter or return to the United States, there are no legally required vaccines. Many countries, however, do have strict entry requirements, and travelers who arrive without proper vaccination certificates may be denied entry, quarantined or possibly vaccinated at the point of entry. Therefore, it is important to determine what vaccines are required before beginning a journey.

Presently, the only legally required vaccinations are those for cholera and yellow fever, and each country has its own requirements for them. In the past, smallpox vaccination was required by many countries, but in 1980 the World Health Organization declared the global eradication of smallpox and on January 1, 1982 smallpox was deleted from the list of diseases subject to regulation.

Yellow Fever

Yellow fever vaccine, containing a live attenuated strain of the yellow fever virus, is one of the most

important and effective vaccines. It is required by some countries before travelers are allowed entrance, particularly when areas to be visited are endemic for yellow fever. If yellow fever exists in the country of destination, the traveler should be vaccinated regardless of the country's regulations (Figs. 33.1 and 33.2). The vaccine is relatively nontoxic and induces long lasting immunity. Reactions, which are generally mild, occur in 1 to 5% of vaccines. These include mild headache, myalgia, low grade fever, or other minor symptoms 5 to 10 days after inoculation. Since yellow fever vaccine is a live attenuated virus, it poses a theoretic risk to the pregnant woman, although teratogenicity has not been encountered. Pregnant women who must travel to yellow fever endemic areas should be vaccinated. It is presumed that the unknown but small risk to the fetus is less than the risk to the mother. If at all possible, the trip should be postponed until after delivery. The vaccine is contraindicated in immunocompromised patients. Since the vaccine strain is grown in chick embryo culture, it should

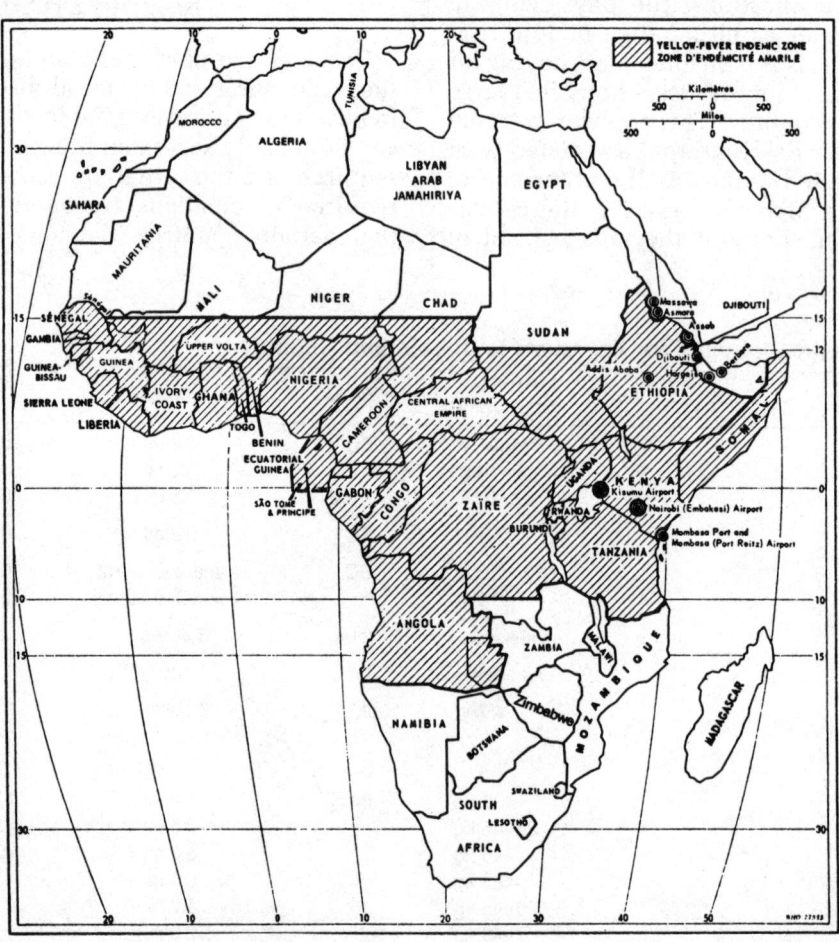

Figure 33.1. Yellow fever endemic zone in Africa. (From *Health Information International Travel, 1983.* Supplement to *Morbidity and Mortality Weekly Report,* vol 32, August, 1983. US Department of Health and Human Services, HHS Publication no. (CDC) 83-8280.)

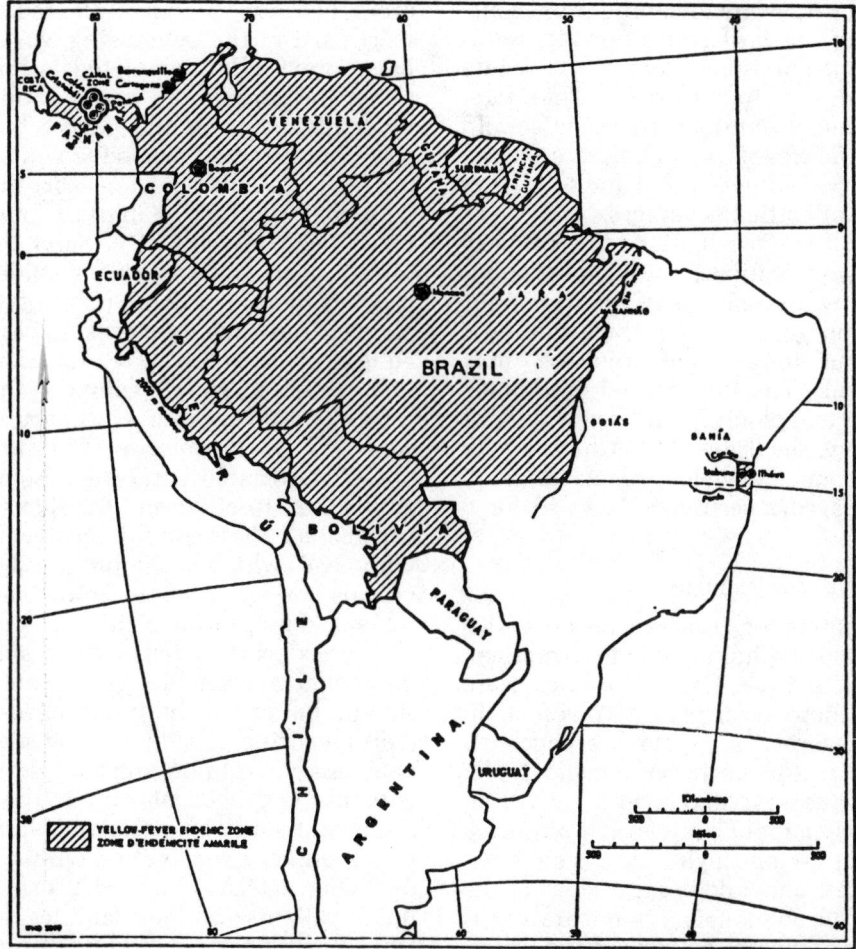

Figure 33.2. Yellow fever endemic zone in the Americas. (From *Health Information for International Travel, 1983.* Supplement to *Morbidity and Mortality Weekly Report*, vol 32, August, 1983. US Department of Health and Human Services, HHS Publication no. (CDC) 83-8280.)

not be given to travelers with known hypersensitivity to eggs. Yellow fever immunization is also not recommended in children less than 1 year old. Yellow fever vaccine is available only through official yellow fever vaccine centers; locations of these centers can be obtained by calling the local health department. The dose of vaccine is 0.5 cc subcutaneously, and it must be given with 1 hour of reconstitution. The vaccine should be stored at 5°C until it is reconstituted. The vaccine gives solid immunity for at least 10 years. If it is contraindicated for a traveler to receive yellow fever vaccine for any of the above reasons, a detailed letter explaining the contraindications should be provided to the traveler.

Cholera

In 1973, the World Health Assembly recommended discontinuing required vaccination against cholera, but vaccination against cholera is still required for entry into a few countries (Table 33.2).

Table 33.2.
Countries That Still Require Cholera Vaccination[a]

(1) Albania II[b]	(8) Malta II
(2) Angola II	(9) Mozambique I
(3) Cape Verde II	(10) Niger II
(4) Korea, Republic of (South) II	(11) Pakistan II
(5) Lesotho II	(12) Pitcairn II
(6) Maldives III	(13) Somalia II
(7) Mali II	(14) Sudan II

[a] As of January 1, 1984.
[b] (I), Vaccination certificate required of travelers arriving from all countries. (II) Vaccination certificate required of travelers arriving from infected areas. (III) Vaccination certificate required of travelers arriving from a country any part of which is infected.

Unless the vaccine is legally required, it is not recommended because, although cholera is widespread around the world, infection in travelers is extremely rare; and the vaccine, a killed vaccine, is of limited effectiveness (8). For travelers following usual tourist routes and using standard precautions in countries endemic for cholera, the estimated attack rate is less than one in a million trips (5). Therefore, rather than recommend immunization, one should emphatically instruct travelers to cholera endemic areas not to eat uncooked vegetables and to always drink boiled water or bottled beverages.

If a traveler requires vaccination, the primary series consists of two injections, but for most countries one injection will satisfy entry requirements. The vaccine can be given both intradermally or subcutaneously, but intradermal injection may cause fewer reactions. The intradermal dose is 0.2 ml for those 5 years and older. For intramuscular or subcutaneous dosing, see Table 33.1. Chlorea vaccination is not recommended for infants under 6 months old. The vaccine certificate is valid for 6 months.

Typhoid Vaccine

Recently, the Centers for Disease Control (CDC) analyzed all cases of typhoid fever in American citizens from 1970 to 1979. Over 900 cases were reported; 62% of those occurred in travelers. In addition, many areas of the world are reporting multiple antibiotic resistance in *Salmonella typhi*, the organism that causes typhoid fever.

Typhoid vaccination, though not legally required, is recommended for certain high risk travelers because typhoid fever is endemic in most areas of the developing world (10). *Salmonella typhi* is transmitted by the ingestion of contaminated food and water. If a traveler to developing countries is likely to stray off of the usual tourist route, stay in small villages, and eat local food, he should be immunized because of the increased risk.

The currently available killed typhoid vaccine provides approximately 70 to 90% protection depending in part on the degree of subsequent exposure. The acetone-dried typhoid vaccine should be used without the paratyphoid component. Paratyphoid antigen offers little protection and is responsible for many of the side effects common with typhoid immunization. Even so, the typhoid vaccine frequently causes pain at the injection site, fever, headache, and malaise for 1 to 3 days. If the traveler has never been vaccinated before, the primary sequence is two inoculations 1 month apart (see Table 33.1 for doses). Booster doses should be given every 3 years. If the traveler does not have time to get both injections in the primary series, it is prudent to give one, since significant immunity results.

A new live oral attenuated typhoid vaccine is being tested and shows great promise, but it is not yet available for routine use.

Polio Vaccine

Status of protection against poliomyelitis should be considered in any traveler visiting developing areas because poliomyelitis remains endemic in most parts of the developing world. Travelers who have previously completed primary series with either the Sabin (oral, live) or Salk (parental, inactivated) vaccine should have a booster dose if the last immunization was given more than 10 years previously. A history of at least three doses of oral polio vaccine (OPV, Sabin) or four doses of inactivated polio vaccine (IPV, Salk) with IPV boosters each 5 years until age 18 is evidence of adequate primary immunization. Such fully immunized people need only one dose of polio vaccine before traveling to high risk areas. If a traveler is only partially immunized, he should complete the primary series.

Adults who require a primary series should receive IPV. IPV is preferred in adults because the risk of OPV-associated paralysis is somewhat higher in adults than in children. If children are not already vaccinated, they should receive a primary series with OPV, which is the preferred vaccine for individuals younger than 18. If an unimmunized adult traveler does not have time to complete a primary IPV series prior to departure, a single dose of OPV may offer reasonable protection. On return, he should be primarily immunized with IPV. Live (OPV) vaccine should not be given routinely to women known to be pregnant, although teratogenicity has not been shown. If the risk of polio is significant and the pregnant woman is unimmunized, primary vaccination with IPV would be prudent. Since OPV is a live virus, immunocompromised patients and their families should not receive OPV; instead they should be immunized with IPV. Table 33.1 summarizes information regarding doses for polio vaccines.

Tetanus and Diphtheria

Tetanus occurs worldwide, but is slightly more common in the tropics. Thus, tetanus immunization should be kept up-to-date in travelers. Boosters need to be given every 10 years regardless of age. Travelers, if they injure themselves, are less likely to seek medical help so that adequate pretravel immunization becomes more important. Diphtheria is endemic in many developing countries, and most cases occur in unimmunized or partially immunized individuals. Therefore, routine immunization with tetanus-diphtheria (Td) should be given rather than tetanus toxoid alone. For primary immunization, persons older than 7 years should receive three doses of Td. The first doses are 1 to 2 months apart and the third 6 to 12 months later. Local reactions may occur within 12 to 48 hours after vaccination. Severe local reactions can occur in adults if the booster is given within a short time of the previous vaccine. Therefore, routine boosters should not be given more often than every 10 years. The only contraindication to Td is a history of hypersensitivity reactions after prior immunization.

Hepatitis A

Hepatitis A continues to be an important risk for travelers to many areas of the developing world. Although the risk is small for individuals who travel on ordinary tourist routes and stay for short periods of time, it may be considerable for those individuals who bypass the tourist routes and stay for extended periods of time. Immune globulin provides passive protection against hepatitis A and should be strongly advised for high risk travelers. Injection of 2 cc for stays of less than 3 months, and 5 cc for stays of 3 to 6 months is usually given. If the traveler will be staying for an extended period of time, he should have repeat immune globulin, in the same doses, every 6 months. Immune globulin should be given very near to the date of departure to ensure longer efficacy. The only side effects are muscle soreness at the injection site. Pregnancy is not a contraindication to immune globulin.

Hepatitis B (See Also Chapters 32 and 42)

The risk of hepatitis B is generally low for the routine traveler. Health care workers who are likely to have contact with blood or secretions from patients in areas endemic for hepatitis B should receive hepatitis B vaccine. The prevalence of hepatitis B virus carriers is 5 to 15% in sub-Saharan Africa, Southeast Asia including China and Indonesia and between 1 to 5% in North Africa, South Central Asia, and Southern Europe. Since hepatitis B can be transmitted through sexual contact, travelers should be counseled appropriately when going to endemic areas. Vaccination or hepatitis B immune globulin (HBIG) prophylaxis may be appropriate for individuals who are likely to have sexual contacts. Primary adult vaccination consists of three intramuscular doses of 1 ml of vaccine. The first two doses are given 1 month apart and the third dose should be given 6 months later (see additional details in Chapter 32).

Rabies

Rabies remains an important public health problem in many areas of the developing world and has occurred in travelers. Rabies transmission occurs when rabies virus is introduced into open cuts or wounds, usually through the bite of an infected animal. Pre-exposure rabies prophylaxis, which consists of three inoculations of human diploid cell killed-virus vaccine (1 ml intramuscularly on days 0, 7, and 21 or 28) is appropriate for long term travelers who will live in endemic areas. Individuals who anticipate animal exposure such as veterinarians, animal handlers, and laboratory workers should also be vaccinated. Persons with continued risk of rabies exposure should receive a booster dose of vaccine (1 ml) every 2 years. Children are especially at risk because of the increased likelihood of contact with stray dogs. The human diploid cell vaccine is more immunogenic and causes fewer reactions than the old duck embryo vaccine. Occasional local reactions and rare systemic reactions such as headaches, myalgias, and dizziness may occur. Pregnancy is not a contraindication to pre-exposure prophylaxis. If the traveler is exposed to rabies, he or she should still seek medical help for post-exposure immunization. Any animal bite should be thoroughly cleansed with soap and water to help reduce the rabies risk.

Tuberculosis (See Also Chapter 29)

Tuberculosis continues to be a worldwide health problem, but the risk to the short term traveler is small. *Mycobacterium tuberculosis* is primarily a respiratory pathogen contracted by inhaling droplet nuclei, but unpasteurized milk products can also spread the disease. Travelers who will be spending extended periods of time in tuberculosis endemic areas should have a tuberculin skin test prior to departure. Bacillus-Calmette-Guérin (BCG) vaccine use is controversial and most U.S. experts do not recommend it. Periodic skin tests in long term travelers are recommended to detect subclinical infections.

Measles, Mumps, Rubella, Influenza (See Also Chapter 32)

The so-called "childhood" viral illnesses are prevalent in the tropics. Prior to travel children should have received routine immunizations against these diseases. Adolescents and adults who have neither had these diseases nor been immunized against them are at risk of becoming infected while traveling. These diseases may be much more serious in adults, and vaccination should be strongly considered. Rubella vaccine is indicated for females of childbearing age without serological evidence of prior rubella infection. Certain travelers may benefit from pretrip vaccination with influenza vaccine. Influenza causes morbidity and mortality throughout the world and poses risk to unvaccinated travelers. The same criteria for selecting candidates for influenza vaccine in the U.S. should be used (see Chapter 32).

Miscellaneous Vaccines: Typhus, Plague, Meningococcal

Typhus vaccine is no longer available, and the disease poses little risk except for those working with louse-infected refugees. No typhus has been reported in an American traveler since 1950. Plague exists in certain rural areas in Africa, Asia, and South America. Vaccination is not recommended for most travelers, but if the traveler will have direct contact with wild rodents in plague-enzootic areas, vaccination should be considered. Local and systemic reactions after plague vaccine occur frequently. Meningococcal meningitis occurs throughout the developing world, often in devastating epidemics. Although cases in American travelers are rare, vaccine may be indicated in travelers going to countries with known epidemics. When vaccination is considered, the bivalent A-C vaccine should be given if the serotype is unknown.

Timing of Vaccines

Many travelers come to see the physician just before their departure. In this situation, all active immunizations can be given concurrently. There is, however, some evidence that cholera vaccine may decrease slightly the efficacy of yellow fever vaccine if the two vaccines are given within 3 weeks of each other. Otherwise, simultaneous administration of multiple vaccines produces good antibody responses to all the antigens. However, when it is possible, multiple vaccinations should be spread out over time and all should be completed by 1 week before arrival in a developing country to decrease the likelihood of reactions and to assure that adequate antibody levels have been attained. When vaccines are administered concurrently, they should be given with separate syringes at different body sites. Killed vaccines can be given at the same time as immune globulin. With live attenuated vaccines (especially polio vaccine), passively acquired antibody may interfere with replication of the vaccine virus and decrease the efficacy of the vaccine. Therefore, if possible, live virus vaccines should be given at least 14 days *before* the administration of immune globulin and probably 3 months *after* administration.

MALARIA PROPHYLAXIS

Malaria is a potentially fatal parasitic disease caused by infection of red blood cells with plasmodia species. It is usually transmitted by *Anopheles* mosquitos, but can be acquired from transfused blood and intravenous drug use. Malaria tends to be more severe in immunologically "virgin" travelers than in residents of endemic areas. The disease is characterized by high fevers, chills, sweats, myalgias, and headache with no obvious focal signs or symptoms of infection. Malaria exists worldwide (Fig. 33.3). The risk of contracting malaria varies from country to country and from season to season depending upon local conditions such as rainfall, altitude, and mosquito density. Since malaria is almost a totally preventable disease in travelers, there should be no deaths in travelers due to malaria. Each year, though, several American travelers still die because of inadequate protection against malaria. Prevention of malaria requires a 2-fold approach: (*a*) to minimize mosquito contact and (*b*) to take appropriate prophylactic medicine.

To avoid mosquito exposure, travelers should sleep in screened rooms and under mosquito nets. *Anopheles* mosquitos feed predominantly from dusk

to dawn. Therefore, travelers who must be out during this time should try to cover exposed body parts with clothing or insect repellant. Long sleeved shirts, long-legged trousers and occasionally a face net should be worn if at all possible. Mosquito repellant containing N,N-diethyl-meta-toluamide (deet) should be applied to exposed skin. Outdoor nighttime activity should be avoided whenever possible.

Even with appropriate mosquito protection, travelers may get bitten by malarious mosquitos. The second approach is therefore to take chloroquine phosphate as a chemoprophylactic agent. Chloroquine, 500 mg of the phosphate salt (300 mg base), should be taken once per week for 2 weeks before entering a malaria endemic zone, for each week while in the zone, and for 6 weeks after departure. Other chemoprophylactic agents such as chloroquine sulfate or amodioquine, are effective, but are not available in the United States. Travelers who take chloroquine prophylaxis should still avoid mosquitos, since compliance with taking the medicine may not always be perfect.

Routine chemoprophylaxis has been complicated by the emergence of chloroquine resistance in *Plasmodium falciparum*. Travelers to areas with known chloroquine resistance, including South East Asia, parts of East Africa, Indonesia, and Oceania, as well as the Amazonian basin (Fig. 33.4), are at risk of contracting chloroquine-resistant malaria if chloroquine alone is used for chemoprophylaxis. Until very recently, it was recommended that travelers to these areas take Fansidar (pyrimethamine, 25 mg, and sulfadoxine, 500 mg) in addition to chloroquine. Because of the risk of adverse reactions to Fansidar, which include erythema multiforme, Stevens-Johnson syndrome, and toxic epidermal necrolysis, these recommendations have been altered (6a). The revised recommendations place increased responsibility on individual travelers and their physicians. Short term travelers (less than 3 weeks) to areas with a high level of transmission of chloroquine-resistant *P. falciparum* malaria, including East Africa and Oceania (Papua, New Guinea, Solomon Islands, Vanuatua, and Irian Jaya) should take chloroquine as routine prophylaxis. In addition, these travelers should be given a single treatment dose of Fansidar (3 tablets) to be taken if they develop a febrile illness compatible with malaria and they are unable to get prompt professional medical care. This is a temporary measure only, and travelers still should be advised to seek medical follow-up as soon as possible. For travelers staying more than 3 weeks in these areas, consideration should be given to using Fansidar, 1 tablet weekly, in combination with chloroquine. If weekly use of Fansidar is prescribed, the traveler should be advised to discontinue it immediately if any side effects occur. There are alternative chemoprophylactic agents, but none has undergone carefully controlled efficacy and safety

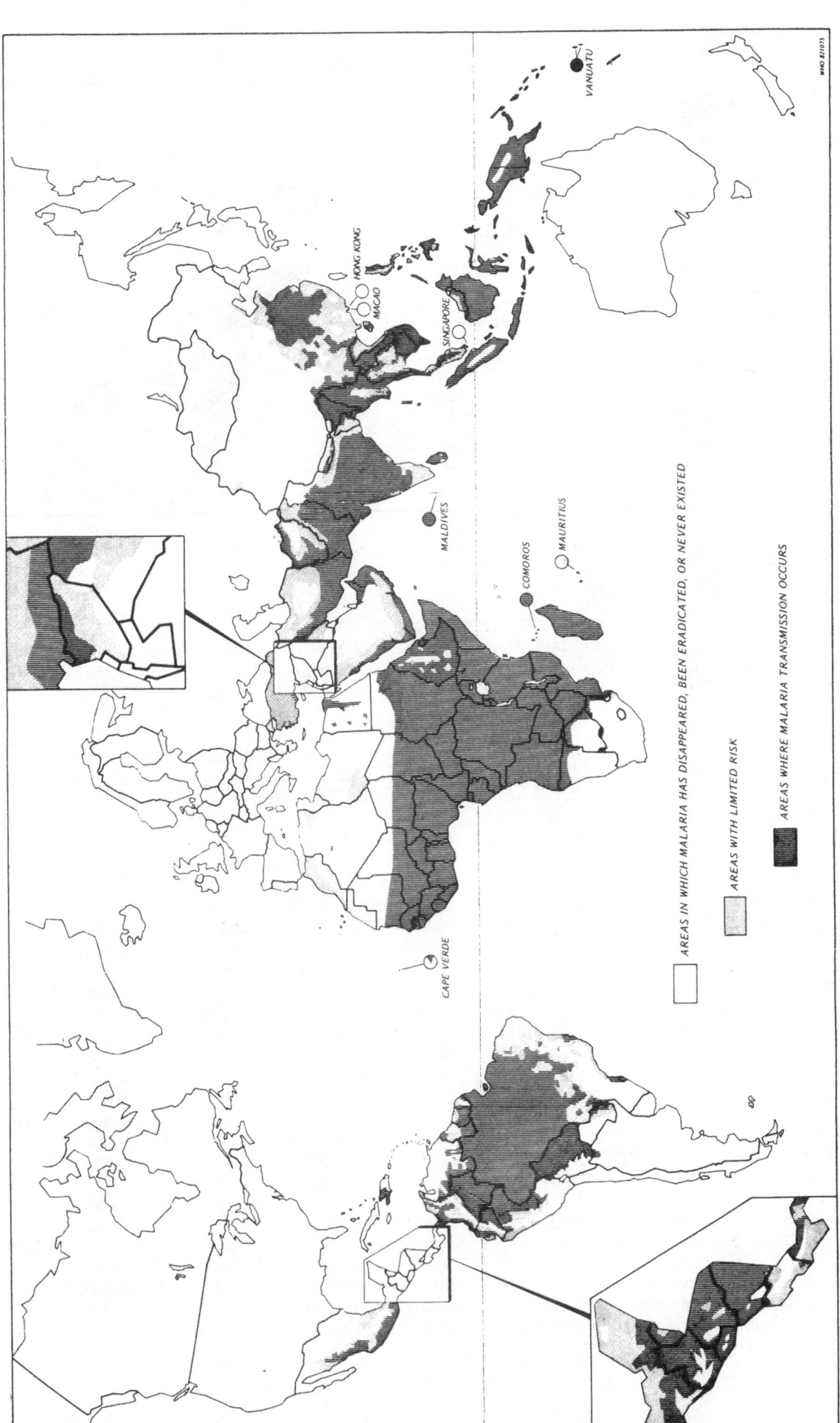

Figure 33.3. Epidemiological assessment of status of malaria, 1982. (From Vaccination Certificate Requirements for International Travel and Health Advice to Travelers. Geneva, World Health Organization, 1984.)

AREAS IN WHICH MALARIA HAS DISAPPEARED, BEEN ERADICATED, OR NEVER EXISTED

AREAS WITH LIMITED RISK

AREAS WHERE MALARIA TRANSMISSION OCCURS

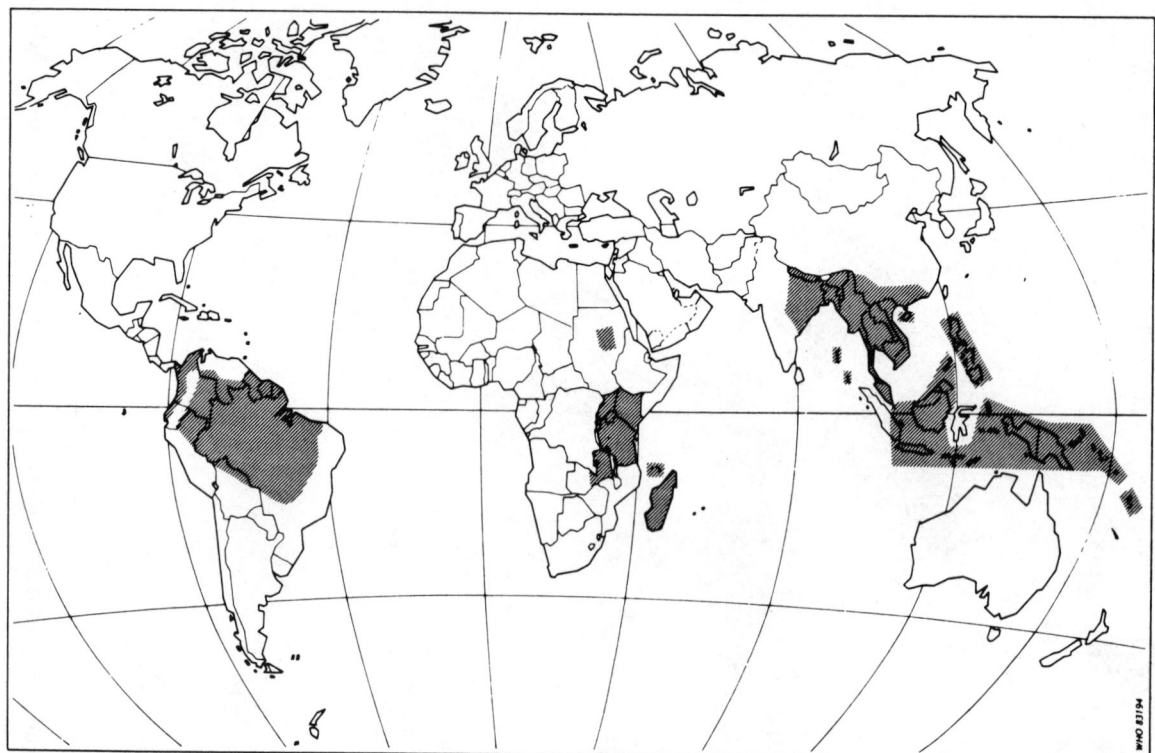

Figure 33.4. Areas with chloroquine-resistant *Plasmodium falciparum*, December 1982. (From *Health Information for International Travel, 1983.* Supplement to *Morbidity and Mortality Weekly Report*, vol 32, August, 1983. US Department of Health and Human Services, HHS Publication no. (CDC) 83-8280.)

studies; therefore, none is available in the United States. Amodiaquine has been shown to be slightly more effective than chloroquine in treating chloroquine-resistant malaria, and it may possibly afford more protection than chloroquine for prophylaxis. There is some preliminary evidence that doxycycline may be effective as a suppressive agent also. Proguanil (Paludrine) has been used both alone and in combination with other antimalarials, but is not available in the United States. It cannot be emphasized enough that personal protection measures against mosquitos must be practiced systematically in these areas. In areas of the world with only low level transmission of resistant malaria, including China, Southeast Asia, South America, and the Indian subcontinent, chloroquine is still the preferred drug for prophylaxis. Certain areas, such as the rural Amazonian basin and the northeast regions of Thailand near the refugee camps, have reported cases of malaria resistant to both Fansidar and chloroquine. The appropriate chemoprophylactic regimen for these areas is controversial. If travelers are going to these areas, an update on current prophylaxis recommendations should be obtained from the Centers for Disease Control, Malaria Branch.

Routine malaria prophylaxis with either chloroquine or Fansidar does not prevent delayed attacks of malaria from *Plasmodium vivax* or *Plasmodium ovale* because these species have an extra-erythrocytic chronic liver phase not eradicated by these two agents. Primaquine is an 8-aminoquinolone drug that is effective against the chronic liver forms of vivax and ovale malaria. For travelers with minimal mosquito exposure and short stays in endemic areas, primaquine is not routinely indicated. Primaquine prophylaxis should be considered in travelers who have had extended stays in areas endemic for either *P. vivax* or *P. ovale* malaria and who have had significant mosquito exposure. Primaquine, 15 mg of base daily for 14 days, is usually given during the last 2 weeks of chloroquine chemoprophylaxis. Primaquine can cause hemolysis in people with glucose 6-phosphate deficiency, and has several other potential side effects, such as headache, nausea, vomiting, and gastrointestinal distress.

Chloroquine when used at recommended dosage for malaria suppression has rarely been associated with serious adverse effects. Occasionally minor side effects such as dizziness, gastrointestinal distress, headache, and blurred vision have been reported but these rarely necessitate discontinuation of the drug. When chloroquine is used for prolonged periods of time in high doses as in the therapy of rheumatoid arthritis, it may be associated with a severe retinopathy. This serious side effect is very rare when chloroquine is used at the relatively low doses for malaria chemoprophylaxis. The risk of retinopathy appears to increase after a cumulative dose of 100 g of base, and periodic retinal examinations should be considered in persons who have taken this much chloroquine.

Fansidar has been associated with severe adverse reactions, including blood dyscrasia, hepatotoxicity, Stevens-Johnson syndrome as well as hypersensitivity reactions (see page 406). There is little published data on the incidence of side effects from prolonged usage of Fansidar, but practical experience suggests that it is safe for at least 2 to 3 years. Both pyrimethamine and sulfadoxine affect the folic acid pathway and the antifolate effects may be exacerbated by poor nutrition, malabsorption, and concurrent usage of antimicrobials.

Chloroquine is felt to be safe in pregnant and lactating women, and should be recommended to pregnant women traveling to malaria endemic zones. In laboratory animals, pyrimethamine has been shown to be teratogenic and therefore Fansidar should not be prescribed to women who are pregnant or may become pregnant. Travel to chloroquine-resistant areas should be avoided if at all possible, and if necessary, extreme precaution should be used to avoid mosquitos. Chloroquine can be made into a liquid form for children (dose is 5 mg/kg).

FOOD AND WATER

Food and water are the most common vehicles for the introduction of infectious agents into the body. It is best for the traveler to the developing world to consider any uncooked food and any product containing unpasteurized milk as possibly contaminated and therefore not safe to consume. Some meats, including beef, can harbor pathogens such as *Trichinella spiralis* and *Taenia solium* and *Taenia saginata*. Raw or uncooked fresh water fish, and crustaceans can transmit liver flukes and tapeworms. Even after foods have been cooked, it is imperative that food be properly stored. Food held at ambient temperatures is a medium in which bacterial pathogens can rapidly multiply. Creamy desserts are often vehicles for *Salmonella* and staphylococcal food poisoning and should be avoided in areas with poor refrigeration (see clinical description, Chapter 26). Fruits that can be peeled are safe as long as they are peeled by the consumer just prior to eating. The travelers should be wary of cheese products made from unpasteurized milk as possible sources of brucella and other enteric pathogens (2). Salads should be avoided because lettuce and leafy vegetables are difficult to clean properly and often harbor infectious parasite eggs, cysts, and bacteria.

Although water may be safe in hotels in large cities, only water that has been adequately boiled and chlorinated should be considered safe to drink.

If the traveler is uncertain about the purity of the water, it should be boiled. Routine chlorination may not kill all parasites. In areas where purified water is not available or where hygiene and sanitation are poor, travelers are advised to drink only the following beverages: (a) those that use boiled water, such as hot tea or coffee; (b) canned or bottled carbonated beverages, including carbonated bottled water and soft drinks; and (c) beer or wine.

Boiling is by far the most reliable method of making water safe to drink. If the water contains sediment or floating matter, it should be strained with a cloth prior to boiling or treating chemically. The water should be boiled vigorously for at least 10 minutes, then allowed to cool to room temperature. If boiling is not possible, water can be chemically disinfected with tincture of iodine or tetraglycine hydroperiodide tablets. Cloudy water should always be strained to remove sediment before adding iodine. The purification tablets can be purchased from a pharmacy or a sporting goods store. The traveler should follow the manufacturer's instructions. If the water is cloudy, the number of tablets should be doubled. If the water is extremely cold, it should be allowed to warm up before dissolving the tablets. Tincture of iodine should be used as follows:

Per Quart or Liter of Water	Timing
Clean water, 5 drops	Let sit 30 minutes
Cloudy or cold water, 10 drops	Let sit several hours

It should be remembered that where water may be contaminated, ice (as well as containers for drinking) should also be considered contaminated. If at all possible, boiled or bottled water should be used for making ice, rinsing drinking vessels, and also for brushing teeth. If boiled or bottled water is unavailable, the hot water tap can be used as a last resort. Although many infectious agents do not grow at these temperatures, hot tap water is by no means completely safe.

DIARRHEA

Diarrhea is a common but not usually a serious health problem for most travelers. Cases occur when fecally contaminated food or water is ingested and, therefore, the precautions mentioned above for food and water should be followed. Even with good personal hygiene and avoidance of suspect food and water, the attack rate for travelers' diarrhea remains quite high. Approximately 75% of episodes are caused by bacterial agents, with greater than 50% due to enterotoxigenic *Escherichia coli*. Since the causative agents can be assumed to be bacterial three-fourths of the time, several strategies to prevent bacterial diarrhea or to treat it early have been studied (3).

Most causes of diarrhea are self limited and may only require rest and replacement of fluids and salts. This can usually be accomplished with fruit drinks or carbonated beverages, but occasionally traveler's diarrhea may be severe and the traveler should be advised to take a few packets of oral rehydration salts (ORT), such as Infalyte or Orlyte, to be mixed with clean water when needed. Severe diarrhea can cause dehydration and can possibly result in significant morbidity. Drinking the oral rehydration solution prevents the dehydration, and increases the sense of well-being even though it does not stop the diarrhea. Commercial ORT products are available in most countries. If no packets are available, a similar solution can be prepared by placing 1 level teaspoon of salt plus 4 level teaspoons of table sugar in a liter of water. The packet is preferable, however, because it provides a more "complete" formula. Any solution remaining after 24 hours should be discarded as it may become contaminated with bacteria.

Early treatment with either doxycycline (100 mg every 12 hours) or trimethoprim-sulfamethoxazole (Bactrim or Septra, 1 double-strength tablet every 12 hours) will limit the length of an episode of traveler's diarrhea to less than 36 hours; both of these antimicrobials are available in generic forms. Generally, these antimicrobials should be started soon after the diarrhea starts and continued for 3 to 5 days. Potential side effects, although uncommon, consist of (a) for trimethoprim-sulfamethoxazole, allergic reactions, skins rashes, and Stevens-Johnson syndrome. b) For doxycycline, photosensitivity, expressed as exaggerated sunburn, and *Candida* vaginitis in women. These small risks and inconveniences may be justified in a traveler who has a limited amount of time and cannot afford 3 to 5 days of a typical traveler's diarrhea.

The use of antimicrobials for prophylaxis has been a controversial issue. Antimicrobials can be taken daily *to prevent diarrhea* (7). Two that are 80 to 90% effective for prophylaxis are doxycycline (100 mg) and trimethoprim-sulfamethoxazole (1 double-strength tablet), taken once daily.

In January 1985, a consensus conference on traveler's diarrhea held at the National Institutes of Health recommended against the use of prophylactic antibiotics. The potential risk of serious adverse reactions to the prophylactic agent was believed to outweigh the benefits. Although the panel found no basis for recommending prophylaxis, they concluded that "some travellers may wish to consult with their physician and may elect to use prophylactic antimicrobial agents for travel under special circumstances, once the risks and benefits are clearly understood" (7a). The usual traveler should not be subjected to the risk of antimicrobials, but if antimicrobials are used they should be limited to those persons traveling to developing countries for

less than 3 weeks, especially individuals with severe medical conditions that could be worsened by diarrhea.

Drugs that inhibit bowel motility such as Lomotil or Imodium may provide temporary relief when diarrhea is especially inconvenient (such as during an 8-hour country bus trip). They provide brief relief of symptoms, but may be contraindicated in diarrhea caused by invasive organisms. Liquid Peptobismol may also be helpful but very large amounts are needed to significantly reduce diarrhea. Also, its use is not without possible complications due to the salicylates it contains. Peptobismol will bind the antibiotic doxycycline and negate its effectiveness, so these two drugs should not be taken together. Kaopectate is not effective in reducing the frequency and volume of diarrhea. At best, it may cause the stool to be somewhat less liquid.

For diarrhea that is very severe, is associated with repeated vomiting, or does not improve after several days, the traveler should be advised to consult a physician rather than attempt self-treatment. He should also see a doctor if (a) there is blood in the stool; (b) there is a fever higher than 101°F, especially if accompanied by shaking chills; or (c) antimicrobial therapy does not provide rapid improvement. Finally, in preparation for possible diarrhea, the traveler should be reminded that toilet tissue is difficult to find in many developing countries, and that it is prudent to take a supply with him.

Additional information regarding the pathogenesis and epidemiology of diarrheal illnesses is contained in Chapter 26.

SCHISTOSOMIASIS

Schistosomiasis is one of the world's major public health problems. Three predominant species exist (*Schistosoma mansoni*, *S. japonicum*, *S. haematobium*) and are found worldwide (see maps, Figs. 33.5, 33.6, and 33.7). Although few travelers are aware of schistosomiasis, it is a relatively common disease in much of the developing world. After infection, the disease may lie dormant, until it causes problems later in life. People contract schistosomiasis by wading or swimming in fresh or estuary water that is contaminated by the parasite. The cercariae (larval stage) can penetrate the skin and pass into the bloodstream without causing any symptoms at the time. Symptoms which may occur with schistosomiasis depend on the stage of the infection. Sometimes, there may be a rash at the site where the cercariae invaded, but this is not common. About 4 or 5 weeks after infection, an episode of fever, cough, and general malaise may occur. Still later (6 months to several years), more severe complications may occur, usually related to liver or urinary tract disease.

In recent years, severe cases of schistosomiasis have occurred in Americans after river rafting in

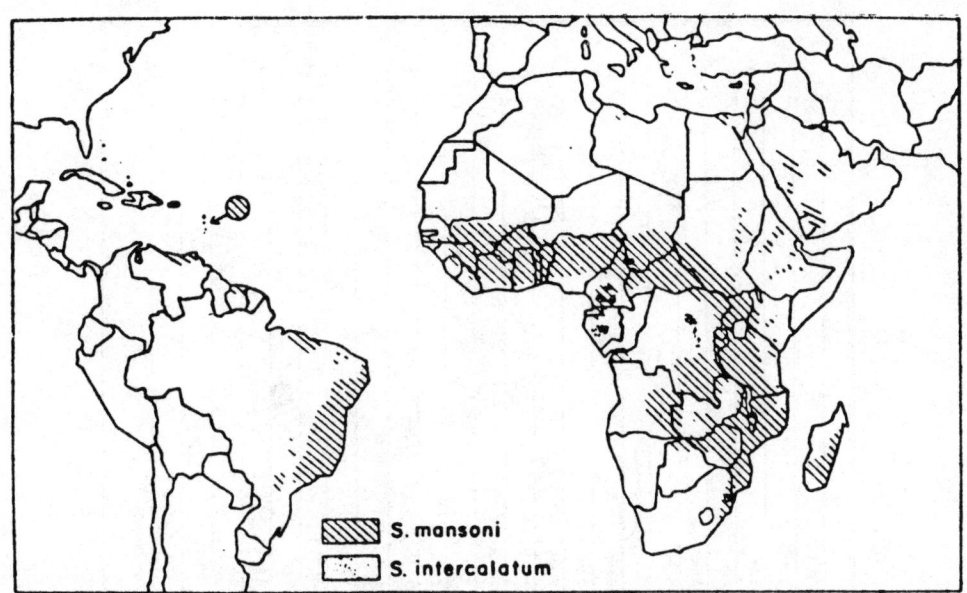

Figure 33.5. Geographic distribution of *S. mansoni* and *S. intercalatum.* (From Warren KS, Mahmoud AAF (eds): *Tropical and Geographical Medicine.* New York, McGraw-Hill, 1983.)

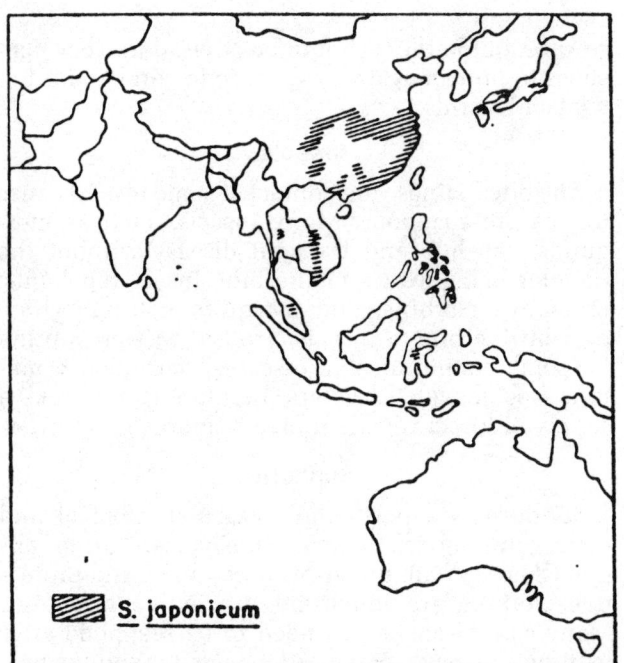

Figure 33.6. Geographical distribution of *S. japonicum.* On the mainland of Indochina, *S. mekongi* is probably the predominant species. (From Warren KS, Mahmoud AAF (eds): *Tropical and Geographical Medicine.* New York, McGraw-Hill, 1983.)

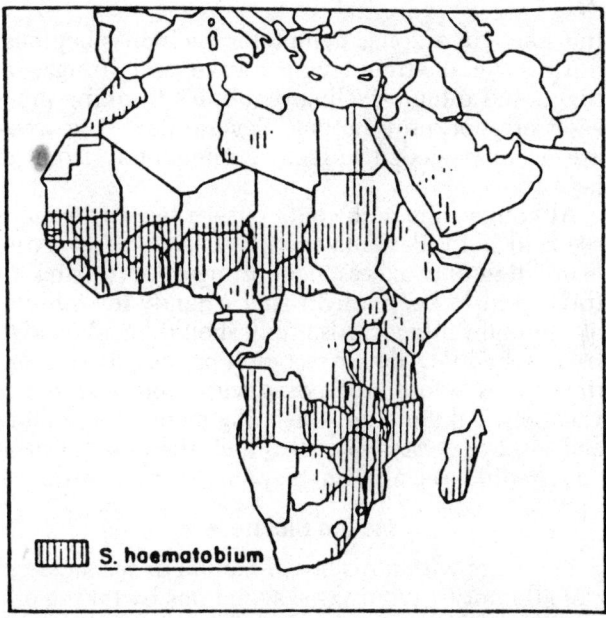

Figure 33.7. Geographical distribution of *S. haematobium.* (From Warren KS, Mahmoud AAF (eds): *Tropical and Geographical Medicine.* New York, McGraw-Hill, 1983.)

MISCELLANEOUS HEALTH CONCERNS

Jet Lag

Ethiopia (4) and after swimming in fresh water in Kenya (1a). Although treatment has improved with the advent of praziquantyl, it is better to advise travelers to avoid fresh water contact in endemic areas and thereby prevent disease acquisition.

Jet lag seems to be nearly universal for travelers traversing several time zones (see Fig. 33.8), though some seem to be more affected than others. More than simple travel fatigue, jet lag occurs when the body's physiological clock has not yet adjusted to

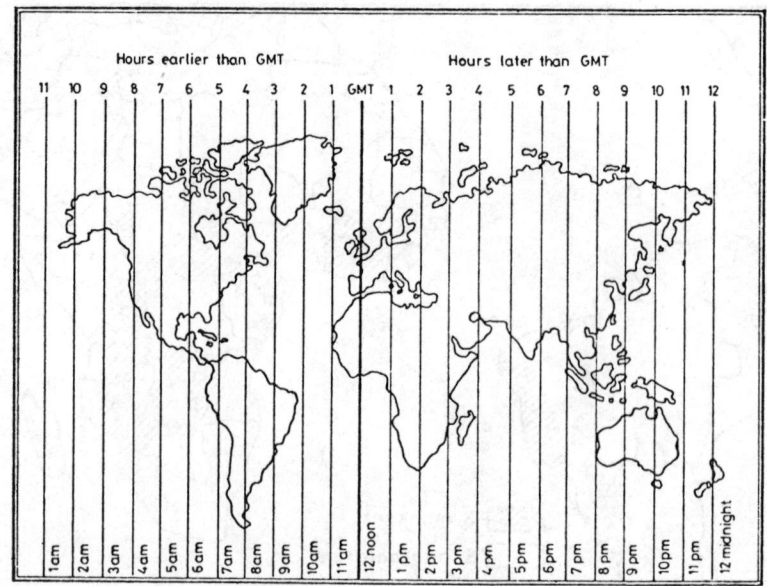

Figure 33.8. Time zones ("jet lag" typically occurs when five or more time zones are crossed). (*GMT*, Greenwich Meridian Time.) (From Walker E, Williams G: ABC of healthy travel: during travel and acclimatization. *Br Med J* 286:865, 1983.)

the new time zone. Symptoms include sleepiness during the daytime, lying awake and hungry at night, and often a feeling that one's thinking processes are not quite normal. Several days to a week are usually needed to recover completely from jet lag.

Although time is the only cure, a few suggestions seem to help. Patients should be advised to avoid overeating and excess alcohol ingestion during air travel and to keep a light snack handy for middle-of-the-night hunger. Also they should be advised to try to schedule a day of rest after passing six or more time zones before proceeding with their business or vacation. Taking a mild sleeping medication before bed for 2 or 3 days may also help them to get back on schedule (see also Chapter 85, "Sleep Disorders").

Motion Sickness

Travelers with a history of motion or sea sickness can attempt to avoid these symptoms by taking one of the antihistamines useful for this problem or transdermal scopolamine. Further details are found in Chapter 81.

Swimming and Bathing

Swimming in contaminated water may result in eye, ear, skin, and some intestinal infections. Wading, washing, and swimming should be avoided in water that is liable to be infested with the snail hosts of schistosomiasis (see above) or with human sewage or with animal urine that may contain *Leptospira*. Generally, only chlorinated pools should be considered safe places to swim in developing countries. Ocean beaches may be safe, if not contaminated by

sewage, but bathers should be advised to wear light shoes to protect against exposure to coral and other contact hazards.

Insects

The bites, stings, and contact of some insects cause unpleasant reactions. Many insects, such as mosquitos, can bite and transmit disease without the traveler being aware of the bite. Insect repellants, protective clothing, and mosquito netting, which prevent the bite of insects, are the best prevention for some communicable diseases, particularly malaria (see above). Travelers therefore should take a supply of insect repellant cream, lotion, or spray.

Sunburn

Sunburn is a particular hazard in tropical and high glare environments. Sunshades, sunscreens (see Chapter 100), broad-brimmed hats, and protective clothing are important preventive measures. Many sunscreen lotions need to be reapplied after bathing or heavy perspiration. For maximum protection, travelers should apply all sunscreen products before going outside. A small percentage of people who take the antibiotic tetracycline (including doxycycline) may develop an exaggerated burn after exposure to the sun—this may be important if this antibiotic is being taken daily for diarrhea prevention.

High Altitude

High altitudes can be a problem for individuals with pre-existing heart or lung disease, and portable oxygen may be advisable for these situations.

Healthy individuals may also be subject to altitude sickness when climbing above 10,000 feet and especially above 15,000 feet. Initial symptoms include dizziness, headache, extreme fatigue, chilliness, nausea, and vomiting. More severe symptoms may also occur, most commonly difficulty in concentrating, extreme shortness of breath, and more severe headache. In most individuals, symptoms are mild and clear within 24 to 48 hours. If symptoms persist or are severe, a return to lower altitude may be required. Administration of oxygen generally relieves acute symptoms. Preventive measures include adequate rest before travel, avoidance of alcohol and tobacco, and decreased physical activity at high altitude.

The carbonic anhydrase inhibitor acetazolamide (Diamox) has been shown to reduce the time needed for acclimatization to high altitudes by 24 to 48 hours, in both simulated and actual climbing situations. Recently, the FDA approved this drug for use in the prevention of altitude sickness (1). The recommended dosage for travelers is 250 mg every 8 to 12 hours, with medication initiated 24 to 48 hours before and continued during ascent. Although its mechanism of action is poorly understood, acetazolamide is known to promote excretion of bicarbonate by the kidneys. This bicarbonate excretion compensates for the respiratory alkalosis seen at high altitudes and this property may contribute to the drug's beneficial effects on acclimatization.

Snakes and Scorpions

Poisonous snakes live in many developing countries, although most travelers will never see them unless they visit a zoo. If travelers will be walking through brush or jungle, or will be walking at night, they should wear good quality leather boots which go above the ankle. Not all snakebites are poisonous and not all poisonous snakebites are fatal, but immediate treatment by a physician is essential. If possible, the traveler should bring the snake for identification.

Scorpion bites are painful, but seldom dangerous, except possibly to infants. Exposure to bites can be avoided by sleeping under mosquito netting and shaking clothing and shoes before putting them on.

Medicines

If travelers are taking prescribed medications, they should obtain an adequate supply before leaving and keep all medications in their luggage.

Many medications are sold without prescription overseas. However, the traveler should be cautious about purchasing medicines. Although medicines made by recognized pharmaceutical companies are generally of high quality, the quality of other medicines may not be guaranteed. The traveler should be advised not to self-medicate; many medicines have serious side effects.

Women and Children

Some medications used commonly in travelers should not be given to pregnant women, in particular doxycycline (impairs tooth development in the infant) and Fansidar (see "Malaria" above). Travel late in pregnancy may precipitate labor. In fact, many airlines will not allow air travel during the final month. Immunizations recommended for children are, in general, the same as those recommended for adults (see above) except that yellow fever vaccine is not usually required under 1 year of age. Routine "baby shots" are even more important for children traveling to developing countries since diphtheria, whooping cough, polio, and measles are relatively common. The dosages of medicines have to be adjusted for children. This is especially important for malaria medications. Because children may be restless on long airline trips, some parents are tempted to sedate their children. This is not recommended, however, because children may react adversely to sedatives.

Miscellaneous Infections

Many people experience a "traveler's cold" during a trip. These are thought to be due to infection with respiratory viruses to which the traveler has no immunity. Travelers should bring their favorite cold remedy and an extra box of tissues with them. Fungal infections, especially "jock itch" and athlete's feet, may also be more common, especially in hot humid environments. Travelers should wear clean dry socks, or sandals when possible and use antifungal powders and ointments as needed. Adventurous travelers should be reminded that sexually transmitted diseases, particularly gonorrhea, are very common in many areas and are frequently resistant to the usual antibiotics.

Long Term Travelers

Recommendations for long term travelers are generally the same regarding food and water, immunizations, malaria prophylaxis, *etc.* In addition, gamma globulin should be given every 6 months and immunizations for typhoid (every 3 years) and yellow fever (every 10 years) should be kept up to date. If the traveler hires people to work in the house, these people should be examined medically before starting work. The employee will benefit from this, and it will minimize the possibility of infections being transmitted to the traveler's family.

Medical Emergencies

If the traveler becomes seriously ill or injured while traveling, the United States consulate can provide advice on where to go for help.

INTERNATIONAL TRAVELERS HEALTH KIT

The following is a suggested first aid and health kit that represents the minimal necessary equipment for the traveler to the developing world:

1. *International Immunization Card* with documentation of vaccines received.
2. Appropriate medication for *malaria prophylaxis.*
3. *Mosquito repellent.*
4. *Water purfication tablets or tincture of iodine.*
5. *Oral rehydration salt packets.*
6. *Antimicrobial medication for treatment or prevention of diarrhea* as arranged with the traveler's physician.
7. *Imodium or Lomotil.*
8. *Sunscreen.*
9. *Bandaids* (for blisters).
10. A spare pair of glasses or at least the lens prescription.
11. Any prescription medication the traveler takes regularly.
12. The traveler's favorite "cold" remedy.
13. Fever thermometer.
14. Aspirin or acetaminophen (paracetamol in most other countries).
15. Astringent or antiseptic.
16. Antifungal powder.

POST-TRAVEL SCREENING

Most persons who acquire viral, bacterial, or parasitic infections in developing countries will become ill within 6 weeks after returning, but certain infectious diseases, such as malaria and schistosomiasis, may not manifest themselves until later. The traveler should be advised to seek medical help for any unexplained symptoms during the 12 months following the end of his trip. When an unexplained late illness occurs, it is necessary to identify all the developing countries which the traveler visited in order to know which infectious disease risks the travel encountered.

For travelers who stay for relatively long periods in the developing world, it is prudent to provide routine screening on arrival home. This should include a complete blood count, liver function tests, tuberculosis skin test, stool examination for occult blood, urinalysis, and stool examination for ova and parasites. If these tests are all normal, the traveler has probably not acquired a serious unrecognized infectious disease, but post-trip surveillance for another 6 months is still warranted.

General References

Health Information for International Travel. Supplement to *Morbidity and Mortality Weekly Report,* DHHS publ no. (CDC) 84-8280 Atlanta, Centers for Disease Control.
   A practical manual, updated yearly.
Schultz MG: Exotic diseases: Ounce of prevention or pound of cure? *Postgrad Med* 62:121, 1977.
   An overview of the risks.
Warren KS, Mahmoud AAF: *Tropical and Geographical Medicine.* New York, McGraw-Hill, 1983.
   An in-depth textbook.
Wolfe, M: Diseases of travelers. *CIBA Clin Symp* 32:2, 1984.
   Well illustrated publication, with practical recommendations concerning common infectious disease problems.

Specific References

1. Acetozolamide for acute mountain sickness. *FDA Drug Bull* 13:27, 1983.
1a. Acute schistosomiasis with transverse myelitis in American students returning from Kenya. *Morbidity and Mortality Weekly Report,* vol 33, p 445, 1984.
2. Arrow PM, Smaron M, Ormiste V: Brucellosis in a group of travelers to Spain. *JAMA* 251:505, 1984.
3. DuPont HL, Sullivan P, Evans DG, *et al*: Prevention of traveler's diarrhea. *JAMA* 243:237, 1980.
4. Istrie GR, *et al*: Acute schistosomiasis among Americans rafting the Omo River, Ethiopia. *JAMA* 251:508, 1984.
5. Monger H, Steffe R, Schar M: Epidemiology of cholera in travelers, and conclusions for vaccination recommendations. *Br Med J* 286:184, 1982.
6. Reid D, Dewar RD, Fallon RJ, *et al*: Infection and travel: the experience of package tourists and other travelers. *J Infect* 2:65, 1980.
6a. Revised recommendations for preventing malaria in travelers to areas with chloroquine-resistant *Plasmodium falciparum. Morbidity and Mortality Weekly Report,* vol 14, p 186, 1985.
7. Sack DA, *et al*: Prophylactic doxycycline for traveler's diarrhea: Results of a prospective double-blind study in Peace Corps Volunteers in Kenya. *N Engl J Med* 298:758, 1978.
7a. Travelers' diarrhea. Consensus Conference. *JAMA* 253:2700, 1985.
8. Snyder JD, Blake PA: Is cholera is a problem for United States travelers? *JAMA* 247:2268, 1982.
9. Steffen R, van der Linde F, Gyr K, Schar M: Epidemiology of diarrhea in travelers. *JAMA* 249:1176, 1983.
10. Taylor P, Polland R, Blake P: Typhoid in the United States and the risk to the international traveler. *J Invest Dermatol* 148:599, 1983.

SECTION 4

Gastrointestinal Problems

CHAPTER THIRTY-FOUR

Disorders of the Esophagus: Dysphagia and Gastroesophageal Reflux

HAROLD J. TUCKER, M.D.

DYSPHAGIA

Difficulty in swallowing, dysphagia, is an extremely reliable indicator of disturbance in oropharyngeal or esophageal function. It should never be dismissed as an "emotional" problem or a symptom of "globus hystericus" (see page 424). The patient frequently says that food is sticking in his chest, often pinpointing the involved area. Occasionally, dysphagia may be accompanied by pain on swallowing, odynophagia, but the two symptoms are quite distinct and may occur independently.

Physiology of Swallowing

Normal swallowing requires the coordination of the skeletal muscles of the pharynx, the cricopharyngeus muscle (the upper esophageal sphincter) and the proximal one-third of the esophagus, with the smooth muscle of the distal body of the esophagus and the lower esophageal sphincter. Thus, the initiation of swallowing is voluntary, but involuntary processes subsequently propel the swallowed bolus through the esophagus into the stomach. The following sequence of events occurs during normal swallowing: relaxation of the upper esophageal sphincter to permit entry of the bolus into the esophagus; closure of the sphincter to prevent esophageal-pharyngeal regurgitation and aspiration; propulsion of the bolus distally by esophageal peristalsis; relaxation of the lower esophageal sphincter (LES), to allow easy entrance of the bolus into the stomach; and prompt closure of the LES to prevent reflux of gastric contents.

Dysphagia may occur from a disturbance of any of the anatomical structures or of the physiological events involved in normal swallowing.

Clinical Evaluation

History

Because of the complexity of the swallowing mechanism, the causes of dysphagia are quite varied. Certain aspects of the history are very helpful in elucidating the underlying disorder. Difficulty in swallowing solids strongly suggests an anatomical obstruction—such as carcinoma, stricture, or esophageal ring, whereas difficulty in swallowing solids and liquids suggests a motility disturbance—such as achalasia, scleroderma, or diffuse esophageal spasm.

The history may also be useful in identifying the region of abnormal function as either pre-esophageal (oropharyngeal) or esophageal (Table 34.1). Symptoms suggestive of pre-esophageal dysphagia include regurgitation of liquid through the nose, aspiration with swallowing, and an inability to propel a bolus of food into the pharynx. The most common causes of this type of dysphagia are neuromuscular conditions, such as bulbar palsy due to brainstem infarcts or tumors, pseudobulbar palsy (usually from bilateral cerebral vascular accidents which have compromised cortical function), polymyositis, and myasthenia gravis. Patients with esophageal dysphagia complain of retrosternal fullness after swallowing and of the feeling that food is stuck at a certain point in the esophagus—often relieved by regurgitation. Esophageal dysphagia is most commonly caused by narrowing of the lumen by either inflammatory or neoplastic strictures. The history, then, indicates whether the dysphagia is due to an anatomical obstruction or to a neuromuscular disturbance, and focuses attention on the region of involvement.

Mild weight loss may be described by patients with any type of chronic dysphagia, due to voluntary decrease in intake of food which often accompanies their symptoms. More severe weight loss, plus anorexia, suggests carcinoma.

Special Studies

To delineate the cause of dysphagia, one or more of the following procedures should be employed:

Table 34.1.
Types of Dysphagia

	Symptoms	Common Causes
Pre-esopha-geal (oro-pharyngeal)	Regurgitation of liq-uid through the nose, aspiration with swallowing, inability to propel a bolus into the pharynx	Neuromuscular conditions: brain-stem lesions, polymyositis, myasthenia, pseudobulbar palsy
Esophageal	Retrosternal ful-ness after swal-lowing	Strictures: inflam-matory or neo-plastic
	Sticking of a bolus at a certain point	Motor disturbance (*e.g.*, achalasia)

radiological studies; esophagoscopy; and esophageal motility studies.

Consultation with a gastroenterologist is recommended for most patients with dysphagia, both for evaluation of the clinical problem and for the performance of esophagoscopy and motility studies.

Radiology

The initial study in most patients with dysphagia should be a *barium swallow*, a procedure which can identify motility disturbances as well as anatomical deformities, and is the easiest procedure for the patient to tolerate (it takes only 15 to 20 minutes and is associated with essentially no discomfort). As with all radiological studies, the radiologist should be informed about the specific disorders that are most suspected. Without this communication, the radiologist may perform a routine barium swallow looking for only carcinoma, stricture, hiatal hernia, or reflux and may not pay specific attention to the motility pattern. Proper radiographic evaluation of esophageal motility requires that the patient be placed in the recumbent position and that the flow of the barium column be monitored. In this way, normal peristalsis can be seen to propel the bolus of barium distally, while in motor disorders the barium may not move distally until the patient is tilted upright. In addition, to observe the rapid activity of pharyngeal contractions and to detect abnormal esophageal contractions, the barium swallow should be recorded on cine film (a cine-esopha-gogram). In this fashion, barium studies often can detect both organic and functional abnormalities leading to dysphagia. However, a negative study does not exclude either anatomical or motor disorders of the esophagus and a positive study seldom permits a specific diagnosis to be made; therefore, a barium swallow should always be followed by endoscopy.

Endoscopy

Esophagoscopy is an essential part of the evaluation of dysphagia. Because of the insensitivity of the barium swallow, endoscopy should be performed in all patients with persistent dysphagia, particularly in those with persistent difficulty in swallowing solid food. Esophagoscopy is complementary to the radiographic examination. The procedure is well tolerated, and can generally be performed on an ambulatory basis. When a lesion is detected by the radiographic test, endoscopy provides the most direct approach to establish the nature of the lesion, whether inflammatory or neoplastic. Biopsies and brushings for cytological evaluation can be obtained under visual guidance. Further, the instrument may disrupt esophageal webs or rings that are causing the dysphagia, and thus may be both a diagnostic and a therapeutic tool. Inability to pass the endoscope through the esophagus into the stomach confirms an anatomical cause of the dysphagia and rules out a motor disturbance (*e.g.*, achalasia). The patient's experience with upper gastrointestinal endoscopy is described in Chapter 35.

Recording of Esophageal Motility

Esophageal manometry is the best procedure for the evaluation of esophageal motor function. This study measures the strength, function, and coordination of both the upper and lower esophageal sphincters and of the body of the esophagus in response to a swallow (Fig. 34.1A). The procedure is well tolerated, takes only about 20 minutes and involves the passage of a narrow triple lumen catheter either through the nose or the mouth into the stomach. Recordings are made of the amplitude and coordination of contractions within the pharynx and esophagus as the catheter is withdrawn. Various motility disturbances can be diagnosed by use of this technique (Table 34.2). Esophageal manometry should be performed in all patients for whom a structural cause for the dysphagia cannot be found.

Specific Causes of Dysphagia

Carcinoma of Esophagus

Cancer of the esophagus should always be suspected as the cause of dysphagia in a patient over the age of 40. The incidence of esophageal carcinoma in the United States is approximately 7500 cases/year. Men, especially black men, are more likely to develop esophageal cancer than are women. Predisposing factors include cigarette smoking, heavy alcohol use, lye strictures, achalasia, Plummer-Vinson syndrome (see below, page 424), and Barrett's mucosa.

In the vast majority of cases, esophageal cancer is of the squamous cell type. These tumors are most common in the middle third of the esophagus. Adenocarcinoma is more likely to be seen when the normal squamous cells of the esophagogastric junction are destroyed by reflux (see below) and are replaced by columnar cells (Barrett's mucosa). Carcinoma of the cardia of the stomach may directly

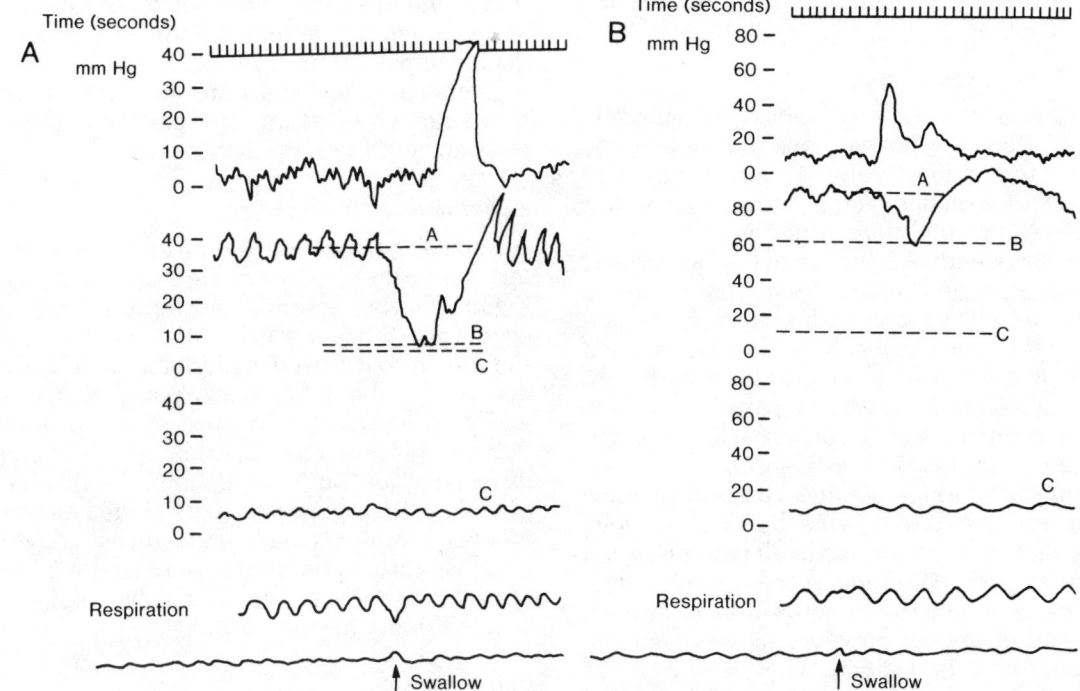

Figure 34.1. *A.* Esophageal manometry tracing in a normal subject demonstrating the esophageal response during a single swallow. Pressure recordings are obtained at 5-cm intervals from the esophagus, lower esophagus, lower esophageal sphincter (LES), and stomach. Prior to the swallow, the LES maintains a high pressure (A) compared to intragastric pressure (C). With a swallow, there is prompt relaxation of the LES (B) toward gastric pressure (C). An esophageal contraction occurs in the esophageal body in response to a swallow (primary peristalsis). The LES returns to its basal level as the esophageal contraction reaches the LES. *B.* Esophageal manometry tracing in a patient with achalasia. The basal LES pressure (A) is abnormally high (>80 in tracing). With a swallow, there is incomplete relaxation of the LES (B), leaving a residual high pressure compared to gastric pressure (C). In the esophageal body, nonperistaltic, repetitive contractions may be found, but there is no normal peristalsis. (Adapted from Cohen S, Lipshutz W: Lower esophageal sphincter dysfunction in achalasia. *Gastroenterology* 61:814, 1971.)

Table 34.2.
Esophageal Motility Study

	Normal Response to Swallow	Achalasia	Diffuse Spasm	Scleroderma	Dermatomyositis
Pharynx	Normal contraction at nadir of relaxation of upper esophageal sphincter	Normal	Normal	Normal	Low
Upper esophageal sphincter	High pressure zone with complete relaxation	Normal	Normal	Normal	Low pressure with partial relaxation
Midbody of esophagus	Peristaltic wave of contraction	Aperistalsis; occasional simultaneous contractions	Some peristalsis with frequent repetititve and simultaneous contractions	Proximal esophagus—normal; distal—loss of amplitude progressing to aperistalsis	Proximal esophagus—low amplitude waves; distal esophagus–normal
Lower esophageal sphincter	High pressure zone with complete relaxation	Hypertonic—incomplete relaxation	Usually normal but may be high with incomplete relaxation	Low pressure	Normal pressure and relaxation

extend into the lower esophagus and obstruct the esophageal lumen.

Diagnosis

The diagnosis of esophageal cancer is generally made only after symptoms have developed, by which time the lesion is already advanced, with involvement of regional lymph nodes. In patients with predisposing conditions, such as achalasia or Barrett's mucosa, earlier detection of the cancer may be achieved by regular (exact frequency yet to be determined) esophagoscopy with cytological brushings of the entire esophagus. Most patients present with dysphagia for several months and with progressive weight loss. Odynophagia (pain on swallowing) may accompany the dysphagia. Occult blood loss is common but hematemesis is unusual.

The diagnostic workup includes a barium swallow and upper endoscopy. After the barium swallow, endoscopy should be performed in all patients. Even if the X-ray is negative, the endoscope can still detect mucosal lesions. When the tumor is already defined by X-ray, endoscopy can supply a tissue diagnosis, which is important in deciding whether surgery or radiation is indicated. Multiple biopsies and directed brush cytologies obtained *via* the endoscope provide a positive tissue diagnosis in over 95% of cases. However, radiological evaluation remains important as it provides useful information concerning the degree of esophageal obstruction, the length of the tumor, and the appearance of the fundus of the stomach. With the combined use of these two techniques, differentiation can be made between cancer of the esophagus and other esophageal lesions—such as peptic stricture of the esophagus, achalasia, severe esophagitis, and esophageal varices.

Therapy

Therapy for esophageal cancer is generally surgery or radiation. The choice between these two forms of therapy depends generally on the cell type and the location of the neoplasm. Adenocarcinoma is less radiosensitive, usually occurs in the distal one-third of the esophagus, and therefore, is better suited for a surgical approach. Squamous cell carcinoma is relatively radiosensitive, and numerous studies suggest that radiation of the lesions in the distal and middle thirds of the esophagus is as effective as is surgery (5) (See Chapter 8 for a discussion of radiotherapy in the treatment of cancer). Surgical resection is more extensive and less well tolerated, the more proximal the tumor. Combination radiotherapy and resection have been reported to improve survival, but greater experience with this approach is needed. With either approach, the prognosis is very poor: 75% are dead within 1 year of diagnosis, and 95% by 5 years. Palliation, *i.e.*, maintenance of an open esophagus so that the patient can swallow food and saliva, should be the minimal aim of therapy. At times, passing dilators through the tumor and inserting prosthetic tubes into the esophageal lumen are helpful adjuncts to provide some degree of palliation.

Therapeutic decisions are best made together by the general physician, the gastroenterologist, the surgeon, and the radiation therapist.

Achalasia

Achalasia (spasm of the lower esophageal sphincter) is a motor disorder of the distal esophagus causing dysphagia for solids and liquids. The condition occurs in all age groups, with a peak incidence in the fourth and fifth decades. The incidence of this disorder is about 1/100,000 population/year. Men and women are equally susceptible to the disease. Patients present most commonly with progressive dysphagia for both solids and liquids and, frequently, with regurgitation of ingested material. Pulmonary symptoms such as nocturnal coughing and even aspiration pneumonia may be the initial mode of presentation. Occasionally, substernal chest pain is associated with the dysphagia.

Pathogenesis

The pathogenesis of achalasia is not known. There have been several studies that have described abnormalities in the myenteric ganglion cells in the distal esophagus (LES zone) and in the body of the esophagus, as well as abnormalities in the vagal nucleus and its peripheral fibers. However, these findings have not been consistent. Pharmacological studies have further supported the concept of denervation of the esophagus. There is an exaggerated response of the LES and of the body of the esophagus to cholinergic stimulation (e.g., in the Mecholyl test) and to the hormone gastrin, consistent with the concept of denervation hypersensitivity. The cause for the neuropathic injury is unknown.

Diagnosis

The routine chest X-ray frequently suggests the diagnosis. The normal gastric air bubble is absent, and an air-fluid level in the dilated esophagus is sometimes seen behind the heart. With a very dilated and tortuous esophagus, the mediastinum appears widened. The typical features on barium esophagogram (Fig. 34.2) include (a) smooth tapered narrowing of the distal end of the esophagus that fails to open properly, (b) retention of barium and secretions in the more proximal esophagus, and (c) absence of peristalsis. The distal narrowing is often described as a "bird beak" or "pen quill" deformity. It is important that the patient be examined while he is upright, to demonstrate the height of the retained barium-filled column.

Esophageal manometry has demonstrated three distinct abnormalities in patients with achalasia: (a) hypertonicity of the LES, (b) failure of the LES to relax following a swallow, and (c) absence of peri-

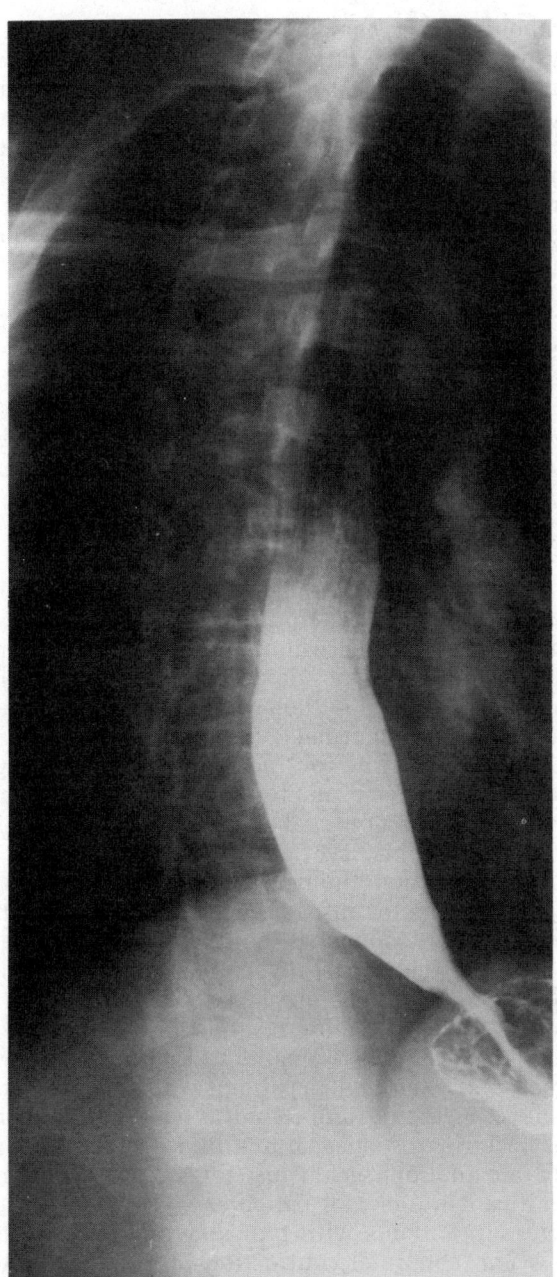

Figure 34.2. Barium swallow in a patient with achalasia. The esophagus is dilated, and the tapered distal segment never opens normally. Under fluoroscopy, no peristalsis is seen, but simultaneous contractions are noted.

stalsis of the entire esophagus. The procedure should be done, if possible, in every patient with the disease so that the results of treatment can be measured against the baseline pressures. In achalasia, the basal LES pressure is elevated, at times to very high levels, and the degree of relaxation is incomplete, generally less than 50% (Fig. 34.1*B*). Thus, there is a constant high pressure zone that impedes the passage of the esophageal contents. Peristalsis is also absent, fur-

ther impairing the propulsion of the bolus distally. At times the esophageal contractions, while not peristaltic or propagative, are of high amplitude and simultaneous, resulting in the chest pain. Injection of a cholinergic agent (Mecholyl test) has been shown to cause a marked increase in the LES pressure in patients with achalasia. However, since this test is not specific for achalasia, is uncomfortable for the patient, and provides little additional information, there is no need to perform it.

Differential Diagnosis

Achalasia must be differentiated from other disorders that lead to obstruction of the passage of food into the stomach. Esophageal strictures, both peptic and neoplastic, and carcinomas at the esophagogastric (EG) junction may result in symptoms and even in a radiographic and manometric picture similar to that of achalasia (7). Thus, it is important that all such patients be evaluated with endoscopy. Failure to pass the endoscope into the stomach indicates an anatomical obstruction (such as carcinoma or stricture) rather than a functional one (such as achalasia). Scleroderma (see below) with its associated esophageal motility disturbance may result in dysphagia with diminished peristalsis seen on X-ray. However, by the time patients with esophageal scleroderma develop stricture and dilation of the esophagus that may mimic achalasia, they usually have other obvious stigmata of scleroderma (particularly tight skin of the face and hands or Raynaud's phenomenon). Further, on esophageal manometry the LES pressure in scleroderma is low rather than high as it is in achalasia (Table 34.2), and the disorder of motility is confined to the smooth muscle portion (distal two-thirds) of the esophagus, with a normally functioning proximal segment. In patients from South America, Chagas' disease may result in a megaesophagus, and present with manometric patterns indentical to that of achalasia.

Therapy

There are two types of therapy for achalasia: pneumatic dilation and surgery. Both forms of therapy are aimed at reducing the pressure gradient between the esophagus and the stomach, thus decreasing the severity of the dysphagia. The aperistalsis and impaired sphincter relaxation persist after therapy. *Pneumatic dilation* is performed by a gastroenterologist in the hospital. The esophagus is aspirated completely prior to the dilation. After premedication with analgesics and sedatives, a bag dilator is passed into the stomach. The dilator is a weighted tube, the distal portion of which includes an inflatable balloon. Under fluoroscopic guidance, the balloon portion is positioned across the area of the LES. It is then inflated for 30 seconds to 2 minutes, causing a forceful disruption of the LES muscle. The dilator is then removed and can be expected to be blood streaked. The patient usually experiences chest pain during the procedure. The major risk of the procedure is esophageal perforation, which occurs in 1 to 5% of dilations. The day following the dilation, the LES pressure may be recorded manometrically to document that the dilation has indeed lowered the basal LES pressure significantly. Satisfactory results, i.e., improvement in dysphagia, weight gain, and decrease in retention of barium, can be expected in about 75% of cases. In successful cases, there is immediate relief of symptoms. The patient is then observed overnight and is discharged the following day. Dilation can be repeated if symptoms of dysphagia recur or worsen, but most patients have only minimal symptoms for many years after therapy.

Surgical therapy involves a thoracotomy with transection of the circular muscle of the LES zone to the level of the mucosa, the Heller myotomy. This surgical approach provides similar satisfactory results, with a success rate of 75 to 80%. The procedure may cause significant reflux esophagitis in as many as 25% of patients. As a result of this troublesome complication, some have advocated combining a fundoplication with the myotomy. Because of the ease to the patients of pneumatic dilation compared to a thoracotomy, and because of the high incidence of reflux after surgery, pneumatic dilation is generally the initial procedure of choice. Surgery should be reserved for (a) failure of repeated dilations to provide symptomatic relief, (b) esophageal perforation secondary to pneumatic dilation, (c) inability to perform dilation because of the shape of the esophagus or the presence of an epiphrenic diverticulum, and (d) inability to exclude carcinoma.

Complications

A major complication of achalasia is esophageal cancer. The incidence of this complication ranges from 6 to 29% in various series (3). The development of cancer in patients with achalasia should not be confused with cancer of the esophagogastric junction presenting with an achalasia-like picture. The cancer that develops in patients with primary achalasia usually occurs many years after the diagnosis of achalasia has been established, is of the squamous cell type, and generally occurs in the midportion of the esophagus. There is no evidence that successful therapy of achalasia prevents the development of cancer. Thus, all such patients should be under surveillance with periodic endoscopy with esophageal cytology (exact frequency yet to be determined but probably of the order of every 1 to 3 years).

Diffuse Esophageal Spasm

Clinical Presentation

Symptomatic diffuse esophageal spasm (SDES) is a disorder characterized by nonperistaltic esophageal contractions, often of high amplitude, that result in dysphagia and substernal chest pain. The disorder is seen equally in both sexes and at all ages (although it appears to be rare in children). The dysphagia is intermittent and is experienced for both solids and liquids. The pain also is intermittent and may, at times, be provoked by certain foods, particularly hot and cold beverages. At other times, the pain occurs spontaneously and may even awaken the patient at night. The pain is highly variable in quality, sometimes described as knife-like, sometimes as dull and crushing; it may radiate to the neck, back, or arms. It may be brief, or it may last for hours. Because of its location, radiation, and "crushing" quality, it is frequently confused with the pain of ischemic heart disease. When no cardiac disease is found, many of these patients are believed to have a psychogenic disturbance. Thus, this condition is often underdiagnosed and is easily confused with other conditions.

Diagnosis

The procedures for the diagnosis of this condition include radiographic studies and esophageal manometry. The *barium swallow*, or preferably the cineesophagogram, may demonstrate nonperistaltic spontaneous and simultaneous contractions (tertiary waves). These abnormal contractions are frequently encountered during routine barium swallow, especially in the elderly, and by themselves do not make a diagnosis of esophageal spasm without the appropriate clinical history. Further, as SDES is an intermittent condition, the barium swallow may be normal or may be too insensitive to detect the motility disturbance. *Esophageal motility* studies are more sensitive (Table 34.2). Provocative agents (Mecholyl, edrophonium) can be employed during the motility studies to identify more clearly those patients who develop chest pain associated with abnormal esophageal contractions (4). In patients who are considered to have angina but are found to have normal coronary arteries, esophageal motility studies can demonstrate an esophageal cause for the chest pain in a significant number of patients, 30 to 40% in most series (1). Patients with typical symptoms of SDES in whom abnormal contractions are demonstrated on a barium swallow do not need esophageal manometry.

Esophageal Spasm Induced by Reflux

In some patients, the esophageal spasm and its symptoms are induced by reflux of gastric acid into the esophagus (see below, page 424); such patients may present with symptoms only of chest pain and/or dysphagia, without any history of heartburn. It is important to recognize acid-induced esophageal spasm, as the therapy for this condition will vary from that of the primary form of SDES. The acid-induced spasm can be suggested by the presence of a low LES pressure on esophageal manometry. During an esophageal motility study, the esophagus can be perfused over a 20-minute period with 0.1% hydrochloric acid (Bernstein test). The patient's subjective sensation in response to the acid infusion is evaluated at the same time as his esophageal contractions are measured. A positive study is characterized by the occurrence of the patient's typical symptoms during the acid perfusion, in association with abnormal esophageal contractions (ideally in the absence of electrocardiographic changes), and by the relief of these symptoms when the acid is cleared from the esophagus by saline infusion. Therapy should be directed at the gastroesophageal reflux primarily (see below, page 424). Therapy for the esophageal spasm (see below) may actually worsen the condition by further lowering LES tone, thus promoting more reflux.

Therapy

Therapy for SDES is aimed at reducing the amplitude and frequency of the abnormal contractions (Table 34.3). The patient should first be reassured that there is an organic cause for this discomfort, but that it is not of cardiac origin. Identification and avoidance of precipitating factors, such as cold beverages, should be recommended. Pharmacotherapy also can be very helpful. Both calcium channel blockers (*i.e.*, nifedipine or diltiazem) and nitroglycerin preparations (6) are very effective in relieving dysphagia and chest pain that are due to esophageal spasm. Positive effects can be demonstrated both manometrically and clinically. Which of these drugs is prescribed is a matter of personal preference of the physician and of the patient. The various preparations that are used and the average doses that are employed are listed in Table. 34.3. The great major-

Table 34.3.
Therapy for Symptomatic Diffuse Esophageal Spasm

Reassurance
  Explain etiology of symptoms; natural history of disease
Avoidance of Precipitating Factors
  Avoid very cold or hot liquids; discuss relationship to stress
Medications
  Calcium Channel Blockers
    Nifedipine, 10–20 mg before meals and at bedtime
  Nitroglycerin
    Isosorbide dinitrate, 5–20 mg sublingually before meals and at bedtime
    Nitroglycerin 0.4–0.6 mg sublingually before meals
  Hydralazine (Apresoline), 25–50 mg three to four times a day
  Anticholinergics
    Propantheline bromide (*e.g.*, Pro-Banthine), 15 mg four times a day
    Dicyclomine (*e.g.*, Bentyl), 10–20 mg four times a day
Dilatation
  Bougienage with a large caliber dilator
  Pneumatic dilatation
Surgery
  Long myotomy

ity of patients will have a satisfactory response to either a calcium channel blocker or to a nitroglycerin preparation. Patients who do not respond to a drug of one class after a reasonable trial (weeks to months depending on the frequency of attacks) should be switched to a drug of the other class. If symptoms still persist, anticholinergics (e.g., propantheline bromide, Pro-banthine) or hydralazine (Apresoline), a potent smooth muscle relaxant, may be useful in relieving spasticity (Table 34.3).

If these pharmacological efforts fail, forceful dilation may be recommended. Dilation is most successful in patients with elevated LES pressures and with dysphagia as the predominant symptom. Chest pain, on the other hand, appears to be less likely to respond to dilation. A long myotomy, cutting the esophageal muscle from the esophogogastric junction to the aortic arch, has been advocated for the rare patient refractory to all of the above measures. Although the reported results of this procedure are impressive, the potential complications are significant and very difficult to manage. Myotomy should be reserved for those few patients with well documented esophageal spasm that is severely disabling and truly intractable. The majority of patients have attacks episodically, learn to avoid precipitating causes, and can be managed successfully medically.

Scleroderma of the Esophagus

The esophagus is involved in as many as 80% of patients with scleroderma. At times the esophageal symptoms are the presenting complaints that lead to the diagnosis. Indeed, the esophagus may demonstrate the characteristic abnormalities even before skin changes occur. The main symptoms of esophageal scleroderma are heartburn and dysphagia. The cause for these symptoms can readily be appreciated by examining the esophageal motility (Table 34.2). In esophageal scleroderma the LES pressure is very low, resulting in free gastroesophageal reflux. In addition, the peristaltic waves initially are of reduced amplitude, progressing later to complete aperistalsis in the smooth muscle portion of the esophagus, sparing the skeletal muscle portion. As peristalsis is impaired, the refluxed acid remains abnormally long in the esophagus, perhaps accounting for the frequent development of an esophageal stricture in this disorder. Thus, the dysphagia may be due to the primary motor abnormality or may signify the development of a peptic stricture.

The pathogenesis of scleroderma is unknown. In the esophagus, the disorder is not simply secondary to replacement of muscle fibers with collagen, since the motility dysfunction can be demonstrated in the absence of histopathological changes. Several studies have suggested a neural defect rather than a primary myogenic disorder.

Scleroderma is a chronically progressive disease for which no specific treatment exists. Therapy of esophageal manifestations is directed at symptomatic relief and prevention of strictures.

Patients with scleroderma, whether or not they have dysphagia or heartburn, should be referred to a gastroenterologist for evaluation of esophageal motility, and to diagnose reflux esophagitis and stricture formation. If reflux is present, the patient should be treated intensively with cimetidine and antacids (see page 426) to try to prevent stricture formation (see below, page 426). Strictures should be dilated by bougienage (see below). Stimulation of the smooth muscle by bethanechol (Urecholine) or metoclopramide (Reglan), to enhance LES tone and improve peristaltic contractions also may be tried (see below, page 426). If muscle atrophy is already present, however, these agents may not be helpful. Antireflux surgery should be avoided if at all possible because the motility disorder may lead to significant dysphagia after fundoplication.

Esophageal Webs and Rings

Dysphagia for solid foods may be caused by esophageal webs or rings. An esophageal *web* is a mucosal structure that protrudes into the lumen, most commonly in the proximal esophagus. The association of an iron deficiency anemia with a proximal esophageal web constitutes the *Plummer-Vinson syndrome*. Esophageal *rings* are located in the distal esophagus and may be either mucosal or muscular; rings can be demonstrated in up to 10% of the population, but rarely cause symptoms.

The ring that occurs at the gastroesophageal junction is referred to as *Schatzki's ring*. The origin of these lesions is unclear, some being congenital and others probably acquired. They are often found in asymptomatic individuals. There is no evidence that gastroesophageal reflux is associated with the development of the Schatzki ring, even in the presence of a hiatal hernia.

Symptoms arise when the ring narrows the esophageal lumen to less than 13 mm. A typical presenting symptom of a patient with an esophageal ring is intermittent dysphagia for solid foods. The patient may point to the area of the ring. At times a bolus of food may become impacted; the patient then regurgitates and subsequently may be able to resume eating without further difficulty. The intermittency of the dysphagia, the chronicity of the condition, and the difficulty in making the diagnosis unless specifically suspected often results in misdiagnosis and inappropriate therapy.

The diagnosis of esophageal ring is best made by *barium swallow*. The lower esophageal ring is best detected when the lower segment of the esophagus is distended as it is during a Valsalva maneuver. Endoscopy is sometimes helpful to differentiate rings from annular strictures secondary to either reflux esophagitis or carcinoma. Cervical webs are frequently missed on conventional radiography but

may be detected with cine studies. The webs are usually detected on the anterior surface of the esophagus, and lateral and oblique films are needed to demonstrate these lesions. *Endoscopy* frequently fails to visualize cervical webs but may disrupt the lesion during blind passage of the instrument into the esophagus. The endoscope may well demonstrate an esophageal ring during air insufflation of the distal esophagus.

Therapy generally involves reassurance with recommendation to chew food well and slowly, as well as mechanical disruption of the ring or web. If the webs are associated with iron deficiency, the treatment of the anemia is believed to cause rapid regression of the web. Bougienage with a large caliber dilator frequently disrupts the lower esophageal ring with complete relief of the dysphagia. The procedure causes transient discomfort but much less pain than does pneumatic dilation. It is ordinarily done by a gastroenterologist in his office. Rarely symptoms may persist after bougienage, and pneumatic dilation (see above) or even surgery may be necessary.

Globus Hystericus

Globus hystericus is a diagnosis frequently made in patients with dysphagia who have no demonstrable organic disease. However, this condition does not produce dysphagia and should not be used to explain away the symptom of dysphagia. Patients with globus describe the sensation of a "lump" in the throat, but they do not actually have difficulty swallowing. At times, these symptoms may be more pronounced with eating. However, when specifically questioned, patients will deny dysphagia, or food "sticking" or being "held up" in this region; and they will state that the symptom is present even when they are not eating. The pathogenesis of this condition is unknown, but hypertonicity of the upper esophageal sphincter, as a primary disorder or as a consequence of esophageal reflux, has been suggested. A psychophysiological disturbance may also be the cause as this symptom is usually seen in anxious patients (see Chapter 13). Reassurance and an explanation of the problem form the basis for treatment. Mild sedation may be helpful. The significance of this disorder is mainly its differentiation from other conditions that produce true dysphagia.

GASTROESOPHAGEAL REFLUX

Symptomatic gastroesophageal reflux is a common clinical condition that may lead to significant morbidity. It is now well established that competency of the LES is the major deterrent against reflux. The presence of a hiatal hernia is not a factor in gastroesophageal reflux as it does not affect the strength of the LES. Therefore, whether or not a hiatal hernia is present, therapy, whether it be medical or surgical, should be directed toward restoration of LES competency.

Pathophysiology

Several abnormalities in LES function have been observed in patients with gastroesophageal reflux. First, the basal LES tone is lower than in normals. Second, the hypotensive LES fails to rise in pressure appropriately with increases in intragastric pressure. Third, in patients with reflux, the response of the LES to a meal is low compared to that of normal subjects (2). These pathophysiological abnormalities help to explain the occurrence of reflux under basal conditions, during periods of increased intra-abdominal pressure, and postprandially when acid secretion is stimulated.

Etiology

Gastroesophageal reflux may occur in several different conditions. *Idiopathic hypotension* of the LES is the most common cause of reflux. The sphincter tone is low and responds poorly to physiological excitatory stimuli. The etiology is unknown, but defects in myogenic, neurogenic, and hormonal function of the LES have been suggested. Patients with *scleroderma* frequently complain of reflux, or present with stricture formation even in the absence of reflux symptoms. Pregnancy is a condition that is commonly associated with reflux, with 30 to 50% of pregnant women experiencing heartburn, usually during their third trimester. Estrogen and progesterone are known to reduce LES tone; and, with increase in intra-abdominal pressure during gestation, reflux frequently results. *Hypothyroidism* may also cause decreased LES tone and reduced peristaltic force, but it rarely is a cause of symptomatic gastroesophageal reflux. *Iatrogenic causes* of reflux are common: anticholinergics, nitrites, tranquilizers, and β-adrenergic agents are all capable of reducing LES pressure. Also smoking cigarettes and eating *certain foods* (e.g., fatty foods and chocolate) reduce LES presure and may induce symptomatic reflux, usually within an hour of ingestion. Other foods, like coffee, alcohol, and citrus fruits, may induce similar symptoms without affecting LES pressure.

Diagnosis

History

Heartburn is the classic symptom of gastroesophageal reflux. Most patients complain of burning substernal pain that radiates upward, often aggravated by meals and by lying down and relieved by sitting up. The exact cause of the pain is not known. A sour taste is another common complaint. *Dysphagia* suggests the presence of a motor abnormality or a stricture (see above). *Odynophagia*, or pain on swallowing, is an infrequent complaint with reflux esophagitis and usually signifies severe disease.

Tests

Various tests are available to confirm the clinical diagnosis. As no single test provides complete information about the cause and consequences of reflux, judicious selection among these tests is required. A comparison of all tests indicates that the combination of esophageal biopsies or acid infusion tests with acid reflux measurements gives about a 90% positive diagnosis. This yield is higher than that of any single test for this disorder.

Performance and selection of these various tests will generally require consultation with a gastroenterologist. For the majority of patients with classic symptoms of gastroesophagel reflux, empiric therapy can be instituted without performing any of these diagnostic procedures. However, in cases with an uncertain diagnosis, or in patients who fail to respond to standard therapy (see below), one or more of these esophageal function tests may be indicated to document the presence and degree of reflux. Certainly before antireflux surgery is performed, unequivocal evidence should be obtained that gastroesophageal reflux is causing the patient's symptoms.

The *acid reflux test* involves the placement of a pH probe in the esophagus several centimeters proximal to the LES and documenting the drop of intraesophageal pH with the occurrence of reflux. The *experience of the patient* during the passage of this probe is the same as it is during the passing of a nasogastric tube. A pH of less than 4 is considered a positive test, documenting the reflux of acid into the esophagus. Similarly, *esophageal manometry* (see page 418) can determine the strength of the LES (normally 12 to 30 mm Hg). In over 80% of patients with reflux, the LES pressure will be low. Abnormal motility can be documented at the same time and scleroderma can even be diagnosed as a cause for the gastroesophageal reflux *via* this technique. During the motility study, the *Bernstein (acid perfusion) test* can be performed. Reproduction of the patient's symptoms *via* infusion of acid and relief of the symptoms with infusion of distilled water is considered a positive test (see page 422). This study confirms that the patient's symptoms can be produced by acid. The *patient's experience* during the performance of the test, which takes 30 minutes or less, is essentially the same as it is during the measurement of esophageal motility (see page 418) except that heartburn may be produced by the infusion of acid.

Radiological studies are useful in identifying the complications of reflux such as esophageal ulcers or stricture but are too insensitive to be relied on to confirm the presence of reflux. As stated above, the presence of hiatal hernia on barium swallow does not diagnose gastroesophageal reflux and should not be incriminated as the cause for the patient's symptoms. Also, the demonstration of reflux by barium swallow does not establish that the patient's symptoms are due to reflux; therefore, the barium swallow cannot be relied upon as a single test to make the diagnosis of reflux. *Endoscopy* may detect ulceration and esophageal strictures. Mucosal biopsies can provide histological evidence of acute esophagitis and of the chronic effects of reflux, even when the endoscopic appearance of the esophagus is normal. Characteristic microscopic changes secondary to reflux include increased thickness of the basal cell zone and proximity of the dermal papillae to the epithelial surface. The presence of polymorphonuclear leukocytes in the squamous lining indicates acute inflammation.

Complications

The complications of reflux include hemorrhage, ulcerations, stricture formation, and development of Barrett's epithelium. Esophagitis is the cause of 5 to 10% of all cases of upper gastrointestinal hemorrhages. Peptic ulcers and strictures must be differentiated from malignancy and from caustic ingestion. The presence of a midesophageal ulcer or stricture should raise the suspicion of Barrett's epithelium (columnar type mucosa that replaces the squamous mucosa damaged by chronic reflux). This type of columnar mucosa contains several different cell types, including parietal cells capable of secreting acid. Of further significance is that this mucosa is a metaplastic response to inflammation and thus may progress to the development of adenocarcinoma. Patients with this type of mucosa should therefore be under surveillance for the development of cancer. There are reports of regression of this abnormal mucosa following successful antireflux surgery.

Therapy

The therapy for gastroesophageal reflux is aimed at reducing the volume and acidity of the gastric contents and at restoring LES competence. The vast majority of patients can be managed successfully with relatively simple therapy. The *initial step* (Table 34.4) consists of dietary and mechanical maneuvers, antacids, and discontinuance of drugs, when possible, and foods that reduce LES tone. Certain foods, such as coffee, citrus juice, and spices, which further irritate the inflamed esophagus and provoke pain, should also be restricted. Patients should be instructed not to lie down after a meal as this promotes greater reflux. Elevation of the head of the bed 6 to 8 inches (not just sleeping on more pillows) and avoidance of tight garments that increase intra-abdominal pressure are also helpful. Antacids, when given in effective doses (see Table 34.4), improve symptoms in 70% of cases. These compounds not only neutralize the acidic gastric contents but, by alkalinizing the stomach, may also increase LES pressure, thus decreasing the frequency of reflux. A combination of antacid plus alginic acid (Gaviscon—

Table 34.4.
Management of Gastroesophageal Reflux

STAGE I:
General recommendations:
Elevate head of bed
Avoid fatty foods, chocolate, alcohol
Avoid citrus fruit juices, smoking, coffee
Avoid tight-fitting garments or activities that increase intra-abdominal pressure
Lose weight
Avoid late night snacks or lying down shortly after a meal
Medications: Antacids—30–45 ml 1 hour *after* meals and at bedtime or antacids plus alginic acid—2 tablets after meals and at bedtime
STAGE II:
H2 antagonists
Cimetidine, 300 mg before meals and at bedtime
Ranitidine, 150 mg twice a day
Bethanechol (25 mg) or metoclopramide (10–20 mg) before meals and at bedtime
STAGE III:
Surgery: fundoplication

chewable tablets or liquid) is reported to be especially helpful because of the ability of the alginic acid to form a foamy gel-like layer on top of the gastric fluid.

The *second stage* of therapy, if necessary, involves the use of drugs that inhibit gastric acid secretion or increase LES pressure. These medications should be instituted if initial measures fail to relieve symptoms. Cimetidine (Tagamet), the H_2 receptor antagonist, markedly reduces acid secretion but has no effect on LES tone in man. Reflux symptoms are greatly decreased with this drug compared to placebo. The required duration of therapy with cimetidine is not established; 4 to 6 weeks of therapy is a reasonable course. Occasionally, in patients with persistent symptoms, it is useful to give 300 mg of cimetidine at bedtime indefinitely. Other H_2 antagonists, like ranitidine, can be expected to be equally effective. Cholinergic drugs, such as bethanechol (Urecholine), increase LES tone and speed the rate of gastric emptying. Symptoms are improved even though cholinergic agents stimulate gastric secretion. Metoclopramide (Reglan), a smooth muscle stimulant, also increases LES tone and may be useful in the treatment of patients with reflux. These agents should be employed in a stepwise fashion before declaring the patient's symptoms refractory to medical management (see Table 34.4).

Surgery is indicated in only 3 to 10% of patients with gastroesophageal reflux. The indications are (*a*) stricture, (*b*) hemorrhage secondary to erosive esophagitis, (*c*) peptic ulcer of the esophagus, (*d*) recurrent aspiration pneumonia secondary to reflux, and (*e*) intractability of symptoms. Before surgery is considered, however, the diagnosis of gastroesophageal reflux should be unequivocal and the patient should have received maximum medical therapy. Operations incorporating a fundoplication around the distal esophagus provide symptomatic improvement in a about 90% of patients. Simple repair of a hiatus hernia has not been equally effective nor is the benefit long lasting. The fundoplication procedure recreates an effective barrier to reflux. Several variations of the fundoplication are available and local surgical expertise generally dictates the specific type of operation that is performed. Complications include dysphagia, which is often only transient, and the "gas-bloat" syndrome from the inability to belch. Antireflux surgery for patients with scleroderma is potentially hazardous as it may markedly exacerbate dysphagia (see above, page 426). Vagotomy is not indicated in the treatment of gastroesophageal reflux.

Hiatus Hernia

Herniation of a part of the stomach through the diaphragm through the normal esophageal hiatus into the thorax is called a *hiatus hernia*. The defect is quite common but the precise prevalence is very much influenced by the zeal of the radiologist during the performance of an upper gastrointestinal series. Estimates of prevalence therefore have ranged from 10 to 30% overall. The defect is twice as common in women as in men and is extremely common in elderly people, affecting perhaps 70 to 80% of the population who are older than age 60. Many physicians still correlate hiatus hernia with reflux esophagitis, but certainly a hernia may exist without producing symptomatic reflux and reflux may occur without hernia. If a patient has clear-cut reflux esophagitis, the treatment of it (see page 426) should not be influenced by the presence of a hiatus hernia. If a patient who does not have reflux is inadvertently discovered to have a hiatus hernia, no

treatment is indicated (in the past needless surgery has been done to reduce a hiatus hernia in patients whose symptoms were not clearly attributable to the defect).

A *paraesophageal hernia*, the hernia of part of the stomach through the diaphragm adjacent to the gastroesophageal junction, is potentially dangerous because about one-third of the time the hernia incarcerates and produces acute obstruction, a surgical emergency.

General References

Cohen S: Motor disorders of the esophagus. *N Engl J Med* 301:184, 1979.

> Excellent review of classification and evaluation of this topic.

Snape WJ Jr, Cohen S: Gastroesophageal reflux: Advances in medical and surgical treatment. In Glass GBJ (ed): *Progress in Gastroenterology*. New York, Grune & Stratton, 1977, vol 3, chap 25, p 695.

> Thorough review of pathophysiology and therapy.

Specific References

1. Brand D, Martin D, Pope C: Esophageal manometrics in patients with angina-like chest pain. *Am J Dig Dis* 22:300, 1977.
2. Farrell RL, Gastell DO, McGuigan JE: Measurements and comparisons of lower esophageal sphincter pressures and serum gastrin levels in patients with gastroesophageal reflux. *Gastroenterology* 67:415, 1974.
3. Just-Viera J, Haight C: Achalasia and carcinoma of the esophagus. *Surg Gynecol Obstet* 128:1081, 1969.
4. London RL, Ouyang A, Snape WJ, et al: Provocation of esophageal pain by ergonovine or edrophonium. *Gastroenterology* 81:10, 1981.
5. Parker E, Moertel C: Carcinoma of the esophagus: is there a role for surgery? *Am J Dig Dis* 23:730, 1978.
6. Swamy N: Esophageal spasm: clinical and manometric response to nitroglycerin and long acting nitrites. *Gastroenterology* 72:23, 1977.
7. Tucker H, Snape WJ Jr, Cohen S: Achalasia secondary to carcinoma: manometric and clinical features. *Ann Intern Med* 89:315, 1978.

Abdominal Pain

MARVIN M. SCHUSTER, M.D.

Abdominal pain is one of the most common presenting complaints of patients to their physicians. In ambulatory practice, it is the fifth most common symptom generally, and the second most common symptom of women (Chapter 1). Many patients complain of having chronic pain that is constant or recurrent; and in this population it is important to consider functional as well as organic causes for the symptom. Acute adominal pain (occurring within 24 hours of the patient seeking help) almost always reflects an organic process. In any case, whether chronic or acute, abdominal pain due to an organic cause is more often a symptom of gastrointestinal disease than nongastrointestinal disease.

The physician's response to the patient with abdominal pain will be influenced by its rapidity of onset, its apparent severity, its location, and by accompanying signs and symptoms (fever, gastrointestinal bleeding, diarrhea, etc) that may suggest a specific process. Although there is no information about the relative frequency of the various causes of abdominal pain, experience suggests that, most often, acute pain is self-limited (abates within hours) and the pain is usually attributed (without proof) to viral gastroenteritis or to dietary indiscretion. Chronic pain, if associated with an organic process, is most often due to peptic, gallbladder or diverticular disease, to chronic relapsing pancreatitis (primarily in alcoholics), or to carcinoma (most commonly pancreatic or colonic). The symptoms and signs that accompany these processes are discussed in a general way in this chapter and more specifically in the chapters devoted to these conditions. Chronic pain, not associated with a demonstrable organic process, is most often due to the irritable bowel syndrome (see Chapter 39).

The significance of pain is determined by two major factors—the characteristics of the pain and the characteristics of the patient. The relative significance of pain to the patient depends on its severity and frequency, the degree to which it interferes with his daily life or sleep patterns, and its meaning to him, both implied and symbolic. Even severe pain can be tolerated for brief periods if it appears infrequently, whereas less severe pain may be less tolerable if it interrupts important activities or disturbs sleep. Pain which has no anticipated end is generally less well tolerated than pain which, even though intense, has a predictable span. The threshold of pain tolerance varies considerably from one individual to another, because of both neurological and psychological factors. When pain suggests to the patient a serious underlying disorder, such as cancer, this concern itself may decrease his tolerance for pain. Also, pain which is primarily organic may be reinforced by the secondary psychosocial gains that it provides.

Elderly patients with abdominal pain require special attention. Even serious underlying conditions may be manifested by minimal subjective complaints and minimal objective signs. For example, the diagnosis of appendicitis and of ruptured appendix is easily missed because pain may not be severe and fever and leukocytosis may be minimal or absent. Therefore careful follow-up of abdominal pain in the elderly warrants repeated abdominal and rectal examination and serial determinations of temperature and laboratory tests (such as white blood cell and differential counts).

Management of any type of pain can be significantly improved by consideration of certain general principles. For example, reassurance that pain can be relieved by medication or surgery can significantly raise the threshold of tolerance. On the other hand, the existence of severe pain sensitizes patients to additional, less intense pain (such as lumbar puncture or venipuncture) and the patient's "overreaction" to the second pain should not be taken to imply that the primary pain is psychogenic. Another common misconception is that alleviation of pain by placebo implies psychogenc origin; in fact, organic pain may be more readily relieved by placebo than is psychogenic pain. A post hoc rationalization which accounts for this phenomenon views the patient with organic pain as a person who wants desperately to get rid of his pain, whereas the person with psychogenic pain may be unwilling "to give it up" because of secondary gain.

TYPES OF ABDOMINAL PAIN

A few general concepts concerning abdominal pain are reviewed here, since their understanding can be quite helpful diagnostically. Pain involving the digestive system can be visceral, parietal, referred, or psychogenic. Metabolically associated and neurogenic pain (see below) is presumed to operate through one or more of these mechanisms.

Visceral Pain

Visceral pain can result from spasm or stretch of the muscle wall of a hollow viscus, from distension of the capsule of a solid organ such as the liver, or from inflammation and ischemia of a visceral structure. Tenderness associated with visceral pain (including sometimes rebound tenderness) is often felt directly over the part of the digestive system that is involved, although (except for the terminal ileum) small bowel tenderness is usually not well localized. Abdominal viscera are insensitive to cutting, tearing, crushing, and burning.

Parietal Pain

The parietal peritoneum, mesentery, and posterior peritoneal covering are sensitive to forces similar to those that affect the viscera, but the omentum and anterior abdominal wall are less sensitive. Parietal tenderness is more localized than visceral tenderness, and rebound tenderness is experienced over the involved area. Parietal pain that is the result of generalized inflammation (peritonitis) encompasses a large area of the peritoneum. A rigid abdomen, associated with pain, usually means that the inflammation is severe.

Referred Pain

Both visceral and parietal pain may be referred to a remote site along shared nerve pathways (dermatomes). Gallbladder pain, for example, typically radiates to the infrascapular area, and right diaphragmatic pain to the right shoulder. Esophageal pain can be confused with the pain of myocardial ischemia because the sites to which the pain radiates may be identical (e.g., neck, left arm, etc). The more severe the visceral pain, the more likely it is to be referred to the back, as for example with esophageal spasm or with cholecystitis. The skin overlying the

dermatome to which the pain is referred may be hypersensitive. Deep palpation of the primary site of the painful organ may intensify the pain, not only locally, but at its referred site, whereas the reverse is not true; deep palpation over the referred site does not usually enhance pain over the primary site.

Abdominal Pain Caused by Metabolic Disease

Metabolic disease may produce intestinal pain by a direct effect on the alimentary tract, as, for example, when intestinal spasm is induced by porphyria, lead poisoning, or familial Mediterranean fever. In hereditary angioneurotic edema, C-1 esterase deficiency may produce intestinal swelling which can result in pain due to partial obstruction or to intestinal spasm. On the other hand, metabolic disorders may secondarily produce gastrointestinal pain; for example, hyperparathyroidism may produce a painful peptic ulcer or pancreatitis. Hyperlipidemia also may evoke pancreatitis, but may be associated with abdominal pain in the absence of this entity.

Neurogenic Pain

Neurogenic abdominal pain (causalgia) is experienced by the patient as a burning sensation along the route of distribution of the nerve and is sometimes associated with hyperesthesia. Usually the spinal root is involved by herpes zoster, carcinoma, arthritis, etc, but peripheral neuropathies due to operative trauma or to diabetes may also produce neurogenic abdominal pain. There is no relationship of neurogenic pain to digestive function (e.g., eating or defecating).

Psychogenic Pain

Psychogenic pain may represent a conversion reaction which results in the perception of pain where no organic dysfunction exists; or it may result from psychophysiological reactions characterized by pathological or physiological responses to psychological stress (see Chapter 12). For example, emotional stress can lead to painful intestinal spasm in patients with irritable bowel syndrome (Chapter 39). This spasm is a measurable physiological event. Similarly, stress may lead to peptic symptoms due to gastric hypersecretion which also can be quantitated. Pain or tenderness that represents a conversion reaction (emotions converted into somatic complaints) may disappear during periods of distraction. Such pain may be inconsistent and incompatible with known neuroanatomy and neurophysiology.

HISTORICAL CLUES TO DIAGNOSIS

Although the successful diagnosis of conditions that present with abdominal pain depends on meticulous pursuit of leads that are provided by history and physical examination, familiarity with standard questions and examination techniques assists in ensuring completeness. Questions relating to local features include the nature and quality of pain, its location, radiation, intensity, timing, duration, and course and the factors which precipitate, aggravate, and alleviate it. Associated symptoms and signs include tenderness, fever and chills, anorexia, nausea and vomiting, diarrhea and constipation, obstruction, borborygmus, rectal bleeding, passing of mucus, jaundice, and genitourinary symptoms. Although aggravation of pain by emotional tension is seen with functional disorders, such as irritable bowel syndrome, the pain of many organic disorders can also be accentuated by stress.

Rapidity of Onset of Pain

The temporal development of abdominal pain is an important factor which guides the physician in the urgency and direction of the evaluation. In particular, pain that develops abruptly, within minutes, and becomes rapidly severe is very ominous (Table 35.1).

In addition, situations in which a silent period follows the initial symptoms are notoriously deceptive problems for the primary physician. For example, a perforated viscus or an intestinal infarction may be characterized by resolution of the intense initial pain hours after perforation or infarction first occurs and by a recurrence of pain several hours later when peritonitis and volume depletion are well established.

Almost always, therefore, if the patient complains of an abrupt onset of severe abdominal pain on the day that he visits the physician, even if the pain has resolved and the abdominal examination is unrevealing, a complete blood count, urinalysis, chest X-ray, plain and upright films of the abdomen, and close surveillance over several hours are imperative and are usually best accomplished in an emergency room.

When the onset of pain is more gradual, there are many more possible causes, and considerable judgment is necessary in deciding about the urgency and direction of the evaluation. The physician will need particularly to be guided by the patient's history, the nature and location of the pain (see below), and by the examination (see below). In all cases follow-up examination is warranted. Newly experienced abdominal pain should never be dismissed, even if it is felt to be innocuous, without follow-up, at least by phone, within a few days. In this way, any important new symptoms will not be missed. It is best for the physician to initiate this follow-up since it will obviate the need for the patient to decide whether a change in symptoms is important enough to trouble the physician.

Nature and Location of Pain (Tables 35.2 and 35.3)

Esophageal pain is generally described as pressing, constricting, or burning. It is usually located in the

Table 35.1.

Causes of Acute Abdominal Pain According to Rapidity of Onset[a]

Intestinal Causes	Extraintestinal Causes
ABRUPT ONSET (INSTANTANEOUS)	
Perforated ulcer	Ruptured or dissecting aneurysm
Ruptured abscess or hematoma	Ruptured ectopic pregnancy
Intestinal infarct	Pneumothorax
Ruptured esophagus	Myocardial infarct
	Pulmonary infarct
RAPID ONSET (MINUTES)	
Perforated viscus	Ureteral colic
Strangulated viscus	Renal colic
Volvulus	Ectopic pregnancy
Pancreatitis	
Biliary colic	
Mesenteric infarct	
Diverticulitis	
Penetrating peptic ulcer	
High intestinal obstruction	
Appendicitis (gradual onset more common)	
GRADUAL ONSET (HOURS)	
Appendicitis	Cystitis
Strangulated hernia	Pyelitis
Low small intestinal obstruction	Salpingitis
Cholecystitis	Prostatitis
Pancreatitis	Threatened abortion
Gastritis	Urinary retention
Peptic ulcer	Pneumonitis
Colonic diverticulitis	
Meckel's diverticulitis	
Crohn's disease	
Ulcerative colitis	
Mesenteric lymphadenitis	
Abscess	
Intestinal infarct	
Mesenteric cyst	

[a] Adapted from Way LW: Abdominal pain and the acute abdomen. In Sleisenger MH, Fordtran JS (eds): *Gastrointestinal Disease.* Philadelphia, WB Saunders, 1978, p 405.

substernal area and, when severe, radiates through to the back. The location of the pain is a good clue to the location of the underlying disease. Although pain from the lower esophageal region may be referred higher, lesions high in the esophagus do not refer to the lower part of the esophagus (see also Chapter 34).

Gastric pain is usually experienced in the subxiphoid area or the left upper quadrant. Although gastritis is perceived as a true pain (often burning or cramping in quality), the distress caused by both duodenal and gastric ulcer is experienced as a gnawing discomfort or as a hunger sensation rather than as pain. The discomfort caused by peptic ulcer is felt on an empty stomach and is relieved by eating. Thus nocturnal pain of peptic ulcer usually awakens the

Table 35.2.
Nature and Location of Gastrointestinal Pain

Organ Involved	Nature of Pain	Location of Pain
Esophagus	Burning, constricting	Upper lesions → high substernal Lower lesions → low substernal or referred upward Severe → back
Stomach	Gnawing discomfort, pain	Epigastric Left upper quadrant
Duodenum	Gnawing discomfort, hunger, pain	Epigastric
Small intestine	Ache, cramp, bloating, sharp	Diffuse Periumbilical Terminal ileum → right lower quadrant
Colon	As above	Lower abdomen Sigmoid → left lower quadrant Rectum → midline and sacrum
Pancreas	Excruciating, constant	Upper abdomen radiating to back
Gallbladder	Severe, later dull ache	Right upper quadrant Radiates to right scapula or interscapular area
Liver	Ache, occasionally sharp	Right lower rib cage Right upper quadrant if liver is enlarged

patient between 1 and 3 A.M. In contrast, pain of gastritis may be aggravated by eating or relieved only momentarily and then subsequently intensified over a period of 10 to 15 minutes. A change from ulcer distress to a burning, boring, or knife-like pain (especially when there is radiation through to the back) is an indication of a complication of ulcer—namely penetration. Pain that is precipitated by meals suggests gastric outlet obstruction (often due to pyloric channel ulcer) or high intestinal obstruction (see also Chapter 36).

Duodenal pain is felt also in the epigastric area or slightly to the right of it, and it, too, may radiate through to the back. When perforation of an ulcer occurs, the pain appears abruptly in the epigastric region and later settles into the right lower quadrant as gastric contents are spilled into the right gutter.

Small intestinal pain is generally diffuse and poorly localized. It is experienced in the periumbilical area and, when severe, radiates through to the back. Pain deriving from the terminal ileum may be localized to the right lower quadrant. Uncommonly it may radiate down the leg. Small intestinal pain is generally crampy, sharp, or aching. Bloating, distension, and dull ache are terms that frequently are associated with prolonged mechanical obstruction or reflex ileus, whereas more acute forms may be manifested by sharp steady pain. Associated fever and chills suggest inflammatory bowel disease.

Colonic pain is better localized, often to the lower abdomen. Sigmoid pain is felt in the left lower quadrant, and rectal pain is often described by the patient as being located over the rectum, usually in the midline. Gas pocketed in the splenic flexure of the colon (seen most commonly in patients with the irritable bowel syndrome) produces left upper quadrant or left chest pain that may be confused with the pain of myocardial ischemia. Temporary relief is obtained by passing gas (see also Chapter 39). Colonic pain generally is crampy or of an aching quality unless perforation occurs, and then it is frequently severe and constant. Associated fever and chills suggest diverticulitis, diverticular abscess, or ulcerative colitis.

Pancreatic pain is excruciating and constant and usually located in the upper abdomen with radiation through to the back, but it may be felt in almost any area of the abdomen. Chronic pancreatic pain (due to inflammation, pseudocyst, or carcinoma) is similar in nature and location to acute pancreatic pain but may be less severe. Pancreatitis is almost invariably associated with vomiting. If vomiting is not present, other diagnoses, such as pancreatic carcinoma, should be considered.

Appendicitis often begins as diffuse abdominal pain that intensifies over a period of hours as it settles in the right lower quadrant. The pain of appendicitis is frequently aggravated by extension of the right leg.

Gallbladder pain generally begins in the right upper quadrant or epigastrium and radiates to the interscapular area or to the right infrascapular area. It is excruciatingly severe, may be aggravated by deep inspiration, and is replaced by a dull, aching sensation that persists for hours after the severe pain subsides. Tenderness can often be elicited by deep palpation under the rib in the area of the gallbladder, especially during deep inspiration. Gallbladder pain

Table 35.3.
Differential Diagnosis of Adominal Pain Due to Gastrointestinal Disorders[a]
A. Character, Location, Production or Relief

Disorder	Character	Location	Produced or Relieved by
Peptic ulcer	Gnawing hunger discomfort, occasionally burning, gastric—within minutes after meals; duodenal—usually several hours after meals	Subxiphoid, may radiate to back	Produced by empty stomach, relieved by food, antacids or H_2 receptor blockers
Penetrating ulcer	Severe boring constant pain	Subxiphoid radiating to back	May awaken patient in early morning hours, may be relieved by antacids or H_2 receptor blockers
Perforated ulcer	Abrupt, severe pain followed within 6 hours by deceptive refractory period with diminishing of pain	Intially epigastric—then right lower quadrant (right gutter)	Initial pain spontaneous, peritonitis aggravated by movement
Small bowel obstruction	Crampy severe pain with partial obstruction, constant pain develops with complete obstruction or stangulation	Generalized periumbilical or localized over strangulation	Relieved by intubation decompression
Large bowel obstruction	Crampy pain initially, constant pain with subsequent distension or strangulation, onset less sudden than upper intestinal obstruction	May be localized or generalized	Occasionally relieved by intubation decompression
Intestinal infarct	Severe, excruciating, abrupt onset	Generalized	Relieved only by surgery
Intussusception	Sudden onset severe crampy pain	Periumbilical	Temporary relief may occur with emesis
Appendicitis	Initially colic then continuous with varying intensity	Initial colic in periumbilical area, subsequently continuous in right lower quadrant, occasional testicular radiation	Aggravated by extension of right leg
Pancreatitis	Severe constant pain	Epigastric, radiation to back or lower abdomen	Often initiated by alcoholic binge or eating after binge, by common duct obstruction, penetrating ulcer, or blunt trauma
Cholecystitis	Constant, severe pain preceding nausea and vomiting; subsidence of pain followed by aching	Right upper quadrant radiating to infrascapular region	Precipitated by heavy meal and aggravated by deep inspiration
Biliary colic	Crampy, severe pain	Epigastrium, radiating to right upper quadrant and subscapular region	Precipitated by heavy meal within 1–3 hours
Diverticulitis	Crampy or continuous pain	Left lower quadrant, may radiate to back	Relieved by anticholinergics and antibiotics
Crohn's disease	Crampy with partial obstruction and continuous pain with inflammatory mass	Periumbilical or right lower quadrant, may radiate to back	May be precipitated by milk. Relieved by defecation or intubation decompression
Ulcerative colitis	Crampy pain usually, may be constant with toxic dilation	Often left lower quadrant or any area of colon, generalized with toxic megacolon or perforation	Precipitated by emotional stress or infection; toxic megacolon by opiates or enemas; relieved temporarily by defecation

B. Abnormal Physical Findings, Associated Signs, and Laboratory Features

Disorder	Abnormal Physical Findigns	Associated Signs and Symptoms	Laboratory Features
Peptic ulcer	Subxiphoid tenderness	Nausea, vomiting, retrosternal burning; weight gain with duodenal ulcer; weight stable or loss with gastric ulcer	Endoscopic or X-ray demonstration of ulcer, possible occult blood in stool or melena and iron deficiency anemia
Penetrating ulcer	Marked subxiphoid tenderness	Writhing, clutching abdomen	Amylase may be elevated
Perforated ulcer	Initially rigid with rebound, during refractory stage tenderness disappears to return later, absence of liver dullness with intraperitoneal air	Patient lies rigidly still, pale perspiring; emesis may be present	Upright film shows free air under diaphragm, leukocytosis

Table 35.3—*Continued*

Small bowel obstruction	Borborygmus, high pitched sound with rushes initially; later quiet abdomen; tenderness may be mild or rebound tenderness may be present	Emesis (may be feculent with lower obstruction), obstipation, may be weak with shock-like appearance	Plain film of abdomen showing air-fluid levels, may show stepladder pattern.
Large bowel obstruction	Initially hyperperistalsis with high pitched rushes, subsequently distension and decrease in bowel signs	Nausea but less vomiting than with high obstruction, obstipation or marked constipation	Large bowel distension with air-fluid levels and no air demonstrated distal to obstruction
Intestinal infarct	Quiet bowel sounds, tenderness present but not commensurate with pain, later rebound tenderness	Shock, bloody diarrhea, melena, vomiting; history of intestinal angina	Leukocytosis, hemoconcentration; bloody fluid on paracentesis; plain film of abdomen may reveal normal gas pattern or no gas due to fluid-filled loops
Intussusception	Tender mass in abdomen, high pitched peristaltic rushes	Intially normal stool after onset, then blood mucus and constipation; vomiting is late; fever after strangulation	Barium enema demonstrates coiled spring appearance of invagination; with ileocecal intussusception, small bowel loop is in colon
Appendicitis	Localized rebound tenderness, hyperesthesia over area	Initially diarrhea, then constipation; nausea, vomiting may be present; fever, tachycardia; rectal tenderness in right perirectal area	Leukocytosis
Pancreatitis	Marked epigastric tenderness, guarding and upper abdominal distension; the pain of chronic pancreatic disease may be less pronounced	Emesis almost invariable, fever, with hemorrhagic pancreatitis purple color in flank or periumbilical region; emesis is less common in patients with chronic pancreatic disease	Marked leukocytosis, hyperamylasemia; serum calcium depression on days 2 and 4, toxic psychosis on days 2 and 4; X-ray may show calcification, localized ileus, or colon cut-off sign; upper gastrointestinal series demonstrates pancreatic enlargement and spicules in C loop of duodenum; may have left pleural effusion
Cholecystitis	Tenderness over gallbladder area especially on deep inspiration; Murphy's sign may be positive	More common in obese women 40 years or older or after pregnancy; high incidence among some American Indian populations	Leukocytosis; plain film may show calcified stone; oral cholecystogram nonvisualized during attacks, TcHIDA nonvisualized; cholangiograms may show radiopaque stones
Biliary colic	As above	As above; jaundice may be present	Radiopaque stones may be seen on plain film; nonvisualization on cholecystogram during colic; subsequently may show radiolucent stones; i.v. cholangiogram may show dilated duct; bilirubin, alkaline phosphatase increase; may have hyperamylasemia
Diverticulitis	Guarding and tenderness in left lower quadrant	Constipation, fever, tachycardia; rectal tenderness on left; may have urinary frequency or dysuria from pericolonic involvement	Leukocytosis, barium enema shows diverticula but may not visualize during acute episode, may show partial obstruction
Crohn's disease	Tender mass in right lower quadrant, borborygmus	Nausea, vomiting, diarrhea, fever; may have perirectal fistula; tender mass in right rectal area, occasional clubbing	Anemia, elevated sedimentation rate; small bowel series shows cobblestone appearance or string sign
Ulcerative colitis	Tender over involved area, distended especially over transverse colon with toxic megacolon	Frequent passage of small amounts of bloody liquid stool; tenesmus with rectal involvement; fever, tachycardia, arthralgia, erythema nodosa; proctoscopy reveals bleeding and friability	Anemia; elevated sedimentation rate; barium enema demonstrates ulcerations, shortening, effacement of colon

*ᵃ Modified from *Handbook of Differential Diagnosis*, vol 2, part 1: *The Abdomen*. Nutley, NJ, Rocom Press, 1974.*

often appears several hours after a heavy dinner. Associated fever and chills suggest ascending cholangitis (see also Chapter 90).

Hepatic pain localizes over the liver, and a tender liver can be demonstrated by palpating the edge during deep inspiration or by fist percussion over the lower right rib cage anteriorly (or over the right upper quadrant if the liver is enlarged).

PHYSICAL EXAMINATION

The patient's *general appearance* provides clues concerning the severity, the duration, and frequently the cause of the underlying condition. The cold, sweat, and pallor of shock along with the marble skin (superficial vessels seen over blanched skin) indicating vasoconstriction are signs of significant hemorrhage. Tachycardia and perspiration are seen in both shock and sepsis, but the skin in shock is cold and clammy while in sepsis it is warm and moist. Signs of sepsis suggest bacterial enteritis, inflammatory bowel disease, intra-abdominal abscess, cholangitis, pancreatitis, peritonitis, or pyelonephritis.

The position assumed by the patient may be characteristic of a particular disorder. A position of truncal flexure often typifies patients with pancreatitis, while patients with gallbladder colic tend to pace or writhe about and appear restless in their unsuccessful attempt to find a comfortable position. This is in sharp contrast to the immobile position assumed by patients with peritonitis who attempt to avoid even the slightest jarring movement.

Inspection of the abdomen is facilitated by using incident lighting to visualize abdominal asymmetry and to outline masses and pulsations. In thin patients with partial obstruction peristaltic intestinal movement may be seen through the abdominal wall, and churning peristalsis may coincide with reports of crampy abdominal pain. Flank discoloration (Gray-Turner sign) or periumbilical discoloration (Cullen sign) results from retroperitoneal or intraperitoneal hemorrhage dissecting into the subcutaneous tissues and may indicate hemorrhagic pancreatitis. A strangulated hernia may protrude visibly from ventral defects, the inguinal area, or into the scrotum where peristaltic contractions may occasionally be appreciated. Patients with subphrenic abscess or gallbladder disease may have inspiratory pain that results in splinting and in avoidance of deep inspiration.

Auscultation should always be performed before palpation so that abdominal sounds may be evaluated before they are altered by palpation. At times borborygmus will be audible without the stethoscope. Specifically one should search for hyper- or hypoperistaltic sounds, for the high tinkles of obstruction, and for bruits suggesting vascular distortion from aneurysms, compression of blood vessels, or invasion of blood vessels (as, for example, invasion of the splenic artery in advanced pancreatic

carcinoma). Although a silent abdomen implies reflex ileus, bowel sounds may also be quiet or markedly diminished late in the course of mechanical obstruction. Whenever obstruction (especially gastric outlet obstruction) is considered, the physician should try to elicit a succussion splash. This is done by placing the stethoscope over the area (e.g., the stomach) and shaking the patient gently but abruptly. A sloshing sound indicates the presence of air and fluid. This finding in the stomach 3 or more hours after eating or drinking indicates delayed gastric emptying or, rarely, marked hypersecretion.

Gentle *percussion* should precede palpation and is an excellent means for detecting rebound tenderness, masses, and tympany (either generalized or localized) over an area of ileus or obstruction. Since air will rise to the area between the liver and the abdominal wall, absence of liver dullness with the patient in a recumbent position is an important finding indicating the presence of free air in the abdominal cavity.

Before *palpation*, it is wise to ask the patient to point to the site of maximum pain. Gentle palpation should at first avoid that site to minimize the chances that muscle guarding will interfere with the examination. Preferably the patient should be lying perfectly flat on his back with knees flexed to facilitate relaxation of abdominal muscles. Guarding may be localized over specific lesions (often inflammatory), or there may be marked rigidity if pain is severe, as in perforation or penetration. Subxiphoid tenderness suggests an active ulcer. Tenderness over the liver, especially when the liver edge is brought down against the examining finger by deep inspiration, suggests inflammation in this organ. With gallbladder disease tenderness is localized to the region of the gallbladder, and with cystic or common duct obstruction a distended viscus can sometimes be felt as well. Right lower quadrant tenderness is found with appendicitis as well as with Crohn's disease involving the ileum or the ileocecal area. A left lower quadrant tender sigmoid cord is felt most commonly with irritable bowel syndrome but can also indicate diverticular disease. A distinct tender mass in the right lower quadrant suggests inflammation (usually Crohn's disease) extending beyond the bowel; a similar finding in the left lower quadrant is suggestive of diverticulitis. Board-like rigidity indicates an intra-abdominal catastrophe, such as perforation or infarction. Pulsatile masses should be differentiated from laterally expansile masses since the former can represent a mass overlying an artery, whereas the latter implies aneurysmal dilation. When localized perforation has occurred, rebound tenderness may be localized over the area. Hyperesthesia may exist over the segmental distribution of the spinal nerve that innervates the particular area of the viscus. This finding is detected by gently rubbing the fingers over the skin of the involved dermatome.

Rectal examination can be extremely helpful in localizing areas of tendernass as well as in palpating masses through the rectum. Periappendiceal abscesses can sometimes be identified in this manner, as can a perforated diverticulum. On digital examination the finger should circumscribe a complete circle examining the entire perirectal area.

Genital and pelvic examination, like the rectal examination, should be performed in all patients with abdominal pain since it can detect hernias as well as genitourinary and other pelvic problems.

If analgesic drugs have been administered, it is useful to re-examine the patient after pain has been relieved to identify masses or localized tenderness that may have been obscured by guarding and rigidity.

LABORATORY TESTS

A complete blood count, urinalysis, and test for occult blood in the stool are required in every person with serious acute abdominal pain (see above), as are a chest-Xray and plain and upright films of the abdomen. Other laboratory tests should be ordered as indicated by the specific findings.

A low hematocrit value or hemoglobin concentration can call attention to intraperitoneal or retroperitoneal bleeding, while hemoconcentration raises consideration of mesenteric vascular occlusion. High white count and high erythrocyte sedimentation rate suggest inflammation or infection. Blood in the urine points to kidney stones as a possible source of pain, while white cells point to infection. Glycosuria may arouse suspicion of a diabetic crisis.

The presence of occult blood in the stool reinforces concern about the gastrointestinal tract as a source of painful symptoms, and may be an early sign of vascular ischemia or intussusception, or a sign of more common lesions, such as peptic ulcer, polyp, or inflammatory bowel disease.

RADIOLOGY

Plain and upright films of the abdomen are helpful in delineating gas patterns which may demonstrate displacement of intestine by intra-abdominal masses or may show localized loops of ileus, such as one sees with pancreatitis or pyelonephritis. Air is distributed more widely in the small bowel in reflex ileus and in intestinal obstruction. In the latter the typical stepladder pattern is often encountered, with slight separation of the loops due to edema of the wall of the small bowel; an upright film demonstrates air-fluid levels in the dilated loops. Absence of air distal to a specific point suggests obstruction at that point. Volvulus can be diagnosed on the plain film which demonstrates a sausage-shaped air or air-fluid-filled viscus coming to an apex. In gastric volvulus the greater curvature is seen above the

lesser curve; and a double air-fluid level is a classic finding, one level being in the lesser curvature of the fundus and the other in the antrum (because of the inverted U-shaped stomach under these conditions). Free air under the diaphragm on the upright film indicates a perforated viscus unless the patient has had recent surgery (at which time air was introduced) or has pneumatosis cystoides intestinalis, in which case a large amount of air may appear subdiaphragmatically from ruptured pseudocysts. The important clue to pneumatosis cystoides intestinalis is the presence of free air in the absence of signs or symptoms of perforation or peritonitis. Radiopaque gallbladder or kidney stones or pancreatic calcification seen on plain film may help to corroborate a suspected diagnosis or point attention toward one of these organs.

Contrast studies are performed for specific indications. For example, an upper gastrointestinal series (see "Patient Experience," page 440) can be performed instead of upper endoscopy (see below) when the history is typical of peptic ulcer and not suggestive of esophagitis, gastritis, or duodenitis (diagnoses which are not well demonstrated by X-ray examination). An upper gastrointestinal series is also helpful when pancreatitis or pancreatic pseudocyst is thought to be the basis of the pain, since the compression on the C loop of the duodenum may suggest these diagnoses. Barium enema (see "Patient Experience," in Chapter 37) can be useful, not only in demonstrating a low site of obstruction but also in reducing an intussusception. When pain is thought to result from gallbladder disease (see Chapter 90) and opaque stones are not visible on plain abdominal film, *ultrasonography* is an excellent means of demonstrating stones in the gallbladder, but is not reliable in detecting ductal stones. An oral cholecystogram may demonstrate radiolucent stones; if the gallbladder fails to be visualized with reinforced dosage, a diseased gallbladder is quite likely. *TcHIDA or PipHIDA radioisotopic studies* may demonstrate obstruction of the common or cystic duct. This technique requires injection of isotope and serial views for 1 hour, while the appearance of isotope in the gallbladder is examined (a sonogram is usually performed beforehand to localize the gallbladder).

Ultrasonography is also useful in showing pancreatic edema or pseudocysts, in evaluating a suspected abdominal aortic aneurysm, and in evaluating a patient who is difficult to examine for an intra-abdominal mass; this technique has the advantage of avoiding irradiation. Sonography is often unsatisfactory in obese persons and in persons with metal abdominal sutures because adipose tissue and metal reflect sound.

Computerized tomography (CT) is a sensitive means of demonstrating masses, infarcted tissue, and cysts but is expensive and exposes the patient to irradiation.

Table 35.4.
Ultrasound and Computerized Tomography (CT) Scanning: Comparison of the Technique and the Patient Experience[a]

Characteristic	Ultrasound	CT
Basis of tissue attenuation	Tissue elasticity, acoustic impedance	Electron density; linear attenuation coefficient
Radiation dose or toxic effect	None known at diagnostic energy levels	8–10 R (skin exposure)
Morphological detail	Good	Excellent
Contrast medium useful	None	Iodinated intravascular and oral agents; diatrizoate meglumine (Gastrografin)
Time for examination	½–1 hour	½–1 hour
Operator skill	Substantial	Minimal
Ease of interpretation	Complex—many artifacts	Straightforward
Preparation	Nothing by mouth after midnight (for pelvis, three glasses of water 1 hour before study and do not void)	Evacuate barium from recent gastrointestinal studies (or wait 1 week)
Cooperation	Lie still, supine	Lie still, supine

[a] Adapted from Ferrucci JT Jr: Body ultrasonography (first of two parts). *N Engl J Med* 300:538, 1979.

Table 35.4 compares the ultrasound and CT technique and the patient experience.

Selective *mesenteric angiography* should be performed in patients suspected of having mesenteric vascular ischemia (particularly in elderly persons with postprandial abdominal pain) or mesenteric vascular occlusion (*e.g.*, in women taking contraceptive medication). This is particularly helpful in older patients since normal arteriographic findings rule out mesenteric vascular disease; on the other hand, occlusion even of two of the three major aortic branches (celiac, superior mesenteric, and inferior mesenteric arteries) may occur without symptoms of mesenteric vascular disease. It may be prudent to hospitalize the patient for this procedure. The patient experience is similar to that described for renal arteriography (Chapter 62).

ENDOSCOPY

Upper gastrointestinal endoscopy requires referral to a gastroenterologist (see below). It should be considered as an ambulatory procedure to clarify or confirm findings in upper gastrointestinal series or to obtain a biopsy for diagnosis (*e.g.*, when cancer is suspected). Endoscopy should be one of the first diagnostic procedures performed when abdominal pain is associated with upper gastrointestinal bleed-

ing (see Chapter 37), but these patients should be hospitalized (see below).

Proctoscopy should be performed in any patient with abdominal pain and rectal bleeding or a change in bowel habits or in any patient in whom inflammatory bowel disease (proctitis, ulcerative colitis, Crohn's disease) is suspected. Moreover, anal lesions such as hemorrhoids and fissures are best demonstrated by proctoscopy. The procedure routinely should precede roentgenographic examination of the lower bowel since the barium enema does not visualize the lower rectum.

Colonoscopy, like upper endoscopy, requires referral to a gastroenterologist (see below). It should be considered in patients with abdominal pain who have occult rectal bleeding (see Chapter 37), in those with suspected diffuse colonic inflammatory disease (ulcerative colitis. Crohn's disease) or suspected ischemic colitis, and in patients with polypoid lesions on barium enema who require biopsy or, often, resection of the lesion. Colonoscopy cannot be performed within a day or two of a barium X-ray of the lower or upper gastrointestinal tract.

Patient experience. In addition to concerns about facts relating to endoscopy, many patients have specific apprehensions and misconceptions which can only be managed appropriately if the patient is encouraged to express them. The most common questions concern the indication for the procedure and the anticipated benefits, and technical details about the procedure itself, including prior preparation, side effects, and risks. Much of the patient's anxiety can be allayed if the referring physician can answer these questions appropriately. The physician may find it helpful to emphasize that recent scientific and technical advances have improved instrumentation so that the new fiberoptic instruments can be passed with relatively little discomfort and that photographs can be taken for detailed study, as well as brushings for cytology and biopsy for histology.

UPPER ENDOSCOPY (ESOPHAGOSCOPY, GASTROSCOPY, DUODENOSCOPY). Preparation varies, but usually the patient will be asked to fast for 8 hours before the procedure and will be given a topical anesthetic by gargle or atomizer spray and also an intravenous or intramuscular sedative or tranquilizer. It is often helpful to reassure patients that the procedure can be and in fact often is performed without any premedication, as, for example, in patients with massive bleeding. Moreover, although the swallowing of tubes sounds like an awesome task, the knowledge that endoscopy is performed in patients of all ages and that children as well as elderly people tolerate the procedure well is also reassuring. The instrument is about the diameter of the fifth finger and introduction produces discomfort rather than pain. The entire procedure seldom lasts more than 20 minutes. Instillation of air, which is necessary to distend the organ so that it can be well visualized, tends to produce a sensation of bloating. This air can be aspirated at the end of the procedure.

The discomfort from upper endoscopy is usually much less than that from a barium enema, and biopsies are painless. A topical anesthetic is administered initially to minimize gagging. During the procedure, the patient experiences the sensation of having something in his throat that he cannot swallow. Bleeding and perforation, the most serious complications, are extremely rare. The procedure is usually performed on an outpatient basis, and since sedation is generally employed, the patient should be accompanied by someone who will be able to take him home following the procedure.

PROCTOSIGMOIDOSCOPY. Whether or not prior preparation is appropriate depends on the suspected pathology. If proctoscopy is performed to detect or biopsy a mass lesion, a laxative is used the day before and a cleansing enema is given on the morning of the procedure. On the other hand, mucosal lesions (such as inflammatory bowel disease) are best demonstrated without preparation (other than a natural bowel movement the morning of the procedure). Most enema preparations tend to produce some mucosal edema that may obscure mucosal lesions. Proctosigmoidoscopy is not painful, but there is an uncomfortable sensation produced by the distention of the rectosigmoid region by the instrument and by air.

FIBEROPTIC SIGMOIDOSCOPY AND COLONOSCOPY. Fiberoptic sigmoidoscopy can generally be performed if a laxative is administered the day before the procedure and if an enema is given on the morning of the procedure. Colonoscopy requires further cleaning, usually necessitating a liquid diet 2 to 3 days before the procedure in addition to laxatives and an enema. Good cleansing is especially important if polypectomy is contemplated. For colonoscopy premedication similar to that used in upper endoscopy (see above) is appropriate, as well as an intravenous analgesic such as Demerol to minimize the discomfort and crampy pain commonly associated with insufflation of air and negotiation of curves. The procedure may take from 30 minutes to over 1 hour. Polypectomy adds additional time as well as additional risk (perforation and bleeding) but generally does not increase discomfort nor involve the additional recovery time that would be required after an abdominal operation to remove polyps.

TREATMENT

The treatment of patients with abdominal pain depends on the severity of the pain, its rapidity of onset, and the nature of the underlying condition, if known. Severe pain with an abrupt or rapid onset frequently reflects a gastrointestinal disorder that will require surgical intervention (see Table 35.1) Hospitalization and consultation with a gastroenterologist and a surgeon should be requested immediately in almost all cases. Less severe pain (pain that does not prevent the patient from ambulating, talking normally, thinking coherently, *etc*) should not be treated aggressively with analgesic drugs until an attempt has been made to establish a diagnosis, since the pain will often abate spontaneously within minutes or hours and will not recur. In such circumstances, no further evaluation is indicated. If the pain recurs or persists and the cause is not obvious, the screening tests described on page 435 should be done. If these tests do not provide a diagnosis, referral to a gastroenterologist is indicated.

As a general rule, analgesic drugs may be prescribed to patients with persistent pain, but opiates should be avoided if possible, because they may aggravate the underlying condition. (For example, morphine may aggravate pancreatitis by producing duodenal and ampullary spasm, thus enhancing pancreatic duct obstruction; and opiates or anticholinergics may produce toxic megacolon in patients with active ulcerative colitis. Furthermore, there is a risk of narcotic addiction in any patient whose pain is likely to be of prolonged duration.)

General References

Ferrucci JT Jr: Body ultrasonography (first of two parts). *N Engl J Med* 300:538, 1979.
> Good review of the clinical uses of sonography, with useful comparison of computerized tomography scanning.

Handbook of Differential Diagnosis. vol 2. part I: *The Abdomen.* Nutley, NJ, Rocom Press, 1974.
> Excellent illustrations by M. F. Netter and good tables.

Hendrix TR, Bulkley GB: Abdominal pain. In Harvey AM, Johns RJ, McKusick VA, *et al* (eds): *Principles and Practice of Medicine.* New York, Appleton-Century-Crofts, 1984.
> Excellent chapter written by a gastroenterologist and a surgeon, organized for the most part as a problem-solving approach for ambulatory and hospitalized patients.

Way LW: Abdominal pain. In Sleisenger MH, Fordtran JS (eds): *Gastrointestinal Disease.* Philadelphia, WB Saunders, 1983.
> Very good discussion organized along classical rather than problem-oriented lines; written by an experienced surgeon.

CHAPTER THIRTY-SIX

Peptic Ulcer Disease

HAROLD J. TUCKER, M.D.

NORMAL GASTRIC FUNCTION

The two primary functions of the stomach are the secretion of various substances that are important in digestion and absorption and the movement of gastric contents downstream into the small intestine.

There are four primary classes of secretory cells: mucus-secreting cells of the cardia, hydrochloric acid-secreting parietal cells of the body (which also secrete intrinsic factor—see Chapter 49), pepsinogen-secreting chief cells of the body, and gastrin-secreting G cells of the antrum. Gastric function is regulated by neural and hormonal influences which determine the rate and amount that the various cells secrete and the rate at which the stomach empties its contents into the duodenum. During the *cephalic phase* of gastric activity, the anticipation of eating initiates cholinergic impulses which, *via* the vagus nerve, stimulate parietal cell secretion of acid and G cell secretion of gastrin (which then also stimulates acid secretion). During the *gastric phase*, distention of the stomach by food causes local nerve endings to stimulate acid and gastrin secretion further—the G cells are also directly stimulated by protein and protein breakdown products and inhibited by acid. During the *intestinal phase* of gastric activity, intestinal hormones (secretin, cholecystokinin, and probably others), the secretion of which is stimulated directly by gastric acid, inhibit the action of gastrin on the parietal cells.

EPIDEMIOLOGY

Peptic ulcer disease is a common clinical entity. However, for unknown reasons the incidence of peptic ulcer disease, both duodenal and gastric, has been declining for the last 20 to 30 years. The current incidence of new cases of duodenal ulcer disease is about 2/1000 men and 0.8/1000 women/year. For gastric ulcer, the incidence is only 0.5 and 0.3/1000/year, respectively. The highest incidence is between the ages of 45 and 65 in men and over the age of 55 in women. The overall prevalence of the disease in the general population remains high (about 10%).

RISK FACTORS

Certain factors are associated with an increased risk of developing peptic ulcer disease (Table 36.1). Genetic factors appear to play an important role. Men (see above) are more prone to both duodenal and gastric ulcers than are women. Duodenal ulcer is 3 times more common in first degree relatives of a patient with a duodenal ulcer than in the general population. Furthermore, certain genetic markers,

Table 36.1.
Risk Factors for Peptic Ulcer Disease

Male sex
First degree relative with duodenal ulcer
Genetic markers:
  Elevated levels of pepsinogen I
  Presence of HLA-B5 antigen
  Decreased red blood cell acetylcholinesterase
Stress
Cigarette smoking
Zollinger-Ellison syndrome
Chronic renal failure—for duodenal ulcer disease only
Chronic obstructive pulmonary disease—for duodenal ulcer
  disease only
Alcoholic cirrhosis—for duodenal ulcer disease only
Drugs: aspirin—for gastric ulcer disease only

such as pepsinogen I, HLA-B5, and red blood cell acetylcholinesterase, can identify groups at increased risk. With the aid of such markers, peptic ulcer disease has been shown to be genetically heterogeneous. In certain families there appears to be an autosomal dominant mode of inheritance, while in others no discernible pattern is found.

The role of *stress* in the pathogenesis of peptic ulcer disease is well recognized but difficult to quantitate. Nevertheless, it is clear that threats to the psychological or physical well-being of some people appear to predispose them to peptic ulceration. Why some people react to stress by developing peptic disease, others by developing another disease (e.g., asthma or hypertension) is unknown (see Chapter 12 for a discussion of psychosomatic illness).

Cigarette smoking has been repeatedly demonstrated to be associated with an increased frequency of duodenal ulcer disease with frequencies ranging between 33 and 100% above that of nonsmokers (3). In addition, there is evidence that cigarette smoking may delay the healing rate of both gastric and duodenal ulcers and increase the frequency of their recurrence. There is no epidemiological evidence that alcohol is ulcerogenic, although it is a known cause of acute gastritis. Coffee, both caffeinated and decaffeinated, is a mild stimulant of gastric acid secretion. Symptoms may be exacerbated by coffee, but a definite causal relationship with ulcer disease has not been demonstrated.

Certain disease states have been associated with an increased risk of peptic ulcer disease. Evidence for such associations must be carefully evaluated in light of the high prevalence of ulcer disease in the general population and the frequent use of ulcerogenic drugs. There is, however, good evidence linking duodenal (but not gastric) ulcer disease with chronic obstructive pulmonary disease, alcoholic cirrhosis, chronic renal failure, and hyperparathyroidism.

*Conditions that lead to increased gastric acid se-*cretion also predispose to ulcer disease. The Zollinger-Ellison syndrome, or gastrinoma (see below), is the best example of such a condition. Extensive small bowel resection may also lead to hyperplasia of antral gastrin-containing cells and result in ulcer disease. Retained antrum following gastric surgery is yet another example of a situation in which there is uninhibited acid production associated with recurrent ulcerations.

Many drugs are reputed to be ulcerogenic, although the evidence is not well established for most of them. Aspirin is one drug that does appear to cause gastric (but not duodenal) ulcers. Experimentally, aspirin disrupts the gastric mucosa both physiologically and anatomically, leading to ulcer formation. Chronic aspirin use has been shown epidemiologically to be linked to an increased frequency of gastric ulceration. Aspirin use also increases the risk of bleeding from peptic lesions (see Chapter 51). Enteric coated or buffered aspirin has no advantage over regular aspirin with respect to these untoward effects.

There is no evidence that other anti-inflammatory agents cause ulcers. Corticosteroids have frequently been linked to the formation of ulcers and to the complications of hemorrhage and perforation. Prospective and retrospective studies of this issue have concluded that steroids do not increase the prevalence of peptic ulcer disease or of its complications (2). The same statement can be made for agents like indomethacin, phenylbutazone, and other anti-inflammatory agents, although many of these drugs may cause erosive gastritis.

PATHOPHYSIOLOGY

The pathophysiology of duodenal ulcer disease differs from that of gastric ulcer disease.

Duodenal Ulcer

Simplistically, duodenal ulcer disease can be viewed as the result of an imbalance between the normal duodenal defense mechanisms and the amount of acid delivered to the duodenum from the stomach. Multiple abnormalities have been identified that result in this imbalance: (a) increased parietal cell mass, (b) increased capacity of parietal cells to secrete acid, (c) increased vagal "drive" to secrete acid, (d) defective inhibition of gastrin release and of gastric secretion following gastric acidification or following a meal (these first four abnormalities result in a considerably increased acid production compared to normal), (e) abnormally rapid gastric emptying, and (f) altered duodenal defense mechanisms.

Duodenal defense mechanisms include neutralization of acid by pancreatic bicarbonate and absorption of acid by duodenal contents. There are some data to suggest that pancreatic bicarbonate secretion is decreased by nicotine. This observation may provide an explanation for the association between smoking and ulcer disease, but its true significance is still uncertain. Pancreatic secretion is otherwise normal in peptic ulcer disease, and there is no increased risk in patients with chronic pancreatitis.

Gastric Ulcer

The current understanding of the pathogenesis of gastric ulceration is less clear. It is generally believed that the basic defect in gastric ulcer formation is the disruption of the gastric mucosal barrier. It has been shown that this barrier can be broken by such irritants as bile, alcohol, and aspirin. These experimental observations help explain the epidemiological data associating alcohol with acute gastritis, and aspirin with gastric ulcers and erosions. Furthermore, in patients with gastric ulcers, radiological and manometric studies have suggested that there is an increased duodenal gastric reflux. This reflux of bile across an incompetent pyloric sphincter results in the disruption of the mucosal barrier. Once the barrier is broken, hydrogen ion may diffuse back into the gastric cells, leading to ulceration via local histamine release, vasodilation, and tissue damage. Thus, according to this concept, gastric ulcer formation requires injury to the gastric mucosal barrier and the presence of some, but not necessarily an excessive amount of, acid.

Another factor that may be involved in the formation of some gastric ulcers is pyloric stenosis, which most commonly occurs secondary to a chronic duodenal ulcer that antedates the formation of a gastric ulcer. With pyloric deformity there may be poor gastric emptying, resulting in stasis and antral distension. This distension leads to increased gastrin release and increased gastric acid production. This hypothesis is supported by the frequent association radiographically of both duodenal and gastric ulcerations. In the Veterans Administration (VA) Cooperative Study of gastric ulcer, over 40% of patients had radiographic evidence of concurrent duodenal ulcer disease (5). Furthermore, patients with gastric ulcers just proximal to the pylorus are frequently found to produce increased amounts of acid, just as patients with duodenal ulcers do.

DIAGNOSIS

History

The most common symptom of peptic ulcer disease is epigastric distress—vague discomfort or a feeling of gnawing hunger—usually in the midline. If actual pain occurs, it is typically aching or burning.

Classically, the distress of duodenal ulcers occurs several hours after a meal and may awaken the patient from sleep; it is relieved within minutes by food, antacids, or vomiting. Typically distress is not present before breakfast. In patients with gastric ulcers, the history is more variable. In some, a similar distress-food-relief pattern exists, while in others there is no relationship with food. Occasionally, the distress is actually exacerbated by food.

Other less frequent symptoms of ulcer disease include nausea, vomiting, and heartburn. However, in some patients with ulcers one or more of these symptoms may occur in the absence of typical ulcer pain. Weight loss occurs in up to 50% of patients with a benign gastric ulcer (and is therefore not a helpful feature in distinguishing a benign from a malignant ulcer). Patients with duodenal ulcer often gain weight because they eat more in an attempt to control their pain.

The history may also suggest certain complications. Pyloric obstruction presents first with early satiety and then with persistent vomiting, frequently of undigested food. A change in the quality of the pain or radiation of the pain to the back or shoulder suggests penetration of the ulcer. A history of melena suggests bleeding. Occasionally, one of these complications is the first clinical manifestation of peptic ulceration.

Physical Examination

The physical examination may provide supportive, although nonspecific, information. Localized epigastric tenderness is common. The presence of a succussion splash 4 hours postprandially is evidence of gastric outlet obstruction. Rectal examination should be included in the initial physical examination to obtain a stool specimen for testing for occult blood.

Radiological Studies

Confirmation of the presence of peptic ulcer disease can be made with barium studies or with endoscopy.

Patient experience. The patient should be told that the upper gastrointestinal series requires him to have a series of X-rays taken after he swallows a bolus of barium, that peristalsis is monitored fluoroscopically during the procedure, and that to coat as much of the stomach and duodenum as possible, he will be X-rayed while he is prone. The entire procedure takes about 20 to 25 minutes.

Endoscopically demonstrable duodenal or gastric ulcers are visible by barium X-ray in up to 80% of cases.

Duodenal Ulcer

The radiographic diagnosis of duodenal ulcer disease depends upon the detection of an ulcer crater. Associated findings include edema and radiation of the duodenal folds adjacent to the ulcer, deformity of the bulb, and spasm. Occasionally the ulcer crater may not be detected because of overhanging edematous folds which prevent filling of the crater with barium, shallowness of the ulcer crater, or an inadequate technique. Air contrast studies enhance the detection rate of shallow ulcers and erosions. Ulcers greater than 3 cm are classified as giant duodenal ulcers. Duodenal ulcers do not carry the risk of malignancy that gastric ulcers do, and therefore follow-up X-rays to confirm healing are generally not needed. In patients with chronic ulcer disease with severe deformity of the bulb, distinction radiographically between old scarring with deformity and new active ulcerations is often very difficult. Comparison with previous films and correlation with the clinical state are needed in these cases.

In the postoperative patient, barium studies are often difficult to evaluate. With conventional studies, anastomotic ulcers are detected in only 50% of cases. The air contrast technique may be of more value in this situation. Distinction between surgical deformity and recurrent ulcerations is often difficult without a previous postoperative study for comparison.

Gastric Ulcer

Radiological studies are valuable in the detection and evaluation of gastric ulcers. The radiographic features characteristic of a benign gastric ulcer include (a) penetration of the ulcer crater beyond the expected course of the gastric lumen; (b) radiating gastric folds converging on the ulcer reaching right up to the ulcer margin; (c) smooth appearance of surrounding mucosa; (d) central location of the ulcer, surrounded by a smooth mound of edematous mucosa; and (e) smooth and round or oval margins of the ulcer crater. The radiation of the gastric folds up to the thin overhanging margin of the ulcer is probably the most reliable sign of benignity. Appreciation of the surrounding gastric mucosa and the radiation of the folds is best achieved with good air contrast technique (Fig. 36.1). (The air contrast study causes distension of the stomach but no real pain.) The size of the ulcer is not helpful as a differential point in an individual case, except that the incidence of malignancy in gastric ulcers increases with increasing size of the ulcer crater. Similarly, location of the ulcer is not of predictive value. Coexistent duodenal ulcer disease (seen in 40% of gastric ulcer patients) considerably decreases the likelihood that a gastric ulcer is malignant, but does not rule it out. Multiple ulcers need to be evaluated and followed individually.

In evaluating a gastric ulcer, the radiologist generally describes it as benign, malignant, or indeterminant. As many as 10% of gastric ulcers may be classified in this last category. Although the radiographic impression of a benign or malignant ulcer is generally very accurate, discrepancies still occur.

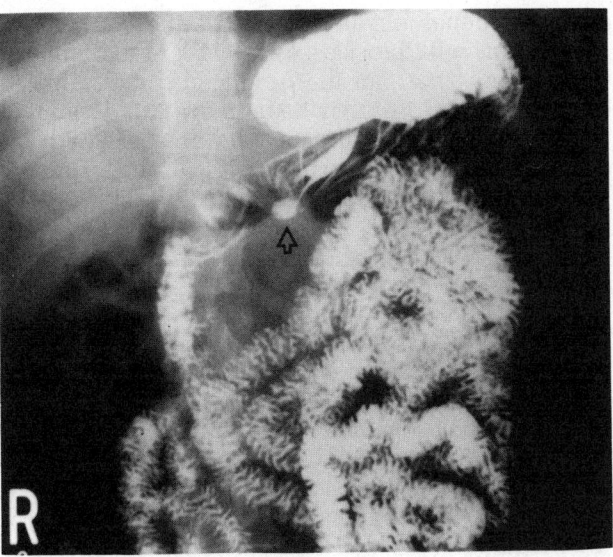

Figure 36.1. X-ray study in a patient with a benign gastric ulcer. The presence of gastric folds radiating to the edge of the ulcer, with no distortion of the surrounding mucosa, is characteristic of a benign gastric ulcer.

The incidence of malignancy in an ulcer diagnosed radiographically as benign ranges from 3 to 7% with higher frequencies when "indeterminant" lesions are included. Air contrast techniques may decrease this error rate. Furthermore, barium studies may miss lesions, particularly when multiple ulcers are present. Even carefully performed radiography will miss up to 20% of ulcers seen by endoscopy. Thus, while a barium study is frequently the initial procedure of choice for gastric ulcers, it must be recognized that its sensitivity is less than that of endoscopy and that it is associated occasionally with erroneous results.

Endoscopy

Endoscopy is of value in the diagnosis of both duodenal and gastric ulcers. It has the advantages of increased sensitivity, the opportunity for obtaining biopsies, and the avoidance of radiation. In certain situations endoscopy may be the preferred initial mode of examination rather than X-ray (see page 436 for a description of the patient's experience with endoscopy).

Duodenal Ulcers

Indications for endoscopy for duodenal ulcer disease include (a) abdominal pain suggestive of peptic ulcer disease with negative X-ray studies, (b) refractory or recurrent ulcer symptoms despite appropriate medical therapy of radiologically visible ulcers, (c) evaluation for anastomotic ulcers, (d) differentiation between old scarring and new active ulcer craters seen on X-ray, (e) acute pyloric obstruction, and (f) upper gastrointestinal bleeding. Uncomplicated duodenal ulcers do not require endoscopic evaluations with biopsies, as the risk of malignancy is extremely low, nor do they need to be followed endoscopically until they heal. In the patient known to have peptic ulcer disease who presents with recurrent typical symptoms, the indications for repeat X-ray studies, endoscopy, or empiric therapy have not been established. The advantages and disadvantages of the various alternatives should be considered for each individual patient.

Gastric Ulcer

There is considerable controversy over the role of endoscopy in patients with gastric ulcer. Clearly, in the patient whose clinical condition or whose radiographic studies suggest a gastric malignancy endoscopic evaluation is indicated. Adenocarcinoma of the stomach, lymphoma, metastatic carcinoma to the stomach (e.g., malignant melanoma), and leiomyosarcoma all may be ulcerated and may be differentiated by endoscopy and biopsy. Even in patients with a benign appearing ulcer, early endoscopy is frequently recommended because of its increased accuracy in distinguishing benign *versus* malignant disease and its increased sensitivity in demonstrating multiple ulcers, gastritis, and coexisting duodenal ulcer disease. Endoscopy with multiple biopsies and directed brushings for cytology can accurately diagnose gastric ulcers in 97 to 99% of cases. However, it can also be argued that routine early endoscopy is unnecessary because (a) newer air contrast radiographic techniques may provide similar degrees of accuracy, (b) the incidence of gastric carcinoma is decreasing, and (c) the prognosis of patients found to have a gastric malignancy may be unaltered even with earlier detection. In addition, as the ultimate determinant of the benign nature of an ulcer is that it heals completely and resolves, some would argue that a late endoscopic evaluation to determine whether there has been complete resolution of the ulcer is the most important one.

It is apparent that judgment and individualization are important. Endoscopy is the most accurate means of distinguishing a benign from a malignant ulcer. In a patient with severe cardiac or pulmonary disease in whom gastric surgery would be almost unthinkable, even for malignant disease, endoscopy for an ulcer that appears benign is unwarranted. Otherwise endoscopy should be performed routinely soon after diagnosis. The mode of follow-up frequently depends on the individual evaluation. In the patient with an ulcer that appears benign by X-ray and by endoscopy, radiological follow-up to complete healing is generally satisfactory. Clearly if the initial ulcer cannot be well visualized on X-ray, endoscopy should be used to follow the healing of the ulcer. In the patient with a suspicious or "indeterminant" lesion by X-ray but without initial endoscopic evaluation, endoscopy should be performed subsequently to confirm complete healing of the ulcer. Malignant ulcers have been found to have resolved on radiographic studies but not on endoscopic evaluation. Finally, ulcers that fail to heal after an appropriate interval should be re-evaluated endoscopically. It should be recognized that because of greater sensitivity of the procedure, the healing rate shown by endoscopy is probably slower than the generally accepted healing rate, defined radiographically as 50% reduction in size of ulcer at 6 weeks and complete healing at 12 weeks.

Gastric Analysis

Gastric secretory studies have enhanced the understanding of the pathophysiology of ulcer disease but are of limited clinical usefulness. While many patients with duodenal ulcer disease can be shown to hypersecrete acid, over one-half of such patients actually have normal levels of acid production. The presence of a hypersecretion, furthermore, does not predict the development of ulcer disease in an individual patient. Dyspepsia with a negative X-ray is not an indication for gastric analysis.

In patients with gastric ulcers, gastric analysis is only rarely helpful. Persistent achlorhydria despite stimulation (with Histalog or pentagastrin) strongly suggests that the ulcer is malignant; but, on the other hand, over 80% of patients with malignancies will have demonstrable acid production following stimulation.

The main indications for gastric analysis are for preoperative evaluation of patients with suspected Zollinger-Ellison syndrome (see below) or in the postgastrectomy patient with recurrent ulcer disease. However, gastric analysis is not useful as an indicator of the type of surgery needed—more acid production does not necessarily require more gastric resection (7).

Gastric analysis requires gastric intubation for about 2 hours. The procedure is performed in the gastrointestinal laboratory of most hospitals (not in the general physician's office). During the first hour, the volume and hydrogen ion activity of gastric secretions are measured and are reported as the basal acid output (BAO) in milliequivalents per hour. Secretion is then stimulated, usually with pentagastrin or Histalog. The former, a synthetic analogue of gastrin, is generally recommended as it has fewer side effects than Histalog (a histamine analogue) and causes peak secretion earlier. Volume and hydrogen ion activity are again measured for the next hour and reported as maximal acid output (MAO). Peak acid output (PAO) is similar to MAO, but refers to the highest acid output following stimulation rather than the total acid output. Mean basal secretion and maximal acid secretion in normals are 2.4 and 25 mEq/hour, respectively, while in patients with duodenal ulcers the mean values are 5 and 43 mEq/hour, respectively.

Serum Gastrin Measurements

Measurements of the level of gastrin in the blood are now readily available and are of use in the evaluation of selected patients with peptic ulcer disease. The fasting basal serum gastrin level is normal (i.e., <150 pg/ml) in patients with duodenal and gastric ulcer disease but is elevated, often to very high levels (usually 1000 pg/ml or more), in patients with the Zollinger-Ellison syndrome (see below). Therefore, fasting gastrin determinations are very useful in screening for this condition. In patients with frequently recurrent ulcers, and in patients refractory to conventional therapy—features suggestive of the syndrome—two or three fasting serum gastrin determinations should be made to rule out this condition since the levels may fluctuate. Also, in all patients undergoing elective ulcer surgery, a preoperative gastrin level should be measured, (see page 453 for a discussion of hypergastrinemia).

NATURAL HISTORY

Both duodenal and gastric ulcers recur extremely frequently. In multiple series, using periodic endoscopic examination after healing of the initial ulcer and cessation of medical therapy, the recurrence rate for duodenal ulcer disease has been 50 to 77% within the first 6 months (9). Some of these recurrences are asymptomatic and detected only endoscopically, but the majority are associated with typical ulcer symptoms. Similarly, for gastric ulcers, the recurrence rate is also high with 30 to 56% recurring within a 2-year period. In the VA Cooperative Study 11% had two recurrences within a 2-year interval. In patients whose index ulcer healed slowly (persisting for over 3 months), the recurrence rate was even higher—67% within 2 years (5). Although first recurrence of a gastric ulcer does not increase the risk for subsequent recurrences, the rate remains high (30 to 40%).

Complications of peptic ulcer disease are also common. Hemorrhage occurs in about 15 to 20% of patients over a 15- to 25-year follow-up, somewhat more frequently in patients with duodenal ulcers than in patients with gastric ulcers. Recurrent hemorrhage is also common, occurring in 30 to 50% of patients with duodenal ulcer disease. The incidence of recurrent hemorrhage after the first, second, or third hemorrhage remains constant at 30 to 50%. In gastric ulcer disease, a second hemorrhage occurs up to 40% of the time and subsequent bleeding occurs in 25% of cases. The age of the patient or the severity of the index hemorrhage does not predict the likelihood of subsequent hemorrhage. Perforations occur in 5 to 10% of patients with peptic ulcer

disease, more commonly in patients with duodenal ulcers. Pyloric outlet obstruction is the least common major complication of peptic ulcer disease, occurring in less than 5% of patients, the vast majority of whom have duodenal ulcer disease.

MEDICAL THERAPY

Medical therapy includes dietary manipulations and restrictions, antacids, and antisecretory agents. Its purpose is to relieve pain, promote healing, and prevent recurrences and complications. Surgical therapy is aimed at reducing the capacity of the stomach to secrete acid (in patients with intractable pain) and at treating severe complications of the disease (massive bleeding, perforation, obstruction).

Diet and Related Restrictions

There is no evidence that modification of the diet is helpful in the treatment of peptic ulcer disease. Bland diets and increased milk consumption have not been shown to be of any benefit. It is more important to identify specific foods, if any, that seem to exacerbate symptoms in the individual patient. For example, caffeinated beverages may mildly stimulate acid secretion and may aggravate symptoms. However, in the absence of such aggravation, there is little benefit from restricting coffee or caffeine as these agents are not usually related to ulcer formation. Patients should be advised to eat regularly, but not to increase the frequency of meals or to use "bedtime snacks" habitually.

Avoidance of alcohol is frequently recommended. However, while alcohol has been shown to cause acute gastritis it is not directly related to ulcer disease. Restriction of alcohol is advisable for the general health of the patient but not specifically because of ulcer disease.

Aspirin, however, should be avoided in all patients with ulcers, or a history of ulcers. Aspirin is associated with gastric ulcer formation and may promote bleeding from both duodenal and gastric lesions. Similar restrictions are often imposed on other anti-inflammatory agents, such as indomethacin, but with less supportive evidence. While it is unclear what effect these agents have in the presence of an acute ulcer, their use is not contraindicated by the simple history of past ulcer disease.

Patients should be strongly advised to discontinue cigarette smoking. Its use has been associated with duodenal ulcer disease and with a decrease in the rate of the healing of both duodenal and gastric ulcers (14).

Antacids

Antacids have long been the mainstay of ulcer therapy. With appropriate dosage, antacids have been shown to be superior to placebo in promoting healing of duodenal ulcers. Although a relatively high percentage of ulcers do heal with placebo therapy over a 4-week period (45%), complete healing with antacid use was found in 78% of patients in one study (11). Interestingly, it does appear that, despite its positive effect on ulcer healing, antacid therapy is no better than placebo in relieving symptoms of duodenal ulcer. Despite widespread acceptance, there is little evidence that antacids relieve symptoms or promote healing of gastric ulcers.

Despite their widespread use, antacids are frequently misused in terms of proper dosage and optimal timing of administration. A wide variety of antacid preparations are commercially available, but not all antacids are the same. Preparations differ in their ability to neutralize acid, in their composition, and in their cost. Table 36.2 lists a comparative analysis of the doses, costs, and sodium content of commonly used antacids based on the acid neutralization effect of 30 ml (1 ounce) of a potent antacid, Mylanta-II. For example, 30 ml of Gelusil provides only one-third of the neutralizing effect of the same volume of Mylanta-II. It is clearly important, therefore, to know which antacid is being used by the patient and to prescribe the appropriate dose. For the majority of patients with duodenal ulcers a dose equal to the neutralizing effect of 1 ounce (30 ml) of Mylanta-II provides effective acid neutralization. Antacid tablets are more convenient to take but a large number of them must be taken to achieve an effect comparable to a relatively small dose of a liquid preparation. For example, 20 Rolaid tablets have the neutralizing capacity of 2 tablespoons of Mylanta II (at a cost of approximately $20 more a month).

The timing of the antacid dose is also of importance in achieving optimal acid neutralization. In patients with duodenal ulcer disease, there is exaggerated and prolonged secretion of acid in response to a meal. Thus, while a meal may buffer the acid, gastric emptying of the meal may be rapid, so that high levels of acid are left to bathe the duodenum. For this reason, frequent meals are also ineffective and may even be harmful, as the postprandial hypersecretion actually exacerbates the ulcer condition. It has been shown, however, that adequate doses of antacid (1 ounce of Mylanta-II or an equivalent), given at 1 and 3 hours following a meal can effectively neutralize gastric secretion for about 4 hours. Giving this dose of antacid at these intervals following a meal and at bedtime results in the high rate of ulcer healing described above. Antacid therapy should be continued for a 4- to 6-week period, after which it may be stopped completely if the ulcer has healed or used on an "as needed" basis if occasional symptoms recur.

Antacids have a number of potential side effects. The most common side effect is *alteration of bowel habits*—an effect that is predictable and inevitable at the doses recommended, depending on the composition of the antacid. Magnesium-containing antacids (e.g., Maalox) result in diarrhea, while aluminum-containing compounds, (e.g., Amphojel) are constipating. Most antacids attempt to balance these two ingredients, but invariably the effect of one predominates. Alternating doses between two different antacids (Mylanta-II and Amphojel) can prevent this problem. It is important to recommend this pattern at the outset rather than run the risk of a patient discontinuing the antacid because of resultant diarrhea or constipation. The patient should be instructed about the rationale for alternating the antacids, and he should balance the frequency of alternating the antacids with the stool pattern desired.

Electrolyte problems have also been noted when antacids are used. *Hypermagnesemia* can occur in patients with renal failure. *Hypophosphatemia* may result from aluminum hydroxide-containing compounds that bind intraluminal phosphate, causing severe muscle weakness and hemolysis of red cells. *Hypercalcemia*, with its consequences, can be seen after prolonged use of calcium-containing antacids (e.g., Tums). These latter antacids are very potent but are not recommended, not only because of the extraintestinal complications of hypercalcemia, but also because of the stimulant effect of hypercalcemia on gastric acid secretion. Thus, although these antacids transiently and effectively neutralize gastric acid, the absorbed calcium subsequently creates a rebound phenomenon of gastric hypersecretion which may exacerbate the ulcer diathesis. For similar reasons, consumption of large quantities of milk is generally not recommended.

Antacids may interfere with the absorption of a variety of drugs. Although the clinical significance of such interference is uncertain, it is probably best to prescribe that drugs be taken 1 hour before or after the ingestion of an antacid.

Table 36.2.
Comparison of Various Antacids[a]

Brand Name	Contents			One Dose[b]		Cost (¢)
	Al	Mg	Ca	Vol (ml)	Na (mg)	
Mylanta-II[c,d]	+	+		30	47.9	20
Maalox	+	+		48	53.8	25
Mylanta[d]	+	+		52	40.6	23
Riopan	+	+		56	7.9	22
Amphojel	+			64	77.0	28
Gelusil	+	+		93	132.7	37
Camalox	+	+	+	35	17.8	16

[a] From Ippoliti A, Peterson W: The pharmacology of peptic ulcer disease. *Clin Gastroenterol* 8:54, 1979.
[b] Dose defined as volume of antacid with neutralizing capability equivalent to 30 ml (1 ounce) of Mylanta-II.
[c] Mylanta-II has twice as much aluminum hydroxide and magnesium hydroxide per unit volume as Mylanta.
[d] Contains simethicone.

A well confirmed problem with antacid therapy is poor compliance, in part because of the high frequency of daily doses, the inconvenience of liquid preparations, and the high cost of recommended antacid regimens (see Table 36.2). Furthermore, since antacids are not prescription drugs, the patient may not have explicit written instructions on the bottle (recommendations on the bottle are often quite different from those needed for ulcer healing). Clearly, when antacids are selected for ulcer therapy, the physician should write down the regimen and should take the time to explain the rationale for what may seem to the patient a very large amount of antacid. As noted below, cimetidine has important advantages over antacids in facilitating patient compliance.

H₂ Antagonists: Cimetidine and Ranitidine

Cimetidine (Tagamet) and ranitidine (Zantac) are both competitive antagonists of the histamine (H₂) receptor on the gastric parietal cells. Thus, they block acid secretion in response to a wide variety of stimuli, including food, cholinergic agents, pentagastrin, histamine, and hypoglycemia. Nocturnal and food-induced acid secretion is reduced by 80% by these drugs. Therefore, they are both extremely effective in the healing of duodenal and gastric ulcers. However, there are some differences in the two drugs that may impact on the decision of which of them to use in an individual patient.

Cimetidine

Cimetidine is effective in the treatment of duodenal and gastric ulcer disease, peptic esophagitis, and Zollinger-Ellison syndrome. It is available in 200-, 300-, and 400-mg tablets or as a liquid, 300 mg/ 5 ml. The usual dose is 300 mg orally four times/ day, but some studies have reported similar degrees of success with 400 mg twice a day. It seems most reasonable to take the medication ½ hour prior to a meal and at bedtime to inhibit the postprandial and nocturnal hypersecretion of acid that is characteristic of peptic ulcer patients. The dose should be modified in patients with renal failure: given every 8 hours in patients with moderate renal impairment (creatinine clearance of 19 to 35 ml/minute), and every 12 hours when there is severe renal impairment (creatinine clearance less than 10 ml/minute).

For patients with acute duodenal ulcer disease, cimetidine should be given for 6 weeks, at which time 85 to 90% of ulcers will have healed. Tapering the dose is not necessary, as there is no evidence for a rebound acid hypersecretion or increased ulcer diathesis after cessation of therapy. Maintenance with 400 mg at bedtime may be instituted in certain circumstances (see below). Antacids may be as effective as is cimetidine but are less convenient to take, are frequently associated with troublesome side effects, and are more expensive. For patients with gastric ulcers, cimetidine should be continued until the ulcer has been documented to have healed completely.

Cimetidine appears to have few significant side effects. However, most studies of toxicity have been short term, and therefore the safety of long term use of the drug has not been clearly established. Several potential side effects have received particular attention. Neutropenia has been of considerable concern, since a previous investigational H₂ receptor antagonist, metiamide, was associated with this potentially life-threatening complication. However, in the making of cimetidine, the thiourea group contained in metiamide and thought to be the cause for the bone marrow toxicity was replaced with a cyanoguanidine group. There are no experimental data to indicate that cimetidine is toxic to leukocytes. Since its widespread use over the past several years, there have been isolated case reports of neutropenia, often not secondary to bone marrow suppression, and of thrombocytopenia associated with use of cimetidine. In the majority of these reports, a direct causal relationship between cimetidine and the hematological abnormality could not be established. Thus, there is little evidence that cimetidine is a bone marrow suppressant, and routine follow-up white blood cell counts and platelet counts are not recommended during cimetidine therapy.

Through its effect on hepatic enzyme activity, cimetidine prolongs the half-life of a variety of commonly used drugs, including diazepam (Valium), chlordiazepoxide (Librium), warfarin (Coumadin), theophylline, propranolol, and phenytoin (Dilantin). Particularly close monitoring of patients taking these drugs is therefore necessary if cimetidine is to be used.

An antiandrogenic effect of cimetidine has been demonstrated in several animal species. Prostatic weight and the size of the testes, prostate, and seminal vesicles have decreased in animals given the drug. In humans, gynecomastia has occurred, most frequently in patients given high doses and/or prolonged therapy, as in patients with Zollinger-Ellison syndrome. Blood levels of testosterone, luteinizing hormone, and follicle-stimulating hormone are normal, but prolactin levels have been elevated. With discontinuation of cimetidine, the gynecomastia generally has slowly resolved.

Numerous nonspecific side effects have been reported during cimetidine usage. These have included diarrhea, headache, fatigue, and dizziness. In a group of patients taking placebo or antacids as necessary, the frequency of these side effects was similar. Mental confusion, however, has been reported with cimetidine, generally in elderly patients with some degree of renal impairment. Cimetidine also commonly causes a mild reversible (less than 0.3 mg/dl) rise in levels of serum creatinine.

Ranitidine

Ranitidine is another H$_2$ antagonist that has more recently been approved for therapy in ulcer disease and hypersecretory states. On a molar basis, it is more potent than cimetidine and its inhibition of gastric acidity lasts longer (8 to 12 hours). Although the drug is metabolized by the liver (unlike cimetidine), a significant portion is also excreted unchanged by the kidney. The usual dose is 150 mg orally, twice a day, but should be reduced to 75 mg twice a day in patients with serious renal disease (serum creatinine greater than 4.0 mg/dl).

Ranitidine is as effective as cimetidine in healing duodenal ulcers and is probably as effective in the treatment of other peptic disorders as well. Since clinical efficacy appears to be similar, the choice between these two drugs then depends more on patient compliance, cost of the drug, and untoward side effects.

Ranitidine is taken twice a day while cimetidine is taken four times a day, making compliance with ranitidine somewhat easier. However, in comparative studies, compliance with the taking of both of these drugs was excellent. Ranitidine, however, is more expensive, costing approximately $40.00 to $45.00/month while cimetidine costs about $30.00 to $35.00/month.

A major potential benefit of ranitidine is its reduction of some of the side effects associated with cimetidine. Ranitidine is believed to have fewer antiandrogen effects, less interference with drug metabolism, and fewer CNS side effects. However, the experience with ranitidine is not as great as it is with cimetidine, and it is likely that the precise incidence of side effects is not yet known.

Many new H$_2$ antagonists are being evaluated currently, and some will soon be commercially available. These agents are designed to be as effective as cimetidine and ranitidine but to have fewer side effects. Whether there will be an advantage in using these new drugs remains to be seen.

Sucralfate

Sucralfate is a complex of aluminum hydroxide and sulfated sucrose. Its mechanism of action appears to be multifactorial: (a) It binds to ulcerated mucosa forming a "protective barrier" on the ulcer base, preventing further erosion. (b) It binds pepsin and inhibits further peptic activity. (c) It has a cytoprotective effect on gastric mucosa, perhaps mediated by prostaglandin release. (d) It binds bile salts, which are irritative to the gastric mucosa. Its systemic absorption is minimal, and it does not inhibit or neutralize gastric acidity.

Sucralfate is an effective drug for the treatment of both duodenal and gastric ulcers. Most studies have demonstrated it to be as effective as cimetidine in healing ulcers, although the total number of patients studied has been small. Perhaps due to its cytoprotective properties, sucralfate has also been reported to be effective in preventing drug- and stress-induced gastritis. Maintenance therapy with sucralfate has also been effective in reducing the frequency of ulcer relapse.

Sucralfate is administered as a 1-g tablet, four times a day (1 hour before meals and at bedtime). As it is minimally absorbed, the dose does not need to be adjusted for patients with kidney or liver disease. (Specifically, aluminum toxicity has not been observed in patients with renal failure.) Constipation is the most frequent side effect, occurring in about 4% of patients. Hypophosphatemia can occur and interference with drug absorption has been reported, for example, with tetracycline and warfarin. Taking other drugs 1 hour apart from sucralfate avoids this potential interaction. There is no evidence that cimetidine or antacids interfere with the effect of sucralfate (or *vice versa*), so these agents may be administered concurrently. As with ranitidine, experience with this promising new drug is still relatively limited, and its full range of indications and side effects remains to be defined. The cost of sucralfate is approximately $30.00 to $35.00/month.

Anticholinergics

The role of anticholinergic drugs in the treatment of duodenal ulcer is uncertain. These agents are capable of reducing basal acid secretion by 50% and stimulated acid secretion by 30 to 50%, with an inhibitory effect lasting 4 to 5 hours. Recent data have suggested that is it not necessary to give near toxic doses of anticholinergics to reduce acid secretion effectively but that a single standard dose of 15 mg of propantheline bromide (Pro-Banthine) achieves an optimal result. Despite this potentially beneficial function, the data on the relief of ulcer symptoms and on the ulcer healing rates with anticholinergics have been conflicting. Currently, anticholinergics are not recommended as first line therapy for duodenal ulcer disease. Rather their main use has been as an adjunct to antacids or to cimetidine. Anticholinergics can enhance the inhibitory effect on acid secretion of cimetidine and prolong the hypochlorhydric state for over 5 hours. Thus, these agents are recommended as additional therapy in patients unresponsive to cimetidine or antacids, in patients with nocturnal pain, and in patients with gastrinoma (Zollinger-Ellison syndrome—see below). If relief of nocturnal pain or prolongation of the effect of antacids or cimetidine is the aim, it seems reasonable to use an anticholinergic drug that may provide a longer duration of effect. Glycopyrrolate (Robinul), 1 to 2 mg, is a typical long acting anticholinergic that may be most appropriate at bedtime.

There is no indication that anticholinergics are helpful in the treatment of gastric ulcer. Indeed, these drugs may inhibit gastric emptying, which may prolong gastric ulcer disease. In addition, anticholinergics may impair pyloric sphincter function, resulting in an increased reflux of bile. Thus, in patients with gastric ulcers, these drugs may actually be harmful and should not be used.

The side effects of anticholinergic therapy include dry mouth, urinary retention, constipation, and aggravation of glaucoma. Gastroesophageal reflux (see above) may also be aggravated. In patients with marked pyloric deformity secondary to chronic ulcer disease, anticholinergic therapy may decrease gastric motility and cause gastric outlet obstruction.

Other Agents

Various new drugs are concurrently under investigation for use in patients with peptic ulcer disease. *Carbenoxalone* has been studied extensively in Europe, and improved healing rates for both duodenal and gastric ulcers have been reported. Aldosterone-like side effects have limited its usefulness. *Bismuth* has been demonstrated to be equally effective in a small number of studies. Its mode of action, like carbenoxalone, is unknown, but binding of pepsin and improvement in mucosal resistance to ulceration are possible mechanisms. *Prostaglandins* are currently being investigated for their protective effect against gastric erosions and ulcerations. *Omeperazole* is an extremely potent inhibitor of acid secretion that need be taken just once a day. Potential side effects are presently being evaluated. *Pirenzipine* is a new anticholinergic agent that appears to be selective for gastric parietal cells; initial studies are very encouraging.

Summary of Medical Therapy: Recommendations

Duodenal Ulcer

At the present time, it is very difficult to state dogmatically that one drug is superior to another in the treatment of peptic ulcer disease. Cimetidine, ranitidine, and sucralfate appear to be similarly effective in the healing of ulcers and in the provision of symptomatic relief. Antacid therapy should be used more for intermittent relief of symptoms than as primary therapy because of its cost and because of difficulties with compliance. Cimetidine is cheaper than ranitidine, is extremely effective, and, despite the concerns, is very safe. Ranitidine is a less well known commodity and is expensive, but it is very convenient. Cimetidine and ranitidine are effective in hypersecretory states and in gastroesophageal reflux, while sucralfate probably is of less benefit in these conditions. Ranitidine or sucralfate may be preferred in elderly patients or in patients with renal failure because of the lower incidence of

mental confusion with these drugs. These drugs may also be preferred to cimetidine when other drugs, such as warfarin or theophylline, are used concomitantly.

Whatever medication is prescribed, patients should be strongly encouraged to avoid cigarette smoking (14). Dietary instructions are simply to avoid those foods that produce symptoms, but bland diets or milk diets are not recommended. For the patient with nocturnal pain, adding an anticholinergic agent such as glycopyrrolate (Robinul, 1 mg) or propantheline bromide (Pro-Banthine, 15 mg) at bedtime may be beneficial. Doubling the dose of antacids at night may also be helpful. This therapy should be continued for 4 to 6 weeks (even if all symptoms have been relieved earlier), by which time ulcers will have healed in over 80% of patients. Follow-up X-ray or endoscopy is generally not indicated, and therapy can be discontinued at this time.

Peptic symptoms are usually relieved within 2 or 3 days. If the patient has failed to respond, re-evaluation is important to be certain that the symptoms are indeed due to ulcer disease. The addition of antacids with cimetidine, or the addition of an anticholinergic drug may be helpful to patients who have continuing peptic disease. Identification of potentially aggravating factors such as stress or continued cigarette smoking should be made. The value of supportive counseling (Chapter 11) and of the short term use of drugs to relieve anxiety (Chapter 13) also should not be forgotten.

Gastric Ulcer

Patients should be instructed to discontinue cigarette smoking and the use of aspirin. Other gastric irritants, such as alcohol, should also be avoided. Antacids or cimetidine should be used in the same doses as recommended for the treatment of duodenal ulcer. Therapy should be continued until complete healing of the ulcer has been documented. Evaluation (X-rays or endoscopy) should be made at 6 weeks following initial identification of the ulcer and, if the ulcer persists, again at 12 weeks. If the ulcer persists despite 3 months of medical therapy, the physician should again make certain, by endoscopy, that the lesion is benign. If the ulcer is felt to be benign, the decision to continue medical therapy is generally based on the patient's clinical condition, the degree of healing that has already occurred, and the risks of complications and recurrences *versus* the risk of surgery.

Maintenance Therapy

Patients with peptic ulcer disease should be made aware that ulcers frequently recur, and that the propensity to form new ulcers persists for a long, but probably not indeterminate, period of time. Theoretically, if one could safely reduce the frequency of these recurrences, one could markedly reduce the morbidity and complication rates of ulcer disease. Cimetidine and anticholinergics have both been investigated in this regard. Several studies have confirmed the preventive role of maintenance cimetidine therapy in doses ranging from 400 mg at bedtime to 400 mg twice a day. The cumulative recurrence rate for patients maintained on placebo, after documented healing of the index duodenal ulcer, was 83% over a 1-year period compared to 18% on cimetidine maintenance therapy (1). Thus, the frequency of symptomatic and asymptomatic, but endoscopically identified, recurrences can be markedly reduced by such therapy. Sucralfate and ranitidine are as effective as is cimetidine in this regard. The long term benefit and safety of such therapy remain unresolved. Anticholinergics, given at full doses, also reduce the incidence of symptomatic recurrences.

Even though maintenance therapy is effective, the indications for it are still unclear. In most studies, patients with recurrent ulcers tend to have severe long-standing ulcer disease. It is certainly possible that in many other patients, the risk of recurrence is relatively low, and the need for preventive measures may not be as great. Long term safety of treatment is still of some concern. Thus, maintenance therapy is probably not indicated in all patients after their first ulcer but should be reserved for the patient with severe disease, manifest by complications (e.g., recurrent hemorrhage) or frequent symptomatic recurrences. In such patients, therapy with, for example, cimetidine, 400 mg at bedtime or twice a day for 1 year, may be indicated. Further evaluation of this problem is still needed.

SURGICAL THERAPY

Surgery is effective therapy for the relief of ulcer symptoms and for the prevention of ulcer recurrence. While certain postoperative problems are common, the vast majority of patients feel significantly better after surgery. Thus, in the appropriate setting, surgery should be considered as a good and effective alternative form of therapy, rather than as a punishment for failure to respond to medical therapy.

Indications

The indications for ulcer surgery are perforation, uncontrolled hemorrhage, gastric outlet obstruction, and intractability. At times, obviously, surgery is performed as an emergency, but often it is performed after a prolonged period of symptomatic ulcer disease. Intractability is probably the weakest indication for ulcer surgery, although it may be the one most commonly used. It should be recognized that intractability may be due to the disease itself, to the

patient's noncompliance with an appropriate medical regimen, or to insufficient medical therapy provided by the clinician. Thorough review with the patient of maximal medical therapy as outlined above will help to delineate the cause for the refractoriness of medical therapy.

Prior to surgery, except for emergency situations, some preoperative assessment should be made to rule out Zollinger-Ellison syndrome (see below) and hypercalcemia.

Types of Operations

Various operations are available for the treatment of ulcer disease. The physician should discuss with the surgeon the various alternatives and reach an agreement about which operation may be best suited for the individual patient. Of course, the final decision is generally made by the surgeon in the operating room after he has evaluated the gastroduodenal area. The patient should also be educated about the rationale for the planned surgical approach and what the expected outcome is.

Duodenal Ulcer

For duodenal ulcer disease, surgery involves a vagotomy plus either a drainage procedure or a concomitant gastric resection. Vagotomy is indicated as it reduces basal acid secretion and reduces the sensitivity of the parietal cells to various stimuli, including gastrin. There are three types of vagal resections: (a) truncal, (b) gastric (selective), and (c) proximal gastric (parietal cell or superselective). *Truncal vagotomy* involves division of the main vagal fibers as they pass through the esophageal hiatus. All other abdominal organs that are innervated by the vagus nerve, in addition to the stomach, are therefore affected by this form of vagotomy. In addition, the vagotomy interferes with antral motility and gastric emptying. Thus, to prevent gastric stasis, a drainage procedure (pyloroplasty) is required in conjunction with this type of operation.

Selective or gastric vagotomy was introduced in order to avoid the unnecessary effect of the truncal vagotomy on extragastric sites. Selective vagotomy is effective in reducing acid secretion. However, as it impairs gastric emptying, a drainage procedure must be employed with this operation also. The loss of control of gastric emptying and the ablation of the pyloric sphincter are themselves major causes for various postgastrectomy complications. As a result the usefulness of selective vagotomy is limited.

Proximal gastric or parietal cell vagotomy is an attempt to inhibit acid secretion only and to avoid significant disruption of normal gastric motility. The operation involves cutting of the vagal branches innervating the body of the stomach but preserving the antral fibers. Thus, with a properly performed operation a drainage procedure is believed to be unnecessary. As a result, this type of operation, which does not involve any gastric resection or formation of an anastomosis, has a very low mortality rate, avoids early postoperative complications, such as suture breakdown and fistulization, and significantly reduces postgastrectomy complications, such as diarrhea and the dumping syndrome (see below). Early experience, or perhaps inexperience, with this procedure has resulted in an ulcer recurrence rate that approaches that of a truncal vagotomy and pyloroplasty—about 6 to 8%—and in some cases even exceeds that level. However, it certainly appears that as surgeons become more experienced and skilled with this procedure, parietal cell vagotomy will become the procedure of choice for ulcer disease.

Currently, two of the most commonly employed operations are *vagotomy plus pyloroplasty* (V + P), and *vagotomy plus antrectomy* (V + A). Some surgeons extend the antrectomy (distal 20% of the stomach) to a hemigastrectomy (resection of 50% of the stomach). The advantages of V + P are that it is technically an easier procedure and is associated with a lower mortality rate (less than 1%). The major disadvantage is a higher ulcer recurrence rate (6 to 8%). Vagotomy plus resection is technically more time consuming and involves formation of an anastomosis; therefore, it may cause a higher immediate postoperative morbidity, as well as a higher mortality rate. However, when performed by an experienced surgeon electively on a stable patient, the reported mortality is only 1% and the recurrence rate is also 1% or less. Thus, in the elderly unstable patient, V + P may be the most appropriate procedure. However, in the young patient, the concern over the rate of recurrent disease is an important consideration, and V + A may then be the most appropriate form of surgery.

Gastric Ulcer

For gastric ulcers the type of surgery is less certain since our understanding of the condition is less clear. In contrast to duodenal ulcer disease a vagotomy may not be indicated in all patients with a gastric ulcer who undergo surgery. However, in patients who have evidence of concomitant duodenal ulcer disease (approximately 10 to 40% of patients with gastric ulcers) and in patients who have pyloric ulcers, which generally behave as duodenal ulcers, a vagotomy is clearly indicated. If the ulcer is within the antrum, an antrectomy or hemigastrectomy that includes the ulcer is frequently the preferred operation. When the ulcer cannot be included in the gastric resection, a full thickness biopsy of the ulcer should be taken for frozen section to rule out malignancy. The recurrence rate for gastric ulcers after these types of operation is very low (1 to 2%).

Following antrectomy or hemigastrectomy, the stomach may be anastomosed to the duodenum (Bilroth I anastomosis) or to the jejunum (Bilroth II).

The type of anastomosis is determined by the surgeon based on the degree of duodenal deformity and on technical considerations.

Postgastrectomy Syndromes

A wide variety of problems develop in the postgastrectomy state (Table 36.3). In 10% of patients, the postgastrectomy complications are severe. Many of these conditions result from the altered physiology created by the surgery. An appreciation of the pathophysiology of these problems is important to their overall management.

Postcibal Symptoms: Pain, Vomiting, Early Satiety; and the Dumping Syndrome

The most common complaints of the postgastrectomy patient are early satiety and postcibal vomiting, frequently accompanied by epigastric pain. These complaints occur commonly (25 to 60% of patients in various series, usually within 3 or 4 months) in both vagotomized and nonvagotomized patients who have undergone either simple drainage procedures or more extensive gastric resections. The exact cause of these problems is not known.

There is evidence to suggest that postcibal complications are related to the entry of fluid into the small bowel. The timing of these symptoms occurs at periods coincident with the transit of solutions from the stomach into the intestine (first 30 minutes following a meal). Distension of the proximal bowel may produce many of the same symptoms. Vomiting, when it occurs, is usually of small volume and is bile stained. Vagotomy inhibits the fundic relaxation that occurs with swallowing food. As the stomach fails to distend, liquids, in particular, are emptied into the small bowel more rapidly, resulting in distension of the intestine as well as in a rapid delivery of hypertonic fluids.

The postprandial complaints may be associated with vasomotor phenomena, such as light-headedness, diaphoresis, and postural hypotension. The

Table 36.3.
Range of Reported Prevalence (Percent) of Various Problems after Ulcer Surgery[a,b]

Problem	V + P	V + A	STG-BII	STG-BI
Gastrointestinal symptoms (excluding diarrhea)	25–65	34–63	3–51	40
Hypoglycemic symptoms	6–12	4–16	1–12	
Diarrhea	16–30	1–43	2–17	18
Weight loss	5–39	10–42	25–44	36
Anemia	3–18	7	9–44	17
Bone disease			1–13	

[a] From Meyer J: Chronic morbidity after ulcer surgery. *Gastrointestinal Disease*. Philadelphia, WB Saunders, 1978, p 960.
[b] V + P, vagotomy plus pyloroplasty; V + A, vagotomy plus antrectomy; STG-BII, subtotal gastrectomy with Bilroth-II anastomosis; STG-BI, subtotal gastrectomy with Bilroth-I anastomosis.

combination of these vasomotor conditions and the above alimentary complaints is commonly referred to as "the dumping syndrome." The pathogenesis of this syndrome is unknown. However, current concepts center around the effect of various hormones (serotonin, gastric inhibitory peptide) which can induce experimentally similar vasomotor phenomena. These hormones may be released by intestinal distension and/or the influx of hypertonic solutions into the jejunum. In addition, hypertonic solutions may draw excess fluid into the intestinal lumen, causing hypovolemia. However, the role that transient hypovolemia plays in the dumping syndrome is uncertain, as prevention of it does not regularly prevent symptoms of the syndrome.

Management of this condition is aimed at slowing gastric emptying and avoiding hypertonic solutions and overdistension of the intestine. The patient should be instructed to eat frequent small meals that are high in protein and low in carbohydrates. It is important that patients do not drink while eating a meal, as liquids accelerate gastric emptying. Lying down after a meal may be helpful because it slows down gastric emptying and may also reduce the intensity of the vasomotor symptoms.

The postcibal complaints must be differentiated from other postoperative causes of epigastric pain and vomiting. Afferent loop obstruction, gastric outlet obstruction, recurrent ulcerations at the anastomosis, and reflux gastritis all must be considered in the patient who complains of postprandial pain and vomiting. *Partial afferent loop obstruction* is an uncommon complication but deserves special attention because it is surgically remediable. Pain occurs as the obstructed afferent limb distends with pancreatic and biliary secretions that are increased in volume following a meal. Vomiting is typically bilious and contains little if any food. The diagnosis can be made by the radiographic demonstration of a dilated limb that is slow to empty. During endoscopy it may be impossible to pass the endoscope into the afferent loop. When the diagnosis is established, surgical revision is necessary.

Gastric outlet obstruction, on the other hand, is usually associated with vomiting of a large volume of undigested food. X-ray studies and endoscopy can demonstrate the nature of the obstruction. It may be caused by scarring or by surgical deformity at the anastomosis as well as by recurrent ulcerations.

Anastomotic ulcers should be considered as a potential cause for postprandial pain and vomiting. They may occur at any time after the operation— even years later. The preoperative history of pain-food-relief no longer applies to anastomotic ulcers. Conventional X-ray studies in the postgastrectomy state usually do not identify these marginal ulcers. Air contrast studies and, preferably, endoscopy are more sensitive in the detection of these recurrent lesions (see page 452).

With loss or bypass of the pyloric sphincter, bile can reflux freely into the stomach, an event that is routinely seen on endoscopy in the patient after gastrectomy. It is believed, with some experimental data as support, that chronic perfusion of the gastric mucosa with bile leads to acute and possibly chronic *gastritis*. However, the correlation between the severity of the symptoms and the severity of the gross and microscopic appearance of the gastritis is very poor. Perianastomotic gastritis is commonly seen on endoscopy whether or not the patient has symptoms. Thus, it is sometimes very difficult to be certain that the symptoms of epigastric pain and bilious vomiting are due to the gastritis seen on endoscopy. When the gastritis is severe as judged by endoscopy and histological evaluation, and no other cause or explanation for the symptoms is apparent, the diagnosis of bile gastritis (alkaline or reflux gastritis) is usually made. Various kinds of treatment have been proposed for this difficult condition. Medical therapy is of unproven value. Most patients are hypochlorhydric, and further effort to reduce acid secretion by cimetidine or antacids is rarely helpful. Amphojel, an aluminum hydroxide-containing antacid (Table 36.2), binds bile salts and has been advocated as potentially useful in this condition, but there are few data to support that contention. Similarly, cholestyramine, a resin which binds bile salts, is of no benefit. In isolated reports, some patients are said to have benefited from metaclopramide (Reglan), a smooth muscle stimulant which improves gastric emptying, but, again, the value of this drug for this condition is uncertain. Surgery has provided the most consistently beneficial results in patients with bile gastritis. Formation of a Roux-en-Y anastomosis with diversion of the bile away from the stomach is often very effective. Thus, in the select patient with a troublesome condition, a second operation to divert the bile downstream may be necessary.

Diarrhea

Chronic diarrhea occurs in 10 to 40% of patients following ulcer surgery, usually within 3 to 4 months of the operation. It is much less common when only a parietal cell vagotomy is performed. In some studies, the severity and prevalence of the diarrhea have decreased with time after the initial surgery, but in the prospective VA study on ulcer surgery there was no difference in the prevalence of the diarrhea at 2 and 5 years postoperatively (12). Multiple factors have been suggested as causes for the diarrhea, and in some patients, several factors may be working in concert. Causes for the diarrhea that are related to the ulcer surgery include (a) increase in fecal bile acids. (b) rapid gastric emptying, (c) rapid intestinal transit, (d) lactose intolerance, (e) development of malabsorption (f) gastrocolic fistula, (g) Zollinger-Ellison syndrome, and (h) inadvertent gastroileal anastomosis. The evaluation of chronic diarrhea in general is discussed in Chapter 38.

Increased loss of bile acids into the colon has been

reported in a number of series of patients after gastrectomy. Bile salts, when they reach the colon, may promote mucosal secretions that lead to diarrhea. Clinically, many postgastrectomy patients with diarrhea have responded to cholestyramine, which binds bile salts. This abnormality in the handling of bile salts has been attributed to the vagotomy and therefore is often referred to as "postvagotomy diarrhea." The mechanism by which the vagotomy alters bile absorption or secretion is unknown.

Rapid gastric emptying may contribute to the diarrhea in several ways. The effects of the delivery of the hypertonic volume to the small intestine have been discussed above in association with the dumping syndrome. In addition, patients with latent lactose intolerance may develop diarrhea as their low level of the intestinal enzyme, lactase, is overwhelmed by the rapid delivery of a lactose load. Thus, lactose-restricted diets may also be beneficial in such patients.

Significant *malabsorption* (greater than 12 to 15% fecal fat excretion) is a rare complication of the postgastrectomy state. Mild degrees of steatorrhea are common, however, resulting from poor mixing of food with pancreatic and biliary secretions, rapid transit, and maldigestion of foodstuffs. Additionally, bacterial overgrowth may occur in the afferent loop. Rarely, a patient with latent celiac disease may be revealed by ulcer surgery.

The evaluation of malabsorption and diarrhea is discussed in detail in Chapter 38. Pancreatic insufficiency may be difficult to diagnose in the setting of a Bilroth II operation and therapeutic trials of pancreatic enzymes may be needed. X-ray studies may disclose a gastrojejunal-colonic fistula that leads to diarrhea and, frequently, to feculent vomiting. The Zollinger-Ellison syndrome (see below) should be considered in any patient with coexisting ulcer disease and diarrhea. When significant malabsorption is present, a bile salt breath test and small bowel biopsy are indicated to look for bacterial overgrowth and for primary bowel disease such as sprue (see Chapter 38).

Therapeutically, any or all of the following may be beneficial, depending on the results of evaluation of the diarrhea: (a) lactose-restricted diet, (b) treatment for dumping syndrome and rapid gastric emptying with small frequent feedings and with liquids taken only between meals, (c) trial of cholestyramine—one scoop (4 g) four times a day, which often can be reduced to a lower dosage once the diarrhea is controlled, and (d) antidiarrheal medications, like Lomotil or Imodium taken with meals to decrease the intestinal rush. The symptomatic treatment of diarrhea is discussed also in Chapter 38.

Weight Loss

Weight loss occurs in 30 to 40% of patients after ulcer surgery. While it is generally believed that weight loss is more common or more significant after subtotal gastrectomy than after vagotomy and drainage, the results of prospective surgical series are conflicting. It is important to recognize, however, that as with most postgastrectomy problems, weight loss is not strictly correlated with a reduction in the size of the stomach.

The most common cause of weight loss is a reduction in caloric intake. Patients may eat less following surgery because of (a) early satiety, (b) symptoms of the dumping syndrome, (c) postprandial abdominal pain, and (d) attempts to avoid postprandial diarrhea. The mechanisms and management of these postprandial problems are discussed above. It is important to review these aspects of the postgastrectomy state with the patient to identify the factors contributing to the weight loss. Encouraging the patient to consume small feedings and even to supplement his diet with high caloric additives, such as Ensure or Precision, may be helpful.

Other causes for significant weight loss include (a) malabsorption, (b) development of a gastrojejunal-colic fistula and (c) development of a carcinoma in the gastric remnant. While malabsorption is common following ulcer surgery, it is usually minimal. Fecal excretion of fat rarely exceeds 15% of oral intake after V + P or even after subtotal gastrectomy with gastrojejunostomy. Nitrogen loss also does not play a significant role. An increase in oral intake by 10% would compensate for the degree of fecal loss of fat and nitrogen. Infrequently, the steatorrhea exceeds 15% and contributes to significant weight loss. Causes for this degree of malabsorption include (a) celiac sprue unmasked by the gastric surgery, (b) pancreatic insufficiency, and (c) bacterial overgrowth. As these conditions require specific therapy, in the patient with significant weight loss (greater than 10% of preoperative weight), malabsorption should be documented by measurement of fecal fat excretion over a 72-hour period. When greater than 12 to 15% excretion is found, patients should be evaluated for these specific causes of malabsorption. Consultation with a gastroenterologist is recommended under these circumstances. A small bowel biopsy and evaluation for bacterial overgrowth (bile salt breath test (Chapter 38), Schilling test (Chapter 38), or quantification of intestinal bacteria) will usually be performed.

Anemia

Anemia may occur following any of the traditional operations used in treatment of peptic ulcer disease; the prevalence is somewhat higher after gastrojejunostomy (9 to 44%) compared to other operations (less than 20%). The anemia occurs gradually, usually several years postoperatively. By far the most common cause is iron deficiency due to chronic blood loss, secondary to recurrent ulcer disease or, more often, to stomal gastritis. Much less commonly, macrocytic anemia, due to folate or vitamin B_{12}

deficiency, occurs—folate deficiency because of poor intake in anorectic patients or to malabsorption (see above); B_{12} deficiency because of loss of intrinsic factor-secreting parietal cells in patients with high subtotal gastrectomies or because of malabsorption due to bacterial overgrowth in the small intestine. (The diagnosis and treatment of macrocytic anemia are discussed in Chapter 49.)

Recurrent Ulcer

Recurrent ulceration following ulcer surgery is uncommon. However, management of this complication is often difficult and frequently requires a second operative procedure. Recurrences commonly occur within the first 2 years after the initial surgery but may occur many years later. The type of initial surgery influences the rate of recurrence, with less than a 1% recurrence rate after vagotomy and resection, 6 to 8% after vagotomy plus pyloroplasty, and up to 36% after resection of less than two-thirds of the stomach without vagotomy. Recurrence rate after parietal cell vagotomy is reported to be anywhere from 0 to 25%. The recurrent ulcers occur near the anastomosis, most commonly on the intestinal side.

The cardinal features of recurrent ulcer are abdominal pain, weight loss, and gastrointestinal bleeding. The pain is often in the left upper quadrant or to the left of the epigastrium. The relationship of the pain to meals is variable; it may actually be exacerbated by eating so that food is avoided and marked loss of weight ensues. Bleeding occurs in two-thirds of patients and may present as an overt gastrointestinal hemorrhage. Nausea and vomiting are frequent nonspecific findings. The recurrent ulcer with its attendant edema may lead to gastric outlet obstruction or even to afferent loop obstruction. A dramatic presentation is that of feculent vomiting with severe diarrhea, indicative of the formation of a gastrojejunal-colic fistula.

The diagnosis can be confirmed by radiographic and endoscopic studies. Single contrast upper gastrointestinal series, however, reveal anastomotic ulcers in only 50% of cases in which they are present. Air contrast X-rays may improve this yield. Endoscopy is the most sensitive technique and distinguishes between recurrent ulcerations and severe gastritis.

An evaluation must be made of the underlying cause of the recurrent ulcer. The most common cause is an inadequate surgical procedure (15). In some patients, an incomplete (or no) vagotomy has been performed, while in others inadequate gastric resection has been done. In cases where the recurrent ulcer develops on the gastric side of the anastomosis, inadequate drainage or gastric emptying should be considered. Zollinger-Ellison syndrome (see below) should always be considered, as over one-fourth of patients with this syndrome have al-

ready undergone at least one ulcer operation before the appropriate diagnosis is made.

In patients with a recurrent gastric ulcer, special consideration should be given to the possibility of a gastric malignancy and endoscopy should be performed routinely.

Both medical and surgical therapy have their place in the management of the postoperative recurrent ulcer. Therapy with antacids is not very successful. However, cimetidine has been demonstrated to heal anastomotic ulcers effectively in a small group of patients (4); the long term course of these patients is still unknown.

A second operation is at times required to control the ulcer disease. The type of reoperation is frequently determined by the initial operation, with risk of recurrences still a problem. As a general rule, repeat vagotomy and gastric resection are required, with more limited operations resulting in a high frequency of a second recurrence. For patients with an initial adequate resection (two-thirds gastrectomy), a repeat abdominal or even a thoracic vagotomy may be all that is needed.

Gastric irradiation may be an alternative for the inoperable patient as it may result in reduction in acid secretion for about 6 months and allow the ulcer to heal. The consultant gastroenterologist should advise the generalist in this regard.

Bone Disease

Defects in bone formation and metabolism may occur after ulcer surgery. Osteomalacia and osteoporosis have been reported, but are rare, following vagotomy and drainage procedures. Fractures are more common in the postgastrectomy patient. Malabsorption of vitamin D and/or calcium is believed to be responsible for the bone disease. Patients generally present with recurrent fractures or with back pain due to a collapsed vertebra. Therapy includes supplemental calcium or vitamin D. While the incidence of symptoms is low, this problem may accentuate other conditions that also lead to osteoporosis such as in postmenopausal women or in patients taking corticosteroids.

Carcinoma in the Gastric Remnant

The development of gastric carcinoma years after ulcer surgery has only recently been recognized. In reported series, the carcinoma develops more than 15 years following the initial surgery (8). It is difficult to ascertain the true risk of this rare complication as many of these patients are now elderly and are therefore at an age when the incidence of gastric carcinoma in the general population is at its peak. It is believed that as a result of gastric surgery there is constant free reflux of bile into the stomach. This enterogastric reflux has been shown in animals to result in alterations in the gastric mucosa, gradually evolving from chronic to atrophic gastritis and then to neoplastic changes. Similarly, in patients, one can demonstrate chronic gastritis around the anastomosis. It is in this area that most of the gastric remnant carcinomas develop. The clinical features include abdominal pain, weight loss, and bleeding. The diagnosis is often difficult because the radiographic appearance of the "normal" gastric remnant frequently consists of hyperplastic folds and irregularity of the anastomosis. Endoscopy with biopsy may be the most helpful means of recognizing the carcinomatous changes. The prognosis is reported to be poor in this type of gastric cancer.

ZOLLINGER-ELLISON SYNDROME

The Zollinger-Ellison syndrome represents dramatically the relationship between gastrin, acid secretion, and ulcer formation. The syndrome results from a non-β islet cell tumor of the pancreas that autonomously secretes gastrin and is therefore called a *gastrinoma*. In the majority of cases there are multiple tumors, most commonly found in the head of the pancreas. They vary considerably in size from several millimeters, often undetectable at surgery, to huge masses that may even be palpable through the abdominal wall. Approximately two-thirds of gastrinomas are malignant in their biological behavior and histological appearance; they can metastasize and be a cause of death, although generally they are slow growing.

With the introduction of readily available measurement of gastrin, the concept of the clinical features of the Zollinger-Ellison syndrome has begun to change. The original description of the syndrome focused on the virulent nature of the ulcer diathesis and on the atypical location for the ulcers. It is now recognized, however, that 75% of ulcers in patients with Zollinger-Ellison syndrome occur in the duodenal bulb and appear as routine single duodenal ulcers. The finding, however, of postbulbar and jejunal ulcerations should alert the physician to the possibility of the syndrome. Over one-quarter of patients undergo ulcer surgery before the diagnosis of the syndrome, which is usually made only when anastomotic ulcers develop. Diarrhea is another frequent symptom, occurring in more than one-third of patients, which may precede the formation of ulcers by several years; however, 7% of patients have diarrhea and never develop an ulcer.

Diagnosis

The diagnosis of the Zollinger-Ellison syndrome should be suspected under the following conditions: (a) failure of medical therapy, resulting in the need for ulcer surgery: (b) giant ulcer; (c) multiple ulcers; (d) postbulbar or jejunal ulcers; (e) anastomotic ulcer; (f) ulcer disease in association with diarrhea (but not diarrhea secondary to drugs); and (g) radio-

graphic or secretory evidence of gastric hypersecretion.

The diagnosis of the Zollinger-Ellison syndrome is usually based on the fasting serum gastrin concentration. Elevations greater than 1000 pg/ml in association with the typical clinical picture are nearly diagnostic of a gastrinoma.

However, in patients with mild elevations of the serum gastrin concentration (i.e., between 150 and 300 pg/ml) and in postoperative patients, differentiation between Zollinger-Ellison syndrome and other causes for hypergastrinemia is important. Consultation with a gastroenterologist is advisable. Other conditions that may lead to hypergastrinemia include (a) retained antrum, (b) G-cell hyperplasia, (c) postvagotomy plus pyloroplasty, (d) small portion of the population with routine duodenal ulcer disease, and (e) pernicious anemia.

Differentiation of these disorders from the Zollinger-Ellison syndrome requires the use of provocative tests, the secretin and calcium infusion tests, generally performed by a gastroenterologist. The secretin test is preferred because it is more reliable and is safer. In both tests, the response of the serum gastrin level to the infusion of a stimulating substance is monitored. In the *secretin test*, the serum gastrin level rises, usually within the first ½ hour, after the injection of secretin in patients with Zollinger-Ellison syndrome, whereas in all other disorders the gastrin level falls or is unchanged.

In the *calcium infusion test*, serum gastrin determinations are made immediately before and then repeatedly for 4 hours after the intravenous administration of calcium. In all conditions, the gastrin level increases. However, in the Zollinger-Ellison syndrome, the response is exaggerated with a greater than 50% rise over basal levels.

Gastric analysis (see above, page 442) may provide further supportive data. Marked hypersecretion is found in both the basal state and following pentagastrin stimulation. Since the stomach is being influenced by an autonomous tumor, further stimulation with exogenous pentagastrin provides little additional stimulation to secretion. Thus, the BAO/MAO ratio is 0.6 or greater in this syndrome. However, there is considerable overlap with normal values so that the gastric secretory data alone cannot be used to make the diagnosis.

Various attempts have been made to localize the gastrinoma in the hope that excision of an isolated tumor would be curative. Unfortunately, such efforts have not been successful since multiple tumors are frequently present; small lesions are undetectable by surgical inspection of the pancreas; and these tumors frequently have metastasized by the time surgical exploration is performed. The use of selective pancreatic venography with measurements of gastrin levels from each venous site may provide an improved method to localize the gastrinoma.

Therapy

Because the tumor mass is rarely localized and curable by local resection, therapy has been directed at the end organ. Total gastrectomy has been the procedure of choice. While there is little evidence to suggest that gastrectomy alters the biological behavior of the gastrinoma, it does prevent the consequences of the hypersecretion of acid. In the past, patients died from this condition most often because of the virulent nature of the ulcer diathesis, including frequent recurrences, diarrhea, and even malabsorption, as well as multiple operations. Complete removal of the end organ prevents these complications.

More recently, medical therapy has been successful in controlling the ulcer disease and the diarrhea. Cimetidine, a histamine (H_2) receptor antagonist, is capable of inhibiting gastric acid secretion in response to a variety of stimuli (see page 445). For most patients with gastrinoma, the standard dose of cimetidine, 1200 mg/day, is sufficient to control acid production. In a small percentage, increased doses of cimetidine or the addition of an anticholinergic drug is needed. Such medically treated patients are, obviously, required to take medications frequently and for many years, probably the rest of their lives. While this may be a major disadvantage in some patients, it is important to recognize that medical therapy can provide an effective alternative to total gastrectomy (10). Even if surgery is performed, medical therapy can provide time to stabilize the patient, to correct nutritional deficiencies, and to allow the surgery to be performed on an elective basis.

DYSPEPSIA WITHOUT ULCERATION

Dyspepsia is a syndrome of persistent or recurrent epigastric discomfort, often related to meals, that is frequently associated with nausea, belching, and bloating. Patients with dyspepsia can be classified into one of two groups: (a) patients whose symptoms, typical of peptic ulcer disease, are intermittent and have a predictable relationship to meals (i.e., reproducibly either relieved by eating (the usual response) or aggravated by it); and (b) patients whose symptoms are atypical in that they are more persistent but are less predictable—sometimes relieved and other times aggravated by eating. In the first group a peptic ulcer or a scarred duodenal bulb can be found in up to 70% of patients. Those patients who have symptoms, in whom there is neither radiographic nor endoscopic evidence of an ulcer (Moynihan's disease) should be treated, and generally respond, like patients with documented peptic disease (see above).

In patients with atypical symptoms (50 to 60% of all dyspeptic patients) an anatomical cause of the condition will be found less than 25% of the time. Women predominate in this group, in contrast to

patients with documented peptic ulcer disease (see page 445). It is recommended that dyspeptic patients whose symptoms do not suggest peptic ulceration be treated symptomatically (see below) and that diagnostic studies (specifically upper gastrointestinal endoscopy—upper gastrointestinal series is much less likely to be helpful in this setting) be avoided unless (a) there is no response to therapy in 7 to 10 days, (b) symptoms abate partially but persist for 6 to 8 weeks, (c) a complication of peptic ulcer disease develops (e.g., bleeding or perforation), or (d) signs of a severe systemic illness develop (6).

Apart from peptic ulcer disease, three conditions are often considered in the differential diagnosis of dyspepsia: gallstones, gastritis, and motility disorders.

Gallstones

Gallstones are commonly found in dyspeptic patients, but since both gallstones and dyspepsia are common problems in the general population, it is difficult to be certain that gallbladder disease is a cause of dyspepsia. Also, there is no evidence that cholecystectomy is effective in relieving dyspeptic symptoms unless there has been an identifiable episode of acute cholecystitis or a history of biliary colic. Perhaps the most common "cause" of the postcholecystectomy syndrome (see Chapter 90) is the mistaken assumption that gallstones were causing dyspeptic symptoms and that cholecystectomy would relieve those symptoms.

Gastritis

Inflammation of the stomach is a diagnosis that is ordinarily made by endoscopic biopsy and that may be associated with dyspepsia. There are several common types of gastritis.

Acute erosive gastritis is characterized by multiple, small, often hemorrhagic erosions, seen most commonly in patients with acute stressful illness or with overingestion of alcohol or of drugs, especially aspirin. Gastrointestinal bleeding is common in patients with this condition and distinguishes it from most other causes of dyspepsia without ulceration; such bleeding is, of course, an indication for hospitalization.

Chronic nonerosive gastritis is subdivided into three groups—superficial gastritis, atrophic gastritis, and gastric atrophy (an end stage with minimal inflammation). This condition, the cause of which is unknown, is quite common, especially with advancing age. Therefore, whether chronic nonerosive gastritis causes dyspepsia is unclear. There is no current treatment that is effective in changing the gastric histology toward normal or in preventing the development in patients with superficial gastritis of atrophic gastritis (a progression, however, that occurs in only about half of such patients (13)). It is not known whether gastric atrophy invariably begins as superficial or atrophic gastritis, although many think that it does (see also page 450 for a discussion of chronic gastritis postgastrectomy).

Patients with atrophic gastritis and gastric atrophy appear to be more likely to develop *gastric cancer*, although the risk is higher in those parts of the world where the incidence of gastric cancer is relatively high. Patients with gastric atrophy are also at slight risk of developing *pernicious anemia* (see Chapter 49) (many patients with pernicious anemia have gastric atrophy, but only a small number of patients with gastric atrophy have pernicious anemia).

Motility Disorders

In patients with documented abnormal gastroduodenal motility (e.g., gastric atony associated with diabetes mellitus—see Chapter 72) dyspeptic symptoms are common. Many people believe that abnormal motility is the underlying problem in all patients with dyspepsia, just as abnormal colonic motility may be associated with the irritable bowel syndrome—see Chapter 39). Therefore, even though there is no evidence that such a disorder exists, antispasmodic drugs are often prescribed to dyspeptic patients in an attempt to relieve "pylorospasm." Also, metoclopramide (Reglan) is sometimes prescribed to improve the rate of gastric emptying, especially in patients who complain of excessive gaseousness and bloating. Neither regimen has been proven to be effective.

Treatment

Since peptic ulcer disease cannot be entirely excluded, even in patients with atypical symptoms in whom a gastrointestinal series and endoscopy have been negative, a trial for 2 to 3 weeks of an antiulcer regimen is indicated initially (see pages 443–447). Antacids, H$_2$ receptor antagonists, or sucralfate may be effective in isolated cases, but there is no way to predict which dyspeptic patient will respond except to say that the more the history suggests peptic ulcer disease, the more likely there will be a response to an antiulcer regimen.

Nausea is best treated with a phenothiazine, even though significant side effects may occur (see Chapter 16). Sedation and anticholinergic symptoms are common but usually abate in a few weeks; drug-induced Parkinson's syndrome is uncommon with the dosages used to treat nausea. Chlorpromazine (Thorazine), 10 to 25 mg 30 to 60 minutes before meals, or prochlorperazine (Compazine), 5 to 10 mg orally 30 to 60 minutes before meals or a 25-mg suppository each morning, is a reasonable regimen. Treatment can be discontinued when symptoms abate.

Belching and *bloating* are most often due to air swallowing (aerophagia). Patients should be told about that since they often are unaware that they are swallowing air. They should be advised that with each swallow, air is also swallowed, and that, therefore, they should try to swallow less often. The following instructions may be useful: (a) Eat slowly and take small bites (b) Drink liquid only at the end of the meal. (c) Do not drink from a straw. (d) Do not chew gum or suck on hard candy. (e) Do not smoke. (f) Avoid apples (they contain large amounts of air), carbonated beverages, and any other food that causes symptoms. (g) Fix loosely fitting dentures. Various over-the-counter measures (e.g., simethicone) are advertised as reducing the amount of gastrointestinal gas, but they are almost always ineffective.

Dyspeptic patients often ask whether a change in their diet will relieve their symptoms. In general, avoidance of fried or greasy foods, chocolate, onions, and acidic fruits (citrus fruits, tomatoes) may be helpful, but there is considerable variation in response. Known gastric irritants, such as aspirin and alcohol, should be avoided also.

In the long run, reassuring the patient that dyspepsia does not reflect a serious underlying illness is one of the most important things that the physician can do.

General References

Ippoliti A, Peterson W: The pharmacology of peptic ulcer disease. *Clin Gastroenterol* 8:53, 1979.
> Discussion of use of various medications. Provides good comparative analysis.

Thomas J, Misiewicz G: Histamine H$_2$-receptor antagonists in the short and long term treatment of duodenal ulcer. *Clin Gastroenterol* 13:501,1984.
> Comprehensive review.

Specific References

1. Bodemar G, Walan A: Maintenance treatment of recurrent peptic ulcer by cimetidine. *Lancet* 1:403, 1978.
2. Conn HO, Blitzer BL: Non-association of adrenocorticoid therapy and peptic ulcer. *N Engl J Med* 294:473, 1976.
3. Friedman G, Siegelaub AB, Seltzer C: Cigarettes, alcohol, coffee, and peptic ulcer. *N Engl J Med* 290:469, 1974.
4. Gugler R, Lindstaedt H, Miederer S: Cimetidine for anastomotic ulcers after partial gastrectomy. *N Engl J Med* 301:1077 1979.
5. Hanscom D, Buchman E: The follow-up period (V.A. Cooperative Study on Gastric Ulcer). *Gastroenterology* 61:585, 1971.
6. Health and Public Policy Committee, American College of Physicians: Endoscopy in the evaluation of dyspepsia. *Ann Intern Med* 102:266, 1985.
7. Johnston D, Pickford IR, Walker BE, Goligher JC: Highly selective vagotomy for duodenal ulcer: do hypersecretors need antrectomy. *Br Med J* 1:716, 1975.
8. Kobayashi S, Prolla J, Kirsner J: Late gastric carcinoma developing after surgery for benign conditions. *Am J Dig Dis* 15:905, 1970.
9. Korman MG, Hetzel D, Hansky J, et al: Relapse rate of duodenal ulcer after cessation of long-term cimetidine treatment. A double blind controlled study. *Dig Dis Sci* 25:88, 1980.
10. McCarthy D: The place of surgery in the Zollinger-Ellison syndrome. *N Engl J Med* 302:1344, 1980.
11. Peterson WL, Sturdevant RAL, Frankl HD, et al: Healing of duodenal ulcer with an antacid regimen. *N Engl J Med* 297:341, 1977.

12. Postlethwait RW: Five year followup: results of operation for duodenal ulcer. *Surg Gynecol Obstet* 137:387, 1973.
13. Siurala M, Salmi HJ: Long-term follow-up of subjects with superficial gastritis or a normal gastric mucosa. *Scand J Gastroenterol* 6:459, 1971.
14. Sontag S, Graham DY, Belsito A, *et al*: Cimetidine, cigarette smoking, and recurrence of duodenal ulcer. *N Engl J Med* 311:689, 1984.
15. Stabile B, Passaro E: Recurrent peptic ulcer. *Gastroenterology* 70:124, 1976.

CHAPTER THIRTY-SEVEN

Gastrointestinal Bleeding

HAROLD J. TUCKER, M.D.

The presence of blood in the stool is always a significant finding that requires thorough investigation. Gastrointestinal bleeding may present as (*a*) occult blood, (*b*) melena (black stool) or intermittent hematochezia (the passage of overtly bloody stool), and (*c*) massive hemorrhage. The last situation requires immediate hospitalization and, often, emergency diagnostic procedures. (The vomiting of blood, also, almost always dictates immediate hospitalization.) Otherwise, the evaluation of gastrointestinal bleeding often can be performed in an ambulatory setting. Table 37.1 shows the common conditions associated with gastrointestinal bleeding.

TESTS FOR DETECTION OF BLOOD IN STOOL

A variety of tests are available to detect blood in the stool. These tests differ in sensitivity and speci-

ficity and therefore differ in their value as indicators of disease. The three commonly used tests for fecal occult blood are the orthotolidine tablet test (Hematest); the dilute alcoholic solution of guaiac test (guaiac); and the modified guaiac slide test (Hemoccult). These tests depend on the peroxidase activity of hemoglobin and reflect the concentration of hemoglobin in the stool. In "normal" subjects, the hemoglobin concentration of the stool is less than 2 mg of hemoglobin/g of stool as measured by tagged red cell assay. Both the guaiac and Hematest assays are extremely sensitive and may be positive at this normal level of fecal hemoglobin concentration. As a result, the false positive rate for these tests is excessively high, 60 and 30%, respectively; that is, evaluation of a patient with a positive stool guaiac test, for example, will be negative 60% of the time.

However, the Hemoccult slide test, because it is less sensitive, has reduced the false positive rate to as low as 1 to 2% (4). If multiple slides (three pairs) are evaluated, the false negative rate for Hemoccult is similar to that of the other tests, approximately 15 to 20%. Therefore, a positive test for occult blood with the Hemoccult slide test is highly specific for significant bleeding although only moderately sensitive. Since colonic cancers and polyps may bleed intermittently, multiple specimens should be evaluated. In patients over the age of 40 with at least one positive slide test, about 15% have carcinoma, and another 30% have polyps greater than 5 mm in length (3); left-sided lesions are detected more often than are right-sided ones. In asymptomatic patients with a positive slide test who have carcinoma, over 80% have lesions limited to the bowel (3). Thus, a

Table 37.1.
Common Causes of Gastrointestinal Bleeding

OCCULT BLEEDING
  Colonic polyps
  Colonic cancer
  Peptic ulcer disease
  Gastric cancer
MELENA
  Duodenal ulcer
  Gastric ulcer
  Gastritis
  Gastric carcinoma
  Esophagitis
HEMATOCHEZIA
  Rectal outlet disorders (hemorrhoids, cryptitis, fissures)
  Colonic polyps
  Colonic cancer
  Diverticulosis
  Inflammatory bowel disease
  Angiodysplasia

positive Hemoccult test for occult blood in the stool requires further investigation.

More reliable methods for detecting fecal blood are under investigation (1).

Laxatives increase both the number of positive and false positive results of the Hemoccult test (probably by an irritant effect on the normal colonic mucosa and on colonic lesions—such as cancer). For this reason, many screening programs have recommended a high bulk diet for several days before the stool is tested in the hope of maximizing the discovery of occult lesions. False negative results are more likely in patients taking high doses of vitamin C. False positive tests may result from peroxidase-rich foods (rare red meat, and uncooked vegetables like broccoli, turnips, and cauliflower) and from iron salicylates and nonsteroidal anti-inflammatory agents. Rehydration of the fecal material also increases the false positive rate and is not recommended.

The optimal number and the timing of the collection of stool samples have not yet been determined. The object is to detect bleeding from lesions that are known to bleed sporadically. Because compliance is a major factor in this screening test, convenience for the patient is important. Therefore, the recommendation is to obtain two different samples from three different stools over a 3-day period once a year. Patients should avoid raw red meat, high doses of vitamin C and aspirin for 3 days before and during the 3 days of testing. Other changes in the diet do not seem to improve the results of the test and do reduce compliance. The stool slides can be stored up to 6 days if necessary without a decrease in the sensitivity of the test.

EVALUATION OF PATIENTS WHO HAVE GASTROINTESTINAL BLEEDING
Choosing Appropriate Tests

The history and physical examination direct the sequence of the various tests used to investigate a patient with gastrointestinal bleeding. The patient's age, the nature of associated symptoms, and the severity of bleeding are all important factors. For example, patients with peptic symptoms (Chapter 36) require an initial evaluation of their stomach and duodenum, while patients with a change in bowel habits require an initial evaluation of their colon. In general, patients under the age of 35 are less likely to have a colonic lesion than are patients over 35. Peptic disease and benign rectal lesions are more evenly distributed in adults of all ages.

In asymptomatic patients with occult fecal blood or in patients with hematochezia but with no other symptoms, the lower bowel should be investigated first. In patients with melena but with no other symptoms, the upper gastrointestinal tract should be investigated first. The more precise sequence in which the tests are done is described below.

Lower Gastrointestinal Tract

Proctosigmoidoscopy should always be the first test done in the evaluation of the lower bowel; it should be followed by an air contrast barium enema (see below). In patients over the age of 35, colonoscopy should be the next test, even if the barium enema is negative.

The finding of hemorrhoids, polyps, or even a rectal cancer on proctoscopy does not obviate the need for a barium study. However, if the pattern of bleeding is consistent with rectal disease (see Chapter 91), if a rectal lesion is seen during proctoscopy, and if the colonic mucosa is well visualized by barium enema and is normal, colonoscopy is not necessary. Also, diverticulosis (see Chapter 40), found on barium enema, should not be considered the cause of intermittent mild hematochezia until colonoscopy has failed to provide another explanation.

Proctosigmoidoscopy

Anorectal lesions either cannot be visualized or are poorly visualized by barium enema. Cryptitis, bleeding hemorrhoids, fissures, and proctitis can only be seen by proctoscopy; and rectal polyps or cancer are much better seen by proctoscopy than by a barium enema. The preparation of the patient for this procedure and the patient's experience during the procedure are described in Chapter 35.

Flexible sigmoidoscopy is a relatively new procedure used to evaluate the descending colon. It is better tolerated and identifies more lesions than does rigid proctosigmoidoscopy. It has limited value, however, in patients with gastrointestinal bleeding, as colonoscopy is still required to evaluate the possibility of more proximal colonic lesions.

Radiological Studies

The barium enema is a valuable test in the detection of colonic lesions. Even in patients with suspected anorectal disease, the barium enema is indicated to rule out other lesions, particularly in patients at high risk for polyps and cancer. The barium enema may also detect diverticula, inflammatory bowel disease, strictures, extraluminal masses or intramural filling defects from endometriosis or from metastatic tumor.

The *double (air) contrast barium* technique is preferred in the search for a colonic source of bleeding. This technique has the advantage over the conventional single contrast barium enema in providing much better detail of the mucosa. One study showed that single contrast technique missed as many as 45% of polyps compared to 12% missed by air contrast (8). Early changes of inflammatory bowel disease are also detectable by this technique. However, because of the risk of perforation, the double contrast barium enema should not be requested in patients suspected of having an obstructing lesion or diverticulitis.

Patient experience. The patient's colon must be cleaned before the study can be performed satisfactorily. A reasonable regimen is the ingestion of 2 to 3 liters of liquids as well as a low residue diet (see Table 38.2, Chapter 38) the day before the examination and administration of a laxative, such as 2 to 4 tablespoons of milk of magnesia at night; on the morning of the examination, a sodium phosphate enema (Fleet) is self-administered. This preparation will be effective in about 90% of patients. Patients who are chronically constipated may need 2 days of preparation.

The patient should be told that the barium will be introduced into his rectum, while he lies on his left side on a hard table, through a lubricated plastic enema tip; often a ballon is then inflated around the tip to seal the rectal ampulla. He will then be told to lie on his back while the barium is allowed to flow in, intermittently, under fluoroscopic observation. Frequently, cramping is experienced during this process. After the colon is filled, several films will be taken, with the patient in various positions. The barium will then be evacuated. The films will be developed and an additional film will be taken after evacuation. The entire procedure takes 45 to 60 minutes.

The *air contrast barium enema* differs from the standard technique in that a smaller amount of very dense barium is introduced followed by insufflation of air. All patients experience cramping during this procedure (usually more than is experienced during the standard barium enema), and atropine may be given to inhibit cramping. The patient will be flatulent for several hours after the procedure.

Colonoscopy

Colonoscopy is indicated in patients with gastrointestinal bleeding of suspected colonic origin in whom proctosigmoidoscopy and barium enema have not provided an unequivocal diagnosis. Some gastroenterologists may choose to do colonoscopy prior to doing a barium enema. In patients with polyps, colonoscopy may also provide a way in which the polyps can be removed without major surgery (see below). An experienced endoscopist can reach the cecum in over 90% of cases. The complications from the procedure are mainly perforation and hemorrhage; the overall complication rate for diagnostic colonoscopy is 0.3 to 0.4%, with a mortality rate of 0.02%. If polypectomy is performed, the morbidity rate increases to 1 to 2%, but the mortality rate remains the same (6).

The sensitivity of colonoscopy in experienced hands is much higher than that of even an air contrast barium enema (see above): only 2% of polyps are not diagnosed. In anemic patients with occult bleeding Tedesco *et al* (7) showed that colonoscopy revealed polyps (greater than 5 mm) or cancer in 15% of patients with negative barium enema examinations and that, in patients with rectal bleeding, 34% had a significant lesion (including 11% with cancer) when the barium enema was reported as negative or simply as showing diverticulosis.

Patient experience. Preparation for colonoscopy usually includes a liquid diet for 2 or 3 days and laxatives and enemas (prescribed by the consultant gastroenterologist). Before the procedure, the patient is sedated intravenously (usually with Demerol and Valium). During the procedure, the patient may experience discomfort when the bowel is distended with air for inspection and as the colonoscope is maneuvered through the bowel lumen. The duration of the procedure is variable, depending on the tortuosity of the colon, the presence of disease, and on the skill of the endoscopist; but, on the average it lasts from 30 to 60 minutes.

Upper Gastrointestinal Tract

The sequence of tests performed in evaluation of the upper gastrointestinal tract depends on the diagnosis that is suspected. Usually an upper gastrointestinal series is done first—especially in patients with suspected peptic disease or carcinoma. On the other hand, if an inflammatory process is suspected (esophagitis or gastritis), endoscopy might be done preferentially. If the patient has melena and an upper gastrointestinal series is negative, or reveals a gastric ulcer (Chapter 36) or a tumor, endoscopy should be the next routine procedure. If the upper and lower gastrointestinal tract have been evaluated in a patient with gastrointestinal bleeding, and the studies have been negative, a small bowel series should be considered to investigate the possibility of

Crohn's disease and other disorders that affect mainly the small intestine.

Radiological Studies

The *upper gastrointestinal series* is valuable in the detection of mass lesions in the esophagus and stomach and in identifying gastric and duodenal ulcerations. It is well tolerated, serves as a permanent guide for follow-up evaluation, and is relatively inexpensive. The air contrast technique affords better mucosal detail than the standard study and should be used in the evaluation of gastric and esophageal erosions. The patient's experience during the performance of an upper gastrointestinal series is described in Chapter 36.

The conventional *small bowel series* is very poor at detecting small lesions of the intestine (such as cancer or a leiomyoma). Disorders like Crohn's disease or lymphoma are more likely to be revealed by X-ray (although a definitive diagnosis will only be made by biopsy). These sources of bleeding are relatively uncommon and should be suspected only when the more frequent conditions (peptic ulcer disease, colonic polyps) have been excluded. The patient should be warned that the small bowel series will require him to spend 1 to 5 hours in the radiology waiting room during which time films will be taken every 30 minutes.

Endoscopy

Upper endoscopy is now a widely used and readily available means of investigating gastrointestinal blood loss. This technique not only is more sensitive than are X-rays but also provides a direct means of obtaining specimens for histological examination. Because of the increased sensitivity, endoscopy is indicated even if barium studies have been negative. Endoscopy is usually recommended only after barium X-rays have been done, however, because it is less well tolerated, is associated with more risk, is more costly than X-rays, and it can be avoided if a diagnosis can be made radiologically. Further, it is technically easier to perform endoscopy if the location of a lesion has already been identified by X-ray studies.

Patient experience. Upper endoscopy is an outpatient procedure that usually takes less than 15 minutes. The patient fasts overnight before the procedure. He is sedated with intravenous medication (Valium and Demerol) and his throat is anesthetized wtih a topical anesthetic. Some gagging is common during passage of the endoscope into the esophagus. Under direct vision, biopsies and cytological brushings can be obtained from suspicious lesions and for histological confirmation. Complications include perforation and bleeding but are extremely uncommon. Newer, smaller caliber endoscopes are now available which have greatly improved patient tolerance of the procedure.

SELECTED LESIONS THAT BLEED

The commonest cause of upper gastrointestinal bleeding—peptic disease—is discussed in Chapter 36. Several common causes of lower gastrointestinal bleeding are discussed in other chapters: benign anorectal disorders (Chapter 92), inflammatory bowel disease (Chapter 38), and diverticulosis (Chapter 40).

Colonic Polyps

Colonic polyps should be suspected in any patient over 30 years of age who has gastrointestinal bleeding. Bleeding may be occult or may occur as intermittent hematochezia. The patient is often totally asymptomatic but may complain of a change in bowel habits, abdominal pain, or of passing mucus per rectum. It is believed that all cancers of the colon (excluding those associated with ulcerative colitis, see Chapter 38) arise from these benign epithelial tumors (5). Thus, the way to prevent colonic cancer is to discover and remove polyps before they have become malignant. Although polyps are most common in the rectosigmoid region, they may be found anywhere in the colon. The detection of a polyp on proctoscopy or on barium enema is an indication for referral to a gastroenterologist.

The risk of polyps becoming malignant is related to their histological type and size. Hyperplastic polyps, the most common type in adults, have no malignant potential. Villous and tubular adenomas, however, carry a definite risk of malignant transformation that increases as they increase in size. The risk that a villous adenoma over 2 cm is cancerous is over 50% (5) (Table 37.2). Fortunately, if the cancer remains confined to the mucosa of the polyp (*carcinoma in situ*), colonoscopic polypectomy is curative. Once the cancer has infiltrated the stalk of the polyp, surgery is indicated. Since the cancerous change in the polyp may be focal, single biopsies of a polyp are not sufficient to exclude the presence of a malignancy.

Once a polyp has been detected, surveillance for additional polyps is essential. In 30% of patients more than one polyp is present at the time of initial investigation. Subsequent development of new polyps occurs in at least 10% of patients. The patient

Table 37.2.
Polyps: Relationship of Size, Histological Type, and Risk of Carcinoma

Histological Type	Size		
	Under 1 cm (%)	1–2 cm (%)	Over 2 cm (%)
Tubular adenoma	1.0	10.2	34.7
Intermediate type	3.9	7.4	45.8
Villous adenoma	9.5	10.3	52.9

should continue to have yearly tests for occult blood in the stool. The finding of a single positive test is an indication for a repeat evaluation. Even when the stools are negative for blood, periodic evaluation of the colon is still recommended. Colonoscopy or air contrast barium enema should be repeated every 3 to 4 years to detect early lesions.

Multiple polyposis syndromes are rare inherited abnormalities which are significant for their malignant potential. Familial polyposis, Gardner's syndrome, and Turcot syndrome all are associated with multiple adenomatous polyps of the colon (Fig. 37.1) and therefore carry a high risk of the development of carcinoma. Gardner's syndrome includes osteomas and soft tissue tumors, and Turcots' syndrome includes tumors of the central nervous system. Familial polyposis and Gardner's syndrome are inherited as an autosomal dominant defect; Turcot syndrome, as an autosomal recessive. The diagnosis of a polyposis syndrome is usually made when the patient is in his twenties, with cancer developing some 20 years later. There is considerable controversy about the therapy of these conditions. Colonic resection is indicated but its extent and timing are not uniformly agreed upon. Ideally, when rectal polyps are present, a proctocolectomy should be

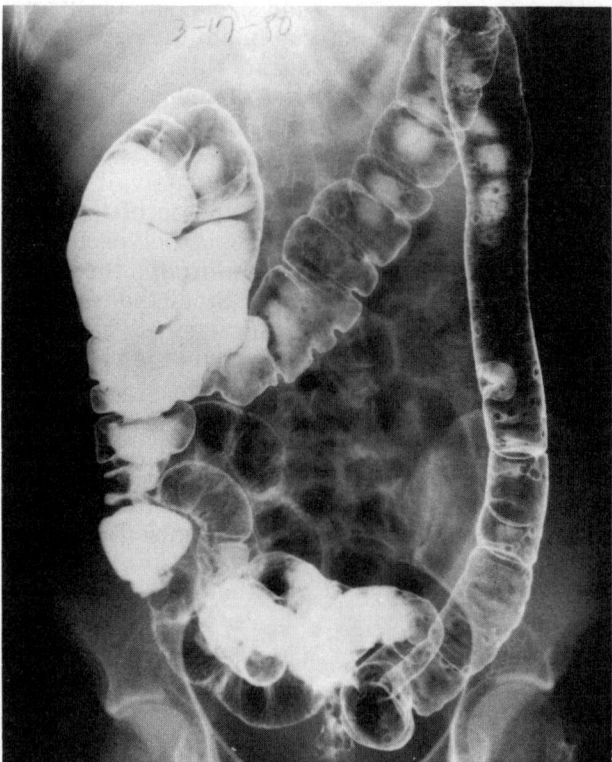

Figure 37.1. Double (air) contrast barium enema performed in a patient with familial polyposis. With this technique, numerous polyps, of varying sizes, may be seen throughout the colon.

performed to eliminate the risk of cancer. However, as the patients are generally quite young, the prospect of an ileostomy (see Chapter 41) and of potential sexual dysfunction is often overwhelming to them. Subtotal colectomy with ileal-rectal anastomosis is better tolerated by the patient, but requires frequent evaluations of the rectum with removal of all new polyps. Even then, the risk of rectal carcinoma remains high. Newer operations involving ileorectal pull-through procedures are being studied with early encouraging results. Consultation with a gastroenterologist and gastrointestinal surgeon is recommended as soon as the diagnosis is made.

Colonic polyposis syndromes should be distinguished from conditions associated with juvenile polyps or hamartomas that are of low malignant potential. The *Peutz-Jeghers syndrome* consists of multiple hamartomas, predominantly of the small intestine, associated with buccal and cutaneous pigmentation. While the malignant potential of the hamartomas is low, duodenal and ovarian carcinomas have been reported in 2 to 5% of patients. Rarely *juvenile polyps* may occur throughout the gastrointestinal tract. In the absence of associated extracolonic manifestations, this syndrome is called *generalized juvenile polyposis*; when accompanied by alopecia, nail bed changes, hyperpigmentation, and malabsorption, it is called the *Cronkhite-Canada syndrome*.

Colonic Cancer

Epidemiology and Etiology

Colonic carcinoma is one of the most common causes of death from cancer in this country. Its incidence is second only to skin and lung cancer. In an attempt to reduce the high incidence and mortality rate of this cancer, efforts are being directed toward identification of risk factors and toward earlier detection of the lesions.

Colon cancer occurs with increasing frequency in older age groups, with a peak incidence in the sixth and seventh decades. Geographic differences in the mortality rates due to this neoplasm have suggested an etiologic role for dietary and environmental factors. The proportion of cancers in the right side of the colon has been increasing in recent years with a commensurate drop in the proportion of rectosigmoid lesions. Currently, about one-third of colon cancers are within reach of the rigid sigmoidoscope, one-third within reach of the flexible sigmoidoscope, and one-third are proximal to the splenic flexure. The three main predisposing causes of large bowel cancer are colonic polyps, familial polyposis, and ulcerative colitis (see above and Chapter 38). The presence of these conditions dictates the need for a strict surveillance program in patients with these conditions, and even, at times, prophylactic surgery to prevent the development of large bowel cancer. (See page 459 for cancer-polyp association, and page 476 for risk of cancer in ulcerative colitis.)

Screening Tests

Because of the high incidence of colon cancer, and its precursor, the colonic polyp, screening tests should be performed routinely in all patients over 30 years old. The most important and cost effective in the *testing of stool for occult blood*. Six stools should be tested consecutively for occult blood annually by use of the Hemoccult slide test, currently the most reliable technique (see page 456). The Hemoccult-II provides a convenient method of checking two different parts of a stool at one time. These slides or cards are convenient for the patient because they can be mailed to the physician's office without a significant loss in the rate of positive reactions. In one study, 80% of patients ultimately found to have colonic cancer after detection of occult blood in their stool in a screening program had disease limited to the bowel (and therefore had a good prognosis).

In addition to multiple tests for occult blood, a *yearly rectal examination* should also be performed in patients over the age of 40. Proctosigmoidoscopy, preferably by use of a flexible sigmoidoscope, should also be performed in 2 consecutive years to ensure a normal rectal and rectosigmoid area. Subsequently, proctoscopy can be performed every 3 to 5 years in the asymptomatic patient who has negative tests for fecal blood. Yearly proctoscopy has not proved to be of sufficient additional value to warrant its cost and discomfort.

Diagnosis

History

Unfortunately, most patients with adenocarcinoma of the colon are diagnosed only after symptoms have developed. Less than 5% are asymptomatic at time of diagnosis, and it is in this group, that the highest chance for cure exists. The major symptoms are abdominal pain (25 to 75%) and a change in bowel habits (20 to 50%), either constipation or diarrhea. Abdominal pain is least common in patients with cancer of the rectum, where even large lesions can be accommodated without producing symptoms. Gross blood in the stool is another common complaint, occurring in 75% of patients with rectal cancer and in 30 to 40% of patients with colonic cancer above the rectum. Unfortunately, this hematochezia is frequently mistakenly attributed to hemorrhoids.

Physical Examination

The findings on physical examination vary according to the location and extent of the lesion. The primary tumor may be palpable as an abdominal mass, particularly in lesions of the right colon where lesions can remain "asymptomatic" for long periods of time. Metastatic disease may be suggested by the presence of a large, hard nodular liver, ascites, peripheral adenopathy, or by palpating a mass in the cul-de-sac on rectal examination. Signs of anemia may be present, particularly in lesions of the cecum and ascending colon that may bleed occultly for months or even years before the diagnosis is made. Most patients will have a positive test for occult blood (at least one) sometime during their course of illness.

Radiological Studies

The diagnosis of colon cancer is made most often on barium enema. Findings may include a polypoid mass, stenosis, either as a stricture or with an "apple-core" appearance, distortion of the mucosa, and localized rigidity of the bowel wall. At times, distortion or fixation of adjacent structures may be seen. The development of a gastrocolic fistula, best seen on barium enema, is also suggestive of a primary colonic neoplasm.

The accuracy of the radiographic diagnosis of colon cancer is excellent, except at opposite ends of the large bowel. The cecum is often difficult to evaluate because of the inability to cleanse the region completely and, at times, to distinguish a "prominent" ileocecal valve or sphincter from a mass. The rectum is also difficult to visualize optimally, as frequently it is obscured by the balloon through which the barium is administered. Thus, proctoscopy is essential in any patient suspected of having a colorectal carcinoma.

Endoscopy

The role of endoscopy varies depending on the location of the tumor. Proctosigmoidoscopy with biopsy is the best and most direct method of diagnosing rectal carcinoma. For lesions above the reach of the sigmoidoscope, the accuracy of a well performed barium enema is so high that colonoscopy to obtain preoperative histological diagnosis is not generally needed. However, it should be recognized that spasm, benign strictures, and even stool can be confused with cancer on radiographic examination and that some polypoid lesions, even if large or sessile, can be removed *via* the colonoscope.

In addition, colonoscopy does have an important role in the evaluation for other colonic lesions (see page 458). The prevalence of coexistent polyps in patients with colon cancer is high, ranging from 10 to 30%. These residual polyps may develop later into carcinoma, accounting for the incidence of a second colon cancer in 5 to 10% of patients with cancer of the colon who have been followed for up to 25 years (5). In addition, synchronous colon carcinomas occur in 3 to 5% of patients. Thus, colonoscopy is helpful in ensuring that the rest of the colon is free of neoplastic lesions. Optimally, colonoscopy should be performed preoperatively; otherwise, it should be done within the first year postoperatively.

Carcinoembryonic Antigen

Carcinoembryonic antigen (CEA) is a normal fetal antigen that is found in the blood of many patients with carcinoma of the colon (about 50% of patients with local disease and about 80% of patients with metastatic disease). It also is found sometimes in the blood of patients with other malignancies or with a variety of benign conditions (including heavy cigarette smoking). Therefore CEA titers are not useful screening tests for the presence of colon cancer.

The assay is helpful, however, in the postoperative managment of patients who have CEA in their blood at the time of diagnosis. Persistently elevated CEA levels postoperatively suggest metastatic disease; falling levels that then rise on follow-up evaluation suggest the re-emergence of the malignant tumor, usually at a remote site.

Therapy

Surgery is the most effective therapy for colon carcinoma. Inoperable low rectal and anal lesions may be treated with radiation. Chemotherapy provides little additional benefit at the present time.

Preoperative Evaluation

Prior to surgery, most patients should undergo evaluation for metastatic disease. Liver function tests should be performed routinely. The role of routine liver scan, computerized tomography, and ultrasound of the liver in the diagnosis of hepatic metastasis remains to be determined. In patients with bowel obstruction or bleeding, surgery may still be needed as palliation, despite the presence of liver metastases. In patients asymptomatic from their bowel lesions, the presence of hepatic metasases should deter surgical intervention. However, abnormal liver function tests alone should not be considered absolute evidence of metastatic disease. A histological diagnosis should be made, if possible. (Needle liver biopsy is a simple way to obtain tissue.) A preoperative CEA level should also be determined as a baseline (see above).

For patients requiring an ostomy, preoperative evaluation by an enterostomal therapist is very helpful, not only to discuss with the patient problems and concerns about the ostomy, but also to mark the proper location of the ostomy preoperatively (see Chapter 41).

Prognosis

The prognosis for colon carcinoma is based on several variables. The major variable is the extent of the tumor, in terms of its invasion through the bowel wall and of its lymph node involvement (Table 37.3). Vessel invasion and the degree of differentiation of the tumor histologically also affect survival. The pathologist's interpretation of the resected specimen is much more meaningful than the surgeon's estimation of "curable."

Table 37.3.
Colon Carcinoma

Classification[a]	Staging and 5-Year Survival	
	Microscopic Findings	Percent 5-Year Survival
A	Disease limited to mucosa	95
B	Tumor extends to serosa	60–70
C	Tumor extends to serosa and nodes involved	<40
D	Distant metastases	<5

[a] Modification of the Duke classification.

Follow-up Care

Most patients undergoing resection of colon cancer do well in the early postoperative period. Diarrhea may be present early, but it is usually transient and is easily controlled with antidiarrheal medication if needed. The patient with a colostomy needs continued followp-up care by the surgeon and the enterostomal therapist to insure proper functioning and handling of the ostomy (see Chapter 38).

The long term follow-up is aimed at detection of recurrence or spread of the cancer and at continued surveillance for new colonic lesions. Most commonly, metastases occur in adjacent nodes with spread to the liver. Physical examinations should be done and liver function tests and CEA levels should be measured every 6 months for 3 to 5 years.

To evaluate for new colonic lesions, or for the infrequent occurrence of tumor at the anastomosis, colonoscopy should be performed within the first 6 to 12 months, postoperatively. If no lesions are found, repeat colonoscopy or air contrast barium enema should be performed about every 3 years. In the interim, yearly evaluation for occult fecal blood loss should be performed with three to six Hemoccult slides. Should any of these slide tests be positive, colonoscopy should be repeated.

Arteriovenous Malformations of Colon

Arteriovenous malformations of the colon may be a source of gastrointestinal bleeding, most often in the elderly. A variety of terms have been used to describe these abnormalities including angiodysplasia, hemangioma, and vascular ectasia. The etiology of the disorder is unknown. While the lesions may occur throughout the gastrointestinal tract, they are found most commonly in the mucosa of the cecum and ascending colon where multiple lesions are often found, ranging in size from 1 mm to over 1 cm. An association of angiodysplasia of the colon with aortic stenosis has been observed repeatedly (2).

The prevalence of angiodysplasia and the frequency with which it causes bleeding are still uncertain. With increasing utilization of selective angiography, the disorder is being recognized more frequently. In one study of patients over the age of 60 without even a history of gastrointestinal bleeding, submucosal vascular ectasis was detected in

53% and mucosal lesions in 27% (2). It was suggested, therefore, that angiodysplasia may be the most common cause of bleeding from the right colon, and may be the most common cause of major lower intestinal bleeding in the elderly.

These dysplastic lesions, when they bleed, usually produce hematochezia. The bleeding is often brisk, and may be massive, but occult blood loss also may occur. Bleeding often stops spontaneously, but commonly recurs. The *diagnosis* is best made by selective arteriography (by which a malformation can be visualized even when the bleeding has stopped) or by colonoscopy. The lesions cannot be detected by barium enema, are not recognizable from the serosal surface by the surgeon, and are often overlooked by the pathologist. Lesions that have bled should be excised, preferably by surgical resection in the involved colon. However, colonoscopic removal or cauterization of discrete mucosal lesions can be performed by an experienced gastroenterologist.

The generalist should be aware of this disorder, especially in elderly patients who present to him with gastrointestinal bleeding in whom initial evaluation (see above) is unrevealing; but the diagnosis will be made only after consultation with a gastroenterologist and a radiologist.

General Reference

Winawer S, Sherlock P: Approach to screening and diagnosis in colorectal cancer. *Semin Oncol* 3:387, 1976.

> Reviews value of various screening tests and provides useful recommendations.

Specific References

1. Ahlquist DA, McGill DB, Schwartz S, *et al*: HemoQuant, a new quantitative assay for fecal hemoglobin. Comparison with Hemoccult. *Ann Intern Med* 101:297, 1984.
2. Boley SJ, Sammartano R, Adams A, *et al*: Nature and etiology of vascular ectasias of the colon. *Gastroenterology* 72:650, 1977.
3. Bond J, Gilbertson U: Early detection of colonic carcinoma by mass screening for occult stool blood: a preliminary report. *Gastroenterology* 72:A8, 1977.
4. Morris D, Hansell J, Ostrow JD, Lee C: Reliability of chemical tests for fecal occult blood in hospitalized patients. *Am J Dig Dis* 21:845, 1976.
5. Muto T, Bussey HJ, Morson BL: The evolution of cancer of the colon and rectum. *Cancer* 36:2251, 1975.
6. Silvis SE, Nebel O, Rogers G, *et al*: Results of the 1974 American Society for Gastrointestinal Endoscopy Survey. *JAMA* 235:928, 1976.
7. Tedesco F, Wayne J, Raskin J, *et al*: Colonoscopic evaluation of rectal bleeding—a study of 304 patients. *Ann Intern Med* 89:907, 1978.
8. Thoeni RF, Menuck L: Comparison of barium enema and colonoscopy in the detection of small colonic polyps. *Radiology* 124:631, 1977.

CHAPTER THIRTY-EIGHT

Constipation and Diarrhea

HAROLD J. TUCKER, M.D.

CONSTIPATION

Definition

Constipation is often defined as the infrequent, difficult passage of stool. However, it may mean different things to different people: that the stools are too infrequent, too difficult to expel, too hard, too small, or that there is a sensation of incomplete evacuation. Of these, frequency of bowel movements is the most readily measured aspect. Several studies have identified that there is a wide variation in the frequency of bowel movements among normal subjects of both sexes and of all ages, ranging from three per day to three per week. Therefore, someone who has less than three bowel movements per week is constipated, by definition. On the other hand, a change in frequency of movements from, say, two per day to three per week may also signify constipation.

Almost always, constipation is due to a delay in transit within the colon. A wide variety of conditions may affect colonic transit (Table 38.1). There may be structural abnormalities that obstruct the passage of intraluminal contents, or there may be conditions that alter colonic motility. Evaluation of patients with constipation must therefore include consideration of a wide variety of possible etiologies. Although it is difficult to be precise about the relative frequencies of these etiologies, in general, chronic constipation (months or longer) is most commonly due to an idiopathic motility disorder (such as in sedentary old people eating a low fiber diet or in patients with the irritable bowel syndrome), to the

use of constipating drugs, and to local rectal problems (fissures, hemorrhoids, and tumors).

Evaluation

History

The history provides the most useful information about the etiology of constipation. It may reveal a gross misconception about normal bowel habits or a neurotic preoccupation with bowel function. It is important to determine whether there is a history of, or suggestion of, a systemic process (e.g., hypothyroidism or scleroderma), a neurological disorder (e.g., cerebrovascular disease or Parkinson's disease), or the taking of drugs (e.g., anticholinergics or antidepressants), all of which are known to affect colonic motility. Most systemic or neurological diseases are almost certain to affect organs outside the gastrointestinal tract so that, in addition to constipation, patients have symptoms that reflect extraintestinal dysfunction. On the other hand, local processes (e.g., strictures or tumors) often produce other gastrointestinal symptoms in addition to constipation, such as abdominal pain or rectal bleeding. Thus, rectal bleeding should always be thoroughly evaluated (see Chapter 37) even though, in constipated patients, it frequently is caused by perianal disease (fissures, hemorrhoids, cryptitis). Abdominal pain, with constipation, is also a prominent feature of the irritable bowel syndrome (see Chapter 39). Most patients with "idiopathic" diet-related, or drug-induced constipation are otherwise asymptomatic except for a "bloated" sensation if constipation is prolonged.

Physical Examination

The physical examination should be focused on the identification of underlying causes of constipation. Rectal examination should be done routinely to look for fissures, hemorrhoids, and inflammation as well as anal stenosis or stricture, secondary to previous surgery or inflammation. The anal sphincter normally is closed. A gaping anal opening or asymmetry of the anal opening may indicate a neurological disorder (spinal cord trauma, peripheral neuropathy) that impairs sphincteric function. After inspection, a careful digital examination should be performed to evaluate the strength of the anal

Table 38.1.
Various Causes of Constipation

IDIOPATHIC (POSSIBLE MECHANISMS):
  Dietary factors—low residue
  Motility disturbances—colonic inertia or spasm (irritable
    bowel syndrome)
  Sedentary living combined with a low residue diet
STRUCTURAL ABNORMALITIES:
  Tumors
  Strictures
  Anorectal disorders—fissures, thrombosed hemorrhoids
ENDOCRINE/METABOLIC:
  Diabetes mellitus
  Hypothyroidism
  Hypercalcemia
  Pregnancy
  Hypokalemia
NEUROGENIC:
  Hirschsprung's disease
  Trauma
  Spinal cord tumors
  Cerebrovascular events
SMOOTH MUSCLE/CONNECTIVE TISSUE DISORDERS:
  Scleroderma
  Amyloidosis
DRUGS:
  Narcotics
  Anticholinergics
  Antacids—aluminum, and calcium-containing compounds
  Antidepressants
PSYCHOGENIC (especially depression)

sphincters, the presence of masses, the consistency of the stool, and the presence of any painful or tender areas.

Endoscopy

Anoscopy and proctosigmoidoscopy should be performed routinely in newly constipated patients in whom the cause is not obvious. Proctosigmoidoscopy can be performed in the office, often without a prior enema. In fact, when the appearance of the mucosa is important (as it is in patients with suspected ulcerative colitis), an enema should be avoided. In contrast, if exophytic bleeding lesions (i.e., polyps) are suspected, a cleansing enema (e.g., Fleet enema) is desirable and is usually administered by the patient at home before the office visit. Anoscopy may be needed to search properly for hemorrhoids or fissures (see Chapter 92). Proctosigmoidoscopy can be performed with the patient in the knee-chest position on a routine examining table, or in the left lateral position. Sigmoidoscopy should be performed to the highest level possible, with limitations imposed by the patient's tolerance of the procedure, the presence of stool, and the length of the instrument (a rigid scope extends to 25 cm while a flexible instrument can be passed to 60 cm). It is important to recognize that even a good air contrast barium enema is not a substitute for sig-

moidoscopy becaue the most distal 15 to 20 cm of the colon are notoriously difficult to evaluate radiographically. The patient's experience during proctosigmoidoscopy is described in Chapter 35.

Inflamed hemorrhoids and fissures, found during sigmoidoscopy, may be caused by constipation, but may also cause pain on defecation, and thus may promote constipation. These are also common causes of bleeding in the chronically constipated patient. A spotty brown pigmentation, *melanosis coli,* is indicative of chronic laxative abuse (see below, page 472), particularly of the anthraquinone family (e.g., cascara). An obstructing lesion, such as a carcinoma or polyp, may also be identified by proctosigmoidoscopy.

A *rectal biopsy* may diagnose amyloidosis, ulcerative colitis, or Crohn's disease, and a deeper, suction biopsy of a rectal valve may diagnose Hirschsprung's disease. Biopsies of the rectal mucosa can be taken safely below the peritoneal reflection (about 12 cm proximal to the anus in men, 8 cm in women). Punch biopsies can be performed by a general physician who has had appropriate training and experience. Suction biopsies should be performed only by a surgeon or gastroenterologist. Rectal biopsy should be painless unless a tender inflamed lesion is biopsied, and, if done properly, the risk of bleeding and perforation, the major complications, is very low.

Radiographic Studies

Radiographic examination is primarily helpful in the detection of obstructing lesions and should be performed in all adult patients who complain of constipation of relatively recent onset (within the preceding 6 months). The plain film of the abdomen may occasionally diagnose an obstructing carcinoma before a barium study has been done. The presence of a megacolon or a volvulus, either of the sigmoid or cecum, also may be easily diagnosed by a plain film. The more recent the onset of constipation, the more likely it is that the *barium enema* (see patient experience, Chapter 37) will yield positive results. Obstructing neoplasms and strictures can be identified by barium studies. Sometimes, patients with Hirschsprung's disease reach adolescence or adulthood without the diagnosis having been made. A narrowed rectal segment on X-ray is a clue to the diagnosis in such cases; it can be best seen when the patient is in the lateral oblique position and the X-ray is taken just as the barium is being instilled. The radiologist may also comment on the motility of the colon, particularly if there is significant spasm or if haustral markings are absent, as seen in patients who use laxatives chronically or who have an atonic megacolon. Repeated barium studies are rarely helpful unless some aspect of the history or physical examination suggests a new development.

Manometry

In patients suspected of having Hirschsprung's disease, *anal manometry* is a very simple and useful test. It is generally available in most medical centers and may be performed by either a gastroenterologist or a surgeon. The test involves insertion of balloon-tipped catheters into the anorectal region. Pressure measurements are made of the internal and external anal sphincter as well as within the rectum. Normally, with sudden distension of the rectum, the internal anal sphincter relaxes and the external sphincter contracts. In Hirschsprung's disease, this rectal anal inhibitory reflex is abnormal, and the internal anal sphincter fails to relax with rectal distension. This test is especially useful in cases of short segment or ultrashort segment Hirschsprung's disease in which the diagnosis is very difficult to establish by rectal biopsy.

Other Studies

Colonic motility tests and transit studies are additional procedures that may provide insight into the pathophysiology of constipation. These studies are generally available only in selected centers where there is specific interest in this problem. They should be performed in the few patients who are severely impaired by constipation and who are refractory to conventional therapy.

Colonic motility studies are generally performed by placing catheters, which monitor intracolonic pressures, in the rectal and sigmoid regions. The study can identify various patterns of colonic activity in patients with constipation. In some, high amplitude phasic contractions are seen spontaneously as well as in response to stimulation. This type of segmental activity is sometimes associated with pain and is believed to cause constipation by impeding the distal flow of luminal contents. In other patients an atonic pattern is found, characterized by a decreased response to stimulation and a loss of resistance to distension (4).

Colonic transit time can be measured by plotting the expulsion of radiopaque markers after ingestion. Daily plain films of the abdomen demonstrate the course of these markers through the gastrointestinal tract. In almost all normal subjects, 20 radiopaque markers will be evacuated within a week. Retention of these markers beyond that time period confirms the presence of constipation. Moreover, the distribution of these markers may have a relationship to the underlying motility disturbance (5).

Treatment

The treatment for constipation should, if possible, be based on the correction of the underlying abnormality. For example, if there is a systemic disease that can be treated (*e.g.*, hypothyroidism) or a constipating drug that can be stopped, this is an ideal situation since it can easily be corrected. The simple use of laxatives as a reflex response to this symptom should be discouraged. Successful therapy must include an open discussion with the patient about the broad limits of normal bowel function and about the patient's own concepts of normal bowel activity.

Bowel Retraining

Bowel retraining is an important initial aspect of therapy for those patients whose constipation does not have an identifiable and remediable cause. The patient should be encouraged to have a regular daily routine with time set aside for having a bowel movement, preferably within 5 to 10 minutes after a meal, to take advantage of the strong stimulus of the gastrocolic reflex. This behavior modification program allows the patient to become more aware of and responsive to the normal urges to defecate. Patients should be advised always to respond to such urges. In the severely constipated patient, a bowel-retraining program may be initiated with the use of enemas or suppositories to enhance bowel activity at the desired time. For enemas, lukewarm tap water should be used since all other solutions may be irritating if used repetitively. The enema should be given within an hour of eating a meal to take advantage of the gastrocolic reflex. For suppositories, glycerin or bisacodyl (Dulcolax) should be used, again just after eating; however, they should not be used for more than a few days because they may eventually be irritating.

Diet

Diet is an important factor in bowel function. Numerous studies have indicated that high fiber diets speed the transit of material through the gastrointestinal tract and increase stool frequency. Several mechanisms may account for this observation: (*a*) fiber may act as a bulk-forming agent; (*b*) fiber may increase the concentration of fecal bile salts, which have a pronounced cathartic effect; and (*c*) fiber, metabolized by colonic bacteria to nonabsorbable volatile fatty acids, may act as an osmotic cathartic. Thus, the low fiber diet generally consumed in this country may account for the large number of patients who complain of constipation. As an initial step, the patient should be placed on a diet rich in fiber conent. As listed in Table 38.2 there are a variety of foods high in fiber suitable for the patient's daily diet.

Laxatives

Despite numerous warnings, laxatives are still popular in the treatment of constipation. The presence of an estimated 700 or more commercially available laxatives and enema preparations attests to the widespread use of these agents. The mechanism of action for most laxatives is poorly understood, and the potential for toxicity is often under-

Table 38.2.
Fiber Content of Various Foods

Type of food	Dietary Fiber per Average Serving
	g
Vegetables	
Beans (navy, lima, kidney, baked)	8.5–10.0
Beans (string)	2.0
Broccoli	3.2
Brussel sprouts	2.3
Cabbage	2.0
Carrots	2.0
Celery	1.0
Corn	2.6
Corn on the cob	5.9
Lettuce	1.0
Potato (baked with skin)	3.0
Potato (french fried)	1.6
Peas, canned	6.0
Rice	0.8
Fruit	
Apple with peel	2.0
Apple juice	0.0
Banana	1.5
Grapefruit (fresh)	0.6
Orange	2.0
Peach	2.0
Raspberries	4.6
Strawberries	1.8
Breads	
Whole wheat	1.3
White, rye, French	0.7
Cereal	
All-Bran (100%)	8.4
Corn Flakes	2.6
Wheaties	2.6
Meats, chicken, liver, fish, lamb	0.0
Cheese, milk, yogurt	0.0

estimated (Table 38.3). Few data are available for comparison among the various laxatives, and the decision to use a particular laxative often is determined by individual preference rather than by objective evidence of efficacy or safety.

There are a number of different mechanisms by which a laxative effect may be achieved. *Bulk-forming agents* are natural or synthetic polysaccharides or cellulose derivatives that exert their laxative effect by absorbing water and increasing fecal mass. Methylcellulose, psyllium seed, and bran are examples of such laxatives. In addition to their hydrophilic properties, these agents are metabolized by colonic bacteria, resulting in accumulation of osmotically active metabolites. These laxatives are extremely effective in increasing the frequency and in softening the consistency of stool. There have been isolated reports of obstruction secondary to hydrophilic agents in patients with esophageal or small bowel strictures. In the majority of cases, however, this type of laxative is highly effective and

the potential for adverse effects appears to be low. However, in patients with an atonic form of constipation, particularly with megacolon, these agents are often ineffective and produce an uncomfortable sensation of bloating and gaseousness at high doses.

Dioctyl sodium sulfosuccinate (Colace) is frequently labeled as a *stool softener* or a wetting agent. Its use as a softener rather than as a true laxative may well be a function of the dosage.

The *saline laxatives* are generally magnesium or sodium salts that are poorly absorbed and therefore act as hyperosmolar solutions. It has been suggested that these compounds (*e.g.*, magnesium sulfate, milk of magnesia, and sodium phosphate) also release cholecystokinin, a hormone which is known to stimulate colonic motility. Complications include hypermagnesemia in patients with renal failure and hypocalcemia from phosphate overdoses.

Stimulant laxatives, such as anthraquinone derivatives (senna, cascara) and diphenylmethane compounds (phenolphthalein, bisacodyl), exert their effects primarily by altering electrolyte transport by the intestinal mucosa and thereby increasing intestinal motor activity. The effect of these agents is claimed to be more specific on the colon. Phenolphthalein, an ingredient found in many over-the-counter preparations, has been associated with severe allergic dermatitis. The chronic use of the anthraquinone derivatives has also been reported to induce damage to the intramural plexus, and thus actually to worsen bowel motility. Agents, such as these that affect electrolyte transport, may result in significant hypokalemia, factitious diarrhea, protein-losing enteropathy, and salt overload. While these agents are undoubtedly effective, their chronic use may lead to significant side effects, and they should be avoided when possible.

Castor oil, previously thought to be a stimulant laxative, is now understood to exert its cathartic effect by alteration of intestinal fluid and electrolyte secretion. Ricinoleic acid, the active ingredient of castor oil, has effects on the small and large intestine similar to that of bile acids: it inhibits absorption of sodium and glucose and stimulates fluid and electrolyte secretion by increasing cellular cyclic adenosine monophosphate (AMP) and by inhibiting sodium-potassium adenosine triphosphatase (ATPase). This increase in intraluminal fluid content may then secondarily affect intestinal motility.

Lactulose (Cephulac or Chronulac syrup) is a semisynthetic disaccharide that is not metabolized by the intestinal enzymes. As a result, water and electrolytes are retained within the intestinal lumen by the osmotic effect of this undigested sugar. In addition, this agent is converted by colonic bacteria to organic acids which may further alter electrolyte transport and/or affect colonic motility. Lactulose is commonly used in patients with hepatic encephalopathy (see Chapter 42). It has also been shown to

Table 38.3.
Laxatives

Classification and Active Ingredient	Examples	Dose	Average Onset of Action	Potential Adverse Effects
BULK				
Psyllium seed	Konsyl Effersylliuum Perdiem (with senna)	1 tsp to 2 tbsp/day	12–24 hours or more	Increased gas and bloating sensation; bowel obstruction if stricture present
Plus dextrose	Metamucil L.A. Formula			
Bran		4+ tbsp/day		
EMOLLIENT (SOFTENERS)				
Dioctyl sodium (or calcium) sulfosuccinate	Colace, Pericolace (with casanthranol)	1–3 caps/day	24–48 hours	Electrolyte imbalance
	Surfak	1 cap/day		
SALINE				
Magnesium salts	Milk of Magnesia, magnesium citrate	2–4 tbsp	3–6 hours or less	Hypermagnesemia, hypocalcemia, hyperphosphatemia in chronic renal failure
Sodium salts	Phospho-Soda	2 tbsp in ½ glass of H_2O		
	Fleet enema	120 ml	2–5 minutes	Dehydration; hyperphosphatemia in chronic renal failure
STIMULANT				
Phenolphthalein	Correctol, Ex-Lax	1–2 tablets (100–200 mg)	6–8 hours	Dermatitis; electrolyte imbalance, melanosis coli
Bisacodyl[a]	Dulcolax	2–3 tabs (10–15 mg)		
Senna	Senokot, Perdiem (with psyllium)	1–4 tsp or 2–4 tabs		
Cascara (Casanthranol)	Pericolace (with dioctyl sodium)	1–2 tabs		
Ricinoleic acid	Castor oil	1–2 tsp		
CO_2	Ceo-two suppositories	1–2	10–30 minutes	
OSMOTIC				
Lactulose[a]	Cephulac, Chronulac	1–2 tbsp/day		Excessive gas production

[a] Requires a prescription.

be an effective laxative in patients with chronic constipation. There is little current information on the relative merits of lactulose *versus* bulk laxatives except that lactulose is relatively expensive and requires 24 to 48 hours to achieve its effect.

Surgery is rarely necessary in the treatment of constipated patients. It is, however, required for resection of an obstructing lesion, and myectomy may be needed for treatment of Hirschsprung's disease. Various procedures have been recommended for patients with megacolon who suffer from recurrent volvulus, ranging from simple tacking down of the loose mesentery to resection of bowel. Finally, in severe cases of intractable constipation, extensive surgery has been advocated varying from resection of redundant sigmoid loops to subtotal colectomy with ileal proctostomy. The exact role and precise indication for this type of surgery remain to be more clearly defined.

General Recommendations

Therapy of constipation should always be directed first at identifying and treating any underlying disorder (Table 38.1). If the constipation is drug induced, the drug should be discontinued (if possible) and be substituted with an alternative that is less constipating. When constipation is "idiopathic" or is due to an irreversible, underlying disorder (e.g., diabetes), or is secondary to a necessary drug, then dietary changes and some form of laxative therapy may be necessary.

In practically all patients with constipation, a high fiber diet or a bulk laxative will be helpful. The amount of dietary fiber and/or bulk laxative that is needed varies from patient to patient and must be titrated individually. As the only significant side effect from this form of therapy is "excessive" gas and a bloated sensation, the dose can be gradually increased until either the constipation is resolved or the side effects become too uncomfortable. For the vast majority of patients, this form of therapy will be successful and appears to be very safe on a chronic basis. No other laxatives need be used.

However, in patients with partial bowel obstruction (as recognized on X-ray), or in those with an atonic form of constipation (e.g., institutional megacolon), the high fiber-bulk laxative approach is not effective. A patient with constipation due to partial obstruction must be treated surgically. A patient with an atonic colon may need a stimulant laxative. Senna compounds, bisacodyl (either as a tablet or a suppository), or enemas are most effective in such cases. Combinations of a stimulant laxative with a bulk agent (e.g., Perdiem) or with a softener (e.g., Pericolace) are reasonable and effective forms of therapy. Bulk agents alone in such cases simply distend the already distended bowel further without improving bowel function.

Special consideration must be given to the bedridden or wheelchair-bound patient. In such patients laxatives may result in incontinence, as the patient may not be able to recognize or respond quickly enough to the sudden urge to defecate. In these circumstances, bulk agents are useful to keep the stool soft, but suppositories or enemas should be used (simple tap water enemas are usually sufficient; also see Table 38.3), with the patient already positioned on the commode. In this fashion, the embarrassment and soilage of fecal incontinence can be avoided, and fecal impactions can be prevented. These enemas or suppositories should be used regularly (daily to every third day) to prevent fecal impactions and "overflow" diarrhea and incontinence.

DIARRHEA

Diarrhea is a troublesome problem which almost everyone has experienced. In the vast majority of cases, the diarrheal illness begins abruptly, lasts only a day or two, and resolves without serious sequelae (see Chapter 26). Only occasionally does the illness continue for more than a week or do symptoms recur after the initial attack. The task facing the clinician is to identify the few patients with a significant underlying disorder that may require a specific therapeutic approach.

Definition

Patients complaining of diarrhea generally have an increase in the frequency and fluid volume of the bowel movement. Stool weight is the best objective measurement of diarrhea, with mean weights in this country ranging normally between 100 and 200 g/day. In the patient with chronic diarrhea, objective documentation of daily fecal output is sometimes necessary (see below). Most cases of significant diarrhea will have in excess of 250 g of stool/day. There is a subset of patients with diarrhea who present with the frequent passage of small volumes of liquid stool. Patients with inflammatory conditions or space-occupying lesions of the rectum may present in this fashion. Patients with the irritable bowel syndrome have stool volumes either within or slightly above the normal range. Patients with secretory forms of diarrhea, or small bowel disorders with malabsorption, frequently pass large volumes of stool, often in the range of 500 to 1000 (or greater) g/day.

Pathophysiology

There are several basic causes of diarrhea: (a) osmotic load within the intestine resulting in retention of water within the lumen, (b) excessive secretion of electrolytes and water into the intestinal lumen, (c) exudation of protein and fluid from the intestinal mucosa, and (d) altered intestinal motility.

Osmotic diarrhea occurs when poorly absorbable material retains fluid within the intestinal lumen. This mechanism operates in patients with malabsorption or with lactose intolerance in which poorly absorbed sugars accumulate within the intestinal lumen and exert a considerable osmotic load. Magnesium-containing laxatives and some magnesium-containing antacids (e.g. Maalox) probably produce diarrhea through a similar mechanism.

Secretory diarrhea is perhaps the best studied pathophysiological type of diarrhea. In such cases, the intestinal mucosa secretes increased amounts of water and electrolytes, under the stimulation of a variety of substances, of which cholera toxin is the prototype (some enterotoxigenic *Escherichia coli* produce diarrhea in the same way (see Chapter 26); other substances include bile acids and long chain fatty acids (postileal resection, Crohn's disease, or a malabsorption syndrome), certain gastrointestinal hormones, and anthraquinone laxatives (see above, page 467). Many of these stimulating agents have been shown to increase intracellular cyclic AMP and to inhibit sodium potassium ATPase. The increase in cyclic AMP leads to increased secretion.

Exudative diarrhea results from the outpouring of protein, blood, or mucus from an inflamed or ulcerated mucosa. Ulcerative colitis, Crohn's disease, salmonellosis, and infiltrative disorders like Whipple's disease and lymphoma are examples of this mechanism.

Motility disorders may lead to diarrhea, although the exact correlation between the abnormal motility and the diarrhea is not completely understood. The *irritable bowel syndrome* (see Chapter 39) is generally believed to be a motor disorder that causes abdominal pain and altered bowel habits, with diarrhea predominating in many patients. Diabetes mellitus may also lead to diarrhea due to neurogenic dysfunction. Other conditions, like scleroderma, can lead to stasis of the bowel with resultant bacterial overgrowth, steatorrhea, and diarrhea.

It is not always possible to identify one particular mechanism to account for diarrhea in a given patient; sometimes more than one mechanism is operative. However, an appreciation of pathophysiology enables the physician to understand better the clinical features of a diarrheal illness and to select appropriate therapy.

Evaluation of Acute Diarrhea

(Acute diarrhea due to infectious agents is discussed in greater detail in Chapter 26). The vast majority of patients who present to the physician with a sudden onset of diarrhea generally have a benign, self-limited illness. These patients will not require an extensive evaluation and can be simply reassured. It is important, however, to recognize that a small percentage of such patients may actually have a significant underlying illness for which specific therapy is needed.

If diarrhea persists for more than 72 hours or if there is gross blood in the stool, an evaluation is indicated. In any case, the patient should always be evaluated (if possible) before medicine is prescribed, since in certain situations even nonspecific antidiarrheal therapy may actually be harmful.

History

The history clearly reveals whether the illness is acute or chronic and also provides major clues to the underlying cause. The sudden onset of loose watery stool is most commonly due to an infectious process, and much less often due to ingestion of drugs or poisons. Infectious diarrhea is likely to affect more than one person. Frequently, no specific bacterial agent is identified and the syndrome is labeled "viral gastroenteritis." Bacteria may cause diarrhea by a direct effect on the bowel or by elaboration of a toxin that produces intestinal dysfunction. Toxin-induced diarrhea, often associated with vomiting, begins within 6 hours of ingestion of contaminated food, whereas bacteria-induced diarrhea

does not begin for 12 to 24 hours. Bloody diarrhea should never be ascribed to "viral" or to toxin-mediated diarrhea; it is more likely to be due to bacterial infection (*Shigella, Campylobacter, Yersinia,* and *Salmonella*), to ulcerative colitis, or to ischemic bowel disease. Information about recent travel should include not only trips out of the country but also camping or fishing trips. Giardiasis, for example, may be carried by beavers who contaminate water supplies and cause both epidemic outbreaks as well as individual cases of acute diarrhea among campers and hikers. Recent use of drugs is a common cause of new onset diarrhea (Table 38.4) which is often overlooked by both the physician and the patient. Some antihypertensives (e.g., methyldopa, hydralazine, reserpine, and guanethidine), magnesium-containing antacids, broad spectrum antimicrobials, and quinidine are commonly used drugs that can lead to diarrhea.

Physical Examination

Physical examination is generally unremarkable. The patient's state of hydration should be estimated, as it is an important measure of the severity of the diarrhea and of the need for hospitalization. Abdominal examination may reveal mild diffuse tenderness. The bowel sounds are clearly active or hyperactive. Rectal examination is essential since diarrhea may be the initial manifestation of obstructing rectal carcinoma; furthermore in the geriatric population, fecal impactions may result in "overflow" diarrhea so that constipating agents may be mistakenly recommended.

Stool Examination

If diarrhea has continued for more than 3 to 4 days, the stool should be examined for the presence of blood, fecal leukocytes, and enteric pathogens. Blood in the stool suggests mucosal disruption and is not a feature of osmotic or secretory diarrhea. Inflammatory conditions like ulcerative colitis and pseudomembranous colitis frequently present with bloody diarrhea.

Fecal leukocytes are best seen by microscopic examination of the liquid portion of the stool after staining with methylene blue or Gram's stain (3). They are not seen in infectious processes that do not invade the mucosa such as "viral enteritis," toxin-mediated diarrhea, cholera, or infection with noninvasive *E. coli* (see Chapter 26). *Salmonella, Shigella,* amoebae, and *Campylobacter,* which are invasive organisms, typically lead to exudation of fecal leukocytes, as does chronic inflammatory bowel disease. In these conditions, in which the mucosal barrier is broken, the course of the diarrheal illness is unpredictable and may even become life threatening. The absence of fecal leukocytes or blood is, therefore, very reassuring and, in these cases, the disease is usually transient.

Table 38.4.
Common Drugs That May Induce Diarrhea

ANTIBIOTICS:
   Clindamycin
   Ampicillin
   Cephalosporin
ANTACIDS: Magnesium-containing
ANTIHYPERTENSIVE AGENTS:
   Guanethidine
   Hydralazine
   Methyldopa
   Propranolol
   Reserpine
CARDIOVASCULAR AGENTS:
   Digitalis
   Quinidine
ANTIMETABOLITES: Colchicine
ALCOHOL
NUTRITIONAL SUPPLEMENTS: Hyperosmolar solutions
   (enteral feedings)
POTENT DIURETICS:
   Furosemide
   Ethacrynic acid

Stool cultures for bacterial pathogens should be obtained on all patients who have fecal leukocytes. Specific isolation techniques are needed to diagnose *Yersinia* and *Campylobacter*, common causes of acute diarrhea, and should be requested. The differentiation on clinical grounds between acute infectious diarrhea secondary to *Salmonella* or *Shigella* and nonspecific acute inflammatory bowel disease is extremely difficult without a stool culture. In the absence of fecal leukocytes, stool cultures are generally negative. Gram stain of the stool is not helpful except in cases of suspected staphylococcal enterocolitis or gonococcal proctitis.

Examination of the stool for parasites such as amoebae and *Giardia* is very important even in the absence of a history of travel since the organism may be passed by personal contact with a carrier. Microscopic examination of the inflammatory exudate of a patient with acute amebic colitis will almost always demonstrate motile trophozoites especially if the slide is prewarmed (e.g., over a light bulb) and then examined immediately. Rectal biopsy may identify the organisms in the exudate. Giardiasis can be detected on examination of fresh stool in only about 50% of patients. If the physician is not proficient in the identification of protozoons in the stool, he must refer the patient to a medical center or must rely on serology or rectal biopsy to diagnose amoebiasis or duodenal aspiration or biopsy to diagnose giardiasis.

Endoscopy

Proctosigmoidoscopy is important in patients with acute diarrhea associated with fecal leukocytes or fecal blood. The proctoscopy should be performed without a prior enema, as enemas may alter the appearance of the mucosa and reduce the chance of detecting intestinal pathogens like amoebae.

Many acute diarrheal illnesses produce a similar, nonspecific mucosal appearance on proctoscopy, but certain findings are suggestive of specific diseases. In viral enteritis, giardiasis, toxin-mediated diarrhea, drug-induced diarrhea, and other conditions not accompanied by fecal leukocytes or blood loss, the proctoscopy is normal. In ulcerative colitis the rectal mucosa is involved in at least 95% of cases, and the mucosa is uniformly abnormal with bleeding and a granular friable appearance. Uncommonly, Crohn's disease affects the rectum and causes discrete aphthoid ulcers with normal intervening mucosa. Amebiasis occasionally produces classical flask-shaped ulcers that may be single or multiple, with normal intervening mucosa; more often, however, it produces a pattern very similar to ulcerative colitis. In shigellosis, multiple small superficial ulcers may be seen, but the appearance may also be indistinguishable from that of ulcerative colitis. Pseudomembranous colitis is identified by the presence of numerous raised yellow plaques covering an inflamed mucosa. Occasionally a carcinoma or large villous adenoma may be detected by sigmoidoscopy. Proctoscopy also provides an extremely opportune time to obtain samples of stool and exudate for culture and microscopic examination. The patient's experience with proctosigmoidoscopy is described in Chapter 35.

Radiographic Studies

Radiography is of very limited value in evaluation of acute diarrhea and may, in fact, be confusing. In patients suspected of having inflammatory bowel disease or ischemic colitis, plain films of the abdomen may demonstrate an irregular appearance to the bowel wall secondary to mucosal edema, often described as "thumbprinting." In the gravely ill patient with fulminant colitis, the X-ray may confirm the presence of "toxic megacolon." In the vast majority of cases of acute diarrhea, a plain film is not needed. Barium studies during the acute phase of the diarrhea are likewise not needed and in certain conditions may even be hazardous, as in patients with severe colitis or ischemic bowel disease. Similarly, a small bowel series during acute "viral enteritis" may be frighteningly abnormal, resembling sprue, and yet may rapidly return to normal after resolution of the acute illness.

Evaluation of Chronic Diarrhea

The approach to patients with either acute diarrhea which lasts longer than 3 to 4 days or chronic diarrhea (lasting longer than 2 weeks) is very much the same. While the *physician* may be reassured, knowing that the majority of such patients do not suffer from any serious progressive or disabling disease, the *patient* requires a specific diagnosis and effective therapy. The differential diagnosis is so varied, and the available tests are so numerous, that the diagnostic workup of chronic diarrhea poses a difficult problem. The following discussion provides a practical approach to this problem.

History

The history is often very helpful in differentiating organic from "functional" diarrhea—i.e., irritable bowel syndrome and painless ("nervous") diarrhea (see Chapter 39). If organic diarrhea is suspected, the physician must determine whether the pathogenic mechanism is osmotic, secretory, motor, or exudative (see above).

In patients with so-called "functional diarrhea," the history of diarrhea often dates back many months or years, although occasionally it can be traced to a specific acute diarrheal illness. Despite the chronicity, no sequelae, such as weight loss, anemia, or hypoalbuminemia, have occurred. The patient typically complains of several watery, at times explosive, bowel movements early in the morning, and then no subsequent movements the rest of the day. Nocturnal bowel movements are rare. The total stool output is usually small, however—often less than 200 g/day and rarely, if ever, greater than 500 g/day. Mucus is present frequently. There is no blood in the stool unless secondary conditions, such as anal fissures, have developed. Postprandial pain is a feature of irritable bowel syndrome but is absent in patients with "nervous" or "painless" diarrhea. The condition frequently waxes and wanes in severity, and stress often exacerbates the symptoms.

The most common cause of chronic secretory diarrhea is *laxative abuse*. It should be suspected in apparently healthy patients with large volume diarrhea, especially if they have *melanosis coli* on proctoscopic examination (see above, page 465). Although such patients may have emotional problems with which the physician must deal (see Chapter 12), often the abuse simply reflects an individual's misconception about how often he should have a bowel movement and his attempt to adhere to that standard.

In patients with organic disease, the history may indicate the part of the intestinal tract that is involved. The passage of a large volume of frothy, malodorous stools without blood suggests small bowel diarrhea, often secondary to malabsorption. The frequent passage of small volumes of poorly formed bloody stools suggests inflammatory, exudative disorders of the colon like ulcerative colitis. The presence of recognizable fat droplets (oil) suggests malabsorption, frequently secondary to pancreatic insufficiency. (Floating stools and undigested food in the stools are not helpful observations as they may be seen in both organic and functional

diarrheal states.) The association of diarrhea with the ingestion of certain dietary products (milk, hyperosmolar solutions) may go unrecognized by the patient unless he is specifically asked. A detailed drug history (see below) is also important since many drugs may cause diarrhea.

Other symptoms may help the physician to arrive at a specific diagnosis. *Arthritis and arthralgias* may suggest the presence of one of several uncommon bowel diseases, e.g., inflammatory bowel disease and Whipple's disease; conversely, diarrhea may be an important feature of Reiter's syndrome (Chapter 71). *Weight loss*, in the absence of anorexia, should suggest malabsorption, hyperthyroidism, or a malignant tumor. *Abdominal pain* may reflect the irritable bowel syndrome (Chapter 39), in which case it is generally in the left lower quadrant or in the suprapubic region, or a disease of the small bowel (e.g., Crohn's disease) in which case it is periumbilical, or in the right lower quadrant.

Physical Examination

The physical examination may reveal additional information about the etiology of the diarrhea. Patients with malabsorption may have evidence of weight loss, peripheral neuropathy (secondary to vitamin deficiency), and carpopedal spasm (secondary to hypocalcemia). Erythema nodosum and pyoderma gangrenosum may be seen in some cases of inflammatory bowel disease. Hyperpigmentation is a feature of Whipple's disease and Addison's disease. Diabetic diarrhea is frequently associated with other evidence of autonomic dysfunction, such as postural hypotension. Nondeforming arthritis is a feature of Whipple's disease and inflammatory bowel disease. Hepatosplenomegaly and lymphadenopathy suggest lymphoma or Whipple's disease. The abdominal examination may reveal an arterial bruit or an aortic aneurysm which suggests ischemic bowel disease. A rectal examination may disclose perianal disease (e.g., abscesses or fistulas, secondary to Crohn's disease) a rectal tumor, or a fecal impaction.

Endoscopy

Proctoscopy should be performed during the initial visit without a prior cleansing enema. Proctoscopic examination of the rectal mucosa and a rectal biopsy (see page 471) may suggest specific etiologies—ulcerative colitis, Crohn's disease, amebiasis, pseudomembranous colitis, Whipple's disease, or amyloidosis. The finding of *melanosis coli* (spotty brownish pigmentation) in a patient complaining of diarrhea indicates laxative abuse. At the time of proctoscopy, stool specimens are obtained for microscopic evaluation and culture. Gonococcal proctitis appears similar to ulcerative proctitis (see below) and requires direct plating on a warm special culture medium (Thayer-Martin) with prompt incubation. Routine stool cultures should be made as well. The stool should be examined for pus cells, blood, fat (Sudan stain), and parasites (see page 471).

After this initial evaluation, the etiology of the chronic diarrhea in most patients is either evident or strongly suspected. It is usually possible to distinguish functional from organic diarrhea; to detect evidence of inflammatory or infiltrative disease; to suspect the presence of malabsorption; to characterize the diarrhea as "small bowel" or "large bowel"; and even to suggest the underlying pathophysiology. Further evaluation is then dictated by the results of this initial workup.

Laboratory Studies

Laboratory studies should be selected to support the clinical impression but rarely are able to make or exclude a specific diagnosis. For example, the erythrocyte sedimentation rate (ESR) may be elevated in a variety of inflammatory diseases that cause diarrhea, but a normal ESR does not exclude inflammatory bowel disease or a connective tissue disorder.

Radiological Studies

A plain film of the abdomen may reveal pancreatic calcifications (indicative of chronic pancreatitis) or a dilated small bowel or an abnormal bowel contour (such as in inflammatory bowel disease).

In the patient over 40 years old, with chronic or recurrent diarrhea, a barium enema is indicated during the initial evaluation. In younger patients, barium studies are unlikely to be useful unless a specific disorder is suspected. The presence of blood in the stool, at any age, is a clear indication for a barium enenma, regardless of the presence of hemorrhoids or fissures. Neoplastic and inflammatory conditions may be diagnosed in this way, and ulcerative colitis and Crohn's disease of the colon can be differentiated in about 90% of cases. When the barium enema is introduced, an attempt should be made to reflux barium into the terminal small bowel to rule out Crohn's disease of the ileum.

The timing of the barium study is important. Barium will interfere with the collection of stool for measurement of volume and fat and with the detection of parasites. A barium enema should be delayed for 1 week following a rectal biopsy to prevent colonic perforation. The patient's experience with the barium enema is discussed in Chapter 37.

A *small bowel series* (see Chapter 37 for a discussion of the patient's experience with this procedure) is helpful in distinguishing mucosal disease (celiac sprue), inflammatory conditions (Crohn's disease), and infiltrative processes (Whipple's disease or amyloidosis). In addition, a small bowel series is indicated in postsurgical patients to clarify the anatomy (e.g., a blind loop or fistulas) and to detect localized areas of dilation and stasis.

Other Studies

A *quantitative stool collection*, while regarded as unpleasant by both the patient and laboratory personnel, is a very informative test. It should be employed early in the evaluation of patients in whom the initial routine workup does not suggest a diagnosis. The test can be performed in the ambulatory setting by having the patient collect all of his stool in a preweighed container (such as a paint can), usually supplied by the clinical laboratory. (He can also defecate into a bedpan or into a special stool collection trap, placed inside a commode, and then transfer the stool to a preweighed container.) The test should be performed before barium studies or other invasive tests in these patients. As mentioned previously, the normal stool weight is less than 250 g/day (or less than 250 ml/day). Most patients with the irritable bowel syndrome will have stool volumes within this range. A stool volume of greater than 1000 ml/day suggests a secretory diarrhea.

The *osmolality and electrolyte* concentration of the specimen can also be measured. In osmotic diarrhea, the measured fecal osmolality is greater than twice the sum of the concentration of fecal sodium and potassium. In secretory diarrhea, the calculated and measured osmolality are the same. *Fecal fat* should also be measured during this collection. Normally less than 7% of ingested fat is secreted in the stool per day (6 to 7 g on an average American diet containing 70 to 100 g of fat). The presence of steatorrhea dictates a different approach to the remainder of the workup (see below). In the absence of excessive fat excretion, or of evidence of an exudative process (e.g., inflammatory bowel disease), high volume diarrhea suggests a secretory process.

In patients suspected of having a secretory diarrhea, further evaluation will generally require hospitalization and consultation with a gastroenterologist. In secretory diarrhea, having the patient ingest nothing by mouth for 48 hours will not alter the volume of diarrhea, whereas in osmotic diarrhea the stool volume will significantly decrease. Causes of chronic secretory diarrhea include hormone-secreting tumors and surreptitious laxative abuse. Evaluation of such patients frequently requires availability of various hormone assays. Familiarity with these uncommon conditions is needed to approach the differential diagnosis judiciously.

Evaluation of Malabsorption

When the quantitative fecal collection demonstrates steatorrhea, the evaluation of the diarrhea should be focused on the cause of malabsorption. Basically malabsorption can result from (a) small intestinal disease, (b) pancreatic disease, (c) hepatobiliary disease, and (d) gastric disease. A series of diagnostic studies is utilized initially to define the organ involved and then to diagnose the specific disease. Consultation with a gastroenterologist is generally recommended to help perform and analyze these various tests.

The *d-xylose test* measures the absorptive capacity of the proximal small bowel. Normally, the sugar is absorbed passively by the intact small intestinal mucosa, enters the blood, and is excreted in the urine. The test is performed in the same manner as an oral glucose tolerance test and can be performed in the ambulatory setting by most clinical laboratories. A 25- or 50-g oral dose of xylose is given, and the patient's urine is collected over the next 5 hours. Blood samples are collected at 1 and 2 hours after ingestion. In disorders of the intestinal mucosa (e.g., sprue, Whipple's disease) xylose is poorly absorbed and low levels are found in the serum and urine. Uncommonly, massive bacterial overgrowth may also produce an abnormal *d*-xylose test that reverts to normal with treatment. Since an abnormal xylose test suggests mucosal disease, a small bowel biopsy should be performed next.

If the *d*-xylose test is normal, pancreatic insufficiency is the most likely cause of steatorrhea. In this case pancreatic calcifications may be seen on an abdominal plain film, and diabetes mellitus is frequently present. Pancreatic insufficiency can be confirmed by measuring pancreatic secretions (secretin test) or by measuring intraluminal contents after a test meal. These tests, performed usually in the gastroenterology laboratory of a medical center, involve intubation of the duodenum with collection of intraluminal contents. Newer methods that do not require intubation but simply a prolonged urine collection, e.g., Bentiromide test, have recently been introduced and are becoming more available. Often, however, if a presumptive diagnosis of pancreatic insufficiency is made, the patient is treated empirically with pancreatic enzymes (e.g., Viokase, 3 to 6 tablets with meals or Pancrease, 2 to 3 tablets with meals); diagnostic and therapeutic decisions should be made in consultation with a gastroenterologist.

Suction biopsy of the small intestine is often useful in the detection of various disorders that may cause malabsorption and/or diarrhea. The procedure can be performed by a gastroenterologist in an ambulatory setting. The biopsy instrument, a small caliber tube, is passed by mouth through the stomach, and positioned fluoroscopically at the duodenal-jejunal junction. The patient is given prior mild sedation (Valium intravenously) and a topical anesthetic is sprayed onto the back of the pharynx. The procedure may last from 15 minutes to 2 or 3 hours depending on the ease of passage of the tube (usually the tube can be passed rapidly). Complications (including perforation and bleeding) are extremely rare. Disorders that may be diagnosed by small bowel biopsy include sprue, Whipple's disease, intestinal lymphoma, amyloidosis, lymphangiectasia, and eosinophilic gastroenteritis. Giardiasis also can be diagnosed by examination of the intestinal mu-

cosa and of the intestinal mucus or fluid by the pathologist or the consulting gastroenterologist.

Disorders of the terminal ileum (Crohn's disease, ileal resection) may also lead to diarrhea and malabsorption. Evaluation should include a *Schilling test* or a *bile salt breath test*. The Schilling test measures vitamin B_{12} absorption, which is abnormal in disorders of the terminal ileum, the site of B_{12} absorption. Absorption is impaired despite the presence of intrinsic factor (see Chapter 49) or the administration of antibiotics.

Similarly, the bile salt breath test measures bile acid absorption which is also abnormal in disorders of the terminal ileum. The patient is given orally a radiolabeled (^{14}C) bile salt. In the presence of terminal ileal disease, the bile salt is malabsorbed, and excess acid reaches the colon, where bacteria deconjugate it and release $^{14}CO_2$ which diffuses across the colon and is excreted in the breath. Therefore, in ileal disease, the level of $^{14}CO_2$ in the patient's expired air is abnormally high. The same abnormality can be seen when there is bacterial overgrowth in the small bowel, so that the bile acid is deconjugated and metabolized there instead of in the colon. Bile acid malabsorption due to bacterial overgrowth is reversed when the patient is given antibiotics. Both the Schilling test and the bile salt breath test are performed by nuclear medicine specialists.

Specific Causes of Chronic Diarrhea

Lactose Intolerance (See Also Chapter 39, Page 483)

Lactose intolerance is the most common form of carbohydrate malabsorption. It results from a deficiency or total absence of the enzyme lactase in the brush border of the intestinal mucosa, which causes maldigestion and therefore malabsorption of lactose. The unabsorbed carbohydrate exerts an osmotic effect which draws water into the intestinal lumen. In the colon, the lactose is metabolized by bacteria to organic acid, CO_2, and hydrogen. The acid contributes to the diarrhea by both an osmotic effect and an irritating effect on the colonic mucosa. Thus, the unabsorbed carbohydrate, if present in sufficient quantities (the critical amount varies widely), may cause diarrhea, gaseousness, bloating, and abdominal cramps.

Lactose intolerance may be present either as an inherited condition or one that develops because of damage to intestinal epithelium (e.g., due to infectious enteritis or sprue). Even in patients with a genetic disorder the onset of the disease is unpredictable and may not occur until adult life. The secondary cases are usually, but not always, reversible if the underlying disease is successfully treated. The severity of the clinical symptoms is highly variable.

In some patients even small amounts of lactose produce severe symptoms, while in others large quantities may be consumed with no or only minimal symptoms. Isolated lactase deficiency is most common in blacks (70 to 75% prevalence) and in many Asians (87% prevalence among Chinese), but may also be found in 5 to 20% of the white population in this country (2). The condition is more pronounced in certain clinical settings: when superimposed on another diarrheal disorder, most commonly irritable bowel syndrome; after gastric surgery, which permits rapid delivery of lactose to the small bowel; and when a patient consumes extra amounts of milk as part of therapy for ulcer disease.

The *diagnosis* of lactose intolerance is suggested by the history and by the response to a lactose-free diet. Nearly a third of patients with symptomatic lactose intolerance, however, may not have made the correlation between the dietary intake and the resulting symptoms, as a wide variety of foods, ranging from bread to instant coffee, contain lactose (see Table 39.2, page 484).

Specific tests for the diagnosis of lactose intolerance include the lactose tolerance test and the hydrogen breath test. The *lactose tolerance test* measures changes in the concentration of serum glucose after ingestion of 50 g of lactose. A rise in glucose of 20 mg/100 ml above fasting is normal. The test has about a 30% false positive rate, and its validity depends on a variety of factors besides simply the presence of the lactase enzyme. The *hydrogen breath test* is easier to perform and is more accurate. Unabsorbed lactose is fermented by colonic bacteria and the resultant hydrogen is absorbed and expired in the breath. In normal subjects after a lactose load, there is only a trace amount of hydrogen in the expired air, whereas in lactose-deficient patients substantial levels are recorded. This test is widely available; it is usually performed by a nuclear medicine specialist or in a gastrointestinal laboratory and requires 2 to 4 hours of the patient's time.

Ordinarily, a 3-week trial of a diet that is free of milk and milk products is a satisfactory therapeutic trial to test the diagnosis of lactose intolerance. The other tests are indicated only in equivocal cases.

Fecal Impaction

Although it is the result of chronic constipation, fecal impaction commonly causes diarrhea. The adults most at risk for impaction are elderly sedentary people—often bedridden. The feces are usually impacted in the rectum or in the rectosigmoid region, but occasionally may extend high up into the colon (rarely, even to the cecum). The leaking of colonic fluid around the impaction, resulting in the passage of frequent small volume watery bowel movements, accounts for the diarrhea. Other symptoms are common but are usually nonspecific: a sense of fullness in the rectum, vague lower abdominal pain, nausea, and headache. On *physical examination*, the firm stool is palpable in the left lower quadrant of the abdomen, which is best examined bimanually (a finger of one hand in the rectum and the other hand on the abdomen). The impaction is *best removed* manually if it is low enough, or through the sigmoidoscope, if it is not. Repeated enemas (e.g., phosphosoda with mineral oil) may be helpful once some of the very hard stool is removed. Common *complications* of impaction include recurrent urinary tract infection (because of compression of the ureters—more common in women), intestinal obstruction, perforation of the colon, and local ulceration.

Ulcerative Colitis

Ulcerative coitis is a chronic inflammatory disorder of colonic mucosa; its cause is unknown. It is recommended that patients with this condition be followed by the general physician in consultation with a gastroenterologist. The disorder may affect patients of any age, including the elderly, with a peak incidence in the third and fourth decades.

The clinical picture of ulcerative colitis is highly variable. The disorder may be limited to the rectum (ulcerative proctitis) or may involve the entire colon. Symptoms may range from occasional rectal bleeding, even without diarrhea, to profuse watery and bloody diarrhea. The severity of the initial presentation and the extent of the disease at the time of the initial attack have been shown to be useful predictors of the eventual course of the disease. Most patients (about 60%) have mild disease, *i.e.*, less than four bowel movements a day without fever, weight loss, or hypoalbuminemia. The vast majority of these patients will have colitis limited to the rectosigmoid region or to the descending colon. About 10 to 15% of patients with ulcerative colitis develop severe pancolitis with accompanying deterioration in their general health. Another 25% have moderate disease with more troublesome diarrhea, often containing blood, accompanied by crampy lower abdominal pain. Patients with moderate or severe disease may also have systemic symptoms of fever, fatigue, and weight loss. The clinical course is characterized by periodic exacerbations which in general respond well to adjustments in medical therapy. The smallest group of patients with ulcerative colitis consists of those with severe disease. This group includes the 1% of patients who present initially with fulminant colitis. In patients with severe colitis, symptoms may suddenly worsen, with profuse diarrhea, rectal bleeding, and high fevers. Plain films of the abdomen may demonstrate a dilated bowel ("toxic megacolon"). Mortality is high in this group of patients.

As there is no specific test for or histopathology of ulcerative colitis, the diagnosis depends on the constellation of symptoms, on the appropriate endoscopic and histological appearance of the colonic mucosa, on the exclusion of other inflammatory conditions, and on the natural history of the disorder. Patients with acute presentations, depending on the circumstances, must be differentiated from patients with bacterial diarrheas (see Chapter 26), amebiasis (see above page 471), Crohn's disease (see below), and ischemic colitis (ischemic colitis presents with acute abdominal pain and the passage of bloody stool; this is a disease of middle-aged or older people who usually have evidence of generalized atherosclerosis).

Treatment

Medical therapy for ulcerative colitis generally includes corticosteroids and sulfasalazine (Azulfidine). Steroids are particularly useful for acute exacerbations, but are not helpful in preventing relapses. Conversely, sulfasalazine is of limited value in the treatment of acute attacks, but has been shown to reduce the frequency of exacerbations and may allow reduction of the dosage of steroids. A minority of patients with ulcerative colitis need continuous steroid therapy. Other drugs, such as cytotoxic agents, require further evaluation before they can be recommended.

Surgery in ulcerative colitis is curative, and patients should be counseled early in their course about the role of surgery in the treatment of this disorder. Patients should be informed about the indications for surgery and the types of operations that are available. Early attention to this issue will enable the patient to accept an operation more readily if it is needed. Surgery for ulcerative colitis involves a proctocolectomy with an ileostomy to which a stomal appliance is attached to assure continence. Construction of a continent ileostomy, a relatively new procedure, avoids the need for a stomal appliance, but the procedure is technically difficult and, in 30% of cases, requires at least one revision. However, as exerience with this operation increases, it may become more popular. Also, early experience with ileorectal pull-through operations suggests that continence can be preserved after this procedure as well and this operation too may be offered more frequently in the future.

Cancer of the Colon

The risk of cancer of the colon is increased 5 to 10 times in patients with ulcerative colitis. The major risk factors are (a) duration of disease—risk increases significantly after 8 to 10 years of disease; (b) extent of colonic involvement—pancolitis carries the highest risk, while the risk in patients with ulcerative proctitis is similar to that of the general population; and (c) age of onset of disease—patients under the age of 25 at the time of onset have the highest risk, independent of the extent of disease. The cancer may be found anywhere in the colon, although most commonly it is within the rectum or

rectosigmoid. It may be multicentric. It is important that the patient know about the risk of cancer since it may influence his decision to undergo colectomy. After they have had the disease for 7 years, high risk patients should have yearly evaluations of the colon by either colonoscopy or air contrast barium enema. In addition, since dysplastic changes of the colonic mucosa have been identified as "precancer" and have been shown to correlate closely with the development of cancer elsewhere in the colon, serial colonic and rectal biopsies should be obtained in high risk patients.

Crohn's Disease

Crohn's disease or regional enteritis is a chronic inflammatory condition of unknown cause involving all layers of the intestine. The condition most commonly affects the terminal ileum, but any area from the esophagus to the anus can be involved. The onset of the disease most commonly is in adolescence and young adulthood.

Presentation

Crohn's disease may be localized initially to the small bowel, involve small bowel and colon, or be confined to the colon only. The inflammatory process usually remains confined to the initial site of involvement unless surgery is performed. Recurrence is the rule following surgery, and the condition may then involve additional segments of bowel. As the inflammatory process persists, the bowel wall becomes thickened and stenotic, leading to bowel obstruction. Fistula formation is characteristic and may spread to involve any contiguous structure. As a result, abscess formation and infection may complicate the clinical course. Diarrhea, abdominal pain, and weight loss are the common symptoms. Unlike the symptomatology in ulcerative colitis, persistent rectal bleeding is not a prominent feature.

The *differential diagnosis* includes disorders of both the small and large bowel. Occasionally the patient presents with fever and acute right lower quadrant pain resembling acute appendicitis. When there is terminal ileal involvement, Crohn's disease must be distinguished from lymphoma and tuberculosis. Colonic involvement may suggest ulcerative colitis (see above), ischemic colitis, or carcinoma (see Chapter 37). The predominant involvement of the distal small bowel and the right colon, the presence of characteristic skip areas, stricturing of the bowel, and fistula formation are helpful diagnostic features that suggest Crohn's disease.

Treatment

Therapy for Crohn's disease is similar to that for ulcerative colitis, depending heavily on corticosteroids and sulfasalazine (Azulfidine). These agents may be effective in treating the recurrent attacks that characterize Crohn's disease, but neither agent has been shown to be effective in preventing relapses. Metronidazole (Flagyl) may prove to be effective for perirectal fistulas. Immunosuppressants, like azathioprine (Imuran), have produced variable results, and their use in this condition is still controversial.

Surgery is sometimes necessary in Crohn's disease to treat the complications of the inflammatory process. Surgery is indicated for (a) resection of fibrotic obstructing lesions, (b) drainage of abscesses, and (c) resection of complicated fistulas. Occasionally the disease is refractory to medical therapy, and the diseased bowel must be resected. It must be recognized that surgery is not intended to be curative, so that removal of normal bowel to achieve wide "disease-free" margins is generally not indicated. Bypass surgery is being performed less often, as there appears to be an increasing frequency of the development of cancer in bypassed segments. In the rare patient whose disease is extensive and unresponsive to medical and surgical intervention, or in whom a short bowel syndrome has developed secondary to the disease and to repeated surgery, long term home parenteral hyperalimentation can be beneficial in providing good nutritional support and even in ameliorating symptoms.

Course

Despite its chronicity and tendency for recurrence. Crohn's disease takes a highly variable course. Prolonged relatively asymptomatic periods occur, even after years of disease activity and after multiple operations. There is a poor correlation between the clinical severity and the radiological appearance of the disease. Mortality from the disease is low. As the natural history is so variable, the physician should approach the patient with Crohn's disease in a positive and hopeful fashion, yet be aware of the potential for significant morbidity. All patients should be followed in close consultation with a gastroenterologist.

Drug-Induced Diarrhea

A variety of commonly used medications may cause diarrhea (Table 38.4). The diarrhea may be a direct result of the pharmacological activity of the drug (e.g., magnesium-containing antacids or colchicine); or the mechanism for the induction of diarrhea may be unknown (e.g., hydralazine or propranolol). The diarrhea may also signify drug toxicity (e.g., digitalis). Certain drugs have repeatedly been associated with diarrhea (antibiotics, antacids, quinidine, digitalis, alcohol), while in other cases (hydralazine, propranolol) the relationship is not well established (1).

Diarrhea associated with antibiotics may range from a mild increase in the frequency and volume of stools to a toxic, life-threatening condition. Diarrhea may develop during the course of antibiotic therapy, after either parenteral or oral use, but may also occur up to 3 weeks after discontinuation of the drugs. The antibiotics most commonly associated with diarrhea are ampicillin, tetracycline, clindamycin, and the cephalosporins.

In the more severe forms of antibiotic-associated diarrhea the diarrhea is bloody and is accompanied by abdominal cramps and fever. Proctoscopy may reveal pseudomembranes which appear as raised plaques on edematous friable mucosa. Histologically these pseudomembranes are collections of fibrin, mucin, and leukocytes. The etiology of pseudomembranous colitis is now believed to be due to the proliferation of Clostridium difficile and the elaboration of its toxin. This organism accounts for the vast majority of cases of pseudomembranous colitis and for about 20% of antibiotic-associated diarrhea in general.

Therapy involves discontinuation of the antibiotics and, in cases of pseudomembranous colitis, administration of oral vancomycin (see Chapter 26). This antibiotic is effective against clostridial organisms, and the response is fairly rapid. Relapses after discontinuation of vancomycin have been reported. Metronidazole may be used in refractory cases, although experience with it in this condition is much more limited than it is with vancomycin. Oral cholestyramine has also been used effectively to bind the toxin. Antidiarrheal medications are contraindicated as they may actually prolong the duration of the disease.

Postsurgical Diarrhea

A variety of surgical procedures may result in diarrhea. Obviously, extensive small bowel resections, e.g., for mesenteric vascular occlusions, result in severe diarrhea and steatorrhea. Management of such patients requires careful attention to nutritional factors and often requires narcotics for control of the diarrhea. Long term home hyperalimentation (available mainly through university centers and requiring special equipment and specially trained personnel) has allowed patients to overcome the severe malabsorption that would accompany massive small bowel resection.

Resection of the ileum is less well tolerated than is resection of the jejunum since the ileum serves as the only site for absorption of bile acids. When the ileal resection is limited (less than 100 cm) the total bile acid pool remains sufficient to prevent significant steatorrhea. However, there is still an excessive loading of bile salts into the colon where they stimulate mucosal secretion and result in diarrhea. Therapy for this form of diarrhea is aimed at binding the fecal bile acids with an agent such as cholestyramine. The dose is 4 g (usually provided by one package or scoopful), given before meals and at bedtime. When ileal resection is more extensive, (greater than 100 cm) the total bile acid pool becomes diminished below the critical level needed for proper digestion and absorption of fat, and steatorrhea develops. The use of cholestyramine in this situation only further depletes the bile acid pool and worsens the steatorrhea and diarrhea. Therefore, dietary fat should be supplied in the form of medium chain triglycerides which do not require bile salts for absorption. Commercial preparations are available (e.g., Portagen), and consultation with a nutritionist as well as a gastroenterologist is recommended.

Diarrhea may also follow *gastric surgery*. At times the vagotomy causes diarrhea by altering intestinal motility and, for unclear reasons, by increasing the concentration of fecal bile salts. Therapy with cholestyramine has been successful in this postvagotomy syndrome. Gastric surgery may also unmask a latent lactase deficiency or, rarely, a latent celiac sprue. The blind loop syndrome with resultant bacterial overgrowth, dumping syndrome, inadvertent gastroileal anastomosis, and gastrocolic fistula are all complications that may result in diarrhea in patients after gastrectomy (see Chapter 36).

Diarrhea occurs rarely following routine cholecystectomy, but, when it does occur, it has been associated with an increased concentration of fecal bile salts. Therapy with cholestyramine is effective. Subtotal colectomy, with an ileal-rectal anastomosis (e.g., for multiple polyposis), frequently results in diarrhea which is usually easily controlled by antidiarrheal medication (see below) and diminishes with time. Segmental colonic resection usually does not result in diarrhea.

Symptomatic Antidiarrheal Therapy

Diarrhea is, after all, merely a symptom, and therapy, if possible, should be directed at the primary underlying process. However, a wide variety of agents are available for symptomatic control of diarrhea. The efficacy of these agents is highly variable, and the mechanism of action of many is poorly understood. Symptomatic treatment should be avoided in patients with acute infectious diarrhea (except in minimal doses to prevent marked discomfort), since early suppression of bowel movements in these conditions prolongs the diarrhea.

Hydrophilic bulk-forming agents, like psyllium seed (Metamucil, Konsyl), have been shown to improve the consistency of ileostomy and colostomy effluent (see Chapter 41). These agents, which paradoxically are also used in treating constipation (see page 467), are particularly useful in patients with painless diarrhea and in patients with irritable bowel syndrome (Chapter 39).

Another group of antidiarrheal medications consists of those classified as *adsorbents* on the premise that these agents adsorb factors within the intestinal lumen which cause diarrhea. Medications of this group include kaolin and pectin (Kaopectate), bismuth salts (Pepto-Bismol), aluminum hydroxide (Amphojel), and cholestyramine (Questran). These agents are generally available over the counter, but their value is not well established. Pepto-Bismol has been shown, however, to be effective in controlling the symptoms of traveler's diarrhea (see Chapter 26). Cholestyramine, as previously mentioned, is effective in treating bile acid-induced diarrhea, as in patients after ileal resection, vagotomy, or cholecystectomy. This drug also may bind other compounds, like digoxin and warfarin, and thereby decrease their absorption.

Opiate and opioid derivatives are probably the most effective antidiarrheal medications. Opiate drugs delay the transit of intraluminal contents through the small and large intestine. A possible central effect cannot be excluded. In patients with extensive small bowel resection tincture of opium or codeine may be the only effective form of therapy. The synthetic agents, diphenoxylate-atropine (Lomotil) and loperamide (Imodium) are effective also and generally are very well tolerated. The atropine in Lomotil contributes little to its antidiarrheal effect and may cause significant toxicity. Imodium has the theoretical advantages of a more favorable ratio of gastrointestinal effects to central nervous system effects and a longer duration of action. Imodium has the practical disadvantage of being relatively expensive, costing about $29.00/100 tablets compared to approximately $18.00 for Lomotil and about $5.00 for generic brands of diphenoxylate-atropine. The development of megacolon, prolongation of symptoms, and worsening of pseudomembranous colitis have all been linked to the injudicious use of these agents in patients with bacterial diarrhea. The potential risk for abuse is theoretically less for Imodium, but has probably been overemphasized for Lomotil.

Another class of drugs that is under intensive investigation is classified as "*antisecretory*." Some of these drugs inhibit the synthesis of prostaglandins, ubiquitous fatty acids which increase intestinal secretion by stimulating adenylate cyclase activity within intestinal cells. (Adenylate cyclase is the enzyme which catalyzes the formation of cyclic AMP, the concentration of which influences certain transport systems in cell membranes.) Other drugs of this class inhibit adenylate cyclase directly. For example, indomethacin (Indocin) inhibits prostaglandin synthesis and has been shown experimentally to inhibit the effect of enterotoxin; and propranolol (Inderal), an inhibitor of adenylate cyclase, suppresses bile acid-induced fluid accumulation in intestinal loops. Certain diuretics, like ethacrynic acid (Edecrin), which act on electrolyte transport, also have been shown to be effective enterotoxin antagonists. While these antisecretory agents are not now recommended for use in antidiarrheal therapy, investigation into their mechanism of action may lead to the development of new effective forms of therapy against diarrhea.

Since there are few data to allow an objective comparison of the various antidiarrheal medications, the choice of drug must be based on efficacy, safety, and cost. For acute self-limited illnesses, drugs like kaolin-pectate and bismuth salts are often tried by patients, even before a physician is consulted. For such patients, diphenoxylate-atropine or loperamide is highly effective. Patients should be instructed to use medication after a diarrheal movement, not to exceed 8 tablets/day. Loperamide may provide longer diarrhea-free intervals with fewer side effects (6).

For patients with chronic diarrhea, the choice of medication is based on the severity of the diarrhea and on its cause. In patients with the diarrhea-predominant form of the irritable bowel syndrome (Chapter 39), hydrophilic agents may be useful. The dose should be titrated to the desired bowel habits, with doses ranging from 1 teaspoon to 2 tablespoons/day mixed in 8 ounces of juice or water. In patients with diarrhea from other causes diphenoxylate-atropine or loperamide should be tried. These medications can be given in divided doses throughout the day. Diarrhea can also be prevented by taking 1 or 2 tablets before engaging in an event associated with diarrhea (meals, examinations, etc).

In more severe cases of diarrhea, narcotics are necessary. Tincture of opium is convenient because it can easily be titrated (by the drop) to control diarrhea at the lowest possible dose. A recommended starting dose is 6 drops every 4 to 6 hours, to be adjusted by 1 or 2 drops per dose depending on the patient's response. Codeine, at a dose of 15 to 30 mg, may also be used with the same dosage schedule.

General References

Fingl E, Freston J: Antidiarrheal agents and laxatives: changing concepts. *Clin Gastroenterol* 8:161, 1979.
Matseshe J, Phillips S: Chronic diarrhea: a practical approach. *Med Clin North Am* 62:141, 1978.
    Provides clear guidelines to the evaluation of this problem and indications for various tests.
Schuster MM: Constipation and anorectal disorders. *Clin Gastroenterol* 6:643, 1977.

Specific References

1. Deren JJ: Iatrogenic diarrhea. *Pract Gastroenterol* 4:25, 1980.
2. Gray GM: Intestinal disaccharidase deficiencies and glucose-galactose malabsorption. In Stanbury JB, Wyngaarden JB, Frederickson DS (eds): *Metabolic Basis of Inherited Disease,* ed 4. New York, McGraw-Hill, 1978, p 1526.
3. Harris JC, DuPont HL, Hornick RB: Fecal leukocytes in diarrheal illness. *Ann Intern Med* 76:697, 1972.
4. Kaufman N, Schuster M: Colonic motility studies differentiate three types of constipation, *Gastroenterology* 76:1166, 1979.
5. Martelli H, Devroede G, Arhan P, et al: Some parameters of large bowel motility in normal man. *Gastroenterology* 75:612, 1978.
6. Palmer KR, Corbett CL, Holdsworth CD: Double blind crossover study comparing loperamide, codeine, and diphenoxylate in the treatment of chronic diarrhea. *Gastroenterology* 79:1272, 1980.

CHAPTER THIRTY-NINE

The Irritable Bowel Syndrome

MARVIN M. SCHUSTER, M.D.

DEFINITION AND EPIDEMIOLOGY

Irritable bowel syndrome (IBS) is the most common gastrointestinal condition encountered in medical practice. The syndrome is diagnosed on the basis of (a) abdominal pain, (b) altered bowel habits, and (c) the absence of detectable organic pathology. A related condition, *painless (or "nervous") diarrhea*, should be considered either as a separate entity, or at best a variant of IBS, because it affects persons with different personality profiles, is more directly and immediately related to emotional stress, and has a different course and prognosis. Symptoms of IBS generally appear during late teenage or in the early twenties and more commonly afflict women than men, the disorder having a female to male predominance of 2:1. The symptoms rarely appear for the first time after the age of 50, and therefore the physician should be extremely reluctant to make this diagnosis in the older patient who has had a recent onset of symptoms. There is some question about whether recurrent abdominal pain of childhood is a form of IBS or leads to IBS in later life.

There are many other terms by which irritable bowel syndrome is known. These include mucus colitis, nervous colitis, spastic colon, nervous colon, irritated colon, and unstable colon. The term "colitis" is especially inappropriate since no inflammation is present and since it is frightening to the patient, who easily confuses it with ulcerative colitis. This misconception imposes unnecessary stress on patients whose condition is readily aggravated by stress. The term irritable bowel syndrome is more appropriate than other terms because it refers to general gastrointestinal irritability, indicating that areas other than the colon may be involved, and it also emphasizes that this is a syndrome and not a specific disease.

PATHOPHYSIOLOGY

The signs and symptoms of irritable bowel syndrome appear related predominantly to exaggeration of normal intestinal motility patterns. In normal subjects the dominant type of motor activity is that of segmenting contractions, which tend to retard the forward movement of intraluminal contents. This impeding activity represents about 90% or more of the wave types recorded in normal individuals. When this type of activity is excessive, constipation ensues. In diarrheal states this activity is markedly diminished or abolished and is replaced by infrequent mass propulsive movements (which may occur five or six times a day during episodes of diarrhea). The symptoms of irritable bowel syndrome (abdominal pain, constipation, diarrhea) are related to excessively strong, spastic contractions either of the segmenting (impeding) or of the propulsive type. The motility pattern of IBS has been described as the paradoxical motility of constipation and diarrhea, but the paradox is a spurious one, if these basic principles are understood.

Motility can be influenced by a number of factors, such as meals, emotionally stressful situations, anxiety, and various drugs (e.g., opiates). In IBS, exacerbation of symptoms by meals (i.e., pain, distension, and occasional diarrhea) is thought to be related to an exaggeration of the normal biphasic postprandial response—the gastroileocolic response, which consists of an early neurogenic (reflex) component during the first 15 to 30 minutes postprandially, and hormonally stimulated contractions that appear after 40 minutes. The hormonal phase may be initiated by gastrointestinal hormones released during feeding. For example cholecystokinin, which is released as food enters the duodenum, can reproduce postprandial symptoms in some patients with IBS, and these symptoms are associated with increased motility. Whether this or other hormones of this type are clinically important is unknown.

DIAGNOSIS

History

Most patients with IBS come to medical attention after their symptoms have been present for months or years. Major complaints are those of pain and altered bowel habits. Which of these two components is emphasized depends on which is the more disturbing to the patient. This, in turn, is determined by the intensity of each symptom, by the patient's reaction to it, and by the disruptive effects of the symptom on the patient's function and activities. For example, some patients are less bothered by abdominal pain which can be hidden from others but are perturbed by urgent diarrhea which interferes with their job or social functions. The pattern of symptoms varies considerably from person to person but remains fairly consistent for a given individual, with changes for an individual occurring predominantly in intensity or frequency of occurrence. Typically, symptoms are intermittent with symptom-free periods lasting days, weeks, or, rarely, months. An occasional patient will have symptoms every day.

Pain

The quality of pain may be described by one patient as crampy, by another as sharp or burning. For most, the pain is relieved temporarily by a bowel movement. One of the most important features that differentiates functional from organic pain is that the pain does not awaken the patient from sleep. It is important that the question concerning this feature is carefully phrased, since there is an important distinction between awakening with pain and being awakened by pain. Patients with IBS who are depressed have early morning awakening, and, after awakening, experience pain; but close questioning can determine that the patient was not awakened by the pain. The location of pain may vary from person to person, but is fairly consistent for a given person. Pain may be localized to any quadrant, although it is more common in the lower abdomen than anywhere else and in the left lower quadrant more common than in the right. Although the pain usually does not radiate, some patients describe transmission into the lower back or down the legs. The distribution of the pain is generally over a wide enough area so that the patient, when asked to point to the location of the pain, does so with the flat of his hand rather than with a finger, and often makes a circular motion covering a broad area. More often than not, the onset of pain does not appear to correlate with any known precipitating stressful event; instead, periods of illness may correlate with general periods of stress over months or years. It is important to determine what life experiences or interpersonal relationships constitute stress for a particular person so that this can be taken into account when establishing a treatment program.

Altered Bowel Habits

The altered pattern of defecation in patients with irritable bowel syndrome may consist of constipation, diarrhea, or more commonly, alternating constipation and diarrhea, with one of the two predominating (Chapter 38 discusses these symptoms in detail). As with pain, the altered pattern of defecation, though variable from person to person, is fairly consistent for a given individual, changing only in periodicity and intensity.

Not infrequently the major disordered bowel function occurs in the morning, with the first stool being normal in consistency followed in rapid succession by increasingly loose stools, sometimes associated with flatulence and sometimes also precipitated by meals. The bowel movements are accompanied by a great deal of urgency and are preceded by cramps which are relieved by defecation. Formed stools are often compressed and of narrow pencil-sized diameter because of the molding effect of rectosigmoid spasm. In other instances spasm of the colon results in the passage of scybalous stools described by the patient as dehydrated pellets. Mucus may cover the stools or be passed separately. Stools may mistakenly be referred to as diarrheal when they consist of frequently passed small quantities of soft fragments that are narrow in caliber. Explosive defecation may result from evacuation of gas along with the stool.

Painless Diarrhea

Patients who present with diarrhea but do not have abdominal pain generally are thought to have a disorder that is different from irritable bowel syndrome, although sometimes painless diarrhea is classified as a variant of the irritable bowel syndrome. Compared to patients with IBS their symptoms are more directly related to a stressful event, follow more immediately upon that stress, and respond more readily and dramatically to alleviation of stress. Also the prognosis is generally better than it is in classical IBS.

Relationship of Symptoms to Meals

Some, but not all, patients with IBS experience exacerbation of their symptoms postprandially (see above). They appear to be a special subset of patients. Some patients report intolerance of specific foods, most commonly milk, caffeine, fried foods, and red wine.

Gas

Intestinal gas derives either from swallowing of air, from bacterial breakdown of poorly digested foods, or from diminished absorption of gas (which may occur during the rapid transit which accompanies diarrhea). Aerophagia is aggravated by frequent swallowing while chewing gum and during nervous states and is induced by a dry throat or by the excessive intake of carbonated beverages including beer. Increased gas production follows eating of legumes (beans, for example) which contain stachyose and raffinose, substances that can only be digested by colonic flora, resulting in release of large amounts of hydrogen in the colon. If patients have milk intolerance because of lactase deficiency, undigested lactose enters into the colon where it is broken down by colonic bacteria, also resulting in gaseous distension.

Although gaseous distension is a frequent complaint, actual measurements have demonstrated that patients with IBS have no more gas than do normal subjects. Instead, they have a decreased tolerance to distension from normal amounts of gas, a factor which may be related to hypermotility of their bowel and to the lowered threshold for distension-induced spasm. Gas, because it tends to rise, usually forms pockets under the splenic flexure, which is the highest portion of the colon in the upright position. This entrapment of air is further facilitated by distal rectosigmoid spasm which impedes its passage. The *splenic flexure syndrome* which ensues is experienced as chest pain that may mimic the pain of myocardial ischemia. A similar *hepatic flexure syndrome* can accompany gas trapped on the right side and may mimic the pain of cholecystitis.

Studies in which air has been instilled into the small bowel have demonstrated that patients with IBS tend to reflux gas more readily into the stomach than do normal subjects, which may explain their complaint of increased belching. This complaint too seems to result from abnormal intestinal motility.

Upper Gastrointestinal Symptoms

One-fourth to one-half of patients with IBS complain of dyspeptic symptoms such as heartburn, "indigestion," pain, and nausea (but rarely vomiting). These upper gastrointestinal symptoms reinforce the concept that the motor abnormality is not restricted to the colon alone.

Significance of Weight Loss and Bleeding

Irritable bowel syndrome *per se* is not associated with either weight loss or gastrointestinal bleeding, and the appearance of either of these two symptoms in patients with IBS should alert the physician to another disorder. However, significant depression accompanying irritable bowel syndrome may explain substantial weight loss, just as anal fissures or hemorrhoids resulting from the altered bowel habits of the syndrome may explain bright red rectal bleeding. Nevertheless, either of these two symptoms warrants a meticulous search for other disorders, including cancer. A sudden change in symptom

pattern after a period of many years also warrants a search for a new disorder.

Psychological Factors (See Table 39.1)

Seventy percent of patients with IBS have abnormal scores on psychological testing. The psychological disturbances that most commonly accompany irritable bowel syndrome are hysteria, anxiety, depression, and cancerphobia. Of these, anxiety is the most readily detected and perhaps the easiest to treat by pharmacological means, by psychological approaches, or by environmental manipulation. Depression is generally masked and is commonly overlooked by patient and physician alike (see Chapter 15). This is in part because somatization, a common manifestation of depression, results in a focus upon complaints that may misdirect the physician's attention from underlying psychological factors. Depression should be suspected in patients who appear preoccupied or sad or who by their report or the report of family members have lost interest in matters that formerly interested them. Cancerphobia may be suggested when the patient compares his symptoms with those of a relative or friend who has had cancer. In addition to determining whether the patient has an unwarranted and excessive fear of cancer, the physician should also seek to elicit from him and from other informants any other fears or concerns that the patient has with respect to himself and his illness.

Physical Examination

Except for an anxious demeanor, patients with IBS usually look remarkably healthy, and physical examination is correspondingly normal with the frequent exception of mildly increased tympany to percussion over one or more areas of the colon and a tender cord-like sigmoid palpable in the left lower quadrant. A palpable sigmoid itself is not an unusual finding, even in normal people, because firm stool may be present in this area, but tenderness is significant. Tenderness may be present in other areas also, particularly in the right lower quadrant, where a squishy cecum may be palpated.

Digital rectal examination is usually unremarkable, but may reveal excessive tenderness. Proctoscopic examination should demonstrate no structural abnormality, but often does reveal rectal and rectosigmoid spasm and excessive tenderness, that precludes advance beyond 12 or 13 cm. At times excessive mucus is encountered.

In patients with symptoms of IBS, the physician should look for signs of hyperthyroidism, masses, adenopathy, and partial intestinal obstruction as well as for abdominal bruits which might signal ischemic intestinal angina in the elderly.

Laboratory Tests

Basic laboratory tests should be carried out to demonstrate the absence of anemia, a normal white

Table 39.1.
Psychological Features of Irritable Bowel Syndrome[a]

Psychopathology	Diagnostic Features	Treatment
Depression	Sad, tearful, hopeless, fatigue, loss of interest, early morning awakening	Antidepressant medication, environmental manipulation
Anxiety	Symptoms increased by stress	Relaxation training; environmental manipulation; learn coping techniques
Gratification from illness behavior	Symptoms often interfere with work or socializing	Treat as a physical deformity; encourage maximum activity; discourage talking to others about illness; recognize chronic nature of disorder
Cancer phobia	Patient or family reports fear; patient describes similarity of his symptoms with a known cancer victim	Adequate early workup, then limit further investigation; discuss openly with patient

[a] After Whitehead WE, Schuster MM: Psychological management of irritable bowel syndrome. *Prac Gastroenterol* 3:32, 1979.

blood cell count and sedimentation rate, the absence of blood, ova, and parasites on three stool examinations, a negative sigmoidoscopy, and (when symptoms are severe enough or prolonged enough to warrant the study) a barium enema negative except for spastic contractions. Effacement of haustra may be seen in the barium enema if there has been prolonged laxative abuse (see Chapter 38). Occasionally a small bowel series will be necessary to rule out Crohn's disease, especially when diarrhea predominates or when there is associated unexplained fever or weight loss. Painful splenic flexure symptoms sometimes require studies to rule out coronary artery disease (see Chapter 57).

The basic principle in the selection and timing of laboratory tests is to perform as early as possible those tests which are necessary to convince both the physician and the patient that organic disease has been ruled out. It is generally imprudent to postpone some tests for a later date or to repeat tests continually, since this behavior arouses the suspicion that the diagnosis is uncertain, that the disease might be progressive, or that a new and more dire consequence, such as cancer or colitis, may be developing.

Differential Diagnosis

Many of the symptoms of irritable bowel syndrome are nonspecific and can be produced by other disorders. A careful travel history should be obtained relative to possible bacterial infection or parasitic infestation, including giardiasis and amoebiasis.

Since patients with *lactose intolerance* often do not associate their symptoms with milk, the failure to find a direct relationship between milk intake and diarrhea should not dissuade the physician from testing for milk tolerance. Lactose intolerance is best ruled out by a therapeutic trial on a lactose-free diet (see sample lactose-free diet, Table 39.2) for 3 weeks,

eliminating all milk and milk products, including butter, cottage cheese, yogurt, and soft cheeses. Aged cheeses, such as Swiss cheese and Jarlsberg, are permissible since most of the lactose in them has been eliminated. Yogurt contains little lactose and may be reintroduced later as tolerated. Acidophilus milk (cultured with *Lactobacillus acidophilus*), contrary to popular misconception, contains the same amount of lactose as does regular milk. However the amount of lactose in milk can be virtually eliminated by adding 12 drops of lactase (Lactaid, Maxilact, or a similar preparation) to a quart of milk, which is then permitted to remain overnight in the refrigerator; this procedure reduces, but does not eliminate entirely, the symptoms of lactose intolerance (3). Also, Lactrase capsules taken just prior to ingestion of milk products will reduce the lactose load substantially. Otherwise, nondairy (lactose-free) substitutes, such as Coffeemate, Cremora, or Mocha Mix, may be used. Margarine may be substituted for butter. If all symptoms disappear on a lactose-free diet, then the diagnosis is that of lactose intolerance. Partial improvement implies that, in addition to irritable bowel syndrome, the patient has lactose intolerance and that some of the symptoms (usually those of gaseous bloating and diarrhea) are due to the intolerance. The therapeutic dietary trial is more useful than a lactose tolerance test, which simply tests the patient's response to a given amount of lactose in a single dose at a particular time (see also Chapter 38, page 474).

Among the other disorders which can mimic symptoms of diarrhea-predominant irritable bowel syndrome are hyperthyroidism, nontropical sprue, carcinoid, Zollinger-Ellison syndrome, medullary carcinoma of the thyroid, diabetic autonomic neuropathy, Addison's disease, and Whipple's disease. Constipation-predominant IBS may be mimicked by hypothyroidism, hyperparathyroidism, diverticular

Table 39.2.
Lactose-Free Diet[a]

Type of Food	Food Allowed	Food to be Avoided
Milk and milk products	Nutramigen and soya bean milk used in place of milk. Nondairy "milk" which does not contain lactose.	All milk or any species and all products containing milk as skim, dried, evaporated, condensed yogurt, cheese,[b] ice cream, malted milk, sherberts.
Meat, fish, fowl	Plain beef, chicken, fish, turkey, veal, pork, ham, liver or other organ meats.	*Creamed* or *breaded* meat, fish, or fowl; sausage products such as weiners, liver sausage; cold cuts which contain milk.
Eggs	All	None
Vegetables	All	Creamed, breaded, or buttered vegetables. Any vegetables to which lactose has been added during processing.
Potatoes and substitutes	White potatoes, sweet potatoes, yams, macaroni, noodles, rice, spaghetti.	Any creamed, breaded, or buttered potatoes or starch and instant potatoes if lactose has been added during processing.
Breads and cereals	Any that do not contain milk or milk products.	Prepared mixes as muffins, biscuits, waffles, pancakes, dry cereals with added skim milk powder. Instant cream of wheat and other instant hot cereals. Read labels carefully.
Fats	Margarines which do not contain milk or milk products. Salad dressings which do not contain milk or milk products. Bacon, salad oils, shortening.	Margarines and dressings containing milk or milk products; butter, cream cheese.
Soups	All except those listed under foods excluded.	Cream soups, chowders, commercially prepared soups which contain lactose.
Desserts	Water and fruit ices; Jello, angel food cake; homemade cakes, pies, cookies made without milk from acceptable ingredients. Ice cream made with nondairy mix.	Commercial cakes and cookies and mixes; custard, puddings, ice cream made with milk; any containing chocolate.
Fruits	All fresh, canned, or frozen that are not processed with lactose.	Any canned or frozen that are processed with lactose.
Miscellaneous	Nuts and nut butter, unbuttered popcorn, olives, pure sugar candy, jelly or marmalade, sugar, Karo, chewing gum.	Gravy, white sauce, coffee, powdered drink, carmels, molasses, molasses candies, instant coffee (Folger's instant coffee and Tang are lactose free).

[a] In all instances labels should be carefully read and any product which contains milk, lactose, dry milk solids, or curds should be omitted. Avoid also whey and sugar substitutes with lactose. For milk products use Coffeemate, soy milk baby formulas, or Lactaid milk.
[b] Swiss, Jarlsberg, Edom, and *sharp* cheddar are the only cheeses allowed.

disease, intestinal obstruction, and colon cancer. Suspicion of any of these disorders justifies the appropriate tests to rule them out. Further evaluation of patients with atypical symptoms of irritable bowel syndrome should be done in consultation with a gastroenterologist.

THERAPY

Natural History

There is evidence that approximately 15% of the general adult population have the irritable bowel syndrome but have not sought medical attention for it (4). It is currently uncertain whether patients who seek medical attention are different from those who do not, and whether this difference, if it exists, is based on the severity of symptoms or on their effect on a particular person. Approximately one-fourth of patients who seek medical treatment for IBS ultimately have a permanent remission. It is unclear whether this represents the natural course of the disease or a response to early treatment of mild disease. The patient who is referred for gastroenterological consultation often has correspondingly more severe and chronic symptoms and generally experiences a more prolonged course.

Although there is little information concerning patients with IBS who present to the primary care physician, it has been shown that the course of patients seen by gastroenterologists follows a fairly consistent pattern that is characteristic for the given individual. In fact, the pattern is so consistent that any significant change should be accepted as a warning of a new superimposed problem warranting further investigation.

General Principles

Since the underlying etiology of IBS is unknown, treatment is symptomatic and relies on education, reassurance, diet, supportive and behavioral therapy, and pharmacotherapy aimed at both the underlying motor disorder and its psychological concomitants. Successful management requires an interest in the patient and his disorder, an understanding on the part of both patient and physician of what is known about IBS, and, above all, a recognition of the chronic nature of the disorder, which implies acceptance of a prolonged cooperative therapeutic endeavor.

Education and Reassurance

Treatment begins with the first interview and physical examination, which should be designed to begin to establish a relationship of mutual interest and confidence and which should be thorough enough to demonstrate to the patient that the physician has taken seriously the complaints and is performing all necessary maneuvers to rule out organic causes. At the same time attention to the details of all contributing factors, including diet, emotional reactions, interpersonal relationships, social interactions, and the patient's fears and concerns, provides ample evidence to the patient that these are important factors for him to consider and with which he must deal. The worst mistake that a physician can make is to downplay the symptoms on the grounds that they exist only in the patient's mind. This is incorrect physiologically and therapeutically; a definite motor disorder exists and can be demonstrated by both myoelectric and motility recordings.

It is important to take the time to explain to the patient the present understanding of the disordered motility (see page 480) and the factors influencing it to emphasize that, although the disorder is chronic, it can be managed by appropriate cooperation between patient and physician. The demonstrated ability of the physician to predict the course establishes that he is knowledgeable and promotes confidence. Furthermore, if the patient knows what to anticipate and understands that treatment can be expected to ameliorate rather than eliminate the disorder, he is better prepared to face recurrence, which otherwise might be disappointing and frightening. Labeling and understanding the abnormal motor activity can be reassuring to the patient and may provide him with the patience required to wait for gradual improvement. At the same time the positive implications of the diagnosis should be underscored, emphasizing that IBS, though often persistent, does not lead to cancer, colitis, or ileitis and does not alter life expectancy.

Diet

Even when the patient keeps a meticulous daily log relating onset of symptoms to life events (including activities, interpersonal relations, and food intake), it is often difficult to make direct associations with any degree of specificity. It is best to explain to those individuals who have postprandial distress that, although some foods may be bothersome, it is usually the act of eating (rather than a specific food) that aggravates the symptoms. Since a lactose-free diet can provide dramatic relief for patients who are lactose intolerant, it is worthwhile trying such a diet in every patient (as stated above). (Those patients who improve on a 2-week lactose-free trial may then add small amounts of lactose-containing foods until symptoms appear. This will establish the level of lactose that can be tolerated by that person). Otherwise the most that can be said about food intolerance is that some people react badly to coffee, carbonated beverages, and spicy sauces, although no convincing evidence exists in this regard. Therefore patients may wish to abstain from these foods for a period, noting whether symptoms recur on at least two occasions when each substance is reintroduced. Any food that is definitely associated with precipitation of symptoms should obviously be avoided, but one should be careful not to create a dietary cripple.

Although the therapeutic role of bran in the treatment of IBS has not been established, some patients with constipation-predominant IBS do derive benefit from a diet comprising at least 14 g of bran. This can be administered as 2 tablespoons of miller's unprocessed bran three times daily. Bran can be obtained from a health food store. Since it looks and tastes like sawdust, it can be camouflaged in cereal, baked in cookies, or taken with a beverage. Studies in another disorder, diverticular disease, show that the effect of bran on transit and motility appears to be specific and is not common to all fibers (1). Therefore lettuce, celery, and fruits may not produce similar results. Bran has been shown to increase the size of stool and the frequency of its passage. Patients should be warned that there might be some increase in flatulence when bran is first administered, but that it will wear off by the end of 3 weeks in 80% of patients. However, 15 or 20% of people find these side effects intolerable even after 3 weeks. Dosage should be titrated for each patient, weighing the beneficial effects against the annoying side effects.

The hydrophilic colloids (bulk agents such as Metamucil, Konsyl, or L.A. Formula containing psyllium seed) may be especially useful in those patients who have alternating constipation and diarrhea. Because of their hydrophilic qualities they tend to bind water and therefore decrease the fluidity of diarrheal stools, while preventing excess dehydration in constipated patients. Initially, 1 to 2 tablespoons of hydrophilic powder are prescribed in conjunction with a meal two to three times a day, and the dose is gradually diminished to once a day (adjusting to the patient's response). It is better to prescribe the agent before or after a meal rather than at bedtime, so that it becomes mixed with the meal as it traverses the gastrointestinal tract. When taken at night the medication can result in the passage of rock-hard stool followed by a gelatinous mass. Patients who are thin should take the bulk agent after meals, since it tends to suppress appetite, whereas obese patients may derive benefit from taking it before meals, thus achieving satiation without caloric content.

Drugs

Although there are ample theoretical grounds for prescribing antispasmodic medication, clinical experience with spasmolytic agents has been disappointing. Nevertheless, some patients improve with antispasmodic drugs, particularly those whose symptoms are induced by meals and those who complain of tenesmus. Well controlled studies are needed to determine whether anticholinergic medication has more than a placebo effect. When used for those whose symptoms are related to meals, anticholinergics should be prescribed 30 to 45 minutes before meals so that the major benefit of the drug will be available at the time of anticipated symptoms. Patients with tenesmus should take the drug on a regular basis, timing the dose so that it is given as close as possible to 1 hour before anticipated symptoms. There is no evidence that one anticholinergic is better than another, but it seems logical to use drugs which have the highest ratio of antispasmodic to antisecretory effect, so that a large dose can be administered to suppress spasm without producing undesirable side effects, such as dry mouth. Mebeverine, a spasmolytic agent with little or no antisecretory effect, is available in most countries outside the United States and is prescribed in doses of 100 to 200 mg four times a day (½ hour before meals if symptoms are meal related). In this country dicyclomine hydrochloride (Bentyl) is given in dosages of 20 to 40 mg, four times a day, as tolerated. The major side effects are tachycardia and orthostatic hypotension. Thus, baseline and follow-up recordings of pulse rate and blood pressure, with the patient seated and standing are very important. Dicyclomine should be prescribed in small quantities to elderly people who are susceptible to orthostatic changes; for example, 10-mg doses on a divided basis, gradually increasing to reach the desired effect as tolerated. If improvement ensues, long term medication for months or years is warranted. Tolerance usually does not develop, but change to a different anticholinergic may be helpful if benefit decreases. A therapeutic trial should be carried out for at least 3 weeks to test the efficacy of the drug.

Significant diarrhea may respond to diphenoxylate-atropine (Lomotil), 1 to 2 tablets every 6 hours while diarrhea persists. The related drug, loperamide (Imodium) has a longer duration of action, and 1 to 2 tablets every 8 hours may be given. Care should be taken to discontinue medication as soon as the diarrhea is controlled in order to avoid inducing constipation, especially in those patients who are prone to have alternating diarrhea and constipation. Patients who have strongly diarrhea-predominant IBS and who do not respond to the above medications may benefit from codeine, 30 to 60 mg every 6 hours, especially if pain is disabling. Because of its potentially addicting qualities, codeine should be prescribed with caution, although addiction is rare when codeine is taken for diarrhea. This is partially because intestinal tolerance to the drug does not develop. The same dose that controls diarrhea at one stage continues to control it subsequently, and escalating doses are not required as they are in patients who have developed central nervous system addiction.

Analgesic medication should be avoided if possible and when needed should be prescribed in the mildest form and lowest dose possible. Aspirin and acetaminophen, however, are rarely effective. Pentazocine (Talwin), 50 to 100 mg, can be given every 6 hours as needed for severe pain, but the number of tablets taken should be monitored. Morphine and codeine (see above) generally should be avoided, especially when constipation exists, because they tend to aggravate spasm; and Demerol should be reserved for extreme pain on unusual occasions.

Gas Control

Most medications designed to alleviate gaseous distension have proven disappointing. However, simethicone (Mylicon), 2 to 4 tablets with meals, or activated charcoal, 4 tablets with meals and at bedtime, can be prescribed as a therapeutic trial. Phazyme 95, 1 to 2 tablets with meals and at bedtime, or similar enzymes, such as Ilozyme, Pancrease, Viokase, Cotazym, *etc*, can also be tried.

Psychological Management (See Table 39.1)

Psychological management begins with the recognition of depression, anxiety, and somatization of affect. Symptoms of IBS often are anxiety provoking and frequently are perpetuated by social reinforcement (secondary gain). Psychological evaluation and management usually can be effectively performed by the interested physician without the need for psychiatric referral. The condition itself is not an indication for psychiatric consultation. Referral should be reserved for those patients who would need expert psychotherapy whether or not they have irritable bowel syndrome.

Psychological management is dictated by answers to the following questions:

1. Is there evidence of anxiety, and are the symptoms aggravated by stress? If so, what are the specific stresses? Stress-induced anxiety can be handled by avoiding or modifying situational factors, and by teaching relaxation techniques (using audiotapes).* Occasionally mild tranquilizing agents are indicated (see Chapter 13).

2. Is the patient depressed? As with anxiety, attempts should be made to determine specific depressing situations, especially to determine whether simple maneuvers can alter them. If not, the patient sometimes can learn new ways of handling situations which cannot be avoided. Tricyclic antidepressants (see Chapter 15) may prove helpful in depression.

3. Does gratification from illness behavior (see Chapter 12) reinforce the illness? Evidence that this is so derives from the history that the illness keeps the patient from job-related or social discomfort and stress. The spouse, family, or friends respond sympathetically to the patient's symptoms, providing further reinforcement. The patient's motivation is generally unconscious, and it is a strategic error to accuse a patient of trying to derive benefit from the illness. Treatment is designed to reduce the amount of gratification that illness behavior evokes. The patient is asked not to discuss his illness with family members, but instead to reserve his complaints for his physician. In return family members are instructed to help the patient by discouraging excessive discussion of his illness and by avoiding overly sympathetic responses. The patient is instructed to view the illness as he would a physical disability which he would like to overcome by pushing his performance to maximum capacity.

4. What misconceptions does the patient have about his illness? The answer to this question can be obtained from questions directed to the patient as well as to his family who may provide information that the patient is reluctant to give. A rational explanation of the patient's disorder is necessary, but the physician should also listen attentively to the patient's irrational fears (of cancer, for example), and he should deal with them as well. Patience is required since these issues may need to be worked through repetitively. A steady, supportive approach is most desirable, as well as a clear demonstration that the physician is acquainted with and sensitive to the patient, his disorder, and his needs. Regular (although not necessarily frequent) follow-up visits supply reassurance to the patient while "p.r.n." (as the need arises) visits are often viewed as abandonment or as an indication of impotence on the part of a physician who feels incapable of providing further help. Furthermore, "as needed" visits lend themselves to greater abuse by the patient who is seeking secondary gains (see also Chapter 12).

PROGNOSIS

Whether treatment alters the prognosis or simply affects the patient's ability to accept or deal with his symptoms has not been established. It is difficult to determine the impact of a specific form of treatment on the natural course of irritable bowel syndrome for a number of reasons. First, each patient is different; some have milder symptoms, some more severe; some have frequent recurrences, some infrequent. Second, patients with painless diarrhea (see page 480) have been included in some of the studies and excluded from others. Prognosis for this group is better than that of IBS patients with pain; and the number of such patients included in any given study markedly influences the results of a particular treatment program. Third, the more serious the associated psychological factors, the more prolonged the course of IBS, no matter what the underlying precipitating factors and presentation. Fourth, physicians are different in their training, interest, background, and approaches. Fifth, various treatment programs have been fashionable from time to time and none has undergone systematic, long term evaluation in a manner that provides useful scientific data. All of these factors underscore the need for organized, individualized, multifaceted management by a physician who is interested, educated, skillful, and compassionate.

General References

Chaudhary NA, Truelove SC: The irritable colon syndrome. A study of the clinical features, predisposing causes, and prognosis in 130 cases. *Q J Med* 31:307, 1962.
> Good clinical review based on analysis of personal experience in a large number of patients.

Schuster MM (ed): Irritable bowel syndrome. *Pract Gastroenterol* 3:3, 4, 5, 6 (May–Dec), 1979.
> In-depth and still up-to-date symposium consisting of 15 articles by leading experts, each focusing on a specific clinical aspect of irritable bowel syndrome.

Thompson WG: *The Irritable Gut*. Baltimore, University Park Press, 1979.

---

* An excellent program was developed by Brudzinski and is sold by BMA Audio Cassettes, 200 Park Ave. South, New York, NY 10003.

A delightfully written overview of functional disorders of the gut including irritable bowel syndrome.

Specific References

1. Eastwood MA, Smith AN, Brydon WG, Pritchard J: Comparison of bran, ispaghula and lactulose on colon function in diverticular disease. *Gut* 19:1144, 1978.

2. Eastwood MA, Smith AN, Brydon WG, Pritchard J: Colonic function in patients with diverticular disease. *Lancet* 1:1181, 1978.
3. Reasoner J, Maculan TP, Rand AG, Thayer WR: Clinical studies with low-lactose milk. *Am J Clin Nutr* 34:54, 1981.
4. Whitehead WE, Winget C, Fedoravicius A, *et al*: Learned illness behavior in patients with irritable bowel syndrome and peptic ulcer. *Dig Dis Sci* 27:202, 1982.

CHAPTER FORTY

Diverticular Disease

HAROLD J. TUCKER, M.D.

DEFINITIONS

The term "diverticular disease" encompasses a variety of clinical states that may differ in their etiology and prognosis. The nomenclature of diverticular disease of the colon is listed in Table 40.1. As can be seen from this classification, *diverticulosis* simply refers to the presence of diverticula (actually, since they contain no muscular wall, pseudodiverticula). *Symptomatic diverticular disease* refers to diverticulosis associated with pain and altered bowel habits in the absence of evidence of diverticular inflammation. *Diverticulitis* is the occurrence of inflamed diverticula, generally implying perforation of a diverticulum. The *prediverticular state* is characterized by the radiographic, pathological, and often clinical features of diverticulosis without the formation of diverticula. The distinction between these entities is more than semantic, as the pathophysiology and natural history of each of these conditions probably vary.

EPIDEMIOLOGY AND PATHOGENESIS

The prevalence of diverticular disease in the United States, although extremely low before the age of 30, increases considerably thereafter so that, currently, 20% of men and women over 40, and 50% over 60, have diverticulosis of the colon. These figures reflect a striking rise in the frequency of the condition over the last 70 years (5% of people over 60 were affected in the early years of this century) that is paralleled by a 25% decrease in total crude fiber in the average American diet. This association has lead to the hypothesis that a low fiber diet increases intraluminal pressure and that the increased pressure leads to herniation of the mucosa through weakened or porous parts of the colonic muscle. In support of this hypothesis is the demonstration of exaggerated contractile responses of the sigmoid colon which contains diverticula, in response to meals and cholinergic stimulation. Thus, both a low fiber diet and disordered colonic motility have been implicated in the pathogenesis of diverticulosis.

This "dismotility" hypothesis, however, has not proved to be applicable to all cases of diverticulosis.

Table 40.1.
Nomenclature of Diverticular Disease of Colon[a]

DIVERTICULOSIS (presence of multiple diverticula):
  Asymptomatic
  Symptomatic (pain, bowel irregularity)
  Complicated by hemorrhage
DIVERTICULITIS (necrotizing inflammation in one or more
      diverticula):
  With microperforation (local inflammation)
  With macroperforation, manifested by abscess, fistula, peri-
      tonitis, obstruction, or hemorrhage
PREDIVERTICULAR STATE: Muscular thickening and
      shortening of colonic wall without recognizable diverticula

[a] Adapted from Almy T, Howell D: Diverticular disease of the colon.
N Engl J Med 302:324, 1980.

It is now recognized that the abnormal motor re-sponse of the sigmoid colon is more closely associ-ated with the symptoms of lower abdominal pain than with the presence of diverticula. Indeed, in patients with asymptomatic diverticulosis, the sig-moid motility pattern is normal, while many sub-jects with similar symptoms but with no diverticula have an abnormal motor response. The history of symptoms of abdominal pain in many patients with diverticular disease is short and does not suggest the presence of any prolonged motility disturbance. Thus, while a motility disturbance may account for some of the symptoms associated with diverticulosis, it alone cannot account for the development of di-verticulosis.

Another aspect in the pathogenesis of this condi-tion is the weakness in the colonic wall through which the mucosa herniates to form the diverticu-lum. The site of herniation occurs at areas of least resistance, most often at points of penetration of intramural vessels through the circular muscle layer. The association of colonic diverticula with scleroderma and with Marfan's and Ehlers-Danlos syndromes suggests that loss of muscle mass or de-fects in collagen may be important factors. Changes in collagen synthesis are known to occur with aging and may explain the increased prevalence of diver-ticular disease in elderly people. Thus, the formation of diverticula may also involve a degenerative proc-ess of the colonic muscle with a change in tensile strength of the colon wall.

ASYMPTOMATIC DIVERTICULOSIS

The majority of patients with diverticulosis de-tected on barium enema are entirely asymptomatic. The diverticula may be localized to the rectosigmoid junction or may involve the entire colon diffusely. The sigmoid colon is involved almost always (95% of the time). Rectal diverticula rarely occur, because of the muscular wrapping of the rectum.

The natural history of diverticulosis is variable.

The majority of patients are asymptomatic; how-ever, diverticulitis does occur in 10 to 25%, and bleeding somewhat less often. In some patients, symptoms develop similar to those of the irritable bowel syndrome (IBS). The association between IBS and diverticulosis is unclear. One study demon-strated an increase in the development of diverti-ulosis in patients with IBS (1). However, in most patients with diverticulosis, there is no history of antecedent IBS (see Chapter 39).

There is little evidence that therapy for asympto-matic diverticulosis is of any value. If the develop-ment of diverticulosis is really related to low fiber intake with resultant increased intraluminal pres-sure during segmental activity, then a high fiber diet may be beneficial. However, there is no evidence that such therapy prevents or even delays the oc-currence of symptomatic diverticular disease or of such complications as diverticulitis or hemorrhage. Maintenance of regular bowel habits without the use of laxatives is probably the best advice for these patients. It is also prudent to alert them to the manifestations of symptomatic diverticular disease (see below) and to urge them to seek medical care promptly should such symptoms develop.

SYMPTOMATIC DIVERTICULAR DISEASE
Diagnosis

Diverticular disease may at times cause abdomi-nal pain and an alteration in bowel habits. The crampy pain is generally in the left lower quadrant, made worse by meals (presumably due to gastrocolic reflex) and at least partially relieved by having a bowel movement or by passing flatus. Bowel habits, usually during the painful episodes, become irregu-lar, with development of constipation, diarrhea, or both in an alternating fashion. These painful attacks are usually episodic rather than continuous.

Physical examination reveals tenderness, at times marked, in the left lower quadrant. A tender sigmoid loop may be palpable, but there is no other palpable mass. The stool should be negative for occult blood, but rectal bleeding may be found due to coincidental rectal outlet disorders such as fissures or hemor-rhoids. Fever is not present.

Proctosigmoidoscopy, if performed during an at-tack (see below), will show a normal colonic mucosa. However, considerable pain and spasm may be caused by the procedure.

The *barium enema* (see Chapter 37, "Patient Ex-perience") is essential both for the diagnosis of di-verticulosis and for excluding other reasons for symptoms. Spasm may be a feature of diverticular disease, but fistulas or a mass suggest diverticulitis, carcinoma, or Crohn's disease.

Therapy

The therapy for symptomatic diverticular disease is based on the assumption that low fiber diets and increased colonic pressure are important pathogenetic fators. Diets high in fiber (see Table 38.2, Chapter 38) are prescribed and have been shown to be effective in improving bowel transit and in relieving symptoms. Commercial preparations of hyrophilic colloids made from vegetable fiber are available and convenient, but are expensive compared to dietary sources (see Table 38.3, Chapter 38). Thus, patients should be instructed about high fiber diets, and, if necessary, be given hydrophilic agents, such as Metamucil, 1 tablespoon/day in a glass of water or juice.

In addition to dietary maneuvers, anticholinergic drugs or antispasmodic drugs may also be helpful. While these agents are not of proven value for this condition, some patients do respond. Dicyclomine (Bentyl), at a dose of 10 to 20 mg before meals and at bedtime, is an often used initial drug. Other more potent anticholinergics may produce adverse side effects and may aggravate the constipation.

The patient should be told that the course of the disease is unpredictable and that attacks will probably be experienced at irregular intervals (months to years) for the rest of his life. There is no reason for the patient to continue to take medication for the condition between attacks, but maintenance of a high fiber diet is reasonable.

DIVERTICULITIS

In general, diverticulitis results from perforation of a diverticulum. The perforation may be grossly evident with fistulization and abscess formation, or it may be only microscopic and well confined. As noted previously, diverticulitis occurs in less than one-quarter of all patients with diverticulosis. Even this estimate is probably exaggerated, as convincing evidence for the presence of inflammation is often lacking. The recurrence rate for diverticulitis treated medically or surgically is about 25% (2).

Diagnosis

The cardinal symptoms of acute diverticulitis are pain and fever. The pain may be severe and abrupt in onset. Complete obstruction may occur with resultant abdominal distension and nausea. Urinary tract symptoms and purulent vaginal discharge may occur because of fistula formation or because of inflammation of contiguous structures. The severity of the symptoms depends on the extent of the peridiverticular inflammation.

Abdominal tenderness and fever are found on *physical examination*. Localized peritonitis may be noted by the marked direct and rebound tenderness over the involved area, generally most pronounced in the left lower quadrant. Rectal bleeding occurs in about 25% of patients and is usually occult. A pelvic mass may be felt on rectal and vaginal examination. *Leukocytosis* is almost always present. Pyuria and/

or hematuria may be found owing to contiguous involvement with the bladder or ureter.

The *differential diagnosis* includes painful diverticular disease, carcinoma of the colon, and inflammatory or ischemic bowel disease. The presence of peritonitis, fever, and leukocytosis rules out simple symptomatic diverticular disease. The other conditions are distinguished from diverticulitis by their clinical course and by proctoscopy and barium enema.

Proctoscopy (see "Patient Experience," Chapter 35) can be performed in patients with acute diverticulitis if the diagnosis is in doubt. The rigid proctosigmoidoscope will, in general, not reach the area containing the diverticula, but can exclude ulcerative colitis and rectal carcinoma. (The consultant gastroenterologist usually will not perform flexible sigmoidoscopy because of the risk of converting a confined infection to an open perforation.)

The timing of the *barium enema* depends on the clinical setting. In general, the barium enema should be delayed for 3 to 6 weeks to allow resolution of the acute inflammation and thereby to reduce the risk of perforation. The X-ray should be performed at this time not so much to make the diagnosis of diverticulitis but to exclude other conditions, such as carcinoma or Crohn's disease.

However, the barium enema can be performed earlier if the diagnosis is uncertain. In such cases, the radiologist must be informed of the potential diagnosis, and he should perform as limited a study as needed to make the definitive diagnosis. The diagnosis of diverticulitis is based on the finding of a mass effect on the contour of the bowel or the extravasation of the barium outside a diverticulum. The presence of spasm or thickening of the bowel wall are not, by themselves, radiographic evidence of diverticulitis.

Therapy

Most patients with diverticulitis should be hospitalized, placed on bowel rest, and given analgesics and antimicrobial drugs (preferably, a combination to which normal aerobic and anaerobic bacteria are sensitive). Selected patients, with mild tenderness and low grade fever, may be treated on an ambulatory basis with oral broad spectrum antibiotics (e.g., tetracycline, 250 mg four times a day).

For the vast majority of patients, this medical therapy will be successful; and in 75% of cases, there will be no recurrence over the next 10 years. However, failure to resolve the acute inflammatory process, recurrent attacks of diverticulitis, and obstructive stricture formation are indications for surgical intervention. It seems reasonable, although not established, that patients should be placed on a high fiber diet following recovery from an acute episode of diverticulitis.

DIVERTICULAR BLEEDING

Diverticulosis is the most common cause of massive lower gastrointestinal bleeding in adults. However, failure to distinguish diverticular hemorrhage from bleeding secondary to *angiodysplasia of the colon* (Chapter 37) has resulted in an overestimate of the incidence of diverticular bleeding. Both diverticulosis and angiodysplasia are common in the older population, and both frequently are found in the ascending colon, a common site of massive lower gastrointestinal bleeding. The exact mechanism for initiating diverticular bleeding is uncertain. There is no evidence that dietary therapy reduces the risk of hemorrhage. Most instances of bleeding occur in patients who are otherwise asymptomatic.

Massive hemorrhage is the most common mode of presentation for diverticular bleeding. However, massive lower gastrointestinal bleeding in a patient known to have diverticula should not automatically be ascribed to diverticulosis: in 30% of cases colonoscopy detects a second lesion (cancer, angiodysplasia) equally capable of causing bleeding (3). Occult bleeding should only be ascribed to diverticulosis after other causes have been excluded by a thorough evaluation (see Chapter 37).

Patients with diverticular hemorrhage require hospitalization for hemodynamic stabilization, diagnosis, and therapy. About 80% of patients will stop bleeding, and only 20 to 25% will bleed a second time.

General References

Almy T, Howell D: Diverticular disease of the colon. *N Engl J Med 302*:324, 1980.

> A good discussion on pathophysiology and classification of diverticular disease. Well referenced.

Specific References

1. Havia T, Manner R: The irritable colon syndrome. A follow-up study with special reference to the development of diverticula. *Acta Chir Scand 137*:569, 1971.
2. Larson D. Masters S, Spiro H: Medical and surgical therapy in diverticular disease. A comparative study. *Gastroenterology 71*:734, 1976.
3. Tedesco F, Waye J, Raskin J, *et al*: Colonoscopic evaluation of rectal bleeding—a study of 304 patients. *Ann Intern Med 89*:907, 1978.

CHAPTER FORTY-ONE

Care of Patients with Colostomy or Ileostomy

MARVIN M. SCHUSTER, M.D.

INTRODUCTION

Ostomies are openings of a portion of the gastrointestinal tract—usually the ileum or the colon—which have been surgically diverted to the abdominal wall. It is estimated that there are in excess of 1 million ostomates (the preferred term for people with ostomies) in North America. Unfortunately the amount of time devoted in medical curriculum and postgraduate training to the care of ostomies is not commensurate with these impressive numbers, and therefore few physicians have the necessary background to be appropriately helpful to the ostomate. This is particularly unfortunate in light of the fact that the partial or total colectomy that results in an ileostomy or colostomy often cures the underlying condition, leaving a healthy patient who is capable of normal function, assuming that he receives appropriate preoperative preparation and postoperative ostomy care.

Ninety percent of ileostomies are performed for ulcerative colitis. Less often, other conditions, such as Crohn's disease of the colon or familial polyposis, require this operation. Most of the patients are young, 75% or more being between the age of 20 and 45 years of age.

In contrast, colostomies are usually performed for cancer of the rectum, and less often for diverticulitis or for neurological impairment or gunshot wounds which have led to incontinence. Both children and young adults with congenital disorders, such as im-perforate anus, may have colostomies, but 80% of patients who have colostomy surgery are over the age of 50.

Appropriate management of the stoma begins before surgery and continues for a short period after successful surgery and for a longer period when old problems persist or new ones arise.

PREOPERATIVE CARE

Ostomy management should begin as soon as ostomy surgery is seriously considered. For preparation of the patient to be most effective, family members should be included, since the approach is best tailored to meet the needs of the patient and the family. Preparation should encompass a brief description of the surgery, emphasizing the benefits to be derived, and of the stoma, stressing the fact that the stoma itself need not interfere with any aspect or future life except for vigorous body contact sports. Emphasis is placed on the fact that modern developments in appliances permit normal functioning and that there is no way that anyone will be able to tell that the clad patient has an ostomy. After these brief introductory comments the patient and family should be given an opportunity to voice their concerns and to ask questions, both during this first discussion and later, when the initial shock has worn off.

Many resources are available during the preoperative stage: the informed physician or surgeon, specially trained stoma nurses or enterostomal therapists (most of whom are nurses who have had specialized training at one of the schools of enterostomal therapy), and members of the visiting committee of the local chapter of the United Ostomy Association. The latter are usually lay ostomates trained as members of the visiting committee, who are specifically selected whenever possible to match the patient in age and sex (and frequently in socio-economic status), so that the patient can identify readily with the visitor. The benefits to be derived from the visiting team cannot be overemphasized; for even the most comforting of professionals cannot be as reassuring to the patient as some kindred soul who has undergone similar surgery, has adjusted to it, and is leading a healthy, productive, and joyful life.

Pamphlets, available through the local ostomy

chapters, can assist the patient in his acceptance of the procedure, provide an optimistic projection for the future, and educate him in the use of ostomy appliances and in colostomy irrigation. In addition, films on preoperative preparation are available; these can be shown in portable projectors so that they can be viewed in the doctor's office, hospital clinic, or the patient's home.* These films are particularly useful when viewed by the patient after the first discussion of the topic, because they not only depict healthy ostomates who discuss their initial and subsequent adjustment, but also provide minimal basic anatomical information and information concerning appliances. Such information not only allays fears and misconceptions, but also provides the basis for logical questions.

What to Tell the Patient about Conventional Ileostomy

Conventional ileostomies require that the patient continuously wear a pouch which is applied to the body using a skin barrier (a wafer-like adhesive) that provides a watertight seal. In this manner the intestinal contents (a better term than stool or waste material) discharge into the pouch, which can be emptied into the toilet simply by unclipping the end of the pouch four or five times a day. The contents are liquid and usually odorless. The pouch is flat and cannot be detected through the clothing or even in a bathing suit. The seal is tight enough so that persons can swim, dive, and participate in dancing and in sports such as skiing or baseball. Modern materials are so effective that the pouch can be worn for a week at a time without being removed.

What to Tell the Patient about a Kock, or Internal Pouch

The Kock pouch or internal pouch (sometimes called "continent ileosotomy") consists of several loops of small intestine sutured to each other and opened so that they form a reservoir pouch (artificial rectum) within the abdomen. This reservoir is connected to the abdominal wall with a short segment of ileum and opens into the abdominal wall much as a conventional ileostomy does, except that it can be placed much lower on the abdomen since it will not require a pouch if it performs well. Between the pouch and the short ileal conduit, a nipple valve is constructed by inverting the ileum into the pouch in such a manner that it prevents leakage and therefore provides continence. In order to evacuate the contents of the pouch the patient inserts a Silastic catheter into it through the ileostomy and the nipple valve. The ileal contents then drain through the catheter into the toilet bowl. Although frequent

---

* One such film is *Ostomy: A New Beginning.* Available from Milner Fenwick, 2125 Greenspring Dr, Timonium, MD 21093. Cost $250.00.

drainage is necessary initially, eventually most patients drain three or four times a day. Because it does not require an external appliance the stoma can be placed near the groin, permitting the wearing of brief attire, such as a bikini.

This type of surgery is not recommended for patients who have Crohn's disease involving the ileum. Moreover, one-third of the operations are not initially successful in providing total continence and therefore require revision, and in some instances more than one revision. These factors need to be taken into consideration when deciding the appropriate form of surgery for the specific patient, especially when patients with conventional ileosotomies ask about the advisability of converting their conventional, well functioning ileosotomy to the "continent ileosotomy." This operation is also not appropriate for people who have neurological disorders that impair manual dexterity and interfere with insertion of the Silastic catheter.

What to Tell the Patient about Colostomy

There are basically four different types of colostomies: the dry colostomy, the wet colostomy, the loop colostomy, and the continent colostomy utilizing the magnetic cap. Most permanent colostomies are *dry sigmoid colostomies* which result from rectal resection, usually for cancer of the rectum. Since only the rectum has been removed, there is no alteration of the usual stool consistency. This is an important feature since it means that patients who have frequent and erratic bowel habits, as for example with irritable bowel, will continue to have these bowel habits and therefore will have unpredictable evacuation. They will most likely have to wear an appliance. Patients who have more regular bowel habits can often develop controlled evacuations by use of irrigation (enemas) which they administer initially daily for proper control, and later in most instances every 2 days. Some colostomates simply wear a small adhesive Band-Aid or gauze pad, although most prefer to wear a small appliance (stoma cap) to protect them against incontinence during those few days a year when they develop the same episodes of diarrhea that affect the general population. Patients who suffer from irritable bowel syndrome (see Chapter 39) or nervous diarrhea before surgery will continue to have similar symptoms after surgery and therefore may not achieve continence during intervals between irrigations.

The *wet colostomy* refers to loose stool that occurs when a colostomy is situated proximal to the splenic flexure. This type of colostomy is usually performed as a temporary bypass and is generally less desirable, since evacuations are more frequent and cannot be controlled by irrigation, and since the contents are malodorous because of colonic bacterial action. A permanent ileostomy is generally preferable to a permanent wet colostomy. The wet colostomy requires an appliance large enough to contain the colonic evacuations.

Loop colostomies and double barrel colostomies are performed as (usually temporary) diverting procedures in the proximal colon. The loop is brought over a glass or plastic rod, and the resultant irregular oblong shape may make a watertight appliance fit difficult.

Research is currently under way toward perfecting a magnetic cap which covers the colostomy in order to provide continence. It is held in place by a magnetic ring sutured around the stoma. The cap is removed when evacuation is desired. At present the procedure is available only at selected centers since there are many complications, and the success rate is less than 50%.

Informed consent for colostomy requires that the patient be made aware of possible postoperative impotence. If impotence does occur, psychological adjustment to it is improved with preoperative counseling. Impotence is uncommon among ileostomates, but some degree of sexual impairment occurs in 80% of colostomates, 50% of whom are totally impotent after surgery. This is due to the wide resection that is necessary for rectal cancer surgery, the major indication for a colostomy, as well as to the advanced age of the colostomate compared to the ileostomate. Patients may be reassured that sexual counseling is available if problems arise and that many couples have found alternative satisfactory means of sexual gratification. In selected patients, it may be appropriate to offer the possibility of penile implants (see Chapter 18). Obviously these concerns are less significant for the female ostomate who does not suffer from impaired performance, although impaired gratification may still be an important factor.

POSTOPERATIVE MANAGEMENT

Only late postoperative problems will be discussed here since the early problems will be managed in hospital. Four major categories of problems are (a) psychological adjustment, (b) sexual adjustment, (c) appliance management, and (d) local and physiological problems. Again, all can be minimized by appropriate preoperative preparation and counseling of the patient and the patient's family by an informed physician working with the appropriate members of the health team.

Psychological Adjustment

A concerted effort should be made postoperatively by the medical team as well as by the family, and particularly the spouse, to restore self-esteem and foster independence. During the early postoperative months men tend to depend on their wives for nursing care, but women seem to prefer help from other women (daughters, mothers, sisters) rather than from husbands. This is explained by the fact that wives express more concern about being physically unacceptable to the husband than *vice versa.* On the other hand, one-fifth of wives have been reported to react by vomiting, fainting, or showing frank expressions of disgust when first exposed to their husband's stoma. This obviously engenders a sense of rejection, degradation, and loss of self-esteem. All too often little consideration is given by the physician to the possibility of such exaggerated responses or their consequences. Attendance at meetings of local ostomy chapters is a good way of preparing the family during the postoperative period. Formal psychotherapy may be needed when depression is severe, when suicidal inclinations appear prominent, or when behavior is bizarre.

Sexual Adjustment

When debilitating illnesses, such as inflammatory bowel disease, have led to decreased libido and impaired sexual function, ileostomy may lead to improved postoperative sexual function and more satisfactory sexual relations. This is less often true when colostomies, performed with proctectomy and radical pelvic dissection, lead to neurological impairment of potency. Even in these circumstances psychological factors may play a major role, as demonstrated by a survey (1) which reported that all men who had had extramarital affairs before surgery terminated these relationships postoperatively, feeling that only their wives would accept them. Also, cessation of relationships involving a female colostomate was invariably initiated by the female and was never reported to be a result of rejection by the husband.

In general, impaired sexual relationships may result from neurological impairment, depression with loss of libido, inhibitions due to a sense of humiliation and embarrassment or, in some unfortunate instances, from rejection by the spouse. An awareness of these possibilities will prepare the physician to assist with preventive or corrective measures. Frank discussions with the male patient may in some instances indicate the advisability of urological referral for prosthesis. Sexual counseling by the attending physician or specially trained counselors may assist in adjustment to alternate forms of sexual gratification.

Appliance Management

Modern improvements have impressively decreased the number of problems that are directly attributable to the appliance.

Skin Problems

Skin breakdown, a problem which used to plague 50% of ileostomates, is now uncommon because of effective skin barriers which have replaced the old cement adhesives. Hypersensitivity to adhesives or the pouch can be diagnosed when the contour of skin reaction conforms to that of the adhesive or the pouch. If hypersensitivity is suspected, a patch test utilizing the arm or trunk distant from the stoma may confirm the suspicion. Skin problems are more common among ileostomates than colostomates because ileostomy effluent contains digestive enzymes. Skin that has been excoriated by ileal leakage should be treated with a cortisone spray, such as Kenalog, and an antifungal powder, such as Mycostatin, neither of which interferes with adherence of the appliance. Ointments and creams should be avoided because they do prevent adhesion. More serious skin problems should be referred to gastroenterologists and to enterostomal therapists experienced with ostomy care. Skin complications for proximal colostomies may be similar to those of ileosotomies.

Odor

Odor problems are more commonly encountered by colostomates than ileostomates because of putrefactive bacteria present in the colon. Some bacterial colonization of the ileum takes place after colectomy, but odor problems occur only occasionally in 50% of ileostomates and more often in about a third. Sudden increase in gas and odor may signify partial intestinal obstruction. Dietary factors such as oils, fat-soluble vitamins, eggs, and onions may be associated with offensive odors and may be diagnosed by careful dietary history or by use of elimination diets. Odors may also be due to malabosorption resulting from small bowel disease or resection. A number of deodorants are available that can be placed into the pouch (Nilodor, Banish, Aspirin and Ostoban powder), and additionally bismuth subcarbonate orally may be helpful.

Leakage

Under ordinary circumstances leakage is rarely seen with new appliances, but may become a problem if pregnancy or postoperative weight gain (as, for example, when a patient has been emaciated from inflammatory bowel disease) may change body contour requiring refitting of the appliance. The stoma may shrink during the first 6 to 8 weeks after surgery, and good follow-up care is vital for at least the first postoperative year. Minimal bleeding at the stoma may occur occasionally and is no cause for alarm. A soft wet cloth should be used to clean the stoma, since dry materials may stick to the surface and cause bleeding. Skin excoriation can occur as a result of perspiration under the pouch, particularly in hot weather. This can be prevented by wearing a cover over the pouch and also by powdering the skin liberally.

Local and Physiological Complications

Ileostomates are much more likely to experience complications of this type than are colostomates and most of these complications appear within the first year after surgery. Obstruction due to volvulus, herniation, or adhesions is the most commonly encountered problem, while prolapse, retraction, and fistula formation are seen less frequently. These problems usually require consultation with a surgeon or gastroenterologist and often need surgical correction. Crampy abdominal pains, abdominal distension, vomiting, and excessive diarrheal discharge suggest the presence of obstruction. Gastroenteritis may mimic some of these symptoms but persists only for several days.

Because of the absence of normal colonic absorptive function, ileostomates may be susceptible to dehydration or electrolyte imbalance (particularly salt depletion), especially in hot weather because of sweating and increased incidence of infectious diarrhea. For this reason ileostomates should be encouraged to increase water and salt intake during the summer unless there are medical contraindications. Antidiarrheal agents, such as deodorized tincture of opium, Lomotil, or Imodium, may be needed during these periods and also should be available during travel to foreign countries where traveler's diarrhea may be a problem.

With these minimal precautions neither ileostomy nor colostomy imposes any dietary restrictions, except that ileostomates should avoid excessive quantities of peanuts or fibrous foods such as bean sprouts, which have been reported to be associated with obstruction. Taken in moderation, however, these foods usually present no problem.

Colostomy Irrigation

Although a few colostomates (having distal colostomy) find that they can have controlled bowel movements by careful dietary manipulations, the vast majority use irrigation to control evacuation. This simply involves the instillation of 1 liter of warm tap water through the colostomy. The replacement of the old irrigating catheter with the blunt cone (which is placed against the stoma to prevent backflow) has virtually eliminated the problems of perforation. Although tepid water is preferred in order to avoid cramping, some patients find cold water more effective. It is normal for patients to have an initial evacuation followed within ½ hour by further excretion; for this reason the patient should be advised to continue wearing the irrigation sleeve (long pouch) with the end closed for ½ hour after irrigation. Cramps experienced during the irrigation may be due to rapid instillation of water, air distension of the bowel resulting from failure to expel the air from the irrigating tip, or from obstruction. Constipation and diarrhea should be handled much in the same fashion as with patients who have intact colons (see Chapter 38), relying on dietary manipulations as much as possible (prunes and bran for constipation and hard cheeses and rice for diarrhea).

General References

Kretschmer KP: The intestinal stoma. *Major Probl Clin Surg* 24: 1975.
  Valuable for both physicians and patients
Schuster MM, Bengel JR: Management of ileostomy and colostomy. In Spittell J Jr (ed): *Clinical Medicine* vol 10, Chap 523. New York Harper & Row, 1982.
  A comprehensive review directed primarily at physicians.

Sparberg M: *Ileostomy Care*. Springfield, IL, Charles C Thomas, 1971.
Walter FC: *Modern Stoma Care*. New York, Churchill Livingstone. 1976.
  The above two references are useful texts for both physicians and patients.

Specific References

1. Dyk RB, Sutherland AM: Adaptation of spouse and other family members to the ostomy patients. *Cancer* 9:123, 1956.

CHAPTER FORTY-TWO

Diseases of the Liver

ESTEBAN MEZEY, M.D.

HEPATITIS

Hepatitis is an inflammatory condition which may be localized in the liver or may be part of a generalized systemic process. Acute hepatitis is usually a self-limited disease. The principal causes of acute hepatitis are viruses, drugs, and alcohol. Chronic hepatitis refers to unresolved hepatitis which has persisted for a period longer than 6 months. Cirrhosis is often the principal consequence of chronic hepatitis.

Acute Hepatitis

Viral Hepatitis

Viral hepatitis is a systemic infection whose principal manifestations are hepatic. The two types of viral hepatitis which are well defined separate entities are type A and type B. Delta (δ) hepatitis (hepatitis D virus) refers to infection by a defective virus-like particle which is dependent on persisting or concomitant infection with type B virus. The term non-A, non-B hepatitis refers to those cases which cannot be identified as either hepatitis A or B and are not caused by other viruses (such as cytomegalic virus or Epstein-Barr virus).

The characteristic features of type A, B, and non-A, non-B hepatitis are shown in Table 42.1. Type A hepatitis, previously known as infectious hepatitis, is more common than the other types. It is usually transmitted by the fecal-oral route and has a particularly high incidence wherever persons come in close contact under poor hygienic conditions. A number of epidemics have been described after fecal contamination of the water or food supply. Ingestion of contaminated shellfish has been associated with sporadic cases as well as with epidemics.

Type B hepatitis, previously named serum hepatitis, is usually transmitted by the parenteral route from blood, blood products, or contaminated needles. However, it has also been shown to be transmitted by the ingestion of contaminated blood, by sexual contact, and from the mother to the fetus. The δ agent is transmitted by the same routes as type B hepatitis [10]. Its incubation period ranges from 3 to 13 weeks. Infection with δ agent may

Table 42.1.
Comparison of Characteristics of Various Types of Viral Hepatitis

Characteristic	Type A	Type B	Type Non-A, Non-B
Hepatitis A antibody	Appearance or increase in titer	Absent No change in titer	Absent No change in titer
Hepatitis B surface antigen	Absent	Present in early stage of illness	Absent
Incubation period	15–50 days	50–160 days	15–160 days
Route of infection	Oral and parenteral	Usually parenteral, also oral or sexual	Usually parenteral
Age preference	Children	Any age	Any age
Seasonal incidence	Autumn-winter, epidemic outbreaks	All year	All year
Severity	Usually mild	Often severe	Often severe
Mortality	0.1%	1.0%	1.0%
Prophylactic value of γ-globulin	Good	Good with hyperimmune hepatitis B globulin	Unclear
Hepatitis B vaccine		90% efficacy	

become manifest as a biphasic pattern of hepatitis when there is simultaneous infection with hepatitis B virus, or as a clinical exacerbation of hepatitis in patients who are carriers of hepatitis B virus with or without chronic liver disease. The δ agent has been implicated in cases of fulminant hepatitis and in worsening of chronic liver disease with more rapid progression to cirrhosis. The incidence of δ hepatitis, however, is unknown.

Type non-A, non-B hepatitis is principally acquired by the parenteral route from blood transfusions or from intravenous drug abuse (4). The importance of nonparenteral routes of infection remains to be determined. Non-A, non-B hepatitis is currently responsible for 90% of transfusion-transmitted hepatitis. The use of commercial blood appears to be the most significant factor in the transmission of this type of hepatitis.

Clinical Presentation

The clinical symptoms of the various types of hepatitis are similar. However, viral hepatitis, type B and type non-A, non-B, is usually more severe and is associated with a higher incidence of morbidity and mortality and late sequelae. The majority of cases of hepatitis are anicteric; patients have a few nonspecific symptoms such as fatigue and nausea; and the disease is often misdiagnosed as a flu-like illness. The correct diagnosis, if suspected, is made by demonstrating bilirubin in the urine and an increase in serum aminotransferases. In icteric disease the symptoms which usually precede jaundice are anorexia, fatigue, abdominal discomfort, and nausea. Erythematous skin rashes, urticaria, and arthralgias may also appear. These initial symptoms are followed within 10 days by the appearance of dark urine, often pruritus, and jaundice. It is at this

stage that most patients seek medical attention. On physical examination a tender palpable liver is found in about 70% of the patients. Posterior cervical lymphadenopathy and splenomegaly may also be present. Jaundice usually increases in intensity in the first few days and then begins to decrease, disappearing completely by 2 to 8 weeks after onset.

Laboratory Features

A mild degree of transient anemia, granulocytopenia, lymphocytosis with the appearance of atypical lymphocytes, and mild hemolytic anemia, with an increase in the reticulocyte count, are commonly found in patients with viral hepatitis. Both direct and total fraction of serum bilirubin rise, the height reached by the total bilirubin being an indication of the severity of the disease. However, total serum bilirubin levels greater than 30 mg/dl are almost invariably due to complicating hemolysis. The serum aminotransferases generally rise before the onset of detectable jaundice, may reach levels as high as several thousand units, and may remain elevated for several weeks. The height reached by the aminotransferases in the serum provides only a rough estimate of the degree of hepatocellular injury and is of no prognostic value. However, a rapid fall in aminotransferases from a high peak value to normal in less than 1 week may be an indication of fulminant hepatitis with massive necrosis and collapse of liver parenchyma. The serum alkaline phosphatase usually rises in the early, cholestatic phase of hepatitis, remains elevated throughout the illness, and is often the last serum enzyme to return to normal levels after clinical recovery. The serum albumin is normal in acute hepatitis. Serum γ-globulins are frequently transiently elevated. The prothrombin time is usually normal and, if prolonged, is usually responsive to the administration of vitamin K. Prolongation of the prothrombin time with no response to vitamin K administration suggests severe hepatitis; and if the prolongation increases, it is indicative of fulminant hepatitis.

Immunological Features

A marked advance in the diagnosis of hepatitis occurred with the discovery in 1964 of an antigenic substance in the blood which was later documented to be associated only with type B hepatitis. This antigen, initially named Australian antigen because it was first detected in the serum of an Australian aborigine, is now designated hepatitis B surface antigen (HB$_S$Ag). In 1973 the hepatitis A antigen was discovered, and the determination of serum antibodies to this antigen began to be used for the identification of type A hepatitis. Delta agent, which is associated with HB$_S$Ag, was discovered in 1977. At present there is no marker available for the identification of non-A, non-B hepatitis.

In acute type A hepatitis fecal excretion of hepatitis A antigen (HA Ag) can be demonstrated a few days before the increase in serum aminotransferases, rising to a peak during maximum serum aminotransferase elevation, and then falling as jaundice appears. Antibody to hepatitis (anti-HA, predominantly IgM) appears in the serum as HA Ag disappears from the stool, and rises rapidly to high levels. Afterwards antibody titers (predominantly IgG) remain detectable for at least 10 years, indicative of immunity against reinfection. Since hepatitis A infection is very common, many healthy individuals have detectable anti-HA in the serum. The prevalence of positive anti-HA is about 30% in the United States and as high as 90% in certain areas of Latin America and Asia (24). Hence, identification of an acute episode of hepatitis as type A requires a high titer of anti-HA of the IgM class or the appearance of or a rise in anti-HA titer in the serum collected during the convalescent as compared with the acute stage of hepatitis.

The hepatitis B virus by electron microscopy appears as a double shelled 42-nm spherical particle originally called the Dane particle. The outer shell of this particle is HB$_S$Ag, while the inner core contains an antigen which has been designated the hepatitis B core antigen (HB$_C$Ag). The inner core also contains double stranded DNA and DNA polymerase activity. In acute type B viral hepatitis HB$_S$Ag first appears in the blood 1 to 2 weeks before, and usually disappears by 2 months after, the onset of clinical symptoms (Fig. 42.1). Radioimmunoassay and reverse passive hemagglutination are the only reliable procedures for detection of HB$_S$Ag. (The hemagglutination technique is slightly less sensitive than the radioimmunoassay.) Antibody to hepatitis B core antigen (anti-HB$_C$) appears in the serum at the onset of clinical symptoms, reaches a peak soon after the maximal level of serum aminotransferase is reached,

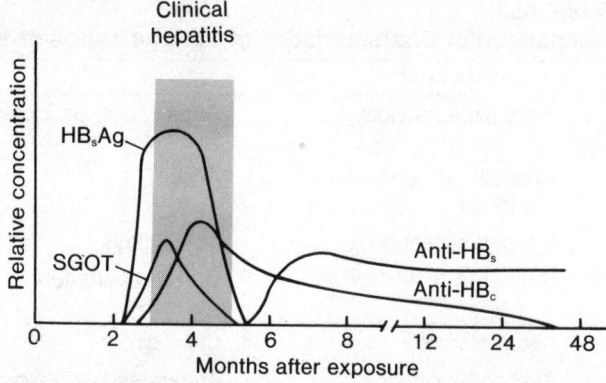

Figure 42.1. Pattern of appearance of hepatitis B surface antigen (HB$_S$Ag) and antibodies to hepatitis B surface antigen (anti-HB$_S$) and to hepatitis B core antigen (anti-HB$_C$) in acute hepatitis B infection. (From Mezey E: Specific liver diseases. In Halsted JA, Halsted CH (eds): *The Laboratory in Clinical Medicine*, ed 2. Philadelphia, WB Saunders, 1981.)

and then falls gradually, becoming undetectable 1 to 2 years after the infection. Antibody to the hepatitis B surface antigen (anti-HB$_S$) usually appears during the convalescence when HB$_S$Ag is no longer detectable and then persists for many years. The presence of HB$_S$Ag, IgM anti-HB$_C$, or a rise in anti-HB$_S$ titer during the acute illness is evidence that the hepatitis is due to the hepatitis B virus (11). Persistence of HB$_S$Ag in the serum beyond 3 months after the infection suggests that the patient has become a chronic carrier of the hepatitis B virus (17). High titers of anti-HB$_C$ but absent anti-HB$_S$ are usually found in association with HB$_S$Ag in the carrier state. The presence of anti-HB$_S$ indicates that the patient has had a prior infection with type B hepatitis and now is immune to reinfection. In 1972 a new antigen termed e antigen was discovered in HB$_S$Ag-positive sera. The e antigen (HB$_e$Ag), although associated only with type B hepatitis, is immunologically distinct from HB$_S$Ag and HB$_C$Ag. HB$_e$Ag appears transiently in the serum during the early phase of acute type B hepatitis. In chronic carriers of HB$_S$Ag the presence of HB$_e$Ag is a marker of active virus replication and correlates with infectivity of the carrier (7). Some studies suggest that the presence of HB$_e$Ag in the chronic carrier is an indicator of progression of acute hepatitis B to chronic hepatitis or cirrhosis.

δ agent is a defective virus-like particle which is composed of a small RNA genome surrounded by δ antigen and a coat of HB$_S$Ag. Acute δ hepatitis agent infection is associated with a brief rise in δ antigen lasting approximately 10 days followed by the appearance of δ antibody (anti-δ). Initially the antibody is of IgM type, lasting 10 to 20 days, followed by the appearance of IgG anti-δ. A characteristic of δ infection is a lowering of HB$_S$Ag titers, probably because it requires hepatitis B virus for its replication.

Hepatitis non-A, non-B has been transmitted to chimpanzees by serum derived from patients with acute and chronic non-A, non-B hepatitis, suggesting that patients can become carriers of the agent responsible for this type of hepatitis. Since there are no serological markers for this hepatitis, the diagnosis remains one of exclusion (4).

At present the practical diagnostic usefulness of the immunological markers for hepatitis is as follows: Hepatitis A infection is confirmed by the demonstration of a rise in anti-HA titer in the serum collected during convalescence as compared with the acute stage of hepatitis, or preferably the presence of anti-HA of the IgM class. Infection with hepatitis B is usually confirmed by the presence of HB_SAg; but if the antigen is absent and it is clinically indicated, the diagnosis can be confirmed by demonstrating IgM anti-HB_C. The determination of anti-HB_S is useful to find out whether or not a person is immune to hepatitis B and a candidate for prophylaxis, a subject which is discussed later in this chapter (page 500). Acute δ infection is diagnosed by the presence of δ antigen or IgM anti-δ, but currently these assays are not routinely available.

Management

Acute viral hepatitis usually resolves completely in 1 to 3 months. There is no specific therapy. Bed rest is indicated initially in the symptomatic patient because it often alleviates the symptoms, although there is no evidence that it changes the overall course of the illness (16). As the patient's symptoms improve, a gradual increase in activity is allowed as tolerated by the patient. Intake of a normal calorie, high protein diet should be encouraged, although it is often difficult for the patient to eat because of nausea and anorexia. However, these symptoms are usually minimal in the morning and, hence, the patient should be encouraged to eat a large breakfast. Strict isolation of the patient to his own room and bathroom is often impractical and probably unnecessary. General hygienic measures, such as washing the hands after contact with the patient and careful handling of stool and blood samples, are mandatory.

Hospitalization is indicated in patients in whom the diagnosis is uncertain, and in those who have severe symptoms of nausea and vomiting, changes in mental status, or a prothrombin time that is prolonged more than 4 seconds above the control value. In addition, it is usually advisable to admit to the hospital patients over the age of 50 years, who tend to have a more severe course of hepatitis than do younger patients, as well as those patients who do not have somebody at home who can observe and help them.

Nausea can be controlled with oral Benadryl, 25 mg three times a day, or by Compazine, 10 mg two to four times a day, without danger of central nervous system depression. No sedatives or tranquilizers should be given because they may precipitate hepatic encephalopathy. Corticosteriods are of no value in the treatment of acute viral hepatitis.

Patients should be followed at intervals varying from 1 to 3 weeks and should not be discharged from ambulatory care until all symptoms have disappeared and all laboratory tests have returned to normal. Patients are advised not to ingest alcoholic beverages until 1 month after all laboratory tests have returned to normal.

An informative booklet for patients, entitled *Viral Hepatitis, Everybody's Problem*, is available from the American Liver Foundation (Cedar Grove, NJ 07009).

Liver Biopsy

Liver biopsies are only indicated if the diagnosis is uncertain or if the clinical course of the disease is prolonged beyond 6 months. A specialist in liver disease should be consulted to evaluate the patient and to perform the liver biopsy.

For liver biopsy the patient is admitted to the hospital. Before admission for this procedure the patient should be demonstrated to have a history of normal hemostasis, a prothrombin time less than 4 seconds above control, and a platelet count greater than 80,000/mm^3. A liver biopsy is contraindicated if there is an infiltrate in the right lower lung, or a right-sided pleural effusion, absent hepatic dullness to percussion, suspected liver hemangioma or abscess, massive ascites, extrahepatic obstruction, or severe anemia (hemoglobin less than 10 g/dl). After application of local anesthesia, the liver biopsy is performed by the intercostal right subcutaneous route using suction with a needle 1.6 mm in diameter. It entails minimal risk when done by a skilled operator. The most common complication is pleuritic pain lasting a few hours after the biopsy, which is noted in about 5% of the cases. The most serious complications are bleeding and bile peritonitis, which occur in less than 1% of cases. The incidence of mortality from liver biopsy is 0.2%

Prognosis

The majority of patients with acute viral hepatitis recover from their illness without any sequelae. The mortality rate from all types of hepatitis is less than 0.1%. The principal cause of death is the development of fulminant hepatitis, which is more common in type B hepatitis. Fulminant hepatitis, which is rare, usually overcomes the patient within 10 days of the onset of the symptoms of hepatitis. Older patients and patients with other medical illnesses, such as diabetes, are more likely to have a prolonged course and higher mortality. The course of hepatitis is not influenced by pregnancy. Indications of a poor prognosis are changes in mental status, a nonpalpable liver which is also small on hepatic scan, or a liver that decreases rapidly in size, and a prothrombin time that is prolonged more than 4 seconds above normal.

Chronic hepatitis and cirrhosis occur in 3 to 5% of patients with type B and in 10–20% of patients with non-A, non-B hepatitis (13). They do not occur after type A hepatitis. These complications should be suspected in patients who continue to have clinical and laboratory evidence of liver disease 6 months following the onset of acute hepatitis (20). Most patients clear the HB$_S$Ag from their serum within 3 months of the onset of the illness. About 10% of patients with type B hepatitis become chronic carriers of HB$_S$Ag. Chronic carriers of HB$_S$Ag with abnormal serum aminotransferases should be evaluated for the development of chronic active hepatitis by liver biopsy. An increased incidence of hepatocellular carcinoma has been found in carriers of HB$_S$Ag.

Differential Diagnosis

A number of other viruses have been reported to cause hepatitis. *Cytomegalic inclusion infection*, usually clinically inapparent in the adult, can present with manifestations of hepatitis in patients being administered immunosuppressive therapy or following blood transfusions in healthy subjects; the diagnosis is made by culture of the urine. *Mononucleosis* (caused by the Epstein-Barr virus) frequently is associated with hepatocellular dysfunction with mild transient jaundice in 5 to 10% of patients. The presence of a heterophil antibody, which is not absorbed by guinea pig kidney, or a positive mononucleosis spot test, confirms the diagnosis (see Chapter 52).

Hepatitis due to *leptospirosis* should be suspected in patients who have been in close contact with rodents; the diagnosis is established by recovery of leptospiras in culture of the blood or by a rise in antibodies in the course of the disease. *Drug hepatitis* (page 501) presents with clinical features which are indistinguishable from viral hepatitis, and a history of drug intake is a most important clue in suspecting the diagnosis. *Alcoholic hepatitis* (page 502) usually develops after recent heavy alcohol ingestion; the serum aminotransferases are rarely elevated more than 10 times above normal and the elevation is primarily in the serum aspartate aminotransferase (AST). In patients with marked cholestasis, as evidenced by persistent elevation of the bilirubin, high serum alkaline phosphatase, and pruritus in association with persistent dark urine and light stools, the diagnosis of extrahepatic biliary obstruction should be entertained. An abnormal sonogram may provide a clue to *extrahepatic obstruction* if the biliary ducts are found to be dilated, and the patient should then be referred to a specialist in liver diseases for further evaluation.

Prevention and prophylaxis of viral hepatitis. General hygienic measures, such as washing the hands after contact with the patient, are the most effective means of preventing the spread of hepatitis from patients to other persons. The patient's dishes and eating utensils can be shared by other persons only if cleaned by heating above 120°C for 15 to 20 minutes in a dishwasher, after the patient has used them. Assignment of the patient to a separate bathroom is ideal, but often impractical. The viruses are present in feces, blood, and other body fluids of the patients. The handling of all of these materials should be done with care. Since the virus appears in the stool during the prodromal period of hepatitis, the precautions mentioned should be taken routinely in environments where there is a high risk of development of hepatitis, such as in institutions for the mentally retarded. The screening of blood for HB$_S$Ag before transfusion has virtually eliminated the development of type B hepatitis following blood transfusions. Hence 90% of post-transfusion hepatitis at present is type non-A, non-B. The development of post-transfusion hepatitis can be reduced further by using voluntary rather than commercial blood donors. Other sources of type B and non-A, non-B which can easily be controlled are contaminated needles, pins used to test sensation, and dental and surgical instruments. All used needles or pins should be discarded in specially labeled bottles containing 40% formalin, which is known to inactivate the hepatitis virus. The preferred method for cleaning surgical and dental instruments is by heat sterilization. The risk that most health workers who are HB$_S$Ag positive pose to their patients is minimal if high standards of hygiene are maintained (12). The exceptions are dentists and surgeons who often develop cuts on their hands while operating. Dentists are urged to wear gloves regardless of whether they are HB$_S$Ag positive to protect themselves and their patients. Patients who have had hepatitis B or hepatitis non-A, non-B and have recovered (clinically and, in the case of hepatitis B, serologically) may be infectious for many years and therefore should not be allowed to donate blood.

Standard immune serum globulin is known to prevent the clinical manifestations of hepatitis A in 80 to 90% of persons when administered early after exposure. However, it does not prevent subclinical infection. It is indicated for close personal contacts of patients with known hepatitis A, inmates of institutions during an epidemic of hepatitis A, and travelers to areas where hepatitis is endemic. It is not indicated for casual acquaintances or co-workers of the patient or for persons who are known to have anti-HA antibody in their serum. The recommended dose of standard immune globulin is 0.02 ml/kg. For continuous protection of persons in hepatitis endemic areas repeated doses of standard immune serum globulin, 0.06 ml/kg, should be given every 6 months.

The role of standard immune serum globulin in the prevention of type B hepatitis is uncertain. *Hep-*

atitis B immune globulin (containing a high titer of anti-HB$_S$) prevents approximately 75% of cases of type B hepatitis in people who have been stuck with needles contaminated by HB$_S$Ag-positive patients, in spouses of HB$_S$Ag-positive individuals, in newborns of HB$_S$Ag-positive mothers, and in the staff of dialysis units (18). It is not indicated for casual or work contacts of patients with type B hepatitis or for persons who have been demonstrated to have anti-HB$_S$. Testing for anti-HB$_S$ should be done routinely before administration of hepatitis B immune globulin provided that the results of the tests can be obtained within 1 week of exposure to the virus. The recommended dose of hepatitis B immune globulin is 0.06 ml/kg, which corresponds to 4 ml for an adult, with the dose repeated in 1 month. An initial dose should be given immediately after a person has been stuck with a contaminated needle and as soon as possible to spouses of HB$_S$Ag-positive individuals. Administration of hepatitis B immune globulin does not interfere with the efficacy of concomitant or subsequent administration of hepatitis B vaccine.

Hepatitis B vaccine is a suspension of highly purified formalin-inactivated HB$_S$Ag particles obtained from chronic HB$_S$Ag carriers. It is administered intramuscularly in an initial dose of 1.0 ml (20 μg of HB$_S$Ag protein) followed by the same dose at 1 and 6 months after initial administration. It has an efficacy of approximately 90% in the development of anti-HB$_S$ and prevention of clinical hepatitis B infection (18). The only side effect of the vaccine is occasional soreness and redness at the injection site. The vaccine is recommended only for susceptible individuals at high risk of contracting hepatitis B infection, which include (a) health care professionals exposed to blood or blood products, including laboratory and blood bank personnel, operating room staff, surgeons, dentists, endoscopists, pathologists, and the staff in oncology, dialysis, and emergency room units; (b) homosexuals and drug addicts; (c) family partners, in particular sex partners, of chronic HB$_S$Ag carriers; (d) patients who frequently receive transfusions of blood or blood products; (e) patients in hemodialysis units; (f) inmates and staff of institutions for the mentally retarded; (g) newborn infants of mothers who have acute type B hepatitis or are chronic carriers of HB$_S$Ag. The vaccine is not routinely recommended for individuals who come in contact with HB$_S$Ag carriers at work or in school. Screening for antibodies to hepatitis B virus prior to vaccination is only cost effective for groups with a very high risk of infection (greater than 20%). For routine screening, either anti-HB$_S$ or anti-HB$_C$ can be tested. However, determination of anti-HB$_C$ is preferred to screen groups at high risk of infection to avoid vaccination of HB$_S$Ag carriers. On occasion anti-HB$_S$ is nonprotective either because it is a nonspecific reactant or protective only to one subtype of HB$_S$Ag. Vaccination of individuals who

have anti-HB$_S$ from previous infection does not cause adverse effects.

Chapter 32 contains additional information regarding (a) primary prevention of hepatitis B with hepatitis B vaccine, (b) postexposure prophylaxis for adults and newborn infants exposed to persons who either have active hepatitis B or are known HB$_S$Ag carriers, and (c) postexposure prophylaxis for adults exposed to persons whose HB$_S$Ag status is not known.

There have been insufficient studies to know whether the incidence of post-transfusion non-A, non-B hepatitis is decreased by the administration of standard immune serum globulin. In any case, elimination of commercial blood donors seems to be a more practical way of preventing post-tranfusion non-A, non-B hepatitis.

Drug-Induced Hepatitis

The liver is the principal organ concerned with drug metabolism; hence, it is not surprising that it is also a principal target for drug toxicity. Every drug has the potential for producing hepatocellular damage. Drug-induced hepatitis results either from direct hepatotoxicity or from an idiosyncratic reaction (host hypersensitivity). *Hepatotoxic reactions* caused by direct toxins such as carbon tetrachloride and inorganic phosphorus are dose dependent and reproducible with a brief interval after exposure to the drug. *Idiosyncratic reactions* are the more common response to drugs. Characteristically, they are not dose dependent, occur in only a small number of individuals who are exposed, and are preceded by a sensitizing period of 1 to 4 weeks of exposure or a history of prior exposure. Drug reactions may be cholestatic, simulate viral hepatitis, or combine features of both processes.

Cholestatic Reactions

Cholestasis is due to a direct dose-related effect of the administration of anabolic steroids and oral contraceptives. Cholestasis occurs in 1 to 2% of patients receiving anabolic steroids, but occurs less frequently after the ingestion of oral contraceptive drugs. Jaundice and pruritus are prominent symptoms. The elevated serum bilirubin is composed principally of the direct fraction. Serum alkaline phosphatase and cholesterol are elevated, while serum aminotransferases are normal or only slightly elevated. Cholestasis disappears soon after withdrawal of the offending drug.

A much larger number of drugs cause cholestasis due to hypersensitivity. Examples are phenothiazine derivatives such as chlorpromazine, antibiotics such as erythromycin, antithyroid drugs such as propylthiouracil and methimazole, hypoglycemic agents such as tolbutamide and chlorpropamide, and cytotoxic drugs such as chlorambucil. Common clinical features of these drug reactions are fever, right upper quadrant abdominal pain, pruritus, skin rash, and eosinophilia. Serum aminotransferases are moderately elevated (less than 10 times above normal). The clinical and laboratory abnormalities usually subside between 2 to 4 weeks after discontinuation of the drug, although on occasion cholestasis persists for months to years. Severe pruritus is treated with cholestyramine (Questran) given in a dose of 4 g three times a day before meals. Relief of pruritus is obtained in 4 to 7 days after starting this medication. Patients with cholestasis should be hospitalized whenever the jaundice persists unchanged or increases 2 to 4 weeks after discontinuation of the drug.

Hepatocellular Reactions

Most agents that produce direct hepatocellular damage are toxins rather than drugs. Acetaminophen, however, is a drug that produces hepatic necrosis in all individuals if ingested in a large dose (greater than 10 g), usually in a suicide attempt. Shortly after ingestion the patient develops nausea and vomiting, but evidence of hepatocellular damage often does not become apparent until 48 hours later when serum aminotransferases rise and the prothrombin time becomes prolonged. The patient's condition then deteriorates; jaundice appears and central nervous system depression may occur. The mortality rate of patients who took an overdose of acetaminophen was found to be 3.5% in one large study (9). Thus patients who are known or are suspected of ingesting toxic amounts of acetaminophen should be hospitalized.

Idiosyncratic hepatocellular reactions have been reported after the administration of a number of drugs, the most common of which are isoniazid, α-methyldopa, phenylbutazone, 6-mercaptopurine, and halothane. Asymptomatic increases in serum aminotransferases, which subside despite continued administration of the drug, have been reported in 5 to 10% of patients taking isoniazid or α-methyldopa (14). Because of the frequent transient nature of the serum aminotransferase elevations, there is no need to monitor this test in asymptomatic patients. However, the development of symptoms of fatigue and anorexia or of nausea and general malaise is an indication for determination of serum aminotransferases; if aminotransferase activity is increased, the drug should be discontinued immediately because this often heralds the onset of severe hepatocellular damage. The incidence of acute hepatitis in patients taking the drugs listed above is 0.1 to 0.3%. Women and older patients are more likely to be affected. The onset of the reaction is between 1 and 10 weeks after the start of therapy. The symptoms, laboratory tests, and findings on liver biopsy are indistinguishable from those of viral hepatitis (see page 496). The hepatitis usually resolves after the drug is discontinued. However, a mortality rate as high as 12% has been reported for severe hepatitis due to isoniazid. Moreover, chronic active liver disease can develop if the drug responsible for the hepatitis is continued. Administration of corticosteriods is not indicated in drug-induced hepatitis.

Alcoholic Hepatitis

This condition is seen most frequently after prolonged heavy alcohol intake. Women are more susceptible to alcoholic liver disease than men and it usually does not develop in men who drink less than 80 g of ethanol/day or in women who drink half this amount (equivalent to 8 and 4 ounces of 86 proof whiskey, respectively). Many of the presenting clinical characteristics of patients with alcoholic hepatitis (such as anorexia, marked fatigue, jaundice, and tender hepatomegaly) are indistinguishable from those of viral hepatitis (see pages 496 to 497). However, patients with alcoholic hepatitis are more likely to have fever and leukocytosis. The elevation of the serum aminotransferases is rarely 10 times above normal, and frequently there is a prolongation of the prothrombin time. The elevation of AST is characteristically higher than that of serum alanine aminotransferase (ALT). Patients with alcoholic hepatitis should be admitted to the hospital and a definite diagnosis established by liver biopsy, if not contraindicated by abnormal hemostatic function. Liver biopsy differentiates alcoholic hepatitis from drug-induced hepatitis and viral hepatitis and gives an indication of any underlying chronic liver disease. The illness is often more severe than in patients with viral hepatitis, and decompensation with hepatic encephalopathy and death can occur. About one-third of patients with alcoholic hepatitis have been shown to progress to cirrhosis, often in a short period of 6 months (6).

Chronic Hepatitis

Chronic hepatitis refers to chronic inflammation of the liver detected by abnormal liver tests or by abnormal liver histology which has persisted for longer than 6 months. The spectrum of chronic hepatitis varies from a benign reversible process to an unrelenting process which often progresses to cirrhosis. Liver histology is essential both for the diagnosis and to establish the severity of the disease and the need for treatment. Two types of chronic hepatitis are recognized by the examination of tissue obtained on liver biopsy: chronic persistent hepatitis, which is a self-limited disease and does not require therapy, and chronic active hepatitis, which is a progressive process associated with increased morbidity and mortality and which often improves with therapy. In chronic persistent hepatitis, liver biopsy reveals portal inflammation often with expansion of the portal areas and focal parenchymal necrosis with preservation of the lobular architecture and slight or absent fibrosis: whereas in chronic active hepatitis there is extension of inflammation and necrosis from the portal area to the hepatocytes adjacent to it (piecemeal necrosis), disruption of the lobular architecture, and increased fibrosis with the formation of intralobular septa of fibrous tissue (bridging) (1).

The principal causes of chronic hepatitis are infection with hepatitis viruses, both type B and type non-A, non-B (not type A), idiopathic (formerly called lupoid hepatitis), and drugs such as isoniazid, α-methyldopa, nitrofurantoin, and oxyphenacetin. In addition, Wilson's disease, α_1-antitrypsin deficiency, and primary biliary cirrhosis may present with clinical and histological features of chronic hepatitis.

Chronic Persistent Hepatitis

Patients with chronic persistent hepatitis are either asymptomatic or have mild nonspecific symptoms such as fatigue. On physical examination there are no peripheral manifestations of chronic liver disease, but there may be mild hepatomegaly. Laboratory tests show mild elevation of serum aminotransferases (2 to 5 times normal), but the remainder of the liver tests are usually normal. Forty percent of the patients have detectable HB_SAg in the serum. The diagnosis is established by liver biopsy and the patient is then reassured about the benign course of his condition. If symptoms and elevation of the aminotransferases persist, a liver biopsy is indicated after 2 to 3 years to rule out a sampling error on the initial liver biopsy. Patients with persistent hepatitis have been shown to have elevated serum aminotransferases for over 10 years without any evidence of progression of the disease.

Chronic Active Hepatitis

The onset of chronic active hepatitis is usually insidious. The patient may be asymptomatic and liver disease may be detected by aminotransferase elevations done on routine testing, or he may present symptoms of general malaise, fatigue, abdominal discomfort, anorexia, and jaundice. In about a third of the patients the disease evolves from a clinically overt episode of acute hepatitis. Physical examination in patients with chronic active hepatitis reveals hepatomegaly and often peripheral manifestations of chronic liver disease, such as spider angiomas, palmar erythema, and gynecomastia. Elevations of serum bilirubin, aminotransferases, and globulins are the most sensitive indicators of the activity of the hepatocellular damage, while decreases in serum albumin and prolongation of the prothrombin time reflect loss of hepatocellular function and a poor prognosis. Older male patients are more likely to have HB_SAg in the serum and to present with an acute onset of illness. On the other hand, HB_SAg-negative patients are more likely to be women and to present with systemic symptoms of acne, amen-

orrhea, arthralgia and arthritis, pleurisy, or intermittent fever. In addition, they may have associated thyroiditis, Sjögren's syndrome, ulcerative colitis, glomerulonephritis, or hemolytic anemia. Laboratory tests on these patients show evidence of immunological hyperactivity: serum γ-globulin is often markedly elevated; lupus erythematosus (LE) cells are present; and there is an increased incidence of elevation of the titer of antinuclear antibodies and smooth muscle antibodies. In addition, antimitochondrial antibodies are found in 15% of these patients.

The clinical course of patients with chronic active hepatitis is quite variable. Patients can be asymptomatic for a long time, have periods of intermittent worsening and remission, or have a progressive course to cirrhosis and death if untreated (19). δ agent is associated with clinical exacerbation of chronic hepatitis and more rapid progression to cirrhosis (10).

Differential Diagnosis

The diagnosis of *Wilson's disease* should be considered in all patients, particularly those under 25 years who present with clinical and laboratory features of chronic hepatitis (22). Wilson's disease is discussed in more detail in the section on cirrhosis (page 505). The diagnosis of *chronic hepatitis due to α_1-antitrypsin deficiency* is suggested by the finding of an absent or low α_1-globulin on serum protein electrophoresis (5). The diagnosis is established by demonstrating a low value of α_1-antitrypsin in the serum by quantitative measurement and by protease inhibitor (Pi) typing (5). The common allele is PiM, while liver disease occurs in about 20% of individuals who are homozygous for the allele PiZ. Liver biopsy reveals PAS-positive cytoplasmic inclusions which are resistant to diastase in both homozygous and heterozygous individuals for the allele PiZ. There is no known therapy for this deficiency, which is transmitted by co-dominant inheritance. The diagnostic characteristics of *primary biliary cirrhosis* are discussed in the section on cirrhosis (page 505). The diagnosis of *drug-induced chronic hepatitis* (page 501) is dependent on a careful history and on the demonstration of improvement of the patient after discontinuation of drugs which are known to produce this illness. In most cases chronic active hepatitis due to drugs will revert to normal after discontinuation of the offending drug (9).

Therapy

Corticosteroids have been shown to be beneficial in symptomatic patients with chronic active hepatitis who are HB_SAg negative. Clinical, biochemical, and histological improvement and even remission have been observed; and mortality rates have been reduced after therapy with corticosteroids (21). Prednisone or prednisolone, 40 to 60 mg, is given initially to suppress the activity of the disease and then tapered slowly, usually over a period of 1 to 3 months, to a maintenance dose of 15 to 20 mg. Symptomatic improvement followed by a fall in serum aminotransferases occurs in the first few weeks. Histological transformation to a lesion of persistent hepatitis will occur in some patients within a 2-year period. Treatment with corticosteroids is discontinued in patients who attain remission. In the remainder of the patients it is not continued beyond 4 years because the prospect of remission diminishes while the risk of side effects increases (2). Asymptomatic patients with chronic active hepatitis who are HB$_S$Ag negative are usually only treated if they have marked elevations of serum aminotransferases (greater than 10 times above normal) and histological evidence of severe liver disease (marked multilobular necrosis and bridging). Administration of corticosteroids to patients with chronic active hepatitis who are HB$_S$Ag positive is contraindicated because it appears to favor replication of hepatitis B virus, resulting in a higher morbidity and mortality (13).

UNEXPLAINED ELEVATIONS OF LIVER ENZYMES IN SERUM

Elevations of serum aminotransferases and alkaline phosphatase are occasionally found in normal subjects or in patients not suspected of having liver disease. In such a situation the abnormality should first be confirmed by repeat testing. Next, it is important to remember that elevated serum aminotransferases and alkaline phosphatase do not necessarily originate from the liver. For example, elevated serum aminotransferases can be due to injury to the heart and striated muscle; if the source of the serum aminotransferases is muscle, the more specific creatine kinase will also be elevated. An isolated increase of serum alkaline phosphatase can originate from liver or bone. The hepatic origin of alkaline phosphatase can be confirmed by demonstration of an elevated 5′-nucleotidase, which, unlike alkaline phosphatase, is present only in the liver and in the epithelium of the bile ducts. By contrast, an elevated serum alkaline phosphatase accompanied by a normal serum 5′-nucleotidase is almost invariably due to bone disease; a very common cause of such an occurrence is a recent bone fracture. Any persistent elevation of serum aminotransferases for longer than 6 months which remains unexplained is an indication for liver biopsy to rule out chronic hepatitis. A persistent elevation of serum alkaline phosphatase in the absence of an elevated serum bilirubin can occur in fatty liver, which is common in the diabetic and obese patient or can be the result of space-occupying lesions, such as granulomas or occasionally metastatic carcinoma. A liver scan is recommended in these cases to rule out metastatic carcinoma, but a liver biopsy is indicated only if the scan shows a space-occupying lesion or if there is clinical suspicion of diseases such as tuberculosis and sarcoidosis that result in hepatic granulomas.

ALCOHOLIC FATTY LIVER

Fatty liver is due to alterations of lipid metabolism caused by alcohol, and therefore occurs in all persons ingesting alcohol in excessive amounts. It is manifested mainly by a feeling of abdominal fullness due to hepatomegaly and mild elevation of the serum aminotransferases (rarely more than 2 times above normal). On occasion marked fatty infiltration is associated with symptoms of malaise, weakness, anorexia, tender hepatomegaly, and even jaundice. These symptomatic patients require admission to the hospital and a liver biopsy to distinguish fatty liver from alcoholic hepatitis and cirrhosis. The treatment of fatty liver consists of bed rest and abstinence from alcohol. With abstinence the abnormal accumulation of fat will disappear in a period of 4 to 6 weeks. As the patient improves, the liver decreases in size and becomes nontender. Serum bilirubin and aminotransferases promptly return to normal. Recurrent episodes of symptomatic fatty liver are common after heavy alcohol ingestion, but there is no evidence that this lesion in itself leads to cirrhosis.

CIRRHOSIS

Cirrhosis is a chronic diffuse liver disease characterized by widespread hepatic fibrosis and nodule formation. The fibrosis is the result of extensive destruction of liver cells, and the nodularity represents regeneration. For clinical purposes cirrhosis can be classified into the following major categories: alcoholic (micronodular), postnecrotic (macronodular), cardiac, biliary, Wilson's disease, hemochromatosis, and schistosomiasis. The two major types of cirrhosis are alcoholic, which is characterized by regular small nodules, and postnecrotic, in which there is extensive scarring of the liver and the presence of irregular nodules of various sizes (23). On occasion cirrhosis of the alcoholic is of the macronodular type; this is more common in chronic alcoholics who no longer drink alcohol. The onset of cirrhosis is usually insidious and associated with nonspecific symptoms, such as fatigue, anorexia, weight loss, nausea, and abdominal discomfort. As the disease progresses, signs of hepatocellular failure become prominent: jaundice, edema, ascites, electrolyte abnormalities, bleeding tendencies, spider angiomas, palmar erythema, gynecomastia, impotence, and loss of axillary and pubic hair. Hepatomegaly and portal hypertension resulting in splenomegaly and a venous collateral circulation are common. The most severe complications of cirrhosis are hepatic encephalopathy, bleeding from esophageal varices, and infection. Patients with alcoholic cirrhosis often present with recurring episodes of hepatocellular failure, precipitated by hepatocellular necrosis and fatty infiltrations induced by alcohol ingestion, which is reversible with clinical improvement after abstinence from alcohol, and after bed rest and optimal nutrition. By contrast, patients with postnecrotic cirrhosis are more likely to present insidiously with evidence of portal hypertension. When hepatocellular failure occurs in these patients, it is usually a terminal event because it is the result of excessive fibrosis and reduced hepatic parenchymal mass rather than of reversible lesions such as necrosis and fatty infiltration found in alcoholic cirrhosis. Rapid deterioration of patients with cirrhosis should raise the suspicion of a complicating hepatocellular carcinoma. Common laboratory findings in patients with cirrhosis include anemia, a normal or slightly decreased white blood cell count, and moderate thrombocytopenia. The most frequent abnormal liver tests are hyperbilirubinemia, a depressed serum albumin, elevated serum globulins, and a prolonged prothrombin time. Liver biopsy is indicated to establish a firm diagnosis in all cases where hemostatic function allows this procedure to be done (see page 499).

Differential Diagnosis

The diagnostic characteristics of some of the other types of cirrhosis are as follows: (a) *Cardiac cirrhosis* develops only after prolonged and severe cardiac failure, usually due to valvular disease, particularly in patients with tricuspid incompetence or in patients with constrictive pericarditis. Jaundice, hepatomegaly, and ascites are prominent features, but the diagnosis can only be established with certainty by liver biopsy. Treatment of cardiac failure, in particular of constrictive pericarditis by pericardiectomy, results in improvement of liver function. (b) *Primary biliary cirrhosis* (3) is a chronic disease of unknown cause which is characterized by progressive intrahepatic cholestasis and is most frequently seen in middle-aged females. The principal manifestations are jaundice with pruritus, hepatomegaly, hypercholesterolemia with the formation of xanthoma and xanthelasma, and steatorrhea due to the decreased delivery of bile acids to the intestine. Antimitochondrial antibodies are found in 95% of these patients, and their presence is virtually diagnostic. Liver biopsy in the early stages reveals injury to the septal and large intralobular bile ducts with surrounding accumulation of the inflammatory plasma cells and lymphocytes and with granuloma formation. In the end stages of the disease cirrhosis develops which is nearly indistinguishable from postnecrotic (macronodular) cirrhosis. (c) *Wilson's disease* is a rare disorder of copper metabolism which is inherited as an autosomal recessive (22). Its symptoms are due to hepatic and neurological dysfunction. In children the principal symptoms are

due to liver involvement, while in adults neurological symptoms tend to predominate. The diagnosis should be suspected in all children or young adults who develop cirrhosis since treatment with copper-chelating agents can arrest the disease and alleviate all symptoms. A characteristic finding which is virtually diagnostic is the presence of Kayser-Fleischer rings, which are greenish-brown rings found in the posterior surface and periphery of the cornea. Since these rings cannot often be seen by the naked eye, it is important to refer all suspected patients to the ophthalmologist for slitlamp examination of the cornea. Serum ceruloplasmin, the copper-binding protein, is reduced in most but not all cases. Histological examination of a liver biopsy is not diagnostic. However, quantitative determination of copper with finding of more than 250 μg/g of dry liver weight or the urinary excretion of more than 50 μg/24 hours is diagnostic. Hospitalization is not required for treatment of Wilson's disease with D-penicillamine. (d) *Hemochromatosis* is an inherited disorder of iron metabolism, resulting in excessive body iron which is principally characterized by cirrhosis, diabetes mellitus, and grayish pigmentation of the skin. Other symptoms are cardiac failure and arrhythmias, peripheral neuritis, arthritis, and testicular atrophy. The iron overload appears to be due to an increased absorption of dietary iron, and the mode of inheritance is autosomal recessive. The disease usually appears in persons over 40 years of age and develops earlier in males, probably because of the menstrual loss of iron in females. The diagnosis is made by demonstrating a high serum iron (greater than 150 μg/dl), a high saturation of iron-binding protein (greater than 50%), and increased serum ferritin, usually in a patient with a family history of the disease (15). (e) *Hepatic schistosomiasis* may occur in persons from tropical areas who have been infected by schistosome cercariae while swimming or walking in infested water. The liver disease is due to the deposition of ova of *Schistosoma mansoni* in the portal areas, with the development of an inflammatory reaction, often with granuloma formation and periportal fibrosis. Jaundice is uncommon in these patients on presentation. The most common laboratory abnormalities are increases in serum alkaline phosphatase and mild elevations of serum bilirbuin and aminotransferases. The diagnosis of active infection is made by demonstrating mobile *Schistosoma* ova on fresh examination of rectal biopsy, and the diagnosis of liver involvement is made by showing the presence of ova capsules on liver biopsy.

Management

The treatment of uncomplicated cirrhosis consists of voluntary restriction of activity if the patient has weakness and fatigue, a diet high in protein but low in salt, and abstinence from alcohol (see Chapter 21). This regimen almost invariably results in improvement of hepatocellular function in patients with alcoholic cirrhosis and occasionally in patients with postnecrotic cirrhosis. Tranquilizers and sedatives should be avoided. Infection and gastrointestinal bleeding, which in addition to alcohol ingestion are frequent precipitating factors of decompensation, should be searched for and treated. Vitamin K, 15 mg parenterally, may improve prolongation of the prothrombin time. Multivitamins and folic acid, 1 mg/day, may be given if the patient's dietary intake does not appear to be adequate or if there is evidence of vitamin deficiencies. Potassium deficiency is frequent and may contribute to the precipitation of hepatic encephalopathy, but its extent is difficult to assess because serum potassium concentration is a poor reflection of the total body potassium. However, when serum potassium falls below 3.5 mEq/liter, the deficit of body potassium is approximately 300 to 500 mEq. This can be replaced over a period of a few days with oral solutions of 10% potassium chloride which provides 40 mEq of potassium/ounce. Fluid retention is treated with sodium restriction (500 mg of sodium chloride/day) and diuretics. The induced diuresis should be slow and result in a loss of no more than 2.27 kg (5 lb) of weight per week because of the danger of precipitating electrolyte depletion and hypokalemia. Diuresis can be initiated by spironalactone, 25 mg orally three times a day. Thiazide diuretics or furosemide can be added to the regimen in gradually increasing doses if diuresis is inadequate. The development of acute hepatic encephalopathy manifested by asterixis or by changes in mental status is an indication that the patient should be hospitalized for evaluation and treatment. Acute and chronic gastrointestinal bleeding is also an indication for hospitalization.

Protein can be restricted in stable cirrhotic patients to 45 g/day without development of a negative nitrogen balance as long as a minimum of 400 g of carbohydrate are ingested a day. A change from animal protein to a vegetable protein diet may also improve hepatic encephalopathy. The exact mechanism whereby vegetable protein is better tolerated is unknown. However, vegetable protein contains smaller amounts of ammonia, methionine, and aromatic acids and also results in alterations of small intestinal and colonic bacterial flora (8). Lactulose is a nonabsorbable synthetic dissacharide which when administered in doses of 20 to 30 g (30 to 45 ml) three to four times a day reduces blood ammonia and improves encephalopathy in over 80% of patients. Lactulose usually is effective only when it also increases the frequency of bowel movements. Other than producing mild abdominal cramps and flatulence, lactulose is devoid of side effects. The mechanism of its action is not well defined, but its effectiveness is related to its ability to trap nitrogen in the stool and decrease ammonia production. Some of the decrease in ammonia production may be due to a decrease in contact time of the stool with colonic bacteria. The beneficial effects of a vegetable protein diet and lactulose on hepatic encephalopathy are additive. Patients with chronic hepatic encephalopathy can be treated with protein restriction and lactulose on an ambulatory basis.

General References

Dienstag JL: Hepatitis A virus: identification, characterization, and epidemiologic investigations. *Prog Liver Dis* 6:343, 1979.
> Excellent review of all aspects of hepatitis A virus, including clinical characteristics of hepatitis A infection and prophylaxis.

Hoyumpa AM Jr, Greene HL, Dunn GD, Schenker S: Fatty liver: biochemical and clinical considerations. *Am J Dig Dis* 20:1142, 1975.
> Discusses various causes, clinical presentation, and management of fatty liver.

Leevy CM, Popper H, Sherlock S: Diseases of the liver and biliary tract. Standardization of nomenclature, diagnostic criteria and diagnostic methodology. Fogarty International Center Proceedings No. 22. DHEW Publication No. (NIH) 76-725, 1976.

Sherlock S: Long incubation (virus B, HAA-associated) hepatitis. *Gut* 13:297, 1972.
> Reviews characteristics of the hepatitis B virus and clinical characteristics of hepatitis B virus infection.

Sherlock S: Hepatic reactions to drugs. *Gut* 20:634, 1979.
> Good basic review of drug hepatitis. Discusses mechanisms of drug injury.

Specific References

1. Boyer JL: Chronic hepatitis—a perspective on classification and determinants of prognosis. *Gastroenterology* 70:1161, 1976.
2. Davis GL, Czaja AJ: Prolonged steroid therapy for severe chronic active liver disease (CALD): a diminishing return? *Gastroenterology* 78:1153, 1980.
3. Dickson ER, Fleming CP, Ludwig J: Primary biliary cirrhosis. *Prog Liver Dis* 6:487, 1979.
4. Dienstag JL: Non-A, non-B hepatitis. II. Experimental transmission, putative virus agents and markers and prevention. *Gastroenterology* 85:743, 1983.
5. Fagerhol MK, Laurell CB: The polymorphism of "prealbumins" and α_1-antitrypsin in human sera. *Clin Chim Acta* 16:199, 1967.
6. Galambos JT: Alcoholic hepatitis: its therapy and prognosis. *Prog Liver Dis* 4:567, 1972.
7. Grady GF, and the U.S. National Heart and Lung Institute Collaborative Study Group: Relation of e antigen to infectivity of HB_sAg-positive inoculations among medical personnel. *Lancet* 2:492, 1976.
8. Greenberger NJ, Carley J, Schenker S, et al: Effect of vegetable and animal protein diets in chronic hepatic encephalopathy. *Am J Dig Dis* 22:845, 1977.
9. Hamlyn AN, Douglas AP, James O: The spectrum of paracetamol (acetaminophen) overdose: clinical and epidemiological studies. *Postgrad Med J* 54:400, 1978.
10. Jacobson IM, Dienstag JL: The delta hepatitis agent: "viral hepatitis, type D." *Gastroenterology* 86:1614, 1984.
11. Krugman S, Overby LR, Mushahwar IK, et al: Viral hepatitis, type B. Studies on natural history and prevention re-examined. *N Engl J Med* 300:101, 1979.
12. LaBrecque DR, Freeman R: Risk of transmitting hepatitis B from staff to patient in a renal dialysis unit. *Gastroenterology* 75:972, 1978.
13. Lam KC, Lai CL, Trepo C, Wu PC: Deleterious effect of prednisolone in HB_sAg-positive chronic active hepatitis. *N Eng J Med* 304:380, 1981.

14. Maddrey WC, Boitnott JK: Drug-induced chronic liver disease. *Gastroenterology* 72:1348, 1977.
15. Powell LW, Halliday JW: The detection of early hemochromatosis. *Am J Dig Dis* 23:377, 1978.
16. Repsher LH, Freebern RK: Effects of early and vigorous exercise on recovery from infectious hepatitis. *N Engl J Med* 281:1393, 1969.
17. Sampliner RE, Hamilton FA, Iseri OA, *et al*: The liver histology and frequency of clearance of the hepatitis B surface antigen (HB$_S$Ag) in chronic carriers. *Am J Med Sci* 277:17, 1979.
18. Seeff LB, Koff RS: Passive and active immunoprophylaxis of hepatitis B. *Gastroenterology* 86:958, 1984.
19. Sherlock S. Chronic hepatitis. *Gut* 15:581, 1974.
20. Sherlock S. Predicting progression of acute type-B hepatitis to chronicity. *Lancet* 2:354, 1976.
21. Soloway RD, Summerskill WHJ, Baggenstoss AH, *et al*: Clinical, biochemical, and histological remission of severe chronic active liver disease: a controlled study of treatments and early prognosis. *Gastroenterology* 63:820, 1972.
22. Sternlieb I, Scheinberg IH: Chronic hepatitis as a first manifestation of Wilson's disease. *Ann Intern Med* 76:59, 1972.
23. Summerskill WHJ, Davidson CS, Dible JH, *et al*: Cirrhosis of the liver. A study of alcoholic and non-alcoholic patients in Boston and London. *N Engl J Med* 262:1, 1960.
24. Szmuness W, Dienstag JC, Purcell RH, *et al*: Distribution of antibody to hepatitis A antigen in urban adult populations. *N Engl J Med* 295:755, 1976.

SECTION 5

Renal and Urological Problems

Proteinuria

JOHN R. BURTON, M.D.

Proteinuria is frequently encountered in ambulatory practice. It may signify a serious underlying disorder or it may be simply an abnormal laboratory finding in an asymptomatic individual with little or no effect on his present or future health.

This chapter will discuss the methods of detection of protein in the urine and describe an approach to the evaluation and management of patients with this problem.

METHODS FOR DETECTING PROTEINURIA

Normally a small amount of protein is present in the urine. There is limited glomerular filtration of albumin and relatively greater filtration of lower molecular weight proteins, with nearly complete tubular resorption or digestion of filtered proteins. There is some tubular secretion, especially of a heavy molecular weight protein called the Tamm-Horsfall protein. The Tamm-Horsfall protein is the only protein identified in the urine that is not found in the plasma, and it forms the matrix that is seen in all urinary casts (6). The quantity of protein in the urine is normally less than 150 mg/24 hours. While this is a small quantity, it may be detected by sensitive screening tests when the urine is physiologically concentrated.

Certain disease states affect the glomeruli and/or the tubules, resulting in increased amounts of proteins in the urine. Office screening for proteinuria is easily accomplished by several accessible and inexpensive semiquantitative methods described in detail below.

All methods have some limitations as shown in Table 43.1, which provides a summary of the false results that are obtained under different conditions. It is clear that a combination of the dipstick test and one of the others may be required for diagnosis. Moreover, *all* methods are sensitive (dipstick detects 20 to 30 mg of protein/dl, sulfosalicylic acid and heat and acetic acid, 5 to 10 mg/dl) so that false positive results may be obtained on concentrated urine.

Dipstick

This is the most practical and easiest test for semiquantitation of urinary proteins. When moistened with urine, the stick becomes yellow when protein is absent. As protein concentration increases, interference with the dye-buffer combination results in an increasingly green color. While simple and inexpensive, the technique has several limitations: (*a*) The dipstick method is primarily sensitive to albumin. Therefore, globulins or parts of globulins (heavy or light chains—Bence Jones protein) may be missed. (*b*) Since the color reaction is pH dependent, false positive reactions may be observed if the urine is alkaline (pH greater than 7.5). This error can be avoided by adding a drop of strong acid (*e.g.*, 1 N HCl) prior to testing to assure that the pH in the urine is less than 7.0. (*c*) High concentrations of salt in the urine will reduce the quantitative estimate of protein. This effect should be considered if the reaction is 1+ or 2+ and the patient is known to eat large quantities of salt. (The dipstick technique is not affected by urine turbidity or by drugs.) Because of these limitations, an alternative method of screening for proteinuria should be available in the physician's office. Either of the methods described below is satisfactory.

Sulfosalicylic Acid (SSA)

Another relatively easy and inexpensive semiquantitative test for proteinuria is protein precipitation with a 3 to 10% solution of sulfosalicylic acid. This solution is added to the urine in an approximate ratio of 8 ml to 2 ml of urine. After inversion and incubation at room temperature for a few moments flocculation is graded on a 0 to 4+ basis. The SSA test is important since it will precipitate globulins

Table 43.1.
Urinary Constituents Which Alter the Results of Protein Screening Tests[a]

Urinary Constituents	Dipstick	Sulfosalicyclic Acid	Heat and Acetic Acid
Radiographic contrast media	No effect	False positive	False positive
Tolbutamide metabolites	No effect	False positive	False positive
Sulfisoxazole metabolites	No effect	False positive	False positive
Highly alkaline urine	False positive	False negative	False negative
High salt concentration	False negative	No effect	No effect
Vaginal or prostatic secretion	No effect	False positive	False positive

[a] Modified from Bradley M, Schumann GB, Ward PCJ: Examination of urine. In Henry JB (ed): *Todd-Sanford-Davidsohn Clinical Diagnosis and Management by Laboratory Methods,* ed 16. Philadelphia, WB Saunders, 1979.

and light chains and, therefore, can reliably detect Bence Jones protein.

SSA is used most frequently in two situations: as a check when the dipstick is negative, if there is a large quantity of salt in the urine or when globulins or light chains are being sought. False positive test results occur, however, if the urine is turbid, and in this situation the urine must be filtered before it is tested. False positive results also occur when the test is done within 3 days of the administration of iodinated radiological contrast media or administration of some drugs (Table 43.1). In addition, the SSA test will detect proteins of prostatic and vaginal origin. The physician should take care to avoid these contaminants by not palpating the prostate before collecting urine from men and by obtaining a clean voided urine specimen from women, which should show no or only a few vaginal cells microscopically.

SSA is available from some pharmacies or from hospital laboratories. It is also marketed as Bumintest tablets by the Ames Company and is available through physician or surgical supply stores. When dissolved in water as directed the tablets will provide a solution containing about 5% SSA.

Heat and Acetic Acid

This method is more time consuming and is recommended as a second method of urine protein testing only when SSA is not available. Glacial acetic acid may be purchased at a photography store and must be diluted for accurate results. The diluted solution, 1 volume of glacial acetic acid to 2 volumes of water, may be stored and used as necessary. The test is performed by heating the top of a test tube containing approximately 10 ml of urine. After the top of the urine begins to boil rapidly, 3 or 4 drops of the diluted acetic acid are added. Reheating to boiling causes a white precipitate to form if protein (either globulin or albumin) is present in the urine specimen. False positive results occur if the specimen is contaminated with prostatic or vaginal secretions or in the presence of certain drugs or radiographic contrast media (Table 43.1). Further, the rapid boiling may mask the visualization of a transient precipitation of Bence Jones protein.

OFFICE ASSESSMENT OF PATIENTS WITH PROTEINURIA

When proteinuria is identified and confirmed, much can be done in the office to diagnose the problem and to minimize referral. First, it is important to define as closely as possible the *onset of proteinuria* by reviewing results of previous urinalysis done for insurance, school, military, employment, or previous health examinations. Occasionally, the patient may notice a foaming of the urine upon voiding when proteinuria is massive. Further, the onset of edema, nocturia, or hypertension may date the onset of a disease associated with proteinuria.

Second, the *physical examination* should be reviewed for the presence of signs that may be associated with the cause of renal disease (such as diabetic retinopathy or large polycystic kidneys) or that may result from renal disease (such as edema) or both (such as hypertension).

Third, a *microscopic urinalysis* should be done. The presence of other abnormalities, such as hematuria, casts, and/or inflammatory cells, will suggest specific patterns of renal disease of which proteinuria may be just a concomitant.

Fourth, an *assessment of renal filtration function* by measurement of serum creatinine or of creatinine clearance is the most important assessment of renal function (see Chapter 47, Chronic Renal Failure).

Fifth, it is important to *quantitate the proteinuria* by examining a 24-hour urine sample or by determining the protein/creatinine ratio, as this will help to classify the disorder (see below) and will assist in the development of the differential diagnosis. The patient will need precise instructions, verbal as well as written, to ensure adequacy of a 24-hour urine collection.

Twenty-Four-Hour Urine Collection for Protein

A container without preservatives, usually a gallon jug, is given to the patient with instructions about the collection process. The 24-hour collection is best done on a day when the patient will be using one toilet; and it is helpful for the patient to place a note on the toilet on the day of collection to remind him to collect all required specimens. On the day of collection the first voided morning specimen is discarded; and then all urine in the next 24 hours, including the *next* morning's first voided specimen, is collected in the container. Once collected, it is not necessary to cool the urine; and it is not critical when the protein determination is done.

Quantitation of urine protein is a precise measurement in a well controlled laboratory, and any value greater than 200 mg/day is considered abnormal. Proteinuria is classified as *non-nephrotic* if the excretion is between 200 mg and 3500 mg in 24 hours and classified as *nephrotic* when the excretion is greater than 3500 mg in 24 hours, regardless of the presence or absence of other manifestations of the nephrotic syndrome (low serum albumin, edema, high serum cholesterol). The simultaneous measurement of urinary creatinine is an index of the adequacy of collection and is helpful. Most individuals who are not wasted and are of average body mass produce between 800 and 1500 mg of creatinine/day.

Protein/Creatinine Ratio

The determination of the protein/creatinine ratio

$$\frac{mg/dl\ of\ protein}{mg/dl\ of\ creatinine}$$

may be useful and eliminates the need for precise volume or time measurements. A ratio of greater than 0.2 mg of protein/mg of creatinine is considered abnormal, and a ratio of greater than 3.5 represents nephrotic range proteinuria. An excellent correlation between the protein/creatinine ratio and the 24-hour urine protein excretion is found when the ratio is determined in an aliquot of urine obtained during normal daytime activity (1). The determination of the protein/creatinine ratio should be utilized whenever there is doubt regarding the adequacy of a 24-hour collection.

NON-NEPHROTIC PROTEINURIA

A physician considering the differential diagnosis of patients with this range of proteinuria should first rule out physiological explanations or problems that are not primarily renal. These are listed in Table 43.2 and can be eliminated by brief questioning and repeat semiquantitative assessment of urine protein. A variety of primary renal and systemic diseases may be associated with non-nephrotic range proteinuria. Also most, if not all, patients with nephrotic range proteinuria (see below) may have, at some time, had non-nephrotic range protein excretion.

Non-isolated Proteinuria

If an abnormality related to proteinuria is discovered during initial evaluation (e.g., hypertension,

Table 43.2.
Cause of Proteinuria Not Due to a Primary Renal Disease

Congestive heart failure
Epinephrine administration
Exercise
Fever
Stress resulting in catecholamine release

hematuria, or renal failure), further investigation may be necessary. The direction and extent of the investigation depend on the nature of the abnormality. Renal biopsy may be indicated, especially if there is hematuria, red blood cell casts, mild renal failure, or evidence of systemic disease (e.g., systemic lupus erythematosus (SLE)). Table 43.3 lists some additional investigations which may be indicated to evaluate abnormalities associated with proteinuria. A telephone consultation with a nephrologist may be helpful in deciding the need for further evaluation.

Isolated Proteinuria in Apparently Healthy Persons

If the initial evaluation is negative except for the presence of isolated proteinuria, the proteinuria may be further classified as persistent (25 to 30% of patients) or intermittent (70 to 75% of patients) (9). The physician can determine which pattern is present by obtaining five or six specimens for semiquantitative analysis over several months. Also, the 24-hour urine protein excretion is almost always less than 1 g in patients with isolated proteinuria.

Persistent Proteinuria

Patients with protein in greater than 80% of urine specimens are defined as having persistent proteinuria. The disorder may be further classified by evaluating the effect of posture. Constant persistent proteinuria is present when the patient is both recumbent and on ambulation; and orthostatic persistent proteinuria is present when the patient is in the upright position only (see below).

Constant Proteinuria

In most patients with constant proteinuria, diverse morphological changes are identified in kidney biopsy specimens. Few long term studies of these patients have been made, but their course is likely to be indolent. Renal failure develops very rarely, although most patients develop abnormal urine sediment, and 50% develop hypertension (3). It is not necessary to perform renal biopsy when there are no other findings, but yearly re-evaluation is appropriate and should include blood pressure measurement, urinalysis, and determination of 24-hour protein excretion and of serum creatinine and creatinine clearance.

Table 43.3.
Selected Investigations Which May Be Appropriate in the Diagnosis of Proteinuria That Is Not Isolated or That Is Nephrotic

Antinuclear antibody, if systemic lupus erythematosus (SLE) is suspected

Antistreptolysin (ASO) titer, if there is a possibility of post-streptococcal glomerulonephritis

Complement (C_3, C_4), if glomerulonephritis is suspected

Complete blood count, to provide a baseline evaluation for subsequent use and to provide a clue to a systemic illness (such as leukemia)

Erythrocyte sedimentation rate, if collagen vascular disease is suspected

Fasting blood sugar, to consider the possibility of diabetes mellitus

Hepatitis B surface antigen, if hepatitis-associated vasculitis may be present

Intravenous pyelogram, to provide evidence for structural renal disease (such as papillary necrosis)

Lupus erythematosus (LE) prep, if SLE is suspected

Serum albumin, if nephrotic range proteinuria is present

Serum electrolytes (Na^+, K^+, Cl^-, HCO_3^-, Ca^{2+}, PO_4^{2-}), to provide a screen for abnormalities subsequent to renal disease

Serum and urine protein electrophoresis, if multiple myeloma is suspected

Uric acid, to screen for urate-related renal disease

Urine culture, if pyuria is present

X-ray of chest, to provide evidence for a systemic disease—for example, sarcoidosis

---

Orthostatic Proteinuria

The phenomenon of regularly reproducible postural proteinuria (also called fixed and orthostatic) has been clarified largely by the work of Robinson *et al* (8), who have followed for several years a number of male military recruits who have had this problem. Orthostatic proteinuria is defined as proteinuria only in the upright position. Its pathogenesis is not known. A simple method of determining the presence of this phenomenon is to have the patient collect two urine specimens. The patient rests quietly for 2 hours and then voids just before retiring in the evening. The patient does not get out of bed for 8 hours, and then upon arising voids completely into a container labeled "recumbent urine." The patient then stays up but is not vigorously active and collects all subsequent urine over the next 8 hours and then voids fully at the end of this collection period. This specimen is labeled "ambulatory urine." The protein concentrations in the urine specimens are then compared. An alternative to this method requires less time but is less quantitative. When this latter test is conducted during moderate fluid restriction, the results are reproducible. On the morning after overnight fluid deprivation, two or more urine specimens are collected consecutively during each of two sequentially assumed body postures: recumbence and ambulation. A semiquanti-

tative test and a measurement of urine concentration to confirm antidiuresis are performed on each sample (9). In patients with orthostatic proteinuria the "recumbent" protein excretion is negligible, whereas proteinuria is found when the patient assumes upright posture.

A renal biopsy is not necessary in the evaluation of a patient with this problem; but, when done as part of a research protocol, minor abnormalities have been defined in approximately half of the individuals while the others have had a biopsy that appeared normal on light microscopy (studies utilizing electron and/or immunofluorescent microscopy have not been done). It would, however, be prudent to follow the patient by measuring urinary protein excretion and serum creatinine or creatinine clearance on a yearly basis even after the proteinuria has cleared (see below).

If fixed and orthostatic proteinuria is documented, the prognosis seems to be excellent. Military recruits with this problem have been followed for 20 years (11). None has developed renal failure, and approximately 80% are no longer proteinuric. Not all patients who were free of protein in the urine at 10-year follow-up remained protein free after 20 years, although none of those patients showed significant deterioration in renal function. Also, a small number of patients re-evaluated 42 to 50 years following the establishment of the diagnosis of postural proteinuria manifest an excellent prognosis (10).

Intermittent Proteinuria

A study of individuals with intermittent isolated proteinuria (protein in less than 80% of specimens) revealed definite abnormalities by light microscopy in the renal tissue of approximately 60% of patients, while approximately 40% had a normal or nearly normal biopsy (7). The significance of these findings is unclear, however, in light of an independent study which retrospectively analyzed the prognostic significance of proteinuria in male college students and found there was no excess mortality 37 to 45 years later; morbidity was not studied (5).

In any case, patients who are found to have asymptomatic intermittent proteinuria and who have no evidence of systemic or renal disease can be given an optimistic prognosis. It is not necessary to perform kidney biopsy in these individuals, but it would be prudent to follow them yearly with measurement of urine protein excretion, a urinalysis, and determination of serum creatinine and creatinine clearance. Should deterioration in function, significant increase in protein excretion, or new abnormalities occur, then reassessment and possibly a renal biopsy are necessary.

NEPHROTIC PROTEINURIA

When a 24-hour protein quantitation reveals greater than 3.5 g of protein or the protein/creatinine ratio is greater than 3.5, nephrotic range proteinuria is established by definition and is indicative of glomerular disease. There are many causes of nephrotic syndrome, but there are relatively few conditions which are seen with significant frequency in a general medical practice (Table 43.4). When nephrotic range proteinuria develops in a patient who has been diabetic for over 10 to 15 years, the renal lesion is almost always diabetic glomerulosclerosis, particularly if the patient also has diabetic microaneurysms in the retina. In this setting, a renal biopsy is usually not necessary. On the other hand, a biopsy is usually necessary to diagnose a specific primary renal disease if a diagnosis cannot be made by other tests (e.g., detection of Bence Jones proteinuria or rectal biopsy for amyloid), or it may be needed to guide therapy or to help determine prognosis (e.g., SLE). Table 43.3 lists some of the laboratory evaluations which may be helpful in determining the cause of renal disease. *Renal vein thrombosis* occurs in a significant number of patients with certain histological patterns of idiopathic nephrotic syndrome. Clues to the development of this complication include pulmonary embolism, sudden deterioration in renal function, marked increase in the level of proteinuria, or the development of hematuria. Suspicion of this complication requires hospitalization of the patient for urgent evaluation. Once nephrotic range proteinuria has been identified, consultation with a nephrologist is appropriate to help decide the extent of the workup, as well as to provide suggestions for treatment (2).

Renal Biopsy

Patient experience. Renal biopsy requires hospitalization for 24 to 48 hours. Generally, in patients without renal failure and no bleeding abnormality, percutaneous biopsy is performed under local anesthesia with fluoro-

scopic or sonographic guidance. This technique permits the nephrologist to sample the lower portion of the kidney and to avoid the hilar vessels and the renal collecting system. With percutaneous biopsy the patient usually experiences minimal discomfort and is able to be out of bed in 12 hours.

The biopsy core is approximately 1 mm in diameter and approximately 10 to 20 mm in length. Usually two such tissue cores are obtained. The risk associated with percutaneous renal biopsy is small if performed by an experienced physician.

Microscopic hematuria is almost inevitable, and usually there is a small hematoma at the biopsy site on the surface of the kidney. However, it is usually of no clinical consequence. Gross hematuria occurs in approximately 5 to 10% of patients, but less than 5% require a transfusion to replace blood loss. Fewer than 1 in 1000 patients requires nephrectomy because of continued massive bleeding, and mortality from biopsy is very rare. A renal arteriovenous fistula may develop after biopsy, but it usually closes spontaneously. Rarely this complication may require treatment if bleeding continues or if hypertension develops (4). Even more rarely, there may be perforation of another viscus.

When percutaneous biopsy is not feasible, open biopsy can be obtained; some surgeons perform this procedure under local anesthesia in selected patients.

Regardless of the technique of obtaining the biopsy, the evaluation of tissue by the pathologist should include light, immunofluorescent, and electron microscopy and it should be done by a pathologist experienced in preparation and interpretation of renal biopsy material.

The physician who has referred to a nephrologist a patient in whom a renal biopsy has been performed should expect communication on the following: the probably diagnosis, based upon all aspects of the microscopic assessment; whether or not specific therapy for the condition is indicated; and what prognostic judgment can be made. Knowledge that guides therapy in disease associated with nephrotic syndrome is continually developing, and current information should be expected from the consultant.

MANAGEMENT OF PATIENTS WITH PROTEINURIA

Non-nephrotic proteinuria requires no special treatment. The physician's major effort is directed at diagnosis, education, surveillance, and at treatment of any underlying disease. However, if the proteinuria is felt to be caused by a drug, it should be discontinued. Proteinuria from drugs may take several months to resolve and occasionally it is permanent.

Some patients with nephrotic range proteinuria are asymptomatic and require no therapy unless the

Table 43.4.
Cause of Nephrotic Syndrome in Adults[a]

MOST COMMON
    Diabetes mellitus—most common
    Idiopathic membranous glomerulopathy—second most common
    Idiopathic lipoid nephrosis—third most common in adults (most common in children)
    Drug toxicity (*e.g.*, nonsteroidal anti-inflammatory agents, captopril, lithium, or gold)
LESS COMMON
    Focal glomerular sclerosis
    Proliferative glomerulonephritis
    Membranoproliferative glomerulonephritis
    Collagen vascular disease
    Amyloidosis

[a] An extensive list of potential causes of nephrotic syndrome can be found in Early LE, Foreland M: Nephrotic syndrome. In Early LE, Gottschalk CW (eds): *Strauss and Welt's Diseases of the Kidney*, ed 3. Boston, Little, Brown, and Co, 1979.

results of the renal biopsy dictate that treatment be given. When either edema or hypoalbuminemia is present, special therapy may be indicated. (In the absence of renal failure, albumin synthesis is either increased or normal in patients with the nephrotic syndrome.) Generally, assurance of an adequate protein intake is accomplished in patients who have nephrotic range proteinuria by the daily administration of 2 to 3 g of protein/kg dry weight (estimated or actual weight before edema developed). This can be accomplished with protein supplements, such as eggnog, milkshakes, or meat protein supplements. High protein intake can be discontinued if remission is obtained.

In the presence of edema, salt restriction to a tolerable level such as a no added salt diet (approximately 2 to 3 g of Na) is appropriate. If the edema is more severe and is unresponsive to sodium chloride restriction, then the cautious use of diuretics may be helpful, beginning with thiazides and then substituting a loop diuretic (furosemide or bumetanide) if necessary. There should not be an attempt to rid the patient entirely of edema which could risk contraction of the circulating volume with serious consequences; the patient may benefit from alternate-day diuretics which will diminish the risk of inducing serious volume contraction. Potassium-sparing diuretics (spironolactone, triamterene, or amiloride) may be added if renal failure is absent and if loop diuretics have not been entirely adequate. If acceptable control is still not achieved, consultation with a nephrologist is appropriate.

Prediction of the course and selection of specific therapy in patients with nephrotic range proteinuria depend on the pathological pattern that is identified in the biopsy. Patients with nephrotic range proteinuria will need regularly scheduled office visits at 1- to 4-month intervals. Usually this follow-up is done by the primary physician and the patient will see the nephrologist only once a year. The office visit provides an opportunity to review the patient's symptoms and to perform a limited physical examination (which, at a minimum, should include weight, volume assessment, and blood pressure) as well as to evaluate the 24-hour urine protein excretion, or a protein/creatinine ratio, the renal function (creatinine or creatinine clearance), and the serum electrolytes if diuretics are being used. Less frequently an assessment of the serum albumin may be necessary.

General References

Abuelo JG: Proteinuria: diagnostic principles and procedures. *Ann Intern Med* 98:186, 1983.
   A well written review of the evaluation of patients with proteinuria.
Bremer BM, Stein JH, eds: *Nephrotic Syndrome.* Vol 9: *Contemporary Issues in Nephrology.* New York, Churchill Livingstone, 1982.
   A comprehensive monograph covering all aspects of the nephrotic syndrome written by a panel of experts.
Pesce A, First MR: Proteinuria: an integrated review. In Camerson S, Glassock RJ, Van Ypersele de Strihov C (eds): *Kidney Disease.* New York, Marcel Dekker, 1979, vol 1.
   A valuable monograph which provides a thorough review of the mechanism and pathophysiology of proteinuria as well as a discussion of disease states.

Specific References

1. Ginsberg JM, Chang BS, Matarese RA, Garella S: Use of single voided urine samples to estimate quantitative proteinuria. *N Engl J Med* 309:1543, 1983.
2. Kassirer JP: Is renal biopsy necessary for optimal management of the idiopathic nephrotic syndrome? *Kidney Int* 24:561, 1983.
3. King SE: Diastolic hypertension and chronic proteinuria. *Am J Cardiol* 9:669, 1962.
4. Leiter E, Gribetz D, Cohen S: Arteriovenous fistula after percutaneous needle biopsy—surgical repair with preservation of renal function. *N Engl J Med* 287:971, 1972.
5. Levitt JI: The prognostic significance of proteinuria in young college students. *Ann Intern Med* 66:685, 1967.
6. McQueen EG, Sidney M: Composition of urinary casts. *Lancet* 1:397, 1966.
7. Muth RG: Asymptomatic mild intermittent proteinuria. *Arch Intern Med* 115:569, 1965.
8. Robinson RR, Thompson AL, Durrett RR: Fixed and reproducible orthostatic proteinuria. VI. Results of a 10-year follow-up evaluation. *Ann Intern Med* 73:235, 1970.
9. Robinson RR: Isolated proteinuria in asymptomatic patients. *Kidney Int* 18:399, 1980.
10. Rytand DA, Spreiter S: Prognosis in postural (orthostatic) proteinuria. Forty- to fifty-year follow-up of six patients after diagnosis by Thomas Addis. *N Engl J Med* 305:618, 1981.
11. Springberg PD, Garrett LE, Thompson AL Jr, et al: Fixed reproducible orthostatic proteinuria: results of a 20-year follow-up study. *Ann Intern Med* 97:516, 1982.

CHAPTER FORTY-FOUR

Hematuria

JAMES K. SMOLEV, M.D., AND JOHN R. BURTON, M.D.

INTRODUCTION

Hematuria, especially microscopic, is a very common finding. The prevalence of the problem varies with age, sex, and health status but probably averages nearly 3 to 4% of apparently healthy adults. Therefore, the general physician often will need to evaluate patients found to have it. This chapter reviews the significance of hematuria including problems that may be confused with this condition, provides a differential diagnosis of hematuria, and suggests guidelines that will help determine the need for and type of consultation that may be appropriate.

SIGNIFICANCE OF HEMATURIA

Normally 1 to 2 million red blood cells are lost in the urine every 24 hours. However, when studied microscopically in centrifuged urine, this amounts to only 1 to 2 red blood cells/high power field. Therefore, the finding of more than 3 or 4 red blood cells/high power field should be considered abnormal, and requires an explanation. Under certain conditions, however, hematuria may be considered normal; for example it will often be found just after pelvic or prostatic examination, bladder instrumentation, catheterization, or after a prostate or renal biopsy or even after vigorous exercise (e.g., up to 18% of male marathon runners have hematuria at the conclusion of the race (8)). Therefore, in these situations repeat urinalyses should be done before other causes of the problem are considered. Also, if a female patient is menstruating or a male patient has a lesion on his foreskin, an evaluation for hematuria should not be undertaken unless bleeding persists after menstruation stops or after the lesion is treated.

Hematuria may be a manifestation of a serious disease, which may be otherwise asymptomatic. For example, Golin and Howard (4) and Carson and coworkers (3) found a tumor of the genitourinary tract in 10% and 12.5%, respectively, of patients studied because of microscopic hematuria. On the other hand, the finding of red urine or red blood cells in the urine may not be significant. For example, as mentioned above, the remarkable increase in the number of red blood cells in the urine after vigorous exercise may not be abnormal unless a repeat urinalysis in several hours under resting conditions also shows hematuria. Certain urinary pigments and other chemicals may simulate gross hematuria but may be excluded by the demonstration of a *normal* microscopic urinalysis and a *negative dipstick* test for blood. Common examples of these agents are anthocyanins (beets), methyldopa (Aldomet) in the presence of toilet bleach, phenolphthalein (laxatives such as Correctol, Feen-A-Mint, Ex-Lax, Phenolox), phenazopyridine (Pyridium), and porphyrin. Moreover, when urine pH is low, crystals of uric acid have a reddish hue but these can be seen by microscopic examination, and both crystals and color will disappear by the addition of alkali (such as a drop of ammonia water) to the urine specimen.

Gross hematuria may alarm a patient because of the perception that he is losing a great deal of blood. Excessive blood loss is unusual and the patient will benefit from reassurance about this; nevertheless, it is important for the physician to appreciate that the amount of hematuria has no correlation with the seriousness of the underlying cause of the problem.

PATTERNS OF HEMATURIA

Hematuria may be gross or microscopic, and it may occur intermittently or continuously. Intermittent hematuria should not, however, be dismissed as relatively insignificant since most serious disorders—including neoplasia—frequently are characterized by intermittent hematuria. Moreover, hematuria from any cause may manifest as gross hematuria on some occasions and at other times as microscopic hematuria.

Microscopic

Microscopic hematuria is identified by microscopic examination of the urine or by observation of a positive dipstick test for blood in the urine.

Dipstick Screening Test (Table 44.1)

Most multipurpose reagent strips have a colorimetric test for pigments; this test may often be the first clue to the presence of hematuria. The test detects hemoglobins and myoglobins and is therefore not specific for blood in the urine. Hemoglobin from intravascular hemolysis and myoglobin released from injured muscles both produce a positive reaction. The dipstick screening technique should not be taken as diagnostic but should always be confirmed by a microscopic urinalysis. Furthermore, since the test requires an oxidation reaction, false positive results may occur in the rare presence of oxidizing agents such as hypochlorite (contamination from bleach in vitro) or peroxidases (from bacteria when the urine is heavily infected). In addition, false negative reactions may occur occasionally because of reduction of the oxidizing potential of the strip if the patient has ingested large amounts of vitamin C or agents which form formaldehyde in

Table 44.1.
Limits of Dipstick Method for Detection of Blood in the Urine

REASONS FOR A POSITIVE TEST
　Hematuria—greater than approximately 10 red blood cells/
　　high power field
　Hematuria with red blood cell lysis
　　From hypotonic urine (specific gravity less than 1.008)
　　From highly alkaline urine (pH greater than 6.5–7.0)
　Hemoglobinuria—from intravascular hemolysis
　Myoglobinuria—from muscle injury
　False positive reactions
　　From hypochlorite (bleach) contamination of container
　　From peroxidase (from heavy growth of bacteria)
REASONS FOR A FALSE NEGATIVE TEST
　Vitamin C—ingestion by the patient of large amounts of
　　vitamin C (>200 mg/day) results in diminished oxida-
　　tion potential of the test material. The dipstick test
　　may miss trace quantities of blood, although usually
　　there is a quantitative decrease in the estimate of
　　blood (such as 3+ to 2+) (9). (This is of concern only
　　if red blood cells are observed but the dipstick test is
　　negative.)
　Formaldehyde—ingestion of bacterial suppressant agents
　　(such as Mandelamine or Hiprex) which produce form-
　　aldehyde in acid urine or contamination of the con-
　　tainer with formaldehyde will diminish the oxidizing
　　potential of the reagent strips. This results in a quan-
　　titative estimate error or, if hematuria is minimal, false
　　negative results.

the urine (such as Mandelamine or Hiprex), or if the urine specimen container has been contaminated with formaldehyde.

The dipstick test is not a useful way to quantitate hematuria. The test is more sensitive to free hemoglobin than to hemoglobin contained in red blood cells. The lower limit of sensitivity is approximately 30 μg/dl of hemoglobin (approximately equivalent to 10 red blood cells/mm^3 of urine (the approximate volume in one high power field). Therefore, with fewer than about 10 red blood cells/high power field, the dipstick test may be negative. On the other hand, if the cells in the urine have lysed because the urine is hypotonic (specific gravity less than 1.008) or because of the presence of highly alkaline urine (greater than pH 6.5 to 7.0), the dipstick will be more sensitive than the microscopic assessment; however, hemoglobin can still not be differentiated from myoglobin under these circumstances.

Gross

The pattern of gross hematuria is helpful in identifying its cause. *Initial hematuria* is the appearance of blood just as urination is initiated, with clearing as voiding continues. It is due to a disease in the urethra. *Terminal hematuria* is the appearance of hematuria just at the conclusion of voiding, and it indicates a disease near the bladder neck or the posterior urethra. *Total gross hematuria* refers to the appearance of blood throughout most of the urinary stream and may result from a disease process in any portion of the urinary tract.

When evaluating patients who have gross hematuria, it is helpful to note any associated symptoms which help to delineate the underlying problem. For example, colic suggests a renal calculus, and irritative symptoms (frequency, urgency, and dysuria) suggest urinary tract infection.

Hematuria confirmed as indicated above should always be considered abnormal, and a thorough evaluation should be planned.

CAUSES OF HEMATURIA

Evaluation of hematuria results in the establishment of a specific diagnosis in 50 to 80% of patients (3,4). Table 44.2 lists causes of hematuria arranged according to the presence of associated findings on urinalysis, and Table 44.3 lists common causes of hematuria that might be suspected based on the patient's age and sex.

APPROACH TO EVALUATION OF PATIENTS WITH HEMATURIA

Using Tables 44.2 and 44.3 as a guide, the physician should review the patient's history, perform a physical examination, and review the urinalysis to determine the direction for subsequent evaluation.

Table 44.2.
Selected Causes of Hematuria and Associated Findings in Urinalysis

Hematuria Alone	Hemturia and Pyuria with Little or No Proteinuria	Hematuria with Casts and/or with Significant Proteinuria (Greater than 1 g/24 Hours)
Disorders anatomically adjacent to the urinary tract:	Infection (anywhere in the genitourinary tract):	Hypertension—especially accelerated
Aortic aneurysm	Bacterial	Arterial emboli
Renal artery aneurysm	Fungal	Glomerulonephritis:
Pelvic or retroperitoneal disease (e.g., lymphoma)	Mycobacterial	Primary
Anticoagulant drugs (an underlying cause unmasked by anticoagulants is present in 80%) (1)	Viral	IgA nephropathy
	Helminthic (schistosomiasis)	Membranoproliferative
Arteriovenous fistula (kidney)		Focal
"Benign essential hematuria"—see text.		Systemic:
Benign prostatic hypertrophy		Systemic lupus erythematosus
Calculi (see Chapter 46)		Polyarteritis nodosa
Diverticula:		Henoch-Schölein
Calyceal		Goodpasture's syndrome
Urethral		Nephrotoxins—examples:
Bladder		Anti-inflammatory agents
Arterial emboli		Lithium
Glomerulonephritis—e.g., IgA nephropathy		Penicillin and its derivatives
Hereditary disorders:		Thrombosis of the renal vein
Alport's disease		
Cystic disease:		
Polycystic disease		
Medullary cystic disease		
Medullary sponge kidney		
Hemoglobinopathy (SS, SA, SC, S Thal)		
Hemangioma		
Arteriovenous malformation		
Neoplasia (benign or malignant)		
Telangiectasia		
Thrombocytopenia		
Trauma		
Urethritis		
Varicosities		

Isolated

Isolated hematuria is best evaluated by obtaining a complete blood count, including a platelet count, and in black or in white patients with a Mediterranean heritage, a hemoglobin electrophoresis (see Chapter 49). Renal function should be assessed by the meaurement of serum creatinine or by creatinine clearance to establish associated renal failure (see Chapter 47). In an individual who is over the age of 50, a neoplastic process should be considered and urine cytology should be evaluated. Approximately 30% of tumors in the upper urinary tract and approximately 50% of bladder tumors will shed identifiable cells into the urine. It is best to obtain specific information from the laboratory about the proper method for collection and transfer to the laboratory and about whether the patient should be hydrated or dehydrated for the procedure. Three separate specimens obtained on different days are considered an adequate initial screen.

If after this evaluation no diagnosis is established, an intravenous pyelogram (IVP) should be performed. If the IVP is normal, a urologist should be consulted for consideration of further evaluation using computerized tomography or cystoscopy.

Based on this initial assessment the urologist may suggest sonography, nephrotomogram, renal scan, or angiography (2). If the patient is having gross hematuria, it is a particularly opportune time for the urologist to perform endoscopy, as it may allow him to visualize the site of the blood loss, which then can become the focus of more definitive evaluation. Cystoscopy is not contraindicated in patients with hematuria who also have a coagulopathy (iatrogenic or otherwise), but biopsy should not be done. Even when only microscopic hematuria is present, the cystoscopist may be able to identify a lesion; or if none is seen, one or the other upper tract may be identified as the bleeding source by testing urine emanating from each ureter with test tape (5). Should the IVP and cystoscopic evaluation be neg-

Table 44.3.
Common Causes of Hematuria Arranged by Age and Sex[a]

Age (years)	Sex	Causes
0–20	Male and female	Acute glomerulonephritis
		Acute urinary tract infection (viral, bacterial)
		Congenital urinary tract anomalies
20–40	Male and female	Acute urinary tract infection
		Calculus
		Sickle cell disease
		Tumor
40–60	Male	Bladder tumor[b]
		Calculus
		Infection
		Renal tumor[b]
	Female	Infection
		Stone
		Bladder tumor[b]
		Renal tumor[b]
Over 60	Male	Benign prostatic hyperplasia; prostate carcinoma[b]
		Bladder tumor[b]
		Renal tumor[b]
	Female	Bladder tumor[b]
		Infection
		Renal tumor[b]

[a] Adapted from Wyker AW, Gillenwater JY: *Method of Urology*, Baltimore, Williams & Wilkins, 1975.
[b] Tumor will account for 50% of patients with gross hematuria that are over 50 years old.

ative, then a nephrologist should be consulted for consideration of further evaluation, which may in certain situations include a percutaneous renal biopsy (see Chapter 43).

Association with Pyuria

If a patient is found to have hematuria associated with pyuria (with or without irritative symptoms), an infectious cause is likely, and routine bacterial cultures should be obtained. If a specific organism is identified, appropriate antimicrobial therapy should be given (see Chapter 27), after which the patient should be followed for several weeks to ensure that hematuria has been eradicated and does not recur. If irritative symptoms (frequency, dysuria, and urgency) suggesting infection have been present and the routine culture is sterile, sexually transmitted disease, especially *Chlamydia* or gonorrhea (see Chapter 27), or less commonly, viral infection or tuberculosis may be present. However, because noninfectious disorders of the bladder (including malignancies) may produce similar symptoms, the physician should ensure that symptoms, especially

in patients over age 50, have abated and that urinalysis is normal on two or three subsequent occasions. When a sexually transmitted infection is considered, but cannot be proven, a course of antimicrobial therapy may be given (see Chapters 27 and 94). *Chlamydia trachomatis* infection, especially, may be manifest by hematuria and pyuria with minimal irritative symptoms. Viral infections should be short lived and nonrecurrent. The confirmation by culture of the diagnosis of tuberculous infection of the urinary tract requires several weeks; an acid-fast stain of the urine is not a reliable indicator because of the regular presence of acid-fast material from smegma bacilli.

Associated with Urinary Casts or Significant Proteinuria

In a situation where hematuria is associated with urinary casts (especially red blood cell casts) or substantial proteinuria (greater than 1 g/24 hours), evaluation for glomerular disease is indicated (see Chapter 43). Direct referral to a nephrologist for evaluation, which in some instances may include percutaneous renal biopsy, is often appropriate.

SURVEILLANCE OF PATIENTS WITH UNEXPLAINED HEMATURIA

By following the approach outlined above, a cause for hematuria will be identified in approximately 50 to 80% of patients (3,4). However, even when this evaluation has not revealed the underlying cause, the physician should not presume the situation to be innocuous, as serious problems (such as tumor) may be identified at follow-up (4). If the complete initial workup is negative, it would be prudent to see the patient every 3 to 6 months. On these occasions the history, physical examination, and urinalysis should be reviewed; in patients over 50, a urine specimen should be sent for cytological examination. If there is continued hematuria that has not been explained after 1 year, the IVP should be repeated and consultation with a urologist should be arranged for consideration for a repeat cystoscopy.

The diagnosis of *benign essential hematuria* is not specific. When the initial evaluation fails to reveal a cause of the hematuria, that hematuria should be labeled "unexplained," and it should not be considered benign until no cause has been identified after 2 years of follow-up. Some of these patients with unexplained hematuria may have a familial glomerular abnormality (7). Should the physician identify a kindred of such patients, a nephrologist should be consulted because a renal biopsy may be indicated.

HEMATOSPERMIA (6)

The presence of blood in the ejaculate of males is an alarming but usually innocuous symptom. This problem occurs most often in men over 40, and most often the episodes recur over several weeks or months. When it occurs in an otherwise asymptomatic man who has a normal physical examination (including rectal examination of the prostate and seminal vesicles) and a normal urinalysis, the patient should be reassured that it is innocuous and that no further workup is necessary. If there is any abnormality, further evaluation for benign prostatic hypertrophy or cancer of the prostate, seminal vesicles, bladder, or urethra should be considered and a urologist should be consulted.

General References

Abuelo JG: Evaluation of hematuria. *Urology* 21:215, 1983.
    A well referenced practical review of the etiology and evaluation of hematuria.
Earl OP: *Manual of Clinical Nephrology.* Philadelphia, WB Saunders, 1982.
    A very practical reference with good sections on urinalysis and hematuria.
Froom P, Riback J, Benbassat J: Significance of microhaematuria in young adults. *Br Med J* 288:20, 1984.
    A study of 1000 males with asymptomatic isolated microhematuria.

Specific References

1. Antolak SJ, Mellinger GT: Urologic evaluation of hematuria occurring during anticoagulant therapy. *Urology* 101:111, 1969.
2. Benson GS, Brewer EO: Hematuria: algorithms for diagnosis. *JAMA* 246:993, 1981.
3. Carson CC, Sergura JW, Greene LF: Clinical importance of microhematuria. *JAMA* 241:149, 1979.
4. Golin LA, Howard RS: Asymptomatic microscopic hematuria. *Urology* 124:389, 1980.
5. Jacobellis V, Fabiano A, Tallarigo C: A new technique to localize the origin of idiopathic microscopic hematuria. *J Urol* 127:475, 1982.
6. Leary FJ, Aguilo JJ: Clinical significance of hematospermia. *Mayo Clin Proc* 49:815, 1974.
7. Rogers PW, Kurtzman NA, Bunn SM, White MG: Familial benign essential hematuria. *Arch Intern Med* 131:257, 1973.
8. Siegel AJ, Hennekins CH, Solomon HS, Van Boeckel E: Exercise related hematuria. *JAMA* 241:391, 1979.
9. Smith BC, Peake MJ, Fraser CG: Urinalysis by use of a multitest reagent strip; two dipsticks compared. *Clin Chem* 23:2337, 1977.

Hypokalemia

JOHN R. BURTON, M.D.

Low levels of potassium in the serum are frequently encountered in ambulatory practice. The consequences are often trivial, but occasionally they are life threatening. Loss of potassium through the gastrointestinal tract and by use of diuretics accounts for the majority of patients with hypokalemia seen in ambulatory practice, but there is an extensive differential diagnosis for this problem. This chapter will review the physiological background of potassium homeostasis, outline the symptomatic consequences of potassium depletion, develop an approach to the differential diagnosis, and discuss the management of patients with hypokalemia.

PHYSIOLOGICAL BACKGROUND

Total body potassium is approximately 50 mEq/kg of body weight. For example, a 70-kg (154 lb) person would have approximately 3500 mEq of total body potassium. Serum potassium reflects, but does not indicate with certainty, total body potassium. Generally a decrease of 1.0 mEq of potassium in the serum reflects approximately a 10 to 20% deficiency of total body potassium.

The balance of potassium is zealously guarded during health. This balance is schematically represented in Figure 45.1. It can be seen from the figure that a relatively small amount of potassium (approximately 2%) exists outside body cells and a large amount (approximately 98%) exists inside cells. This asymmetry of distribution of potassium is determined by (a) the relative permeability of cell membranes to sodium and potassium, (b) sodium-potassium-ATPase activity within membranes, (c) electrochemical forces, (d) hydrogen ion activity of extracellular fluid, (e) insulin (independent of glucose transport), (f) epinephrine, and (g) aldosterone. Accordingly, acute changes in serum potassium concentration due to cellular shifts without a change in total body potassium are affected by changes in one or more of these factors. The electrocardiogram is a useful way of assessing the relative intra- to extracellular potassium ratio. Figure 45.2 schematically represents changes in the electrocardiogram as potassium concentration is changed.

The delicate balance of potassium is largely modulated by the excretion of potassium by the kidneys. Ninety percent of ingested potassium (usual intake is between 60 and 100 mEq/day) is excreted in the urine; the remainder is excreted in the intestinal tract. The skin is usually an insignificant site of potassium loss. In temperate climates less than 5 mEq/day of potassium are lost in sweat. However, with profuse sweating dermal losses of potassium may approach 25 to 30 mEq/day.

Renal potassium excretion is a distal tubular function since potassium excretion is freely filtered by the glomerulus and then nearly completely resorbed by the proximal tubule. Excretion is regulated by (a) the rate of urine flow bathing and the quantity of sodium delivered to the distal tubular cells; (b) the concentration of potassium in the distal tubular cells; (c) the level in the blood of aldosterone, a hormone which stimulates excretion of potassium by the kidney, increasing its concentration in the tubular cells; and (d) the relative electrochemical forces between tubular fluid and tubular cells. (The more negative the charge of the urinary fluid the greater the electrochemical force attracting potassium from the cells to the tubular fluid.) Although

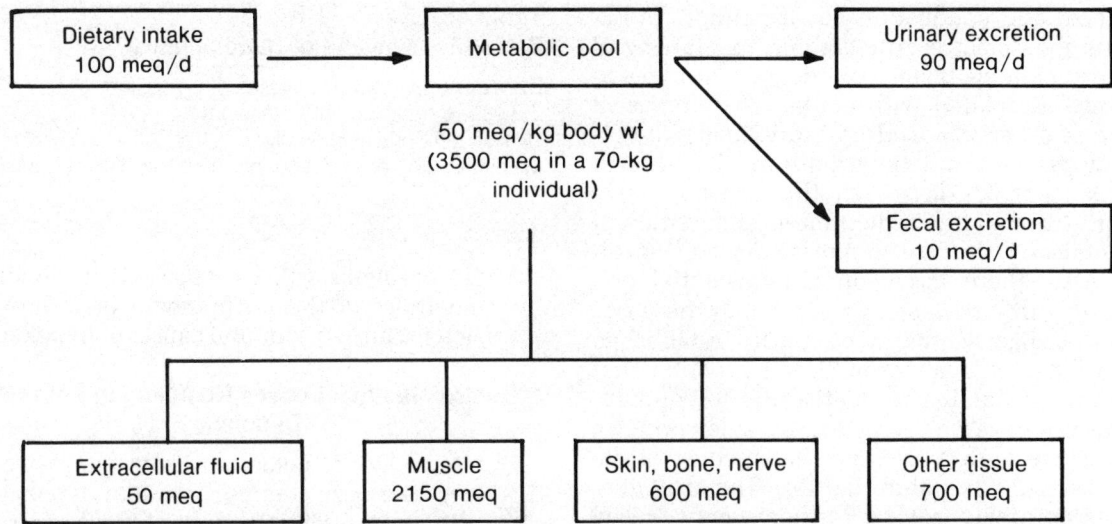

Figure 45.1. Balance of potassium. (Adapted from Kliger AS, and Hayslett JP: Disorders of potassium. In Brenner BM, Stein JH (eds): *Acid-Base and Potassium Hemostatis.* New York, Churchill Livingstone, 1978.)

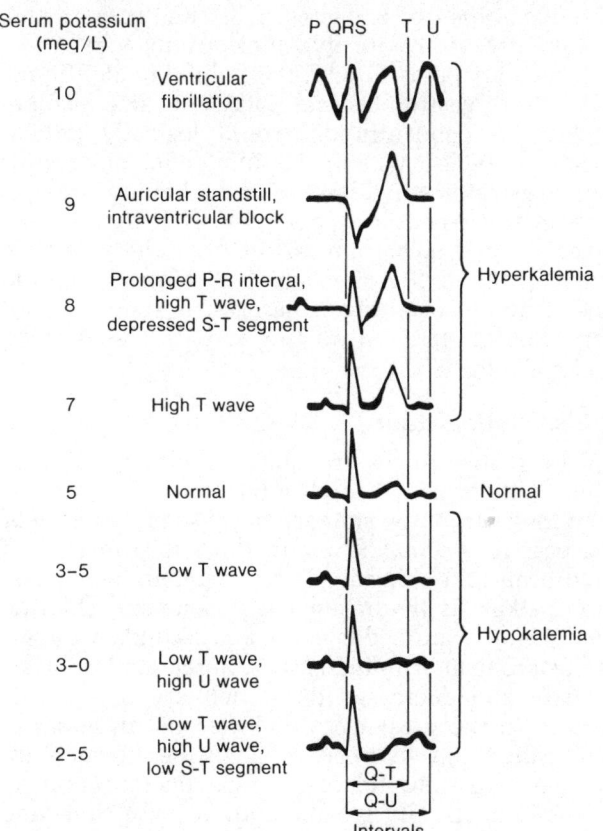

Figure 45.2. Electrocardiogram in assessment of potassium. (Adapted from Burch GE, Winsor T: *A Primer of Electrocardiography*, ed 6. Philadelphia, Lea & Febiger, 1972, p 128.)

potassium balance is delicate, conservation is not nearly as efficient as it is with respect to sodium. Generally, 5 to 15 mEq of potassium /day are lost in the urine even with no potassium intake.

Although the intestinal tract accounts for approximately 10% of potassium excretion normally, when uremia is present, the gastrointestinal tract excretes increased amounts of potassium and may account for one-third of the total potassium excreted.

CONSEQUENCES OF POTASSIUM DEPLETION

Most often the practitioner detects mild hypokalemia in an asymptomatic individual. Almost as often the symptoms of the problem that has led to potassium depletion are prominent—for example, vomiting or diarrhea. However, there are a variety of less frequent symptomatic, and potentially serious, consequences of severe potassium depletion with which the practitioner should be familiar.

Skeletal muscle, which has a very high cellular potassium content, manifests potassium depletion by symptoms ranging from mild weakness (usually manifest by proximal muscle weakness—manifesting as difficulty climbing stairs or a rubbery feeling in the legs) to paralysis, including failure of respiratory musculature. Muscles depleted of potassium are also at risk from an ischemic insult. For this reason a potassium-depleted individual performing physical exercise may develop myonecrosis and occasionally myoglobinuric acute renal failure.

Cardiac muscle may show patchy microscopic necrosis in states of chronic potassium depletion; and as a result, not infrequently conduction abnormalities develop. Severe hypokalemia (less than 2.5 mEq/liter) has been recognized as a cause of cardiac ventricular ectopy, and this is especially true following acute myocardial infarction or following epinephrine administration (18). Hypokalemia in general causes a state of hyperpolarization in cardiac cells predisposing to ventricular ectopy, re-entry phenomena, and conduction abnormalities. Utilizing continuous electrocardiographic monitoring of ambulatory patients, even mild degrees of hypokalemia were associated with cardiac arrythmias in one-third of otherwise healthy individuals who received diuretics for mild hypertension (5). Although no deaths occurred, these arrhythmias were markedly diminished by the reduction or elimination of hypokalemia by the use of potassium-sparing diuretics. Also, there has been circumstantial evidence that antihypertensive agents may have resulted in cardiac deaths in men with established electrocardiographic abnormalities by noting that the expected reduction in deaths due to coronary artery disease was not achieved by a lowering of blood pressure with a regimen that included thiazides or thiazide-like diuretics (14). Hypokalemia-related arrhythmias may be further aggravated by magnesium losses. Myocardial cells are also more sensitive to digitalis preparations in the face of potassium depletion. Digitalis toxicity may occur at nontoxic plasma levels when hypokalemia is present (1). Postural hypotension is seen with severe potassium depletion and may develop after only several days of severe potassium deficiency.

Potassium depletion affects the musculature of the *gastrointestinal tract*, resulting in decreased motility with clinical manifestations of ileus (constipation and distension).

In the *kidney*, *chronic* potassium depletion results in microscopic changes of vacuolar formation in the distal nephron. Renal function is impaired with *severe* potassium deficiency, and mild degrees of renal failure occur. The patient with chronic potassium depletion is also unable to concentrate and acidify the urine normally, although this condition takes several weeks to manifest maximally.

Various *vague symptoms* have been attributed to hypokalemia, including muscular cramps, agitation, depression, fatigue, and weakness. Chronic potassium deficiency may be associated with *precipitation or worsening of diabetes mellitus* by reducing insulin secretion without significantly changing insulin sensitivity (4, 17). Also, potassium deficiency inhibits glycogen storage and synthesis. Potassium depletion also is associated with precipitation of *hepatic encephalopathy* in patients with severe liver disease and a tendency to hepatic failure. Finally, potassium depletion may be associated with a rise in plasma cholesterol concentration but the significance of this is not yet known.

DIFFERENTIAL DIAGNOSIS

The four mechanisms that may lead to hypokalemia are listed in Table 45.1. Gastrointestinal potassium loss and diuretics account for the vast majority of patients seen in ambulatory practice with a low serum potassium concentration.

Table 45.1.
Basic Mechanisms of Hypokalemia

Excessive gastrointestinal loss of potassium
Excessive renal loss of potassium
Diminished potassium intake
Maldistribution of extracellular and intracellular potassium

These problems will be discussed in detail, and the remainder of the chapter will provide a brief approach to the less common causes of hypokalemia.

Gastrointestinal Losses Resulting in Potassium Deficiency

Excessive loss of potassium from the gastrointestinal tract is a very common cause of hypokalemia. This is usually associated with clinical contraction of the extracellular fluid volume, which will be readily detected on physical examination with evidence of weight loss, a lower than usual jugular venous pressure, a decrease in skin turgor, and, frequently, orthostatic hypotension and tachycardia. The urinary potassium level is helpful in identifying the site of gastrointestinal potassium loss. Urinary potassium concentration would logically be expected to be low when potassium deficiency results from gastrointestinal losses and the kidney attempts maximally to conserve potassium. That is true, however, only if potassium is lost from the intestinal tract distal to the stomach. Gastrointestinal fluid losses due to vomiting or nasogastric suction result in urinary potassium wasting and associated metabolic alkalosis.

Chloride Depletion

The gastric juices are rich in hydrochloric acid (but contain only 5 to 10 mEq/liter of potassium), and losses from the stomach because of vomiting or nasogastric suction result in the loss primarily of hydrogen and chloride. These losses induce metabolic alkalosis (hydrogen ion deficiency), chloride deficiency, volume depletion, and secondary hyperaldosteronism. The increased filtered load of bicarbonate and decreased distal delivery of chloride result (in the presence of aldosterone) in losses of potassium and hydrogen. The urine in such instances will show relatively high concentrations of potassium, usually greater than 40 mEq/liter, and an acid pH.

Bicarbonate Depletion

Fluid loss from the gastrointestinal tract below the stomach results in a low urinary potassium and frequently a systemic acidosis secondary to gastrointestinal bicarbonate loss. This situation is commonly seen in patients who have acute and chronic diarrhea or who have malabsorption syndromes.

Colonic Losses

The colon may excrete large quantities of potassium. Usual colonic content contains approximately 40 mEq/liter, but on occasion colonic mucus may contain up to 90 mEq/liter. There are isolated reports of diarrhea secondary to *laxative abuse* resulting in potassium depletion, but there are no data available to indicate how commonly this occurs. Most practitioners will witness it only occasionally. *Enemas* also may result in significant potassium depletion but only if patients are receiving multiple enemas frequently.

Patients with a *villous adenoma* of the colon often develop hypokalemia because of excess excretion of potassium by the tumor. They usually notice the passage of large quantities of mucus with their bowel movements, although the stool itself may appear normal. Therefore, the diagnosis of villous adenoma should be considered when loss of potassium from the gastrointestinal tract is suspected but there is no immediately obvious explanation. Villous adenoma usually, but not always, occurs in elderly patients.

Diuretics

Diuretics that act proximally in the nephron accelerate potassium excretion by increasing the amounts of sodium and water that are delivered to the distal tubules. There, sodium is resorbed, but, as a result, increased amounts of potassium and hydrogen ions are excreted. Furosemide, ethacrynic acid, and bumetanide as well as the thiazides and chlorthalidone, are diuretics that act in this way and may cause hypokalemia. The fall in serum potassium concentration usually reaches a nadir within 7 days after initiation of most diuretics unless an intercurrent problem develops that induces additional loss of potassium (e.g., diarrhea). Clinically, the degree of potassium depletion is most dependent upon sodium ingestion (see below). Some diuretics are associated more than others with greater hypokalemia: thiazide and thiazide-like diuretics on the average are associated with a fall in the plasma potassium concentration of approximately 0.62 mEq/liter and the longer (e.g., chlorthialidone or metolazone) more than the shorter (e.g., hydrochlorothiazide) acting agents are more potent kaluretic agents; comparatively, furosemide causes less potassium depletion with an average fall in potassium concentration of only 0.3 mEq/liter (13). The use of multiple (non-potassium-sparing) diuretics acting at different nephron sites (e.g., furosemide and a thiazide) almost always results in significant hypokalemia.

Diuretics in Nonedematous Patients

Patients who take diuretics but who are not edematous (for example, a patient with mild hypertension who is being treated with a thiazide diuretic) are not usually severely depleted of potassium. Less than 5 to 7% of such individuals develop a deficiency of total body potassium manifest by a serum potassium concentration less than 3.0 mEq/liter (3). Levels below 3.0 mEq/liter, when confirmed should suggest three possible explanations: (a) *Excess salt intake.* A high intake (10 to 15 g/day) of sodium chloride in a patient who is taking a potassium-wasting diuretic will increase the amount of sodium delivered to the distal nephron, accelerating potassium excretion and leading to potassium depletion. Moderate salt restriction (5 to 6 g/day) during diuretic treatment precludes increased distal delivery of sodium and thereby protects against this mechanism for excessive potassium loss (16). (b) Severe salt restriction (1 to 2 g/day) may result in accelerated kaluresis and more pronounced hypokalemia because of resultant renin-aldosterone stimulation (secondary aldosteronism) (9). (c) An unrecognized *potassium-wasting state* (see below). Both primary and secondary aldosteronism may be revealed by excessive hypokalemia following the introduction of potassium-wasting diuretics. These states should be suspected, particularly if the potassium value of the untreated individual was in the low or low normal range. Additional discussion of these states is found later in this chapter (page 528).

Metabolic alkalosis is seen in nonedematous patients who are taking diuretics. Many of the potent potassium-wasting diuretics induce a net loss of hydrogen ion, causing a rise in serum bicarbonate. Further, the excretion of urine containing relatively large amounts of sodium and chloride and relatively little bicarbonate contracts the extracellular fluid and results in a rise in plasma bicarbonate concentration. Alkalosis develops, which then is propagated by chloruresis and subsequent chloride deficiency and which can be corrected only by a chloride-containing salt as discussed below (page 527).

Diuretics in Edematous Patients

Edematous patients receiving diuretics frequently develop a severe depletion of total body potassium, probably for several reasons: (a) because of a high rate of secretion of aldosterone and enhanced resorption of sodium by the kidney; (b) decreased potassium intake because of poor appetite; and (c) decreased total body stores of potassium because of intercurrent illness, disease, and malnutrition. This situation most commonly occurs in patients with severe congestive heart failure, cirrhosis with ascites, or the nephrotic syndrome. Metabolic alkalosis is also very frequently present and in this instance, just as in the situation associated with hydrochloric acid loss from the stomach, it is impossible to correct the potassium deficiency without correction of the associated chloride deficiency (see page 527). That may be done only by providing potassium chloride.

Monitoring Potassium in Patients Receiving Diuretics

Before administration of oral diuretics, serum potassium should be measured. If it is normal, serum potassium should be measured approximately 1 week after the initiation of or increase in dose of the diuretic. Most of the patients who tend to develop hypokalemia will have done so by 7 days. Subsequent to that initial follow-up, a yearly assessment is probably adequate in the nonedematous patient unless other indications for measurement of serum potassium arise. In edematous patients with associated secondary hyperaldosteronism there is a greater stimulus for potassium depletion, and monitoring should be more frequent.

Diet and Potassium Supplements in Patients Taking Potassium-Wasting Diuretics

A typical daily diet in the United States contains 60 to 100 mEq of potassium. When initiating diuretic therapy in the presence or absence of edema, it is sensible to review the dietary habits of the patient to ensure an ingestion of approximately 100 mEq of potassium/day. Some judgment in this matter is important since a high potassium diet may provide too great a caloric or sodium load. There are a variety of foods relatively high in content of potassium (Table 45.2). Many have found it helpful to issue to a patient, who has just been started on diuretics, a list of such foods to assure that the patient knows how to plan a 100 mEq/day intake. The current admonishment to take diuretic tablets with a glass of orange juice (12 mEq of potassium) or a banana (9 mEq of potassium) is relatively insignificant dietary advice.

There is controversy over which patients on diuretics should be given potassium supplements (3, 6). The controversy stems primarily from two issues: dispute regarding the significance of the known effect of a mild decrease in extracellular potassium concentration on the development of cardiac arrhythmias (5, 15), and dispute regarding the risk of potassium supplements in ambulatory patients. The controversy has been fueled more recently by the finding that potassium supplementation in hypertensive patients with diuretic-induced hypokalemia resulted in a slight fall in mean blood pressure in a small group of patients (7a, 7b). This study will need confirmation especially in light of the fact that the majority of experimental evidence in animals suggests that potassium depletion results in a fall in blood pressure. Probably it is reasonable to say that not every nonedematous patient who is taking a potassium-wasting diuretic should be given potassium supplementation, but that supplementation should be restricted to certain situations (Table 45.3).

The practitioner is frequently faced with patients who, having started on diuretics, complain of minor symptoms such as fatigue and muscular aches or weakness and who have a very slight fall in their potassium levels. Studies have failed to relate such symptoms to potassium deficiency. However, potassium supplements are often prescribed in this situation as a trial and discontinued if symptoms do not abate.

The volume depletion and loss of potassium that may complicate diuretic therapy often can be minimized or eliminated by using *diuretics every other*

Table 45.2.
Some Common Potassium-Rich Foods

Food Source	Average Portion	Potassium	Sodium
VEGETABLES		*mEq*	*mEq*
Artichoke	1 large	22.0	3.7
Beans			
Cooked dried	½ cup	10.7	—
Lima	⅝ cup	10.8	—
Brussels sprouts	7 medium	7	—
Corn	1 ear	5.0	—
Potato			
White	1 boiled	7.3	—
Sweet	1 boiled	7.7	—
Tomato	1 medium	9.4	—
Fresh			
Canned	½ cup	5.6	3.3
Squash—winter	½ cup boiled	11.9	—
MEATS			
Hamburger	1 patty	9.8	1.7
Rib roast	2 slices	11.2	2.5
Fish, *e.g.* haddock	1 medium fillet	8.0	7.7
Clams	4 large	6.0	1.7
Oysters	6 medium	3.1	3.1
FRUITS			
Apple	1 medium	2.8	—
Applesauce	⅓ cup	1.7	—
Apricots	3 medium	7.2	—
Avocado	½ pitted	15.5	—
Banana	1–6 inch	9.5	—
Cantaloupe	¼ medium	6.4	—
Dates	10 pitted	16.6	—
Fruit cocktail	½ cup	4.3	—
Grapefruit	½ medium	3.5	—
Melon	¼ small	6.4	—
Orange	1 small	7.7	—
Peach	1 medium	5.2	—
Pear	1 medium	6.7	—
Plum	2 medium	7.7	—
Prunes, dried	10 medium	17.8	—
Raisins	1 tablespoon	2.0	—
Strawberries	10 large	4.2	—
Watermellon	1 slice	15.4	—
JUICE			
Grapefruit	1 cup	10.4	—
Orange	1 cup	12.4	—
Pineapple	1 cup	9.2	—
Prune	1 cup	15.0	—
Tomato	1 cup	13.7	20.9
Vegetable	1 cup	14.1	21.7
NUTS			
Peanuts—roasted	1 tablespoon	3.0	—
Peanut butter	2 tablespoons	2.0	—
Mixed nuts	3½ oz	2.0	—
MILK			
Buttermilk	8 oz	8.0	14
Skim milk	8 oz	8.5	6
Whole milk	8 oz	9.0	5

Table 45.3.
Indications for Potassium Supplementation in Patients Who Are Administered Potassium-Wasting Diuretics

Potassium concentration falls below normal (<3.5 mEq/liter) or

Potassium level is normal, no renal failure is present, and:
1. A digitalis preparation is administered simultaneously
2. A patient also has diabetes mellitus
3. A patient also had a tendency to develop hepatic encephalopathy
4. A patient also has a concurrent problem that in itself may be associated with potassium depletion (e.g., malabsorption syndrome, exogenous or endogenous mineral or glucocorticoid excess)
5. A patient has a known risk for myocardial infarction (e.g., a patient with angina, cardiomegaly and persistent ECG abnormalities even though he may not be taking a digitalis preparation)

day. The regimen has value when the diuretics are administered for control of edema. Their effectiveness as antihypertensive agents requires that they be administered daily.

If prescription of potassium is indicated, a variety of potassium salts are available (Table 45.4). When potassium salts are given prophylactically, as in the nonedematous patient who has some risk of potassium depletion, any potassium salt may be prescribed and is selected on the basis of palatability and cost.

On the other hand, in the patient who has developed hypokalemia after taking diuretics, potassium supplementation must be provided by administration of potassium *chloride*. Volume contraction and chloride depletion with high aldosterone production increase avidity of the distal nephron for sodium so that there is increased excretion of potassium and hydrogen ions. The potassium deficiency cannot be corrected until the chloride depletion is corrected exactly analogous to the situation in which hypokalemia is associated with vomiting or nasogastric suction. Potassium chloride is available in 10 to 20% solutions. It should be noted that hypokalemia cannot be corrected by diet alone since the anions most often accompanying potassium in foods are phosphate and citrate: chloride is necessary. (But simply liberalizing the use of NaCl in the diet may defeat the original purpose and effect of the diuretic).

In the 10% solution, each 15-ml dose contains 20 mEq of potassium. The aim should be to administer 60 mEq of potassium supplement/day. Potassium chloride is a relatively inexpensive medication with minimal side effects, except for hyperkalemia when it is inappropriately prescribed (to patients with renal failure or with the simultaneous administration of a potassium-sparing diuretic). Its palatability and occasional gastrointestinal irritation (nausea, vomiting, or errosive gastritis) are its greatest limit-

ing factors. Often, patients find potassium salts more tolerable when chilled and taken with tomato juice (100 ml contain 8 mEq of sodium).

Potassium chloride embedded in wax matrix tablets (such as Slow-K) or as microencapsulated particles (such as Micro-K Extentabs) does not have the bad taste that limits the use of the liquid by many patients. Although more costly, it is safe and has only occasionally been reported to be associated with small intestinal ulceration and bleeding. In the past these latter complications occurred frequently with enteric coated potassium chloride tablets and led to their disuse.

In edematous patients, since potassium depletion is much more common than it is in patients without edema, supplementation at the initiation of diuretic therapy is indicated.

After initiating the administration of potassium salts, the potassium level should be checked in 2 to 4 weeks and then, if normal, at 3-month intervals in the edematous patient and approximately at 6- to 12-month intervals in the nonedematous patient.

Potassium-Sparing Diuretics

Often potassium salts are not effective in correcting the potassium depletion associated with the administration of potassium-wasting diuretics. In this instance a potassium-sparing diuretic, such as spironolactone, triamterene, or amiloride, is indicated and the administration of potassium salt should be discontinued. This situation mostly occurs in patients who have primary or secondary aldosteronism. The potassium-sparing agents prevent the distal tubular excretion of large quantities of potassium. The dose of each drug is adjusted according to the response of the serum potassium. Their maximum activity is generally seen 2 or 3 days after their initiation, so that dose adjustments can be made

Table 45.4.
Commonly Available Potassium Salts

Source	Potassium Concentration
SOLUTIONS[a]	
Potassium chloride	
5% (generic)	10 mEq/15 ml
10% (generic, Kaochlor 10%, Kaon Cl-10, Klor-10%, Klorvess 10%)	20 mEq/15 ml
20% (generic, Kaon Cl-20)	40 mEq/15 ml
Potassium citrate (Polycitra-K)	30 mEq/15 ml
Potassium gluconate (generic, Kaon Elixir)	20 mEq/15 ml
EFFERVESCENT GRANULES OR TABLETS	
Potassium chloride (Klorvess)	20 mEq/packet
TABLETS	
Potassium chloride (K-Tab, Kaor-Cl, Slow-K, Micro-K, Extencaps)	6, 7, 8 and 10 mEq/tablet
Potassium gluconate (Kaor)	5 mEq/tablet

[a] Available with or without sugar and in different flavors. Taste generally improved by chilling.

every 3 or 4 days until a dose is obtained which controls the serum potassium concentration. Careful surveillance of the serum potassium concentration, once stable, at approximately 4- to 12-week intervals, is important, to avoid the dangerous complication of hyperkalemia. Amiloride (Midamor) and triamterene (Dyrenium) have the advantage of requiring only a single daily dose and are not associated with gynecomastia in men, a potential side effect of spironolactone (Aldactone). These agents should be avoided, except in consultation with a nephrologist, in patients with renal failure. Triameterine should not be used in patients with history or urinary calculus disease (see Chapter 46).

Less Common Causes of Hypokalemia

The less common causes of hypokalemia seen in ambulatory practice are dietary deficiency, excess urinary potassium loss due to one of a number of syndromes, and maldistribution of body potassium. The approach to diagnosing one of these problems is based upon historical information, physical examination, urinary potassium levels, acid-base status, and activity or renin in the peripheral blood. An unexpectedly low serum potassium value should always be confirmed by repeat testing two or three times before initiating a further workup.

Deficient Potassium Intake

There is a wide distribution of potassium in foods. Therefore, it is unusual for dietary potassium deficiency to occur unless the patient fails to eat adequately for a prolonged interval. Alcoholic patients and patients with terminal malignancy may become hypokalemia in this manner. Also, if a patient is catabolic with an excess loss of tissue potassium, an unsupplemented diet may be relatively deficient in potassium. Dietary deficiency of potassium, particularly in the elderly, may contribute to diuretic-induced hypokalemia. Dietary deficiency is established by history, clinical evidence of malnutrition, the absence of other obvious causes of hypokalemia, and correction of the deficiency with a balanced diet with or without potassium supplements. In such patients, the urinary output of potassium should be less than 10 to 20 mEq/day when they are hypokalemic; there is usually an obligate loss of this amount every day.

Excessive Losses of Potassium in Urine

In the presence of hypokalemia, an unexplained excessive loss of potassium in the urine (greater than 20 mEq/liter) is a diagnostic challenge. The differential diagnosis in this situation is complex, but it can be simplified by assessing the acid-base status of the patient as outlined in Table 45.5.

Excessive Production of Mineralocorticoid Hormones

Mineralocorticoid hormone excess is a less common cause of hypokalemia, but the evaluation of the patient is complex and requires the careful determination of the concentration in the serum of several hormones. It is imperative in this situation to have the support of a laboratory skilled in hormonal measurement; otherwise, definitive workup is impossible. Certain basic diagnoses may be made in an office, however, which may minimize the need for referral of patients to a center experienced in evaluation of abnormalities of aldosterone production.

Table 45.5 outlines the diagnostic possibilities related to the concentration of serum bicarbonate and of renin in the serum. Before approaching the diagnostic possibilities the practitioner needs to obtain an accurate history, identify normal or high blood pressure, and establish the presence or absence of edema.

It is mandatory to measure plasma renin and/or aldosterone activity under defined conditions of salt balance and position, and since many medications influence aldosterone or venous renin activity (Ta-

Table 45.5.
Hypokalemia Secondary to Renal Loss

Determine that patient is not using a potassium-losing diuretic
Consider when there is no suggestion of dietary inadequacy or gastrointestinal symptoms that could explain potassium loss
Document by identifying a spot urine potassium concentration of greater than 20 mEq/liter or a urine potassium excretion of greater than 20 mEq/24 hours
Classify on the basis of the plasma bicarbonate concentration
HIGH BICARBONATE
  Measure peripheral renin activity under proper conditions (see text):

Low Renin	*High Renin*
1. Primary aldosteronism (occasional)	1. Secondary aldosteronism (common)
a. Adenoma (more occasional)	a. Associated with edema-forming state
b. Idiopathic hyperplasia (less occasional)	b. Diuretic use associated with volume depletion
c. Aldosterone-producing carcinoma (very rare)	c. Renovascular hypertension
d. Glucocorticoid-remediable aldosteronism (very rare)	d. Accelerated hypertension
e. Congenital adrenal enzymatic defect (very rare)	e. Renin-secreting tumor
f. Exogenous hormone— gluco- or mineralocorticoid (occasional)	2. Bartter's syndrome (rare)
2. Licorice excess (rare)	
3. Liddle's syndrome (very rare)	

LOW BICARBONATE
  Rental tubular acidosis (occasional)
  Diabetic ketoacidosis (common)
NORMAL BICARBONATE
  Magnesium deficiency (occasional)
  Osmotic diuresis (occasional)
  Leukemia (rare)

Table 45.6.
Some Drugs Known to Affect Peripheral Renin Activity[a]

Antihypertensives:
  α-Methyldopa
  β-Blockers
  Clonidine
  Diuretics
  Ganglionic blockers
  Hydralazine
  Labetalol
  Minoxidil
  Prazosin
  Reserpine
α-Agonists (catecholamines)
α-Blockers:
  Chlorpromazine (Thorazine)
  Haloperidol (Haldol)
  Ergot alkaloids, *e.g.*, bromocriptine (Parodel) or ergotamine
    and caffeine (Cafergot)
  Phenoxybenzamine (Dibenzyline)
  Phentolamine (Regitine)
  Estrogens
  Glucocorticoids
Protaglandin inhibitors:
  Aspirin
  Other nonsteroidal anti-inflammatory agents
Theophylline preparations

[a] The following reference will provide a more thorough account of these interactions: Schambelan M, Stockigt JR: Pathophysiology of the renin-antiotensin systems. In Brenner BM, Stein JH (eds): *Hormonal Function and the Kidney.* New York, Churchill Livingstone, 1979.

ble 45.6), all such drugs should be discontinued for 2 weeks before measuring these hormones. Further, spironolactone is particularly potent and has been documented to interfere with renin measurement for as long as 6 months after it has been discontinued (11). Also, oral contraceptive pills may have a prolonged influence on renin metabolism, and they should be discontinued for 6 months before measuring renin activity.

A number of protocols have been developed to evaluate the renin-aldosterone axis (7, 8, 12, 19).

In physician's offices, complex protocols to measure renin and/or aldosterone activity are not practical, but the *plasma renin* may be obtained if measured under proper conditions. A useful procedure for stimulation of renin production is outlined in Table 45.7.

If the renin is low, indicating suppression, further evaluation of a sophisticated nature is required to establish and to localize excess primary aldosterone or other corticoid hormone production. For this, referral to a center experienced in these measurements is suggested. If, on the other hand, a high peripheral renin is found, then secondary hyperaldosteronism is present.

Primary Hyperaldosteronism

The symptomatic findings of primary hyperaldosteronism—in addition to hypertension—are related to potassium depletion and occur only when such depletion is severe: weakness, paralysis, tetany, arrhythmias, polyuria, polydipsia. Patients with primary hyperaldosteronism almost always have spontaneous hypokalemia. Less than 10% have normal levels of potassium; and these few patients will manifest hypokalemia, often profound, if potassium-wasting diuretics or large amounts of sodium chloride are administered. Both of these circumstances result in increased delivery of sodium to the distal nephron where, under the influence of excessive aldosterone, sodium is resorbed and potassium and hydrogen ions are excreted, resulting in hypokalemia and metabolic alkalosis.

Attempts to uncover patients with primary aldosteronism should be limited to situations in which—if the condition is found to be present—surgery would be undertaken. Such cases include young individuals and those with hypertension that is not easily managed medically. It must be borne in mind, however, that most patients with primary aldosteronism can be treated with the aldosterone antagonist, spironolactone (Aldactone) other potassium-sparing diuretics or with spironolactone in combination with a non-potassium-sparing diuretic (see below).

Table 45.7.
Protocol for Stimulation of Renin Production

1. Discontinue medications known to affect renin
2. No added salt diet for 1 week
   a. If there is doubt concerning dietary compliance, a 24-hour urine Na should confirm less than 100 mEq excretion/24 hours (10)
3. On day of study stimulate renin by following either method a or b:
   a. The patient should take furosemide (Lasix), 40 mg orally at 6–8 A.M. (19)
      The patient may rest for 1–2 hours and then assume the upright posture (slow walking) for an additional 2–3 hours or
   b. The patient should be given furosemide (Lasix), 40 mg intravenously (7)
      The patient should ambulate for 30 minutes following the injection.
4. Collection of specimen:
   a. Collect the peripheral venous specimen in an EDTA (*i.e.*, not a heparin) tube (the patient may sit down for the phlebotomy)
   b. The specimen should be quickly taken to the laboratory or chilled in the refrigerator (4–5°C) if there will be a delay before delivery to the laboratory (a delay beyond overnight should be avoided)
   c. In the laboratory the plasma is separated and frozen to −20°C until the assay can be performed

Initial screening for primary aldosteronism is best performed by careful determination of serum potassium on multiple (at least three) occasions. During these times the patient should not have received diuretics for at least 2 to 3 weeks and should not be ingesting a low sodium diet. If definite hypokalemia is shown to be present, plasma renin activity should then be measured. Plasma renin is suppressed in primary aldosteronism, but is also low or undetectable in many normal persons. Suppressed renin is not demonstrated unless the value remains low following a stimulation test. Screening for suppressed renin is performed as outlined in Table 45.7. If hypokalemia and low renin activity coexist, further evaluation will include determination of urinary or plasma aldosterone. Referral to an endocrinologist or nephrologist with expertise in this area should be made at this point (or after a trial of spironolactone; see below). Determinations of aldosterone under nonstandardized conditions (lack of control of sodium intake) are uninterpretable. Further, many commercial laboratories are unreliable in terms of the accuracy or validity of their hormone measurements.

When hypokalemia, suppressed renin, and aldosterone excess have been unequivocally established, localization procedures are undertaken by the consultant (computerized tomography (CT); selective arteriography; retrograde venography; selective venous sampling for aldosterone; adrenal scanning with radioiodine-labeled cholesterol). These procedures also serve to distinguish adenomas from hyperplasia. Adenomas as small as 0.5 cm have been localized in this way; their excision has led to cure of hypertension. If evidence for bilateral hyperplasia is found, surgery is not undertaken, since in such cases bilateral adrenalectomy is necessary, despite which most patients do not experience relief of hypertension. Some of these patients may have a form of hyperaldosteronism caused by increased secretion of an aldosterone-stimulating glycoprotein (2); a few patients may have a glucocorticoid-remediable form of hyperaldosteronism; rarely, a congenital enzymatic block may cause the problem. Patients with bilateral hyperplasia are best managed medically. After obtaining a renin determination in the workup (see above), a trial of spironolactone (Aldactone) is useful with all patients. Large doses (400 to 600 mg daily) are necessary, and several weeks may be needed for a response. Failure of spironolactone to normalize the blood pressure while normalizing the hypokalemia strongly suggests that—regardless of the anatomical basis for the aldosterone excess—surgery would not be curative of the hypertension. Such a situation is to be expected in hyperplasia and in a minority of cases of solitary adenoma. Also, the normalization of blood pressure with the administration of spironolactone does not by itself prove the presence of an aldosterone-producing tumor. A useful review of all aspects of primary aldosteronism has been provided by Melby (see "General References").

Secondary Hyperaldosteronism

Hypokalemia is often associated with secondary hyperaldosteronism. Secondary hyperaldosteronism is characterized by a large potassium deficiency with metabolic alkalosis, excess urinary potassium loss, and high peripheral renin.

Secondary hyperaldosteronism is most often seen in *edema-forming states* in patients with heart failure, cirrhosis, or nephrotic syndrome.

Accelerated hypertension is associated with hypokalemia and metabolic alkalosis in approximately 20% of patients, due to high renin production from the bilateral renal ischemia.

Fifteen percent of patients with *renovascular hypertension* have hypokalemia. The hypokalemia is secondary to unilateral renal ischemia and high renin production with secondary hyperaldosteronism. Similarly, but rarely, *renin-secreting renal tumors* may result in hypokalemic metabolic alkalosis from renal potassium losses and are associated with a high peripheral renin and thereby a secondary high aldosterone concentration.

Bartter's Syndrome

This rare disorder presents with severe hypokalemic metabolic alkalosis and excess urinary potassium and chloride losses. Blood pressure is normal; edema is absent. Renin and aldosterone activities are markedly elevated and are the reason for the electrolyte abnormalities. The cause of this disorder is unknown.

Maldistribution of Potassium

Alkalosis is associated with a shift of potassium from extracellular fluid into cells. This shift occurs regardless of whether the alkalosis is induced on a metabolic or respiratory basis. It is not associated with severe total body potassium depletion but is nevertheless associated with sensitivity to digitalis. *Hypokalemic periodic paralysis* is a rare disorder characterized by spontaneous episodes of paralysis that also may be precipitated by a variety of stimuli including the administration of insulin, glucose, or ACTH. Hyperthyroidism may rarely result in this syndrome, especially in Japanese. Although a fall in serum potassium is regularly demonstrated during the paralysis, balance studies indicate an increase in total body potassium, implying a shift of potassium from extracellular to intracellular fluid.

Vitamin B_{12}, when administered initially in the therapy of anemia due to vitamin B_{12} deficiency, may cause severe shifts of potassium as metabolic activity is increased in hematopoietic cells. When unrecognized and untreated, fatal hypokalemia has been demonstrated in this setting. Careful observation of serum potassium concentration in this situation will alert the practitioner to appropriate therapy.

Soluble barium salts (carbonate, chloride, hydroxide, nitrate, acetate, sulfide) are associated with hypokalemia by creating a maldistribution of potassium. This is extraordinarily rare, but occurs episodically with poisoning from some rodenticides, depilatories, and fireworks. Epidemics secondary to barium chloride contamination of table salt have occurred in two recorded instances. Barium sulfate is not soluble and is not a cause of hypokalemia.

General References

Brenner BM, Stein JH (eds): *Acid-Base and Potassium Homeostasis.* New York, Churchill Livingstone, 1978.
> Provides a well referenced source on disorders of potassium metabolism.

Melby JC: Primary aldosteronism, Nephrology Forum. *Kidney Int* 26:769, 1984.
> A good review of primary aldosteronism.

Nardone DA, McDonald WJ, Girard DE: Mechanisms in hypokalemia: clinical correlation. *Medicine* 57:435, 1978.
> This paper presents a logical approach to the diagnosis of hypokalemia based on the site of potassium loss and associated acid-base status.

Narins RG (ed): *Controversies in Nephrology and Hypertension.* New York, Churchill Livingstone, 1984.
> Excellent discussions of the pros and cons of routine potassium administration with diuretic therapy.

Streeten DHP, Tomycz N, Anderson GH: Reliability of screening methods for the diagnosis of primary aldosteronism. *Am J Med* 67:403, 1979.
> Reviews the methods for screening for primary aldosteronism in 1036 consecutive referred hypertension patients.

Specific References

1. Aronson JK, Grahame-Smith DG, Wigley FM: Monitoring digoxin therapy: the use of plasma digoxin concentration measurements in this diagnosis of digoxin toxicity. *Q J Med* 47:111, 1978.
2. Carey RM, Sen S, Dolan LM, *et al*: Idiopathic hyperaldosteronism: a possible role for aldosterone-stimulating factor. *N Engl J Med* 311:94, 1984.
3. Harrington JT, Isner JM, Kassirer JP: Our national obsession with potassium. *Am J Med* 73:155, 1982.
4. Helderman JH, Elahi D, Andersen DK, *et al*: Prevention of the glucose intolerance of thiazide diuretics by maintenance of body potassium. *Diabetes* 32:105, 1983.
5. Holland OB, Nixon JV, Kuhnert L: Diuretic-induced ventricular ectopic activity. *Am J Med* 70:762, 1981.
6. Kaplan NM: Our appropriate concern about hypokalemia. *Am J Med* 77:1, 1984.
7. Kaplan NM, Kem DC, Holland OB, *et al*: The intravenous furosemide test: a simple way to evaluate renin responsiveness. *Ann Intern Med* 84:639, 1976.
7a. Kaplan NM, Carnegie A, Raskin P, *et al*: Potassium supplementation in hypertensive patients with diuretic-induced hypokalemia. *N Engl J Med* 312:746, 1985.
7b. Kassirer JP, Harrington JT: Fending off the potassium pushers. *N Engl J Med* 312:785, 1985.
8. Kowarski AA, Edwin CM, Akesode AP, *et al*: The integrated concentration of plasma renin activity and aldosterone in essential hypertension. *Johns Hopkins Med J* 142:35, 1978.
9. Landmann-Suter R, Struyvenburg A: Initial potassium loss and hypokalemia during chlorthalidone administration in patients with essential hypertension: the influence of dietary sodium restriction. *Eur J Clin Invest* 8:155, 1978.
10. Laragh JH, Baer L, Brunner HR, *et al*: Renin angiotensin and aldosterone system in pathogenesis and management of hypertensive vascular disease. *Am J Med* 52:633, 1972.
11. Lowder SE, Liddle GW: Prolonged alteration of renin responsiveness after spironolactone therapy. *N Engl J Med* 291:1243, 1974.
12. Lyons DF, Kem DC, Brown RD, *et al*: Single dose captopril as a diagnostic test for primary aldosteronism. *J Clin Endocrinol Metab* 57:892, 1983.
13. Morgan DB, Davidson C: Hypokalemia and diuretics: an analysis of publications. *Br Med J* 905, 1980.
14. Multiple Risk Factor Intervention Trial Research Group: Multiple Risk Factor Intervention Trial. *JAMA* 248:1465, 1982.
15. Papademetriou V, Fletcher R, Khatri IM, Freis ED: Diuretic-induced hypokalemia in uncomplicated systemic hypertension: effect of plasma potassium correction on cardiac arrhythmias. *Am J Cardiol* 52:1017, 1983.
16. Ram CVS, Garrett BN, Kaplan NM: Moderate sodium restriction and various diuretics in the treatment of hypertension. *Arch Intern Med* 141:1015, 1981.
17. Rowe JW, Tobin JD, Rosa RM, Andres R: Effect of experimental potassium deficiency on glucose and insulin metabolism. *Metabolism* 29:498, 1980.
18. Struthers AD, Whitesmith R, Reid JL: Prior thiazide diuretic treatment increases adrenaline-induced hypokalemia. *Lancet* 1:1358, 1983.
19. Wallach L, Nyarai I, Dawson KG: Stimulated renin: a screening test for hypertension. *Ann Intern Med* 82:27, 1975.

CHAPTER FORTY-SIX

Urinary Stones

JOHN R. BURTON, M.D., AND JAMES K. SMOLEV, M.D.

Urinary stones are very common in the United States. The physician will encounter such patients frequently and will therefore need to be familiar with the evaluation and management of this common problem. Although urological intervention or nephrological consultation may occasionally be required, the vast majority of patients with stones can be evaluated, treated, and followed by the primary care physician. This chapter will review the various manifestations of stone disease; the types of urinary stones; the evaluation of patients with stones; the acute and chronic management of patients with urinary stones, and, finally, when to obtain consultation for these patients.

PRESENTATION OF URINARY STONE DISEASE

Physicians will encounter patients who have urinary stone disease in one of five clinical settings: (a) a patient with acute colic, (b) a patient with persistent or recurrent urinary tract infection, (c) a patient with isolated hematuria, (d) a patient with no symptoms in whom a stone is discovered incidentally on an X-ray taken for other purposes, or (e) a patient who gives a history of having had a stone.

Acute Colic

Presentation

Most patients with urinary stones will have at some time an acute episode of colic. The stone, if obstructing, causes ureteral spasm, resulting in severe intermittent pain. The location of the pain depends on the location of the stone in the ureter but is most often felt in the flank; and then as the stone moves distally, pain radiates in a characteristic pattern around the groin and into the testicles in the male or into the labia majora in the female. Nausea, vomiting, paralytic ileus, and other gastrointestinal symptoms that often suggest a primary gastrointestinal problem may be associated with pain. Examination reveals an uncomfortable, restless patient. There may be costovertebral tenderness as well as deep tenderness in the abdomen. More importantly, there are no signs of peritoneal irritation present (guarding, rebound, or rigidity). Fever is not present unless urinary tract infection has developed in the obstructed urinary tract.

Urinalysis almost always demonstrates microscopic (or gross) hematuria. The presence of pyuria is important since chronic bacterial infection may be associated with the development of urinary stones; however, pyuria may be absent even if infection is present during complete ureteral obstruction.

Management

The aim of management of a patient with colic should be (a) relief of discomfort, (b) surveillance for infection, and (c) determination of whether stones will pass spontaneously or will require surgical removal. The abdominal X-ray is useful in monitoring the site and progression of the stone. Approximately 90% of renal stones are radiodense and will be seen on a good quality X-ray. The size and position of the stone will help to decide the urgency of subsequent studies, such as an intravenous pyelogram (IVP). In general, stones that are less than 5 mm will pass spontaneously; those between 5 and 10 mm have a 50% chance of passing spontaneously; and those greater than 10 mm usually require surgical removal. The common sites where stones become lodged are (a) the renal calyx, (b) the ureteral pelvic junction, (c) in the ureter at the pelvic brim where the ureter begins to pass over the iliac vessels, (d) in the lower third of the ureter, and (e) at the ureterovesical junction. If there is doubt about whether calcification seen on the plain X-ray is within the urinary tract, an oblique view may help. It is also important to review old abdominal films taken for any reason to see if a stone was present at that time. An intravenous pyelogram should also be obtained as soon as possible in the patient with colic, as it will help to establish the diagnosis, especially in patients with radiolucent stones, and it will provide certain important information (see below) that will aid in management.

Several factors will help the physician decide whether to hospitalize a patient with renal colic, to obtain urgent urological consultation, or to manage the patient at home. First, the patient with nausea and vomiting cannot be assured of an adequate fluid intake or of adequate oral analgesia and should be admitted to a hospital. Second, fever suggests infection proximal to an obstructing stone, and urgent urological consultation should be obtained. Third, if an IVP reveals any of the following findings, urgent urological consultation should be obtained: (a) a nonfunctioning kidney (completely obstructed ureter), (b) a partially obstructed ureter from a solitary kidney, and (c) urine extravasation. Fourth, if the stone is greater than 10 mm, spontaneous passage is very unlikely and urological consultation should be obtained.

Most patients can be managed at home by the general physician. Forced hydration of 2 to 3 liters of fluid/24 hours is necessary to maintain a good urinary flow and to help in moving the stone. When the patient is voiding, all of the urine voided during the period of intermittent colic should be collected, and strained through an old stocking, a fine knit screen, or a filter paper so that the passed stone may be saved and analyzed. It is important to prescribe analgesic medication such as meperidene (Demerol) 75 to 150 mg every 3 to 6 hours to control the discomfort. A phenothiazine (e.g., Phenergan, 25 mg) given with the Demerol will provide additional relief. The patient should be instructed to contact his physician and admission to a hospital and urgent urological consultation should be arranged should fever, pain, not easily controlled or persisting beyond a few days, or vomiting develop (see above). The physician will want to follow the patient by arranging for a weekly X-ray of the abdomen to determine the progression of the stone. If by 6 weeks the stone has not passed it is unlikely that spontaneous passage will occur, and urological consultation should be obtained. Because of the demands of their occupation or for social reasons, some patients will want to consider surgical removal of the stone earlier, and therefore will request urological consultation sooner.

Stones that pass from the ureter into the bladder generally pass with ease through the urethra. In the event of a bladder outlet obstruction, a stone may be retained in the bladder (*bladder stone*) where it may grow and in time become an infection stone (see below).

An occasional patient who has acute ureteral colic will give a history of allergy to radiological dye. In this instance, an ultrasonic study of the collecting system of the kidney may help in deciding about the presence of obstruction or the presence of a solitary kidney. If this is unavailable, then urological consultation should be obtained so that either an antegrade (i.e., via a catheter passed percutaneously into the renal pelvis) or retrograde pyelogram can be considered. These methods are safe for individuals who have given a history of allergy to IVP dye.

It is important for the physician to recognize that occasionally a patient with a history strongly suggestive of renal colic may have another cause for the pain. A dissection of the aorta, acute back strain or lumbar disc disease, the passage of blood clots in the ureters as in sickle cell disease or renal infarct, as well as malingering should be considered. A malingerer is often difficult for the physician to identify but usually may give a classic history of acute renal colic to a physician who he is seeing for the first time and may also relate a history of allergy to IVP dye. Often these patients will have blood (obtained from a fingerstick or oral injury) in the urine specimen they give to the physician.

When a patient is referred to a urologist for *stone removal*, there are several options. Lower ureteral stones may be removed using a basket which is inserted through a cystoscope. This procedure is very similar to cystoscopic examination but requires general or spinal anesthesia and hospitalization. Stones located more proximally may require removal by open ureterolithotomy, open pyelolithotomy or, in the case of a staghorn calculus, nephrolithotomy. However, operative ureteroscopes are now available which may reduce the need for open ureterolithotomy. Also, newer closed techniques (as opposed to open surgery) have become increasingly available and have the distinct advantage of decreasing postoperative morbidity. Some urologists are now performing percutaneous nephrosotolithomy. This procedure requires an angiogram to visualize the kidney then antegrade percutaneous puncture to provide access to the renal collection system (Fig. 46.1). A stone may be extracted intact or it may first need to be crushed or to be fragmented utilizing shock waves (ultrasonic lithotripsy). In a limited number of centers in the United States studies are beginning utilizing *extracorporeal shock wave lithotripsy*. This procedure requires that a patient be positioned with the utmost precision in a water bath (to permit undisturbed energy transfer) and then the focusing of shock waves (Fig. 46.2) on the calculus. The stone is fragmented into small particles, which theoretically will then pass spontaneously. The indications for these newer techniques are under investigation. Both require hospitalization and are performed under spinal or general anesthesia.

Other Patterns of Stone Presentation

Urinary stones usually produce symptoms that suggest acute colic, at least at some time in their course. When stones are discovered in patients who do not have colic (see page 532), these patients demand the same evaluation and management (see below) as do patients who have passed a stone associated with colic.

TYPES OF STONES AND THEIR CAUSES

There are four main types of urinary calculi: (*a*) calcium oxalate or phosphate, (*b*) uric acid, (*c*) struvite—triple phosphate—(magnesium, ammonium phosphate), and (*d*) cystine. Calcium stones are by far the most common. Table 46.1 shows the classification of stone-forming patients by the type of stone passed.

It is important for the clinician caring for a patient with stone disease to be familiar with the metabolic disorders these patients may have. This understanding will be helpful in planning a diagnostic evaluation and specific therapy (see below). This is particularly true in the evaluation of the patient with the most prevalent stone type—calcium.

Calcium Stones

Table 46.2 shows the metabolic and clinical disorders in calcium stone formers. This table shows that in almost 80% of patients who have had a calcium stone the cause is known. The approach to these disorders is discussed below.

Uric Acid Stones

Uric acid stones are caused by the high insolubility of undissociated uric acid (pK of 5.7—i.e., 50% of uric acid is undissociated at pH 5.7, 90% is undissociated at pH 4.7). Three factors are associated with uric acid stone formation: (*a*) hyperuricosuria, (*b*) highly acid urine, and (*c*) low urinary volume. The prevalence of uric acid stones in the general population is very low (Table 46.3). On the other hand, uric acid stones are very prevalent in patients who have gout, asymptomatic hyperuricemia, or hyperuricosuria. Many patients will have passed uric acid stones long before a gouty attack has occurred. It is known that many patients with gout produce

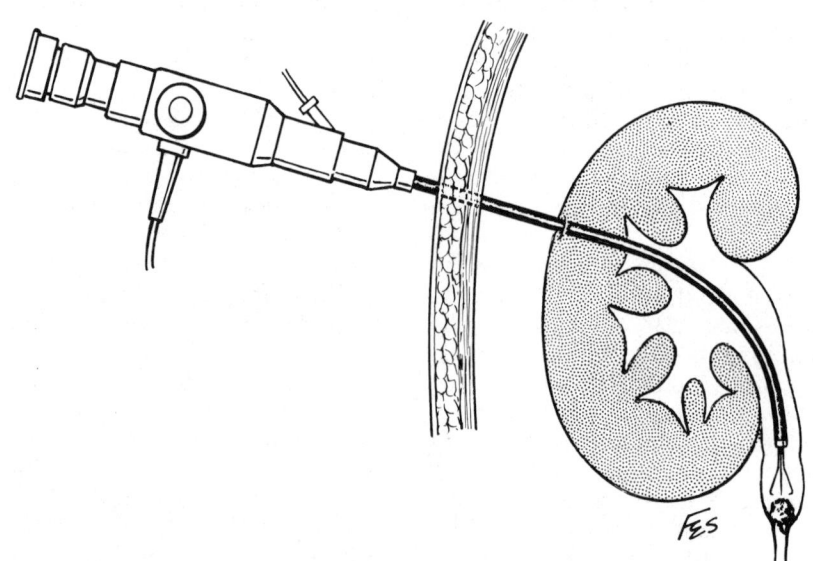

Figure 46.1. Percutaneous removal of a small stone using a flexible nephroscope. (From Roth RA: Residual stones. In Roth RA, Finlayson BF (eds): *Stones: Clinical Management of Urolithiasis.* Baltimore, Williams & Wilkins, 1983.)

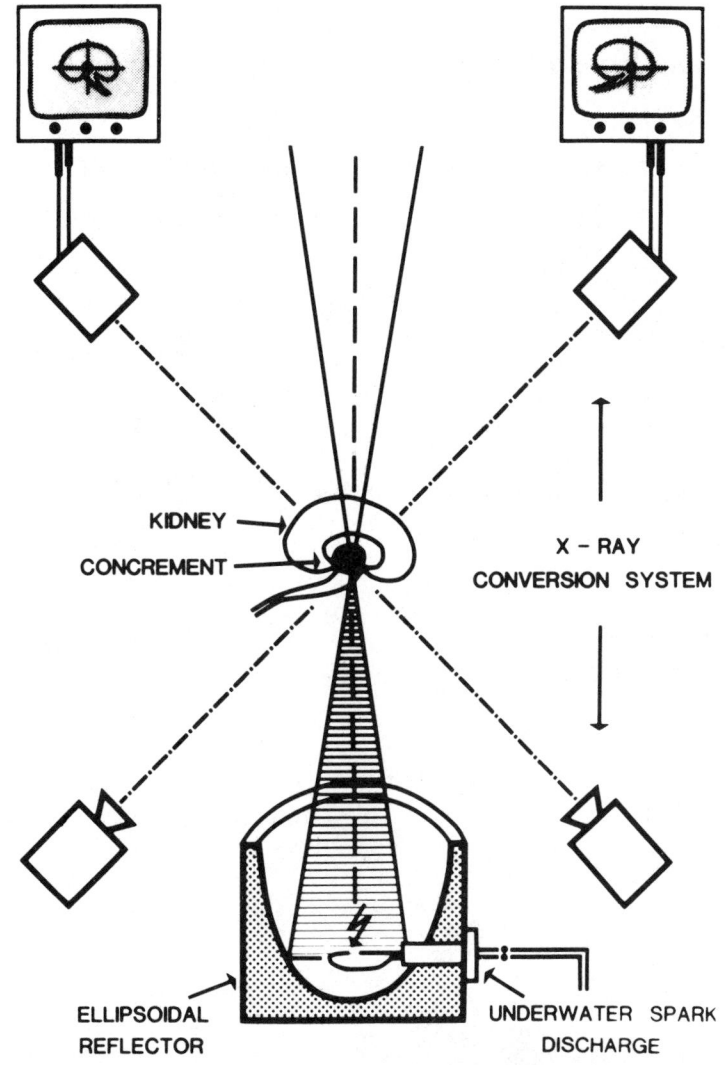

KIDNEY

CONCREMENT

X – RAY
CONVERSION SYSTEM

ELLIPSOIDAL
REFLECTOR

UNDERWATER SPARK
DISCHARGE

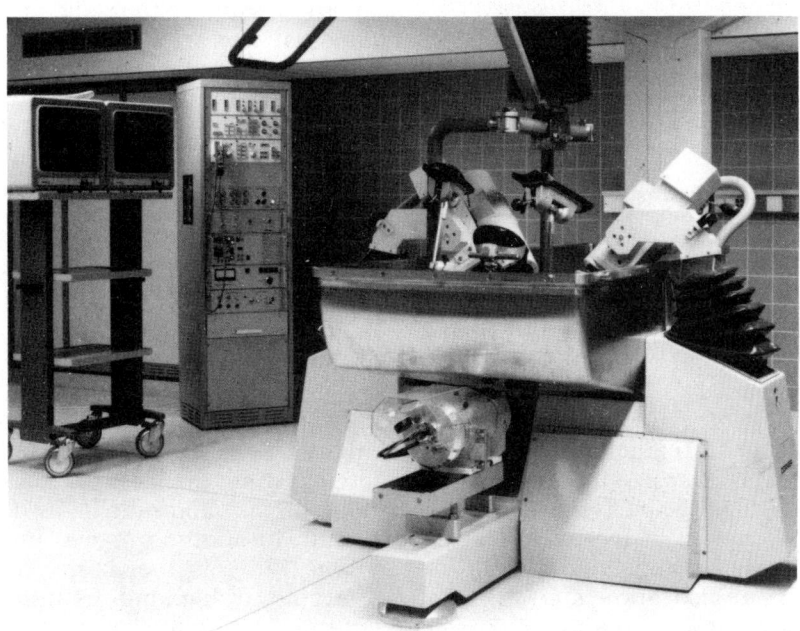

Figure 46.2. Schematic drawing of the technical arrangement (*top*) and photograph of the actual apparatus (*bottom*) for extracorporeal shock wave lithotripsy. (From Chaussey C, Schmidt E, Jocham D: Nonsurgical treatment of renal calculi with shock waves. In Roth RA, Finlayson BF (eds): *Stones: Clinical Management of Urolithiasis.* Baltimore, Williams & Wilkins, 1983.)

Table 46.1.
Classification of Stone-Forming Patient by Type of Stone Passed[a]

	Coe Series 519 Patients	Combined Series 1870 Patients
Calcium oxalate (with or without phosphate)	88.6[b]	63.2[b]
Calcium phosphate	2.1	7.4
Calcium and uric acid	4.2	
Uric acid	1.5	5.4
Cystine	0.6	2.5
Struvite	3.0	21.5

[a] From Coe FL: *Nephrolithias: Pathogenesis and Treatment.* Chicago, Year Book Medical Publishers, 1978.
[b] All values expressed as percentages of patients in each category.

Table 46.2.
Metabolic and Clinical Disorders in 460 Consecutive Calcium Stone Formers[a]

	No. of Patients	(%)
Idiopathic hypercalciuria	95	(20.7)
Marginal hypercalciuria[b]	53	(11.5)
Hyperuricosuria[c]	67	(14.6)
Hypercalciuria and hyperuricosuria[c]	54	(11.7)
Hyperuricemia	26	(5.7)
Primary hyperparathyroidism	24	(5.2)
Renal tubular acidosis[e]	17	(3.7)
Inflammatory bowel disease[f]	21	(4.6)
Medullary sponge kidney	7	(1.5)
Sarcoidosis	3	(0.7)
No disorder found	93	(20.2)
Total	460	

[a] From Coe FL: *Nephrolithiasis: Pathogenesis and Treatment.* Chicago, Year Book Medical Publishers, 1978.
[b] Urine calcium > 140 mg/g of creatinine but less than 250 mg/24 hours in women and 300 mg/24 hours in men.
[c] Urine uric acid above 800 mg (men) and 750 mg (women), in at least one of two 24-hour urine collections.
[d] Marginal hypercalciuria not included.
[e] Distal, hereditary form.
[f] Regional enteritis, ulcerative colitis, granulomatous ileocolitis.

an abnormally high fraction of their daily acid load as titratable acid rather than as ammonium and therefore have an unusually low average urinary pH. Further, patients with chronic diarrhea or patients with excessive fluid loss from the skin may have highly concentrated urine, which will predispose to uric acid calculus formation. Patients who have myeloproliferative disease and those who have solid tumors that are undergoing lysis may have excessive uric acid excretion, which may be associated with uric acid stones and tubular plugs of urate. Patients with gout also have more calcium stones than does the general population (10). The association may result from crystallization of uric acid, which then forms a nidus for calcium deposition.

Table 46.3.
Prevalence of Uric Acid Stones in Various Populations

Population	Lifetime Incidence (%)
General population	0.01
Patients with gout	22
Hyperuricosuria in primary gout[a]:	
<300 mg/24 hours	11
300–699 mg/24 hours	21
700–1100 mg/24 hours	35
>1100 mg/24 hours	50
Hyperuricemia in men[b]:	
7–8 mg/dl	12.7
8–9 mg/dl	22
>9 mg/dl	40

[a] From Yüu T, Gutman AB: Uric acid nephrolithiasis in gout. *Ann Intern Med* 67:1133, 1967.
[b] From Hall AP, Barry PE, Dawber TR, McNamarea PM: Epidemiology of gout and hyperuricemia. *Am J Med* 42:27, 1967.

Struvite Stones (Infection Stones)

It is generally believed that infection stones form primarily as a consequence of the hydrolysis of urea and the production of ammonium by the bacterial enzyme urease. The production of ammonia leads to a highly alkaline urine which promotes the precipitation of magnesium, ammonium, and phosphate. These are the components of the infection-induced or struvite stone. The majority of urea-splitting organisms are *Proteus* species; however, *Pseudomonas, Klebsiella, Staphylococcus,* and some *Escherichia coli* strains are capable of producing urease. Struvite stones do not form *de novo* but almost always are a complication of another primary stone disease where infection has become superimposed, and they are especially likely to grow into *staghorn calculi* (large stones which cannot pass the ureteropelvic junction and which form a cast of all or a portion of the pelvicalyceal system).

Cystine Stones

Cystine stones are rare and the general physician will encounter this problem very infrequently and then most likely in young patients, as the onset is usually in childhood. The stone forms because of crystallization of cystine when the urine is supersaturated with this substance, which occurs when there is a defect in renal tubular resorption of filtered cystine. This is a particularly virulent form of stone disease and may be associated with staghorn calculi. In addition to cystinuria, there is usually urinary loss of other basic amino acids, including ornithine, lysine, and arginine. The disorder is an inherited autosomal recessive trait, although some heterozygous patients have excess cystine excretion, as is shown in Table 46.4. Cystine is much less soluble in acid urine than it is in alkaline urine, and

Table 46.4.
Urinary Cystine Excretion

Normal individuals	<100 mg
Heterozygotes for cystinuria	150–300 mg
Homozygotes for cystinuria	>600 mg

cystine stones generally, therefore, will form when urine is acid and cystine excretion is greater than 400 mg/24 hours.

NATURAL HISTORY OF URINARY STONE DISEASE

Urinary calculus disease is a chronic illness. Once a stone has formed, there is a tendency for recurrence and management (see below) should be tailored to the stone activity, to the type of stone, and to any associated metabolic abnormality.

Stone activity—the number of stones formed and the change in size of existing stones—is an important, although at times difficult, determination to be made. It requires a yearly review of stones passed and removed, as well as an evaluation by abdominal X-ray of increase in size of known stones or the appearance of new stones. The activity of urinary calculi depends on a number of factors: stone type, associated metabolic abnormality, treatment received (both specific and nonspecific), and age. Precise rates of recurrence, therefore, cannot be given with real accuracy.

Since calcium stone formers make up the largest population of patients with stones, there is more information about recurrences in this group. In solitary calcium stone formers (history of passing a single stone) there is a recurrence in half of the patients by 5 years and in two-thirds of the patients with 9 years, with a peak recurrence at about 2 years and a second smaller peak at 8 years after passage of the initial stone (Fig. 46.3).

Because of this high recurrence rate it is suggested that evaluation for associated metabolic abnormalities be undertaken in each patient who has formed a calcium stone or if the stone type is unknown. If a passed stone is known to be uric acid, struvite, or cystine, recurrence is also likely and a metabolic evaluation should be undertaken; since calcium stones may be mixed with these types, the evaluation should be comprehensive.

DIAGNOSTIC WORKUP OF PATIENTS WITH URINARY STONE DISEASE

Evaluation of patients with stone disease can be accomplished entirely in an ambulatory setting. This evaluation depends on history, physical examination, and certain laboratory measurements.

History

A history is important in determining the activity of stone disease (see above) as well as in providing clues to the nature of the stone. *Family history* may provide a clue to cystine stones, uric acid stones (gout), and some calcium stones (*e.g.*, those associated with renal tubular acidosis). *Dietary history* may reveal excessive intake of calcium, purine, and/or oxalate (see below). The *eating habits* are important. For example, if a patient takes only one large meal a day, there may be a sudden surge of uric acid that requires excretion in a highly acid urine, resulting in predisposition to uric acid calculi. High protein meat diets may be associated with excess ingestion and excretion of acid and thereby may be connected with stone disease. An approximate daily fluid intake is also an important part of the history. Some individuals may ingest as little as 500 to 700 ml/day and thus have concentrated urine most of the day. *Medication history* is important. For example, aspirin in high doses (more than 5 g/day, especially if the urine is also alkaline) and probenecid are associated with increased uric acid excretion and may be a predisposition to uric acid calculi. Further, calcium-containing antacids (*e.g.*, Camalox, Bisodol, Titralac, Tempo, or Tums) as well as vitamin D may be associated with hypercalciuria and calcium stone formation. Acetazolamide (Diamox) may be associated with development of chronically alkaline urine and a higher incidence of calcium calculi. Triamterene and its metabolites have been found as the nidus in urinary calculi (and occasionally it may be the only ingredient). For this reason, a history of the use of triamterene preparations (Dyazide or Dyrenium) should be sought (4) and use of these medications discontinued in patients with a history of urinary calculus. Moreover, certain medications, such as thiazides or allopurinol,

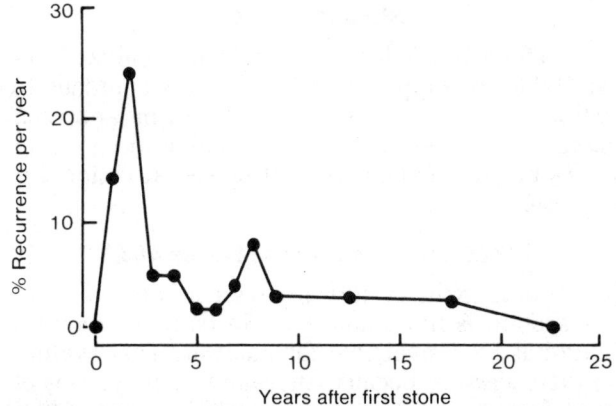

Figure 46.3. Rate of stone recurrence in patients who have formed a single calcium stone. (From Coe FL: *Nephrolithiasis: Pathogenesis and Treatment.* Chicago, Year Book Publishers, 1978.)

will interfere with calcium and uric acid excretion, respectively, and interfere with results of testing in a patient who is being evaluated for renal stone disease. *Occupational history* is important in that the environmental temperature (and therefore fluid losses) and/or the accessibility to fluids are factors influencing stone formation by promoting decreased output of highly concentrated urine.

Physical Examination

Physical examination (when there is no colic) occasionally will give clues to specific problems. For example, band keratopathy (stippled calcification of the perimeter of the cornea, which may require a slitlamp for visualization) may be seen in hyperparathyroidism, or there may be signs of sarcoidosis, hyperthyroidism, inflammatory bowel disease, neoplasia, or gouty arthritis. Most often, however, the examination is normal.

Urinalysis

The urinalysis provides a simple assessment that may give specific direction to the determination of the cause of the urinary calculus. It is important that the urinalysis is complete, including the determination of pH. The pH is usually acid in patients with a uric acid or a cystine stone and is invariably alkaline in patients with struvite stones. Also, the pH may suggest the presence of renal tubular acidosis: The first voided morning urine is usually acid, so that finding a urine pH > 6.0 in this specimen suggests the possibility of renal tubular acidosis. The microscopic analysis may show crystals or evidence of infection. Crystals of cystine have the appearance of a benzene ring and are highly suggestive of cystinuria. Other crystals are more variable and are not diagnostic. Oxalate crystals appear in urine normally, and their identification should not suggest a disorder.

Stone Analysis

If a stone is available it should be analyzed because the stone type will determine the approach to evaluation and treatment. Stones can be analyzed inexpensively at commercial laboratories, and stones may be mailed without preservative for this purpose.

Laboratory Assessment (Table 46.5)

A thorough laboratory analysis as described in this section is important even in patients where a stone has been available for analysis. This evaluation is necessary because there are many causes of stone formation: For example, struvite stones often start as some other primary stone type—most often calcium; and patients with pure uric acid or cystine stones occasionally have other types as well. Patients will usually comply with the testing necessary

Table 46.5.
Laboratory Assessment of Patients with Urinary Calculi[a]

Measure	Day of Testing			
	1	2	3	4
24-hour urinary volume	✓	✓	✓	✓
24-hour urinary calcium[b]	✓			✓
24-hour urinary uric acid[c]		✓	✓	
24-hour urinary creatinine	✓			✓
Urinalysis	✓			
Urine cystine screen (cyanide-nitroprusside test)	✓			
Urine culture (if pyuria)	✓			
Urine pH (taken on first voided morning specimen collected under mineral oil)	✓			
Serum calcium	✓			
Serum phosphorus	✓			
Serum uric acid	✓			
Serum chloride	✓			
Serum bicarbonate	✓			
Serum creatinine	✓			
Serum urea nitrogen	✓			

[a] During evaluation patients should follow their usual diet and life habits except on day 4 (second urinary calcium determination) when a 1-g calcium intake should be ensured (see page 539).
[b] The 24-hour urine container should contain 15 ml of concentrated HCl (with warning to avoid contact).
[c] The 24-hour urine container should contain a few crystals of thymol to retard bacterial overgrowth.

for proper evaluation of a metabolic disorder if they understand the relative ease with which it may be accomplished, the high rate of recurrent calculi, and the importance of specific therapy for different metabolic problems (see below).

Laboratory assessment of patients who have formed urinary calculi is relatively simple and noninvasive and can be easily performed in the office. It is important that this initial evaluation be accomplished *without* the patient modifying his diet or habits so that an underlying process associated with urinary calculus disease will not be masked.

An *intravenous pyelogram*, if not done previously as part of the evaluation of an episode of acute colic, should be done in an attempt to search for underlying structural disease (such as anatomical abnormality of the lower tract or medullary sponge kidney).

In addition to the laboratory assessment outlined in Table 46.5, *parathyroid hormone* should be measured if hypercalcemia and hypercalciuria are documented and if other causes of hypercalcemia are ruled out (see Chapter 74). Urinary *oxalate* should also be determined when hyperoxaluria is expected clinically (Table 46.6), although oxalate determination is not always a reliable analysis and hyperoxaluria is uncommon; therefore, it is not a routinely performed measurement.

Table 46.6.
Situations Where Hyperoxaluria May Be Expected

Hereditary overproduction—usually virulent stone disease with frequent recurrences and nephrocalcinosis often occurring before age 12 years
Methoxyflurane anesthesia—immediately following
Ethylene glycol ingestion—immediately following
Chronic inflammatory bowel disease affecting the ileum, ileal resection, or small bowel bypass
Cellulose phosphate ingestion—during entire period of ingestion
Oxalate gluttony (tea, spinach, rhubarb)

Hypercalciuria

While calcium excretion varies somewhat with intake of calcium and of protein, generally the upper limits of calcium excretion for individuals eating a normal diet are 250 mg/24 hours for women and 300 mg/24 hours for men. Patients with hypercalciuria without hypercalcemia deserve special attention because they are seen quite commonly and because of the variable pathogenesis of their stones. Table 46.7 lists the causes of hypercalciuria that may be unassociated with hypercalcemia.

Most patients will have idiopathic hypercalciuria either from a *renal leak* (renal hypercalciuria) or *excessive gastrointestinal absorption* (absorptive hypercalciuria) of calcium. In the latter, which occurs more commonly, there is excess gastrointestinal absorption (and then excretion) of calcium after the ingestion of calcium. The differentiation of renal from absorptive hypercalciuria requires the use of an *oral calcium tolerance test* (1, 5), which, because of its complexity, is not routinely recommended in an office practice, although there is controversy about this (see Narins, "General References"). However, it is important to be aware that some patients with absorptive hypercalciuria may have normal calcium excretion if they inadvertently restrict their calcium intake on the day of the urine collection. Therefore, it is advantageous to ensure that the patient has at least a 1-g intake of calcium on the fourth day of urine collection (second urine calcium determination)—Table 46.5. This calcium intake may be ensured by having the patient drink 1 quart of whole milk (approximately 250 mg of calcium/8 ounces) or, if milk is not tolerated or not desired, calcium glubionate (Neo-Calglucon Syrup, available from a pharmacy without a prescription), 1 tablespoon three times a day (345 mg of calcium/tablespoon). It is easiest if the physician dispenses this from office stock because the test requires that the patient ingest a relatively small amount. Some patients with hypercalciuria, especially the absorptive type, will benefit by restriction of calcium in the diet (see below).

PREVENTIVE TREATMENT OF URINARY CALCULUS DISEASE
General Measures

It is important to educate patients who have formed stones about the nature of urinary calculi, their natural history, the importance of regular surveillance, and the effectiveness of therapy.

Diet

Specific diet restriction is discussed under the various stone types (see below).

Fluid Intake

Regardless of the type of stone that has been formed, a patient should maintain a high intake of fluids to ensure a urinary output of 3 to 4 liters/day. This high urinary output prevents supersaturation and the high flow rate may wash out small crystalline formations before they produce any obstructive symptoms.

Patients with recurrent stone disease require a high fluid intake throughout the day and night (6). This can be accomplished by having the individual drink 3 liters through the day and then take 1 or 2 glasses of water before retiring. This should result in a nocturnal diuresis necessitating voiding 3 to 4 hours later, at which time a further ingestion of 1 or 2 glasses of water will continue the diuresis until morning. Although annoying to the patient, once the habit is formed it is a small nuisance compared to the benefit of preventing subsequent stone formation.

Habits

Patients should be counseled to avoid dehydration and consequently concentrated urine when participating in sports, during travel, or work.

Table 46.7.
Causes of Hypercalciuria That May Not Be Associated with Hypercalcemia

Idiopathic hypercalciuria
Administration of loop diuretics (furosemide, ethacrynic acid, or bumetanide)
Excessive salt ingestion
Exogenous adrenal corticosteroids
Cushing's syndrome
Paget's disease of bone
Immobilization
Progressive bone disease
Malignant tumors
Hyperthyroidism
Sarcoidosis
Renal tubular acidosis
Other causes of metabolic acidosis
Medullary sponge kidney
Severe phosphate deprivation

Specific Therapy for Calcium Stone Formers

Calcium is present in the vast majority of urinary calculi, and hypercalciuria is the most frequent disorder uncovered during the evaluation of patients with urinary calculus disease. In addition to the general measures described above, there are several specific therapies.

The decision, however, to use specific therapy (especially pharmacological therapy) must be made on an individual basis. The rate of stone recurrence for a large population of patients may not apply to an individual patient. It is prudent to use only general therapeutic measures until there is an increase in stone activity. At this time a decision should be made about adding such specific therapy as might be appropriate from the workup.

Restricted Calcium Diet

This is suggested in the patient who has been found to have hypercalciuria. A severely calcium-restricted diet is not generally advocated and may have limitations because of the induction of chronic negative calcium balance and its potential for subsequent bone disease, an issue especially important in white women (see Chapter 77). Generally a calcium-restricted diet is obtained by limiting intake of milk and milk products, in which case the calcium intake may fall from 1500 to 2000 mg to 400 to 700 mg/day.

Thiazide Diuretics

Thiazide administration has been shown to result within a day or two in up to a 90% reduction in stone formation. It causes a fall in urinary calcium excretion by as much as 50 to 60%. It also increases (by action on the tubular transport mechanism) magnesium and zinc excretion, which may be important in the inhibition of calcium crystallization. Thiazides are useful in the treatment of nearly all types of calcium stone formers and are an ideal theoretical choice in the treatment of renal hypercalciuria. They should be avoided in patients with hypercalcemia (e.g., those with hyperparathyroidism or sarcoidosis).

The dose of thiazide to be used for the prevention of urinary calculi is uncertain. The incidence of side effects was nearly 35% in one early study (9) utilizing a dose of hydrochlorothiazide of 50 mg twice a day, the regimen that usually resulted in maximal hypocalciuria. Most side effects were seen soon after initiation of the drug. Considering these two facts, it is now suggested that intolerance of thiazides can be limited to less than 10% of patients by the following regimen: Hydrochlorothiazide, 25 mg/day for the first week, then an increase by 25 mg/week until the maintenance dose of 50 mg twice a day is reached. The dose is reduced to 25 mg twice a day if side effects develop (9). Chapter 45 provides a discussion of the management of the hypokalemic

complications of thiazides. However, it should be emphasized here that, should a potassium-sparing diuretic be added, it should not be triamterene because of the association of this agent with the formation of urinary calculi.

Orthophosphate (Inorganic Phosphate)

The administration of inorganic phosphate may result in the complete cessation of new urinary calculi formation in 90% of patients (7). However, because of the large doses required and the high incidence of side effects, the use of inorganic phosphate is still controversial. Its method of action may be to decrease calcium absorption directly by forming unabsorbable complexes in the gastrointestinal tract (therefore making it ideal for treatment of patients with absorptive hypercalciuria), but also to some extent by increasing plasma phosphate. This, in turn, leads to a fall in the ionized calcium, resulting in increased parathyroid hormone production, a subsequent fall in the glomerular filtation rate, and an increase in renal tubular calcium absorption. Further, the increased plasma phosphate may inhibit the renal production of 1,25-dihydroxyvitamin D_3, a substance which increases calcium absorption. Increased phosphate absorption may also decrease stone formation by increasing urinary pyrophosphate, which inhibits crystal formation.

There are risks associated with using orthophosphates. The excess stimulation of parathyroid hormone could result in bone disease, and increase in plasma phosphate concentration could lead to renal disease. Further, many patients have had intolerable diarrhea, nausea, or vomiting.

The inorganic phosphate salts are prescribed primarily as a mixture of sodium and potassium phosphate (e.g., K-Phos), 1 g four times a day. Its use is probably best restricted to patients in whom thiazides are contraindicated or not tolerated. The administration of these agents, however, is not recommended without at least a telephone consultation with a nephrologist or urologist.

Cellulose Phosphate

This is an ion exchange resin that became available in this country in 1983. Cellulose phosphate (Calcibind) 2.5-g packets, is mixed with water, juice, or a soft drink and is started usually at a dose of 5 g taken within 30 minutes of each meal. The patient should be on a moderately restricted calcium diet (no milk or milk products) and still excrete in the urine greater than 300 mg of calcium/day. It is important to monitor the 24-hour urinary calcium excretion and to decrease the dose of cellulose phosphate when the calcium excretion is less than 150 mg/day. Its use is especially promulgated for the treatment of absorptive hypercalciuria because it increases the fecal excretion of calcium by binding dietary calcium and also by binding calcium that has been secreted by the gastrointestinal tract. The decreased absorption of calcium by the bowel results in a fall in urinary calcium excretion with an associated increase in urinary phosphate excretion. This agent may result in chronic negative calcium balance and subsequent bone disease. Cellulose phosphate also binds magnesium, and hypomagnesemia may develop but can be corrected with magnesium supplementation. Its use, because of the quantity required, may be unacceptable to many patients, and it frequently causes unacceptable diarrhea and/or occasional offensive stools. Its use is not recommended without consultation with a nephrologist or urologist.

Patients with Calcium or Uric Acid Stones Who Are Found to Have Hyperuricosuria

Patients with calcium stones who have hyperuricosuria or those who have mixed calcium and uric acid stones should be treated in the same way as if they had pure uric acid stones.

If purine gluttony is present hyperuricosuria can be modified by dietary restriction of purine-rich food, such as liver, kidney, and fish roe. Gluttony, however, is not often the problem, and other means are necessary.

Uric acid stone formation can be markedly modified by increasing the urinary pH; increasing the pH of the urine from 4.5 to 5.5 or 6.5 increases uric acid dissociation from 15% to 40% and 80%, respectively. Alkalinization can be accomplished by the administration of sodium bicarbonate several times a day. However, because sodium bicarbonate frequently causes gas and gastrointestinal discomfort, citrate salts (Polycitra solution containing 2 mEq base/ml) are more palatable, and therefore preferable. Most patients require 10 ml three times/day, but the dose should be adjusted as necessary based on the results of regular urine pH testing. The metabolism of citrate results in the generation of bicarbonate. During the initial week of treatment and periodically thereafter, the patient should be taught to measure his urinary pH several times a day to ensure proper alkalinization (urine pH > 6.5). If neither citrate nor bicarbonate is practical, the urine pH may be increased by using acetazolamide (Diamox), 250 to 500 g, four times a day.

Should these agents not be effective in controlling recurrence of uric acid stones, if the urine pH cannot be kept above 6.5, or if uric acid excretion is above 650 mg, allopurinol (which decreases uric acid production) may be used and is very effective in reducing stone recurrence. Allopurinol (Zyloprim) should be initiated at a dose of 200 mg once a day and raised to a level that controls uric acid excretion to below 500 or 600 mg/24 hours (doses greater than 300 mg are divided in two daily doses). Complications from allopurinol are usually minor (minor skin rash, drug fever, or precipitation of an acute gouty attack); the drug should be discontinued whenever a skin rash or fever occurs because diffuse fatal systemic vasculitis has been reported. Allopurinol also has been reported to be associated, although rarely, with the acceleration of cataract formation, with cholestatic hepatitis, and with leukopenia. The use of allopurinol is especially important as a preventive measure in patients who have excess uric acid excretion because of a myeloproliferative disease or in anticipation of tumor lysis. Also, when allopurinol is not entirely satisfactory, a thiazide (see above) alone or in combination with allopurinol is beneficial in reducing the frequency of recurrence.

Hyperoxaluria

In this group of patients the aim is lower oxalate excretion. Treatment depends to some extent on the cause of hyperoxaluria, and frequently a telephone consultation with a nephrologist may be helpful in managing a patient with this complex problem. The consultant may consider the use of cholestyramine in a dose of 8 to 16 g/day, in addition to increased calcium supplementation and a low oxalate diet. In patients who have had ileal resection, pyridoxine deficiency may develop. This deficiency results in the reduction of the transamination of glyoxylate to glycine and hyperoxaluria results. In this situation the use of this vitamin (150 to 400 mg every 24 hours) may provide benefit.

Cystinuria

This group of stone formers generally have particularly virulent disease and are best managed in consultation with a nephrologist. Generally it is necessary to raise urinary pH in a manner similar to the method used in patients with uric acid stones (see above) and, if stone activity continues, to use D-penicillamine, which forms complexes with cystine and prevents its precipitation.

Struvite or Infection Stones

Infection stones are particularly virulent. Untreated patients with infected staghorn calculi frequently develop sepsis and require urgent nephrectomy. Further, when the disease is bilateral there is an associated 25% mortality rate in 5 years (8). In view of this morbidity and with the recent advance in surgical techniques for controlling infection stones, early urological referral is suggested. The goal of surgery in such patients is to remove the stone totally. This may be done by a variety of surgical approaches. The operative mortality for these procedures in skilled hands is less than 1%. Application of hypothermia combined with a technique permitting the kidney to be bivalved has permitted great success in total stone removal with preservation of renal function. There is, however, still a relatively high recurrence rate. Also, percutaneous nephrostolithotomy may be used for smaller stones. This procedure usually requires that the stone be broken up by a shock wave probe (ultrasonic lithotripsy) (see page 534). In another treatment the stone may be perfused and dissolved by an acid solution (Renacidin) using a percutaneous catheter placed antegrade into the pelvis of the kidney (3).

In addition to the surgical treatment of stone disease, medical therapy is an important adjunct. Associated metabolic abnormalities should be sought and treated. Specific antimicrobial therapy is necessary in conjunction with surgery, and, where stones cannot be removed surgically, suppressive therapy with antimicrobials may decrease the incidence of septicemia. The use of oral agents which prevent infecting bacteria from splitting urea (urease inhibitors) has been shown to decrease recurrence of some struvite stones by preventing the formation of highly alkaline urine resulting from the ammonium produced by urea-splitting organisms. Acetohydroxamic acid (Lithostat) became available in 1983 for use as an adjunct to antimicrobial therapy and surgery in patients with struvite stones. Acetohydroxamic acid, 250 mg, three to four times a day or a total dose of 10 to 15 mg/kg/day (but never more than 1.5 g/day) should be used only when the patient is infected with urea-splitting organisms as evidenced by a high urinary pH. Because of its teratogenic effects, it is contraindicated in women who are pregnant. Also it is not effective in the presence of moderate renal failure (creatinine ≥ 2.5 or creatinine clearance < 20 ml/minute). Experience with the drug is still limited, and the general physician should prescribe it only after consultation with a urologist.

Urinary Calculi in Patients without an Identifiable Metabolic Disorder

Approximately 10 to 15% of stone formers found after evaluation not to have a metabolic disorder may respond to thiazides and/or allopurinol as outlined above (2).

General References

Coe FL (guest ed): Nephrolithiasis. In Brenner BM, Stein JH (eds): *Contemporary Issues in Nephrology*, New York, Churchill Livingstone, 1980, vol 5.
> This is a review monograph covering all aspects of urinary stone disease and provides an extensive documentation of the literature.
Narins RG (ed): *Controversies in Nephrology and Hypertension*. New York, Churchill Livingstone, 1984.
> Contains a thorough and well referenced discussion on the extent of the workup for hypercalciuric patients with stone disease.
Roth RA, Finalayson B (eds): *Stones: Clinical Management of Urolithiasis*. Baltimore, Williams & Wilkins, 1983.
> A multiauthored monograph that is well referenced and which covers all aspects of stone disease, including the newer treatments utilizing shock waves.

Specific References

1. Broadus AE, Dominguez M, Bartter FC: Patholphysiological studies in idiopathic hypercalciuria: use of an oral calcium tolerance test to characterize distinctive hyperalciuria subgroups. *J Clin Endocrinol Metab* 47:751, 1978.
2. Coe FL: Treated and untreated recurrent calcium nephrolithiasis in patients with idiopathic hypercalciuria, hyperuricosuria, or no metabolic disorder. *Ann Intern Med* 87:404, 1977.
3. Dretler SP, Pfister RC, Newhouse JH: Renal stone dissolution via percutaneous nephrostomy. *N Engl J Med* 300:341, 1979.
4. Ettinger B, Oldroyd NO, Surgel F: Triamterene nephrolithiasis. *JAMA* 244:2443, 1980.
5. Pak CYV, Kaplan RA, Bone H, et al: A simple test for the diagnosis of absorptive, resorptive and renal hypercalciurias. *N Engl J Med* 292:497, 1975.
6. Pak CY, Sakhaee K, Crowther C, Krinkley L: Evidence justifying a high fluid intake in treatment of nephrolithiasis. *Ann Intern Med* 93:36, 1980.
7. Thomas WC Jr: Use of phosphates in patients with calcureous renal calculi. *Kidney Int* 13:390, 1978.
8. Wojewski A, Zajaczkowski T: The treatment of bilateral staghorn calculi of the kidneys. *Int Urol Nephrol* 5:249, 1974.
9. Yendt ER: Medical management of calcium stones. In Roth RA, Finlayson B (eds): *Stones: Clinical Management of Urolithiasis*. Baltimore, Williams & Wilkins, 1983, chap 7, pp 187–209.
10. Yü T, Butman AB: Uric acid nephrolithiasis in gout. Predisposing factors. *Ann Intern Med* 67:1133, 1967.

CHAPTER FORTY-SEVEN

Chronic Renal Failure

GARY R. BRIEFEL, M.D.

INTRODUCTION

Renal insufficiency, either as a primary event or complicating another illness, is a common clinical problem, and the general physician will regularly be required to manage patients who have impaired kidney function. This chapter will review the epidemiology, evaluation, manifestations, clinical course, and management of patients with chronic renal failure. In addition, the chapter provides guidelines describing when consultation with a nephrologist is necessary; it also contains a discussion about dialysis and renal transplantation.

The healthy *kidney* performs a wide variety of functions that contribute to the maintenance of the internal environment of the body. In addition to its role in maintaining the balance of water and electrolytes, the kidney has important endocrine and metabolic functions. It produces hormones responsible for normal bone formation (1,25-dihydroxyvitamin D_3), red blood cell production (erythropoietin), and blood pressure control (renin, prostaglandins). The kidney is responsible for degrading a number of polypeptide hormones, including parathyroid hormone, insulin, gastrin, and prolactin among others. Also, the kidney serves as a major excretory route for many toxic metabolic wastes as well as for a wide variety of drugs or their breakdown products.

In parallel with the progressive destruction of renal mass that occurs with many chronic kidney diseases, patients pass through a sequence of clinical stages before reaching *end-stage renal failure* (the point when dialysis is required). The divisions between these stages may vary between individuals; nevertheless, these distinctions are useful in predicting the kinds of abnormalities that are to be expected for any given degree of renal dysfunction. During the stage of *renal impairment*, the blood urea nitrogen (BUN) and serum creatinine concentrations are often within the normal range, despite a fall of the glomerular filtration rate (GFR) to as low as 50 ml/minute. Signs and symptoms, if present during this stage, are usually attributable to the underlying disease (e.g., diabetes, hypertension). As renal function declines further (GFR 20 to 50 ml/minute), the BUN and serum creatinine levels become noticeably increased and some metabolic abnormalities appear (e.g., metabolic acidosis, carbohydrate intolerance, reduced synthesis of 1,25-dihydroxyvitamin D_3). Also at this point, the kidney's ability to respond to acute changes in body fluid and electrolyte composition is reduced. In this stage of *renal insufficiency*, although the BUN concentration is increased (*azotemia*), symptoms attributable to the retention of nitrogenous wastes are absent. However, the patient may begin to experience symptoms related to anemia (fatigue), loss of urine-concentrating ability (polyuria), or volume expansion (dyspnea and/or edema). When the GFR falls below 20 ml/minute (serum creatinine concentration usually > than 5 mg/dl) the patient enters the stage of *renal failure*. This stage is associated with a further reduction in the kidney's ability to maintain homeostasis and is characterized by multiple biochemical abnormalities (e.g., hypocalcemia, hyperphosphatemia, metabolic acidosis, fluid overload). The term *uremia* is employed to describe the entire set of signs, symptoms, and metabolic disturbances that occurs in advanced kidney failure (GFR < 10 ml/minute, serum creatinine concentration usually > than 8 mg/dl), and which may affect virtually all organ systems. Examples of some uremic manifestations include nausea, vomiting, anorexia (gastrointestinal tract), lassitude, reversal of the sleep cycle (nervous system), heart failure, hypertension (cardiovascular system), pruritis (skin), and infertility (endocrine system).

EPIDEMIOLOGY OF CHRONIC RENAL FAILURE

There are currently over 70,000 patients on dialysis in the United States, and many more living with successful kidney transplants. Since 1974, the year Medicare coverage was extended to patients with chronic renal failure who needed dialysis, the incidence of end-stage renal failure has increased from 71/million population/year to over 100/million/year in 1983 (9). In actual numbers, 20,000 new patients require dialysis each year. The incidence of end-stage renal disease has been noted to be 30 to 40% higher in males than females and to peak between the ages of 65 and 74 years (Fig. 47.1). The rate has also been estimated to be from 3 to 4 times greater in blacks than in whites due in part to the higher prevalence of hypertension in blacks.

The reported distribution of patients entering the End-Stage Renal Disease program by primary diagnosis is as follows: primary hypertensive disease, 23.4%; diabetic nephropathy, 21.8%; glomerulonephritis, 19.7%; interstitial nephritis, 6.4%; polycystic kidney disease, 5.9%; etiology unknown, 8.8%; miscellaneous, 14% (9).

CLASSIFICATION

Kidney diseases are often classified according to whether they produce acute or chronic renal failure.

Acute renal failure is defined as a deterioration of glomerular filtration that occurs over hours or days, whereas the course of *chronic renal failure* often runs from months to years. Many of the diseases that cause acute renal failure are reversible, and recovery is often complete (e.g., aminoglycoside nephrotoxicity). Recovery from those diseases that produce chronic renal failure is less common. It should be emphasized that some illnesses producing acute renal failure may not be entirely reversible and can progress to end-stage renal disease (e.g., Goodpasture's syndrome, acute cortical necrosis). Conversely, some of the chronic forms of renal disease can improve with therapy and may, therefore, never progress to the point of requiring dialysis treatments (e.g., membranous glomerulonephritis or the nephropathy of systemic lupus erythematosus).

The causes of kidney failure may be further subdivided into those with prerenal, renal, or postrenal components. *Prerenal azotemia* is caused by factors that produce a decrease in renal perfusion. Diminished perfusion may result from anatomical lesions such as might occur with renal artery stenosis, but more commonly it is related to pathological states of decreased cardiac output (heart failure), vasodilatation (septic shock), or volume depletion (vomiting or excessive diuretic use). Prerenal azotemia due to volume depletion, for example, may often be superimposed on existing chronic renal failure due to other causes. *Postrenal azotemia* is caused by lesions that occur distal to the kidney parenchyma involving the renal pelvis, ureters, bladder, or urethra. Common examples of such lesions would include prostatic enlargement, nephrolithiasis, or retroperitoneal cancers.

Most of the diseases that cause chronic renal failure directly involve the *kidney parenchyma* and are classified according to the anatomical region that is primarily affected (Table 47.1). *Glomerular lesions* can be due to proliferation of endothelial or mesangial cells (e.g., postinfectious glomerulonephritis), thickening of the basement membrane (e.g., membranous glomerulopathy, diabetic nephropathy), glomerulosclerosis (e.g., focal sclerosis), or combinations of the three (e.g., membranoproliferative glomerulonephritis). Any of the diseases that cause glomerular lesions, if sustained, can lead to what is termed *chronic glomerulonephritis*. Clinically, glomerular diseases are often associated with hypertension, edema, renal insufficiency, hematuria, and nephrotic range proteinuria.

Diseases that primarily affect the *tubulointerstitial* areas of the kidney are characterized morphologically by interstitial inflammation, fibrosis, and tubular atrophy. In the past these lesions were often equated with bacterial infections of the kidney (pyelonephritis), but most are thought currently to be due to toxins (e.g., analgesics, heavy metals), metabolic derangements (e.g., hyperuricemia, hypercalcemia), or immunological disorders (e.g., methicillin

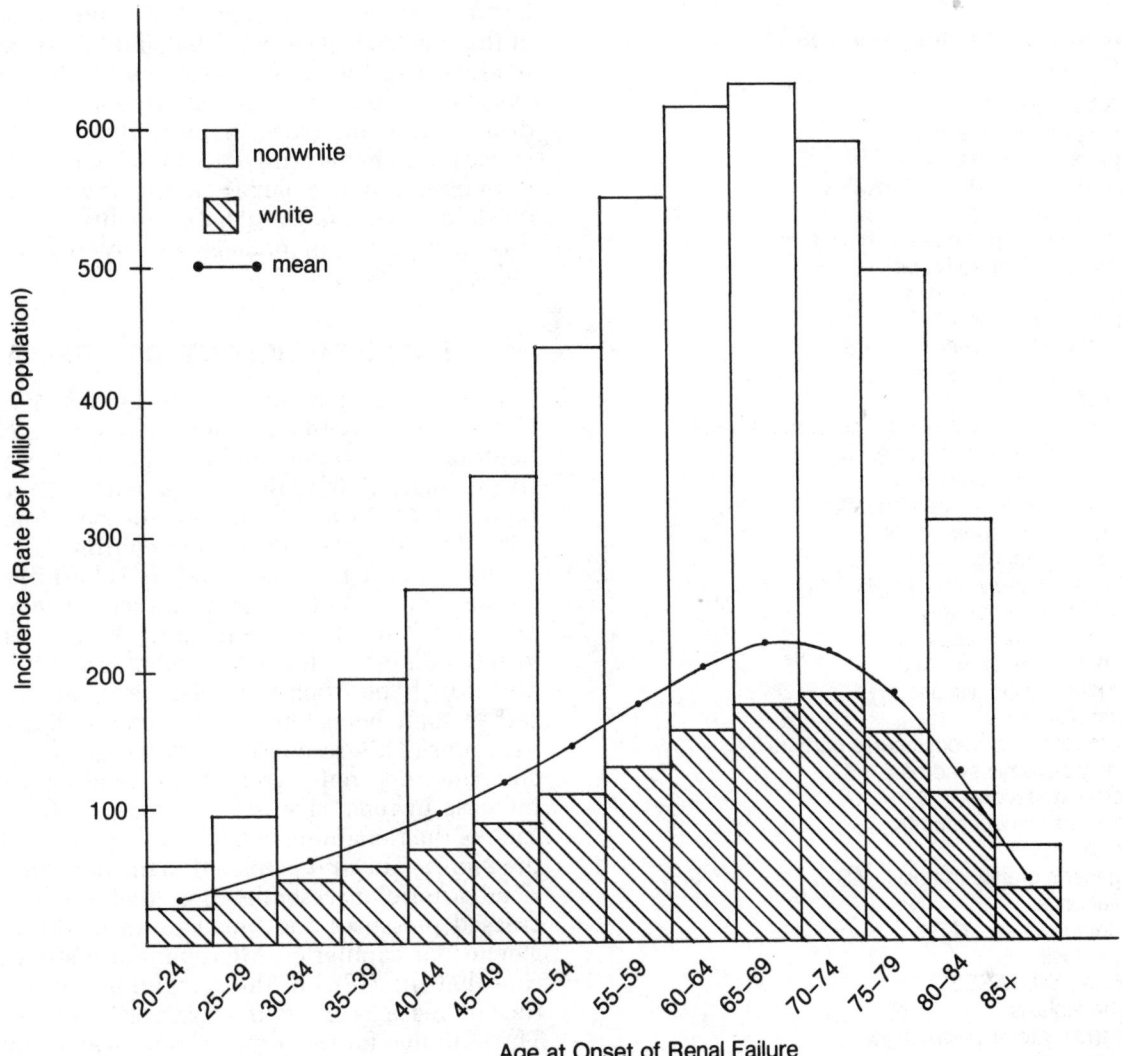

Figure 47.1. The curves show the incidence (rate/million) of patients entering the End-Stage Renal Disease Program (starting dialysis) for whites, nonwhites, and the population as a whole. (Adapted and redrawn from Eggers PW, Connerton R, McMullan M: The Medicare experience with end stage renal disease: trends in incidence, prevalence, and survival. Working Paper Series. Department of Health and Human Services, Health Care Financing Administration, Office of Research and Demonstrations, May 1983.)

interstitial nephritis). The glomeruli are only secondarily involved in the tubulointerstitial diseases. Polycystic and medullary cystic kidney diseases represent a subgroup of the tubulointerstitial nephropathies and are characterized pathologically by the presence of a multitude of thin walled cysts derived from tubular epithelium. Patients with interstitial forms of kidney disease are not usually hypertensive or edematous, and they often produce large volumes of urine with high sodium contents. Typically, glycosuria, non-nephrotic range proteinuria (< 3 g/day), sterile pyuria, and hyperchloremic metabolic acidosis are present.

Lesions of the *renal vessels* may be located in the main renal arteries (e.g., atherosclerosis, fibromuscular dysplasia), medium-sized arteries or arterioles (e.g., polyarteritis nodosa, scleroderma), or the renal veins (e.g., renal vein thrombosis). Renal insufficiency is a result of a reduction in blood flow to the glomeruli. Involvement of the renal vessels is often a part of a systemic illness that also affects vessels in other areas of the body. The clinical features of the renal vasculitides are very similar to those of glomerulonephritis (see above) except that nephrotic range proteinuria (> 3 g/day) is uncommon.

A number of renal diseases can variably affect one or more of the kidney's anatomical regions. For instance, renal involvement in multiple myeloma may take the form of a diffuse thickening of the glomerular basement membrane, or more frequently

Table 47.1.
Classification of Kidney Diseases That Result in Renal Failure[a]

PRERENAL DISEASES
    Renal artery stenosis
    Hepatorenal syndrome   S
RENAL PARENCHYMAL DISEASES
    Glomerular diseases
        Membranous glomerulonephritis (GN)   I
        Membranoproliferative GN   I
        Focal glomerulosclerosis   I
        Rapidly progressive GN   I
        Goodpasture's syndrome   I,S
        Lupus nephritis   I,S
        IgA nephropathy   I
        Alport's syndrome—hereditary nephritis   H,S
        Diabetic glomerulosclerosis   M,S
    Tubulointerstitial diseases
        Chronic pyelonephritis with reflux
        Analgesic nephropathy   N
        Radiation nephritis   N
        Polycystic kidney disease   H,S
        Sickle cell nephropathy   S
        Heavy metal nephropathy   N
        Gouty nephropathy   M,S
        Medullary cystic disease   H
    Vascular diseases
        Thrombotic thrombocytopenic purpura   S
        Hemolyic-uremic syndrome   S
        Scleroderma kidney   S
        Hypertensive nephropathy   S
        Vasculitis   I,S
        Wegener's granulomatosis   I,S
    Miscellaneous
        Myeloma kidney   N,S
        Amyloidosis   S
POSTRENAL DISEASES
    Nephrolithiasis
    Bilateral ureteral obstruction
    Bladder outlet obstruction

[a] H, hereditary; I, immunologically mediated; M, metabolic; N, nephrotoxic; S, part of a systemic disorder.

it causes a tubulointerstitial nephropathy. Systemic lupus erythematosus is another example of a disease that can produce either glomerular or tubulointerstitial damage.

One can further subclassify renal diseases as to whether they are congenital, part of a systemic disorder, primary to the kidney, or by the mechanism of injury. The *congenital* or *hereditary* diseases most often encountered are polycystic kidney disease and Alport's form of hereditary nephritis. Diabetes mellitus and hypertension are the two most common *systemic* disorders producing chronic renal failure, and together they are listed as the etiology of approximately 45% of the patients entering dialysis programs. *Immunological* injury to the kidney can be in the form of glomerular immune complex deposition, as in systemic lupus erythematosus, or antiglomerular basement membrane antibody disease,

best exemplified by Goodpasture's syndrome. Most of the immunologically mediated diseases predominantly affect the vessels or glomeruli, but can also cause damage to the tubulointerstitial areas as in a drug-induced interstitial nephritis (e.g., methicillin). *Drugs* (e.g., phenacetin) or *toxins* (e.g., heavy metals) most often produce damage to the interstitium. *Metabolic* disorders (e.g., diabetes mellitus, gout, oxalosis) can result in damage to any region of the kidney.

PATHOPHYSIOLOGY OF UREMIA

The course of many chronic kidney diseases is characterized by the progressive loss of functioning nephrons. The kidney undergoes a number of adaptive changes that allow most patients with chronic renal failure to have few signs or symptoms until 80% of the original number of nephrons is lost.

The kidney's response to injury is best illustrated by the events following uninephrectomy. On a gross anatomical level, the remaining kidney becomes visibly enlarged. This enlargement is a result of the physical hypertrophy of the residual nephrons rather than being due to the production of new nephrons. This response to renal injury is termed compensatory renal growth. Correlating with the increase in renal size is an increase in the GFR of each of the remaining nephrons. The mechanism for the increase in GFR is related to the development of renal arteriolar vasodilatation that results in increased pressures and blood flows in the residual glomerular capillaries. Micropuncture studies indicate that the GFRs of the remaining normal nephrons increase 2- to 3-fold over their baseline values. The stimulus for this process is not yet known. It is also not entirely clear whether the adaptive process that occurs in a healthy kidney following surgical ablation of the contralateral kidney is similar to that which occurs in diseases that diffusely affect the nephron population, such as glomerulonephritis.

The ability of the impaired kidney to maintain the concentrations of individual components of the body's fluids within normal limits is variable. The concentrations of substances that are simply filtered and neither secreted nor resorbed by the tubule, such as urea and creatinine, begin to rise relatively early in the course of renal impairment (GFR 50% of normal). In contrast, the serum concentration of phosphorus, which is under the influence of parathyroid hormone (PTH), is kept within the normal range until more than 80% of renal function is lost. This is because in renal failure increased PTH activity progressively reduces the amount of phosphorus resorbed by the tubule (normally 80% of filtered phosphorus is resorbed) in parallel with the reduction in renal mass. Once the GFR falls below 20% of normal, this mechanism can no longer keep pace, and the serum phosphorus level begins to rise. Other solutes, such as sodium and potassium, are even better regulated, and their concentrations are maintained within the normal range until the GFR is less than 5 ml/minute.

Eventually the reserve capacity of the kidney is overwhelmed, and a number of signs, symptoms, and metabolic abnormalities appear that are characteristic of uremia (Table 47.2). Uremia is a complex syndrome that results from the failure of the kidney to fulfill its excretory, endocrine, and metabolic functions. In the patient with end-stage renal disease virtually every organ system is affected to some degree. The mechanisms for only some of the abnormalities that appear in uremia are well understood. Efforts to explain the metabolic consequences of renal failure by the retention of toxic wastes are only partially satisfying. Because urea is easily measured, it is the putative toxin that has been most thoroughly examined. Other nitrogenous waste products (e.g., ammonia, guanadinosuccinic acid), "middle molecules" (polypeptides of intermediate molecular weight), and a variety of organic and inorganic compounds have been implicated in the

Table 47.2.
Major Physiological and Clinical Abnormalities of Uremia

Fluid and electrolyte abnormalities
    Volume expansion
    Hyperkalemia
    Hypocalcemia
    Hyperphosphatemia
    Metabolic acidosis
Endocrine-metabolic abnormalities
    Vitamin D deficiency
    Hyperparathyroidism
    Carbohydrate intolerance
    Impotence and infertility
    Hypertriglyceridemia
Hematological-immunological abnormalities
    Impaired platelet function
    Abnormal T and B cell function
    Anemia
Cardiovascular abnormalities
    Hypertension
    Accelerated atherosclerosis
    Pericarditis
Dermatological abnormalities
    Pruritis
    Increased pigmentation
    Acne
Gastrointestinal abnormalities
    Nausea and vomiting
    Anorexia
    Pancreatitis
Neuromuscular abnormalities
    Peripheral neuropathy
    Seizures
    Coma
    Asterixis
    Myoclonus

pathogenesis of uremia. Each of these toxins, individually or together, potentially could interfere with a specific cellular metabolic function and give rise to a manifestation of uremia.

It is clear that not all of the manifestations of uremia can be attributed to the retention of metabolic waste products. There are a number of well described endocrine and metabolic derangements of equal significance in the pathogenesis of uremia. A deficiency of certain hormones results when the failing kidney is no longer able to produce them in adequate quantities (e.g., erythropoietin, 1,25-dihydroxyvitamin D_3). Other hormones, normally degraded or metabolized by the kidney may be present in excess (e.g., parathyroid hormone, insulin, prolactin). Alternatively, the damaged kidney may elaborate an excess of hormone (e.g., renin). Hormone levels or activity may also be altered as a consequence of abnormal protein binding (e.g., thyroid hormone), peripheral resistance (e.g., insulin, parathyroid hormone), or loss of feedback control (e.g., luteinizing hormone).

The complexity of the multiple endocrine derangements present in uremia is best illustrated by the example of PTH. PTH levels rise progressively throughout the course of renal failure in order to maintain normal concentrations of calcium and phosphorus. Further elevations in the level of PTH are due to the failure of the diseased kidney to metabolize PTH and also because in uremia there is a resistance to the action of PTH on bone. The trade-off for the maintenance of calcium-phosphorus balance during the early part of renal insufficiency is the development, later in the patient's course, of secondary hyperparathyroidism. In addition to producing bone lesions (osteitis fibrosa cystica), some nephrologists believe that increased levels of PTH are partly responsible for impairment of neurological function, anemia, and impotence in uremic patients. Similar derangements in other endocrine systems may be found to be responsible for some of the other manifestations of the uremic syndrome.

DIAGNOSIS OF CHRONIC RENAL FAILURE

Presentation

Kidney disease can most easily be recognized when it is associated with a clearly defined abnormality, the most common being proteinuria, hematuria, and urinary tract obstruction. The recognition of one of these abnormalities is helpful in focusing the ensuing diagnostic evaluation. Frequently, the presence of renal disease is discovered during the evaluation of a systemic disease of which renal dysfunction is only a part (e.g., diabetes mellitus, hypertension).

Due to the remarkable reserve and adaptive capabilities of the kidney, symptoms of uremia do not appear until glomerular filtration is reduced to 10 to

15% of normal. Therefore, unless clearly overt signs of renal involvement are present (e.g., gross hematuria), many patients will progress to advanced renal failure asymptomatically. In other patients whose renal insufficiency is detected early in its course by routine blood tests, specific findings on history and physical examination may also be absent. Special laboratory testing in these patients frequently permits establishment of a definitive diagnosis. The complete evaluation may vary from brief, in the patient with advanced renal failure and markedly shrunken kidneys, to extensive, in the patient who may have potentially reversible disease of recent onset. Most of the evaluation can be performed on an ambulatory basis.

History and Physical Examination

Findings in the history and physical examination can provide useful information that helps to establish the nature of the kidney disease, estimate its duration, and determine its effect on the patient. One of the major goals in evaluating the patient with recently identified renal failure is to distinguish those patients with primary kidney diseases from those whose renal failure is due to familial, congenital, or systemic illnesses.

First the *family history* should be reviewed for the presence of polycystic kidney disease, Alport's syndrome, medullary sponge kidney, hypertension, diabetes mellitus, or renal failure. The presence of a hereditary form of renal disease in the family should help to establish the etiology of the patient's kidney problem. Next, there should be a careful review of the *past medical history* with a particular emphasis on discovering the presence of a systemic illness that can cause renal failure (e.g., hypertension, diabetes mellitus, collagen vascular disorders). Patients should be asked whether they have experienced symptoms related to the presence of skin rashes, arthritis, Raynaud's phenomenon, hemoptysis, and sinusitis, to name a few. In the absence of symptoms related to a systemic illness one needs to question the patient about symptoms associated with abnormalities of the urinary tract. Dysuria, frequency, renal colic, hesitancy or urinary incontinence would point to an abnormality of the lower urinary tract as the cause of the patient's renal dysfunction.

In addition to the symptoms that may prove useful in establishing a diagnosis, there are a number of symptoms (e.g., nausea, vomiting, fatigue, nocturia, itching, restless leg), that are nonspecific. These "uremic" symptoms are present in most patients with advanced renal failure.

Since symptoms of renal failure often do not appear until late in the course of renal failure, it is sometimes difficult to pinpoint the time of onset of the disease. Important clues can occasionally be found when records of past physical examinations performed for work, insurance, or military purposes are reviewed.

Since drugs may either be the cause of renal dysfunction (e.g., heroin, analgesics, aminoglycosides) or may aggravate pre-existing renal insufficiency (e.g., diuretics, nonsteroidal anti-inflammatory drugs) (Table 47.3), there should be a complete inventory of past and current drug use.

The *physical examination* should be focused in a search for signs of systemic illnesses and for renal structural abnormalities. These might include high blood pressure, hypertensive or diabetic retinopathy, vascular bruits, vasculitic skin rashes, gouty tophi or ocular abnormalities (e.g., band keratopathy of hypercalcemia). Enlarged kidneys to palpation may be found in patients with polycystic disease or hydronephrosis. A pelvic or rectal examination should be performed to evaluate causes of lower urinary tract obstruction, such as prostatic or cervical cancer. When obstruction or neurogenic bladder is suspected, the bladder should be catheterized after the patient voids in order to measure a residual volume (see Chapter 6 for technique). A residual volume that is larger than approximately 100 ml should raise concern for bladder outlet obstruction (see Chapter 45) or neuropathic bladder (most commonly seen in diabetics). Signs of heart failure, pericarditis, or neuropathy are most often related to the stage of renal failure and are not helpful in establishing an etiology.

Laboratory Investigation

Laboratory testing of patients with chronic renal insufficiency serves to establish the severity and

Table 47.3.
Some Commonly Used Drugs That May Adversely Affect Renal Function[a]

ANTIBIOTICS
  Aminoglycosides (ATN)
  Penicillins (IN)
  Tetracyclines (increased azotemia and acidosis)
ANALGESICS
  Aspirin (PN and reduction in RBF)
  Phenacetin (PN and IN)
  Nonsteroidal analgesics (IN, nephrotic syndrome, and reduced RBF)
DIURETICS
  Thiazides (volume depletion and IN)
  Furosemide (volume depletion and IN)
MISCELLANEOUS
  Radiocontrast materials (ATN)
  Methysergide (retroperitoneal fibrosis causing obstructive uropathy)
  Penicillamine (NS)
  Gold (NS)
  H_2 receptor antagonists (interfere with secretion of creatinine and produce false elevations of the serum creatinine concentration)
  Captopril (precipitates renal failure in patients with renovascular disease)

[a] ATN, acute tubular necrosis; PN, papillary necrosis; IN, interstitial nephritis; NS, nephrotic syndrome; RBF, renal blood flow.

etiology of the kidney disease, as well as to determine the presence of complicating abnormalities.

Diagnostically, the *urinalysis* can often provide important information. Red blood cells can be seen with any renal disorder. Red blood cell casts are most indicative of a glomerular or vascular lesion. White blood cells, with or without casts, are found in the interstitial nephropathies, including, but not limited to, bacterial pyelonephritis. Hyaline or granular casts are not indicative of a specific pathological process.

The urine dipstick is only a rough guide to the amount of proteinuria. Therefore, a 24-hour urine specimen should be obtained to quantify proteinuria and to calculate the creatinine clearance (see below). Alternatively, a protein/creatinine ratio may be determined in an aliquot of urine as described in Chapter 43. The finding of nephrotic range proteinuria (greater than 3 g/day) usually indicates a glomerular lesion, whereas lesser amounts are seen in some glomerular or vascular disorders and in most interstitial forms of nephritis (Chapter 43). When proteinuria is found in patients over 40 years of age, the possibility of multiple myeloma should be considered, and such patients should be evaluated with serum and urine electrophoreses.

The following tests should be ordered when an immunological disease is suspected: measurement of the serum complement levels (C3 and C4), performance of a lupus erythematosus preparation, and screening for the presence of antistreptococcal antibodies, antinuclear antibodies, rheumatoid factor, and cryoglobulins. Hepatitis B surface antigen (see Chapter 42) can be demonstrated in the blood of some patients with membranous glomerulopathy and in some forms of vasculitic renal disease. This antigen should also be screened for in any patient being referred for chronic dialysis or transplantation, since precautions to prevent the spread of hepatitis will need to be taken, if the test is positive.

The severity of anemia roughly parallels the blood urea nitrogen, as shown in Figure 47.2. The absence of anemia in patients with renal insufficiency should suggest either recent onset, the presence of polycystic kidney disease, or hydronephrosis. Both polycystic kidney disease and hydronephrosis can be associated with normal or elevated hematocrit values. The peripheral blood smear should be examined carefully for abnormalities associated with diseases that can produce renal failure. Rouleaux formation may be present in multiple myeloma, while leukopenia may be associated with collagen vascular diseases. A microangiopathic hemolytic anemia can be seen in patients with thrombotic thrombocytopenic purpura, the hemolytic-uremic syndrome, postpartum renal failure, accelerated hypertension, or scleroderma.

Measurements of the concentration of blood glucose, serum electrolytes (Na, K, Cl, CO_2, Ca, PO_4), uric acid, and liver tests (alkaline phosphatase, bili-

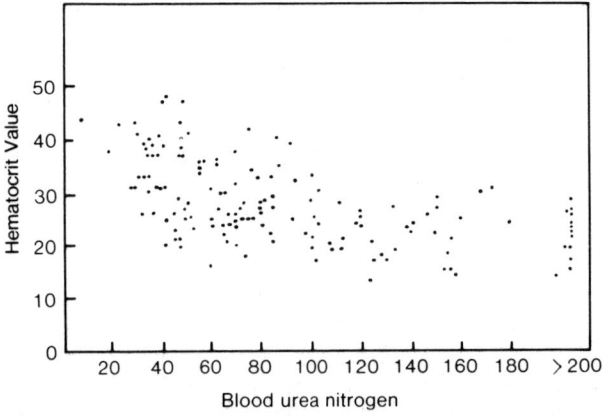

Figure 47.2. The relationship of blood urea nitrogen concentration to the hematocrit value in patients with chronic renal failure (From Erslev AJ: Erythrocyte function of the kidney. In Wesson LG (ed): *Physiology of the Human Kidney*. New York, Grune & Stratton, 1969, p 521.)

rubin, serum transaminases) are helpful in monitoring the patient. The presence of hypercalcemia may suggest a tumor or hyperparathyroidism. The uric acid level is usually elevated in patients with renal insufficiency, but a level greater than 12 mg/dl may indicate the presence of primary hyperuricemia or of a myeloproliferative disorder.

The estimation of severity of renal disease is best accomplished by obtaining a measurement of the serum creatinine concentration and/or creatinine clearance. The serum creatinine concentration is a better indicator of renal function than is the level of BUN, since the latter is affected by such nonrenal factors as diet, intestinal bleeding, liver function, and protein catabolism. The general relationship between the serum creatinine concentration and the GFR is shown in Figure 47.3. In the early stages of renal insufficiency the serum creatinine concentration is an insensitive indicator of functional impairment since it may remain in the normal range (less than 1.5 mg/dl) until GFR has decreased by as much as 50%. It is not until the GFR falls from 50 to 25% of normal that the serum creatinine concentration rises from 2 to 4 mg/dl. Therefore, most of the loss of functioning nephrons occurs at levels of serum creatinine that would be considered to be only modestly elevated. Once the GFR is reduced to 20 to 30% of normal, the curve expressing the relationship between serum creatinine and the GFR rises steeply. Absolute changes in the serum creatinine concentration when there is end-stage renal disease are therefore relatively less significant, when related to losses of GFR, than those seen in early renal insufficiency.

The amount of muscle mass (creatinine is produced by muscle, and its production rate directly parallels the muscle mass) must also be taken into account when evaluating the serum creatinine concentration. For example, (Fig. 47.3), a muscular patient who produces 1.5 g of creatinine/day will have a GFR of 30 ml/minute when his serum creatinine concentration is 5 mg/dl, while an emaciated patient who produces only 0.5 g of creatinine/day will have a creatinine clearance of only 10 ml/minute at the same level of serum creatinine. In addition, relying on serum creatinine concentrations alone may lead one to underestimate the extent of disease in advanced renal insufficiency when creatinine production may be decreased and extrarenal routes of creatinine excretion become more significant.

For these reasons, calculation of the creatinine clearance provides a more accurate reflection of renal function than does the serum creatinine concentration. The creatinine clearance is a close approximation of the GFR. The formula used for calculating clearance is UV/P divided by 1440, where U is the urine creatinine in mg/dl, V is urine volume in ml/day, P is the plasma creatinine concentration in mg/dl, and 1440 is the number of minutes in 24 hours. The result is expressed in ml/minute; the normal creatinine clearance is approximately 100 to 140 ml/minute in men and 85 to 125 ml/minute in women. A correction can be made for body surface area, but in adults this is not needed for usual clinical purposes. A 24-hour urine collection is used to determine daily creatinine production (UV). To confirm the adequacy of this collection, the expected daily creatinine production may be estimated by multiplying body weight in kilograms by 20 for men and by 15 for women. For example, the expected daily creatinine production in a 70-kg male patient would be 70 × 20 = 1400 mg, or 70 × 15 = 1050 mg for a female patient. This estimation, however, will no longer be valid when severe renal failure (GFR < 20 ml/minute) causes a fall in the production of creatinine. In performing the 24-hour urine, the patient should be instructed to choose a convenient time to begin the collection—usually upon rising in the morning. At this time the patient voids and discards the urine but collects all subsequent urine until the same time the following day when the patient again voids and adds that specimen to the collection. The blood sample for measurement of creatinine is generally obtained at the end of the collection period but may be drawn at any time during the collection. When performing a 24-hour urine collection is impractical, one can estimate the creatinine clearance by using nomograms which are based on the patient's serum creatinine, weight, and age (see page 562).

It is important to understand that changes in GFR (reflected by an increasing serum creatinine concentration or a falling creatinine clearance) are not necessarily related to permanent changes in intrinsic kidney function and may be due to other factors (see below, page 553).

A gradual deterioration of GFR with age has been well documented and occurs even in the absence of overt renal disease (18). The following equation may be used for estimating the creatinine clearance in men.

$$\text{GFR (ml/minute)} = 133 - 0.64 \times \text{age (years)}$$

The clearance for women age 50 or greater is approximately 5 to 10 ml/minute less than for males. Thus, at age 70, for example, an individual may have lost 30% of his or her previous GFR due to aging.

Renal Imaging Techniques

Anatomical and functional evaluation of the kidney can be obtained through a variety of tests, all of which need not be performed on any individual patient. Renal imaging techniques in chronic renal failure should be used to (a) establish renal size, (b) detect remediable lesions, and (c) determine etiology.

Renal sonography is a reliable means of estimating kidney size and will also detect the presence of significant hydronephrosis. Because of the risk of radiocontrast dye toxicity in patients with renal impairment, the sonogram should be used in place of the intravenous pyelogram (IVP) as the initial imaging technique in most instances. Normal kidney length as measured by sonography is from 9 to 10 cm, with the left kidney being 0.5 cm larger than the right. An abdominal X-ray to include kidneys, ureters, and bladder (KUB), with tomograms if necessary, is the simplest and least expensive test for estimating renal size but will not detect the presence of hydronephrosis. Normal kidney length as measured by X-ray is approximately 12 to 13 cm or roughly the same as three to four lumbar vertebrae and discs. The kidneys appear longer when meas-

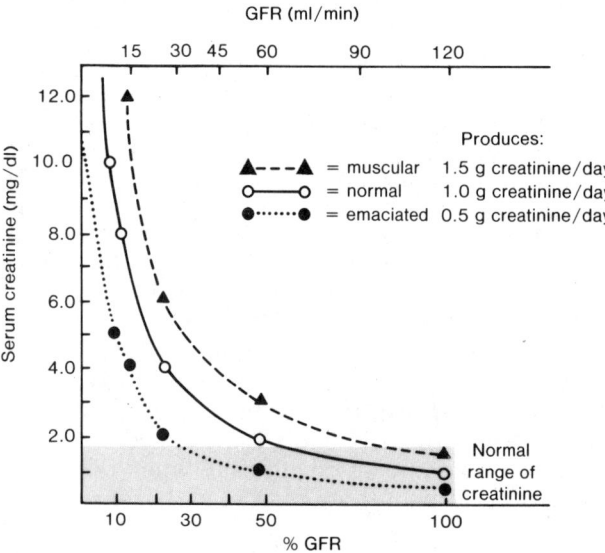

Figure 47.3. The relationship of the serum creatinine concentration to glomerular filtration rate in patients with different muscle mass.

ured by X-rays due to a projection effect. Small kidneys by either technique usually indicate advanced chronic renal disease. However, normal or large kidneys may be seen in chronic renal failure (e.g., diabetes mellitus, amyloidosis).

Hydronephrosis, due to obstruction, should be ruled out in every patient with chronic renal insufficiency. Patients with end-stage renal disease who have small kidneys and no evidence of hydronephrosis require no further radiological evaluation. If the screening sonogram reveals the presence of hydronephrosis, subsequent evaluation of the obstructed kidney may include a retrograde pyelogram, a computerized tomographic (CT) scan, or a sonographically guided percutaneous antegrade pyelogram. The advantage of the latter technique is that it allows for the placement of a simultaneous percutaneous nephrostomy tube for drainage.

The IVP is most useful in determining the etiology of renal failure in those diseases that produce gross anatomical abnormalities, such as chronic pyelonephritis, nephrolithiasis, polycystic kidneys, obstruction, or papillary necrosis. The IVP is not useful in patients with parenchymal disorders that are not associated with gross anatomical defects. Although IVPs can be performed in patients with advanced renal failure by combining the use of high dose contrast materials with tomography (7), there is a significant risk of producing acute renal failure, particularly in elderly or diabetic patients (8). The risk of dye-induced acute renal failure is present not only with IVPs, but whenever contrast materials are administered (e.g., arteriograms or oral cholecystograms). Therefore, the use of radiocontrast materials of any kind should be avoided in patients with renal failure, especially if they are elderly and/or have diabetes mellitus, unless important information that cannot be obtained by alternative means is needed (e.g., localizing the site of ureteral obstruction). Further, since the decline in renal function from radiocontrast materials appears to be partially preventable by avoiding volume depletion, patients should be instructed to maintain salt and fluid intake both before and following the examination.

The renal arteriogram and CT are not routinely performed in patients with chronic renal failure and contribute mainly to the evaluation of vascular or mass lesions. The renal radioisotope scan is of limited usefulness in evaluating chronic renal insufficiency, as it provides functional rather than anatomical information. The data provided are dependent on the radioisotope used. However, the technetium scan, which allows for estimation of renal perfusion, may be useful to determine the viability of an obstructed kidney or one with staghorn calculi.

Renal Biopsy

Once the baseline data have been accumulated, a nephrologist should be consulted, at least by telephone, to help in interpreting the information and to decide whether a renal biopsy is indicated. The renal biopsy provides pathological information and for many disease entities is the most specific diagnostic test available. The biopsy should be considered when the diagnosis is uncertain, to estimate prognosis, and to help demonstrate renal involvement of a systemic illness. Most renal biopsies can be performed percutaneously, under local anesthesia, but do involve a brief hospitalization (see Chapter 43). If the kidneys are very small or if renal failure is advanced, a biopsy is usually not done.

MONITORING THE PATIENT WITH RENAL INSUFFICIENCY

The interval between visits is determined by the stage of renal insufficiency, the rate of progression, and the presence of complicating disorders. Early in the course, patients should have office visits scheduled every 3 to 4 months for monitoring of their symptoms, signs (e.g., weight, blood pressure, edema, etc), and laboratory data (e.g., serum creatinine concentration, BUN, electrolytes, complete blood counts, urinalysis, and creatinine clearance). As renal failure progresses, visits will have to be spaced more closely, usually at 1-month intervals until dialysis becomes necessary. Once the GFR falls below 10 ml/minute, clinical decisions are based more on the presence of symptoms or specific electrolyte abnormalities, such as hyperkalemia or acidosis, than on further changes in the creatinine clearance. Drug dosages should be reviewed at each visit and adjusted according to the degree of renal dysfunction (see below). When the creatinine clearance falls below 5 ml/minute, many patients develop potentially serious electrolyte imbalances and usually require weekly visits for careful monitoring.

COURSE AND PROGNOSIS

The underlying renal disease largely determines prognosis. Many renal diseases have characteristic rates of progression. For example, patients with polycystic kidney disease typically have very indolent courses and some never progress to end-stage renal failure. More aggressive courses, with advanced renal failure developing within months to a year, are more likely to occur in patients with diseases such as rapidly progressive glomerulonephritis, systemic sclerosis, or malignant hypertension. However, most renal diseases fall into an intermediate group, with end-stage renal failure developing within 1 to 5 years after the initial diagnosis.

Using the serum creatinine concentration alone to monitor the progression of renal disease in a patient is often misleading due to the nonlinear relationship between it and the GFR (see above). Because 24-hour urine collections are often impractical or improperly done, alternative means to predict and monitor the progression of chronic renal failure have been proposed. The formula which appears to be most useful and valid is the plot of the *reciprocal of the serum creatinine over time* (Fig. 47.4). In many, but not all, patients this plot will be linear, with the slope reflecting the rate of progression and the x intercept the time of end-stage renal failure. It has been suggested that the slope is constant for a given individual and that any deviation reflects the effects of therapy or the presence of a superimposed process. Mathematical formulations such as this may be useful, but must be interpreted only in conjunction with the remainder of the clinical and laboratory information.

THERAPY

Goals

The goals of therapy fall into four major categories. The first is to treat the underlying renal disease, if possible (e.g., corticosteroids for membranous nephropathy). The second is to slow the progression of renal deterioration by modifying the known or suspected factors that are thought to aggravate the primary process (e.g., treatment of hypertension). The third goal is to treat the specific complications of renal disease (e.g., acidosis) as they occur and also

attempt to prevent the long term complications of uremia before they can become fully established (e.g., secondary hyperparathyroidism). Finally, the patient should be referred to a dialysis and transplantation center prior to the need for dialysis (see below).

Specific Treatments

Once a diagnosis is established, a nephrologist should be consulted, in order to decide whether effective therapy is available for the patient's renal disease. In general, the earlier in the course a treatment is started, the more likely it is to be successful in halting or reversing the disease. When the patient's renal disease is advanced or the effectiveness of the treatment is not well established, it is often advisable to forgo potentially toxic therapies, as the hazards often outweigh the benefits.

Many of the immunologically mediated renal diseases (e.g., membranous nephropathy, Wegener's disease, Goodpasture's syndrome, lupus nephritis) may respond to treatment with corticosteroids, cytotoxic agents, or plasmapheresis. For others, there is no proven effective therapy (e.g., immunoglobulin A nephropathy, membranoproliferative glomerulo-

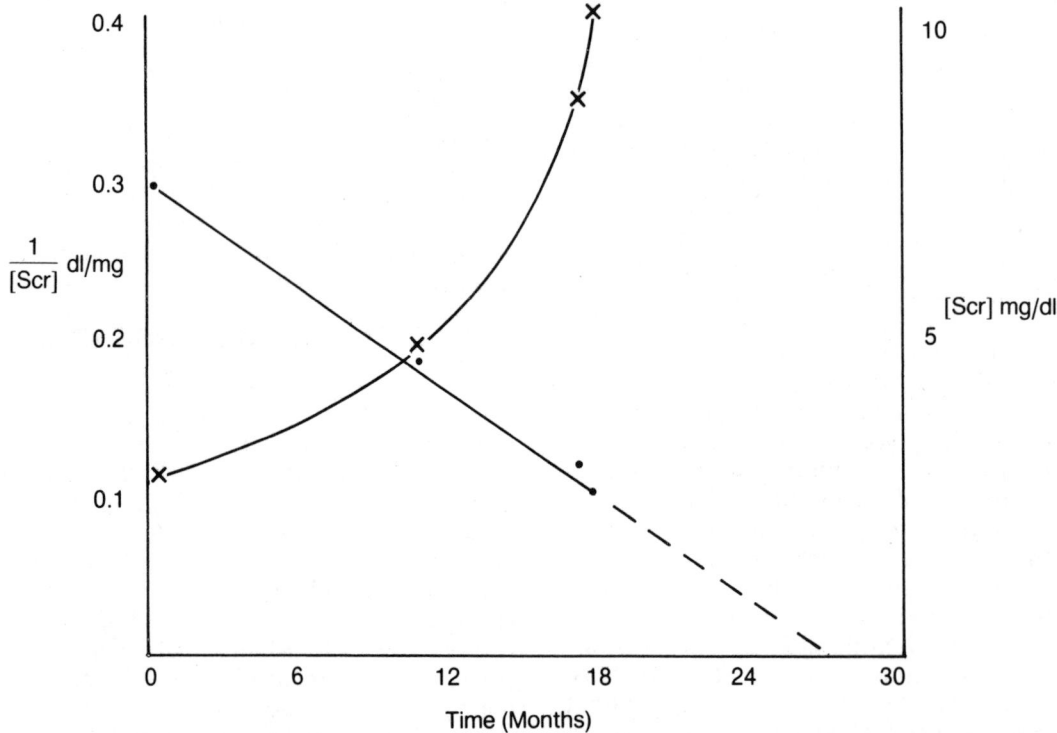

Figure 47.4.   The relationship between serum creatinine concentration ([*Scr*]) and the reciprocal of serum creatinine concentration (*l*/[*Scr*]) over time in a patient during an 18-month period. The linear relationship between the reciprocal of serum creatinine concentration over time suggests that nephrons are being lost at a constant rate. This kind of plot can also be used to monitor the course of renal failure. By extending the line derived from observed data it is possible to make a rough estimate (– – –) as to when dialysis will be necessary. [Scr] = ×—×; $\frac{1}{[Scr]}$ = ·—··

nephritis). Those patients with immunologically mediated renal diseases who require therapy should be under the care of a rheumatologist or nephrologist.

When the renal disease is associated with a metabolic disorder, such as occurs in gout or diabetes mellitus, it is reasonable to treat the underlying abnormality (e.g., hyperuricemia, hyperglycemia). Treatment directed at metabolic control may slow the course of renal deterioration, but it is not likely to result in significant reversal of established disease. In fact, the cause and effect relationship between hyperuricemia and renal failure in patients with gout is debatable (19).

When a drug (e.g., methicillin, indomethacin) or other toxic substance (e.g., heavy metal) is identified as the cause of renal failure, the offending agent should be withheld or avoided. A trial of corticosteroids may be given to patients with drug-induced interstitial nephritis, but this treatment is still controversial and the decision should be made in conjunction with a nephrologist.

It has been demonstrated that the vascular lesions in the kidney due to malignant hypertension may resolve slowly and usually only partially with control of blood pressure. In some patients this will correlate with significant improvement in the GFR.

Obstructing lesions of the urinary tract may require surgical excision (e.g., benign prostatic hypertrophy) or urinary diversion (e.g., retroperitoneal fibrosis) in order to preserve or improve renal function. Other patients can be managed more conservatively (e.g., intermittent straight catheterization of the bladder) if the lesion is not amenable to surgical therapy (e.g., neurogenic bladder).

Treating Reversible Causes of Deterioration of Renal Function

Progressive deterioration in renal function may be due to continued disease activity or intercurrent insults to the kidney. Therefore, before any change in serum creatinine concentration is attributed to the natural progression of the underlying renal disease, several alternative possibilities should be considered (Table 47.4).

Table 47.4.
Causes of Renal Functional Deterioration

Volume depletion (salt and water depletion)
Congestive heart failure
Drug nephrotoxicity
Ureteral or urethral obstruction
Orthostatic hypotension
Microcrystal deposition (*e.g.*, acute hyperuricemia)
Hyperphosphatemia-hypercalcemia
Hypertension
Radiocontrast materials (oral and parenteral)
Glomerular hyperperfusion

Extracellular volume depletion is probably the most common cause for a fall in GFR. It may be related to an intercurrent illness associated with anorexia, fever, gastrointestinal losses of sodium and water, excessive salt restriction, or diuretic use. The usual clinical signs of volume depletion (e.g., low jugular venous pressure, orthostatic hypotension, tachycardia, and decreased skin turgor) may be absent, and a therapeutic trial of salt administration may be required to establish the diagnosis. Weight loss between office visits is usually the most important diagnostic clue to the presence of volume depletion. The urinary sodium concentration or urine osmolality, usually helpful in establishing the diagnosis of volume depletion, are of little value in the patient with chronic renal failure since concentrating and salt-conserving ability in these patients is often impaired.

Patients with decompensated *congestive heart failure* may also present with superimposed prerenal azotemia. Optimal treatment of heart failure may improve renal function in these patients (see Chapter 61).

Drugs given for treatment of various other disorders can be related to worsening of renal failure (Table 47.3). A careful review of both prescribed and over-the-counter medications is, therefore, necessary whenever assessing unexpected changes in kidney function. It should be noted that ibuprofen (Advil) is now available without a prescription. Of the drugs prescribed in the ambulatory setting, diuretics and nonsteroidal anti-inflammatory agents (NSAIDs) are probably the most common offenders. Diuretics can aggravate pre-existing renal failure by inducing intravascular volume depletion, and less commonly by producing an interstitial nephritis. Careful monitoring of the blood pressure, weight, BUN, and serum creatinine concentration will help to detect early signs of prerenal azotemia in patients receiving diuretics. Withholding diuretic therapy for several days usually allows intravascular volume and GFR to return to baseline values. The NSAIDs can also cause a deterioration in kidney function either by causing a reversible reduction of renal blood flow or by producing an interstitial nephritis. At this time it cannot be said that one nonsteroidal compound is safer to use in the patient with renal insufficiency than another. It is, therefore, best to avoid them altogether once the GFR is less than 50 ml/minute.

Obstruction, because of its reversibility, should always be considered in patients with a fall in the GFR. This is particularly true in elderly men predisposed to prostatic hypertrophy or in diabetics who may have autonomic neuropathy affecting bladder emptying. Drugs that reduce bladder tone (e.g., antidepressants, antispasmodics, and antiparkinsonian drugs with anticholinergic properties) should always be considered as causes of obstruction. If obstruction is a consideration, the patient should be tested for a postvoid residual (see Chapter 6 for technique).

Hypertension, present in many patients with renal insufficiency, may also aggravate pre-existing kidney failure. Although treatment of hypertension may produce a transient worsening of kidney function, long term control of hypertension slows the progression of renal insufficiency (see Chapter 62).

Orthostatic hypotension, due to drugs or to autonomic neuropathy, can cause a worsening of renal failure. Drugs, and other causes of this problem, are summarized in Table 81.7. Orthostatic hypotension should be managed by adjusting or stopping the drugs and/or prescribing the practical measures summarized in Table 84.8.

Microcrystal deposition in the kidneys has been suggested by some as a cause of progressive deterioration in patients with azotemia. Serum uric acid concentrations are often elevated in patients with renal insufficiency. There is no evidence, however, that reducing the serum uric acid concentration will prevent further deterioration when the original kidney disease was not due to gout. Allopurinol is not used therefore unless it is needed to control symptomatic gout. Several experiments have shown that restriction of phosphorus intake may prevent progression of renal insufficiency, possibly by preventing a rise in the calcium/phosphorus ratio that can lead to renal calcification.

Once a certain level of renal impairment has been attained, further deterioration seems to be inevitable, even when the original insult is transient and when other causes of additional damage have been excluded. An excellent example of this phenomenon is the course of renal disease following ureteral reimplantation in patients with vesicoureteral reflux and mild renal insufficiency. Even in the absence of continuing reflex or infection, some of these patients will, in time, develop proteinuria and progressive renal insufficiency. Renal biopsies in these patients have revealed the lesion of glomerulosclerosis.

The mechanism that has been postulated to explain the progressive nature of renal disease is related to the "adaptive" changes that occur in the kidney following irreversible nephron injury (5). According to this hypothesis, following a reduction in nephron mass, renal vasodilatation occurs and leads to hyperperfusion of the remaining nephrons. These changes are considered to be adaptive because they result in increased glomerular filtration rates. However, experiments have shown that this state of *hyperperfusion*, if sustained, can in itself be harmful (Fig. 47.5). Glomeruli of nephrons exposed to prolonged hyperperfusion become sclerotic, begin to

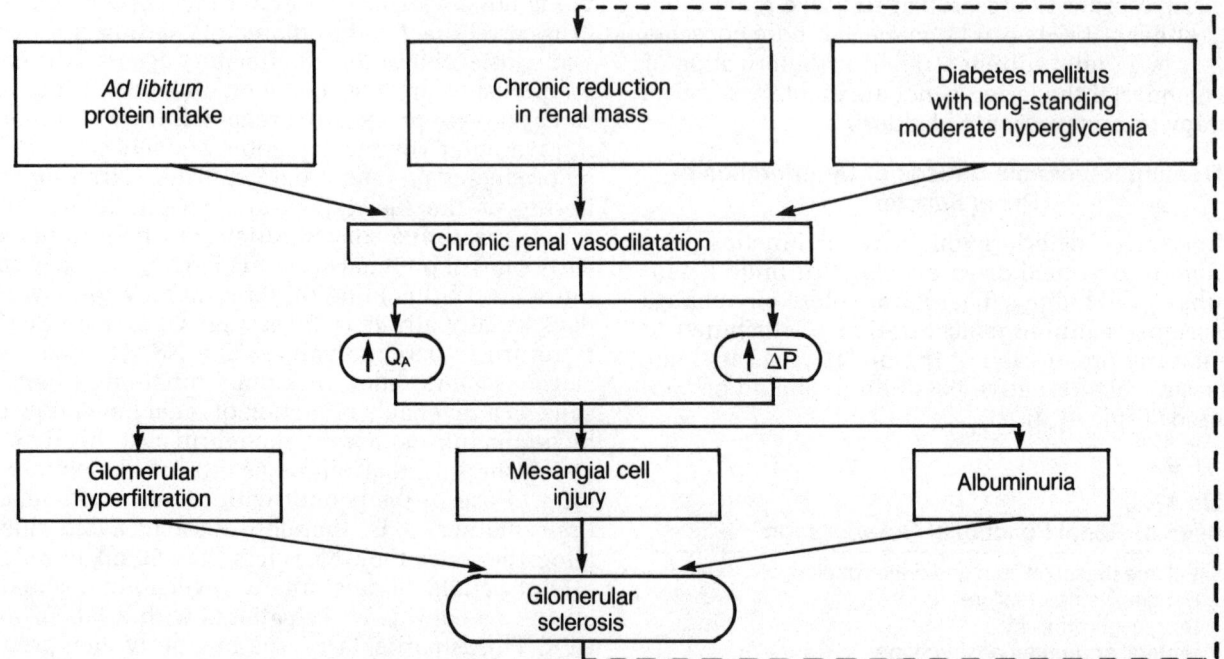

Figure 47.5. The proposed sequence of events whereby a chronic reduction in kidney mass and the consequent increase in glomerular pressures and flows leads to progressive renal damage. Q_A, blood flow; $\overline{\Delta P}$, transcapillary hydraulic pressure. (Redrawn from Brenner BM, Meyer TW, Hostetter TH: Dietary protein intake and the progressive nature of kidney disease: the role of hemodynamically mediated glomerular injury in the pathogenesis of progressive glomerular sclerosis, aging, renal ablation, and intrinsic renal disease. *N Engl J Med* 307:652, 1982.)

leak protein, and eventually are destroyed. As more and more nephrons are lost, the stimulus for hyperperfusion of the residual nephrons is increased and the process becomes self-perpetuating. Evidence is gathering that many diseases that produce limited kidney damage (e.g., patchy cortical necrosis, analgesic nephropathy, radiation nephritis) may progress to end-stage disease by this mechanism. Fortunately, experiments have shown that the degree of hyperperfusion can be attenuated by the limitation of protein intake in the diet. This observation has led to the hypothesis that dietary restriction of protein (see below) in patients with chronic progressive renal diseases may be able to slow or halt the deterioration of kidney function that until now seemed to be inevitable.

Dietary Management

The major goals of dietary management in the patient with chronic renal insufficiency are to optimize intravascular volume, correct electrolyte abnormalities, relieve uremic symptoms, and prevent or slow the progression of kidney disease (Table 47.5).

The volume of the intravascular space is directly related to salt balance, which is in turn regulated by the kidney. As renal function declines, the ability of the kidney to maintain salt balance in response to changes in sodium intake becomes limited, especially when the changes occur abruptly. The intravascular volume may be depleted if the intake of

Table 47.5.
Dietary Management of Renal Failure

Therapy	Goals
Salt 4–6 g/day	Maintain intravascular volume
Fluid 1–3 liters/day	Avoid dehydration
Potassium if [K] > 5.5 mEq/liter restrict intake to 2–2.4 g/day	Prevent hyperkalemia
Protein Restrict intake to 0.55–0.6 g/kg/day (50% rich in essential amino acids)	Relieve uremic symptoms Retard progression of renal failure
Calories provide 35–45 kcal/kg/day	Maintain nutrition
Calcium provide 1–1.5 g/day	Maintain [Ca] = 9–10 mg/dl
Vitamins multivitamin + folate	Replace vitamins lacking in protein-restricted diet
Phosphorus restrict intake to 600–900 mg/day	Prevent secondary hyperparathyroidism

salt is reduced (e.g., excessive salt restriction, anorexia) or if there are losses of salt (e.g., vomiting, diarrhea, diuretics). A reduction in intravascular volume can lead to a further increase in the BUN and serum creatinine concentrations above the baseline values (prerenal azotemia). Conversely, the intravascular volume will increase if the intake of salt is suddenly augmented (dietary indiscretion) and the patient can develop hypertension, edema, and/or heart failure.

Most patients with chronic renal insufficiency maintain sodium balance on a 4- to 6-g *salt* intake. Patients with congestive heart failure or hypertension may need further limitation of salt intake (2 g of salt), whereas the rare patient with severe "salt-wasting" nephropathy may require salt supplements to prevent volume depletion. Most of these latter patients have some form of interstitial renal disease.

Salt intake should be adjusted so as to maintain intravascular volume at the level that maximizes the GFR for any given degree of renal failure. Assessing the state of the intravascular volume can be aided by obtaining serial body weights (rapid changes in weight are usually due to fluid gains or losses), by the physical examination (e.g., orthostatic change of pulse and blood pressure, jugular venous pressure, skin turgor, edema), and by measuring changes in the BUN and serum creatinine concentrations (increases in the level of BUN are proportionately greater than that of the serum creatinine concentration in states of volume depletion). It is often useful to establish an "*ideal*" weight. This is the weight at which the patient has optimal renal function without overt signs of volume overload. For some patients, those with congestive heart failure or nephrotic syndrome, for example, a small amount of edema is acceptable, since worsening of azotemia may develop when further diuresis is attempted. Whenever there is a significant change in the GFR, the state of the intravascular volume and the ideal weight should be re-evaluated.

When the glomerular filtration rate falls as a result of volume depletion, it is necessary to restore the intravascular volume. This can be accomplished either by adding salt to the diet or by prescribing sodium chloride (600 mg four times a day) or sodium bicarbonate tablets (600 mg four times a day) until the patient's weight and GFR return to baseline values. If oral replacement is not practical (e.g., persistent vomiting) the patient should be hospitalized for intravenous therapy.

If volume overload develops or persists despite salt restriction, diuretics can be used to increase salt excretion (Table 47.6). Since the thiazide diuretics, with the exception of metalazone (Zaroxalyn), lose their effectiveness when the GFR falls below 30 ml/minute, it is often necessary to use a loop diuretic, such as furosemide (Lasix) or bumetanide (Bumex).

Table 47.6.
Diuretics in Renal Failure

Drug	Dose	Route of Excretion	Comments
Thiazides (Hydrochlorthiazide)	50–200 mg/day	Renal	May induce volume depletion and hyperuricemia. Loses effectiveness if GFR < 30 ml/minute but may be used in combination with loop diuretics in advanced renal failure.
Metalozone (Zaroxalyn)	5–20 mg/day	Renal	May induce volume depletion and hyperuricemia. Effective when GFR > 10.
Furosemide (Lasix)	20–400 mg/day	Renal	May induce volume depletion and hyperuricemia. Effective when GFR > 5. May produce ototoxicity and rarely interstitial nephritis. May increase nephrotoxicity of antibiotics.
Bumetanide (Bumex)	1–10 mg/day	Renal	May induce volume depletion and hyperuricemia. Side effects include ototoxicity and muscle pains and may also increase the risk of antibiotic nephrotoxicity.
Ethacrynic acid (Edecrin)	Avoid	Hepatic	Usually avoided in renal failure since the risk of ototoxicity is significantly higher than with furosemide or bumetanide.
Spironolactone (Aldactone) Triamterene (Dyrenium) Amiloride (Moduretic)	Avoid	Hepatic	Avoid when GFR < 50 ml/minute due to the risk of inducing serious hyperkalemia.

Another loop diuretic, ethacrynic acid (Edecrin), has been associated with an unacceptable level of ototoxicity and should not be used in patients with renal insufficiency. The potassium-sparing diuretics spironolactone (Aldactone), triamterene (Dyrenium), and amiloride (Moduretic) are also best avoided in patients with significant renal failure, due to the risk of inducing serious hyperkalemia.

Potassium restriction is usually unnecessary until the late stages of renal failure (GFR < 15 ml/minute), except in the small number of patients with the syndrome of hyporeninemic-hypoaldosteronism (see below), but careful monitoring of serum potassium levels is indicated nonetheless. If hyperkalemia develops, potassium restriction to between 2 and 2.4 g/day (40 to 50 mEq) is necessary. This can generally be accomplished by instructing the patient to reduce the intake of fresh fruits, citrus juices, beans, and vegetables (see also Chapter 45, Table 45.2, for a list of the potassium content of common foods). Patients who are on sodium-restricted diets must also be informed that many salt substitutes are unacceptable because they are often composed of potassium salts.

The association of hyperkalemia and hyperchloremic metabolic acidosis in patients with mild to moderate renal insufficiency (GFR > 25 ml/minute) should lead one to consider the presence of the *hyporenin-hypoaldosterone* syndrome (16). This syndrome occurs most frequently in azotemic patients with hypertension, diabetes mellitus, or interstitial nephritis. This disorder probably has many causes, but it is due in part to a suppression of the renin-aldosterone axis. The diagnosis is usually made on clinical grounds, after excluding other reasons for hyperkalemia (e.g., high potassium intake or drugs

that reduce the renal excretion of potassium), but can be more firmly estabished by the demonstration of a low plasma renin concentration that fails to rise after stimulating the patient with furosemide (Lasix), 40 mg orally, and upright posture for 2 hours. The patient should also have no evidence of glucocorticoid deficiency (random cortisol concentration of 15 to 25 μg/ml; see also Chapter 74). Since, in the absence of aldosterone, potassium excretion by the kidney is dependent on an adequate urine flow rate (1.5 to 2 liters/day), patients with this syndrome are at risk for developing severe hyperkalemia during periods of salt restriction or of volume depletion. Normotensive patients may be treated with a mineralocorticoid (fluorohydrocortisone (Florinef), 0.1 mg tablets, ½ to 1 tablet/day). Alternatively, if hypertension is present or develops following the administration of the mineralocorticoid, the patient may be treated with a combination of furosemide (Lasix) (40 to 80 mg twice a day) plus sodium bicarbonate (600 mg four times a day). The furosemide is used to promote a good urine flow rate, whereas the sodium bicarbonate helps to prevent salt depletion and also is of use in correcting the associated metabolic acidosis. The goal of therapy is to keep the serum potassium concentration within the normal range. Since therapy is frequently complicated, these patients are best managed in conjunction with a nephrologist or endocrinologist.

Although diluting and concentrating abilities are impaired in renal failure, most patients are able to ingest 1 to 3 liters of fluid/day without developing hyponatremia. If hyponatremia occurs, fluids should be limited to less than 1.5 liters/day in order to prevent water intoxication.

Protein-restricted diets are indicated for patients

with advanced renal failure (GFR < 15 ml/minute) who develop nausea, vomiting, or other symptoms attributable to uremia. Since many of the end products of protein metabolism have been implicated in the causation of the uremic syndrome, therapy consists of reducing protein intake to about 0.6 g/kg of body weight/day (approximately 40 g of protein/day in a 70-kg individual). Normal protein intake in the United States exceeds 70 g/day. Half of the protein intake should be in the form of meats, fish, eggs, or milk, since these foods are rich in essential amino acids. In order for the patient on a protein-restricted diet to maintain adequate nutritional balance, total caloric intake must be adjusted to provide 35 to 45 kcal/kg/day. This can be accomplished by increasing the intake of fats and carbohydrates.

Since protein-restricted diets are often deficient in *vitamins*, *calcium*, and *phosphorus*, patients should receive a daily vitamin supplement (e.g., Pramilet) and 1 to 1.5 g of elemental calcium/day (a single 600-mg calcium carbonate tablet provides 250 mg of elemental calcium). The reduction in dietary phosphorus is desirable (see below), and therefore phosphorus supplements are not given.

If symptoms such as nausea and vomiting related to uremia persist or the clearance falls below 5 ml/minute, the patient should be started on dialysis. Further restriction of protein intake is possible, but should only be attempted for limited periods and under the direct supervision of a nephrologist. With the present availability of dialysis, little is to be gained by trying to maintain a very symptomatic patient on a highly restricted diet. Proper planning for patients with progressive renal disease should prevent referral of debilitated, malnourished, and neuropathic patients to a dialysis center.

There is currently considerable interest among nephrologists about the use of protein-restricted diets to retard the progression of renal disease in order to delay or even obviate the need for dialysis (4). Protein restriction has been shown in experiments to reduce the degree of compensatory hypertrophy following renal injury and to forestall the development of glomerular sclerosis, proteinuria, and progressive renal failure (see page 554). Several studies have been published describing the effects of various protein-restricted diets, with or without concomitant phosphorus restriction, on the course of patients with renal insufficiency (serum creatinine concentration between 2 and 6 mg/dl) (13, 14). The results of these studies lend support to the hypothesis that protein restriction can, in fact, slow the rate of renal deterioration ordinarily expected in this group of patients (Fig. 47.6). Further studies are needed to clarify the exact indications, the time of initiation, the composition, and the potential long term benefits/complications of protein-restricted diets. Nevertheless, it seems reasonable, in the absence of more specific therapy, to advise patients with moderate renal insufficiency (serum creatinine

between 2 and 6 mg/dl) to reduce their protein intakes to about 40 g/day (13).

Considering the complexity of such diets and the need for individualization of salt, mineral, protein and potassium intake, consultation with a dietician or a nephrologist proficient in prescribing renal diets is suggested. Constant encouragement and supervision of dietary therapy are needed. The success of dietary treatment often depends on the involvement of family members as well as an enthusiastic dietician.

Calcium and Phosphorus

Renal osteodystrophy is a general term that encompasses osteitis fibrosa, osteomalacia, and a variety of other bone lesions that occur in patients with kidney failure. The pathophysiological factors that lead to osteodystrophy originate in the early stages of renal failure, although clinical manifestations generally do not develop until the patient is on dialysis.

The pathophysiology of renal osteodystrophy is complex but can be briefly summarized as follows. PTH secretion increases during the early stages of renal failure (GFR > 30 ml/minute) for two major reasons: (a) to keep the serum phosphorus concentration within normal limits; PTH acts to increase the rate of phosphorus excretion by the remaining nephrons and thereby prevents the rise in serum phosphorus concentration that would otherwise occur during the course of renal failure; (b) to maintain a normal serum calcium concentration. Small, but significant, decreases in serum-ionized calcium concentrations can result from equally small increases in the serum phosphorus level as well as from diminished gastrointestinal absorption of calcium. Decreased calcium absorption in renal failure is predominantly a consequence of an intestinal defect (related to vitamin D deficiency), but may in part be due to diminished intake because of anorexia or protein restriction. PTH serves to maintain serum calcium concentrations in the normal range largely by mobilizing calcium from the bones.

The increased rate of PTH secretion is successful at keeping serum calcium and phosphorus levels within the normal range until the GFR is less than 30 ml/minute. In more advanced renal failure hypocalcemia and hyperphosphatemia develop. The most important consequence of prolonged *secondary hyperparathyroidism* is the development of bone disease (osteitis fibrosa cystica).

Osteomalacia, in renal insufficiency, is due partly to the failure of the diseased kidney to convert 25-hydroxyvitamin D_3 to its more active form, 1,25-dihydroxyvitamin D_3. The active form of vitamin D is necessary for normal bone mineralization. Although the serum levels of vitamin D are normal in patients with GFRs above 30 ml/minute (since this level is not elevated), this state may represent a relative deficiency of the hormone. Absolute defi-

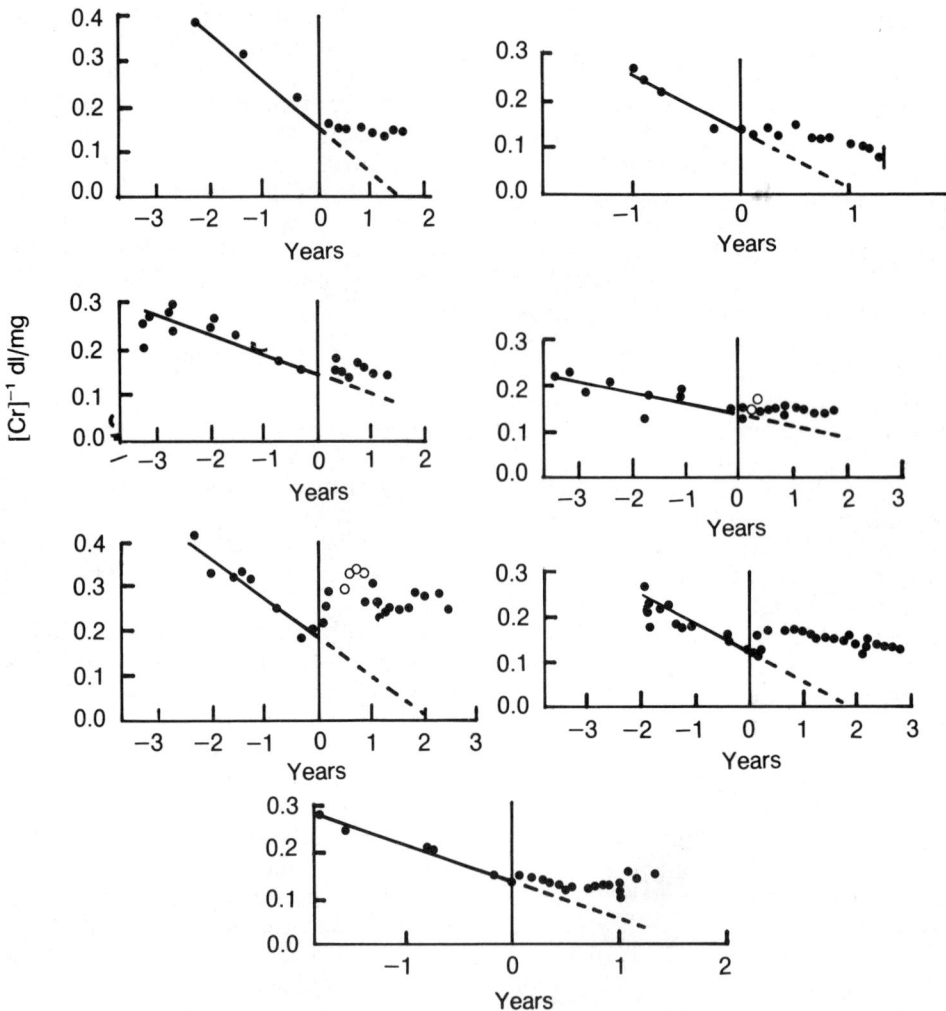

Figure 47.6. Data showing how the rate of progression of renal failure, as determined by a plot of the reciprocal of serum creatinine concentration over time, in seven different patients, was affected by the institution at time 0 of a low phosphorus, low protein diet. A decrease in the slope reflects stabilization of renal function. The *dashed line* indicates the projected course. (Data redrawn from Mitch WM, Walser M, Steinman TI, *et al*: Effect of a keto acid-amino acid supplement to a restricted diet on the progression of chronic renal failure. *N Engl J Med* 311:623, 1984.)

ciencies of vitamin D are found once the GFR falls below 30 ml/minute. Abnormal collagen synthesis, the titration of bone buffers, and the accumulation of aluminum in the bone matrix have also been implicated in the pathogenesis of osteomalacia.

Patients with renal insufficiency should have periodic (see above for frequency) measurements of calcium, phosphorus, magnesium, and alkaline phosphatase. Routine measurements of PTH levels are not indicated unless the patient is hypercalcemic, since virtually all patients with renal insufficiency will have increased levels. Levels of PTH, when measured by the carboxy-terminal assay, will be uniformly high, since the kidney is responsible for the elimination of that fragment. Therefore, determination of PTH levels, when necessary, should

be by an assay that measures the intact or N-terminal hormone. Bone X-rays or biopsies are not routinely obtained in the patient not yet on dialysis, unless the patient has symptomatic bone disease.

The clinical features of deranged calcium and phosphorus metabolism, including bone pain, fractures, and proximal myopathy, are not often seen until after the patient is on dialysis. Nevertheless, therapy to correct these abnormalities should begin during the early stages of renal failure (Table 47.7).

Based on a knowledge of calcium, phosphorus, and vitamin D alterations in early renal insufficiency described above, it is possible to outline a plan of therapy directed at reducing the incidence and severity of renal osteodystrophy in late renal insufficiency. The goals of therapy are to limit the

Table 47.7.
Steps in the Management of Calcium and Phosphorus Balance in Patients with Renal Failure

Therapy	Goals
GFR 50–30 ml/minute	
Calcium supplements (1–1.5 g/day) (see text)	Maintain serum calcium concentration at 9–10 mg/dl
Vitamin D (Rocaltrol 0.25–1.0 μg/day)	Maintain serum calcium concentration at 9–10 mg/dl
GFR < 30 ml/minute	
Restrict phosphorus intake (600 mg/day)	Maintain serum phosphorus concentration at 2.5–4.5 mg/dl
Phosphorus-binding antacids (aluminum carbonate or aluminum hydroxide taken with meals)	Maintain serum phosphorus concentration at 2.5–4.5 mg/dl

rise in PTH secretion that usually accompanies renal failure and to prevent the development of osteomalacia. These goals can be achieved by maintaining a positive calcium balance, by providing vitamin D, and by reducing phosphorus intake.

Since *calcium* absorption is diminished in patients with renal insuffiiency, the first step in treatment is to assure an adequate intake of calcium. This is particularly important if the patient is on a protein-restricted diet that often contains only 300 to 400 mg of calcium (normal calcium intake is 800 to 1000 mg/day). Supplements in the form of calcium carbonate (generic), 600 mg four times/day, will provide 1000 mg of elemental calcium/day. Calcium lactate (generic), 300 mg (2 tablets four times/day), can be substituted if the carbonate is not tolerated due to constipation or bloating.

Vitamin D supplementation in patients with GFRs between 50 and 30 ml/minute has been demonstrated to induce positive calcium balance, reduce levels of PTH, and heal bone lesions (11). It is reasonable, therefore, to begin routine vitamin D administration when the GFR falls below 50 ml/minute. One should start at the lowest dose of the vitamin D preparation selected and raise the dose every 4 weeks until the serum calcium is in the upper range of normal. Vitamin D therapy should not be used when serum calcium or phosphorus levels are greater than 10.5 and 6 mg/dl, respectively, because of the possibility of inducing metastatic calcification. If the serum phosphorus level is elevated, as is common in a patient whose GFR is below 30 ml/minute, it is necessary to first reduce the level of phosphorus to normal prior to initiating either calcium or vitamin D therapy (see below). Due to the frequency with which hypercalcemia develops in patients receiving vitamin D preparations, it is suggested that serum calcium levels

be monitored weekly (until the serum calcium concentration stabilizes) following a change of dosage, and monthly thereafter.

The serum phosphorus concentration will often rise following institution of vitamin D therapy because both calcium and phosphorus absorption are increased. If dietary phosphate restriction (600 mg/day) (see below) is not sufficient to maintain serum phosphorus levels within the normal range, phosphate binders must be used (see below). Avoidance of hypercalcemia or hyperphosphatemia by careful monitoring should prevent the fall in GFR reported in some patients with advanced renal insufficiency taking vitamin D.

The form of *vitamin D* used is important since preparations (e.g., vitamin D_2 or D_3) that require final activation by the kidney have proven to be ineffective in the usual doses. The most commonly used vitamin D preparations that do not require renal activation are 1,25-dihydroxyvitamin D_3 (Rocaltrol) and dihydrotachysterol (DHT). When given orally both Rocaltrol (0.25 to 1.0 μg/day) and DHT (0.125 to 0.5 mg/day) are effective in improving calcium absorption and raising serum calcium levels in azotemic patients. Studies comparing the effectiveness of DHT and Rocaltrol have not been performed, although the latter, because it is the native hormone, has possible advantages. Both can produce hypercalcemia, but due to its shorter half-life the hypercalcemia induced by 1,25-dihydroxyvitamin D_3 tends to be of shorter duration. Despite their effectiveness in promoting positive calcium balance, none of the vitamin D sterols has been consistently shown to reverse osteomalacia.

Restriction of dietary phosphorus to 600 to 900 mg/day (normal intake is 1 to 1.8 g/day) should be initiated when the serum phosphorus level first becomes elevated. This degree of phosphorus restriction can be achieved by restricting the intake of protein and dairy products. Despite restriction of phosphorus intake, the serum phosphorus level often becomes elevated when the GFR falls below 30 ml/minute. At this juncture it is necessary to start treatment with phosphate binders. Oral antacids containing aluminum hydroxide (Alternajel or Amphojel) or aluminum carbonate (Basaljel) bind phosphate in the intestine and thereby reduce phosphate absorption. These binders are available in liquid, tablet, and capsule forms. Liquids are the most effective but the least well tolerated preparation (they may produce nausea, bloating, and/or constipation). Stool softeners may be used to counter the constipation but occasionally osmotic laxatives such as lactulose or sorbitol may be required (see Chapter 38). Other medications (Table 47.8) should not be given simultaneously with phosphate binders since their absorption may be adversely affected. The initial dose of antacid should be 1 or 2 tablespoons or tablets/capsules given with meals; the dose

Table 47.8.
Drugs Whose Bioavailability Is Altered by Phosphate Binders

DECREASED
  Digoxin
  Oral anticoagulants
  Tetracycline
  Anticholinergics
  Aspirin
  Chlorpromazine
INCREASED
  Penicillin
  Pseudoephedrine

should be increased (at 2-week intervals) until the serum phosphorus concentration is normal (2.5 to 4.5 mg/dl). Serum phosphorus concentration should be monitored every 1 to 2 months to avoid the syndrome of phosphate depletion (low serum phosphorus) that may result in muscle weakness, osteomalacia, and fractures.

Aluminum-containing antacids should also be used for the treatment of gastritis or ulcers since magnesium toxicity can occur in patients with chronic renal failure who take magnesium-containing antacids, such as Maalox or Mylanta (see also Chapter 36, Table 36.2). However, it has been demonstrated that aluminum from the antacids is absorbed and can accumulate in the brain and bones of a patient with renal failure. This aluminum accumulation has been implicated in the pathogenesis of the *dialysis dementia syndrome* (myoclonus, seizures, and dementia) as well as some forms of osteomalacia that develop in some patients with end-stage renal failure. In patients in whom aluminum-related syndromes are thought to be a problem, calcium carbonate should be used in place of the aluminum-containing antacids.

Acidosis

A mild *hyperchloremic* (*normal anion gap*) *metabolic acidosis* develops commonly in patients with early renal insufficiency. This occurs because production of ammonia by the failing kidney results in the retention of hydrogen and chloride ions. However, the acidosis in moderate renal insufficiency is generally not severe enough (serum bicarbonate > 18 mEq/liter) to warrant therapy. It should be realized that the *hypochloremic* (*with an abnormal anion gap*) *acidosis* commonly associated with renal failure does not generally appear until the GFR has fallen below 20 ml/minute.

A patient whose level of serum bicarbonate has fallen below 18 mEq/liter has a seriously reduced buffer reserve and runs the risk of severe acidosis during periods of stress (e.g., from infection or volume depletion). If protein restriction (see above, page

567), which reduces exogenous acid load, is insufficient to restore buffering capacity, base in the form of sodium bicarbonate, 600 mg four times a day, may be given, provided edema is not a problem. Should sodium bicarbonate not be tolerated because of gastrointestinal complaints (belching and bloatedness), calcium lactate, 300 mg (generic), 2 tablets four times a day, may be given (lactate metabolism results in the generation of bicarbonate). The physician should attempt to maintain the serum bicarbonate level above 18 mEq/liter.

Hypertension

Hypertension (see also Chapter 62) may be the consequence of or the cause of renal failure. Regardless of its etiology, hypertension always requires treatment. Antihypertensive therapy in patients with mild to moderate renal insufficiency is similar to that in patients with normal renal function and hypertension. A salt-restricted diet (e.g., 2 g/day) may be attempted as a first step. Loop diuretics, such as furosemide or bumetanide, can be added when salt restriction is insufficient or when nondiuretic drugs (e.g., Apresoline, captopril) lead to secondary salt retention. Thiazides are generally avoided in patients with GFRs below 30 ml/minute because they often lose their diuretic effect. Potassium-sparing diuretics (spironolactone, triamterene, amiloride) should not be used in patients with significant renal impairment due to the increased risk of developing hyperkalemia.

Methyldopa, hydralazine, prazosin, clonidine, calcium channel blockers, and β-blockers are all useful in patients with chronic renal insufficiency (see Chapter 62). There is no consistent relationship between the pharmacokinetic properties of an antihypertensive drug and its effect on lowering the blood pressure. Therefore, one must titrate the dose to the level of blood pressure. Many vasodilating drugs induce a state of fluid and salt retention and must be used in conjunction with a diuretic in order to be effective. As renal function deteriorates, the use of larger doses of diuretics will often be necessary to control hypertension. There is often a fine line between effective blood pressure control and hypotension when potent diuretics and antihypertensives are being used; therefore, careful monitoring of the blood pressure (both supine and upright) and of serum creatinine concentration is necessary. It is not unusual for patients with hypertensive renal disease to show a temporary decrease in renal function when blood pressure control is instituted, followed by improvement in function. With the use of such potent drugs as minoxidil or captopril (for detailed discussions of these drugs see Chapter 62), bilateral nephrectomy (which results in a severe anemia and the requirement for dialysis) for the treatment of refractory cases of hypertension can generally be avoided. Long term control of hypertension may be important in reducing the risk of atherosclerosis in patients on dialysis.

Anemia

A normochromic, normocytic anemia develops in patients with chronic renal failure, and its severity is proportional to the degree of renal insufficiency (Fig. 47.2). The hematocrit value will generally fall to between 15 and 25% in a patient with advanced renal failure. The anemia of renal failure results mainly from shortened red blood cell survival and an inability of the bone marrow to compensate because of decreased erythropoietin production and/or effect. Other causes of anemia (e.g., iron deficiency) must also be considered.

All patients should be placed on a multivitamin regimen which includes folate, to replace the vitamins lacking in the restrictive diets. Perinatal vitamins (e.g., Pramilet, Stuart-Natal) are often used because they contain both folate and iron. Blood transfusion, when necessary, should not be withheld for fear of sensitizing a potential transplant recipient. Patients who have received multiple blood transfusions have higher rates of retention of functioning transplanted kidneys than do those who have not received transfusions (15). Iron deficiency is almost universal in patients on hemodialysis but may also occur in the predialysis patient, particularly if multiple blood samples have been taken or if there is bleeding. Iron deficiency is best diagnosed in patients with chronic renal failure by measuring the level of serum ferritin. The serum iron and iron-binding capacity are often low in patients with renal failure and are not reliable in establishing the state of iron stores. The values of serum ferritin that are associated with normal iron stores are higher in patients with renal failure than they are in those without kidney disease. Therefore, the laboratory should be consulted in order to interpret serum ferritin levels properly in the uremic individual. The treatment of iron deficiency is the same in azotemic patients as it is in any other patient (see Chapter 49).

Anabolic steroids, which stimulate erythropoietin production, have been shown to be useful in increasing red cell mass in patients on dialysis. Although anabolic steroids may also increase the red blood cell mass slightly in uremic patients not yet on dialysis, they lead to significant side effects, especially severe salt retention, and are therefore not recommended for such patients.

DRUG MANAGEMENT IN RENAL FAILURE

The incidence of adverse drug effects is increased in patients with renal failure, a fact that is largely attributable to the alterations in pharmacokinetics that occur as renal function declines. Adverse drug effects, in this group of patients, can be divided into those that are due to abnormal drug metabolism (e.g., increased incidence of digitalis toxicity) and those that are due to an effect on renal function that is part of the anticipated pharmacological action of the drug (e.g., reduction in GFR with thiazides or nonsteroidal anti-inflammatory drugs (3). In renal failure, drug bioavailability, volume of distribution, and protein binding may be abnormal; however, the most significant derangement is the prolongation of half-life of many drugs or their metabolites. Therefore, it is necessary to have a basic understanding of how a drug's administration should be modified when renal failure is present. This information is available from several sources (1, 2).

Since even over-the-counter preparations (aspirin, ibuprofen, magnesium-containing antacids) have the potential for causing toxicity, patients should be reminded to telephone their physician before using nonprescription drugs. Whenever possible drugs that require no modification of dosage or that do not affect kidney function adversely should be substituted for those with a greater potential for inducing toxicity. The avoidance of drugs with marginal efficacy will help to reduce the frequency of adverse effects.

A complete review of the topic of drug usage in renal failure may be found elsewhere (2). Guidelines are provided below for the drugs most commonly prescribed in ambulatory practice (see Tables 47.9 and 47.10).

Before initiating therapy with a drug that requires dose modification in renal failure, it is necessary to have an accurate estimation of GFR. Predicting the GFR from the serum creatinine level alone is not recommended; rather one should either measure the creatinine clearance directly or use one of the for-

Table 47.9.
Some Commonly Used Drugs That Require Dosage Reduction in Renal Failure (GFR < 30 ml/minute)

Cardiovascular drugs
  Digoxin (Lanoxin)
  Nadolol (Corgard)
  Atenolol (Tenormin)
  Procainamide (Pronestyl)
  Disopyramide (Norpace)
Antihypertensive drugs
  Captopril (Capoten)
  Clonidine (Catapres)
  Guanethidine (Ismelin)
H₂ receptor antagonists
  Cimetidine (Tagamet)
  Ranitidine (Zantac)
Hypoglycemic drugs
  Insulin
Drugs used in the treatment of gout
  Allopurinol (Zyloprim)

Table 47.10.
Some Commonly Used Drugs That Should Be Avoided in Patients with Renal Failure (GFR < 30 ml/minute)

Antimicrobials
  Cephaloridine (Loridine)
  Tetracyclines
  Nitrofurantoin (Macrodantin)
  Nalidixic acid (Negram)
Analgesics
  Aspirin
  Nonsteroidal agents (Motrin, Nalfon, *etc*), meperidine (Demerol)
Diuretics
  Potassium-sparing diuretics (Aldactone, Moduretic, Dyrenium)
  Ethacrynic acid (Edecrin)
  Thiazides (Diuril, *etc*)
Antacids
  Magnesium-containing antacids (Maalox, Mylanta, *etc*)
Hypoglycemic drugs
  Acetohexamide (Dymelor)
  Chlorpropamide (Diabinase)
Drugs used in the treatment of gout
  Phenylbutazone (Butazolidine)
  Sulfinpyrazone (Anturane)
  Probenecid (Benemid)

mulas for estimating GFR, e.g.:

creatinine clearance

$$= \frac{(140 - age) \text{ (body weight in kg)}}{72 \times \text{serum creatinine}}$$

Depending on what modifications are required for a particular drug, an appropriate loading and maintenance dose can be chosen. A loading dose must be given whenever rapid achievement of therapeutic drug levels is desired. Maintenance doses are adjusted either by lengthening the interval between administrations or by reducing the size of each dose. The use of nomograms or tables does not guarantee that adverse drug effects will not occur. The monitoring of serum drug levels is therefore often helpful, particularly when using drugs with low toxic/therapeutic ratios. Finally, the list of drugs should be reviewed periodically and the patient questioned specifically about side effects.

Antimicrobials

When renal impairment is not advanced (GFR > 30 ml/minute), no change is necessary for most of the commonly used antimicrobials in the dosages employed in ambulatory practice (e.g., penicillins, cephalosporins, erythromycin, chloramphenicol). The administration of tetracyclines, however, with the exception of doxycycline, is not recommended in the patient with impaired renal function as these drugs tend to aggravate uremia. When treating uri-

nary tract infections in patients with GFRs below 50 ml/minute the urinary antiseptic drugs, such as nitrofurantoin (Macrodantin) or naladixic acid (Negram), should not be used because they are ineffective and there is an increased risk of systemic toxicity associated with the retention of metabolites. Antimicrobials such as ampicillin and the cephalosporins that are secreted by the renal tubular cells achieve a high urine concentration, even when the glomerular filtration rate is very low. Given without dosage reduction, they are effective in the therapy of urinary tract infections in patients with advanced renal failure. Trimethoprim-sulfamethoxazole in usual doses is also effective in patients with impaired renal function.

Analgesics

The following analgesics require no dosage modification in renal failure: acetaminophen, codeine, pentazocine (Talwin), and propoxyphene (Darvon). Aspirin and all the other NSAIDs should be avoided in patients with a creatinine clearance below 50 ml/minute, as they can cause significant reductions of GFR and/or hyperkalemia (6). The use of meperidine (Demerol) in advanced renal failure is hazardous due to the accumulation of its metabolites, which may induce seizures (even in patients without an underlying seizure disorder).

Sedatives, Hypnotics, and Tranquilizers

In the patient with renal failure, no alteration in dosage is necessary for the benzodiazepines (e.g., Valium, Librium, Dalmane), short acting barbiturates (e.g., Seconol, Nembutal), neuroleptics (e.g., Haldol), phenothiazines (e.g., Thorazine), and tricyclic antidepressants (e.g., Elavil), since all are chiefly metabolized by the liver. However, the phenothiazines and tricyclics must be used with caution since they have significant anticholinergic properties and, accordingly, may cause urinary retention. All of the psychoactive drugs are capable of causing excessive sedation in patients with advanced renal failure.

Antacids and H₂ Receptor Antagonists (See Also Chapter 36)

Many of the commonly prescribed or over-the-counter antacids contain magnesium compounds as a major constituent, and magnesium absorption with toxicity may occur when the GFR falls below 30 ml/minute. Therefore, the patient should be instructed to use antacids that are based on aluminum (as opposed to magnesium). However, there is concern that, with prolonged ingestion, signifiant amounts of aluminum will be absorbed and accumulate in the tissues of patients with renal failure. Although this accumulation has the potential for producing toxicity, there is as yet no satisfactory alternative to the aluminum-containing antacids.

The dosage of the H_2 receptor antagonists, cimetidine and ranitidine, must be reduced to 75% and then 50% as the creatinine clearance falls below 50 and 30 ml/minute, respectively. Both can cause an increase in serum creatinine levels, probably due to inhibition of the tubular secretion of creatinine.

Cardiovascular Drugs
(See Also Chapters 59 and 61)

Both the loading and maintenance doses of digoxin must be reduced once the GFR falls below 50 ml/minute (12). The loading dose of digoxin should be reduced by 75% and the maintenance dose by 50% once the GFR falls below 50 ml/minute. Despite the use of nomograms and the monitoring of drug levels, digoxin toxicity remains a problem in the uremic patient. Therefore, whenever feasible, other treatments for heart failure should be tried before resorting to digoxin.

There are now available to the physician a large variety of β-blocking agents, each with slightly different pharmacological or pharmacokinetic properties. The most important consideration in patients with renal failure is the route of excretion. The dosages of propranolol (Inderal), metoprolol (Lopressor), labetalol (Normodyne), and pindolol (Timolol), which are all metabolized by the liver, are unchanged even in advanced renal failure. Atenolol (Tenormin) and nadolol (Corgard) are both excreted largely by the kidney, but can still be used effectively in patients with renal failure by initiating treatment at 50% of the customary dose. All β-blocking agents should be used with caution in patients with impaired renal function as they reduce cardiac output and may thereby aggravate azotemia.

The dosage interval should be increased by 2- to 4-fold when giving procainamide (Pronestyl) and disopyramide (Norpace) to avoid toxicity in patients with renal failure. Monitoring blood levels of the drug, and in the case of procainamide, its active metabolite (N-acetylprocainamide), is important in guiding therapy. Quinidine does not require dosage modification, even in advanced renal failure.

The use of antihypertensive drugs in patients with renal failure is discussed in Chapter 62, Table 62.7.

Hypoglycemic Agents (See Also Chapter 80)

The half-life of insulin is prolonged in renal failure, and therefore attention to dosage is required in the diabetic with developing renal insufficiency in order to avoid hypoglycemia. Except for tolbutamide, the oral hypoglycemic agents (acetohexamide, chlorpropamide) have active metabolites that accumulate in renal failure and may produce prolonged hypoglycemia. Therefore, non-insulin-dependent diabetic patients taking oral hypoglycemic agents should be converted to tolbutamide once the GFR falls below 50 ml/minute.

Anticonvulsants

The dose of phenytoin (Dilantin) is essentially unchanged in renal failure since an increased volume of distribution and a shortened half-life are offset by reduced protein binding. Since the unbound fraction of phenytoin is increased, the therapeutic and toxic effects of Dilantin occur at lower levels in patients with renal failure than they do in patients without kidney disease (Fig. 47.7).

Drugs Used in the Treatment of Gout

Colchicine may be used for the prophylactic treatment of symptomatic gout in usual dosages (0.6 to 1.2 mg/day). The dose of allopurinol must be reduced to 200 mg/day in patients with GFRs below 50 ml/minute and to 100 mg/day when the GFR is below 30 ml/minute. The uricosuric agents probenecid (Benemid) and sulfinpyrazone (Anturane) are ineffective when the GFR falls below 50 ml/minute and should therefore not be used. Phenylbutazone (Butazolidin) should not be used in patients whose GFRs are below 50 ml/minute since it can cause sodium retention and also because many of its active metabolites depend on renal excretion. Indomethacin (Indocin) is almost entirely metabolized by the liver, and therefore it does not accumulate in patients with even advanced renal failure. However, patients who receive indomethacin for the treatment of acute gout must have their BUN and serum creatinine concentrations monitored carefully, as indomethacin can cause a transient worsening of renal function.

CHRONIC RENAL FAILURE AND COEXISTING DISORDERS

Nonrenal diseases often occur in patients with uremia. In some, such as patients with systemic lupus erythematosus or diabetes mellitus, the renal disease is part of a generalized illness that affects many other organ systems. Others may have diseases unrelated to the kidneys, such as coronary artery disease, chronic obstructive pulmonary disease, or malignancy. The coexistence of multiple disorders often complicates management. For example, angina in patients with coronary artery disease may be aggravated by the anemia of chronic renal failure.

Diabetes Mellitus

Up to 50% of insulin-dependent diabetics and a substantial portion of non-insulin-dependent diabetics develop chronic renal failure, and patients with diabetes account for up to 30% of many dialysis populations. The mechanism whereby diabetes affects the kidney is predominantly through a microvasculopathy producing nodular glomerulosclerosis. In man a relationship between poor glucose control

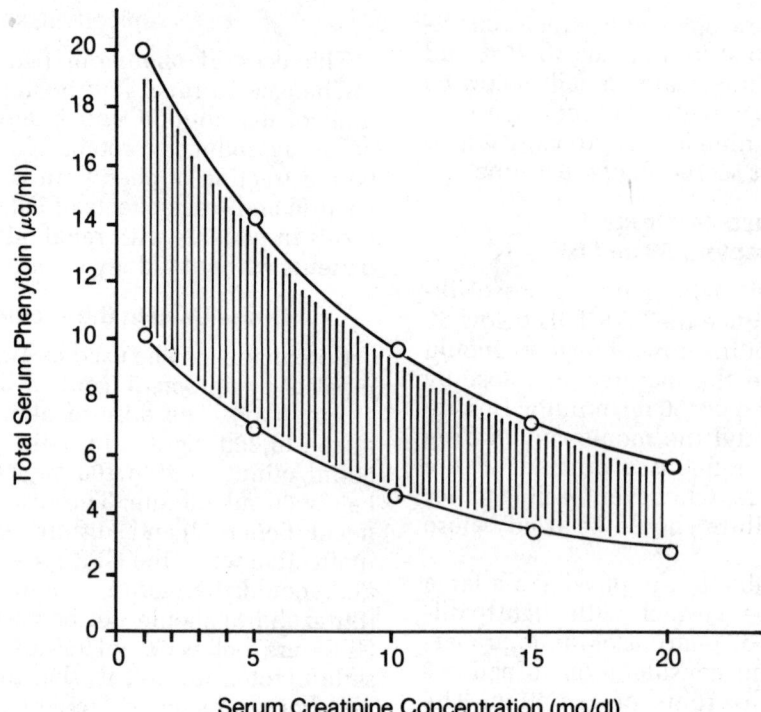

Figure 47.7. The range of total serum phenytoin concentrations in patients with varying degrees of renal failure that provide therapeutic levels of free drug. (Redrawn from Reidenberg NM, Affrime M: Influence of disease on binding of drugs to plasma proteins. *Ann NY Acad Sci* 226:115, 1973.)

and the development and progression of renal disease is suspected but has not been unequivocally established (Chapter 72). It has been suggested that the increased GFR and renal blood flow seen during the early stages of diabetic nephropathy may have pathophysiological significance (Fig. 47.5). This state of renal hyperperfusion, in part, can be reversed with strict glucose control. Control of systemic hypertension in the later stages of diabetic nephropathy has also been shown to reduce the rate of renal deterioration. The onset of renal disease (in type I diabetes) usually develops after 10 to 15 years of diabetes and is initially manifest by proteinuria. Renal insufficiency soon follows, and there is usually a rapid decline in kidney function leading to end-stage renal failure within another 1 to 2 years. The natural history for patients with type II diabetes has not been as well defined.

Renal disease may reduce the requirement for insulin, an effect related at least in part to decreased hormone degradation in the renal tubules as nephrons are progressively lost. Some oral hypoglycemic agents, notably chlorpropamide and acetohexamide, also have prolonged half-lives in uremic patients. As a consequence of these pharmacological abnormalities, the first overt manifestation of renal disease in some diabetics is the occurrence of hypoglycemia. Therefore, the dose of insulin or oral hypoglycemic drugs should be regularly assessed in the patient with renal impairment.

Diabetes, *per se*, is not a contraindication to performing dialysis or transplantation, although the course of diabetics is more complicated than that of patients with isolated renal failure. The form of therapy best suited for these patients with end-stage renal failure is uncertain. Hemodialysis, peritoneal dialysis, and transplantation each have proponents. The diabetic patient should be reminded that dialysis and transplantation are supportive therapies for renal dysfunction and will not improve their diabetes. The referring physician should also remember that the course of these patients is less favorable than that of patients with kidney disease without diabetes (see below, "Dialysis and Transplantation"). The microvasculopathy that destroys the kidney also affects the retinal and peripheral vessels. Since blindness and peripheral vascular disease are important causes of morbidity and mortality in the dialysis and transplant population, it is critical for these patients to have appropriate attention to eye (see Chapter 72) and foot (see Chapter 102) (10).

Heart Disease

Patients with congestive heart failure and/or angina often require more frequent monitoring as renal function declines. Diuretics may lose their effectiveness, or as anemia worsens patients with ischemic heart disease may become more symptomatic. In this situation transfusions are often necessary if there has been an inadequate response to antianginal therapy.

Patients with renal failure have been noted to have an accelerated rate of atherogenesis. This may be explained by the presence of hypertension, glucose intolerance, hypertriglyceridemia, and reduced levels of high density lipoproteins in this group of patients.

Malignancy

Renal failure is not an uncommon occurrence in patients dying with a malignancy as a result of hypercalcemia, sepsis, or drug nephrotoxicity. In many of these patients it would be inappropriate to prolong their lives by initiating dialysis. However, patients with multiple myeloma or other neoplasms that may have a good prognosis might benefit from dialysis. Dialyzing patients with neoplastic diseases should be recommended, therefore, only after careful discussion with the patient, his family, an oncologist, and a nephrologist.

SYMPTOMATIC THERAPY OF ADVANCED RENAL FAILURE

Patients with advanced renal failure (GFR < 10 ml/minute) invariably develop a variety of uremic symptoms. Gastrointestinal disturbances, such as nausea, anorexia, and vomiting, are frequent. Treatment involves further restriction of protein (see page 556), and/or antiemetics (e.g. Compazine). Itching is often a bothersome problem of unknown etiology. Reduction of serum phosphorus to normal levels, skin lubricants (see Chapter 100), and antihistamines (e.g., Benadryl, 25 to 50 mg four times/day) are all worth 1- to 3-week trial periods. Ultraviolet light therapy may also be helpful, but this requires consultation with a dermatologist performing this form of therapy. Fatigue, dyspnea, and chest pain may be due to worsening anemia or volume overload and should respond to blood transfusions or diuretics. Neuromuscular symptoms, such as myoclonus, restless legs, and disturbed sleep, are signs of advanced uremia and should serve as warnings that more severe abnormalities (e.g. seizures, coma) may soon develop. The persistence of these symptoms despite the best conservative medical management is an indication for dialysis regardless of the BUN or serum creatinine concentration. Although there are no absolute laboratory criteria defining the time at which dialysis should be initiated, a serum creatinine concentration of greater than 10 to 12 mg/dl or a creatinine clearance of less than 5 ml/minute is commonly accepted as an indication. Delay in starting dialysis can lead to patients developing severe peripheral neuropathy, malnutrition, and/or pericarditis from which complete recovery might not be possible.

DIALYSIS AND TRANSPLANTATION

In 1983 over 70,000 patients were being maintained on dialysis in the United States. Most facilities provide hemodialysis, peritoneal dialysis, and transplantation (or referral to a transplant center) for patients with end-stage renal failure (Table 47.11). Either form of dialysis therapy can be performed at a center or at the patient's home. Some patients will choose dialysis as a permanent form of treatment, while others will undergo dialysis temporarily until they receive a kidney transplant. Although dialysis does not correct all of the metabolic abnormalities of chronic renal failure, it has enabled thousands of patients to lead productive lives.

Hemodialysis

The hemodialysis procedure involves circulating the patient's blood through a machine that corrects electrolyte abnormalities and has the capability of removing excess fluid and toxic metabolic wastes. In the case of slowly progressive renal failure, provisions for dialysis should be concluded months in advance of need. The goal of dialysis therapy is to maintain health at a level consistent with a relatively normal life style. Therefore, it is not advisable to wait for signs and symptoms of far advanced uremia (e.g., pericarditis, seizures, coma, or bleeding) to appear before initiating dialysis. The patient should be referred to a nephrologist associated with a dialysis center when the creatinine clearance approaches 20 ml/minute. In this way the patient may be familiarized with the various forms of therapy offered at that facility and become acquainted with the staff.

Before actually starting dialysis, it is necessary to provide some kind of vascular access to allow for the repeated venipunctures required for this form of therapy. The preferred access is the arteriovenous fistula, which is usually created at the wrist of the

Table 47.11.
Treatments for End-Stage Renal Failure

Hemodialysis
  Home
  Hospital based
  Satellite or self-care (*e.g.*, those not situated in a hospital)
Peritoneal dialysis
  Continuous ambulatory peritoneal dialysis (CAPD)
  Intermittent peritoneal dialysis (IPD)
Renal transplantation
  Living donor transplant
  Cadaveric transplant

nondominant arm. The creation of a fistula can be performed, in most instances, under local anesthesia and often in an outpatient surgical unit. Since there is often a 1- to 2-month maturation period necessary before the fistula can be used, arrangements for the creation of the fistula should be made early, and always before the GFR falls to less than 10 to 15 ml/minute. If the patient's vessels are inadequate to support the creation of an arteriovenous fistula, an alternative would be to insert a synthetic (Dacron, Gortex) graft under the skin of the forearm. The synthetic graft can generally be used within 3 weeks of placement. The most common complications after placement of a fistula or graft are clotting and infection.

Hemodialysis is performed in most centers two to three times/week, and each session lasts about 4 hours. Except for needle insertion, the procedure, per se, is not painful; but some patients do experience muscle cramps, headaches, nausea, or syncope during or just after dialysis. *Hospital-based dialysis* should be reserved for those patients who require intensive monitoring. *Home dialysis* is encouraged for those patients with good home situations who have willing and able partners. Home dialysis patients have the advantage of more flexible schedules and a greater sense of control than do hospital-based patients and, therefore, have the greatest chance of maintaining their previous life style. The remainder of the patients can be treated at *outpatient dialysis centers.*

As a group, hemodialysis patients have an 80% survival rate for the first year, and at 5 years the survival rate falls to about 55%. Home dialysis patients, who are generally healthier, do better than those with coexistent diseases (e.g., diabetes mellitus, 20% 5-year survival rate) or the elderly (30% survival rate at 5 years for those starting dialysis over the age of 60 years). The development of the long term complications of chronic renal failure, including progressive neuropathy, osteodystrophy, cardiovascular disease, and an array of endocrine disturbances, reflects the fact that dialysis does not correct all of the metabolic disturbances of uremia.

Peritoneal Dialysis

Peritoneal dialysis procedures involve the instillation of dialysis fluid through a catheter into the abdominal cavity. Fluid and toxic solutes are transferred across the mesenteric capillary bed into the dialysis fluid, which is then removed through the catheter. Recent improvements in the techniques of peritoneal dialysis have increased its popularity among patients. Peritoneal dialysis, until recently, required 12- to 16-hour periods of being connected to an automatic cycling machine, two to three times/week (*intermittent peritoneal dialysis,* IPD). Even then, its simplicity and freedom from hemodynamic complications made this form of therapy attractive,

particularly to the elderly or to those with heart disease. Currently, *continuous ambulatory peritoneal dialysis* (CAPD) has nearly replaced the older machine-based therapy. In this technique the patient constantly carries 2 liters of dialysis solution in his abdomen (17). The fluid is exchanged four times a day, every day. However, since fluid movement is determined by gravity, and no machine is necessary, the patient is able to perform dialysis at home, at work, or virtually anywhere. This degree of freedom is one of the most attractive aspects of CAPD. Its other attributes, at least theoretically, are the greater removal of larger molecular weight substances than that provided by hemodialysis, and the continuous nature of the dialysis that eliminates the large swings in the concentration of electrolytes, creatinine, *etc* that occur with the more intermittent forms of therapy. Also the abdominal catheter for CAPD can be placed at the time of the first dialysis and does not require a maturation period. The major difficulty associated with peritoneal dialysis is the development of peritonitis. The incidence in the typical patient is about one infection every 8 months, but these infections generally respond to antimicrobials and continued peritoneal dialysis; often treatment of peritonitis does not require hospitalization. However, the peritoneal dialysis catheter may need periodic replacement.

Comparative survival statistics between hemodialysis and peritoneal dialysis are difficult to interpret due to significant population selection biases. Whether hemodialysis or peritoneal dialysis is used depends on the center to which the patient is referred and on patient preference. At most dialysis facilities the patient will have a choice and may change dialysis modes if the outcome of one is unsatisfactory.

Renal Transplantation

Of all available therapies, a successful renal transplant provides for the most complete correction of the uremic syndrome. Unfortunately, many transplanted kidneys are lost because of immunological rejection. Innovations in antirejection therapy, such as the use of the potent immunosuppressant drug cyclosporine or of monoclonal antibodies, appear to be improving the rate of graft survival.

The success of renal transplantation depends greatly on the antigenic similarity between donor and recipient. Except in the cases of identical twins (where rejection does not occur) the best results are found in living related donor, HLA antigen identical, sibling transplants. In this instance, kidney survival is greater than 90% at 1 year and 75% at 5 years. More commonly performed are 2 HLA antigen matched, sibling to sibling, or parent to child organ transplants with a success rate of 75% at 1 year and 55% at 5 years. Patient survival for non-HLA identical living related donor transplants is over 90% at both the 1- and 5-year intervals. The majority of patients do not have the potential for living related donors (less than 25% of patients are able to receive living related donor transplants) and must await a cadaveric transplant which, despite the best tissue typing, has a significantly lower success rate of 55% at 1 year and 30% at 5 years. The use of cyclosporine in some centers has raised the 1-year kidney survival rate for cadaveric transplants to 75%. Patient survival rates for cadaveric transplants are 90% at 1 year and 75% at 5 years. Comparison of survival statistics between cadaveric transplants and dialysis patients is complicated because of selection bias. Transplant patients tend to be younger, have better myocardial function, and have fewer coexisting illnesses than their dialysis counterparts. If these factors are taken into account then no significant difference in the survival rate can be found between patients receiving cadaveric kidney transplants or those being treated by dialysis.

Patients with uncomplicated renal transplants require at least a 3- to 4-week hospitalization. It is hoped that the use of cyclosporine will substantially reduce this time. After transplantation (except for those performed between identical twins), the patient requires lifelong immunosuppression, usually with prednisone and azathioprine (Imuran). The patient must understand that there is always the risk of rejection and the possibility of graft failure with a return to dialysis. Although there is no doubt that a successfully functioning transplant restores health better than any other therapy, patients on immunosuppressive therapy have considerable risks—corticosteroid complications, malignancies, or serious infections.

Since the primary physician is most familiar with the patient, he can be of great value in advising which forms of therapy might coincide best with the patient's expectations. Frequently, patients will have a better understanding of their choices if they visit a dialysis or transplant unit and talk with patients or staff. They can also be referred to support groups, such as the National Association of Patients on Hemodialysis and Transplantation (NAPHT, 565 Northern Blvd, Great Neck, NY 11021). These groups offer great help in allaying fears and providing information. The decision to suggest a renal transplant is most clear-cut in adolescents or young adults who wish to pursue an active, vigorous life, to have a job, and to have intact sexual functions. This is particularly so if a well matched living donor is available. Elderly patients or those with extensive multisystem disease may not be able to tolerate the vigors of transplantation. For others, a period of dialysis and assessment of the patient's adjustment to this therapy will often help in determining whether to continue dialysis or to consider transplantation. The patient who adjusts well to dialysis can often be fully rehabilitated and can maintain a job as efficiently as the patient with a successful renal transplant. At the present time it appears that quality of life is the most important criterion determining which form of therapy is selected, since survival appears to be similar in patients undergoing either cadaveric transplantation or dialysis.

CONCLUSION

The personal financial impact of chronic renal failure and the cost of hemodialysis and transplantation, which initially were prohibitively expensive, have been minimized for patients and their families by the extension of the Medicare program to patients under the age of 65 with end-stage renal failure. Nevertheless, patients often have to leave their jobs because of chronic illness or because of the time requirements of therapy.

Despite advances in dialysis and transplantation in recent years, the best hope for patients with chronic renal diseases lies in prevention and appropriate therapy in the early stages of renal insufficiency. These objectives must be accomplished by the patient's primary physician.

General References

Campbell JD, Campbell AR: The social and economic costs of end-stage renal disease. *N Engl J Med* 299:386, 1978.
> A patient's view of the effects of living with renal failure.

Friedman EA (ed): *Strategy in Renal Failure*. New York, John Wiley & Sons, 1978.
> Readable and comprehensive review of the management of uremic patients. Sections on dialysis and transplantation of patients with systemic diseases.

Guttmann RD: Renal transplantation. I and II. *N Engl J Med* 301:975, 1038, 1979.
> A complete discussion of transplantation.

Massry SG, Goldstein DA, Molluche HH: Current status of the use of 1,25-$(OH)_2$-d_3 in the management of renal osteodystrophy. *Kidney Int* 18:409, 1980.
> An excellent editorial review on renal osteodystrophy and the rationale and method of treatment.

Roxe DM: Toxic nephropathy from diagnostic and therapeutic agents. *Am J Med* 69:759, 1980.
> This article provides a brief review of diagnostic and therapeutic drugs which cause nephrotoxicity, and reviews the mechanism of toxicity.

Specific References

1. Anderson RJ, Schrier RW (eds): *Clinical Use of Drugs in Patients with Kidney and Liver Disease*. Philadelphia, WB Saunders, 1981.
2. Bennett WM, Muther RS, Parker RA, et al: Drug therapy in renal failure: dosing guidelines for adults. Part 1 and Part 2. *Ann Intern Med* 93:62, 286, 1980.
3. Bennett WM, Plamp C, Porter GA: Drug related syndromes in clinical nephrology. *Ann Intern Med* 87:582, 1977.
4. Bergstrom J: Discovery and rediscovery of low protein diets. *Clin Nephrol* 21:29, 1984.
5. Brenner BM, Meyer TW, Hostetter TH: Dietary protein intake and the progressive nature of kidney disease: the role of hemodynamically mediated glomerular injury in the pathogenesis of progressive glomerular sclerosis, aging, renal ablation, and intrinsic renal disease. *N Engl J Med* 307:652, 1982.
6. Clive DM, Stoff JS: Renal syndromes associated with nonsteroidal antiinflammatory drugs. *N Engl J Med* 310:563, 1984.

7. Cunningham JJ: Excretory urography in acute and chronic renal failure. Current concepts and techniques. *Urology* 5:303, 1975.

8. D'Elia JA, Gleason RE, Alday M, *et al*: Nephrotoxicity from angiographic contrast material: a prospective study. *Am J Med* 72:719, 1982.

9. Eggers PW, Connerton R, McMullan M: The Medicare experience with end stage renal disease: trends in incidence, prevalence, and survival. Working Paper Series. Department of Health and Human Services, Health Care Financing Administration, Office of Research and Demonstrations, May 1983.

10. Friedman EA, L'Esperance JR (eds): Clinical management of diabetes mellitus. In *The Diabetic-Renal-Retinal Syndrome*. New York, Grune and Stratton, 1980.

11. Healy M, Malluche HH, Goldstein DA: Effects of long term therapy with 1,25 (OH)₂D₃ in patients with moderate renal failure. *Arch Intern Med* 140:1030, 1980.

12. Jelliffe RW, Brooker G: A nonogram for digoxin therapy. *Am J Med* 57:63, 1974.

13. Maschio G, Oldrizzi L, Tessitore N, *et al*: Effects of dietary protein and phosphorus restriction on the progression of early failure. *Kidney Int* 22:371, 1982.

14. Mitch WM, Walser M, Steinman TI, *et al*: Effect of a keto acid-amino acid supplement to a restricted diet on the progression of chronic renal failure. *N Engl J Med* 311:623, 1984.

15. Opelz G, Terasaki PI: Prolongation effect of blood transfusions on kidney graft survival. *Transplantation* 22:380, 1976.

16. Phelps KR, Lieberman RL, Oh MS, Carroll HJ: Pathophysiology of the syndrome of hyporeninemic hypoaldosteronism. *Metabolism* 29:186, 1980.

17. Popovich RP, Moncrief JW, Nolph KD, *et al*: Continuous peritoneal dialysis. *Ann Intern Med* 88:449, 1978.

18. Rowe JW, Andres R, Tobin JD *et al*: Age-adjusted standards for creatinine clearance. *Ann Intern Med* 84:567, 1976.

19. Yu T, Berger L, Dorph DJ, Smith H: Renal function in gout. Factors influencing the renal hemodynamics. *Am J Med* 67:766, 1979.

CHAPTER FORTY-EIGHT

Bladder Outlet Obstruction

JAMES K. SMOLEV, M.D.

INTRODUCTION

The bladder, bladder outlet, prostate, and urethra may be affected by a wide variety of conditions that result in symptoms of urinary obstruction or bladder irritability. These disorders are very common, especially in older men.

Benign prostatic hyperplasia (BPH) is the commonest cause of bladder outlet obstruction in males over 50 years of age. Autopsy studies have shown that 50 to 60% of men over 50 have significant enlargement of the prostate due to BPH and the prevalence increases with age. A number of other conditions may also cause symptoms of bladder outlet obstruction in the male: urethral stricture; carcinoma of the prostate; neurogenic bladder; bladder calculus; prostatitis; bladder neck contracture; and carcinoma of the bladder. Also, functional obstruction, seen in both women and men, may result from chronic bladder distension, debilitating disease, psychogenic retention, or medications.

The primary physician can usually arrive at a working diagnosis and determine the need for a referral—either urgently or electively—by review of the patient's history, physical examination, and several laboratory tests.

HISTORY

Bladder outlet obstruction is characterized by symptoms of urinary hesitancy, diminished force and caliber of the stream, and postvoid dribbling. Urinary frequency and nocturia result from a diminished bladder capacity caused by bladder muscle hypertrophy. The hypertrophy results in increased intravesical pressure during voiding, thereby providing compensation for the obstruction. In time, however, the bladder will decompensate, which will lead to the presence of residual urine, infection, hematuria, hydronephrosis, and renal failure.

Patients with urethral stricture usually have a history of prior urethral trauma, instrumentation (most commonly, indwelling Foley catheter), or urethritis and, in association with symptoms of bladder outlet obstruction, may notice a split urine stream. Carcinoma of the prostate may present with obstructive symptoms which are often of a shorter duration than those seen in patients with BPH, in whom symptoms of outlet obstruction (see above) may progress over several years. Recent onset of back or bone pain, anorexia, or weight loss suggests malignancy. *Neurogenic bladder* should be suspected when other symptoms of neurological disease are present, when disorders of bowel or sexual function coexist with bladder outlet obstruction, or when a systemic disease which causes neurological bladder dysfunction (such as diabetes mellitus or tabes dorsalis) exists.

A history of current and recently used *medications* (Table 48.1) is mandatory in the evaluation of the patient with symptoms of bladder outlet obstruction. Anticholinergic agents (antispasmodic and antiparkinsonian drugs) as well as many antidepressant drugs depress bladder muscle contractility; sympathomimetic agents (such as ephedrine) increase bladder outlet resistance. A diuresis (such as from a diuretic, glucosuria, or a large, brisk fluid intake) may overstretch a partially compensated detrusor muscle and cause acute urinary retention.

Table 48.1.
Phamacological Agents with Known Influence On Bladder Function

DRUGS WHICH INCREASE BLADDER TONE AND CONTRACTILITY:
  Bethanecol (Urecholine)
DRUGS WHICH DECREASE BLADDER CONTRACTILITY:
  Anticholinergic drugs (*e.g.*, Pro-Banthine or Donnatal)
  Tricyclic antidepressent drugs
DRUGS WHICH INCREASE BLADDER OUTLET RESISTANCE:
  Antiparkinsonian drugs (*e.g.*, Levodopa or Sinemet)
  Sympathomimetic drugs (*e.g.*, Actifed, Brethine, Dexedrine, Isuprel, Novafed, Sudafed, Triaminic)
DRUGS WHICH INCREASE URINARY VOLUME:
  Diuretics

It is important to distinguish *bladder outlet obstructive symptoms*—hesitancy, decreased stream, postvoid dribbling—from *irritative bladder symptoms*—frequency, urgency, nocturia. Although anatomical or functional obstruction may produce both types of symptoms, only irritative symptoms are seen with cystitis (see Chapter 27), bladder stones (see Chapter 46), and bladder carcinoma. Finally, the differentiation of polyuria from urinary frequency, and nocturia from enuresis (involuntary bedwetting) can be made by appropriate questioning.

PHYSICAL EXAMINATION

The physical examination of the patient with symptoms of bladder outlet obstruction should be thorough, with special emphasis on the urinary tract.

The *abdominal examination* may reveal several findings: a distended bladder from retention, renal tenderness (from infection or hydronephrosis) or a renal mass (from hydronephrosis), inguinal herniae from straining at urination when outlet obstruction is present. In the male, the *examination of the penis* may reveal phimosis or urethral meatal stenosis that could cause obstruction. The *examination of the epididymides* may show evidence of acute or chronic infection, which is a complication of bladder outlet obstruction. A brief *neurological examination*, particularly of the anal sphincter tone, genital and perineal sensation, and motor, sensory, and reflex activity of the lower extremities may disclose abnormalities that suggest a neurogenic bladder as the cause of the patient's symptoms.

A careful *rectal examination of the prostate* is important in evaluating the patient with suspected BPH or prostate carcinoma even though there are certain limits: rectal palpation permits examination only of the posterior lobes of the prostate and BPH most commonly involves the unpalpable lateral and median lobes; moreover, the size of the prostate gland as estimated by rectal examination is not directly related to the degree of urinary obstruction.

The most important information obtained from the rectal examination is the *consistency* of the prostate gland. In patients with prostate enlargement, BPH can be differentiated from prostatic carcinoma with over 75% certainty based on the rectal examination. The patient may be examined when he is in the decubitis, knee-chest, or standing-bending position. The patient should void as fully as possible before the examination since a full bladder will distort the size of the prostate. To prevent anal sphincter spasm, appropriate time should be used to explain the procedure to the patient. Using ample lubricant, the anal sphincter should be slowly and gently dilated by gradual insertion of the finger through the anus, asking the patient to bear down slightly. This examination will permit the determination of shape and consistency of the prostate as well as the presence of tenderness and of the adequacy of sphincter tone.

The normal prostate is palpable 2 to 5 cm from the anal verge through the anterior rectal wall. The examining finger can normally reach over the top (base) of the prostate, as well as over each lateral border. A median sulcus is appreciated in the midline. The posterior lobes of the prostate can be compared in size, configuration, and consistency with the tip of the nose.

BPH not only often results in obliteration of the median sulcus, but also the examining finger may not reach the base of the gland. The consistency of the gland in BPH is smooth and rubbery—very similar to the thenar eminence of the hand. The gland is not tender unless prostatitis is present. BPH may be characterized by symmetrical or asymmetrical enlargement and by distinct nodules called spheroids. The clinical differentiation between carcinoma and asymmetric or nodular BPH is based on the degree of induration or hardness of the gland.

Classically, prostatic carcinoma is characterized by a rock hard nodule or mass involving one or both posterior lobes. Palpation of the zygomatic arch of the face offers a similar consistency to prostatic carcinoma. However, not all hard nodules will be found on biopsy to be cancer. In approximately 30 to 40%, there will be granulomatous prostatitis, prostatic calculi, spheroids of BPH, or nodularity resulting from transuretheral prostatic resection.

If the physician is suspicious of prostatic carcinoma, it is important to determine the extent of the local lesion—single nodule, diffuse involvement, or extension outside the capsule—and to refer the patient to a urologist.

PRELIMINARY LABORATORY ASSESSMENT

At this juncture in the evaluation of the patient who has symptoms of bladder outlet obstruction that are felt to be due to BPH, the general physician must determine the need and urgency for urological consultation. A urinalysis, urine culture (if pyuria is present), and measurement of serum creatinine or creatinine clearance will provide the information necessary to make this decision.

If the patient does not have hematuria, urinary tract infection, or renal failure and if the diagnosis of BPH is likely, further evaluation will depend on whether the patient is a candidate for surgery (Table 48.2). If there is no indication for surgery, then no further evaluation is necessary at this juncture.

UROLOGICAL INVESTIGATION

When surgery is a consideration and a patient is referred to a urologist, several further assessments are frequently made.

Table 48.2.
Indications for Surgery in Patients Who Are Thought to Have Benign Prostatic Hyperplasia

Acute urinary retention[a]
Epididymitis (especially if recurrent)
Gross hematuria
Recurrent urinary tract infections
Renal failure secondary to obstruction[a]
Chronic symptoms which are intolerable.

[a] Necessitates urgent urological referral.

Radiology

Intravenous pyelography (IVP) is usually performed to determine whether there is hydronephrosis or other structural disease of the urinary tract. Besides assessing the upper tract, this study may demonstrate bladder trabeculations or significant residual urine. The pelvic and vertebral bones can also be evaluated and may provide a clue to the presence of metastatic prostatic cancer.

If a patient has a history of an allergic reaction to intravenous contrast material, there are several alternative methods for studying the urinary tract. *Renal ultrasound* is useful in the detection of significant obstruction. Depending on the agent used, a *renal scan* may be used to evaluate renal blood flow or delayed excretion suggesting obstruction. A *retrograde pyelogram* done in conjunction with cystoscopy (see below) will provide visualization of dilated ureters. The dye used during this procedure is not absorbed and can be used safely in allergic patients.

If an IVP is felt to be mandatory in a patient with a history of previous mild to moderate reaction, there is approximately a 35% chance of reaction. A decision to perform a study in this instance must be made on an individual basis and in consultation with the radiologist and urologist, and the protocol suggested in Chapter 23 should be followed. If the history suggests a urethral stricture, a *retrograde urethrogram* may be performed. This procedure requires urethral catheterization, instillation of contrast material, and then the obtaining of an X-ray while the patient is voiding. There is no need for anesthesia during this procedure, and there is only minimal discomfort during insertion of the cathether.

Instrumentation

A urologist will gain considerable information in the evaluation of a patient with symptoms of bladder outlet obstruction by performing several invasive procedures. Because these procedures may be associated with the development of infection, they should not be done casually.

Bladder Catheterization for Postvoid Volume

Inserting a urethral catheter (see Chapter 6) immediately after a patient has voided will determine the amount of residual urine (greater than 100 ml is abnormal), as well as help to determine if there is a urethral stricture. If a neurogenic bladder is suspected as a cause of the patient's symptoms, the patient should be referred to a urologist for a consultation and the performance of a cystometrogram and possibly a cystourethroscopy.

Cystometrogram

A cystometrogram is easily performed by a urologist in his office. The procedure is similar to a catheterization for residual urine (see above). After the catheter is placed, a sterile solution is used to fill the bladder and to record and classify the detrusor response to the increasing volume.

Cystourethroscopy

Patient experience. Cystoscopy may easily be done in a urologist's office under local anesthesia. When performed under these conditions, the patient will often perceive a feeling of suprapubic pressure as the bladder is being filled with the irrigating fluid, but the degree of discomfort is usually slight. Examination of the entire urethra, prostate, and bladder takes just a few minutes. However, if a retrograde pyelogram is performed, another 15 minutes may be required. Following cystoscopy, patients will often experience marked dysuria. The patient should have been advised about this and informed that it may be relieved by voiding while sitting in a bathtub filled with warm water or by taking phenazopyridine (Pyridium), 100 mg three times a day for a day or two. Hematuria following cystoscopy is also common and may persist for 2 or 3 days. The patient should be informed of this possibility, reassured that it is benign, and advised to force fluids (2 to 3 liters/day) should it occur. Infection in the urinary tract occurs only rarely following cystoscopy. Occasionally, acute urinary retention occurs from edema of the prostate subsequent to instrumentation. If this complication occurs, the insertion of an indwelling catheter and hospitalization are necessary. An uncommon long term complication of cystoscopy is urethral stricture. The use of newer, smaller instruments is likely to eliminate this complication.

The urologist learns a great deal from the cystoscopic examination. The entire urethra is seen. The size of the prostate, the degree of occlusiveness, trabeculation in the bladder, and diverticula are all directly visualized. This information is most important in helping the urologist decide the need for and the type of surgery.

TREATMENT OF BLADDER OUTLET OBSTRUCTION

Benign Prostatic Hypertrophy

The only currently available treatment for BPH is prostatectomy. Rarely, because of operative risk, the urologist may not be able to perform surgery and urinary retention may have to be treated with a catheter, usually placed in a suprapubic position into the bladder. In the future, pharmacological therapy that diminishes the size of an obstructing gland may be available.

The urologist removes the obstructing prostatic tissue either transurethrally (TURP) or by one of the open operative approaches (suprapubic or perineal). The particular approach used will depend on a combination of the condition of the patient, the size and configuration of the prostate gland, and the urologist's experience. In general, glands which are very large are removed by open prostatectomy and smaller glands by TURP.

Transurethral Resection of the Prostate

TURP is the most commonly used procedure in the treatment of BPH. It requires hospitalization for 4 to 7 days; general or spinal anesthesia is used.

Complications have been minimized by the use of smaller more efficient instruments, by improved lighting and by irrigating fluids. Nevertheless, bleeding, infection, and plasma hypo-osmalality (from absorption of irrigation fluid) occur. Long term complications of TURP include *urethral stricture* (see below), *bladder neck contracture*, and *incontinence*.

A frequent consequence of TURP is *retrograde ejaculation*—a situation characterized by the ejaculation of semen into the bladder rather than externally through the urethra. This phenomenon occurs because the bladder neck is resected as part of the TURP and, therefore, cannot subsequently contract as is necessary to produce antegrade ejaculation. Retrograde ejaculation results in sterility but does not usually affect orgasms. This consequence should be discussed with sexually active patients and their partners before prostatectomy. TURP should not produce organic erectile impotence; however, psychogenic impotence may follow genitourinary surgery. The management of psychogenic impotence is described in Chapter 18.

Most patients can resume normal physical and sexual activity in approximately 4 weeks following TURP. Complete healing of the prostatic fossa, however, usually takes 2 to 3 months, and therefore during this period a urinalysis may reveal white and red blood cells.

Open Prostatectomy

Open prostatectomy requires a slightly longer hospitalization and recovery period. This approach is used when, in addition to having a large prostate, the patient has a coincidental bladder condition, that can be repaired at the same time (e.g., bladder diverticulum or bladder stone). Organic erectile impotence occurs occasionally, especially when the perineal approach has been used. If this complication occurs, an evaluation should be performed (see Chapter 18) before attributing the impotence to the surgery and presuming it to be irreversible.

It is very important for a patient undergoing any

form of prostatectomy for BPH to understand that the entire prostate gland is not removed. Because of the presence of residual prostate tissue, these patients have a risk equal to that of the general population of developing prostatic carcinoma. Rectal examinations should be done every 12 months, therefore, to detect changes which may suggest malignancy. Also, because residual prostatic tissue remains, recurrent symptoms or complications from prostatic hypertrophy may develop later. The frequency of recurrence depends primarily on the extent of the initial surgery and therefore is highly variable.

Urethral Stricture

A urethral stricture may be treated either with urethral dilation, transurethral incision of the stricture, or open urethral surgery. The method selected depends on the length and location of the stricture, the patient's overall health, and the urologist's experience.

Prostatic Carcinoma

The therapy of prostatic carcinoma is somewhat controversial but may be approached on the basis of the stage of the disease (Table 48.3).

Stage A prostatic carcinoma is disease unsuspected on rectal examination of the prostate, but which is discovered at the time of prostatectomy done for obstructive symptoms. In this instance, the urologist will initiate a metastatic evaluation for carcinoma of the prostate by obtaining a serum acid phosphatase determination, bone scan, and intravenous pyelogram.

In the situation of stage A disease, controversy exists regarding the most accurate method of further classification. Studies (4) have shown that first level lymph nodes (the obturator and iliac nodes) are positive in from 12 to 50% of prostatic cancers that are found only on pathological examinations. Because of this, the procedures of lymphangiography, computerized tomography (CT) scanning, and open surgical lymphadenectomy all have advocates as well as detractors.

If there is no evidence for lymph node involvement, the prostatic tissue that has been resected should be re-examined to determine the percentage of the tissue involved by carcinoma. If less than 5% of the available tissue is cancer—and if it is well differentiated—then *stage A_1 disease* is present, and no further therapy is required. Careful follow-up by a urologist every 3 to 6 months for 3 years and then yearly is necesssary to determine recurrence by performing rectal examination and perhaps cystoscopy. If a larger percentage of the tissue is cancer, or if it is less well differentiated, the classification is *Stage A_2*, and most authorities recommend definitive radiotherapy as the treatment (7). Radiation cystitis and proctitis occur with this form of treatment in approximately 30% and 25%, respectively; but frequently symptoms can be controlled with treatment. Some urologists recommend radical prostatectomy for those under age 60 with well differentiated stage A_2 carcinoma of the prostate (6).

Stage B carcinoma is defined as disease limited to the prostate gland and is detected clinically either as a nodule or as diffuse hardness of a lobe. If less than one lobe is involved and if the patient is under 70 years of age and has no contraindicating medical diseases, he is a candidate for curative radical prostatectomy. In the hands of a urologist experienced in this type of surgery, the complication of incontinence can be minimized. A recent modification of the traditional radical prostatectomy permits the removal of all cancerous tissue yet spares the pelvic nerves which control erection; there is preservation of pre-existing potency in greater than 90% of patients (6).

Most extensive localized prostatic cancer, *Stage C*, is best treated by definitive radiotherapy (4). If bladder outlet obstruction is also present, the patient may also need a TURP, and this occasionally will need to be repeated.

Metastatic or *stage D* prostatic cancer is best managed by hormonal therapy when symptoms require treatment. Studies by the Veterans Administration Cooperative Urological Research Group (VACURG) have shown that hormonal therapy initiated at the time of diagnosis does not prolong survival compared to hormonal therapy initiated only in response to symptoms (such as bone pain) (2, 3). Diethylstilbestrol (1 to 3 mg/day) and orchiectomy give similar results, producing an 85 to 90% partial symptomatic response rate in previously untreated patients. The duration of response is on the average 18 months, although prolonged remissions have been documented. There is no advantage to combining orchiectomy and estrogen therapy. Generally, estrogen therapy, which causes salt and water retention, should be avoided in patients who also have an

Table 48.3.
Staging of Prostatic Carcinoma

Stage	Description
A	Clinically undetectable; found on pathological examination after prostatectomy
A_1	Focal; well differentiated
A_2	Diffuse; poorly differentiated
B	Limited to prostate on rectal examination
B_1	Solitary nodule; < 1.5 cm; one lobe
B_2	One whole lobe or both lobes
C	Locally extending outside of prostatic capsule or seminal vesicles
D	Distant metastases

Table 48.4.
Survival with Appropriately Managed Prostatic Carcinoma

Stage	% Survival	
	5-Year	15-Year
A₁	Normal life expectancy	
A₂	50%	
B₁ᵃ	85–90%ᶜ	50%
B₂ᵇ	20%	1%
C	50%	
D	50% (3 year)	

ᵃ Radical surgery.
ᵇ Untreated.
ᶜ Survival is better than stage A₂ probably because the cancer can be detected on examination and may therefore be detected earlier; also A₂ is a larger, more poorly differentiated cancer, than B.

edema-forming illness (such as severe congestive heart failure or nephrotic syndrome) not controlled by diuretics. New approaches to the hormonal control of prostatic carcinoma are under investigation. The intention of these studies is to identify agents which have equal or better efficacy than the more traditional orchiectomy or estrogen therapy, with fewer side effects. Good results have been reported (5) with the gonadotropin-releasing hormone analogue, leuprolide, but the expense, the need for daily injections, and the uncertainty about the durability of response limits its current usefulness. Investigation is under way to evaluate cytotoxic chemotherapy in all stages of prostatic carcinoma (1), but to date this approach has been unrewarding.

Much of the controversy in the diagnosis and treatment of prostatic cancer results from the inability to assess accurately the influence of prostate cancer on longevity. Prostate cancer occurs in older men who often have coexisting diseases that influence longevity. Also, the natural history of the disease is not well understood. The best estimates for survival with various stages of prostatic cancer with the treatments discussed above are listed in Table 48.4.

Urinary Incontinence (See Also Chapter 6)

Urinary incontinence is a common problem of the elderly and of younger women. It may be a manifestation of urinary outlet obstruction. The evaluation of incontinence is discussed in Chapter 6. In general, younger patients with incontinence are best referred to a urologist for evaluation and definitive treatment, which is usually surgical. Elderly patients with urinary incontinence are usually managed by the general physician; therefore, their treatment is discussed extensively in Chapter 6, Geriatric Patients.

General References

Catalona WJ, Scott WW: Carcinoma of the prostate. In Walsh PC, Perlmutter AD, Gittes RF,, Stamey TA (eds): *Campbell's Urology*, Philadelphia, WB Saunders, 1985.
Walsh PC: Benign prostate hyperplasia. In Walsh PC, Perlmutter AD, Gittes RF, Stamey TA (eds): *Campbell's Urology*, Philadelphia, WB Saunders, 1985.
    Both chapters provide an in-depth review of their respective subjects.

Specific References

1. Anderson T: Chemotherapy of urologic cancer—principles and practice. In Javadpour N (ed): *Principles and Management of Urologic Cancer*. Baltimore, Williams & Wilkins, 1979.
2. Bailar JC, Byar DP: Estrogen treatment for cancer of the prostate: early results with three doses of diethylstilbestrol and placebo. *Cancer* 26:257, 1970.
3. Byar DP: The Veterans Administration Cooperative Urologic Research Group's studies of cancer of the prostate. *Cancer* 32:1126, 1973.
4. Catalona WJ, Scott WW: Carcinoma of the prostate: a review. *J Urol* 119:1, 1978.
5. The Leuprolide Study Group. Leuprolide versus diethylstilbestrol for metastatic prostatic cancer. *N Engl J Med* 311:1281, 1984.
6. Walsh, PC, Lepor H, Eggleston JC: Radical prostatectomy with preservation of sexual function: anatomical and pathological considerations. *Prostate* 4:473, 1983.
7. Whitmore WF Jr, Batata M, Hilaris B: Prostate irradiation: iodine-125 implantation. In Johnson DE, Samuels ML (eds): *Cancer of the Genitourinary Tract*. New York, Raven Press, 1979.

SECTION 6

Hematological Problems

CHAPTER FORTY-NINE

Anemia

LARRY WATERBURY, M.D.

GENERAL CONSIDERATIONS

Anemia, a reduction of the proportion of red cells or of hemoglobin in the blood, is a condition, like hypoxia or jaundice, which always reflects a primary underlying disease. Although there are sometimes symptoms (e.g., shortness of breath on exertion) or signs (e.g., pallor) which are associated with anemia, the diagnosis of the condition is essentially dependent on one or more laboratory measurements—such as the hematocrit value (the amount of red cells in a volume of blood) or the hemoglobin concentration. In general, anemia is defined in a man as a condition in which the hematocrit value is less than 42% or the hemoglobin concentration less than 14 g/100 ml and in a woman as a hematocrit value less than 37% or a hemoglobin concentration less than 12 g/100 ml. When anemia is diagnosed, other measurements, described below, are important in establishing the cause of the process and in leading the clinician to appropriate therapy.

Most of the routine complete blood counts (CBC) obtained in clinical practice in this country are determined by automated counting methods (Table 49.1). The CBC usually reports the hemoglobin concentration (Hgb), hematocrit value (Hct), red blood cell count (RBC), white cell count, mean corpuscular volume (MCV), mean corpuscular hemoglobin (MCH), and mean corpuscular hemoglobin concentration (MCHC). One commonly used automated system (Coulter) measures the hemoglobin, RBC, and MCV, and from these variables calculates the hematocrit value, MCH, and MCHC. With the use of the automated counters the indices (MCH, MCHC, MCV), especially the MCV, are precise, accurate measurements which can be utilized in approaching the diagnostic workup of anemia. The calculated Hct value is a few percentage points lower than that obtained by centrifugation (packed cells trap plasma, distorting the ratio of red cells to plasma).

APPROACH TO EVALUATION OF ANEMIA

The routine data base which should be obtained for every anemic patient includes the hematocrit value, hemoglobin concentration, MCV, MCHC, and reticulocyte count (Table 49.2). A smear of the peripheral blood should be obtained by fingerstick or from unanticoagulated blood on the tip of a venipuncture needle. (Anticoagulants distort the mor-

Table 49.1.
Representative Normal Values (Coulter S)

	Men	Women
Hemoglobin, g/dl of blood	14–18	12–16
Hematocrit value, %	42–54	37–47
Mean corpuscular volume, MCV, fl	82–98	82–98
Mean corpuscular hemoglobin, MCH, pg	27–32	27–32
Mean corpuscular hemoglobin concentration, MCHC, g/dl of red blood cells	31.5–36	31.5–36

Table 49.2.
Routine Data Base for Anemic Patients

Hematocrit value
Hemoglobin concentration
Mean corpuscular volume
Mean corpuscular hemoglobin concentration
Reticulocytic count (and calculation of reticulocytic index)
Evaluation of a peripheral blood smear (fingerstick)

Table 49.3.
Reticulocyte Index

$$\text{Reticulocyte index} = \text{reticulocyte count} \times \frac{\text{patient Hct}}{\text{normal Hct}}$$

Example: reticulocyte count 6%, hematocrit 15%

$$\text{Reticulocyte index} = 6 \times \frac{15}{45} = 2\%$$

phology of the blood cells.) The smear may be stained in the physician's office or transported to an outside laboratory to be stained and interpreted. On the basis of all of these data, and a complete history and physical examination, the physician can progress a long way toward an etiological diagnosis of the anemia. Three questions should be asked:

1. *What is the MCV?* With the use of the automated counters the MCV is a direct measurement of red cell size. The normal range varies with individual laboratories but is approximately 82 to 98 femtoliters (fl). Actually it is helpful to use a broader normal range of 80 to 100 fl to classify the anemia as microcytic (MCV less than 80 fl), normocytic (MCV 80 to 100 fl), or macrocytic (MCV greater than 100 fl). Microcytic and macrocytic anemias have very limited differential diagnoses, and therefore by simply noting the MCV the physician can limit greatly the diagnostic approach when the anemia is microcytic or macrocytic.

2. *What is the basic mechanism of the anemia?* There are only three ways patients become anemic: (a) decreased effective production of red cells by bone marrow, (b) bleeding, or (c) hemolysis. The most helpful laboratory measurement in defining the mechanism of anemia is the reticulocyte count. The *reticulocyte count* is used to assess the appropriateness of the response of the bone marrow to anemia. The normal reticulocyte count is approximately 1%, representing the 1% of new cells which are released into the circulation from the bone marrow daily (the ordinary red cell life span being in the range of 100 days). Under the stimulus of erythropoietin, in the anemic patient the bone marrow should be able to triple acutely its output of new cells; when anemia is chronic and severe, the bone marrow may be able to increase its output of cells to 8 to 10 times normal. This increased bone marrow activity is reflected in an appropriately elevated reticulocyte count. The reticulocyte count must be adjusted for the level of anemia to obtain a value known as the *reticulocyte index* (Table 49.3), a more accurate reflection of erythropoiesis. In patients with bleeding or hemolysis the reticulocyte index should be at least 3%, whereas in patients with anemia due to decreased production of red cells the reticulocyte index is less than 3%, and usually less than 1.5%.

In addition to the reticulocyte index serial hematocrit values over a few days or weeks may provide the physician with clues to the mechanism of the anemia. Total shutdown of production in the marrow in the absence of bleeding or hemolysis will result in a fall in the hematocrit value of only 3 or 4 percentage points/week. If the value has fallen more rapidly, bleeding or hemolysis must have taken place. Anemia with an appropriate reticulocyte response in the absence of bleeding usually means hemolysis.

3. *Does the patient have another problem that is commonly associated with anemia?* Table 49.4 lists anemias commonly associated with various clinical characteristics and diseases. For this purpose race and sex are also taken into consideration. Women are more frequently iron deficient than are men, and black patients are more likely than are whites to have hemoglobinopathies or glucose 6-phosphate dehydrogenase deficiency.

In summary, the initial data base should enable the physician to classify the anemia on the basis of the MCV, to categorize the basic mechanism of the anemia, and to consider possible causes based upon the patient's problem list. This initial assessment should then suggest the appropriate further diagnostic workup.

ANEMIA WITH A LOW MCV

Table 49.5 lists those anemias commonly associated with a low MCV. For the most part the diagnosis rests between iron deficiency anemia and thalassemia. Occasionally the anemia of chronic inflammation and, even more rarely, sideroblastic anemia are microcytic, although more often they are normocytic or, in the case of sideroblastic anemia, sometimes macrocytic.

Iron Deficiency Anemia

Although dietary iron deficiency does occur in the infant and during the rapid growth phase of adolescence, in this country iron deficiency generally occurs only as a result of bleeding. Iron deficiency from menstruation and from pregnancy is extremely common in women; but iron deficiency in a man or in a postmenopausal woman should be considered to be due to gastrointestinal bleeding until proven otherwise.

Table 49.4.
Anemias Associated with Various Clinical Characteristics

FEMALE: Iron deficiency
BLACKS: Glucose 6-phosphate dehydrogenase (G-6-PD) deficiency, hemoglobinopathies, thalassemia
MEDITERRANEAN ORIGIN: G-6-PD deficiency, thalassemia
FAR EAST ORIGIN: Hemoglobinopathies, thalassemia
VIRAL INFECTIONS: Immune hemolysis. Decreased production
BACTERIAL INFECTION:
  Anemia of inflammation
  Microangiopathic hemolysis
  Oxidative hemolysis (G-6-PD deficiency)
  Other hemolytic mechanisms
MALIGNANCY:
  Microangiopathic hemolysis
  Immune hemolysis
  Decreased production
ALCOHOLIC LIVER DISEASE:
  Bleeding
  Hypersplenism
  Folate deficiency
  Decreased production
  Sideroblastic anemia
  Iron deficiency
  Hemolysis
HYPER-HYPOTHYROIDISM:
  Decreased production
  Pernicious anemia
  Iron deficiency
RENAL FAILURE:
  Decreased production
  Hemolysis
  Bleeding
AORTIC VALVE REPLACEMENT: Microangiopathic hemolysis
MALIGNANT HYPERTENSION: Microangiopathic hemolysis
RHEUMATOID SYNDROMES:
  Anemia of inflammation
  Iron deficiency
  Immune hemolysis
COLLAGEN VASCULAR DISEASE:
  Immune hemolysis
  Anemia of inflammation
DRUGS:
  Aldomet: Immune hemolysis
  Quinine/quinidine: Immune hemolysis
  Penicillin: Immune hemolysis (rare)
  Butazolidin/chloramphenicol: Dose-related marrow depression; idiosyncratic aplastic anemia
  Gold: Aplastic anemia
  Antituberculosis drugs: Sideroblastic anemia
  Dilantin: Megaloblastic anemia (folate); pure red cell aplasia
  Sulfa: G-6-PD hemolysis

Diagnosis (7)

The history and physical examination may yield information that suggests the presence of iron deficiency. Such information includes a history of multiple past pregnancies in a woman; strange dietary habits such as the eating of ice, starch, or clay (pica); any past history of gastrointestinal bleeding, a sore tongue, brittle and ridged fingernails, spoon nails, and cheilosis. The physical findings are seen only in patients with long-standing and severe iron deficiency.

Table 49.5.
Causes of Anemia with Low Mean Corpuscular Volume

Iron deficiency
Thalassemia
Anemia of chronic inflammation (occasionally)
Sideroblastic anemia (rarely)

Most of the body's iron is incorporated in hemoglobin, but approximately one-third of it is stored in reticuloendothelial sites, primarily in the spleen, liver, and bone marrow. In patients with slow continued bleeding the reticuloendothelial iron stores supply the bone marrow's requirement for iron until the stores are depleted. It is at this point that iron deficiency anemia begins to develop. In iron deficiency cell size (MCV) correlates with the degree of anemia, so that very mild iron deficiency anemia may be associated with normal sized cells (10). The MCV progressively decreases as the anemia becomes more severe, but the MCHC usually remains normal until the hematocrit value falls below 30%. As the anemia becomes more marked, the red cells also become progressively more distorted (poikilocytosis). Table 49.6 illustrates the relationship between the hematocrit value, the MCV, and the degree of red cell distortion (poikilocytosis) seen in iron deficiency anemia of varying degrees of severity.

Often the diagnosis of iron deficiency is obvious after the initial history, physical examination, and standard laboratory evaluation. If not, a number of other tests may be useful; The *reticulocyte index* is inappropriately low for the degree of anemia. The *serum iron concentration* (SI) is low but is usually low also in patients with acute and chronic inflammation and malignancy. Furthermore, an acute infectious process such as pneumococcal pneumonia will cause an immediate drop in the serum iron even though the patient is not iron deficient. Classically, the *total iron-binding capacity* (TIBC) is elevated. It is a measure of the serum transferrin, the iron transport protein which supplies bone marrow reticulocytes with iron. However, many iron-deficient patients have a normal TIBC, and it may be low in cases of chronic inflammation or of malignancy whether or not iron deficiency is present. The *bone marrow iron stain* is the most definitive way to prove a diagnosis of iron deficiency, since iron stores are depleted when iron deficiency anemia is present and are normal or elevated in patients with microcytic anemia due to other causes.

Table 49.6.
Representative Data Base at Various Stages in the Slow Development of Severe Iron Deficiency Anemia[a]

Hct	42	42	35	27	19
MCV (82–98 fl)	92	88	82	75	68
MCHC (32–36 g/dl)	33	33	33	31	29
SI (65–175 μg/dl)	70	60	35	20	20
TIBC (250–375 μg/dl)	300	300	300	400	450
Serum ferritin (10–200 μg/ml)	60	30	5	3	1
Peripheral smear	Normal	Normal	Normal	1+ poikilocytosis 1+ hypo-chromia	4+ poikilocytosis 4+ hypo-chromia
Bone marrow iron stores	Present	Absent	Absent	Absent	Absent

[a] Hct, hematocit value; MCV, mean corpuscular volume; MCHC, mean corpuscular hemoglobin concentration; SI, serum iron; TIBC, total iron-binding capacity. Numbers in parentheses are the range of normal values.

Serum ferritin may be helpful in the assessment of body iron stores (12). Ferritin is a water-soluble complex of iron and a binding protein, apoferritin. The serum ferritin concentration reflects the status of the reticuloendothelial stores and, in general, is a more specific test than the serum iron and iron-binding capacity in the diagnosis of iron deficiency. A low serum ferritin concentration almost always reflects iron deficiency. A very elevated serum ferritin concentration usually signifies iron overload, as in the patient who has received multiple transfusions. There are, however, a number of clinical situations in which the serum ferritin may be spuriously normal or even elevated in the presence of iron deficiency anemia (Table 49.7). In these situations it may be difficult to make a definitive diagnosis of iron deficiency without a bone marrow iron stain.

Treatment

After institution of oral iron therapy, the reticulocyte response is maximal at around 7 to 10 days. The hematocrit value begins to rise after about 1 week, and in the uncomplicated case a normal hematocrit value is reached in a few weeks. However, it takes many months of therapy for patients subsequently to replete their iron stores. In the menstruating woman with iron deficiency anemia, treatment for a year may be necessary; and in the man with iron deficiency anemia, treatment for 6 months is frequently indicated. Iron deficiency is very common in menstruating women, especially in those with heavy menstrual periods and a history of multiple pregnancies. Some may require constant iron therapy to maintain a normal hematocrit value. Standard treatment with oral iron consists of 1 tablet of iron (e.g., ferrous sulfate, 300 mg, which contains 60 mg of elemental iron) three times daily on an empty stomach (1 hour before meals). If it is difficult for patients to take the noontime dose, it is reasonable to omit it. There are numerous preparations of iron other than ferrous sulfate, but there is usually no justification for recommending any of them unless a reduction in the dose of elemental iron is

Table 49.7.
Inappropriately Normal or Elevated Serum Ferritin Levels

Acute liver disease
Cirrhosis
Hodgkin's disease
Acute leukemias
Solid tumors (occasionally)
Fever
Acute inflammation
Renal dialysis patients
Recent treatment with iron

required (see below). Generally time-release spansules and enteric coated preparations are to be avoided. They are costly, and absorption is variable. Preparations containing iron, including ferrous sulfate, can be obtained without prescription. The most vigorously promoted iron preparation, Geritol, costs the patient approximately 5 times as much as ferrous sulfate for an equivalent dosage of elemental iron. The addition of ascorbic acid to iron preparations to increase absorption is not worth the cost.

Side effects. Approximately 15% of patients have gastrointestinal side effects from oral iron, most commonly constipation, but abdominal cramping and diarrhea are also seen. When such side effects develop, the physician may elect to administer iron only once a day, or he may instruct the patient to take his iron with meals instead of on an empty stomach. Taking iron with food will decrease iron absorption by approximately 50%, but absorption will still be sufficient to replenish the body's iron if treatment is continued long enough. If symptoms still continue after these alterations in dose and schedule, it is helpful to decrease the individual dose of oral iron. If the dose is decreased to less than 40 mg of elemental iron, symptoms will frequently abate. This can be done by using pediatric liquid preparations, which are usually well tolerated. If these adjustments in the dosage and schedule of oral iron administration are made, *parenteral iron* is rarely indicated. Parenteral therapy is indicated, however, in patients with small and large bowel inflammation, rapid gastrointestinal transit, or malabsorption, and when the patient has severe iron deficiency and noncompliance has been repetitively proven. Iron dextran is the most commonly used form of parenteral iron and is usually given in 2.0-ml (100-mg) doses intramuscularly or intravenously. If the intravenous route is chosen it must be given slowly (no more rapidly than 1.0 ml/minute). Guidelines for the dosage of parenteral iron are provided in the *Physicians' Desk Reference*, but may be grossly calculated from age and hemoglobin concentration (see Table 49.8). Injections should be given daily until the calculated required dose has been administered. Side effects from parenteral iron include pain and rash at the injection site, staining of the skin, fever, and rare anaphylactoid reactions.

Thalassemia

In the normal adult there are three hemoglobins present in mature red cells: A, the major component, and two minor components, A_2 and F (fetal). Each hemoglobin molecule consists of four heme groups and four globin chains; the globin chains in each molecule are of two different types. All three hemoglobins have two α-globin chains but differ in the second set (β, δ, γ) of globin chains (Table 49.9). Anemia is due to a combination of decreased hemoglobin production and, usually, mild hemolysis.

Thalassemia is an inherited defect in globin chain production. β-Thalassemia (19) is seen in the United States primarily in black patients or those of Mediterranean (Greek and Italian) origin. The genetics of α-thalassemia are complicated, and the disorder appears to have a wider racial distribution than does

β-thalassemia but it is especially common in American blacks (17). Most patients have inherited only one defective gene (heterozygotes) and are clinically asymptomatic but may have marked red cell microcytosis. The diagnosis is important as the entity is frequently confused with iron deficiency anemia resulting in lifelong repetitive workups for gastrointestinal bleeding and inappropriate treatment with iron. Patients with homozygous β-thalassemia usually do not survive into adulthood; homozygous α-thalassemia is not compatible with life.

Diagnosis

Table 49.10 lists the typical data base for the patient with heterozygous α- or β-thalassemia. The combination of a low MCV and a mild anemia should alert the physician to the diagnosis, since in iron deficiency the degree of microcytosis parallels the severity of the anemia (see above). This discrepancy between the MCV and the Hct value, plus the frequent presence of coarsely stippled red cells on peripheral smear should result in the presumptive diagnosis of heterozygous thalassemia.

In the forms of β-thalassemia most commonly seen in the United States there is a decreased production of β chains with a compensatory increase in the production of δ chains, resulting in a decreased production of hemoglobin A and an increased production of hemoglobin A_2. This increase can be assessed by electrophoresis of the hemoglobin and is a definitive diagnostic test for β-thalassemia. Less commonly, in this country, increases in hemoglobin F may be seen in patients with β-thalassemia. Hemoglobin F must be assayed by a separate special technique (alkali denaturation test).

The α-thalassemias are more difficult to diagnose since a decreased production of α chains will affect the relative concentrations of all of the normal adult hemoglobins. A definitive diagnosis of one of the α-thalassemia syndromes may be quite difficult and may require family studies or techniques available only in research laboratories. However, the diagnosis of presumptive α-thalassemia in the setting of an appropriate data base (hematological values consistent with the diagnosis in the absence of iron deficiency and of β-thalassemia) is reasonable even in the absence of laboratory confirmation. Microcytosis

Table 49.8.
Representative Total Body Iron Deficits at Various Body Weights and Hemoglobin Concentrations

Patient Weight	Iron Deficit at Various Hemoglobin Levels			
	4 g/dl	6 g/dl	8 g/dl	10 g/dl
lb				
100	2250	1750	1400	1000
120	2650	2100	1650	1150
140	3050	2500	1950	1350
160	3550	2850	2200	1550
180	3950	3200	2500	1750

Table 49.9.
Globin Chain Composition of Normal Adult Hemoglobins

		Percentage of Total in Normal Adults
Hgb A	$\alpha_2\beta_2$	97
Hgb A_2	$\alpha_2\delta_2$	2
Hgb F	$\alpha_2\gamma_2$	1

Table 49.10.
Heterozygous Thalassemia: Typical Data Base[a]

Hct	37%
MCV	69 fl
MCH	20 pg
MCHC	32 g/dl
Reticulocyte count	2.5%
Red blood cell morphology	Microcytosis, poikilocytosis, stippling
Ferritin	Normal or increased

[a] Abbreviations are as in Table 49.6.

in black patients living in the United States is more likely due to one of the α-thalassemia syndromes than to iron deficiency.

Patient Education

It is important for the physician to explain to patients with heterozygous thalassemia that the clinical features of their condition mimic iron deficiency. The patient should be put on guard against repetitive diagnostic workups for iron deficiency. The physician should emphasize the benign nature of the illness and that the anemia, being mild, usually does not cause any symptoms. He should caution the patient against taking oral iron since thalassemic patients actually have an increase in iron stores. Genetic counseling is important; a couple, both heterozygous for β-thalassemia, have a 25% chance of having a child with homozygous thalassemia. Furthermore, the genetic defect for thalassemia and those for hemoglobin S and C are alleles. Hemoglobin S-thalassemia may be a severe disease.

Miscellaneous

The *anemia of chronic disease* and the *anemia of malignancy* may be associated with a low MCV (although the MCV is usually normal). These entities are discussed below in the section dealing with normocytic anemia (page 591). *Sideroblastic anemias* (characterized by increased iron stores and by ringed sideroblasts in the bone marrow) are occasionally microcytic, and some hemoglobinopathies are associated with a low MCV (hemoglobin E). The former are best treated in consultation with a hematologist; the latter are rare in this country.

ANEMIA WITH A HIGH MCV

The physician should recognize that an MCV greater than 100 fl is abnormal and an attempt should be made to explain the abnormality. Table 49.11 lists conditions associated with an elevated MCV (9). For the most part, the diseases associated with an elevated MCV are liver disease, the megaloblastic anemias (including drug-induced megaloblastosis), and the refractory anemias with hypercellular bone marrows (preleukemia, sideroblastic anemia). Occasionally an elevated MCV measured by

Table 49.11.
Differential Diagnosis of Mean Corpuscular Volume Greater Than 100 fl

Spurious
Reticulocytosis (marked)
Liver disease
Alcoholism
Refractory anemia (preleukemia, sideroblastic anemia)
Drugs
Megaloblastic anemias
Normal variant

the automatic counter is *spurious*, caused by red cell antibodies or by marked rouleaux formation in patients with a very high erythrocyte sedimentation rate. Since young red cells are large, patients with a marked *reticulocytosis* may have an elevated MCV.

Liver Disease

Chronic hepatocellular and obstructive liver disease results in loading of cholesterol in the lipid portion of the red cell membrane, so that the cell increases in size. Thus the MCV is frequently elevated but is usually not greater than 110 fl. On smears, cells appear to be round and centrally targeted, without significant variation in shape. This morphological abnormality is not a cause for anemia. However, patients with liver disease frequently have other reasons to be anemic (bleeding, hemolysis, folic acid deficiency). The severe alcoholic often has an elevated MCV even in the absence of overt liver disease or of marked megaloblastosis (6). Presumably the elevated MCV results from either periodic episodes of alcoholic liver disease, or from folic acid deficiency, or both. Owing to poor diet, the alcoholic frequently becomes folic acid depleted. In addition, alcohol interferes with folic acid metabolism.

Megaloblastic Anemia (15)

Table 49.12 lists the various etiologies of megaloblastic anemia related to vitamin B_{12} or folic acid deficiency. The body's stores of B_{12} are such that a diet without B_{12} (one in which animal protein was completely excluded) would not result in B_{12}-in-

Table 49.12.
Causes of Megaloblastosis Due to Vitamin B_{12} and Folic Acid Deficiency

B_{12}
  Pernicious anemia (acquired and congenital)
  Gastrectomy
  Ileal resection
  Crohn's disease and tropical sprue
  Fish tapeworm infestation
  Blind loop syndrome
  Nutritional deficiency (vegans diet, rare)
  Familial selective malabsorption (Imerslund's syndrome)
FOLIC ACID
  Dietary (old age, the alcoholic, chronic disease)
  Malabsorption (sprue)
  Hemodialysis
  Severe exfoliative skin disease (*e.g.*, psoriasis)
  Drugs:
    Interference with absorption or utilization (Dilantin, alcohol)
    Dihydrofolate reductase inhibitors (methotrexate, trimethoprim)
  Increased requirements:
    Pregnancy
    Infancy
    Hemolysis (*e.g.*, sickle cell anemia)

duced megaloblastosis for several years; therefore, dietary B_{12} deficiency is extremely rare. By far, the most common etiology of B_{12} deficiency is pernicious anemia, an acquired defect of the gastric mucosa resulting in deficient formation of intrinsic factor, a substance which binds ingested B_{12} and allows its absorption in the terminal ileum. Patients with pernicious anemia are usually elderly and complain of sore mouth, indigestion, and constipation or diarrhea. Neurological problems, including peripheral neuropathy, dorsal column dysfunction (loss of vibratory and position sense in the lower extremities), and changes in affect, are common. The anemia develops so slowly that patients frequently present with very low hematocrit values and yet remarkably good cardiovascular compensation for their anemia. Such patients usually have an expanded total blood volume and are prone to develop heart failure if given transfusions. B_{12} deficiency from other causes (Table 49.12) is less common. Patients who have had total gastrectomy or ileal resection or who have ileal disease (Crohn's disease, tropical sprue) are likely to develop B_{12} deficiency and should receive prophylactic B_{12}. B_{12} deficiency after partial gastrectomy is uncommon.

In contrast to B_{12} the body's stores of folic acid are depleted rapidly when patients eat a diet deficient in folate. (The main sources of folate in the diet are leafy vegetables, fruits, nuts, and liver.) Folic acid deficiency, therefore, is most often dietary. For example, pregnant women have an increased need for folate, and without prenatal care may develop folate deficiency, as may patients whose dietary intake is severely restricted because of chronic disease or multiple surgical procedures. Intestinal malabsorption due to any cause is also a common cause of folate deficiency. Finally, a number of drugs may be associated with folate deficiency: Dilantin interferes with folate absorption; alcohol interferes with folate utilization; and methotrexate and trimethoprim-sulfamethoxazole (Bactrim, Septra) interfere with folate metabolism. Also some chemotherapeutic agents used in the treatment of cancer and to induce immunosuppression in patients with a variety of disorders (e.g., psoriasis, systemic lupus) cause megaloblastosis (e.g., hydroxyurea, cytosine arabinoside, 6-mercaptopurine, Imuran) by inhibiting the synthesis of nucleic acids.

Diagnosis

The morphology of the peripheral blood and bone marrow is the same in patients with folic acid and B_{12} deficiencies. With a severe megaloblastic anemia the MCV is frequently markedly elevated. An MCV of greater than 120 fl is almost always due to a megaloblastic anemia. The red cells in the peripheral blood are characterized by marked variation in size and shape. The common cell is a macro-ovalocyte (large egg-shaped cell). One may also see How-

ell-Jolly bodies (nuclear fragments), Pappenheimer bodies (iron granules), and nucleated red blood cells. The nuclei of the neutrophils are frequently hypersegmented, and commonly there is a neutropenia and thrombocytopenia. The bone marrow is typically markedly cellular, revealing characteristic megaloblastic changes of all cell lines. The bone marrow iron stain usually reveals increased numbers of iron-containing nucleated red cells (sideroblasts).

Folic acid and B_{12} assay. Classically in B_{12} deficiency (pernicious anemia), the serum B_{12} level is quite low (less than 100 pg/ml) and the serum folate level is high. Spuriously normal B_{12} levels may occasionally be seen in B_{12} deficiency, and spuriously low levels may be seen without B_{12} deficiency in some patients with folic acid deficiency (see Table 49.13). The serum folate assay has little clinical usefulness in the workup of a megaloblastic anemia secondary to folic acid deficiency. The red cell folate concentration does reflect chronic folate deficiency, although it may be falsely low in some patients with B_{12} deficiency (Table 49.13).

The Schilling test. The Schilling test is a measure of B_{12} absorption and requires the measurement of total radioactivity excreted during a 24-hour period after the ingestion of radioactive B_{12}. This test is primarily useful in cases where the data are confusing and/or in patients already treated with B_{12}, where the serum levels are no longer helpful. The Schilling test requires a cooperative patient who is able to collect a 24-hour urine sample. The test includes the following steps: After voiding, the patient takes 0.5 μCi of ^{60}Co or ^{57}Co cyanocobalamine by mouth. A 24-hour urine collection is initiated; at 2 hours 1 mg of B_{12} is given by injection (the flushing dose) and the percentage of the radioactive B_{12} excreted in 24 hours is determined. Normally 7% or more of the dose is excreted in 24 hours. Incomplete collection will result in a spuriously low Schilling test and a false diagnosis of B_{12} malabsorption. In addition, if there is severe megaloblastic anemia, there are changes in the gastrointestinal mucosa which will affect B_{12} absorption. For example, the

---

Table 49.13.
B_{12} and Folate Assays

Serum B_{12} Concentration
1. Spuriously low in some patients with folate deficiency.
2. Spuriously low in some pregnant patients.
3. May be elevated for weeks after one injection of B_{12}.
4. Increased in myeloproliferative syndromes.

RBC Folate Concentration
1. Reflects chronic folate deficiency.
2. Falsely low in some patients with B_{12} deficiency.
3. Falsely high in reticulocytes.

Serum Folate Concentration
1. A measure of recent dietary intake of folate.
2. May be low, normal, or elevated in B_{12} deficiency.

Schilling test may be abnormal in folic acid deficiency until the megaloblastic process is treated for a week or two (see Table 49.14).

Table 49.15 outlines a stepwise approach to the use of the laboratory in differentiating between folic acid and B_{12} deficiency in a patient with a megaloblastic anemia.

Other laboratory features. Megaloblastic anemias are essentially hemolytic in that there is marked destruction of abnormally formed cells within the marrow (ineffective erythropoiesis) which frequently results in indirect hyperbilirubinemia and an elevated serum lactate dehydrogenase. The serum iron is usually elevated, and the reticulocyte index is inappropriately low.

Gastric achlorhydria is present in pernicious anemia, and antibodies to gastric mucosal cells and to intrinsic factor are frequently present, as are other autoantibodies, especially antithyroid and antiadrenal antibodies. There is an increased prevalence of thyroid disease (hypo- and hyperthyroidism and euthyroid goiter) in patients with pernicious anemia.

Treatment

The usual treatment for B_{12} deficiency is monthly intramuscular administration of 100 μg of B_{12} for the rest of the patient's life. Many physicians will treat patients daily while they are in the hospital, particularly if they have neurological signs; however, there is little evidence that this practice is more efficacious.

One to 5 mg of folic acid daily is adequate treatment for patients with folic acid deficiency. Treatment should be given at least until a normal hematocrit level is reached and should be continued if the patient is not eating an adequate diet or if the underlying disease persists (malabsorption, for example). Patients with a chronic hemolytic state, such as sickle cell anemia, patients on hemodialysis (folic acid is dialyzable), and pregnant patients, should receive prophylactic treatment. Whether or not patients are hospitalized depends on the severity of their symptoms and signs, the severity of their anemia, and, in the case of folate deficiency, the nature of their underlying disease.

With appropriate treatment of megaloblastic anemia there is a rapid reticulocytosis which reaches a peak at about 7 to 10 days; the hematocrit value begins to rise in about 1 week; in uncomplicated cases it will rise at a rate of 4 to 5 percentage points/week. The leukopenia and thrombocytopenia respond dramatically, and white blood cell and platelet counts may return to normal in a day or two. There is a variable response of the neurological complications of B_{12} deficiency. "Megaloblastic madness" usually abates dramatically. Dorsal column problems and peripheral neuropathies will usually improve, but more slowly. Cortical spinal tract signs are usually refractory to treatment.

The serum potassium concentration frequently falls with treatment of megaloblastic anemia, and there are case reports of fatal cardiac arrhythmias because of hypokalemia. Therefore it is important to monitor the serum potassium and to supplement it as needed (see Chapter 45).

The Myelodysplastic Syndromes (14)

These syndromes are acquired disorders of bone marrow stem cells seen in elderly patients which at presentation may mimic a megaloblastic anemia. However, the morphological features of the bone marrow and usually the peripheral smear, are different (Table 49.16). There are characteristic morphological white cell changes, the serum B_{12} and folic acid levels are high, and the patients do not respond to folic acid or B_{12}. In the bone marrow ringed sideroblasts (red cell precursors containing granules of iron which form a ring around the nuclei) are common, as are megaloblastoid changes. Approximately 25% of patients develop acute nonlymphocytic leukemia, usually within a year, but sometimes only after several years.

Table 49.14.
Causes of a Falsely Positive Schilling Test

1. Incomplete urine collection
2. Renal failure
3. Some patients with megaloblastic anemia before treatment
4. Gastric antibodies to intrinsic factor
5. Defective intrinsic factor
6. Drugs (alcohol, colchicine, neomycin, cholestyramine)
7. Pancreatic insufficiency

Table 49.15.
Differentiating between Folate and B_{12} Megaloblastosis

Etiology by History	RBC Folate	Serum B_{12}	Interpretation	Further Testing
Suggests folate	↓	Nl or ↑	Folate deficiency	None
Suggests folate	↓	Sl ↓	Folate deficiency	Recheck B_{12} after folate Rx for 1 week
Suggests B_{12}	Nl or ↑	↓	B_{12} deficiency	None
Suggests B_{12}	↓ (serum folate usually ↑)	↓	B_{12} deficiency	May confirm with Schilling test

All other combiantions → Schilling test.

Table 49.16.
Laboratory Features in Three Conditions Associated with an Elevated Mean Corpuscular Volume

	Liver Disease	Megaloblastic Anemia	Myelodysplastic Syndrome
MCV	Usually <115 fl	Maybe >115 fl	Usually <115 fl
White blood cells (WBCs)	Variable	Frequently decreased	Frequently decreased
Platelets	Variable	Frequently decreased	Frequently decreased
Red blood cell (RBC) morphology	Targets, no anisocytosis or poikilocytosis	Marked anisocytosis and poikilocytosis, macro-ovalocytes	Marked anisocytosis and poikilocytosis, may mimic megaloblastic anemia
Nucleated RBCs	Not common	Common	Common
WBC morphology	Normal	Hypersegmented nuclei of neutrophils	Abnormal mononuclear cells, no nucelar hypersegmentation of neutrophils
Platelet morphology	Normal	Normal	Frequently large and degranulated
Serum folate	Depends on diet	Decreased in folate deficiency, elevated in B$_{12}$ deficiency	Normal or elevated
Serum B$_{12}$	Normal	Decreased in B$_{12}$ deficiency, may be slightly decreased in folate deficiency	Normal or elevated

ANEMIAS WITH NORMAL MCV AND APPROPRIATE RETICULOCYTE INDEX (HEMOLYSIS AND BLEEDING)

Anemias due to bleeding and hemolysis are associated with an appropriate bone marrow response manifested by an appropriate reticulocyte index. The MCV is usually normal; however, if the reticulocyte count is high, the MCV may be slightly elevated. The diagnosis of hemolysis is suggested by an anemia with a reticulocyte index of at least 3% in the absence of overt bleeding. It should be remembered that bleeding is far more common than hemolysis and that bleeding in certain body sites (e.g., retroperitoneal bleeding in patients taking anticoagulants or bleeding into the site of a hip fracture) may be associated with a marked drop in hematocrit value and a high reticulocyte count, without external evidence of blood loss. Furthermore, the correction of anemias which are due to decreased bone marrow production may also give a data base which mimics hemolysis (e.g., patients with an appropriate reticulocyte response after being treated with iron, folic acid, or B$_{12}$, or after alcohol withdrawal).

Approach to Hemolysis (21)

It is appropriate to attempt to prove that hemolysis is occurring before obtaining diagnostic tests in a search for specific etiologies. The diagnostic approach to hemolysis varies, depending upon whether hemolysis is primarily *intravascular* or *extravascular*.

Intravascular Hemolysis

Table 49.17 lists hemolytic mechanisms associated with intravascular destruction of red cells. Almost all of them require that the patient be hospitalized and that, if possible, diagnostic testing and treatment

Table 49.17.
Clinical States Associated with Intravascular Hemolysis

Acute hemolytic transfusion reactions
Severe and extensive burns
Physical trauma (*e.g.*, march hemoglobinuria)
Severe microangiopathic hemolysis (*e.g.*, aortic valve prosthesis)
Glucose 6-phosphate dehydrogenase deficiency
Paroxysmal nocturnal hemoglobinuria
Clostridial sepsis

be planned in consultation with a hematologist. In intravascular hemolysis red cell lysis occurs within the vascular space, resulting in hemoglobinemia. The plasma becomes visibly red or brown (methemoglobinemia) at a low concentration of hemoglobin (around 30 mg/100 ml). Free hemoglobin initially binds to haptoglobin (a binding protein produced in the liver). Once haptoglobin is saturated, free hemoglobin passes through the glomerulus and hemoglobinuria occurs. Some of the hemoglobin in the renal tubules is absorbed by the renal tubular cells which slough into the urine several days later and stain positively for iron (urine hemosiderin). The latter test, therefore, is helpful in documenting the presence of intravascular hemolysis several days after it has occurred. Table 49.18 suggests an appropriate data base when hemolysis is suspected in those clinical states associated with intravascular hemolysis.

Extravascular Hemolysis

Most hemolysis occurs extravascularly within cells of the reticuloendothelial system. A diagnosis of extravascular hemolysis is more difficult to prove than that of intravascular hemolysis. There is no

Table 49.18.
Appropriate Further Data Base When Intravascular Hemolysis Is Suspected

Observation of the color of the serum/plasma
Observation of the color of the urine
Measurement of free plasma hemoglobin
Heme pigment test of the urine if there are no red cells in the urine sediment
Measurement of serum haptoglobin
Iron stain of urine sediment for hemosiderin several days after a presumed hemolytic event

Table 49.19.
Most Common Causes of Extravascular Hemolysis

Autoimmune hemolysis
Delayed hemolytic transfusion reactions
Hemoglobinopathies
Hereditary spherocytosis
Hypersplenism
Hemolysis with liver disease

hemoglobinemia, hemoglobinuria, or hemosiderinuria. Haptoglobin is partially saturated because there is a slight leakage of free hemoglobin into the circulation. There may be indirect hyperbilirubinemia, but this is an extremely insensitive sign of hemolysis. There is an increase in fecal and urine urobilinogen, but these substances are also difficult to quantitate. Other tests of hemolysis, such as red cell survival, are difficult, and the results are not known for several days. The physician must frequently be satisfied with only a presumptive diagnosis of extravascular hemolysis. Therefore, when extravascular hemolysis is suspected, it may be appropriate to obtain tests diagnostic of specific disease states based on a knowledge of the patient's other problems and on the baseline data base (Table 49.19).

Information from the peripheral smear. In hemolytic states the peripheral smear frequently reveals only evidence of the response of the bone marrow to hemolysis (large polychromatophilic or finely stippled red cells). It does not, as many physicians believe, always reveal fragmented red cells. Occasionally, however, the smear may give further clues about the specific etiology of the hemolysis as indicated below.

Spherocytes. Spherocytes are seen in small numbers in many hemolytic states. When present in large numbers they suggest either hereditary spherocytosis, autoimmune hemolysis, or one of the hemoglobin C hemoglobinopathies.

Elliptocytes. In large numbers these suggest a diagnosis of hereditary elliptocytosis.

Fragmented cells (schistocytes). Sharply pointed fragmented cells (helmet cells, spiculated cells, triangle cells) are seen in microangiopathic states (see page 587).

Spiculated cells. Sometimes these cells are seen in patients with severe liver disease and hemolysis (usually in a terminal stage of liver disease). Spiculated cells are also one type of schistocyte found in the blood of patients with microangiopathic hemolysis.

"Bite" cells (blister cells). Such cells are sometimes seen in patients with oxidative hemolysis (e.g., glucose 6-phosphate dehydrogenase deficiency). In "bite" cells all of the hemoglobin appears to be pushed to one side of the cell.

Poikilocytosis and the hemoglobinopathies. In patients with sickle cell disease and in the various other sickle cell syndromes the peripheral smear is frequently diagnostic (see below).

Hemolysis with a Positive Coombs' Test (18)

Once the physician suspects hemolysis, the diagnostic testing should be guided by the patient's problem list. Because of the relatively common occurrence of immune hemolysis and the important therapeutic implications of such a diagnosis, it is desirable to obtain a Coombs' test at this stage in the workup.

Positive Direct Coombs' Test

The direct Coombs' test is done by mixing the patients cells with Coombs' antiserum containing antibody to IgG and to complement. If the test is positive, the physician should first ascertain from the laboratory personnel that the positive result is attributable to antibody and/or complement on the red cell surface. If this is in the case, it is important to determine whether the antibody is an *alloantibody* or an *autoantibody*.

Alloantibodies are antibodies induced by prior transfusion or, in a woman, by placental transfer of fetal red cells. The antibodies are directed against specific minor red cell antigens, and it is important to identify them in the event that future transfusions are necessary. Ordinarily the antibody is primarily present in the patient's plasma and is identified by an antibody screen (indirect Coombs' test). However, a direct Coombs' test would also be positve due to the presence of alloantibodies if the patient had recently been transfused with cells that were still circulating and sensitized by the antibody.

In a patient with hemolysis, if there has not been a recent transfusion, a positive direct Coombs' test generally implies the presence of an autoantibody. In this situation the antibody may be present in the serum as well as on the surface of the red cells. Table 49.20 describes the differences between allo- and autoantibodies. Autoantibodies are classified as either *warm antibodies* or *cold antibodies*. Warm antibodies are usually IgG and cannot be identified by direct agglutination of red cells, but require a Coombs' test. Cold antibodies, however, are usually IgM, cause direct agglutination of red cells in the cold, and result in a positive Coombs' test because

Table 49.20.
Comparison of Alloantibody and Autoantibody

	Alloantibody	Autoantibody
Direct Coombs'	Frequently negative; may be positive if sensitized foreign red cells are still circulating	Positive
Indirect Coombs' Antibody screen (panel)	Positive Specificity is seen	Positive or negative Panagglutination, no specificity seen

of fixation of complement to the red cell, which is identified by nonspecific Coombs' antiserum.

Hemolysis Due to Warm Antibodies

Table 49.21 lists the conditions commonly associated with autoimmune hemolysis resulting from a warm antibody. Patients may develop such antibodies secondary to one of a number of conditions, including infections (particularly viral), collagen vascular disease (systemic lupus erythematosus, SLE), lymphoproliferative diseases, other malignancies, and secondary also to the effect of drugs. The most common drug causing a positive Coombs' test is α-methyldopa (Aldomet) (22). A positive Coombs' test is not usually observed unless the patient has been taking high doses of Aldomet for a long period of time; in such circumstances a positive Coombs' test is not uncommon, but hemolysis is rare.

Idiopathic autoimmune hemolysis is a relatively infrequent disease; sometimes it precedes the development of SLE or lymphoma. Patients usually present with anemia, which may be severe. On physical examination the spleen is slightly enlarged in 50% of patients, and mild jaundice and fever are not uncommon. The peripheral smear shows a marked polychromatophilia, spherocytosis, and, frequently, a markedly elevated reticulocyte count. Autoimmune hemolysis which is temporary, e.g., caused by drug administration or by viral infections, usually requires no treatment (although if a drug is implicated, it should be discontinued). The process gradually remits over the course of 3 to 4 weeks. Patients receiving Aldomet, who do not have hemolysis but do have a positive Coombs' test, need not discontinue use of the drug. Patients with chronic primary autoimmune hemolysis should be referred to a hematologist, who usually prescribes corticosteroids, which are usually effective if first given in reasonably high doses and slowly tapered as the anemia improves. Occasionally splenectomy is required for refractory cases. In patients with secondary chronic autoimmune hemolysis treatment of the underlying disease is the most important therapy.

Cold Agglutinin Hemolysis

The most common etiology of autoimmune hemolysis due to a cold antibody is viral or mycoplasma pneumonia (13). Severe hemolysis is rare. Chronic cold agglutinin hemolysis secondary to a collagen vascular disorder or to a lymphoprolifera-

Table 49.21.
Autoimmune Hemolysis Due to a "Warm Antibody": Differential Diagnosis

IDIOPATHIC
SECONDARY
  Infection (particularly viral)
  Drugs
    Aldomet
    Penicillin
    Quinine/quinidine
  Collagen vascular disease (systemic lupus erythematosus)
  Lymphoproliferative disorders
  Miscellaneous (thyroid disease, malignancy, *etc*)

tive disease is frequently more refractory to treatment with steroids and splenectomy than is the case with warm antibody hemolysis. Transfusion therapy may be a problem in such cases since the antibody is a panagglutinin and reacts with all blood types; therefore, a compatible cross-match may be impossible to obtain. Ordinarily the IgM antibody in cold agglutinin hemolysis is not significantly hemolytic, and transfusions may be attempted cautiously when absolutely necessary (20).

Hemolysis with Fragmented Red Cells on Peripheral Smear (3)

Table 49.22 lists those conditions associated with hemolysis and the presence of fragmented red cells on peripheral smear. The peripheral blood is characterized by the presence of sharply pointed poikilocytes (schistocytes). Such cells are quite characteristic and are clearly differentiated from abnormally shaped red cells seen in other conditions. The hemolysis may be severe, and in such cases is usually intravascular, resulting in hemoglobinemia, hemoglobinuria, haptoglobin saturation, and, subsequently, hemosiderinuria (page 000). Red cell fragmentation may occur after insertion of a prosthetic aortic valve. Rarely this may be associated with clinically significant hemolysis. More frequently red cell fragmentation is due to arteriolar lesions (fibrin, inflammation, etc) which cause damage to red cells as they pass through the damaged vessel. When fragmented red cells are accompanied by thrombocytopenia, one should consider the possibility of *disseminated intravascular coagulation* (Chapter 50) and of the syndrome known as *thrombotic thrombocytopenic purpura*. This latter syndrome is usu-

Table 49.22.
Hemolysis with Fragmented Red Cells on
Peripheral Smear: Differential Diagnosis

Aortic valve prosthesis
Arteritis (malignant hypertension, polyarteritis, *etc*)
Disseminated intravascular coagulation
Thrombotic thrombocytopenic purpura
Hemolytic uremic syndrome
Malignancy
Giant hemangiomas
Renal transplant rejection
Eclampsia

ally accompanied by fever, by neurological defects which characteristically fluctuate, and by some degree of renal failure. The mortality rate is high, and patients suspected of suffering from this condition should be hospitalized immediately and treated in consultation with a hematologist. The hemolytic uremic syndrome is a related (perhaps identical) syndrome, more common in children, characterized by the prominence of renal failure over other organ dysfunction.

Hemolysis with Enlarged Spleen (Hypersplenism) (8)

It is important to remember that not all large spleens cause "cytopenias" and that the degree of cytopenia does not necessarily correlate with the size of the spleen. Thrombocytopenia and leukopenia are more common than is anemia. Splenomegaly, from almost any cause, may result in hypersplenism, but the syndrome is seen most often in patients who have chronic liver disease and congestive splenomegaly. Splenomegaly is sometimes seen in patients with hemolysis from other mechanisms, such as autoimmune hemolysis or hereditary spherocytosis. Rarely, splenectomy is necessary because of severe cytopenias resulting from hypersplenism. Occasional patients with Felty's syndrome (see Chapter 70) are benefited by splenectomy, as are some patients with chronic leukemia or lymphoma.

Glucose 6-Phosphate Dehydrogenase (G-6-PD) Deficiency (2)

G-6-PD deficiency is seen primarily in black patients in the United States. Inheritance is sex linked. Ten percent of black males are affected (hemizygotes), as are 20% of black females (heterozygotes). In the affected black patients hemolysis due to G-6-PD deficiency is an acute intravascular hemolytic event usually precipitated either by infection or by an oxidant drug. Drugs known to precipitate hemolysis include sulfonamides, nitrofurantoin, and primaquine. Caucasian type G-6-PD deficiency is seen primarily in patients from Mediterranean countries and usually is more severe than the African type,

sometimes causing chronic persisting, partially compensated, hemolysis.

Diagnosis after a hemolytic event may be difficult, especially in the female heterozygotes. Screening tests for G-6-PD deficiency (available from most commercial and hospital laboratories) may be normal at this time, and even the affected hemizygote black male may have a normal screening test for several weeks after hemolysis (young cells have more G-6-PD activity). Ocassionally a characteristic cell ("bite cell") is seen in the peripheral blood during a hemolytic event.

Although the frequency of the genetic defect is high, the incidence of severe hemolysis with provocation (infection, drugs) is low. Ordinarily routine screening before treatment with a known oxidant drug (e.g., sulfonamide) is not advocated.

Sickle Cell Disorders (1)

Approximately 10% of the black population in the United States carry the sickle cell gene. The gene is also present to a lesser extent in Greeks, Italians, Arabians, and persons from India. Hemoglobin S results from a mutation in the β-globin chain in hemoglobin which, when oxygen tension is reduced, causes the formation of rigid elongated tactoids that distort red cell shape and increase red cell rigidity. The clumping together of sickled cells leads to tissue ischemia and infarction. A number of common inherited disorders involving hemoglobin S are listed below.

Sickle Cell Trait

Most people who are heterozygous for hemoglobin S (sickle cell trait) are completely well and are not anemic. The peripheral smear appears normal, although sickling is seen if the blood is deoxygenated. Hemoglobin electrophoresis reveals approximately 40% hemoglobin S and 60% hemoglobin A, whereas hemoglobins A_2 and F are present in normal concentration.

Most patients with sickle trait lead a normal life. However, rare clinical events attributable to the presence of sickle cell hemoglobin do occur. For example, splenic infarction at high altitudes (>10,000 feet) has been reported. (Oxygen pressures in commericial aircraft are high enough that individuals with sickle cell trait may fly with impunity.) Occasionally infarctions occur in other more vital organs during vigorous exercise. All individuals with sickle cell trait have renal tubular dysfunction resulting in hyposthenuria; and on occasion severe hematuria may occur due to hypertonicity in the renal medulla, resulting in sickling and leading to ischemia and tubular infarction. Persons with sickle cell trait have a higher incidence of renal infections, especially during pregnancy.

It is important to identify patients with sickle cell

trait so that they may be given genetic counseling. A couple, both heterozygous for hemoglobin S, should be informed that they have a 25% chance of having a child with sickle cell anemia. There are a few centers in this country where prenatal diagnosis of sickle cell anemia by amniocentesis is now possible; presumably the technique will be more widely available in the near future.

Sickle Cell Anemia (Hemoglobin SS) (1, 5)

Sickle cell anemia exists in approximately 0.25% of the black population in the United States. The disease is usually severe, resulting in significant morbidity as well as in a shortened life expectancy. One of the most disturbing features of the illness is the painful ("thrombotic") crisis, a recurrent episode of severe pain, usually in the limbs and the abdomen, due to small infarctions in multiple sites. Patients have a lifelong, often severe, anemia, with hematocrit values which range from the high teens to the midthirties (average—midtwenties). The primary mechanism of the anemia is extravascular hemolysis, so that there is a chronic reticulocytosis and a chronic indirect hyperbilirubinemia. The patients usually have a leukocytosis, the white count rising occasionally as high as 30,000 to 40,000/ml during a painful crisis. A mild thrombocytosis is also common. The peripheral smear shows markedly distorted red cells including characteristically sickled cells. Upon electrophoresis only hemoglobin S with a variable amount of hemoglobin F (no hemoglobin A) is detected.

The multiple and repetitive episodes of organ ischemia due to sickling result in a host of abnormalities. The bones characteristically appear abnormal on X-ray, revealing areas of old infarction which mimic the changes of osteomyelitis. The medullary spaces are usually widened due to the marked compensatory expansion of bone marrow. The spine frequently takes on a distorted appearance, and aseptic necrosis of the femoral (and, rarely, humeral) head is common, sometimes requiring joint replacement. Many adult patients are tall with long, thin extremities. Puberty is frequently delayed. Splenomegaly usually disappears by age 8 due to repeated infarctions of the spleen. An adult with sickle cell anemia is essentially autosplenectomized. This lack of splenic function contributes to the propensity for infections, related especially to a decreased ability to resist pneumococcal infections. *Gallstones* (pigment stones) are common, and sicklers do develop cholecystitis, which may be extremely difficult to differentiate clinically from a syndrome of intrahepatic cholestasis secondary to sickling in the hepatic sinusoids. There is some hazard to *surgery* (see Chapter 90), but patients with recurrent abdominal pain consistent with cholecystitis, who have gallstones, should probably have elective cholecystec-

tomy. *Pregnancy* in women with SS disease is complicated by increased risk of pyelonephritis, pulmonary infarction, antepartum hemorrhage, prematurity, and fetal death. With time, patients develop *cardiomegaly* and chronic myocardial disease related to repetitive microinfarctions of the heart. Murmurs are frequent and may suggest rheumatic or congenital heart disease. Patients with sickle cell anemia develop *venous thromboses* and pulmonary embolism. They also develop thromboses *in situ* in the lungs followed, after many years, by chronic scarring and fibrosis. Pulmonary thrombosis/embolism may lead to pulmonary hypertension and heart failure. Cerebral vascular accidents are common, including infarction and intracerebral and subarachnoid hemorrhage. Seizures are frequent as well. Up to 75% of patients with sickle cell anemia develop *leg ulcerations* which may be chronic and extremely difficult to heal. Sickle cell patients are very prone to serious *retinopathy*, which rarely may lead to blindness, due to plugging of small retinal capillaries and subsequent neovascularization. It is important for these patients to be examined yearly by an ophthalmologist, because some of the problems can be prevented by photocoagulation of abnormal new retinal vessels.

SC Disease

The genes which code for hemoglobin S and hemoglobin C are alleles. The C hemoglobin mutation is relatively common in blacks (about 2% prevalence), and patients doubly heterozygous for S and C constitute aprroximately 0.15% of that population. The syndrome is very similar to that of SS disease but is usually somewhat more mild. In contrast to sickle cell anemia, the spleen is palpable in 50% of adult patients.

S-Thalassemia

Patients doubly heterozygous for hemoglobin S and β-thalassemia trait have a syndrome similar to sickle cell anemia but usually much more mild. Characteristically the MCV is low, and target cells are more prominent on smear than they are in SS disease. The spleen may be palpable, and the hemoglobin electrophoresis reveals 70 to 80% hemoglobin S and smaller amounts of hemoglobin A and F (the reverse of the pattern in sickle cell trait).

Treatment

Painful "thrombotic" crisis. Painful crises are frequently severe and may last for a few hours to several days and occasionally for several weeks. They may be associated with high fever and with neutrophilia, which makes it difficult but important to differentiate crises from infection. There is no specific therapy. The patient is usually treated with narcotics and with hydration. Since patients can become addicted to narcotics because of the repetitive episodes of severe pain, it is important to limit strictly the amount of narcotics given them in ambulatory practice. When pain is severe and persistent, hospitalization is indicated.

Infection. As mentioned above, patients with sickle cell anemia are prone to infections, especially with the pneumococcus. Patients with sickle cell anemia should receive pneumococcal vaccine (see Chapter 32) and should be encouraged to seek medical help at the first evidence of infection or fever.

Hemolytic and aplastic crises. Acceleration of hemolysis is quite unusual. If hematocrit values drop significantly below baseline, it is most likely to be because of decreased marrow production, associated with infection. Such episodes are much more common in children. If they occur, hospitalization and tranfusion are often necessary. Patients with chronic severe hemolysis have an increased requirement for folic acid, and folic acid deficiency may occur, resulting in reticulocytopenia and more severe anemia. Therefore, daily folic acid therapy (1 mg) is reasonable for all patients with sickle cell anemia.

Thrombosis/embolization. When patients with sickle cell disease develop deep vein thrombosis or pulmonary embolism, they should be treated with anticoagulants as would any patient with such problems (see Chapter 51). However, venography should be avoided because of the danger of the development of leg ulcers in any patient with SS hemoglobin whose lower extremities are traumatized. It is frequently difficult to distinguish pulmonary thrombotic/embolic problems from pneumonia.

Leg ulcers. Leg ulcers are often large and are particularly refractory to treatment. Skin grafting is usually only temporarily helpful and frequently does not seem to be worth the time and discomfort involved. It is important to keep the ulcers clean, to elevate the legs frequently, and to use surgical stockings and elastic wraps (see Chapter 88).

Hematuria. Patients with sickle cell trait, sickle cell anemia, SC disease, and sickle cell-thalassemia all are prone to bouts of severe hematuria related to sickling and to medullary ischemia precipitated by the hypertonicity of the renal medulla. Bleeding can occur for days or even weeks. Maintenance of a high urine flow is important in order to prevent clots from causing obstruction, and usually the hematuria stops spontaneously.

Priapism. Priapism is common in SS and SC disease and usually results in permanent impotence once it has resolved. If urological intervention is to be attempted, it must be done within a few hours of the onset of the priapism. It is frequently only temporarily helpful. Once impotence has occurred, penile protheses are frequently quite helpful.

Recommendations for Preventive Care

1. *General.* It is important to remember that patients with sickle cell disorders have a lifelong chronic illness and will require frequent and recurrent use of the health care system. The patient needs one general physician who is familiar with him. The availability of emergency care 24 hours a day is also exceedingly important.

2. *Infection.* There should be rapid evaluation of fever, chills, or other signs of infection. The patient should be immunized with the pneumococcal vaccine (see Chapter 32). Because heart murmurs and cardiomegaly are common, it is often difficult to know if a patient with sickle cell anemia has rheumatic heart disease. If the physician is in doubt, it is reasonable for him to prescribe prophylactic antibiotics before dental procedures, *etc* (see Chapter 86).

3. *Narcotic abuse.* As mentioned above, analgesics should be given in doses sufficient to relieve pain during a thrombotic crisis. However, the use of narcotics on an ambulatory basis should be avoided if at all possible, since addiction can occur. Easy access to the physician should obviate the need to give the patient a supply of narcotics to take in case of pain.

4. *Folic acid.* Patients should receive 1 mg of folic acid daily.

ANEMIAS WITH NORMAL MCV AND AN INAPPROPRIATELY LOW RETICULOCYTE INDEX

Mild normocytic anemias without appropriate reticulocyte responses are among the most common problems seen in clinical practice. Before considering possible etiologies and embarking on a diagnostic workup, it is important for the physician to be sure that the hematocrit value/hemoglobin concentration is reproducibly low. Moreover, the normal values for the laboratory should be known. For example, in some laboratories a hematocrit value of 35% in a woman is normal. One should also consider the variation in normal values related to age, sex, pregnancy, *etc.* Finally one should be sure that volume overload is not the etiology. Marked volume shifts may result in swings in hematocrit value of 6 or 8 percentage points. Table 49.23 lists the differential diagnosis of a normocytic anemia with an inappropriately low reticulocyte count.

Anemia of Renal Failure (11)

Patients with uremia are anemic primarily because of decreased production of erythropoietin. The red cell morphology on smear is usually normal, but occasionally spiculated cells (burr cells) may be seen. An occasional patient may have a microangiopathic peripheral smear (see page 000). There may be a mild thrombocytopenia, and the nuclei of the neutrophils may be hypersegmented even in the absence of folic acid deficiency. The hematocrit value depends on the degree of renal failure (see Fig. 47.3, Chapter 47). Anemia is unusual if the creatinine is less than 3 mg/100 ml. The hematocrit value

Table 49.23.
Anemia with a Normal Mean Corpuscular Volume and Low Reticulocyte Index: Differential Diagnosis

Renal failure
Anemia of chronic disease (inflammatory disease and malignancy)
Anemia of hypoendocrine states (hypothyroidism, *etc*)
Mild (early) iron deficiency
Combined iron deficiency and megaloblastic anemia
Sideroblastic anemia
Aplastic anemia
Bone marrow infiltration (myelophthisis)
Bleeding or hemolysis plus one of the above

seen in patients with renal failure on dialysis is extremely variable (from the low teens, requiring transfusion, up to the midthirties). It is important to remember that patients in renal failure may also be anemic because of iron deficiency (secondary to blood loss) or because of folate deficiency (since folic acid is dialyzable). Some patients with glomerulonephritis or arteritis may have a microangiopathic hemolytic anemia.

Anemia of Chronic Disease (4)

Any chronic inflammatory disease (e.g., rheumatoid arthritis) or malignant neoplastic disease may cause mild to moderate anemia, unrelated to blood loss or hemolysis. (If the hematocrit value is less than 25%, another explanation should be sought.) Red cell morphology is usually normal but occasionally the MCV may be less than 80 fl, requiring differentiation of the process from other causes of a microcytic anemia (see page 579). The serum iron and the total iron-binding capacity are low; the percent saturation may be just as low as it is in iron deficiency ($\leq$10%). The serum ferritin is normal or elevated, and bone marrow iron stores are normal or increased.

In addition to chronic infections, an *acute* infection or inflammation will cause a drop in serum iron, reticulocytopenia, and a decrease in bone marrow red cell production. If present for 1 week or more, therefore, an acute inflammatory process may result in a fall in the hematocrit value of several percentage points.

Mild Early Iron Deficiency

Although severe iron deficiency results in microcytic anemia (see pages 578–581), in the early stages mild iron deficiency may result in anemia with a normal peripheral smear and a normal MCV. Diagnosis can usually be made by measurement of serum ferritin or by a bone marrow iron stain. In addition, a patient with severe iron deficiency, when it accompanies a macrocytic anemia such as a megaloblastic anemia (as in an alcoholic patient with iron deficiency and folic acid deficiency), may have a severe anemia which is normocytic. The reticulo-

cyte count is inappropriately low until alcohol is withdrawn and iron and folate are administered.

Anemia in the Elderly (16)

Old age *per se* is not an explanation for a significant normocytic anemia. Hematocrit values in healthy patients in their seventies are only slightly lower than they are in the normal general adult range (Table 49.1). However, it is in elderly patients that frustrating, mild, unexplained, normocytic anemias occur. In such patients the following possible explanations should be considered: (*a*) fluid overload, (*b*) blood loss from phlebotomy if the patient has been hospitalized recently, and (*c*) any recent inflammatory disease (viral or bacterial infection, inflammatory joint problem) which may depress bone marrow production and, if present for several days, may result in a drop in hematocrit value. If none of the above explanations seems appropriate, and there is no reason to suspect an underlying problem to explain the hematocrit value, it is reasonable simply to follow the hematocrit value without further diagnostic workup. If it is known that the anemia is relatively recent (e.g., if there is a record of a normal hematocrit value 3 months previously), then other efforts should be made to explain the anemia. For example, the possibility of occult gastrointestinal bleeding with early iron deficiency, and of the anemia of chronic disease (has there been a recent weight loss, fever, *etc*?) should be entertained.

General Reference

Williams WJ, Beutler E, Erslev AJ, Lichtman MA (eds): *Hematology*, ed 3. New York, McGraw-Hill, 1983.
    The currently standard text.

Specific References

1. Abramson H, Bertles JF, Wethers DL (eds): *Sickle Cell Disease*. St Louis, CV Mosby, 1973.
2. Beutler E: Glucose-6-phosphate dehydrogenase deficiency: diagnosis; clinical and genetic implications. *Am J Clin Pathol* 47:303, 1967.
3. Brain MC: Microangiopathic hemolytic anemia. *N Engl J Med* 281:833, 1969.
4. Cartwright GE: The anemia of chronic disorders. *Semin Hematol* 3:351, 1966.
5. Charache S: Treatment of sickle cell anemia. *Annu Rev Med* 32:195, 1981.
6. Colman N, Herbert J: Hematologic complications of alcoholism: overview. *Semin Hematol* 17:164, 1980.
7. Cook JD: Clinical evaluation of iron deficiency. *Semin Hematol* 19:6, 1982.
8. Dameshek W: Hypersplenism. *Bull NY Acad Med* 31:113, 1955.
9. Davidson RJL, Hamilton PJ: High mean red cell volume: its incidence and significance in routine hematology. *J Clin Pathol* 31:493, 1978.
10. England JM, Ward S, Down MC: Microcytosis, anisocytosis and the red cell indices in iron deficiency. *Br J Haematol* 34:589, 1976.
11. Erslev AJ: Management of anemia of chronic renal failure. *Clin Nephrol* 2:174, 1974.
12. Halliday JW, Powell LW: Serum ferritin and isoferritins in clinical medicine. *Prog Hematol* 11:229, 1979.

13. Jacobson LB, Longstreth GF, Edgington TS: Clinical and immunologic features of transient cold agglutinin hemolytic anemia. *Am J Med* 54:514, 1973.
14. Koeffler HP, Golde DW: Human preleukemia. *Ann Intern Med* 93:347, 1980.
15. Lindenbaum J: Status of laboratory testing in the diagnosis of megaloblastic anemia. *Blood* 61:624, 1983.
16. Lipschitz DA, Udupa KB, Milton KY, Thompson CO: Effects of age on hematopoiesis in man. *Blood* 63:502, 1984.
17. Pierce HI, Kurachi S, Sofroniadou K, Stamatoyamopoulos G: Frequencies of thalassemia in American blacks. *Blood* 49:981, 1977.
18. Pirofsky G: Clinical aspects of autoimmune hemolytic anemia. *Semin Hematol* 13:251, 1976.
19. Rawley PT: The diagnosis of beta-thalassemia trait: a review. *Am J Hematol* 1:129, 1976.
20. Rosenfield RE, Jagathambal: Transfusion therapy for autoimmune hemolytic anemia. *Semin Hematol* 13:311, 1976.
21. Waterbury L: *Hematology for the House Officer*. Baltimore, Williams & Wilkins, 1984, p 29.
22. Worrledge SM: Immune drug-induced hemolytic anemias. *Semin Hematol* 10:327, 1973.

CHAPTER FIFTY

Disorders of Hemostasis

PHILIP D. ZIEVE, M.D.

In healthy man a number of different processes interact to ensure that blood is maintained in a fluid state until the integrity of a blood vessel wall is compromised; at that point, a plug is rapidly formed to prevent exsanguination. Three major systems are involved in this regard: the vasculature itself, the blood platelets, and the coagulation system.

EVALUATION OF PATIENTS

The history is the most important aid in determining whether or not a patient has a hemorrhagic diathesis. Patients with either congenital disorders of hemostasis or acquired disorders of long standing will almost certainly have had unexpectedly excessive bleeding in response to minor trauma or to surgery. The clinician should ask specifically whether the patient has required transfusion following an operative procedure or a seemingly minor trauma.

Bleeding due to trauma to the vasculature is overwhelmingly more common than bleeding due to defective hemostasis. Therefore, patients who present, for example, with gastrointestinal or genitourinary hemorrhage are more likely to have a lesion, such as a peptic ulcer, a carcinoma, a diverticulum, or a tumor of the kidney or of the bladder that has bled than a disorder of hemostasis. Similarly, nose bleeds, bleeding gums, or excessive menstrual flow most likely reflect local (usually benign) problems. Furthermore, even if patients have hemostatic dysfunction, they are likely to bleed from local lesions, the propensity to bleed of which has been accentuated by the hemostatic abnormality.

Specific disorders of hemostasis may be suspected strongly on the basis of the patient's history and

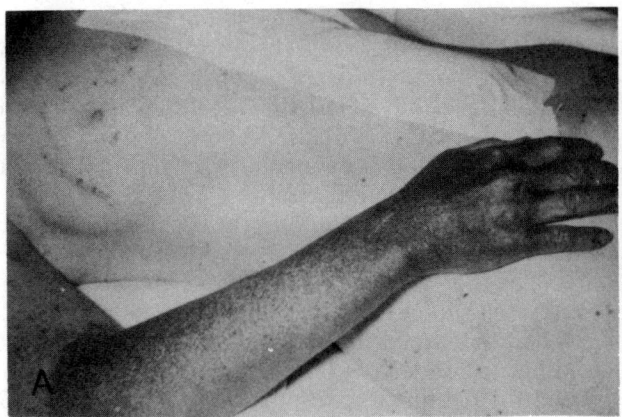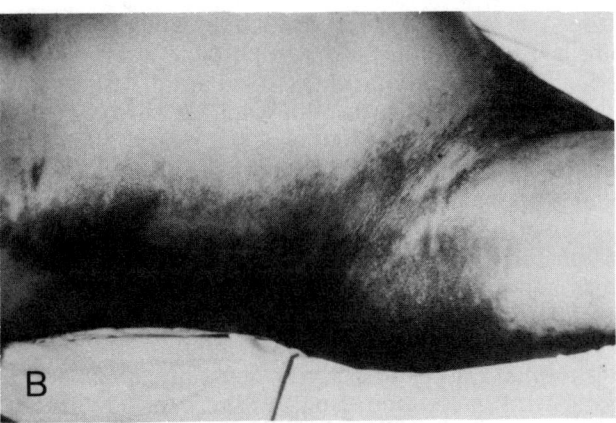

Figure 50.1. Bleeding due to thrombocytopenia compared to bleeding due to abnormal coagulation. *A.* Immune thrombocytopenic purpura. *B.* Hemophilia A.

(From Zieve PD, Levin J: *Disorders of Hemostasis.* Philadelphia, WB Saunders, 1976.)

because of characteristic findings on physical examination (see Fig. 50.1 and below), but in almost all instances laboratory tests are required before a specific diagnosis can be made. Screening tests, procedures which are extremely sensitive to alterations in hemostasis, are ordinarily relied upon first in a patient with a suspected hemorrhagic diathesis (Table 50.1). If any of these tests is abnormal or if the clinician strongly suspects that a disorder of hemostasis exists even if the tests are not abnormal, more specific tests are indicated; these are best performed in consultation with a hematologist. A number of years ago, the bleeding time and the clotting time were the most common tests performed to screen patients for possible disorders of hemostasis. Although both of these have lost favor because of their lack of sensitivity, the bleeding time, as mentioned below, despite its limitations is still the only readily performed procedure to detect *qualitative* abnormalities of blood platelets (see page 598).

DISORDERS OF BLOOD VESSELS

Vascular disease (Table 50.2) is diagnosed uncommonly as a cause of a hemorrhagic diathesis, in part because, except for trauma, disorders of the vasculature that result in untoward bleeding are relatively rare (2), and in part because there is no reliable screening test to detect generalized vascular dysfunction. The primary hemorrhagic manifestation of vascular disease is purpura, a confluent purplish discoloration of the skin due to extravasation of blood from cutaneous and subcutaneous blood vessels. Although patients with an abnormal vasculature may occasionally experience bleeding from relatively large blood vessels, most commonly they bleed into the skin or mucous membranes. Because purpura is a common response to minor trauma, it

Table 50.1.
Laboratory Evaluation of Hemostatic Function

System	Screening Tests	Specific Tests
Blood vessels	None	Depends on suspected underlying disorder (see the text)
Platelets—quantitative	Scanning of a stained smear of the peripheral blood	Platelet count
Platelets—qualitative	Bleeding time	Platelet aggregation Platelet release reaction
Coagulation	Partial thromboplastin time, prothrombin time, thrombin time	Factor assays

Table 50.2.
Bleeding Due to Vascular Disease

Cutaneous	Mucocutaneous
Senile purpura	Amyloidosis
Steroid purpura	Myeloma
Autoerythrocyte sensitization	Macroglobulinemia
Cryoglobulinemia	Vitamin C deficiency
Hyperglobulinemia of Waldenström	Hereditary hemorrhagic telangiectasia

cannot in itself be taken as evidence of an underlying hemorrhagic diathesis.

Cutaneous Lesions

Unexplained bruises, especially in the lower extremities, are common and usually are not associated with an underlying disease process. A history of "easy bruisability" therefore is not likely, in itself, to lead to a diagnosis of a disorder of hemostasis. Similarly, *senile purpura*, which occurs characteristically on the dorsum of the hand and the extensor surfaces of the forearms, does not represent a generalized hemorrhagic diathesis, but results from the loss of connective tissue support to intracutaneous blood vessels, which then are easily traumatized and bleed within the substance of the skin. Identical lesions are seen sometimes in patients with *Cushing's syndrome* or in patients who have received corticosteroid therapy.

Allergic purpura (Henoch-Schönlein purpura) (4) represents a hypersensitivity reaction to an antigenic stimulus which usually cannot be identified (although occasionally a drug or a bacterial infection can be incriminated as a provocative agent). Characteristically patients develop a symmetrical petechial rash, most prominent on the extremities. The lesions are slightly raised, distinguishing them from the petechiae of thrombocytopenia. No hemostatic dysfunction is associated with this condition; the cutaneous manifestations of the disorder are part of a widespread vasculitis, the manifestations of which also may include arthralgias (sometimes with evidence of joint effusions) fever, malaise, abdominal pain, gastrointestinal bleeding, and renal disease due to a focal glomerulonephritis which occasionally may progress to chronic renal failure. There is no specific treatment for this condition, although if the patient is taking a drug that is suspected to be a sensitizing agent, it should be discontinued. Most patients recover spontaneously within 3 or 4 weeks, but sometimes signs and symptoms of the disease continue for up to a year. Patients should be reassured while they are symptomatic that unless they have evidence of progressive renal disease, they will ultimately recover.

Autoerythrocyte sensitization (15) is a disorder characterized by apparently spontaneous painful ecchymoses, usually on the lower extremities and anterior trunk. The disorder is named as it is because of a belief at one time that it arose as the result of a hypersensitivity response to the patients' red cells or red cell stroma, and in fact the lesions can sometimes be produced by injection of red cells into the skin of these patients. It has become apparent, however, that virtually all patients with the disorder, most of whom are women, are severely psychoneurotic and in some instances frankly psychotic; and many people believe now that the lesions are self-inflicted.

Cryoglobulinemia (6) either as a special feature of dysproteinemia, (see below) or as a benign primary abnormality, sometimes associated with immune complex disease, may also cause purpuric bleeding, especially on the lower extremities, the ear lobes, or the tip of the nose. Patients with immune complex disease may have associated renal failure.

The diagnosis of cryoglobulinemia may be made by placing a sample of the patient's serum in a refrigerator overnight and then inspecting the serum to see whether a white gel or precipitate has formed which disappears when the specimen is warmed. The blood for this test should be drawn in a warm syringe, and then it should be allowed to clot and retract in a 37°C water bath.

Hyperglobulinemic purpura of Waldenström (8) is a rare condition characterized by purpura, especially of the lower extremities, an elevated erythrocyte sedimentation rate, mild anemia, and a polyclonal increase in the blood of a mixture of IgG and anti-IgG immunoglobulins. The disease is more common in women and, particularly after the age of 40, may be associated with an underlying collagen vascular disorder. The primary condition is untreatable, but is generally benign.

Mucocutaneous Lesions

Some patients with vascular disease are prone to bleed from the oral, nasal, or gastrointestinal mucosa, as well as from the skin. Such patients may present to their physicians, not only with cutaneous hemorrhage, but with bleeding gums, epistaxis, hematemesis, or melena.

Primary amyloidosis (5). Mucocutaneous bleeding may be a symptom of primary amyloidosis because of the deposition of amyloid within the walls of blood vessels. Periorbital bleeding and bleeding in skin folds are especially common. The skin in the areas of hemorrhage sometimes appears thickened because of palpable amyloid deposits within it. Patients suspected of having this disorder should have skin biopsies with appropriate staining as well as serum and urine electrophoresis in an attempt to make a specific diagnosis.

Dysproteinemia (14). Either myeloma or macroglobulinemia may be associated with untoward bleeding, either because of increased viscosity of the blood or because the coating of blood vessels and platelets with the abnormal protein interferes with normal hemostatic function. Abnormal coagulation is also common in patients with these disorders. Patients suspected of having dysproteinemia should have samples of their serum and urine examined by electrophoresis in an attempt to demonstrate a monoclonal protein. If the diagnosis of dysproteinemia seems likely on the basis of this test and of the clinical presentation, consultation with a hematologist or oncologist is appropriate.

Vitamin C deficiency (7). There are three situations in which symptomatic vitamin C deficiency (scurvy) might be seen in this country: in chronic alcoholics, in food faddists, and in chronically ill or debilitated patients. Since humans, unlike most animals, are unable to synthesize vitamin C, they are dependent upon exogenous sources, such as fruits or leafy vegetables. People who cannot or will not eat an adequate diet of foods which contain the vitamin are subject to the manifestations of scurvy. The signs and symptoms of scurvy are largely attributable to the formation of defective connective tissue, because of the human body's absolute dependence on vitamin C for the synthesis of normal collagen. Mucocutaneous bleeding is common in patients with vitamin C deficiency, who present characteristically with large ecchymoses on their extremities, with bleeding gums, and, very suggestive of this disorder, perifollicular hemorrhages which appear commonly on the lower extremities and anterior trunk. Sometimes patients with vitamin C deficiency develop hemarthroses similar to those seen in patients with severe coagulation disorders. All of the manifestations of scurvy are readily reversed by administration of vitamin C, so that although the disorder is uncommon it should be considered in patients with compatible signs and symptoms. Vitamin C deficiency can be confirmed by assay of the blood, but this is usually unnecessary since, if the diagnosis is suspected, a therapeutic trial of vitamin C is innocuous.

Hereditary hemorrhagic telangiectasia (13). This is an inherited abnormality of blood vessels (an autosomal dominant condition) in which there is dilation of abnormally thin walled venules and capillaries. The dilations result in characteristic telangiectases which are small, flat, red or purple lesions that blanch on pressure. They occur throughout the body but can be seen externally most commonly on the lips, the tongue, the mucous membranes of the nose, and the hands. Lesions of larger blood vessels also occur in this disease, most commonly pulmonary arteriovenous fistulas which develop in up to one-third of patients and which may cause "high output" heart failure. The mucocutaneous lesions may bleed excessively when traumatized. Recurrent epistaxis is the most common symptom of patients with the disorder, but the most troublesome problem is recurrent gastrointestinal bleeding, which is notoriously difficult to manage. Accessible lesions can ordinarily be treated by local compression. There is no pharmacological agent which will alter the course of the condition, but symptoms are quite variable; many patients experience relatively little difficulty during the course of their life.

DISORDERS OF PLATELETS

Platelets provide a cellular defense against the loss of blood from traumatized vessels, especially where blood flow is relatively rapid, as it is on the arterial side of the circulation and in the left heart. Platelets are particularly effective in sealing leaks from small arterioles and capillaries; when platelets are abnormal, either quantitatively or qualitatively, it is these vessels which bleed most prominently. The platelet plug is initiated by the exposure of platelets to subendothelial collagen which is exposed by injury to the vascular intima. The absorption of a protein, von Willebrand factor (VWF—see below, page 600), to specific receptor sites on the platelet surface is important in the mediation of this process. Thereafter, aggregating agents, such as thrombin and adenosine diphosphate, cause the accretion of platelets at that site, eventually forming an adhesive plug which within minutes prevents the further flow of blood. Eventually the plug is replaced by fibrin laid down by the activation of the coagulation mechanism, which occurs simultaneously with the initiation of platelet plug formation.

Thrombocytopenia is one of the most common acquired disorders of hemostasis. The normal platelet count is between 150,000 and 400,000/mm^3, but the platelet count ordinarily must be reduced below 50,000/mm^3 before untoward bleeding is observed, and even then bleeding usually does not occur unless the patient is traumatized. So-called spontaneous bleeding is unlikely unless the platelet count is reduced below 20,000/mm^3. The characteristic lesion of thrombocytopenia is the petechia, a small purpuric hemorrhage occurring on the skin or mucous membranes, especially at sites of elevated capillary pressure, such as the lower extremities, the forearm after inflation of a blood pressure cuff, or the face after prolonged crying or coughing. In fact, if capillary pressure is raised high enough, or if capillaries are damaged after sunburn, for example, petechiae may be seen in otherwise normal people. Although cutaneous bleeding may be the first clue to the diagnosis of thrombocytopenia, morbidity from the disorder is more likely to result from gastrointestinal or genitourinary hemorrhage. As previously mentioned (see page 592), if bleeding from these sites occurs, the patient should be examined at an appropriate time to determine whether an organic lesion, such as a carcinoma of the colon or of the kidney, has bled in association with defective hemostasis. The most feared complication of thrombocytopenia is intracerebral bleeding which, although it occurs infrequently, is still one of the major causes of death in patients with the disorder.

Evaluation of Thrombocytopenic Patient

The best screening test for the evaluation of the numbers of platelets in the blood is observation of a stained smear of the peripheral blood. With relatively little experience it is easy to determine whether the platelet count is unusually low or high. In un-anticoagulated blood, at least one clump of platelets should be seen, on the average, in every oil immersion field. In anticoagulated blood, one platelet should be seen for every 10 to 20 red cells. If a quantitative abnormality is suspected, a precise platelet count can be obtained. Such tests as the bleeding time and the measurement of clot retraction are much less useful as screening tests for detecting *quantitative* abnormalities of platelets.

However, the bleeding time, despite its limitations, is still the best screening test to evaluate *qualitative* abnormalities of platelet function (see below, page 598).

Patient experience. The bleeding time should be done by use of a commercially available, spring-loaded, disposable device (Simplate) which makes a small incision in the forearm. The examiner should puncture the skin with a disposable lancet. A blood pressure cuff should be inflated to 40 mm Hg above the elbow during the test. The time between the instant the puncture is made and the point at which blood from the wound can no longer be adsorbed onto a piece of filter paper is the bleeding time. The patient should be warned of the very transient sharp pain that he will experience when the wound is made and of the small scar, usually inapparent, that may form when the wound heals.

In ambulatory practice the physician will most often encounter patients with platelet counts lower than normal in whom the precise pathophysiology of thrombocytopenia is not clear.

Many patients are found to have thrombocytopenia during the course of routine hematological studies performed to obtain baseline data, or as part of an evaluation of an apparently unrelated condition. If the platelet count is over 50,000/mm³ in such circumstances, and the history, physical examination, and other hematological evaluation, do not suggest that an underlying disease is present which urgently requires diagnosis and treatment, the clinician is probably justified in simply following the patient with serial platelet counts (performed monthly until it is determined how stable the counts are). If the counts do not decrease further, and if no other evidence of a disease process emerges, there is no need to stress the patient with further diagnostic procedures.

Symptomatic thrombocytopenia due to *decreased production* of platelets is usually observed in conjunction with processes, such as aplastic anemia, leukemia, or disseminated tuberculosis, that affect other hematological cell lines. In contrast, severe thrombocytopenia due to *increased destruction* of platelets does not necessarily indicate the presence of a disease process that is affecting parts or systems of the body other than the blood platelets or their precursors. In order to be reasonably certain, however, about the pathophysiology of thrombocytopenia it is necessary to perform an aspiration of the bone marrow and to evaluate the numbers of megakaryocytes on a properly stained smear. That requires referral to a hematologist. Patients who have thrombocytopenia because of diseases involving the bone marrow will have reduced numbers of megakaryocytes; if the underlying disease process is severe, it is likely that abnormalities of production of, or qualitative changes in, other cell lines also will

be noted. On the other hand if the patient is thrombocytopenic because of increased destruction of platelets, the numbers of megakaryocytes will be increased and the marrow will otherwise appear normal (although increased erythroid activity might be seen in those patients who are bleeding). If the practitioner decides that a bone marrow aspirate is indicated because of the severity of the thrombocytopenia (ordinarily less than 20,000 to 30,000 platelets/mm³), because of evidence of a hemorrhagic diathesis at higher platelet counts, or because of a suspicion of a generalized underlying disease affecting the bone marrow, referral to a consultant in hematology is warranted. Depending on the nature of the underlying disease, it would then be appropriate for the hematologist to initiate and maintain therapy, or to refer the patient back to the primary physician.

Decreased Production of Platelets (Table 50.3)

Decreased production of platelets is a common mechanism for thrombocytopenia in ambulatory patients. Apparent suppression of thrombopoiesis is often associated with *viral infections*, such as benign upper respiratory infections, infectious mononucleosis, and childhood exanthems. In most cases, bone marrow aspirates show megakaryocytes in normal or reduced numbers, although they sometimes appear morphologically abnormal. At other times increased numbers of megakaryocytes are seen, suggestive of a destructive process (perhaps immunological) to which the marrow has responded with increased production of platelets. In general, patients with benign viral infections are not likely to have severe thrombocytopenia and so are not at major risk of bleeding. The process ordinarily dissipates as the infection resolves.

Certain *drugs* predictably produce thrombocytopenia by affecting thrombopoiesis. Among these, cytotoxic agents are unlikely to be administered by the general internist. Chloramphenicol suppresses hematopoiesis and if given for a long period of time

Table 50.3.
Thrombocytopenia Due to Decreased Production of Platelets

GENERALIZED DISORDERS OF HEMATOPOIESIS
Aplastic anemia[a]
Invasive processes: leukemia, metastatic carcinoma, disseminated infection (*e.g.*, tuberculosis)[a]
Folate or vitamin B_{12} deficiency[a]
Drugs: cytotoxic agents, chloramphenicol, alcohol
SPECIFIC DISORDERS OF THROMBOPOIESIS
Certain infections (usually viral)[b]
Certain drugs (in most cases, cause and effect have not been demonstrated)

[a] Not discussed in the text.
[b] Processes most likely to be seen in ambulatory practice.

(usually more than a few weeks) may produce pancytopenia. It is unlikely that the practitioner would prescribe chloramphenicol for long periods in ambulatory practice, but if he does, he should be aware that the process is reversible when the drug is discontinued, in contrast to the much rarer cases of aplastic anemia caused by chloramphenicol which do not appear to be dose related and are probably not reversible.

Although thiazide diuretics have been reported to produce mild to moderate thrombocytopenia commonly, in fact a clear-cut cause and effect relationship has not been demonstrated unequivocally. In the reported studies platelet counts have fallen several weeks after the beginning of therapy, sometimes associated with morphologically abnormal megakaryocytes. Rarely, however, thiazides have been clearly implicated in immunologically induced destructive thrombocytopenia (see below). Thiazide diuretics also are a common cause of allergic purpura (see page 594), but patients with this condition have normal platelet counts.

Conceivably a large number of drugs are capable of producing thrombocytopenia by suppressing thrombopoiesis. Therefore, if patients are symptomatic from thrombocytopenia or have counts below 50,000/mm³ and the cause of thrombocytopenia is not known, the practitioner would be advised to discontinue administration of all drugs that are not considered absolutely essential.

Management

Unless thrombocytopenia is severe or unless patients have demonstrated a hemorrhagic diathesis, treatment is not necessary. Clearly, if drugs are incriminated in the process, they should be discontinued, if possible. If it is expected that thrombocytopenia will be transient (as, for example, in patients being treated with cytotoxic therapy for an underlying malignancy), treatment with platelet transfusions sometimes is indicated. Also, some patients with chronic diseases of the bone marrow, such as aplastic anemia, may require more regular platelet transfusion. In any event, patients who are considered candidates for platelet transfusions should be followed by hematologists or oncologists as well as by the primary physician.

Increased Destruction of Platelets (Table 50.4)

Destruction of platelets as a cause of thrombocytopenia is infrequently seen in ambulatory practice but, when seen, is most likely to have an immunological basis. *Autoimmune thrombocytopenia* (3), the most common of the antibody-induced disorders associated with a low platelet count, is a diagnosis made in a practitioner's office by exclusion. Such patients characteristically present with petechial bleeding. Physical examination reveals no other ev-

Table 50.4.
Thrombocytopenia Due to Increased Destruction of Platelets

IMMUNOLOGICAL
Autoimmune[a]
Isoimmune: neonatal and post-transfusion[b]
Drug-induced: quinidine, quinine, gold, heroin
NONIMMUNOLOGICAL
Infections[b]
Drug-induced: alcohol[a]
Mechanical injury[b]

[a] Processes most likely to be seen in ambulatory practice.
[b] Not discussed in the text.

idence of disease; in particular, the spleen is usually not palpable. An acute disease, often preceded by benign viral infection, is seen more commonly in children and, by definition, lasts less than 6 months. The chronic illness (formerly called ITP, idiopathic thrombocytopenic purpura) lasts longer than 6 months and is seen more often in women than men (ratio of 3 or 4 to 1). It sometimes is associated with an underlying lymphoproliferative disorder, a collagen vascular disease, especially systemic lupus erythematosus, and, more rarely, with autoimmune hemolytic anemia. Recently, there has been an increased incidence of immune thrombocytopenia in homosexual men (12), many of whom appear to have at least some of the characteristics of the acquired immune deficiency syndrome (see Chapter 52). Autoimmune thrombocytopenia has been shown to be due to an antibody adsorbed to the surface of circulating platelets which results in their premature destruction by the reticuloendothelial system.

A large number of drugs (11) have been associated with thrombocytopenia on an immunological basis. The most common are quinidine and quinine, but even these agents are implicated rarely. However, if a patient presents to the practitioner with severe thrombocytopenia due to increased destruction of circulating platelets, it is important to ask what drugs the patient is taking and to consider stopping them if there is any question of their being involved in the process. In recent years it has been demonstrated that occasional patients with rheumatoid arthritis treated with gold salts will develop thrombocytopenia that has an immunological basis; in fact, this process appears to be much more common than the generalized suppression of hematopoiesis occasionally associated with the administration of gold. In addition, several cases have been reported where heroin addicts have thrombocytopenia of an immune type, apparently produced by heroin (or an adulterant used with it).

It is not unusual for *alcoholics* to develop thrombocytopenia, usually to a moderate degree, after a binge. Alcohol appears to damage platelet membranes, causing their premature destruction, and also to inhibit compensatory increase in platelet production by marrow megakaryocytes. Once the binge is over, the platelet count returns to normal (or transiently higher than normal) in 4 to 5 days. Alcoholics of long standing who have developed cirrhosis of the liver and portal hypertension may have chronic thrombocytopenia because of increased sequestration of platelets in their spleens.

Management

Patients who are thrombocytopenic because of increased destruction of platelets also should be treated in consultation with a hematologist. If the patient presents with untoward bleeding, or if platelet counts are lower than 20,000/mm^3 and immediate consultation is not available, the practitioner would be justified in beginning treatment with the equivalent of 60 mg of prednisone a day and hospitalizing the patient while awaiting expert advice. Modification of the steroid dose, and decisions about splenectomy or other kinds of therapy should be made in conjunction with an experienced hematologist.

After treatment, approximately 90% of patients with chronic autoimmune thrombocytopenia ultimately have a permanent remission to the point where their platelet counts are high enough to support normal hemostasis without continued therapy. The rest require the continuing care of a hematologist.

Increased Sequestration of Platelets

Patients with large spleens often have thrombocytopenia because of redistribution of platelets within a larger splenic pool, most commonly because of congestive splenomegaly associated with portal hypertension. Splenectomy reverses thrombocytopenia, but should only be considered if there is a clear-cut hemorrhagic diathesis and if the underlying disease responsible for the enlarged spleen permits an operation to be performed.

Increased Utilization of Platelets

Patients with disseminated intravascular coagulation (10) characteristically have thrombocytopenia almost always in association with multiple defects in coagulation. Such patients often present acutely ill because of the underlying disease which has incited the hemostatic disorder. For example, in patients with various complications of pregnancy, disseminated carcinoma, or in some patients with septicemia, hemostatic mechanisms have been activated because of exposure of the circulating blood to thromboplastic material. The hemorrhagic diathesis is manifest most commonly by widespread bruising, petechiae, and mucous membrane bleeding, occasionally, but not often, associated clinically with evidence of venous or arterial thrombosis. In addition to thrombocytopenia, patients present with disordered coagulation, which can be identified by measuring the prothrombin time, the partial thromboplastin time, and the concentration of fibrinogen in the plasma, and by the demonstration of increased titers of fibrinogen and fibrin degradation products in the plasma or serum. These products are formed by the fibrinolysis of fibrin by plasmin, the major proteolytic enzyme of the blood. Patients who are strongly suspected of having disseminated intravascular coagulation or in whom the diagnosis has been made should be hospitalized for further treatment and to identify and treat the underlying disease.

Qualitative Disorders of Platelets (1)

A number of inherited abnormalities of platelets have been identified which result in impaired hemostasis even though platelet counts are often within normal limits. In general the hemorrhagic diathesis associated with these conditions is milder than it is in patients with severe thrombocytopenia. Practitioners are unlikely to see these patients in their practice, but in patients who have unexplained bleeding, such as frequent epistaxis or recurrent gastrointestinal hemorrhage, with apparently normal coagulation and normal or slightly reduced platelet counts, it is reasonable to perform a bleeding time, which is almost always abnormal in patients with qualitatively abnormal platelets. Similar abnormalities may be acquired in patients with various disease states, most commonly *uremia*; in fact, patients with chronic renal failure who have a tendency to bleed often improve after hemodialysis. Perhaps the most common acquired qualitative disorder of blood platelets occurs after the ingestion of *small doses of aspirin*, which regularly prolongs the bleeding time and interferes with platelet aggregation and with the release of certain intracellular platelet constituents. Although untoward bleeding is unusual in patients who have taken aspirin, the drug may intensify a pre-existing tendency to bleed.

Thrombocytosis

Platelet counts above 400,000, unless associated with a myeloproliferative disorder, such as polycythemia vera, myeloid metaplasia, or chronic granulocytic leukemia, are not in themselves associated with an increased risk of morbidity from excessive bleeding or clotting. They may, however, signify the presence of an underlying disease which requires attention. If on a routine evaluation there are a large number of platelets on the patient's peripheral blood smear, the practitioner should ask for a platelet count. If thrombocytosis exists, the most common causes are inflammatory disease and solid tumor malignancies. Since there are, however, a large number of conditions that have at least on occasion been associated with an elevated platelet count, there is no reason for the practitioner to perform more than his usual comprehensive history and physical examination and any laboratory tests suggested by these examinations in an attempt to explain the thrombocytosis.

Patients with myeloproliferative disorders, if they have thrombocytosis, almost always also have large distorted platelets on smear and other hematological abnormalities typical of the particular disease. The great majority of those patients will also have splenomegaly. The treatment of thrombocytosis associated with myeloproliferative disease should be made in consultation with a hematologist.

COAGULATION DISORDERS

The generation of a solid fibrin clot from circulating soluble fibrinogen is the body's major defense against the loss of blood from the vasculature, especially from blood vessels larger than the capillary, arteriole, and venule. Coagulation is initiated by the exposure of proteins to an altered blood vessel surface, most commonly after trauma, and to thromboplastic substances to which the blood is exposed normally also when blood vessels are injured. Thereafter a series of enzymatic reactions occurs that results in the conversion of fibrinogen by the proteolytic enzyme, thrombin, to fibrin. There are two converging pathways of coagulation which are important in this mechanism: the first, the so-called intrinsic pathway, which begins with surface activation of coagulation proteins, and the second, the so-called extrinsic pathway, which begins with the exposure of the blood to tissue thromboplastin. The best screening tests to detect abnormalities of clotting are the partial thromboplastin time, which tests the intrinsic and the final common pathway, and the prothrombin time, which tests the extrinsic and the final common pathway. Both of these tests are reliably performed by hematology laboratories. The clotting time is an insensitive test and should not be relied upon as a screening procedure to detect abnormalities in this system.

There are enzymatic mechanisms which oppose coagulation and which prevent unwarranted widespread clotting of the blood when a blood vessel is injured. These mechanisms, although clearly important physiologically, are rarely recognized clinically; but a few cases have been reported of patients with an increased tendency to thrombosis and low levels of activity of one of the various protease inhibitors which normally circulate in the blood and which regulate coagulation. The best characterized of these inhibitors is antithrombin III, which inhibits the activity of a number of coagulant proteins as well as that of thrombin, and protein C, a vitamin K-dependent protein which catalyzes the proteolysis of activated factors V and VIII (see also Chapter 51, page 601). The fibrinolytic system generates the proteolytic enzyme, plasmin, which adsorbs to the clots and results in their ultimate dissolution. Bleeding as

the result of increased endogenous fibrinolytic activity is essentially unheard of, and the practicing physician need not be concerned with this possibility. There has been interest in recent years in stimulating fibrinolysis by the infusion of activating enzymes in the treatment of thrombotic disease, but the therapy, which may result in bleeding, requires hospitalization.

Patients who have a deficiency of one or more of the coagulation proteins are more likely to have extensive soft tissue bleeding or major hemorrhage in response to trauma than are patients with disorders of the vasculature or of blood platelets (petechiae (see page 595) are never a sign of abnormal coagulation). Congenital disorders of coagulation are relatively rare; the most common of them is hemophilia A (factor VIII deficiency) an X-linked disorder that affects only 1 of 10,000 males in the population. Congenital disorders are ordinarily readily diagnosed because of the history of lifelong bleeding and because, in the case of hemophilia, of a history of characteristic hemorrhage into joints and soft tissues. Patients who have a severe hemorrhagic diathesis because of a congenital abnormality of clotting almost always have markedly low levels of the deficient coagulation protein. Therefore, screening tests such as the partial thromboplastin time are almost always abnormal and provide clues to the presence of the disorder. It is unlikely that the practitioner will encounter such patients since most of them are diagnosed in childhood and are treated by experienced hematologists thereafter. If the clinician should encounter such a patient, however, whom he suspects of having a congenital disorder of coagulation, but who has not previously been diagnosed, referral to an appropriate center would be warranted.

Von Willebrand's disease (16) is an inherited abnormality of hemostasis (autosomal dominant) in

Table 50.5.
Advise to Be Given Patients with a Disorder of Hemostasis

Take only medicine prescribed by your doctor. Do not take aspirin or cold remedies. You may take Tylenol instead of aspirin for pain, colds, *etc.*

Do not drink any alcoholic beverage.

Avoid any activity that might expose you unnecessarily to trauma—for example, contact sports.

Wear a bracelet (prescribed by the physician), identifying you as a "bleeder" and giving the name of your disorder.

Call your physician:

Whenever you experience any abnormal bleeding (including excessive menstrual bleeding);

Before you visit your dentist;

Before seeing any other physician;

If you are hospitalized for any reason, without his knowing it.

which there is a reduction in the concentration and/ or the structure of a protein, the von Willebrand factor (VWF), which ordinarily binds to platelets and mediates their adhesion to subendothelial collagen in the course of platelet plug formation (see above, page 595) (16). Normally VWF forms a complex with antihemophilic globulin (factor VIII), the protein which is deficient in the blood of patients with classic hemophilia. It seems likely that VWF acts as a carrier of factor VIII so that patients with von Willebrand's disease often have reduced levels of factor VIII.

The qualitative disorder of platelets is reflected in a prolonged bleeding time and decreased platelet adhesiveness. The platelets of these patients characteristically do not aggregate in vitro when exposed to the obsolete antibiotic ristocetin. The course of the disease as well as the extent of the laboratory abnormalities are quite variable from one patient to another, but in general the hemorrhagic diathesis is milder than it is in hemophilia A. Patients bleed most commonly from their gastrointestinal tract; it is not unusual that symptoms of the disease are not apparent until the patient is an adult. The bleeding time and the partial thromboplastin time are useful screening tests, but any patient suspected of having the disorder should have plasma factor VIII assayed as well. The diagnosis and treatment of patients with von Willebrand's disease require the ongoing participation of a qualified hematologist.

Acquired disorders of coagulation are more common than congenital ones. By their nature they are more likely to be associated with multiple defects in hemostasis such as are seen in patients with disseminated intravascular coagulation (see above, page 598) or in patients taking anticoagulant drugs (see Chapter 51). The diagnosis and management of these problems are discussed on those pages.

ADVICE TO PATIENTS WHO HAVE A DISORDER OF HEMOSTASIS

Table 50.5 lists some rules to give patients who have hemostatic dysfunction (also see Table 51.2 Chapter 51). It is also important that the patient knows the name of his disease and its clinical manifestations.

General References

Ratnoff OD, Forbes CD (eds): *Disorders of Hemostasis.* New York, Grune & Stratton, 1984.
    A recent, well edited review.
Williams WJ, Beutler E, Erslev AJ, Lichtman MA (eds): *Hematology.* New York, McGraw-Hill, 1983.
    The currently standard text.

Specific References

1. Bellucci S, Tobelem G, Caen JP: Inherited platelet disorders. In Brown EB (ed): *Progress in Hematology.* New York, Grune & Stratton, 1983, vol 13, p 223.
2. Bick RL: Vascular disorders associated with thrombohemorrhagic phenomena. *Semin Thromb Hemostasis* 5(3):167, 1979.
3. Burns TR, Saleem A: Idiopathic thrombocytopenic purpura. *Am J Med* 75:1001, 1983.
4. Cream JJ, Gumpel JM, Peachey RDG: Schönlein-Henoch purpura in the adult. A study of 77 adults with anaphylactoid or Schönlein-Henoch purpura. *Q J Med* 39:461, 1970.
5. Glenner GG: Amyloid deposits and amyloidosis. *N Engl J Med* 302:1283, 1333, 1980.
6. Grey HM, Kohler PF: Cryoimmunoglobulins. *Semin Hematol* 10:87, 1973.
7. Hodges RE, Hood J, Canham JE, et al: Clinical manifestations of ascorbic acid deficiency in man. *Am J Clin Nutr* 24:432, 1971.
8. Kyle RA, Gleich GJ, Bayrid ED, Vaughn JH: Benign hypergammaglobulinemic purpura of Waldenström. *Medicine* 50:113, 1971.
9. Mammen EF: Congenital coagulation disorders. *Semin Thromb Hemostasis* 9:1, 1983.
10. Merskey C, Johnson AJ, Kleiner GJ, Wohl H: The defibrination syndrome: clinical features and laboratory diagnosis. *Br J Haematol* 13:528, 1967.
11. Miescher PA: Drug-induced thrombocytopenia. *Semin Hematol* 10:311, 1973.
12. Morris L, Distenfeld A, Amorosi E, Karpatkin S: Autoimmune thrombocytopenic purpura in homosexual men. *Ann Intern Med* 96:714, 1982.
13. Osler W: On multiple hereditary telangiectases with recurring haemorrhages. *Q J Med* 1:53, 1907.
14. Perkins HA, MacKenzie MR, Fudenberg HH: Hemostatic defects in dysproteinemias. *Blood* 35:695, 1970.
15. Ratnoff OD: The psychogenic purpuras: a review of autoerythrocyte sensitization, autosensitization to DNA, "hysterical" and factitial bleeding, and the religious stigmata. *Semin Hematol* 17:192, 1980.
16. Zimmerman TS, Ruggeri ZM, Fulcher CA: Factor VIII/von Willebrand factor. In Brown EB (ed): *Progress in Hematology.* New York, Grune & Stratton, 1983, p 279.

CHAPTER FIFTY-ONE

Thromboembolic Disease

PHILIP D. ZIEVE, M.D.

Patients with acute vascular occlusions, whether they be venous or arterial, almost always require hospitalization for initial diagnosis and treatment. The responsibility of the clinician in his office, therefore, is initially to recognize the problem and arrange for hospitalization in an appropriate facility and ultimately to manage the patients once discharged from the hospital.

VENOUS THROMBOEMBOLISM

Presentation

The majority of patients who present to the physician with venous occlusion have formed clots in the veins of the lower extremities. The primary pathological process is stasis of blood (such as might be seen in people who are chronically ill, obese, or for other reasons lead sedentary lives).

Occasionally, an underlying malignancy, not always apparent, is associated with venous (and/or arterial) thromboembolic disease (14, 23). More rarely, an inherited deficiency of a naturally occurring anticoagulant (e.g., protein C, an inhibitor of activated coagulation factors V and VIII (6) or antithrombin III, an inhibitor of thrombin as well as of several other activated coagulation factors (16)) is implicated in the genesis of recurrent thrombosis. Also, some patients with systemic lupus erythematosus or another collagen vascular disease develop an anticoagulant against a complex of activated factor X, factor V, and phospholipid that, rather than causing a tendency to bleed, is associated with recurrent thrombosis (4). This "lupus anticoagulant" can be suspected when patients with a collagen vascular disease are found to have a prolonged prothrombin time and partial thromboplastin time.

Patients with venous occlusion usually present with swelling, pain, and tenderness of the affected extremity, although swelling alone and, more rarely, pain or tenderness alone may be the presenting symptom. Embolism to the lungs of clots from veins of the lower extremities is the major complication experienced by patients with venous thrombosis and is the primary reason why diagnosis and treatment are urgent. On the basis of history and physical examination alone, however, it is virtually impossible to distinguish thrombosis of the deep veins of the lower extremities from other processes. At least half the time other diagnoses (especially musculoskeletal injury) prove to be responsible for these signs and symptoms (20). Since it is clots in the deep veins that impose the risk of pulmonary embolism, it is extremely important to make this distinction so that rational treatment can be instituted. Therefore, patients suspected of having thrombosis of the deep veins or of having had pulmonary embolism without clinical evidence of peripheral thrombosis *must* undergo specific diagnostic studies so that appropriate therapy for venous thromboembolism may be instituted. The most reliable diagnostic test is contrast venography. If characteristic filling defects are seen in radiographs of the veins after injection of contrast material, the diagnosis is established (Fig. 51.1). However, because of the potential morbidity of the procedure (see below), other tests have been recommended. The three most popular are impedance plethysmography, Doppler ultrasonography, and scanning of the extremities after injection of radioiodinated fibrinogen. The latter, because it is not very sensitive to clots in proximal veins, which are more likely to embolize than are distal clots, is not recommended for routine use. Both plethysmography and ultrasonography may be falsely positive in patients with venous stasis; both procedures are more sensitive in detecting proximal than distal clots. Either of these tests may be substituted for venography if the following conditions are met: (a) thrombophlebitis is suspected on clinical grounds, and plethysmography or ultrasonography is positive; and (b) the vascular laboratory has established that the results of the procedure have a high correlation with those of venography. If thrombophlebitis is suspected but plethysmography and/or ultrasonography is negative, venography must be done. Once a definite diagnosis of deep venous thrombosis is

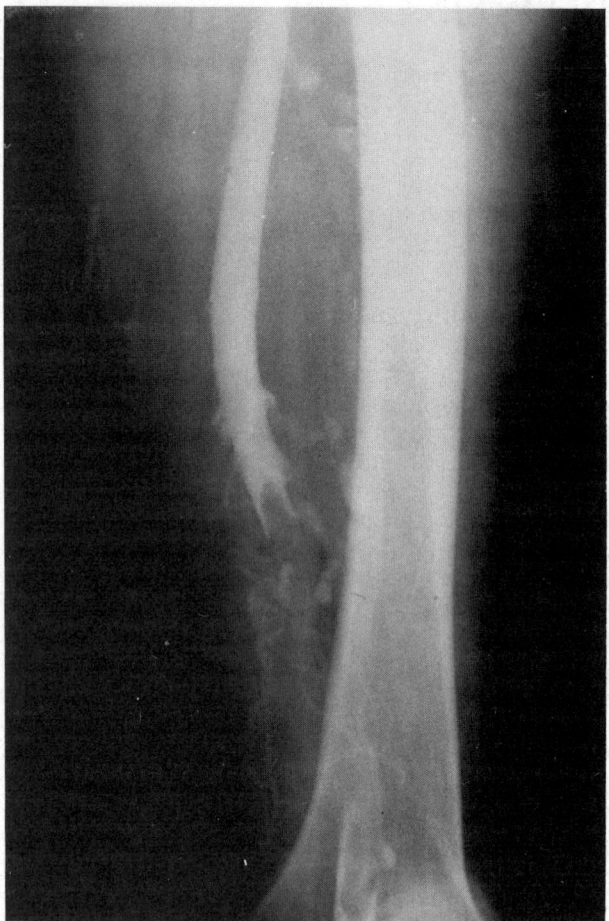

Figure 51.1. Venogram showing clots of deep veins of thigh.

made, the patient must be hospitalized for treatment.

Patient experience. Impedance plethysmography is performed by inflating a pneumatic cuff at the midthigh to occlude venous return and then rapidly deflating it. The changes in blood volume are measured by changes in electrical resistance detected by a pair of electrodes attached to the cuff. There is no discomfort associated with this procedure other than the mild transient sensation of increased pressure during the few seconds of inflation.

Venography is performed after injection of a contrast medium into a dorsal vein of the foot. The patient should be warned that the procedure commonly is associated with unpleasant burning or cramping in the lower extremity while the dye is being injected. In addition, up to one-quarter of patients develop a painful swelling of the leg and ankle which begins 2 to 12 hours after the study, intensifies for 12 to 24 hours, and then begins to subside. The pathogenesis of this delayed reaction is unclear; no specific therapy, therefore, is indicated. There is a risk that venography itself will cause thrombosis; the incidence of deep vein thrombosis, proved by repeat venography, is probably in the range of 3 to 13%, and of superficial thrombosis, 6 to 25% (3).

If patients present with signs and symptoms of pulmonary embolism (see Chapter 53), the first diagnostic procedure should be a ventilation/perfusion scan of their lungs. If the scan is negative or read as "low probability" and the patient has signs and symptoms of venous occlusion of the lower extremities, further diagnostic studies should be done, as described above, to establish that diagnosis. If the lung scan is interpreted as indeterminate or high probability, the patient should be hospitalized—in the first instance for pulmonary angiography and in the second, for treatment. In many instances, however, the clinician will elect to admit the patient to the hospital on the basis of the clinical presentation and then obtain all necessary diagnostic procedures.

Treatment

The most important therapy for patients with thromboembolic disease of the lower extremities is anticoagulation, instituted to prevent extension of the clot. The larger the clot, the more likely it is to break off and become an embolus. Anticoagulation is usually instituted in the hospital with heparin which is administered on the average for 10 days, the approximate time for clots to become adherent to the vessel wall. Heparin is utilized because its onset of action is immediate and because of an unsubstantiated impression that it is a more effective anticoagulant than are coumarin compounds, the other major class of available anticoagulant drugs.

Coumarin Compounds

Coumarin compounds are the drugs commonly used in the anticoagulation of ambulatory patients. Ordinarily patients who have been hospitalzed for diagnosis and initial treatment of venous thromboembolic disease are given a coumarin compound while heparin is being administered so that by the time that drug is discontinued, the full effect of the coumarin has become established. Coumarins interfere with the synthesis of vitamin K-dependent clotting factors (factors II, VII, IX, and X) by the liver. Their effect is not fully realized, therefore, until they have been given for approximately 5 days. The administration of warfarin, the commonly used coumarin, usually is initiated in doses of 10 mg a day and then adjusted depending upon the therapeutic response, which is monitored by use of the prothrombin time, a reproducible, dependable test performed reliably by most clinical laboratories. The goal of anticoagulant therapy with coumarin is to maintain the prothrombin time 1½ to 2 times the control value since it is within this range that a reasonable therapeutic effect is achieved and the risk of untoward bleeding is relatively small. It has been suggested that administration of warfarin in a dosage sufficient to prolong the prothrombin time only 1¼ control is also effective (19), but additional confirmatory studies are necessary before this regimen, associated with a considerably reduced risk of bleeding, can be recommended. During the first several weeks of administration of warfarin, the prothrombin time should be measured at least every few days until it is determined that the proper dosage schedule has been achieved. Thereafter it is appropriate to measure the anticoagulant response monthly. At the same time it is prudent to examine the patient's urine and stool for occult blood and to assess his hematocrit value or hemoglobin concentration.

During the course of anticoagulation with coumarin compounds patients should be instructed to avoid predictable trauma such as might be expected from playing contact sports or from working in an environment associated with a high risk of injury. The physician should not give intramuscular injections to the anticoagulated patient; subcutaneous injections, done properly, are safe. Venipunctures are also safe, but the wound should be compressed for 10 to 15 minutes after the needle is withdrawn. Arterial punctures are contraindicated as outpatient procedures, where prolonged compression and observation of the puncture site are impractical.

Factors affecting response. There are a number of factors that might alter the patients responsiveness to warfarin following a period of stability (Table 51.1). Rarely the amount of vitamin K ingested in the patient's diet might be altered drastically, increasing the potency of warfarin if less vitamin K is ingested and decreasing it if considerably more is ingested. Significantly decreased ingestion of vitamin K is almost always associated with a markedly decreased intake of food—for example, in patients who are anorexic because of illness or who have instituted severe dietary restrictions in an attempt to lose weight. The effect of reduction in intake of vitamin K will be most pronounced in those patients who are concomitantly receiving antibiotics, which will inhibit the synthesis of vitamin K by normal flora of the intestinal tract. Because the vitamin K-dependent clotting factors are synthesized in the liver and because coumarins are metabolized by the liver, patients who develop intercurrent hepatic illness (hepatitis, for example) should be watched carefully for enhanced effective anticoagulation. In such a circumstance, the clinician would be wise to measure prothrombin times more frequently, but would not be required to discontinue warfarin unless bleeding ensued or the prothrombin time became significantly prolonged over the baseline therapeutic control.

One of the major problems confronting the clinician in dealing with a patient taking coumarin anticoagulants is the possibility of drug interaction. A number of pharmacological agents will potentiate the anticoagulant effect of coumarins and a few will inhibit it (24). The major drugs implicated are listed in Table 51.1. The clinician should be cautious, however, when initiating any new forms of therapy or discontinuing old ones in a patient who is receiving courmarin anticoagulants. Prothrombin times should be checked more frequently for several weeks to be sure that the pharmacological response to coumarin has not been altered. In general, the likelihood of a potentiated response is much higher than that of an inhibitory one, so that there is greater risk of an increased susceptibility to bleeding than of an inhibition of anticoagulation. The clinician should also be careful about the use of drugs, such as aspirin, which have an effect on hemostasis that might be enhanced by warfarin or that may produce bleeding by injuring the gastric mucosa. Other nonsteroidal anti-inflammatory agents (see Chapter 70) may be safer than aspirin, but all of them have at least a potential for compromising hemostasis (few data are available) and should be used cautiously.

Complications. It has been reported that there is a major risk in the use of coumarin compounds (and/or heparin) in pregnant patients (15). Major hemorrhagic complications occur in the fetus as well as teratogenic effects unrelated to the anticoagulant action. It has been recommended, therefore, that pregnancy be avoided in women who are being treated with anticoagulant drugs since a normal infant can be expected only about two-thirds of the time.

By far the major complication experienced by patients taking coumarin anticoagulants is hemorrhage (9, 10). Minor episodes, such as small bruises and bleeding gums following brushing of the teeth, are relatively common but ordinarily do not require a change in the dose schedule of the anticoagulant. Occult rectal bleeding, minor bleeding from hemorrhoids, microscopic hematuria, and menorrhagia will be encountered in less than 10% of patients. When bleeding of this kind is observed, it is essential to make every attempt to establish the site of bleeding by the use of appropriate diagnostic studies. If prothrombin times have been maintained within the therapeutic range, the rapidity and extent of bleeding will dictate to the clinician whether the antico-

Table 51.1.
Some Factors That May Affect a Patient's Response to Warfarin

Enhanced Response	Reduced Response
Vitamin K deficiency	Barbiturates
Liver disease	Cholestyramine
Drugs:	Glutethimide (Doriden)
Cimetidine	Griseofulvin
Clofibrate	Rifampin
Disulfiram (Antabuse)	Spironolactone
Metronidazole (Flagyl)	
Phenylbutazone	
Quinidine	
Anabolic steroids	
Heparin	

agulant drug should be discontinued, at least temporarily. Major genitourinary or gastrointestinal bleeding sufficient to lower the hematocrit value or hemoglobin concentration, or bleeding of any degree in the central nervous system, dictates prompt discontinuation of the anticoagulant and immediate hospitalization for further diagnosis and treatment. It would be prudent for the physician to administer 25 to 50 mg of vitamin K_1 (AquaMephyton) intravenously at a rate no greater than 5 mg/minute while arranging for hospitalization. (The prothrombin time will begin to shorten in 4 to 6 hours and, in most patients, will be in a safe range in 12 to 24 hours.) Major hemorrhage is often associated with an independent organic process, such as a peptic ulcer, a carcinoma of the colon, or a cerebrovascular lesion; bleeding of this kind is likely to occur even when the prothrombin time is in the so-called therapeutic range.

Advice for management of patients who are taking a coumarin compound and who are to undergo a surgical procedure is provided in Chapter 86.

Rarely, patients administered a coumarin anticoagulant will develop, within 10 days, hemorrhagic infarcts in their skin (often in women's breasts) with eventual sloughing of necrotic tissue. Under such circumstances, the drug must be stopped immediately.

Table 51.2 provides information useful for patients at the onset of anticoagulation or at the time that the patient is discharged from hospital. Selection of

Table 51.2.
Advice to Be Given Patients Taking a Coumarin Anticoagulant

Take *only* medicines prescribed by your doctor. DO not take mineral oil, laxatives, aspirin, (or any product such as a cold remedy, that contains aspirin), or another proprietary anti-inflammatory agent (currently only ibuprofen—Advil or Nuprin—is available), or any multivitamin preparation that contains vitamin K. You may take acetaminophen (*e.g.*, Tylenol) instead of aspirin for pain.

Take your coumarin at the same time each day.

Avoid wide variation in the kinds and amounts of food you eat, especially fish, broccoli, spinach, cabbage, kale, or cauliflower.

Do not drink more than 1 or 2 glasses of beer or wine or the equivalent of more than 30 ml of whiskey/day.

Avoid any activity that might expose you unnecessarily to trauma—for example, contact sports.

Call your doctor immediately whenever:
  You experience any abnormal bleeding;
  Before you visit your dentist;
  Before seeing any other physician;
  If you cannot keep your scheduled appointment;
  Before leaving on a trip;
  If you are hospitalized, for any reason, without his knowing it.

patients who are able to follow these rules will diminish considerably the incidence of hemorrhagic complications in patients taking anticoagulant drugs (also see Table 50.5, Chapter 50).

Heparin

Since heparin must be administered parenterally, it is not a drug that can be conveniently used by outpatients. If, however, because of unacceptable side effects unrelated to its anticoagulant effect, a coumarin cannot be used, the practitioner should instruct the patient or his family in the use of subcutaneous heparin, administered twice a day in doses designed to maintain the partial thromboplastin time (PTT, like the prothrombin time, a reliable, easily obtained test) at 1½ times control. Once a dosage regimen is established (usually 10,000 units twice a day), it probably is not necessary to measure the PTT again unless the patient develops bleeding or recurrent thrombosis. It has been demonstrated that prevention of recurrent thromboembolism is comparable to that achieved by the use of warfarin and that the risk of bleeding, surprisingly, may be lower (18). So-called low dose heparin (5000 units twice a day) is probably inadequate prophylaxis (17).

In recent years it has been recognized that heparin—especially bovine heparin—causes thrombocytopenia in 5 to 10% of patients to whom it is administered (21). The mechanism of this phenomenon is unclear, although an immunological process may be involved. The onset is usually within a week or two of initiation of therapy, and therefore the problem is likely to be recognized in hospital. A small proportion of these thrombocytopenic patients develop, paradoxically, arterial thrombosis. Platelet counts under 40,000 to 50,000/mm^3, thrombocytopenic bleeding, or arterial thrombosis dictate that the heparin be discontinued and that an alternative form of therapy for venous thromboembolic disease be sought (21). Heparinized ambulatory patients who exhibit untoward bleeding or clotting should be hospitalized, and a platelet count should be done as part of their evaluation. However, routine platelet counts are probably not cost effective in the follow-up of patients receiving heparin.

Prolonged use of heparin (4 months or more) in doses in excess of 10,000 units/day has been reported to cause osteoporosis; spontaneous spinal and rib fractures have been observed. The risk of this complication developing is unknown; until more data are accumulated, treatment with heparin for longer than 3 months is at least relatively contraindicated.

Heparin (especially the bovine preparation) also commonly causes reversible elevation of aminotransferase activity, without other evidence of hepatic dysfunction (11). As yet no pathological correlation with this reaction has been identified.

Aspirin

Although aspirin (see below) has been recommended in the prophylaxis of venous thromboembolism, there is no consensus that it is useful; and there is no justification for prescribing it as treatment of venous thrombosis.

Course

Patients who are being treated with coumarin anticoagulants have a recurrence rate of venous thromboembolism of 10 to 40 episodes/1000 patient months (8). One month after discharge from hospital, the rate stabilizes at approximately 10 episodes/1000 patient months and remains in that range or slightly lower thereafter. The beneficial effect of anticoagulant therapy in such patients is most pronounced during the first 2 months after discharge from hospital; after 3 months the recurrence rate is the same whether the patient is anticoagulated or not, thereby providing a rationale for discontinuing therapy after 3 months in patients who are not at high risk because of continuing stasis (8). Patients who maintain risk factors for thromboembolic disease (chronic venous stasis for whatever reason) may, barring complications of drugs, be considered for more prolonged periods of treatment. Although there is no reliable information in this regard, it is reasonable to continue therapy for high risk patients indefinitely unless a contraindication—such as major bleeding—develops.

Patients who have sustained thromboses of the deep veins of the lower extemities should be advised to avoid prolonged sitting or standing in one position, should be encouraged to elevate their legs for two to three periods of 30 minutes each day, and to wear elastic stockings to promote venous return. Although the effectiveness of these maneuvers has not been established, there is little or no risk associated with any of them, and they may be of some value. At such time when a decision is made to discontinue anticoagulation therapy, it may be terminated abruptly without fear of an increased risk of early recurrence of venous thrombosis; the so-called "rebound phenomenon" has never been demonstrated.

Some patients, after repeated attacks of thrombosis of the veins of the lower extremities, will develop chronic changes in those veins with loss of competence of the valves and hemorrhage of small tributary veins leading to chronic edema and discoloration of the legs and ankles (25). Sometimes painful stasis ulcers also will develop that make it very difficult for the patient to move about. The treatment of this postphlebitic syndrome is the promotion of venous return from the lower extremities by the use of support stockings during the day and by elevation of the lower extremities for several hours each day. In those patients who have developed

ulcers, bed rest with persistent elevation of the extremity above the level of the heart is recommended and, if necessary, administration of appropriate antibiotics. On such a regimen, the ulcers will invariably heal, although they may recur if the patients are not careful to continue to follow prescribed conservative therapy (see Chapter 88).

ARTERIAL THROMBOEMBOLISM

Unlike clots that form in the venous circulation, arterial thrombosis is primarily initiated by platelet plug formation, begun by the adherence of ambient platelets to altered surfaces in arterial vessels or in the left heart. Symptoms and signs of thrombosis appear more abruptly than do those of venous occlusion and commonly are associated with necrosis of tissue that had been fed by the now obstructed vessel. Heparin and coumarin anticoagulants, both experimentally and clinically, are of little use in preventing the formation of such clots or in preventing their propagation. There is a great deal of interest, therefore, in the use of drugs that interfere with platelet plug formation and that might be useful in the prophylaxis of arterial thromboembolism. Although a number of agents have been tested, only three—aspirin, dipyridamole, and sulfinpyrazone—can reasonably be expected to be efficacious, and even these agents have not been clearly established as useful.

Aspirin

This drug, the most commonly used therapeutic agent in the world, has for some years been recognized to interfere with platelet function and therefore to inhibit platelet plug formation. It is now recognized that aspirin interferes with the formation of a very potent aggregating substance, thromboxane A_2, formed in platelets by the metabolism of prostaglandins. Aspirin inhibits the rate-limiting enzyme in this reaction, cyclooxygenase; as the result, the aggregation of platelets by collagen or connective tissue is inhibited and the release of substances, which themselves stimulate platelet aggregation, is impaired. Presumably as a result of the impairment, the bleeding time in patients taking even a single tablet of aspirin a day is prolonged.

Aspirin inhibits not only prostaglandin synthesis in platelets but also the formation by vascular endothelium of prostacyclin, a potent inhibitor of platelet aggregation. There is no good information on the proper dose of aspirin to be administered to achieve an optimum effect (presumably at the point where there is maximum inhibition of thomboxane A_2 synthesis and minimum inhibition of prostacyclin synthesis) (13).

Unless aspirin is administered to patients with an underlying hemostatic disorder (including the administration of an anticoagulant drug—see above), a hemorrhagic diathesis is unusual. However, it has been well established that aspirin has a toxic effect on the mucosa of the gastrointestinal tract that may result in bleeding or may increase the likelihood of hemorrhage from pre-existent peptic ulcerations.

There have been a number of studies performed to assess the efficacy of aspirin as a prophylactic agent in patients with atherosclerotic heart disease and cerebrovascular disease. To date there is no conclusive evidence that the drug is of any use in patients who have have sustained a myocardial infarction in preventing either reinfarction or death (2). There is one well designed multicenter study, however, that showed, in a 12-week trial, considerable reduction in the incidence of myocardial infarction or of death in men with unstable angina given 324 mg of aspirin a day (22), but more data are needed before it will be known whether this therapy is justified. On the other hand, it has become a routine in most centers to administer dipyridamole (75 mg three times a day) and aspirin (325 to 975 mg every day) indefinitely to patients who have undergone coronary artery bypass surgery, largely as the result of one well controlled study which showed a significant reduction for at least a year or more postoperatively of vein-graft occlusion (7). Whether dipyridamole is important to this regimen (see below) is unknown.

There are several studies which suggest a beneficial effect of aspirin (1000 to 1200 mg/day) in preventing subsequent strokes as well as death from cerebrovascular disease in patients who had had transient (5, 27) or completed (5) "cerebral ischemic events." In one of these studies (27) the benefit was limited to men, in the other (5) the positive effect was seen in both men and women. Until more definitive studies are reported, it would be reasonable for the clinician to administer aspirin in a dosage of 1000 to 1300 mg/day indefinitely to patients who have experienced transient ischemic attacks or completed thromboembolic strokes.

Finally, there is suggestive but inconclusive evidence of a positive effect of aspirin in preventing embolization in patients who have undergone implantation of prosthetic heart valves.

Dipyridamole

Dipyridamole (Persantine) was developed as a vasodilating agent, but subsequently was discovered to inferfere with platelet plug formation in vivo. The drug can be shown in vitro to inhibit phosphodiesterase, the enzyme which breaks down cyclic adenosine monophosphate (AMP) within blood platelets and other cells. Cyclic AMP is a potent inhibitor of platelet aggregation, and dipyridamole presumably exerts its effect by maintaining higher levels of cyclic AMP within platelets. There is no evidence in vitro, however, that dipyridamole inhibits the aggregation of platelets or the release reaction, nor is the bleeding time in vivo prolonged by this drug. Experimental studies have revealed no evidence that dipyridamole is of use in patients with ischemic heart disease or cerebrovascular disease. In patients who have prosthetic heart valves there is some suggestion that embolization may be prevented by dipyridamole, but few data have been obtained. At present, therefore, there is no justification for the use of dipyridamole in clinical practice to prevent arterial thromboembolism. In some studies dipyridamole and aspirin have been administered together (e.g., see above), and it is conceivable that some synergism may be attained in this manner since the drugs have different mechanisms of action. However, again there is no information to recommend the use of this combination.

Sulfinpyrazone

Sulfinpyrazone (Anturane) was developed as a uricosuric agent but, like aspirin, has been discovered to inhibit prostaglandin (and therefore thromboxane A_2) synthesis in vitro. Unlike aspirin this biochemical effect is quite transient and is therefore dependent upon continued administration of the drug. Sulfinpyrazone has no effect on the aggregation of platelets or on the bleeding time. There has been no demonstration of a positive effect of this drug as a prophylactic agent in patients with cerebrovascular disease (27); neither is there any study to indicate that sulfinpyrazone is of use in patients with prosthetic heart valves. However, a large collaborative randomized double blind study has been

Table 51.3.
Evidence of Effects of Drugs on Thromboembolic Disease

Drug	Ischemic Heart Disease	Prosthetic Heart Valves	Cerebrovascular Disease
Aspirin	Inconclusive	Suggestive but inconclusive evidence of positive effect in preventing embolization only	Positive effect
Dipyridamole	Not yet demonstrated	Few data; may prevent embolization	No effect
Sulfinpyrazone	Unclear	No data	No effect

reported demonstrating that sulfinpyrazone reduces considerably the incidence of sudden death for 7 months after myocardial infarction (26). Thereafter no effect of the drug could be demonstrated. The design of this study was challenged by the Food and Drug Administration, but the data were analyzed by an independent group and the conclusions were reaffirmed (1). Additional experiments will undoubtedly be necessary to establish definitively the efficacy of sulfinpyrazone in patients who have had an acute myocardial infarction. If sulfinpyrazone is administered, the most common adverse reactions of which the clinician should be aware are "peptic" symptoms best treated by administering the drug concomitantly with antacids.

SUMMARY

Table 51.3 summarizes the evidence for the use of agents which interfere with platelet function in the treatment and prophylaxis of thromboembolic disease.

General References

Deykin D: Current status of anticoagulant therapy. *Am J Med* 72:659, 1982.
  A concise, sensible review.
Eichner ER: Platelets, carotids, and coronaries. Critique on antithrombotic role of antiplatelet agents, exercise, and certain diets. *Am J Med* 77:513, 1984.
  A well referenced critical review, somewhat biased toward the use of aspirin.
Hirsh J, Genton E, Hull R (eds): *Venous Thromboembolism*. New York, Grune & Stratton, 1981.
  A comprehensive, well referenced text.

Specific References

1. Anturan Reinfarction Trial Policy Committee: The Anturan reinfarction trial: reevaluation of outcome. *N Engl J Med* 306:1005, 1982.
2. Aspirin Myocardial Infarction Study Research Group: A randomized, controlled trial of aspirin in persons recovered from myocardial infarction. *JAMA* 243:661, 1980.
3. Bettmann MA, Paulin S: Leg phlebography: the incidence, nature, and modification of undesirable side effects. *Diagn Radiol* 122:101, 1977.
4. Boey ML, Colaco CB, Gharavi AE, et al: Thrombosis in systemic lupus erythematosus: striking association with the presence of circulating lupus anticoagulant. *Br Med J* 287:1021, 1983.
5. Bousser MG, Eschwege E, Haguenau M, et al: "AICLA" controlled trial of aspirin and dipyridamole in the secondary prevention of athero-thrombotic cerebral ischemia. *Stroke* 14:5, 1983.
6. Broekmans AW, Veltkamp JJ, Bertina RM: Congenital protein C deficiency and venous thromboembolism: a study of three Dutch families. *N Engl J Med* 309:340, 1983.
7. Chesbro JH, Fuster V, Elveback LR, et al: Effect of dipyridamole and aspirin on late vein-graft patency after coronary bypass operation. *N Engl J Med* 310:209, 1984.
8. Coon WW, Willis PW III: Recurrence of venous thromboembolism. *Surgery* 73:823, 1973.
9. Coon WW, Willis PW III: Hemorrhagic complications of anticoagulant therapy. *Arch Intern Med* 133:386, 1974.
10. Davis FB,, Estruch MT, Samson-Corvera EB, et al: Management of anticoagulation in outpatients. *Arch Intern Med* 137:197, 1977.
11. Dukes GE, Sanders SW, Russo J, et al: Transminase elevations in patients receiving bovine or porcine heparin. *Ann Intern Med* 100:646, 1984.
12. Fields WS, Lemak NA, Frankowski RF, Hardy RJ: Controlled trial of aspirin in cerebral ischemia. *Stroke* 8:301, 1977.
13. Fitzgerald GA, Oates JA, Hawiger J, et al: Endogenous biosynthesis of prostacyclin and thomboxane and platelet function during chronic administration of aspirin in man. *J Clin Invest* 71:676, 1983.
14. Gore JM, Applebaum JS, Greene HL, et al: Occult cancer in patients with acute pulmonary embolism. *Ann Intern Med* 96:556, 1982.
15. Hall JG, Pauli RM, Wilson KM: Maternal and fetal sequelae of anticoagulation during pregnancy. *Am J Med* 68:122, 1980.
16. Harpel PC: Blood proteolytic enzyme inhibitors: their role in modulating blood coagulation and fibrinolytic enzyme pathway. In Colman RW,, Hirsh J, Marder VJ, Salzman EW (eds): *Hemostasis and Thrombosis: Basic Principles and Clinical Practice*. Philadelphia, JB Lippincott, 1982, p 738.
17. Hull R, Delmore T, Genton E, et al: Warfarin sodium *versus* low-dose heparin in the long-term treatment of venous thrombosis. *N Engl J Med* 301:855, 1979.
18. Hull R, Delmore T, Carter C, et al: Adjusted subcutaneous heparin *versus* warfarin sodium in the long-term treatment of venous thrombosis. *N Engl J Med* 306:189, 1982.
19. Hull R, Hirsh J, Jay R, et al: Different intensities of oral anticoagulant therapy in the treatment of proximal-vein thrombosis. *N Engl J Med* 307:1676, 1982.
20. Hull R, Hirsh J: Advances and controversies in the diagnosis, prevention, and treatment of venous thromboembolism. In Brown EB (ed): *Progress in Hematology*. New York, Grune & Stratton, 1981, vol 12, p 73.
21. King DJ, Kelton JG: Heparin-associated thrombocytopenia. *Ann Intern Med* 100:535, 1984.
22. Lewis HD, Davis JW, Archibald DG, et al: Protective effects of aspirin against acute myocardial infarction and death in men with unstable angina. *N Engl J Med* 309:396, 1983.
23. Sack GH, Levin J, Bell WR: Trousseau's syndrome and other manifestations of chronic disseminated coagulopathy in patients with neoplasms: clinical, pathophysiologic, and therapeutic features. *Medicine* 56:1, 1977.
24. Standing Advisory Committee for Haematology of the Royal College of Pathologists: Drug interaction with coumarin derivative anticoagulants. *Br Med J* 285:274, 1982.
25. Strandness DE, Langlois Y, Cramer M, et al: Long term sequelae of acute venous thrombosis. *JAMA* 250:1289, 1983.
26. The Anturane Reinfarction Trial Research Group: Sulfinpyrazone in the prevention of sudden death after myocardial infarction. *N Engl J Med* 302:250, 1980.
27. The Canadian Cooperative Study Group: A randomized trial of aspirin and sulfinpyrazone in threatened stroke. *N Engl J Med* 299:53, 1978.

CHAPTER FIFTY-TWO

Selected Illnesses Affecting Lymphocytes: Mononucleosis, the Acquired Immune Deficiency Syndrome, Chronic Lymphocytic Leukemia, and the Undiagnosed Patient with Lymphadenopathy

LARRY WATERBURY, M.D., AND PHILIP D. ZIEVE, M.D.

A number of illnesses affect the lymphoreticular system, some of them benign (such as most cases due to viral infection), some of them malignant (e.g., lymphoma). The diagnosis is sometimes readily apparent from the clinical presentation, but at other times extensive studies are necessary before a precise diagnosis can be made. This chapter reviews three conditions that affect lymphatic organs and lymphocytes: the mononucleosis syndrome, the acquired immune deficiency syndrome, and chronic lymphocytic leukemia. All of these are conditions in which the general physician will be involved in the diagnosis and treatment of the patient.

INFECTIOUS MONONUCLEOSIS

There are four infectious diseases, caused by herpesviruses, which affect humans: infectious mono-nucleosis (Epstein-Barr virus (EBV)), cytomegalovirus (CMV) infections, herpes simplex infections (Chapters 94 and 100), and varicella/zoster infections (Chapter 100).

Epidemiology and Pathogenesis

The EBV is the cause of infectious mononucleosis (4), an acute febrile illness that primarily affects teenagers and young adults (the age group between 15 and 25 years). Infection with the virus is extremely common; for example, over 50% of college students of both sexes have antibodies to it; and each year 12 to 13% of college students who do not have antibodies to EBV develop them (most of them in the course of clinical mononucleosis) (16). Because of the ubiquity of exposure relatively early in life, infectious mononucleosis is rare in people over the age of 30 and, when it does occur, may present atypically (see below). The virus seems to be spread by oral contact, first infecting the throat, then B lymphocytes, which generate a T cell response that results in the atypical lymphocytosis that is a hallmark of the disease.

EBV has also been cultured from tumor cells of patients with Burkitt's lymphoma and with nasopharyngeal carcinoma, and such patients also have antibodies to the virus in their blood. It seems likely, therefore, that EBV has a role in the development of these neoplasms.

Signs and Symptoms

Clinical illness usually begins after a 1- to 2-month incubation period. Classically patients present with pharyngitis, lymphadenopathy, splenomegaly, and marked atypical lymphocytosis. Table 52.1 lists the relative frequency of the characteristic signs and symptoms associated with the illness. Pharyngitis can be extremely severe and is frequently accompanied by an exudate which may be foul smelling. Rarely it may be so severe that it leads to respiratory obstruction. Of the relatively few patients who do not present with pharyngitis (especially children), most simply have a nonspecific febrile illness associated with malaise. Other patients present with

Table 52.1.
Signs and Symptoms of Infectious Mononucleosis

Common Symptoms		Common Signs		Less Common Signs and Symptoms	
Malaise	100%	Adenopathy	100%	Jaundice	10%
Sore throat	85%	Fever	90%	Arthralgia	5%
Warmth, chilliness	70%	Pharyngitis	85%	Skin rash	5%
Anorexia	70%	Splenomegaly	60%	Diarrhea	5%
Headache	50%	Bradycardia	40%	Photophobia	5%
Cough	40%	Periorbital edema	25%		
Myalgia	25%	Palatal enanthem	25%		

mild jaundice and a syndrome that mimics infectious hepatitis. Posterior cervical adenopathy is characteristic of almost all patients, and there is frequently generalized lymph node enlargement as well; approximately 60% have an enlarged spleen. Some patients may experience a protracted course with nonspecific symptoms, lymphadenopathy, and splenomegaly that persist for weeks. Most patients are significantly improved by the end of 3 weeks.

Patients usually present to the physician at the end of the first week of a nonspecific illness characterized by malaise, and perhaps by anorexia, mild headache, and low grade fever. Adenopathy, splenomegaly, and pharyngitis usually appear at about this time and slowly resolve over the following weeks. However, as noted below, the classical laboratory features of the illness may not be present until the second or third week of the clinical illness. Patients over 40 years of age tend to have more prolonged fever and less adenopathy than do young adults (8).

Laboratory Features

The hematocrit value is usually normal, although occasionally mild hemolysis and, rarely, a severe autoimmune hemolytic anemia are seen. The peripheral white cell count is usually elevated, reaching its height during the second and third weeks of the clinical illness. Early in the course there may be a severe absolute neutropenia, and occasionally the absolute neutrophil count is less than 500/μl. The differential count of the white cells is characterized by an absolute lymphocytosis with large numbers (over 10% of the total white cell population) of atypical lymphocytes (large lobulated or indented nuclei and vacuolated and/or bluish cytoplasm). The platelet count is normal to slightly decreased in the majority of patients; severe thrombocytopenia may occur rarely. Slight increases in the activity of hepatic enzymes are common but never reach the height seen in viral hepatitis; older patients, however, tend to have more marked hepatic dysfunction, and in this group jaundice is common (8).

Serological Features

Diagnosis is based upon the presence of typical clinical features and characteristic serological tests.

Table 52.2.
Serological Evidence of Epstein-Barr Virus (EBV) Infection (4)

1. IgM antibody to viral capsid antigen (IgM anti-VCA). Appears early in primary infection and disappears within 3 to 6 months.
2. IgG antibody to viral capsid antigen (IgG anti-VCA). Appears slightly later than IgM anti-VCA and remains detectable for life.
3. Antibodies to the early antigen (EA) complex of EBV of the diffuse (D) type (anti-D). Anti-D antibodies appear early in primary infection and disappear by 2 to 3 months.
4. Antibodies to EB nuclear antigen (anti-EBNA). Anti-EBNA appears very late (months) after primary infection and is detectable for life.

A number of different EB virus antibodies have been identified (7). They are summarized in Table 52.2. *Immunoglobulin M antibody to viral capsid antigen (IgM anti-VCA)* appears within 1 to 6 weeks after onset of infection and disappears within 3 to 6 months; a rising titer during the first few weeks of clinical illness is the most useful, generally most easily available, serological evidence of recent primary infection. Antibodies to the early antigen (EA) complex of EBV of the diffuse (D) type (known as *anti-D antibodies*) also appear early in primary infection and disappear by 2 to 3 months, but anti-D antibody testing is much less available than IgM anti-VCA testing (7). *Heterophil antibodies* are elevated in most patients; the highest titers are reached during the first week of clinical illness. Differential absorption studies are necessary to identify the presence of those heterophil antibodies that are specific for infectious mononucleosis (the antibodies are absorbed by bovine red cells but not by guinea pig kidney). A number of rapid macroagglutination slide tests are commercially available (13). Most utilize horse red cells, which are more sensitive than sheep red cells in the detection of heterophil antibodies. Some kits utilize differential absorption techniques as well. In general, the slide kits are quite sensitive to the detection of heterophil antibodies but may yield positive results also in other conditions associated with such antibodies (serum sickness, viral hepatitis, cytomegalovirus infections, other viral illnesses, leukemia).

In patients with classic symptoms of infectious mononucleosis a positive mononucleosis slide test is sufficient serological confirmation for the diagnosis for clinical purposes. Some 5 to 10% of patients with clinical infectious mononucleosis and serological evidence of recent primary EBV infection are heterophil antibody negative. Another 5 to 10% of patients with clinical features of infectious mononucleosis have another illness (cytomegalovirus infection, toxoplasmosis, etc).

Complications (3)

Severe complications of infectious mononucleosis are rare but do occur. They include neurological problems (encephalitis, meningitis, peripheral neuropathy, Guillain-Barré syndrome), bacterial superinfection, and splenic rupture. The latter has accounted for a number of deaths, especially since the diagnosis is easily missed. The physician should be suspicious of such a diagnosis if there is a recent history of sudden, brief, sharp abdominal pain. Occasional deaths have been seen also with severe pharyngitis and airway obstruction. All of these complications are even more rare when the mononucleosis syndrome is caused by an infectious agent other than the EB virus (see below). The pharyngitis in infectious mononucleosis may closely resemble that of exudative streptococcal pharyngitis, and all patients should have throat cultures to rule out bacterial infection.

Recently, two studies have been reported of patients who had serological and clinical evidence of *chronic EB virus infection* of more than 1 year's duration (10, 19). Some of these patients had episodic, and others, persistent symptoms. There was no clear-cut epidemiological distinction between these patients and patients with self-limited disease, but in contrast to patients with self-limited mononucleosis (see Table 52.1), adenopathy and pharyngitis were somewhat less common (approximately 60% of patients) and splenomegaly was unusual (4 to 22% of patients). Chronic fatigue and depression were dominant complaints. There was no indication in any of these patients of a major immunological or a more virulent illness (i.e., an opportunistic infection or a neoplasm). The prevalence of protracted EB virus infection is not yet known.

Treatment

There is no specific treatment for infectious mononucleosis, and all that is usually necessary is supportive care. There is no evidence that prolonged bed rest is helpful. It is reasonable for patients to avoid strenuous activities until they feel strong enough to participate. Contact sports should be avoided if the spleen is tender or significantly enlarged. Since splenomegaly may persist for months, however, it seems unreasonable to avoid contact sports until the spleen is no longer palpable. Although contacts do occasionally develop infectious mononucleosis, there is no evidence that the disease is highly infective and patients should not be rigidly restricted from interpersonal contacts. (However, the patient continues to shed the virus for several months after onset of the illness).

Surgery, of course, is indicated for splenic rupture (15). Corticosteroids are usually reserved for patients with severe pharyngitis and impending airway obstruction, in which situation they are usually dramatically effective. Ordinarily a high dose (such as 40 to 60 mg of prednisone daily) is given initially, with rapid tapering of treatment by 1 week to 10 days.

Other Causes of the Mononucleosis Syndrome

Cytomegalovirus Infection (CMV)

Although CMV infections may cause devastating clinical illness in the newborn (*in utero*) and in the immunocompromised host, infection in the noncompromised adult causes a clinical syndrome essentially indistinguishable from infectious mononucleosis except that exudative pharyngitis is very unusual in CMF infection. Unlike exposure to EBV, which has occurred in most adults in the United States by age 25, primary CMV infections usually occur at an older age, making CMV mononucleosis the most common cause of the mononucleosis syndrome in patients over 25 to 30 years of age. Up to 50% of people over the age of 40 have antibodies to CMV, although most do not have a history of infection. Diagnosis usually depends on the demonstration of at least a 4-fold rise in CMV complement fixing antibodies over a 4- to 6-week period. When available, the demonstration of IgM antibodies to CMV antigens or the demonstration of cytolytic antibodies to CMV antigens is more useful in proving recent primary infection (Table 52.3).

Toxoplasmosis

Acute toxoplasmosis may also cause a clinical syndrome that resembles infectious mononucleosis, but pharyngitis does not occur and splenomegaly and lymphadenopathy are usually not as prominent. Diagnosis usually depends on a constellation of serological findings indicative of recent primary infection (see Table 52.3).

Other Infections

Other infections may mimic infectious mononucleosis. These include hepatitis A, hepatitis B, non-A-, non-B hepatitis, rubella, and adenovirus infection. Sometimes an etiological agent cannot be identified even after extensive serological testing. Table 52.4 suggests a stepwise plan for the serological evaluation of patients with the mononucleosis syndrome.

Table 52.3.
Etiologies Other Than EBV for the Mononucleosis Syndrome—Serological Diagnosis of Recent Infection

CMV	Four to 8-fold rise in complement fixation titer. Elevated IgM or cytolytic antibodies to CMV antigen, if available, are more helpful.
Toxoplasmosis	Dye Test (DT) or immunofluorescent antibody (IFA) titers of > 1:1000 plus an IgM-IFA titer of > 1:64.
Hepatitis A	Elevated titer of IgM antibody to hepatitis A antigen (IgM anti-HAAg). (See Chapter 42.)
Hepatitis B	Elevated hepatitis B surface antigen (HB$_S$Ag). Chronic carrier state identification will require follow-up measurement of HB$_S$Ag, HB$_e$Ag, and lack of rise of anti-HB$_S$. (See Chapter 42.)
Rubella	The hemagglutination inhibition antibody (HIA) titer is the most widely used. The antibody is first detected after onset of the rash, and the titer rises rapidly for 1 to 2 weeks thereafter. If one does not catch this rise with acute and convalescent sera, the titer usually remains high for several months, so a single high titer is not meaningful. However, a low titer (< 1:16) 2 weeks after the rash is strongly against the diagnosis.

Table 52.4.
Stepwise Serological Testing in the Diagnosis of the Etiology of the "Mononucleosis Syndrome"

1. Typical clinical features with a positive heterophil slide test. This essentially establishes a diagnosis of infectious mononucleosis, usually due to EBV. *Recommendation*: No further testing is needed.
2. Typical clinical features with a negative heterophil slide test at the time the patient first presents to the physician. *Recommendation*: Draw acute serum samples (save frozen in two containers) for pertinent serological testing for EBV, toxoplasmosis, CMV, hepatitis A, hepatitis B, and rubella (see Table 52.3). Repeat heterophil slide test during the third week of clinical illness. If positive, no further testing is necessary. If negative, repeat EBV serology (at least 2 weeks post acute sample) and send with one of the acute serological samples for EBV IgM anti-VCD testing (and anti-D testing if available). If the EBV serologies are diagnostic of recent infection, no further testing is necessary.
3. Typical clinical features, negative slide test at week 3 of clinical illness, and negative EBV serology (IgM anti-VCD or anti-D). *Recommendation*: Draw convalescent sera for testing for toxoplasmosis, CMV, hepatitis A, hepatitis B, and rubella and send with acute sera for appropriate serological testing (Table 52.3).
4. Typical or atypical clinical features with negative serologies for all of the above. Consider other etiologies (leukemia, lymphoproliferative disease, granulomatous disease, collagen vascular disease, *etc.*) *Recommendation*: Consider lymph node biopsy and other tests (*e.g.*, bone marrow aspiration and/or biopsy.)

ACQUIRED IMMUNE DEFICIENCY SYNDROME (AIDS)

Since 1981 there has been an epidemic in this country of a syndrome characterized by a defect in celllar immunity that leads to a remarkable susceptibility to certain opportunistic infections and to a propensity to develop an otherwise rare neoplasm, Kaposi's sarcoma, and less often, other lymphomas. The defect has not been preceded by a disease known to produce immunosuppression, nor has it been attributable to the administration of immunosuppressive drugs.

The Centers for Disease Control (CDC), therefore, have established the following criteria for diagnosis of the syndrome:

1. Kaposi's sarcoma in a patient younger than 60
   or
   An unexplained opportunistic infection that is at least moderately predictive of a deficiency of cellular immunity (e.g., *Pneumocystis* pneumonia, disseminated cytomegalovirus or herpes simplex infection, disseminated atypical mycobacterial infection, disseminated fungal infection)
   and
2. Absence of a known cause of immune deficiency (such as a lymphoreticular neoplasm or immunosuppressive therapy).

Epidemiology

Male homosexuals are by far the largest group of people who have proved to be susceptible to the development of AIDS. In this country, over 70% of the reported cases have been in this group. Of the rest, approximately 17% of cases have developed in heterosexual men and women who have been intravenous drug abusers; 5%, in Haitian emigrants (of both sexes) to the United States (many of whom have probably not been homosexuals or drug abusers); and 1%, in hemophiliacs who have received concentrates of antihemophilic factor (5). There have also been scattered cases in female sexual contacts of men who had AIDS, in children born to women who had AIDS, and in nonhemophiliac people of all ages who had received random blood transfusions within 5 years of developing the syndrome and who had no other apparent risk factors.

The homosexuals who have developed AIDS have, compared to appropriate controls, been much more likely to have multiple sexual partners (a median of 68 a year), to have attended bathhouses seeking partners, to have inserted their tongue or hand into their partner's rectum during sex, and to have had syphilis, non-B hepatitis, and/or parasitic diarrhea (9).

Approximately 60% of the reported cases of AIDS have been detected in New York City and its environs and in San Francisco; but relatively high attack rates have been reported in Miami and in Los Angeles (9).

Outside the United States cases have been reported from Haiti, from Western Europe, and from central Africa, where the syndrome appears to be endemic (some cases have been reported in Europe among immigrants from central Africa).

The commonest specific disease associated with AIDS is *Pneumocystis* pneumonia, occurring in 51% of reported cases; 25% of reported cases have had Kaposi's sarcoma; 16% have had other opportunistic infections; and 7% have had both *Pneumocystis* pneumonia and Kaposi's sarcoma (9).

Pathogenesis

Because of the populations that are at risk, it has appeared likely that an infectious agent, transmitted by sexual contact or by exposure to blood products, is responsible for the immunodeficiency that is the hallmark of the syndrome. It now appears that that agent is a human T cell leukemia virus (HTLV-III), which is an RNA retrovirus that specifically infects helper T lymphocytes and kills them (11). Virtually all patients with AIDS have antibodies to this virus (as do 65 to 85% of healthy people among the populations most susceptible to development of the syndrome: male homosexuals and intravenous drug abusers). The incubation period after exposure to the virus, before clinical expression of disease, is probably 3 to 5 years.

Signs and Symptoms

The initial symptoms of AIDS are nonspecific: severe malaise, increased fatigability, low grade fever, anorexia, weight loss, and night sweats. These complaints often develop insidiously over a number of months. Patients with such symptoms, in the populations at risk, are said to have "pre-AIDS." The proportion of this population that will ultimately develop AIDS is unknown. If a specific opportunistic infection develops, there will be symptoms specific to that illness (e.g., odynophagia in patients with *Candida* esophagitis, chronic diarrhea in patients with cryptosporidiosis, chronic cough, dyspnea, and chest pain in patients with *Pneumocystis* pneumonia, or neurological dysfunction in patients with toxoplasmosis or cryptococcosis of the central nervous system).

The physical examination usually reveals a patient who appears chronically ill and who shows signs of considerable loss of weight. Whitish plaques of oral candidiasis may be noted on the mucous membranes of the mouth and oropharynx. Generalized lymphadenopathy, in about 20% of patients, precedes for a number of months the development of the full blown syndrome, but many people with "pre-AIDS" have generalized adenopathy as well as abnormalities of their lymphocyte population and may never develop AIDS (1). Again, findings specific to an opportunistic infection or to Kaposi's sarcoma (papular or nodular lesions, usually red-brown or blue, on the skin and/or mucous membranes, characterized histologically by vascular proliferation and the presence of spindle-shaped neoplastic cells) ultimately become manifest.

Laboratory Findings (14)

The anemia of chronic disease (see Chapter 49) develops in almost all patients. Lymphopenia (absolute lymphocyte counts less than 1500/mm³, often less than 500/mm³) is very common and is due to a marked reduction in the number of helper T cells. That reduction is reflected in a reversed helper (OKT4) to suppressor (OKT8) T cell ratio (normally greater than 1.2) of 0.7 or less (the reversed ratio is not diagnostic of AIDS; it is common in patients with "pre-AIDS" as well). Those ratios currently are measured only in specialized immunology laboratories. The prevalence of antibodies to a variety of viruses (e.g., CMV, EBV, herpes simplex) is high in populations at risk, whether or not they have AIDS. Tests for detection of HTLV-III are now commercially available, but they are used primarily for the screening of blood donors.

Autoimmune thrombocytopenia occurs with apparently increased frequency in sexually active homosexual men (20); about one-third of these people ultimately develop AIDS (sometimes years later); in those who do not, the course and treatment of the illness are the same as in other populations (see Chapter 50); but the disease apparently is different from classic autoimmune thrombocytopenic purpura in that there are immune complexes, rather than antiplatelet antibodies, adsorbed to the platelet surface.

Other laboratory findings, including biopsies, serologies, and cultures, depend on which infection and/or neoplasm has developed.

Treatment and Course

Patients with established AIDS (see criteria above) should be hospitalized and treated aggressively for whatever opportunistic infection or neoplasm they have developed. Patients with "pre-AIDS," manifest by nonspecific symptoms and suppression of helper T cells, can only be followed closely so that, if they develop a specific illness, they can be treated properly. Counseling by the physician is important in managing the understandable anxiety that such patients often express (see Chapter 13, The Anxious Patient).

Neither patients with AIDS nor patients with pre-AIDS should engage in sexual activity or donate blood. There is no evidence that nonsexual contacts, including physicians, need take special precautions in dealing with these patients.

It is to be expected that all patients who develop the complete syndrome will die within 2 to 3 years.

Support by the physician of both family and patients is important during this difficult period (see Chapter 13, The Anxious Patient and Chapter 19, Dying, Death, and Bereavement). It is particularly important that the social stigma associated with the illness is minimized and that the patient not be isolated from his friends and family.

CHRONIC LYMPHOCYTIC LEUKEMIA

Chronic lymphocytic leukemia (CLL) is a disease characterized by the monoclonal proliferation of lymphocytes (usually B cells), which, unlike normal lymphocytes, often are unable to synthesize immunoglobulin.

Clinical Features

CLL is the most common type of leukemia that is encountered in the United States. It is primarily a disease of older men (17) in that two-thirds of patients are 60 or older and 2 to 3 times as many men are afflicted as are women. A mild tendency for the disease to segregate in families suggests that genetic factors may play a role in its acquisition (2).

Many patients are asymptomatic when diagnosed (see below), but complaints of malaise and of increased fatigability are common. Ultimately most patients develop generalized lymphadenopathy and splenomegaly.

A persistent absolute lymphocytosis (greater than 10,000/μl for 3 months or longer) is the hallmark of the disease; lymphocyte counts as high as 200,000 to 300,000/μl may be seen occasionally. Other tests (bone marrow aspiration, lymph node biopsy) are ordinarily not necessary to establish the diagnosis.

As the disease progresses, hypogammaglobulinemia, anemia, granulocytopenia, and thrombocytopenia may develop. Autoimmune disorders (autoimmune hemolytic anemia and thrombocytopenia and pure red cell aplasia) develop in 10 to 15% of patients.

Treatment and Course

The survival of patients with CLL correlates best with the stage of their disease at diagnosis (12). For example, asymptomatic patients with only an absolute lymphocytosis have an essentially normal life expectancy. Patients with lymphadenopathy alone have a median survival of 6 to 8 years, and patients with anemia or thrombocytopenia have a median survival of 2 to 3 years.

Treatment does not influence survival but can be very helpful in decreasing the severity of signs and symptoms in the later stages of the disease. Thus, stable, asymptomatic patients with or without lymphadenopathy and/or splenomegaly do not require treatment. On the other hand, patients with marked constitutional symptoms (weight loss, severe malaise) or with symptomatic anemia or thrombocytopenia should be treated, usually with an oral alkylating agent (chlorambucil or cyclophosphamide) and with prednisone. Various treatment schedules are utilized, dependent primarily on the preference of the therapist. However, side effects may be minimized if therapy is given in short courses (an alkylating agent on day 1, prednisone on days 1 to 4) every 2 to 3 weeks. Patients with autoimmune hemolysis and thrombocytopenia require more aggressive treatment with corticosteroids, and splenectomy is sometimes necessary in severely anemic or thrombocytopenic patients who are unresponsive to corticosteroids. A hematologist or medical oncologist should be consulted at the time of diagnosis of CLL and should be involved in the care of patients who require treatment.

THE UNDIAGNOSED PATIENT WITH LYMPHADENOPATHY: WHEN TO RECOMMEND LYMPH NODE BIOPSY

Lymphadenopathy is a common physical finding that is associated with multiple disease processes. The decision about when to biopsy an enlarged lymph node is one of the more difficult in clinical medicine (6). The problem most often arises in younger patients. Older patients with localized lymphadenopathy, unexplained by infection or inflammation, should be assumed to have cancer until proven otherwise, and the biopsy decision, therefore, is usually an easy one. However, lymphadenopathy in children and in young adults is usually due to inflammation, and biopsy is usually not diagnostic. The clinician is often concerned in such circumstances about the possible harm from a delay in the diagnosis of a malignancy (Hodgkin's disease or non-Hodgkin's lymphoma most commonly) or a granulomatous condition (tuberculosis, sarcoid, etc) for which specific treatment is indicated. However, considerable harm may result from unnecessary biopsy. There is, for the patient, both psychological and physical discomfort from the procedure, and most important of all there is frequently uncertainty about the interpretation of the biopsy of a "reactive" node. The histology of reactive nodes, especially those encountered in the mononucleosis syndrome, can be difficult to interpret. Reed-Sternberg cells (ordinarily pathognomonic of Hodgkin's disease) can be seen in the nodes of patients with infectious mononucleosis, and reactive nodes can sometimes look like and be interpreted as diagnostic of Hodgkin's disease or of non-Hodgkin's lymphoma. Because of these problems, the physician should avoid, if possible, performing a biopsy of a lymph node in a patient with the mononucleosis syndrome. However, since patients with systemic lymphoma, Hodgkin's disease, miliary tuberculosis, etc may have symptoms suggestive of the infectious mononucleosis syndrome (fever, anorexia, weight loss, malaise,

Table 52.5.
When to Recommend Lymph Node Biopsy in the Teenager and Young Adult

Features against early biopsy
1. Mononucleosis syndrome, especially when proven serologically.
2. Ear-nose-throat symptoms (earache, sore throat, coryza, tonsillar or dental infection).
3. Lymph nodes less than 2 cm in diameter.
4. Normal chest X-ray, especially when associated with one of the above.

Features for early biopsy
1. Systemic illness with atypical features of the mononucleosis syndrome and without serological proof of a cause of the mononucleosis syndrome (see Table 52.4).
2. Lymph nodes greater than 2 cm in diameter and an abnormal chest X-ray, absence of ear-nose-throat symptoms, or no proof of a typical mononucleosis syndrome.
3. Localized supraclavicular lymphadenopathy. This may be seen in the mononucleosis syndrome but in its absence is suggestive of mediastinal (right supraclavicular) or abdominal (left supraclavicular) granulomatous or neoplastic disease.

etc), one of the main reasons to pursue, by serological studies (see above, page 609), a specific etiology for the syndrome is to attempt to make a diagnosis without having to do a biopsy.

If a specific diagnosis cannot be made on the basis of serological studies, there are relatively few criteria upon which the clinician can rely in order to decide whether a biopsy is indicated. However, one helpful recent retrospective study reported that in the age range of 9 to 25 years three variables were important in determining whether a lymph node biopsy might be diagnostic of an illness requiring specific treatment (18): (a) the size of the node to be tested by biopsy, (b) the presence or absence of ear-nose-throat symptoms, and (c) the presence or absence of an abnormality on chest X-ray. Nodes greater than 2 cm in diameter were more likely to contain important histological information than were smaller nodes. An abnormal chest X-ray (adenopathy, infiltrate) in a patient with peripheral adenopathy correlated with useful biopsy information. Patients with lymphadenopathy but without any ear-nose-throat symptoms were more likely to have a diagnostic lymph node biopsy. Table 52.5 summarizes some of the features that can be utilized by the physician, especially in the young patient, to help decide about the advisability and timing of a lymph node biopsy.

General References

Fauci AS: Acquired immunodeficiency syndrome: epidemiologic, clinical, immunological and therapeutic considerations. *Ann Intern Med* 100:92, 1984.
    A comprehensive review.
Niederman JC: Infectious mononucleosis. In Hoeprich PD (ed): *Infectious Disease*, ed 3. Philadelphia, Harper and Row, 1983, p 1205.
    A concise authoritative review.
Rundles RW: Chronic lymphocytic leukemia. In Williams WJ, Beutler E, Erslev AJ, Lichtman MA (eds): *Hematology*, ed 3. New York, McGraw-Hill, 1983, p 981.
    A detailed, well referenced review.

Specific References

1. Abrams DI, Lewis BJ, Beckstead JH, *et al*: Persistent diffuse lymphadenopathy in homosexual men: endpoint or prodrome? *Ann Intern Med* 100:801, 1984.
2. Conley CL, Misiti J, Laster AJ: Genetic factors predisposing to chronic lymphocytic leukemia. *Medicine* 59:323, 1980.
3. Dorman JM, Glick TH, Shannon DC, *et al*: Complications of infectious mononucleosis. *Am J Dis Child* 128:239, 1974.
4. Evans AS, Niederman JC, McCollum RW: Seroepidemiologic studies of infectious mononucleosis with EB virus. *N Engl J Med* 279:1121, 1968.
5. Fauci AS: Acquired immunodeficiency syndrome: epidemiologic, clinical, immunological and therapeutic considerations. *Ann Intern Med* 100:92, 1984.
6. Greenfield S, Jordan MC: The clinical investigation of lymphadenopathy in primary care practice. *JAMA* 240:1388, 1978.
7. Horwitz CA, Henle W, Henle G, *et al*: Heterophile-negative infectious mononucleosis and mononucleosis-like illness. *Am J Med* 63:947, 1977.
8. Horwitz CA, Henle W, Henle G, *et al*: Infectious mononucleosis in patients aged 40 to 72 years: report of 27 cases, including 3 without heterophil-antibody responses. *Medicine* 62:256, 1983.
9. Jaffe HW, Keewhan C, Thomas PA, *et al*: National case-control study of Kaposi's sarcoma and *Pneumocystis carinii* pneumonia in homosexual men. Part 1. Epidemiologic results. *Ann Intern Med* 99:145, 1983.
10. Jones JF, Ray CG, Minnich LL, *et al*: Evidence for active Epstein-Barr virus infection in patients with persistent, unexplained illness: elevated anti-early antigen antibodies. *Ann Intern Med* 102:7, 1985.
11. Popovic M, Samgadharan MG, Read E, Gallo RC: Detection, isolation, and continuous production of cytopathic retrovirus (HTLV-III) from patients with AIDS and pre-AIDS. *Science* 224:497, 1984.
12. Rai KR, Sawitsky A, Cronkite EP, *et al*: Clinical staging of chronic lymphocytic leukemia. *Blood* 46:219, 1975.
13. Rippey JH, Bowman HE: Infectious mononucleosis test performance on CAP survey specimens. *Am J Clin Pathol* 72:363, 1979.
14. Rogers MF, Morens DM, Stewart JA, *et al*: National case-control study of Kaposi's sarcoma and *Pneumocystis carinii* pneumonia in homosexual men. Part 2. Laboratory results. *Ann Intern Med* 99:151, 1983.
15. Rutkow IM: Rupture of the spleen in infectious mononucleosis. *Arch Surg* 113:718, 1978.
16. Sawyer RN, Evans AS, Niederman JC, McCollum RN: Prospective studies of a group of Yale University freshmen. I. Occurrence of infectious mononucleosis. *J Infect Dis* 123:263, 1971.
17. Skinnider LF, Tan L, Schmidt J, Armitage G: Chronic lymphocytic leukemia. A review of 745 cases and assessment of clinical staging. *Cancer* 50:2951, 1982.
18. Slap GB, Brooks SJ, Schwartz JS: When to perform biopsies of enlarged peripheral lymph nodes in young patients. *JAMA* 252:1421, 1984.
19. Straus SE, Tosato G, Armstrong G, *et al*: Persisting illness and fatigue in adults with evidence of Epstein-Barr virus infection. *Ann Intern Med* 102:7, 1985.
20. Walsh CM, Nardi MA, Karpatkin S: On the mechanism of thrombocytopenic purpura in sexually active homosexual men. *N Engl J Med* 311:635, 1984.

SECTION 7

Pulmonary Problems

CHAPTER FIFTY-THREE

Common Pulmonary Problems: Cough, Hemoptysis, Dyspnea, and Chest Pain

PHILIP L. SMITH, M.D., AND EUGENE R. BLEECKER, M.D.

Patients who develop acute respiratory diseases usually present with symptoms that result in the rapid diagnosis and treatment of the underlying disorder. On the other hand, chronic diseases of the lung that cause slowly progressive symptoms may go undetected unless incidentally discovered as part of a general medical evaluation that includes routine chest roentgenogram and screening pulmonary function tests. This chapter will discuss four common pulmonary symptoms with which the general physician is often confronted: cough, hemoptysis, dyspnea, and noncardiac chest pain.

COUGH

Cough is an important defense mechanism that clears the airways of both secretions and inhaled particles. Although it is often associated with other respiratory symptoms, cough may be the major symptom that prompts a patient to seek medical advise. A cough is composed of three phases: a deep inspiration, closure of the glottis accompanied by a rapid increase in pleural pressure, a final opening of the glottis, and an explosive release of pressure.

A brief understanding of the anatomy of the re-flexes that are involved will aid in the evaluation and treatment of cough. Initially there may be stimulation of mucosal neural receptors located throughout the nasopharynx, larynx, trachea, and bronchi down to the level of the terminal bronchioles. Stimulation of the same receptors in the nasopharynx may cause sneezing, whereas stimulation of tracheal and bronchial receptors also may cause bronchospasm. After activation of the receptors, impulses are conducted along afferent pathways in the 9th and 10th cranial nerves to the cough center in the medulla. The reflex is completed through efferent pathways which cause forceful contraction of the diaphragm and other expiratory muscles. While many different stimuli activate these receptors, all essentially initiate cough by some form of mechanical or chemical irritation. Additional factors, such as acute inflammation of the airways, may disrupt the bronchial mucosa, increase its permeability and expose the receptors. The accompanying increases in respiratory secretions will lead to cough. Environmental pollutants, such as cigarette smoke, can directly stimulate the receptors without necessarily provoking an inflammatory reaction. Finally, although stimulation of irritant receptors may cause reflex bronchoconstriction, the bronchospasm itself, through reflex pathways, induces cough.

Acute Cough Syndromes

Table 53.1 shows the common and uncommon causes of cough. Generally cough that occurs as a symptom of acute inflammatory disease, such as tracheitis and tracheobronchitis, is limited by the length of the illness. In contrast, cough that is triggered by mild bronchospasm may persist for weeks to months following a viral upper respiratory tract infection (see below). Usually viral infections and atypical pneumonias are associated with nonproductive coughs, while bacterial infections are associated with significant sputum production. Younger patients tend to have a more productive cough associated with pneumonia, while older individuals, especially those with chronic obstructive pulmonary disease, may retain secretions because of airway collapse during coughing. When a productive cough follows a typical viral syndrome, it may also signal the development of a superimposed bacterial bron-

Table 53.1.
Causes of Cough

Causes	Examples
COMMON CAUSES	
Acute	
Inflammation	Tracheitis, bronchitis, pneumonia
Irritation	Air pollutants
Bronchospasm	Postrespiratory infections
Chronic	
Inflammation	Bronchitis, pollution, cigarettes, bronchiectasis, aspirated foreign body
Irritation	Cigarettes, cancer
Bronchospasm	Asthma, postrespiratory infection
LESS COMMON CAUSES	
Irritation	Aortic aneurysm, chronic aspiration, auditory canal stimulation (cerumen, hair)
Inflammation	Sarcoid, alveolitis
Psychogenic	

chitis or pneumonia. High concentrations of industrial pollutants, such as insoluble gases (for example, SO_3 or NO_2), which are not removed in the upper airway can cause either a nonproductive or a productive cough secondary to chemical irritation.

Chronic Cough Syndromes

Coughing that is persistent is more bothersome than the acute cough syndrome described above. Clearly the most common cause of coughing is cigarette smoking. Such coughing is usually dry and hacking and is worse in the morning. The number of cigarettes smoked bears little relationship to the development of cough except at very high levels of cigarette consumption (three to four packs/day) (15). Perhaps because they inhale more deeply, smokers of marijuana may complain of a persistent cough after smoking only one to two cigarettes daily. By definition, all patients with bronchitis have productive coughs. As opposed to patients with bronchogenic and mediastinal tumors, who often complain of coughing, patients with metastatic tumors or with nodules that arise peripherally outside of the airways or beyond irritant receptors seldom present with cough. In nonsmokers, the most common cause of chronic cough is postnasal drip resulting from chronic sinusitis or allergic rhinitis (15). It is very important to recognize that airway obstruction in smokers as well as nonsmokers can be associated with a chronic dry cough. This in fact, may be the only manifestation of obstructive airway disease and need not be associated with dyspnea, wheezing, or large changes in pulmonary function.

Other less common causes of chronic cough include any process that stimulates the neural receptors in the pleura and pericardium (5). Even im-

pacted cerumen in the external auditory canal can elicit a chronic cough. If a complete history and physical examination have revealed no positive findings, it is often tempting to attribute chronic cough to a psychogenic etiology; however, this is an extremely rare cause of coughing and has most often been reported in children. Characteristically, psychogenic cough is not productive, it subsides during sleep and is clearly related to emotional stress (7).

Evaluation

Evaluation of the acute and chronic cough syndromes is similar. Usually a history and physical examination will yield a presumptive diagnosis. Informaton should be obtained about the circumstances surrounding the development and duration of the cough, environmental exposure, smoking history, and any past history of obstructive airway disease. A history of constant swallowing or of throat clearing suggests postnasal drip, even though the patient may deny many other symptoms associated with sinusitis.

Although the physical examination seldom provides a specific diagnosis, it may provide important clues. Careful examination of the ears, nose, throat, and lower respiratory tract is of paramount importance. Cobblestoning in the oropharynx represents lymphoid hyperplasia, which is commonly seen in patients with chronic sinusitis, but this is a nonspecific finding that can be found in other conditions not necessarily associated with cough. Examination of the chest may reveal rhonchi caused by the loose secretions that result from acute or chronic infection. Occasionally a localized wheeze suggests a bronchogenic tumor, whereas generalized wheezing at end expiration confirms the diagnosis of obstructive lung disease. (However, a normal physical examination cannot exclude a diagnosis of airway obstruction.) Finally, the physical examination allows the physician to observe the quality and severity of the cough. A harsh cough associated with loose secretions is characteristic of tracheobronchitis resulting from viral upper respiratory infection. When little or no coughing occurs in the course of the visit, the patient should be asked to cough so that the physician can see whether the cough is productive or is associated with wheezing. This is also useful since some patients, especially women, refuse to admit to expectoration of sputum and often unconsciously swallow their secretions.

If a diagnosis is not obvious after a history and physical examination, laboratory testing is indicated. A complete blood count and microscopic examination of a "wet prep" of the sputum should be performed. Sputum with eosinophilia, as seen in asthma, may appear purulent, and if it is not examined microscopically, the patient may be treated inappropriately with antibiotics. A chest roentgenogram will demonstrate virtually all acute infections that involve the pulmonary parenchyma as well as some of the rarer causes of chronic cough, such as aortic aneurysm and sarcoidosis. The roentgenogram also will demonstrate atelectasis associated with a bronchogenic tumor or with an aspirated foreign body. Patients with coughing due to viral and bacterial tracheobronchitis, asthma, or cigarette smoking will usually have a normal chest roentgenogram. Hyperventilation, which suggests underlying obstructive pulmonary disease, may be observed, in which case a spirogram should be obtained to document airway obstruction (see below). However, patients with reversible obstruction may have only intermittent bronchospasm, and between attacks their pulmonary function may be normal.

If no specific diagnosis has been made after this evaluation, the patient should be seen periodically for 1 to 2 months before other invasive diagnostic procedures are attempted. When the chest roentgenogram is normal, bronchoscopy seldom provides additional useful information. Although a proximal bronchogenic tumor can be hidden on a chest roentgenogram by the mediastinal shadows, patients with these tumors often have associated hemoptysis (see below) (15).

Confirmation that bronchospasm and hyperreactive airways are the causes of persistent coughing can be obtained by bronchoprovocation tests with pharmacological agents, such as histamine or methacholine. These tests are not usually necessary (see Chapter 55) and, to obtain them, the patient will need to be referred to a pulmonary specialist who has appropriate laboratory facilities to perform them. These procedures should be done only after a medical history, physical examination, and laboratory studies, including routine spirometry, have been completed since they are not indicated in patients with obvious spasmodic asthma or with significant obstructive airway disease. The main purpose of bronchoprovocation is to confirm the presence of hyperreactive airways in patients with an equivocal history and laboratory studies. Often, routine spirometry that is consistent with early airways obstruction (see chapter 55) may provide adequate supporting evidence for the physician to initiate a diagnostic trial with bronchodilators.

Therapy

The specific therapy of the various acute inflammatory and irritating processes likely to cause coughing is discussed in detail in individual chapters dealing with these topics.

In general, viral tracheobronchitis requires only symptomatic therapy since coughing will usually spontaneously subside in 2 to 4 weeks. Patients with persistent coughing and a history compatible with allergic airways disease (rhinitis, extrinsic asthma), intermittent (intrinsic asthma) or chronic obstructive airways disease, as well as those with broncho-

spasm and coughing following a viral upper respiratory tract infection should have a diagnostic and therapeutic trial with bronchodilators. Therapy with bronchodilators should be started after a spirogram is obtained to document airflow obstruction or after appropriate bronchoprovocation studies (see above). Treatment should begin with an inhaled long acting specific β_2-sympathomimetic agonist (metaproterenol, terbutaline, fenoterol) and later, if necessary, an oral methylxanthine can be added. A detailed therapeutic approach to the pharmacological treatment of bronchospasm is presented in Chapter 55.

Cessation of cigarette smoking and avoidance of a polluted environment may be the most important aspects of the therapy of both acute and chronic cough. In one study of 200 patients with a chronic cough, 50% had relief within 1 month of cessation of cigarette smoking while eventually 77% of these patients had complete resolution of their cough (14). Thus, the patient who continues to smoke and to complain of cough is particularly frustrating since it is often difficult to convince him that as few as one to two cigarettes/day cause airway irritation and inflammation.

If a patient has impacted cerumen in the auditory canal, removal of the irritation provides immediate relief. Obviously, if a patient has an aortic aneurysm or a bronchogenic tumor associated with a cough, these problems must be dealt with before the cough will abate. The treatment of postnasal drip (chronic sinusitis) is dealt with in Chapter 28.

After specific therapy has been initiated (or if the underlying process is not treatable), the use of antitussives should be considered. In spite of the enormous demands made for antitussives, there are few situations in which these preparations are absolutely necessary. Moreover, the expectoration of sputum is a major goal in the therapy of inflammatory lung disease. Therefore, when antitussives are needed in patients with productive coughs, it is usually better to attempt cough reduction (not total suppression), primarily to allow patients to sleep. In the United States there are several hundred cough and decongestant preparations usually sold as combination products. Understandably, the Food and Drug Administration has made efforts recently to eliminate ineffective preparations from the marketplace.

Antitussives act on the cough reflex either by anesthetizing the peripheral irritant receptors or by increasing the threshold of the cough center. Table 53.2 summarizes the most useful active non-narcotic oral antitussives, their site of action, and their recommended dosages.

Probably the two most effective "non-narcotic" antitussives are dextromethorphan and benzonatate. Dextromethorphan is chemically derived from the opiates; however, it is classified as non-narcotic because it has no sedative or analgesic effects and,

Table 53.2.
Non-Narcotic Antitussives[a]

Drug	Brand Name	Usual Dose	Site of Action	Comment
Benzonatate	Tessalon	100–200 mg four times a day	Peripheral	Considered most effective peripheral agent
Dextromethorphan	Many preparations	15–30 mg four times a day	Central	Considered most effective central agent
Noscapine	Tusscapine	15–30 mg four times a day	Central	
Levopropoxyphene	Novrad	100 mg four times a day	Central	

[a] Most of these drugs are available as proprietary medications.

therefore, has little potential for abuse. Dextromethorphan is the most commonly used antitussive and suppresses cough centrally. It is metabolized by the liver and should be avoided in patients with significant hepatic insufficiency. Occasionally, the drug will cause nausea or dizziness, and overdosages of more than 200 mg will lead to central nervous system depression. Benzonatate is a peripherally acting anesthetic similar to tetracaine. Its only side effects are mild dizziness, vertigo, and occasional nausea. If the drug is accidentally chewed, both unpleasant taste and prolonged oral anesthesia will occur. Overdosage has been associated with central nervous system stimulation resulting in tremors followed by profound central nervous depression. It is reasonable to treat patients initially with dextromethorphan and, if intolerable cough persists, to substitute benzonatate. Two other useful oral antitussives, noscapine and levopropoxyphene, are less commonly used but are alternatives if neither dextromethorphan nor benzonatate can be taken.

If non-narcotic antitussives are ineffective, then codeine should be tried. Many clinicians will prescribe codeine preferentially to patients with persistent cough because it is a more potent cough suppressant than the non-narcotic agents. Codeine is effective in doses of 10 to 20 mg administered every 3 to 6 hours. The common side effects—nausea, vomiting, constipation, dry mouth, and sedation—are usually not experienced when these recommended doses are employed.

Topical anesthetics can be used as cough suppressants, but they are weak, usually ineffective, and may cause hypersensitivity reactions. These weak anesthetics primarily anesthetize the irritant and pain receptors in the oral pharynx and are contained in many over-the-counter gargles and throat lozenges. If they are abused or used in excessive doses, the gag reflex will be abolished and the risk of pulmonary aspiration will be increased.

The use of expectorants and humidification of the airways in patients with respiratory disease is discussed in Chapter 55.

HEMOPTYSIS

Hemoptysis is defined as the expectoration of blood; it can range from the coughing of minimal amounts of blood-tinged sputum to the coughing of large amounts of blood with clots. Distinguishing between hemoptysis and hematemesis is not difficult since expectorated blood usually is bright red, frothy, has an alkaline pH, and is often mixed with sputum containing macrophages and white blood cells. Frequently, patients with hemoptysis will complain of a tickling or bothersome irritation in their chest, and occasionally they will be able to localize these sensations to one lung. On the other hand, hematemesis is characterized by blood that is darker brown, has an acid pH, and is mixed with food particles; often there is a history of alcoholism, drug abuse, or previous gastrointestinal disease. When either massive hemoptysis or hematemesis occurs, the distinction is not difficult since the physician can easily differentiate coughing from vomiting. Sometimes blood from a lesion in the sinuses or in the upper aiwway will be aspirated and later expectorated, making it appear that the bleeding occurred in the lower respiratory tract. Thus, a careful history and physical examination must be performed to avoid inappropriate treatment. The patient should be instructed always to collect and save his bloody sputum so that the hemoptysis can be quantified. Nevertheless, a history of hemoptysis should not be ignored if a patient cannot produce a specimen on command since the symptom can be intermittent.

The various pulmonary causes of hemoptysis are summarized in Table 53.3. Published reports about the relative probabilities of the various causes of hemoptysis reflect the type and location of the reporting institution. Studies from large urban centers note a greater incidence of infectious etiologies, such as tuberculosis (8); those from the Veteran's Administration find primarily lung cancer and bronchitis; and studies from predominantly referral institutions report a higher incidence of unusual causes. Similarly, the etiology of hemoptysis found in an ambulatory setting will also depend on the patient population served by the medical practice.

In the typical ambulatory practice, blood streaking of the sputum is caused by bronchitis or bronchiectasis 30 to 60% of the time, and by lung cancer 20 to 30% of the time. When the entire sputum is bloody, carcinoma or bronchiectasis is more likely than bronchitis. However, with the more liberal use

Table 53.3.
Pulmonary Causes of Hemoptysis

COMMON	
Inflammatory	Bronchitis, bronchiectasis, tuberculosis, pneumonia, lung abscess
Neoplasm	Lung cancer
Vascular	Pulmonary embolus/infarction
LESS COMMON	
Inflammatory/ immunological	Goodpasture's syndrome, idiopathic pulmonary hemosiderosis, cavitary disease (with a "fungus ball"), parasites, broncholithiasis, cystic fibrosis
Neoplasm	Bronchial adenoma, metastatic cancer
Vascular	Arteriovenous malformation, sequestration, mitral stenosis, anticoagulation
Chest trauma	

of antibiotics and the appropriate decline in the use of diagnostic bronchography, structural bronchiectasis resulting from recurrent infection is probably underdiagnosed while bronchitis (chronic productive cough) is overdiagnosed. Active cavitary tuberculosis is now a less common cause of hemoptysis than it once was, but "dry" bronchiectasis, the result of old tuberculous infection, is still frequently found. Bronchogenic carcinoma that originates in a major bronchus often presents with hemoptysis resulting from an associated infection, erosion of the tumor through the bronchial mucosa, or bleeding of a friable tumor. Usually blood from pneumonia or a lung abscess is mixed with "pus," and the sputum appears red-brown or red-green. Hemoptysis from pulmonary emboli occurs in approximately 30% of cases of documented emboli associated with an infarction of the lung (1). Interestingly, even with the advent of the fiberoptic bronchoscope, the cause of hemoptysis remains undiagnosed 5 to 15% of the time (16).

Less common causes of hemoptysis are also listed in Table 53.3, but again this ranking reflects to some extent the location of a practice since mycetomas within fungus cavities (6) and parasitic diseases that cause hemoptysis, for example, will be much more frequently seen in endemic areas of the country. While the more common presentation of bronchial adenomas is atelectasis with cough and fever, these vascular tumors do cause hemoptysis also. Metastatic tumors tend to enlarge within the lung parenchyma; thus bleeding as the initial presentation is exceedingly rare. Chronic mitral stenosis that is associated with poorly controlled congestive heart failure and pulmonary hypertension will lead to bleeding of the bronchial veins and to blood-tinged sputum. Hemoptysis can occur in patients treated with warfarin or heparin, especially those who have associated lung disease such as bronchitis or cancer, even if the anticoagulation is carefully controlled. Occasionally blunt chest trauma will produce hemoptysis in an otherwise healthy individual.

Evaluation

The diagnostic evaluation of hemoptysis is aimed at localizing the site and quantifying the amount of bleeding, beginning with a history and physical examination, followed by an examination of the chest roentgenogram. If the source of hemoptysis is an intrathoracic structure, the patient, may be able to localize the site of bleeding to the right or left lung (a tickling sensation is sometimes experienced on the affected side). An attempt should then be made to quantitate the amount of hemoptysis since patients who have expectorated more than 25 to 50 ml of bright red blood during a 24-hour period require hospitalization. Although rare, massive hemoptysis of more than 600 ml of blood during a 24-hour period represents a medical emergency, since survival of the patient is dependent on rapid diagnosis and on surgical therapy (10). Other useful data that should be elicited during a medical history include a prior history of tuberculosis or of chronic bronchitis, evidence of systemic symptoms compatible with a pulmonary neoplasm, or a recent history of an acute pulmonary infectious process or of chest trauma. A history of mitral valvular heart disease or of travel with possible exposure to parasites should alert the physician to these less common causes of bleeding.

During the physical examination, extrathoracic sources of bleeding from structures such as the nasal passages, sinuses, and pharynx should be sought. Localized wheezing or rales suggest disease confined to one side of the chest, information that may be particularly useful when the chest roentgenogram is normal. Next, sputum should be repeatedly collected and examined to quantify the severity of the hemoptysis (8) and to observe whether or not there are clots, which suggest slower bleeding.

Evaluation of the chest roentgenogram is critical since all acute inflammatory diseases, such as active tuberculosis, pneumonia, and lung abscess, will produce obvious pulmonary infiltrates. In addition, 85% of neoplasms and most pulmonary emboli with an associated infarction will also show localized pulmonary lesions. However, localization of the bleeding source is frequently precluded by bilateral aspiration of blood or by the presence of bilateral pulmonary disease on chest roentgenogram. Patients with bronchitis or bronchiectasis often have normal films. If the bronchiectasis is a result of old tuberculosis, however, apical scarring may suggest the diagnosis; otherwise, there may be increased lower lobe markings or infiltrates if there is recurrent infection. Bronchitis is a clinical diagnosis made in patients with a productive cough, although differentiation of bronchitis from bronchiectasis is difficult by history and chest roentgenogram alone. Bronchography can be used to distinguish these entities, but the complications of this procedure do not warrant its diagnostic use unless bleeding is recurrent and severe, and unless surgical resection is being considered. Furthermore, the medical management of both bronchitis and bronchiectasis is the same.

The primary diagnostic entity that must be excluded in patients with the first episode of hemoptysis is lung cancer (see Chapter 56). Tumors that cause hemoptysis typically arise in central bronchi, and the diagnosis is usually made with a chest roentgenogram and bronchoscopy. Since 15% of patients with lung tumors who present with hemoptysis may have a normal chest roentgenogram (16), most pulmonologists recommend bronchoscopy, bronchial brushings, and bronchial washings in patients presenting with their first episode of hemoptysis. However, some have advocated simply observing patients less than 40 years old who have a normal chest roentgenogram and hemoptysis of less than 1 week's duration since they have a relatively small chance of having a pulmonary malignancy (11). Unfortunately, the published data supporting this approach are small, but this approach may be more readily adopted, considering the recent attempts to control the costs of health care. An alternative is to obtain three sputum cytologies followed by bronchoscopy if the cytologies are positive. Bronchoscopy is possible in selected ambulatory patients (see Chapter 56 for a description of the patient's experience during this procedure). In patients with positive sputum cytologies or with an abnormal chest roentgenogram consistent with lung cancer, the evaluation should proceed as outlined in Chapter 56.

Rare vascular causes of hemoptysis should be considered when common causes seem unlikely. Mitral stenosis causes hemoptysis only after years of pulmonary hypertension, venous congestion, and gross cardiomegaly; therefore, the physical examination and chest roentgenogram will usually suggest the diagnosis. Arteriovenous malformations can be diagnosed with a chest roentgenogram that demonstrates two visible vessels, and can then be confirmed by computerized axial tomography or by angiography.

If the evaluation, including history and physical examination, sputum cytology, chest roentgenogram, and bronchoscopy, is unrevealing, additional procedures, such as computerized axial tomography, may be useful in selected cases.

Therapy

Not every patient with hemoptysis needs admission to the hospital for diagnosis and treatment. Nevertheless, all patients over 40 years old with their first episode of hemoptysis do need a thorough investigation. Also, patients with significant hemoptysis (8, 10) (more than 25 to 50 ml of blood/day) require hospitalization and rapid diagnostic evaluation. If there is evidence of airways obstruction, treatment with bronchodilators may relieve coughing and thereby reduce hemoptysis. Patients with

the diagnosis of bronchitis or of bronchiectasis can usually be treated on an ambulatory basis with antibiotics, such as tetracycline or ampicillin, 1 to 2 g a day for 10 days. Blood streaking of the sputum usually resolves within 2 to 3 days, but a full course of antibiotic therapy should be completed. When hemoptysis is due to pneumonia, lung abscess, or tuberculosis, no specific therapy is needed other than treatment of the underlying condition (see Chapters 28 and 29). Arteriovenous malformations often stop bleeding spontaneously; but if the bleeding does persist, angiography will be necessary to document the extent of the malformation followed by either therapeutic embolization (13) or by surgical removal. Mitral stenosis that results in hemoptysis indicates severe pulmonary hypertension and is often too far advanced to allow surgical correction, but cardiological consultation should be obtained in order to evaluate and to maximize the medical therapy of left heart failure.

Cough suppressant therapy can be important in the acute phase of hemoptysis since this allows clots to form and to occlude the area of bleeding. However, it must be cautioned that oversedating the patient can lead to aspiration and asphyxiation if significant bleeding persists. Cough suppressants are primarily needed either when there is active bleeding or when clots are being frequently expectorated. On the other hand, blood streaking of the sputum does not require cough suppression. Furthermore, in patients with pneumonia or lung abscess, where blood is mixed with purulent expectorations, cough suppressant therapy is contraindicated since pulmonary drainage is an important part of the treatment.

DYSPNEA

Breathing is an unconscious act that usually occurs effortlessly; yet even a normal person becomes aware of his breathing during deep sighs or during moderate to severe exercise. Dyspnea, the abnormal, uncomfortable sensation of breathlessness, is difficult to define since patients often cannot accurately perceive or quantitate the feeling. Similar to an individual's threshold for the recognition of pain, the complaint of dyspnea is dependent both on the individual's limit for discomfort and on the specific circumstances which provoke shortness of breath. Thus, dyspnea must be defined in terms of what is abnormal for a particular individual in the context of his level of fitness and of the amount of activity that is associated with breathlessness. Some patients become dyspneic with relatively small measurable alterations in ventilation, while others, such as patients who are hyperventilating with Kussmaul breathing, may not complain of dyspnea. Fortunately, a reasonable correlation exists between the degree of dyspnea and objective measurements of physiological dysfunction.

Often the actual complaint of dyspnea may not be expressed as such, and it may vary depending on the type of precipitating illness as well as on whether it developed abruptly or over a longer period of time. Thus, the asthmatic may complain of acute shortness of breath or of a "tightness" in his chest, while the patient with an acute pulmonary embolism may state that his breath has suddenly been taken away, and he cannot "get enough air" even though he ventilates easily. In contrast, the patient with emphysema who has modified his life style may dismiss the sensation of breathlessness as part of his advancing age.

Normal Ventilation

There is no single mechanism responsible for dyspnea. Since dyspnea is the result of a variety of diverse influences acting alone or together, a brief discussion of the control of ventilation may help the practicing physician understand the complexity of dyspnea and the reason why this sensation often does not immediately respond to correction of obvious physiological abnormalities. Normally ventilation is coupled to the individual's metabolic demands as reflected in the oxygen consumption and carbon dioxide elimination necessary to meet a given level of activity. These needs are sensed by peripheral (carotid and aortic bodies) and central (medullary) chemical chemoreceptors that respond to the O_2, CO_2, and pH of blood and cerebral spinal fluid. The acute stimulation of these receptors provokes changes in minute ventilation. In addition, the control and regulation of the rate and pattern of breathing are influenced by the reflex effects of activation of neural receptors that lie in the lung parenchyma, airways, blood vessels, respiratory muscles, and chest wall. For example, receptors in the chest wall and diaphragm will respond to increased stiffness (decreased compliance) in the lung that occurs with fluid accumulation or with interstitial fibrosis. In addition, interstitial edema may activate "C" fibers located in the alveolar interstitium and may reflexly cause dyspnea in patients with pulmonary edema. Other receptors located in the airway epithelium cause rapid, shallow breathing, coughing, and bronchospasm when irritating substances are inhaled. Finally, the central nervous system alone can cause large alterations in breathing that lead to hyperventilation in association with anxiety attacks (see Chapter 13). This discussion should help in understanding, for example, why the correction of arterial hypoxemia alone in a patient with an asthmatic attack usually does not relieve the sensation of breathlessness. In this situation, dyspnea results from the complex interaction of both chemical and neural stimuli to breathe, coupled with an individual's response to these signals. Correction of only one of these problems, therefore, is not sufficient to abolish dyspnea.

Evaluation

The causes of dyspnea are diverse and include essentially all diseases that result in significant functional impairment of either the respiratory system (gas exchange and/or pulmonary mechanics) or the cardiovascular system (circulatory and/or cardiac function) as well as any hematological abnormality that impairs oxygen delivery. Table 53.4 summarizes the general disease categories that are likely to cause abnormal breathlessness.

In ambulatory practice the major causes of dyspnea are obstructive airways disease and arteriosclerotic and hypertensive heart disease, either alone or in combination. The prevalence of symptomatic

Table 53.4.
Causes of Dyspnea

Dyspnea	Acute	Chronic
COMMON		
Pulmonary:		
Obstructive airways disease	Asthma, bronchitis	Bronchitis, emphysema
Restrictive lung disease	Pneumothorax	Pleural effusions, cancer
Inflammatory	Pneumonia	
Vascular	Pulmonary embolism	
Cardiac	Left heart failure, acute myocardial infarction	Left heart failure
Other	Psychogenic	Obesity, anemia
LESS COMMON		
Pulmonary:		
Upper airway obstruction	Epiglottitis, aspiration (foreign body)	
Restrictive lung disease		Diffuse, interstitial lung disease, diaphragm paralyses, kyphoscoliosis
Cardiac		Pericarditis
Other	CO intoxication	Thyrotoxicosis, anemia

lung disease in a specific geographic region or socioeconemic group is further modified by the prevalence of cigarette consumption, urban pollution, and occupational exposure to inhaled toxic substances. Furthermore, the clinical circumstances and sequence of events in which dyspnea occurs will aid in its evaluation. For example, the etiology of dyspnea is obvious in a teenager with seasonal asthma who develops shortness of breath and wheezing during a picnic in late summer (ragweed season). Often an upper respiratory tract infection will trigger pulmonary decompensation and dyspnea in patients with long-standing chronic obstructive lung disease. Upper respiratory airway obstruction in epiglottitis or foreign body aspiration can lead to acute severe dyspnea. Pleural effusions commonly occur with advanced lung cancer or as a complication of pulmonary infections and will cause dyspnea when they are large and involve more than half of one hemothorax. Congestive heart failure is often associated with typical anginal chest pain, and dyspnea will develop slowly or rapidly depending on whether there is acute or chronic cardiac decompensation. Psychogenic dyspnea or the hyperventilation syndrome has a rapid onset and is usually found in emotionally disturbed or anxious patients (see Chapter 13). Patients with severe chronic anemia tend to complain of dyspnea more often than do patients with anemia secondary to acute blood loss, in whom orthostatic dizziness and syncope are more common.

One of the first steps in evaluating a patient who complains of dyspnea is deciding whether the symptoms reflect an acute or chronic event since the more serious causes of dyspnea tend to present abruptly. In general, dyspnea of sudden onset is easier to evaluate, but the workup must proceed quickly to determine whether the patient should be admitted to the hospital for more intensive evaluation and therapy. On the other hand, the evaluation of chronic dyspnea can usually be accomplished more slowly in an ambulatory setting.

Evaluation of Dyspnea of Sudden Onset

In a young patient, the medical history and physical examination alone will often suggest a presumptive diagnosis, such as asthma, pneumonia, or pneumothorax. These diseases present with clinical findings including wheezing, localized rales and rub, evidence of pulmonary consolidation, or a unilateral decrease in breath sounds. In general, bronchitis does not cause dyspnea in a healthy individual unless bronchospasm, as manifested by wheezing, is also present. Acute left ventricular failure or angina with cardiac decompensation will cause acute dyspnea and may be associated with distended neck veins, an S_3 gallop, diffuse or basalar rales, wheezing, and pedal edema (see Chapter 61). Unfortunately,

some of these clinical findings, such as distended neck veins and wheezing, can be observed in patients with acute exacerbations of obstructive airways disease. Frequently patients with cardiopulmonary disease present with a mixture of these physical findings; therefore, further laboratory examination is necessary. The chest roentgenogram and electrocardiogram are the two most useful tests that help to distinguish acute cardiac from pulmonary disease. Also, a spirogram will document the presence and severity of functional pulmonary disease and serves as a guide in the therapy of bronchospasm (see Chapter 55). All acute inflammatory pulmonary disease causing significant dyspnea will appear as localized or diffuse parenchymal infiltrates on a chest roentgenogram. A significant pneumothorax can be easily missed, and diagnostic accuracy will be improved with an expiratory film. The development of acute hyperinflation on a chest roentgenogram indicates severe bronchospasm. In contrast, congestive heart failure will produce interstitial or alveolar fluid accumulation often associated with an increase in size of the cardiac silhouette. Besides the chest roentgenogram, an electrocardiogram must be examined for cardiac arrhythmias or ischemic changes. Even without a history of chest pain, an electrocardiogram still should be obtained to exclude the diagnosis of a silent myocardial infarction.

Pulmonary Embolism

Pulmonary embolism is a major life-threatening cause of acute dyspnea, but the diagnosis can be difficult. Its evaluation requires a systematic approach with a logical sequence of diagnostic testing.

The incidence of pulmonary embolism is high in patients with a recent history of peripheral venous disease, prolonged immobilization, chronic obstructive lung disease, or congestive heart failure. In a multicenter study (1) 60% of patients with pulmonary embolism were men, and, of the women under age 45 who had pulmonary emboli, 75% were found to be using oral contraceptives (see Chapter 93). In this same study, the most frequent symptoms present at the time of diagnosis were dyspnea and chest pain, which were found in over 80% of patients. Hemoptysis, cough, and apprehension were seen less frequently. The physical examination is usually not helpful in the diagnosis, especially since many of the patients have underlying respiratory and cardiovascular diseases that may, in themselves, produce abnormal physical findings: tachycardia, tachypnea, an accentuated second pulmonic heart sound, *etc.*

Most laboratory tests are not useful in the diagnosis of pulmonary embolism (12). Chest roentgenograms are frequently abnormal, but the findings are nonspecific (localized infiltrates, atelectasis, an elevated hemidiaphragm, or a pleural effusion). The arterial gas tensions are also often abnormal (reduced PaO_2 and $PaCO_2$) but are not helpful diagnostically, in part because of considerable variation and in part because of the high prevalence of cardiopulmonary diseases that alter both the PaO_2 and $PaCO_2$.

The most useful procedure in the screening of patients for pulmonary embolism is a ventilation/perfusion (V/Q) scan of the lungs. (A perfusion scan alone will not always permit the probabilities of embolism to be established accurately.) Whether or not the patient is hospitalized before having the scan depends on the severity of the presentation.

Patient experience. There is little discomfort associated with a lung scan. The patient should be instructed that he will inhale an oxygen and xenon mixture for 3 to 4 minutes, followed by a venous injection of radioactive labeled technetium. Several different projections are then recorded on a scanner while the patient is lying on a table.

The V/Q scan is 100% sensitive, but it can be nonspecific depending on the configuration, location, and number of perfusion defects seen (9). If the V/Q scan is normal, the diagnosis of an acute pulmonary embolus is excluded. In general, 5 to 7% of patients with a low probability scan, 20 to 30% of patients with a moderate probability scan, and 80 to 90% of patients with a high probability scan have a pulmonary embolism. However, it must be emphasized that the use of these probabilities is dependent on strict adherence to accepted published criteria for interpreting lung scans (2) and on the experience of the individual nuclear medicine laboratory. Patients with low, moderate, or high probability scans should be hospitalized for further diagnostic studies (angiography) and/or anticoagulation with heparin (see Chapter 51). Patients with acute dyspnea and simultaneous symptoms and signs of peripheral venous thrombosis (less than 40% of patients with pulmonary emboli) should undergo venography to confirm the diagnosis (see Chapter 51). If venography is positive, the patient should be hospitalized for initiation of anticoagulant therapy.

The resolution of pulmonary emboli varies and can occur as early as 1 to 2 weeks in patients who have had small emboli. With larger emboli and in those patients with underlying cardiopulmonary disease, there may be angiographic evidence of emboli that persist for 2 or 3 months (3). If chest pain occurs after discharge, a repeat lung scan (and perhaps, depending on the results, angiography) is necessary to determine whether embolization has recurred.

Evaluation of Chronic or Progressive Dyspnea

The evaluation of chronic, progressive dyspnea can be a simple or complicated process depending on the responsible disease. In contrast to acute dyspnea, chronic dyspnea usually is more difficult to diagnose and often requires more extensive diagnostic procedures; therefore, the evaluation should proceed in a logical sequence to avoid initially expensive and invasive laboratory testing. The first step is a careful history. Because shortness of breath is appropriate to certain levels of activity depending on the fitness of the individual, the physician must decide whether the patient's symptoms are abnormal and over what period of time they have developed. Many patients with chronic cardiopulmonary disease adapt to the insidious onset of dyspnea by subconsciously changing daily habits and avoiding physical activity. To quantitate the degree of dyspnea, the physician must determine what specific activity causes dyspnea and must compare the patient's abilities to perform work with an appropriate peer group and with his baseline performance. Thus, the complaint of dyspnea in a 35-year-old who normally runs 5 miles and now becomes short of breath after running only 2 miles should not be ignored.

Initial laboratory testing should include a chest roentgenogram, which may reveal advanced degrees of obstructive pulmonary disease, the presence of diffuse interstitial lung disease, or cardiovascular disease manifested by either cardiomegaly or by signs of congestive heart failure. An electrocardiogram is necessary to look for evidence of ischemia, arrhythmias, or hypertrophy of cardiac chambers. Pulmonary function should be assessed initially with a spirogram, because this test categorizes the two most common pulmonary diseases—namely, obstructive or restrictive lung disease (see Chapter 55). A normal spirogram virtually excludes significant parenchymal or airways disease. Although patients with classic asthma may have a normal spirogram during symptom-free periods, more commonly there is evidence of slight reduction in the baseline forced expiratory volume, as a percentage of forced vital capacity. Additional specialized procedures that aid in the diagnosis of asthma are discussed in Chapter 55. Finally, initial laboratory testing should include a hemoglobin determination or hematocrit value to determine whether a patient is severely anemic or polycythemic.

If an obvious cause of dyspnea is not found after these initial investigations, additional more specialized tests, which may not be readily available to all physicians, may be necessary. It is important to understand when these tests are appropriate and how they are performed. They can usually be obtained by referral of patients to hospital pulmonary function or cardiac diagnostic laboratories, and through consultation with pulmonary or cardiac subspecialists.

1. *Complete pulmonary function tests.* In addition to baseline spirometry (see Chapter 55) other pulmonary function tests include the measurement of total lung capacity and functional residual capacity,

which quantitate the degree of hyperinflation or restriction. The single breath diffusion capacity measures the amount of alveolar capillary surface area available for gas exchange. Thus, the diffusion capacity is reduced in patients with pulmonary emboli and other vascular occlusive diseases as well as in patients with emphysema. In contrast, an elevated diffusion capacity is found in conditions that elevate the pulmonary blood volume—for example, erythrocytosis or early congestive heart failure. These additional tests should only be considered if spirometry is abnormal. The experience of the patient during the performance of these tests is described in Chapter 55.

2. *Arterial blood gas analysis.* Initially, an arterial blood gas determination should be performed to document the presence of hypoxemia or hypercapnia and to characterize the acid-base status. Several general points require emphasis: First, a normal resting arterial blood gas does not exclude significant pulmonary disease. In fact, many patients with severe chronic obstructive lung disease have normal resting arterial $PaCO_2$ and pH with only a slight reduction in PaO_2. Therefore, during an evaluation of dyspnea, a blood gas should always be used in conjunction with other assessments of pulmonary function. Second, arterial blood gases drawn after completion of exercise in a dyspneic patient may not provide useful information about exercise-induced changes in blood gases since abnormalities in gas exchange that occur during exercise usually reverse immediately. Third, for reasons discussed above, measurement of blood gases should not be used as a definitive screening procedure to exclude the diagnosis of pulmonary embolism.

3. *Cardiovascular testing.* The use of specialized noninvasive cardiovascular evaluation, including echocardiograms and gated heartpool nuclear scanning to assess right and left ventricular function or the presence of valvular heart disease, is discussed in Chapters 60 and 61.

4. *Exercise testing.* If a patient is dyspneic on exertion and baseline testing of cardiopulmonary function, as described above, is normal or only mildly abnormal, exercise testing should be considered.

In general, there are two types of exercise tests available. The first is a standard *cardiac stress test* where the patient exercises and is then observed for the development of chest pain and for electrocardiographic ischemic changes (Chapter 57). In referral centers, this cardiac stress test has been modified to permit functional evaluation of cardiac performance during exercise by using radioisotope scanning techniques with thallium (Chapter 57). The second type of exercise testing is a *cardiopulmonary stress test* in which cardiac function, pulmonary gas exchange, ventilation, and physical fitness are quantitated at specific work loads. The two types of tests are similar, but the patient should be told that the cardiopulmonary test requires, in addition to the exercise, breathing into a mouthpiece and measurement of oxygenation by either an oximeter or by means of an indwelling arterial line. Such complicated invasive cardiopulmonary stress testing is justified and useful in order to determine whether dyspnea is due to (a) cardiac or pulmonary disease, (b) exercise-induced asthma, or (c) poor physical fitness. One can use this type of evaluation to assess the effects of, for example, anti-inflammatory drugs (e.g., corticosteroids), administered to patients with acute interstitial lung disease, or of supplemental oxygen given to patients with severe hypoxemia. Furthermore, the test can measure the ability of a patient with underlying cardiopulmonary disease to achieve work loads appropriate for activities of daily life. This type of testing is particularly useful in evaluating patients for disability compensation, since static pulmonary function and noninvasive cardiac testing may not accurately predict the functional state of a given patient during actual working conditions. These tests require expert interpretation by cardiologists or pulmonologists. Most cardiologists do not perform full cardiopulmonary stress tests. Cardiac stress testing will relate information on the presence of angina, arrhythmias, or myocardial ischemia during exercise. On the other hand, most pulmonologists may not be well trained in the sophisticated interpretation of electrocardiographic changes during exercise. Nevertheless, it is usually possible for the referring physician to determine the most likely etiology for dyspnea and to make the appropriate referral. In large hospital centers with combined cardiopulmonary laboratories, simultaneous consultation and exercise testing by cardiologists and pulmonologists may be available.

This approach to the evaluation of dyspnea will almost always answer the questions necessary for diagnosis of the underlying condition and for establishment of a therapeutic regimen in patients with dyspnea. At times, a patient with circulatory abnormalities may need a brief hospital admission for additional invasive cardiac catherization studies to assess the state of the pulmonary vasculature or the degree of cardiac dysfunction. For example, it may be necessary to insert a Swan-Ganz catheter into the pulmonary circulation and to measure directly pulmonary arterial pressures and pulmonary capillary wedge pressures to learn whether a patient with severe obstructive lung disease and cor pulmonale also has significant functional left ventricular failure which requires treatment.

Therapy

There are no specific therapeutic modalities for treatment of dyspnea. Treatment of this symptom is primarily aimed at therapy of the underlying cardiac, pulmonary, or hematological disorders that cause abnormal breathlessness.

NONCARDIAC CHEST PAIN

Chest pain is a particularly frightening symptom because of the widespread knowledge and concern about heart disease; however, nonspecific musculoskeletal pain is more common than angina, especially in patients less than 40 years old (4). Most patients with chest pain can be evaluated and treated in an ambulatory setting; a few patients require referral to a specialist. The common noncardiac cause of chest pain will be discussed in this section which should be read in conjunction with Chapter 57.

Afferent neural impulses responsible for thoracic pain are carried by the sympathetic chain, vagus, and phrenic nerves. Visceral structures which include the lung, diaphragm, heart, and esophagus all lie within the thoracic cage and have overlapping innervation. Chest pain arising from these different organs will often have similar referral patterns; therefore, irritation of the diaphragmatic pleura, diaphragm, or pericardium, due to either thoracic or abdominal disease, causes chest pain that radiates to the shoulder. In addition, patients may have difficulty localizing pain from the deeper anatomical structures within the chest, while diseases involving the superficial structures, muscles, and ribs will be more easily localized. Since there is no sensory innervation of the lung parenchyma, alveolar or interstitial disease does not cause chest pain unless the pulmonary vasculature, bronchi, or pleura are involved.

Table 53.5 lists selected common and less common causes of chest pain. Fleeting, sharp, or lance-like chest pain is probably the most common complaint

Table 53.5.
Causes of Chest Pain

COMMON CAUSES	
Chest wall (musculoskeletal)	Nonspecific (smokers, nonsmokers with increased exertion)
	Costochondritis (Tietze's syndrome)
Cardiac	Angina
Pulmonary	Tracheitis, cough, pleuritis, pneumonia
Neurological	Radicular pain of cervical spine disease
LESS COMMON CAUSES	
Chest wall (musculoskeletal)	Thoracic outlet syndrome, herpes zoster, fractured rib, tumor
Cardiac	Aneurysm, pericarditis
Pulmonary	Pneumothorax, pulmonary embolus, pulmonary hypertension, cancer
Gastrointestinal	Stomach disease, duodenal ulcer, abdominal infection, peritonitis, esophageal reflux

in patients who do not have evidence of organic heart disease. Smokers complain more frequently than nonsmokers of both angina-like and nonangina-like chest pain. This has resulted in use of the term "tobacco angina" to describe two distinct types of chest pain in smokers (4). There are smokers with pre-existing angina whose pains clearly are precipitated by smoking. There is also a second, larger group of smokers who have normal or diseased hearts, and who complain of intermittent atypical chest pain that is not necessarily associated with smoking a cigarette. This chest pain is not relieved by nitroglycerin or provoked by exercise. It gradually disappears within weeks to months, sometimes years after the cessation of smoking; and it is assumed that it is not due to myocardial ischemia.

Musculoskeletal pain is very common in young individuals who increase their exercise abruptly (including the patient who acutely hyperventilates as part of an anxiety state—see Chapter 13). A history of unusual exertion with increased breathing plus tenderness of intercostal muscles usually suffices to make this diagnosis.

Pain caused by tracheitis or tracheobronchitis is a distinctive substernal burning sensation that is precipitated by coughing and is most often associated with viral respiratory infections. This is in contrast to the sharp, stabbing, pleuritic chest pain that is experienced with pneumonia. The latter is clearly localized to the chest wall and arises from stretching the inflamed parietal pleura during breathing or coughing.

Other causes of chest pain include costochondritis (Tietze's syndrome), which is an anterior localized pain associated with tenderness over one or more costochondral junctions; herpes zoster, which commonly causes unilateral aching and/or itching, limited to one dermatome, which may precede by several days the eruption of vesicles; rib fracture or bone metastases, which are more chronic and pleuritic in nature; and cervical spine disease with referred pain to the chest. Acute stabbing chest pain can occur with a spontaneous pneumothorax, which occurs primarily in young men or in older patients with obstructive pulmonary disease. Frequently, a small (<20%) pneumothorax is not accompanied by significant dyspnea in otherwise healthy individuals. Pleuritic chest pain associated with pulmonary emboli results from infarction of parenchymal lung tissue with irritation of the parietal pleura and almost always is associated with dyspnea; and in most patients, the chest roentgenogram will show an infiltrate. The pain associated with pulmonary hypertension is heavy and aching and often similar to that of cardiac ischemia (see Chapter 57). Gastrointestinal disorders, such as reflux esophagitis or gastric or duodenal ulcer, are usually distinguished from cardiopulmonary chest pain by their association with eating, and by their relief by antacids (Chapters 34 and 36).

Evaluation

Many of the common causes of noncardiac chest pain can be diagnosed by a thorough history and physical examination. Since discrete anatomical structures must be involved in order to cause noncardiac chest pain, the physical examination is more useful in the diagnosis of noncardiac chest pain than it is in the diagnosis of dyspnea and hemoptysis. Inspection of the chest wall may reveal the characteristic unilateral eruption of herpes zoster along a dermatome. Light palpation over the chest wall will elicit pain and crepitus from fractured ribs. Mild pressure over the costochondral junctions anteriorly will reproduce the pain of Tietze's syndrome. (In general, cardiac pain is not worsened by pressure over the chest wall.) In pneumonia or pulmonary infarction a distinct friction rub can be heard directly over the specific area of chest pain. With pericardial involvement a friction rub that varies with respiration or with the cardiac cycle is usually present. A thorough abdominal examination is important because diseases involving the abdominal visceral organs can cause referred chest pain that is indistinguishable from that produced by involvement of the thoracic structures. Often laboratory studies and a chest roentgenogram will not be necessary for the diagnosis of these common causes of chest pain.

Therapy

The treatment of chest pain requires therapy of the underlying disease process, as well as analgesic drugs for the pain itself. Nonspecific chest pain found in normal people requires reassurance; however, angina-like pain in smokers ideally requires, first, diagnostic testing to exclude ischemic heart disease, followed by discontinuing cigarette smoking for both diagnosis and therapy. Tracheal irritation is limited to the duration of the viral illness but can be treated by cough suppression and bronchodilators (see under "Cough"). Tietze's syndrome is treated with standard anti-inflammatory agents and heat. While the pain of herpes zoster is often severe, it may be controlled with mild narcotics such as codeine, 30 to 60 mg every 4 to 6 hours. Unfortunately, chest pain experienced in pulmonary hypertension does not respond to treatment with non-narcotic analgesics, and narcotics in sedative doses are required if the hypertension does not improve with treatment and if the pain is severe.

Pleuritic pain in patients with pneumonia or pulmonary embolus responds to specific therapy of the inflammatory process. Nevertheless, narcotics may be needed to reduce splinting of the chest wall and thereby to prevent atelectasis. Codeine (60 mg) is usually adequate therapy, but the physician must consider the undesired cough suppressant action of this drug in inflammatory lung disease. In situations where pain is extreme an intercostal block may be useful. This is performed by local infiltration of the inferior surface of the rib near the spine with 5 to 10 ml of lidocaine (1 to 2%). Although this therapy only lasts from 4 to 6 hours, local block in combination with the administration of narcotics often provides more long term control of pleuritic chest pain.

General References

Burki NK: Dyspnea. *Clin Chest Med* 1:47, 1980.
    A good discussion of the mechanisms of dyspnea.
Fishman AP: *Pulmonary Diseases and Disorders.* New York, McGraw-Hill, 1982, vols 1 and 2.
    The standard text of pulmonary medicine.
Hinshaw HC, Murray MF: *Diseases of the Chest.* Philadelphia, WB Saunders, 1980.
    A practical approach to pulmonary medicine
Hyers TM (ed): Pulmonary embolism and hypertension. *Clin Chest Med* 5, no. 3, 1984.
    Excellent monograph on epidemiology, pathophysiology, diagnosis, and treatment.
Jones NL, Campbell EJ: *Clinical Exercise Testing,* ed 2. Philadelphia, WB Saunders, 1982.
    The standard text on this subject.
Ziment I: *Respiratory Pharmacology and Therapeutics.* Philadelphia, WB Saunders, 1978.
    An exhaustive review of this subject.

Specific References

1. Bell WR, Simon TL, DeMets DL: The clinical features of submassive and massive pulmonary emboli. *Am J Med* 62:355, 1977.
2. Biello DR, Mattar AG, McKnight RC, Siegel BA: Ventilation-perfusion studies in suspected pulmonary embolism. *AJR* 133:1033, 1979.
3. Dalen JE, Banas JS Jr, Brooks HL, et al: Resolution rate of acute pulmonary embolism in man. *N Engl J Med* 280:1194, 1969.
4. Friedman GD, Siegelaub AB, Doles LG: Cigarette smoking and chest pain. *Ann Intern Med* 83:7, 1975.
5. Irwin RS, Rosen MJ, Braman SS: Cough: a comprehensive review. *Arch Intern Med* 137:1186, 1977.
6. Kaplan J, Johns CJ: Mycetomas in pulmonary sarcoidosis: non-surgical management. *Johns Hopkins Med J* 145:157, 1979.
7. Kravitz H, Gomberg RM, Burnstine RC, et al: Psychogenic cough tic in children and adolescents. *Clin Pediatr* 8:580, 1969.
8. Lyons HA: Differential diagnosis of hemoptysis and its treatment. Basics of RD, published by The American Lung Association, 1976.
9. McNeil BJ, Hessel SJ, Branch WT, et al: Measures of clinical efficacy. III. The value of the lung scan in the evaluation of young patients with pleuritic chest pain. *Nucl Med* 17:163, 1976.
10. Rogers RM, Bedrossian C, Coalson JJ, et al: The management of massive hemoptysis in a patient with pulmonary tuberculosis. *Chest* 70:519, 1976.
11. Snider GL: When not to use the bronchoscopy for hemoptysis. *Chest* 76:1, 1979.
12. Szucs MM Jr, Brooks HL, Grossman W, et al: Diagnostic sensitivity of laboratory findings in acute pulmonary embolism. *Ann. Intern Med* 74:161, 1971.
13. Terry PB, Barth KH, Kaufman SL, White RI Jr: Balloon embolization for treatment of pulmonary arteriovenous fistulas. *N Engl J Med* 302:1189, 1980.
14. Wynder EL, Kaufman PL, Lesser RL: A short-term follow-up study on ex-cigarette smokers. *Am Rev Respir Dis* 96:645, 1967.
15. Wynder EL, Lemon FR, Mantel N: Epidemiology of persistent cough. *Am Rev Respir Dis* 91:679, 1965.
16. Zavala DC: Diagnostic fiberoptic bronchoscopy: techniques and results of biopsy in 600 patients. *Chest* 68:12, 1975.

CHAPTER FIFTY-FOUR

The Abnormal Chest Roentgenogram

PHILIP L. SMITH, M.D., AND EUGENE R. BLEECKER, M.D.

The general physician will often, in the course of evaluation of a patient, be faced with the interpretation of an abnormal chest roentgenogram. Many physicians have the capability of taking chest roentgenograms in their office; others use the facilities of consultant radiologists. A knowledge of the significance of chest roentgenographic findings will allow the physician to plan more specific radiographic and diagnostic procedures.

It is essential that a chest roentgenogram always be compared with any previous available roentgenogram since changes may have been present for many years and therefore not require further evaluation. Also, depending on the appearance of the abnormality, it may be most appropriate simply to plan follow-up serial films.

SPECIFIC PATTERNS INDICATIVE OF AN ABNORMAL CHEST ROENTGENOGRAM

This section will review common abnormalities that indicate the presence of pulmonary disease that requires further evaluation.

Air Bronchogram (Fig. 54.1)

Normally, bronchi beyond the mainstem division cannot be seen; however, when lung tissue surrounding a bronchus is devoid of air because of either collapse or consolidation, an air bronchogram can be seen. The presence of an air bronchogram distinguishes a collapsed or consolidated part of the lung from an extrapulmonary density such as a pleural effusion. However, an air bronchogram is not present in every collapsed or consolidated lung because bronchi may fill with secretions or exudate. Therefore, its absence is less significant than its presence.

Silhouette Sign (Fig. 54.2)

The obliteration on a chest roentgenogram of the margin of a normally opaque structure in the chest by an abnormal pulmonary density is called the silhouette sign. If the physician has knowledge of thoracic anatomy and of spatial relations, he can use the silhouette sign to localize abnormalities within the lung parenchyma. Outlines of organs that are in contact with parenchymal infiltrates will be obliterated because the normal air interface is eliminated. On the other hand, intrathoracic lesions that are not anatomically contiguous will not interfere with the outlines of other nearby structures. For example, obliteration of the cardiac border localizes an abnormality to the right middle lobe or the lingular segment of the left upper lobe (Fig. 54.2). In contrast, an infiltrate that overlaps but does not obliterate the cardiac border is posterior and represents a lower lobe lesion. Lower lobe abnormalities obliterate diaphragmatic borders while obliteration of the left border of the aortic knob, a posterior structure, occurs with lesions of the apical posterior segment of the left upper lobe.

Collapse (Fig. 54.3)

The collapse or diminution in volume of the whole lung, a lobe, or a segment of one of the lobes can be an important clue to the presence of asymptomatic pulmonary disease, such as bronchial carcinoma, or it may be the cause of a symptom, such as dyspnea in an asthmatic patient with mucous plugging. The primary mechanisms that cause pulmonary collapse are (a) bronchial obstruction either due to an intrinsic bronchial mass or to an extrinsic or intrinsic stenosis of the bronchus, (b) compression of the lungs from a large pleural effusion or from a pneumothorax, (c) peripheral bronchial plugging with subsequent pulmonary collapse, and (d) contraction of the

lung secondary to chronic inflammatory disease. The signs of collapse are related to anatomical landmarks within the lung and are manifest by displacement of the septa in the lung, loss of aeration within the pulmonary parenchyma, and crowding of the vascular and bronchial lung markings. Other signs that are suggestive of collapse reflect the secondary effects of loss of lung volume such as elevation of the diaphragm, shift of the mediastinal structures toward the collapsed area, diminution in the size of a hemithorax, compensatory hyperinflation, hilar displacement, and tracheal deviation. These latter signs are much more difficult to interpret in patients with underlying lung disease in whom many of these signs may exist in the absence of collapse.

Pleural Effusion (Fig. 54.4)

Small amounts of free fluid within the pleural space will obliterate the costophrenic or costocardiac angles. Because the density of pleural fluid is greater than the density of the lung, a subpulmonic collection will displace laterally the crest of the diaphragm. An increased density between the stomach gas bubble and pulmonary tissue may also indicate the presence of fluid within the pleural space. The diagnosis of a large pleural effusion is not difficult because fluid within the pleural space on an upright chest roentgenogram will form a concave density across the chest cavity; decubitus roentgenograms will demonstrate free pleural fluid in the dependent hemithorax. If the patient is recumbent, the pleural fluid will layer over the entire hemithorax, causing the lung to appear opaque.

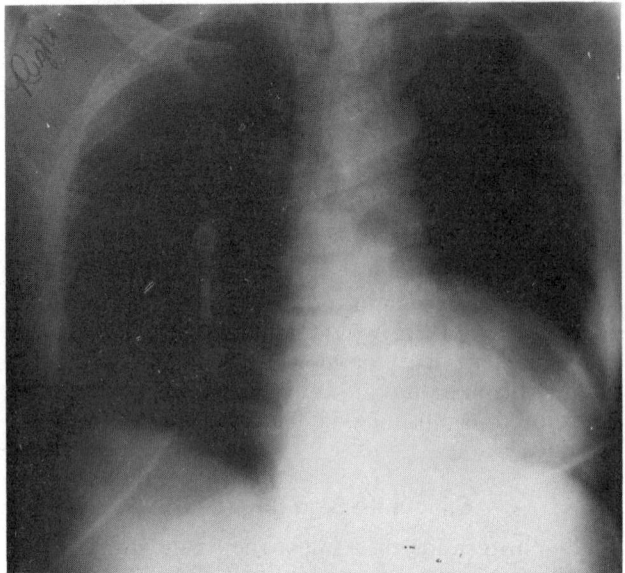

Figure 54.1.   Air bronchogram. Patient presented with fever and sputum production; the initial roentgenogram demonstrates a branching air bronchogram seen behind the heart on the left, which is consistent with a lower lobe infiltrate.

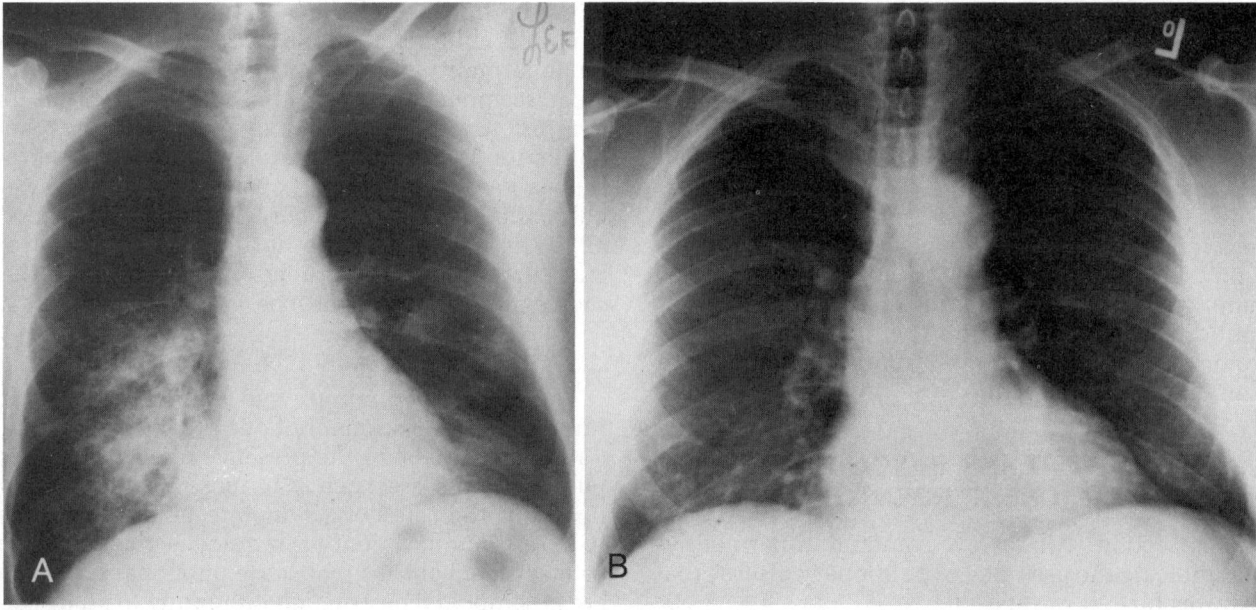

Figure 54.2.   Silhouette sign. In this figure, a right middle lobe infiltrate obscures the border of the heart (A). A previous X-ray is shown for comparison (B).

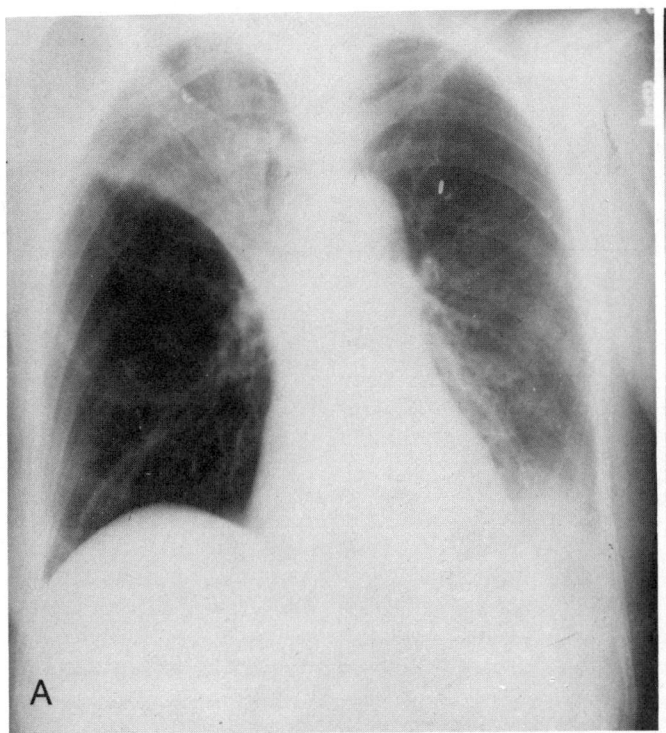
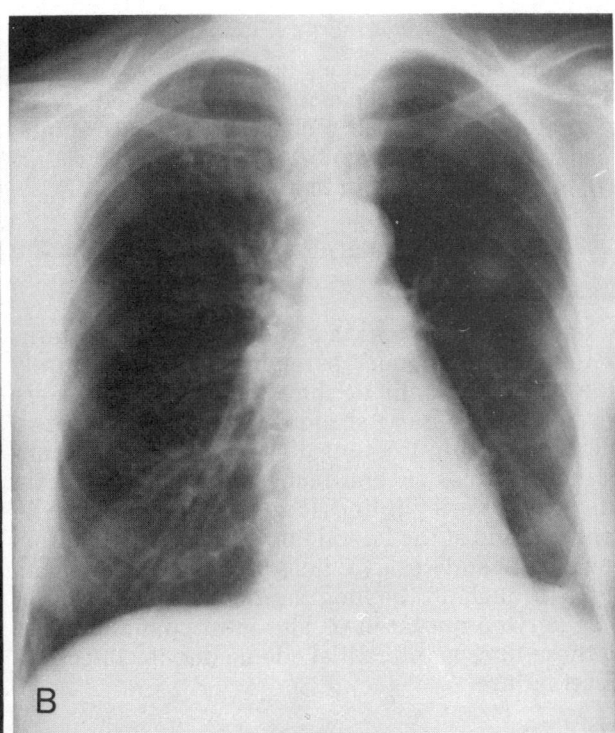

Figure 54.3. Collapse. This demonstrates collapse of the right upper lobe and partial collapse of the left lower lobe in a patient complaining of cough and increased sputum (A). The right middle lobe fissure is displaced upwards and there is blunting of the left hemidiaphragm. Note that there is no air bronchogram in either collapsed segment. Aggressive physical therapy was initiated and within 24 hours there is resolution of the collapse on the right and almost complete resolution on the left (B).

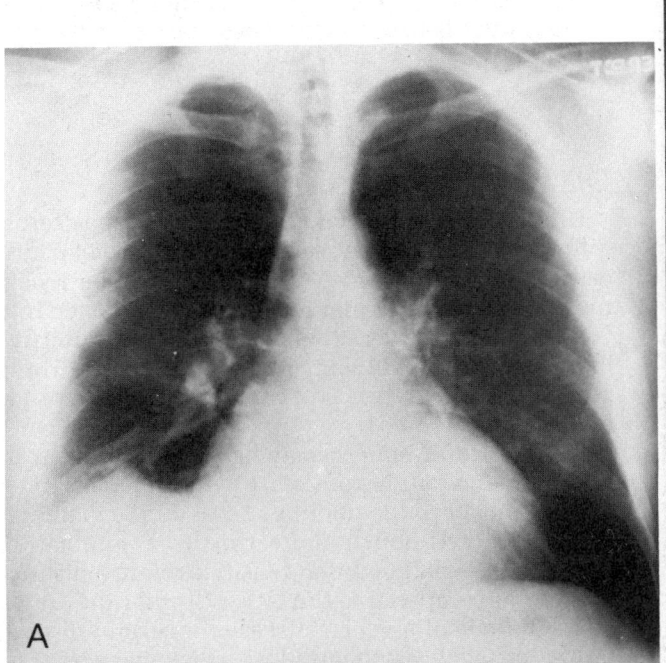
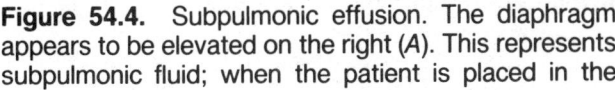
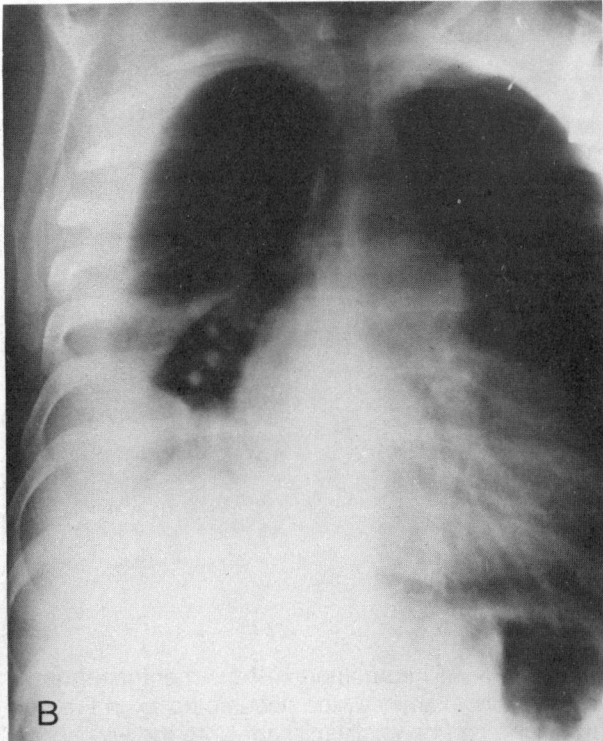

Figure 54.4. Subpulmonic effusion. The diaphragm appears to be elevated on the right (A). This represents subpulmonic fluid; when the patient is placed in the right lateral decubitis position (B), fluid layers on the right and tracks in the minor fissure and along the apex and diaphragm.

Pneumothorax (Fig. 54.5)

A small collection of air is difficult to see within the pleural space. This diagnosis is aided by an expiratory chest roentgenogram that accentuates the amount of air within the pleural space by reducing the volume of air in the lung.

Abnormal Pulmonary Parenchymal Patterns

Septal

Normally lung markings reflect vascular patterns within the pulmonary parenchyma and are rarely due to the bronchi or the lymphatics. There are three types of linear shadows that represent septal markings within the lung: Kerley A lines, thin non-branching lines several inches long radiating from the hilum; Kerley B lines (Fig. 54.6), up to 1 inch in length found at the lateral lung bases, radiating from the pleura; and Kerley C lines, fine interlacing structures throughout the lung parenchyma that produce a spiderweb appearance. The most common cause of these lines is interstitial edema due to congestive heart failure.

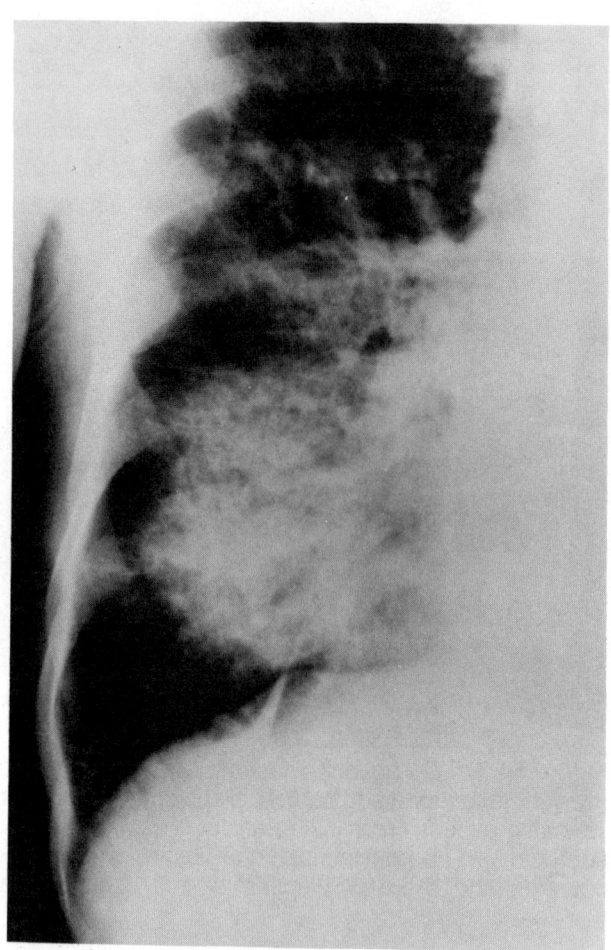

Figure 54.6. Kerley B lines. A close view of the right lower lung in a patient with congestive heart failure demonstrates horizontal linear lines that run to the edge of the lung.

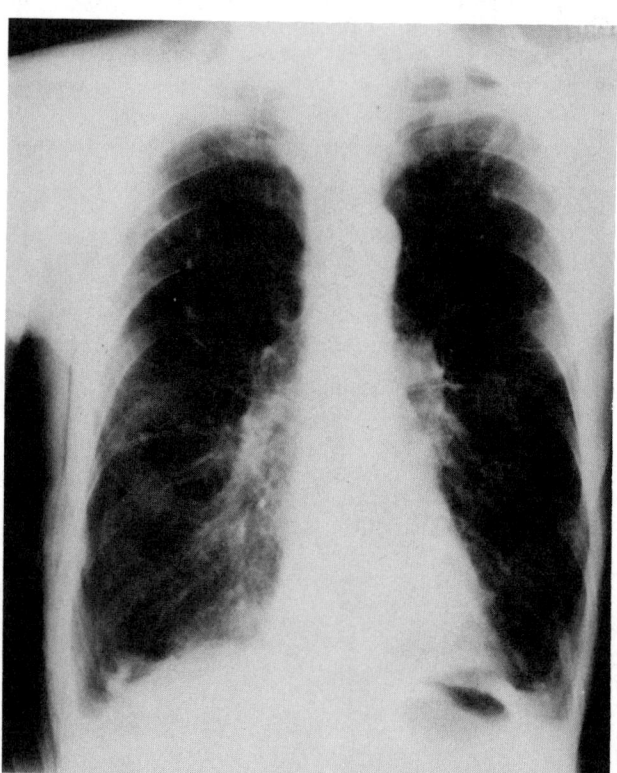

Figure 54.5. Pneumothorax. If the roentgenogram is not carefully examined, the pneumothorax in the right lower lung can be easily missed. Note the widespread bullae throughout the lung.

Diffuse

Diffuse lung disease takes on two general patterns: diffuse interstitial disease and diffuse alveolar disease. *Alveolar infiltrates* (Fig. 54.7A) can be recognized by their fluffy margins, their coalescence into "rosette" formations, their occasional "butterfly" configuration, involving hilar and central lung zones, and the presence of air bronchograms or air alveolograms.

An *interstitial pattern* may be primarily linear or reticular and often consists of multiple, discrete, noncoalescent round nodules, 1 to 5 mm in diameter (Fig. 54.7B). Although there can be a summation effect, these small nodular densities retain a distinct identity as compared to the larger, fluffier infiltrates characteristic of alveolar disease. In certain disease processes, such as tuberculosis, histoplasmosis, or healed viral pneumonia, these nodules may calcify

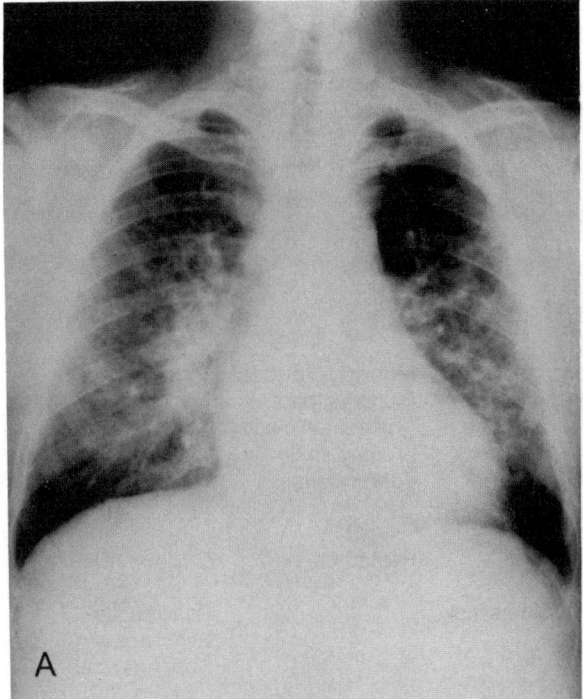
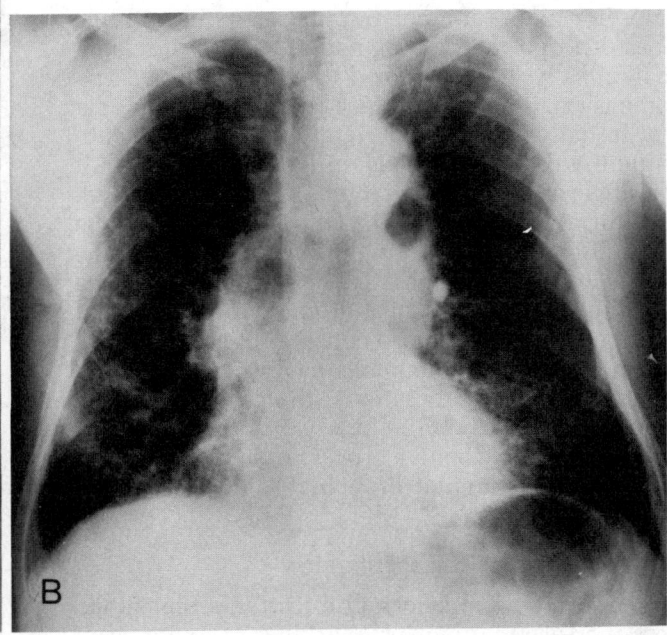

Figure 54.7. *A.* Alveolar patterns. This patient has progressive dyspnea after inhaling fumes from an automobile accident. Compared to *B*, little air is visible in the infiltrate because fluid is filling the alveoli. *B.* Interstitial pattern. This demonstrates bilateral interstitial infiltrates in a patient with progressive dyspnea and with fibrosis on biopsy. Compared to *A*, there is a lacy reticular appearance with accentuation of the air spaces by the fibrosis.

and thus appear more dense. The presence of honeycombing is pathognomonic of interstitial disease and pulmonary fibrosis. It can be identified on a chest roentgenogram as round or oval, irregular air spaces that have a reasonably uniform diameter of 1 to 10 mm and are arranged in grape-like bunches, thus giving the impression of a beehive.

COMMON PROBLEMS IN PATIENTS WITH ABNORMAL CHEST ROENTGENOGRAMS

In this section three general disease categories will be discussed in which the chest roentgenogram provides the basis for diagnosis and further evaluation. A general approach will be outlined including the initial evaluation that should be completed by the physician before referral to a pulmonary specialist or a thoracic surgeon. Frequently, this diagnostic evaluation can be completed in an ambulatory setting, with or without consultation.

Recurrent or Slowly Resolving Bacterial Pneumonias

Obstructing pulmonary carcinoma must be considered in any patient who has a slowly resolving pneumonia. Most patients with bacterial pneumonia respond rapidly to antibiotic therapy, and their chest roentgenogram will return to normal over 3 to 6 weeks (see Chapter 28). Patients with chronic obstructive lung disease (Chapter 55) who have difficulty mobilizing their bronchial secretions and patients with superimposed congestive heart failure or with necrotizing pneumonia may have significant pulmonary infiltrates that persist for 8 to 12 weeks (1). If the patient shows symptomatic improvement with a decrease in both the amount and purulence of sputum, a decrease in fever, and slow but progressive roentgenographic clearing, further evaluation during this period is usually not warranted. If roentgenographic abnormalities persist and if there is other evidence of poor response to therapy or if the pneumonic infiltrate is found in an asymptomatic individual, further evaluation to exclude pulmonary carcinoma is warranted (see Chapter 56).

Patients with recurrent pneumonias (3) also must be evaluated for the possibility of lung cancer. More frequently, these patients have associated chronic diseases such as underlying airways disease, congestive heart failure, diabetes mellitus, or bronchiectasis. In evaluating patients with recurrent pneumonia, it is vital to review all previous chest roentgenograms to document the anatomical location and the characteristics of the recurrent pneumonic infiltrate. In general, if a pneumonia recurs in multiple lobes or in pulmonary segments that are unrelated anatomically, the likelihood of bronchogenic carcinoma is small. For example, a recurrent pneumonia that initially involves the right upper lobe and subsequently the lower lobe is unlikely to be the result of a single obstructive carcinoma. On the other hand, an infiltrate that occurs first in the right lower lobe and subsequently in the right middle lobe could be caused by a single mass lesion that occludes the bronchus intermedius. In addition to the anatomical location, it is important to consider the time during which recurrent pneumonias have occurred. If the interval is more than 3 years, the possibility of an underlying obstructing lung cancer is unlikely. However, chronic benign processes, such as a benign tumor or a congenital bronchial abnormality, are still possible.

Apical Infiltrates

Frequently roentgenographic patterns that range from increased pulmonary markings or minor scarring to cystic or cavitary disease in the upper lobes will be interpreted by a radiologist as showing old granulomatous lung disease with possible active tuberculous infection. The evaluation of these patients includes questioning about previous tuberculous lung disease (including the type and duration of antituberculous therapy) and an assessment of the reactivity of the tuberculin skin test. Comparison with old chest roentgenograms is mandatory because the activity of an old granulomatous infection of the lung cannot be determined from an isolated chest roentgenogram. Frequently, old chest roentgenograms demonstrate that no change has occurred. The evaluation and treatment of patients with tuberculosis are discussed in Chapter 29.

Superior sulcus tumors, usually adenocarcinomas, form in the apex of the lung and may be difficult to distinguish initially from pleural thickening or old granulomatous disease; later in the course, roentgenograms may reveal erosion by tumors of adjacent ribs (see also Chapter 56, page 671).

Pleural Effusion

In general, when a pleural effusion is seen on a chest roentgenogram, it is important to examine the fluid. The major exception to this rule is the patient who develops acute pulmonary edema associated with a rapidly developing pleural effusion that resolves with therapy for congestive heart failure (see Chapter 61). The physician should be able to perform a thoracentesis in order to determine the etiology of the effusion (Table 54.1). The fluid should be collected in both a heparinized and a nonheparinized tube so that cytological examination can be

Table 54.1.
Causes of Pleural Effusion

Effusion	Common	Uncommon
Vascular	Congestive heart failure[a] Pulmonary infarction	
Metabolic		Hypoproteinemia[a] Cirrhosis[a] Nephrotic syndrome[a] Glomerulonephritis[a]
Malignancy Infection	Metastatic disease Bacterial (parapneumonic and empyema) Tuberculous	Mesothelioma Mycoplasma (and other atypical pneumonias) Fungal Viral
Trauma	Hemothorax	Chylothorax
Gastrointestinal		Pancreatitis Esophageal rupture Subphrenic abscess
Collagen vascular disease		Systemic lupus erythematosus Rheumatoid arthritis
Miscellaneous		Asbestos exposure Drug hypersensitivity Postmyocardial infarction syndrome Meig's syndrome[a] Lymphoma and lymphatic abnormalities

[a] Usually transudative pleural effusion.

performed, if necessary. Most pleural effusions are clear and straw colored, and deviations from this norm are useful diagnostically. For example, a bloody effusion suggests pulmonary infarction or tumor, a lime-green effusion suggests tuberculosis, and a viscous fluid with feculent odor strongly suggests an anaerobic empyema.

Pleural fluids can either be classified as transudates or exudates (2). An exudate is characterized by a pleural fluid protein concentration that is greater than 50% of the concentration of serum protein. Because of their high protein content, exudative pleural effusions usually have a specific gravity of more than 1.015, or a protein concentration of greater than 3 g/100 ml. A cell count and pleural fluid cytology should be performed since polymorphonuclear leukocytes in pleural fluid suggest acute inflammation and infection, while a predominance of lymphocytes suggests tuberculosis or malignancy. The presence of more than 5% pleural mesothelial cells usually excludes the diagnosis of tuberculosis. Low pleural fluid glucose concentrations occur in infections as well as in rheumatoid arthritis. If pleural effusion is bloody or appears infected, the patient should be hospitalized for further diagnostic studies and for therapy (pleural fluid pH, pleural biopsy, *etc*).

Pneumothorax

There are three major types of pneumothorax: (*a*) spontaneous. (*b*) iatrogenic, and (*c*) traumatic. Of these, the general physician is most commonly faced with a spontaneous pneumothorax either in a young healthy individual or in the older patient with underlying pulmonary disease. In the former, a subpleural apical bleb ruptures into the pleural space, causing varying amounts of air to collect. This is most commonly seen in 20- to 30-year-old males and is usually unrelated to activity, although 20% may admit to severe coughing at the time. In the older patient, emphysema with concomitant bullous disease is frequently associated with pneumothoraces. Pleuritic chest pain is a major manifestation of small pneumothoraces (10 to 20%), while dyspnea predominates in patients with larger collections of air.

After the diagnosis of pneumothorax is made, the generalist must decide whether the patient needs observation (ambulatory or inpatient) or consultation with a thoracic surgeon for insertion of a chest tube. Needle aspiration to expand the lung is discouraged since further laceration can occur. In general, patients with underlying lung disease must be hospitalized and must have a chest tube inserted since the leak seldom seals spontaneously. On the other hand, a young patient who is not in distress may remain at home and be followed by a physician with repeat roentgenograms as long as the pneumothorax does not enlarge. There should be obvious shrinking of the space within 3 to 5 days, and eventually the lung should totally re-expand.

Diffuse Pulmonary Disease

While there are numerous causes of diffuse interstitial pulmonary disease, there are few causes of diffuse alveolar lung disease. Therefore, the distinction between an alveolar and an interstitial process is important. Unfortunately, it is not always possible to distinguish between the two entities and there may be a mixture of both. Moreover, a disorder that begins as an interstitial process can often merge into an alveolar process, such as early congestive heart failure progressing to severe pulmonary edema.

The causes of diffuse *alveolar* filling disease of the lung are shown in Table 54.2. The three most frequent causes are infection, edema, and hemorrhage

Table 54.2.
Causes of Diffuse Alveolar Pulmonary Disease

Disorder	Common	Uncommon
Infection (pus) Edema (fluid)	Pneumonia Cardiac and noncardiac pulmonary edema	
Hemorrhage (blood)		Anticoagulation Trauma Hemoptysis with aspiration Goodpasture's syndrome Idiopathic pulmonary siderosis
Cells	Sarcoidosis	Bronchoalveolar cell cancer "Eosinophilic" infiltrative disorders
Foreign material		Lipoid pneumonia Contrast media Alveolar proteinosis

and are characterized by rapid progression and regression. In contrast, diffuse interstitial lung disease develops more slowly. Therefore, the time course for the development of pulmonary symptoms and roentgenographic abnormalities is an important aspect in the differential diagnosis of diffuse lung disease.

While *interstitial* lung disease (Table 54.3) can be idiopathic, the primary goal in the evaluation is to determine whether a treatable disease is present. The initial medical history, physical examination, and laboratory testing should be oriented toward evaluating the patient for the presence of a pneumoconiosis secondary to occupational exposure, pulmonary involvement associated with collagen vascular disease, sarcoidosis, and granulomatous (tuberculous) infections of the lung. Once the more common causes of interstitial lung disease are excluded, the less common causes must be considered before the diagnosis of idiopathic pulmonary fibrosis is made. Often this process will require consultation with a pulmonary specialist who will guide this evaluation. Specialized pulmonary function testing, including lung volume determination, diffusion capacities, and cardiopulmonary exercise testing (see Chapter 53), are necessary in addition to routine spirometry. In many of these patients transbronchial biopsy using a fiberoptic bronchoscope may be recommended. The findings in lung biopsy are often useful in guiding therapy in patients with collagen vascular pulmonary diseases, sarcoidosis, idiopathic pulmonary fibrosis, and infectious disease. If the tissue obtained with transbronchial biopsy is inadequate for diagnosis, consultation with a thoracic surgeon for open thoracotomy and pulmonary biopsy may be indicated.

Table 54.3.
Causes of Diffuse Interstitial Pulmonary Disease

Disorder	Common	Uncommon
KNOWN CAUSES		
Infection		Miliary tuberculosis
		Fungal
		Viral and atypical pneumonia
		Pneumocystis infection
Collagen vascular disease	Scleroderma	
	Rheumatoid arthritis	
	Systemic lupus erythematosus	
Occupational (pneumoconiosis)	Asbestosis	
	Silicosis	
	Coal miner's pneumoconiosis	
Hypersensitivity and drug reactions	Extrinsic allergic alveolitis	Nitrofurantoin
		Cytotoxic drugs
Physical agents		Radiation
Vascular	Early heart failure	
Neoplastic		Lymphoma
		Lymphatic metastasis
UNKNOWN CAUSES		
Idiopathic pulmonary fibrosis	Sarcoidosis	Eosinophilic granuloma

Solitary Nodule

This radiological finding always requires evaluation. A detailed discussion of the problem is to be found in Chapter 56.

General References

Felson B: The chest roentgenologic workup—what and why? Convenient methods. Published by the American Thoracic Society. Basics of RD 8(5), 1980.

    A concise selective review.

Felson B: *Chest Roentgenology*. Philadelphia, WB Saunders, 1973.

    An extensive basic approach to chest roentgenology.

Fulmer JD (ed): Interstitial lung disease. *Clin Chest Med* 3, no. 3, 1982.

    Excellent review.

Light RW (ed): *Pleural Disease*. Philadelphia, Lea and Febiger, 1983.

    An exhaustive review of this subject.

McLoud TC (ed): Chest radiology. *Clin Chest Med*. 5: no. 4, 1984.

    Excellent monograph on old and new techniques used in the diagnosis of thoracic disease.

Proto AV: The chest radiologic workup—special studies. The American Thoracic Society. Basics of RD 9(1), 1980.

    A concise review of special roentgenographic studies of the chest.

Specific References

1. Jay SJ, Johanson WG Jr, Pierce AK: The radiologic resolution of *Streptococcus pneumoniae* pneumonia. *N Engl J Med* 293:798, 1975.
2. Light RW, MacGregor I, Luchsinger PC, Ball WF: Pleural effusions: the diagnostic separation of transudates and exudates. *Ann Intern Med* 77:507, 1972.
3. Winterbauer RH, Bedon GA, Ball WC Jr: Recurrent pneumonia. Predisposing illness and clinical patterns in 158 patients. *Ann Intern Med* 70:689, 1969.

CHAPTER FIFTY-FIVE

Obstructive Airways Disease

EUGENE R. BLEECKER, M.D., AND PHILIP L. SMITH, M.D.

Obstructive diseases of the airways are the most common forms of pulmonary disease encountered in ambulatory practice. They include asthma (intermittent episodic bronchospasm), chronic obstructive bronchitis (bronchitis complicated by progressive airways obstruction), and emphysema (destruction of pulmonary parenchyma with associated obstructive lung disease). Although these diseases may differ in their clinical presentation, etiology, and prognosis, they all share the common feature of reduced expiratory airflow. Usually, patients with obstructive lung disease present with acute intermittent dyspnea at rest or with the insidious onset of progressive dyspnea during exercise. On the other hand, the diagnosis of early obstructive airways disease can only be made in asymptomatic patients by demonstrating a decrease in forced expiration that is objectively measured with a spirometer (Fig. 55.1) (35). Furthermore, since the severity of airways obstruction often does not correlate with clinical symptoms such as wheezing and dyspnea, objective tests of pulmonary function are needed both to establish the initial diagnosis as well as to follow the clinical course of the disease (Table 55.1). To understand the pathophysiological disturbances found in these patients and to assess the severity and prognosis in an individual patient, a review of some basic principles of airway mechanics is important.

PATHOPHYSIOLOGICAL ABNORMALITIES IN OBSTRUCTIVE LUNG DISEASE

To quantitate the amount of air leaving the lungs over a period of time, a forced expiration is performed into a spirometer which records the volume and speed of expiration. The factors that determine the speed and volume of a forced expiration are schematically represented in Figure 55.2. The lung is an elastic structure enclosed by the rigid chest wall with a potential cavity, the pleural space, located between. During normal respiration, the inspiratory muscles contract, and both pleural and alveolar pressures become negative, causing air to flow into the lungs. With expiration, air leaves the lungs as a result of their tendency to deflate when the respiratory muscles relax. Normally, as expiratory effort is increased, pleural pressure, which surrounds the intrathoracic airways, rises and com-

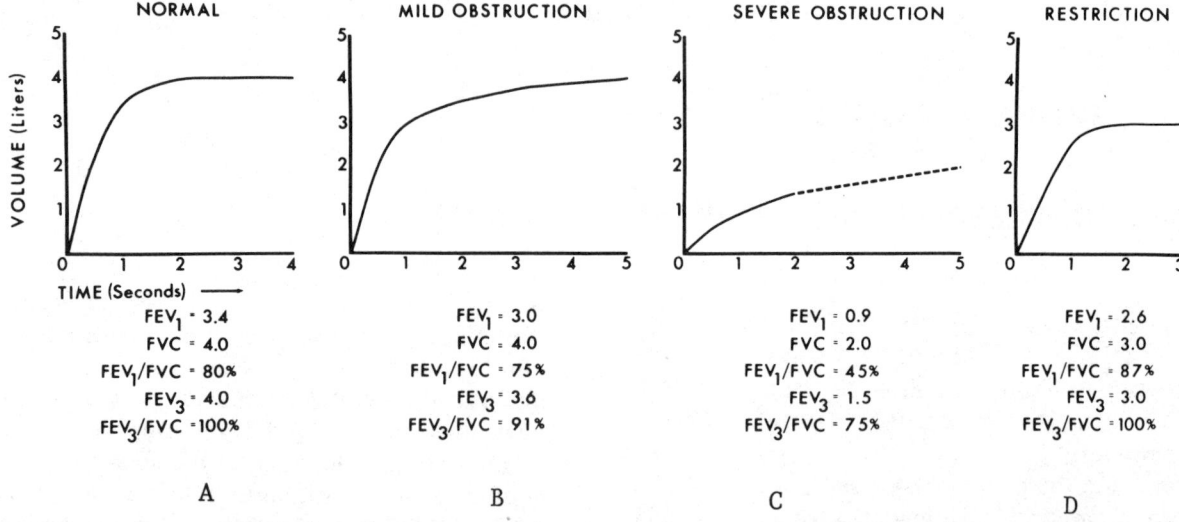

Figure 55.1. Spirographic tracings of forced expiration. Exhaled volume is plotted against time. The forced vital capacity (FVC) is represented by the total volume expired. One-second forced expiratory volume (FEV$_1$) is the volume of air expired during the first second. Three-second forced expiratory volume (FEV$_3$) is the volume of air expired during 3 seconds. *A.* Normal spirogram. *B.* Spirogram from a patient with mild obstructive airways disease. The curve does not develop a normal plateau and FEV$_3$/FVC percentage is reduced. *C.* Spirogram from a patient with severe obstructive defect. If the spirogram were incorrectly terminated after 2 seconds, the FVC would be artificially reduced (see the text). When it is performed correctly (*dotted lines*) it is obvious that there is airway obstruction and that there is no restrictive disease. *D.* Spirogram showing restrictive pulmonary disease (FEV$_1$/FVC is normal but FVC is reduced).

presses them (Fig. 55.2). This tendency for airways to collapse is opposed by the elastic properties of the lung that stabilize the bronchi and keep the airways open. Although slight airway compression occurs in normal subjects during a maximal expiratory effort, there is a marked tendency for airways to collapse in patients with emphysema in whom the structural components of the lung are destroyed.

Figure 55.3 diagrammatically illustrates airway morphology and the supporting elastic structures in the lung and shows how asthma, chronic bronchitis, and emphysema produce decreased expiratory airflow. In these diseases, forced expiration is limited by several factors (Table 55.2). In asthma, there is initial bronchospasm often followed by mucosal edema and retained secretions. During an acute asthmatic attack, bronchial smooth muscle may narrow and even close the airways, causing air trapping and subsequent hyperinflation. In bronchitis, the onset of airflow obstruction may be insidious with initial mucous gland hyperplasia and retained bronchial secretions, especially in the peripheral airways (< 2 mm). In addition, the presence of bronchial infection may lead to airway hyperresponsiveness to various inhaled agents (8), causing further smooth muscle bronchospasm. Finally, in emphysema, airways may collapse during normal tidal breathing because of destruction of the structural elements of the lungs.

PULMONARY FUNCTION TESTING IN OBSTRUCTIVE AIRWAYS DISEASE

Spirometry

Spirometry (Fig. 55.1) is the most useful pulmonary function test to assess airflow limitation in asthma and obstructive pulmonary disease. This test is performed in all pulmonary testing facilities and relatively inexpensive spirometers are also readily available (2, 23). Physicians who treat a significant number of patients with chronic obstructive airways disease should have a spirometer in their offices. Ideally, a spirometer should provide a graphic record of the patient's forced expiration, which should be maintained for at least 4 to 5 seconds in order to measure both forced expiratory volume during the first second (FEV$_1$), and the forced vital capacity (FVC, the total volume that can be exhaled after a maximal inspiration). An electrical spirometer is less desirable, but if one is used, a graphic record is still necessary to evaluate the quality and reproducibility of the patient's effort. Calibration must be performed frequently with a calibrating syringe to document accurately the measurements made with the spirometer (52). The American Thoracic Society has published guidelines for the use of spirometers (2). Three reproducible tracings should be made and the FEV$_1$ or another measurement of expiratory flow (maximal or midmaximal expiratory flow rates)

Table 55.1.
Indications for Pulmonary Function Testing in Obstructive Airways Disease

To establish the presence and severity of airway obstructon
To evaluate objectively the reversibility of airways obstruction and the results of therapy
To assist in the differentiation between emphysema and other forms of airways obstruction
To serve as a basis to predict the course and prognosis of chronic obstructive disease
To evaluate work potential (see Chapter 9) or operative risks (see Chapter 86)

should be calculated. Airway obstruction can be quantitated in three ways: measurement of absolute FEV_1, the FEV_1 as a percentage of predicted, using readily available nomograms: and the ratio of FEV_1/FVC. Severe obstruction is usually present when the FEV_1 is less than 1.0 liter, than 25% predicted, or than 25–40% of the FVC. The ratio of the FEV_1/FVC is used to evaluate airways obstruction since pure restrictive ventilatory defects cause an equal reduction in the FEV_1 and the vital capacity; and the FEV_1/FVC ratio, therefore, will be normal (Fig. 55.1D). A reduction of the FEV_1/FVC ratio below 75% indicates the presence of airflow obstruction. Since patients with obstructive lung disease empty air from their lungs slowly (Fig. 55.1, B and C), their spirograms do not show a normal plateau. Therefore, if expiration is not prolonged, the FVC will be artificially reduced and the diagnosis of airway obstruction may be overlooked. For example, if a patient with obstructive airways disease exhales for only 2 seconds, the spirogram will be artificially truncated, (Fig. 55.1C). If it were stopped at 2 seconds, the FVC would be recorded as 1.1 liters, the FEV_1 as 0.9 liter, and the FEV_1/FVC as 78%. When it is correctly performed and expiration is prolonged for 4 to 6 seconds (Fig. 55.1C, *dotted line*), the actual FVC is measured as 2.0 liters and the FEV_1/FVC ratio (0.9/2.0) is 45%. Therefore, if the spirogram were not examined, an erroneous diagnosis of restrictive, rather than severe obstructive, lung disease would be made.

Patient experience. There is little discomfort associated with spirometry in normal individuals or in patients with mild to moderate obstructive airways disease. After a nose clip is applied, the patient is instructed to take a deep inspiration, immediately followed by a forceful expiration that should continue for at least 4 seconds. Forced expiration can occasionally result in coughing and, extremely rarely, cyanosis and hypoxemia in patients with severe airways disease and resting hypoxemia.

The peak expiratory flow rate can be measured in patients with asthma by use of inexpensive peak flow meters, which do not provide a printed record or a measurement of vital capacity. This peak flow meter can be used by a patient at home to monitor lung function serially during therapy (see below).

Complete Pulmonary Function Tests

Other pulmonary function tests that are useful in the detailed assessment of obstructive airways disease include the measurement of lung volumes, diffusion capacity, and arterial blood gases both at rest and during exercise (see Chapter 53, under "Dyspnea"). The measurement of *lung volumes* quantitates the degree of hyperinflation that may be found either in patients with long-standing airway obstruction or in patients with acute asthma. Occasionally, initial clinical and symptomatic improvement in airways obstruction during recovery from an asthmatic attack will be reflected by a decrease in the degree of hyperinflation (59). Lung volume measurements are also useful in the evaluation of patients with restrictive pulmonary diseases. The *single breath diffusion capacity* for carbon monoxide

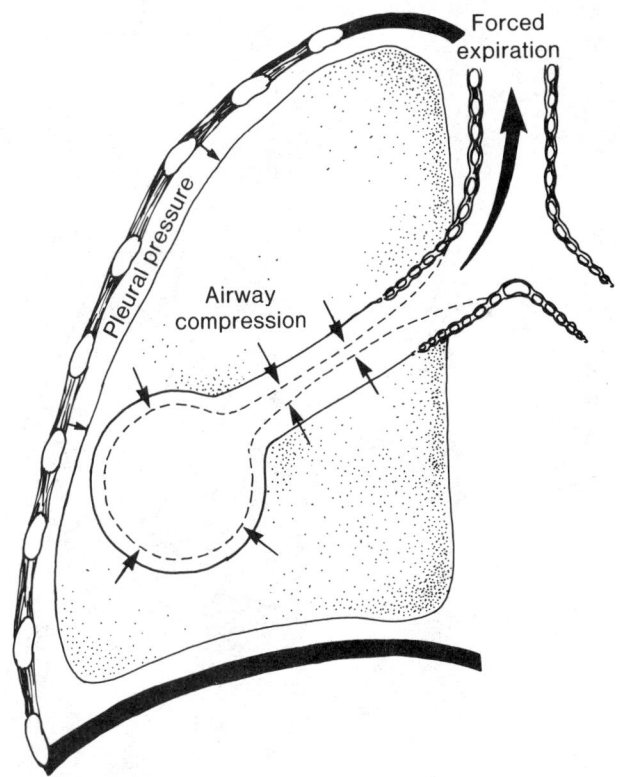

Figure 55.2. A schematic representation of the lungs and chest wall during a forced expiration. With maximal forced expiration, pleural pressure increases and becomes positive. At the point where pleural pressure exceeds intraluminal airway pressure, the airways are compressed. The structural components of the lung stabilize the airways, hold them open, and oppose their tendency to collapse during expiration (see the text).

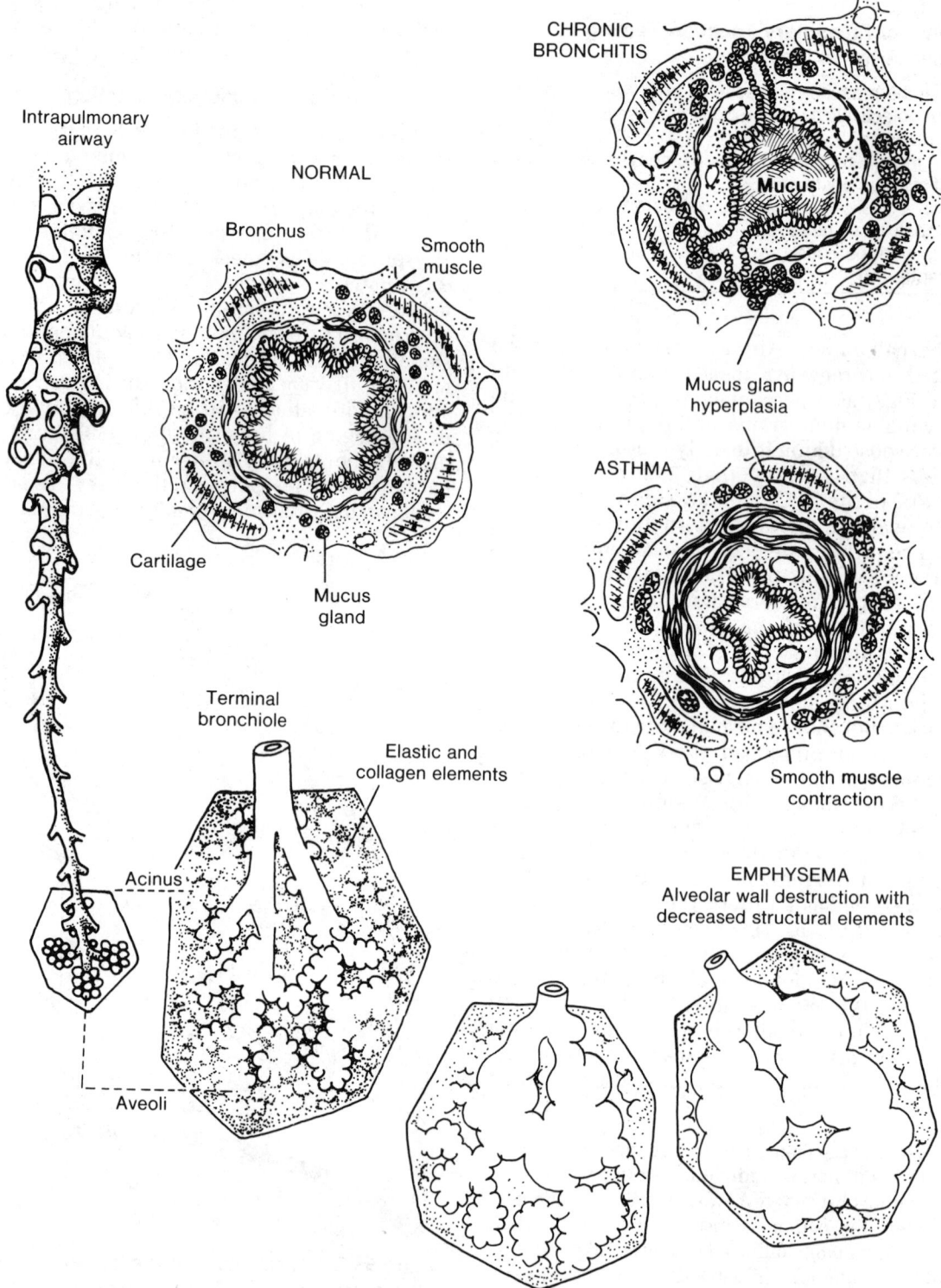

Figure 55.3. Schematic representation of the morphology of normal airways and lung parenchyma and the changes produced in these structures by asthma, chronic bronchitis, and emphysema (see the text).

reflects the amount of functional alveolar capillary surface area available for gas exchange. Diffusion capacity is reduced not only in pulmonary fibrosis and congestive heart failure but also in emphysema. The findings of expiratory airflow limitation, hyperinflation, and a reduced diffusion capacity often correlate with the pathological diagnosis of anatomical emphysema (24) (Fig. 55.8).

Patient experience. There is no discomfort or risk during the measurement of lung volumes, but it is necessary that a patient be able to remain seated for 6 to 8 minutes, breathing a mixture of air and helium. Severely obstructed patients whose vital capacity is less than 1 liter cannot perform a single breath diffusion capacity since they must inspire and hold at least a 1-liter inspiratory volume for 10 seconds.

Other pulmonary function tests, such as the measurement of pulmonary compliance or airway resistance using a body plethysmograph, are sophisticated tests that are not usually helpful in the routine management of patients with obstructive airways disease. Flow volume curves provide similar information to routine spirometry; however, the apparatus for this test is more complicated, is difficult to calibrate accurately, and is expensive. Nevertheless, many testing facilities use flow volume curves rather than spirometry. Flow volume curves are specifically useful in the evaluation of extrathoracic airway obstruction and some examples of these curves obtained in upper and lower airway obstruction are illustrated in Figure 55.4 (25).

Early Detection of Airways Disease

The early diagnosis of chronic obstructive lung disease depends on sensitive pulmonary function tests that correlate with the presence of peripheral airway obstruction (< 2 mm). Anatomically, these airways lack significant cartilage, have a smooth muscle wall that contains large numbers of mucus-secreting goblet cells, and rely entirely on the sur-

Table 55.2.
Mechanisms of Airway Obstruction

Smooth muscle spasm
Mucosal edema and inflammation
Mucous gland hyperplasia
Increased bronchial secretions
Airways collapse
Airways hyperreactivity to inhaled substances (cigarette smoke, dust, histamine)

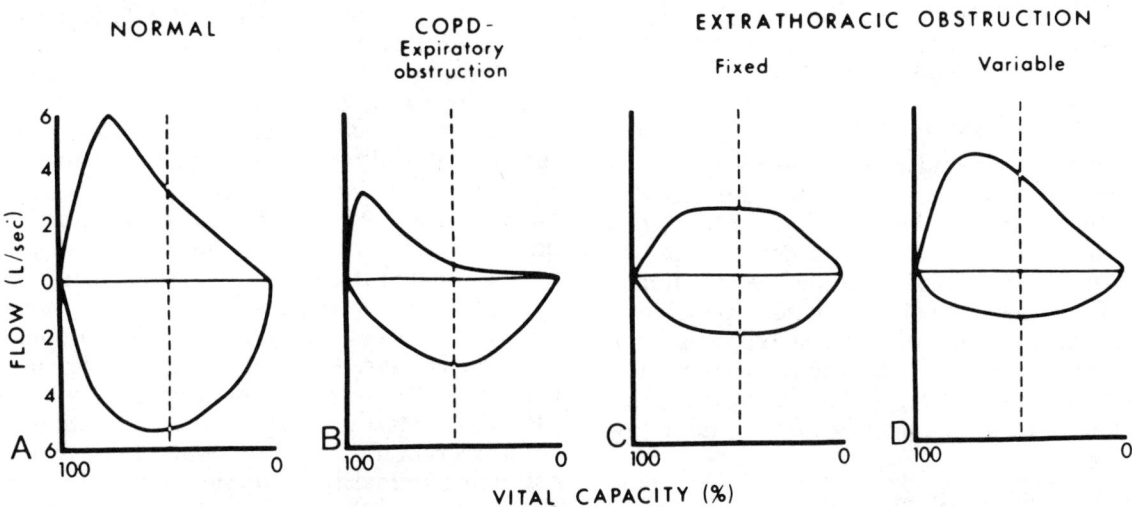

Figure 55.4. Flow volume curves (loops) of maximal forced expiration (*upper*) and maximal inspiration (*lower*). Expiratory and inspiratory flow is plotted against lung volume expressed as a percentage of vital capacity. The *dotted line* can be used to compare flow rates at 50% of the vital capacity where inspiratory flow rates normally exceed expiratory flow rates. *A.* Normal flow volume curves. *B.* Flow volume curves illustrating expiratory airflow obstruction showing decreased flow rates at all points in lung volume throughout maximal expiration. *C.* Fixed extrathoracic airway obstruction (cancer or fracture of the larynx) produces a pattern where there is a decrease and flattening of both inspiratory and expiratory flow volume curves. Inspiratory flow rate at 50% of the vital capacity is equal to similar expiratory flow rate. *D.* Variable extrathoracic obstruction (vocal cord paralysis) produces a pattern where there is a decrease and flattening of maximal inspiratory flow volume curves. Inspiratory flow rates at 50% of the vital capacity are less than similar expiratory flow. (Modified from Hyatt RE, Black LF: The flow-volume curve: a current perspective. *Am Rev Respir Dis* 107:191, 1973.)

rounding lung parenchyma for structural support. Correlations of the pathological findings in the lungs of patients with early bronchitis and emphysema (24, 54) show abnormalities in these peripheral airways. Early peripheral airways disease may be predicted by a spirogram in which the FEV_1 is relatively normal (80% of predicted and the FEV_1/FVC ratio is 75%) but in which the FVC does not reach a plateau normally within 4 seconds, thereby indicating slowly emptying parts of the lungs (29). This can be further shown by measuring the forced expiratory volume after 3 seconds, the FEV_3, which is normally 98 to 100% of the FVC (FEV_3/FVC ratio: Fig. 55.1).

ASTHMA (INTERMITTENT OBSTRUCTIVE AIRWAYS DISEASE)

Definition

Asthma is difficult to define; for many physicians it simply implies wheezing from any cause. More specifically, asthma is a heterogeneous clinical syndrome that is characterized by intermittent dyspnea and wheezing resulting from widespread narrowing of the intrapulmonary airways. Unlike other causes of airflow obstruction, the key features in asthma are reversibility of airway obstruction with relatively symptom-free periods between attacks and increased responsiveness of the airways to a wide variety of inhaled stimuli. The prevalence of asthma in the United States is estimated to be 3% of the population or almost 9 million people.

Types of Asthma

The above definition of asthma describes only the clinical characteristics of this heterogeneous disease. Asthma can also be classified according to precipitating factors, namely, the presence or absence of an allergic etiology. On the basis of clinical findings, more than half of an asthmatic population can be assigned to one of the five types that are listed in Table 55.3, although even these, as well as the rest of the asthmatic population, show considerable overlap in the clinical features of their disease.

Nonallergic Intrinsic Asthma

The most common type of asthma is not due to allergy, but to poorly defined intrinsic factors. These asthmatics have persistent hyperreactivity of the airways to multiple nonallergic stimuli (see below).

Table 55.3.
Types of Asthma

Nonallergic intrinsic asthma
Allergic extrinsic asthma
Nonallergic extrinsic asthma
Asthma associated with chronic obstructive lung disease
Exercise-induced asthma

Although some intrinsic asthmatics have allergies that occasionally trigger an acute asthmatic attack, the usual clinical course of their disease does not correlate with their allergic hypersensitivities. Instead, asthmatic attacks may be related to infection, exercise, inhaled irritants, or psychological stimuli. Although intrinsic asthmatics may have significant eosinophilia in their blood and sputum, unlike patients with allergic asthma (see below), their serum IgE levels are normal. Asthmatic symptoms may begin at any age, but often start during adulthood. Commonly, patients may date the onset of asthma to an acute upper respiratory tract infection. While intrinsic asthmatics may improve with appropriate therapy after their first attack, they subsequently develop chronic symptomatic asthma. Frequently the clinical manifestations of their disease are severe and have a tendency to persist throughout the year, showing variations in severity rather than complete symptomatic remissions. Some of these patients have chronic bronchitis that either complicates or precipitates asthmatic attacks (see below).

Asthma and airways hyperreactivity. A characteristic feature found in all asthmatics is airways hyperreactivity, an exaggerated degree of bronchospasm induced by various inhaled agents (8). These agents include immunological mediators, such as histamine and some prostaglandins; cholinergic agents, such as methacholine; and various irritants, such as dust, cigarette smoke, and cold air (exercise-induced asthma). The presence of increased nonspecific airways reactivity is thought to correlate with the severity of asthmatic symptoms such as coughing and intermittent wheezing. Some patients with chronic obstructive lung disease also show increased airways reactivity. Neural reflex mechanisms may be partially responsible for bronchospasm induced by the inhaled irritants. These substances activate irritant receptors whose afferent pathways travel in the vagus nerves. Subsequent reflex bronchoconstriction is caused by activation of efferent vagal pathways. These same parasympathetic mechanisms mediate the cough reflex and control bronchial secretions. Some patients have symptoms consisting primarily of airways irritability such as persistent coughing (see Chapter 53, under "Cough"). They have airways hyperreactivity to inhaled agents (methacholine) and their symptoms improve after treatment with bronchodilators (32). These patients probably have mild intrinsic asthma.

Allergic Extrinsic Asthma

In 5 to 10% of asthmatics, clinical asthma is primarily caused by specific allergic factors. These stimuli include seasonal exposure to the pollens of gasses, ragweed, and trees or to other specific allergens, such as animal dander, dust, or some occupational agents. Allergic asthmatics frequently note the onset of recognizable symptoms early in life and relate a family or personal history of asthma or of other allergic diseases (allergic rhinitis, eczema, and urticaria). Many allergic extrinsic asthmatics also have attacks triggered by multiple nonallergic causes.

In these allergic patients, the intradermal injection of a specific allergen causes a wheal and flare reaction; inhalation of this same antigen causes airways obstruction. When a susceptible individual is exposed to an allergen, specific IgE or reaginic antibody is produced. This antibody sensitizes mast cells and basophils (3) and re-exposure to that allergen initiates a sequence of biochemical reactions within these sensitized target cells (type I immunological reaction) (see Chapter 23, Fig. 23.1). These reactions cause the formation, release, and synthesis of histamine and other vasoactive substances which cause contraction of bronchial smooth muscle, alter vascular permeability, and attract inflammatory cells to the reaction site. In addition, these substances cause the pathophysiological changes found in an allergic asthmatic attack (3).

The release of these mediators is inhibited by increases in cellular cyclic AMP (adenosine 3':5'-monophosphate) and facilitated by increases in cyclic GMP (guanosine 3':5'-monophosphate). β-Sympathomimetic agonists (such as isoproterenol) directly increase cyclic AMP, and theophylline preparations (such as aminophylline) inhibit the activity of phosphodiesterase, an enzyme that catalyzes the breakdown of cyclic AMP, thereby suppressing mediator release. Cholinergic stimulation, on the other hand, may enhance the release of mediators by increasing levels of cyclic GMP. These interactions are the basis for the pharmacological treatment of allergic asthma.

Nonallergic Extrinsic Asthma Due to Specific Agents

In some patients, exposure to inhaled or ingested agents causes asthma that does not seem to be caused by the irritant effects of the inhaled substances, nor is it mediated by classic immunological reactions. However, recent studies have shown that some of these substances (toluene-2,4-diisocyanate (TDI) or phthalic acid anhydride) may cause their effects through immunological mechanisms. They may act as haptens and combine with serum albumin to form a complete antigen that provokes an IgE-mediated asthma attack (28). When the exposure to these agents occurs in industrial settings, the reversible bronchospasm they produce is called "occupational asthma." Examples of these agents include metal fumes and salts (chromium, nickel, ammonium), wood (oak and western red cedar), vegetable, grain, and coffee bean dusts (flour—baker's asthma), industrial chemicals used in manufacturing processes of plastics, polyurethane foams (TDI, phthalic acid anhydride, epoxy resins, solder-

ing fluxes), pyrolysis products of plastics (meat wrapper's asthma), enzymes (*Bacillus subtilis* detergents), as well as exposures during the manufacture of pharmaceutical agents (penicillin, pancreatic enzymes) (10) (see Chapter 7 and General References under "Asthma").

Aspirin and other drug sensitivity. Other agents such as aspirin, nonsteroidal anti-inflammatory drugs (indomethacin and phenylbutazone), and tartrazine (yellow dye no. 5), a common coloring agent used in many foods and drugs, precipitate bronchospasm in 5 to 10% of all asthmatics (51) and urticaria in susceptible individuals (Chapter 23). While the precise mechanisms through which these ingested substances trigger asthma are unknown, it is felt that they are probably not initiated through classic IgE-mediated immunological reactions. Asthmatics with aspirin sensitivity are more commonly female and have associated nasal polyps and sinusitis. Bronchospasm occurs within 2 hours of the aspirin ingestion, and severe reactions may be accompanied by vascular shock and, rarely, death. Therefore, asthmatics should avoid taking these substances, and challenges with these agents should be performed with extreme care. Table 23.12, Chapter 23, lists both prescription and nonprescription compounds that contain aspirin.

Asthma Associated with Chronic Obstructive Lung Disease

There are patients with chronic obstructive airways disease (chronic obstructive bronchitis or emphysema) whose disease is characterized by intermittent "asthmatic" attacks. A small number of these patients give a history of typical childhood asthma or of other allergic diseases. The importance of this somewhat artificial grouping is to emphasize that, although the prognosis in these patients is determined by their chronic obstructive lung disease (see below), the pathophysiology and treatment of an acute exacerbation of bronchospasm are similar to those of typical asthma.

Exercise-Induced Asthma (Cold Air)

Most asthmatics, regardless of etiology, develop wheezing and dyspnea after moderate to severe exercise, especially in cold environments (7). Some forms of exercise, such as running or bicycle riding, are more asthmogenic than others, such as swimming, where ambient air is usually warm and humid. Recently it has been shown that the production of postexertional asthma is directly related to increased heat loss from the pulmonary airways during exercise-induced hyperventilation. The mechanisms by which these stimuli trigger bronchospasm are not completely understood, but they may act directly on airway smooth muscle or may produce bronchoconstriction by altering the osmolarity of respiratory secretions. Thus, in experimental situations, exercise-induced bronchospasm can be prevented by having an asthmatic breathe air that is humidified and heated to body temperature (34). The response to exercise or breathing of cold air represents another instance of airways hyperreactivity in asthma (14). In some mild asthmatics, attacks of exercise-induced bronchospasm represent the primary clinical manifestation of their disease. Also, an elderly intrinsic asthmatic complaining of dyspnea on exertion outdoors on a cold winter day may actually be experiencing exercise-induced asthma rather than cardiac or pulmonary decompensation.

Clinical Presentation of Asthma

Usually asthmatic attacks are episodic, lasting hours to several days, separated by symptom-free periods during which airflow obstruction is absent or mild. Although the patient notes wheezing and coughing productive of white mucoid sputum during a mild asthmatic attack, he can perform ordinary tasks without difficulty. During more severe asthmatic attacks, however, he will experience exertional dyspnea that persists even at rest. Frequent coughing reflects airway hyperirritability. *Status asthmaticus* refers to a very severe and persistent asthmatic state that does not substantially improve despite intensive therapy.

Evaluation of Mild or Asymptomatic Asthma

History

A complete medical history is essential in the initial evaluation of patients with bronchial asthma to determine the overall severity, the specific factors which precipitate or aggravate symptoms, and the therapeutic modalities that are effective in an individual patient. The medical history should also establish the frequency and severity of asthmatic attacks as well as a description of exercise tolerance during symptom-free periods. If the asthmatic attacks are associated with bronchitis, the frequency, quantity, and duration of sputum production should be documented. The occurrence of seasonal exacerbations should alert the physician to the possibility of environmental factors such as ragweed or grass allergy (see Chapter 23, Fig. 23.3). A history of cough and wheezing precipitated by exposure to cigarette smoke suggests the presence of nonspecific airways reactivity. On the other hand, a personal history of cigarette smoking is so unusual in asthma that it is more likely that such a patient actually has chronic obstructive pulmonary disease. The severity of exercise-induced bronchospasm should be elicited, especially in adolescents and young adults, in whom the presence of postexercise asthma may interfere with normal social and physical development.

Physical Examination

Tachypnea, tachycardia, and a pulsus paradoxus (a drop in systolic blood pressure of greater than 15 mm Hg with inspiration) should be looked for. The upper airways should be examined for the presence of sinusitis, nasal polyps, or evidence of allergic rhinitis (boggy, pale nasal mucosa, conjunctivitis). During the rest of the physical examination particular emphasis should be placed on breathing pattern, the use of accessory muscles of ventilation, and the presence of rhonchi and rales during auscultation of the chest. If wheezing is not heard during quiet breathing, a maximal timed forced expiratory maneuver should be performed by asking the patient to blow out all of the air in his lungs as fast as possible after a maximal inspiration. This will frequently induce wheezing not present during quiet breathing; and by timing the forced expiration, a simple index of airways obstruction is obtained. Normal subjects are able to perform a forced expiration in less than 4 seconds, but with airflow obstruction the duration of expiration is greater than 5 or 6 seconds.

Laboratory Testing

In mild asthmatics spirometry is useful to document baseline normal pulmonary function during a symptom-free period. In those patients with more severe asthma, spirometry provides an objective measure of severity and serves as a guide for therapy. For a transient time after the initial improvement from an acute attack, significant residual abnormalities in airways function often persist (35). Depending on the individual asthmatic, these residual abnormalities in airways function either resolve or persist with varying severity. It is possible that this subclinical airways obstruction can serve as a focus for future recurrent asthmatic attacks. In asthmatics without superimposed chronic obstructive airways disease, blood gas analysis is indicated only to assess severe asthmatic episodes (see below). In older patients (> 40 years), especially those with evidence of persistent airways obstruction or associated cardiovascular disease, baseline spirometry, an electrocardiogram, and a chest roentgenogram should always be obtained.

A complete blood count (CBC) with differential and sputum examination should be performed in asthmatics who have clinical findings of an acute infectious process. Eosinophils can make sputum appear grossly purulent; therefore, microscopic examination of the sputum in an asthmatic is necessary in order to avoid inappropriate use of antibiotics. Besides eosinophils, sputum may also contain Charcot-Leyden crystals (pointed elongated eosinophilic crystals) and Curschmann's spirals (mucous casts of small bronchioles) (19). If parenchymal pulmonary infection is suspected because of the presence of fever, purulent sputum, and physical findings such as rales and consolidation, a chest roentgenogram and sputum culture are indicated.

Skin testing (Chapter 23) is indicated when a specific allergen is suspected and confirmation of that suspicion is necessary for proper management (see below, page 647). Common allergens that cause allergic asthma include ragweed pollens, various grasses, extracts of trees, molds indigenous to specific localities, and animal danders (cat, dog). Skin testing is most easily obtained by referral to an allergist. Total serum IgE is usually only moderately elevated in patients with allergic asthma, and its measurement is not indicated in the routine clinical management of this disease. Specific serum IgE, measured by the radioallergosorbent test (RAST), provides information similar to that provided by allergy skin testing. Therefore, the RAST is helpful only when skin testing cannot be performed.

Bronchial Challenge Procedures

Diagnostic testing with *exercise or inhalation challenge* with pharmacological agents is occasionally useful to confirm the presence of hyperreactive airways in patients with questionable symptoms. These tests involve inhaling gradually increasing concentrations of either histamine or methacholine and observing spirometric changes in airflow obstruction (13, 14). Similarly, an exercise challenge can be performed and pulmonary function can be quantitated during the first 30 minutes after maximal exercise. When positive, these tests can cause some mild to moderate distress in an asymptomatic asthmatic since a 20 to 30% reduction in FEV_1 is used as an end point for the diagnosis of hyperreactive airways. For example, an exercise challenge might help to confirm the diagnostic impression of exercise asthma in a young patient who complains of excessive coughing and dyspnea after physical exertion (14). These challenges require referral to a pulmonary function laboratory which is able to perform provocative testing. Inhalation challenge with specific antigen is almost never indicated since it does not distinguish allergic nonasthmatic patients (grass and ragweed hay fever) from asthmatics with these specific allergies (8). An exception is inhalation challenge in suspected occupational exposure when it may be important to establish the relationship between symptoms and a specific incriminating substance.

Acute Asthma

In order to understand fully the basis for the symptoms, signs, and laboratory findings that correlate with severe asthma, a review of the pathophysiology of acute bronchospasm is indicated.

Pathophysiology of Acute Asthma

Obstruction to expiratory airflow in acute asthma is initially caused by bronchial smooth muscle spasm that is followed, as the attack persists, by bronchial wall edema, inflammatory cell infiltration, and mucous plugging of the airways. With progressively more severe asthma ($FEV_1 < 1.5$ liters), the asthmatic is forced to compensate for bronchoconstriction in order to permit gas exchange to take place. He does this by breathing at high lung volumes, since, as the lungs enlarge to total lung capacity, the airways are mechanically opened. Unfortunately, breathing in a hyperinflated state requires a marked increase in the inspiratory muscle forces and results in varying degrees of dyspnea and fatigue. A reduction in vital capacity correlates with the degree of hyperinflation, and, in very severe attacks, the vital capacity may be only slightly larger than the asthmatic's tidal volume. Therefore, the severity of the asthmatic attack is highly correlated with the two simple measures of forced expiration, the FEV_1 and the FVC (Fig. 55.1) (35, 46).

Another major physiological change that occurs during a severe asthmatic attack is the development of pulmonary hypertension due to the direct effects of hypoxia and the mechanical effects of hyperinflation on the pulmonary vasculature. These changes are manifested by electrocardiographic abnormalities such as acute right axis deviation, "p" pulmonale, and right ventricular strain. In addition, during breathing in acute asthma the marked swings in pleural pressure are associated with hyperinflation that affects left ventricular function and accounts for the development of pulsus paradoxus. A summary of these pathophysiological changes is listed in Table 55.4.

Evaluation of an Acute Asthmatic Attack

Unfortunately, subjective symptoms such as dyspnea and wheezing do not correlate with severity of asthma (35), and the physician must rely on objective physical findings and laboratory tests to evalu-

Table 55.4.
Pathophysiological Changes in Acute Bronchial Asthma

Expiratory airflow obstruction (FEV_1 and expiratory airflow are reduced)

Breathing at high lung volumes to prevent airway closure at resting lung volumes (vital capacity is reduced)

Pulmonary hypertension (P pulmonale and right ventricular strain on ECG)

Large fluctuations in pleural pressure with respiration (pulsus paradoxus)

Ventilation-perfusion mismatch (arterial blood gases show hypoxemia always, hypocapnea (low $PaCO_2$) usually, and hypercapnea (high $PaCO_2$) only in very severe asthma)

ate an acute asthmatic attack (Table 55.5). During the physical examination, the findings of a pulsus paradoxus and the use of accessory muscles of ventilation with sternocleidomastoid contractions correlate with the development of severe airflow ob-

Table 55.5.
Objective Evaluation of Acute Asthma

Vital signs: tachycardia and pulsus paradoxus
Physical examination: use of accessory muscles of respiration with sternocleidomastoid contractions
Spirometry: reduced FEV_1 and increase in FEV_1 after administration of a bronchodilator
Chest X-ray: hyperinflation
ECG: acute cor pulmonale
Arterial blood gases (low PaO_2, low or high $PaCO_2$)
Sputum smear and culture: eosinophils or evidence of infection

Table 55.6.
Indications of Severe Asthma Necessitating Immediate Hospitalization (Acute Respiratory Failure)

$FEV_1 < 0.7$, $FVC < 1.2$ (absent bronchodilator response)
$PaO_2 < 50$ mm Hg, $PaCO_2 > 40$ mm Hg
Disturbance of consciousness, obvious exhaustion
Silent chest
Pulsus paradoxus > 15 mm
Pneumothorax or pneumomediastinum

struction, hyperinflation, and a marked reduction in FEV_1 (< 40% predicted or 1.25 liters) (35, 46).

When physical findings are present that suggest severe asthma, objective pulmonary function measurements should be performed in every asthmatic who is old enough to cooperate. An FEV_1 less than 1 liter or 25% predicted correlates with severe hypoxemia ($PaO_2 < 60$ mm Hg) (38). Spirometry can then be used to monitor the course of the asthmatic attack as well as the response to bronchodilator treatment. An absent bronchodilator response suggests status asthmaticus. If these physical findings and objective tests do not improve with therapy, the patient should be sent to the emergency room for treatment. The findings listed in Table 55.6 indicate severe respiratory failure in status asthmaticus and the patient requires immediate hospitalization.

A chest roentgenogram is indicated in those patients with acute asthma who do not improve readily with initial treatment or in those in whom pulmonary infection is suspected. The chest roentgenogram should be inspected for atelectasis due to mucous plugging of the airways, for pulmonary infiltrates due to infectious processes that could precipitate or complicate an asthmatic attack, and for a pneumothorax or a pneumomediastinum. Furthermore, the presence of acute hyperinflation on a chest roentgenogram indicates a severe asthmatic attack (Fig. 55.5). The significance of electrocardiographic abnormalities consistent with acute cor pulmonale

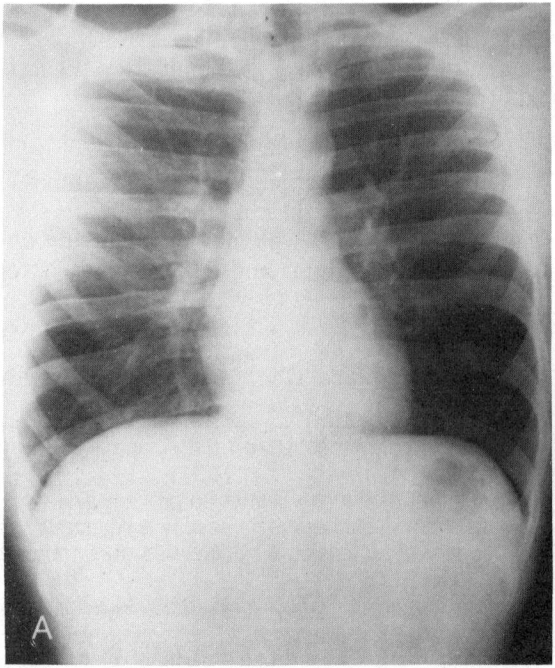
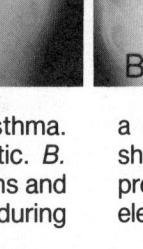
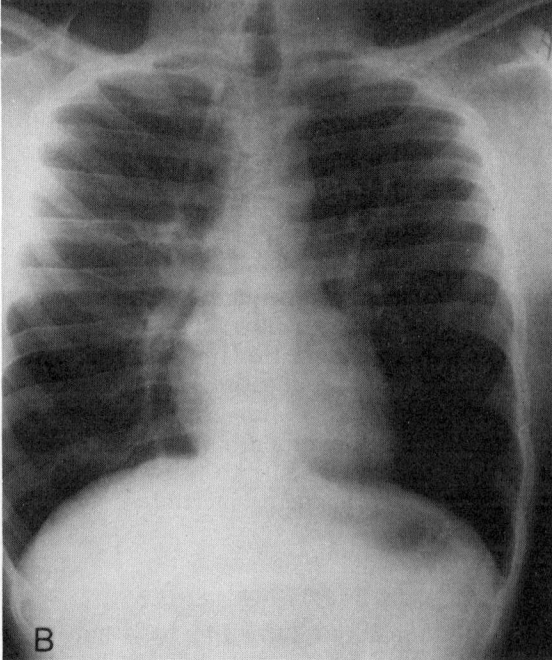

Figure 55.5.   Acute hyperinflation in severe asthma. *A.* Normal chest roentgenogram in an asthmatic. *B.* Acute hyperinflation (lowered flattened diaphragms and widened intercostal spaces) in the same patient during a severe asthmatic attack. Pulmonary function tests showed a marked reduction in FEV_1 (0.8 liter, 18% predicted) and FVC (2.1 liters, 38% predicted) and an elevated total lung capacity (7.3 liters, 112% predicted).

and pulmonary hypertension has been discussed. The measurement of arterial blood gases should be performed when physical findings and spirometry ($FEV_1 < 1.25$ liters or 40% predicted) suggest a severe asthmatic attack. Arterial hypoxemia develops during acute episodes of bronchial asthma (38), and in the very severe attack ($FEV_1 < 0.7$ liter or 10 to 15% predicted) hypoxemia can be life threatening. Usually in mild to moderately severe asthmatic attacks alveolar hyperventilation is maintained and arterial CO_2 tensions are reduced. In asthma an arterial CO_2 tension that rises into the normal range or becomes elevated predicts imminent respiratory failure.

Differential Diagnosis

Because of its characteristic clinical presentation, acute bronchial asthma is easily differentiated from the other cardiopulmonary diseases that present with cough, wheezing, and dyspnea. In middle-aged and elderly patients one must consider acute left ventricular failure with "cardiac asthma," pulmonary embolism, or an infectious exacerbation of chronic obstructive pulmonary disease. Occasionally patients only complain of persistent coughing and deny wheezing or dyspnea. These patients often have pulmonary function tests which reveal mild obstruction, have bronchial hyperreactivity, and improve with bronchodilator treatment (35).

Airflow limitation produced by obstruction in the upper airways (larynx, trachea) caused by a foreign body, tumor, secretions, edema, inflammation, or tracheal malacia can sometimes be confused with lower airway obstruction. In upper airway obstruction, there may be a history of goiter, hoarseness, or prior endotracheal intubation. Physical examination usually reveals inspiratory stridor (wheezing during inspiration). Inspiratory flow volume curves (25), performed in a pulmonary function laboratory, show a reduction in inspiratory flows and a specific diagnostic pattern (Fig. 55.4). Direct or indirect laryngoscopy may visualize an anatomical abnormality.

Treatment of Asthma

Since asthma has multiple etiologies, its management requires a combined therapeutic approach that should attempt to maintain pulmonary function in a near normal state as well as to prevent recurrent asthmatic attacks (Table 55.7). Precipitating factors in an individual asthmatic must be identified and avoided. Clinical manifestations, including bronchospasm and pulmonary infections, must be effectively treated, while medical complications should be prevented.

Avoidance of Precipitating Factors

As indicated above, numerous, often apparently unrelated, factors precipitate or worsen clinical asthma. Some of these stimuli are easily defined and controlled, while in other asthmatics the exact etiologies of an attack are difficult to determine with

Table 55.7.
Treatment of Asthma

GENERAL MEASURES
    Control of environmental factors:
        Cigarette smoke, air pollutants
        Occupational exposures
        Control of environmental temperature and humidity
    Control of allergy to specific inhaled or ingested agents
    Control of emotional and psychological factors
    Control of respiratory infections
SPECIFIC TREATMENT
    Pharmacological
        Smooth muscle spasm—bronchodilators: local/systemic
        inflammation (corticosteroids)
    Mechanical airways obstruction—mucus:
        Hydration—local/systemic
        Physical therapy
        Mucolytic agents: to be avoided
    Infection: appropriate antibiotics
    Hypoxemia: humidified oxygen
    Sedation: to be avoided

certainty. Knowledge of the triggers of asthma is of prime importance in its evaluation and treatment.

Environment. Asthmatics should avoid exposure to irritating dusts, sprays, or aerosols, both at home and at work. For example, passive exposure of asthmatics to cigarette smoke, especially in enclosed spaces such as cars, airplanes, or poorly ventilated rooms, will cause worsening of airway function. The exact role of air pollutants in provoking asthma is still not completely known. However, it is known that ozone, sulfur dioxide, and nitrogen dioxide exposure can increase nonspecific airways reactivity in normal subjects and can cause symptoms and bronchospasm in asthmatics (8). Often occupational factors are not immediately obvious since asthmatic symptoms may occur several hours after leaving the workplace (coughing and dyspnea awakening the patient from sleep). Since direct challenge with suspected provoking agents is not always practical and is often dangerous, the etiology of an asthmatic's symptoms may be indirectly ascertained by systematically avoiding specific, potentially provoking factors. At home, the control of environmental temperature and humidity is accomplished with an air conditioner that will also help to filter pollens and air pollutants. The filter should be changed regularly to avoid the accumulation of sensitizing airborne molds and fungi. In rare circumstances, removal to a more favorable climate may be indicated to control chronic asthma (see page 664).

Allergy. Desensitization consists of injections of increasing concentrations of an antigen to which the asthmatic is sensitive, thereby inducing blocking antibody (IgG antibody that interferes with the antigen-antibody reaction). It is indicated when there are a limited number of allergens, demonstrated by skin testing, that appear to be etiologically related to an individual's asthma (27). Desensitization therapy is expensive, time consuming, and not always effective. Therefore, before it is started, every attempt should be made to eliminate or reduce specific allergen exposure. At times, only a reduction in exposure to a known allergen can be effected. For example, if it is not possible to remove a household pet from the home of an allergic asthmatic patient, the pet should be excluded from the patient's bedroom. Down-filled pillows and shag rugs that accumulate dust should not be used.

Emotion. Asthmatic attacks can be produced and reversed in some patients by appropriate verbal suggestion (37). For example, less bronchodilation is produced by isoproterenol if the asthmatic is told he is being treated with a bronchoconstrictor rather than a bronchodilator. Therefore, the expectations of the asthmatic patient as well as of those treating him have a significant influence on the therapeutic efficacy of any given therapeutic regimen. Despite these considerations, all asthmatic patients must receive adequate medical treatment and symptoms should not be ignored because they may have psychogenic etiologies.

In some asthmatics, emotional factors play a much greater role in modulating the course of their disease and often cause difficult therapeutic problems. In addition, asthma can be a chronic, debilitating disease that in itself will stress the asthmatic and his family. Usually supportive measures initiated by a sympathetic physician, as well as by the patient's family members and friends, will avoid the need for psychiatric care. Occasionally, supportive psychotherapy will be useful, especially when counseling is available from a professional who is experienced in treating psychosomatic illnesses. In selected patients, mild sedatives (see Chapter 13) may be an adjunct to the total treatment regimen, but preferably other means should be used to help a patient cope with the anxiety caused by his disease. He should be assured of the concern of those around him, as well as of the constant availabilty of adequate emergency care. Sedation is specifically contraindicated in severe (Table 55.6) asthmatic attacks since sedating a severely ill, exhausted asthmatic can result in acute respiratory failure (38) and even death.

An important adjunct to the psychosocial management of childhood asthma is the encouragement of a general exercise program. Asthma should not be an automatic excuse preventing participation in physical education and sports. With appropriate premedication, asthmatics can participate in most activities. Some activities may be less asthmogenic than others (see "Exercise-Induced Asthma" above) (7). It is important not to isolate the asthmatic from his peers by unnecessary restrictive measures.

Infections. Upper respiratory tract infections can cause transient increases in nonspecific airways reactivity with persistent coughing, and occasional bronchospasm in nonasthmatics (Chapter 28, Respiratory Infections, and Chapter 53, under "Cough"). In fact, these reactions may be so severe and persistent that these "nonasthmatics" require treatment with bronchodilators. Therefore, it is not surprising that most asthmatics have attacks triggered by respiratory infections.

If there is clinical evidence of an acute bacterial respiratory infection associated with an asthmatic attack, antibiotic therapy should be initiated. Usually, the initial drug of choice is either tetracycline or ampicillin, administered for 7 to 10 days, unless the sputum smear or culture dictates the use of a different antibiotic regimen.

Pharmacological Treatment

Pharmacological therapy is the primary therapeutic modality used to treat reversible bronchospasm in asthma and in chronic obstructive lung disease (55). The five drug categories generally available include (a) sympathomimetics, (b) theophylline preparations, (c) antiallergic drugs, (d) anticholinergics, and (e) corticosteroids. Detailed knowledge of the mechanism of action and side effects of these drugs is important for every physician who takes care of patients with reversible airways disease. The selection of an appropriate drug regimen is complicated by the many preparations available for most of these agents. Specific combinations, dosage, and route of delivery will often be determined by whether these drugs are used for preventive therapy in stable asthmatics or for the emergency treatment of acute asthma.

Sympathomimetic agents.. This group of drugs may be functionally divided into agents that have α- and β-sympathomimetic activities. More recently, β agonists have been further divided into those with β_1 and β_2 selective actions (Table 55.8). The undesirable side effects of β agonists are due to their β_1 actions which stimulate the cardiovascular system, causing tachycardia and, possibly, arrhythmias. The β_2 actions of these drugs increase cyclic AMP levels in mast cells and bronchial smooth muscle, thereby inhibiting mediator release and directly dilating the airways smooth muscle.

Epinephrine has both α- and β-adrenergic effects, while *isoproterenol* is a potent β_1- and β_2-sympathomimetic agent. Besides lack of specificity, these older sympathomimetics have a shorter duration of action because they are rapidly metabolized by catechol-*ortho*-methyltransferase (COMT), an enzyme present in high concentrations in the gut. Therefore, these drugs can only be administered by an aerosol or parenteral route and their duration of action is shorter. Two proprietary medications, Bronchaid and Primatine Mist, are metered dose inhalers that deliver 0.23 and 0.20 mg of epinephrine, respectively. Newer β_2-sympathomimetic agonists (metaproterenol, terbutaline, albuterol, fenoterol) are not

Table 55.8.
β-Sympathomimetic Agonists

Generic Name	Trade Name	B$_2$ Selectivity		Onset of Action	Inhalation Peak Effect	Duration of Effect	Dosage Form
				min	*min*	*hours*	
Isoproterenol	Isuprel Mistometer	$\beta_2 =$	β_1	1–5	5–15	1–2	Metered dose inhaler, 131 μg/puff Nebulized solution, 1:100, 1:200
Isoetharine	Bronkosol Bronkometer	$\beta_2 >$	β_1	5	5–15	2–3	Metered dose inhaler, 340 μg/puff Nebulized solution, 1%
Metaproterenol[a]	Alupent	$\beta_2 >>>$	β_1	1–5	30–60	2–5	Metered dose inhaler, 0.65 μg/puff Nebulized solution, 5% Tablets, 10 and 20 mg
Terbutaline	Brethine Bricanyl Brethaire	$\beta_2 >>>$	β_1	1–5	30–60	2–5	Metered dose inhaler, 200 μg/puff Injection, 1 mg/ml Tablets, 2.5 and 5 mg
Bitolterol	Tornalate	$\beta_2 >>>$	β_1	3–5	30–60	4–8	Metered dose inhaler, 370 μg/puff
Albuterol	Proventyl Ventolin	$\beta_2 >>>>$	β_1	5–15	60–90	3–6	Metered dose inhaler, 90 μg/puff Tablets, 2.4 and 4.8 mg
Fenoterol[b]	Berotec	$\beta_2 >>>>$	β_1	1–5	60	4–8	Metered dose inhaler, 200 μg/puff

[a] Available as a proprietary product.
[b] Pending release in the United States.

metabolized by COMT and thus have a longer duration of action than isoproterenol. These agents have progressively greater β_2 selectivity and potency as shown in Table 55.8. Improved effectiveness of the newer β-sympathomimetic aerosol preparations has made them an integral part of the treatment of reversible airways obstruction. Unfortunately, these agents still retain some β_1 cardiac side effects and, furthermore, when administered systemically, all cause skeletal muscle tremor, a specific β_2 side effect. This annoying symptom may occur even when oral treatment with terbutaline or metaproterenol is begun at reduced doses, but it frequently improves with continued therapy (2 weeks). *Ephedrine* is widely used because it is well absorbed orally, but its side effects include stimulation of the cardiac and central systems, thereby limiting its usefulness. The need to counteract these side effects has led to fixed dose combination tablets which contain ephedrine, a sedative, and a theophylline preparation. These drug combinations, although convenient and popular, do not meet the specific needs of an individual and usually do not deliver an adequate therapeutic dose of any of its components. Since newer β_2 agonists (metaproterenol and terbutaline) are well absorbed orally, they should replace ephedrine.

For the ambulatory treatment of asthma, the new β_2-sympathomimetic agonists can be used as aerosols to prevent asthmatic attacks caused by known trigger factors, such as exercise, cold air exposure, or inhaled irritants. When therapy with an inhaled agent is begun, all patients should be shown how to use a metered dose inhaler, and thereafter their technique should be checked periodically. Illustrations showing the correct technique are usually included in the package insert. This process should be performed as follows. The patient should shake the inhaler before use. Then at the end of a normal exhalation or at functional residual capacity, the inhaler should be held up to the open mouth and triggered at the beginning of a slow gradual inspiration to total lung capacity; slow, not rapid, inspiration should be particularly emphasized to the patient. That breath should be held for approximately 5 or more seconds. A second inhalation of the drug can be taken immediately, or the patient can wait 15 minutes before the second dose. This allows for deeper penetration of the aerosol into the lung since the first breath should dilate the airways. In patients who require continuous treatment for either short periods during an exacerbation or chronically because of persistent bronchospasm, two inhalations are taken every 6 to 8 hours. Recently, some physicians have been prescribing the use of inhaled sympathomimetics at more frequent intervals (every 3 to 4 hours). Although this treatment is usually safe, it should not be used in patients with cardiac disease (33).

Often acute asthmatic attacks are initially treated in the physician's office, but when they are severe (Tables 55.5 and 55.6), treatment should be started in the office and the patient should then be sent to an emergency room. In an acute asthmatic attack, subcutaneous epinephrine (0.1 to 0.3 ml of 1:1000) or inhaled isoproterenol (two inhalations of 131 μg/metered dose/breath) are effective therapeutic regimens (20, 33, 48). These medications can be repeated three times at 30-minute intervals in young patients without heart disease. However, since both of these drugs have significant cardiac side effects, there is a trend to replace them with a specific β_2-sympathomimetic agonist. *Metaproterenol, terbutaline, and albuterol* are available for aerosol administration and *fenoterol* will soon be released for aerosol administration (Table 55.8) (42). Terbutaline is currently available for parenteral administration and may be preferred to parenteral epinephrine because of its sustained action. However, repeat administration of parenteral terbutaline should be performed cautiously since this drug has a long duration of action and in high doses still produces unwanted cardiac side effects.

Theophylline preparations. Numerous theophylline preparations are available for the treatment of reversible airways disease. The physician should become familiar with two of these compounds, choosing an inexpensive short acting agent (such as generic aminophylline) and a long acting preparation (such as LaBid, Phyllacintin, Somophyllin-CRT, Sustaire, or Theo-Dur) (43). In the future, the ophylline preparations with a longer duration of action (24 hours) may be marketed, but further experience is necessary before they can be recommended routinely. The toxic side effects of theophylline include stimulation of the central nervous system, nausea, vomiting, and inotropic and chronotropic cardiac actions. Toxic levels of these drugs cause grand mal seizures, cardiac arrhythmias, and even death (56). For the most part, gastrointestinal side effects are related to serum levels of theophylline and not to the direct effects of oral theophylline on the gut mucosa. Absorption from the gastrointestinal tract and metabolism of theophylline in the liver vary and may require adjustment of dosage in different individuals. The dose of theophylline should be reduced in patients with liver disease, congestive heart failure, or a history of seizures. Several drugs (e.g., cimetidine, propranolol, and erythromycin) depress the metabolism of theophylline. Adolescents and heavy smokers often metabolize this drug more rapidly and may require increased doses. Ideally, peak plasma theophylline levels should be maintained between 10 and 20 μg/ml. At higher plasma levels, there is an increase in serious side effects, such as central nervous system irritability and cardiac tachyarrhythmias. In many ambulatory patients, the measurement of serum the-ophylline levels is usually not indicated, especially when there is a good therapeutic response and no evidence of side effects. However, in patients with altered theophylline clearance (liver or cardiac disease) or in those in whom high doses are required to achieve therapeutic effects, monitoring the serum theophylline level is important. Blood should be sampled 1 to 2 hours after a drug dose to establish the peak serum level.

Initial therapy with oral aminophylline should start with 200 mg administered three or four times/day; however, some patients may require ultimately as much as 1200 to 1600 mg daily. The dose can be increased every 2 to 5 days while the patient is observed for therapeutic and toxic effects. The new, long acting theophylline preparations, although more expensive, appear to be useful because patient compliance is improved since these preparations are usually taken only twice a day. However, three daily doses are required in individuals who metabolize theophylline rapidly. Frequently, therapeutic levels are achieved with lower doses. Treatment should begin with 200 mg twice a day and the dose should be increased by a 100-mg increment/a day every 2 to 3 days. Many patients complain of nervousness, mild gastric distress, and headache when any of the theophylline preparations are started. These distressing side effects usually resolve during continued therapy (2 to 4 weeks).

Antiallergic drugs. Cromolyn (Intal) is a drug that does not act as a bronchodilator and, although its exact mechanism of action is unknown, it may stabilize mast cells, preventing immunological release of mediators (6), or may improve nonspecific airways reactivity. It is administered as an inhaled dry powder, usually three to four times a day, which occasionally causes coughing and mild bronchospasm in some asthmatics. Because of these irritant properties, it is contraindicated in acute asthmatic attacks, and it may be necessary to administer a nebulized sympathomimetic bronchodilator before cromolyn during routine use. Recently a nebulized cromolyn solution without irritant side effects has become available, and a metered dose inhaler in canister form is scheduled for release in the United States.

Cromolyn is an effective prophylactic agent in some allergic and nonallergic asthmatic patients and is specifically useful in patients with significant exercise-induced asthma. Acute administration of 20 mg before exercise may prevent exericise-induced bronchospasm. It is usually used chronically in allergic asthmatics with known factors that specifically trigger asthma such as animal dander. Its effectiveness in patients with other forms of reversible obstructive airways disease is difficult to predict, but when effective, some severe asthmatics may be able to reduce systemic steroid requirements (see below). Some physicians are using cromolyn for the initial therapy of chronic allergic asthma. Initially it should be administered for a trial period of 2 to 4 weeks. Symptoms and objective pulmonary function tests (spirometry) should be used to assess its efficacy. Patients for whom cromolyn is prescribed should understand that its effect is to prevent but not to treat an asthma attack. This is important because many patients associate the use of inhaled medications with the symptomatic treatment of acute asthma.

Pretreatment with *antihistamines* does not prevent or reduce bronchospasm produced by inhaled specific antigen. Therefore, antihistamines should not be used to treat airways obstruction in allergic asthmatics. However, these drugs can be used to control allergic or vasomotor rhinitis (Chapter 23) in patients who also have asthma.

Anticholinergic agents. One of the first forms of treatment for asthma was inhalation of anticholinergic agents. A rationale for the use of these drugs is that airway tone is maintained by the parasympathetic nervous system; inhaled anticholinergic agents block postganglionic efferent vagal neural control of airway tone and cause bronchodilation. Another reason is that anticholinergic agents also block reflex bronchospasm (see "Asthma and Airways Hyperreactivity," page 642). Use of these agents was abandoned until recently because of unwanted side effects such as drying of respiratory secretions, reduced bronchial mucociliary transport, blurred vision, urinary retention, and cardiac and central nervous system stimulation. Atropine is the most potent anticholinergic agent, but when inhaled some of it is absorbed systemically. Although atropine is frequently used to treat bronchospasm, it is not officially approved for use as a bronchodilator by the Food and Drug Administration. When atropine is used, a total dose of 0.8 to 1.6 mg (atropine sulfate parenteral solution) is inhaled from a hand nebulizer (DeVilbiss) every 4 to 8 hours. Some asthmatics, and many patients with chronic obstructive bronchitis, improve airways function with atropine treatment, and it may be tried in combination with or as an alternative to inhaled sympathomimetic agents (31). Recently, a new compound, ipratropium (Sch 1000 or Atrovent), a quaternary ammonium compound, has become available for experimental use. It will soon be released commercially and is available at present from Boehringer-Ingelheim, Ltd. for individual patients whose bronchospasm is improved only by inhaled atropine. Its major advantage is that it is not absorbed systemically during inhalation therapy (11, 53). The exact role of these agents in the treatment of obstructive airways disease will be determined only after they are widely available.

Corticosteroids. Corticosteroids are effective agents for treating reversible obstructive airways disease, but their exact mechanism of action is unknown. They cause bronchodilation and reduction in bronchial inflammation and improve the response to β-sympathomimetic agents. The onset of their therapeutic effects is delayed and does not begin for 6 to 12 hours (33, 36). Steroids may be administered as "*burst*" *therapy* in which high doses (40 to 80 mg of prednisone) are started and tapered rapidly (10 to 20 mg a day) over a 7- to 10-day period. "Burst" therapy is used to treat severe asthma attacks or acute severe exacerbations of bronchospasm in patients with reversible chronic obstructive lung disease. The major side effects from "burst" therapy are steroid-induced abnormalities in glucose metabolism. However, when corticosteroids are used to treat severe obstructive airways disease for *prolonged periods*, they may produce many other unwanted systemic side effects (Cushing's syndrome, adrenal pituitary suppression, osteoporosis, *etc*). In addition, the patient's ability to deal normally with infectious processes is impaired. Since reactivation of tuberculosis can occur during chronic corticosteroid treatment, any patient with a positive purified protein derivative skin test should receive simultaneous INH (isoniazid) prophylaxis. Acute adrenal insufficiency may occur during stressful medical or surgical illnesses (Chapter 74). Whenever chronic steroid therapy is begun in an ambulatory setting, objective pulmonary function tests are required to evaluate its therapeutic effectiveness since some patients will feel better due to the euphoria produced by steroids but have unchanged pulmonary function. The lowest effective dose should be employed and, if possible, alternate-day steroid therapy should be attempted. This should be done by decreasing the dose of prednisone by 5 mg every 2 to 3 days and measuring the FEV_1 periodically (weekly). When symptoms of bronchospasm worsen, the tapering process should be slowed. If bronchospasm improves after prolonged treatment, then further reduction or elimination of prednisone therapy may be possible. Aerosolized steroids (see below) or cromolyn may be useful to help reduce or even eliminate the need for systemic steroids in some patients.

Nonabsorbable corticosteroid aerosols (beclomethasone: Vanceril, Beclovent) are available. The technique for inhaler use described on page 649 should be reviewed with the patient who is beginning to use an aerosolized steroid. The use of these agents often permits a reduction or, if the patient is taking 20 mg of prednisone or less a day, even the elimination of oral steroid therapy. Treatment may also be initiated with these inhaled agents. Side effects from aerosolized steroid preparations are negligible but include the development of oral candidiasis, which is prevented by rinsing the mouth with water immediately after inhaling the steroids or treated by gargling with small doses of an antifungal agent, e.g., mycostatin. The usual dose of beclomethasone is 84 μg (two breaths) inhaled three to four times a day; the maximum dose, in severe asthmatics, is 20 inhalations (840 mg) a day. Whenever inhaled steroid therapy is started, the dose of oral steroids should be decreased slowly (5 to 10 mg weekly) in patients who have been treated with systemic corticosteroids for long periods of time. If patients being treated with beclomethasone have an acute exacerbation of asthma, treatment with oral prednisone should be reinstituted.

General Approach to Pharmacological Therapy of Reversible Airways Disease

The purpose of this section is to integrate some of the principles of the pharmacological treatment of bronchospasm that have been discussed separately under specific drug categories (55).

Occasional Symptomatic Use of Bronchodilators

During remission or in patients with very mild asthma ($FEV_1 > 70\%$ predicted), the occasional symptomatic use of aerosolized specific β_2-sympathomimetic agonists usually controls intermittent episodes of bronchospasm (Fig. 55.6). Alternatives to aerosol therapy are the use of theophylline derivatives or oral preparations of β_2-sympathomimetic agonists (metaproterenol, terbutaline). Such occasional use of bronchodilators can control intermittent episodes of bronchospasm and prevent bronchospasm from specific known stimuli (exercise, cold air, irritants). Also cromolyn can be used intermittently to treat exercise-induced asthma.

Chronic Bronchodilator Therapy

There are two choices for initial continuous therapy in patients with reversible obstructive airways disease who cannot be managed with occasional intermittent bronchodilators. One choice is to treat these patients with aerosolized β_2-sympathomimetic agents. Ordinarily these drugs are effective and have

fewer systemic side effects than theophylline preparations (33, 48). However, many physicians use theophylline as the drug of choice for chronic bronchodilator therapy. Those patients whose bronchospasm is not controlled with a single bronchodilator require combination therapy. Recent questions have arisen about potential unwanted cardiac side effects during combination therapy with theophylline and oral β_2-sympathomimetics in patients with cardiovascular disease (40). In patients with known cardiac disease, oral theophylline preparations should be combined with *inhaled* specific β_2-sympathomimetics (58).

The role of anticholinergic agents in the treatment of bronchospasm still needs to be determined. There are patients with chronic obstructive bronchitis who respond poorly to aerosolized β-sympathomimetics but show significant bronchodilation with inhaled atropine (31). Cromolyn provides effective prophylactic treatment for allergic and exercise-induced asthma. In allergic patients, this drug must be used continuously. Systemic corticosteroids should be reserved for status asthmaticus and for severe chronic asthma that does not respond to conventional therapy.

Acute Asthmatic Attacks

Less severe acute asthmatic attacks can be treated either with aerosolized β_2-sympathomimetics or oral theophylline preparations. If there are objective signs of a severe asthma (Tables 55.5 and 55.6), traditional regimens such as subcutaneous injections of epinephrine or inhaled isoproterenol are more effective than are theophylline preparations (48). The addition of theophylline seems indicated in the treatment of *severe* acute asthma ($FEV_1 < 1.0$ liter) (20). More recently, systemic therapy with subcutaneous injections of terbutaline is being substituted for epinephrine. Also, the new selective β_2-sympathomimetic agents may be preferable to inhaled isoproterenol.

Depending on individual reliability, patients with reversible airways obstruction should be instructed what medications (usually a sympathomimetic aerosol or an oral theophylline compound) they can use for self-treatment before they must contact the physician (30). For example, an intelligent young adult asthmatic should know that he can use an inhaled β-sympathomimetic agonist more frequently (every 2 to 4 hours) and can take an extra dose of aminophylline to self-treat a mild asthma attack. If he does not improve after a 4-hour period, then he should call his physician.

Other Specific Therapeutic Measures in Asthma

Respiratory Therapy

During acute asthmatic attacks, there is increased water loss from the respiratory tract and a tendency,

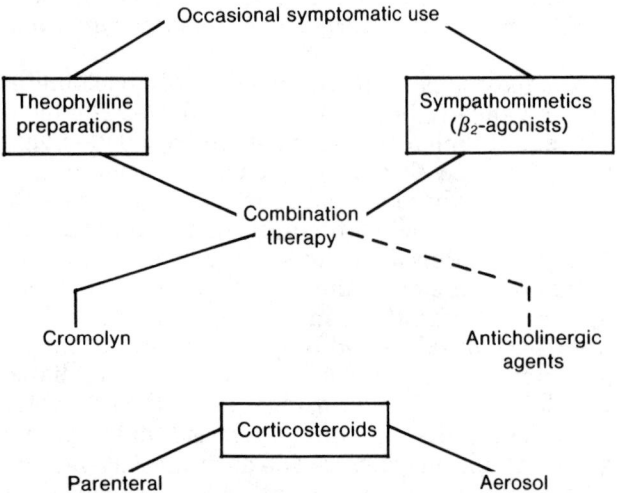

Figure 55.6. Approach to the pharmacological treatment of reversible airways disease (see the text).

especially in young children, for patients to become dehydrated. Usually oral rehydration is adequate. During the winter months when ambient room air is dry, a home humidifier will effectively increase the water content of the air. Care should be taken to clean these humidifiers to prevent the accumulation of molds or fungi. Rarely dehydration is so severe that parenteral or nebulized humidification becomes necessary. Ultrasonic aerosols which are hypo- or hypertonic and inhaled mucolytic substances from ultranebulizers irritate the airways and produce bronchospasm and coughing. Therefore, these forms of respiratory therapy should be avoided. Finally, there is no scientific basis for the use of intermittent positive pressure breathing ventilators (IPPB) either as a form of respiratory therapy or as a means of delivering bronchodilators (39).

Oxygen

In rare cases when asthmatics with objective evidence of severe asthma (Tables 55.5 and 55.6) are treated in the physician's office, the administration of humidified oxygen may be indicated. If the patient does not improve, he should be sent to an emergency room. In the usual uncomplicated young asthmatic without chronic hypoventilation and CO_2 retention, there is little risk of causing respiratory failure by blunting the hypoxic ventilatory control. Only enough oxygen (28 to 35% venturi mask or 2 liters/minute nasal cannula) should be administered to improve arterial PO_2 into a normal range (65 to 80 mm Hg).

Medical Complications of Reversible Airways Disease

There are a number of medical complications of asthma that may impair the patient's response to the usual therapeutic regimens (Table 55.9). In general, these complications should be sought if there is not an appropriate therapeutic response.

Table 55.9.
Medical Complications of Reversible Airways Disease

COMPLICATIONS OF BRONCHODILATORS
Paradoxical fall in arterial oxygenation
Paradoxical bronchospasm
Cardiac arrhythmias
ATELECTASIS
PULMONARY INFECTIONS
Bronchitis
Pneumonia
AIR IN EXTRAPULMONARY SPACES
Penumothorax (tension)
Pneumomediastinum
ALLERGIC BRONCHOPULMONARY ASPERGILLOSIS

Complications of Pharmacological Treatment

In severe asthma, bronchodilators may cause a paradoxical fall in arterial oxygenation by altering the pulmonary homeostatic mechanisms that match ventilation and perfusion in the lungs. These falls in arterial oxygenation are small (5 to 10 mm Hg) and are easily treated with supplemental oxygen. Although this paradoxical hypoxemia is an indication for oxygen administration, it is not an indication to withdraw bronchodilator therapy.

Very rarely, the propellants used to aerosolize sympathomimetic and corticosteroid agents may provoke paradoxical bronchospasm. If an asthmatic complains of coughing and wheezing after using one of these aerosols, a different preparation should be employed.

Sympathomimetics and theophylline preparations stimulate cardiac activity and may cause arrhythmias, especially when used in therapeutic doses, in the presence of moderate hypoxemia or in elderly patients with pre-existing cardiac disease (40). However, arrhythmias can also be triggered by bronchospasm and hypoxemia during acute airways obstruction. In these situations, reversal of bronchospasm and improvement in gas exchange often improve the arrhythmias.

Mechanical Airways Obstruction

Mucus impaction in the airways may lead to microatelectasis or to the collapse of a pulmonary segment or of an entire lobe of the lung. Patients with major lobar collapse should be hospitalized. Frequently, the symptoms and physical signs of atelectasis are obscured during acute asthmatic attacks by wheezing and dyspnea. Therefore, atelectasis is best diagnosed with a chest roentgenogram (see Chapter 54). Usually, atelectasis will improve after treatment of bronchospasm, hydration, and physical therapy (coughing, chest percussion, and postural drainage). Bronchoscopy to remove an obstructing mucus plug is rarely needed. In fact, in a patient with reactive airways disease and acute bronchospasm, it may even worsen bronchospasm and provide only temporary improvement of atelectasis.

Infection

While pulmonary infections often precipitate asthmatic attacks, bronchitis and pneumonia (see Chapter 28) may develop as a complication of asthma. Development of purulent sputum during the course of a prolonged or persistent asthmatic attack requires re-evaluation for superimposed infection, with a sputum smear and then appropriate antibiotic therapy.

Extrapulmonary Air

Rarely, air can accumulate abnormally in the extrapulmonary spaces. The presence of a pneumomediastinum is best detected by a chest roentgenogram, but it is frequently associated with subcutaneous air in the neck, thorax, and groin (palpable crepitus). Although no specific therapy is indicated, the patient should be hospitalized for careful observation because air may dissect into the pleural space. A pneumothorax can only be detected effectively by a chest roentgenogram and if a pneumothorax develops during an acute attack, regardless of its size, the patient should be hospitalized since the subsequent development of a tension pneumothorax can be life threatening.

Allergic Bronchopulmonary Aspergillosis

Rarely, allergic bronchopulmonary aspergillosis complicates chronic asthma (50). These patients have airways obstruction that does not improve with usual therapeutic measures; they have febrile episodes associated with a cough productive of purulent sputum containing dark brown plugs, and a chest roentgenogram that shows focal bronchiectasis and mucus impaction. They often have pulmonary infiltrates that change location during serial roentgenographic studies. These patients usually have blood eosinophilia and serum precipitins as well as immediate and delayed skin reactions to *Aspergillus* antigen. Early treatment with corticosteroids may improve bronchospasm, and it prevents progression to irreversible bronchiectasis. If this diagnosis is suspected, consultation with a pulmonologist or an allergist is advisable.

Course and Prognosis of Asthma

The course and prognosis of pure bronchial asthma are not well understood. Traditionally, it is thought that uncomplicated asthma developing during childhood or early adult life is not a risk factor for progressive fixed obstructive pulmonary disease. However, there is also evidence that airways hyperreactivity and allergy are found more frequently in patients with severe obstructive pulmonary disease, so that these factors may be risks for the development of chronic airways obstruction. Further epidemiological studies are necessary to define these relationships (5, 9, 29).

In general, when bronchial asthma begins at an early age, it usually improves, although the estimation of the rate of remission from childhood asthma varies in different studies from 30 to 70% (26). After a spontaneous remission, some childhood asthmatics will experience a recurrence of symptomatic asthma during adulthood. These latter patients, as well as patients with adult onset intrinsic asthma, often have asthma that is persistent and severe. Other patients who had a history of bronchial asthma during childhood, which seemed to resolve spontaneously, develop chronic progressive airways obstruction later in life. Additional risk factors, such as chronic cigarette smoking and exposure to urban and industrial air pollution, complicate their disease

(see page 644). Furthermore, it is unknown whether their history of bronchial asthma and associated airways hyperirritability are additional risk factors for the development of fixed obstructive lung disease.

Although death from asthma, or one of its complications, is rare, it does occur with a recorded incidence in the United States of 1 in 100,000 or approximately 2,000 deaths during the course of a year. Deaths in young asthmatics are usually preventable since they are caused by one of the medical or therapeutic complications that have been discussed. For example, in England in the early 1970s, increased mortality from bronchial asthma coincided with the marketing of high dose isoproterenol inhalers. It was postulated that these patients developed cardiovascular toxicity and arrhythmias from isoproterenol overdosage by the repeated use of these inhalers (16). Often acute respiratory failure and death in status asthmaticus are attributable to sedation of seemingly anxious patients whose respiratory drive is easily depressed because of fatigue and exhaustion. Asthmatics who manifest the objective signs of severe asthma (Tables 55.5 and 55.6) should receive rapid emergency treatment and should be hospitalized if they do not improve rapidly. Asthma can worsen as quickly as it can improve with appropriate therapy.

Management of the Pregnant Asthmatic (57)

Most studies suggest that pregnancy has an unpredictable effect on asthma, with most patients experiencing no change in their disease and a small percentage either improving or experiencing deterioration. However, asthma may affect the outcome of pregnancy with a reported 2-fold increase in perinatal mortality and a small increase in the risk of infant prematurity. While the incidence of these complications is slight, prolonged asthmatic attacks produce hypoxemia and acid-base disturbances that can cause serious fetal complications. Therefore, prompt treatment of severe asthmatic attacks is important, and this may require the use of drugs which, at least theoretically, may produce some adverse effects on maternal and fetal function.

In general, management of the pregnant asthmatic is the same as is the treatment of the nonpregnant asthmatic (see "General References," Weinberger). *Theophylline and sympathomimetic agents* are generally safe for the fetus but may cause uterine smooth muscle dilatation and may, thereby, inhibit labor. While the newer inhaled specific β_2-sympathomimetic drugs are not officially approved for use during pregnancy, there are no reports of adverse fetal effects caused by any of these agents. In contrast, drugs such as *epinephrine*, which have α-adrenergic properties, can reduce uterine and placental blood flow due to vasoconstriction and, at least theoretically, may impair fetal circulation.

While *cromolyn* also has not been approved for use during pregnancy, animal studies have not documented adverse effects in the fetus. Commonly used corticosteroid preparations, such as prednisone and prednisolone, cross the placenta poorly, and therefore fetal adrenal steroid production is not compromised when the mother receives these drugs. However, systemic corticosteroids do suppress maternal adrenal function, and supplemental steroids are frequently required to treat maternal stress during labor. Inhaled steroids have not been officially approved for treatment of pregnant asthmatics, but it would appear, because of their reduced systemic absorption, that their potential for affecting the fetus is negligible.

CHRONIC AIRWAYS OBSTRUCTION: CHRONIC OBSTRUCTIVE BRONCHITIS AND EMPHYSEMA

Patients with advanced chronic airways obstruction have a clinical course characterized by progressive loss of pulmonary function that eventually leads to respiratory failure and death. Usually management of these patients focuses upon the treatment of exacerbations of airways obstruction and pulmonary infection, basically providing palliative support for the complications of this disease. However, before the development of irreversible progressive air flow obstruction, there is a period when functional impairment and pathological abnormalities are potentially reversible. Therefore, this discussion will emphasize not only the therapy of symptomatic obstructive lung disease, but also the identification of susceptible individuals at a time when the development of irreversible airways disease is preventable.

Chronic progressive airways obstruction is most commonly caused by chronic obstructive bronchitis and emphysema. Chronic bronchitis is defined in clinical terms but has certain pathological correlates. In contrast, emphysema, a specific morphological diagnosis, has associated clinical correlates, pulmonary function abnormalities, and characteristic roentgenographic patterns. In their pure forms, these two diseases represent distinct processes with different pathological features and clinical manifestations. However, clinically they usually coexist (54).

It is very difficult to estimate the prevalence of chronic bronchitis and emphysema in the United States since there is often an insidious onset of respiratory symptoms and many patients are not diagnosed until relatively late in the course of their disease. However, as much as 15 to 25% of the adult population has a history compatible with chronic bronchitis. How many of these have clinical airways obstruction is unknown. Autopsy series show that approximately 60% of adult men and 15% of adult women have some evidence of emphysema.

Definitions

Chronic Bronchitis

Chronic bronchitis is defined as a clinical syndrome characterized by cough and sputum production that occurs on most days for at least a 3-month period during 2 consecutive years. Most often these symptoms are due to chronic bronchial irritation that is precipitated by agents such as cigarette smoke and air pollution. This results in hyperplasia of globet cells and mucus-secreting glands and in chronic mucus hypersecretion. By definition this excessive production of mucus is not due to specific diseases such as bronchiectasis, tuberculosis, or heart disease. Morphological changes that correlate with the clinical diagnosis of chronic bronchitis are initially found in small airways (< 2 mm) and later progress to involve other parts of the tracheal bronchial tree (Fig. 55.3). The hypertrophied mucus glands occupy a greater proportion of the bronchial wall, which is inflamed, edematous, and eventually fibrotic. The lumina of peripheral airways are frequently filled with mucopurulent secretions (54).

Simple chronic bronchitis. A large proportion of patients who smoke develop chronic bronchitis. Most of these patients cough up a small quantity of mucoid sputum each morning. They either ignore this chronic cough or willingly accept it as a minor complication of cigarette smoking. Some of these patients will have intermittent episodes of purulent sputum production and occasional mild wheezing associated with upper respiratory tract infections. Many of these patients do not have a demonstrable impairment of expiratory airflow or an increased rate of decline in pulmonary function.

Chronic obstructive bronchitis. At the other end of the spectrum is a disease characterized by progressive airflow obstruction and chronic mucopurulent sputum production. The bronchi, normally sterile, are chronically infected. The factors that protect certain individuals and place others at risk for the development of airflow obstruction are not completely understood (see below). It is known that those who are susceptible to the effects of cigarette smoking and chronic bronchopulmonary infection have a progressive course, with accelerated loss of lung function that leads to pulmonary disability and eventual respiratory failure (Fig. 55.7).

Emphysema

Pulmonary emphysema is defined in anatomical terms and is a diagnosis that is made with certainty only by a pathologist. It is morphologically defined as permanent abnormal dilation and destruction of the alveolar ducts and air spaces distal to the terminal bronchioles. Each component of this definition is important. The enlargement must be permanent; therefore, the temporary overdistension of the lung that occurs in asthma cannot be regarded as

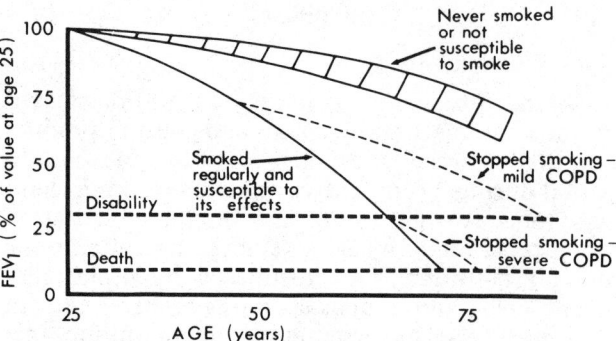

Figure 55.7. Effect of risk factors from smoking on the loss of lung function (FEV_1). The *upper curves* are derived from subjects who do not smoke or are not susceptible to the effects of smoking. They lose lung function gradually throughout adult life (15 to 30 ml/year). *Lower curves* show accelerated loss of lung function in subjects who are susceptible to the effects of cigarette smoke. At age 65 there is respiratory disability since FEV_1 has decreased to 25 to 30% of predicted (1 to 1.2 liters) and further functional deterioration will eventually cause death due to complications of respiratory insufficiency. If that subject stops smoking, life may be prolonged but a respiratory death will still eventually result. If intervention is initiated earlier in life (40 to 50 years) when there is mild COPD, accelerated loss of lung function is reversible and a respiratory death will be avoided. Although this figure illustrates theoretical loss of FEV_1 for an adult cigarette smoker, susceptible smokers will lose lung function at different rates, thereby becoming disabled at different ages. (Modified from Fletcher C, Peto R: The natural history of chronic airflow obstruction. *Br Med J* 1:1645, 1977.)

emphysema. The enlargement must be abnormal; thus the changes that occur with normal aging cannot be considered to be true emphysema. Perhaps the most important concept is that there should be accompanying disruption of alveolar walls. Since the pathological definition of emphysema is nonspecific, it is necessary to classify emphysema into anatomical subtypes. The most important, clinically, are centrilobular and panlobular emphysema (54).

Centrilobular emphysema. This form is generally considered to represent the commonest type of emphysema. In centrilobular emphysema there is mainly destruction of the respiratory bronchioles and alveolar ducts which become confluent to form emphysematous spaces. Deposits of carbonaceous material are found in these areas. The distal alveolar sacs are often spared. The emphysematous lesions are located in the proximal acinar space at the center of the lobules between the conducting airways and the alveolar sacs. The major clinical association of centrilobular emphysema is chronic obstructive bronchitis due to cigarette smoking where pathological abnormalities in the peripheral airways are the

rule. Early disease with patchy pulmonary involvement does not cause roentgenographic abnormalities. But when it is far advanced, pathological and roentgenographic examination shows that centrilobular emphysema is primarily located in the upper lung fields.

Panlobular emphysema. This less common form of emphysema is characterized by uniform involvement of the pulmonary lobule with morphological destruction of the distal structures and alveolar capillary membrane. Panlobular emphysema is less commonly associated with chronic bronchitis and cigarette smoking, tends to occur in the lower lung fields, is more frequently associated with the formation of cysts and bullae, and is found in patients with hereditary α_1-antitrypsin deficiency (see below) and with bronchiolar obliteration. Frequently the two major forms of emphysema occur in combination, with centrilobular emphysema in the upper lung zones and panlobular in the lower. However, pathological distinction is difficult to make when severe disease exists.

Other forms of emphysema include paraseptal emphysema, which is associated with spontaneous pneumothorax, and irregular emphysema, which is found in patients with diffuse pulmonary fibrosis.

Etiology

There are many risk factors and proposed etiologies associated with the development of chronic obstructive airways disease. They are listed in order of relative importance in Table 55.10. Knowledge of these factors is important in understanding those measures that may alter the progression and thus prevent the development of irreversible chronic airways obstruction.

Age

The average nonsmoking adult shows a yearly decline of 15 to 30 ml in FEV_1 with increasing age. Thus an FEV_1 of 4 liters in a 25-year-old would be expected to fall to almost 3 liters by age 65 (Fig. 55.7) (21). However, this normal loss of lung function is not associated with pulmonary disease. Additional

Table 55.10.
Risk Factors and Airways Obstruction (Approximate Order of Relative Importance)

AGE
INHALED IRRITANT AND NOXIOUS AGENTS
   Smoking
   Urban and industrial air pollution
HEREDITY
   Familial incidence
   α_1-Antitrypsin deficiency
SEX (MALE > FEMALE)
SOCIOECONOMIC STATUS
AIRWAYS HYPERREACTIVITY

risk factors add to the effects of this loss of pulmonary function and act synergistically to cause clinical airways obstruction (15, 29).

Inhaled Irritant and Noxious Agents

The common factor that exists in the great majority of patients with chronic airways obstruction is exposure to inhaled irritant and noxious agents.

Cigarette smoking. Cigarette smoke represents the most obvious and widespread pulmonary contaminant. Since 1940 when cigarette consumption in the United States increased to present high levels (10 lb of cigarettes *per capita*), there has been a progressive rise in the incidence and death rate from obstructive pulmonary disease and lung cancer. Various studies have shown that there is pathological evidence of either chronic bronchitis or emphysema in patients with more than a 40-pack year history of smoking (defined as number of years smoking X packs of cigarettes/day). Furthermore, the risk of dying from chronic lung disease is from 3 to 14 times greater in smokers than in nonsmokers.

The deleterious effects of cigarette smoke may be specific or may be due to nonspecific effects of inhaled irritants on the tracheal bronchial tree. For example, stimulation of mucus secretion may result in the loss of normal mucociliary clearance mechanisms. If infection develops, inflammatory cells release proteolytic enzymes that may cause destruction of the pulmonary parenchyma by overwhelming the lungs' protective defenses. Moreover, smoking also depresses the phagocytic function of the alveolar macrophage, increasing the tendency for respiratory infections (4).

Specifically, cigarette smoking seems to have a significant effect on loss of lung function, and patients who smoke heavily decrease their FEV_1 by an average of 40 to 60 ml/year. A patient whose FEV_1 was 4 liters at age 25 would have an FEV_1 of 2 liters by the age of 65 (Fig. 55.7) (21). Unfortunately, some smokers lose lung function even more rapidly and approach a loss in FEV_1 of 60 to 80 ml/year. Nevertheless, patients who stop smoking may resume the normal 30 ml/year rate of decline within 1 year after the cessation of cigarette smoking. In some patients who continue to smoke, the rapid decline in lung function causes clinical obstructive pulmonary disease (Fig. 55.7) (15, 29).

Urban and industrial air pollution. The effects of air pollution from exposure to urban or industrial environments on the development of chronic obstructive airways disease are unknown. Photochemical oxidant air pollutants include ozone and nitrogen dioxides which are formed by the effect of solar radiation on automobile and truck emissions. Low concentrations of sulfur dioxide and other particulate matter from the burning of fossil fuels are also present in an urban environment where there are also trace amounts of miscellaneous substances (ar-

senic, asbestos, cadmium, hydrogen sulfide, lead, and mercury). Periods of atmospheric inversions with increased environmental levels of air pollutants have been associated with exacerbations and even death in patients with cardiopulmonary disease. The sequelae of high exposures to these agents are airway inflammation, pulmonary parenchymal damage, and obstructive pulmonary disease. Furthermore, recent studies of low level exposures to all three of these agents demonstrate that they cause transient airways hyperreactivity in normal subjects and an exacerbation of respiratory symptoms in asthmatics (8). Therefore, it is probable that air pollution and cigarette smoking act synergistically to trigger symptomatic exacerbations and pulmonary function abnormalities in patients with chronic obstructive pulmonary disease. However, it is not known to what extent exposure to low levels of urban and industrial air pollutants contributes to the etiology and progression of pulmonary disease.

Heredity

Familial incidence. First degree relatives of patients with chronic obstructive airways disease have abnormal lung function and an increased rate of decline of their FEV_1. This relationship holds even when other risk factors, such as smoking, are controlled. The relationship of this finding to the well known familial aggregation of asthma, allergy, and airways hyperreactivity is poorly understood (see below) (29).

α_1-*Antitrypsin deficiency.* While diseases such as cystic fibrosis are obvious inherited causes of obstructive lung disease that begins in childhood, α_1-antitrypsin deficiency is a rare genetic abnormality that causes liver disease in children and panlobular emphysema in adults. α_1-Antitrypsin deficiency should be suspected when emphysema develops without a history of chronic bronchitis or smoking in patients below the age of 45 or when multiple family members develop obstructive lung disease at an early age. Serum antiproteolytic activity is determined by the Pi (inhibitor) phenotype. Normal individuals have two M genes and are considered MM phenotypes, whereas patients with α_1-antitrypsin deficiency have two Z genes or a ZZ phenotype. Homozygous α_1-antitrypsin deficiency is found in only 1 in 4000 people, but at least 60% of ZZ phenotypes will develop severe emphysema during adulthood. These individuals also have a high incidence of cirrhosis, and the combination of lung and liver disease with an onset in early to middle adult life may indicate the presence of this syndrome. It is postulated that a deficiency of α_1-antitrypsin activity makes the lung vulnerable to damage by the endogenous proteolytic enzymes released by inflammatory cells. Inheritance is co-dominant so that the heterozygote, MZ, as well as several other mixed genotypes have intermediate levels of circulating antitrypsin. Recent evidence suggests that partial deficiency (heterozygote) is not a risk for the development of obstructive lung disease even when other factors such as smoking are present. The diagnosis of this condition is discussed below (page 660).

Sex

Male sex seems to be an important predisposing factor for the development of obstructive airways disease. Even in nonsmoking young males, there is still accelerated loss of lung function compared to nonsmoking premenopausal females. After menopause, women appear to have a more rapid decline in FEV_1 than similarly age-matched male controls (15, 29). In addition, the acute and chronic physiological effects of cigarette smoking are different in men. In young men, cigarette smoking causes changes in peripheral airways function, while similar changes are not produced by cigarettes in premenopausal women. This is especially interesting since the earliest pathological abnormalities of chronic bronchitis are in the peripheral airways. The reasons for these sex differences are unknown, but they may relate either to the protective effects of female sex hormones or to the deleterious effects of androgens.

Socioeconomic Status

People from lower socioeconomic groups seem to decrease FEV_1 at a faster rate than those from higher economic groups. While the risk factor is still found after controlling for the effects of smoking, sex, and age, it may well relate to increased exposure of the respiratory tract to airborne pollutants in urban environments or to industrial exposures to noxious agents (15).

Airways Hyperreactivity

Recent studies of first degree relatives of patients with obstructive lung disease show that those with hyperirritable airways lose lung function at accelerated rates (9) as do patients with significant chronic airways obstruction who are hyperreactive to inhaled agents (methacholine) (5). It is not known whether this airways hyperirritability develops as a consequence of obstructive lung disease or is a risk factor *per se*. Allergy may also influence this relationship since allergic factors are associated with hyperreactivity and have been found with increased frequency in patients with far advanced obstructive lung diseases (29).

Clinical Presentation

History

Usually, patients with emphysema present with dyspnea and those with chronic obstructive bronchitis, with cough and sputum production. These two diseases are so interrelated that most patients have manifestations of both. It is useful, however, to recognize the characteristic features of these syndromes. These are summarized in Table 55.11. Although these two types represent extremes of a clinical spectrum, occasional patients are seen who qualify as having relatively pure emphysema (type A) or bronchitis (type B).

The usual patient with chronic airways obstruction has a long history of a chronic cough with mucopurulent sputum production. The onset of dyspnea is insidious but progressive. Frequently, these patients attribute their poor exercise tolerance to the effects of age or sedentary life style and their chronic cough to the effects of smoking. Often they develop clinically apparent airflow obstruction (wheezing) during upper respiratory tract infections, and the recovery period from these respiratory infections is prolonged. Eventually, dyspnea becomes so severe that it interferes with routine activities and medical attention is sought. In other patients, a respiratory tract infection triggers airway obstruction and acute respiratory failure. Milder forms of obstructive airway diseases are often diagnosed as incidental findings during a routine physical examination, a preoperative evaluation, or a medical evaluation for an unrelated disease. Occasionally, patients with chronic airways obstruction (emphysematous type) will be seen because of progressive weight loss that may initially suggest the presence of an occult malignancy.

When the diagnosis of advanced obstructive airways is well established, its course is relentlessly progressive. In patients with bronchitis, daily cough and sputum production usually increase, becoming more purulent and tenacious during infectious exacerbations. Some patients have difficulty clearing respiratory secretions during attacks of airflow obstruction. In these patients, the production of scant, viscous, purulent sputum may precede the development of respiratory failure. Wheezing and dyspnea are often persistent features of severe disease. Chronic hypoxemia causes cor pulmonale, and the patient will note peripheral edema and weight gain. Some patients will experience asthmatic episodes that periodically worsen their baseline airways obstruction. Usually, these are associated with respiratory infections, but they may be triggered by any of the stimuli that precipitate an acute asthmatic attack.

Physical Examination

In individual patients, physical findings depend on the severity and type of chronic obstructive airways disease (Table 55.11). Vital signs may be normal or show tachypnea and a pulsus paradoxus (see page 646) during severe bronchospasm. In milder forms of obstructive lung disease ($FEV_1 > 1.2$ liters), auscultation of the chest may be unremarkable or may reveal either rhonchi due to mucus within the

Table 55.11.
Clinical Findings in Emphysematous and Bronchitic Varieties of Chronic Airways Obstruction

Findings	Type A (Emphysema)	Type B (Bronchitis)
CLINICAL PRESENTATION:		
Dyspnea	Early onset, severe progressive	Insidious onset, intermittent during infection
Cough	Onset after dyspnea	Precedes onset of dyspnea
Sputum	Scant and mucoid	Copious and purulent
Respiratory infection	Rare	Frequent
Body weight	Thin, weight loss	Normal or overweight
Respiratory insufficiency	Late manifestation	Frequent episodes
PHYSICAL EXAMINATION:		
Cyanosis	Absent	Often present
Plethora	Present	Absent
Chest percussion	Hyperresonant	Normal
Chest auscultation	Distant breath sounds, end expiratory wheezing	Rales, rhonchi, wheezes
Cor pulmonale	Often terminal	Common
LABORATORY EVALUATION:		
Hematocrit value	Normal	Occasional erythrocytosis
Chest roentgenogram	Hyperinflation with increased anteroposterior diameter and flat diaphragms. Attenuated vascular markings, bullous changes, small vertical heart	Increased bronchovascular markings with normal to enlarged heart and evidence of old inflammatory disease
PHYSIOLOGICAL EVALUATION:		
Spirometry	Irreversible expiratory obstruction, airway closure	Expiratory obstruction, reversible component
Total lung capacity and residual volume	Marked increase	Mild increase
Lung elastic recoil	Marked reduction	Near normal
Diffusion capacity	Marked decrease	Normal or slight reduction
PaO_2		
Rest	Slightly decreased (65–75 mm Hg)	Marked decrease (45–65 mm Hg)
Exercise	Often falls	Variable (decrease to increase)
$PaCO_2$	Normal or low (35–40 mm Hg)	Normal or elevated (40–60 mm Hg)
Pulmonary hypertension	None to mild, worsens during exercise	Moderate to severe variable exercise response
PATHOLOGY	Widespread emphysema, may be panlobular	Chronic bronchitis with or without mild centrilobular emphysema

airways or wheezing if bronchospasm is prominent. Breath sounds may be distant in patients with severe emphysema. Frequently, the diagnosis of airways obstruction is best made during the physical examination by performing a timed FVC. After inspiring to total lung capacity, the patient should perform a complete maximal expiration through an open mouth. This maneuver usually produces audible wheezing in patients with chronic obstructive airways disease, while in patients with severe emphysema whose airways collapse, faint wheezing may be all that is heard. In everyone with significant expiratory airflow obstruction, the timed FVC will be prolonged beyond 4 to 5 seconds. Many other respiratory findings occur with progressively severe disease and primarily reflect pulmonary hyperinflation. These include an increased anteroposterior diameter of the chest, widened intercostal spaces, hyperresonance, a decreased area of cardiac dullness, and low diaphragms. The same signs of severity found in patients with asthma, such as use of accessory muscles of respiration, occur in individuals with chronic airways obstruction during acute attacks of bronchospasm (Tables 55.5 and 55.6).

When cor pulmonale develops there is often cyanosis, a right ventricular heave, a holosystolic murmur along the left sternal border, an S_3 gallop, and varying degrees of hepatomegaly and peripheral edema. Neck veins will be distended and a large V wave with a Y descent is visible as pulmonary hypertension worsens, causing tricuspid valve dilation and insufficiency.

Laboratory Testing

Pulmonary function testing. The most characteristic functional defect in patients with chronic obstructive bronchitis and emphysema is decreased forced expiratory flow. This obstructive defect is best measured with a spirogram, which should be employed in the diagnosis and assessment of severity in chronic obstructive airways disease as well as for the evaluation of specific therapeutic regimens (see page 638 for the patient experience during this procedure). It is also useful in predicting the prognosis, course, operative risk (see Chapter 86), and work potential (Table 55.1) (12, 17). In general, it is unusual for patients with an FEV_1 of approximately 2 liters, or 60% of predicted, to experience significant dyspnea during normal physical activities. On the other hand, reduction of the FEV_1 below 1.2 liters or 40% of predicted is associated with dyspnea on mild exertion and significant disability. The severity of hyperinflation will be reflected by a reduction in vital capacity as well as by increases in lung volumes (59). Residual volume is usually elevated and, in emphysematous patients, total lung capacity is increased. When emphysema is present, the diffusion capacity of the lung is reduced, reflecting the loss of functional alveolar capillary membrane available for gas exchange. The presence of significant airways obstruction, hyperinflation, and a reduced diffusion capacity for carbon monoxide correlates with the pathological finding of emphysema (Fig. 55.8) (24, 54).

Arterial blood gas analysis. In evaluating and treating patients with significant chronic obstructive airways disease ($FEV_1 < 1.2$ liters), baseline arterial blood gas analysis is necessary to measure the level of oxygenation and adequacy of alveolar ventilation. When the FEV_1 is greater than 1.2 liters, resting arterial blood gases are usually relatively normal or show only mild hypoxemia. With more severe airways obstruction ($FEV_1 < 1.0$ liter), the degree of hypoxemia and hypercapnea will depend on the ventilation perfusion abnormalities and pulmonary homeostatic mechanisms. Since hypoxemia correlated only roughly with the severity of airways obstruction as reflected by spirometry, arterial blood gases must be measured to evaluate the degree of resting hypoxemia in order to guide the treatment of cor pulmonale (see below). In addition to hypoxemia, it is important to know whether the patient has a chronically elevated arterial $PaCO_2$ indicating alveolar hypoventilation. The diagnosis of acute respiratory failure in patients with severe obstructive lung disease is usually made by finding either an acute fall in arterial oxygenation (absolute $PaO_2 < 55$ mm Hg) and/or an acute increase in $PaCO_2$ tension of more than 10 mm Hg with associated acute respiratory acidosis. Such acute changes usually require hospitalization and intensive treatment.

Other laboratory tests. Normally, the mucopurulent sputum produced by patients with chronic obstructive bronchitis is infected with a mixed bacterial flora including *Streptococcus pneumoniae* and *Haemophilus influenzae*. Other pathogens may be present, depending on the frequency and type of broad spectrum antibiotic treatment. Sputum culture is usually indicated only when there is parenchymal pulmonary infection (pneumonia), and specific treatment will depend on the predominant organism seen on Gram stain and cultured from the sputum. A complete blood count will document erythrocytosis, which indicates significant hypoxemia, and eosinophilia, which may suggest allergic or asthmatic etiologies. A white blood count and differential count are helpful in the evaluation of pulmonary infection. An electrocardiogram may show arrhythmias, atrial hypertrophy (P pulmonale), and evidence of pulmonary hypertension (persistent S waves in the lateral precordial leads).

Patients who develop emphysema at an early age (45 or younger) with a history of cigarette smoking or chronic bronchitis, give a familial history of emphysema, or have roentgenographic evidence of panlobular emphysema should be screened with serum protein electrophoresis during symptom-free periods. If the α_1-peak is absent, then an α_1-antitrypsin level should be measured (available from a commercial laboratory). α_1-Antitrypsin is an acute phase reactant and should not be measured during periods of infection. If both the α_1-peak and antitrypsin level are low, then genetic phenotyping should be obtained if possible. This is important (29) for prognosis and genetic counseling. However, phenotyping is only done in a few medical centers in this country.

Roentgenographic Findings

As many as 50% of patients with significant chronic airways obstruction will have normal or near normal chest roentgenograms. In the others, there will be a variety of findings which are relatively nonspecific. Despite this, a chest roentgenographic examination is important both in the diagnosis and in the overall management of patients with airways obstruction. Specifically it is useful as a baseline study for the future evaluation of radiological abnormalities as well as to exclude other associated pulmonary diseases, such as pneumonia, atelectasis, or a pneumothorax.

Bronchitis. In patients with chronic obstructive bronchitis, there may be increased tubular markings, especially at the lung bases, that suggest thickening and disease of the bronchi. These patients may have increased vascular markings, evidence of pulmonary hypertension, and right heart enlargement, but their roentgenograms usually do not show marked hyperinflation or cystic or bullous changes.

Emphysema. The diagnosis of emphysema can often be made from a chest roentgenogram when severe morphological changes in the lung result in obvious roentgenographic findings (Fig. 55.8). In milder cases of emphysema, it is difficult to make a specific diagnosis. Many of the findings that are

A

	Actual	Predicted	% Predicted	Post BD[a]	Post/Pre BD[a]
SPIROMETRY					
FVC	2.32 liters (L)	3.99 L	58	2.50	107
FEV$_1$	0.98 L	3.17 L	30	1.15	117
FEV$_1$/FVC %	42	79.4		46	
LUNG VOLUMES					
(He dilution)					
TLC	7.82 L	6.29 L	124		
VC	2.86 L	3.99 L	71.7		
FRC	5.64 L	3.72 L	152		
RV	4.96 L	2.30 L	215		
DIFFUSING CAPACITY					
(single breath)					
DLCO[c] ml	11.6	24.4	47.5		
ARTERIAL BLOOD GASSES[b]					
PaO$_2$	56 mm Hg				
PaCO$_2$	48 mm Hg				
PH units	7.38				

[a] Bronchodilator.
[b] At rest, sitting, breathing room air.
[c] Diffusion capacity for carbon monoxide.

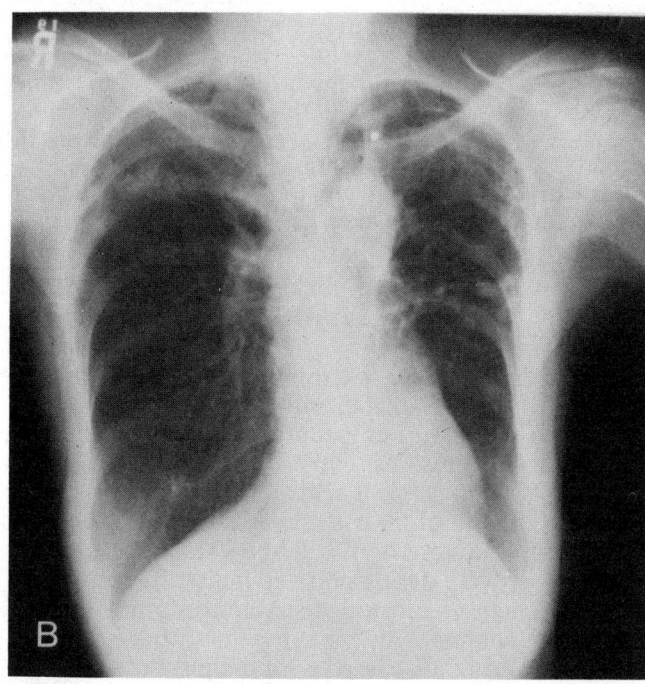
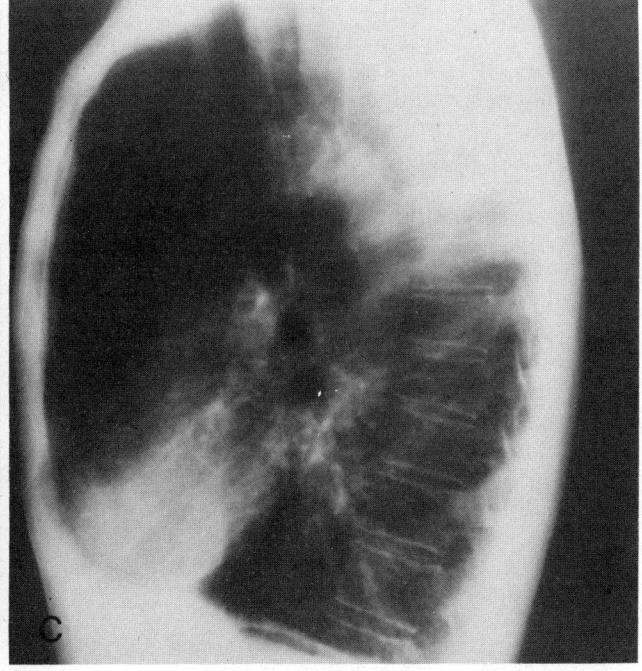

Figure 55.8. *A.* Typical pulmonary function test results in a patient (male, 60 years old, 161 lb, 69 inches tall) with severe chronic obstructive pulmonary disease and probable emphysema. Forced expiration demonstrates a severe obstructive ventilatory defect with an immediate response to aerosolized bronchodilators. Spirograms do not reach a plateau, indicating slowly emptying areas of lungs. Lung volumes show an elevated total lung capacity (*TLC*) and residual volume (*RV*) indicating hyperinflation consistent with obstruction, suggesting early airway closure. Single breath CO diffusion capacity is reduced, indicating loss of effective alveolar capillary surface area for gas exchange. Reduced diffusion capacity and airway obstruction are consistent with the presence of emphysema. Arterial blood gases show an elevated carbon dioxide tension indicating hypoventilation, a mild compensated respiratory acidosis, and low oxygen tension with desaturation. This patient with chronic airflow obstruction is hyperinflated, has a reduced diffusion capacity suggesting emphysema, and has hypoxemia associated with chronic CO$_2$ retention. His chest roentgenogram (*B* and *C*) is compatible with emphysema and shows hyperinflation and bullous changes with loss of vascular lung markings (see the text). *VC,* vital capacity; *FRC,* functional residual capacity.

associated with emphysema only reflect hyperinflation, which occurs in asthma or during a bronchospastic exacerbation in patients with chronic obstructive bronchitis. The changes characteristic of hyperinflation include an increased radiolucency of the lungs, an increase in the anteroposterior diameter of the thorax, an enlarged retrosternal air space, and a low and flat diaphragm which makes a greater than 90° angle with the sternum on the lateral views (Fig. 55.8). Changes in vascular markings in the lung fields are often subtle and difficult to detect, especially when there is congestion of the pulmonary veins or parenchymal infection. Regional or generalized loss of vascularity in the peripheral lung fields with rapid tapering of the proximal branches of the pulmonary artery occurs more frequently in panlobular emphysema, especially in the lower lung fields. Centrilobular disease tends to show increased bronchovascular markings, especially in the lung bases. The pulmonary parenchyma needs to be examined carefully for the presence of cysts or bullae, although frequently these structures cannot be distinguished from the hyperlucent lung fields. Occasionally, an upper lobe bulla will be mistaken for a pneumothorax and a chest tube will be inserted inappropriately. Therefore, it is necessary to obtain a good quality baseline chest roentgenogram of every patient with moderate to severe obstructive airways disease. Although not indicated in the routine diagnosis of bullous disease, both chest tomography and computerized axial tomographic (CT) scanning of the lung will visualize cystic spaces in the pulmonary parenchyma.

Cardiac evaluation. The heart frequently appears small and is located in a vertical position. In the diagnosis of ventricular failure, the usual radiological criteria for cardiac enlargement are not valid. Often one must look for subtle findings of a change in cardiac size by reviewing serial chest roentgenograms. More recently, noninvasive diagnostic tests which include biplane echocardiography and gated heart pool scanning have become available to evaluate the function of both the left and the right ventricles (see Chapter 60).

MANAGEMENT OF THE AMBULATORY PATIENT

General Measures

The primary goal in managing the ambulatory patient with obstructive airways disease is to prevent progression of the disease. When there is severe fixed airflow obstruction, therapeutic goals include improving symptoms and decreasng pulmonary disability by treating any reversible components of bronchospasm, heart failure, and infection. It is clear that prevention and prompt treatment of exacerbations in chronic airways obstruction will improve the quality and duration of life.

The successful management of this chronic disease requires a comprehensive approach either by the physician or by a medical team that includes a therapist, vocational counselor, and visiting respiratory nurse clinicians as well as active participation by the physician. Studies have shown that patients consider their physician to be very influential. Whatever preventive and therapeutic measures are selected, they will be more effective if the physician actively coordinates and supports them. For example, it seems that physicians advise their patients to stop smoking only when there are findings consistent with overt lung disease such as objective evidence of abnormal chest roentgenograms, pulmonary function tests, or evidence of respiratory infection. Furthermore, in smoking cessation programs only 25% of participants said their physician actively participated and on further questioning most indicated that their physician would have been influential in affecting the outcome of the program (see Chapter 20).

If possible, the nurse, respiratory therapist, and physician should work together as a team, instructing the patient and his spouse. Ideally, general instruction should include information about pulmonary anatomy and physiology as well as basic information about the etiology and prognosis of chronic airways obstruction. This instruction can be given in individual as well as in group sessions and should be supplemented with visual aids and booklets which are published by the American Thoracic Society and available for distribution through the local (state) and national lung associations.

Even if therapeutic interventions do not markedly improve respiratory function, appropriate adaptation of a patient's life style and recreational activities is worthwhile. For example, while exercise programs do not improve pulmonary function, they physically condition sedentary patients, making them able to participate in a wider range of activities (see below). In patients with severe disease resulting in curtailment of their usual recreational activities, counseling on alternative hobbies and activities may help to prevent depression and maintain useful family interactions. Although sexual dysfunction is extremely common in these patients, this important aspect is rarely discussed with the physician. Sexual activity is often made easier by the use of supplemental oxygen or pretreatment with a bronchodilator. Alternatives include making the nondyspneic person the more active partner or the use of different positions (see Petty in "General References"). If the patient's disease precludes ambulation, then follow-up patient care is often best performed by home visits. The respiratory nurse clinician with the aid of the patient's spouse can facilitate this type of care. When the disease becomes terminal, the nurse and the physician can counsel the patient and his family about the possibility of dying at home (see Chapter 19). The physician should allay the patient's fears of suffocation and struggling since death is often peaceful, with the patient eventually dying in a coma secondary to CO_2 retention. Furthermore, one needs to discuss with the patient and his family whether resuscitative attempts such as intubation and prolonged mechanical ventilation in an intensive care unit are appropriate and desirable. During this period, support from the physician, family, and clergy is vital. The patient may often be made comfortable with therapeutic modalities that include fluids, oxygen (see below), and sedation, if necessary.

Preventive Management

The *early diagnosis* of very mild peripheral airways disease is made with sophisticated pulmonary function testing that is not generally available. Furthermore, it is questionable whether physicians can motivate patients with subclinical asymptomatic disease to modify their life style. However, there is a period when mild to moderate airways obstruction is easily diagnosed using a spirogram (Fig. 55.1) and modification of the patient's habits and treatment with bronchodilators, if indicated, may prevent the development of irreversible obstructive lung disease (Fig. 55.7). The routine screening with spirometry of patients at risk (greater than 35 years of age who have a significant smoking history or chronic bronchitis) will identify many patients with significant obstructive lung disease. For example, in our laboratory, approximately 35% of healthy Baltimore firemen between the ages of 25 and 45 who had screening spirometry as part of a physical examination exhibited at least mild degrees of airflow obstruction. Prevention of the development of irreversible airways obstruction may well depend on behavior modification in such patients. Smoking cessation and the avoidance of industrial irritants will be better accepted by the patient when he knows the results of objective testing and the prognostic significance of these abnormalities. It is probable that the course of obstructive lung disease can be favorably altered by a systematic program (smoking cessation and bronchodilator therapy) in patients under 50 years of age with an FEV_1 more than 2 liters (29).

Important to any preventive regimen is complete *cessation of cigarette smoking*. This is especially true in any patient with homozygous PiZZ (α_1-antitrypsin deficiency). There are many smoking cessation programs and regimens that have been used with varying success rates. In evaluating the results of these programs, objective methods to assess their efficacy must be used (blood carboxyhemoglobin levels, sputum thiocyanate levels). Furthermore, the follow-up period must be long enough to judge that their effectiveness was not transient. At present, objective evaluation of these programs shows that only approximately 15 to 20% of subjects are able to abstain from smoking for 1 year. Strategies and methods for the physician to utilize in programs for smoking cessation are discussed in Chapter 20.

While *pulmonary infections* cannot be specifically linked to the progression of obstructive airways disease, the effective treatment of bacterial exacerbations is important since acute respiratory failure can be precipitated if exacerbations are not promptly treated. Furthermore, vaccination with anti-influenza and antipneumococcal vaccines may be useful in preventing pneumonia which can be devastating in patients with severe obstructive lung disease (see Chapter 32).

Reduction of Secretions

Removal of Secretions

In patients with chronic airways obstruction and mucus hypersecretion, therapeutic interventions are aimed at the reduction and removal of respiratory secretions. Pulmonary secretions are normally cleared from the lung by mucociliary clearance and coughing. In obstructive airways disease, both of these mechanisms are impaired (see Chapter 53, under "Cough"). Often coughing is not effective because of airway collapse during forced expiration. Postural drainage and chest percussion can remove mucus secretions from the airways and these measures should be used by the ambulatory patient whenever there is persistent hypersecretion. Patient instruction in postural drainage and chest percussion can be obtained by referral to a respiratory therapy department, or the physician can learn these principles by referring to the literature such as is given under "General References" (Respiratory Therapy). In addition, the mobilization of secretions is aided by pretreatment with two breaths of an aerosolized bronchodilator (β_2-sympathomimetic, see page 000). Often the best times for this type of respiratory therapy are before retiring at night and after arising in the morning. Thus the patient may be able to sleep more restfully and also may be aided in clearing secretions that have accumulated during the night. If significant pulmonary hypersecretion is not present, these measures are not indicated (22).

Avoidance of Irritants

Respiratory secretions will be stimulated both directly and reflexly by inhaled irritants. Furthermore, these substances cause bronchospasm which prevents mobilization of secretions. Therefore, smoking, urban and industrial pollutants, and other irritating inhaled substances must be avoided. This includes avoiding "passive smoking" by inhaling ambient air that is contaminated with tobacco smoke since this has been shown to increase airways obstruction in asthmatics.

Alteration of Sputum Character

It has never been effectively proven that oral hydration will thin respiratory secretions and improve pulmonary function in obstructive lung disease (see "General References"—Conference on Scientific Basis of Respiratory Therapy). Nevertheless, most physicians still recommend that patients without significant heart failure should drink approximately 1 liter of fluid daily.

Mucolytic agents are irritating substances that cause direct and reflex bronchospasm. Furthermore, liquefaction of bronchial secretions in patients who are unable to mobilize them adequately with effective coughing may be deleterious.

Even if bronchial secretions are thick and viscous, treatment with a bland aerosol (normal saline) has not been shown to be effective. For example, patients with cystic fibrosis with thick bronchial secretions do not show improvement in clinical status after bland aerosol treatment (47).

Treatment of Infection

Most patients with chronic bronchitis have a course that is characterized by intermittent infection with mucopurulent sputum. Treatment of these acute infectious exacerbations with a broad spectrum antibiotic that is active against *S. pneumoniae*, *H. influenzae*, and other common pathogens is indicated. Usually, a 7- to 10-day course of either ampicillin, tetracycline, or trimethoprim-sulfamethoxazole is administered. In intelligent, cooperative patients, antibiotic therapy may be initiated by the patient when he notes a change in sputum character or color. In general, continuous antibiotic therapy should be avoided unless there is evidence of persistent chronic infection or bronchiectasis.

Physical Therapy and Rehabilitation

Intermittent Positive Pressure Breathing (IPPB)

Historically, IPPB machines have been used for both physical therapy and the delivery of bronchodilators. However, there is no scientific basis for the use of IPPB machines. In fact, IPPB may induce transient pulmonary overdistension that is harmful in these patients who are already hyperinflated (22, 39). IPPB may be useful in the delivery of medications to patients who are so severely obstructed that they are unable to take a deep breath from a freon-powered metered dose inhaler or hand bulb nebulizer (DeVilbiss). This circumstance is rare in ambulatory practice. Many patients who already have IPPB machines at home are so psychologically dependent on this form of physical therapy that the physician may decide that the use of such a machine should be continued. The administration of oxygen through any IPPB machine is contraindicated, because the oxygen mixture setting which supposedly delivers 40% oxygen usually administers much higher concentrations.

Breathing Exercises

There is scientific evidence that pursed lip breathing may help an emphysematous patient maintain airways stability during expiration (see Petty, "General References"). Diaphragmatic exercises may give the patient a sense of well-being and may improve diaphragmatic muscle function. These breathing exercises are usually taught by a respiratory therapist. Specific details about them are available in the medical literature (22).

Exercise Rehabilitation

Exercise retraining programs do not improve pulmonary function, but they do seem to improve exercise tolerance and skeletal muscle function. Probably this is due to the nonspecific effects of training in sedentary poorly conditioned patients. Furthermore, after exercise training the patient may be able to perform a given level of exercise at a lower oxygen consumption and a lower minute ventilation. Community-based exercise training programs are more frequently available for cardiac rehabilitation (see Chapter 58). Occasionally, these may be adapted to the needs of patients with chronic obstructive pulmonary disease. If no organized programs are available, the physician should consider instructing his patients in an informal program of graded increases in physical activity (see (22) and "General References").

Change in Environment

In selected circumstances environmental change may be important therapeutically. Some patients seem to improve when they move from cold winter climates to either warm humid or warm dry climates. There is no evidence that the course of obstructive lung disease is altered by such environmental changes. Perhaps some of these patients improve by escaping from urban industrialized areas with air pollution. When such a move is contemplated, its social and economic effects must be carefully weighed by the patient and his family. Environmental changes are more important in patients with hypoxemia who live at altitudes above 4000 feet where atmospheric oxygen tensions are less than 120 mm Hg compared to 150 mm Hg at sea level. A move to a low altitude may improve hypoxemia and decrease pulmonary hypertension. Since the adverse psychological consequences of such a move may outweigh its medical benefits, those patients may do as well remaining at high altitude by using treatment with low flow oxygen (see below). Travel in an airplane or vacationing in high altitude areas may be contraindicated in patients with severe hypoxemia. Since airplane cabins are maintained at a pressure equivalent of 5000 feet, low flow supplemental oxygen should be administered throughout flight to patients with arterial PaO_2 under 55 mm Hg. Also, vacations in high altitude locations (above 4000 feet) should be avoided in patients with severe chronic hypoxemia (PaO_2 less than 55 mm Hg).

Treatment of Bronchospasm

Initial and maintenance therapy of bronchospasm is outlined in detail in the discussion of asthma in this chapter. In patients with chronic reversible airways disease, the principles of pharmacological treatment are similar to those used in asthma; however, the response of patients to bronchodilators is usually not as marked. Some patients (Fig. 55.8) increase their FEV_1 only by 10 or 15%, but the response of only a few hundred milliliters may provide significant improvement in exercise tolerance. A poor response to inhaled bronchodilators during laboratory testing does not preclude improvement after chronic therapy with pharmacological agents. Such patients should have a repeat assessment of their lung function after a period of 1 to 2 months. If there is still no response to high doses of bronchodilators, patients with severe bronchospasm (FEV_1 < 1.2 liters) should be given a therapeutic trial with corticosteroids (see below). When there is no objective or symptomatic improvement, bronchodilators may be discontinued, although some physicians recommend continued maintenance therapy to prevent bronchospastic exacerbations. There is some evidence that patients who do not respond to inhaled β-sympathomimetic agonists may improve airways function with inhaled anticholinergic agents (see page 651). Also, combinations of these two agents have been used successfully to treat patients with chronic bronchitis and obstructive lung disease (18). Very rarely, patients with a history of allergy or childhood asthma may improve with cromolyn (6).

If exercise tolerance is severely impaired by dyspnea, or if there is a poor or absent response to standard bronchodilators, a trial with *corticosteroids* is indicated (see page 651). A favorable response to steroids occurs more frequently in patients with reversible airways disease when there is blood or sputum eosinophilia or when there is a previous history of allergy or asthma. Usually, a trial of systemic corticosteroids such as prednisone (40 mg/day) is maintained for 3 to 6 weeks. Before, during, and after therapy, objective evaluation of lung function with spirometry is mandatory. Usually, systemic steroids are used in these trials because they are more effective than aerosolized preparations. If there is improvement, the steroid dose should be reduced while the patient is monitored with serial spirometry. Aerosolized corticosteroid agents can be used to supplement standard bronchodilators, can be used with systemic steroid therapy, or can even be substituted if the effective dose of oral prednisone is less than 20 mg/day. Prednisone doses less than 5 mg/day are not therapeutic and should be discontinued, or aerosolized steroid agents should be substituted.

Treatment of Heart Failure

Cor Pulmonale

In severe chronic airways obstruction (FEV_1 < 1.0 liter) pulmonary hypertension and cor pulmonale (Table 55.12) are caused by chronic hypoxemia (PaO_2 < 50 mm Hg). This severe hypoxemia also causes erythrocytosis, renal function abnormalities, impaired cognitive function, emotional instability, and dyspnea at rest and during exercise. Chronic low flow oxygen therapy is indicated when severe oxygen desaturation persists despite appropriate treatment (Table 55.13) (1, 22, 41). Other supplementary measures include the use of diuretics, salt restriction, and phlebotomy when the hematocrit value exceeds 60. When oxygen therapy is effective, erythrocytosis and peripheral edema usually improve. Since chronic therapy with oxygen is costly (approximately $3000 to $4000/year for 2 liters of O_2 for 24 hours), it should be used judiciously. Furthermore, when high concentrations of oxygen are ad-

Table 55.12.
Treatment of Heart Failure

COR PULMONALE
   Oxygen
   Salt restriction, diuretics, KCl
   Phlebotomy
PULMONARY VASCULAR CONGESTION (LEFT VENTRICULAR FAILURE)
   Salt restriction, diuretics, KCl
   Digitalis (?) (increased sensitivity to digitalis in cor pulmonale)

Table 55.13.
Low Flow Oxygen Therapy in Obstructive Airways Disease

INDICATIONS
   Pulmonary hypertension and cor pulmonale
   Erythrocytosis
   Neuropsychological status
   Exercise intolerance
COMPLICATIONS
   Cost
   Respiratory depression
METHODS OF DELIVERY
   Source of oxygen (compressed air tank, O_2 generator, portable O_2 source)
   Nasal cannula/Venturi mask
DURATION OF THERAPY
   Intermittent—low flow oxygen when resting PaO_2 > 55 to 60 mm Hg with:
      Exercise-induced dyspnea and hypoxia; relieved by oxygen: documentation by exercise testing
      Nocturnal-dyspnea, restlessness, or insomnia: documented and relieved by oxygen
   Continuous—PaO_2 < 55 to 60 mm Hg after treatment
      Cor pulmonale and congestive heart failure
      Diminished cognitive function
      Persistent erythrocytosis

ministered to severely hypoxemic patients with elevated levels of arterial $PaCO_2$, there may be depression of the respiratory drive, causing acute hypercapneic respiratory failure. Only enough oxygen to raise the resting arterial PaO_2 above 60 to 65 mm Hg is required.

The source of oxygen will be determined by the duration of daily therapy, the flow of oxygen required, and the mobility of the individual patient. For example, oxygen from a large compressed air tank or from an oxygen generator can be delivered to a sedentary patient who does not leave home. If tanks are used, one can be placed in the bedroom and the other in the area of the living quarters where the patient spends most of the day. The use of a costly portable oxygen apparatus is not indicated for a sedentary patient. On the other hand, a patient with exercise-induced hypoxemia who wants to continue to remain active may require a portable oxygen apparatus. Oxygen may be administered through a nasal cannula or through a Venturi mask. While the mask will deliver a complete range of specific oxygen concentrations (24 to 35%), nasal cannulas are usually preferred because they can be used during meals and do not interfere with coughing. A 1-liter flow rate through a nasal cannula delivers approximately 24 to 26% inspired oxygen concentrations, while a 2-liter flow rate delivers approximately 28 to 30%.

The duration of oxygen therapy must be individualized for each patient. If the resting arterial PaO_2 is greater than 55 to 60 mm Hg, intermittent oxygen therapy should be considered for exercise-induced dyspnea or during nocturnal periods when there is evidence of restlessness or insomnia. In these situations, the effect of exercise (see Chapter 53, under "Dyspnea") or sleep (see Chapter 85, Sleep Disorders) on arterial oxygenation must be documented. One cannot predict whether these moderate degrees of resting hypoxemia will worsen, stay the same, or improve during exercise. The clinical implications of arterial oxygen desaturation during sleep are not fully understood. Many patients with obstructive lung disease and moderate hypoxemia ($PaO_2 < 55$ to 60 mm Hg) have worse hypoxemia during sleep. If these changes are documented, low flow oxygen should be employed to prevent the development of cor pulmonale. Continuous therapy with low flow oxygen is indicated when the arterial PaO_2 is less than 55 to 60 mm Hg. In these situations, oxygen administration for at least 12 to 15 hours a day improves survival and reverses pulmonary hypertension (1, 22, 41). Usually erythrocytosis will improve and repeated phlebotomies are not necessary.

Left Heart Failure

The diagnosis of left ventricular failure in patients with severe chronic obstructive lung disease is often difficult. Noninvasive cardiac testing may help to diagnose the presence of left ventricular dysfunction (see "Laboratory Testing" above). The treatment of left heart failure should begin with diuretics and salt restriction. Frequently slight pulmonary vascular congestion is sufficient to cause respiratory decompensation in these patients. The role of digitalis is very controversial, and it should be used as a last resort (see Chapter 60). Many patients with endstage cor pulmonale have cardiac arrhythmias, especially multifocal atrial tachycardia, which are worsened by digitalis. Therefore, throughout the course of digitalis treatment, careful evaluation for toxic side effects is necessary.

Course and Prognosis of Chronic Airways Obstruction

It has been emphasized that lung function deteriorates with advancing age, and risk factors, especially cigarette smoking, accelerate this loss of pulmonary function (Fig. 55.7) (21). Some subjects are more susceptible to these risk factors and lose lung function more rapidly. When the FEV_1 falls below 50% of predicted, its decline seems to be accelerated, and unless progression is prevented, irreversible obstructive lung disease results. Pulmonary disability occurs when the FEV_1 is between 1 and 1.6 liters or about 25% of predicted (see Chapter 9, Table 9.2).

Once obstructive airways disease is established, there is a tendency for the disease to worsen. In a general way, the prognosis of patients with airways obstruction can be estimated from their FEV_1 (12, 17). In moderate obstructive airways disease when the FEV_1 is more than 1.25 liters, the 5-year survival is similar to that determined by the patient's age and sex. If the FEV_1 remains above 1.25 liters, these patients continue to have near normal expected survival (12, 17). If there is evidence of cardiac disease, resting tachycardia, or if the FEV_1 is between 0.75 and 1.25 liters, 5-year survival decreases to approximately 66% of normal. This figure is further reduced to 33% if the FEV_1 is less than 0.75 liter or there is evidence of cardiac disease, tachycardia at rest, hypercapnea, or a very low pulmonary diffusion capacity for carbon monoxide (emphysema). There are obvious exceptions to these general estimates of prognosis (44) since the short and long term response to bronchodilator therapy may alter the progression of airways obstruction. However, it is very useful for the physician to have a general understanding of the prognosis of different levels of airways obstruction based on objective measurement of pulmonary function.

The progressive course of obstructive pulmonary disease should not justify withholding treatment from these patients. There is little doubt that symptoms as well as the quality of life can be markedly improved and life can be prolonged. Figure 55.9 illustrates the response to treatment and subsequent loss of pulmonary function in two patients with

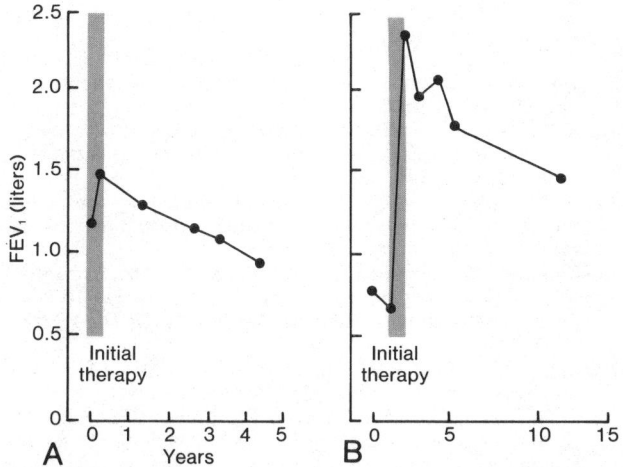

Figure 55.9. Response to treatment and subsequent loss of pulmonary function in two patients with severe chronic airways obstruction. *A.* In this patient, initial therapy increased FEV₁ by 300 ml. However, from this improved FEV₁, there is still progressive deterioration of pulmonary function leading to an eventual respiratory death. *B.* This patient was lost to follow-up for 1 year and FEV₁ deteriorated during that period. He had a better therapeutic response with marked improvement in pulmonary function. Although there was still progressive loss of lung function, from the new baseline FEV₁, respiratory disability was prevented during the 15-year follow-up period. (Modified from Burrows B: *Lung Biology in Health and Disease* (Petty TL, ed). New York, Marcel Dekker, 1978, vol 9.)

severe obstructive airways disease. In patient A, initial therapy increased FEV₁ (300 ml), but after this response, lung function deteriorated progressively, leading to eventual respiratory failure and death. The second patient was lost to follow-up for 1 year and his FEV₁ deteriorated during this period. However, with therapy, there was marked improvement in pulmonary function. Although after treatment there was still progressive loss of lung function, respiratory disability was prevented during a 15-year follow-up period.

Expiratory airflow obstruction seems to be the major cause of disability and increased mortality in patients with chronic obstructive bronchitis and emphysema. There is considerable evidence that early changes in lung function can be detected and diagnosed with a spirogram (Fig. 55.1*B*). Serial measurements, perhaps at yearly intervals, in subjects who are at high risk for the development of chronic obstructive lung disease (cigarette smoking, chronic bronchitis, α_1-antitrypsin deficiency, air pollution, *etc*) would objectively demonstrate an abnormal rate of deterioration and provide the physician with essential diagnostic information. The effectiveness of preventive treatment of early obstructive lung dis-

ease would obviously depend on the physician's ability to modify those factors that are important in the etiology of airways disease in an individual patient. Therefore, a screening spirogram with measurements of FEV₁, FEV₃, and FVC is an important initial step in preventing the development of progressive irreversible airways obstruction.

General References

Normal and Abnormal Physiology

Murray JF: *The Normal Lung.* Philadelphia, WB Saunders, 1976.
    This very readable textbook provides a more extensive discussion of pulmonary mechanics, circulatory physiology, and acid-base balance.
West JB: *Respiratory Physiology: The Essentials,* ed 2. Baltimore, Williams & Wilkins, 1979.
West JB: *Pulmonary Pathophysiology: The Essentials,* ed 2. Baltimore, Williams & Wilkins, 1981.
    These two concise handbooks are excellent reviews of the essentials of pulmonary physiology and pathophysiology.

General Textbooks of Pulmonary Disease

Fishman AP: *Pulmonary Diseases and Disorders.* New York, McGraw-Hill, 1980.
Fishman AP (ed): *Update: Pulmonary Diseases and Disorders.* New York, McGraw-Hill, 1982.
Hinshaw HC, Murray JF: *Diseases of the Chest.* Philadelphia, WB Saunders, 1980.
Guenter CA, Welch MH (eds): *Pulmonary Medicine,* ed 2. Philadelphia, J.B. Lippincott, 1982.
    These four textbooks of pulmonary disease provide excellent extensive discussion of obstructive pulmonary disease.

Asthma

Bailey WC (ed): Asthma. *Clin Chest Med* 5: no. 4, 1984.
    Comprehensive multiauthored review of all aspects of bronchial asthma.
Bienenstock J (ed): *Immunology of the Lung and Upper Respiratory Tract.* New York, McGraw-Hill, 1984.
    This book reviews the immunological basis of lung disease.
Brooks SM, Lockey JE, Harber P (eds): Occupational lung diseases. I. *Clin Chest Med* 2: no. 2, 1981.
Brooks SM, Lockey JE, Harber P (eds): Occupational lung diseases. II. *Clin Chest Med* 2: no. 3, 1981.
Morgan WKC, Seaton A (eds): *Occupational Lung Diseases,* ed 2. Philadelphia, WB Saunders, 1984.
    These three textbooks form a comprehensive review of occupational asthma and lung disease, providing a basis to approach the diagnosis and therapy of disease related to industrial and environmental factors.
Patterson R (Chairman), Sogn DD (Executive Secretary) (eds): *Asthma and the Other Allergic Diseases.* NIAID Task Force Report, NIH Publication no. 79-387. Washington, DC, US Government Printing Office, May 1979.
    This task force report by the National Institute of Allergy and Infectious Diseases provides an extensive discussion of asthma and allergic diseases.

Chronic Obstructive Airways Disease

Hugh-Jones P, Whimster W: The etiology and management of disabling emphysema. *Am Rev Respir Dis* 117:343, 1978.
    State-of-the-art review about the etiology and management of emphysema.
Petty TL (ed): Chronic obstructive pulmonary disease. In *Lung Biology in Health and Disease.* New York, Marcel Dekker, 1978, vol 9.
    This textbook is a comprehensive multiauthored review of

all aspects of the diagnosis and the management (including respiratory therapy) of obstructive pulmonary diseases.
Snider GL (ed): Emphysema. *Clin Chest Med* 4: no. 3, 1983.

Epidemiology and Course of Chronic Obstructive Airways Disease

Epidemiology of Respiratory Diseases Task Force Report. NIH #81-2019. Bethesda, MD. National Institutes of Health, October 1980.
National Institutes of Health publication that reviews the epidemiology and etiology of chronic respiratory diseases.
Fletcher C, Peto R, Tinker C, Speizer FE (eds): *The Natural History of Chronic Bronchitis and Emphysema*. New York, Oxford University Press, 1976.
Macklem PT, Permutt S: The lung in the transition between health and disease. In *Lung Biology in Health and Disease*. New York, Marcel Dekker, 1979, vol 12.
Rom WN (ed): *Environmental and Occupational Medicine*. Boston, Little, Brown, and Co, 1983.
Extensive theoretical and practical multiauthored review of the epidemiology, etiology, and course of chronic obstructive lung disease.

Respiratory Therapy and Pharmacological Treatment

Lertzman MM, Cherniack RM: Rehabilitation of patients with chronic obstructive pulmonary disease. In *Lung Disease—State of the Art 1976–1977*. New York, American Lung Association, 1978, pp 399–419.
State-of-the-art review discussing respiratory therapy and rehabilitation.
Proceedings of the Conference on the Scientific Basis of Respiratory Therapy, Temple University Conference Center at Sugarloaf. Philadelphia, May 2–4, 1974. *Am Rev Respir Dis* 110:193, 1974.
Excellent critical review of the scientific basis of oxygen, aerosol, physical, and intermittent positive pressure breathing therapy.
Shapiro BA, Harrison RA, Trout CA: *Clinical Application of Respiratory Care*, ed 2. Chicago, Year Book Medical Publishers, 1979.
Textbook with discussion of specific modes of respiratory therapy.
Ziment I: *Respiratory Pharmacology and Therapeutics*. Philadelphia, WB Saunders, 1978.
Extensive review of pharmacological treatment of obstructive lung diseases.

Specific References

1. Anthonisen NR: Long-term oxygen therapy. *Ann Intern Med* 99:519, 1983.
2. ATS Statement—Snowbird Workshop on Standardization of Spirometry. American Thoracic Society, Medical Section of the American Lung Association. *Am Rev Respir Dis* 119:831, 1979.
3. Austen KF, Orange RP: Bronchial asthma: the possible role of the chemical mediators of immediate hypersensitivity in the pathogenesis of subacute chronic disease. *Am Rev Respir Dis* 112:423, 1975.
4. Ayres SM: *Cigarette Smoking and Lung Diseases: An Update*. New York, American Thoracic Society, 1975, vol 3, no. 5.
5. Barter CE, Campbell AH: Relationship of constitutional factors and cigarette smoking to decrease in 1-second forced expiratory volume. *Am Rev Respir Dis* 113:305, 1976.
6. Bernstein IL, Johnson CL, Ted CS: Therapy with cromolyn sodium. *Ann Intern Med* 89:228, 1978.
7. Bleecker ER: Exercise-induced asthma. Physiologic and clinical considerations. *Clin Chest Med* 5:109, 1984.
8. Boushey HA, Holtzman MJ, Sheller JA: Bronchial hyperreactivity. *Am Rev Respir Dis* 121:389, 1980.
9. Britt EV, Cohen B, Menkes H, et al: Airways reactivity and functional deterioration in relatives of COPD patients. *Chest* 77:260, 1980.

10. Brooks SM: Bronchial asthma of occupational origin. *Scand J Works Environ Health* 3:53, 1977.
11. Brown IG, Chan CS, Kelly CA, et al: Assessment of the clinical usefulness of nebulized ipratropium bromide in patients with chronic airflow limitation. *Thorax* 39:272, 1984.
12. Burrows B, Earle RH: Course and prognosis of chronic obstructive lung disease: a prospective study of 200 patients. *N Engl J Med* 280:396, 1969.
13. Chatham M, Bleecker ER, Norman P, et al: A screening test for airways reactivity. An abbreviated methacholine inhalation challenge. *Chest* 82:15, 1982.
14. Chatham M, Bleecker ER, Smith PL, et al: A comparison of histamine, methacholine, and exercise airway reactivity in normal and asthmatic subjects. *Am Rev Respir Dis* 126:235, 1982.
15. Cohen BH, Menkes HA, Bias WB, et al: Multiple factors in airways obstruction. *Chest* 77S:257, 1980.
16. Conolly ME, George CF, Davies DS, Dollery CT: Acquired resistance to beta stimulants: a possible explanation for the rise in the asthma death rate in Britain. *Chest* 63:16S, 1973.
17. Diener CF, Burrows B: Further observations on the course and prognosis of chronic obstructive lung disease. *Am Rev Respir Dis* 111:719, 1975.
18. Elwood RK, Abboud RT: The short-term bronchodilator effects of fenoterol and ipratropium in asthma. *J Allergy Clin Immunol* 69:467, 1982.
19. Epstein RL: Constituents of sputum: a simple method. *Ann Intern Med* 77:259, 1972.
20. Fanta CH, Rossing TH, McFadden ER Jr: Emergency room treatment of asthma. *Am J Med* 72:416, 1984.
21. Fletcher C, Peto R: The natural history of chronic airflow obstruction. *Br Med J* 1:1645, 1977.
22. Fox MJ, Snider GL: Respiratory therapy: current practice in ambulatory patients with chronic airflow obstruction. *JAMA* 241:937, 1979.
23. Gardner RM, Hankinson JL, West BJ: Evaluating commercially available spirometers. *Am Rev Respir Dis* 121:73, 1980.
24. Gelb AF, Gold WM, Wright RR, et al: Physiologic diagnosis of subclinical emphysema. *Am Rev Respir Dis* 107:50, 1973.
25. Hyatt RE, Black LF: The flow-volume curve: a current perspective. *Am Rev Respir Dis* 107:191, 1973.
26. Johnstone DE: A study of the natural history of bronchial asthma in children. *Am J Dis Child* 115:212, 1968.
27. Lichtenstein LM: An evaluation of the role of immunotherapy in asthma. *Am Rev Respir Dis* 117:191, 1978.
28. Maccia CA, Bernstein IL, Emmett EA, Brooks SM: In vitro demonstration of specific IgE in phthalic anhydride hypersensitivity. *Am Rev Respir Dis* 113:701, 1976.
29. Macklem PT, Permutt S: *The Lung in the Transition between Health and Disease*. New York, Marcel Dekker, 1979.
30. Maiman LA, Green LW, Gibson G, MacKenzie EJ: Education for self-treatment by adult asthmatics. *JAMA* 241:1919, 1979.
31. Marini JJ, Lakshminarayan S: The effect of atropine inhalation in "irreversible" chronic bronchitis. *Chest* 77:591, 1980.
32. McFadden ER: Exertional dyspnea and cough as preludes to acute attacks of bronchial asthma. *N Engl J Med* 292:555, 1975.
33. McFadden ER: Aerosolized bronchodilators and steroids in the treatment of airway obstruction in adults. *Am Rev Respir Dis* 122:89, 1980.
34. McFadden ER, Ingram RH: Exercise-induced asthma. Observations on the initiating stimulus. Seminars in Medicine of the Beth Israel Hospital, Boston. *N Engl J Med* 301:763, 1979.
35. McFadden ER, Kiser R, DeGroot WJ: Acute bronchial asthma: relations between clinical and physiologic manifestations. *N Engl J Med* 288:221, 1973.
36. McFadden ER, Kiser R, deGroot WJ, et al: A controlled study of the effects of single doses of hydrocortisone on the resolution of acute attacks of asthma. *Am J Med* 60:52, 1976.
37. McFadden ER, Luparello T, Lyons HA, Bleecker ER: The mechanism of action of suggestion in the induction of acute asthma attacks. *Psychosom Med* 31:134, 1969.

38. McFadden ER, Lyons HA: Arterial-blood gas tension in asthma. *N Engl J Med* 278:1027, 1968.

39. Murray JF: Review of the state of the art in intermittent positive pressure breathing therapy. *Am Rev Respir Dis* 110:193, 1974.

40. Nicklas RA, Whitehurst VE, Donohoe RF, Balacz T: Concomitant use of beta adrenergic agonists and methylxanthines. *J Allergy Clin Immunol* 73:20, 1984.

41. Nocturnal Oxygen Therapy Trial Group: Continuous or nocturnal oxygen therapy in hypoxemic chronic obstructive lung disease. A clinical trial. *Ann Intern Med* 93:391, 1980.

42. Pennock BE, Rogers RM, Ryan BR, Ayers IN: Aerosol administration of fenoterol hydrobromide (Th 1165a) in subjects with reversible obstructive airways disease. *Chest* 72:731, 1977.

43. Piafsky KM, Ogilvie RI: Dosage of theophylline in bronchial asthma. *N Engl J Med* 292:1218, 1975.

44. Postma DS, Burema J, Gimeno F, *et al*: Prognosis in severe chronic obstructive pulmonary disease. *Am Rev Respir Dis* 119:357, 1979.

45. Rebuck AS, Gent M, Chapman KR: Anticholinergic and sympathomimetic combination therapy of asthma. *J Allergy Clin Immunol* 71:317, 1983.

46. Rebuck AS, Read J: Assessment and management of severe asthma. *Am J Med* 51:788, 1971.

47. Rosenbluth M, Chernick V: Influence of mist tent therapy on sputum viscosity and water content in cystic fibrosis. *Arch Dis Childhood* 49:606, 1974.

48. Rossing TH, Fanta CH, Goldstein DH, *et al*: Emergency therapy of asthma: comparison of the acute effects of parenteral and inhaled sympathomimetics and infused aminophylline. *Am Rev Respir Dis* 122:365, 1980.

50. Safirstein BH, D'Souza MF, Simon G, *et al*: Five-year follow-up of allergic bronchopulmonary aspergillosis. *Am Rev Respir Dis* 108:450, 1973.

51. Samter M, Beers RF: Intolerance to aspirin. *Ann Intern Med* 68:975, 1968.

52. Shigeoka JW, Gardner RM, Barkman HW: A portable volume/flow calibrating syringe. *Chest* 82:598, 1982.

53. Storms WW, Dopico GA, Reed CE: An anticholinergic bronchodilator. *Am Rev Respir Dis* 111:419, 1975.

54. Thurlbeck WM: Aspects of chronic airflow obstruction. *Chest* 72:341, 1977.

55. Webb-Johnson DC, Andrews JL: Bronchodilator therapy (two parts). *N Engl J Med* 297:476, 1977.

56. Weinberger M, Hendeles L, Bighley L: The relation of product formulation to absorption of oral theophylline. *N Engl J Med* 299:852, 1978.

57. Weinberger SE, Weiss ST, Cohen WR, *et al*: State of the art. Pregnancy and the lung. *Am Rev Respir Dis* 121:559, 1980.

58. Wolfe JD, Tashkin P, Calvarese B, Simmons M: Bronchodilator effects of terbutaline and aminophylline alone and in combination in asthmatic patients. *N Engl J Med* 298:363, 1978.

59. Woolcock A, Read J: Lung volumes in exacerbations of asthma. *Am J Med* 41:259, 1966.

CHAPTER FIFTY-SIX

Lung Cancer

PHILIP L. SMITH, M.D., AND EUGENE R. BLEECKER, M.D.

EPIDEMIOLOGY

Lung cancer represents one of the most common malignant diseases facing Americans, especially with the increase in the elderly population and the increase in environmental pollutants. The death rate of this disease now approaches 120,000/year in the United States with even higher rates elsewhere in the world (8). Although there is a predominant male to female ratio, recent statistics demonstrate a distinct rise in the incidence of lung cancer in women commensurate with their increased consumption of cigarettes (Fig. 56.1).

Cigarette smoking (see Chapter 20) still remains the most important cause of lung cancer. The risk of developing cancer increases proportionately with the amount of smoking as is reflected by (a) the number of cigarettes smoked, (b) the number of years smoking, (c) the degree of inhalation, and (d) the "tar" and nicotine content of cigarettes smoked. Smoking of filter cigarettes or cigarettes with lower amounts of tar reduces lung cancer mortality rates, but these rates are still significantly higher than those of nonsmokers (19). In addition, exposure to various carcinogens such as asbestos, radioactivity, and the pollutants in the urban environment have led to an increased incidence of bronchogenic and pleural tumors (mesothelioma). Furthermore, smoking in combination with substances such as asbestos appears to act synergistically, probably due to the chronic effects of multiple irritants on the bronchial epithelium (10).

Although lung cancer has been classified into different cell types (Table 56.1), squamous cell can-

cer has offered the best opportunity to study the evolution of the disease. In both animals and humans the initial change is basal cell hyperplasia, followed by a change in cell shape which leads to cells that become atypical in appearance and, eventually, ends in localized cancer cells (carcinoma in situ). If the irritation stops at any point, it is postulated that these cellular changes may either arrest or revert to a normal state if the basement membrane has not been involved. This hypothesis is supported clinically by both a decrease in the death rate and in the amount of carcinoma in situ seen in ex-smokers (2, 9).

SCREENING PROGRAMS

Since lung cancer is presumed to take years before it advances to a clinically detectable stage, it would seem plausible that screening programs could detect nascent cancer. Since 1950 there have been several clinical trials designed to evaluate the early detection of lung cancer by sputum cytology and chest roentgenology (3, 8), but none of these studies has shown a statistically significant reduction in the overall mortality from the disease. A recent multicenter study (see Early Lung Cancer Detection—"General References") did show that annual screening with chest roentgenology and sputum cytology improves detection of lung cancer and increases the chances that the tumor can be resected. However, except in one center, there was no increase in survival of these high risk patients (men who were heavy smokers and over age 45). Therefore, at present, it seems reasonable to screen with an annual chest roentgenogram and sputum cytology only high risk patients *who are concerned* about the risk of developing lung cancer.

DIAGNOSTIC PROCESS

Symptoms

Most clinicians will evaluate patients for lung cancer after they have become symptomatic and/or have roentgenographic evidence of carcinoma. The most common presenting symptom is cough, followed by dyspnea, hemoptysis, and chest pain (see Chapter 53) (4). Hemoptysis is more commonly seen in patients with carcinomas that arise centrally in large airways and that either erode through the bronchus or become friable and bleed. Hemoptysis

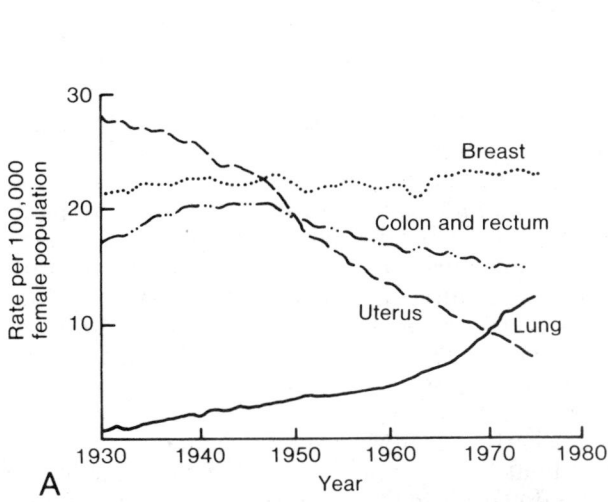

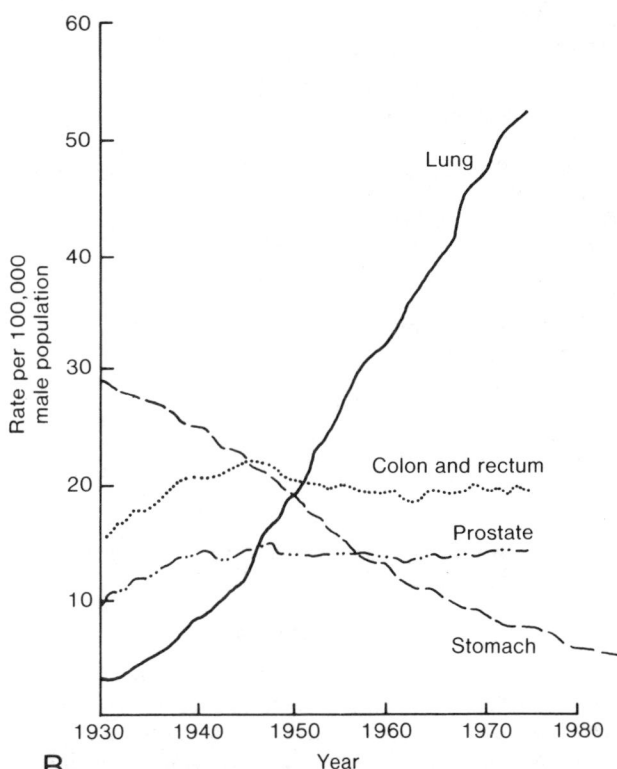

Figure 56.1. Age-adjusted cancer death rates from the four most common primary sources in United States women (*A*) and men (*B*), 1930 to 1975. Lung cancer will be the most common cause of death from malignancy in women by the 1990s if the present rate continues. (Data from the US National Center for Health Statistics and the US Bureau of the Census. Adapted from Hinshaw HC, Murray JF: *Diseases of the Chest.* Philadelphia, WB Saunders, 1980.)

Table 56.1.
Histological Classification of Lung Cancer

Class	Percentage of Cases
I. Squamous cell (epidermoid) carcinoma	30–35
II. Adenocarcinoma	30–35
III. Small cell anaplastic carcinoma (oat cell carcinoma)	20
IV. Large cell undifferentiated carcinoma	15

associated with a negative chest roentgenogram will occur in approximately 10 to 15% of patients with lung cancer (22). Dyspnea usually occurs when there is a large mass, associated pneumonia, or pleural effusion. Pain is most common when there is extension of the tumor beyond the lung parenchyma either into the adjacent mediastinum or into the thorax. In general, patients who are symptomatic at presentation have a poorer prognosis, and those who present with pain have the worst prognosis. Nevertheless, patients who are symptomatic for a longer time before their clinical presentation have a better prognosis than those who present with rapid onset of local and systemic symptoms, regardless of tumor type (7). Pain from a superior sulcus tumor (Pancoast

tumor) is often misdiagnosed as arthritis, and as a result, the patient may complain of shoulder pain for months before the correct diagnosis is made. Tumors that have metastasized outside the lung parenchyma can present with a multitude of symptoms depending on the organ involved. For example, the *superior vena cava syndrome* (facial swelling, distension of the veins of the neck, conjunctival injection, headache, convulsions) is occasionally seen in patients with tumors that involve the venous drainage to the right heart; or a *Horner's syndrome* (miosis, ptosis, enophthalmos, and reduced sweating) is seen in patients with tumors that invade the sympathetic nerve chain. Dysphagia, bone pain, or seizures may be seen when there is involvement of the esophagus, the skeleton, or the nervous system, respectively.

As opposed to these common clinical manifestations approximately 1 to 5% of patients with lung cancer present with various paraneoplastic signs or syndromes (Table 56.2). In general, neurological manifestations are seen in patients with more advanced lung cancer, while connective tissue manifestations, such as hypertrophic osteoarthropathy, may antedate the diagnosis of tumor by as much as 2 years. Virtually any tumor may be associated with extrapulmonary symptomatology, although small

Table 56.2.
Paraneoplastic Syndromes

NEUROMUSCULAR SYNDROMES
  Encephalopathy
  Myelopathy
  Neuropathy—sensory, sensory motor
  Myopathy—myasthenia, Eaton-Lambert
CONNECTIVE TISSUE
  Hypertrophic pulmonary osteoarthropathy
  Scleroderma
ENDOCRINE-METABOLIC
  Cushing's syndrome
  Carcinoid syndrome
  Inappropriate antidiuretic hormone (ADH) syndrome
VASCULAR/HEMATOLOGICAL
  Thrombophlebitis
  Purpura/Anemia

cell and squamous carcinomas are most commonly responsible.

Physical Examination

The physical examination of the lungs is often unrevealing in patients with lung cancer unless obstruction of a major bronchus has occurred. However, the general physical examination may detect signs of extrapulmonary metastasis or of a paraneoplastic syndrome.

Laboratory

Chest Roentgenogram

The laboratory diagnosis of cancer begins with an examination of the chest roentgenogram. While a roentgenogram does not diagnose the lesion, it serves as a focal point for subsequent procedures and for the sequence in which they will be performed. Centrally located lesions associated with atelectasis or pneumonia are most commonly squamous cell carcinomas. Adenocarcinomas and large cell carcinomas tend to arise as peripheral nodules and, therefore, are not associated with atelectasis or pneumonia. On the other hand, small cell tumors most commonly present with hilar adenopathy, often with no primary tumor visible on roentgenogram. Squamous cell carcinoma is the most frequently cavitating tumor, but even with this tumor, cavitation is uncommon. Cavitation represents either tumor necrosis, which usually occurs in lesions larger than 2 cm, or infection that develops into a lung abscess distal to the tumor. The solitary pulmonary nodule is discussed in detail below (pages 674 to 675).

Approximately 15% of patients with lung cancer will present with a negative chest roentgenogram (22). This will occur predominantly in patients with hemoptysis from squamous cell carcinoma that arises proximally but is obscured by mediastinal tissues. Therefore, patients with their first episode of hemoptysis and a negative chest roentgenogram should be referred to a chest physician for further evaluation and for possible bronchoscopy (see Chapter 53).

Cytology

The frequency of diagnosis of lung cancer from cytology submitted from spontaneously expectorated sputum or from bronchoscopy is dependent on the cell type and the location of the tumor. Squamous cell tumors shed cells into the airways and cytologies are positive approximately 80% of the time, whereas patients with a peripheral adenocarcinoma will have positive cytologies less than half the time. Screening sputum cytologies should be done before hospital admission. However, the completion of the diagnostic evaluation during hospitalization should not be delayed in situations where sputum cytological examination is not readily available. In general, spontaneously expectorated sputum is the material most often submitted for cytological examination. Patients should be instructed to produce a deep sputum sample by inhaling to total lung capacity in order to produce a forceful cough. Three to five early morning specimens should be collected in a tight-fitting container, and if they cannot be submitted daily to the laboratory within 2 to 3 hours of collection, a fixative should be added so the specimens can be pooled and submitted together. Saccomanno's solution, which contains 50% alcohol and approximately 7% carbowax, is one of the best fixatives; it can be prepared by the laboratory (14) and stored by the physician. More than five samples does not increase the incidence of a positive diagnosis of cancer. If the patient is not producing sputum, induction by the inhalation of an aerosolized solution of saline can be helpful. The patient inhales, for 15 to 30 minutes, normal saline or a balanced salt solution (Hanks' BSS) that is aerosolized by an ultrasonic nebulizer (DeVilbiss 3583). In general, sputum induction is not a routine office procedure and should be done by experienced personnel. In addition to the sputum collected immediately after induction, there is good material produced on the following morning. The addition of chest vibration or percussion does not improve the yield from sputum cytology. In cases where there is obstruction of the bronchus as evidenced by the physical examination or the chest roentgenogram, it is reasonable to start collecting sputum after therapy, including antibiotics and perhaps bronchodilators, which may re-establish airway patency and allow sputum to be produced.

Bronchoscopy

Bronchoscopy will generally be necessary either to diagnose patients suspected of having cancer or to determine resectability in those patients with positive sputum. Patients deemed inoperable may

not need bronchoscopy. The fiberoptic bronchoscope has greatly aided in the diagnosis of lung
cancer since smaller lesions can now be approached
even though the lesion may not be visualized
through the bronchoscope. Those lesions seen at
bronchoscopy yield a diagnosis by biopsy and brushing in greater than 90% of cases. Fluoroscopy will
be necessary to guide the biopsy forceps and brush
in those patients whose cancers present as peripheral nodules beyond the vision of the bronchoscope.
Depending on the experience of the operator and
the size and location of the tumor, a positive diagnosis will be made on 30 to 70% of peripheral lesions.
With recent advances in technique it is now possible
to obtain transbronchial needle aspirates of paratracheal, subcarinal, and peribroncheal lymph nodes.
Using this approach, even tumors located near the
apex of the lung or near the pleura may be successfully examined by biopsy and staged (11).

Patient experience. In order to reduce expense, bronchoscopy may be performed on an ambulatory basis by a
pulmonologist or a thoracic surgeon. The patient is told
that he will have to fast (including liquids) 12 hours prior
to bronchoscopy and that he will not be able to eat for
approximately 4 hours after its completion when the effects of topical anesthesia wear off. The only discomfort
the patient will experience is coughing caused by irritation of the trachea and main bronchi. There is usually no
pain associated with this procedure. Risks include bleeding and pneumothorax in 5 to 15% of patients in whom
transbronchial biopsy is attempted. However, death is rare
and almost always is associated with a transbronchial
biopsy which has caused significant bleeding.

Needle Biopsy

If a diagnosis of a lesion still has not been made,
transpulmonary needle biopsy of the lung can be
performed. This technique is most useful when a
mass or a nodule is located peripherally near the
pleura or in the apex of the lung. It is especially
helpful in the diagnosis of metastatic carcinoma
since these tumors are difficult to diagnose by bronchoscopy, particularly when they are less than 2 cm
in size. The technique and experience of the operator are of paramount importance in the success of
transpulmonary needle biopsy, and it is necessary
that an individual at a given institution establish his
own record for sensitivity and specificity for this
procedure. In our own institution, the positive predictive value of the procedure is 90%. When the
pathology report indicates nonspecific inflammatory
changes on two separate attempts, there is less than
5% chance of malignancy, and under these circumstances we will consider following certain types of
lesions by chest roentgenograms every few months
and not doing further diagnostic procedures unless
the lesions enlarge or cavitate. Needle biopsy does
not ordinarily require hospitalization.

Patient experience. The patient should be informed that
he will feel a mild pressure with the introduction of the
needle. Otherwise, there is no significant pain. Bleeding
and pneumothorax occur in 30% of patients in whom
biopsies are performed, but only 10% of them require
insertion of a chest tube. Contraindications to the procedure include large blebs that are in the direct path of the
needle, a patient with an uncontrollable cough, in which
case general anesthesia may be necessary, and contralateral pneumonectomy, in which case the production of a
pneumothorax would be devastating. In addition, there is
a relative contraindication to needle biopsy in patients
with pulmonary hypertension since they have an increased risk of bleeding. However, biopsies can be performed in patients with emphysema, although they have
a greater risk of pneumothorax.

Mediastinoscopy

Rarely, mediastinoscopy will be necessary to
make the diagnosis of lung cancer. More commonly,
the procedure is performed to "stage" the tumor (see
below). In either case, the patient must be hospitalized for the procedure. An anterior cervical or parasternal incision is made under general anesthesia,
and biopsies are taken of any palpable lymph nodes.
There is less than a 1% mortality and approximately
a 5 to 10% complication rate that includes infection,
pneumothorax, and bleeding.

Recently the technique of transbronchial (see
above) needle aspiration has been developed. It has
allowed the fiberoptic bronchoscopist to sample
lymph nodes in the mediastinum for the simultaneous diagnosis and staging of lung cancer. The
procedure can be done during fiberoptic bronchoscopy under local anesthesia; therefore, hospitalization may not be required. In our institution this
technique has eliminated the need for mediastinoscopy in many circumstances.

Extrapulmonary Metastasis

At the time of initial diagnosis, approximately 30%
of patients will have evidence of metastatic disease
(4). In that event workup of the primary lesion ceases
since metastatic cancer is a contraindication to any
type of "curative" surgery. Approximately 60% of
patients die as a result of bone, brain, or liver metastasis, depending on the cell type (6). Adenocarcinoma and small cell carcinoma tend to metastasize
earlier in their course than does epidermoid cancer.
Except for small cell carcinoma, extensive evaluations for metastatic liver, brain, and bone disease
are discouraged unless the following conditions exist: (a) if liver function tests are abnormal, a liver
scan should be performed; and if positive, a needle
biopsy is indicated; (b) if bone pain is present, a bone
scan will be the most sensitive test for detecting an
abnormality. A skeletal roentgenographic survey is
much less sensitive but is a reasonable alternative
if scanning is not available; (c) if the neurological

examination reveals focal defects suggestive of intracerebral metastases, a computerized axial tomographic (CT) scan should be obtained. In the case of small cell carcinoma, an extensive metastatic evaluation is always prudent, even in the absence of symptoms, since this type of tumor metastasizes early and is only responsive to chemotherapy or irradiation.

Staging

Regardless of the diagnostic sequence chosen for an individual patient, the process should lead to an accurate histological diagnosis and to accurate clinical staging. This information is essential for planning treatment and for understanding the prognosis, as discussed below. Table 56.1 lists the four histological types of lung cancer. Tables 56.3 and 56.4 summarize the criteria for the clinical stages proposed by the American Joint Committee for Cancer Staging (16).

Table 56.3.
Tumor-Node-Metastases (TNM) System for Lung Cancer

T—Primary tumor
  T0: No evidence of primary tumor
  TX: Malignant cells in secretions but no radiographic or bronchoscopic evidence of tumor
  T1: Tumor less than 3.0 cm in greatest diameter, located beyond a lobar bronchus.
  T2: Tumor larger than 3.0 cm in diameter or any size with extension to hilum. At bronchoscopy tumor is at least 2.0 cm from the carina. No pleural effusion. Atelectasis or obstructive pneumonia, if present, involves less than an entire lung
  T3: Tumor of any size extending to chest wall, diaphragm, mediastinum, within less than 2.0 cm of carina (bronchoscopy) or with effusion or atelectasis of entire lung
N— Regional lymph nodes
  N0: None involved
  N1: Metastasis to ipsilateral hilar region
  N2: Mediastinal nodes involved
M—Distant metastases
  M0: None
  M1: Any metastases to distant sites

Table 56.4.
Stages of Lung Cancer[a]

Occult carcinoma: TX, N0, M0
Invasive carcinoma
  Stage 1: T1, N0, M0; T1, N1, M0; T2, N0, M0
  Stage 2: T2, N1, M0
  Stage 3: T3 with any N or M; N2 with any T or M; M1 with any T or N.

[a] See Table 56.3 for explanation of notations.

SOLITARY NODULES

Clinical

As opposed to patients with mass lesions on chest roentgenogram, those who present with solitary nodules are usually asymptomatic. Solitary pulmonary nodules or "coin" lesions have been variously described as circumscribed densities ranging in size to 6 cm. Since lesions of 6 cm can hardly be classified as coin lesions, the term solitary pulmonary nodule is more appropriate to denote a lesion less than 6 cm in diameter. Until recently, most small pulmonary nodules were resected. Predictably, many benign lesions were removed; therefore, major efforts have been made to improve preoperative diagnostic accuracy.

Laboratory

Chest Roentgenogram

When evaluating an asymptomatic patient with a solitary pulmonary nodule, one should begin with a careful examination of the chest roentgenogram. The obvious first question facing the clinician is whether the nodule is benign or malignant since the diagnosis of a benign lesion will allow the physician to avoid unnecessary and extensive evaluations. There are specific roentgenographic features that will permit the physician to follow the patient with a reasonable assurance that a lesion is benign.

Growth. At one time, if old chest roentgenograms were available and a lesion had not changed in size for 2 years, it was automatically assumed to be benign. It is now appreciated that, occasionally, such lesions are, in fact, malignant so that no further evaluation is necessary (17) only if it can be documented that a lesion has not grown in 5 years. Prospectively, a doubling time (double in volume) between 10 and 500 days suggests that the lesion is malignant, while doubling times of longer than 18 months are usually associated with benign lesions. This type of measurement is not simple, and when no old films (at least 5 years old) are available, waiting for a lesion to grow may result in spread of the tumor. Therefore, observing a new lesion for growth is not recommended.

Calcification. Calcification represents one of the most reliable signs that a nodule is benign. The following patterns of calcification indicate a benign lesion: (a) a central dense calcified nidus, (b) a diffuse or irregular nodular deposit (i.e., the popcorn type calcification that occurs in hamartomas), (c) calcifications scattered throughout the lesion, and (d) a laminated pattern of calcium deposited in concentric layers throughout the lesion, a pattern that is found in granulomas. Finally, a few specks of calcium are not a reliable sign that a lesion is benign.

Small amounts of eccentrically placed calcium visualized in a nodule can occur with scar carcinoma.

The roentgenographic diagnosis of calcification is often arbitrary and depends on interpretation. Siegelman et al (18) have reported the use of the CT scan to assess density and to distinguish benign from malignant lesions by grading the density of the nodule. More dense tissue has higher absorption and, therefore, higher CT density attenuation. Thus, while calcium diffusely spread throughout a lesion may go undetected on a standard chest roentgenogram, it results in a CT scan with a high attenuation number that allows separation of benign from malignant lesions. This method may prove useful in the ambulatory assessment of the solitary pulmonary nodule.

Shape/size. The shape and configuration of a lesion do not provide help in deciding whether the nodule is benign or malignant. While malignant lesions tend to have poorly defined, fuzzy borders, are often lobulated, and sometimes notched, none of these signs is diagnostic of a malignant growth. For that matter, a discretely circumscribed, round, sharply defined nodule is not always benign. Although size itself offers little aid in deciding whether a lesion is benign or malignant, larger nodules are more frequently malignant and offer a poor prognosis (see Table 56.5). Until recently, most nodules less than 1 cm were felt to have such a small chance of being malignant that surgery was frequently thought unnecessary. However, this impression is not true, as can be seen in Table 56.5. This is partly due to case selection but also to more sensitive radiographic techniques that allow visualization of smaller, less dense lesions.

Table 56.5.
Comparison of Nodule Size and Malignancy

	No. of Tumors		
	Study A[a]		% Malignant
Centimeters	Benign	Malignant	
>4	0	5	100
3–4	0	6	100
2–3	4	13	70
1–2	18	28	50
0–1	11	6	47
	Study B[b]		
>4	9	56	87
3–4	20	59	75
2–3	91	105	50
1–2	225	78	34
0–1	104	8	5

[a] Adapted from Siegelman SS, Zerhouni EA, Leo FP, et al: CT of the solitary pulmonary nodule. *AJR* 135:1, 1980.
[b] Adapted from Steele JD: The solitary pulmonary nodule. Report of a cooperative study of resected asymptomatic solitary pulmonary nodules in males. *J Thorac Cardiovasc Surg* 46:21, 1963.

Age. Although malignant solitary nodules can occur at any age, they are almost never seen (0.5%) in patients less than 30 years of age; therefore, lesions in this age group can simply be observed. However, a semiannual chest roentgenogram should be obtained for at least the first 2 years of follow-up.

Metastasis to Lung

Approximately 7% of solitary pulmonary nodules represent metastatic disease (1, 15). Those patients presenting with a solitary pulmonary nodule due to metastatic disease will almost always have a prior history of cancer. Only 20% of metastatic nodules occur in patients with occult disease. Furthermore, there is no evidence that extensive metastatic work-ups will uncover these occult tumors (15). Ordinarily, of 100 solitary pulmonary nodules, seven will be of metastatic origin, but only one or two will represent occult malignancies. Based on these statistics, it is unwise to look for an extrapulmonary primary tumor before precise diagnosis of the solitary nodule is undertaken. A complete medical history, physical examination, and laboratory evaluation, including urinalysis, liver function tests, and screening for occult blood from the gastrointestinal and genitourinary tract, will be adequate to uncover most metastatic disease to the lung. If any of these tests is positive, the possibility of an extrapulmonary neoplasm should be investigated further.

Staging

The actual sequence in evaluating a solitary pulmonary nodule is similar to that already outlined for bronchogenic carcinoma. Cytology will be positive in less than 20 to 30% of patients who present with peripheral nodules. Bronchoscopy will increase the yield if the lesion is greater than 1 cm. At our institution transbronchial needle biopsy is being used more frequently in the evaluation of the solitary pulmonary nodule in an effort to obtain tissue prior to thoracotomy. Using transbronchial forceps biopsy with transbronchial needle aspiration, it is now possible to diagnose and stage lesions prior to thoracotomy (21). In situations where reliable transbronchial or transpulmonary needle biopsy is not available, physicians will need to proceed directly to thoracotomy for diagnosis. The staging of a solitary pulmonary nodule is not as complicated if the lesion is peripheral and is less than 2 cm. These patients are usually asymptomatic, and if initial screening is negative and if the tissue type is not small cell carcinoma, then curative resection can be attempted. If the lesion is located centrally or is greater than 2 cm, mediastinoscopy or transbronchial needle aspiration of mediastinal or paratracheal nodes should be performed to exclude an inoperable tumor.

COURSE/MANAGEMENT

Prognosis

Even with treatment, the prognosis and course of lung cancer are dismal. The present overall 5-year survival for treated and untreated cancer of the lung is 5 to 10%. Seventy-five percent of tumors are unresectable based on clinical evidence of far advanced disease at the time of presentation. Furthermore, less than 50% of those considered clinically resectable (see below) can have their tumor removed when staging procedures are completed. However, even with earlier diagnosis and increased resectability, the overall prognosis appears little altered (see "General References," Early Lung Cancer Detection). Thus, of 100 patients with lung cancer, only 25 will undergo complete staging. Of these, 11 will be resectable and only 8 to 10 will be alive in 5 years. In general, if the tumor is unresectable, the median survival is 2 to 3 months. However, even in patients with unresectable cancer, the 2-year survival is 4% for cancer limited to one hemithorax (13). As with other cancers, survival is correlated with the histological type of tumor and the stage at the time of presentation (Table 56.6). Squamous cell carcinoma and adenocarcinoma are associated with the best prognosis, while small cell carcinoma is associated with the poorest. Within the respective cellular groupings, those with more undifferentiated cell types tend to have the worst prognosis. Except for small cell carcinoma, tumor type becomes relatively unimportant if the carcinoma presents as a small nodule less than 1 cm. Frequently tumors contain more than one cellular element, and depending on the amount of tissue available and the number of specimens examined histologically, disagreement among pathologists frequently occurs. In addition, even the same pathologist, after reviewing different microscopic slides from the same tumor, may reclassify the tumor.

Table 56.6.
Two-Year Survival Rates (Percentage Alive) for Bronchogenic Carcinoma[a]

Cell Type	Stage		
	1	2	3
Squamous	46	39	11
Adenocarcinoma	45	14	7
Large	42	12	12
Small	6	5	3

[a] Adapted from the American Joint Committee for Cancer Staging and End Results (1974) (16). See Table 56.4 for definition of stages. This represents 2155 cases of histologically proved cancer. The staging was based on (a) physical examination, (b) chest roentgenogram, or (c) surgical procedures—bronchoscopy, mediastinoscopy, thoracentesis, biopsies.

Treatment

Surgical resection remains the only proven therapy for non-small cell carcinoma. Attempts at "curative" radiation of any solitary pulmonary nodule are currently unacceptable. Irradiation of larger tumors is considered appropriate for the palliation of atelectasis associated with bronchial obstruction and for relief of symptoms associated with paraneoplastic syndromes. In certain instances irradiation is recommended to patients who have stage I or II disease but who are considered inoperable (see below). Chemotherapy for small cell carcinomas often improves the quality and duration of life (5). However, chemotherapy of lung cancer is in constant evolution and thus patients with such tumors should be referred to an oncologist for definitive therapy (see Chapter 8).

Operability and Resectability

Before proceeding to lung resection, two questions face the clinician: (a) operability: is the patient able to withstand an operation and resection? and (b) resectability: can the tumor be resected? The determination of resectability should be made in consultation with a pulmonary physician and a thoracic surgeon. Whether a tumor can be removed is determined from information derived from bronchoscopy, mediastinoscopy, and, finally, visualization of the tumor at thoracotomy. Unfortunately, only a small number of tumors are resectable at the time of presentation, although a higher percentage of these patients will be alive at 5 years.

The determination of whether a patient is operable should begin as soon as the patient is suspected of having cancer since an inoperable patient can be spared an extensive workup that includes staging procedures. Factors such as age, coexistent medical conditions, and nutritional status are discussed in detail elsewhere (Chapter 8). While there are relatively few absolute criteria that preclude resection of the lung, patients with an FEV_1 less than 1 liter and a pCO_2 greater than 50 mm Hg are poor candidates for any kind of resection. By using both the ventilation/perfusion lung scan and the spirogram, one can predict the amount of functional lung remaining after pneumonectomy, although this prediction is more difficult in patients undergoing lobectomy or segmentectomy. If the predicted postoperative FEV_1 is greater than 800 ml, resection can be performed on patients who otherwise might not have been considered operable candidates. It is important to realize that a normal blood gas does not exclude significant pulmonary disease since patients with emphysema and advanced obstructive lung disease can maintain relatively normal arterial blood gases (see Chapter 55). This underscores the need for obtaining the FEV_1 early in the evaluation, but a word of caution is necessary. Frequently, the initial evaluation reveals pulmonary function that precludes operation; however, after aggressive therapy, including bronchodilators for bronchospasm, antibiotics for infection, percussion and drainage for excessive secretions, and discontinuation of cigarette smoking, a marked improvement may be achieved so that a resection can be attempted.

Operable Patients

The course of lung carcinoma after curative resection is variable depending on the functional lung remaining. Often immediately postoperatively there is a significant amount of unsuspected bronchospasm, which improves with conventional treatment. Most patients with postoperative bronchospasm have underlying bronchitis with preoperative evidence of bronchospasm on spirogram; therefore, routine spirometry, before lung resection, is recommended. In addition spirometry postoperatively will aid in assessing whether there has been worsening of bronchoconstriction. After resection there appears to be some chronic compensatory hyperinflation of any remaining lung parenchyma; therefore, in time, pulmonary function can improve 20 to 30% over the immediate postoperative function and is often associated with improved exercise capability. Normal activities can be resumed within several weeks of surgery, depending on pulmonary reserve (see Chapter 86). Routine follow-up at least every 3 to 4 months for the first 2 years after resection is advised in order to detect metastasis, local recurrence, or a second primary. Yearly sputum cytology and chest X-ray are recommended in patients who continue to smoke (see page 670).

Inoperable Patients

If the patient is inoperable or the tumor is unresectable, and significant tumor remains or recurs, ambulatory treatment is directed at symptomatic relief. Dyspnea resulting from recurring pleural effusions can be effectively relieved in an ambulatory setting by repeated thoracentesis; chest tube drainage and sclerosing of the pleura can be employed (on referral to an oncologist or pulmonary physician) for more chronic resolution. Bone pain from metastasis often responds to local irradiation better than it does to narcotic sedation. Chest wall pain is the most difficult symptom to treat, but local intercostal blocks add to the analgesic effects of narcotics. Pneumonia often occurs when bronchogenic tumors obstruct major bronchi, and therapy with antibiotics alone is usually insufficient. In this situation, palliative irradiation may reduce the tumor size and temporarily allow drainage of the bronchus. Hemoptysis and the superior vena cava syndrome also may respond to radiotherapy. Consultation with an oncologist is useful for the primary physician when

patients have residual tumor and are difficult to manage. Additional discussion of the care of the patient with incurable cancer is found in Chapter 8.

General References

Early lung cancer detection: Summary and conclusions. John Hopkins Medical Institutions, Mayo Foundation, Memorial Sloan-Kettering Cancer Center, University of Cincinnati Medical Center, and the National Cancer Institute. *Am Rev Respir Dis* 130:565, 1984.
> Summary of data from the most recent multicenter screening study for early detection and management of lung cancer.

Matthay RA: Symposium on recent advances in lung cancer. *Clin Chest Med* 3: 1982.
> Superb current symposium by experts on epidemiology, history, management, and treatment of lung cancer.

Mittman C, Bruderman I: Lung cancer: to operate or not ? *Am Rev Respir Dis* 116:477, 1977.
> A general review of the preoperative evaluation of the patient with lung cancer.

Siegelman SS, Stitik FP, Summer WR: *Pulmonary System: Practical Approaches to Pulmonary Diagnosis.* New York, Grune & Stratton, 1979.
> Provides useful, detailed clinical information on procedures used to diagnose pulmonary disease.

Specific References

1. Adkins PC, Wesselhoeft CW Jr, Newman W, Blades B: Thoracotomy on the patient with previous malignancy: metastasis or new primary? *J Thorac Cardiovasc Surg* 56:351, 1968.
2. Auerbach O, Stout AP, Hammond EC, Garfinkel L: Bronchial epithelium in former smokers. *N Engl J Med* 267:119, 1962.
3. Bailar JC III: Screening for lung cancer—where are we now? *Am Rev Respir Dis* 130:541, 1984.
4. Boucot KR, Cooper DA, Weiss W, Carnahan WJ: The natural history of lung cancer. *Am Rev Respir Dis* 89:519, 1964.
5. Carney DN, Minna JD: Small cell cancer of the lung. *Clin Chest Med* 3:389, 1982.
6. Cox JD, Yesner RA: Adenocarcinoma of the lung: recent results from the Veterans Administration lung group. *Am Rev Respir Dis* 120:1025, 1979.
7. Feinstein AR, Wells CK: Lung cancer staging. A critical evaluation. *Clin Chest Med* 3:291, 1982.
8. Guidelines for the Cancer Related Checkup: CA 30:1980.
9. Hammond EC: Evidence of the effects of giving up cigarette smoking. *Am J Public Health* 55:682, 1965.
10. Hammond EC, Selikoff IJ: Relations of cigarette smoking to risk of death of asbestos-associated disease among insulation workers in the United States (Biological Effects of Asbestos. Lyons, France). *IARC Sci Publ* 8:312, 1973.
11. Haponik EF, Summer WR, Terry PB, Wang KP: Clinical decision-making with transbronchial lung biopsies: the value of nonspecific histology. *Am Rev Respir Dis* 125:524, 1982.
12. Hinshaw HC, Murray JF: *Diseases of the Chest.* Philadelphia, WB Saunders, 1980, pp 463–523.
13. Hyde L, Wolf J, McCracken S, Yesner R: Natural course of inoperable lung cancer. *Chest* 64:309, 1973.
14. Koss LG: *Diagnostic Cytology and Its Histopathologic Bases,* ed 2. Philadelphia, Lippincott/Harper, 1979, vol 2.
15. Lawhorne TW Jr, Baker RR, Carter D: Adenocarcinoma of the lung presenting as a solitary pulmonary nodule. *Johns Hopkins Med J* 133:82, 1973.
16. Mountain CF, Carr DT, Anderson WA: A system for the clinical staging of lung cancer. *AJR* 120:130, 1974.
17. Nathan J: Management of solitary pulmonary nodules. An organized approach based on growth rate and statistics. *JAMA* 227:1141, 1974.
18. Siegelman SS, Zerhouni EA, Leo FP, *et al:* CT of the solitary

pulmonary nodule. *AJR* 135:1, 1980.

19. *Smoking and Health: A Report of the Surgeon General.* Washington, DC, US Department of Health, Education, and Welfare, 1979.

20. Steele JD: The solitary pulmonary nodule. Report of a cooperative study of resected asymptomatic solitary pulmonary nodules in males. *J Thorac Cardiovasc Surg* 46:21, 1963.

21. Wang K, Brower R, Haponik E, Siegelman S: Flexible transbronchial needle aspiration for staging of bronchogenic carcinoma. *Chest* 84:571, 1983.

22. Zavala DC: Diagnostic fiberoptic bronchoscopy. *Chest* 68:12, 1975.

SECTION 8

Cardiovascular Problems

CHAPTER FIFTY-SEVEN

Angina Pectoris*

NISHA CHIBBER CHANDRA, M.D., AND PHILIP D. ZIEVE, M.D.

Chest pain is one of the most frequent complaints of patients to physicians in an ambulatory practice. The major early objective in the diagnosis of such patients is the separation of noncardiac from cardiac pain. Chapter 53 describes the various causes of noncardiac pain and their distinguishing characteristics. This chapter describes the diagnosis and treatment of the commonest cause of cardiac pain, transient myocardial ischemia. Chapter 58 describes the posthospital medical care and rehabilitation of patients who have had a myocardial infarction.

Ischemic heart disease due to atherosclerosis is one of the most prevalent ailments in the Western world; in the United States, it remains the leading nontraumatic cause of disability and death, even though, due to increased public awareness and health education, the mortality from ischemic heart disease has declined over 20% from 1968 to 1980. Most lay people recognize that chest pain may be an important symptom of ischemic heart disease and may be a prodrome of myocardial infarction (a "heart attack") and of sudden death. Hence patients with chest pain will often seek prompt medical attention. It is essential that physicians know how

---

* Dr. Gustav C. Voigt contributed to this chapter in the first edition of this book.

to respond to these people in order to make appropriate diagnostic and therapeutic decisions.

In the approach to the patient with chest pain, a detailed history and physical examination must not be replaced by sophisticated noninvasive or invasive cardiovascular procedures. Such procedures are often painful, risky, usually expensive, and are often overutilized. A detailed history and physical examination permit the physician to tailor these studies to meet more specifically the needs of the patient, thereby increasing the efficiency and yield of such procedures.

PATHOPHYSIOLOGY

Normally, the myocardium produces most of its energy by means of aerobic metabolism. When totally deprived of oxygen, the heart stops beating within a few minutes. Oxygen demands (Table 57.1) are a function of the amount of work that cardiac muscle is called upon to perform. That work, in turn, is a function of the *heart rate*, of the *tension* of the walls of the left ventricle, and of the *contractility* of the myocardium (39). Tension (T), described by the Laplace relationship ($T = P \cdot \div r\ 2h$), is directly proportionate to the ventricular blood pressure (P) and volume (r = radius of the ventricular cavity), and is inversely proportionate to the thickness (h) of the ventricular wall. Contractility essentially is the amount of work that the myocardium can do under a given load, and, in the normal heart, is influenced primarily by the peripheral vascular tone (generated by the sympathetic nervous system) and by the intra- and extracellular electrolyte concentration of cardiac muscle. These interrelationships, which affect the heart's ability to do work, are also important in the pathophysiology of heart failure (see Chapter 61).

In practical terms these concepts reveal why the heart is more prone to ischemia when its rate is increased (e.g., by exertion or emotional stress), when left ventricular tension is increased (e.g., by increased blood pressure or by ventricular dilation), or when myocardial contractility is increased (e.g., by the sympathetic discharge that accompanies exertion or emotional stress).

Oxygen supply (Table 57.1) is dependent on the oxygen content of the blood and on the volume of blood flowing through the coronary arteries per unit

Table 57.1.
Some Factors That Influence Myocardial Metabolism

Oxygen Demand	Oxygen Supply
Heart rate	Oxygen content of the blood
Tension (T) of the wall of the left ventricle[a]	Volume of blood flowing through the coronary arteries per unit of time
a. Ventricular blood pressure (P)	
b. Radius (r) of the ventricular cavity	
c. Thickness (h) of the wall	
Contractility of the myocardium	

[a] $T = P \cdot r \div 2h$ (see the text).

of time. Normally, the myocardium extracts as much oxygen as it can from coronary blood; this is reflected in a low coronary sinus blood oxygen saturation (approximately 35%) and a wide arteriovenous oxygen concentration difference across the coronary circulation. Therefore, an increased demand for myocardial oxygen can only be met by an increase in coronary blood flow. This flow occurs primarily during diastole and is determined by two major factors: coronary perfusion pressure (aortic diastolic pressure (during systole the coronary arteries are squeezed and deliver much less blood to the myocardium) minus coronary sinus pressure) and coronary vascular resistance. However, there is little change in total coronary flow over a wide range of coronary perfusion pressures because of flow autoregulation (27). Hence, changes in coronary blood flow occur primarily as a result of changes in coronary vascular resistance. Coronary vascular resistance, in turn, is determined by the degree of collateralization and the patency of the coronary blood vessels; when the vessels are narrowed by spasm or by an atherosclerotic plaque, coronary resistance increases and oxygen demands may not be satisfied.

If the myocardium receives insufficient oxygen to satisfy its metabolic demands, the resultant ischemia usually results in pain, arrhythmia, or left ventricular dysfunction. Transient myocardial ischemia causes transient chest pain—*angina pectoris*; prolonged ischemia causes more prolonged chest pain, most commonly because of *myocardial infarction*. The character of the pain is the same in both situations. Also, when ischemic, the heart is much more susceptible to arrhythmias, which can, in themselves, produce symptoms. The treatment of ischemia is directed at reducing myocardial oxygen demand and at increasing coronary blood flow.

RISK FACTORS

Both genetic and environmental factors influence the development of atherosclerotic heart disease. Recent research has been targeted at defining the

role of these factors in the premature development of cardiovascular disease. The recognition of these risk factors is especially important insofar as they may be modified to prevent disease. In this regard, it is noteworthy that recently the Lipid Research Primary Preventional Trial has conclusively shown that a reduction in plasma cholesterol lowers the incidence of coronary artery disease (28). A pamphlet entitled *Risk Factors and Coronary Disease: A Statement for Physicians* is available from the American Heart Association (2); it summarizes the various risk factors that have been identified and makes recommendations for dealing with them (Tables 57.2 and 57.3).

It is difficult to assign a specific risk to a particular factor because often the risk is proportionate to the degree of exposure (e.g., the number of cigarettes smoked a day or the concentration of cholesterol in the blood) and because the various factors interact in a complicated way to compound the risk of disease in a given patient. However, an active attempt should be made to attenuate the risk associated with those factors that can be modified. The importance of abstinence from tobacco and control of blood pressure and plasma lipids in high risk patients cannot be overemphasized. Table 57.3 lists the proposals of the American Heart Association in this regard and indicates also those which are most likely to be effective in the primary prevention of coronary artery disease.

Although it is not a risk factor *per se*, recent myocardial infarction is a powerful predictor of new angina; almost 50% of patients with no prior history of angina will develop typical angina in the first year after myocardial infarction.

DIAGNOSIS

History

Onset of Ischemic Pain

Many patients with ischemic cardiac pain can document the circumstances and sometimes the date and time of their first pain. This is not so true in patients with pain of neuromuscular or gastrointestinal origin unless trauma or some catastrophe, such as a bowel perforation, has occurred. The ability of the patient to describe the first experience with chest pain is useful, therefore, in differential diagnosis.

Character and Location of the Ischemic Pain

The discomfort of myocardial ischemia is variously described; some describe it as squeezing, crushing, burning, or smothering, whereas others describe it as a shortness of breath or simply a feeling of heaviness. A sharp pain is unlikely to be of cardiac origin, but the patient should be asked to characterize it further, if he can, since "sharp" to some pa-

Table 57.2.
Risk Factors for Coronary Artery Disease

Factor	Comment	Documentation
Blood pressure (Chapter 62)	Risk is directly proportionate to increase of systolic or diastolic blood pressure	Excellent
Blood lipids (Chapter 75)	Risk is directly proportionate to increase in concentration of total cholesterol and of low density lipoprotein (LDL) and inversely proportionate to concentration of high density lipoprotein (HDL)	Excellent
Diabetes mellitus (Chapter 72)	Risk is 2 times control in diabetic men, 3 times control in diabetic women	Excellent
Cigarette smoking (Chapter 20)	Proportionate to number of cigarettes smoked per day (3 times control at a pack or more per day)	Excellent
Oral contraceptives (Chapter 93)	Risk is much greater in women over age 35	Excellent
Personality type	A competitive, driving person (so-called type A personality) is more prone to coronary artery disease	Good
Sedentary living	Individuals who do not exercise regularly may have a greater risk of myocardial infarction than do individuals who exercise regularly	Poor
Diet[a] (Chapter 75)	High lipid content of diet may potentiate coronary artery disease	Poor in humans Excellent in animals

[a] Alcohol and caffeine—though claimed by some in the past to be independent risk factors—have not been established to be so. However, obesity, by increasing the severity of hypertension, hyperlipidemia, and diabetes, may have an important influence on the development of coronary artery disease.

Table 57.3.
Primary Prevention of Coronary Artery Disease: Recommended Actions[a]

DEMONSTRATED RISK FACTORS THAT CAN BE MODIFIED
  Discontinue cigarette smoking
  Control hypertension
  Control blood lipids
  Monitor use of oral contraception
DEMONSTRATED RISK FACTORS THAT CANNOT OR PROBABLY CANNOT BE MODIFIED
  Identify ECG abnormalities
  Identify type A behavior
  Identify diabetes and gout
FACTORS THAT ARE NOT ESTABLISHED RISKS
  Encourage regular physical activity
  Monitor intake of alcohol and coffee

[a] Modified from American Heart Association: Risk factors and coronary disease: a statement for physicians. *Circulation* 62:449A, 1980.

tients means "severe" rather than knife-like or piercing.

Typically, the discomfort is midline and substernal; it often radiates to the shoulder, arm, hand, or fingers—usually to the left. Radiation down the inside of the arm into the fingers supplied by the ulnar nerve is classic. Pain may radiate also into the neck, the lower jaw, or the intrascapular region. Occasionally, the patient may have pain only in a referred location and experience no chest discomfort at all. The atypical pain may be such that the patient may actually consult his dentist because he ascribes pain in the lower jaw that is due to myocardial ischemia to a toothache. In addition, the pain of myocardial ischemia is diffuse and cannot be easily localized: rarely is the patient able to point with one finger to the location of the pain; when pain can be localized in this way, it is likely to be noncardiac in origin (see Chapter 53).

Initiation of Ischemic Pain

The most important diagnostic feature of the discomfort of myocardial ischemia is its relationship to exertion, to emotional stress, or to other situations that may either increase myocardial oxygen demand or decrease myocardial oxygen supply. The cause of atypical pain, pain in an unusual location or of an unusual character, may be clarified by this relationship. Pain that is experienced at rest, if it is due to cardiac ischemia, suggests unstable angina (page 700), variant angina (page 700), or myocardial infarction.

Anxiety is an important and often overlooked provoking factor in many patients. Myocardial oxygen demand may be increased by anxiety to an extent and duration greater than that produced by exercise, resulting in prolonged pain. This is important in understanding environmental factors in a patient with angina. The common cycle of anxiety producing chest pain and the pain in turn producing more anxiety should be recognized as an important mechanism of prolonged pain.

Angina is more likely to occur during cold or windy weather because of increased peripheral vascular resistance and consequently increased myocardial work and perhaps because of cold-activated reflexes that produce a decrease in coronary flow. In some patients a specific diurnal pain pattern may be evident with angina occurring only with an early daily activity, such as an early morning shower or a walk from a car to a place of work. It is important to recognize this pattern because it has specific therapeutic implications. Sometimes ischemic discomfort will follow a heavy meal, perhaps because of the shunting of blood to abdominal viscera and because of increased sympathetic tone.

Nocturnal angina may be a consequence of left ventricular failure or represent unstable angina. Similarly, patients who describe breathlessness and chest pain with exertion may have angina as a consequence of transient left ventricular failure (42).

Occasionally a patient will develop typical angina pectoris with work that involves the hands, arms, and shoulders, whereas the same patient may be able to walk at a brisk pace indefinitely without pain. It has been postulated that this phenomenon is due to the fact that smaller muscles use relatively more oxygen and that the use of smaller muscles in the upper extremities often involves isometric activity (increase in muscle tone with little shortening of muscle fibers), which increases peripheral arterial resistance. This increase in afterload (the resistance to ejection of blood from the heart) increases left ventricular systolic pressure, left ventricular work, and hence myocardial oxygen demand. In contrast, walking or the use of large leg muscles is not isometric; the increase in cardiac output and blood flow to the legs is accomplished in a setting of arterial dilation and a consequent decrease in peripheral resistance and afterload. It is important to establish these relationships for diagnosis and therapy.

Increase in carboxyhemoglobin level is an important though seldom recognized cause of angina in some persons. Commonly this may occur through exposure to high carbon monoxide (CO) levels in heavy traffic or through inhalation of CO in tobacco smoke. These two situations, both with implications for patient management, can be identified by careful history taking.

Relief of Ischemic Pain

Since angina is due to a discrepancy between oxygen supply and demand, relief of pain is achieved by increasing coronary blood flow or by decreasing oxygen demand. Cessation of effort or relief of anxiety decreases oxygen demand, and an-

gina begins to disappear within minutes thereafter. So called "walk through angina" is uncommon. Most people must stop or at least slow the activity responsible for precipitating the pain before it is relieved. A history of relief of pain by sublingual nitroglycerin is also useful. However, the patient must be told that the use of nitroglycerin in this way is a diagnostic trial and that the prescription of nitroglycerin does not necessarily mean coronary artery disease. On the other hand, the physician and the patient both need to know that the relief of chest pain by nitroglycerin is not specific for myocardial ischemia. For example, the pain of esophageal spasm is commonly relieved by nitroglycerin (see Chapter 34). A placebo effect may relieve chest discomfort due to other causes as well.

Duration of Ischemic Pain

Angina pectoris responds promptly to measures directed at reducing myocardial oxygen demand (cessation of effort usually) or possibly at increasing coronary blood flow. Pain is usually relieved within 5 minutes; if it persists beyond 20 minutes, a myocardial infarction is likely and the patient should be hospitalized.

Physical Examination

The examination of a patient who complains of possible ischemic cardiac pain should be done with particular attention to uncovering circumstantial evidence that would support a diagnosis of cardiovascular disease: high blood pressure, evidence of abnormal lipid metabolism such as xanthomas (Chapter 75), funduscopic changes reflecting long-standing hypertension or diabetes, or evidence of peripheral vascular disease (Chapter 87).

Several physical findings suggest ischemic heart disease. A systolic bulge may be felt at the apex of the heart, especially when the patient lies in the left lateral decubitus position. A third or fourth heart sound (S_3 or S_4) may be heard. There may be a paradoxic split of the second heart sound caused by a delay in aortic valve closure because of a decrease in contractility of the left ventricle.

The opportunity to examine a patient during an episode of chest pain should not be missed. The examination should be done promptly, while someone else connects the electrocardiograph machine, before the pain resolves. Physical findings (e.g., S_4, paradoxical splitting of S_2, or a murmur of mitral insufficiency—see Chapter 60) may be present transiently during an episode of chest pain; in such instances, they provide stronger evidence of ischemic heart disease than they would if found incidentally, when the patient was asymptomatic. The blood pressure should also be recorded if the patient is examined while he is experiencing chest pain; transient hypertension during an ischemic attack is seen commonly. A similar phenomenon can be observed during exercise stress testing when a hypertensive response is often documented before symptomatic or electrocardiographic evidence of ischemia. Hypotension detected during myocardial ischemia is an ominous sign and likely indicates global ischemia produced by left main coronary artery disease or severe triple vessel disease. This is important to recognize because early arteriography and bypass surgery should be considered in such patients.

Electrocardiogram

A 12-lead standard electrocardiogram (ECG) should be obtained in any patient with suspected ischemic cardiac pain.

The most reliable ECG sign of chronic ischemic heart disease is a Q wave (8), recorded by those leads of the ECG which are measuring electrical activity of a part of the myocardium that has been infarcted (Fig. 57.1A). Nonspecific ST-T wave changes, abnormalities of conduction (except for left bundle branch block—see below), and arrhythmias do not help to establish the diagnosis of myocardial ischemia. ST depression with a flat or down-sloping ST segment, however, is indicative of subendocardial ischemia (Fig. 57.1B). It is seldom present in the ECGs of patients with ischemic heart disease unless they are experiencing angina at the time the tracing is being recorded. On the other hand, these "ischemic"

changes are seen commonly when a patient with ischemic heart disease is exercised to a point where he develops chest pain. Such ECG changes, appearing with exercise or pain and resolving with rest or with the resolution of pain, are strongly indicative of myocardial ischemia. Hence the necessity of repeating the ECG at rest or after the chest pain has been resolved cannot be overemphasized. ST elevation at rest (Fig. 57.1C) suggests variant angina (see below) or myocardial infarction. T wave inversion in an ECG taken at rest is a nonspecific finding unless it is seen only when a patient is experiencing angina.

Listed below are some important general guidelines in regard to using the ECG for evaluating chest pain. It is important to caution that some exceptions to these guidelines do exist.

1. A patient who has not had a previous myocardial infarction and who has had angina pectoris for less than a year will usually have a normal ECG, if the ECG is done at a time when the patient is not experiencing chest pain. The finding of a normal resting ECG in such a patient is not good evidence against the diagnosis of coronary artery disease. Fifty percent of all patients with known coronary artery disease will have a normal resting ECG (29).

2. A patient with a normal resting ECG will usually have ischemic ECG changes during an episode of angina. Also such patients will usually have a positive exercise stress test (see below). The absence

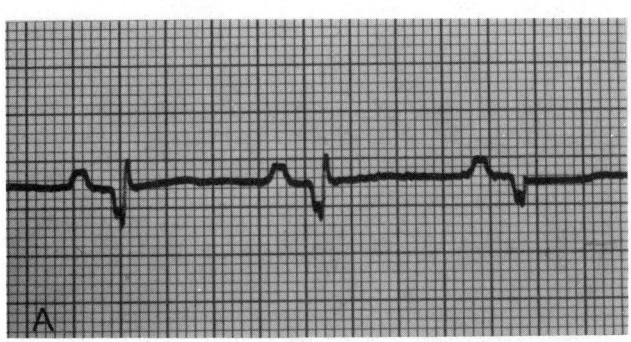
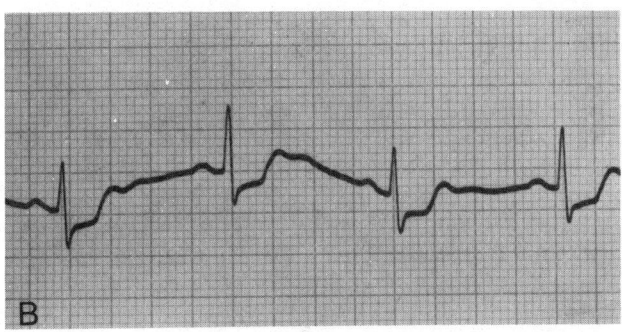
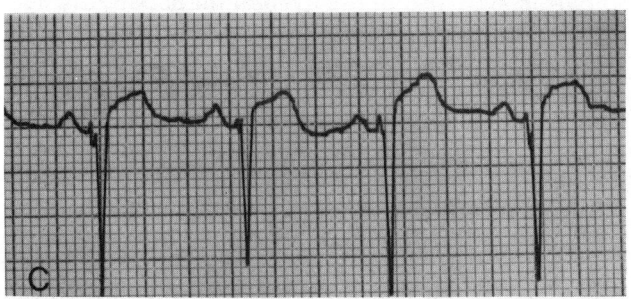
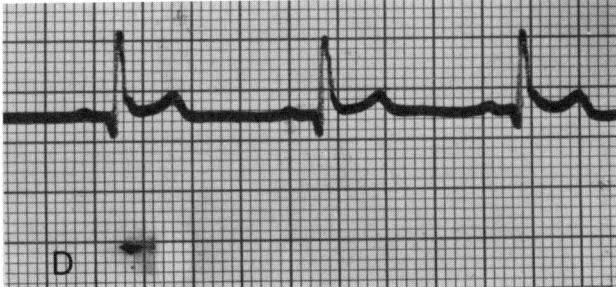

Figure 57.1. Electrocardiographic strips of patients with suspected ischemic heart disease. *A.* Q waves suggestive of chronic myocardial disease. *B.* ST de-pression developing after exertion. *C.* ST elevation during coronary artery spasm (variant angina). *D.* early repolarization (a normal variant).

of changes in such circumstances suggests that the pain may not be cardiac.

3. Patients with long-standing angina pectoris (10 years or more) usually have abnormal resting ECGs. They often have evidence of previous myocardial infarction, left ventricular hypertrophy, conduction abnormalities, or nonspecific ST-T changes.

4. A patient with a baseline abnormal resting ECG, due to previous infarction, left ventricular hypertrophy, bundle branch block, *etc*, may develop no new ECG changes during an attack of angina. Similarly such patients can have an acute myocardial infarction with no changes in their ECG.

5. An abnormal resting ECG, in the absence of other evidence, does not justify a diagnosis of ischemia or of coronary artery disease. Although there is a high degree of statistical correlation between an abnormal ECG and coronary artery disease, the vast majority of people in whom this correlation exists have other evidence of coronary artery disease, such as clinically documented infarction, typical angina pectoris, heart failure, cardiac enlargement, or arteriographically proven disease. When one sees a patient with a negative cardiac history, a normal cardiovascular examination, and an abnormal ECG, it is likely that the ECG abnormalities are due to some form of cardiac pathology other than coronary artery disease or that there is no cardiac disease. The QRS abnormalities of infarction are conduction abnormalities which may have many causes (16), although the most common is infarction. Thus, a pattern suggesting old infarction can be seen in patients without coronary artery disease and may be due to healed myocarditis, to an infiltrative disease such as amyloidosis or sarcoidosis, or to Wolff-Parkinson-White syndrome (see Chapter 59). Similarly ST segment elevation suggesting acute infarction may be seen in the resting ECG of healthy persons with so-called "early repolarization." This pattern (see Fig. 57.1*D*) is found most often in young adult males, usually in the midleft chest leads but also in right chest leads and in limb leads. The ST elevation may reach 4 mm but there is no ST depression in reciprocal leads and the ST elevation usually normalizes during exercise. The presence of nonspecific ST-T abnormalities in an otherwise well person should not be regarded as evidence of heart disease in the absence of other confirmatory findings. Nonspecific ST-T abnormalities *per se* are rarely diagnostic of anything and that is why they are called "nonspecific."

6. There is a high degree of correlation between left bundle branch block and organic heart disease (see Chapter 59), especially coronary artery disease. Right bundle branch block, on the other hand, is seen commonly in the absence of other cardiac abnormalities. It is presumed that right bundle branch block in the absence of other evidence of cardiac disease is congenital; in many instances it is a totally benign finding.

7. Although studies suggest a possible relationship between arrhythmias and cardiac disease, particularly coronary artery disease, these results must be interpreted with caution. One is not justified in making a diagnosis of heart disease because of an arrhythmia in a patient who appears otherwise healthy. This should not be interpreted to justify a cavalier attitude toward arrhythmias. However, there are some people with lifelong arrhythmias such as atrial fibrillation, complete heart block, ventricular premature beats, and paroxysmal ventricular tachycardia, who have no other evidence of disease and whose life expectancy is not obviously shortened. (Arrhythmias are dealt with in more detail in Chapter 59.)

Exercise Stress Tests

The role and the value of exercise stress testing are misunderstood by many health care providers. The exercise stress test is relatively safe and relatively inexpensive; when used in the context of the total clinical picture, it contributes valuable information about the patient with chest pain and/or with other cardiac symptoms.

The rationale behind exercise stress testing is simple. By increasing the work performed by the patient, cardiac work is increased. This increase in work results in an increase in myocardial oxygen utilization which demands an increase in coronary blood flow. If narrowed or obstructed coronary arteries prevent the required increase in coronary blood flow, ischemia may occur and be manifest as chest pain and/or ECG changes.

Various stress test techniques are available, but the most frequently used and best standardized ones require the patient to walk on a treadmill while permitting a controlled increase in work load by increasing the rate and inclination of the device. Exercise on a bicycle ergometer is also commonly used. A bicycle ergometer may also permit a patient to exercise with his arms instead of his legs. This is particularly useful in patients who cannot use the treadmill, because of claudication, arthritis, or amputation, and also in the evaluation of patients who have chest pain predominantly or exclusively with work that involves the arms and shoulders.

The stress test should be performed in a facility that permits monitoring during exercise, has a direct writing instrument to record and document the ECGs, and has equipment and staff trained to deal with arrhythmias and other cardiac emergencies. With properly selected patients and with an appropriately equipped laboratory and a trained staff, an exercise stress test is a safe procedure with reported mortality rates in the range of 0.01% (37).

It is important to recognize that the exercise stress

test is not just a technical procedure. Both the safety of the procedure and the information obtained are greatly enhanced when the team performing the study has sufficient clinical information to understand questions posed regarding the patient's therapy and the limitations of his disease on his life style.

Ordinarily a patient exercises until a predetermined heart rate is attained. This is usually 80 to 90% of the maximum heart rate predicted on the basis of the patient's age (see Table 58.6, Chapter 58). This goal can be modified according to the pre-exercise evaluation of the patient, keeping in mind the needs of the patient and of his physician. For example, in a young person in whom there is a low probability of ischemic heart disease, attempting to reach the maximum heart rate or exercising the patient to the point of exhaustion is reasonable and adds to the sensitivity of the study. A negative study under such circumstances is yet stronger evidence against myocardial ischemia. On the other hand, there is no obligation to reach the maximal heart rate or a high work load in an older patient in whom a negative study (no chest pain and no ischemic ECG changes) is clinically meaningful at a lesser work load. In such cases, the physician might decide that if the patient does not have angina and/or ischemic ECG changes at a work load approximating that patient's normal daily activity, further exercise stress testing is clinically of little value. The physician has thus obtained the necessary information about the patient's cardiovascular physiology to be able to tailor therapy.

Criteria

Criteria for a positive stress test vary among laboratories. Referring physicians must understand these criteria and the purpose for which they are being utilized. Depression of the ST segment with a flat, horizontal, or down-sloping ST segment is the typical ischemic change sought as "positive" electrocardiographic evidence of ischemia (Fig. 57.1B). If 0.5-mm ST depression is used as a criterion of positivity, the laboratory will produce results that are more sensitive but less specific—that is, there will be a higher proportion of false positive results. Conversely, if 2.0-mm ST depression is the criterion, the results will be more specific but less sensitive—that is, there will be a higher proportion of false negative studies. Most laboratories use 1.0-mm ST depression as a criterion of positivity, a compromise that provides a reasonable degree of specificity while avoiding a level of sensitivity that results in an overdiagnosis of ischemic heart disease. On the average, this common criterion results in false positive tests about 10% of the time (i.e., specificity is 90%) and false negative tests about 30% of the time (i.e., sensitivity is 70%). In evaluating the results of exercise

stress testing it is important to keep in mind Bayes' theorem: the predictive accuracy (number of subjects with true positive tests divided by the number of positive tests) of any diagnostic test is directly related to the sensitivity of the test (the percentage of patients with the disease in whom the test is positive), the specificity of the test (the percentage of patients without the disease in whom the test is negative), and the prevalence of the disease in the population studied. This relationship exists whenever the specificity of any test is less than 100%. In populations which have a high prevalence of disease, the predictive accuracy will be very high even when sensitivity and specificity are low. Conversely, the predictive accuracy will be very low in groups of patients with a low prevalence of disease even when the procedure has high specificity and high sensitivity. Therefore, the predictive accuracy of an exercise stress test is dependent upon the characteristics of the population studied. In men with classic angina pectoris or previous myocardial infarction, a positive exercise stress test will accurately predict the presence of occlusive coronary artery disease about 85% of the time (44). On the other hand, in asymptomatic patients with positive ST segment responses to exercise stress testing, the predictive accuracy is much lower. About 60% or more of these patients may have false positive tests (44); that is, arteriographic studies will not demonstrate significant coronary artery disease.

Indications for Exercise Stress Testing

In general, exercise stress testing is used for diagnostic or prognostic purposes or to assess the effectiveness of therapy:

1. *To clarify the etiology of chest pain.* This is probably the most common reason for recommending an exercise stress test in an ambulatory population. In some practices exercise stress tests will be recommended for many patients in order to provide reassurance that chest pain is not due to cardiac ischemia. In such cases factors influencing sensitivity and specificity of the test must be kept in mind.

2. *To assess prognosis* in patients with known ischemic heart disease. A positive stress test after minimal exertion likely indicates severe triple vessel disease or left main coronary artery disease. Similarly a positive submaximal stress test in patients following myocardial infarction identifies a high risk population (see Chapter 58). Serial stress tests, at 6-month or 1-year intervals, can also be used to follow patients with stable angina. A deterioration in performance (angina or ischemic changes on the ECG at a lower work load) strongly suggests worsening coronary artery disease. Occasionally, the physiological significance of an anatomical lesion (e.g., 30 to 50% left anterior descending coronary artery stenosis) noted at coronary arteri-

ography may be questionable. In such a patient a positive stress test in the appropriate ECG leads (*i.e.*, V1 to V4 in this example), would clearly define the critical nature of the anatomical lesion.

3. *To decide whether a patient should have coronary arteriography.* Patients with positive stress tests after minimal exertion, as above, should undergo early coronary arteriography. The referring physician might decide, for example, that a patient with good exercise tolerance who has chest pain associated with 1-mm ST depression in leads II, III, and AVF after maximum exercise will be treated medically, whereas the patient who has chest pain associated with several millimeters of ST depression in many leads after relatively minimal exercise should undergo coronary arteriography.

4. *To evaluate functional capacity of patients* in order to recommend appropriate activities and to assess the ability of the patient to return safely to work. It may be helpful for the physician to know how much activity is necessary to produce evidence of ischemia in a given patient so that he can advise the patient about specific limitations in his activities. The physician should also ask the patient whether he has already done "stress tests" on himself—*i.e.*, trials of various activities to determine which produce angina (most patients have done this). This information, together with the results of the stress test, should then be used by the physician for making specific recommendations regarding exercise and activity.

Some physicians feel that an exercise stress test is appropriate in an apparently healthy middle-aged person who wishes to undertake a new physically stressful activity. For example, a preliminary exercise stress test is considered an appropriate part of the evaluation of a person who wishes to begin mountain climbing or serious running, especially if that person has previously led a largely sedentary life style; the caveats regarding predictive accuracy should be recalled when interpreting stress tests in such persons. Table 58.4 in Chapter 58 lists the metabolic equivalents (METs) of a number of common activities. Stress test data reported in terms of METs achieved before symptoms appear are useful for the physician in counseling the patient regarding safe levels of exercise.

5. *To evaluate patients after myocardial infarction or coronary artery surgery* in order to determine appropriate exercise prescriptions and to define postmyocardial infarction therapy. This is discussed in more detail in Chapter 58.

6. *To ascertain the effects of medical or surgical management of coronary artery disease*, particularly when baseline studies have been performed. The exercise stress test documents objectively whether or not a patient has improved, and, if he has, to what extent. The documentation of improvement with a stress test is often reassuring to the patient.

7. *To document the response of a patient with a cardiac arrhythmia* to exercise and to document the response of the arrhythmia to therapy (see Chapter 59).

Contraindications to Exercise Stress Testing

There are a number of contraindications to stress testing:

1. *The recent onset of unstable angina pectoris* (see below) or recent myocardial infarction is a relative contraindication to exercise stress testing. Most of these patients should not be subjected to maximal exercise stress tests. However, modified submaximal stress tests can be performed with a reasonable degree of safety in selected patients as early as day 10 postmyocardial infarction (43). The information thus obtained may be invaluable for making recommendations concerning physical activity and further therapy.

2. *Uncontrolled hypertension* is a relative contraindication and depends upon the level of blood pressure and upon the degree of end organ impairment.

3. *Exercise stress testing should not be performed in patients with severe uncontrolled congestive heart failure* because of the risk of acute pulmonary edema, of hypotension due to low cardiac output, and of serious arrhythmias.

4. Significant *ventricular arrhythmias* are a relative contraindication to exercise stress testing. However, it may be difficult to know before the test whether a given ventricular arrhythmia is significant, since patients with frequent multifocal premature ventricular contractions may show a decrease or an increase in ectopic activity when stressed; if ventricular ectopy increases with exercise, the test should be terminated.

5. Suspected severe *valvular disease*, particularly obstructive valvular disease such as mitral stenosis, aortic stenosis, or subvalvular aortic outflow obstruction, may impose serious risks to patients who are exercised. This is because the heart may be unable to increase cardiac output in response to an increased demand. In such patients the usual increase in blood pressure with exercise significantly increases ventricular afterload, and thus reduces perfusion. Again, however, modified stress tests can probably be performed with a reasonable degree of safety in appropriately selected patients.

6. Exercise stress testing should be performed with caution in a *variety of other conditions*. Exercise testing is contraindicated in patients with myocarditis, acute pericarditis, severe pulmonary hypertension, recent pulmonary embolism, atrial fibrillation with an uncontrolled ventricular response, intercurrent acute systemic illness, or significant infection. Patients with a high degree of atrioventricular block should be exercised cautiously since they may not be able to increase their

heart rate appropriately. Patients taking medications such as reserpine and a β-blocking agent, particularly when these have been instituted recently, may be at some risk because these drugs limit the response of heart rate or blood pressure to exercise. Patients with severe chronic pulmonary disease may have difficulty when exercised, such as increased bronchospasm, increased hypoxemia, and cardiac arrhythmias. However, exercise stress tests in such patients, with concomitant pulmonary function studies and blood gas analyses, can provide useful information (see Chapter 55).

7. *Neurological or orthopaedic disease* may make it difficult for the patient to engage in an exercise stress test. Modifications of stress testing, by use of a bicycle ergometer, for example, can sometimes circumvent these problems.

Patient experience. The patient will be told that he will spend a total of 1 to 1½ hours at the stress test laboratory; that he should not eat for at least 2 hours before the test; that the preceding meal should be light and should not contain butter, cream, coffee, tea, or alcohol; and that he should wear clothes and shoes that are comfortable to walk in. He will also be told which of his regular medicines he should take on the day of the test (if he has not been told at the time the appointment was made, he should be instructed to telephone the stress test laboratory to inquire about his medications several days in advance). Before testing, ECG leads are applied to the chest and a blood pressure cuff is applied to one arm. The test consists of walking on a treadmill; the speed and the slope of the treadmill are increased during the test. Alternatively, the test may consist of pedaling on a bicycle ergometer. The patient should be told that he will be asked to exercise to a point where he finds it uncomfortable; but that if he experiences chest pain, severe shortness of breath, claudication, or severe light-headedness, the test will be terminated. He should be told that he will not be asked to exercise to a degree inconsistent with his age and physical condition. The duration of the test will be determined by the time it takes to reach a maximum heart rate (usually no more than 10 to 15 minutes).

If radioactive scanning is included in the stress test, the patient will receive an intravenous injection containing thallium-201 at the time of maximum exercise and will have cardiac scanning immediately after exercising and again 3 hours later.

Office Stress Testing (Master's Test)

The use of submaximal office stress testing has decreased greatly in recent years. Popularized by Master and modified by many others, such studies have been replaced by maximal and near maximal stress testing in specifically equipped and staffed laboratories as described above. The utility and safety of doing any sort of exercise stress test in the office setting are questionable. Master's two-step exercise test is much less sensitive than a treadmill exercise test; it will often be negative in patients with clinically evident ischemic heart disease simply because the work load is insufficient to increase myocardial work significantly in many patients.

Radioisotopic Imaging

Thallium-201 is the isotope most used for clinically assessing myocardial regional blood flow. The rationale for using thallium is based on its ability to substitute biologically for ionic potassium; healthy myocardial cells rapidly extract thallium-201 shortly after it is injected; uptake is proportionate to regional perfusion. Low energy emissions permit recording of the myocardial pattern of radioactivity. Areas of infarcted myocardium have no thallium uptake and hence show diminished or absent activity, so-called "cold spots." Perfusion defects are also seen in transiently ischemic myocardium, however, these defects disappear or "fill in" as the ischemic episode resolves, i.e., during the reperfusion scan (20).

Thallium-201 scans are commonly performed as part of an exercise stress test. Thallium is injected intravenously at the time of peak exercise, and scintigraphic images obtained shortly thereafter depict regional myocardial perfusion at the time of peak stress. Scintigraphic images taken 3 hours later show redistribution of isotope. A "filling in" of a "cold spot" defined on the stress images is likely indicative of transient ischemia. On the other hand, a persisting "cold spot," or one with only partial redistribution, is likely due to infarction.

Thallium scanning with exercise stress testing is more sensitive and more specific for detection of occlusive coronary artery disease than exercise stress testing alone (36). It is not reasonable, however, to recommend that all patients undergoing exercise testing should incur the additional expense of a thallium scan. The use of thallium with exercise stress testing is of particular value in those conditions which render ECG interpretation difficult or impossible—for example, left bundle branch block, Wolff-Parkinson-White syndrome, and patients who are more likely to have "false positive" results of exercise stress tests, such as young patients (usually women), patients with mitral valve prolapse, or patients with a baseline grossly abnormal ECG due to infarction, left ventricular hypertrophy, or digitalis.

Besides its value in evaluating selected patients for exercise-related ischemia, thallium-201 scanning is also useful for detecting evidence of a recent or remote myocardial infarction (e.g., in patients with nonspecific ECG changes and a history of a clinical event too remote to be evaluated by measurement of cardiac enzymes). A resting defect on a thallium-201 scan is more sensitive than an ECG Q wave for identifying an old infarction. Recent data also suggest that submaximal thallium exercise stress testing postmyocardial infarction is more sensitive than conventional stress testing alone in identifying high risk patients (15).

Coronary Arteriography

Figure 57.2 shows diagrammatically the coronary arteries and their branches as they appear on coronary arteriography. This technique provides direct information about the presence of coronary artery disease and defines the distribution and severity of obstructive coronary lesions. Coronary arteriography is usually performed in conjunction with detailed intracardiac hemodynamic monitoring and a left ventriculogram. The addition of the latter two procedures allows for the detailed evaluation of valvular lesions and of overall left ventricular function. Coronary angiography has greatly expanded our understanding of the prognosis of coronary artery disease and it has become a major tool for decision making in the individual patient.

Indications

Our expanding clinical experience together with the changing spectrum of therapeutic options make it difficult to define firm guidelines for the use of coronary arteriography. There are certain indications for coronary arteriography that are generally accepted. However, some physicians believe that coronary arteriography should be performed in all (or almost all) patients with angina or myocardial infarction and others who believe that it should only be used as a last resort. It is essential that a referring physician not abdicate his responsibility to a patient through the process of referral for catheterization and arteriography. In addition, the morbidity and mortality of the procedure in the chosen laboratory

should also be known. Ideally, each laboratory should systematically and periodically analyze its performance so that its results and risks are known to referring physicians.

The principal indications for coronary arteriography are:

1. *To determine the operability of patients who have failed maximal medical therapy* (see below). This indication is clear-cut since surgery offers an excellent chance for clinical improvement. In patients with good left ventricular function there is about an 80% chance of operability, and a > 90% likelihood of a significant reduction in angina following surgery.

2. *To detect left main or severe three-vessel coronary artery disease.* Patients with these lesions can often be clinically identified on the basis of the history and/or stress test performance (see above). In addition, patients who are postmyocardial infarction, with a positive early submaximal exercise stress test, represent a high risk population who are likely to have severe triple vessel disease. Both these patient populations have a high 1-year mortality and should undergo early arteriography. Demonstration of left main or severe triple vessel disease in such patients, is an indication for early coronary bypass surgery.

3. *To permit decisions concerning management in young patients with coronary artery disease* who desire to continue an active or stressful life style; ideal recommendations regarding therapy and prognosis can only be made with knowledge of coronary anatomy. This is particularly true if exercise stress testing or radioisotope imaging suggests that there is a large amount of myocardium at risk for infarction.

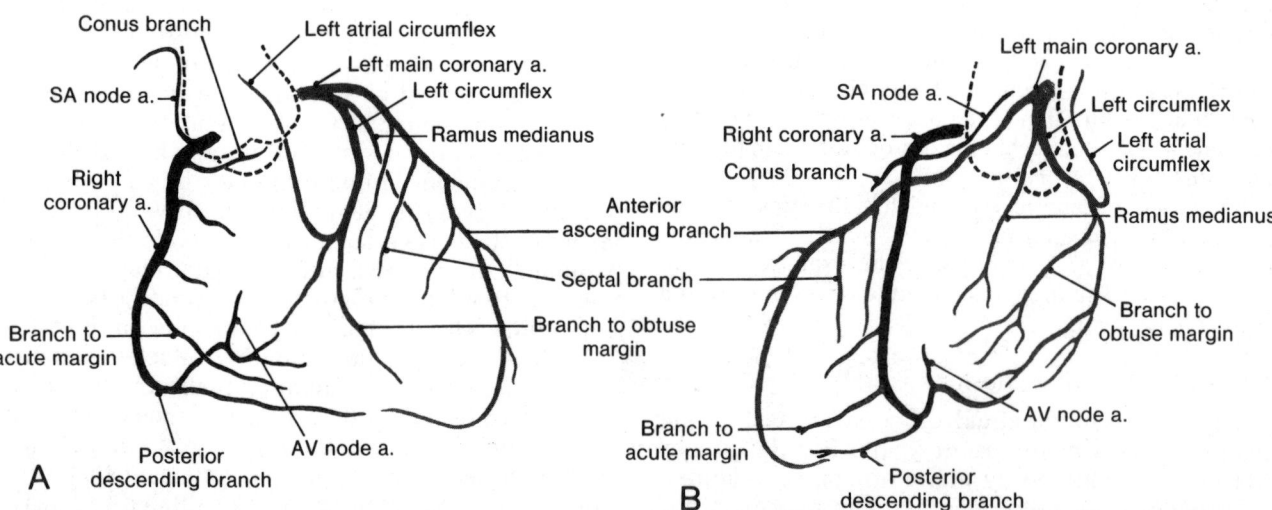

Figure 57.2. Anatomical representation of the coronary arteries. These vessels are represented as they would be seen on the angiogram. No attempt to convey the third dimension has been made. Careful study of the changes in position of the various branches with rotation of the heart is essential to intelligent interpretation of arteriograms. *A.* Anteroposterior. *B* Lateral. (From Abrams HL, Adams DF: The coronary arteriogram. First of two parts. Structural and functional aspects. *N Engl J Med* 281:1276, 1969.)

4. *To evaluate patients who are being considered for noncoronary cardiac surgery,* such as replacement of an aortic valve, and who may benefit from preoperative assessment of coronary anatomy. Armed with this knowledge a surgeon may elect to bypass significant, though clinically silent, coronary lesions or be prepared to bypass these coronary lesions if there are problems with left ventricular function during or immediately following cardiac surgery.

5. *To evaluate left ventricular performance.* If large segments of myocardium contract poorly or if overall ventricular performance is poor (as judged by measurement of ejection fraction or of left ventricular end-diastolic volume, see below), the risk of cardiac surgery is increased (30). On the other hand, in patients with severe angina, arrhythmias, or heart failure, identification of a distinct ventricular aneurysm or a specific valvular lesion offers the potential for surgical correction.

Technique and patient experience. Usually the patient is hospitalized the night before the catheterization. The procedure is not painful and the patient remains awake throughout the study. One hour before the procedure he is given a sedative, usually diazepam (Valium), 10 mg orally. What happens next depends upon the technique that is used. There are two commonly used techniques; both are performed under fluoroscopic control.

By the Sones technique, an incision is made, under local anesthesia, over the right brachial artery, and the catheter is threaded through a small incision into the artery and then *via* the subclavian and brachiocephalic arteries into the aorta near the coronary sinuses. By the Judkins technique, a special catheter is inserted percutaneously into the femoral artery and then threaded up the aorta to the coronary sinuses. The tip of the catheter is moved into either the right or left sinus; contrast medium is injected; and then, under direct fluoroscopic visualization, the orifices of the right and left coronary arteries are injected sequentially with contrast medium. The patient is asked to hold his breath during the few seconds of the injection. The catheter used in the Judkins technique is designed to enter easily either the right or left artery, so that after one arterial system is visualized adequately, the catheter must be withdrawn and the complementary catheter inserted.

After the coronary circulation has been visualized, ventricular pressures are measured and dye is injected directly into the left ventricular cavity to observe ventricular contraction. During ventriculography, aneurysms and valvular lesions, such as mitral regurgitation, can also be assessed. (Another special catheter is introduced in the Judkins technique for this phase of the study). Ejection fraction (the ratio of stroke volume to end-diastolic volume) is measured, then the catheter is withdrawn, and (if the Sones technique has been used) the incisions are sutured.

During this procedure the patient feels slightly woozy from the sedation: there is no pain except for occasional mild midsternal burning or a sensation of hot flushing when the dye is injected. The patient is usually discharged from the hospital the following day. (See also *Heart Catheterization,* an illustrated brochure published for patients by the American Heart Association.)

Complications of Coronary Arteriography

The major complications of coronary arteriography are death, myocardial infarction, and stroke. The minor complications include false aneurysms, arterial thrombosis, bleeding, transient impairment of renal function, allergy to contrast material (see Chapter 23), arrhythmias, and hypotension.

The risks of complications following coronary arteriography are related to the experience of the laboratory performing the studies and to the types of patients being studied. Risks tend to be lower in young, otherwise healthy patients and higher in older patients with poor left ventricular function, particularly those with associated peripheral vascular disease. The incidence of side effects, especially impairment of renal function, is also higher in diabetics. Risks are lower in those laboratories doing a large number of procedures, and the low risk is related to the experience and proficiency of the team performing the study. In laboratories doing six or more procedures a week the overall mortality and the risk of myocardial infarction and of stroke should be of the order of 0.1(%). Another way of evaluating the skill and proficiency of a laboratory is to look at the incidence of studies that have to be repeated because of inconclusive results following the original study. It should not be necessary to repeat more than 1 to 2% of studies. A newly established facility may take some time to reach a critical volume of coronary arteriographic studies before which there may be a higher risk of major and minor complications as well as an increased incidence of repeated studies.

Interpretation of Coronary Arteriography

There is often considerable variation among observers in the interpretation of coronary arteriograms. If there is 70% or more obstruction of a coronary artery, a significant impairment of coronary blood flow, even at rest, may be expected. A 50% narrowing may produce no significant decrease in flow at rest, but may produce serious physiological impairment when there is an increase in myocardial oxygen demand. Sometimes the consulting cardiologist will utilize the combined results of stress testing or thallium stress testing and arteriography to decide whether a given coronary occlusion may be significant enough to consider bypassing. For example, marked anterior ST depression and chest pain during an exercise stress test may indicate that there is a severe decrease in flow through a left anterior descending coronary artery even when the arteriogram demonstrates a lesion that obstructs 50% or less of the lumen.

PROGNOSIS

Mortality

The crude annual mortality rate after the onset of angina in persons without known infarction is about 5% (25). In contrast, the crude first year mortality rate ranges between 10 and 30% for patients with unstable angina, 10% for patients surviving 30 days after myocardial infarction, and 5 to 10% for patients with stable angina of 2½ years' duration (3, 25, 32).

Stress testing (see above) helps to detect those patients with angina who have relatively good or relatively poor prognoses. Patients with typical symptoms of ischemia who have positive exercise stress tests have an annual incidence of subsequent events and mortality which is higher than patients who have negative stress tests (12). Symptomatic patients with equivocal tests will have intermediate risks. The prognosis is worse when ST depression is more down sloping, when the ST depression occurs earlier during exercise, when the degree to which the ST segments are depressed increases, and when the ST depression persists longer after termination of exercise. This information may be helpful in selecting patients for further studies, such as coronary arteriography.

Coronary arteriography (see above) identifies with considerable precision those subsets of patients with relatively poor or relatively good prognoses, regardless of clinical manifestations of their coronary artery disease. The same anatomical spectrum of disease is found in patients with angina of various degrees, in patients with myocardial infarction without angina, and in patients with myocardial infarction plus angina of various degrees (34). Such patients have a similar distribution of significant lesions in the left main (about 10%), left anterior descending (about 80%), left circumflex (about 65%), and right coronary (about 70%) arteries. However, longitudinal studies of patients following arteriography have disclosed that the distribution of disease correlates with the risk of dying of the disease (22). In the first year after diagnosis, there is about a 30% mortality in patients with left main coronary artery disease and about a 15% mortality in patients with three-vessel disease (left anterior descending plus left circumflex plus right coronary artery disease). The first year mortality is about 10% for patients with two-vessel disease, 8% with one-vessel disease when that vessel is the left anterior descending coronary artery, and about 5% when single vessel disease involves the circumflex or right coronary artery (5). Long term studies show an annual mortality of about 10% in patients with three-vessel disease, about 7% in patients with two-vessel disease, and about 2% in patients with one-vessel dis-

ease (5). The higher first year mortality may be related to the events which prompted arteriographic studies in the first place.

Chapter 58 provides additional information about prognosis for subsets of patients with unstable angina or recent myocardial infarction.

Morbidity

Although angina may spontaneously remit after it has been present for a long interval (either as a consequence of myocardial infarction or of collateral circulation), the usual course is one of periodic symptoms and, for many patients, progressive disease (gradually worsening angina, unstable angina, myocardial infarction, congestive heart failure, arrhythmias, or sudden death) (25). Within 5 years of the onset of angina, about one in four men and one in eight women will have had a myocardial infarction (25).

The impact of angina upon a patient's functional capacity depends upon the nature of his usual activities and upon the status of his disease. As described below, pharmacological and nonpharmacological measures can have an important impact upon changing these limitations of activity, even though such measures usually have no impact upon the overall mortality. Many patients with angina can continue to engage in most if not all of their usual activities following therapy. (Table 9.1, Chapter 9, lists the criteria that qualify a person with ischemic heart disease for Social Security benefits.)

TREATMENT OF ANGINA PECTORIS

A useful booklet, *Living with Angina*, can be obtained from the American Heart Association. It will help the patient better understand his illness and the rationale behind its treatment.

Medical Treatment

The basic objective in treating patients with angina pectoris is to relieve or prevent pain by improving the relationship between myocardial oxygen demand and supply. This objective can be attained by increasing coronary blood flow and/or by decreasing myocardial oxygen demand. Angina that occurs with exercise is due usually to an increase in myocardial oxygen demand that cannot be met because of fixed arterial obstruction. A decrease in or cessation of the work that produced angina usually results in a prompt reduction in myocardial oxygen demand. Thus, rest or a decrease in the level of activity may relieve angina in 1 to 2 minutes. When anxiety is a contributing or provoking factor, it may take longer for myocardial work to decrease and the episode of angina may be prolonged.

The major advance in the medical management of angina in recent years has been the demonstration that long acting nitrates, β-blocking agents, and calcium channel blockers can decrease the frequency of anginal attacks and can increase the exercise tolerance and work capacity of many people who suffer from angina. In general, the duration or intensity of exercise before angina is doubled when these drugs are used optimally. Table 57.4 lists practical information about the drugs used most often in the treatment of angina.

Nitrates

Traditionally, nitroglycerin and related compounds have been the mainstay of treatment of patients with angina pectoris. Initially these agents were thought to increase coronary blood flow by producing coronary artery dilation. Although nitrates may increase coronary blood flow in patients with spasm or may increase collateral flow to obstructed vessels, evidence suggests strongly that the mechanism of action of nitrates in most patients is due not to an increase in blood flow but to a decrease in myocardial oxygen demand. These compounds produce dilatation of the venous circulation which in turn reduces venous return and decreases ventricular volume. The decrease in ventricular volume improves the efficiency of the heart and decreases wall tension. These effects ultimately reduce myocardial oxygen demand. Nitrates also produce, to a lesser degree, arterial dilatation, and thereby reduce the resistance to ventricular ejection. This effect further decreases myocardial oxygen demand by reducing left ventricular work. Thus, the beneficial antianginal effect of nitrates is due primarily to peripheral vasodilatation.

Sublingual nitroglycerin is still the drug of choice for the relief and prevention of discrete episodes of angina pectoris in most patients. In many patients with mild or infrequent angina, nitroglycerin is often the only medication required for the prevention or relief of pain. The initial dose should be small (0.4 mg) in order to minimize unpleasant side effects (flushing, headache, light-headedness) in those patients in whom higher doses may be unnecessary.

Patients should be taught that it is important that their pain be relieved as soon as possible. Since many patients experience some premonitory symptoms before the development of chest pain, they should be instructed to take nitroglycerin whenever such symptoms appear. Use of nitroglycerin in this way may do more than simply prevent ischemic pain. Angina often produces some anxiety, which may increase heart rate, left ventricular contractility, and hence myocardial oxygen demand. Thus, ischemia may be increased and the severity and the duration of pain may be prolonged. Additionally, some patients, during periods of ischemia, develop serious arrhythmias, hypotension, or incipient heart failure, which the prompt administration of nitroglycerin may abort (42). If pain is not relieved by 2 to 3 tablets of nitroglycerin (the patient should wait

for 3 minutes before taking another tablet) or if tablets must be taken more often than every 30 to 60 minutes, the patient should be instructed to call his physician immediately, because of the danger of impending myocardial infarction. Since nitroglycerin may lose potency on storage, the physician should advise patients not to keep tablets longer then 3 to 4 months after opening the bottle, and that if pain is not relieved and usual side effects are also not experienced, the problem may be due to a change in the drug rather than to a change in cardiac status. Prophylactic use of nitroglycerin is of particular value in patients who have mild or moderate angina in response to specific and reproducible stress. For example, the patient who develops angina after walking from a car to a place of work can be taught to take nitroglycerin after the car is parked, to wait a few minutes, and then to walk to work, thereby preventing pain altogether. The use of prophylactic nitroglycerin before sexual intercourse may also prevent angina and may alleviate the anxiety that is naturally associated with sexual activity when angina is anticipated.

It is important to teach the patient to use sublingual nitroglycerin correctly. The patient should take it while he is sitting to maximize the vasodilating effect (reduced in the supine position) and to avoid the possible untoward effects of hypotension (increased in the standing position). When initiating treatment with sublingual nitroglycerin, it is advisable to administer the first dose in the office so that the patient can experience the side effects and receive reassurance from a physician or nurse that this is an expected response. Patients who start taking nitroglycerin at home may otherwise become so frightened by side effects that they may delay taking it or may avoid its use altogether. The most common side effects are flushing and headache; both may diminish with increasing usage of the drug.

Long acting nitrates. Long acting nitrates have an important role in the control of angina. As shown in Table 57.4, long acting nitrates are available in a variety of preparations. Careful studies of small numbers of patients have confirmed the clinical efficacy of two preparations—nitroglycerin ointment and isosorbide tablets (10, 35). Both of these preparations produce about a 50% increase in the exercise time before symptoms appear. These effects last from 4 to 6 hours after drug administration. Patients restudied on an average of 6 months after beginning isosorbide tablets maintained the same increase in exercise tolerance (10). The dose of nitrate needed to improve symptoms may be relatively high; fortunately, available preparations permit a great deal of flexibility in dose adjustment, as shown in Table 57.4.

In selecting among available preparations, the major considerations should be the known efficacy and convenience of a particular nitrate for the patient.

Table 57.4.
Selected Drugs Used in the Treatment of Angina[a]

Class	Brand Name	Available Strengths	Usual Starting Dose	Usual Maximum Dose	Onset	Duration
NITRATES						
Nitroglycerin Sublingual[b]	Nitrostat and others	0.15-, 0.30-, 0.40-, 0.60-mg tablets, sublingual	1 tablet (0.4 mg) at time of, or in anticipation of pain	2–3 tablets at time of pain	30 sec	3–5 min
Topical						
Ointment	Nitro-Bid, Nitrol	2% ointment	½ inch every 4–6 hr as needed	4–5 inches every 3–4 hr	30–60 min	3–6 hr
Patch[c]	Transderm Nitro, Nitro-Dur and Nitrodisc	2.5-, 5-, 10-, 15-mg/24 hr rated release	5 mg	2–3 patches that deliver 15 mg/24 hr	30 min	24 hr
Long acting						
Erythrityl[b] tetranitrate	Cardilate	5-, 10-, 15-mg tablets oral or sublingual; 10-mg tablets, chewable	5 mg sublingually in anticipation of pain or 10 mg orally or chewed three times a day	100 mg a day in divided doses	5 min (sublingual and chewed)	4 hr
Isosorbide[b] dinitrate	Isordil, Sorbitrate and others	5-, 10-, 20-mg tablets, oral; 40-mg tablets or capsules, oral	10 mg every 4–6 hr	60–80 mg every 4 hr	15–30 min	4–6 hr
β-ADRENERGIC BLOCKERS[b]						
Propranolol[b(soon)]	Inderal	10-, 20-, 40-, 80-mg tablets, oral	10–20 mg three or four times a day	320 mg a day in divided doses	1–1.5 hr	4–6 hr
Nadolol	Corgard	40–80-, 120-mg tablets, oral	40 mg once a day	240 mg	1–2 hr	24 hr
CALCIUM CHANNEL BLOCKERS						
Nifedipine	Procardia	10-mg capsule	10 mg three or four times a day; 10 mg at time of pain if sublingual	40 mg every 6 hr	20–30 min	8 hr
Verapamil	Calan	80-, 120-mg tablets	80 mg three or four times a day	120 mg four times a day	30–45 min	6–8 hr
Diltiazem	Cardiazem	30-, 60-mg tablets	30 mg four times a day	60 mg every 6 hr	30–45 min	6–8 hr

[a] Other drugs, other doses of the drugs listed, and combinations of different drugs are marketed. The drugs and dosages shown are the ones most often used. Table 59.3 (page 724) provides information on the pharmacology of all six of the currently available β-blockers.
[b] Generic available.
[c] The brand name of these preparations is followed by a number (5, 10, 15, 20). It is important to know whether that number refers to milligrams per 24 hours (Transderm-Nitro or Nitrodisc) or to square centimeters of the patch (Nitro-Dur).

Using these criteria, isosorbide is probably the best choice for ambulatory patients. The disadvantages of nitroglycerin ointment are that it is messy to apply, that it is difficult to apply similar amounts evenly each time, and that skin irritation may occur after prolonged use. Its major advantage is that it can be removed promptly if a patient develops a significant side effect (e.g., severe hypotension) shortly after application. Many patients are treated in the hospital with nitroglycerin ointment; if its disadvantages become apparent after discharge, substitution of isosorbide is the best plan.

Recently a topical nitrate preparation for once a day use has also become available. It provides controlled release of 5, 10, 15, or 20 mg/day of nitroglycerin through a semipermeable membrane applied to the skin by means of an adhesive tape. It has two advantages compared to nitroglycerin ointment: It is not messy to use and it delivers a standardized dose. However, recent data suggest that constant serum levels of nitrate predispose to the development of tolerance. A tachyphylactic effect has been conclusively demonstrated in patients with heart failure treated with the nitroglycerin patch (1, 38), and it seems likely that a similar effect occurs in patients with angina. Hence patients who develop increasing angina while using this product may benefit from being changed to an oral nitrate regimen or to the nitrate ointment. (Tachyphylaxis has not been demonstrated in patients using nitrate ointment, probably because constant serum levels of nitrate are not achieved for as long a time.)

The side effects of all long acting nitrates are similar to those produced by sublingual nitrates. Many patients will have already experienced the headache produced by sublingual nitroglycerin before being treated with a long acting preparation.

Because of persistent headache, some patients are unable to take long acting nitrates, although in most patients this is not a problem. Because long-acting nitrates can produce orthostatic hypotension, and occasionally syncope, it is very important to check a patient's orthostatic blood pressure response before and after initiating treatment with or increasing the dose of a long acting nitrate. Two relative contraindications to long acting nitrates are a history of migraine or cluster headache and demonstrated orthostatic hypotension before initiation of treatment.

β-Blocking Agents

The introduction of β-blockers heralded a new era in the medical treatment of angina. Six β-blockers are currently available in the United States. Though all are approved by the Food and Drug Administration for use in hypertension, only timolol and propranolol are approved for use following myocardial infarction, and only propranolol and nadolol are approved for use in angina. The others (atenolol, pindolol, metoprolol, and timolol), though used to treat angina in England and Europe, are under evaluation for use in patients with angina in the USA. These agents vary in their cardioselectivity, their metabolism, and, to some degree, their side effects (see below and Chapters 59 and 62).

In many respects β-blockade is an ideal approach to the treatment of angina. It decreases heart rate, decreases contractility, and in many patients systemic blood pressure. These effects alone or in combination significantly reduce myocardial oxygen consumption and thus prevent the frequency and/or severity of angina in most patients.

An added benefit for patients with ischemic heart disease is that β-blockade often effectively prevents arrhythmias (see Chapter 59). It may decrease or eliminate premature ventricular contractions (PVCs), and the ventricular rate in patients with atrial fibrillation may also be decreased. Control of PVCs is beneficial to patients with ischemic heart disease because such patients are at increased risk for ventricular tachycardia or ventricular fibrillation, particularly during an episode of ischemia (7). Furthermore, when PVCs are frequent, the number of hemodynamically effective ventricular contractions is diminished, which in turn decreases coronary as well as peripheral perfusion. In patients who are in atrial fibrillation, decreasing the ventricular response improves left ventricular dynamics by decreasing heart rate, increasing diastolic filling period, and decreasing myocardial oxygen consumption.

The dose of a β-blocker can be rapidly increased over hours or days until the desired effect is obtained. The heart rate is the best guide to maximal treatment; sinus bradycardia at a rate at rest between 50 and 60 beats/minute is a reasonable goal. However, it must be noted that the ideal dose is one that not only results in sinus bradycardia at rest but also "blocks" an increase in heart rate with exercise. It should be recognized that the dose necessary to produce this effect and that necessary to relieve angina pectoris may vary considerably (see Table 57.4).

Since β-blocking agents decrease myocardial contractility, they must be used cautiously in patients with heart failure. If failure increases (sometimes expressed first as decreased exercise tolerance), reducing the dose of the β-blocker and/or adding digitalis (9) may improve cardiac compensation and at the same time reduce the severity or frequency of anginal attacks. If it is approved for the treatment of patients with angina, pindolol may be the β-blocker of choice in such circumstances. It is the only available β-blocker with intrinsic sympathomimetic activity and has, therefore, less negative inotropic effect than the other β-blockers. Often, it can be safely used in patients with reduced left ventricular function.

Extreme caution must be exercised while using all β-blockers in patients with second or third degree block (Chapter 59) since life-threatening bradycardia can be precipitated in such patients.

The nonselective β-blockers (propranolol, nadolol, pindolol, timolol) are contraindicated in patients with intrinsic asthma. A history of allergic asthma or of bronchospasm during pulmonary infections should therefore be sought in all patients for whom β-blockers are being considered. Furthermore, patients with chronic obstructive lung disease may develop increased bronchospasm from β-blockers even if they have no history of allergic or intrinsic asthma; therefore, in such patients a selective β-blocker with minimal β_2-blocking effects should be used. Metoprolol and atenolol are both relatively cardioselective and can often be safely used in such patients and in patients with peripheral arterial disease, particularly Raynaud's disease, in whom nonselective β-blockers may exacerbate symptoms. However, even these agents have β_2-blocking effects at moderate and high doses and should be used cautiously in these situations.

Impotence, though it occurs in 1% or less of the susceptible population, is perhaps the major reason why the use of β-blockers is limited in middle-aged men. It can sometimes be overcome by prescribing a β-blocker with poor lipid solubility and thus less penetration of the nervous system, e.g., atenolol instead of propranolol. Atenolol also is less likely to cause depression or to alter sleep patterns, occasional side effects of other β-blockers.

Several of the newer β-blockers can be administered once or twice a day, a feature which significantly promotes patient compliance. They have been shown to be effective at this schedule and in comparison studies nadolol (administered once a day) and propranolol (administered four times a day) have been shown to be equivalent for control of angina. Since some of the β-blockers are excreted entirely by the kidneys, the interval between doses should be increased in patients with renal insufficiency who are taking those preparations (see Table 59.3, page 724). Also, following the abrupt cessation of therapy with certain β-blocking agents exacerbation of angina and sometimes myocardial infarction have been reported. Hence patients should be instructed *never* to stop therapy abruptly; all β-blockers should be gradually tapered if therapy is to be discontinued.

Calcium Channel Blockers

Calcium channel blockers have added a new dimension to the treatment of angina. These drugs reduce the influx of calcium into the slow channels of the myocardium and smooth muscle (see Chapter 59) and thereby cause several important hemodynamic effects (40): (a) dilatation of coronary arteries and prevention of coronary vasospasm and (b) production of systemic vasodilation, thus effectively reducing preload and afterload. They have been shown to be effective in the treatment of both stable and unstable angina (14, 33). Three calcium channel blockers are currently available in the United States (Table 57.4). Although all three are effective in the treatment of angina, knowledge of their specific effects permits selection of the most appropriate drug.

Nifedipine is the one most often prescribed for patients with angina. It is a potent coronary and systemic vasodilator and therefore reduces the need of the myocardium for oxygen. It is usually given by mouth but for a rapid effect in patients unresponsive to nitroglycerin, a 10-mg capsule can be punctured and the contents taken sublingually. The common side effects of nifedipine are dizziness, flushing, headache, nausea, diarrhea, and, because of systemic vasodilatation, peripheral edema. The major adverse effect is severe hypotension, which, in association with a reflex tachycardia, can actually intensify myocardial ischemia in an occasional patient. All side effects can usually be controlled by a reduction in dosage of the drug. Nifedipine (and other calcium channel blockers) should be used cautiously in patients taking digoxin since excretion of digoxin may be inhibited and digitoxicity may be induced.

Verapamil is most often prescribed for the treatment of arrhythmias but it too is an effective antianginal agent and is unlikely to cause hypotension. However, it has a more potent negative inotropic effect than does nifedipine and, unlike nifedipine, significantly retards atrioventricular conduction. Therefore, it should not be used in patients with compromised left ventricular function or with sinus bradycardia, sick sinus syndrome, or atrioventricular block (see Chapter 59). In these situations, nifedipine is a safer choice. Verapamil might reasonably be prescribed to a patient with a supraventricular arrhythmia who also has angina.

Diltiazem also significantly retards atrioventricular conduction, but it has less of a negative inotropic effect than does verapamil and, in contrast to nifedipine, is unlikely to cause hypotension or other side effects of vasodilation (flushing, headache, edema, etc). Therefore, some cardiologists prefer it to nifedipine in the treatment of patients who do not have an abnormal atrioventricular conducting system.

Initiating and Adjusting Long Acting Drugs for Angina

Either a nitrate preparation or a β-blocker can be tried initially (Table 57.4). If the patient fails to improve, the dose can be increased weekly until a response is achieved. If the type of treatment selected initially fails to help at a maximally tolerated dose, the other agent can be added or substituted.

Since nitrates and β-blockers decrease myocardial oxygen demand by different mechanisms, the continued use of the two types of therapy is quite reasonable.

A number of relative contraindications to either long acting nitrates or β-blockers have been mentioned above; these contraindications are important in selecting the initial treatment in some patients.

A good argument can be made for administering a β-blocker to most patients with angina, especially younger patients desirous of an active life style unless there is a specific contraindication. In patients who have infrequent or mild episodes of angina relieved promptly by rest or by sublingual nitroglycerin, however, a β-blocker may add little benefit. In patients with more frequent or more severe episodes of angina, it is reasonable to initiate treatment with a β-blocker and to prescribe sublingual nitroglycerin for the relief of discrete episodes of pain. If a β-blocker is effective in reducing or eliminating angina pectoris, additional preparations may be unnecessary. In patients with maximal effects from β-blockade who continue to have pain, addition of a long acting nitrate preparation or a calcium channel blocker may bring symptoms under better control.

Because of the known risk of precipitating worsening angina when a β-blocker is abruptly discontinued and because of indirect evidence for a similar problem when long acting nitrates are abruptly discontinued, these drugs should always be tapered over 3 to 7 days when they are being stopped. Clearly, it is very important to warn all patients of this problem so that they do not casually stop and start these drugs; a corollary to this is the importance of explaining that these drugs are being prescribed chiefly to prevent symptoms, so that patients whose symptoms remit do not conclude that they can try stopping medication themselves.

The potency of β-blockers and of calcium channel blockers in the treatment of angina is about the same. In general, β-blockers are prescribed first to patients with predictable angina (chest pain reproducible after a given effort) who are likely to have fixed obstruction of their coronary arteries—unless there is a specific contraindication, such as chronic obstructive lung disease. A calcium channel blocker (usually nifedipine) is prescribed to patients who have variable chest pain, in whom coronary artery spasm (see "Variant Angina," below) may be playing a role.

Since patients who fail to improve after maximal medical management for angina pectoris are considered candidates for coronary arteriography and possible surgery, it is important to define *maximal medical therapy*. In practical terms, administration of a β-blocker in increasing doses, until side effects militate against further increase, in conjunction with a dose of long acting nitrates increased to the point where side effects begin to become intolerable, together with maximal doses of calcium channel blockers, would be considered to constitute maximal medical management in most patients. If a β-blocker and a calcium channel blocker are used together, the dose of both may have to be lower than if either is used alone, because of an additive adverse effect on left ventricular function. Similarly, if a nitrate and nifedipine are used together, severe hypotension is more likely and the doses may have to be reduced. If side effects limit the addition of the third drug, the combination of a β-blocker and calcium channel blocker is likely to be more effective than a β-blocker and a long acting nitrate.

Other Therapeutic Considerations

There are a number of other important considerations in the treatment of patients with angina.

Hypertension is often present in patients with angina. There is a linear relationship between left ventricular work and myocardial oxygen demand. Left ventricular systolic pressure increases in response to an increase in peripheral vascular resistance. Both systolic and diastolic hypertension can increase myocardial oxygen demand. The physician should always attempt to reduce resting blood pressure to normal in patients with chronic hypertension, including those with isolated systolic hypertension. A reduction in blood pressure from 160/100 to 130/85 mm Hg may achieve a reduction of 15 or 20% in myocardial oxygen demand. This can be of crucial importance in reducing the frequency and severity of angina pectoris in the hypertensive patient. Although any sympatholytic antihypertensive agent is reasonable in the hypertensive patient with angina (see Chapter 62), β-blockers are an excellent choice in such patients since they have other antianginal properties and may also control hypertension without diuretics in some patients.

It is important to achieve a maximal level of pulmonary compensation in patients with angina and coexisting *lung disease* (see Chapter 55). Chronic hypoxemia and acidosis and the increased work of breathing in patients with pulmonary disease increase myocardial oxygen demand and decrease myocardial oxygen delivery, or both. Abstinence from cigarettes, avoidance of environmental pollutants, and the judicious use of bronchodilators are also important in the overall management of such patients. In heavy smokers without clinical lung disease, a decrease in smoking may also decrease susceptibility to angina by eliminating the inhalation of carbon monoxide in tobacco smoke (see Chapter 20). Carbon monoxide exposure in heavy traffic should also be avoided in patients whose angina is precipitated in this setting.

The physician should never overlook the possibility of *hyperthyroidism* (Chapter 73) in patients with angina, particularly in those with increasing angina. Often, particularly in the older patient, other obvious signs of hyperthyroidism may not be present. For example, hyperthyroidism may be manifest only by an increased frequency or severity of angina, an increase in heart rate in people with atrial fibrillation, or by increasing heart failure.

Anemia also requires serious consideration, particularly when the hemoglobin concentration falls below 7 g/dl. This is the point at which cardiac output must increase to maintain peripheral oxygen delivery at rest. Angina due to severe anemia is often seen in patients with ischemic heart disease and chronic renal failure.

Heart failure (see Chapter 61) in patients with angina should always be treated. The real possibility that latent heart failure exists in patients with angina decubitus or nocturnal angina should be considered. Diuretics or the use of digitalis may be effective in such patients and may reduce the frequency and severity of angina or eliminate angina altogether. Nifedipine and diltiazem are often ideal therapeutic agents for such patients since their reduction of preload and afterload helps to decrease left ventricular end-diastolic pressure, lower peripheral vascular resistance, and thus improve left ventricular function.

Physical conditioning can improve the exercise tolerance of patients with stable angina (26). For interested patients, referral to a physician-supervised exercise program is the best plan. In recent years, most large communities have developed such programs for patients with coronary artery disease. Chapter 58 describes the physiological basis of physical conditioning and describes a supervised exercise program for cardiac patients. The booklet entitled *Exercise Testing and Training of Individuals with Heart Disease or at High Risk for Its Development; A Handbook for Physicians*, available from the American Heart Association, provides additional information on this subject.

In addition to recommending exercise programs for selected patients, the physician should counsel patients with angina about physical activities that may increase their symptoms and should always ask them to raise any matters of concern about their regular activities. The energy requirements for a broad range of activities are summarized in Table 58.4 in the following chapter.

Percutaneous Transluminal Coronary Angioplasty

Percutaneous transluminal coronary angioplasty (PTCA) (18) has introduced an important option for the treatment of coronary artery disease that cannot be controlled by the administration of drugs. This technique has the ability to restore near normal coronary flow in diseased native coronary arteries, without the cost and morbidity of bypass surgery. It involves the compression of a critical coronary lesion against the wall of the affected coronary artery by means of an inflatable balloon mounted on a special catheter. Patients are identified as candidates for PTCA after cardiac catheterization has clearly delineated coronary anatomy and after it has been determined that bypass surgery would otherwise be indicated. PTCA was initially used to treat patients with single vessel, proximal, discrete, noncalcific coronary lesions. However, in skilled hands, triple vessel coronary lesions, if they do not straddle branch vessels, can be successfully dilated also (11). Though there are no absolute contraindications to the procedure, patients with arterial dissection or with eccentric and long stenotic lesions are poor candidates and have a higher risk of complications during PTCA. These patients are best treated with surgery.

Patients who are appropriate candidates for PTCA undergo the procedure either immediately following cardiac catheterization or at a subsequent time, depending on the clinical situation and on the needs of the particular patient. The catheter is usually introduced through a femoral artery under local anesthesia. A brachial approach can also be used but requires a cutdown. The coronary orifice is reached with a preshaped guiding catheter through which the balloon catheter with the balloon decompressed is inserted. The balloon is positioned halfway across the lesion, and translesional pressure gradients are measured. (Most significant coronary lesions cause a significant pressure drop across the lesion.) Under fluoroscopic control the balloon is dilated with increasing pressures until there is no more indentation of the balloon or until the previously recorded pressure gradient is essentially abolished and dye injections through the guiding catheter show normal flow and a sufficiently patent coronary artery. Steerable catheters have recently been designed and have significantly widened the spectrum of lesions that can be successfully treated by PTCA. The dilatation results in an actual intimal tear and occasionally a coronary dissection may occur. Therefore, a cardiac surgical team is ordinarily on standby during the procedure. Barring complications, the patient's experience during PTCA, and the time of the procedure is the same as it is for coronary angiography (see above). The incidence of major side effects (in addition to dissection, myocardial infarction, and sudden death) is related to the skill and experience of the operator and can be as low as 2 to 4% (4). Overall, the procedure is successful 60 to 80% of the time. Following successful angioplasty, patients are maintained on aspirin and persantine (see Chapter 51) along with a calcium channel blocker. Whether the calcium channel blocker needs to be maintained after hospital discharge, is the subject of several current trials. Patients can usually be discharged on the second hospital day and it is advised that they undergo regular stress tests at 3-, 6-, and 12-month intervals. The long term results of coronary angioplasty are favorable. Though the recurrence rate of stenotic lesions in most centers is about 30%, most recurrences can be successfully treated a second time by the same procedure (19). The vast majority of recurrences occur within the first 8 months after PTCA. Therefore, a lack of symptoms at 8 to 9 months usually indicates an excellent long term prognosis.

PTCA is a especially attractive therapeutic option in younger patients (40 to 50 years of age) in whom coronary bypass grafts, given the current state of the art, could be expected to remain patent for only 10 to 12 years. Also the comparative cost and morbidity of PTCA *versus* bypass surgery make the former more attractive if the therapeutic benefit is likely to be the same. Patients can often return to gainful employment 1 week after PTCA *versus* 3 to 6 months postbypass surgery (23, 24).

Surgical Management

Coronary artery bypass surgery is one of the most common surgical procedures performed in this country today. Our knowledge concerning the indications for the surgery and the effects of revascularization procedures on the coronary circulation and on morbidity and mortality is still developing. It is accepted generally that patients with incapacitating angina pectoris who have good left ventricular function and who have failed maximal medical therapy should be considered as candidates for coronary arteriography and subsequent surgery. It has been demonstrated that patients with left main coronary artery disease or its equivalent benefit symptomatically and have increased longevity following surgical intervention designed to increase coronary blood flow (41). Recommendations regarding surgery for patients with other lesions depend upon the consultant cardiologist's overall assessment of the patient.

The two surgical methods used today consist of saphenous vein bypass graft or implantation of an internal mammary artery into the native coronary artery circulation. The technique that is used is often based on the surgeon's preference and experience. A well illustrated brochure, *Coronary Artery Bypass Surgery*, which explains the procedure and the patient's experience, is available from the American Heart Association.

Patients with good left ventricular function have a 1 to 2% mortality rate from surgery. In addition, about 10% of patients will develop evidence of myocardial infarction during the perioperative period. The risk of complications from myocardial infarction in these patients however, is small since the infarct occurs at a time when myocardial oxygen need is diminished because of cardiopulmonary bypass. Also, the infarct occurs in a setting where complications such as arrhythmias are recognized and treated promptly. Nevertheless, it does represent a risk of loss of functioning myocardium. Perioperative infarction is more likely to occur in older patients and in patients with severe disease distal to a proximal obstruction.

About 60% of properly selected patients initially will have complete (or nearly complete) relief of angina pectoris, and another 20% will have a significant decrease in angina (31). There will be a demonstrable increase in exercise tolerance following surgery in about 60 to 80% of such patients.

Historically, up to 50% of patients have developed recurrent angina within 5 years of bypass surgery (13a). The diagnosis of recurrent angina should be confirmed by exercise stress testing. Initial treatment is the same as it is for patients who have not had bypass surgery: nitrates, β-blockers, or calcium channel blockers. Patients who prove to be unresponsive to medical treatment should undergo coronary angiography in an effort to delineate new lesions that possibly could be amenable either to percutaneous angioplasty or to repeat bypass surgery. In an attempt to prevent formation of such lesions it is now common practice to administer aspirin and persantine to patients postbypass (see Chapter 51, page 606).

The *postpericardiotomy syndrome* develops in approximately 30% of patients after bypass surgery, usually within 2 to 4 weeks (but sometimes as early as a few days or as late as 6 months after the operation.) The syndrome is characterized by fever, pleuritic chest pain, and, often, by pleural and pericardial effusions. Large effusions may require drainage, but most patients respond to diuretics and to a nonsteroidal anti-inflammatory agent (e.g., indomethacin, 25 to 50 mg three times a day for 1 to 2 weeks). Patients who are refractory to such treatment usually respond to prednisone, initially 60 mg a day for 2 to 3 days with tapering of the dose over 7 to 10 days. Recently, it has been suggested that graft occlusion is more likely in patients with postbypass pericarditis. Constrictive pericarditis is a late rare complication of the postpericardiotomy syndrome; when it occurs, pericardial stripping is often necessary.

Whether bypass surgery prolongs survival in patients without left main coronary artery disease or its equivalent is not entirely clear (6). The published studies do not provide a definitive answer in this regard. However, patients with severe triple vessel disease and poor left ventricular function likely have a better prognosis following surgery as compared to a group treated with conventional medical treatment. Until additional data are available, surgery should be recommended primarily to improve the quality of life of patients who have failed a medical regimen and who have demonstrable high risk lesions.

Sixty percent of patients who either were working just prior to bypass surgery or who discontinued work because of cardiac symptoms return to work after surgery. Early ambulation is advisable and the role of cardiac rehabilitation, as early as 6 to 8 weeks postoperatively, cannot be overemphasized (see detailed discussion, Chapter 58).

UNSTABLE ANGINA

Unstable angina is a term used to describe pain due to cardiac ischemia that is becoming more intense, is occurring more frequently—often provoked by diminishing effort (perhaps even at rest)—and is being relieved less readily by nitroglycerin. The syndrome has also been called *crescendo angina* and *preinfarction angina*. Sometimes unstable angina will develop in a patient with previously stable, reasonably controlled angina; at other times, it will develop in a patient with recent onset of ischemic symptoms. During the episode, the ECG shows ST elevation or depression and/or T wave inversion which revert to normal when the pain has abated. Because of the increased risks of myocardial infarction and of sudden death and because of the need for aggressive medical therapy, patients with unstable angina should be hospitalized. Aggressive medical treatment with β-blockers, calcium channel blockers, and intravenous nitroglycerin is usually implemented. Coronary arteriography is indicated as soon as possible in all patients, especially those in whom pain is not controlled by medical therapy, to determine their suitability for coronary bypass surgery or PTCA (see above).

The prognosis of these patients after hospital discharge is described in Chapter 58.

VARIANT ANGINA

Variant angina (Prinzmetal's angina) is, in a sense, unstable in that it occurs usually at rest but, unlike typical angina, does not occur on exertion or in response to emotional stress. Attacks of pain are experienced often at the same time each day, frequently awakening the patient early in the morning. During the attacks, there is ST segment elevation which reverts to baseline when the attack is over; there are also, in about one-third of the patients, transient atrioventricular blocks and/or arrhythmias (including ventricular tachycardia or fibrillation). Unlike unstable angina, pain is usually promptly relieved by sublingual nitroglycerin.

It is now clear that coronary artery spasm (21) often plays a major role in the pathogenesis of variant angina. Two groups of patients have been identified. By far the larger group (85% of patients) have fixed, often proximal, obstruction of a major coronary artery; angina in this group frequently is associated with spasm of the artery near the site of obstruction. The variant syndrome in this group of patients commonly follows months or years of stable typical angina pectoris or follows a myocardial infarction.

The smaller group with variant angina (15% of patients) have normal coronary arteries but have spasm of one of the arteries, thereby reducing blood supply to the myocardium, resulting in ischemic pain. These patients are usually younger and are predominantly women. There is usually no history of typical angina or of myocardial infarction in these patients, and infrequently a history of a systemic arteritis syndrome may be obtained. The ST elevation observed during the anginal attack is a manifestation of coronary artery spasm. It can often be confirmed by arteriography, either by the spontaneous occurrence of arterial spasm and chest pain during the procedure or by induction of arterial spasm by the administration of ergonovine. It is important to perform arteriography in such patients since those with normal coronary arteries are obviously not candidates for bypass surgery or PTCA and most respond favorably to treatment with calcium channel blockers. Calcium channel blockers are the drugs of choice in such patients. If used without calcium channel blockers, β-blockers may potentiate coronary artery spasm because of unopposed α-adrenergic vasoconstriction. However a recent double blind study of patients with rest angina showed that β-blockers, when added to nifedipine and nitrates, significantly reduced the number of episodes of angina in treated patients as compared to a control group on treatment with nifedipine and nitrates alone (17).

General References

Cohn PF, Braunwald E: Chronic ischemic heart disease. In Braunwald E (ed): *Heart Disease.* Philadelphia, WB Saunders, 1984 p 1334.
> A complete discussion of the diagnosis and management of angina pectoris.

Diamond GA, Forrester JS: Analysis of probability as an aid in the clinical diagnosis of coronary-artery disease. *N Engl J Med* 300:1350, 1979.
> A review of the application of Bayes' theorem to this problem.

Heberden W: Commentaries on the history and cure of diseases. Available from the New York Academy of Science, New York, Hofner, 1962.

Specific References

1. Abrams J, Gerety B, Schroeder K, Raizada V: Lack of hemodynamic effects of transdermal nitroglycerin discs. *Circulation* 70 (suppl II):188, 1984.
2. American Heart Association: Risk factors and coronary disease: A statement for physicians. *Circulation* 62:449A, 1980.
3. Block WJ, Jr, Grumpacher EL, Dry TJ, Gage RP: Prognosis of angina pectoris. *JAMA* 150:259, 1952.
4. Bredlau CE, Gruentzig AR, Douglas JS, King SB: Acute complications of percutaneous transluminal coronary angioplasty (PTCA)-initial experience in 3000 consecutive patient attempts. *Circulation* 70 (suppl II):106, 1984.
5. Bruschke AVG, Proudfit WL, Sones FM, Jr: Progress study of 590 consecutive nonsurgical cases of coronary disease followed 5–9 years: I. Arteriographic correlations. *Circulation* 47:1147, 1973.
6. Chalmers TC, Proudfit WL, Feinstein AR, DiBona GF: Sym-

posium: the scientific uses and abuses of the clinical trial: treatment of chronic stable angina with saphenous vein by-pass grafting. Randomized Veterans Administration Cooperative Study. *Clin Res* 26:229, 1978.

7. Chiang BN, Perlman LV and Ostrander LD: Relationship of premature systoles to coronary heart disease and sudden death in the Tecumseh epidemiologic study. *Ann Intern Med* 70:1159, 1969.

8. Cohn PF, Gorlin R, Vokonas PS, *et al*: A quantitative clinical index for the diagnosis of symptomatic coronary-artery disease. *N Engl J Med* 286:901, 1972.

9. Crawford MH, LeWinter MM. O'Rourke RA, *et al*: Combined propranolol and digoxin therapy in angina pectoris. *Ann Intern Med* 83:449, 1975.

10. Danahy DT, Aronow WS: Hemodynamics and antianginal effects of high dose oral isosorbide dinitrate after chronic use. *Circulation* 56:205, 1977.

11. Dorros G, Singh S, Janke LM: Coronary angioplasty in multivessel coronary disease. *Circulation* 70 (suppl II): 107, 1984.

12. Ellstad MH, Wan MKC: Predictive implications of stress testing: follow-up of 2700 subjects after maximum treadmill stress testing. *Circulation* 51:363, 1975.

13. Gazes PC, Mobley EM Jr, Faris HM, Jr, *et al*: Preinfarction (unstable) angina—a prospective study. Ten years followup. Prognostic significance of electrocardiographic changes. *Circulation* 48:331, 1973.

13a. Gersh BJ, Kronmal, RA, Schaff HV, *et al*: Long-term (5 year) results of coronary bypass surgery in patients 65 years or older: A report from the coronary artery surgery study. *Circulation* 68 (suppl II):190, 1983.

14. Gerstenblith G, Ouyang P, Achuff SC, *et al*: Nifedipine in unstable angina. A double-blind randomized trial. *N Engl J Med* 306:885, 1982.

15. Gibson RS, Watson DD, Craddock GB, *et al*: Prediction of cardiac events after uncomplicated myocardial infarction; a prospective study comparing predischarge exercise thallium-201 scintigraphy and coronary angiography. *Circulation* 68:321, 1983.

16. Goldberger AL: Recognition of ECG pseudo-infarct patterns. *Mod Concepts of Cardiovasc Dis* 49:13 (March), 1980.

17. Gottlieb SO, Weisfeldt ML, Ouyang P, *et al*: Propranolol for unstable angina in the era of calcium antagonists: a double blind randomized trial. *Circulation* 70 (suppl II):48, 1984.

18. Gruentzig A: Transluminal dilatation of coronary artery stenosis. *Lancet* 1:263, 1978.

19. Hall DP, Gruentzig AR: Recurrence rate after double-vessel dilatation. *Circulation* 70 (suppl II):107, 1984.

20. Hamilton GW: Myocardial imaging with thallium-201: the controversy over its clinical usefulness in ischemic heart disease. *J Nucl Med* 20:1201, 1979.

21. Hilles LD, Braunwald E: Coronary-artery spasm. *N Engl J Med* 299:695, 1978.

22. Humphries JO, Kuller L, Ross RS, *et al*: Natural history of ischemic heart disease in relation to arteriographic findings. A twelve year study of 224 patients. *Circulation* 49:489, 1974.

23. Jang GC, Block PC, Cowley MJ, *et al*: Comparative cost analysis of coronary angioplasty and coronary bypass surgery: results from a national co-operative study. *Circulation* 66 (suppl II):124, 1982.

24. Jang GC, Gruentzig AR, Block PC, *et al*: Work profile of patients following coronary angioplasty or coronary bypass surgery: results from a national cooperative study. *Circulation* 66 (suppl II):123, 1982.

25. Kannel WB, Feinleib M: Natural history of angina pectoris in the Framingham study: prognosis and survival. *Am J Cardiol* 29:154, 1972.

26. Kennedy CC, Spiekerman RE, Lindsay MI Jr, *et al*: One-year graduated exercise program for men with angina pectoris. *Mayo Clin Proc* 51:232, 1976.

27. Kirk ES, Jennings RB. Pathophysiology of myocardial ischemia. In Hurst JW (ed): *The Heart*, ed 5. New York, McGraw-Hill, 1982, p 976.

28. Lipid Research Clinics Program: The lipid research clinics coronary primary prevention trial results. II. The relationship of reduction in incidence of coronary heart disease to cholesterol lowering. *JAMA* 251:365, 1984.

29. Mattingly TW, Robb GP, Marks HH: Stress tests in the detection of coronary disease. *Postgrad Med* 24:4, 1958.

30. Mitchel BF, Alivizatos PA, Adam M, *et al*: Myocardial revascularization in patients with poor ventricular function. *J Thorac Cardiovasc Surg* 69:52, 1975.

31. Mundth ED, Austen WG: Surgical measures for coronary heart disease. *N Engl J Med* 293:13, 75 and 124, 1975.

32. Norris RM, Caughey DE, Mercer CJ, Scott PJ: Prognosis after myocardial infarction. Six-year follow-up. *Br Heart J* 36:786, 1974.

33. Ouyang P, Brinker JA, Mellits ED, *et al*: Variables predictive of successful medical therapy in patients with unstable angina: selection by multivariate analysis from clinical, electrocardiographic, and angiographic evaluations. *Circulation* 70:367, 1984.

34. Proudfit WL, Shirley EK, Sones FM Jr: Distribution of arterial lesions demonstrated by selective coronary arteriography. *Circulation* 36:54, 1967.

35. Reicheck N, Goldstein RE, Redwood DR, Epstein ST: Sustained effects of nitroglycerin ointment in patients with angina pectoris. *Circulation* 50:348, 1974.

36. Ritchie JL, Zaret BL, Strauss HW, *et al*: Myocardial imaging with thallium-201: a multicenter study in patients with angina pectoris or acute myocardial infarction. *Am J Cardiol* 42:345, 1978.

37. Rochmis P, Blackburn H: Exercise tests: a survey of procedures, safety, and litigation experience in approximately 170,000 tests. *JAMA* 217:1061, 1971.

38. Silber S, Krause KH, Theisen K: Nitrate-tolerance: dependence on dosage intervals? *Circulation* 70 (suppl II):189, 1984.

39. Sonnenblick EH, Strobeck JE: Derived indexes of ventricular and myocardial function. *N Engl J Med* 296:978, 1977.

40. Stone PH, Antman EM, Muller JE, Braunwald E: Calcium channel blocking agents in the treatment of cardiovascular disorders. II. Hemodynamic effects and clinical applications. *Ann Intern Med* 93:886, 1980.

41. Takaro T, Hultgren HW, Lipton MJ, *et al*: The V.A. cooperative randomized study of surgery for coronary arterial occlusive disease. II. Subgroup with significant left main lesions. *Circulation* 54 (suppl III):107, 1976.

42. Taylor SSH: Reversible left-ventricular failure in angina pectoris. *Lancet* 2:902, 1970.

43. Theroux P, Waters DD, Halphen C, *et al*: Prognostic value of exercise testing soon after myocardial infarction. *N Engl J Med* 301:341, 1979.

44. Weiner DA, Ryan TJ, McCabe CH, *et al*: Exercise stress testing. Correlations among history of angina, ST-segment response and prevalence of coronary-artery disease in the coronary surgery study (CASS). *N Engl J Med* 301: 230, 1979.

Postmyocardial Infarction Care, Cardiac Rehabilitation, and Physical Conditioning

MAHMUD A. THAMER, M.D., KERRY J. STEWART, Ed.D., AND
L. RANDOL BARKER, M.D.

EPIDEMIOLOGY OF MYOCARDIAL INFARCTION

Care of the patient who has survived a myocardial infarction (MI) is a common problem in ambulatory practice. There are roughly 7 million survivors of myocardial infarction in the United States at any time. Each year, approximately 1 million persons are added to this group, and about 1 million die (3). About two-thirds of the survivors have had uncomplicated MIs and, therefore, have relatively good long term prognoses.

The majority of persons who have MIs are under the age of 60. It is estimated that in the United States one man in five will have an MI before the age of 60 and that one in 10 to 15 men in this age group will die of atherosclerotic heart disease. These risks are 2 to 3 times lower in women (27). The higher male mortality rates from coronary artery disease (CAD) are particularly striking among young white males. In 1979, the male to female ratios of mortality from CAD were 5.2 at ages 35 to 44 and 2.4 at ages 65 to 74; among nonwhites, the respective ratios were 2.8 and 1.6 (17).

Two epidemiological observations underscore the importance of ambulatory care in reducing mortality due to CAD.

1. About three-quarters of all deaths from CAD occur outside the hospital.

2. In the past decade, the number of people dying of CAD in the United States has decreased about 17% (28); this decrease seems to be largely due to changes which have occurred outside the hospital (i.e., reduction in CAD risk factors and prehospital and postdischarge management of acute MI).

PROGNOSIS OF MYOCARDIAL INFARCTION AND UNSTABLE ANGINA

Patients discharged following hospitalization in coronary care units (CCU) may be divided into three broad categories: those who have had a confirmed MI, those who have had unstable angina, and those who have had cardiac arrest without a confirmed MI. The different prognoses for patients in these three categories have been delineated in the past decade.

Survivors of Myocardial Infarction

Mortality

The overall first year mortality for hospital survivors of an MI is about 5 to 10%. Thereafter, the annual mortality remains between 3 and 5% for the next 15 years. These figures are the same for patients surviving transmural or subendocardial MIs (Fig. 58.1). Most of the deaths in the first year occur during the 3 months following discharge, and they occur chiefly in patients with one or more of the high risk characteristics listed in Table 58.1.

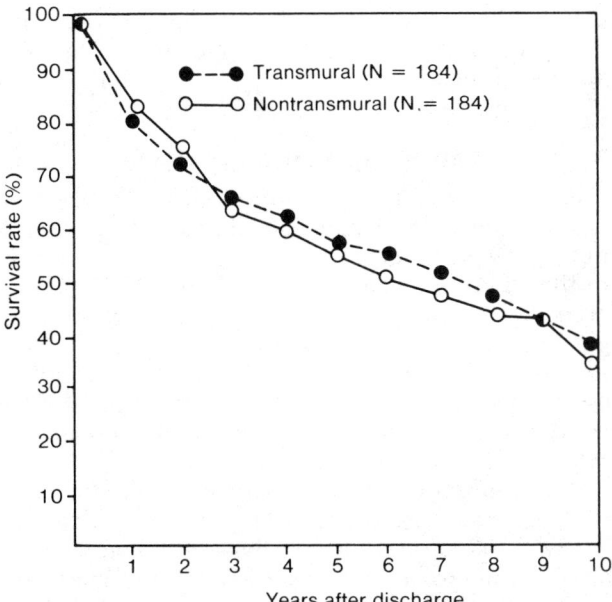

Figure 58.1. Survival rates in matched samples of transmural and nontransmural myocardial infarction patients discharged alive in metropolitan Baltimore, 7/1/66 to 6/30/67 and 1/1/71 to 12/31/71. (From Szklo M, *et al*: Nontransmural MI: prognostic implications, *Primary Cardiology* 6:76, 1980.)

Table 58.1.
Characteristics Associated with Increase in Mortality following Discharge of Patients Who Have Had Myocardial Infarction (MI)[a]

ADMISSION CHARACTERISTICS
    Congestive heart failure (chest X-ray or Killip classification)
    History of hypertension (2, 22)
    Extent of left ventricular ischemia (radionuclide scintigraphy, cardiac enzymes)
CHARACTERISTICS AT DISCHARGE
    History of a previous MI
    Early (within 10 days) post-MI angina, with transient ST-T changes (24)[b]
    Ejection fraction ≤ 40% (radionuclide ventriculography, arteriography)
    Complex ventricular arrhythmia[c] (Holter monitor)
    Proximal left or three-vessel coronary artery occlusive disease (arteriography)
    Positive limited early post-MI ECG stress test (within 2–3 weeks after MI) (29)
CHARACTERISTICS FOLLOWING DISCHARGE
    ECG abnormalities, especially S-T segment depression, ≥ 3 months after MI (6)
    Cigarette smoking (33)

---

[a] Numbers in parentheses are references.
[b] Mortality risk highest when ECG shows "ischemia at a distance," *i.e.*, transient ischemic S-T changes in a myocardial location which is different from the location of the patient's MI.
[c] Multifocal premature ventricular contractions (PVCs), runs of two or more sequential ectopic ventricular beats, or PVCs with R on T pattern.

The classification of acute MI developed by Killip according to the presence and severity of congestive heart failure (CHF) on admission to the CCU is one of the most useful prognostic indices. Class I patients have no evidence of CHF on admission; class II patients have mild CHF; class III patients present with pulmonary edema; and class IV patients present with shock. Figure 58.2 shows the strikingly different survival rates among persons in these four classes, ranging from a 2-year survival rate of about 80% in class I to less than 20% in class IV (22).

Of the other characteristics listed in Table 58.1, the most powerful predictors of mortality during the first year following an MI are one or more of the following: a history of a previous MI; the development of early (within 10 days) post-MI angina accompanied by transient ST segment or T wave changes; an ejection fraction of 40% or less, late hospital phase (predischarge) complex ventricular arrhythmia, left main or three-vessel coronary artery occlusive disease; and a positive submaximal stress test within the first month following an MI. The incidence of sudden death in patients discharged from hospital with *both* left ventricular (LV) dysfunction (ejection fraction < 40%) and frequent PVCs (> 10/hour) is 11 times that of otherwise similar patients with neither of these findings. On reclassification of survivors 6 months after MI with regard to the presence or absence of frequent PVCs and LV dysfunction, these factors are no longer associated with increased risk of sudden coronary death over a further follow-up period of up to 18 months (20).

Morbidity

Postinfarction angina occurs during the year following an MI in approximately 75% of persons who had angina before their MI, and in about 50% of

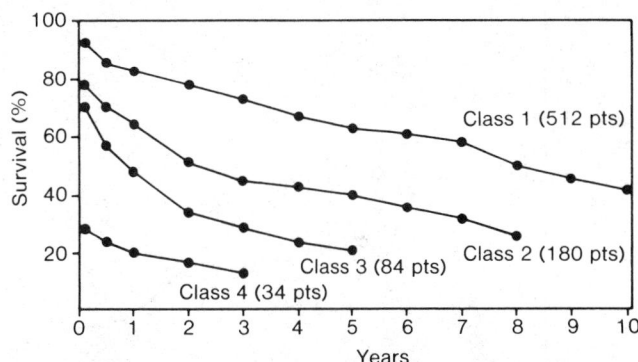

Figure 58.2. Survival after acute myocardial infarction based upon Killip classification (810 patients admitted to the Duke Medical Center Coronary Care Unit from 1967 to 1978). (From: Rosati RA, Harris PJ): In Fries J, Ehrlich GE (eds): *Prognosis; Contemporary Outcomes of Disease.* Bowie MD, The Charles Press Publishers, 1981.)

those who did not have it before their MI (32). In patients who are free of angina or other cardiac symptoms in the hospital, limited (target heart rate of 130 beats/minute or limiting symptoms or ischemic signs) electrocardiogram (ECG) stress testing before discharge increases the ability to predict whether or not a patient will develop angina. Angina during the years following an MI occurs in 86% of patients with positive stress tests (96% of patients with both a positive early post-MI stress test and a previous history of angina) and in 36% of those with negative stress tests (only in 26% of patients with both a negative stress test and no previous history of angina) (32). Additionally, cardiac patients whose limited, early post-MI stress testing shows ischemic ST changes (≥ 0.1 mV exercise-induced ST depression and/or limited work capacity (≤ 5 METs) have 2 or more times the risk of recurrent myocardial infarction and of death over the ensuing year (25, 29, 30).

Other medical complications include congestive heart failure, life-threatening arrhythmias, systemic emboli, and post-MI syndrome.

The psychological and social sequelae during the year following an MI depend both upon the severity of the patient's MI and upon his premorbid psychosocial situation. Of survivors of MIs, 10 to 20% are never able to return to their former occupational and recreational activities, while the other 80 to 90% are able to do so within 2 to 6 months. Based upon extensive observations, Cassem has developed a hypothetical profile of emotional and behavioral reactions to an MI (Fig. 58.3); in this scheme, depression or maladaptive behavior related to pre-existing personality traits will be present in 10% or more of patients during the period following discharge from the hospital. Persistent denial, anxiety,

depression, and dependency after an MI are associated with a decrease in the rate of return to work and usual social activities, regardless of the patient's physiological status.

Patients with Unstable Angina

Patients discharged from the CCU with the diagnosis of unstable angina (see Chapter 57 for definition) have a prognosis which is, in general, similar to that of patients with a completed MI (5 to 10% crude 1-year mortality). Patients with unstable angina also have an 8% 6-month risk and a 12% 1-year risk of developing myocardial infarction, which is essentially similar to the rate of recurrent MI for patients discharged with the diagnosis of completed MI.

In an individual patient with unstable angina, a more precise prognosis can be given when the distribution of coronary artery disease is known. Coronary catheterization has shown that left main coronary artery disease is more common in patients discharged with the diagnosis of unstable angina than in those discharged with the diagnosis of completed MI (15 versus 5%, respectively). Another 10% have diffuse coronary artery disease, 10% have normal coronary arteries (and are presumed to have coronary artery spasm as the etiology of their chest pain), and the remaining 65% are more or less equally divided between single, double, and triple coronary vessel disease (21). This information is of clinical importance because of the demonstrated superiority of surgical over medical treatment of left main coronary artery disease. The prognoses associated with each of the above patterns and the management of unstable angina are described below (page 718) and in Chapter 57.

Survivors of Cardiac Arrests Who Have Not Had a Myocardial Infarction

The first year mortality of all survivors of out-of-hospital cardiac arrest who have not had an MI is about 25%, with about three-quarters of deaths occurring within the first 6 months after hospital discharge. This is approximately 3 times the mortality rate of survivors of out-of-hospital cardiac arrest who subsequently show completed MIs. In a study of 234 survivors of out-of-hospital cardiac arrest, followed for over 4 years, the rate of recurrence of ventricular fibrillation or of sudden death in patients without an acute MI was 31% compared with 5% for out-of-hospital survivors of cardiac arrest who subsequently evolved electrocardiographic changes of acute MI. The median time to recurrent circulatory arrest was 20 weeks. More than 70% of the episodes of ventricular fibrillation were unexpected, occurring during sleep or during the usual activities of daily living (23).

Therefore, the survivors of non-MI ventricular fibrillation constitute a highly unstable group of

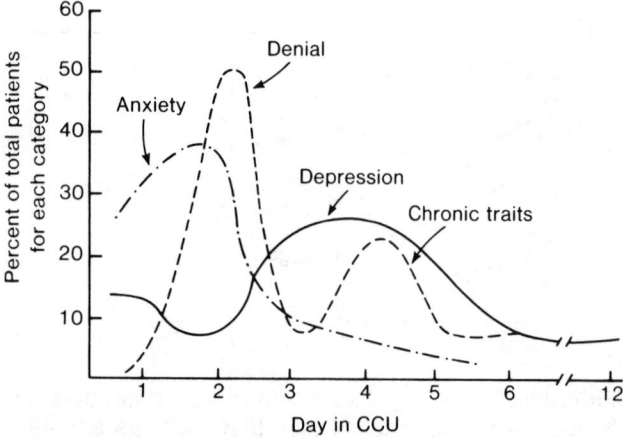

Figure 58.3. Hypothetical patterns and frequencies of emotional and behavioral reactions of coronary care unit (CCU) patients. (Adapted from Cassem NH, Hackett TP: Psychiatric consultation in a coronary care unit. *Ann Intern Med* 75:9, 1971.)

patients requiring aggressive and highly individualized management. The multiplicity of recent advances in electrophysiology, investigational antiarrhythmics, automatic implantable defibrillators and the many innovative surgical approaches to the medically intractable but symptomatic ventricular dysrhythmia dictate prompt referral of such high risk patients to a consulting cardiologist.

REHABILITATION AND MANAGEMENT FOLLOWING MYOCARDIAL INFARCTION

The majority of patients discharged after MI can expect to return to most of their usual activities within 2 to 6 months. For a smaller number of patients, complications of their MI make this outcome impossible. In either situation, an organized plan for care should be followed (Table 58.2). This plan should include the education of the patient and his family, so that they can participate effectively in the rehabilitation process, and should assure optimal monitoring and medical treatment of the patient by the physician and cardiac rehabilitation specialists.

Although, to date, only smoking cessation (33) and

Table 58.2.
Plan of Care for Survivors of Myocardial Infarction following Hospital Discharge

PATIENT EDUCATION (OBJECTIVES FOR ALL PATIENTS)[a]
 Understands disease process (damage to the heart which heals in a few months, leaves a scar)
 Understands likely prognosis
 Understands and follows progressive activity schedule[b]
 Understands approximate timetable for return to work[b]
 Understands importance of controlling major risk factors (smoking, hypercholesterolemia, hypertension) and takes action to control them
 Knows how to recognize principal cardiac symptoms (angina, tachycardia, heart failure, hypotension) and understands how to use sublingual nitroglycerine
 Participates in group classes following discharge[c]
MEDICAL MANAGEMENT
 All patients
  Review in-hospital course for prognostic characteristics (see Table 58.1) and for medications prescribed at discharge
  Assess and reinforce above patient education
  Check periodically for complications of infarction (see Table 58.5)
  Check for behaviorial-psychiatric complications
  Check ECG 2–3 months following discharge
 Selected patients
  β-Blocker treatment (when not contraindicated)
  Referral for physical conditioning[b]

 [a] Essential to *include the patient's spouse* in all aspects of education.
 [b] Serial exercise stress tests may be utilized to plan progressive activity (see the text).
 [c] If programs are available in the community (see details on page 706).

β-blockade (11) have been shown convincingly to be assocated with an improved prognosis after an MI, the comprehensive approach to care summarized in Table 58.2 is appropriate for most patients. It is likely that the efficacy of other aspects of care will be confirmed in the future. For example, a preliminary study has shown that the treatment of hypertension and hypercholesterolemia combined with physical conditioning probably reduces the chance of sudden death during the first 3 years following an MI (15). So far, the superiority of surgical over medical treatment in improving survival in any subset of patients with coronary artery disease—with the singular exception of left main disease—remains controversial (4).

Patient Education

Nowadays, most hospitals initiate education about myocardial infarction as soon as the patient is clinically stable. The educational program is often the responsibility of a cardiac rehabilitation nurse. Patient education should cover the following: the nature of coronary heart disease; cardiac symptoms; cardiac drugs; modification of major risk factors (smoking, hypertension, and hyperlipidemia); and guidelines for resumption of physical activities (includes sexual activity) and return to work. It should be emphasized that myocardial infarction is a manifestation of a disease process that has been going on for many years. Many patients will attribute their MI to what they were doing at the moment it actually occurred. The patient must understand that the MI would have occurred regardless of what he was doing that particular day and that the likelihood of a recurrence may best be diminished by following prescribed medical therapy and making life style changes. These matters may be discussed in a general sense, usually in a group setting.

Individualized information should be provided in a *predischarge conference* at which the patient and his spouse are encouraged to ask questions. The conference should include review of any adverse prognostic features identified before discharge (Table 58.1); the medications prescribed at discharge; discussion of specific plans for cardiac rehabilitation, diet, and smoking modification; a chance for ventilation about emotional stress-laden issues; and realistic appraisal of expectations of return to work. Because of the high frequency of postinfarction angina (see pages 703–704), it is especially important to describe this symptom to patients who have never had it and to point out to all patients that it may occur with the increased activity recommended for the coming weeks. Every patient should be given sublingual nitroglycerin, and the correct use of this drug should be reviewed (see Chapter 57).

Because patients may not retain the information they hear in the hospital, it is important to *provide this information in writing* and to assess and reinforce patient understanding of it after discharge. The patient education booklet *After a Heart Attack* (available from the American Heart Association) gives a useful general account of the disease process, prognosis, coronary risk factors, and rehabilitation process. Risk factor modification is discussed in detail in Chapter 20 (practical approaches to smoking cessation), Chapter 62 (treatment of hypertension), and Chapter 75 (low cholesterol diet).

Many community hospitals have developed *group classes* for survivors of MIs and their spouses. Typically, patients and their spouses are invited to participate in a number of weekly meetings during the first or second month after discharge. Sessions are usually led by a nurse, a social worker, or a cardiologist with the objective of having participants raise questions about the recovery period so that they provide mutual support by sharing experiences with each other. Additional resources available in many communities are patient-run "heart clubs" and physician or allied health professional-supervised physical conditioning programs (see "Physical Conditioning" below). There are also several nationally distributed newsletters for patients with coronary artery disease (e.g., The Coronary Club Bulletin, 3659 Green Road #200, Cleveland, OH 44122. Telephone: (216) 292-7120).

Postdischarge Appointments

In general, each patient who has had an MI should be encouraged to telephone his physician at least once during the first week at home, to discuss any questions which arise, and an office visit should be scheduled within 2 to 3 weeks. Before this visit, the physician should review the patient's hospital summary to determine whether adverse prognostic features were present and to identify the medications prescribed at discharge. The visit should be divided between an assessment of the patient's progress in his rehabilitation (physical activity level, diet and smoking modifications, emotional status, understanding of the overall plan of care, expectation about return to work) and an assessment of his medical status (manifestations of ischemia and heart failure, blood pressure status, and review of current medications). Two or more additional office visits, similar to the first visit, should be scheduled during the 3 months following an MI, and the patient should be encouraged to telephone at any time about symptoms or questions. At about 6 to 8 weeks post-MI, a maximal exercise stress should be considered, as this can provide helpful therapeutic and prognostic information regarding the disease. The stress test is also used to assess functional capacity, and is very helpful in guiding the return to work process. At about 3 months, an ECG should be obtained; it will constitute the patient's new "baseline" ECG with which future tracings should be compared.

Activity Schedule

Table 58.3 contains a practical summary (for use by the patient) of symptom recognition and of a schedule of progressive physical activities for the first 2 to 3 months after MI. Table 58.4 lists a broad array of activities corresponding to the recommended energy levels during the recuperation period and thereafter. Resumption of activities with different energy requirements should be gradual; in particular, the duration of certain activities should be brief at first, with gradual increase, according to how the individual patient feels. The schedule in Table 58.3 can be given to most patients. A more aggressive plan can be tailored for the individual patient if an early physical conditioning program, guided by early stress testing, is available. Similarly, stress test-guided conditioning can also be planned for patients after the first 2 to 3 months of convalescence from an MI. Programs that enroll patients 2 months after MI are widely available. Local affiliates of the American Heart Association commonly maintain lists of local exercise programs. A comprehensive discussion of exercise conditioning for cardiac patients can be found later in this chapter (see "Physical Conditioning," page 712).

Return to Work

Since the majority of patients have their first MI during their active working years, they are commonly concerned about returning to work. A tentative timetable for return to work should be discussed with the patient early after discharge. A number of factors should be taken into consideration. Generally, failure to return to work following an MI is due to psychological rather than physical limitations (see "Psychological Problems," below). Telling the patient, soon after discharge, that he should expect to return to work will help to prevent disability due to psychological factors. Obviously, the type of work is always an important consideration. Patients whose occupations involve mental stress and hectic schedules should be advised to return to work on a part time basis at first, leaving plenty of time for rest and relaxation. For patients whose work involves significant physical exertion, the timing of return to work can be based upon the information contained in Tables 58.3 and 58.4 and guided by the results of exercise stress testing (see below). From Table 58.4, it is evident that most occupations require an energy level of 6 METs or less. Occupational activities classified as heavy work, such as digging ditches, require energy expenditure of 7 or more METs. Certain activities may produce an increased work load on the heart because of psychological stress (e.g., driving a vehicle) or because they entail significant isometric exercise (e.g., carpentry, plumbing, shoveling, operating pneumatic tools, or carrying objects heavier than 30 lb).

Table 58.3.
Activity Schedule and Symptom Recognition for Patients Convalescing from Myocardial Infarction

GENERAL POINTS

All activities, including sitting and lying down, require energy. The amount of energy required to perform a specific activity is expressed as METs. One MET is your resting energy requirement. As activities become more strenuous, the amount of energy required (METs) also increases, as does the work load imposed on your heart.

The schedule recommended in this program is based on the number of METs needed for various activities. Some specific recommendations are given for each of the first 3 months following your return to home. Table 58.4 gives the energy requirements for a wide variety of additional activities. If the table omits your favorite activities, ask your doctor about them.

Warnings: Generally the following activities impose an added strain on your heart and should be avoided, especially during the first 3 months after a heart attack:

1. Taking very hot or cold showers or baths.
2. Holding your breath while exercising, lifting or straining.
3. Working in a bent or stooped position or with arms held above your head.
4. Work that requires continuous tensing of your muscles.
5. Working or exercising during very hot, cold, humid, or windy weather (in bad weather, plan your regular exercise at a nearby shopping mall).
6. Working or exercising during the first hour after a meal or after consuming alcohol.
7. Consuming excessive amounts of alcohol (*e.g.*, more than 1–2 ounces of whiskey, 2–3 beers, 1–2 glasses of wine).
8. Walking or exercising on a hill or an inclined surface.
9. Any activity which creates emotional stress or worry for you.

A. RECOMMENDED ACTIVITY SCHEDULE[a]

First Month (1–3 METs)

From Discharge to 1 Week

Regular exercise: walk 5 minutes at a leisurely pace once/day on a level surface.

Some specific advice: this week, primarily get used to being at home. Occupy yourself with sit-down activities such as watching television, playing cards, sewing, painting, sketching, *etc.* Avoid lifting objects heavier than 5 lb or doing activities which require reaching above your head. You may go up and down the stairs. However, take your time and limit the number of times you need to climb them. Do all of the things you were doing in the hospital. Get up and get dressed each day. You may be surprised at how tired and weak you feel. This is natural. Be sure to take rest periods when you need them, particularly after meals, before you exercise or climb the stairs.

Week 2

Regular exercise: walk 5 minutes at a leisurely pace twice/day.

Some specific advice: continue all of your previous activities, and add others, such as taking rides in the car (however, no driving yet), cooking a meal, washing clothes in a machine (have someone else remove them), making your bed, attending a relaxing movie, going out to dinner, going shopping with your family (let others lift things from the shelves to the basket and carry the groceries), shooting pool, playing shuffle board, throwing a softball underhand, playing a piano or organ.

Weeks 3 and 4

Regular exercise: advance gradually to walking 10 minutes at leisurely pace twice/day during 2 weeks.

Some specific advice: continue your previous activities and others, such as going to church, sweeping floors, polishing furniture, driving the car (beginning with short drives, avoiding heavy traffic).

Second Month (3–5 METs)

Regular physical exercise: progressively increase leisurely walking from 15 minutes once a day at a slightly faster pace to 30 minutes once or twice a day.

Some specific advice: the attached table of activities lists the approximate energy requirements of each. You may gradually increase your activities, by adding additional activities and spending more time at them; consult the attached table for activities requiring 5 METs or less (or more).

RECOGNIZING HEART SYMPTOMS

Your heart will give you warning signs if it is not ready for increased activity. Here are some guidelines to use:

Pulse: Locate your pulse and count the number of times it beats for 15 seconds and multiply that number by 4. This is your heart rate for 1 minute. Take your pulse before you begin your walk or any new activity and at the end of the activity. Contact your doctor before resuming exercise if:

1. There is an increase of 20 heart beats or more/minute in postexercise pulse over pre-exercise pulse.
2. If your heart rate exceeds 120/min.[b]
3. If you detect abnormal heart action: pulse becoming irregular, fluttering or jumping in chest or throat, very slow pulse rate, sudden burst of rapid heartbeats.

Chest Pain: Contact your doctor before resuming exercise if you experience pain or pressure in the chest, arm, or throat precipitated by exercise or following exercise. Remember to take your nitroglycerine and rest if you do experience pain.

Dizziness: Contact your doctor before resuming exercise if you become dizzy, light-headed, or faint during exercise.

Breathing difficulty: Contact your doctor before resuming exercise if you become short of breath during or after a new exercise, or if you awaken from sleep short of breath.

---

[a] Pace of these activities may be scaled up or down by results of early post-MI stress test when available.
[b] These figures may be markedly modified by results of early stress test and/or medication.

Table 58.4.
Energy Requirements of Certain Activities[a]

Activity Level	Self-Care or Home	Occupational	Recreational	Physical Conditioning
Very light (3 METs or less)	Washing, shaving, dressing Desk work, writing, washing dishes Driving auto[b]	Sitting (clerical, assembling) Standing (store clerk, bartender) Driving truck[b] Crane operator[b]	Shuffleboard Horseshoes Bait casting Billiards Archery[b] Golf (cart)	Walking (level at 2 mph) Stationary bike (very low resistance) Very light calisthenics
Light to moderate (3–5 METs)	Clean windows Raking leaves Weeding Power lawn mowing Waxing floors (slowly) Painting Carrying objects 15–30 lb[c]	Stocking shelves (light objects)[c] Light welding Light carpentry[c] Machine assembly Auto repair Paper hanging[c]	Dancing Golf (walking) Sailing Horseback riding Volleyball Tennis (doubles) Sexual intercourse[b] (see details in the text)	Walking (3–4 mph) Level bicycling (6—8 mph) Light calisthenics
Moderate (5–7 METs)	Easy digging in garden Level hand lawn mowing Climbing stairs (slowly) Carrying objects 30–60 lb[c]	Carpenty (exterior home building)[c] Shoveling dirt[c] Pneumatic tools[c]	Badminton (competitive) Tennis (singles) Snow skiing (downhill) Light backpacking Basketball Football Skating (ice and roller) Horseback riding (gallop)	Swimming (breast stoke)
Heavy (7–9 METs)	Sawing wood[c] Heavy shoveling[c] Climbing stairs (moderate speed) Carrying objects 60–90 lb[c]	Tending furnace[c] Digging ditches[c] Pick and shovel[c]	Canoeing[c] Mountain climbing[c] Fencing Paddleball Touch football	Jog (5 mph) Swim (crawl stroke) Rowing machine Heavy calisthenics Bicycling (12 mph)
Very heavy (9 METs)	Carrying loads upstairs[c] Carrying objects 90 lb or more Climbing stairs (quickly) Shoveling heavy snow[c] Shoveling 10/minute (16 lb)	Lumber jack[c] Heavy laborer[c]	Handball Squash Ski touring over hills[c] Vigorous basketball	Running (6 mph) Bicycle (13 mph or steep hill) Rope jumping

[a] From Haskell WL: Design and implementation of cardiac conditioning programs. In Hellerstein HK (ed): *Rehabilitation of the Coronary Patient.* New York, John Wiley & Sons, 1978, p 203.
[b] May cause added psychological stress that will increase load on the heart.
[c] May produce disproportionate myocardial demands because of use of arms or isometric exercise.

In order to evaluate objectively the impact of the patient's expected physical exertion upon his heart, ECG stress testing (see "Patient Experience," Chapter 57) and Holter monitoring, during simulated or actual occupational activities, can be obtained after the first 2 or 3 months of convalescence.

Patients with myocardial infarctions complicated by poorly controlled angina, CHF, or arrhythmias should be evaluated in conjunction with a consulting cardiologist (see "Medical Complications," below) before a plan for return to work and other activities is recommended. Some of these patients will qualify for permanent medical disability (see criteria for disability due to coronary artery disease, Chapter 9, Table 9.1) or for job retraining through vocational rehabilitation (see Chapter 9).

Sexual Activity

It is safe for patients who are symptom free during usual activities of daily living to resume sexual intercourse within 4 to 6 weeks of their MI. Available data suggest that the energy requirement approximates 3 METs during foreplay and afterplay and 5 METs at climax (14). These are equivalent to the oxygen demands of a brisk walk around the block or of climbing one flight of stairs. In a study of patients after MI, coitus accounted for less than 1% of sudden deaths. These usually occurred during extramarital affairs in which the men were considerably older than their companions, and frequently were inebriated at the time of intercourse (31).

When counseling patients about resumption of sexual activity, the physician should give specific advice and should also encourage questions. The pamphlet *Sex and Heart Disease*, available from the American Heart Association, is a helpful adjunct to counseling. Frequency of sexual intercourse can be similar to the frequency before the patient's MI. Sexual foreplay without completion of intercourse can be recommended to patients who wish to resume sex cautiously. In general, sexual activity can be resumed in the position which was most gratifying before the MI; however, the patient should avoid positions in which he supports his weight on his arms, as this requires an isometric type of work (see "Physical Conditioning," below) and may put extra stress on the heart. Sexual activity should be engaged in when both partners are relaxed. It is best to abstain from intercourse for 2 or 3 hours after eating a large meal since eating increases the work of the heart.

Inability to return to a previous pattern of sexual activity may be due to angina precipitated by intercourse, to new medications, or to psychological stress associated with the recent MI. If an otherwise stable patient develops angina during intercourse, he should be advised to take sublingual nitroglycerin just before sexual activity. The evaluation and management of drug-induced and psychological sexual dysfunction are discussed in Chapter 18.

Psychological Problems

It is normal for patients to experience *anxiety and depression* during the first few weeks after discharge from the CCU. Some of these symptoms are due to misconceptions about the nature and prognosis of myocardial infarction, and they respond to clarification of the facts. Most patients do well when encouraged to ventilate their concerns and when reassured that their response is normal. A small supply of a minor tranquilizer (see Chapter 13) can be prescribed to be used if needed. As noted earlier ("Patient Education"), participation in group classes and group exercise programs can also help patients adjust to changes in their lives following myocardial infarction.

Another common psychological complication of MI is an *inappropriate fear of physical activity* of any kind, *i.e.,* the so-called cardiac cripple. Early participation in supervised physical activity including the treadmill test and exercise conditioning have been shown to enhance the patients's self-confidence and ability to perform physical tasks (10). Having the spouse observe the early treadmill test establishes confidence in the spouse that his/her

partner is not a cripple. In some medical centers, selected spouses are offered an opportunity to walk on the treadmill as well. This serves to establish a reference point for estimating ability to engage in activity. Exposure to a wide range of activities in the months following an MI is important since self-confidence is task specific (9, 10). Most cardiac exercise programs (see below) emphasize activities using the legs, such as walking and jogging. While this increases self-confidence in tasks requiring leg work, it does little for arm self-confidence. To increase arm self-confidence, patients must be exposed to arm exercises as well (9, 12). This is especially important for patients who plan to return to work which requires upper body and arm efforts. Of course, the physician must evaluate the patient to determine if this type of activity is appropriate for the patient.

Another common problem is *denial of illness* persisting beyond the first few days in hospital. The behavior associated with persistent denial may create substantial risks. This is especially true of patients who are extremely competitive and are used to controlling most of the circumstances of their lives (1). They are typically determined to return to work as soon as possible and will refuse cardiac rehabilitation on the basis that they can do it better on their own. This behavior arouses anxiety, fear, and concern in the spouse and family and may lead to significant marital conflict. An open discussion with patient and spouse, with each acknowledging the other's concerns, can often lead to resolution of these conflicts and more appropriate behavior from each partner.

At times it is useful to teach patients to *use various forms of feedback* to guide their activities. Specifically, patients are taught to (*a*) use a target heart rate based on an exercise stress test; (*b*) observe themselves and how they feel, with the basic instruction to rest if fatigue or any cardiac symptoms occur during exercise, and to call the physician if symptoms persist after using nitroglycerin; and (*c*) view the spouse as a source of feedback. In most cases, the spouse's observation of how the patient looks is remarkably accurate. If she says he looks tired or does not look right she is probably right. By having the patient agree to consider her comments as well meaning and for his benefit, he will usually comply with her advice. Thereafter, the number of reminding behaviors from the spouse is reduced progressively, and the rehabilitation process can proceed with greater enthusiasm from both partners. With more difficult patients, or where there is pre-existing marital strife, the consultation of a psychiatrist or psychologist may be helpful in managing adjustment problems.

Some patients have relatively *severe psychological and behavioral problems* after MI which may interfere with their rehabilitation. The most common problem is persistent depression, which may have characteristics of a major or minor depressive illness or may present as an adjustment disorder characterized by anxiety, depression, somatization, or a mixture of these responses. The diagnosis and management of these problems are discussed in Chapters 12 (somatization and adjustment disorder), 13 (anxiety), and 15 (depression).

Medical Prophylaxis

Cholesterol-lowering agents, β-adrenergic blocking-agents, and anticoagulants and platelet inhibitors have all been tested as medical measures to prevent recurrent MI. Only β-blocking drugs have been shown convincingly to improve the prognosis in these patients, with a significant reduction in mortality and in the reinfarction rate. The benefits from β-blockers appear to be related to the general class action of β-blockade and do not seem to be related to any specific cardioselectivity, membrane stabilization activity, or intrinsic sympathomimetic activity. The benefits are seen in all ages and in all types of MI. However, older patients (> 60 years) and patients with complicated MI (as long as the complications do not constitute contraindications to use of β-blockers) seem to show greater benefits than other subsets. The overall magnitude of benefit from the use of β-blockers seems to be about a one-third reduction in mortality and about the same magnitude of reduction in reinfarction. The duration of benefit seems to last for at least 2 years after MI with treatment commencing within 1 to 4 weeks posthospital discharge. The contraindications to the use of β-blockers include CHF, asthma, and bradycardia. The recommended dose of the β-blocker is the amount required to produce significant attenuation of heart rate and blood pressure response to exercise without producing significant side effects. In assessing the clinical usefulness of β-blockers following MI, one should keep in mind that, although the magnitude of reduction in mortality and reinfarction

achieved by β-blockers appears to be large in a relative sense (30% reduction in mortality and morbidity), it is, nevertheless, quite small in an absolute sense (decrease in expected mortality from about 9 to 6% or only a 3% reduction, and decrease in reinfarction from about 12 to 8% or only a 4% absolute reduction) (11).

Medical Complications

Table 58.5 lists the principal medical complications of MI, the procedures which may be useful in diagnosing or evaluating them, and potential therapies. In general, the use of sophisticated and costly procedures to evaluate these complications should be coordinated by a consulting cardiologist.

Postinfarction Angina

As pointed out in the discussion of prognosis above, this is a very common problem in survivors of MIs. The medical management of angina is described in detail in Chapter 57. Because protection of the heart from transient ischemia may be especially important during recovery from an MI, the prescription of long acting nitrates or β-blockers and calcium blockers to prevent angina is advisable in most patients who develop angina within the first 3 months following MI. Careful clinical observations and serial stress testing are most useful in adjusting the dose, the combination, and the duration of the antianginal therapy. Because of the poor prognosis associated with angina occurring very early after an MI (24), patients with this problem should be referred to a cardiologist for consideration of coronary catheterization and bypass surgery.

Postinfarction Congestive Heart Failure

A small proportion of patients develop chronic congestive heart failure (CHF) after MI. This complication usually develops before discharge from the hospital. Nowadays, many patients have their left ventricular ejection fraction measured as part of

Table 58.5.
Medical Complications of Myocardial Infarction

Complications	Diagnostic Procedures for Selected Patients[a]	Management Approaches
Angina or other evidence of reversible ischemia	ECG stress testing; radionuclide stress testing; coronary arteriography	Standard antianginal therapy (see Chapter 57); coronary artery bypass for selected patients; physical conditioning
Congestive heart failure	Radionuclide ventriculography and/or echocardiography (ejection fraction, segmental dysfunction, rupture, ventricular aneurysm)	Standard therapy for heart failure (see Chapter 61); surgery in a few selected patients
Arrhythmias	Holter monitor; ECG stress testing, electrophysiological study in selected patients	Standard antiarrhythmic therapy (see Chapter 59); surgery or implanted defibrillator in selected patients
Postmyocardial infarction syndrome (Dressler's)	Echocardiography (pericardial effusion)	Aspirin or other anti-inflammatory agents
Systemic emboli	Echocardiography (intracardiac thrombus)	Anticoagulant therapy (see Chapter 51); surgery in selected patients

[a] Should be coordinated and intepreted by consulting cardiologist.

their evaluation before discharge, so that those at increased risk of developing new CHF after discharge are known. The regimens described in Chapter 61 should be utilized in treating the CHF of patients after MI. In patients whose CHF is difficult to control, the combination of "preload" reduction with long acting nitrates and "afterload" reduction with captopril, a calcium channel blocker, or hydralazine, in doses titrated for the individual patient, is often helpful. A small proportion of patients with persistent CHF may have segmental or global left ventricular dysfunction, or significant mitral regurgitation which may improve significantly after cardiac surgery.

Postinfarction Arrhythmias

A substantial number of survivors of MIs are found to have complex ventricular arrhythmias (see Table 58.1) on 24-hour ambulatory ECG monitoring, which is performed routinely after the first week of hospitalization in many hospitals. It has never been shown convincingly that antiarrhythmic therapy improves the prognosis of such patients; however, because of the poor prognosis associated with ventricular arrhythmias, it is current practice to attempt to control them medically and to confirm control by Holter monitoring and/or serum antiarrhythmics level before or shortly after discharge. The drugs utilized to control arrhythmias are discussed in detail in Chapter 59. Once medical control of arrhythmias has been established, the patient should be treated for 3 to 6 months. If ECG monitoring shows no arrhythmia after this period, antiarrhythmic treatment can be stopped and the patient can be checked 1 week later for recurrent arrhythmia. As mentioned earlier in this chapter, recent work suggests that ventricular irritability and left ventricular dysfunction are independent risk factors for the occurrence of sudden cardiac deaths during the 6 months after MI and that the combination of both of these risk factors is particularly ominous, resulting in an incidence of sudden death which is 11 times that of patients with neither of these risk factors (20).

The use of antiarrhythmic agents in the posthospital management of patients with the combination of complex ventricular arrhythmias and low ejection fractions documented at the end of their stay in the hospital seems prudent, although efficacy has not been established definitively.

Postmyocardial Infarction (Dressler's) Syndrome

It is estimated that 3 to 4% of patients develop this complication, usually within 1 to 6 weeks after a myocardial infarction. The syndrome is characterized by the pain of pericarditis (substernal pain, relieved by leaning forward and increased with inspiration); presence of a friction rub; fever; a pericardial effusion (which can best be demonstrated by echocardiography) and often a unilateral or bilateral pleural effusion.

The principal considerations in the differential diagnosis are pulmonary embolism and recurrence or extension of the recent MI.

When a patient develops the symptoms of Dressler's syndrome, he should be hospitalized immediately, and serial ECGs, cardiac enzymes, and a lung scan should be obtained. If these tests do not show pulmonary embolism, a new MI, or another explanation of the symptoms, the clinical diagnosis of Dressler's syndrome can be made. Echocardiographic evidence of a pericardial effusion and an elevated erythrocyte sedimentation rate may also be present.

Dressler's syndrome usually responds to salicylates or to indomethacin; in patients who do not respond to these drugs, prednisone gives prompt relief of symptoms. Once the diagnosis is secure and symptoms are controlled, the patient can be discharged. The anti-inflammatory drug chosen in hospital should be administered for 1 to 2 months. Prednisone should be tapered off according to the schedule described in Chapter 74. Patients who have recurrent symptoms when anti-inflammatory treatment is discontinued should resume treatment for another month or longer.

Arterial Embolization

This complication occurs in 5 to 10% of post-MI patients. The emboli seem to originate from mural thrombi which are typically seen in the left ventricular apex adjacent to akinetic or dyskinetic wall segments noted in the course of acute transmural anterior MI. About 30 to 40% of acute transmural MIs with akinetic or dyskinetic left ventricular apex show mural thrombi on the echocardiogram. Early development of left ventricular aneurysm (within 2 days of acute anterior transmural MI) carries high risk of death within 1 year that is independent of ejection fraction (19). Anticoagulation (see Chapter 51) in patients demonstrating mural thrombi seems prudent, although its effect on reducing subsequent morbidity and mortality has not been established.

Shoulder-Hand Syndrome

This syndrome, characterized by pain and stiffness of the shoulder and pain and swelling of the hand, may occur during the first 1 to 2 months following an MI. It usually affects the left side. This syndrome rarely occurs when patients are mobilized early after an MI. Management of the shoulder-hand syndrome is described in Chapter 83, Cerebrovascular Disease.

Referral for Cardiological Consultation

Selected patients who have had an MI, especially relatively young persons, and patients with uncontrolled angina refractory to medical therapy, with a markedly positive exercise stress test, with a ventricular aneurysm with CHF refractory to medical therapy, with evidence for "ischemia at a distance" (see footnote to Table 58.1 for definition), or with mechanical complications such as ventricular septal defect (suggested by holosystolic murmur and thrill at the left sternal border) or papillary muscle rupture (suggested by refractory CHF and holosystolic apical murmur) may benefit from cardiac surgery, either by having their symptoms reduced or their prognosis improved. Such patients should be referred promptly to a cardiologist, to assure optimal medical therapy and to obtain an opinion about the advisability and the timing of cardiac surgery. The initial evaluative procedure chosen by the consultant may be one or more of the noninvasive procedures listed in Table 58.5 or cardiac catheterization. Post-MI patients presenting with CHF and severe diffuse left ventricular dysfunction should probably continue to be treated conservatively because of the hitherto unsatisfactory results of coronary artery bypass grafting. Cardiac transplantation offers a glimmer of hope to a very small, highly selected subset of such patients, but the operation remains basically experimental.

Noncardiac Surgery

Noncardiac surgery carries a very high risk during the first 3 to 6 months following an MI (see Chapter 86 for details).

PHYSICAL CONDITIONING

Regular exercise, with the goal of attaining the physiological adaptation known as the conditioning effect, is safe and beneficial for most patients after MI, just as it is for healthy persons. The basic principles of exercise training are applicable to persons with and without heart disease. In addition to the cardiovascular principles related to exercise, principles regarding the musculoskeletal system are important (see Chapter 67).

General Principles

The body will respond and adapt to the kind and amount of physical demands placed upon it. The response is *specific*, meaning that the greatest changes are observed only in those areas upon which demands are placed. For exercise to bring about an improvement in physical fitness, it must *overload* the muscles or organ system involved in the exercise. To overload is to exercise at a greater intensity than the intensity to which one is accustomed. The overload must be applied gradually, in stages, for maximum effectiveness and safety. This is known as *progressive resistance. Threshold of training* refers to the amount of exercise that must be done to produce fitness improvements. The factors that must be considered when establishing the

right amount of exercise are:

1. *Type of activity.* The effects of exercise are specific to the type of activity engaged in and the particular body function it exercises. Thus, if the objective is to improve cardiovascular endurance, then exercise that increases oxygen consumption and heart rate is required. If the objective is to improve strength, then exercise with increasing amounts of resistance is required. There is little carry-over of the effects of an exercise from one component of fitness to another. Activities for cardiovascular fitness entail rhythmic repetitive movements of large muscles groups against relatively small resistance. Such activities are of low intensity and can be performed for a long time. They include walking, jogging, swimming, cycling, rowing, jumping rope, skating, running, and cross-country skiing. These activities increase the demand for oxygen, which is the reason they are called "aerobic" activities. They are also referred to as dynamic activities. On the other hand, sustained, slow movement activity, frequently involving relatively small muscle groups, against high resistance is known as static activity. Examples are weight lifting, push-ups, sit-ups, isometrics, carrying heavy packages, and hand grip. Most activities requiring lifting and straining, such as shoveling, have a large static component. In such activities there is increased peripheral vascular resistance with subsequent increase in blood pressure but relatively little increase in heart rate or cardiac output. Such exercises do not bring about enhancement in oxygen extraction, hence they are generally not aerobic. These activities should generally be avoided by patients in the first few months following MI. However, gradual involvement in activities such as weight lifting may be beneficial and desirable, especially in blue collar workers since their jobs require static efforts.

2. *Intensity.* Exercise intensity is set at a level which requires more effort than normal activity. This level is usually set at 70% of predicted maximal oxygen uptake, a level which is attained when the heart rate reaches approximately 80% of the age-predicted maximum rate. Optimal conditioning occurs when a person sustains this rate during an aerobic activity. Table 58.6 lists target heart rates for healthy persons in various age groups. Lower levels of aerobic exercise also produce a partial conditioning effect. Exercise prescription for patients with heart disease will be discussed later in this chapter.

3. *Duration.* Exercise must be performed for a sufficient amount of time to be effective. Duration can be varied in several ways: (*a*) increase repetitions while maintaining the same rate, such as in weight training; (*b*) increase the distance covered at the same rate, such as in walking or jogging; (*c*) reduce the number of rest periods between different exercises; or, (*d*) reduce the rest time during a rest

Table 58.6.
Target Heart Rates for Healthy Persons, by Age (Approximately 80% Maximum Predicted Heart Rate)[a]

Age	Heart Rate
20–29	170
30–39	160
40–49	150
50–59	140
60–69	130

[a] From Parmely JF, Jr, Blair S, Gazes PC, *et al* (eds): Proceedings of the National Workshop on Exercise in the Prevention, Evalution, and Treatment of Heart Disease. *J South Carolina Med Assoc* 65 (suppl 1): December, 1969.

period. Studies in exercise physiology have suggested that the total work done during an exercise session (*i.e.*, duration × intensity) may be more important in eliciting improvements than intensity or duration alone. Therefore, a long, low intensity workout may be equivalent to a short, high intensity workout if the total work is the same. A long, low intensity workout may be more suitable for beginninners and for middle or older aged individuals since it would reduce the risk of injury. For cardiovascular fitness, duration should be at least 20 minutes at the target heart rate.

4. *Frequency.* This factor refers to the number of times per week exercise is to be done. Exercise must be performed regularly, and for most types of exercise three to five times/week are desirable. However, two to three times/week are probably more sensible for the beginner since many musculoskeletal injuries occur at the start of a program due to overuse. This can increase to three to five times/ week as adaptation takes place.

The *principal hemodynamic adaptation* to aerobic exercise in patients with heart disease takes place in the peripheral vascular and muscular systems. Trained muscles can extract more oxygen from a given blood flow and there is a better distribution of the cardiac output. Heart rate and blood pressure are lower at rest and at a given submaximal work load. As a result, the patient can do more work with less cardiac effort, *i.e.*, less myocardial oxygen demand. This is extremely beneficial to cardiac patients who have limited blood supply through the coronary arteries. Angina may occur at the same threshold, *i.e.*, the same double product (heart rate × systolic blood pressure), but it is at a higher level of body work or MET level. METs (metabolic equivalents) are used to rate the energy requirement of different physical activities. One MET is 3.5 ml of O_2/kg of body weight/minute and is equivalent to oxygen requirement at rest; 2 METs are twice the resting requirements, *etc.* The higher the MET level attained during exercise testing, the more fit the individual is considered to be. In patients with coronary artery disease, the increase in exercise capac-

ity achieved with regular exercise is similar to that achieved with medications such as the β-blockers and nitrates. In healthy people who practice aerobic exercise there are also changes in the heart itself, including increase in diastolic volume, increase in ejection fraction at rest and to a greater extent during exercise, and enhancement of contractility. Few studies have shown any of this central effect in cardiac patients. However, there is evidence suggesting that cardiac patients may achieve these changes if they train hard and long enough (8). Improvement in coronary collateral circulation or myocardial perfusion as a result of training has not been demonstrated in cardiac patients.

Hormonal and Metabolic Effects of Training

In addition to the effect of training on the muscular and cardiovascular systems, aerobic exercise is associated with beneficial changes in a number of other systems: there is increased vagal tone, lowering of catecholamines, decrease in serum triglycerides, increase in the ratio of high to low density lipoprotein, reduction in adipose tissue, and augmentation in plasma fibrinolytic activity.

Conditioning in Healthy Persons

Healthy individuals can develop their own physical conditioning programs, utilizing the self-instruction programs described by Cooper (5), Zohman (34), or others. The objective of conditioning programs is to reach an exercise level at which the body is achieving about 70% of maximal predicted oxygen uptake, a level which is attained when the heart rate reaches approximately 80% of the maximum predicted rate (Table 58.6). As stated previously, optimal conditioning in healthy persons occurs with aerobic activity at the target heart rate for 20 minutes, at least three times/week. Lower levels of aerobic exercise also produce a partial conditioning effect in healthy persons.

Selected individuals should consult their physicians before beginning a conditioning program. In general, persons over the age of 35 and those with major risk factors for atherosclerosis should have a physical examination and a resting ECG. Exercise stress tests should be considered for individuals in a number of categories, as summarized in Table 58.7.

Table 58.7.
Individuals for Whom Stress Testing Should Be Considered When Beginning Exercise Programs

Status	Test or Training Mode
Healthy, under 35	No special test
Healthy, over 35	Stress test[a]
Coronary prone, all ages	Stress test
Coronary stricken, all ages	Stress test

[a] Tests performed by paramedical personnel to assess baseline exercise capacity.

Nondiagnostic fitness tests for apparently healthy individuals are usually available at health clubs, YMCAs, wellness centers, and community colleges. When supervised and interpreted by qualified allied health professionals, these tests can provide the basis for the exercise prescription. Fees are usually nominal and are included in the overall package for exercise sessions.

Physical Conditioning in Patients following Myocardial Infarction

Benefits of Conditioning

Cardiac patients who exercise regularly and who have become conditioned show favorable changes in psychometric tests, better control of angina, and enhancement of physical working capacity.

Psychometric testing has confirmed that exercise conditioning is associated with improvement in self-image and with a lightening of mood. Patients also show less anxiety, denial, and dependency; they appear to be better able to deal with day-to-day stresses; and they feel healthier and participate more actively in leisure time activities.

Because of the peripheral cardiovascular adaptations described earlier, angina pectoris occurs at higher exercise levels. This increased anginal threshold allows the patient to do more work; and at any given level of work, the patient feels more comfortable since the work represents a lower percentage of a now higher maximal capacity. Rating of perceived exertion (RPE) is a scale that measures how hard any given level of work feels. The scale is shown in Table 58.8. The RPE is administered during exercise testing. The patient is asked to rate the

Table 58.8.
Rating of Perceived Exertion (RPE) Scale
Perceived Exertion[a]

6	
7	Very, very light
8	
9	Very light
10	
11	Fairly light
12	
13	Somewhat hard
14	
15	Hard
16	
17	Very hard
18	
19	Very, very hard
20	

[a] The rating of perceived exertion scale (RPE) developed by Borg. (From Borg G: Subjective effort in relation to physical performance and working capacity. In Pick HL (ed): *Psychology: From Research to Practice.* New York, Plenum, 1978, p 333.

work at each stage of the test. After conditioning, the RPE is lower at any given stage and is associated with a lower heart rate and blood pressure at that stage (13). RPE is also a useful way to prescribe exercise. This approach focuses on how the patient actually feels and correlates closely with the target heart rate and/or desired MET level. For most cardiac patients, a prescription at 13 to 14 on the RPE scale is both safe and effective for cardiovascular conditioning.

The effect of exercise training on longevity in patients after MI has not been established definitively. However, in the National Exercise and Heart Disease Project (NEHDP), the 3-year mortality rates for control and exercise groups were 7.3 and 4.6%, respectively, and the 3-year rates for recurrent MI for control and exercise groups were 7.0 and 5.3%, respectively (26). The number of participants (n = 651) was not large enough to establish these results as significant.

Risks of Conditioning

With proper selection, supervision, monitoring, and precautions, physical conditioning for cardiac patients has proven to be remarkably safe. Cumulative data from over 1.5 million man-hours of exercise, done predominantly 3 months after MI, show that the risks of ventricular fibrillation, acute MI, and death are 1/10,000 to 1/32,000, 1/253,000, and 1/100,000 to 1/212,000 man-hours of exercise, respectively (7). There is no comparable large series in the literature on exercise conditioning early after MI. In the authors' experience, with over 200 MI patients, beginning an exercise program at an average of 10 days after hospital discharge, there have been no untoward events during exercise over a 2-year period. These patients exercise three times/week, for an average of 6 to 8 weeks at a conditioning heart rate of about 80% of what they safely achieved on a previous post-MI stress test, usually performed before hospital discharge.

Cardiovascular Medications and Conditioning

Many patients enrolling in exercise programs are taking one or more medications. Many of these medications alter the cardiovascular response to exercise. Patients enrolled in a conditioning program should always be stress tested (see below) while taking their regular medications, and the effects of their drugs must be considered in interpreting test results. For example, β-blockers attenuate the heart rate response to exercise. Thus, heart rate is less useful as an end point for stress testing or as a parameter for the patient to monitor during exercise conditioning. In a patient on β-blockers, symptoms, ECG changes, fatigue, and RPE are used as end points during stress testing. These parameters are also useful for establishing the exercise prescription in patients on certain medications. Table 58.9 sum-

Table 58.9.
Effect of Various Classes of Medications on Hemodynamic Status during Exercise[a,b]

Drug	Peak Heart Rate	Peak Systolic Blood Pressure
ANTIHYPERTENSIVES		
Hydralazine	↑	↓
Minoxidil	↑	↓
Clonidine	↓	↓
Guanethidine	↓	↓↓
Methyldopa	↓	↓
Prazosin	↑	↓
NITRATES	↑	↓
ANTIARRHYTHMICS	=	↓
β-BLOCKERS	↓	↓
DIGITALIS[c]	=	↑
CALCIUM BLOCKERS		
Nifedipine	↑	↓
Diltiazem	=	↓
Verapamil	↓	↓

[a] Expanded from Powles ACP: The effect of drugs on the cardiovascular response to exercise. *Med Sci Sports Exercise* 13:252, 1981.
[b] ↓, decreased; ↑, increased; =, no discernible effect.
[c] Patients with congestive heart failure.

marizes the effects of a number of commonly prescribed cardiac drugs on the hemodynamic response to exercise. Persons taking a variety of drugs have been evaluated and have participated safely in physical conditioning programs. In fact, the majority of patients in the NEHDP were taking one or more medications. The most common drugs were nitrates, diuretics, and tranquilizers; but over 10% were taking β-blockers, antiarrhythmics, digitalis, or antihypertensives. There is some controversy regarding the effect of β-blockers on the response to training. It has been suggested that β-blockers may attenuate the beneficial effects of training. In one study, patients not on β-blockers improved 56% more in muscle strength than patients on β-blockers. However, in the same study, β-blockade had no effect on treadmill performance (16). Clearly, further research in this area is needed.

Referral for Conditioning

The decision to refer a patient for physical conditioning after MI depends on the patient's clinical status, his motivation, and the availability of well supervised and staffed programs designed for such patients. Medically supervised programs, offering ECG monitoring and the immediate availability of emergency care, often accept patients within 2 weeks of hospital discharge. If such a program is not available, the activity schedule shown in Table 58.3 is appropriate. After 3 months, where there is no supervised program available, patients with uncomplicated MI can be advised to increase their exercise level gradually, using the results of a stress test to establish target heart rates or RPE.

Before beginning a conditioning program, the pa-

tient should have an ECG stress test (see Chapter 57 for a description of the patient's experience), the results of which are used in planning the exercise program. In general, the conditioning target heart rate is 70 to 85% of the maximum heart rate safely achieved on the stress test. Figure 58.4 shows the results of such a stress test, performed 3 weeks after an MI in a patient who was evaluated just prior to enrollment in a supervised exercise program.

Contraindications

A patient should not be enrolled or should be discontinued from a conditioning program if the following problems are present: poorly controlled angina, severe dyspnea at low work loads, moderate to severe uncontrolled hypertension (diastolic > 110 mm Hg), complex arrhythmias, atrial fibrillation with a rapid ventricular response, second or third degree heart block, significant valvular or congenital heart disease, significant orthopaedic or pulmonary limitations, chronic alcoholism, or recent acute physical or mental illness.

Exercise Programs

Exercise sessions should be supervised by personnel trained in exercise physiology and cardiopulmonary resuscitation, with immediate availability of monitoring and resuscitative equipment. Programs that accept patients 2 to 3 weeks post-MI should have equipment for continuous ECG monitoring. Sessions are usually held three times a week on nonconsecutive days. The total duration of an average session is about 45 minutes. The pattern for a workout is illustrated in Figure 58.5. During the stimulus phase, the patient exercises at an intensity that elicits a heart rate or rating of perceived exertion (RPE, see above) that falls within the prescribed target zone. Figure 58.6 shows recommendations for exercise intensity based on heart rate response during an exercise stress test. Exercising near the 70% level, for 20 to 30 minutes, will promote fitness, and beginners should be instructed to maintain intensity near this level. Experienced exercisers can advance to the 85% level if a more intense workout is desired. The stimulus, or period at the target heart rate, is preceded by 5 to 10 minutes of warm-up and is followed by 5 to 10 minutes of cool-down (Fig. 58.5). Warm-up and cool-down should include stretching and range of motion calisthenic exercises (see illustration in Chapter 67). Warm-up provides for gradual acceleration of the heart and circulation; it is beneficial to joints and muscles and helps to prevent musculoskeletal injuries. Cool-down provides for gradual deceleration of the cardiovascular system and prevents pooling of blood in the muscles when exercise stops abruptly. Pooling can lead to a precipitous drop in venous return and, consequently, postexercise hypotension. A decrease in circulating blood to the brain, heart, and gastrointestinal system

```
PATIENT: J T  ID#: 00 00 00   DATE:  6 / 6 / 81
REFERRING PHYSICIAN: CCU


*****************************PATIENT DATA****************************


AGE: 34   SEX: MALE   HGT: 68   WGT: 162  INDICATION: EARLY S/P MI
PRESENT SYMPTOMS: NONE
CCU ADMISSION DATE:  5 / 12 / 81    DX: INFERIOR MI
PRIOR EST:  4 / 14 / 75      RESULTS: NEGATIVE EXERCISE STRESS TEST
MEDS: NITROPASTE
RISK FACTORS: SMOKING FAMILY HX


************************PRE-EXERCISE SCREENING**********************


SUPINE: HR: 62 BP: 114 / 78      STANDING: HR: 66 BP: 112 / 80
RESTING EKG:AXIS/PATTERNS:    INFERIOR MI
RESTING EKG:RHYTHM:           NORMAL SINUS RHYTHM
POST-HYPERVENTILATION:        NO SIGNIFICANT CHANGES


***************************EXERCISE RESULTS************************


REASON FOR STOPPING TEST: TARGET HEART RATE ATTAINED
EXERCISE PROTOCOL: MODIFIED NAUGHTON      TOTAL TIME: 14 MIN, 30 SEC
PEAK SPEED: 3 MPH  ELEVATION: 10 % GRADE   METS:  7   NYHA CLASS: 1
PHYSIOLOGICAL DATA: PREDICTED MAX HR:  186   90% MAX HR:  167
PEAK HR:  132       THIS WAS ADEQUATE FOR THE WORK PERFORMED
PEAK BP:  150       THIS WAS ADEQUATE FOR THE WORK PERFORMED
THE RATE-PRESSURE PRODUCT WAS:  19800

     EXERCISE EKG:ST-T CHANGES:
THERE WERE NO SIGNIFICANT CHANGES NOTED.

     EXERCISE EKG:RHYTHM:
THERE WERE NO ARRHYTHMIAS NOTED.

     SYMPTOMS:
THERE WERE NO SYMPTOMS REPORTED.

     CONCLUSIONS:
1.   ADEQUATE, NEGATIVE EARLY POST MI STRESS TEST.
2.   ACCELERATED DIASTOLIC BLOOD PRESSURE RESPONSE TO EXERCISE.
     RECOMMENDATIONS:
A.   MAY START MONITORED EXERCISE PROGRAM.
B.   CONSIDER BETA BLOCKADE IN VIEW OF #2 ABOVE.
```

Figure 58.4. *A.* Example of a formal report of an exercise stress test useful for planning rehabilitation following myocardial infarction (see data Fig. 58.6*B*).

may result in dizziness, fainting, ischemia, arrhythmias, nausea, and other symptoms.

As discussed earlier, training is specific to the muscles used in a particular exercise. Therefore, a training session should consist of a variety of activities designed to provide a well rounded workout. Exercises for both the legs and arms should be incorporated into the session. Aerobic training of the legs can be achieved through bicycling, walking, jogging, and aerobic dance. The arms can be trained with shoulder wheels, rowing machines, and arm ergometers. Swimming, cross-country ski machines, and combination arm-leg cycles are excellent for exercising both lower and upper extremities at the same time. For selected cardiac patients, circuit weight training can be used to improve both aerobic capacity and upper and lower body strength (16). In circuit weight training, the patient moves from weight machine to weight machine, performing for 30 seconds at 40% of maximal capacity, with 30 seconds of rest between each exercise, for a total of 20 minutes. This type of exercise combines elements of dynamic and static forms of exercise. Patients selected for this type of exercise should be preconditioned in a traditional program of walking and jogging for at least 3 months, and achieve at least 6 METs on a treadmill test without symptoms or ischemic electrocardiographic changes.

Protocol

Stage	Bruce Treadmill*	Mets	Mod. Naughton Treadmill*	Mets	BP	HR	Comments
1	1.7/0	2	2/0	2	140/100	87	NO SYMPTOMS; NO EKG CHANGES
2	1.7/10	5	2/3.5	3	145/105	92	NO SYMPTOMS; NO EKG CHANGES
3	2.5/12	7	2/7	4	140/115	98	NO SYMPTOMS; NO EKG CHANGES
4	3.4/14	10	2/10.5	5	140/110	108	NO SYMPTOMS; NO EKG CHANGES
5	4.2/16	13	2/14	6	150/120	128	NO SYMPTOMS; NO EKG CHANGES
6			3/10	7	145/95	132	FATIGUE; NO EKG CHANGES
7			3/12.5	8			
8			3/15	9			
9			3/17.5	10			
10							

*Miles per hr/percent elevation

Recovery

Min	BP	HR	Comments
0	145/95	132	NO SYMPTOMS; NO EKG CHANGES
2	114/85	94	NO SYMPTOMS; NO EKG CHANGES
4	112/80	88	NO SYMPTOMS; NO EKG CHANGES
6	112/84	75	NO SYMPTOMS; NO EKG CHANGES
8	112/84	78	NO SYMPTOMS; NO EKG CHANGES
10	110/82	84	NO SYMPTOMS; NO EKG CHANGES

Target Heart Rate _____130_____

Figure 58.4. *B.* Data from stress test reported in Figure 58.6*A.*

Termination of Supervised Training

Criteria for terminating supervised exercise training and transfer to nonsupervised maintenance programs are not clearly established. ECG monitoring for 6 to 8 weeks, and longer, during early exercise programs is generally recommended. Clinical stability and functional capacity above 7 to 8 METs (Table 58.4) are generally accepted exit criteria.

After a few months of supervised exercise, repeat stress testing is useful for measuring the change in physical working capacity and for adjusting more accurately the optimal exercise training intensity.

Long Term Compliance

Unfortunately, long term compliance with formal exercise programs is less than desirable. Patients must be made to understand that it is necessary to exercise regularly, at the proper intensity, fre-

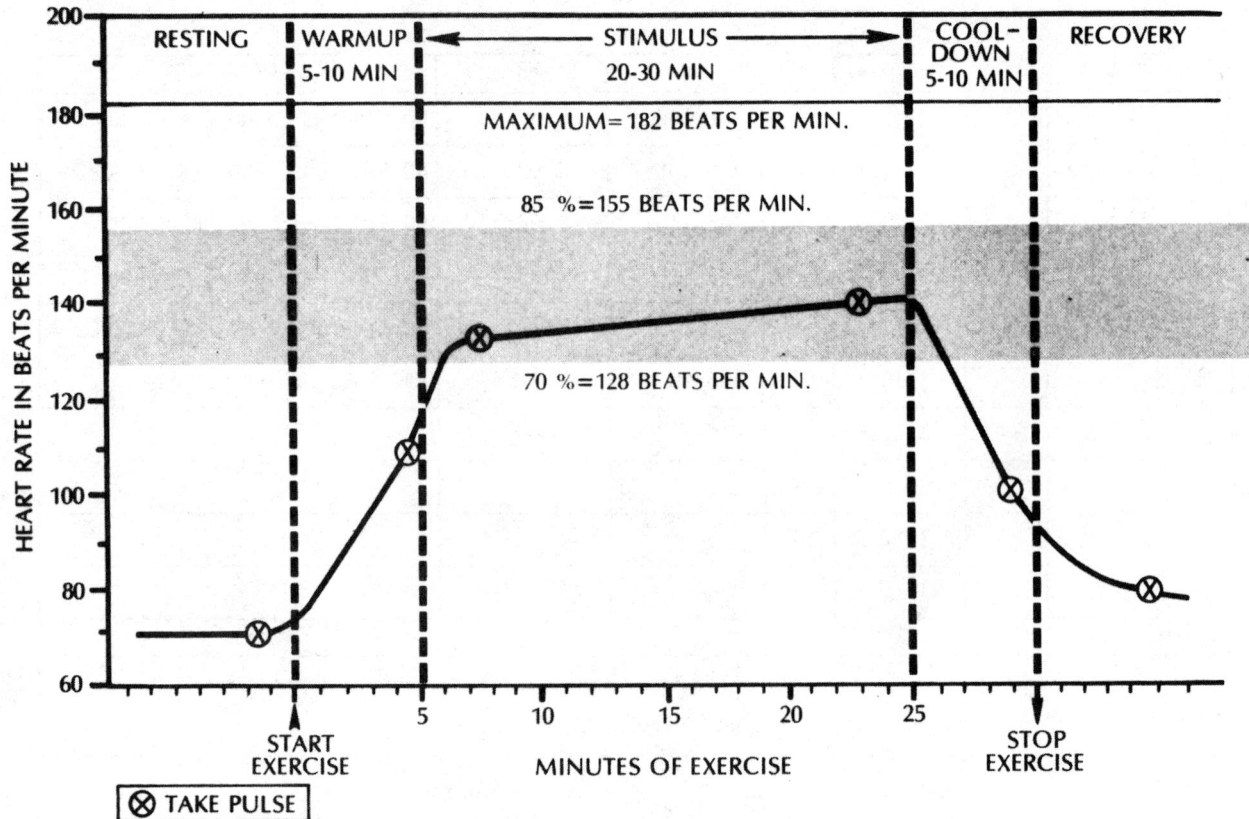

Figure 58.5.   The exercise training pattern.

quency, and duration, if physical fitness is to be maintained. Measurable deterioration in the conditioning effect occurs after missing only a few weeks. The time required to retrieve lost ground seems to be directly related to the length of time without exercise and to the degree of physical fitness achieved before cessation of exercise. Exercise must become a part of the patient's weekly routine, and not something that is done only during the recovery from MI.

HOME CARE FOR ACUTE MYOCARDIAL INFARCTION

A controlled trial in Great Britian has shown that for patients with uncomplicated acute MIs the outcome is similar whether the patient is cared for in the home or in an intensive care unit (18). The authors concluded that home care was ethically acceptable for such patients. Because hospital care is the norm for an acute MI in the United States, it is unlikely that home care will gain significant acceptance here. However, for an occasional older person who presents with a stable acute MI and objects to hospitalization, or for a person who consults his physician several days following an infarct, initial management at home may be appropriate.

The scheme for rehabilitation after MI described in this chapter can be adapted to these situations.

MANAGEMENT OF UNSTABLE ANGINA AFTER DISCHARGE FROM HOSPITAL

Of patients admitted to a hospital with unstable angina, 15 to 30% will continue to have pain despite vigorous medical management. Patients in this subgroup have a 25 to 45% 1-year mortality rate. Therefore, most are evaluated for and referred for coronary artery bypass surgery, an intervention which relieves or eliminates symptoms in the majority and improves the prognosis for those with left main coronary artery disease.

For the 70 to 85% of patients whose unstable angina responds to medical therapy, elective coronary arteriography should be planned within 1 to 2 months of discharge (see "Patient Experience," Chapter 57). For the approximately 10 to 15% of these patients who have significant left main coronary artery disease, coronary artery bypass surgery is recommended, as this seems to improve the patient's longevity. Whether bypass surgery increases longevity in other subsets of coronary artery disease remains a moot point (4).

To date, the rehabilitation of the medically man-

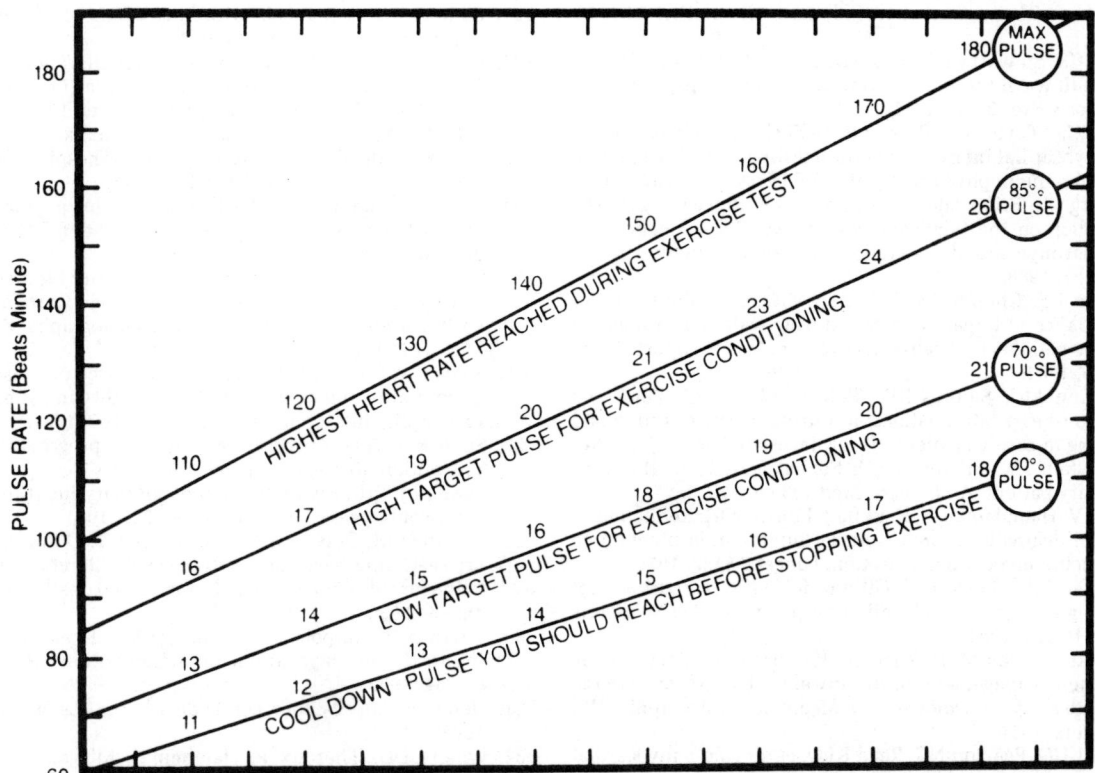

Figure 58.6. Target pulse rates for 10-second counts that should be measured the first 10 seconds after exercise. To convert the count to beats per minute, multiply by 6. To determine a patient's target pulse rate range, identify the highest rate safely achieved during the most recent exercise test on the top line (maximum pulse line); then locate the corresponding values on the 85 and 70% lines directly below. These two values represent the limits of target rate range for exercise conditioning (From Haskell WL: Design and implementation of cardiac conditioning programs. In Wenger NK, Hellerstein HK (eds): *Rehabilitation of the Coronary Patient.* New York, John Wiley & Sons, 1978, p 209).

aged patient with unstable angina has not been studied as systematically as the rehabilitation of the patient after MI. These patients should receive education similar to that recommended for patients after MI regarding the nature of coronary artery disease, the recognition of symptoms, and the control of risk factors (see page 705). Because these patients do not have an ischemic injury which takes 2 or more months to heal, they can usually be permitted to return to their usual activities more rapidly than patients who have had an MI. This is true particularly if their angina is well controlled and a stress test shows minimal or no changes due to ischemia.

Additional information regarding the medical management of unstable angina is found in Chapter 57.

General References

American Heart Association: *Exercise Testing and Training of Individuals with Heart Disease or at High Risk for its Development: A Handbook for Physicians.* Dallas, American Heart Association, 1975.

Long C (ed): *Prevention and Rehabilitation in Ischemic Heart Disease.* Williams & Wilkins, Baltimore, 1980.

   Reviews in depth all aspects of prevention and rehabilitation of the patient with coronary artery disease.

Specific References

1. Baile WF, Engel BT: A behavioral strategy for promoting treatment compliance following myocardial infarction. *Psychosom Med* 40:412, 1978.
2. Battler A, Karliner JS, Higgins CB, et al: The initial chest X-ray in acute myocardial infarction, a prediction of early and late mortality and survival. *Circulation* 61:1004, 1980.
3. Braunald E: Treatment of the patient after myocardial infarction. *N Engl J Med* 302:290, 1980.
4. Braunwald E: Editorial perspective: Effect of coronary artery bypass grafting on survival. *N Engl J Med* 309:1181, 1983.
5. Cooper KH (ed): *The New Aerobics.* New York, Bantam Books, 1970.
6. The Coronary Drug Project Research Group: The prognostic importance of the electrocardiogram after myocardial infarction. *Ann Intern Med* 77:677, 1972.
7. Council on Scientific Affairs, American Medical Association: Physician-supervised exercise programs in rehabilitation of patients with coronary heart disease. *JAMA* 245:1463, 1981.
8. Ehsani AA, Heath GH, Hagberg JM, et al: Effects of 12 months of intense exercise training on ischemic ST-depression in

patients with coronary artery disease. *Circulation* 64:1116, 1981.

9. Ewart CK, Stewart KJ, Keleman MH, *et al*: Psychologic impact of circuit weight testing and training in cardiac patients. *Med Sci Sports Exer* 2:139, 1984.

10. Ewart CK, Taylor CB, Reese LB, DeBusk RF: Effects of early postmyocardial infarction exercise testing on self-perception and subsequent physical activity. *Am J Cardiol* 51:1076, 1983.

11. Furberg CD, Friedwald WT, Eberlein KA: Proceedings of the workshop on the implications of recent Beta-Blocker trials for postmyocardial infarction patients. *Circulation* 67 (suppl):1, 1983.

12. Gillilan RE, Chopra AK, Kelemen MH, *et al*: Prediction of compliance to target heart rate during walk-job exercise in cardiac patients by a self-efficacy scale. *Med Sci Sports Exerc* 16:115, 1984.

13. Gutmann MC, Squires RW, Pollack ML, *et al*: Perceived exertion-heart rate relationship during exercise testing and training in cardiac patients. *J Cardiovasc Rehabil* 1:52, 1981.

14. Hellerstein HK, Friedman EH: Sexual activity in the post-coronary patient. *Arch Intern Med* 125:987, 1970.

15. Kallio V, Hamalainen H, Hakkila J, Luurila OH: Reduction in sudden deaths by a multifactorial intervention programme after acute myocardial infarction. *Lancet* 2:8152, 1979.

16. Kelemen MH, Stewart KJ, Gillilan RE, *et al*: Circuit weight training in a cardiac rehabilitation program. *Med Sci Sports Exerc* 16:128, 1984.

17. Levy RI, Feinlab M: Risk factors for coronary artery disease and their management. In Braunwald E (ed): *Heart Disease: A Textbook for Cardiovascular Medicine*. Philadelphia, WB Saunders, 1984.

18. Mather HG, Pearson NG, Read KLQ, *et al*: Acute myocardial infarction: home and hospital treatment. *Br Med J* 1:334, 1971.

19. Meizlish JL, Berger HJ, Plankey M, *et al*: Functional left ventricular aneurysm after acute myocardial infarction. *N Engl J Med* 16:1001, 1984.

20. Mukharji J, Rude RE, Poole WK, *et al.* and the MILIS Study Group: risk factors for sudden death after acute myocardial infarction: two-year follow-up. *Am J Cardiol* 54:31, 1984.

21. Plotnick GD: Approach to the management of unstable angina. *Am Heart J* 98:243, 1979.

22. Rosati RA, Harris PJ: Acute myocardial infarction. In Fries JF, Ehrlich GE (eds): *Prognosis: Contemporary Outcomes of Disease*. Bowie, MD, Charles Press Publishers, 1981.

23. Schaffer WA, Cobb LA: Recurrent ventricular fibrillation and modes of death in survivors of out-of-hospital ventricular fibrillation. *N Engl J Med* 293:259, 1975.

24. Schuster EH, Bulkley B: Early postinfarction angina, ischemia at a distance and ischemia in the infarct zone. *N Engl J Med* 305:1101, 1981.

25. Schwartz KM, Turner JD, Sheffield LT, *et al*: Limited exercise testing soon after myocardial infarction. Correlation with early coronary and left ventricular angiography. *Ann Intern Med* 94:724, 1981.

26. Shaw LW: Effects of a prescribed supervised exercise program on mortality and cardiovascular morbidity in patients after a myocardial infarction. *Am J Cardiol* 48:39, 1981.

27. Stamler J: Acute myocardial infarction-progress in primary prevention. *Br Heart J* 33:145, 1971.

28. Stamler J: Primary prevention of coronary heart disease: the last twenty years. *Am J Cardiol* 47:722, 1981.

29. Starling MR, Crawford MH, Kennedy GT, O'Rourke RA: Exercise testing early after myocardial infarction: predictive value for subsequent unstable angina and death. *Am J Cardiol* 46:909, 1980.

30. Theroux P, Marpole DGF, Bourassa MG: Exercise stress testing in the postmyocardial infarction patient. *Am J Cardiol* 52:664, 1983.

31. Ueno M: The so-called coitus death. *Jpn J Legal Med* 17:330, 1963.

32. Waters DD, Theroux P, Halphen C, Mizgala HF: Clinical predictors of angina following myocardial infarction. *Am J Med* 66:991, 1979.

33. Wilhelmsson C, Vedin JA, Elmfeldt D, *et al*: Smoking and myocardial infarction. *Lancet* 1:415, 1975.

34. Zohman LR: *Beyond Diet: Exercise Your Way to Fitness and Heart Health*. Englewood Cliffs, NJ, Mazola Products, Best Food, 1974.

CHAPTER FIFTY-NINE

Arrhythmias

SHELDON H. GOTTLIEB, M.D., PHILIP D. ZIEVE, M.D., AND
GUSTAV C. VOIGT, M.D.

Contraction of the heart is normally the result of a well orchestrated electromechanical system. The orderly function of the system is maintained by the domination of the heart rate by a single pulse generator known as the *pacemaker*, by the relatively fast and uniform conduction of the electrical signal *via* specialized *conduction pathways*, and by the relatively long and uniform duration of the electrical signal relative to its velocity of conduction through these pathways, thereby assuring uniform electrical excitation and contraction of the heart. An *arrhythmia* is any disturbance in the normal sequence of impulse generation and condition in the heart.

Arrhythmias may occur in the absence of heart disease or may be symptoms of severe disease. They must be evaluated in the context of the clinical situation in which they occur. A precise etiological diagnosis and an understanding of the pharmacology of the medications used are necessary to treat arrhythmias effectively.

PHYSIOLOGY OF IMPULSE GENERATION AND CONDUCTION

The Action Potential

Muscle contraction is stimulated by an electrical impulse, the action potential. In skeletal muscle, the action potential is transient, and the electrical activity is essentially dissipated before the beginning of contraction. In cardiac muscle, however, the action potential is sustained and lasts almost as long as the contraction itself (Fig. 59.1). In this way, the action potential not only stimulates contraction of the heart but also determines the duration and intensity of contraction. Furthermore, as long as the action potential is maintained, the heart cannot be stimulated to contract again.

The action potential is generated by depolarization and repolarization of the muscle cell (Fig. 59.2). In the resting state the intracellular concentration of potassium is high and that of sodium is low compared to the extracellular fluid. These gradients are maintained by metabolic activity within the cell membrane. The resting membrane potential is strongly negative (*i.e.*, there is an electrochemical gradient across the membrane so that the inside of the membrane is negatively charged compared to the outside of the membrane). If an electrical stimulus is applied, the membrane becomes very permeable to sodium ions, which rapidly leak into the cell (phase 0). The membrane is thus depolarized (loses its negative charge) and, in fact, is transiently positively charged (overshoot). Repolarization occurs relatively slowly as first chloride (phase 1) and then, after a plateau (phase 2), potassium ions (phase 3)

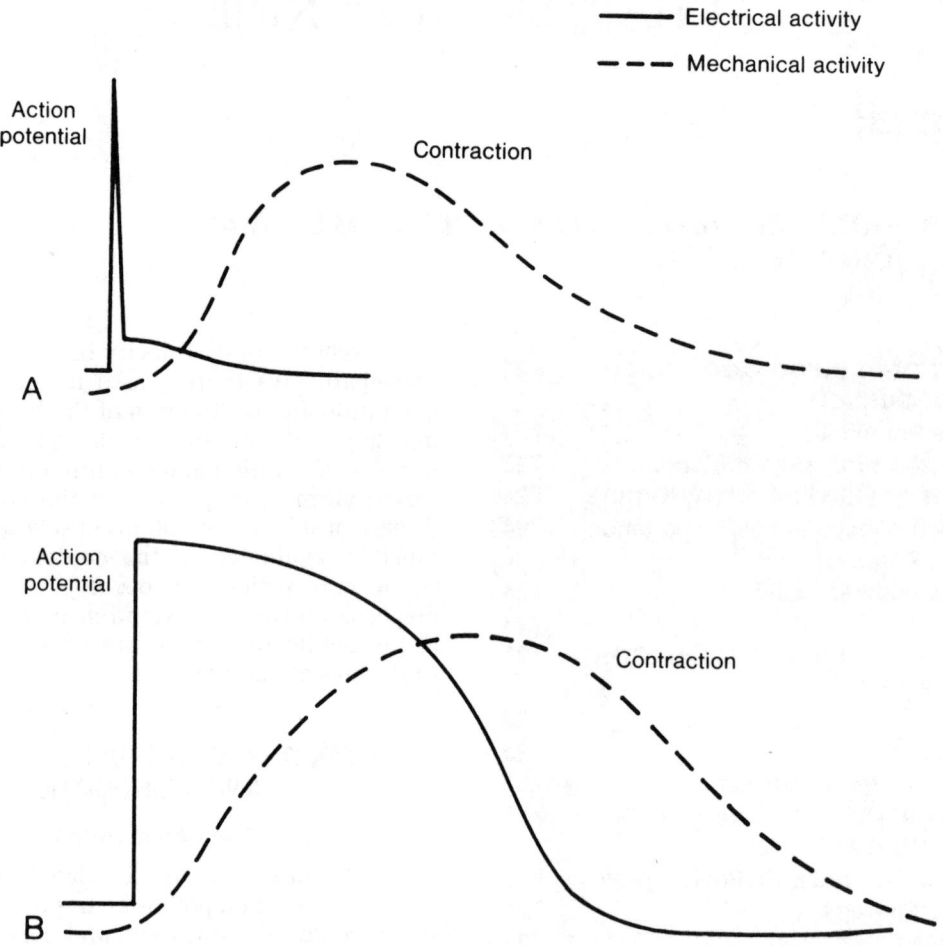

—— Electrical activity

- - - Mechanical activity

Figure 59.1. Comparison between relative time scales of electrical (*continuous curve*) and mechanical (*interrupted curve*) activity in skeletal (*A*) and cardiac (*B*) muscle. (From Noble D: *The Initiation of the Heart Beat*. Oxford, Clarendon Press, 1975 (19).)

move back into the cell to restore the resting potential (phase 4).

Relationship to the ECG

In the heart the phases of rapid depolarization and overshoot correspond to the QRS complex of the electrocardiogram; phase 2 corresponds to the ST segment; and phase 3, to the T wave (Fig. 59.2). During phase 2 the membrane is absolutely and in phase 3 relatively refractory to propagation of another electrical impulse.

Fast and Slow Currents

Although in most cardiac tissue, excitation is propagated by the rapidly depolarizing sodium current (so that the action potential is conducted rapidly), excitation of the sinoatrial node and the proximal part of the atrioventricular node is propagated by a slowly depolarizing current generated by the influx of calcium ions into the cell. Also, in diseased cardiac muscle, the sodium current may be in-

hibited and depolarization may occur entirely *via* the slow calcium current; therefore the action potential may be conducted very slowly. This difference in conduction velocity between cells depolarized by the sodium *versus* the calcium current has important implications in both the generation and the treatment of arrhythmias (see below).

Pacemaker Generation

In most cardiac cells, an action potential will not be generated until an electrical stimulus is applied. In pacemaker cells, slow spontaneous depolarization occurs until a threshold is reached whereupon phase 0 rapidly ensues (Fig. 59.2); this process is called *automaticity*. In the absence of heart block, the heart rate will be controlled by the pacemaker cells that depolarize most rapidly, because then the action potential is conducted rapidly throughout the heart and initiates rapid depolarization of other cells, even if they already have begun spontaneous slow depolarization. Automaticity is affected by the rate of

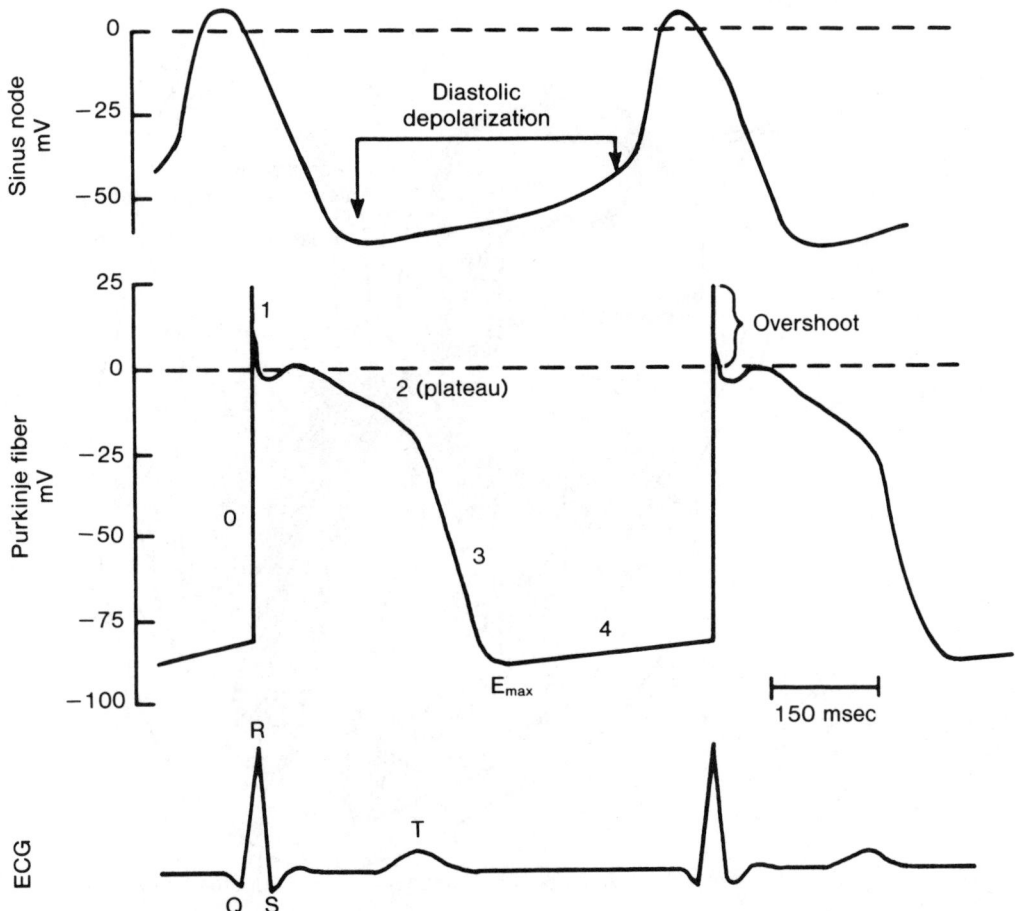

Figure 59.2. Transmembrane potentials from the sinus node and a Purkinje fiber. Note the spontaneous diastolic depolarization in the upper panel, characteristic of pacemaker fibers. The numbers in the *middle panel* are explained in the text. The *lower panel* shows the correlation of the time sequence of changes in the action potential and that of the surface electrocardio- gram. Alterations in depolarization will be reflected in changes in the QRS duration of the surface record; those in repolarization will be associated with altera- tions in the Q-T interval. (From Singh BN, Collett JT, Chew CYC: New perspectives in the pharmacologic therapy of cardiac arrhythmias. *Prog Cardiovasc Dis* 22:243, 1980 (23).)

slow spontaneous depolarization and by the thresh- old potential. Automaticity is enhanced by increased sympathetic tone, decreased vagal tone, increased catecholamine concentration in the blood, thyroid hormone, and digitalis. It is suppressed by decreased sympathetic tone, increased vagal tone, decreased thyroid hormone concentration, and various drugs (e.g., the drugs used in the treatment of arrhyth- mias).

Impulse Generation and Conduction (Fig. 59.3)

Sinoauricular Node

The sinoauricular (SA) node is composed of pace- maker cells located at the junction of the right atrium and the superior vena cava. The cells of the SA node spontaneously depolarize more rapidly than any other cells within the heart and the SA node therefore controls the heart rate.

Atrial Fibers

The action potential generated by the SA node traverses the atrium rapidly along discrete bundles of specialized conduction tissue known as *internodal fibers*. A specialized bundle of tissue connects the right and left atrium and the contractions of the atria are therefore nearly synchronous.

Atrioventricular Node

The internodal fibers terminate in the atrioven- tricular (AV) node cells which lie at the junction of the right atrium and the interventricular septum just above the tricuspid valve and through which the action potential is conducted slowly. Electrical delay in the AV node allows the mechanical activity of the atria (which is slower than their electrical activity) to be synchronized with the mechanical activity of the ventricles. The AV node serves as a protective "gate" and will not respond to extremely

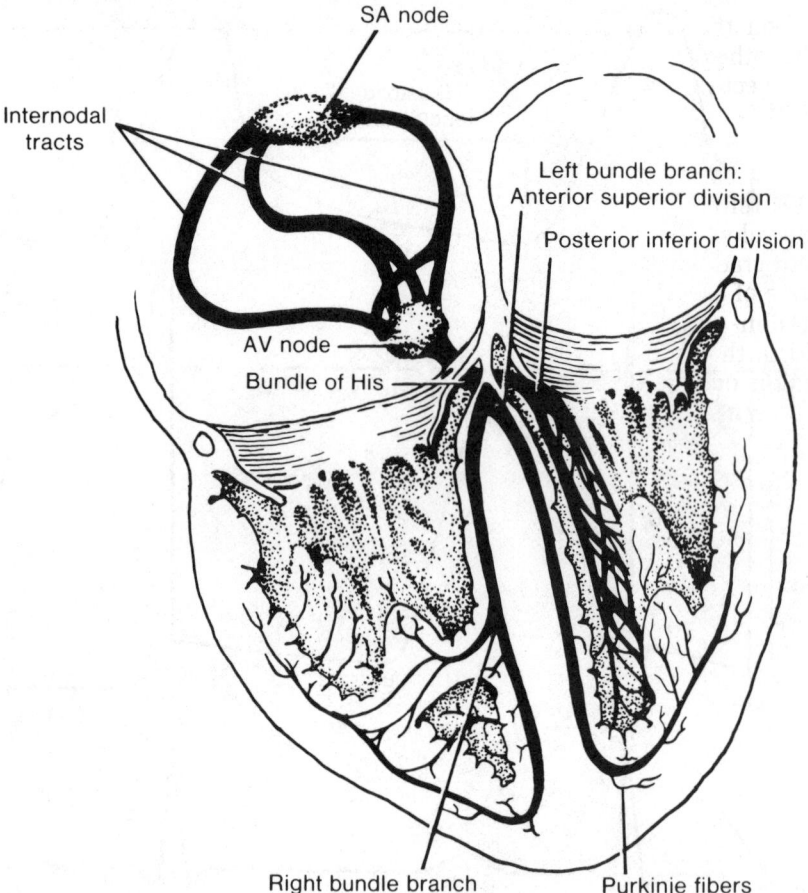

Figure 59.3.   Anatomy of impulse conduction. *SA*, sinoatrial; *AV*, atrioventricular. (From Greene HL, Humphries JO: Cardiac arrhythmias. In Harvey AM, Johns RJ, McKusick VA, *et al* (eds): *Principles and Practice of Medicine*. New York, Appleton-Century-Crofts, 1980 (12).)

rapid impulses generated in the atria, thereby protecting the ventricles from too rapid stimulation. The AV node may function as a subsidiary pacemaker if the SA node fails to pace.

Bundle of His

When the action potential leaves the AV node, it enters the specialized conducting fibers known as the bundle of His. The main bundle of His divides into three branches: the right bundle branch which runs along the right ventricular surface of the septum, the anterior superior branch which runs along the left ventricular surface of the septum, and the posterior inferior branch which runs along the posterior wall of the left ventricle. The action potential is conducted through the bundle branches and into the myocardium by a widespread network of smaller fibers known as *Purkinje fibers*.

MECHANISM OF CARDIAC ARRHYTHMIAS

There are three basic causes of disturbance in the rhythm of the heart: suppression of initiation or propagation of the action potential, ectopic pacemaker activity, and re-entry of the action potential into a pathway through which it has already passed. More than one of these mechanisms may be operative in producing a particular arrhythmia, e.g., ectopic supraventricular tachycardia in a patient with sinus node dysfunction.

Suppression of Initiation or Propagation of Action Potential

A disease process that interferes with pacemaker activity within the SA node or with the movement of the electrical impulse through the normal conduction pathways of the heart results either in abnormal slowing of the heart rate (bradyarrhythmia) and/or in one of the various forms of heart block.

Ectopic Pacemaker Activity

Enhanced automaticity of a part of the cardiac conduction system may result in the initiation of an impulse more rapidly than is normally generated by the SA node. If that happens episodically, occasional premature contractions will occur, the nature of which will depend on the location of the ectopic pacemaker. On the other hand, if there is rapid sustained firing of the ectopic focus, a tachyarrhythmia will be produced.

Re-entry

Alterations in the refractory period of adjacent pathways and of the velocity of the impulse through them may allow retrograde conduction of the action potential through one of the pathways. The forward (antegrade) conduction of the impulse is usually delayed or blocked in the pathway through which retrograde conduction occurs. The retrograde impulse then re-enters an adjacent pathway and is

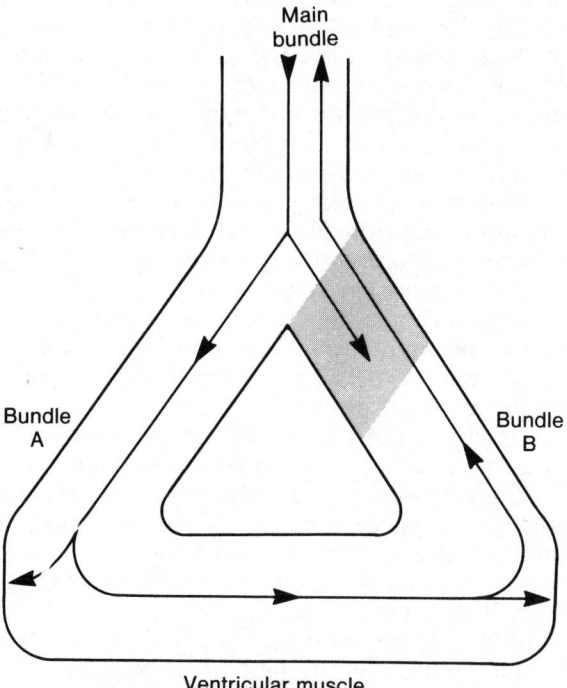

Figure 59.4. Sequence of activation of a loop of Purkinje fiber bundles (A and B) and ventricular muscle (VM) during re-entry. A region of unidirectional conduction block is indicated by the *darkly shaded area* in branch B. Conduction cannot occur through this area in the antegrade direction (from B to VM), but only in the retrograde direction (from VM to B). Slow conduction is present through the loop. The bottom of the figure shows a possible electrocardiographic pattern which may result from this type of re-entry. (From Wit AL, Rosen MR, Hoffman BF: Electrophysiology and pharmacology of cardiac arrhythmias. II. Relationship of normal and abnormal electrical activity of cardiac fibers to the genesis of arrhythmias. B. Re-entry, Section I. *Am Heart J* 88:664, 1974 (25).)

conducted forward again (Fig. 59.4). Sustained re-entry implies either unusual pathways for conduction of the action potential or poorly functioning and hence slowly conducting myocardium. Slow calcium currents (see above) may play an important role in sustained re-entry. Most premature contractions and most tachyarrhythmias are re-entrant rhythms.

DIAGNOSIS OF ARRHYTHMIAS: GENERAL CONSIDERATIONS

History

Arrhythmias may or may not cause symptoms. Symptoms, when they do occur, are due to an appreciation of the irregular rhythm (palpitations) or to a reduction in cardiac output (light-headedness, dizziness, syncope, shortness of breath, or chest pain). It is important to establish whether there are any factors that seem to trigger symptoms (e.g., drinking coffee, smoking, exercise, emotional stress) and whether there are symptoms of an underlying disease that may be associated with arrhythmia (e.g., heart failure, ischemic heart disease, thyrotoxicosis). The patient should be questioned specifically about the taking of stimulant drugs either illicitly (see Chapter 22) or as an ill conceived attempt to lose weight (see Chapter 76) and about the taking of prescription drugs which may cause arrhythmias (digitalis, theophylline, diuretics, β-blockers, tricyclic antidepressants, and antihypertensives).

Palpitations are heartbeats that are sensed—usually because the beats are fast or irregular. However, they do not necessarily imply a significant arrhythmia and they may represent only sinus tachycardia in an otherwise healthy individual. Palpitations are usually described by patients as sensations of beating, flip-flopping, or as a throbbing in the chest. They are often localized to the area of the apex beat, but rapid supraventricular tachycardias are commonly felt substernally or in the neck. Some people seem to sense the compensatory pause (see below) following an extra heart beat, but some may sense the extra beat itself. Often the contraction following an extra beat is more powerful than a normal beat (so-called postextrasystolic potentiation), and this stronger beat may be the one that is felt. Supraventricular beats are more commonly sensed as palpitations than are ventricular beats; and in fact potentially dangerous runs of ventricular tachycardia are commonly asymptomatic.

Light-headedness, dizziness, and syncope are common symptoms of significant arrhythmias. These symptoms and the conditions associated with them are discussed in detail in Chapter 81.

Physical Examination

An arrhythmia is best revealed on physical examination by inspection of the jugular pulse, by palpation of the arterial pulse, and by auscultation of the heart.

Conditions associated with arrhythmia—e.g., heart failure (Chapter 61), chronic obstructive lung disease (Chapter 55), or valvular heart disease (Chapter 60)—can often be recognized by characteristic physical findings.

Inspection of the jugular venous pulse reveals atrial activity. If there is atrioventricular dissociation or complete heart block, so-called cannon waves may be seen intermittently in the jugular veins; they are due to ejection of blood back into the veins when the right atrium contracts against a closed tricuspid valve. Cannon waves that coincide with the arterial pulse may reflect supraventricular tachycardia. If there is atrial fibrillation, there are no atrial waves visible in the jugular pulse.

Palpation of the arterial pulse establishes the ventricular rate—at least of conducted beats—and rhythm. In conjunction with the jugular pulse, it may provide more specific information as well about the nature of an arrythmia.

Auscultation of the heart also establishes the ventricular rate and rhythm and the intensity of S_1, the most useful heart sound in the evaluation of arrhythmia. For example, variation in the intensity of S_1 during a regular tachycardia suggests AV dissociation; variation during a regular bradycardia suggests second or third degree heart block. The intensity of S_1 is also a function of the P-R interval. A loud S_1 suggests a short P-R interval and is also heard in patients with mitral valve prolapse; a soft S_1 suggests a long P-R interval, due, for example, to digitalis toxicity or to electrolyte abnormalities.

Use of the Electrocardiogram

It is essential to obtain an ECG when evaluating a patient who has an arrhythmia. Without it, with few exceptions, a specific diagnosis is impossible. Usually a surface resting ECG is all that is needed. Occasionally, ambulatory (Holter) monitoring or an exercise ECG is indicated to detect a sporadic arrhythmia or an arrhythmia that is induced by stress. Even less commonly, a complex arrhythmia cannot be diagnosed accurately by standard ECG, and an intracavity (His bundle) ECG must be obtained by catheterization in order to make a precise diagnosis.

Surface Resting ECG

There are a number of features of the standard ECG which must be assessed:

Atrial activity. Atrial activity is best assessed in leads 2, 3, aVf, and in V_1. The presence of P waves must be identified. If P waves are present, their configuration and their relationship to QRS complexes must be established. Normally the P-R interval is between 0.12 and 0.20 second, and each QRS complex is preceded by a P wave. If P waves are not present, other evidence of atrial activity (fibrillation or flutter waves) should be sought.

Ventricular activity. The duration of the QRS complexes (normally less than 0.10 second) should be measured and the regularity of ventricular activity should be assessed. A basically regular rhythm may be interrupted by so-called premature beats—QRS complexes that appear before the next regular beat is expected. If premature beats are present, it should be noted whether or not they have a fixed relationship to the preceding normal beat and whether or not their configuration is the same as the regularly occurring complexes.

Ambulatory ECG (16)

The ambulatory (Holter) ECG records on magnetic tape the electrical activity of the heart—usually for a 24-hour period, although some models record for 48 hours. The recording device is small and does not interfere with virtually any of the patient's activities (except bathing and swimming). The technique is useful in the following circumstances:

1. Assessing whether suspicious symptoms—e.g., palpitation, light-headedness, dizziness, or syncope—in a patient with a normal resting ECG are due to an episodic arrhythmia;

2. Assessing whether episodic, but potentially life-threatening, arrhythmias are occurring in a patient with known heart disease (e.g., mitral valve prolapse or ischemic heart disease);

3. Assessing the efficacy of antiarrhythmic therapy or the function of a cardiac pacemaker.

The great majority of episodic arrhythmias are detected during 24 hours of Holter monitoring. If symptoms are very infrequent, however, it may be necessary to record the ambulatory ECG for 48 to 72 hours. It is important to ask the patient to keep a record of symptoms during the time that he is being monitored in order to determine whether those symptoms are, in fact, attributable to arrhythmia.

Exercise ECG

This technique is described in detail in Chapter 57. It is a useful test in the evaluation of patients who have symptoms suggestive of an arrhythmia during or after exercise or those with premature ventricular contractions—to determine if they become more or less frequent during or after exercise (see below, page 739).

GENERAL PRINCIPLES IN MANAGEMENT OF ARRHYTHMIAS

Once it has been established that a patient has a particular arrhythmia, the physician must decide whether treatment is necessary. That decision will be influenced by the effect of the arrhythmia on cardiac output, the potential for thromboembolic complications, the potential for degeneration of the arrhythmia into a more dangerous rhythm, and the relative risk of the treatment *versus* the relative risk of the arrhythmia to the patient's well-being and survival. It must also be determined whether the arrhythmia is constant or intermittent and whether it is secondary to a noncardiac process (e.g., hypoxia, electrolyte imbalance, fever) or a cardiac process (e.g., heart failure, pericarditis, digitalis intoxication), the correction of which will restore a normal cardiac rhythm.

If the physician determines that specific therapy is indicated, he must decide which of the various possible regimens is appropriate: one or more of the various antiarrhythmic drugs, a cardiac pacemaker, electrical conversion of the arrhythmia, or a combination of these.

Pharmacology of Antiarrhythmic Drugs

There are three major classes of antiarrhythmic drugs. *Membrane-active antiarrhythmic drugs* affect cell membrane properties such as rate of depolarization, conduction velocity, action potential duration, and refractory period. *β-Adrenergic blocking drugs* affect sympathetically mediated excitability, and *calcium channel blocking drugs* affect calcium-mediated slow channel currents in the myocardium.

Table 59.1 shows some of the characteristics of the antiarrhythmic drugs that can be conveniently used to treat an ambulatory patient. Because lidocaine (Xylocaine) can only be administered parenterally and has a short half-life, it is limited to hospital use and is not included in the table. All of the drugs that are included can also be given parenterally (usually intravenously) but, again, this route of administration is limited almost exclusively to hospital use.

Most antiarrhythmic drugs have a low toxic:therapeutic ratio and some are exceedingly toxic (Table 59.2). The safe and effective use of antiarrhythmic drugs depends on a careful assessment of the etiology and physiology of an arrhythmia and a knowledge of the pharmacology of the drugs that are used. Doses must, therefore, be individualized, and drug levels should be checked periodically (at first, after a steady state has been reached—see Table 59.1—and then one to three times a year, depending on the patient's response). Levels should be obtained approximately 4 hours after an oral dose of a drug that is taken every 6 to 8 hours, and approximately 8 to 12 hours after an oral dose of a drug that is taken once a day.

Digitalis, the other major drug used in the treatment of arrhythmias, acts indirectly as an antiarrhythmic agent by increasing vagal activity, thereby increasing the refractory period of the specialized conduction tissue of the atria and slowing the velocity of the action potential through the AV node.

Table 59.1.
Characteristics of Antiarrhythmic Drugs

Drug	Common Brand Name	Effects on ECG	Half-life (hr)	Time to Steady State (day)	Available Strength (mg)	Usual Oral Dose	Maximum Daily Dose (mg)	Therapeutic Plasma Levels
Quinidine	Generic	Prolongs QRS, Q-T, and (±) P-R	6	1–2	200 (sulfate) 342 (gluconate)	200–600 mg every 6–8 hours	2400	3–7 μg/ml
Procainamide	Pronestyl	Prolongs QRS, Q-T, and (±) P-R	3–4	1	250, 500 500, 750 (sustained-release)	500–1000 mg every 3–4 hours or every 6 hours (sustained release)	8000	3–8 μg/ml[a]
Disopyramide	Norpace	Prolongs QRS, Q-T, and (±) P-R	6–9	1–2	100, 500	150 mg 4 times daily	1200	2–4 μg/ml
Tocainide	Tonocard	Shortens Q-T	15	1.5–3	400, 600	400–600 mg every 8 hours or 600 mg every 12 hours	3200	4–10 μg of base/ml
Phenytoin (diphenylhydantoin)	Dilantin	Shortens Q-T	24–36	3–5	100	300–400 mg a day	800	10–20 μg/ml
Propranolol	Inderal	Prolongs (±) P-R, shortens Q-T	6	1	10, 20, 40, 60, 80	10–40 mg every 6 hours	640	50–100 ng/ml
Verapamil	Calan, Isoptin	Prolongs P-R	4.5–12	1–2	80, 120	80–120 mg every 8 hours	480	125–400 ng/ml

[a] It may also be important to measure, expecially in patients in cardiac or renal failure, the level of the active metabolite of procainamide, *N*-acetylprocainamide (NAPA).

Table 59.2.
Adverse Effects of Antiarrhythmic Drugs

Drug	Cardiac		Noncardiac	
	Common	Uncommon	Common	Uncommon
Quinidine	Decreased digoxin excretion (may precipitate digitoxicity)	Ventricular arrhythmias, myocardial depression, hypotension	Nausea, diarrhea, tinnitus, vertigo, rash, fever	Hepatic dysfunction, thrombocytopenia, hemolytic anemia
Procainamide	None	Myocardial depression	Nausea, vomiting	Agranulocytosis, lupus-like syndrome
Disopyramide	Myocardial depression, (should be used with caution in patients with severe or poorly compensated congestive heart failure)	Severe hypotension in absence of known heart disease	Anticholinergic effects—especially urinary retention, dry mouth, blurred vision, constipation, aggravation of narrow angle glaucoma	Acute psychoses, cholestasis
Tocainide	None	Ventricular arrhythmias	Dizziness, paresthesias, tremor, nausea, vomiting, sweating	Rashes, convulsions
Phenytoin (diphenylhydantoin)	None	Heart block	Cerebellar-vestibular effects, especially ataxia, nystagmus, vertigo; nausea, lethargy, seizures, rashes	Pseudolymphoma, megaloblastic anemia, peripheral neuropathy
Propranolol[a]	Bradycardia, myocardial depression	Anginal syndrome may worsen if drug suddenly discontinued	Fatigue, nausea, vomiting, depression, impotence, potentiates bronchospasm in patients with asthma	Peripheral vascular insufficiency, hyperglycemia, alopecia
Verapamil	Bradycardia, prolongation of P-R interval, peripheral edema	Precipitation of congestive heart failure or pulmonary edema, severe hypotension, heart block	Dizziness, headache, constipation, nausea	Confusion, sleep disorders

[a] Other β-blocking agents have the same adverse effects, although bronchospasm and peripheral vascular insufficiency may be less likely with use of β-specific agents (see Table 59.3).

General considerations in the use of digitalis including dosages, choice of a preparation, and recognition and treatment of toxicity are discussed in Chapter 61.

Membrane Active Drugs

Quinidine. In addition to its direct effects on the heart, quinidine blocks parasympathetic stimulation by the vagus nerve and may enhance AV conduction (and the ventricular rate) in some patients. For this reason patients with supraventricular tachyarrhythmias should be digitalized to suppress AV conduction before they are given quinidine. Quinidine also is a moderately potent inhibitor of α-adrenergic activity.

Several preparations of quinidine are available; quinidine sulfate is the recommended preparation on the basis of cost, but quinidine gluconate has fewer gastrointestinal side effects. A sustained release preparation containing gluconate (Quinaglute, Duraquin) may be preferred in some patients because it can be given every 8 to 12 hours.

Table 59.1 shows the time necessary to reach a steady state after administration of usual doses of quinidine. If a faster effect is desired, loading doses may be given (e.g., 300 mg every 3 hours for three

doses); in this circumstance hospitalization is advisable, both to monitor the effect of the drug and because the arrhythmia presumably is more dangerous.

Quinidine is used most often to prevent recurrence of supraventricular and ventricular tachyarrhythmias. It is also moderately effective but is no longer the first approach in the conversion of atrial flutter or fibrillation to normal sinus rhythm. The uses of the drug in specific situations are discussed below.

TOXICITY. There are a number of possible toxic effects of quinidine. The most common are gastrointestinal, especially diarrhea, and occur often within hours of administering the drug. Cinchonism (tinnitus, headache, visual disturbances) occurs occasionally. Hypersensitivity reactions (e.g., rash arthralgias, immune thrombocytopenia, or hemolytic anemia) are rare. These reactions often necessitate substitution of another antiarrhythmic drug.

Cardiac toxicity is usually dose related, often signaled by a prolongation of the Q-T interval; Q-T prolongation of 50% or more beyond baseline is an indication for reduction of the dose of quinidine. Serious toxicity is manifest by a high degree of AV block, ventricular tachycardia or fibrillation—all emergency situations that may require cardiorespiratory support and warrant immediate hospitalization. Occasionally, patients taking quinidine die suddenly, sometimes with relatively low plasma levels of the drug. Patients with prolonged Q-T intervals before institution of therapy with quinidine may be more prone to sudden death and therefore probably should not be given the drug.

If patients taking quinidine are asymptomatic, ECGs need be recorded no more frequently than once a year; if they are symptomatic (e.g., complain of exertional chest pain, light-headedness, shortness of breath, etc), more frequent tracings should be obtained (perhaps every 3 or 4 months, although no firm guidelines can be recommended).

DRUG INTERACTIONS. Since patients prescribed quinidine are commonly being treated with digitalis as well, it is especially important to recognize that digoxin levels may increase significantly in patients given quinidine. The precise mechanism is unclear, but quinidine appears to decrease the excretion of digoxin by the kidneys, and therefore it is important to monitor serum digoxin concentrations when quinidine is first prescribed and to alter the dose of digoxin to prevent digitoxicity.

Quinidine is an α-adrenergic blocker and, if it is prescribed with vasodilators (e.g., nitrates, nifedipine, hydralazine, prazosin) or with potent diuretics (e.g., furosemide) may cause symptomatic (especially postural) hypotension.

Drugs that are metabolized by hepatic microsomal enzymes may alter the pharmacokinetics of quinidine, and conversely, quinidine may alter the kinetics of one of these drugs. For example, phenytoin may accelerate the metabolism of quinidine, shortening its effect, and quinidine may inhibit the metabolism of warfarin, prolonging its effect.

Procainamide. The suppressive effects of procainamide on the electrical activity of the heart are the same as those of quinidine; but, unlike quinidine, procainamide has very little effect on vagal or on α-adrenergic activity.

The drug has been thought to be most useful in preventing recurrence of ventricular arrhythmias, although in somewhat higher doses (4 to 8 g/day instead of the more usual 2 to 6 g/day) it is as effective as quinidine in preventing the recurrence of atrial arrhythmias and in converting atrial flutter or fibrillation to normal sinus rhythm.

TOXICITY. The noncardiac toxicity of procainamide is different from that of quinidine. Gastrointestinal symptoms occur less often; and when they do, nausea and vomiting are more common than is diarrhea. Fever or granulocytopenia occurs occasionally.

Fifty percent of people taking procainamide develop antinuclear antibodies (ANA) within 3 months and 90% within 12 months (4). Twenty to 30% of patients with ANA develop a lupus-like syndrome characterized by serositis (pleuritis, pericarditis, synovitis), fever, hepatomegaly and a positive lupus erythematosus preparation. Unlike classical systemic lupus erythematosus, vasculitis is not a manifestation of drug-induced lupus, so that renal disease, for example, does not occur; and, most important, the syndrome abates, usually within months, when the drug is discontinued. The major threat of the syndrome is hemorrhagic pericarditis, and one must watch for signs and symptoms of pericardial tamponade.

Disopyramide. Disopyramide has direct membrane effects very much like quinidine and, like quinidine, blocks parasympathetic activity. It is licensed for the treatment of specific ventricular arrhythmias: unifocal or multifocal premature ventricular contractions and ventricular tachycardia. Disopyramide is used in ambulatory practice primarily for patients with one of these ventricular arrhythmias who cannot tolerate quinidine or procainamide.

The noncardiac toxicity of disopyramide is due mainly to its anticholinergic effects; these include dry mouth, blurred vision, urinary hesitancy, and constipation. Nausea, vomiting, and diarrhea are less common than they are after administration of quinidine or procainamide. The cardiac toxicity of the drug is, in part, similar to that of quinidine in that it can prolong the Q-T interval and produce ventricular tachycardia. Disopyramide may also cause or intensify heart failure or cause profound hypotension in patients who have compromised left ventricular function; it should be administered cautiously to such patients and stopped immediately if adverse reactions occur.

Phenytoin. Phenytoin decreases automaticity and the duration of the action potential in the Purkinje fibers of the myocardium. Its use is limited in the treatment of arrhythmias. Its primary value is in the treatment of complex arrhythmias associated with digitoxicity, and therefore it is seldom prescribed as an antiarrhythmic agent in ambulatory practice. Occasionally, patients will be discharged from hospital and will be taking phenytoin for control of a ventricular arrhythmia that has proved resistant to other drugs (or that has only been controlled by lidocaine, a drug that cannot be used on an ambulatory basis). Such patients are best followed in conjunction with a cardiologist.

Phenytoin toxicity is discussed in detail in Chapter 80.

New membrane-active drugs. A number of new membrane-active antiarrhythmic agents have been under investigation for several years (20). One of them, tocainide, has recently been approved by the Food and Drug Administration for use in the United States and several others (mexiletine, encainide, flecainide, lorcainide, and amiodarone) are likely to be approved within the next few years.

Tocainide is an analogue of lidocaine but can be given orally and has high bioavailability. It is used to suppress ventricular ectopy and in the approximately 60% of patients who respond to it, the number of premature ventricular contractions is reduced by 90% (20). In this regard it is no more effective than are quinidine, procainamide, or disopyramide, but, unlike those drugs, is much less likely to induce a life-threatening ventricular arrhythmia and sudden death and, therefore, may prove to be especially useful in ambulatory practice.

Amiodarone is a very potent antiarrhythmic drug that, unlike the other new drugs, prolongs the refractory state of all cardiac tissues and effectively suppresses both supraventricular and ventricular arrhythmias (28). It has a half-life of up to 2 months and, especially in high doses, is associated with a number of troublesome side effects, including photosensitivity, hypothyroidism, gastrointestinal upset, corneal microdeposits, and pulmonary interstitial fibrosis. Therefore, its role in the treatment of ambulatory patients must still be clarified so that, if it is approved for use, it should be prescribed only in consultation with a cardiologist.

Sympathetic Blocking Agents

These drugs block the effects of cathecholamines (which may potentiate the development of arrhythmias) and slow conduction in the atria, AV node, and myocardium.

β-Blockers are used primarily to lower the ventricular response in patients with atrial tachyarrhythmia; occasionally, in the process, they will convert paroxysmal atrial tachycardia, atrial flutter or fibrillation to normal sinus rhythm. In addition, ventricular arrhythmias initiated by exercise or ischemia (see Chapter 59) or associated with the prolonged Q-T syndrome (see below) may be prevented by these drugs. *β*-Blockers appear to be synergistic with digoxin, and relatively low doses of propranolol

and digoxin, for example, may be very effective in controlling heart rate in patients with atrial fibrillation, or in maintaining normal sinus rhythm in patients who have been cardioverted.

Toxicity. *β*-Blockers sometimes, by blocking sympthetic tone, precipitate heart failure in patients with poor ventricular function (an effect that can be overcome by digitalis), and they are contraindicated in patients with bronchial asthma. Gastrointestinal side effects (primarily nausea and diarrhea) occur occasionally. Most *β*-blockers may cause hair thinning in occasional patients; this effect appears to be reversible when the dose is reduced or the drug is discontinued. Peripheral vascular disease is occasionally exacerbated by nonselective *β*-blockers, in which case a relatively cardioselective *β*-blocker, such as metoprolol or atenolol, should be used.

The properties of the currently available *β*-blocking agents are listed in Table 59.3. Propranolol is the preparation prescribed most commonly. However, it crosses the blood-brain barrier and may cause such side effects as depression and sleep disturbances. Atenolol is long acting, does not cross the blood-brain barrier, and is relatively cardioselective. It appears to have fewer side effects than propranolol. It is not yet clear if any of the other available *β*-blockers offers significant advantages over these preparations. There is no current clear-cut cost advantage in choosing one of these drugs over another.

Calcium Channel Blockers (1, 24)

Calcium channel blockers (see above, page 722) are effective and useful drugs for controlling supraventricular arrhythmias. Conduction through the AV node is dependent on calcium-mediated currents. By blocking these currents, calcium channel blockers may control the ventricular response in atrial fibrillation and may convert to sinus rhythm supraventricular arrhythmias dependent on conduction through the AV node. Verapamil is the only

Table 59.3.
Currently Available *β*-Blockers[a]

	Atenolol (Tenormin)	Metoprolol (Lopressor)	Nadolol (Corgard)	Pindolol (Visken)	Propranolol (Inderal)	Timolol (Blocadren)
β-Blocking plasma levels	200–500 ng/ml	50–100 ng/ml	50–100 ng/ml	50–100 ng/ml	50–100 ng/ml	5–10 ng/ml
Elimination half-life (hr)	6–9	3–4	14–24	3–4	3.5–6	4
Active metabolites	No	No	No	No	Yes	No
Predominant route of elimination[b]	RE (mostly unchanged)	HM	RE	RE (~40% unchanged and HM)	HM	RE (~20% unchanged and HM)
β₁-blockade potency ratio (propranolol = 1.0)	1.0	1.0	1.0	6.0	1.0	6.0
Relative *β₁* selectivity	+	+	0	0	0	0
Available strengths (mg)	50, 100	50, 100	40, 80, 120, 160	5, 10	10, 20, 40, 60, 80	10
Usual maintenance dose	50 to 100 mg every day	50 to 100 mg twice daily	40 to 50 mg every day	5 to 20 mg 3 times daily	40 to 80 mg 4 times daily	20 mg twice daily

[a] Modified from Frishman WH: Beta-adrenoceptor antagonists: new drugs and new indications. *N Engl J Med* 305:500, 1981.
[b] RE, renal excretion; HM, hepatic metabolism.

calcium channel blocker approved for control of supraventricular arrhythmias, although diltiazem also appears to be effective. Verapamil may be useful in an ambulatory setting for the conversion of paroxysmal atrial tachycardia (PAT) to sinus rhythm. Doses of 80 to 120 mg orally may be used safely in patients known to have PAT; conversion to sinus rhythm usually occurs in ½ to 1 hour; alternatively, a dose of 5 to 10 mg intravenously may convert PAT in minutes. If the drug is not effective, referral to a hospital emergency room or a similar facility should be considered. Oral verapamil in doses of 80 to 120 mg every 8 hours may be used for prophylaxis against supraventricular arrhythmias. Verapamil may also be used in doses of 80 to 120 mg every 8 hours for control of heart rate in patients with atrial fibrillation. Diltiazem in doses of 30 to 60 mg every 6 hours may also be effective. These drugs are not effective for control of ventricular arrhythmias. Verapamil is metabolized by the liver and should be used with caution in patients with impaired liver function.

Toxicity. The most common side effects of calcium channel blockers are headache, light-headedness, dizziness, hypotension, and constipation. Verapamil interferes with renal clearance of digoxin and may precipitate digitoxicity. Verapamil is a moderate myocardial depressant and prolongs the P-R interval and should be used with caution in patients with cardiomyopathy, or in those receiving concomitant β-blocker therapy.

Pacemaker Therapy

Implantable electrical pulse generators (pacemakers) are the treatment of choice for patients with symptomatic bradyarrhythmias and heart block. In addition, specialized types of pacemakers may be used to terminate tachyarrhythmias by generating a current pulse which interferes with re-entrant tachycardias (so-called *overdrive pacing*). The decision to implant a pacemaker and the type of unit to use must be determined in consultation with a cardiologist. In general, patients in atrial fibrillation will require ventricular demand pacemakers. Most patients in sinus rhythm will be best served by a multiprogrammable atrioventricular sequential unit. The modest increase in cost and complexity of the atrioventricular sequential units appear in practice to be more than offset by the improved physiological response of patients over long term follow-up. Pacemakers are less than 1 cm thick, weigh less than 70 g, and may function for 10 to 15 years. Pacemaker leads are easily implantable via a percutaneous transvenous technique and rarely become dislodged even during vigorous activity. Symptoms are relieved in a majority of patients who are symptomatic due to bradyarrhythmias and conduction block (see below).

Patient experience. The units are implanted subcutaneously under local anesthesia in the pectoral area and the pacemaker lead is inserted *via* the cephalic vein or directly with the use of a special introducer into the subclavian vein and lodged in the apex of the right ventricle. The procedure takes about 1 ½ hours; the patient experiences some discomfort when the anesthetic is injected and, often, an unpleasant sensation when the tissues are manipulated to create a pocket for the pacemaker unit.

After the procedure, patients, depending on their age and condition, are discharged from the hospital within 3 to 7 days. Patients with sedentary jobs may return to work approximately 2 weeks after pacemaker insertion, but patients with more active jobs should be kept off work for approximately 6 weeks to allow the wound to heal completely. After that, there is little or no discomfort and the unit feels like part of the chest wall. Patients may exercise if they wish but should avoid extreme exertion (for example, doubles tennis rather than singles; jogging rather than hard running).

Patients with implanted pacemakers require careful, long term follow-up. They must be seen approximately every 3 months, and the function of the pacemaker must be assessed with a 12-lead ECG yearly and a rhythm strip at each visit. The ECG documents that the complexes have not changed, implying that the pacemaker lead has not shifted position; and the sensing and pacing functions of the pacemaker are determined with the rhythm strip. Long term follow-up is usually done in conjunction with a cardiologist.

It is important that the make of the pacemaker, its registration number, and its rate be entered into the patient's record and that the patient keep the registration card for the pacemaker on his person in the event of malfunction of the instrument or of an emergency intercurrent problem.

Cardioversion

The electrical conversion of atrial or ventricular tachyarrhythmias is done by the application of a short burst of direct current to the chest wall. The shock is synchronized with the QRS complex of the ECG to avoid applying it during the vulnerable period of the cardiac cycle when ventricular tachycardia or fibrillation might be induced.

Cardioversion is a more reliable technique for the conversion of tachyarrhythmias than is the administration of antiarrhythmic drugs. It may be required on an emergency basis if a patient has developed severe heart failure, hypotension, or ischemia as a result of an arrhythmia. Otherwise the procedure should be planned with the cardiologist who will attempt the conversion.

Digitalis should be withheld for 1 day before the procedure to ensure that an excess amount of drug is not circulating, and quinidine, 400 mg every 6 hours, should be given for 1 day before the procedure to minimize the development of arrhythmia at the time of the conversion. (Some patients will convert to sinus rhythm after administration of quinidine.) It is not clear whether patients to be subjected to cardioversion should be treated with anticoagulants. It seems reasonable, however, to give anticoagulants to patients in chronic heart failure, who have a history of prior embolism, or who have mitral stenosis. Anticoagulation (see Chapter 51) in these circumstances should be maintained for 2 weeks before and 2 weeks after the procedure; many cardiologists maintain anticoagulation indefinitely in these patients.

Patient experience. Cardioversion is done in a hospital with an anesthesiologist in attendance and with resuscitation equipment available. The patient is sedated, usually with 5 or 10 mg of intravenous diazepam or with intravenous Surital (thiamylal, a very short acting barbiturate), given to effect. Normally the patient cannot recall afterward the details of the procedure. For atrial fibrillation, cardioversion is attempted at 100 watt-seconds; the energy level is doubled repetitively and other shocks are administered until there is conversion or until a level of 400 watt-seconds is reached, after which the procedure must be terminated. Complications—embolism or a new arrhythmia—are unusual. After cardioversion, the patient is observed for a day or two and his rhythm is monitored, and then he is discharged. Quinidine is usually administered chronically in an attempt to prevent recurrence of the arrhythmia.

SPECIFIC ARRHYTHMIAS

Sinus Tachycardia

Definition and Etiology

In adults the normal sinus rate is 60 to 100 beats/minute. Sinus tachycardia, a sinus rhythm at a rate greater than 100 beats/minute is usually a physiologic rhythm in that the rate is ordinarily appropriate to the physiological state of the patient—a state that requires an increased cardiac output to meet increased metabolic demands. The maximum sinus heart rate that can be attained varies with age, but usually does not exceed 140 beats/minute unless demands are excessive (vigorous exercise, for example). The common factors that stimulate an increase in the rate of sinus rhythm, other than exercise, are fever (an increase of approximately 10 beats/minute for each Fahrenheit degree rise in body temperature), emotional stress, heart failure, and a variety of drugs that affect the autonomic nervous system (e.g., caffeine, aminophylline, amphetamine, alcohol, antidepressants, phenothiazines, etc).

Physical Findings

A regular rapid pulse and heart rate are detected, although there may be a slight variation in rate—so-called sinus arrhythmia. S_1 is normal and the jugular pulsations are normal.

Electrocardiogram

A P wave precedes each QRS complex; the P-R interval is normal for the rate (0.16 to 0.17 at rates over 130/minute); and the P wave vector is normal (upright P waves in II, III, and aVf).

Treatment

In most cases persistent sinus tachycardia need not be treated; it is the underlying condition that requires therapy. Digitalis, especially, should not be used to treat a patient with sinus tachycardia unless he is in heart failure.

In the occasional patient with an unexplained sinus tachycardia in whom a thorough evaluation fails to reveal an underlying cause, and in whom tachycardia is symptomatic, the use of small doses of propranolol may be justified. Treatment should be initiated with 10 mg, two or three times a day. Recent experience has documented that low dose propranolol may also be helpful in treating the anxiety and tachycardia associated with anticipated stressful situations. Used only as necessary, doses of 20 to 40 mg of propranolol an hour before a public speaking engagement, for example, may help to relieve the associated anxiety and tachycardia experienced by some people.

Sinus Bradycardia

Definition and Etiology

Sinus bradycardia is a heart rate below 60 beats/minute. Impulse generation in the sinus node is often slow in well conditioned people (e.g., long distance runners, heavy laborers). Inappropriately low sinus rates are commonly due to increased vagal tone such as is seen in association with pain, vomiting, or vasovagal syncope. A hypersensitive carotid sinus, more common in elderly people, may also result in marked bradycardia when the sinus is compressed by a tight collar or by the patient's tensing his neck. Parasympathomimetic drugs, such as neostigmine, tranquilizers, phenothiazines, and digitalis and sympatholytic drugs, such as reserpine or methyldopa, also may produce sinus bradycardia. Vagally induced bradycardia may be severe and result in asystole (and loss of consciousness) when the stimulus is marked or prolonged or occurs in a hypoxic patient.

Physical Findings

A regular slow pulse and heart rate are detected. S_1 is normal and the jugular pulsations are normal.

Electrocardiogram

A P wave precedes each QRS complex; the P-R interval is normal for the rate (0.20 to 0.21) and the P wave vector is normal (upright P waves in II, III, and aVf).

Treatment

Asymptomatic sinus bradycardia discovered as an incidental finding does not require treatment. However, patients who present with symptoms of light-headedness or syncope and are found to have sinus bradycardia may have underlying sinus node disease or may be subject to paroxysms of tachycardia and bradycardia, the so-called "sick sinus syndrome" (see below). Patients with sinus bradycardia and symptoms should be evaluated with an ambulatory ECG to determine whether they are suffering from this condition. In any case, patients with symptomatic sinus bradycardia, not due to a drug, are best treated with permanent pacemaker implantation.

Sick Sinus Syndrome

Definition and Etiology

The term sick sinus syndrome refers to a heterogeneous group of arrhythmias involving defective impulse generation by the sinus node and/or abnormal impulse conduction in the atria and AV node. The syndrome is characterized by periods of inappropriate sinus bradycardia (often severe with rates between 25 and 40/minute) which may precede or follow supraventricular tachyarrhythmias and by varying degrees of sinoatrial block including, sometimes, sinus arrest. The rubrics "bradycardia-tachycardia syndrome" or "tachycardia-bradycardia syndrome" are sometimes used, depending upon whether bradycardia precedes or follows a tachyarrhythmia.

The sick sinus syndrome is caused by degenerative fibrotic changes within the sinus node. It is often associated with similar abnormalities in other parts of the cardiac conduction system that result in varying degrees of atrioventricular and intraventricular block. These pathological changes are much more common in patients over the age of 60; although their precise cause is unknown, they are often associated with hypertensive or ischemic heart disease.

Symptoms and Signs

Many patients are asymptomatic. When symptoms do occur, they are produced either by spontaneous sinus arrest or by the tachyarrhythmia itself (palpitations). If there is coexistent left ventricular dysfunction or coronary artery disease, symptoms of heart failure or of ischemia may occur.

The physical examination is often normal unless the patient is examined during an episode of brady- or tachyarrhythmia in which case the findings will depend on the type of arrhythmia that is present (see below). Sometimes light carotid sinus massage will produce symptomatic bradyarrhythmia in a patient with sick sinus syndrome who is in normal sinus rhythm.

Electrocardiogram

The ECG may be normal or may simply reveal sinus bradycardia. Often, there are varying degrees of sinoatrial block, characterized by varying P-P intervals on the ECG. Sometimes sinus arrest occurs, manifest by absent P waves and associated, usually, with a junctional escape rhythm. Some patients have slow atrial fibrillation reflecting a concomitant AV conduction abnormality (see above). The ECG changes of the various atrial tachyarrhythmias are described below in the discussions of these entities.

If there is a history of unexplained syncope or of palpitations and the resting ECG is normal, ambulatory ECG monitoring is indicated (see above, page 726).

Treatment and Course

The treatment of choice for patients with the sick sinus syndrome who are symptomatic from bradyarrhythmias is permanent pacemaker implantation (see above, page 731). Otherwise symptoms are often progressive. Patients with relatively minor symptoms (e.g., light-headedness or dizziness) often will find that they feel significantly better after pacemaker therapy. Vagolytic drugs (atropine, for example) or β-adrenergic agonists (e.g., isoproterenol) are only of transient benefit.

Tachyarrhythmias associated with the syndrome are often not prevented by electrical pacing. However, pacing does allow the use of such drugs as digitalis and propranolol which depress the sinus node and increase the likelihood of sinus arrest or asystole. It is reasonable, after a pacemaker is implanted, to administer propranolol, 10 mg four times a day, and to increase the dose to 40 mg four times a day in an attempt to prevent tachyarrhythmias. If propranolol is not effective, digoxin should be administered as well. If tachyarrhythmias continue, consideration should be given, in conjunction with the consulting cardiologist, to the use of an antiarrhythmic drug (see above).

Patients with sick sinus syndrome have an incidence, unaffected by pacemaker therapy, of arterial embolization of approximately 10%/year (8). However there is no evidence yet to support the use of anticoagulant or antiplatelet drugs (aspirin or persantine) in this condition.

A high mortality rate is associated with the sick sinus syndrome in elderly people, usually because of coexistent atherosclerotic vascular disease (2, 26). Nearly half of patients over the age of 60 die within 2 years of pacemaker implantation (26).

Premature Atrial and Junctional Contractions

Definition and Etiology

Premature atrial and junctional contractions (PACs and PJCs) are commonly seen in patients who are otherwise well. They often are induced by the same stimuli that produces sinus tachycardia, especially caffeine or nicotine. However, in patients with congestive heart failure or chronic pulmonary disease PACs or PJCs may progress to atrial fibrillation or flutter.

Symptoms and Signs

Usually patients are unaware of premature atrial or junctional contractions. Occasionally they will note the PAC or PJC as a palpitation; and the physician, on listening to the heart or palpating the arterial pulse, will be aware of a slight irregularity in the cardiac rhythm.

Electrocardiogram

Premature atrial contractions are reflected in the ECG by a premature morphologically abnormal P wave followed by a premature morphologically normal QRS complex. Often these impulses are not conducted (Fig. 59.5) in which case, if the P wave is buried in the preceding T wave, a false diagnosis of sinus arrest may be made. At other times the premature impulse may be aberrantly conducted, the result of relative refractoriness of one of the bundle branches (usually a right bundle branch pattern is seen following the premature atrial beat).

Premature junctional contractions are reflected in the ECG by a retrograde P wave (negatively deflected in leads II, III, and aVf) which may follow, be hidden in, or precede a morphologically normal but premature QRS complex.

Treatment

Patients with premature contractions who are otherwise well do not require treatment.

Rarely, it may be necessary to prescribe digoxin or propranolol to reduce the frequency of PACs or to prevent their conduction to the ventricles in patients who have annoyingly frequent palpitations. In patients with underlying cardiac or pulmonary disease, digitalization may prevent the progression of PACs to atrial fibrillation. Quinidine or procainamide is also effective in the control of PACs, but the risk associated with the use of these drugs usually is not warranted (see above, pages 728–729).

Paroxysmal Supraventricular Tachycardia

Definition and Etiology

Supraventricular tachycardias (SVTs) are rapid heart rates (120 to 220 beats/minute) triggered by a premature impulse generated anywhere between the sinus node and the AV junction. Most of these arrhythmias are due to re-entry (see page 725)— usually in the AV node, occasionally through an accessory pathway or in the atria. Less often they are initiated by an ectopic atrial pacemaker.

About half the time, patients with SVTs have an otherwise normal heart (14). The common forms of heart disease associated with SVT are the pre-excitation syndrome (see below, page 745), mitral valve prolapse (see Chapter 60), and atrial septal defect (see Chapter 60). Nonparoxysmal atrial tachycardia with block (due to gradually accelerated automaticity of an ectopic atrial focus) is a common manifestation of digitalis toxicity.

Symptoms and Signs

Patients are almost always aware of a suddenly rapid heart rate; usually there are no other symptoms, but if there is coexistent heart disease, patients may complain of shortness of breath or of ischemic

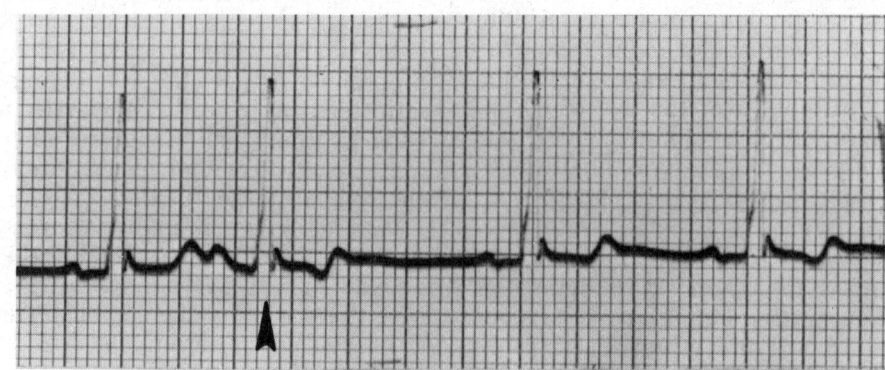

Figure 59.5. A premature atrial contraction (*arrow*). Note the normal configuration of the premature QRS complex.

chest pain. Often the patient will be able to terminate the arrhythmia abruptly by a Valsalva maneuver or by coughing. Frequently, polyuria will be experienced for as long as the arrhythmia lasts.

Attacks often occur spontaneously but may be precipitated by physical or emotional stress, caffeine, or nicotine. They may be as short as a few seconds and as long as several weeks. The frequency of the attacks is also quite variable; some people have attacks every day; some, only a few times during their entire life.

On examination, the physician will note a rapid regular arterial pulse and heart rate—often faster than that measured in patients with sinus tachycardia and usually not associated with the same stimuli. When the atria and ventricles contract simultaneously, cannon waves will be seen in the jugular veins.

Electrocardiogram

Paroxysmal SVT is characterized by a rapid regular heart rate. There is a fixed relationship of the P wave to the QRS complex. If the impulse is generated in the AV node, the P wave may be buried in the QRS complex but the process can be identified by the normal appearance of the QRS complex and by the regularity of the rate. When the P wave is visible, it may follow the QRS complex (some nodal re-entry rhythms, all accessory pathway re-entry rhythms) and will be inverted in leads II, III, and aVf. It may also precede the QRS complex and may appear morphologically normal (atrial re-entry or ectopic rhythm), in which case the diagnosis can only be made (by ECG) if the rate is high enough to make sinus tachycardia unlikely. The P wave also may be hidden in the T wave; but, again, the regularity of the rate and the usually normal duration of the QRS complex establish the diagnosis.

If SVT occurs in association with an AV conduction abnormality, the ventricular rate will be slower than the atrial rate. The arrhythmia can be diagnosed by the rapid regular atrial rate. Various degrees of block may occur (see below)—for example, 2:1 AV block in which the atrial rate is twice the ventricular rate (Fig 59.6).

Sometimes in patients with SVT there are coexistent bundle branch or intraventricular conduction abnormalities, and prolonged abnormal QRS complexes may occur. If P waves are not visible, the only way to distinguish this arrhythmia from ventricular tachycardia is by comparison with an ECG taken when the rate was slow (in which the abnormal QRS complexes will still be seen) and by the regularity and rate (ventricular rates greater than 160 beats/minute are unlikely to represent ventricular tachycardia). If SVT occurs in a patient with an accessory AV conduction pathway (see below), conduction may be aberrant and it may not be possible with a surface ECG to distinguish the arrhythmia from ventricular tachycardia. If there is any ques-

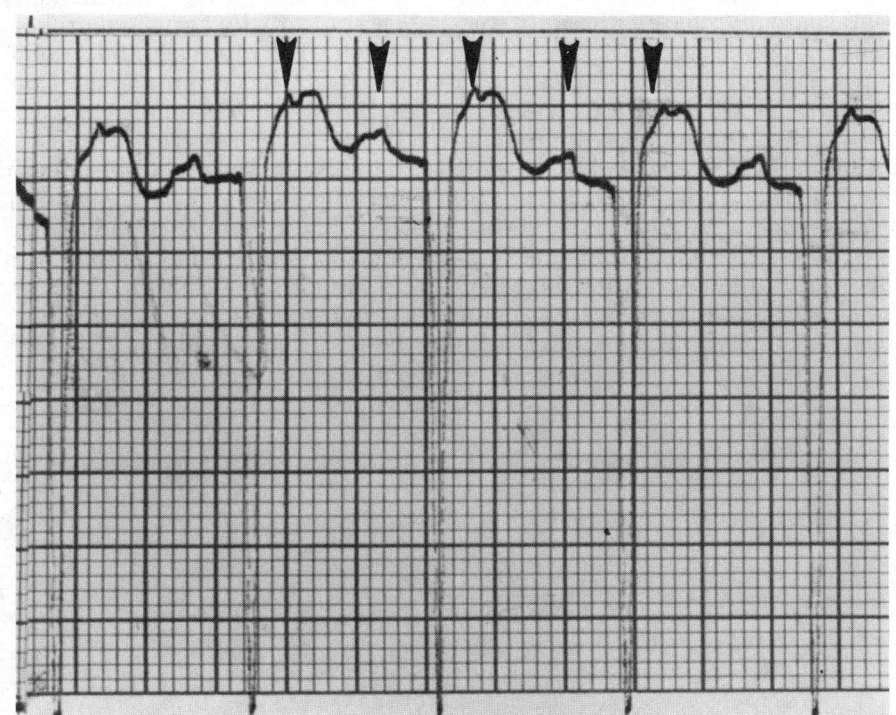

Figure 59.6.   Supraventricular tachycardia with 2:1 AV block. The *arrows* point to consecutive P waves.

tion about which of these diagnoses is correct, urgent consultation with a cardiologist is in order.

Treatment and Course

Therapy of paroxysmal SVT always starts with attempts to increase vagal tone. As mentioned above (see "Symptoms and Signs") the patient often has learned to do this himself. If the arrhythmia persists despite the patient's efforts, the physician should first apply carotid sinus massage. This must be done after auscultation of the carotid arteries to ensure that there are no bruits; if there are, carotid sinus massage is contraindicated. The carotid sinus is at the point of maximum impulse of the carotid artery in the neck. The right sinus should be massaged first for up to 20 seconds; if that has no effect, the left sinus should be massaged; the two sinuses should never be massaged simultaneously. During massage, the patient's ECG should be monitored continuously, and resuscitation equipment should be available.

If carotid sinus massage fails, pharmacological therapy is indicated. This is best done in an emergency room or in a similar facility. If that is not logistically possible, the drug of choice is verapamil, 5 to 10 mg intravenously; it usually converts the arrhythmia to normal sinus rhythm within 5 minutes. If, after administration of verapamil, SVT persists, propranolol (1 mg intravenously every 5 minutes until conversion occurs or until 0.1 mg/kg has been given), digoxin (0.5 mg intravenously), or phenylephrine (0.5 to 1.5 mg intravenously) may be given. One of these drugs is usually successful; rarely electrical cardioversion is necessary.

Chronic administration of digoxin, verapamil, or a β-blocker (see above) is indicated for prevention of recurrent attacks of SVT in patients with frequent symptomatic episodes. Digoxin is probably the drug of choice in otherwise healthy individuals (because it need be taken only once a day and is inexpensive) and in patients with heart failure. Verapamil or β-blockers may be useful in patients with hypertension or with hypertrophic cardiomyopathy. If the attacks recur despite prophylaxis, cardiology con-

sultation is again indicated for advice about the use of antiarrhythmic agents and for possible diagnostic electrical pacing with intracardiac ECG to determine the precise nature of the arrhythmia and the regimen most likely to prevent it.

The *course* of patients with SVT is dependent on its cause. If the arrhythmia occurs in patients who are otherwise healthy, there is no morbidity between attacks and essentially no effect on survival. If it occurs in patients with underlying cardiac or pulmonary disease, there is a real but undefined risk of heart failure, myocardial ischemia, or sudden death during an episode. Otherwise, survival is dependent on the nature and severity of the underlying disease.

If SVT occurs in association with an AV conduction abnormality (commonly 2:1 block), and the patient is taking digitalis, the drug should be withheld and serum potassium concentration should be measured. If the patient is hypokalemic, potassium repletion is, of course, in order; usually this can be accomplished by administration of oral potassium salts (*i.e.*, 20 mEq three times a day—see Chapter 45). Patients with refractory digitoxic arrhythmias with block should be hospitalized for more aggressive treatment. If SVT with atrioventricular block is not due to digitoxicity, it should be treated in the same way as SVT without block.

Multifocal Atrial Tachycardia

Multifocal atrial tachycardia is a chaotic supraventricular arrhythmia characterized electrocardiographically by varying morphology of the P waves, varying P-R intervals, and a rapid heart rate, usually 100 to 200 beats/minute; QRS morphology is normal and every QRS complex is preceded by a P wave (Fig. 59.7). The arrhythmia is usually seen in patients with serious underlying disease, especially decompensated chronic obstructive pulmonary disease, and is better treated by, for example, improving ventilatory function than by attempting directly to suppress the rhythm. Digitalis will not alter this arrhythmia (which is usually well tolerated) and therefore should not be administered.

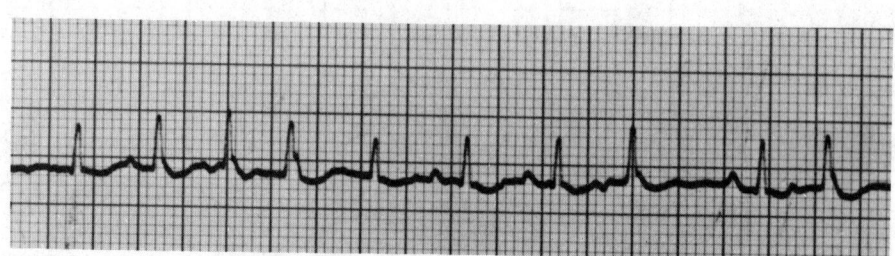

Figure 59.7. Multifocal atrial tachycardia. Note the variation in the morphology of the P waves and in the duration of the P-R intervals.

Atrial Fibrillation

Definition and Etiology

Atrial fibrillation is defined electrophysiologically as rapid uncoordinated generation of electrical impulses by the atria. It is usually triggered by a premature atrial contraction (see above) which, by reentry, generates multifocal impulses at a rate of 300 to 500/minute. These impulses enter the AV node randomly; and, because of the slower rate of conduction of the AV node, not all of them are conducted. Therefore, the ventricular rate is slower than the atrial rate and is irregular. In untreated patients with normal AV conduction the ventricular rate is between 150 and 200 beats/minute.

Atrial fibrillation may occur paroxysmally in people, even in young adults, who have no other evidence of heart disease. In such cases it often is associated with the same stimuli that produce other atrial arrhythmias (sinus tachycardia, premature atrial contractions, paroxysmal supraventricular tachycardia): physical or emotional stress, alcohol, nicotine, or caffeine. The major noncardiac illness associated with atrial fibrillation is hyperthyroidism; and in the presence of a fast ventricular response refractory to digitalis, atrial fibrillation may be the first clue to the diagnosis.

There are many forms of heart disease that predispose to the development of atrial fibrillation; the commonest are hypertensive, atherosclerotic, and rheumatic (especially when it involves the mitral valve), but almost every kind of myocardial disorder has been associated with it. Also, the tachyarrhythmic component of the sick sinus syndrome (see above) may be atrial fibrillation.

Symptoms and Signs

The most common symptoms of atrial fibrillation are palpitations and fatigue. If the ventricular response is fast (as it often is at onset of arrhythmia), patients often complain of feeling "strange," weak, or faint as well. Since atrial contraction normally provides 20% of the total cardiac output, patients with incipient heart failure, ischemic heart disease, or valvular heart disease may develop symptoms (and signs) of those disorders (especially on exertion) when cardiac output is reduced as the result of atrial fibrillation.

Atrial fibrillation is characterized by an irregularly irregular heartbeat and pulse with variation in intensity of the sounds (including murmurs) on both auscultation and palpation. It is prudent to look for signs of diseases known to be associated with atrial fibrillation (e.g., hypertension, mitral stenosis, and hyperthyroidism)—especially since those signs may be subtle or altered by the arrhythmia.

Electrocardiogram

The ECG shows rapid irregular fibrillatory atrial activity at rates between 300 and 500/minute; no P waves are present. The ventricular rhythm is irregularly irregular, at rates which at onset are usually between 150 and 200/minute—unless there is coexistent disease in the AV node, in which case slower rates are likely (Fig. 59.8).

The QRS complex is usually morphologically normal. Occasionally there is aberrant conduction of an impulse in the ventricles, following a beat that has been preceded by a long pause. The aberrant beat usually has a right bundle branch block configuration. This so-called Ashman phenomenon is due to prolonged refractoriness of the (usually) right bundle branch after the long pause. It is important to distinguish these aberrant beats from ventricular premature beats. Apart from their typical relationship to a preceding long R-R interval, aberrant beats are often triphasic (RSR') and their initial vector is the same as that of the normally conducted beats; neither of these features is characteristic of ventricular premature beats.

Treatment and Course

The approach to the treatment of atrial fibrillation should always include a search for underlying or

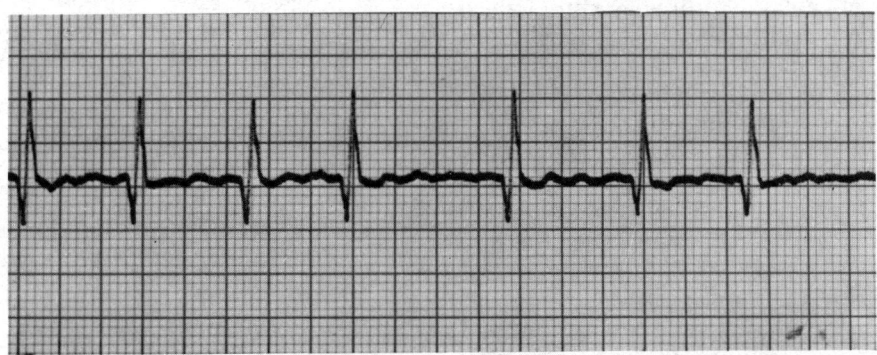

Figure 59.8. Atrial fibrillation. The ventricular rate is 90 to 100 beats/minute, indicative (since digitalis had not been administered) of an associated disorder of atrioventricular conduction.

precipitating factors. Treatment of the arrhythmia has two objectives: to slow the ventricular rate if it is fast and to convert the patient to sinus rhythm if possible.

Paroxysmal atrial fibrillation in a patient who does not have underlying heart disease often will revert to normal sinus rhythm once precipitating factors (e.g., stress, alcohol, nicotine) are removed. Specific treatment is indicated in the following circumstances: a rapid ventricular response associated with symptoms (e.g., extreme fatigue, syncope, angina, or shortness of breath); the presence of known underlying severe heart disease (e.g., aortic stenosis, severe mitral stenosis, ischemic heart disease, chronic congestive failure)—these patients are unlikely to revert to normal sinus rhythm spontaneously; persistent atrial fibrillation—especially if the resting ventricular rate is greater than 110 beats/minute or if the rate after moderate exercise (climbing a flight of stairs, for example) is greater than 150 beats/minute.

Symptomatic patients and patients with underlying severe heart disease are best admitted immediately after onset of the arrhythmia to the hospital for cardioversion or for pharmacotherapy. Patients with persistent atrial fibrillation of less than 6 months' duration, particularly if there is no left atrial enlargement, should be hospitalized for elective cardioversion. Patients with atrial fibrillation that has lasted longer than 6 months or patients with large left atria are likely to be refractory to cardioversion. In general, cardioversion restores normal sinus rhythm in approximately 90% of patients but the relapse rate is high—50% in 1 year and 90% in 3 years (13)—unless the underlying disorder can be corrected or atrial fibrillation has been of short duration.

Asymptomatic or mildly symptomatic patients who have a rapid ventricular response should be treated with digitalis with a goal of a resting ventricular rate between 60 and 90 beats/minute and a rate after modest exercise of below 150 beats/minute. A loading dose by mouth of 0.75 to 1.0 mg of digoxin followed by 0.25 mg a day is ordinariy sufficient. If rapid digitalization is desired, it is best to hospitalize the patient and to administer intravenous digoxin. Approximately 20% of patients will convert to normal sinus rhythm after receiving digitalis.

If digitalization slows the rate but the ventricular response is still too high, verapamil, 80 mg three to four times a day, or small doses of propranolol (10 to 20 mg four times a day) will often lower the rate further (see above, pages 730–731, for a general discussion of the use of these drugs).

Patients who cannot or will not be cardioverted should receive an antiarrhythmic drug after they are digitalized (quinidine is ordinarily the first choice and will cause a return to normal sinus rhythm in about one-third of patients).

If the ventricular response is slow in untreated patients, there is an associated disorder of AV conduction. Such patients do not require specific therapy for the arrhythmia unless they are hemodynamically compromised (i.e., in refractory heart failure) and their heart rate is under 60 to 70 beats/minute, in which case implantation of a pacemaker may be indicated.

Patients with atrial fibrillation are at increased risk of arterial embolization, especially if they have mitral stenosis and/or large left atria. For example, the Framingham study reported that, over a 24-year period, patients with chronic atrial fibrillation with and without rheumatic heart disease had a 17- and 5-fold increase, respectively, in the incidence of stroke (27). Overall the incidence of arterial embolization in patients with chronic atrial fibrillation is about 10% a year (8). It is the practice to give all patients the anticoagulant warfarin before elective cardioversion (see above, page 731), and, although there are no good studies to support it, many physicians routinely treat with anticoagulants any patient with chronic atrial fibrillation if there are no contraindications. It seems reasonable to recommend anticoagulation for all patients who have had even one episode of arterial embolization as well as for patients with mitral stenosis or those who have paroxysmal atrial fibrillation as part of the sick sinus syndrome (see above, page 733).

Apart from the morbidity and mortality associated with atrial embolization, the *prognosis* of patients with atrial fibrillation depends on whether there is underlying heart disease and, if there is, what the nature of it is.

Atrial Flutter

Definition and Etiology

Atrial flutter is a relatively coordinated rapid atrial activity due to re-entry of premature atrial impulses. Atrial beats are generated at about 300/minute. Usually there is a 2:1 AV conduction block so that the ventricular response is abut 150/minute and, unlike atrial fibrillation, both atrial and ventricular responses are regular. Atrial flutter is almost always seen in patients who have underlying disease: ischemic heart disease, rheumatic heart disease, congestive cardiomyopathy, atrial septal defect, mitral valve disease, chronic obstructive pulmonary disease, and thyrotoxicosis—the same diseases often associated with atrial fibrillation. In contrast to atrial fibrillation, however, atrial flutter is not often seen in patients who are otherwise healthy.

Symptoms and Signs

Patients are usually aware of a rapid heart rate; whether or not other symptoms develop depends on the severity and nature of the underlying heart disease.

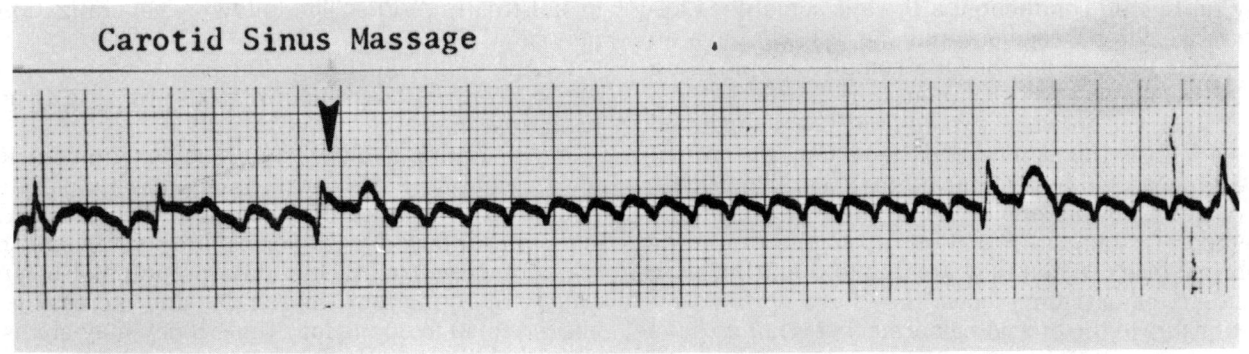

Figure 59.9. Atrial flutter. The flutter waves are clearly revealed after carotid sinus massage (*arrow*).

A regular rapid heart rate and atrial pulse are detected. Sometimes the flutter waves are visible in the jugular pulse. An S_4 is occasionally audible (in distinction to atrial fibrillation).

Electrocardiogram

The ECG shows rapid regular sawtooth flutter waves at about 300/minute (Fig. 59.9); P waves are absent. The ventricular response is regular, usually at about 150/minute and the QRS complex is ordinarily morphologically normal. If the AV node is diseased, higher degrees of AV block may be seen—usually a multiple of 2 (4:1, 8:1, *etc*). Aberrant conduction (see "Atrial Fibrillation") is unusual.

If the diagnosis is unclear, carotid sinus massage may help to distinguish atrial flutter from other paroxysmal supraventricular tachyarrhythmias. It usually causes an abrupt temporary slowing of the rate; and flutter waves, which may have been difficult to detect at a higher rate, will be visible in the electrocardiogram, most commonly in leads II, III, aVf, and V_1.

Treatment and Course

Atrial flutter is an unstable rhythm and usually converts spontaneously to normal sinus rhythm or to atrial fibrillation. Because the rhythm is unstable and because patients usually have underlying heart disease, they are best hospitalized for observation and treatment. Unlike the situation in patients with atrial fibrillation, it is often difficult to lower the ventricular rate with digitalis in patients with atrial flutter. Nevertheless, digitalization is reasonable—especially if hospitalization must be delayed—since some patients will convert to normal sinus rhythm by administration of digoxin alone.

If there is no contraindication, however, electrical cardioversion is the treatment of choice if atrial flutter persists, even if there is a high degree of AV block. Almost every patient can be converted to normal sinus rhythm, usually after application of a much lower current than is necessary to convert atrial fibrillation.

Digitalis (*i.e.*, digoxin, 0.25 mg a day) should be administered to prevent recurrences of atrial flutter. If digitalis is not effective alone, propranolol, 20 to 40 mg every 6 hours, or quinidine, 200 to 300 mg every 6 hours, should also be prescribed. All of these drugs are much more effective in preventing recurrence of flutter than they are in converting it to normal sinus rhythm.

Ventricular Premature Beats

Definition and Etiology

Ventricular premature beats (VPBs) are impulses generated in the ventricles, usually as the result of re-entry of an impulse conducted down from the atria through the AV node, but sometimes as the result of the firing of an ectopic (parasystolic) focus.

Occasional VPBs occur in many healthy people sporadically during their life, more frequently in older people. However, often VPBs are associated with underlying organic heart disease, e.g., ischemic heart disease, cardiomyopathy, or mitral valve prolapse. The frequency of VPBs may be increased in people both with and without heart disease by caffeine, alcohol, sympathomimetic drugs, tricyclic antidepressants, phenothiazines, hypokalemia, hypoxia, and excitement. VPBs are a common manifestation of digitoxicity. Exercise usually abolishes ventricular patient activity in normal people; an increase in the number of VPBs after exertion is highly suggestive of underlying heart disease.

Symptoms and Signs

Patients may not be aware that they have had a VPB, but often they experience a palpitation—either sensing the premature beat itself or the more forceful normal beat that follows it after a compensatory pause.

Electrocardiogram

The ECG shows a premature ventricular response with a morphologically abnormal, often bizarre, wide QRS complex. No P wave precedes a VPB but, by retrograde conduction, a P wave sometimes follows it. The ST segment and the T wave have an opposite vector from the QRS complex. Typically, a VPB is followed by a compensatory pause, *i.e.*, the R-R interval between two normal beats separated by a VPB is the same as that between two normal beats separated by another normal beat (Fig. 59.10).

When VPBs are due to re-entry, they have a fixed temporal ("coupled") relationship to the preceding normal beats. When they are due to the firing of an ectopic (parasystolic) focus, they have no fixed relationship to the preceding normal beats but do have a regular pattern (*i.e.*, the ectopic intervals are constant or are multiples of a constant). Ectopic beats may occasionally fuse with normal beats, producing a complex that is intermediate between the two (Fig. 59.11).

Treatment and Course

Ventricular premature beats in patients with otherwise normal hearts are not harmful. However, there is an increased incidence of sudden death and of myocardial infarction in patients with VPBs who have underlying ischemic heart disease (15). It has not been demonstrated that suppression of VPBs in these latter patients alters their course (9). Since all antiarrhyhmic agents have potentially serious side effects (see above, page 728), the physician must consider for each patient the relative risks of treating

or not treating VPBs. The following generalizations may be useful:

1. Apparently healthy young people with asymptomatic ventricular premature beats probably do not need treatment.

2. Apparently healthy young people with ventricular premature beats causing symptomatic palpitations also probably do not need to be treated. If symptoms interfere with normal life style in spite of reassurance, a trial of low dose propranolol beginning with 10 mg four times a day and increasing if needed to 40 to 80 mg four times a day may abolish VPBs and relieve symptoms. Propranolol commonly produces a sensation of sluggishness in young people, and often they will not continue the medication. In that case, atenolol (Tenormin)—a long acting β-blocker, 50 mg every morning, will often give symptomatic relief with good compliance.

3. Patients with known ischemic heart disease and symptomatic ventricular arrhythmias, especially symptomatic multiformed premature ventricular beats, should be treated. A history of recurrent ventricular tachycardia or ventricular fibrillation is always an indication for chronic antiarrhythmic therapy. Quinidine remains the drug of choice in initial doses of 200 mg four times a day. The dose should be titrated to serum levels of 3 to 7 μg/ml just before the next dose (the level should be measured every 3 or 4 days until the desired concentra-

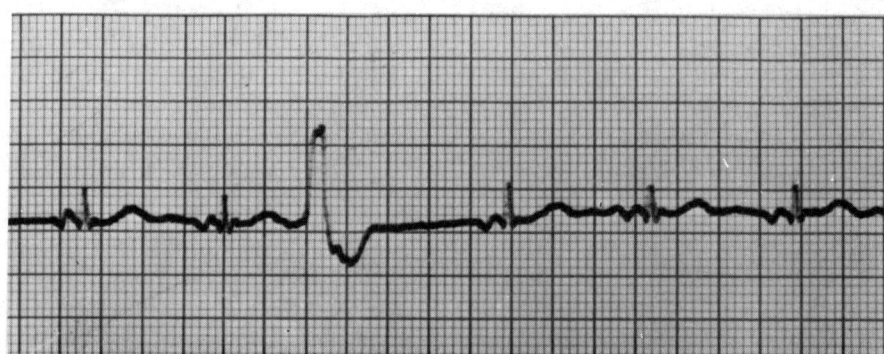

Figure 59.10.   Premature ventricular beat. Note that the R-R interval between the two normal beats separated by the PVB is the same as that between two normal beats separated by another normal beat.

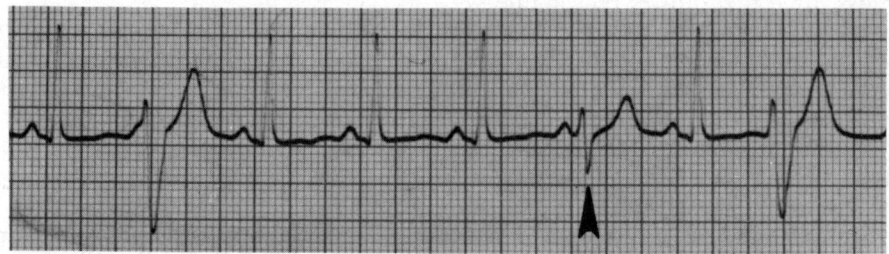

Figure 59.11.   Premature ventricular beats due to the firing of an ectopic focus. The *arrow* points to a fusion beat.

tion is attained). In patients who do not tolerate quinidine, sustained-release procainamide (Procan-SR), 500 to 750 mg every 6 hours, should be tried. The efficacy of the antiarrhythmic therapy should be assessed by an ambulatory ECG (see above, page 726).

4. When ventricular arrhythmias occur in the setting of congestive heart failure, an attempt should be made to achieve a maximal state of cardiac compensation before instituting antiarrhythmic therapy. Hemodynamic compensation may decrease or eliminate ventricular premature beats so that specific antiarrhythmic therapy is not needed. Disopyramide is a myocardial depressant and is specifically contraindicated in patients whose hearts are enlarged and hypocontractile. Furthermore, patients in severe chronic heart failure are more likely to experience problems such as hypokalemia, alkalosis, hypoxemia, and digitalis toxicity, thus increasing the risk of serious side effects from antiarrhythmic agents.

5. Patients with recurrent symptomatic VPBs, recurrent ventricular tachycardia, or ventricular fibrillation may be best managed with a drug regimen which is selected using intracardiac electrophysiological techniques to assess the response to the drugs. This approach requires hospitalization and consultation with a cardiologist.

6. If VPBs have been suppressed for a year and if patients are asymptomatic, it is reasonable to discontinue antiarrhythmic therapy and to obtain an ambulatory ECG 1 week later. If the arrhythmia does not recur, the therapy need not be reinstituted. However, this issue is controversial and consultation with a cardiologist may be advisable prior to the stopping of the therapy.

Heart Block

Heart block, a delay or failure of conduction of the cardiac impulse, is categorized electrocardiographically.

Right Bundle Branch Block (RBBB) (Fig. 59.12)

A delay or block of conduction through the right bundle branch causes a modest prolongation of the QRS complex (> 0.12 second). The initial QRS vector is unaffected since this is accounted for largely by left ventricular depolarization. The right ventricle is activated by a spread of the action potential from the left ventricle, which is seen best in leads I and V_6 where the S waves are wide and slurred and in V_1 where there is a double peak (R-R') of the R wave. RBBB is sometimes seen in the ECGs of patients who have otherwise normal hearts. More often it is associated with an underlying congenital or acquired disorder, e.g., interatrial septal defect and hypertensive or ischemic heart disease. Patients with newly acquired RBBB have an increased risk of cardiovascular morbidity and death from cardiovascular disease (21).

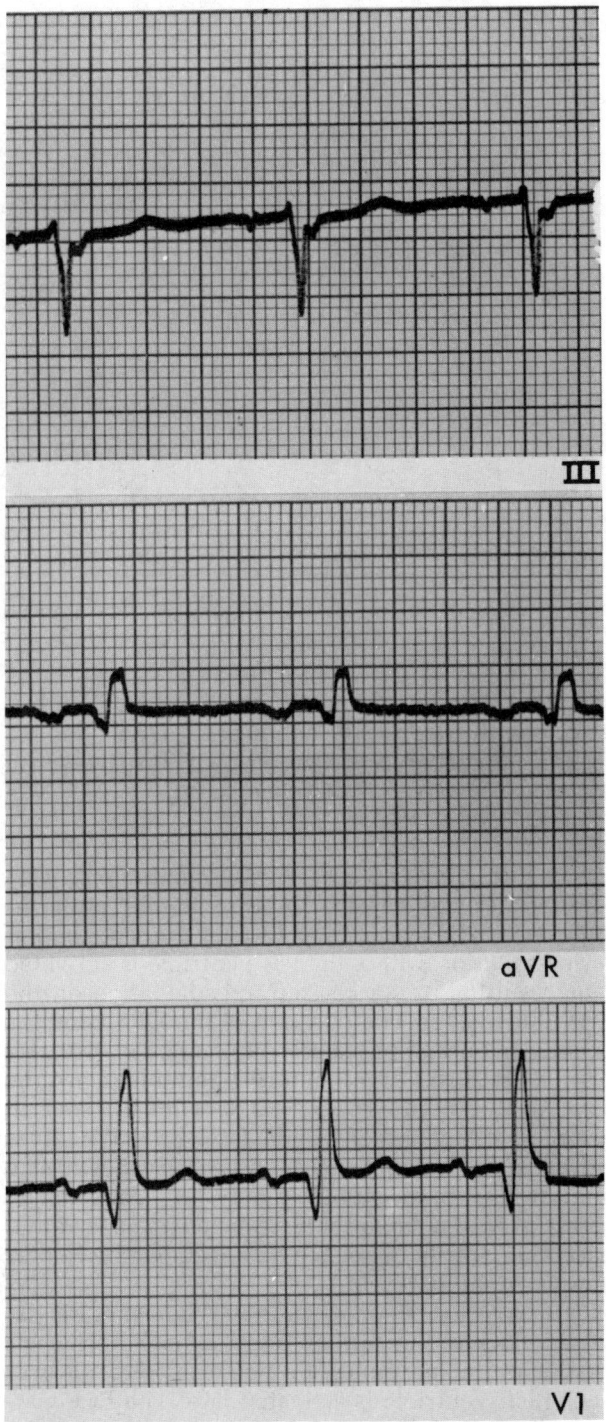

Figure 59.12.   Right bundle branch block and left anterior hemiblock (bifascicular block).

Left Bundle Branch Block (LBBB) (Fig. 59.13)

A delay or block of conduction through the left bundle branch causes a marked prolongation of the QRS complex (0.14 to 0.16 second). The entire sequence of ventricular depolarization is affected so that the QRS complex is widened and the QRS axis is directed to the left and posteriorly. Abnormal

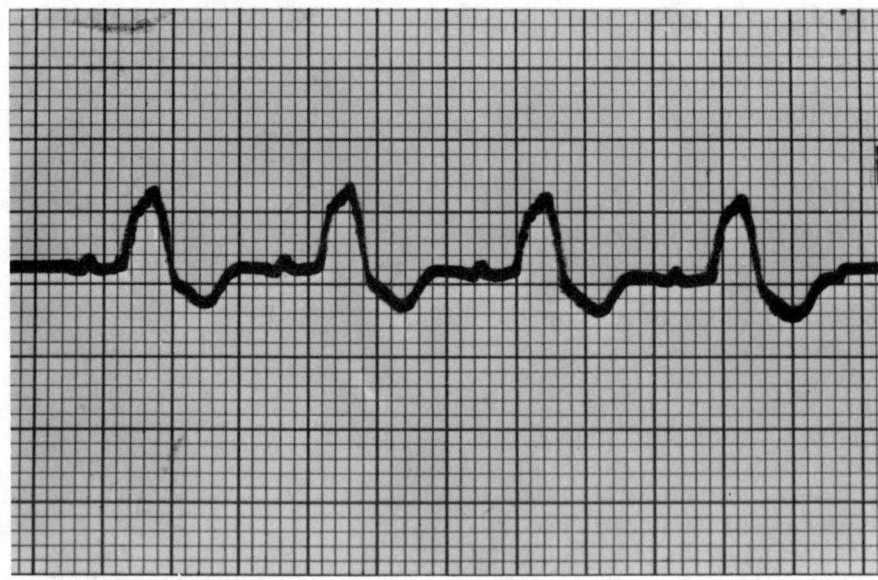

Figure 59.13.   Left bundle branch block.

repolarization is reflected in the T wave, which is always in the opposite direction of the QRS complex.

LBBB almost always signifies heart disease—usually degenerative disease or ischemia.

Hemiblocks

Left anterior hemiblock (LAH). When there is delay or block of the cardiac impulse in the anterior-superior portion of the left bundle branch, the anterior-superior wall of the left ventricle is activated late, resulting in marked left axis deviation on the ECG (Fig. 59.12). The duration of the QRS complex is usually normal or slightly prolonged (< 0.10 second). The causes of left anterior hemiblock are the same as those of LBBB. LAH is occasionally seen in patients with no discernible heart disease. Whatever the cause, LAH is not in itself a poor prognostic sign and, at least in an ambulatory setting, requires no specific therapy (in hospital, some physicians would pace temporarily patients who developed LAH after a myocardial infarction).

Left posterior hemiblock (LPH). When there is delay or block of the cardiac impulse in the posterior portion of the left bundle branch, the posterior wall of the left ventricle is activated late. The ECG pattern of LPH is characterized by marked right axis deviation (> +110°). The causes of LPH are the same as those of LAH and LBBB. Because the posterior portion of the left bundle branch is larger and better perfused than is the anterior-superior portion, LPH is less common than is LAH and usually indicates more extensive left ventricular disease.

Bifascicular Block

Right bundle branch block with LAH (manifest by a RBBB pattern and left axis deviation—Fig. 59.12)
or RBBB with LPH (manifest by a RBBB pattern and right axis deviation) indicates that only one pathway remains to maintain passage of the cardiac impulse from the atria to the ventricles. If bifascicular block is detected in an ambulatory setting, especially if there is a history of syncope or of light-headedness, a cardiologist should be asked to advise whether electrophysiological studies (page 726) and/or pacemaker implantation is indicated. The risk that unselected patients with bifascicular block will develop complete heart block is 5 to 6% a year (18). There is conflicting evidence, however, about the course of patients, generally, with bifascicular block; some report no increased morbidity (17); others, a considerably shortened survival (6, 7). Although there is not a consensus about how to deal with the problem, the prognosis seems to be related to the extent of the underlying disease.

First Degree Heart Block

Definition and etiology. The P-R interval normally varies with heart rate, but should not exceed 0.21 second in people in normal sinus rhythm. First degree AV block is defined as a prolonged P-R interval. The block may be due to a prolongation of conduction in any of the structures between the SA node and the bundle of His. Most commonly, when the QRS duration is normal, a long P-R interval is due to a delay in conduction in the AV node. When first degree block coincides with left bundle branch block, it is likely that there is a delay in conduction in the His bundle. A prolonged P-R interval with right bundle branch block may be due to a block in the AV node or in the bundle of His.

A prolongation of the P-R interval is usually due to degenerative, ischemic, or inflammatory changes in the AV conduction systems. It is commonly seen in older people without other evidence of heart disease, in patients who have had an inferior wall myocardial infarction, or in association with myocarditis (including acute rheumatic fever). Drugs, such as digitalis, which affect vagal activity also may produce a first degree AV block.

Symptoms and signs. First degree AV block in itself does not produce symptoms or abnormal physical findings except a first heart sound that is reduced in intensity (see Chapter 60).

Treatment and course. Patients with first degree AV block who are asymptomatic and who have no other evidence of heart disease need not be treated. If patients with first degree block complain of lightheadedness or dizziness, an ambulatory ECG should be obtained (see above, page 726) since some of these patients may have episodic higher degrees of block.

Second Degree AV Block

Definition and etiology. Second degree AV block is present when some but not all P waves are followed by QRS complexes. Second degree AV block is due to conduction delay or block either in the AV node or in the conduction system below the AV node. The site of the block has important therapeutic implications (see below).

Mobitz-I or Wenckebach second degree AV block (Fig. 59.14). Second degree AV block within the AV node results in the Wenckebach phenomenon, characterized by progressive lengthening of the P-R interval for several cycles until the P wave is blocked completely; and the sequence begins again, often with a normal P-R interval in the beat that follows the blocked P wave. In the absence of disease elsewhere in the conducting system, the QRS complex is normal. The "degree of Wenckebach" is characterized by the ratio of the number of P waves to the number of QRS complexes in each cycle of block. In other words, if block occurs after every third P wave, it is called 3:2 Wenckebach.

Since conduction through the AV node is influenced by vagal tone, type I—second degree AV block may be precipitated by anything that increases vagal tone. It therefore is sometimes seen as a transient phenomenon in people with no other evidence of heart disease. Otherwise, it is produced by the same processes that are associated with first degree AV block.

Mobitz-II second degree AV block (Fig. 59.15). Mob-

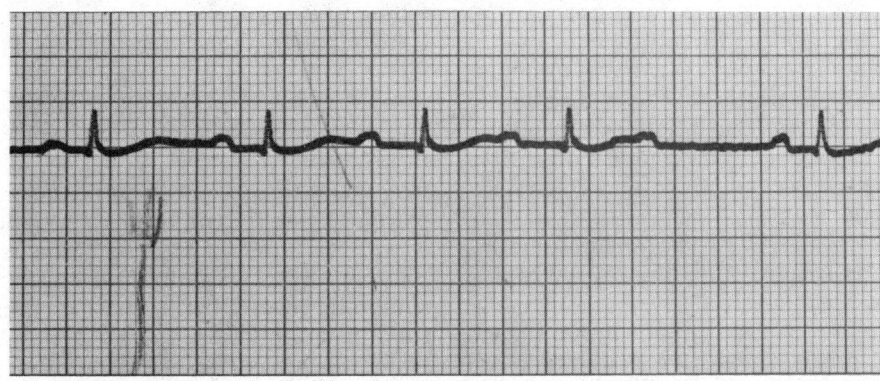

Figure 59.14. Mobitz-I or Wenkebach second degree atrioventricular block.

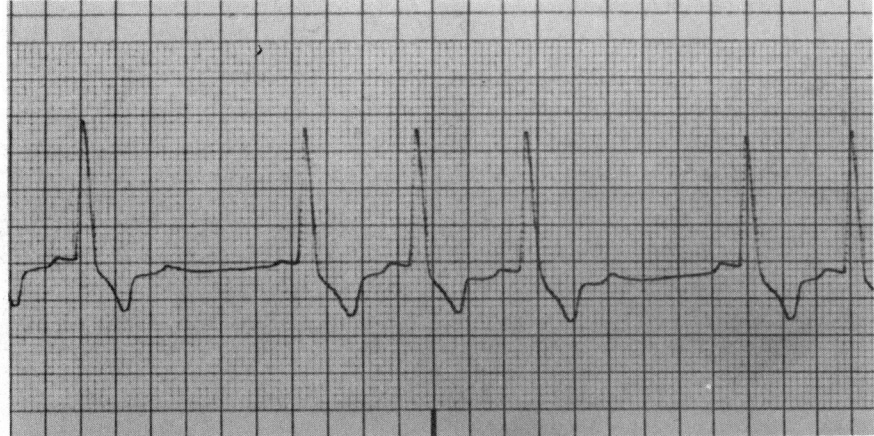

Figure 59.15. Mobitz-II second degree atrioventricular block.

itz-II block is defined as intermittent failure to conduct a P wave due to block below the level of the AV node. The P-R interval of the conducted beat prior to a blocked P wave is usually normal. The block may be intermittent or may occur in a fixed 2:1 or 3:1 ratio. Coexistent bundle branch block is commonly seen. Progression to higher degrees of block or to asystole may occur rapidly.

Vagal influences have little effect on conduction below the AV node so that changes in vagal tone do not influence Mobitz-II block. However, the block may be precipitated by medications such as propranolol, which decrease conduction through the bundle of His. The common causes of Mobitz-II block are degenerative or ischemic changes within the His-Purkinje system.

Symptoms and signs.

MOBITZ-I SECOND DEGREE AV BLOCK. Patients are often asymptomatic but if vagal tone is increased (e.g., by digitalis or propranolol), profound bradycardia may ensue, sometimes with rates below 30/minute. Such patients may complain of light-headedness, syncope, or extreme fatigue.

Physical findings are subtle; irregularity of the heart rhythm and arterial pulse may be noted when a beat is dropped. The first heart sound of the last beat before the dropped beat will be softer than that of the first beat after the pause (because of the variation in P-R interval—see Chapter 60).

MOBITZ-II SECOND DEGREE AV BLOCK. Symptoms and physical findings are similar to those of patients with Mobitz-I block except that they are not influenced by changes in vagal activity and the intensity of the first heart sound is constant.

Treatment and course.

MOBITZ-I SECOND DEGREE AV BLOCK. Asymptomatic patients need not be treated since the risk of rapid progression of the block and of asystole is slight. Symptomatic patients usually have pronounced bradycardia. If so, medications such as digitalis or propranolol, which may be increasing the block, should be discontinued. If such medications are essential to the patient's management, a cardiac pacemaker should be implanted (see page 731).

MOBITZ-II SECOND DEGREE AV BLOCK. Because of the risk of rapid progression of the block and of asystole, all patients, even if asymptomatic, should be treated with a permanent cardiac pacemaker.

Patients with a history of light-headedness or dizziness who have new bundle branch block should be suspected of having had Mobitz-II block. This suspicion often can be confirmed with the use of an ambulatory ECG (page 726). An intracardiac ECG (page 726), if necessary, may also show prolonged conduction through the His bundle. Patients with a known history of coronary artery disease and with new or increased bundle branch blocks who have a clear-cut history of syncope must be thought to have had Mobitz-II block or complete heart block until proven otherwise.

Third Degree (Complete) Heart Block

Definition and etiology. Complete heart block occurs when there is total failure of conduction of impulses from the atria through the AV junction to the bundle of His (or, more rarely, if all three fascicles below the His bundle are diseased). The life of the patient then depends upon the escape of a ventricular pacemaker. A rhythm generated in the upper portion of the His bundle may have a QRS configuration nearly identical to that of normally conducted impulses and will have a rate between 40 and 60 beats/minute (Fig. 59.16). It is more likely to be a stable rhythm than is a rhythm generated by a lower pacemaker. If the pacemaker is located more distally in the conducting system, the ventricular rate decreases; the QRS morphology becomes wider and more bizarre; and the risk of asystole increases. In children or young adults, complete heart block may occur due to congenital defects in development of the AV cushion or of the conduction system itself; escape rhythms are, in such cases, usually generated relatively high in the bundle of His. In older people complete heart block is most commonly due to degenerative and fibrotic changes in the conduction system (5). It is also seen sometimes in association with infiltrative disease of the myocardium (e.g., sarcoid or amyloid), inflammatory processes (e.g., rheumatoid arthritis), and myocardial infections (tuberculosis, syphilis, *etc*) or ischemic heart disease. Occasionally digitalis toxicity may produce complete heart block.

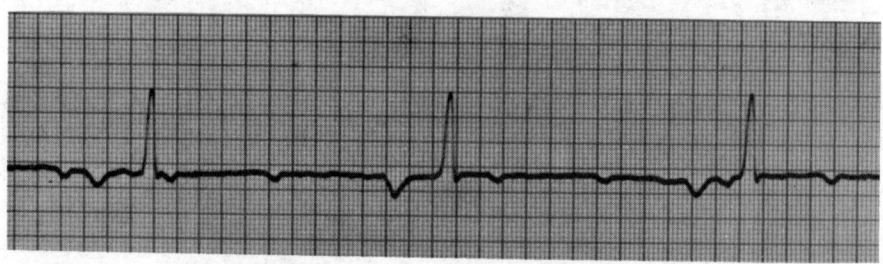

Figure 59.16.   Third degree heart block.

Symptoms and signs. A major symptom of complete heart block is sudden loss of consciousness (a Stokes-Adams attack), the result of asystole or of tachyarrhythmia (ventricular tachycardia or fibrillation). The asystole is due to failure of the ventricular pacemaker; the tachyarrhythmia, to escape of another focus when the idioventricular rate falls too low (a variant of the bradycardia-tachycardia syndrome—see page 733). If the heart begins to pump effectively again within seconds—as it usually does—the patient promptly regains consciousness and is alert and oriented. If perfusion of vital organs is delayed, seizure-like activity (ordinarily not generalized) and even death may ensue. If they are unconscious for more than a few minutes, patients may not become fully alert for some hours.

Complete heart block in patients with underlying myocardial disease may cause symptoms of heart failure (see Chapter 61) primarily because of further reduction in cardiac output as the result of bradycardia.

Physical findings of heart block are all attributable to the dissociation between atrial and ventricular contraction: variation in the intensity of the first heart sound, variation in systolic blood pressure, variation in the intensity of heart murmurs and of third and fourth heart sounds, and the appearance of cannon waves in the jugular pulse. The heart rate, of course, is slow.

Treatment and course. The treatment of complete heart block is permanent pacemaker implantation. The life expectancy of treated patients with complete heart block who have no other evidence of cardiac or systemic disease is excellent and approaches that of their age-matched cohort. Patients with complete heart block due to coronary disease have a prognosis which is determined by the extent of their underlying coronary artery disease and by their myocardial function.

Pre-excitation Syndrome

Definition and Etiology

The atria and ventricles are electrically isolated from each other by the AV groove, and the electrical signal from the atria is conducted to the ventricle *via* the AV node and conducting system. If the AV groove is short circuited by muscle fibers, if muscle fibers from the atria enter the His bundle below the AV node, or if muscle fibers from the His bundle bypass the bundle branches, a variable portion of the right or left ventricle will be depolarized early. These short circuiting fibers are known as accessory atrioventricular, atrionodal, or nodoventricular fibers, depending on their location (Fig. 59.17).

The classic example of pre-excitation is the *Wolff-Parkinson-White (WPW) syndrome* which is due to accessory atrioventricular connections. This syndrome is characterized electrocardiographically by a short P-R interval followed by a wide QRS complex, which is a fusion beat between the area of the ventricle which is pre-excited and the area of the ventricle excited *via* normal conduction pathways (Fig. 59.18). The portion of the complex due to pre-excitation is called the delta wave because of its resemblance to the Greek capital letter Δ. If the accessory bundle connects the atria with the left ventricle, the electrocardiographic pattern resembles right bundle branch block (type A WPW). If, on the other hand, the connection is with the right ventricle, the pattern resembles left bundle branch block (type B WPW); the negative delta wave in lead II in this situation may be taken for a Q wave, and the mistaken diagnosis of remote myocardial infarction may be made.

If the atrial fibers insert into the bundle of His and short circuit the AV node, the P-R interval is short, but no delta wave is seen since below the AV node conduction occurs along the usual pathways. This syndrome is known as the *Lown-Ganong-Levine (LGL) syndrome.* A number of other variants of pre-excitation have been described but are much rarer than these two relatively common disorders (11).

The ECG manifestations of pre-excitation may vary from time to time within a given individual since, if conduction occurs through the normal anatomical pathways, rather than through accessory fibers, no pre-excitation will be seen on the ECG. When pre-excitation is facilitated because of disease in the AV node or because of drugs that suppress conduction through the AV node (e.g., digitalis or propranolol) abnormalities on the ECG will be seen.

Re-entrant supraventricular arrhythmias are common in patients with pre-excitation syndromes (estimates vary from 13% to 60%—usually paroxysmal supraventricular tachycardia, but atrial fibrillation and flutter also occur (3). The morphology of the QRS complex during the tachyarrhythmia will depend on the direction in which the re-entrant tachycardia occurs. If re-entry occurs antegrade through the AV conducting system and retrograde through an accessory pathway, then the QRS duration during the tachyarrhythmia may be normal since the ventricle is depolarized in a normal direction through its normal specialized conducting tissue. If the circuit is established in the opposite direction, the QRS complex will be wide, with a bundle branch block pattern, because most or all of the ventricle will be depolarized by way of the accessory pathway, and the arrhythmia easily can be confused with ventricular tachycardia.

Symptoms and Signs

The pre-excitation syndrome may be an incidental finding on an ECG or it may come to the attention of the physician because of symptoms. Other symptoms of tachyarrhythmia will depend on the nature

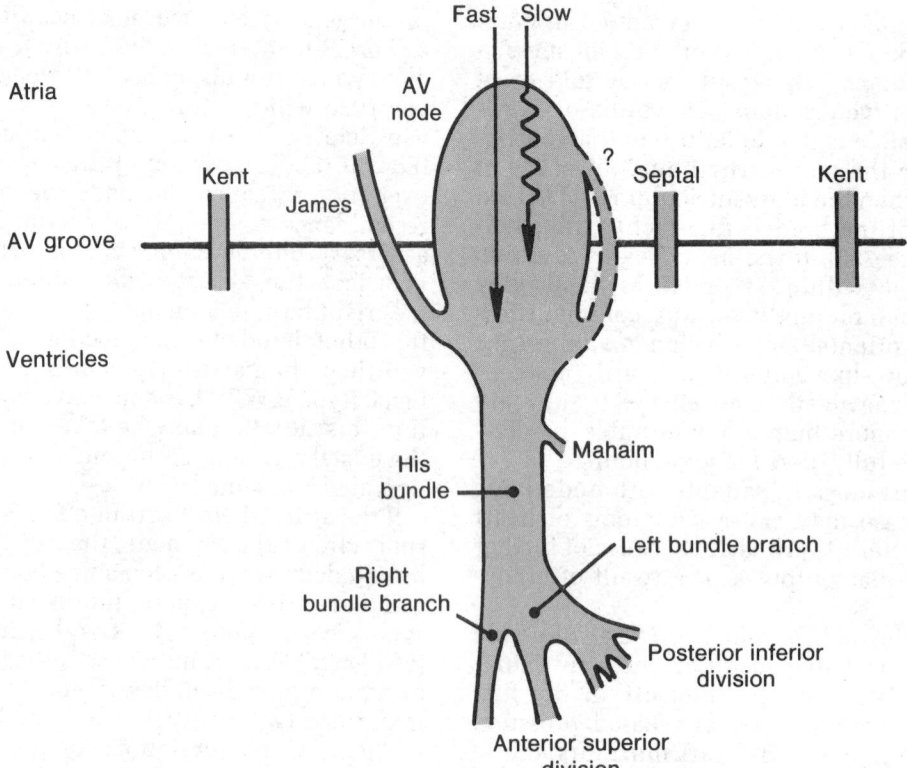

Figure 59.17. Schematic diagram of possible accessory conduction pathways. Accessory atrioventricular (AV) muscle bundles (Kent) are located in either the right or left AV groove or in the septum close to the AV node. Dual AV node pathways are represented by the fast and slow symbols. Accessory nodoventricular muscle bundles or accessory fasciculoventricular bundles (Mahaim) originate in the lower AV node, His bundle, or bundle branches. Atrio-Hisian or atriofascicular bundles (James) insert into the AV node, often the lower AV node. The pathway labeled ? is a hypothetical intranodal bypass which could explain some short P-R syndromes. (From Greene HL: Accessory atrioventricular conduction syndromes: a review. *Johns Hopkins Med J* 139:13, 1976 (11).)

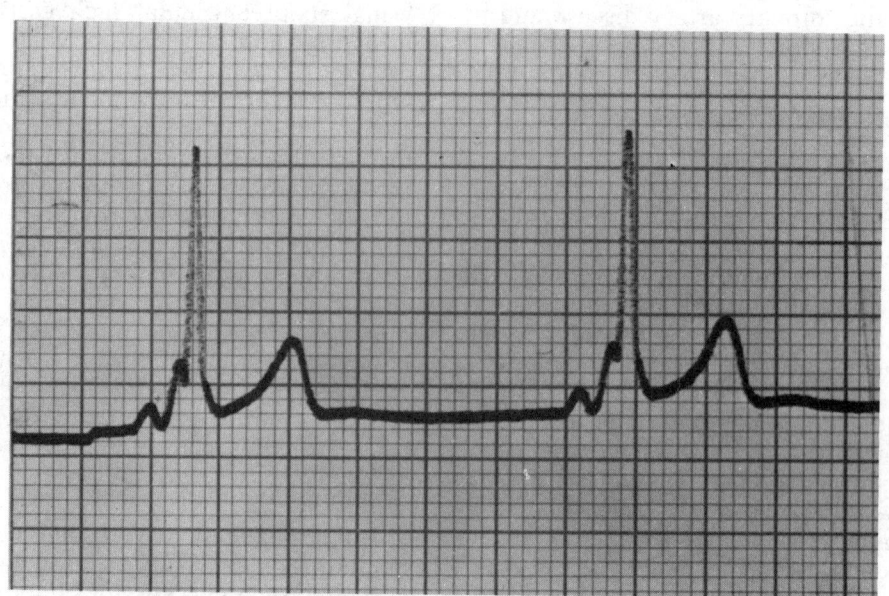

Figure 59.18. The Wolff-Parkinson-White syndrome.

of the arrhythmia and on the presence or absence of underlying heart disease.

There are no physical findings due to pre-excitation other than occasionally a loud S_1, except during periods of tachyarrhythmia; and then the findings depend on the type of arrhythmia that is present.

Prevalence

Pre-excitation syndromes are not rare. The prevalence of pre-excitation is between 1 and 30/1000 people (11). Accurate prevalence rates are difficult to obtain since short P-R intervals with normal QRS durations are commonly seen in people without arrhythmias so that no studies are done to determine whether a bypass tract exists.

Pre-excitation syndromes occasionally may be associated with certain forms of congenital heart disease. Pre-excitation of the WPW type is associated with Ebstein's anomaly of the tricuspid valve, corrected transposition of the great vessels, and hypertrophic cardiomyopathies.

Treatment and Course

Asymptomatic patients need not be treated; their survival is the same as that of the normal population.

Patients with symptomatic supraventricular arrhythmias who, during the arrhythmia, have normal QRS complexes—indicating conduction over the normal pathways—are best treated with propranolol, 10 to 40 mg four times a day. If that approach fails, digitalis is a reasonable alternative (0.25 mg of digoxin/day). Occasionally it will be necessary to administer quinidine or procainamide. The use of these drugs is discussed on pages 728 to 729. Verapamil is not a useful drug for patients with pre-excitation syndromes. It does not directly affect refractoriness of accessory pathways and may reflexly increase conduction through the accessory pathway, thereby increasing the ventricular response in patients in atrial fibrillation.

Patients with symptomatic arrhythmias who, during the arrhythmia have wide QRS complexes, indicating conduction over the accessory pathways, should be hospitalized if possible for treatment with intravenous lidocaine or with quinidine or procainamide. Suppression of arrhythmic attacks thereafter should be attempted first with quinidine and then, if necessary, with procainamide or propranolol. *It is important that the physician be aware that digitalis is contraindicated in this situation.* By increasing the refractoriness of the AV junction, it may enhance conduction through the accessory pathway and induce a dangerously rapid ventricular response.

Patients with frequent arrhythmias, refractory to treatment and to suppression, may be candidates for an operation to transect the accessory pathway—identified during surgery by epicardial mapping. It has been reported that 90% of such operations are successful in preventing further arrhythmia (10), but currently few centers are able to do them.

The *course* of patients with pre-excitation syndromes is unpredictable—some have no or very infrequent arrhythmic attacks; others, despite therapy, have them frequently. Some patients have minimal symptoms during attacks, and others are incapacitated.

The long term survival of patients with pre-excitation who are subject to arrhythmic attacks is related to the severity of the arrhythmia. Patients with occasional palpitations or with easily controlled bouts of paroxysmal ventricular tachycardia are at low risk. Patients with bouts of atrial flutter or fibrillation and a rapid ventricular response are at considerable risk of ventricular fibrillation and of sudden death.

It is important that asymptomatic patients with pre-excitation who wish to engage in strenuous work have stress electrocardiography (Chapter 57 describes the technique and the patient's experience with it). Patients who develop tachyarrhythmias on exercise or have a documented history of tachyarrhythmias should not undertake strenuous exertion.

Long Q-T Interval Syndrome

An inherited syndrome has been described in which delayed repolarization is expressed as a long Q-T interval (>0.45 second). In some families the inheritance is autosomal recessive and is associated with nerve deafness; in others, the inheritance is autosomal dominant and hearing is normal. The long Q-T interval predisposes to re-entry ventricular tachyarrhythmias which often cause syncope and may cause sudden death (22). The Q-T interval should be measured routinely in the ECG of people who complain of syncope for which there is no explanation.

The most effective treatment of symptomatic patients is β-blockade with propranolol; if this does not suppress arrhythmic attacks, excision of the left stellate ganglion may be curative by interrupting sympathetic innervation of the heart. It is not known whether patients with long Q-T intervals who are asymptomatic benefit from propranolol, but certainly treatment is reasonable if there is a family history of sudden death. An exercise ECG is indicated in patients with negative personal and family histories to determine whether arrhythmias can be induced by exertion.

General References

Schamroth L: How to approach an arrhythmia. *Circulation* 47:420, 1973.
    A practical approach to the analysis of arrhythmias.
Treatment of cardiac arrhythmias: *Med Lett* 25:21, 1983.
    A brief synopsis of the treatment of the most common arrhythmias.
Zipes DP: Genesis of cardiac arrhythmias: Electrophysiological considerations and management of cardiac arrhythmias. In Braunwald E (ed): *Heart Disease. A Textbook of Cardiovascular Medicine.* Philadelphia, WB Saunders, 1984, pp 605, 648.
    A comprehensive description, exhaustively referenced.

Specific References

1. Antman EM, Stone PH, Muller JE, Braunwald E: Calcium channel blocking agents in the treatment of cardiovascular disorders; I. Basic and clinical electrophysiologic effects. *Ann Intern Med* 93:875, 1980.
2. Aroestz JM, Cohen SI, Markin E: Bradycardia-tachycardia syndrome; results in twenty-eight patients treated by combined pharmacologic therapy and pacemaker implantation. *Chest* 66:257, 1974.
3. Berkman NL, Lamb LE: The Wolff-Parkinson-White electrocardiogram: a follow-up study of five to twenty-eight years. *N Engl J Med* 278:492, 1968.
4. Blomgren SE, Condemi JJ, Bignall MC, Vaughn JH: Antinuclear antibody induced by procainamide. A prospective study. *N Engl J Med* 281:64, 1969.
5. Davies M, Harris A: Pathological basis of primary heart block. *Br Heart J* 31:219, 1969.
6. Denes P, Dhringra RC, Wu D, et al: Sudden death in patients with chronic bifascicular block. *Arch Intern Med* 137:1005, 1977.
7. Dhingra RC, Denes P, Wu D, et al: Prospective observations in patients with chronic bundle branch block and marked H-V prolongation. *Circulation* 53:600, 1976.
8. Fairfax AJ, Lambert CD, Leatham A: Systemic embolism in chronic sinoatrial disorder. *N Engl J Med* 295:190, 1976.
9. Furberg CD: Effect of antiarrhythmic drugs on mortality after myocardial infarction. *Am J Cardiol* 52:32C, 1983.
10. Gallagher JJ, Pritchett ELC, Sealy WC: The preexcitation syndromes. *Prog Cardiovasc Dis* 20:285, 1978.
11. Greene HL: Accessory atrioventricular conduction syndromes: a review. *Johns Hopkins Med J* 139:13, 1976.
12. Greene HL, Humphries JO: Cardiac arrhythmias. In Harvey AM, Johns RJ, McKusick VA, et al (eds): *The Principles and Practice of Medicine.* New York, Appleton-Century-Crofts, 1980.
13. Jensen JB, Humphries JO, Kouwenhoven WB, Jude JR: Electroshock for atrial flutter and atrial fibrillation: follow-up studies on 50 patients. *JAMA* 194:1181, 1965.
14. Josephson ME, Kastor JA: Supraventricular tachycardia: mechanisms and management. *Ann Intern Med* 87:346, 1977.
15. Kannel WB, Boyle JT, McNamara P, et al: Precursors of sudden coronary death: factors related to the incidence of sudden death. *Circulation* 51:606, 1975.
16. Kennedy HL, Caralis DG: Ambulatory electrocardiography. *Ann Intern Med* 87:729, 1977.
17. Kulbertus HE, deLeval-Rutten F, Duboir M, et al: Prognostic significance of left anterior hemiblock with right bundle branch block in mass screening. *Am J Cardiol* 41:385, 1978.
18. Lister JW, Kline RS, Lesser ME: Chronic bilateral bundle branch block: long-term observations in ambulatory patients. *Br Heart J* 39:203, 1977.
19. Noble D: *The Initiation of the Heart Beat,* Oxford, Clarendon Press, 1975, p 9.
20. Pottage A: Clinical profiles of newer class I antiarrhythmic agents—tocainide, mexiletine, encainide, flecainide and lorcainide. *Am J Cardiol* 52:24C, 1983.
21. Schneider JF, Thomas HE, Kreger BE, et al: Newly acquired right bundle branch block. The Framingham study. *Ann Intern Med* 92:37, 1980.
22. Schwartz PJ, Periti M, Malliani A: The long Q-T syndrome. *Am Heart J* 89:378, 1975.
23. Singh BN, Collett JT, Chew CYC: New perspectives in the pharmacologic therapy of cardiac arrhythmias. *Prog Cardiovasc Dis* 22:243, 1980.
24. Stone PH, Antman EM, Muller JE, Braunwald E: Calcium channel blocking agents in the treatment of cardiovascular disorders; II. Hemodynamic effects and clinical applications. *Ann Intern Med* 93:886, 1980.
25. Wit AL, Rosen MR, Hoffman BF: Electrophysiology and pharmacology of cardiac arrhythmias. II. Relationship of normal and abnormal electrical activity of cardiac fibers to the genesis of arrhythmias. B. Re-entry, Section I. *Am Heart J* 88:664, 1974.
26. Wohl AJ, Laborde NJ, Atkins JM, et al: Prognosis of patients permanently paced for sick sinus syndrome. *Arch Intern Med* 136:406, 1976.
27. Wolf PA, Dawber TR, Thomas HE, Kannel WB: Epidemiologic assessment of chronic atrial fibrillation and risk of stroke: the Framingham study. *Neurology* 28:973, 1978.
28. Zipes DP, Prystowsky EN, Heger JJ: Amiodarone: electrophysiologic actions, pharmacokinetics and clinical effects. *J Am Coll Cardiol* 3:1059, 1984.

CHAPTER SIXTY

Common Cardiac Disorders Revealed by Auscultation of the Heart

BARBARA B. BELL, M.D., EDWARD P. SHAPIRO, M.D., AND PHILIP D. ZIEVE, M.D.

HEART SOUNDS

First Heart Sound (S₁)

The first heart sound is a high frequency ("clicky") sound produced by closure of the atrioventricular (AV) valves, *i.e.*, M_1 (mitral valve closure) followed by T_1 (tricuspid valve closure). Mitral valve closure is louder than tricuspid valve closure.

Abnormally wide splitting of the first heart sound is produced by delays in closure of the tricuspid valve as in patients with right bundle branch block, ventricular ectopic beats, idioventricular rhythm, or left ventricular pacing. In mitral stenosis, mitral valve closure may be so delayed that tricuspid valve closure may actually precede mitral valve closure.

A loud first heart sound indicates a mobile valve. *Increased intensity of the first heart sound* is associated with a rapid ventricular upstroke, which occurs when the ventricles are presented with an increased volume (*e.g.*, ventricular septal defect and atrial septal defect) or with a wide open AV valve at the end of diastole, which occurs when there is shortening of the AV filling time (*e.g.*, atrial tachycardia and conditions associated with a short P-R interval) and when AV filling time is prolonged (*e.g.*, mitral stenosis).

Reduced intensity of the first heart sound may indicate an immobile valve (*e.g.*, severe mitral regurgitation or stenosis) or a long P-R interval.

Second Heart Sound (S₂)

The second heart sound is produced by closure of the semilunar valves, *i.e.*, A_2 (aortic valve closure) followed by P_2 (pulmonic valve closure). Normal splitting of the second heart sound occurs at the height of inspiration, when the splitting may be as wide as 0.10 second and is due to the increase in stroke volume in the right heart with the increase in venous return with inspiration. The two components of the second heart sound are synchronous and virtually single during expiration.

Abnormally wide splitting of S_2 without change in expiration is characteristic of an atrial septal defect or of anomalous pulmonary venous return. S_2 is widely split but variable in patients with pulmonary stenosis. In the presence of severe aortic stenosis, A_2 is delayed beyond P_2, resulting in wide splitting during expiration with no splitting during inspiration (reversed or paradoxical splitting). Paradoxical splitting of the second heart sound also occurs in the presence of a left bundle branch block, severe hypertension, or severe left ventricular failure.

Increased intensities of A_2 *and* P_2 are features of aortic and pulmonary hypertension, respectively. A_2 or P_2 is of reduced intensity when the aortic or pulmonic valve is immobile or severely thickened.

Gallops

The identification of a gallop sound affords valuable information concerning diagnosis, prognosis, and treatment. Gallops are diastolic sounds and appear to be related to the two periods of filling of the ventricles: the rapid filling phase (the S_3 or ventricular diastolic gallop) and the presystolic filling phase related to atrial systole (S_4 or atrial gallop).

The *atrial gallop sound or* S_4 is a low frequency presystolic sound and is found in patients with primary myocardial disease, coronary artery disease, systemic or pulmonary hypertension, or severe aortic or pulmonic stenosis. The atrial gallop is an indication of severity of the underlying disorder and, as the patient's condition improves, the sound may become fainter or disappear. With ventricular hypertrophy an S_4 is a fixed finding of no prognostic significance.

The ventricular gallop sound or S_3 is a low frequency sound. It occurs with the same timing as the normal physiological third sound, approximately 0.14 to 0.16 second after the second heart sound. The third sound is a normal finding in children and young adults up to the age of 30. An S_3 gallop is a feature of severe cardiac decompensation, whatever the underlying cause (hypertension, coronary artery disease, rheumatic heart disease, *etc*) and is an indication of a relatively poor prognosis.

Ejection Sounds ("Clicks")

Ejection sounds are produced at the time of ejection of blood from the left ventricle into the aorta or from the right ventricle into the pulmonary artery. The sound may originate in a thickened valve or in a dilated great vessel. The *aortic ejection sound* is located in the area of aortic auscultation—namely, from the second right intercostal space in a straight line to the cardiac apex, and occurs 0.05 second after M_1. It is a high frequency sound, often called a "click." In the presence of systemic hypertension, the aortic ejection sound is an indication of severity. It disappears as hypertension improves. Aortic ejection clicks may also be heard in patients with aortic stenosis, aneurysm of the ascending aorta, and aortic insufficiency.

Pulmonic ejection sounds (or clicks) are frequently localized to the second left intercostal space and may increase in intensity with expiration. They occur immediately after M_1. Pulmonic clicks are a feature of valvular pulmonic stenosis and also of pulmonary hypertension.

A *midsystolic clicking sound*, with or without a late systolic murmur, may indicate mitral valve prolapse (see below).

Opening Snaps

An opening snap occurs because of a stenotic, but still mobile, mitral or tricuspid valve. The mitral opening snap is best heard between the pulmonic area and the cardiac apex. It occurs 0.04 to 0.12 second after S_2 in early diastole. It is heard in patients with a thickened mitral valve. The earlier the snap, the more severe the stenosis. The tricuspid opening snap is best heard at the lower left or right sternal border and occurs immediately after S_2 in early diastole.

Murmurs

Evaluation of a heart murmur is one of the most common tasks which confronts a physician conducting a physical examination. Virtually all normal people have a systolic murmur during some period of their lives. On the other hand, a murmur may be a sign of serious underlying cardiac or noncardiac disease. It is important that the physician be able to distinguish the innocent murmur from those that reflect an underlying disorder and that he be able to select appropriately the tests, when necessary, that will lead to the precise diagnosis and to the proper management.

General Characteristics of Murmurs

A murmur is a series of audible vibrations produced by turbulence in the circulation. These vibrations can be characterized by intensity, pitch, shape, quality, and timing in the cardiac cycle, precordial location of maximal intensity, and radiation.

The *intensity or loudness of a murmur* is, by convention, graded on a scale of 1 to 6. A grade 1 murmur is audible only after concentrated auscultation. A grade 2 murmur is faint but readily audible. A grade 3 murmur is prominent but not loud. Grade 4 murmurs are loud and are frequently, but not always, associated with a palpable thrill. A grade 5 murmur is very loud. A grade 6 murmur is heard with the stethoscope held 1 cm above, but not actually touching, the chest wall.

The *pitch of a murmur* refers to the frequency of the sound—from high to low. High frequency murmurs usually reflect high velocity and/or high pressure.

The *shape of a murmur* refers to the change in intensity throughout the duration of the sound: for example, crescendo (increasing in intensity), decrescendo (decreasing in intensity), or constant.

The *quality of a murmur* refers to the nature of the sound: harsh, blowing, musical, cooing, rumbling, *etc*. Although these terms are not precise, they are useful in identifying various benign and significant conditions, as will be seen below.

The *timing of a murmur* is particularly important in establishing the cause of the sound—first, whether the murmur is systolic, diastolic, or continuous, and second, whether it is heard in early, middle, or late systole or diastole. Murmurs that last throughout systole are called holosystolic. Late diastolic murmurs are sometimes called presystolic.

The *location of a murmur* refers to that site on the chest wall where the sound is loudest. The *direction of radiation* refers to the other sites where the murmur, though less intense, can still be heard; those sites may be outside the chest (the back or neck, for example). Aortic murmurs may be heard anywhere in a straight line from the second right interspace to the apex. Pulmonic murmurs are heard best at the second left intercostal space; tricuspid murmurs, at the lower left sternal border; and mitral murmurs, at the cardiac apex radiating into the axilla.

There are two kinds of systolic murmurs—ejection and regurgitant murmurs. The ejection systolic murmur may be an innocent flow murmur or it may reflect organic heart disease. The regurgitant murmur may be due to dilation of the annulus of the valve in an otherwise normal heart or may represent organic heart disease.

The *ejection murmur* is a crescendo/decrescendo (or "diamond-shaped") murmur caused by the turbulence of blood flowing through either the aortic or pulmonic valve. The murmur is most commonly midsystolic and ends before the second or closing sound (S_2) of the valve from which the murmur was generated; that is, aortic ejection murmurs end before A_2 and pulmonic ejection murmurs end before P_2. The loudness of the murmur depends in part on the pressure gradient across the valve and in part on other factors, such as thickness of the chest, the cardiac output, *etc*; the shape depends on the acceleration and deceleration of blood flow across the valve as systole proceeds. When diastole is prolonged, for example, by premature ventricular contraction or by atrial fibrillation, ejection murmurs become louder because of the passage of a large volume of blood through the valve. In general, the larger the cardiac output, the louder the murmur. Increases in cardiac output due to hypermetabolic states, such as anemia, fever, or thyrotoxicosis, will increase the loudness of the murmur. Decreases in cardiac output, such as congestive heart failure, will decrease the loudness of the murmur.

Regurgitant murmurs are murmurs produced by backward flow of blood from a high pressure chamber to a compartment of lower pressure. Intensity may be constant as in mitral regurgitation, tricuspid regurgitation, or ventricular septal defect or may be decrescendo as in aortic and pulmonary regurgitation.

Innocent Murmurs

Innocent murmurs are a series of vibrations that are produced in the absence of significant abnormalities of cardiac anatomy or function (Table 60.1).

The innocent murmur can usually be distinguished from significant murmurs by the absence of other physical, radiological, or electrocardiographic evidence of disease. Also, innocent murmurs are usually in early or midsystole, are grade 1 or 2 in intensity, and vary with respiration and/or position. Occasionally, echocardiography (see below) is done to clarify the etiology of a murmur, but more elaborate studies, such as stress tests, radionuclide stud-

ies, and cardiac catheterization, are employed only after it has been decided that a murmur is not innocent and that a more precise diagnosis is necessary.

The most common innocent systolic murmur of childhood and young adulthood that is clearly recognizable as benign based on the characteristics of the murmur alone is the musical or *vibratory midsystolic murmur* (best heard at the lower left sternal border) that is caused by the vibration of the leaflets of the pulmonary valve.

The *venous hum* is a continuous murmur, loudest in the neck, caused by altered flow through the jugular veins. It can be eliminated by turning the patient's head, compression of the internal jugular vein on the side where the murmur is heard, or placing the patient in the supine position.

The *pulmonic ejection systolic murmur* is a systolic crescendo/decrescendo murmur generated by the flow of blood through the pulmonary valve. It is loudest in the left second intercostal space or at the midleft sternal border.

Similarly, the *aortic ejection systolic murmur* is an early systolic murmur generated by the flow of blood through the aortic valve. It is loudest in the right second intercostal space or at the apex of the heart. This innocent or flow murmur, due to sclerosis of the aorta and/or aortic valve, is the most common benign systolic murmur in the middle-aged or elderly patient and may have a cooing quality. An ECG and an echocardiogram may be necessary to rule out left ventricular hypertrophy and aortic stenosis.

Benign flow murmurs commonly are heard in *pregnant women*. Because of the normally increased stroke volume at 28 to 30 weeks of gestation, diastolic filling sounds and systolic ejection murmurs of turbulent flow are common. In pregnant patients also, an S_3 may be prominent enough to be confused with the mid-diastolic murmur of mitral stenosis. The S_3 of pregnancy may be distinguished from the murmur of mitral stenosis, however, by the absence of an opening snap and by the accompanying hyperdynamic apical movement. An echocardiogram is indicated in some patients to make a precise diagnosis.

In the pregnant patient it is critical to compare the femoral and brachial pulses and the blood pressures in the presence of a heart murmur, since coarctation of the aorta may present with a soft heart murmur and, if left undiagnosed, rarely may result in aortic dissection or rupture.

Table 60.1.
Benign or Innocent Systolic Murmurs

Vibratory ejection systolic murmur
Continuous murmur of venous hum
Pulmonic ejection systolic murmur
Aortic ejection systolic murmur
Murmur associated with pregnancy

Clinical Applications of Echocardiography (19)

Echocardiography is a valuable adjunct to the clinical assessment in patients suspected of cardiovascular disease. This technique utilizes high frequency pulsed sound waves to record echoes of cardiac structures as they move within a beam of sound directed into the chest. Sometimes the cardiologist will use phonocardiography in combination with echocardiography to time the various normal and abnormal heart sounds more precisely.

A piezoelectric crystal is used to transmit a short pulse of ultrahigh frequency sound (1 to 8 mHz) into the tissues of the chest. To record an M-mode electrocardiogram, the pulse transducer is placed at one point on the chest wall and rocked to inscribe an arc that will encompass several areas of the heart sequentially. It serves as a source of the sound beam and as a receiver of the echoes. A two-dimensional echocardiogram is recorded using a pulse transducer that is automatically rocked across an arc (mechanical two-dimensional echocardiography) or one which contains multiple piezoelectric crystals directed along the arc (phased array two-dimensional echocardiography). These techniques provide a simultaneous view of the cardiac structures, which is recorded on videotape. These procedures are of no discomfort to the patient; however, he must be able to lie flat for 20 minutes for performance of the test.

Echo spikes arise from the chest wall, right ventricular wall, interventricular septum, mitral leaflets, posterior left ventricular wall, aorta, and left atrium (Fig. 60.1). The size and function of these structures are analyzed and patterns of specific diseases may be recognized.

Two-dimensional echocardiography provides a simultaneous view of these structures and reveals, therefore, their function more precisely than does M-mode or *one-dimensional echocardiography.* Where possible, both modes should be used for optimal visualization of the heart (19). Two-dimensional echocardiography is particularly helpful in assessing left ventricular function in patients with ischemic heart disease where regional structure and function are most important. The noninvasive nature of the test and its ease of performance make two-dimensional echocardiography extremely useful for assessing patients with acute cardiac decompensation. One-dimensional echocardiography is most useful in situations where visualization of rapidly moving structures is important (e.g., mitral leaflet flutter as the result of aortic regurgitation) and in situations where repeated measurements of dimensions of cardiac structures are important.

The echocardiogram is diagnostic in cases of pericardial effusion, idiopathic subaortic stenosis, mitral valve stenosis or prolapse, aortic regurgitation, intracardiac masses, cardiomyopathy, and Ebstein's anomaly of the tricuspid valve. The technique is helpful in cases of aortic stenosis, infectious endocarditis, cardiac tamponade, atrial septal defect, other forms of congenital heart disease, such as ventricular septal defect, tetralogy of Fallot, bicuspid aortic valve, and any other structural abnormality of the heart.

Doppler echocardiography is a new technique that is useful in defining the presence and extent of valvular disease and in quantifying cardiac output. High frequency sound is directed at a column of

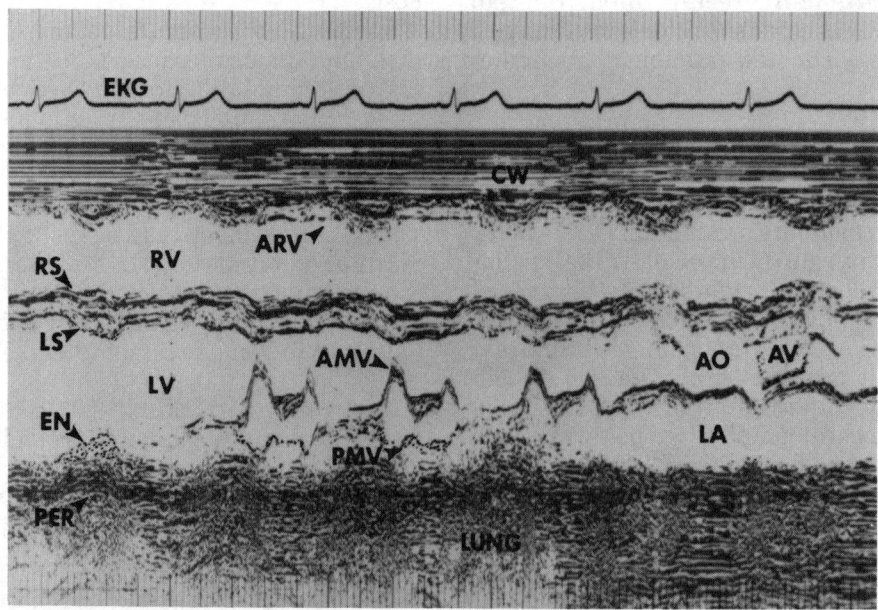

Figure 60.1. Normal one-dimensional echocardiogram. The tracing was taken as the transducer was scanned from the apex to the base of the heart. *AO,* aorta; *AMV,* anterior leaflet of the mitral valve; *ARV,* anterior wall of the right ventricle; *AV,* aortic valve opening; *CW,* chest wall; *EN,* posterior left ventricular endocardium; *LA,* left atrium; *LS,* left ventricular septum; *LV,* left ventricle; *PER,* pericardium; *PMV,* posterior mitral valve leaflet; *RS,* right ventricular septum; *RV,* right ventricle.

moving red blood cells, and the reflected sound is analyzed for changes in frequency, which indicate the direction and velocity of flow. In valvular stenosis a high velocity jet of blood is detected distal to the stenosis; the higher the transvalvular gradient, the higher the velocity of the jet. Valvular regurgitation can be detected by reverse flow. Instruments for Doppler echocardiography are not yet universally available.

SELECTED DISORDERS ASSOCIATED WITH ABNORMAL HEART SOUNDS

Aortic Stenosis

Stenosis of the aortic valve obstructs the flow of blood into the aorta and therefore raises the left ventricular pressure above the aortic pressure. The pressure gradient across the valve reflects the severity of the stenosis. The elevated pressure results in a concentric hypertrophy of the left ventricle. Symptoms develop when the left ventricle can no longer compensate for the pressure load; the heart fails and the cardiac output declines.

Aortic stenosis may occur at any one of several levels. The most common obstruction (75% of patients) is at the aortic valve, although subvalvular and supravalvular aortic stenosis may present with symptoms and signs of severity similar to those of valvular disease. It is particularly important to differentiate fixed aortic outflow obstruction from idiopathic hypertrophic disease which is a functional disorder (see Table 60.2 and below).

Etiology and Epidemiology (21)

In patients below the age of 30, aortic stenosis is most likely to be due to a congenitally stenotic unicuspid valve. Between the ages of 30 and 65, a bicuspid aortic valve, which has become calcified and gradually more rigid over the years, is the most common cause of aortic stenosis. (One or 2% of the general population have a bicuspid aortic valve, and 50% of these valves have calcified by age 50). Rheumatic valvular disease accounts for only 6 to 27% of cases of isolated aortic stenosis in patients between the ages of 30 and 70 years. Over the age of 65, degeneration and sclerosis of the valve account for most cases of aortic stenosis. Except in the elderly, in whom the prevalence is the same in both sexes, isolated aortic stenosis is 3 to 4 times more common in men.

Natural History and Symptoms

Patients with aortic stenosis are usually asymptomatic until relatively late in the course of their disease. Mild to moderate obstruction does not compromise left ventricular function greatly, and even patients with severe stenosis may compensate for years before they develop symptoms. Symptoms ordinarily develop late in the sixth decade after which, if the lesion is not corrected, the average patient dies in about 4 years.

The earliest symptoms are easy fatigability and excessive dyspnea after unusual exercise. Syncope or near syncope with effort (see Chapter 81), angina (see Chapter 57), and dyspnea on unusual exercise (see Chapter 53) are indicative of severe valvular obstruction. Patients with heart failure survive less long (2 years) as a rule than do patients with syncope (3 years) or with angina (5 years) (22). Sudden death occurs in about 15% of symptomatic patients and, particularly worrisome, in about 5% of asymptomatic patients (22).

Physical Findings

Patients with aortic stenosis usually have a loud (grade 3 to 4) systolic ejection murmur. The maxi-

Table 60.2.
Comparison of Valvular Aortic Stenosis and Hypertrophic Cardiomyopathy

	Valvular Aortic Stenosis	Hypertrophic Cardiomyopathy
Symptoms	Dyspnea, angina, syncope or near syncope	Dyspnea, angina, syncope or near syncope
Signs	Systolic ejection murmur loudest at aortic area or at apex; louder if patient squats	Systolic ejection murmur loudest at left lower sternal border; louder if patient stands or performs a Valsalva maneuver
	A_2 may not be audible	A_2 is usually audible
	S_4 is common	S_4 is very common
	Ejection sounds are common	Ejection sounds are uncommon
	Carotid upstroke is delayed	Carotid upstroke is brisk
ECG	Left ventricular hypertrophy (LVH) and strain pattern	LVH and strain pattern; Q waves in inferior and lateral leads are common
Chest X-ray	LVH is a late sign	LVH may occur but unpredictably
	Aortic valve is always calcified (may be seen only on fluoroscopy)	Aortic valve is not calcified
	Ascending aorta may be dilated	Ascending aorta is not dilated
Echocardiogram	Characteristic echos of valvular calcification and of valvular stenosis	Disproportionate septal hypertrophy, systolic anterior displacement of mitral valve

mum intensity of the murmur is at the second right intercostal space and/or at the cardiac apex. At the apex the murmur often has a musical cooing quality. There is usually a thrill in the suprasternal notch or in the second right intercostal space. However, the loudness of the murmur may not correlate with the severity of stenosis. Also, if cardiac output is reduced, as in congestive heart failure, or if the diameter of the chest is increased, the intensity of the murmur may be less than it otherwise would be. A late peak to the murmur does suggest severe obstruction, but this is difficult to appreciate with a stethoscope, and absence of the peak does not mean that obstruction is not severe. Augmentation of the murmur when the patient suddenly squats and diminution of the murmur when the patient stands or performs a Valsalva manuever are characteristic of aortic stenosis.

The systolic murmur, although it may not be loud, is an invariable sign of aortic stenosis; other cardiac sounds are dependent on the nature of the stenotic lesion. An early systolic ejection click is commonly heard when the valve is still mobile. The second aortic sound (A_2) is often not audible when the valve is rigid so that S_2 has only one component (P_2). Paradoxical splitting of the second heart sound, in the absence of left bundle branch block, is a sign of severity. A small pulse pressure (< 30 mm Hg) also indicates severe obstruction (in elderly people, the pulse pressure may be normal despite severe stenosis). A slowly rising pulse—best assessed by palpation of a carotid artery—is characteristic. Under the age of 40, an S_4 is another sign of severe obstruction; over the age of 40, S_4 is common because of the high prevalence of hypertensive and ischemic heart disease and does not correlate with severity of stenosis.

The regurgitant early diastolic murmur of aortic insufficiency is heard in 30 to 40% of patients with aortic valve stenosis.

Laboratory Evaluation

An ECG, a chest X-ray, and an echocardiogram should be obtained routinely in a patient suspected of having aortic stenosis.

Electrocardiogram. The ECG is usually normal until stenosis becomes severe, at which point left ventricular hypertrophy (Fig. 60.2 and Table 60.3) and nonspecific ST depression and T wave inversion are common— but not invariable. In older patients, particularly, an abnormal ECG cannot be relied upon to reflect severity since there are often other reasons why it might be abnormal.

Chest X-ray. Calcification of the aortic valve is always present in patients with aortic stenosis who are older than 35 to 40; but often fluoroscopy is necessary to reveal it. Poststenotic dilation of the

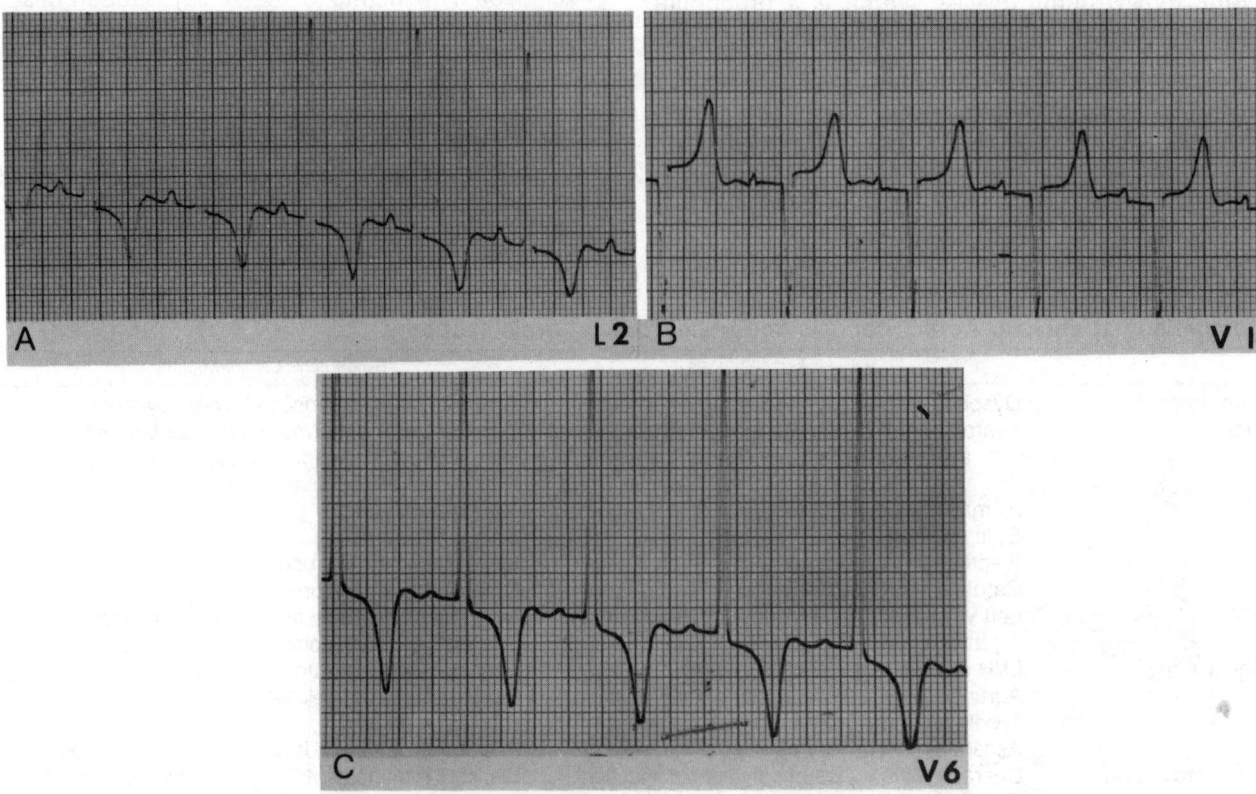

Figure 60.2.   ECG of a patient with left ventricular hypertrophy (see Table 60.3).

Table 60.3.
Principal Electrocardiographic Features of Left Ventricular Hypertrophy[a]

Electrocardiographic Criteria	Point System for Diagnosis[b]
Negative components of P in V$_1$ ≥ 1 mm and ≥ 0.4 second	3 points
QRS	
Largest limb lead R or S ≥ 20 mm or largest chest lead S before transition or R after transition ≥ 30 mm	3 points
OR	
Largest S before transition plus largest R after transition = 45 mm:	
Frontal plane axis ≥ −30°	2 points
Duration in extremity lead ≥ 0.09 second	1 point
Intrinsicoid deflection ≥ 0.05 second	1 point
ST-T	
In general, opposite QRS:	
Without digitalis	3 points
With digitalis	1 point

[a] Modified from Horan LG, Flowers NC: Electrocardiography and vectorcardiography. In Braunwald E (ed): *Heart Disease: A Textbook of Cardiovascular Medicine.* Philadelphia, WB Saunders, 1980, p 229 (11).
[b] Interpretation of point score: 6 points, left ventricular hypertrophy; 5 points, probable left ventricular hypertrophy; 4 points, possible left ventricular hypertrophy. If only voltage criteria are met, ECG may be designated as borderline, and the statement should be made that "left ventricular hypertrophy is suggested only by voltage and should be excluded by other clinical means."

ascending aorta is also commonly seen. The heart size and configuration are usually normal until the disease is far advanced.

Echocardiogram. Echocardiography reveals multiple diastolic echoes of aortic valve leaflets, due to valvular calcification, and, sometimes, an eccentric diastolic closure line. An increase in ventricular wall thickness on echocardiography implies severe obstruction, if there is no other cause for hypertrophy. Doppler echocardiography (see above, page 752) can provide an estimate of the transaortic gradient and may be helpful in distinguishing aortic stenosis from aortic valve sclerosis, in which no gradient is present.

Management

Asymptomatic patients should be reassessed every 12 months so that signs of progressive disease can be detected promptly. Reassessment should include interval history, pertinent physical examination, ECG, chest X-ray, and echocardiogram.

Patients should be cautioned to avoid undue exertion since acute heart failure, arrhythmia, and sudden death are more likely under such circumstances.

The risk of subacute bacterial endocarditis is increased in patients with aortic stenosis and is unrelated to the severity of the stenosis (the risk is unchanged after aortic valve surgery—see below) (17). Therefore, antibiotic prophylaxis (see Chapter 86) is necessary before dental and surgical procedures.

Atrial arrhythmias are uncommon; if they occur, they must be treated aggressively (see Chapter 59) because they are more likely to cause angina, heart failure, or syncope than in a patient without aortic stenosis. β-Blocking agents are probably best avoided because they may compromise left ventricular function further. If heart failure develops, it should be treated with digitalis and diuretics (see Chapter 61), but great care must be taken to avoid volume depletion which may reduce cardiac output to a point where serious underperfusion of vital organs occurs.

Table 60.4 lists the indications for referral of a patient with aortic stenosis to a cardiologist. In general, referral is indicated if the diagnosis is unclear, if the patient is symptomatic, or if an asymptomatic patient has evidence of severe obstruction. Cardiac catheterization (see Chapter 57) is the definitive technique for assessing the severity and site of aortic stenosis. It should be performed in all symptomatic patients and in asymptomatic patients who have signs of severe disease. Hemodynamically significant stenosis is usually associated with a gradient of 50 mm Hg or greater (unless cardiac output is reduced, in which case the gradient may be much lower even if there is severe stenosis). The effective aortic valve orifice in patients with severe obstruction is usually less than 0.5 cm/m^2 of body surface area (compared to 1.6 to 2.6 cm in normal people). At the time of catheterization, angiography is also done to assess left ventricular function, the patency of the coronary arteries, and the degree, if any, of aortic and mitral regurgitation.

The cardiologist is likely to recommend replacement of the stenotic aortic valve with a prosthesis in all symptomatic patients and in asymptomatic

Table 60.4.
Indications for Referral of Patients with Aortic Stenosis

If there is a question about the diagnosis
If the patient is symptomatic
If the asymptomatic patient has signs of severe obstruction:
    Physical signs:
        Small pulse pressure (< 30 mm Hg)
        Late peak to systolic murmur
        Diminished A$_2$
        Paradoxical splitting of A$_2$
    ECG
        Left ventricular hypertrophy
        ST depression, T wave inversion
    Chest X-ray: Concentric left ventricular hypertrophy
    Echocardiogram:
        Concentric left ventricular hypertrophy
        Calcification of aortic valve in patients under 60

patients with signs of severe obstruction who are found to have a large gradient or evidence, on angiography, of left ventricular dysfunction.

Operative mortality in patients without left ventricular failure is 5 to 10%; in patients with left ventricular failure it is 10 to 25%. The patient's postoperative health and long term survival are dependent on a number of factors (age, general health, left ventricular function, etc), but overall the 5-year survival is approximately 80 to 85%, and the 10-year survival is approximately 70 to 75%. Most patients experience a considerable improvement in their sense of well-being and in their exercise tolerance (17). When patients die, however, their death is usually due to a cardiac complication (heart failure, myocardial infarction, or sudden death). (For further details regarding the long term course/management of the patient with a prosthetic valve see below, page 765.)

Hypertrophic Cardiomyopathy

Hypertrophic cardiomyopathy (formerly called idiopathic hypertrophic subaortic stenosis—IHSS) is a disease of cardiac muscle in which the ventricular septum is thickened disproportionately compared to the free wall of the left ventricle (asymmetric septal hypertrophy). The left ventricle is hypercontractile and during systole ejects essentially all of its blood, leaving a "clenched fist" with very high wall stress. The asymmetric hypertrophy distinguishes this condition from those, such as hypertension and aortic stenosis, that cause secondary hypertrophy of the heart muscle (Table 60.2). A common, but not invariable, feature of the disease is obstruction to the left ventricular outflow tract.

Etiology and Epidemiology

The etiology of hypertrophic cardiomyopathy is unknown, although there is evidence that it is usually inherited. Some patients become symptomatic when they are young adults, but the diagnosis is sometimes not made until much later in life. Men and women are equally likely to be affected. Most people with the disease are asymptomatic, and the proportion of affected people who have become symptomatic is unknown.

Natural History and Symptoms

The most common symptom of hypertrophic cardiomyopathy is dyspnea, but patients also complain frequently of angina (with or without evidence of occlusive coronary artery disease) and of syncope or near syncope. These symptoms are much more likely to be induced by exertion than to occur spontaneously.

Most symptomatic patients have a relatively stable, protracted course, but once marked symptoms develop, some patients become rapidly worse, with progressive heart failure, angina, or arrhythmias.

Over a 5-year period in one study, most surviving patients (83%) were either stable or improved (26). The most troublesome feature of the illness is its propensity to cause sudden death. The incidence of sudden death is about 3 to 4%/year in patients with hypertrophic cardiomyopathy, but some families have a particularly high incidence. Unfortunately, there is no way to identify in any given patient an increased risk of sudden death; in fact, death may be the first manifestation of the disease.

Physical Findings

The characteristic signs of the disease are a sustained left ventricular apical impulse, a loud S_4, and a harsh systolic ejection murmur, loudest at the left lower border of the sternum and often accompanied by a thrill. The location of the murmur helps to distinguish the condition from valvular aortic stenosis. Other distinguishing features are as follows: the second heart sound (A_2) is usually audible; a diastolic murmur is rare; the pulse pressure is normal; ejection sounds are uncommon; and, most important, the upstroke of the carotid pulse is brisk. In addition, the murmur of hypertrophic cardiomyopathy is augmented when the patient stands or performs a Valsalva maneuver and is diminished when the patient squats—the opposite of the findings in patients with aortic stenosis.

Laboratory Evaluation

An ECG, chest X-ray, and echocardiogram should be obtained routinely in patients suspected of having hypertrophic cardiomyopathy.

Electrocardiogram. The ECG is abnormal in the majority of patients and is always abnormal in patients with obstruction. Typically, there is evidence of left ventricular hypertrophy (Fig. 60.2 and Table 60.3) and there is nonspecific ST depression and T wave inversion. Q waves are often seen in the inferior and lateral leads, reflecting septal hypertrophy.

Chest X-ray. The left ventricle is sometimes enlarged, but unpredictably so. In contrast to aortic valvular stenosis, the aortic valve is not calcified and the ascending aorta is not dilated.

Echocardiogram. Echocardiography is diagnostic; it demonstrates a thickened ventricular septum, hypertrophied out of proportion to the posterior wall of the left ventricle. Also, the mitral valve apparatus is displaced anteriorly during systole, and the aortic leaflets may close suddenly in early systole and reopen as systole continues. (These abnormalities of the aortic valve may only be present after the patient is administered amyl nitrate.)

Management

The goal of therapy is to reduce the hypercontractile state of the left ventricle. Currently this is best done by means of the calcium channel blocker, verapamil (80 to 120 mg four times a day) unless the patient has signs or symptoms of heart failure. Alternatively, a β-blocker may be prescribed (e.g., propranolol, 10 to 40 mg four times a day). Angina, especially, is often relieved by treatment, but dyspnea also may be decreased as a result of a slower heart rate and of more time for the ventricle to fill. Although it is not clear that the risk of sudden death is reduced by therapy, most patients are symptomatically improved or at least stabilized by treatment.

Drugs which increase ventricular contractility or decrease ventricular volume are best avoided if possible—digitalis, vasodilators, β-adrenergic stimulants, and diuretics. Patients, even if asymptomatic, should avoid undue exertion (e.g., running).

There is an increased risk of endocarditis in patients with hypertrophic cardiomyopathy and they should therefore receive antibiotic prophylaxis before dental and surgical procedures (see Chapter 86).

Surgical removal of a portion of the hypertrophied septum should be considered in severely symptomatic patients. Such a decision should be made in consultation with a cardiologist and a cardiac surgeon. Although the operative mortality is relatively high (5 to 10%), symptoms are usually relieved in patients who survive. In one series the incidence of sudden death appeared to be reduced after operation (26).

Atrial Septal Defect

Atrial septal defect of the ostium secundum type (in the midportion of the septum) is one of the most common congenital cardiac diseases that is diagnosed in adults. It causes, until late in the course (see below), a left to right atrial shunt with a volume overload of the right ventricle and overperfusion of the lungs.

Etiology and Epidemiology

The defect is more common in females; the reported female to male ratio ranges from 1.5 to 3.5:1. Occasionally the defect is associated with other cardiac abnormalities. For example, 10 to 20% of patients with an atrial septal defect have mitral valve prolapse (12).

Natural History and Symptoms

Patients with atrial septal defect are usually asymptomatic until their third or fourth decade. Thereafter, symptoms invariably develop—usually dyspnea or exertion, fatigue, and palpitations—the result of heart failure and of supraventricular arrhythmias. Less commonly, symptoms of pulmonary embolism (Chapter 53) or paradoxical embolism (e.g., a stroke) occur. Virtually all patients are symptomatic by age 60. In fact, three-quarters of untreated patients are dead by age 50 and 90% by age 60. Increased pulmonary blood flow eventually produces pulmonary vascular disease and, conse-

quently, pulmonary hypertension in about 15% of patients (5). When this happens, the left to right shunt first decreases and then reverses; it is at that point that cyanosis develops. Coexistent atherosclerotic or hypertensive cardiovascular disease may complicate the course of older patients with atrial septal defect and may make diagnosis and treatment more difficult.

Physical Findings

Atrial septal defect usually causes a wide fixed split of the second heart sound, the result of late closure of the pulmonic valve, and a soft blowing systolic pulmonic ejection murmur. A low-medium frequency mid-diastolic flow rumble across the tricuspid valve is common. The precordium may be hyperdynamic with a palpable S_3. If pulmonary hypertension has developed (see below), clubbing and cyanosis may be observed, and P_2 will be accentuated. Signs of right ventricular failure (edema, distended neck veins, hepatomegaly) are common late in the disease.

Laboratory Evaluation

An ECG, a chest X-ray, and an echocardiogram should be obtained routinely in a patient suspected of having an atrial septal defect.

Electrocardiogram. The ECG displays an incomplete right bundle branch block or rSR^1 in lead V_1 90 to 95% of the time with a vertical frontal plane axis or right axis deviation. Atrial fibrillation occurs commonly in symptomatic patients; atrial flutter and paroxysmal atrial tachycardia occur less often.

Chest X-ray (Fig. 60.3). The chest X-ray in this disease is almost invariably abnormal and shows increased pulmonary vascularity with a prominent main pulmonary artery and increased heart size. The right pulmonary artery is usually more prominent than the left because of differential flow due to the jet effect.

Echocardiogram. The echocardiogram demonstrates right ventricular enlargement and paradoxical motion of the ventricular septum with respect to the posterior wall of the left ventricle. These findings are also seen with other lesions that cause volume overload of the right ventricle, such as tricuspid and pulmonic regurgitation, and partial anomalous pulmonary venous return.

Management

If a patient is suspected of having an atrial septal defect, he should be referred to a cardiologist for definitive diagnosis. The cardiologist will usually perform cardiac catheterization (see Chapter 57 for a description of the patient experience). All patients, even if they are asymptomatic, should have their defect repaired if pulmonary blood flow is more than 1½ times systemic blood flow. The operative mortality is less than 2%, although some degree of per-

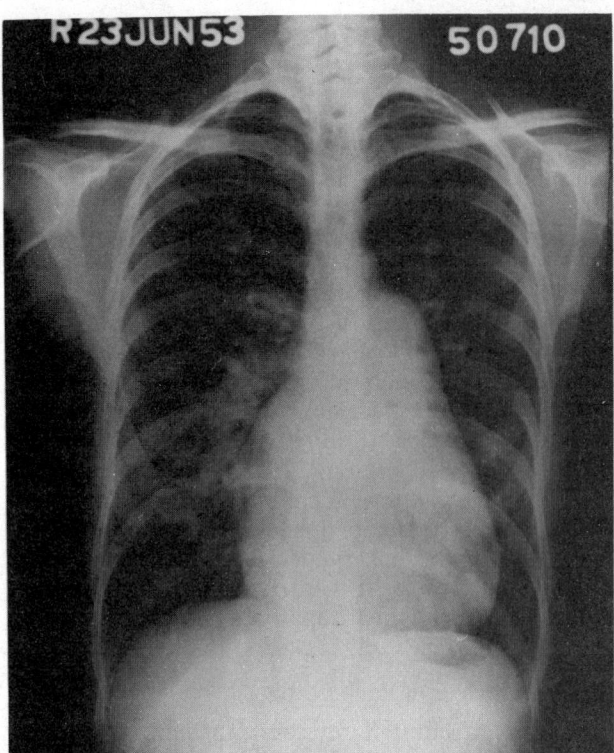

Figure 60.3.   Chest X-ray of a patient with atrial septal defect (see the text).

sistent right or left ventricular dysfunction is common in adults. If severe pulmonary hypertension has developed (pulmonary pressure equal to or greater than the systemic pressure), corrective surgery is contraindicated, but patients with lesser degrees of pulmonary hypertension may still benefit from repair of the defect. Survival after corrective surgery is influenced by the age of the patient and the degree of persistent cardiac dysfunction. Patients with otherwise normal hearts have normal survival rates after successful repair of the atrial defect and usually can resume normal activity.

Endocarditis prophylaxis is unnecessary for patients with atrial septal defect.

Mitral Regurgitation (3)

Mitral regurgitation may develop because of an abnormality of any part of the mitral valve apparatus: the valve leaflets, the chordae tendineae, the papillary muscles, or the annulus. Such abnormality may result in either acute or chronic signs and symptoms, depending on the nature of the lesion.

An incompetent mitral valve allows regurgitation into the left atrium of blood from the left ventricle. The reduced load on the ventricle reduces the tension in the ventricular muscle and allows it to utilize more energy in contraction. Therefore, in patients with chronic mitral regurgitation, cardiac output remains normal for years until, because of age or

intercurrent disease, the ventricle no longer can compensate, and heart failure ensues. In patients with acute mitral regurgitation, ventricular compensation is inadequate and heart failure develops abruptly.

Chronic Mitral Regurgitation

Etiology and Epidemiology

Chronic mitral incompetency in adults may occur in association with a great variety of disorders. Rheumatic fever, despite the marked decline in its incidence in recent years, still is the cause of 25% of cases—usually in association with some degree of mitral stenosis. Otherwise, chronic mitral regurgitation is most often due to papillary muscle necrosis—the result of ischemic heart disease, to an inherited (e.g., Marfan's syndrome or mitral prolapse—see below) or an acquired (e.g., systemic lupus erythematosus) disorder of connective tissue, to idiopathic calcification of the valve—primarily a disorder of the elderly, or to congenital maldevelopment of the mitral apparatus.

Natural History and Symptoms

Patients with chronic mitral regurgitation may remain asymptomatic for many years—even, if the regurgitation is not severe, for their entire lives. Characteristically, when symptoms do develop, they appear gradually over years as the left ventricle slowly loses its ability to compensate for the loss of more than half of its stroke volume back into the left atrium. Dyspnea and fatigue are the usual symptoms of left ventricular failure. Supraventricular arrhythmias, especially atrial fibrillation, are likely to develop if left atrial enlargement becomes marked, compromising somewhat the heart's ability to compensate. Acute pulmonary edema occasionally occurs but is uncommon. Sometimes severe pulmonary hypertension develops without much enlargement of the left atrium. Early surgical correction of the lesion in patients with pulmonary hypertension and signs of right ventricular hypertrophy is important.

In a series of unselected patients with mitral regurgitation, 80% treated medically survived 5 years, and 60% survived 10 years (20). Moderately to severely symptomatic patients do less well; in one report 46% of patients with chronic rheumatic mitral insufficiency survived 5 years (17).

Physical Findings

A high pitched holosystolic murmur, loudest at the apex, is characteristic of chronic mitral regurgitation (patients with mild regurgitation may have only a late systolic murmur). The holosystolic murmur is constant in intensity and radiates always to the axilla and sometimes to the back and to the base of the heart. It is best heard when the patient is in the left lateral decubitus position. The murmur is

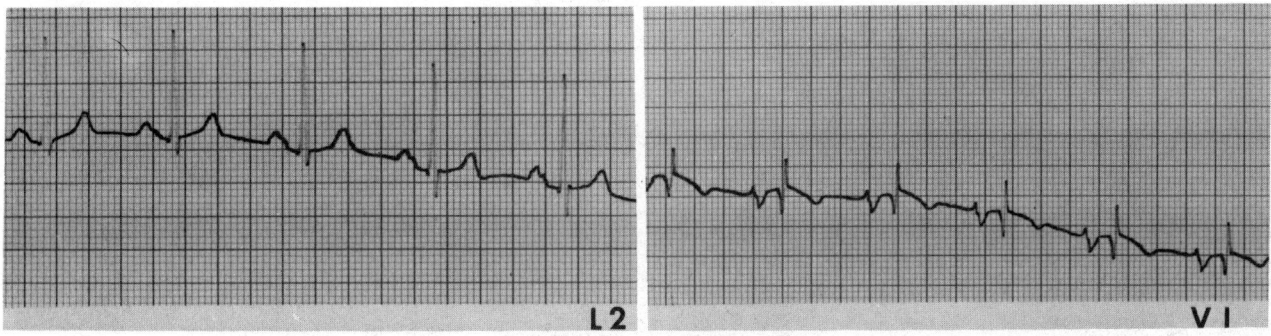

Figure 60.4. ECG of a patient with left atrial hypertrophy (see Table 60.5).

Table 60.5.
Principal Electrocardiographic Features of Left Atrial Hypertrophy[a]

P wave:	
Axis	+45° to −30°
Amplitude (II, III, aVf) duration	> 0.11 second (broad)
Component (V₁)	
Early	Positive but inside normal
Late	Negative, ≥ 0.04 area units[b]

[a] Modified from Horan LG, Flowers NC: Electrocardiography and vectorcardiography. In Braunwald E (ed): *Heart Disease: A Textbook of Cardiovascular Medicine.* Philadelphia, WB Saunders, 1980, p 223 (11).
[b] Area units = mm-seconds. One small block on standard ECG paper = 0.04 mm-second.

Table 60.6
Electrocardiographic Criteria of Right Ventricular Hypertrophy in Adults without Conduction Defects Known NOT to Have Infarction[a]

Sign	Points[b]
Ratio reversal (R/S V₅:R/S V₁ ≤ 0.4)	5
qR in V₁	5
R/S ratio in V₁ > 1	4
S in V₁ < 2 mm	4
R in V₁ + S in V₅ or V₆ > 10.5 mm	4
Right axis deviation > 110°	4
S in V₅ or V₆ ≥ 7 mm and each ≥ 2 mm	3
R/S in V₅ or V₆ ≤ 1	3
R in V₁ ≥ 7 mm	3
S₁, S₂, and S₃ each ≥ 1 mm	2
S₁ and Q₃ each ≥ 1 mm	2
R′ in V₁ earlier than 0.08 second and ≥ 2 mm	2
R peak in V₁ or V₂ between 0.04 and 0.07 second	1
S in V₅ or V₆ ≥ 2 mm but < 7 mm	1
Reduction in V lead R/S ratio between V₁ and V₄	1
R in V₅ or V₆ < 5 mm	1

[a] Modified from Horan LG, Flowers NC: Electrocardiography and vectorcardiography. In Braunwald E (ed): *Heart Disease: A Textbook of Cardiovascular Medicine.* Philadelphia, WB Saunders, 1980, p 226 (11).
[b] Interpretation of point score: 10 points, right ventricular hypertrophy; 7 to 9 points, probable right ventricular hypertrophy or hemodynamic overload; 5 to 6 points, possible right ventricular hypertrophy or hemodynamic overload. These criteria do not take into account serial ECG comparisons. Such additional data may alter the interpreter's impression of the likelihood of fixed enlargement or dynamic overload.

diminished when the patient stands or performs a Valsalva maneuver and is intensified when he squats. If regurgitation is severe, the precordium is usually hyperdynamic and there is an S₃ gallop. S₁ is soft. If pulmonary hypertension has developed, an S₄ gallop, a loud P₂, and a right ventricular heave may be appreciated. Signs of right ventricular failure—edema, hepatomegaly, distended neck veins, hepatojugular reflux—may also be seen late in the course of this disease.

Laboratory Evaluation

An ECG, chest X-ray, and echocardiogram should be obtained routinely if a patient is suspected of having mitral regurgitation.

Electrocardiogram. The ECG shows evidence of left atrial enlargement (Fig. 60.4 and Table 60.5) and, if present, of atrial fibrillation. The pattern of left ventricular hypertrophy (Fig. 60.2 and Table 60.3) is often seen as well, primarily in patients with severe disease. A pattern of right ventricular hypertrophy (Table 60.6) indicating pulmonary hypertension is less common and, when seen, is cause for great concern.

Chest X-ray. Left ventricular and left atrial enlargement are common. On a posteroanterior (PA) film, elevation of the left bronchus and prominence

of the left atrial appendage are the earliest signs of left atrial enlargement; a double density posteriorly is seen when the left atrium is grossly enlarged (Fig. 60.5).

Echocardiogram. Echocardiography demonstrates left atrial and left ventricular enlargement and hyperdynamic motion of the left ventricle, especially the septum. Two-dimensional echocardiography usually can define the etiology of the valvular disease, *i.e.,* rheumatic, prolapsing, ischemic, *etc.* However, in contrast to mitral stenosis, aortic stenosis, or aortic regurgitation, there are no specific echocardiographic signs of mitral regurgitation. Therefore, even if there is clear auscultatory evidence of mitral regurgitation, the echocardiogram may show

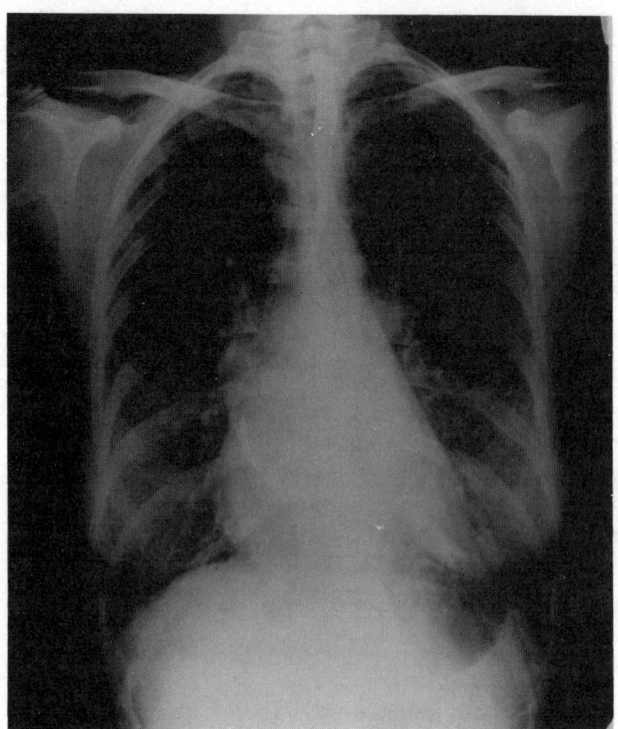

Figure 60.5. Chest X-ray of a patient with left atrial enlargement. Note the straight left heart border and the calcification of the wall of the left atrium.

only the left atrial enlargement. Doppler echocardiography (see above, page 752) may be more helpful in this regard.

Management

Patients who do not have severe disease can be managed medically. Antibiotic prophylaxis against bacterial endocarditis should be administered before all dental and surgical procedures (Chapter 86). If atrial fibrillation is present, restoration of sinus rhythm should be attempted unless the left atrium is greatly enlarged or unless mitral regurgitation has been present for many years. (A detailed discussion of the treatment of atrial fibrillation is to be found in Chapter 59). If heart failure develops, it should be treated by use of the measures described in Chapter 61. Afterload reduction by use of an arteriolar vasodilator may be particularly useful in this condition; by lowering peripheral resistance, ejection of blood into the aorta, rather than back into the left atrium, is favored.

When, despite therapy, patients become more than mildly symptomatic or if the diagnosis is unclear, referral to a cardiologist is indicated (Table 60.7). It is likely that cardiac catheterization and angiography (see Chapter 57) will be done to confirm the diagnosis, to establish the severity of the lesion, to evaluate the function of the left ventricle and, often, the patency of the coronary arteries. At this

Table 60.7.
Indications for Referral of Patients with Mitral Regurgitation

Progressive dyspnea or fatigue
Development of supraventricular arrhythmia
A mildly symptomatic or an asymptomatic patient with progressive cardiac enlargement
Uncertainty about the diagnosis
Acute mitral regurgitation
Patients with mitral valve prolapse who have symptomatic arrhythmias, symptomatic mitral regurgitaion, infectious endocarditis, or transient ischemic attacks

point a decision will be made about the value of operative repair of the lesion. Unless the patient has severe noncardiac disease or unless left ventricular function is so severely reduced that the patient would not tolerate an operation, replacement of the defective valve with a prosthesis is very likely to be recommended. The operative mortality reported from various centers is 3 to 10%.

The health and survival of patients who have undergone successful valve replacement depends on a number of factors (also see below, page 765). Advanced age (over 60), the presence of concomitant mitral stenosis, poor left ventricular function (ejection fraction under 50%), and severity of symptoms preoperatively (New York Heart Association class III or IV—see Chapter 61) are adverse factors which reduce long term postoperative survival. In general, patients with mitral regurgitation on the basis of ischemic heart disease do less well than do patients with rheumatic heart disease. Nevertheless, even patients with one or more adverse risk factors live longer, on the average, with a prosthetic valve than they would without one (9), and most patients are able to be more active than they were before surgery. The overall 10-year survival for patients who have undergone successful mitral surgery is approximately 70% (9). Postoperatively, anticoagulation with warfarin is used routinely to prevent thromboembolic complications (see Chapter 51).

Acute Mitral Regurgitation

Etiology and Epidemiology

Acute mitral incompetence is most often due to rupture of the chordae tendineae, the cords that connect the valve cusps to the papillary muscles of the left ventricle. Most of the time the cause of the rupture is myxomatous degeneration of the valve (see "Mitral Valve Prolapse," below), although occasionally rheumatic fever or acute left ventricular dilation can be incriminated. Much less commonly, acute mitral regurgitation will be caused by papillary muscle rupture or dysfunction (complications of myocardial infarction) or by perforation of a mitral cusp as the result of bacterial endocarditis. The disorder is primarily encountered in middle-aged and elderly patients.

Natural History and Symptoms

Because the left atrium is suddenly presented with a volume load to which it cannot rapidly accommodate, acute pulmonary edema is much more common in patients with acute, compared to chronic, mitral regurgitation. The primary symptom of pulmonary edema is severe dyspnea at rest.

Physical Findings

A harsh holosystolic murmur of constant intensity, loudest at the apex, is characteristic; if a posterior cord has ruptured, the murmur may radiate to the base of the heart, and may mimic the murmur of aortic stenosis. Sometimes an early or midsystolic, or even a crescendo-decrescendo, murmur is heard. An S_3 gallop is almost always heard and an S_4 gallop is common. Unlike the situation in patients with chronic mitral regurgitation, S_1 is normal or even loud. Signs of left-sided heart failure (rales) and of right-sided failure (edema, distended neck veins, *etc*) are also common.

Laboratory Findings

Chest X-ray. The chest X-ray shows marked pulmonary congestion. The left atrium and the left ventricle are minimally enlarged. These findings are the opposite of those found in patients with chronic mitral regurgitation.

Echocardiogram. Chamber enlargement is usually not seen; but increased systolic motion of the valve is common; and if the chordae have ruptured, the flailing chordae or marked prolapse of the leaflets into the left atrium may be visualized by two-dimensional echocardiography.

Management

Patients suspected of having suffered acute mitral regurgitation should be hospitalized immediately for diagnosis, for treatment of acute heart failure, and for consideration for early operative repair.

Mitral Valve Prolapse (6)

Etiology and Epidemiology

Systolic prolapse of a leaflet of the mitral valve into the left atrium has proved to be a very common phenomenon, affecting over 5% of the population (14). Women are more likely to be affected than are men, although reported sex ratios vary considerably. The exact nature of this abnormality is not entirely clear, but in most cases the condition appears to be inherited (autosomal dominant), with reduced penetrance in men and in children.

Histological study of prolapsing valves removed at operation shows "myxomatous degeneration," a proliferation of the spongiosa layer of mucopolysaccharides into the fibrosa layer of collagen, resulting in a weakness in the supporting structure of the valve. This abnormality is also seen in a number of known disorders of connective tissue, including Marfan's syndrome and Ehlers-Danlos syndrome. However, echocardiographic prolapse is also frequently reported in patients with documented coronary artery disease, asymmetric septal hypertrophy, and atrial septal defect, and these cases may represent "secondary prolapse" in which the valve is normal but changes in ventricular geometry cause prolapsing of the leaflets. In these "secondary" cases the click and associated symptoms (see below) are usually not present.

Natural History and Symptoms

Most patients are asymptomatic and the condtion is identified during a routine physical examination. Less often, patients complain of palpitations, chest pain, or dyspnea. The palpitations reflect arrhythmias (see below) or, more commonly, just an awareness of sinus tachycardia. The chest pain sometimes mimics angina (or, in fact, is angina if there is concomitant ischemic heart disease) but more often is sharp lancinating pain in the left chest, unrelated to exertion, and the cause of it is unknown.

In the great majority of patients the syndrome is benign. However, in about 15% of patients (16) significant mitral regurgitation occurs, and patients may complain of dyspnea, due to left ventricular failure.

It is now recognized that patients with mitral valve prolapse are at risk for embolic strokes. In a recent study 40% of patients under 45 who had had a stroke had mitral valve prolapse compared to 6.8% of matched controls (1).

The most feared complication of mitral valve prolapse, sudden death, is quite rare. The risk is higher in patients with a family history of sudden death or in patients with a prolonged Q-T interval on their ECG (see below).

Physical Findings

The characteristic finding in patients with mitral prolapse is a midsystolic click, best heard at the lower left sternal border, due to sudden tensing of the prolapsed valve. It occurs later than the systolic ejection sound heard commonly in association with systemic hypertension (see page 750). Very often the click is followed immediately by a crescendo late systolic murmur which continues until A_2.

The physical findings may vary from time to time in any given patient and may also vary with the position of the patient. In those relatively rare instances where chronic mitral regurgitation has developed, the typical physical findings—including the holosystolic murmur—of this condition will be encountered (see above).

The mitral valve prolapse syndrome is commonly associated with skeletal abnormalities, such as scoliosis and pectus excavatum, suggesting that valve prolapse may be only one component of a generalized disease of connective tissue.

Laboratory Findings

Electrocardiogram. The ECG is usually normal, especially in asymptomatic patients. Symptomatic patients may show nonspecific ST-T wave changes, usually in the inferior leads, and, sometimes prolongation of the Q-T interval.

A variety of arrhythmias may occur in patients with mitral valve prolapse. The commonest are premature ventricular contractions (PVCs) and paroxysmal supraventricular tachycardia. When patients are exercised, it has been reported that many of them develop frequent PVCs and that up to 40% develop atrial arrhythmias (8).

Echocardiogram. The M-mode echocardiogram is usually diagnostic in this condition. It shows late systolic or holosystolic prolapse of one or both leaflets of the mitral valve. Sometimes, however, the M-mode echocardiogram shows no abnormalities despite the typical cardiac findings. These patients probably have minor degrees of prolapse.

Management

Asymptomatic patients need no treatment but should be reassessed by interval history, physical examination, and echocardiogram every few years. Those patients who have a systolic murmur should receive prophylaxis against bacterial endocarditis before dental or surgical procedures (see Chapter 86). (Patients who have only a click probably do not need prophylaxis.)

Patients with palpitations should have ambulatory electrocardiographic monitoring to determine the severity of their arrhythmia, and therapy should be prescribed on the basis of the type of arrhythmia that is present (see Chapter 59). A β-blocking agent is often a drug of choice in the treatment of these patients and also in those with mitral prolapse who complain of chest pain (e.g., propranolol, usual dose 10 to 40 mg, four times a day or atenolol, usual dose 25 to 50 mg a day). The mechanism of action of the drug in the relief of pain is unknown but possibly may be explained by the fact that many untreated patients have been shown to have increased blood levels of norepinephrine and to have increased sympathetic (and vagal) tone.

Patients with symptomatic mitral regurgitation should be treated as described above (page 760).

Referral to a cardiologist is recommended at any time patients become symptomatic from arrhythmia, chronic mitral regurgitation or thromboembolism.

Mitral Stenosis

Stenosis of the mitral valve obstructs the flow of blood out of the left atrium and therefore raises the left atrial pressure above the left ventricular diastolic pressure. The pressure gradient across the valve is a measure of the severity of the stenosis. Because of the increase in left atrial pressure, there is an increase in pressure in the pulmonary blood vessels. The pulmonary congestion accounts for most of the symptoms of the disease.

Etiology and Epidemiology

By far the most common cause of mitral stenosis in adults is rheumatic fever (although a history of rheumatic fever can be elicited in only 50% of patients with pure mitral stenosis). Pure mitral stenosis occurs in 40% of all patients with rheumatic heart disease. The rest of the time there is associated mitral regurgitation, aortic valve disease, and, uncommonly, tricuspid valve disease. Two-thirds of patients with rheumatic mitral stenosis are women.

Natural History and Symptoms

On the average, there is a latent period of nearly 20 years between an attack of acute rheumatic fever and the development of symptomatic mitral stenosis (25). Thus, symptoms usually do not develop before the fourth decade. The severity of symptoms is quite variable: some people, in fact, are never symptomatic; some are mildly symptomatic indefinitely; and some develop progressively severe cardiopulmonary decompensation. Of the patients with progressive disease, it has been estimated that an average of 7 years elapses between the onset of symptoms and the development of total disability (class IV cardiac status—see Chapter 61). In one series the 5-year survival from that point in patients treated medically was only 15% (18).

Pulmonary congestion causes many of the symptoms of mitral stenosis: dyspnea, orthopnea, and paroxysmal nocturnal dyspnea. If left atrial pressure rises acutely because of a sudden stress, frank pulmonary edema may occur. Hemoptysis due to rupture of small bronchial veins or to pulmonary edema is not unusual.

As the disease progresses, pulmonary hypertension develops followed by symptoms of right heart failure: edema, distended neck veins, a tender liver, and ascites. At this point, the flow of blood into the left heart is limited, and the pulmonary arterioles hypertrophy, diminishing the risk of pulmonary edema. Low cardiac output is responsible for the fatigue which is a common complaint of patients at this stage.

Atrial fibrillation (Chapter 59) complicates the course of 40 to 50% of patients with mitral stenosis. The 20% reduction in blood flow across the mitral valve by the loss of left atrial contraction may intensify symptoms of heart failure and of fatigue.

At some time in their course, 20% of patients with mitral stenosis experience symptomatic thromboembolism—most often to the brain; 80% of these patients are in atrial fibrillation.

Physical Findings

A mid-diastolic rumbling murmur with presystolic accentuation is characteristic of mitral stenosis. It is best heard at, and is often limited to, the cardiac apex. To hear it, it may be necessary to turn the patient to the left lateral position and to have him expire fully. Sometimes the patient must be exercised before the murmur is audible. The murmur is best heard with the bell of the stethoscope pressed lightly against the chest. A loud first heart sound (S_1) and opening snap (see above, page 750) usually accompany the murmur when the valve is mobile.

Late in the course, signs of pulmonary hypertension (a loud P_2 and a right ventricular heave) and of right heart failure may be found.

Laboratory Findings

Electrocardiogram. The ECG shows left atrial enlargement (Fig. 60.4 and Table 60.5) in 90% of patients who are in sinus rhythm. With the development of pulmonary hypertension, signs of right ventricular hypertrophy appear (Table 60.6).

Chest X-ray. Left atrial enlargement (see page 759 and Fig. 60.5) is seen in virtually all patients with symptomatic mitral stenosis, but the size of the left atrium does not correlate with the severity of stenosis. Late in the course right ventricular and right atrial hypertrophy will be seen as well. Symptomatic patients are also likely to show radiological signs of pulmonary congestion—the severity of which will determine the findings that are seen (Chapter 61).

Calcification of the mitral valve is not unusual in patients with long-standing mitral stenosis, but this is better visualized by fluoroscopy than by a plain X-ray.

Echocardiogram. Mitral stenosis can be easily diagnosed by echocardiography. Mitral valve thickening can be seen; there is reduced excursion of the anterior leaflet of the valve and abnormal anterior motion of the posterior leaflet during diastole (it normally moves posteriorly). The severity of the stenosis can be accurately assessed by two-dimensional and Doppler echocardiography (see page 752).

Management

Asymptomatic patients need no treatment except prophylaxis for bacterial endocarditis when they are to undergo dental or surgical procedures (Chapter 86). Newly diagnosed adult patients with mitral stenosis do not ordinarily require prophylaxis for β-hemolytic streptococcal infection unless they have had an attack of rheumatic fever within the last 5 to 10 years or are in a population where β-hemolytic streptococcal infection is more prevalent (e.g., military personnel or hospital workers). Patients who have received prophylaxis throughout childhood should continue to receive it indefinitely. When prophylaxis is necessary, the best regimen is 1 to 2

million units of benzathine penicillin G intramuscularly once a month.

Mildly symptomatic patients should be treated with diuretics and sodium restriction (see Chapter 61 for a detailed discussion of the treatment of heart failure). Digitalis, since it does not affect the hemodynamic abnormality, is not useful in this situation unless rapid atrial fibrillation or flutter develops. The treatment of atrial fibrillation is discussed in detail in Chapter 59, but it should be recognized that there is a 1 to 2% incidence of systemic thromboembolism at the time of conversion of atrial fibrillation to normal sinus rhythm in patients with mitral stenosis. The conversion, whether pharmacological or electrical, should be done in the hospital. Patients with persistent sinus tachycardia who are not in heart failure may safely be treated with propranolol (10 to 40 mg, four times a day) to lower their heart rate.

Warfarin anticoagulants should be administered to patients with mild mitral stenosis who have had one or more episodes of systemic or pulmonary thromboembolism (see Chapter 51), who are in atrial fibrillation, or who have echocardiographic evidence of left atrial enlargement. All patients with moderate or severe mitral stenosis should be anticoagulated.

Table 60.8 lists the reasons to refer patients with mitral stenosis to a cardiologist. In general referral is indicated to confirm the diagnosis, to assess the severity of the process, and to consider whether or not to recommend operative repair or replacement of the mitral valve. The cardiologist is likely to perform a cardiac catheterization to measure the size of the mitral orifice and to decide whether to recommend surgery for a patient with moderate or severe stenosis. However, the age of the patient, the presence of severe noncardiac disease, and the presence of other cardiac lesions (e.g., severe ischemic heart disease) will influence the recommendation. Patients with pulmonary hypertension or evidence

Table 60.8.
Indications for Referral of Patients with Mitral Stenosis[a]

Progressive dyspnea or recurrent attacks of pulmonary edema
Symptomatic disease of the aortic and/or tricuspid valve
Women, whether symptomatic or not, who wish to become pregnant
Patients whose symptoms have developed recently who have no history of rheumatic fever (to rule out an atrial myxoma)
Patients with chronic obstructive lung disease
Patients with angina pectoris
Patients with evidence of pulmonary hypertension (including right ventricular hypertrophy)

[a] Modified from Brandenburg RO, Fuster V, Guiliani ER: Valvular heart disease. When should the patient be referred? *Practical Cardiol* 5:50, 1979 (2).

of right ventricular hypertrophy should be referred even if asymptomatic.

The relatively poor prognosis of medically treated patients with progressive disease (see "Natural History and Symptoms" above) dictates that such patients, unless there are specific contraindications, should be offered surgery. The preferred procedure will depend on the anatomy of the valve at the time of operation. If possible a *mitral commissurotomy* will be performed. The operative mortality of this procedure is low (1 to 3%), and the long term results are excellent for a number of years. However, after commissurotomy, 10% of patients within 5 years and 60% within 10 years require reoperation because of restenosis or because of the development of symptomatic mitral regurgitation or of symptomatic aortic stenosis (10). If a prosthetic valve is implanted, the operative mortality is 3 to 10%; the course of patients who survive surgery depends on a number of factors (see below, page 765), but certainly is better than that of symptomatic patients treated medically.

Aortic Regurgitation (7)

An incompetent aortic valve allows regurgitation into the left ventricle of blood ejected into the aorta. In order to compensate for the increased volume load, the left ventricle dilates and hypertrophies so that the effective stroke volume may for a long time be normal. Eventually, however, the left ventricle cannot maintain the work load, and clinical signs and symptoms of heart failure ensue.

Etiology and Epidemiology

Aortic regurgitation may be due to disease of the aortic valve cusps and/or to dilation of the aortic root.

Rheumatic fever is still the most common cause of chronic aortic valvular incompetence, although it now accounts for many fewer cases than it did 20 to 30 years ago. Bacterial endocarditis is the most common cause of acute aortic valvular incompetence. Congenital aortic valvular incompetence or traumatic rupture of a cusp of the aortic valve is relatively uncommon.

Chronic aortic regurgitation due to dilation of the aortic root is most commonly due to syphilitic aortitis (see Chaper 30), although, again, the incidence has dropped considerably. Other, relatively rare, causes include rheumatoid arthritis, ankylosing spondylitis, Reiter's syndrome, and congenital disorders of connective tissue (Marfan's syndrome, Ehlers-Danlos syndrome, and osteogenesis imperfecta). Acute aortic regurgitation due to dilation of the aortic root is most commonly due to a dissecting aneurysm—usually associated with medial necrosis of the aorta. Dissection is associated with systemic hypertension in approximately 50% of cases. Occa-

sionally a primary disorder of connective tissue, such as Marfan's syndrome, can be incriminated.

Aortic regurgitation in general is more common in men than women, but there are specific exceptions (rheumatoid arthritis, for example).

Natural History and Symptoms

Patients with *chronic aortic regurgitation* remain asymptomatic sometimes for up to 20 years or have only mild dyspnea on exertion. When symptoms do develop (progressively more severe dyspnea, orthopnea, paroxysmal nocturnal dyspnea and, less often, angina), they reflect an ominous deterioration in the condition.

Patients with *acute aortic regurgitation* develop fulminant pulmonary edema because of the inability of the left ventricle to compensate for the sudden volume load and for the abrupt rise in left ventricular end-diastolic pressure. Marked dyspnea and weakness may be experienced virtually overnight and in most cases within 2 or 3 months. Other symptoms depend on the underlying cause: fever, for example, if it is endocarditis; severe pain in the chest or back, if it is a dissecting aneurysm.

Physical Findings

Patients with *chronic aortic regurgitation* have a characteristic high frequency early diastolic decrescendo murmur, best heard at the aortic area and at the left sternal border. The duration (but not the intensity) of the murmur correlates with the severity of the lesion so that the murmur is holodiastolic in patients with severe aortic regurgitation. Often there is an accompanying harsh systolic ejection murmur as well, heard at the base of the heart. Severe aortic regurgitation may also cause a loud apical diastolic murmur (the Austin Flint murmur), simulating the murmur of mitral stenosis. Unlike the situation in true mitral stenosis, however, S_1 in patients with aortic regurgitation is sometimes soft, the result of premature closure of the mitral valve, and there is no opening snap. If aortic regurgitation is moderate or severe, the pulse pressure is ordinarily wide, reflecting peripheral vasodilation. The combination of an increased systolic pressure and a reduced diastolic pressure (sometimes as low as 30 mm Hg) produces characteristic changes in the peripheral pulse (waterhammer pulse, "pistol-shot" sounds heard over the femoral artery, etc) and a typical bobbing of the head with each heartbeat.

Patients with *acute aortic regurgitation* often show signs of left- and right-sided heart failure. The regurgitant diastolic murmur is lower pitched and shorter than it is in patients with chronic aortic incompetence; S_1 is often absent and S_3, uncommon with chronic regurgitation, is usually present. The pulse pressure is normal—the result of intense peripheral vasoconstriction.

Laboratory Findings

Electrocardiogram. The ECG also reflects the severity and duration of aortic regurgitation. Patients with chronic disease show the ECG pattern of left ventricular hypertrophy (Fig. 60.2 and Table 60.3), whereas patients with acute disease do not (although they commonly do show nonspecific ST-T wave changes).

Chest X-ray. The size of the heart in patients with aortic regurgitation depends on the duration and severity of the disease. Patients with chronic severe disease have very large left ventricles, but patients with acute regurgitation may have no cardiac enlargement at all.

Echocardiogram. Echocardiography is useful in the assessment of left ventricular function, the degree of hypertrophy of the left ventricle, and of the degree of dilation of the aortic root. Fluttering of the anterior leaflet of the mitral valve during diastole is characteristic of moderate to severe aortic regurgitation and also indicates mobility of the mitral valve (a useful sign in ruling out significant mitral stenosis). Premature mitral valve closure is helpful in confirming very severe aortic regurgitation.

Management

Asymptomatic patients need not be treated, but should be assessed once or twice a year by interval history, physical examination, and chest X-ray. Yearly ECGs and echocardiograms should also be obtained. Prophylaxis for bacterial endocarditis is indicated when patients are to undergo dental or surgical procedures (Chapter 86).

If symptoms of heart failure develop, digitalis and diuretics should be prescribed. Also afterload reducing agents may be effective in otherwise unresponsive patients (see Chapter 61).

Table 60.9 lists the reasons to refer patients with aortic regurgitation to a cardiologist. In general, referral is indicated in patients with chronic disease to confirm the diagnosis and to consider whether or not to recommend aortic valve replacement for

Table 60.9.
Indications for Referral of Patients with Aortic Regurgitation[a]

Uncertainty about the diagnosis
Symptomatic chronic aortic incompetence (dyspnea, fatigue, angina)
Acute aortic incompetence
Asymptomatic patients with evidence of severe chronic aortic incompetence: widened pulse pressure, holodiastolic murmur, left ventricular hypertrophy, progressive cardiac enlargement

[a] Modified from Brandenburg RO, Fuster V, Guiliani ER: Valvular heart disease. When should the patient be referred? *Practical Cardiol* 5:50, 1979 (2).

symptomatic patients and for asymptomatic patients with physical findings of severe disease (widened pulse pressure, holodiastolic murmur, increasing left ventricular enlargement). All patients with suspected acute aortic regurgitation should be seen by a cardiologist as soon as possible. The cardiologist is likely to perform cardiac catheterization (see Chapter 57) to assess the severity of the lesion, the presence of other valvular disease, and the function of the left ventricle. Recently radionuclide angiography has provided the cardiologist with a convenient noninvasive technique for making these measurements easily (see Chapter 61).

Patients with chronic aortic regurgitation do well until they become symptomatic. Thereafter, 50% of patients are dead within 2 years (15). Thus, valve replacement is warranted in all symptomatic patients, preferably before severe left ventricular dysfunction develops. The operative mortality is 5 to 10%, but of the patients who survive surgery, 50% live 10 years or more (24) and their quality of life is usually significantly improved (see below).

The Patient with a Prosthetic Valve

Although patients usually demonstrate clear improvement in symptoms and prognosis after valve replacement, they should not be considered cured. Despite refinements in design, no valve currently available is free of potential serious complications, which, since they may occur many years after surgery, dictate careful long term follow-up of all patients who have prosthetic valves.

Many varieties of mechanical and tissue valves have been developed. The most commonly used mechanical valves are the Starr Edwards ball-in-cage series, the Bjork-Shiley tilting disk valve, and most recently, the St. Jude valve, which has two semicircular tilting leaflets. The most common tissue valves are the Hancock and Carpentier-Edwards valves which are constructed of porcine aortic valve leaflets that have been fixed in glutaraldehyde.

Potential Complications

Thromboembolic phenomena are perhaps the most frequent life-threatening complications of prosthetic valves and may present as sudden stroke, myocardial infarction, or peripheral arterial occlusion. Alternatively, thrombus may accumulate around the valve ring and prevent proper valve motion, resulting in gradual or sudden obstruction of flow and the development of severe congestive heart failure. Thomboembolic events have been more common with prosthetic valves in the mitral than in the aortic position, and they are much more frequent with the mechanical valves than with the tissue valves (4). Despite treatment with full anticoagulation, the incidence of thromboembolic complications with most mechanical valves is about 1 to

2%/year. The incidence is lower with the newer St. Jude valve.

Perivalvular leakage resulting in regurgitation occasionally develops in the postoperative period and may require reoperation.

Prosthetic valve endocarditis develops in 2 to 3% of patients (27) and may present as a febrile illness, a new murmur of valvular regurgitation or stenosis, hemodynamic deterioration, or embolization. Because the infection is at the site of a foreign body, the prognosis for recovery with standard antibiotic therapy is worse than in native valve endocarditis. Recurrence after one trial of medical therapy is generally an indication for replacement of the valve. Prognosis is worse in infections that develop within 60 days of surgery (72% mortality), in which contamination may have occurred at operation, than in those that develop later (45% mortality), where transient bacteremia may be the source of infection.

As long term follow-up data accumulate, late valvular degeneration may become a significant problem after tissue valve implantation. Histological studies have revealed fibrin deposition, tears in the leaflets, and calcification that commonly results in some degree of valvular stenosis (13) and/or regurgitation 5 to 10 years after operation. In some cases where clinical deterioration occurs, reoperation is required. This process is greatly accelerated in children, but also occurs commonly in young adults (age less than 35).

Physical and Laboratory Findings

Auscultatory findings after valve replacement are variable. In general, the ball-in-cage valves produce loud opening and closing clicks. In the aortic position, therefore, there is a prominent systolic "ejection" click, and S_2 is loud and metallic. In the mitral position, S_1 is loud and there is a prominent systolic opening click after S_2, which is similar in timing to the opening snap of mitral stenosis. With the Bjork-Shiley valve the closing sounds are loud but the opening sounds are variable. Porcine valves are the most physiological, and like a native valve, the closing sounds are audible but opening sounds are rare. All valves in either position produce systolic ejection murmurs. Diastolic flow murmurs are common with the Bjork-Shiley valve in the mitral position.

It is important to document the baseline physical examination repeatedly so that the significance of any changes that occur in association with new symptoms can be assessed. The most reliable sign of prosthetic valve dysfunction is the loss or muffling of the opening and closing clicks. New regurgitant murmurs may occur. Congestive heart failure may develop.

The two-dimensional echocardiogram may show abnormal, delayed, or intermittent leaflet motion. Changes from previous studies are helpful so all patients should have a baseline echocardiogram after valve replacement. Tissue valves are well visualized and can be readily assessed by echocardiography. However mechanical valves are usually not well seen, and most of the signs of mechanical valve dysfunction are neither sensitive nor specific. The new technique of Doppler echocardiography (see above, pages 752 to 753) is extremely helpful (28) in accurately detecting and quantifying new valve gradients and regurgitation.

Management

Management of the patient with a prosthetic valve should begin before the valve is implanted; the selection of the proper type of valve for the individual patient is crucial. A tissue valve is most appropriate for the patient who is likely to be noncompliant with anticoagulation or who is at high risk for bleeding complications. This includes alcoholics; patients with psychiatric problems, unexplained syncope, or previous gastrointestinal bleeds; the elderly; and patients whose occupation puts them at high risk of injury. Women of childbearing age who desire future pregnancies should receive tissue valves (see below), but they should be made aware that valve replacement may have to be repeated in 8 to 10 years. Young men, or women who do not anticipate pregnancy and who will tolerate anticoagulation may be better off with the more durable mechanical valves so that reoperation may not be necessary (the ball-in-cage valves, the oldest type in current use, have lasted up to 20 years). These decisions are usually made by the cardiac surgeon after discussing the options with the patient, but it is important that the practitioner communicate his opinions to the surgeon well in advance.

All patients with mechanical valves in the aortic or mitral position must be fully anticoagulated with Coumadin indefinitely (see Chapter 51). Antiplatelet agents (see Chapter 51) are not adequate to prevent thromboembolic complications. If an elective surgical procedure is planned, Coumadin may be safely discontinued 3 days prior to surgery and resumed afterward. Reversal of anticoagulation with vitamin K is not recommended.

Patients with tissue valves in the aortic position should be anticoagulated for 6 weeks after operation only, so that endothelialization of the valve may occur. Coumadin should then be discontinued. There is controversy over whether tissue valves in the mitral position require long term anticoagulation. Most cardiologists would not anticoagulate indefinitely unless atrial fibrillation is present, left atrial enlargement is detected on echocardiogram (a common finding in mitral valve disease), or a previous thromboembolic episode has occurred. Strict antibiotic prophylaxis against endocarditis is indicated. Table 86.9 (page 1243) lists regimens recommended by the American Heart Association before and after various procedures. Note, however, that parenteral rather than oral regimens should always be used in patients with prosthetic valves, and that streptomycin or another aminoglycoside should be added for procedures involving the mouth or respiratory tract.

Prosthetic valve dysfunction is an indication for referral to a cardiologist, who will usually recommend cardiac catheterization (see Table 60.10 for all of the reasons to refer a patient with a prosthetic valve to a cardiologist).

Pregnancy in a patient with a prosthetic valve. Pregnancy poses a serious problem in patients with mechanical prosthetic valves. The ingestion of Coumadin during pregnancy results in a definite increase in the incidence of fetal death and birth defects (see Chapter 51). The spontaneous abortion rate is approximately 30%, probably because Coumadin crosses the placenta barrier and predisposes the fetus to intrauterine hemorrhage. Between 8 and 16% of the liveborn infants will have various birth defects, most commonly nasal hypoplasia with stippled epiphysis (a specific Coumadin embryopathy), but including optic atrophy, microcephaly, and mental retardation.

On the other hand, the risk of thromboembolism is greater during pregnancy, and discontinuation of anticoagulation greatly increases the danger of systemic embolism. In one recent study (23) systemic embolism was seen in 31% of such patients despite antiplatelet therapy. Most of the patients had Starr-Edwards valves.

There is no consensus of opinion regarding the management of early pregnancy when a prosthetic valve is in place. Some authors have recommended substituting full dose heparin, which does not cross the placenta, for Coumadin during the first trimester of pregnancy. However, such therapy requires prolonged hospitalization and the incidence of fetal death appears to be high with this regimen as well (see Chapter 51). In our institution many pregnant patients with prosthetic valves are treated with low dose subcutaneous heparin, which the patient learns to administer herself. The safety and efficacy of this regimen are not clearly established (see Chapter 51). Many clinicians strongly counsel patients with prosthetic valves to avoid pregnancy. Patients with prosthetic valves, especially the mechanical valves, should be well aware of the risks if pregnancy is contemplated.

The proper management of anticoagulation at the end of pregnancy is more clearly defined. If Coumadin has been given, it should be replaced by heparin 2 weeks before delivery is expected. Heparin can then be stopped at the onset of labor, to prevent peripartum hemorrhage.

The best approach to these problems is to urge the surgeon to place a tissue valve rather than a mechanical valve in every patient in whom future pregnancy is possible.

Table 60.10.

Indications for Referral of Patients with Prosthetic Valves

Progressive symptoms of congestive heart failure
Progressive cardiac enlargement
Change in prosthetic heart sounds
Pregnancy, or the desire to become pregnant
Embolization
Endocarditis

General References

Braunwald E (ed): *Heart Disease: A Textbook of Cardiovascular Medicine*, ed 2. Philadelphia, WB Saunders, 1984.
 Encyclopedic review of cardiac physical examination, heart sounds, and cardiac graphic techniques.
Constant J: *Bedside Cardiology*. Boston, Little, Brown, 1976.
 The best teaching text for understanding the physiological basis of heart sounds and how to hear and describe them.
Tavel ME: The systolic murmur—innocent or guilty? *Am J Cardiol* 39:757, 1977.
 Concise characterization of the most commonly heard murmur in an ambulatory practice.

Specific References

1. Barnett JHM, Boughner DR, Taylor DW, et al: Further evidence relating mitral valve prolapse to cerebral ischemic events. *N Engl J Med* 302:139, 1980.
2. Brandenburg RO, Fuster V, Guiliani ER: Valvular heart disease. When should the patient be referred? *Practical Cardiol* 5:50, 1979.
3. Braunwald E: Mitral regurgitation: physiologic, clinical, and surgical considerations. *N Engl J Med* 281:425, 1969.
4. Cohn LH, Koster GK, Mee RBB, Collins JJ Jr.: Long term followup of the Hancock Bioprosthetic Heart Valve. A six-year review. *Circulation* 60 (suppl 2):93, 1979.
5. Craig RJ, Selzer A: Natural history and prognosis of atrial septal defect. *Circulation* 37:805, 1968.
6. Devereux RB, Perloff JK, Reichels N, Josephson ME: Mitral valve prolapse. *Circulation* 54:3, 1976.
7. Goldschlager N, Pfeifer J, Cohn K, et al: The natural history of aortic regurgitation. A clinical and hemodynamic study. *Am J Med* 54:577, 1973.
8. Gooch AS, Vicencio F, Markanlov V, Goldberg H: Arrhythmias and left ventricular asynergy in the prolapsing mitral leaflet syndrome. *Am J Cardiol* 29:611, 1972.
9. Hammermeister KE, Fisher L, Kennedy JW, et al: Prediction of late survival in patients with mitral valve disease from clinical, hemodynamic, and quantitative angiographic variables. *Circulation* 57:341, 1978.
10. Heger JJ, Wann LS, Weyman AE, et al: Long-term changes in mitral valve area after successful mitral commissurotomy. *Circulation* 59:443, 1979.
11. Horan LG, Flowers NC: Electrocardiography and vectorcardiography. In Braunwald E (ed): *Heart Disease: A Textbook of Cardiovascular Medicine*. Philadelphia, WB Saunders, 1980.
12. Leachman RD, Cokkinos DV, Cooley DA: Association of ostium secundum atrial septal defects with mitral valve prolapse. *Am J Cardiol* 38:167, 1976.
13. Lipson LC, Kent KM, Rosing DR, et al: Long term hemodynamic assessment of the porcine heterograft in the mitral position. Late development of valvular stenosis. *Circulation* 64:397, 1981.
14. Markiewicz W, Stoner J, London E, et al: Mitral valve prolapse in one hundred presumably healthy young men. *Circulation* 53:464, 1976.
15. Massell BF, Ameccua FJ, Czohiczer G: Prognosis of patients with pure or predominant aortic regurgitation in the absence

of surgery. *Circulation* 34 (suppl 2):164, 1966.

16. Mills P, Rose J, Hollingsworth J, *et al*: Long-term prognosis of mitral-valve prolapse. *N Engl J Med* 297:13, 1977.

17. Munoz S, Gallardo J, Diaz-Gorrin JR, Medina O: Influence of surgery on the natural history of rheumatic mitral and aortic valve disease. *Am J Cardiol* 35:234, 1975.

18. Oleson KH: The nautral history of 271 patients with mitral stenosis under medical treatment *Br Heart J* 24:349, 1962.

19. Popp RL, Rubenson DS, Tucker LR, French JW: Echocardiography: M mode and two-dimensional methods. *Ann Intern Med* 93:844, 1980.

20. Rapaport E: Natural history of aortic and mitral valve disease. *Am J Cardiol* 35:221, 1981.

21. Roberts WC: Anatomically isolated aortic valve disease: a case against its being of rheumatic etiology. *Am J Med* 49:151, 1970.

22. Ross J Jr, Braunwald E: Aortic stenosis. *Circulation* 38 (suppl 5):61, 1968.

23. Salazar E, Zajarias A, Gutierrez N, Iturbe I: The problems of cardiac valve prostheses, anticoagulants and pregnancy. *Circulation* 70 (suppl 1):169, 1984.

24. Samuels DA, Curfman GD, Friedlich AL, *et al*: Valve replacement for aortic regurgitation: long-term follow-up with factors influencing the results. *Circulation* 60:647, 1979.

25. Selzer A, Cohn K: Natural history of mitral stenosis: a review. *Circulation* 45:878, 1972.

26. Shah PM, Adelman AG, Wigle ED, *et al*: The natural (and unnatural) history of hypertrophic obstructive cardiomyopathy. *Circ Res* 34 (suppl 2):179, 1974.

27. Watanakunakorn C: Prosthetic valve endocarditis. *Prog Cardiovasc Dis* 22:181, 1979.

28. Weinstein IR, Marbarger JP, Pérez JE: Ultrasonic assessment of the St. Jude prosthetic valve: M-mode, two dimensional, and Doppler echocardiography. *Circulation* 68:897, 1983.

CHAPTER SIXTY-ONE

Heart Failure

SHELDON H. GOTTLIEB, M.D.

DEFINITION

The amount of blood which the heart pumps per minute (the *cardiac output*) is normally precisely adjusted to the metabolic needs of the body. The cardiac output may increase by 2 or 3 times as an individual goes from sleep to exercise. An increase in cardiac output may occur within the space of one heartbeat by a sudden decrease in vagal tone which causes an increase in *heart rate*. After several seconds of exercise, sympathetic tone increases, which causes a further increase in cardiac output by increasing the heart rate and the amount of blood pumped per heart beat (the *stroke volume*). The increased cardiac output soon brings about an increase in the amount of blood returning to the right side of the heart (the *venous return*); also the heart further increases its output in response to the stretch in the heart muscle resulting from the increased volume of venous return (the *Frank-Starling* prin-

ciple). If the heart is not able to pump enough blood to meet the metabolic needs of the body, compensatory mechanisms are brought into play by the heart, kidney, lung, and peripheral vascular system. These adjustments cause symptoms and signs recognized as the syndrome of *heart failure. Acute heart failure,* manifest usually by pulmonary edema (recognized by the abrupt onset of extreme breathlessness and evidence of alveolar edema by physical and radiological examination), warrants immediate hospitalization for diagnosis of the underlying and/or precipitating cause and for treatment. However, *chronic heart failure* is usually a problem that can be managed in an ambulatory setting.

EPIDEMIOLOGY OF HEART FAILURE

The *incidence* of heart failure is approximately 0.3/1000/year below age 45, remains constant at approximately 3/1000/year in the middle-age groups, and increases to 8/1000 in patients above the age of 70 (13). The incidence among men is approximately twice that among women (13).

The *prevalence* of heart failure increases greatly in patients above 60 years old (Fig. 61.1). Above the age of 70, women with congestive heart failure outnumber men. This is true in spite of the higher incidence in men and probably reflects the earlier mortality among men from coronary artery disease. Estimates of the prevalence rate for heart failure in patients above the age of 65 vary from approximately 20 to 65/1000 (8).

PHYSIOLOGY OF HEART FAILURE

The Heart as a Pump

Length Tension Relation: Frank-Starling Mechanism and Preload

As heart muscle is stretched, it develops increased tension. The relationship of length to tension defines the *compliance* of heart muscle; the inverse of compliance is *stiffness*. If the ventricle is distended with blood, pressure is developed within the cavity. A higher pressure is needed to distend the ventricle to a given volume in a less compliant, *i.e.*, stiffer, ventricle. The pressure needed to stretch the ventricle to a given end-diastolic volume is called the *preload*, or left ventricular end-diastolic pressure (LVEDP).

The relationship between the volume of the ventricle just prior to contraction and the force developed during contraction defines the *Frank-Starling law of the heart.* If the LVEDP is plotted against *stroke work* (the stroke volume times the mean blood pressure), a *ventricular function curve* is defined (Fig. 61.2). It can be seen from this relationship that the normal ventricle is compliant and will develop an adequate amount of force during contraction with a relatively low preload. However, the failing ventricle requires a high preload in order to increase its stroke work (Fig. 61.2). The implications of this relationship are discussed below.

Afterload

Afterload is the dynamic resistance against which the heart contracts. It determines the degree of stress within the myocardium. Systolic blood pressure closely approximates and is clinically the most useful indicator of afterload. Afterload determines the ease or speed of ventricular contraction and hence the *ejection fraction* (that portion of the ventricular volume that is ejected with each beat) (Fig. 61.3).

Contractility and Inotropic State

The relationship of preload to stroke work defines the *functional state* of cardiac muscle (see above).

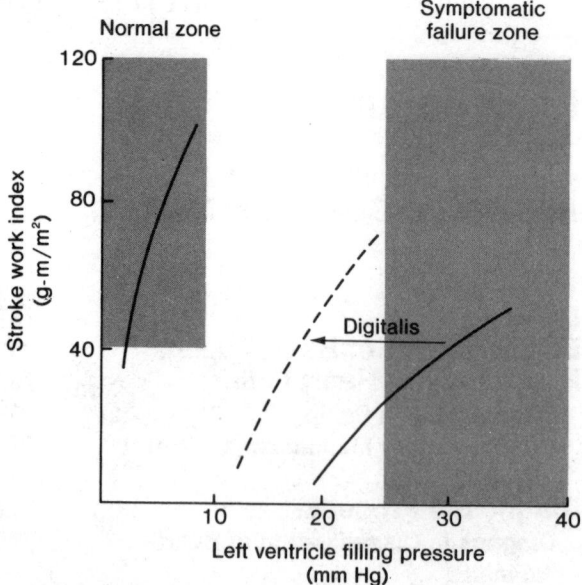

Figure 61.2. Ventricular function curves showing the relationship between left ventricular filling pressures and stroke work. The relative position of the curve defines the *inotropic state* of the heart. Note that for a given curve, *i.e.*, a given inotropic state, the *function* of the heart, or the amount of work the heart is capable of performing, varies with the left ventricular filling pressure. (Adapted from Weisfeldt ML: Congestive heart failure: pathophysiology and the evaluation of ventricular function. In Harvey AM, Johns RJ, McKusick VA, *et al* (eds): *The Principles and Practice of Medicine.* New York, Appleton-Century-Crofts, 1984.)

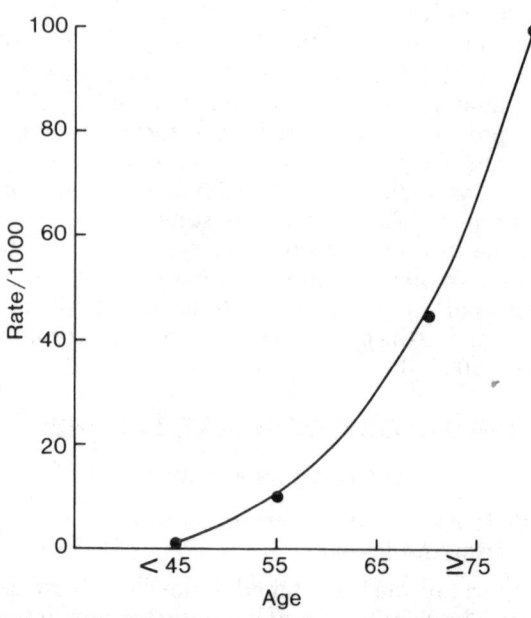

Figure 61.1. The prevalence of heart failure reported from physicians' offices as a function of patient age. Note the marked increase in the sixth and seventh decades. Between 10 and 20% of patients older than age 60 followed regularly by a physician will have a history of heart failure. (From McKee P, Castelli W, McNamara P, Kannel W: The natural history of congestive heart failure: the Framingham study. *N Engl J Med* 285:1441, 1971.)

The relative position of the curve defines the *inotropic state* of the muscle (see Fig. 61.2). For example, infusing the heart with an inotropic substance such as digitalis causes the ventricular function curve to shift to the left, to perform a higher stroke work at a given preload. In other words, the *contractility* of the heart is increased.

Interrelationship between Preload, Afterload, and Inotropic State

The interrelationship between the preload, afterload, and inotropic state is summarized in Figure 61.3 (see also reference 16). If preload is kept constant, an increase in afterload will cause a depression in ventricular function. Thus, if afterload or blood pressure increases, ventricular function or ejection fraction decreases. That causes the ventricular end-diastolic volume, or preload, to increase, restoring the ventricular function to baseline. A further increase in afterload leads to a further depression in ventricular function, which again may be restored by increasing preload, *i.e.*, by increasing left ventricular end-diastolic pressure. Eventually, a limit is reached beyond which preload cannot be

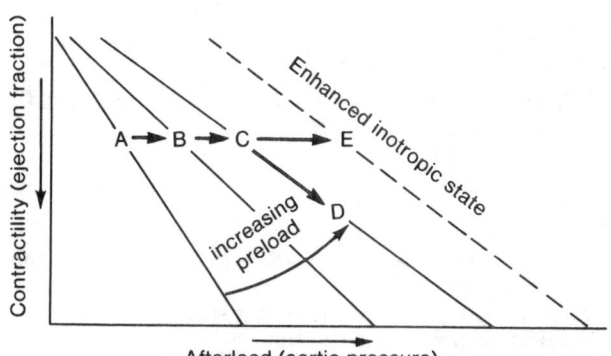

Figure 61.3. The interrelationship between preload, afterload, and inotropic state. The three *solid lines* are a family of curves at different levels of preload but with inotropic state kept constant. Taken together, they represent *ventricular function* as a function of both *preload* and *afterload*. Note that if preload is kept constant, an increase in afterload will cause a decrease in *contractility* as measured by the *ejection fraction*, but that when afterload is decreased to 0, the curves converge, because the *inotropic state* of the muscle is unchanged. As afterload increases, contractility may be maintained by increasing preload (shifting from *point A* to *B* to *C*). When preload reaches the point (*C*) at which an increase will cause pulmonary congestion, (the *preload reserve*) any further increase in afterload will decrease contractility (*point C* to *D*). Contractility may then be increased only by measures, such as digitalization, which enhance the inotropic state (*point D* to *E*). Patients are most sensitive to changes in afterload when their filling pressures are at the preload reserve. (Adapted from Ross J Jr: Afterload mismatch and preload reserve: a conceptual framework for the analysis of ventricular function. *Prog Cardiovasc Dis* 18:255, 1976.)

increased, as noted on the figure. This is the left ventricular filling pressure, the *preload reserve*, above which the pulmonary capillary oncotic pressure is exceeded, fluid passes into the alveoli, and pulmonary congestion occurs. Any increase in afterload which occurs when the preload reserve is reached will cause a decrease in ventricular function. The preload reserve varies with the compliance of the ventricle. If heart muscle is made stiffer or less compliant by a chronic disease process such as hypertension or aortic stenosis, or by an acute process such as ischemia, a higher filling pressure will be necessary to set the level of ventricular function by means of the Frank-Starling principle; and the preload reserve will be reached sooner. The only way to improve ventricular function when the preload reserve is reached is either to decrease the afterload or to change the inotropic state, or contractility, of the muscle. The clinical significance of these interrelationships will be discussed at greater length under "Management."

Biochemical Basis for Decreased Contractility in the Failing Heart

The contractile unit of heart muscle is the sarcomere, which consists of fibers of protein called *actin* and *myosin*. Actin and myosin interact with each other by interlocking protein cross bridges called *troponin*. The interlocking mechanism is facilitated by adenosine triphosphate (ATP) and magnesium. An inhibitory protein, *tropomyosin*, is present on the myosin fibers. Tropomyosin inhibits the interaction between actin and myosin and allows the muscle to relax. Calcium inhibits the tropomyosin complex, frees the troponin cross-bridges, and allows actin and myosin to interact and to develop tension. Calcium is therefore necessary for myocardial contraction to take place. Large amounts of calcium are stored within the heart in a distinctive network of *sarcoplasmic reticulum*. *Excitation contraction coupling* takes place in heart muscle when an action potential, *via* mechanisms not yet understood, causes a release of calcium from the sarcoplasmic reticulum, thereby initiating contraction. In heart failure, there appears to be decreased energy available for cardiac contraction and slow transport of calcium into the sarcoplasmic reticulum following contraction, leading to a delay in relaxation of cardiac muscle. Clinically this is noted as an increase in resistance to filling or, in other words, the *diastolic compliance* of the myocardium is reduced in heart failure.

Compensatory Mechanisms in Heart Failure

Heart Rate

If stroke volume remains constant, an increase in heart rate will cause a proportionate increase in cardiac output in patients in heart failure.

Hypertrophy and Dilation

Left ventricular hypertrophy and dilation may allow compensation to be achieved for many years. The stress in the wall of the heart varies with the radius of the ventricular cavity. If the heart is subjected to a volume load, it dilates in order to accommodate the load and to increase its ability to eject the load (the Frank-Starling principle—see above). However, ventricular dilation causes an increase in ventricular wall stress, which serves as a stimulus to ventricular hypertrophy. The hypertrophy is *eccentric*, so-called because it causes the left heart border to move laterally. Eventually the heart becomes both dilated and hypertrophied and the ratio of wall thickness to cavity size returns to normal, which returns wall stress to normal; therefore a state of compensated ventricular dilation is achieved. The response to a pressure overload is different. An increase in wall stress in the absence of volume overload leads to *concentric* hypertrophy; wall stress per unit area returns to normal but the cavity size is unchanged.

Redistribution of Cardiac Output in Heart Failure

There is a marked increase in peripheral vascular resistance in heart failure, and that causes a redistribution of cardiac output. In less severe failure, where the resting cardiac output is normal, redistribution occurs only during exercise. In severe heart failure, where the resting cardiac output is significantly decreased, redistribution occurs at rest. The decrease in blood flow is most marked in the kidneys and the skin. Decreased renal blood flow causes a release of *renin* from the juxtaglomerular apparatus and therefore plasma *angiotensin* activity is increased. Angiotensin is a potent vasoconstrictor and acts both directly on smooth muscle and indirectly by increasing release of norepinephrine from vascular nerve endings. The increase in angiotensin activity leads to an increase in aldosterone production, which causes an increase in sodium resorption from the distal tubule of the nephron, thereby increasing plasma volume. The renal resorption of sodium is also facilitated by the decrease in cardiac output and in glomerular filtration rate, which causes an increase in the fraction of sodium resorbed in the proximal tubule of the nephron.

DIAGNOSTIC PROCESS

There is no one symptom, sign, or laboratory test which is pathognomonic of heart failure. Diagnosis must therefore be based on a process of clinical inference. The significance of symptoms and signs must be evaluated with regard to the patient's overall condition and to where the patient appears to be in the natural history of his disease. In ambulatory practice, a patient will often present to a new physician with the diagnosis of "heart failure" and will be taking medicine for this condition. In this situation, the physician should satisfy himself that the diagnosis of heart failure is correct before accepting it and maintaining treatment.

Diagnostic Classification of Heart Failure

Etiology of Heart Failure

When the diagnosis of heart failure is made, it is essential to decide upon the most likely etiology, since the prognosis and the treatment of heart failure vary greatly depending upon its cause.

Heart failure is due to one of three basic mechanisms: an increased work load to which the heart cannot accommodate; a disorder of the myocardium so that it is unable to accommodate normal work loads; or a restriction of ventricular filling so that an adequate stroke volume cannot be achieved. Table 61.1 lists selected examples of these conditions. In this country systemic hypertension is the most com-

Table 61.1.
Causes of Heart Failure[a]

INCREASED WORK LOAD TO WHICH THE HEART CANNOT ACCOMMODATE
  High output states:
    Hyperthyroidism[b]
    Anemia[b]
    Systemic arteriovenous fistulas[b]
    Certain dermatological disorders (*e.g.*, psoriasis, erythroderma)[b]
  Valvular regurgitation or left to right shunts[b]
  Increased impedance to ejection:
    Systemic hypertension[b]
    Pulmonary hypertension
    Pulmonic or aortic stenosis[b]
DISORDER OF MYOCARDIUM SO THAT THE HEART IS UNABLE TO ACCOMMODATE NORMAL WORK LOADS
  Cardiomyopathies
  Myocardial infarction
RESTRICTION OF VENTRICULAR FILLING
  Pericardial constriction or effusion[b]
  Mitral and tricuspid valvular stenosis[b]
  Increased ventricular stiffness:
    Infiltrative myocardial disease (*e.g.*, amyloid)
    Ventricular hypertrophy
    Hypertrophic cardiomyopathy

[a] Adapted from Weisfeldt ML: Congestive heart failure: pathophysiology and the evaluation of ventricular function. In Harvey AM, Johns RJ, McKusick VA, *et al* (eds): *The Principles and Practice of Medicine.* New York, Appleton-Century-Crofts, 1984.
[b] Indicates causes of heart failure which are potentially treatable by specific therapy.

mon condition associated with heart failure (75% of cases), followed by ischemic heart disease, with or without hypertension (40% of cases) (8).

The most common precipitating causes of heart failure (Table 61.2) are noncompliance with medication or diet in a patient with previously compensated heart failure, acute myocardial infarction, and uncontrolled hypertension. In patients for whom the precipitating cause is not obvious, it is important to consider arrhythmia (Chapter 59) and pulmonary embolism (Chapter 53). In addition, it is important to inquire about psychosocial stress, which has been shown to precede the onset of symptoms in as many as 50% of patients hospitalized for heart failure (15).

Functional Classification of Heart Failure

The amount of exercise which a patient can perform without symptoms of heart failure determines his *functional class.* The functional classification scheme of the New York Heart Association is useful in categorizing patients (Table 61.3). Correctable disease may be present despite severe symptoms so that the functional classification provides useful prognostic information only within selected subsets of patients. Functional class is best determined by questioning the patient regarding his performance

Table 61.2.
Precipitating Causes of Heart Failure

FACTORS DECREASING MYOCARDIAL EFFICIENCY
  Myocardial infarction
  Ischemia
  Arrhythmia
  Hypoxia
  Alcohol and other toxic substances
  Recent initiation of a β-blocking drug
  Discontinuation of a cardiac glycoside
  Myocardial depressant drugs (*e.g.*, disopyramide (Norpace), adriamycin)
  Pericardial tamponade
  Myocardial infections (*e.g.*, bacterial endocarditis, myocarditis, parasitic infection)
  Vasculitis
FACTORS INCREASING CARDIAC LOAD
  Uncontrolled systemic hypertension
  Noncompliance with low salt diet
  Psychological stress
  Exercise, especially in extremes of heat or humidity
  Discontinuing diuretics, antihypertensive drugs, or afterload reducing agents
  Drugs which retain or contain sodium
  Infection
  Anemia
  Pulmonary embolism
  Thyrotoxicosis
  Acute valvular dysfunction

Table 61.3.
New York Heart Association (NYHA) Functional Classification of Cardiac Patients

Class I: No limitation. Ordinary physical activity does not cause undue fatigue, dyspnea, palpitation, or angina. Prognosis is good.
Class II: Slight limitation of physical activity. Such patients will be comfortable at rest. Ordinary physical activity will result in fatigue, palpitation, dyspnea, or angina. Prognosis is good with therapy.
Class III: Marked limitation of physical activity. Less than ordinary activity will lead to symptoms. Patients are comfortable at rest. Prognosis is fair with therapy.
Class IV: Inability to carry on any physical activity without discomfort. Symptoms of congestive failure or angina will be present even at rest. With any physical activity, increased discomfort is experienced. Prognosis is guarded despite therapy.

during daily activities. For example, a patient may be asked how many stairs he can climb before he has to stop and rest, or how heavy a load he can carry, and what work activities have had to be modified.

History

The most common symptom of heart failure is *dyspnea*. Dyspnea means uncomfortable breathing. It is not the shortness of breath experienced by normal people when they exercise or by anxious people when they hyperventilate (see also Chapter 53). Dyspnea in heart failure is a symptom of increased LVEDP leading to pulmonary venous and capillary congestion. The increase in pulmonary congestion causes an increased stiffness of the lungs and a decrease in the vital capacity. The work of breathing increases and breathing becomes rapid, shallow, and forced.

Orthopnea is dyspnea in the recumbent position. It is frequently experienced by patients with heart failure, although it may also be a symptom of patients with obstructive lung disease or with obesity. Blood normally pools in the lower extremities when a person is upright. When the patient who is in heart failure lies down, there is an increase in venous return to the heart that leads to an increase in pulmonary congestion because of the inability of the compromised left ventricle to accept and to pump the increased load. The severity of orthopnea is assessed by the number of pillows the patient must use to be able to breath comfortably in the recumbent position.

Patients in heart failure with dyspnea and orthopnea often have a dry hacking *cough*; at times this is the patient's most troublesome symptom. The cough usually improves concomitantly with improvement in other symptoms.

Paroxysmal nocturnal dyspnea is characteristic of poorly compensated chronic heart failure. Patients commonly complain of paroxysmal dyspnea approximately 2 hours after falling asleep. It is often associated with bad dreams or nightmares and is relieved by sitting up or by getting out of bed and sitting in a chair. Because the dyspnea often is associated with wheezing, it must be distinguished from the nocturnal shortness of breath sometimes experienced by people with obstructive lung disease (see Chapter 55).

Fatigue is a common complaint of patients in heart failure. It is frequently described as a general sense of weakness or of lassitude. Some patients may complain of fatigue rather than dyspnea. In this setting fatigue is a symptom of low cardiac output, often due to overdiuresis following the aggressive use of potent diuretics.

A history of *edema* and/or *weight gain* (from retention of salt and water) is often elicited from patients in heart failure. Many will also give a history of having taken digitalis in the past for a "heart problem."

Chest pain due to myocardial ischemia is common in patients in heart failure (see Chapter 57). Patients with pre-existing poor left ventricular function may rapidly develop marked left ventricular dysfunction when their hearts become ischemic, or they may develop paroxysmal mitral regurgitation due to acute papillary muscle dysfunction. This may happen in association with exercise in patients with stable ischemic heart disease or may occur paroxysmally and at rest in patients with unstable ischemic heart disease or in patients who may be experiencing spasm of the coronary arteries (see Chapter 57). Paroxysmal dyspnea associated with exercise-induced ischemia is sometimes referred to as an "anginal equivalent." The symptomatic response to nitroglycerin does not by itself differentiate between dyspnea due to ischemia and dyspnea due to chronic congestive heart failure; sublingual nitroglycerin rapidly relieves congestion due to either condition (see below).

Nocturia, a common symptom of heart failure, often occurs early in the illness. It is due to the redistribution in cardiac output that occurs in the recumbent position, restoring in part blood flow to the kidney that, in the upright position, has been diverted to other organs (see above).

Decreased cardiac output by itself or in association with cerebrovascular disease may lead to *impairment in mental function,* ranging from mild confusion to overt psychosis. The most common neuropsychiatric complaints, however, are mild chronic anxiety and depression; these may be the presenting complaints, especially in elderly patients with previously undiagnosed heart failure.

Symptoms of congestion of the gastrointestinal system are common in patients with chronic, poorly compensated heart failure. Chronically increased right heart pressures cause passive congestion of the liver with swelling and discomfort in the right upper quadrant of the abdomen. In extreme cases there will be marked anorexia and weight loss due to gastrointestinal congestion. Some patients may attribute those symptoms to the somewhat unpalatable low salt diet to which they must adhere.

Physical Findings in Heart Failure

The physical findings in heart failure depend upon which compensatory mechanisms are utilized to adjust the cardiac output to the metabolic needs of the body. Findings vary depending upon whether the heart failure is *compensated or uncompensated.*

Uncompensated Heart Failure

In chronic uncompensated or poorly compensated heart failure there will be signs of an attempt at cardiac compensation (increased heart size and heart rate) and signs of increased renin, angiotensin, and aldosterone activity (vascular redistribution and evidence of cardiac, pulmonary and peripheral congestion). Congestion is manifest by a ventricular gallop sound (S_3), rales, jugular venous distention, hepatojugular reflux, and peripheral pitting edema.

Increased heart size may be recognized by inspection, palpation, and percussion of the precordium. The precordium should be palpated with the patient in the supine and in the left lateral position. The location, quality, and size of the point of maximal impulse (PMI) should be noted. The PMI of an eccentrically enlarged heart is displaced laterally and caudally and is heaving and diffuse. The PMI of a concentrically enlarged heart is not displaced but may be thrusting or sustained. The heart border should be percussed, and its position relative to the PMI should be noted.

Sinus tachycardia, defined as a resting heart rate in an adult greater than 100 beats/minute, is a relatively sensitive but nonspecific sign of heart failure; it is a compensatory mechanism to increase cardiac output (see below). *Pulsus alternans,* a regular rhythm in which contractions are successively strong and weak, is most common in patients with increased resistance to left ventricular ejection (e.g., systemic hypertension) and is due to repetitive changes in stroke volume because of incomplete recovery of contractibility by the failing heart.

The second pulmonic sound (P_2) is often accentuated in patients in left ventricular failure, because of increased pulmonary artery pressure. Paradoxic splitting of the second heart sound, an indication of prolonged left ventricular ejection time, may be heard in patients with chronic heart failure and is often associated with a left bundle branch block.

The *ventricular or S_3 gallop sound* is the most sensitive and specific sign of heart failure (9). The S_3 gallop sound is heard approximately 0.16 to 0.19 second after the second heart sound (S_2) and is due to sudden restriction of filling in a relatively noncompliant left ventricle. It is usually heard directly over the PMI and may be audible only when the patient is in the left lateral position. The sound is low pitched and often may be sensed by the cadence of the heart's sounds rather than specifically heard. The cadence closely approximates the word "Kentucky," pronounced KYN-TUC'-KY. The middle syllable is accentuated to represent the loud second heart sound due to increased pulmonary artery pressure in patients in heart failure. The timing of the last syllable closely approximates the timing of the third heart sound when the word is repeated 100 times/minute.

Rales are high pitched sounds (similar to the sound of a clump of hair rubbed between the fingers) produced by the sudden filling with air of fluid-filled alveoli. They are a sign of moderately to severely decompensated left heart failure.

Neck vein distention and hepatojugular reflux are relatively insensitive but specific findings of heart failure. In chronic heart failure, right ventricular filling pressures will usually increase as the LVEDP increases. With time the right ventricle becomes increasingly more stiff and unable to accept a sudden volume load.

Neck vein distention is assessed while the patient is semirecumbent with the head turned slightly away from the examiner. Ideally the internal, rather than the external, jugular vein is inspected since the latter contains valves and may not reflect accurately the right heart pressure. Internal jugular venous distention is seen as a broad based filling in the anterior cervical triangle. However, since the external jugular venous system is often more easily identified, it may be used as an index of the pressure in the superior vena cava if the physician examines the neck properly. If the external jugular is compressed in the supraclavicular fossa, and the examining finger then strips the vein cephalad, blood will rise in the more proximal portion of the vein and the height of this volume of blood reflects the central venous pressure. The physician may choose an arbitrary reference point (such as 10 cm anterior to the posterior axillary line at the sternal angle—this approximates in many the level of the right atrium) and measure the column of blood above this point without regard for the angle of elevation of the thorax. The value of this observation is that accurate serial assessments are possible, permitting the physician to confirm worsening failure (increasing jugular venous pressure) or to recognize a too vigorous diuretic response (abnormally low jugular venous pressure).

Hepatojugular reflux is elicited by having the patient lie supine and semirecumbent at 45°. The patient is asked to breathe normally and is warned that the examiner will apply pressure over the right upper quadrant of the abdomen. Patients so warned will comply and will not hold their breath or perform a Valsalva maneuver which will make the sign impossible to elicit. The sudden increase in venous return causes right ventricular end-diastolic pressure and right atrial pressure to rise; and this will be seen as jugular venous distention.

Peripheral pitting edema is a relatively common, although not a specific, sign of heart failure. It occurs in the dependent portions of the body, which in ambulatory patients means the feet and lower legs. Edema in heart failure is due to increased resorption of salt and water by the kidney. Because pitting edema in the lower extremities becomes detectable only when the leg volume increases by about 10%, an increase in weight may precede pitting edema as an early objective manifestation of decompensated heart failure in ambulatory patients.

Because of low cardiac output and vascular redistribution, patients may have a slightly cyanotic cast to their skin and a drawn colorless look to their face. Their extremities may be cool and their nailbeds may be cyanotic.

Compensated Heart Failure

In contrast to the findings in patients with acute or chronic uncompensated heart failure there may be few or no specific physical findings in compensated patients other than signs of increased heart size. A presystolic gallop or fourth heart sound (S_4) can be heard in most patients with long-standing high blood pressure or ischemic heart disease who are in normal sinus rhythm. The fourth heart sound is thought to be due to atrial contraction into a stiff ventricle. A soft systolic murmur, approximately grade 1 to 2, is commonly heard at the PMI in patients with chronic compensated heart failure. This murmur usually represents minor degrees of mitral insufficiency. The mitral regurgitation is not usually clinically significant but if the murmur is loud or if the patient complains of frequent episodes of paroxysmal dyspnea, a marked increase in mitral regurgitation associated with myocardial ischemia should be suspected, and an attempt should be made to listen to the murmur while the patient is symptomatic.

Laboratory Diagnosis

Chest X-Ray in Heart Failure

The chest X-ray is the most useful diagnostic procedure for the evaluation of suspected heart failure (9). The radiological signs of heart failure are cardiac enlargement and pulmonary congestion.

There are a number of factors that influence heart size on the chest X-ray. These include body build, the depth of inspiration when the film is taken, and the chambers that are enlarged. Nevertheless, determination of the ratio of the transverse diameter of the heart to the greatest diameter of the chest, the *cardiothoracic ratio*, is a reliable and valid measurement of heart size and should be part of the data base of every patient who is thought to have or to have had heart failure. The normal cardiothoracic ratio is less than 0.5.

The pulmonary vasculature should be examined and signs of vascular redistribution, caused by pulmonary venous hypertension, and of enlarged hilar vessels, caused by acute or chronic pulmonary hypertension, should be noted.

Normally, the lower lobes of the lungs are better perfused than the upper lobes. The earliest radiological sign of pulmonary congestion is reduction of blood flow to the lower lobes due to compression of vessels by extravascular fluid which has gravitated to the lung bases. In early heart failure, there is simply an equalization of the size of the vessels to the upper and lower lobes; but as congestion increases, the vessels to the upper lobes become more prominent, the so-called "cephalization" of flow. More severe failure is manifest by signs of interstitial edema and ultimately by alveolar edema and pleural effusion (Chapter 54).

Electrocardiogram

There are no ECG changes that are diagnostic of heart failure. The ECG may, however, reflect an underlying disease (e.g., left ventricular hypertrophy due to hypertension; Q waves or ST-T wave changes due to infarction) or the presence of an unstable rhythm (such as rapid atrial fibrillation) that has caused heart failure.

Patients with well compensated concentric or eccentric hypertrophy of the heart may show only relatively minor nonspecific ST-T wave changes. Grossly abnormal changes are seen in patients who have both dilation and hypertrophy of the left ventricle. The most common manifestations of left ventricular hypertrophy are left axis deviation, increased QRS voltage, and ST-T wave changes. Although there are numerous ECG criteria for left ventricular hypertrophy (LVH), a clinically useful criterion is the index of Lewis: net positivity in lead 1 plus net negativity in lead 3 equals 2.0 mV or more (see also Table 60.3, Chapter 60). Also, an R wave greater than 11 mm in aVL is highly specific for LVH. However, LHV should never be diagnosed on the basis of voltage changes alone; ST-T wave changes should be present in order to make the diagnosis.

Conduction abnormalities are common in patients in heart failure, especially left bundle branch block. Left bundle branch block may be an early sign of congestive cardiomyopathy, especially when it occurs in young patients. It is nearly always a sign of organic heart disease.

Left atrial enlargement is diagnosed by the presence of a negative P wave with an area of greater than 1 mm^2 in lead V$_1$. It commonly is seen in the ECG of a patient with acute heart failure and disappears as the patient is treated.

Right ventricular hypertrophy is most reliably diagnosed in adults by a shift of the QRS axis toward the right greater than 90° (see also Table 60.6, Chapter 60). The QRS axis normally shifts toward the left with age.

Certain ECG changes suggest a decreased ejection fraction, especially in patients with heart failure due to ischemic heart disease. These include (a) Q waves in leads 1, aVL, and V$_1$ through V$_4$ with persistently upward coving of the ST segments in the precordial leads (seen in patients with extensive anterior wall infarctions with aneurysms); and (b) deep Q waves in both inferior and precordial leads with QRS duration greater than 0.1 second (suggesting ischemic cardiomyopathy).

Low voltage (less than 10 mm in all leads) is commonly due to pericardial effusion, hypothyroidism, or infiltrative disease of the heart (e.g., amyloid), but also may be seen in patients with severe emphysema or marked obesity.

Echocardiogram

The echocardiogram, either one- or two-dimensional, is a reliable technique for determining ventricular size and thickness, the presence of valvular and other structural abnormalities, and the presence or absence of pericardial effusion. In one study, echocardiography supplied a specific diagnosis in 31% of patients who presented with cardiomegaly and/or heart failure of unclear etiology (12). The physician should consider echocardiography, therefore, for patients with suspected valvular or pericardial disease or for patients in whom the cause of heart failure is unclear. (The use of echocardiography in the diagnosis of valvular heart disease is discussed more fully in Chapter 60).

Ejection fraction can be obtained by one-dimensional echochardiography by estimating end-systolic and end-diastolic volumes by measurement of the minor axis of the left ventricle; however, two-dimensional echocardiography is necessary to estimate the ejection fraction in patients with ischemic heart disease in whom there may be nonuniform contraction of the left ventricle.

Radionuclide Angiography

Radionuclide antiography ("gated blood pool scan") is a technique for visualizing the cardiac chambers throughout the cardiac cycle. As most commonly performed, pyrophosphate is injected to bind with the patient's red blood cells. One-half hour later technetium-99m is injected intravenously to bind with the red blood cell-pyrophosphate complex. The intracardiac blood pool is scanned in multiple images with a scintillation camera which is synchronized (gated) with the ECG. A computer interfaces with the image from the scintillation camera, divides the cardiac cycle commonly into 16 equal segments, and displays on a television screen in a continuous loop the images obtained sequentially so that a moving image of the heart is seen. The technique is painless and exposes the patient to approximately the same amount of radiation as three plain films of the chest. The cost of radionuclide angiography is approximately 7 times that of an ECG.

The test has several advantages over any other method currently available for determining cardiac function. It is safe, essentially painless, requires no special preparation of the patient, and good images may be obtained even in patients who are obese or who have severe chronic lung disease. Studies have demonstrated excellent correlation of the images obtained with radionuclide angiography compared with ventricular contrast angiography (14).

Radionuclide angiography is an effective tool to differentiate between dyspnea due to cardiac and pulmonary causes, to evaluate left ventricular wall motion abnormalities including ventricular aneurysm, to evaluate left ventricular function reflected in the ejection fraction, to confirm the clinical diagnosis of cardiomyopathy, and to detect hypertrophic cardiomyopathy and atrial myxoma. Radionuclide angiography is especially useful in establishing the prognosis of patients after myocardial infarction. Patients with an ejection fraction of less than 40% are particularly prone to increased morbidity and mortality (14).

The general physician will not ordinarily consider radionuclide angiography without the advice of a cardiologist. However, the technique is an accurate way to complement the clinical assessment of myocardial function in a patient with heart failure.

Cardiac Catheterization

Cardiac catheterization (see Chapter 57) should be considered in any patient in chronic heart failure in whom an etiological and anatomical diagnosis has not been made by noninvasive techniques. In a study of patients with chronic congestive heart failure in whom the etiology of the disease was not apparent, 28% were found to have coronary artery disease. Many of these patients had diabetes mellitus (3). Cardiac catheterization also may be the only way to diagnose occult valvular or pericardial disease or septal defects (see Chapter 60). Consultation with a cardiologist should be obtained before cardiac catheterization is recommended.

Exercise Testing

It is often difficult to determine the functional status of patients claiming Social Security disability or workmen's compensation, and functional limitation is frequently over- or underestimated. Studies have shown that the most precise determination of functional classification is given by exercise testing (6). The protocol used should be one in which the level of exercise is increased in small increments (see Chapter 57). The test should be obtained in consultation with a cardiologist and only if functional classification cannot be satisfactorily determined by clinical means.

MANAGEMENT

The goal of therapy is not merely to control symptoms but to treat specifically the underlying causes of heart failure if possible (see Table 61.1). If the underlying disease cannot be effectively treated, an attempt should be made to increase the capacity of the heart to do work and/or to decrease the amount of work that the heart has to do. Table 61.4 shows the various measures that can be utilized to accomplish these goals in ambulatory patients. These measures are discussed in detail below.

General Principles

Life Style

It is not always possible to improve the function of the failing heart, but it usually is possible to decrease the metabolic needs of the body by encouraging a patient to stop smoking, to avoid emotionally stressful situations and people, and to get an adequate amount of rest. The physician must have a thorough understanding of the patient's work environment and the relationship of the patient to his spouse and family. The patient is more likely to change his life style and priorities if the practitioner discusses the recommended therapy with both the patient and his family. The ambulatory patient should be encouraged to exercise, but to take care to avoid exertion to the point of causing further symptomatic cardiac decompensation. Sometimes this simply means performing the same activities more slowly.

There is a decreased stimulus to renin, angiotensin, and aldosterone production during supine rest, and even severely disabled patients may be able to lead socially useful and satisfying lives if they take a nap in the afternoon and in the early evening or before social or business engagements. Strict bed rest is rarely necessary.

It is important that the temperature and humidity of the patient's home and work environment be controlled as much as possible. Patients should be encouraged to have air conditioners for the summer months to reduce the extra demand placed on the heart by hot humid weather.

Diet

There is little evidence that a severely salt-restricted diet is of benefit in the long term in controlling heart failure in patients who respond well to moderate doses of diuretics. It is a common experience, however, that sudden increases in salt intake may precipitate acute heart failure in patients who have moderately well compensated but relatively severe heart failure. Holiday seasons are particularly dangerous in this regard, probably also because of the increased activity and emotional stress during these times. The physician must be aware of the various types of food that the patient is likely to eat. Most ethnic groups have certain foods that are pre-

Table 61.4.
Measures Used in Ambulatory Treatment of Heart Failure

INCREASING CAPACITY OF HEART TO DO WORK
  Digitalis
  Antiarrhythmic drugs (Chapter 59)
  Pacemaker (Chapter 59)
DECREASING AMOUNT OF WORK THAT HEART
        HAS TO DO
  Rest
  Low sodium diet
  Diuretics
  Vasodilator drugs
  Home oxygen

pared during festive occasions and many of these foods have a high salt content. Examples include "down-home cooking" among black people, which is characterized by use of fatback or salt pork, and many foods prepared by traditional Jewish, Italian, or Polish cooks. Many patients attempt to substitute condiments in place of salt and are not aware that ketchup, hot sauce, *etc* have high salt concentrations. A no added salt diet, which contains approximately 2 to 4 g of sodium, will suffice for most patients in compensated heart failure. Patients with poorly compensated heart failure may require a diet that contains 500 mg to 1 g of sodium. The physician must take the time to discuss diet sympathetically and meticulously with the patient or should refer the patient to a competent dietician. Guidelines for planning these diets and a list of foods to be avoided by patients being treated for heart failure are given in Table 62.9 of Chapter 62 (page 806).

Patients with heart failure may wish to know if they can continue to drink *alcoholic beverages*. In any patient with a cardiomyopathy apparently related to prolonged heavy alcohol use, total abstinence from alcohol may be essential to the management of heart failure. In other patients moderate alcohol use (e.g., wine with meals or a cocktail before dinner) is reasonable.

Drugs Which Promote Positive Sodium Balance

A number of drugs can promote a positive sodium balance: (a) renal sodium retention may be caused by corticosteroids, estrogens, and nonsteroidal antiinflammatory agents other than aspirin, and (b) some antacid preparations contain a significant amount of sodium (see Table 36.3, Chapter 36). Patients with heart failure should not receive these drugs, or, if the drugs are necessary, the patients should be monitored for and treated for increased symptoms of heart failure.

Drug Therapy (Table 61.5)

Heart failure is the result of mismatch between preload, afterload, and inotropic state; each of these factors may be adjusted by use of appropriate measures. Preload may be adjusted by the use of diuretic therapy, salt restriction, and venodilator therapy. Afterload may be adjusted by the control of hypertension and by the use of arteriolar dilating drugs. The inotropic state of the heart may be adjusted by the use of digitalis or by other oral inotropic agents (see page 781).

Diuretic Drugs

Diuretic drugs are used when it is not possible to treat the underlying cause of heart failure or when signs and symptoms of heart failure persist despite treatment of the underlying condition. Diuretics reduce symptoms of circulatory congestion by increasing sodium and water excretion. If the contractility of the heart is depressed, the ventricular function curve is relatively flat and preload may be reduced with little change in ventricular function unless the reduction is excessive (Fig. 61.2). The goal of diuretic therapy is to reach the patient's *dry weight*. Physiologically, this is the weight at which signs of peripheral congestion are substantially relieved and at which the left ventricular filling pressure remains at the preload reserve (i.e., function is optimized *via* the Frank-Starling principle). Clinically, this is the weight at which peripheral edema is substantially resolved, and a significant increase in diuretic dose is necessary to achieve further weight loss. If the heart has dilated because of fluid overload, the decrease in ventricular wall stress (i.e., afterload) and the improvement in ventricular contraction pattern brought about by a decrease in heart size following diuresis often lead to a prompt restoration of ventricular function.

Table 61.5.
Characteristics of Selected Diuretic Drugs[a]

Generic Name	Brand Name	Available Preparations	Usual Daily Dose (mg)	Frequency of Dose/Day	Onset of Effect	Peak Effect	Duration
Chlorothiazide	Diuril	500-mg tablet	500–1000	1–2	1 hour	4 hours	6–12 hours
Hydrochlorothiazide	Generic, Hydro-Diuril, Esidrix	25/50/100-mg tablet	25–100	1–2	2 hours	4 hours	12 hours or more
Chlorthalidone	Generic, Hygroton	50/100-mg tablet	50–100	1	2 hours	6 hours	24 hours
Metolazone	Diulo, Zaroxolyn	2.5/5/10 mg tablet	2.5–10	1	1 hour	2 hours	12–24 hours
Furosemide	Lasix	20/40/80 mg tablet	20–160	1–2	1 hour	1–2 hours	6 hours
Ethacrynic acid	Edecrin	50-mg tablet	50–100	1–2	30 minutes	2 hours	6–8 hours
Bumetanide	Bumex	0.5/1 mg tablet	0.5–2	1	30 minutes to 1 hour	1–2 hours	4 hours
Triamterene	Dyrenium	100-mg capsule	100–300	1–2	2 hours	6–8 hours	12–16 hours
Spironolactone	Aldactone	25 mg tablet	50–400	1–2	Gradual onset	2–3 days after initiation of therapy	2–3 days after cessation of therapy
Amiloride	Midamor	5-mg tablet	5–10	1	2 hours	6–10 hours	24 hours

[a] Modified from Frazier H, Yager H: The clinical use of diuretics. *N Engl J Med* 288:246, 455, 1973 (7).

There are three classes of diuretics in common use: thiazides (hydrochlorothiazide) and thiazide-like agents (metolazone), the so-called loop diuretics (ethacrynic acid, furosemide, and bumetanide), and the potassium-sparing diuretics (spironolactone, triamterene, and amiloride) (Table 61.5) (see also Chapter 45).

The thiazides act on the distal convoluted tubule (diluting segment) of the nephron; although their mechanism of action is unknown, they inhibit sodium transport and they cause a moderate increase in the excretion of sodium, chloride, and water. Potassium and hydrogen losses are accentuated because of the increased delivery of solute to the even more distal portion of the nephron where potassium secretion occurs and is modulated by aldosterone. Thiazide-like agents such as metolazone may act on both the diluting segment and the more distal segments of the nephron and may be particularly effective in patients with very low renal blood flow. The loop diuretics inhibit tubular resorption of chloride and sodium in the thick ascending limb of the loop of Henle. These diuretics are potent and result in a substantial increase in the excretion of sodium, chloride, and water. Like thiazides, the loop diuretics increase the delivery of solute to the more distal portion of the nephron where potassium and hydrogen secretion is accentuated.

Potassium-sparing diuretics by themselves are only weak diuretics. However, they may be especially useful in combination with a thiazide or loop diuretic in preventing hypokalemia or when a patient becomes refractory to the more potent diuretics. The effect of thiazides and loop diuretics may be dampened by the resorption of sodium in the distal segment since they act proximal to the portion of the distal nephron where aldosterone influences sodium resorption. Spironolactone is structurally similar to aldosterone and competitively inhibits aldosterone binding to cellular receptors. Triamterene and amiloride block sodium resorption and potassium excretion but do not compete with aldosterone or even depend on its presence to be effective. These diuretics may cause life-threatening increases in the serum potassium level. Patients must not receive potassium supplementation while taking them. Also, patients with renal failure are at increased risk for developing hyperkalemia if given these diuretics. In any patient serum potassium must be monitored carefully when these agents are used.

Use of diuretic drugs. Diuretic therapy should start with the lowest effective dose of a thiazide compound. Generic hydrochlorothiazide is the drug of choice. It is inexpensive, effective, and the tablet is small and easy to swallow. Many patients with mild heart failure may effectively control symptoms by use of the drug every other day or three times a week. Patients with progressive disease may become resistant gradually to the effect of thiazides and may require doses of 100 mg of hydrochlorothiazide a day for control of edema and dyspnea. Patients become resistant to thiazides when there is significant renal failure (such as when the serum creatinine is > 2 to 4 mg/dl) or when renal blood flow is decreased markedly, as it may be in severe heart failure. There is no evidence that if one thiazide has failed, another will be effective. Metolazone, however, may be effective in such circumstances, even in patients with very low renal blood flow.

When a patient becomes resistant to thiazide or has complications of thiazide therapy (see below), the loop diuretics—furosemide, ethacrynic acid, or bumetanide—should be prescribed. These drugs are often effective in relatively low doses. Furosemide is the most popular of the three drugs because gastrointestinal and ototoxic side effects are more common with ethacrynic acid, especially in higher doses, and because bumetanide is only relatively recently available (bumetanide is, however, the least ototoxic of the loop diuretics). Furosemide should be started at a dose of 20 mg daily and increased as necessary for control of symptoms. A single dose should be administered each day, usually in the morning, although patients in severe failure may sleep better at night if the dose is given in the late afternoon.

Doses of furosemide as high as 1000 mg a day may be necessary in patients with severe heart failure, especially if there is associated renal failure. When more than 160 to 240 mg a day are required, however, the patient becomes at risk for ototoxicity and the physician should reconsider whether the etiology of heart failure has been accurately determined and whether correctable causes of heart failure have been dealt with. If so, it is at this point (if not previously prescribed for potassium control) that a potassium-sparing diuretic—spironolactone or triamterene—should be added to the drug regimen. Triamterene is probably the drug of choice since it has a more rapid onset of action and may be less expensive than spironolactone if more than 3 tablets/day of spironolactone are required. Since these medications will ordinarily be used in patients who have received potassium supplementation (although such supplementation should be discontinued prior to the administration of a potassium-sparing diuretic) and who may have renal failure, the patient's electrolyte concentration must be carefully monitored when these medications are started, when the dose is adjusted, or when there is a change in the severity of the heart failure. Potassium supplementation should be stopped when the drugs are prescribed, and the level of serum potassium should be measured again 1 week later. The usual dose of triamterene is 100 mg, one to three times a day; and of spironolactone, 25 to 100 mg, once or twice daily. The addition of a thiazide diuretic in modest doses (50 mg of hydrochlorothiazide or 5 mg of metolazone) may markedly potentiate the effect of loop diuretics, leading to a rapid mobilization of fluid and thereby allowing these patients to be managed in an ambulatory setting. Careful monitoring of electrolyte levels is essential and the diuretic dose should be reduced when the desired effect is achieved.

Side effects of diuretics.

HYPOKALEMIA (see Chapter 45). The thiazide and loop diuretics have marked kaliuretic effects and, especially in edematous patients, hypokalemia is a common complication of the use of diuretic therapy. Hypokalemia may lead to fatigue/depression and muscle cramps and frequently precipitates digitalis toxicity. The indication for and use of potassium salts in patients taking diuretics is fully dicussed in Chapter 45.

CONTRACTION OF THE EXTRACELLULAR VOLUME. Diuretics are therapeutically effective by causing a net loss of sodium, chloride, and water. If the response is excessive, depletion of the extracellular fluid compartment (the maintenance of which depends on sodium and chloride) will occur. This may have catastrophic consequences such as hypotension (or postural hypotension) with precipitation of ischemia due to changes in cerebral, coronary, or renal blood flow. This complication is especially common when loop diuretics are used, but may occur following the use of thiazides or of combination diuretics. The physician should monitor the patient carefully, therefore, for evidence of excessive contraction of extracellular volume by assessment of his weight, the presence or absence of edema, the degree of fullness of the neck veins, and by assessment of the blood pressure and pulse. Not infrequently a dose of a diuretic that initiated diuresis will need to be reduced once cardiac compensation has improved.

ACID-BASE DISTURBANCE. By their different actions on the nephron, diuretics have an effect on acid-base balance. The thiazides and the loop diuretics are often associated with the generation and maintenance of a metabolic alkalosis. This usually requires no therapy. To correct the alkalosis, the associated volume and potassium deficiency would have to be corrected. If the volume were replenished, the effect of the diuretic would be negated. Therefore usually only potassium chloride supplements are given (see Chapter 45). If the alkalosis is thought to be detrimental, for example in patients with respiratory failure, then either the diuretic should be discontinued or acetazolamide (Diamox) should be added to the regimen to diminish hydrogen ion excretion. The addition of acetazolamide (250 to 375 mg once a day—two to three 125-mg tablets) will increase potassium excretion even more, so that special attention should be paid to potassium supplementation. The infrequency and complexity of this situation are such that a telephone consultation with a nephrologist before initiation of therapy with acetazolamide is appropriate.

Potassium-sparing diuretics may be associated with diminished hydrogen ion excretion and therefore with a mild metabolic acidosis. This is usually of no consequence and requires no treatment.

HYPONATREMIA. The loop diuretics and the thiazides may be occasionally associated with hyponatremia by impairing free water clearance, and therefore caution is especially appropriate in patients who tend to consume relatively large quantities of fluid. These diuretics also may be associated with hyponatremia when the extracellular volume has become contracted (a potent stimulus to the release of antidiuretic hormone) and fluid intake has not been restricted. In both of these instances, water restriction is mandatory. Usually this hyponatremia may be corrected by water restriction of less than 1 liter/day, but occasionally more severe restriction is necessary. Finally, the thiazides may be rarely associated with hyponatremia in euvolemic patients who also are severely potassium depleted. This situation resembles clinically the syndrome of inappropriate secretion of antidiuretic hormone, although the exact mechanism of this complication is not fully known. The drug must be withdrawn should this complication develop.

HYPERURICEMIA. Thiazides, loop diuretics, and triamterene commonly elevate the concentration of serum urate by blocking urate secretion by the proximal renal tubules and/or by enhancing resorption through contraction of extracellular volume. Symptomatic gout, however, is not usual, nor is the elevation of uric acid likely to cause renal injury or stone formation. Therefore, unless gout does occur, treatment is not necessary.

HYPERGLYCEMIA. Thiazides and, less commonly, loop diuretics may cause glucose intolerance. Hypoglycemic therapy may be required (or changed, in diabetics already receiving a hypoglycemic agent) if the diuretic is to be continued (see Chapter 72).

OTOTOXICITY. Loop diuretics may impair hearing, usually reversibly, especially if large doses are taken or if the patient has renal insufficiency.

OTHER EFFECTS. Thiazides are occasionally associated with a hypersensitivity-induced small vessel vasculitis (Chapter 50), with thrombocytopenia (Chapter 50), and with hypercalcemia (Chapter 74). Furosemide in high doses has been associated with the development of interstitial nephritis and renal failure, especially in patients with marked proteinuria. Spironolactone, a weak androgen antagonist, commonly causes gynecomastia and may reduce libido or even cause impotence; these side effects resolve within a few months of discontinuing the drug.

When diuretics have not adequately controlled the signs and symptoms of congestive heart failure, the physician should consider additional medication.

Inotropic Agents: Digitalis

Inotropic drugs may help to restore cardiac compensation by increasing the inotropic state, or contractility of cardiac muscle, thereby increasing the ejection fraction at a given preload and afterload, as described above (see page 770). The only inotropic drugs currently available for oral use are the digitalis glycosides, but a new class of nondigitalis oral inotropic agents may soon be released for clinical use.

The digitalis drugs appear to improve contractility by increasing the delivery of calcium to the contractile apparatus of the heart. Digitalis inhibits sodium-potassium ATPase, and it is postulated that this results in increase of influx of both calcium and sodium into the myocardial cell.

Indications for the use of digitalis drugs. Despite more than 200 years of clinical experience with digitalis preparations, the indications for digitalis therapy remain controversial, and there are conflicting reports regarding the utility of digitalis preparations in acute and chronic heart failure. Digitalis preparations may improve ventricular performance by moderating the heart rate of patients in atrial fibrillation or atrial flutter and by increasng ventricular contractility in some patients who are in heart failure. However, the degree to which digitalis preparations increase ventricular contractility is modest; the toxic to therapeutic ratio is small, and the drug must be pushed to near toxic limits in many cases before significant clinical effect is seen. Furthermore, the indiscriminate use of digitalis as a first line medication for control of heart failure has led to its use in many patients in whom heart failure is not due primarily to a decrease in the inotropic state of myocardial muscle. These include patients whose heart failure is due to valvular heart disease or to systemic hypertension, patients in whom heart failure is due to restrictions to ventricular filling (e.g., hypertrophic cardiomyopathy or pericardial tamponade), and patients in whom symptoms of fatigue are due to a decreased cardiac output induced by excessive diuresis.

Recommendations for use of digitalis compounds.
1. Digitalis glycosides should be prescribed only for patients in congestive heart failure with dilated hearts (a cardiothoracic ratio > 0.5 suggests dilation; echocardiography, however, is the most precise way of demonstrating cardiac chamber size and thickness) and in whom the symptoms of heart failure appear to be due to a decreased inotropic state of heart muscle (usually reflected by an ejection fraction of less than 40 to 45%). It is also a useful drug for certain types of arrhythmias (see Chapter 59).
2. The practitioner should become familiar with the purified glycoside, digoxin, and should use it exclusively. It is well absorbed, can be used parenterally if necessary, and has an intermediate duration of action (half-life of 36 to 48 hours). The Burroughs Wellcome preparation of digoxin, Lanoxin, is the preferred digoxin preparation, because of variable absorption of many other brands. A newly released formulation of Lanoxin, Lanoxicaps (0.05-, 0.10-, and 0.20-mg capsules) may be even more dependably absorbed and may be useful when careful titration of the dose is important. Digitalization is best accomplished in an ambulatory patient by daily administration of the drug at the maintenance dosage (see below). Within four or five half-lives of the drug (approximately 7 days) full digitalization is ordinarily achieved.
3. The effect of digitalis on the patient's condition should be monitored and reassessed periodically. If there is no objective decrease in heart size within 1 or 2 months or increase in exercise capacity after a trial of digitalis therapy, the drug should probably be discontinued (before doing that, however, serum digoxin concentration (see below) should be measured to be certain that adequate blood levels are being attained). Digitalis should be used cautiously in older patients and in any patient known to have impaired renal function. There is no evidence that elderly patients are intrinsically more sensitive to digitalis compounds, but they have a smaller body mass, often have impaired renal excretion of the drug, and have higher serum levels for a given oral dose of the drug.
4. The average dose of digoxin is 0.25 mg/day (of Lanoxicaps, 0.20 mg/day). In patients older than 65 years or in patients with known impairments of renal function, doses of 0.125 mg/day should be prescribed.
5. Digitalis may interact with other medications. It has recently been shown that the administration of quinidine causes a decrease in excretion of digoxin which may lead to digitalis toxicity (11); similar effects have been seen when digitalis is prescribed along with either of the calcium channel blockers, verapamil or diltiazem. The use of thiazides and the loop diuretics may lead to digitalis toxicity either because of increased retention of these drugs secondary to decreased renal blood flow or (and) because of increased sensitivity to digitalis as the result of hypokalemia. Cholestyramine and neomycin and some antacids impair digoxin absorption and may result in a subtherapeutic effect.

Recognition and treatment of digitalis toxicity. Digitalis toxicity commonly is caused by administration of too much digitalis or by overdiuresis (often with associated hypokalemia), by intercurrent development of renal insufficiency, or by administration of drugs which interfere with digitalis excretion. Digitalis toxicity is especially common in older patients in an ambulatory practice. Approximately 10% of patients in the seventh and eighth decades being seen regularly by a physician will be taking digitalis (10).

The manifestations of digitalis toxicity are protean and may be difficult to recognize in older patients and in patients whose normal baseline level of function is not familiar to the practitioner. They include changes in the cardiovascular system, the gastrointestinal tract, and the central nervous system. The most frequent cardiac manifestations of digitalis toxicity are progressive slowing and regularization of the heart rate (i.e., development of a nodal rhythm) of patients in atrial fibrillation, and frequent premature ventricular contractions (PVCs). Digitalis toxicity should be suspected in any older patient who is taking digitalis and has PVCs or any patient in atrial fibrillation whose heart rate falls below approximately 60 and becomes regular. Since digitalis both increases automaticity and decreases conduction through the AV node, paroxysmal atrial tachycardia (PAT) with block may be seen. The peripheral pulse in PAT with block is usually 100 to 120 beats/minute (see Chapter 59). Cardiac toxicity may occur in the absence of other signs or symptoms of digitalis overdose.

Gastrointestinal side effects are common manifestations of digitoxicity. They include anorexia, mild nausea, and occasionally vomiting and diarrhea.

Digitalis may cause changes in the sensorium ranging from mild confusional states to frank delirium and psychosis. In an older patient it may be difficult to determine, without stopping the drug, whether these symptoms are due to primary cerebral disease or to digitalis excess.

The diagnosis of digitalis toxicity is based on clinical and laboratory findings. If symptoms compatible with digitalis toxicity are present, especially in an elderly patient who is also taking a diuretic, the drug should be stopped immediately. The patient should be examined in approximately 3 days and the symptoms should be reassessed. If symptoms have abated, a presumptive diagnosis of digitoxicity is warranted.

At the time of presentation, it is reasonable to measure the serum digoxin concentration. That is done in many commercial and hospital laboratories by use of a radioimmunoassay. It is important that the quality control of the laboratory be known, to ensure reliability of the procedure. An adequately digitalized patient will have a serum digoxin concentration of approximately 0.7 to 1.4 ng/ml; most toxic patients have concentrations above 2.0 ng/ml. However, if a patient has symptoms compatible with digitalis toxicity and his serum digoxin level is within the normal range, toxicity has not been ruled out since at therapeutic levels hypokalemic (or hypercalcemic) patients may become digitoxic. Most patients with digitoxicity can be managed by temporary withdrawal of the medication and by reinstitution of it at a lower dose. Often, diuretic therapy must also be modified and/or potassium supplements administered. However, patients with symptomatic arrhythmias are best hospitalized for a few days so that they can be monitored closely.

Any patient who has become digitalis-toxic should have the indications for digitalis therapy carefully reviewed. In many cases the drug may be stopped without any apparent change in the patient's condition.

Vasodilator Therapy

A major advance in the treatment of heart failure in the past 10 years has been the introduction into clinical practice of vasodilator therapy. In ambulatory practice, vasodilator drugs should be considered for patients whose heart failure cannot be controlled by diuretics and digitalis.

Physiological rationale for vasodilator therapy. The syndrome of heart failure is not due to left ventricular dysfunction *per se*, but to the compensatory responses triggered by the inadequate response of the left ventricle to stress (see above, page 771). The net result is an increase in both left ventricular preload, and afterload. These compensatory mechanisms probably developed in the course of evolution to protect against circulatory collapse due to blood loss. In the setting of left ventricular dysfunction, however, these potentially lifesaving compensatory mechanisms lead to a further deterioration of cardiac function. The judicious use of vasodilator agents may promptly optimize cardiac function and may improve the functional state of patients with chronic heart failure.

The hemodynamic effects of *venodilator drugs* and diuretics are essentially the same. Both classes of drugs cause a decrease in preload, thereby relieving symptoms of vascular congestion (see Fig. 61.2). Venodilators are most useful in patients with severe heart failure in whom preload reserve is exceeded during exercise, leading to an increase in LVEDP and to pulmonary vascular congestion. This may occur in association with ischemia in patients with ischemic heart disease or in association with advanced disease in patients with cardiomyopathy or with valvular heart disease. These drugs should not be used in patients with heart failure due to restriction to ventricular filling (e.g., hypertrophic cardiomyopathy) and should be used with caution in patients with aortic stenosis in whom a reduction in preload may lead to a marked decrease in cardiac output.

Arteriolar vasodilators increase cardiac output by decreasing afterload (i.e., decreasing ventricular wall stress during contraction), thereby allowing the myocardium to contract more efficiently and increasing the ejection fraction and cardiac output (see Fig. 61.3). These medications are most effective in patients with severe peripheral and central congestion, who have signs of peripheral hypoperfusion, such as cool hands and peripheral cyanosis.

It is important to note that arteriolar vasodilators increase cardiac output only if preload remains near the preload reserve (see Fig. 61.3) (16). With afterload reduction the left ventricle unloads more efficiently, and volume shifts from the central to the peripheral venous circulation, thereby lowering preload. If preload drops significantly, cardiac output cannot be maintained, and the blood pressure falls. Thus, in an ambulatory setting, vasodilators must be used with caution, and often with a concomitant adjustment of diuretic dosage.

Four classes of vasodilators are available: drugs that act directly on smooth muscle, drugs that act by blocking the α-adrenergic system, drugs that act by blocking calcium channels, and drugs that block angiotensin converting enzyme (4) (Table 61.6). The choice of an appropriate agent and the effective use of that agent depends upon an understanding of the physiological properties of these drugs.

Smooth muscle dilators. Nitroglycerin in various formulations is an effective venodilator at the low end of the dose range and a mixed veno- and arteriolar dilator at higher doses. The practitioner should be familiar with the use of nitrates in four forms (see also Chapter 57): a short acting sublingual nitrate, long acting nitrates taken orally, nitroglycerin in a petrolatum base (Nitrol Paste), and nitroglycerin dermal patches (Transderm TNG, Nitro-Dur, Nitrodisc). *Sublingual nitroglycerin* is generally used in a dose of 0.4 mg. The medication is sensitive to body heat, light, and moisture and must be kept in a sealed brown glass or plastic container. Patients should be encouraged to purchase new sublingual

nitroglycerin every 6 months to be sure that the medication is active. Sublingual nitroglycerin may be used liberally to control symptoms of pulmonary congestion during normal physical activity such as walking up stairs, shopping, and so forth. Small bottles of 25 tablets may be prescribed and should be kept in strategic locations about the patient's home, car, and workplace. The use of oral forms of *long acting nitroglycerin* has been controversial because of reports of variable blood levels resulting from hepatic metabolism of these drugs. However, it has been shown that high doses of oral nitrates will overwhelm the hepatic enzyme systems and achieve high and sustained blood levels (1). An effective medication is isosorbide dinitrate (generic, Isordil, Sokate) in doses of at least 20 mg orally, four times a day. If symptoms have not improved within a few days, the dosage should be increased. Doses as high as 40 to 60 mg orally, four times a day, may be used safely depending upon the patient's blood pressure response. Before and after each increase in the dose, the patient should be checked for orthostatic hypotension. If there is a drop of more than 15 to 20 mm Hg systolic blood pressure, 3 minutes after going from the supine to standing position, the dosage should be decreased slightly. *Nitroglycerin, 2% in a petrolatum base,* gives effective long acting venodilation but is messy and may be difficult for some patients to apply. It is best used under an occlusive polyethylene wrapping. The usual dose is 1 to 4 inches, four times daily. Again, titration of the dose depends on whether or not heart failure is improved and on whether orthostasis develops. *Nitroglycerin*

Table 61.6.
Vasodilators Useful in Treating Heart Failure

Site of Action	Drugs	Venodilation/ Arteriolar Dilation	Available Tablet Strength	Usual Dose	Effectiveness After 1 Year
Smooth muscle	Isosorbide dinitrate (Isordil)	+++/+	10, 20, 40 mg	20–60 mg every 6 hours	?
	Topical nitroglycerine			2% paste, 1–4 inches every 6 hours Dermal patches, 10–30 cm²/day	
	Hydralazine (Apresoline)	0/+++	10, 25, 50, 100 mg	25–50 mg every 6 hours	?
	Hydralazine plus long acting nitrate	+++/+++		As above, in combination	+++
α-Adrenergic blockade	Prazosin (Minipress)	++/++	1, 2, 5 mg	3–5 mg every 6 hours	+
Calcium channel blockers	Nifedipine (Procardia)	+/+++	10 mg	10–30 mg every 6 hours	?
	Verapamil (Calan, Isoptin)	+/++	80, 120 mg	80–120 mg every 8 hours	?
Angiotensin I converting enzyme inhibitors	Captopril (Capoten)	++/+++	12.5, 25, 50 mg	6.25–50 mg every 6 hours	+++

dermal patches give sustained high blood levels of nitrate over 24 hours. Most patients respond to a 10-cm^2 patch, although up to 40 cm^2 may be necessary in some patients.

The most common side effects of nitrate therapy are headache and nausea. Skin irritation is occasionally seen with the use of nitrol paste or dermal patches. Headache can usually be controlled by aspirin or acetaminophen, and it usually abates after several days of nitrate therapy. Gastrointestinal side effects can occasionally be eliminated by switching to a different preparation of long acting nitroglycerin or switching to nitroglycerin patches. Rubbing alcohol should be used to remove nitroglycerine dermal patches.

Hydralazine is an effective direct arteriolar vasodilator. In properly selected patients and when used in effective doses, hydralazine may increase the cardiac output as much as 2-fold. This improved cardiac output may persist chronically in patients who respond initially.

Hydralazine for afterload reduction must be used cautiously in ambulatory patients. Doses of hydralazine less than 200 mg/day are rarely effective. If the patient's preload is not near maximum, hydralazine may cause a marked fall in blood pressure. In an ambulatory setting it is safest to start hydralazine in a dose of 10 mg and to observe the patient in the office for approximately 2 hours for signs of orthostatic hypotension. The patient can then be given a dose of 25 mg every 6 hours and observed the following day. If orthostatic hypotension or tachycardia is not observed, the dose is increased to 50 mg every 6 hours. At an effective dose the patient's handshake, previously cool, becomes warm and firm, and the patient experiences a general sense of increased well-being and of decreased fatigue. The increased cardiac output may lead to an increase in renal blood flow, and diuretics often become more effective. If signs of peripheral vasodilation are not achieved, the dose of hydralazine should be increased to as high as 100 mg, four times a day. The major complication of hydralazine is a lupus-like syndrome. However, this syndrome usually does not become apparent until 18 to 24 months of treatment with hydralazine in doses above 200 mg/day. Because of the severity of their heart disease, most patients who require such large doses of hydralazine for afterload treatment of congestive heart failure will not live long enough to develop a lupus-like syndrome. Additional information about the properties of hydralazine and other vasodilators is provided in Chapter 62.

In severe heart failure it may be desirable to achieve both venous and arteriolar dilation simultaneously. This may be done by the use of hydralazine and a long acting nitrate such as isosorbide dinitrate, in doses as described above.

Sympathetic blockers. Prazosin (Minipress) is an α-sympathetic blocker with both veno- and arteriodilatory actions and may be useful as a single agent with both preload and afterload reducing properties. The usual dose of prazosin is 2 to 5 mg every 6 hours, although some patients may require larger doses for effective afterload reduction. The effect of prazosin is often only apparent during exercise, and many patients appear to develop tachyphylaxis to the drug. Additional information about prazosin is found in Chapter 62.

Calcium channel blockers. These drugs interfere with contractility of smooth muscle by blocking the entry of calcium into muscle cells, resulting in vasodilation, especially of the arterioles. All of the currently available calcium channel blockers also cause cardiac depression. *Nifedipine,* 10 to 30 mg every 6 to 8 hours, may be the most effective of this class of drugs in patients with ischemic cardiomyopathy, due to its anti-ischemic and vasodilatory properties. In this situation afterload reduction is predominant and the negative inotropic effect is relatively slight. *Verapamil* is an arteriolar vasodilator that has a significant antihypertensive effect. It may be particularly useful, in doses of 80 to 120 mg three times a day, in patients with heart failure due to a restriction to cardiac filling caused by hypertrophic cardiomyopathy with hypercontractility but should not be used, because of its negative inotropic effect, in patients with congestive cardiomyopathy. Common side effects of calcium channel blockers include headache, hypotension, nausea, and constipation.

Angiotensin converting enzyme inhibitors. The only angiotensin converting enzyme inhibitor currently released for clinical use is captopril (5). As discussed above (page 772), the syndrome of heart failure is due in large part to the stimulation of the renin-angiotensin-aldosterone system by the kidney. Captopril blocks the conversion of angiotensin I to angiotensin II, a potent vasoconstrictor and a regulator of aldosterone production. Captopril causes a marked decrease in angiotensin II levels approximately 30 minutes after adminstration (2). It is thus an effective vasodilator and also blocks aldosterone-mediated salt and water retention. Captopril appears to be the most effective vasodilator currently available and it retains its effectiveness in long term use.

Captopril may be used in an ambulatory setting. In patients with obvious signs of circulatory congestion a dose of 12.5 mg should be given and the blood pressure checked in 1 hour. The usual effective dose for heart failure is 12.5 to 50 mg three times a day. Patients who are hyponatremic or at their dry weight should be started at 6.25 mg (one-half of a 12.5-mg cross-scored tablet) and their diuretic dose adjusted (because the danger of symptomatic hypotension is greater in such situations). Because of its antialdosterone effect, potassium supplementation may need to be decreased, and potassium levels should be monitored a week or two after initiation of captopril therapy. Side effects, the most common of which are skin rash and altered taste, are rare, but in such cases the drug may need to be discontinued. Neutropenia, a reported complication, is rare with the low doses used to treat heart failure. Proteinuria and worsening renal failure are occasionally seen in patients with significant pre-existing renal disease.

General recommendations for use of afterload reduction therapy in an ambulatory setting.

1. Select patients whose heart failure is due to decreased left ventricular function, with evidence of both central and peripheral congestion.

2. Captopril appears to be the most effective agent for long term use in an ambulatory setting. When medication cost is an important issue, hydralazine plus a long acting nitrate (isosorbide dinitrate, nitroglycerin ointment or patch) may be used at approximately one-half the cost of full dose captopril.

3. Patient weight should be measured and signs of circulatory congestion (jugular venous distention and hepatojugular reflux) should be assessed each time the physician sees the patient. Symptomatic postural hypotension is a frequent complication of vasodilator therapy in patients in whom diuresis has been excessive.

β-Blocker Therapy

β-Blockade may be useful in the treatment of heart failure due to the following conditions: thyrotoxicosis, severe hypertension responsive to β-blockade therapy, hypertrophic cardiomyopathy, and in patients with failure due to recurrent ischemia. The combination of β-blockade therapy with nitrate therapy may be effective in patients with ischemic cardiomyopathy and chest pain. In all cases, β-blockade therapy is given until the resting heart rate falls below 70 beats/minute and does not show a significant increase with mild to moderate exercise. This usually requires relatively high doses of propranolol (e.g., 160 mg daily in divided doses). Lower doses may be effective in patients with depressed hepatic blood flow or function due to congestive heart failure. β-Blockade therapy should not be used in patients with uncompensated or poorly compensated heart failure and should be used with caution, if at all, in patients with bronchospasm.

Importance of Control of Hypertension in Patients in Heart Failure

Hypertension increases ventricular wall stress, and therefore the afterload on the heart, and reduces the cardiac output, especially as the heart begins to fail. It is essential, therefore, that hypertension be controlled in patients in heart failure. This subject is discussed in detail in Chapter 62.

Home Oxygen Therapy

Patients with severe end-stage heart failure and arterial oxygen desaturation at rest due to low cardiac output or to concomitant pulmonary disease may often feel more comfortable with the use of home oxygen. Patients who require home oxygen therapy because of congestive heart failure rarely survive for more than 6 months to a year. The most efficient way to administer oxygen therapy at home is by means of tanks delivered to the house. This form of therapy is paid for in part, by Medicare, Medicaid, and most private insurance plans. The physician should obtain an arterial blood gas determination to confirm the hypoxia before oxygen is prescribed.

Anticoagulation Therapy

Patients in severe chronic congestive heart failure are at great risk for pulmonary and peripheral emboli. The incidence of peripheral arterial embolization in these patients may be as high as 10%/year. A patient with a markedly dilated left ventricular cavity or a patient with a left ventricular aneurysm, especially if in atrial fibrillation, should be considered for treatment with coumarin anticoagulants (see Chapter 51). However, Coumadin therapy may be hazardous in patients in severe heart failure who have wide swings in prothrombin time due to liver dysfunction. In such circumstances, the prothrombin time should be checked more frequently, perhaps every few weeks.

Electrophysiological Control of Heart Failure

Patients with persistent bradycardia due to sick sinus syndrome or complete heart block and patients with persistent tachyarrhythmias may develop heart failure. The treatment of these problems is discussed in Chapter 59.

Operative Correction of Mechanical Problems Causing Heart Failure

Any patient who is in heart failure because of a mechanical derangement of myocardial function should be considered for operative correction and consultation with a cardiologist should be obtained. The most commonly encountered correctable problems in patients with chronic congestive failure include valvular heart disease, atrial septal defect (Chapter 60), and ischemic heart disease with ventricular aneurysm.

The possibility of a ventricular aneurysm should be considered in any patient with known ischemic heart disease and heart failure. Patients with known ventricular aneurysm who are uncomfortable performing their usual daily tasks should be referred for cardiological consultation and consideration of coronary artery bypass graft surgery with aneurysmectomy. As noted above, radionuclide angiography and two-dimensional echocardiography are the best methods currently available for the noninvasive detection of ventricular aneurysms.

Coronary Artery Bypass Graft Surgery and Congestive Heart Failure

Patients with chronic congestive heart failure and angina pectoris (Chapter 57) should be sent for cardiological consultation. Some of these patients will benefit by coronary artery bypass graft surgery, an aneurysmectomy, or an infarctectomy.

Community Health Services

Many community health services are available to help the physician deal with the patient and the patient deal with his illness.

Home Visits

In two situations, home visits by the patient's physician or by a visiting nurse should be considered in the management of a patient in heart failure: (a) when the patient has repeatedly returned to the office with heart failure due to dietary neglect or to failure to use his medications correctly and (b) when the homebound patient's symptoms are so severe (NYHA class IV, Table 61.3) that he is unable to come for an office visit without becoming exhausted.

Information Booklets

The American Heart Association has useful free booklets explaining low salt diets and has other booklets explaining the management of congestive heart failure to the patient and his family. The booklets may be obtained from a local office of the American Heart Association.

Exercise Programs (Chapter 58)

Graduated regular exercise may benefit some patients with mild chronic heart failure, both physically and psychologically. However, there is no evidence that myocardial function can be improved by exercise. Isometric exercise is contraindicated in any patient in heart failure because of the extra work this demands of the heart. Exercise may be contraindicated entirely in left heart failure due to valvular heart disease and in most patients with functional class III or class IV congestive heart failure.

PROGNOSIS

The prognosis in heart failure is related to the etiology of the heart failure, the functional status of the patient, the initial reponse to treatment, the compliance of the patient, and the patient's age. Most patients in chronic congestive heart failure die suddenly, presumably from ventricular arrhythmia

or from complications of cerebral and peripheral emboli.

In the Framingham study, which included heart failure from all causes, the probability of dying within 5 years of onset of heart failure was 62% for men and 42% for women. The etiology of heart failure in most of these patients was hypertension and ischemic heart disease. The mortality from ischemic heart disease complicated by congestive heart failure is related to ventricular function; patients with an ejection fraction of less than 40% have a particularly poor prognosis and may have a mortality rate of 10 to 20%/year (17). Patients with heart failure due to regurgitant valvular lesions have a mortality in the same range. Heart failure complicating uncorrected aortic stenosis is a particularly ominous sign and the majority of these patients die also within 3 years (Chapter 60).

In general, prognosis is related to the age of the patient and to his functional class (page 772), although there are few studies available in which functional class was accurately determined and prognosis was calculated on a stratified sample. Patients who are functional class II have an annual mortality of approximately 8%. Patients who are functional class III have a slightly higher annual mortality. Patients who are functional class IV rarely live longer than 18 months to 2 years. It is important that the practitioner not venture a prognosis to the patient and family until an optimal level of response to therapy has been achieved.

The mortality from congestive heart failure does not seem to have decreased in the last several years with newer forms of therapy, although these enable patients with chronic heart failure to be more comfortable in their final years of life.

General References

Braunwald E (ed): *Heart Disease: A Textbook of Cardiovascular Medicine.* Philadelphia, WB Saunders, 1984.
    The current standard text. Exhaustively referenced.
Cohn J, Franciosa J: Vasodilator therapy of cardiac failure. *N Engl J Med* 297:27, 254, 1977.
    Excellent review of newer concepts of therapy of heart failure.
Franciosa J: Hypertensive left heart failure: pathogenesis and therapy. *Hosp Pract* 77:Feb, 1981
    Excellent account of the pathogenesis and treatment of the most frequently encountered form of heart failure.
Perloff J, Lindgren K, Groves B: Uncommon or commonly unrecognized causes of heart failure. *Prog Cardiovasc Dis* 12:409, 1970.
    Exhaustive but readable review of commonly unrecognized causes of heart failure.

Specific References

1. Abrams J: Nitroglycerin and long-acting nitrates. *N Engl J Med* 302:1234, 1979.
2. Atlas SA, Case D, Yu ZY, Laragh JH: Hormonal and metabolic effects of angiotensin-converting enzyme inhibitors: possible differences between enalapril and captopril. *Am J Med* 77(2a):13, 1984.
3. Boucher C, Fallon J, Johnson R, Yurchak P: Cardiomyopathic syndrome caused by coronary artery disease. III. Prospective clinicopathological study of its prevalence among patients

with clinically unexplained chronic heart failure. *Br Heart J* 41:613, 1979.

4. Cohn J: Unloading the heart in congestive heart failure. *Am J Med* 77:67, 1984.

5. Davis R, Ribner H, Keung E, *et al*. Treatment of chronic congestive heart failure with captopril, an oral inhibitor of angiotensin-converting enzyme. *N Engl J Med* 301:117, 1979.

6. Franciosa J: Functional capacity of patients with chronic left ventricular failure. *Am J Med* 67:460, 1979.

7. Frazier H, Yager H: The clinical use of diuretics. *N Engl J Med* 288:246, 455, 1973.

8. Gibson T, White K, Klainer L: The prevalence of congestive heart failure in two rural communities. *J Chronic Dis* 19:141, 1966.

9. Harlan W, Oberman A, Grimm R, Rosati R: Chronic congestive heart failure in coronary artery disease: clinical criteria. *Ann Intern Med* 86:133, 1977.

10. Klainer L, Gibson T, White K: The epidemiology of cardiac failure. *J Chronic Dis* 18:797, 1965.

11. Leahey E, Reiffel J, Giardina E, Bigger T: The effect of quini-dine and other oral antiarrhythmic drugs on serum digoxin. *Ann Intern Med* 92:605, 1980.

12. Markiewica W, Peled B, Hammerman H, *et al*: Contribution of M-mode echocardiography to cardiac diagnosis. *Am J Med* 65:802, 1978.

13. McKee P, Castelli W, McNamara P, Kannel W: The natural history of congestive heart failure: the Framingham study. *N Engl J Med* 285:1441, 1971.

14. Nichols A, McKusick K, Strauss H, *et al*: Clinical utility of gated cardiac blood pool imaging in congestive left heart failure. *Am J Med* 65:785, 1978.

15. Perlman L, Ferguson S, Bergum K, *et al*: Precipitation of congestive heart failure: Social and emotional factors. *Ann Intern Med* 75:1, 1971.

16. Ross J Jr: The failing heart and the circulation. *Hosp Practice* 18:151, 1983.

17. Schulze RA Jr, Strauss HW, Pitt B: Sudden death in the year following myocardial infarction: relation to ventricular premature contractions in the late hospital phase and left ventricular ejection fraction. *Am J Med* 62:192, 1977.

CHAPTER SIXTY-TWO

Hypertension

L. RANDOL BARKER, M.D.

INTRODUCTION

In the National Ambulatory Medical Care Survey, management of hypertension was named as the principal reason for approximately 10% of office visits to internists (see Chapter 1, Table 1.3) and approximately 6% of visits to general and family practitioners (Table 1.4). The ambulatory management of this important condition is a longitudinal process requiring skill in enlisting the patient's cooperation and in selecting, monitoring, and adjusting treatment.

EPIDEMIOLOGY

Hypertension has been studied extensively by epidemiologists and clinicians in recent years. The findings from these studies provide the rationale for the care of the individual patient. Because the patient with high blood pressure is usually asymptomatic, an understanding of the risks attending this condition and of the benefits of treatment is especially important.

Prevalence

As shown in the data from the Health and Nutritional Examination Survey (Fig. 62.1), the prevalence of hypertension, defined as a systolic blood pressure of ≥ 160 mm Hg or a diastolic blood pressure of ≥ 95 mm Hg, increases with age, and hypertension is more common in black subjects at all ages. These crude data, based on blood pressure measurement on a single occasion, overestimate the prevalence of sustained hypertension. On repeat exami-

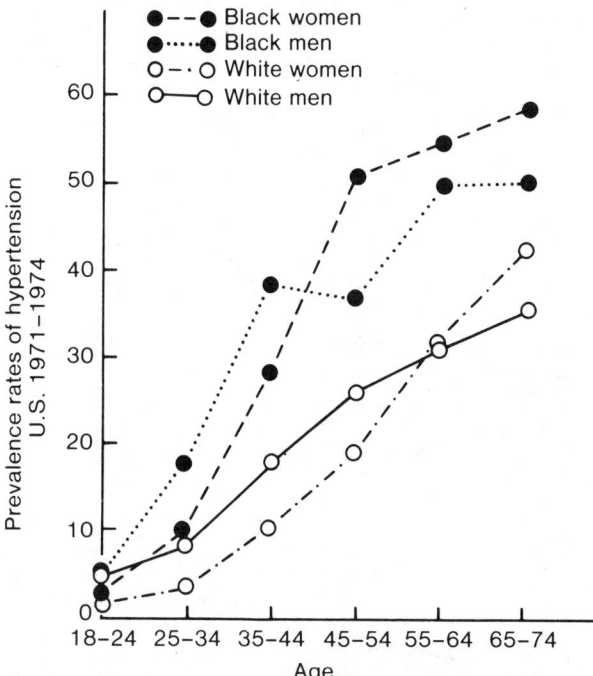

Figure 62.1. The prevalence of hypertension in the United States, defined as a systolic blood pressure of at least 160 mm Hg or a diastolic blood pressure of at least 95 mm Hg. Data from the Health and Nutrition Examination Survey, 1971 to 1974. (From *Advance Data*, Vital and Health Statistics of the National Center for Health Statistics, no. 1, October 18, 1976.)

nation, from 10 to 30% of patients presumed to be hypertensive will be found to have a normal blood pressure, defined as < 140 mm Hg over < 90 mm Hg, and another 10 to 30% will be found to have borderline hypertension, defined as a pressure between 140/90 and 160/95 (8).

For clinical purposes, hypertension is usually defined as sustained diastolic blood pressure of ≥ 90 mm Hg. Of those individuals with sustained diastolic hypertension, approximately 70% have *mild hypertension* (diastolic 90 to 104 mm Hg), 20% have *moderate hypertension* (diastolic 105 to 114 mm Hg), and only 10% have *severe hypertension* (diastolic ≥ 115 mm Hg). These prevalence data indicate that the practicing physician will have to make decisions much more often for patients with mild hypertension than for those with moderate or severe hypertension. The data also explain why the absolute number of morbid events attributable to hypertension in any community is greater in the population of patients with mild hypertension, although the risk of morbid events is much lower in this group than in the other two groups. The following additional blood pressure categories were defined in 1984 by the Joint National Committee on Detection, Evaluation, and Treatment of High Blood Pressure (21): *High normal* (diastolic 85 to 89), *borderline*

isolated systolic hypertension (systolic 140 to 159, diastolic < 90), and *isolated systolic hypertension* (systolic ≥ 160, diastolic < 90). The prevalence of these patterns has not been established, but each is probably as common as mild hypertension.

Risks

For the patient and the physician, the single most important concept in approaching hypertension is that high blood pressure increases the risk of symptomatic cardiovascular disease during the patient's entire life.

This concept has been elucidated by the longitudinal observations on subjects in the *Framingham study*. Adult subjects ranging in age from 45 to 74 years entered the study in 1951 through 1953 and were followed for 18 years. For practical purposes, the Framingham subjects (at entry) can be likened to patients making their first office visit to a physician, at ages ranging from 45 to 74. Based on the average of blood pressures taken on three separate visits, these subjects were subgrouped into those with normal blood pressure, borderline hypertension, and hypertension. During 18 years of follow-up, each new cardiovascular event (myocardial infarction, congestive heart failure, or cerebrovascular accident) was detected. The published analyses provide the practicing physician with a valuable profile of the long term risks associated with high blood pressure (and other cardiovascular risk factors).

One table (Table 62.1) and one figure (Fig. 62.2) from the Framingham study have been selected to emphasize the following messages for the physician and his patient:

1. In any interval of follow-up after initial evaluation, the annual risk of major cardiovascular events is much higher for older patients, as a function of both age and blood pressure at entry.

Table 62.1.
Risk of Cardiovascular Events According to Blood Pressure Status, Men and Women, 45 to 74 (Framingham Study: 18-Year Follow-up)[a]

Age	Average Annual Incidence/1000 Population					
	Men			Women		
	Normal[b]	BHBP[c]	HBP[d]	Normal[b]	BHBP[c]	HBP[d]
45–54	8.3	14.6	23.4	2.4	5.0	8.9
55–64	15.5	29.3	44.4	6.2	14.2	22.7
65–74	16.4	31.9	52.3	8.3	24.9	33.2
45–74[e]	12.4	21.1	35.3	5.7	10.4	18.8

[a] Adapted from Kannel WB: Hypertension in Framingham. In Paul O (ed): *Epidemiology and Control of Hypertension*. Miami, Symposia Specialists, 1975.
[b] Normal, ≤ 140/90.
[c] Borderline, 141/91 to 159/94.
[d] High, ≥ 160/95.
[e] Age-adjusted rates.

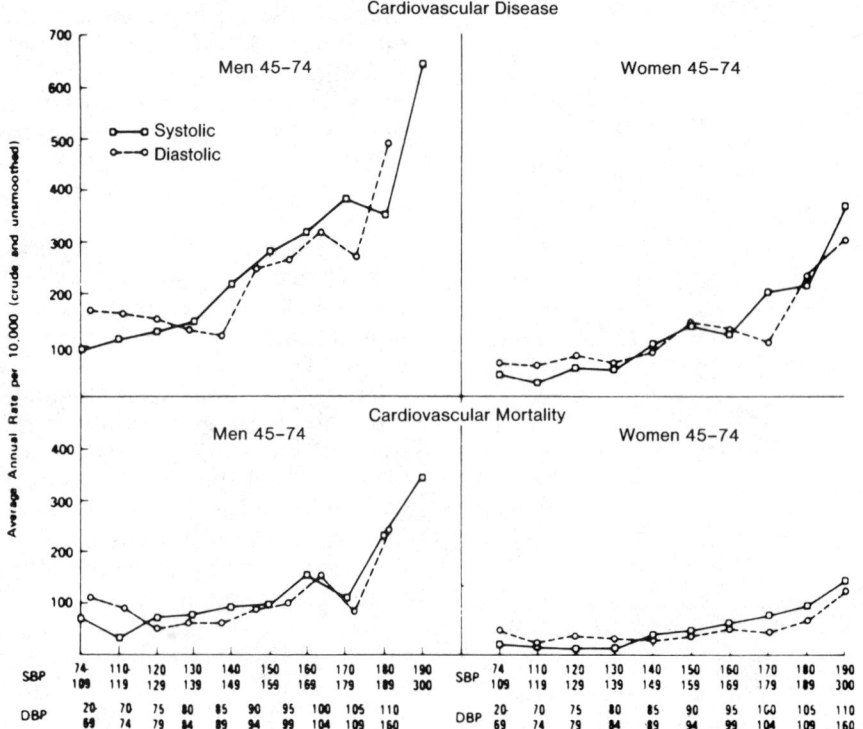

Figure 62.2. The incidence of cardiovascular morbidity (*top*) and mortality (*bottom*) during 18 years' follow-up of the Framingham cohort, plotted according to systolic and diastolic blood pressure at the time of entry for men and women ages 45 to 74. (From Kannel WB, Sorlie P: Hypertension in Framingham. In Paul O (ed): *Epidemiology and Control of Hypertension.* Miami Symposia Specialists, 1975.)

2. Risks rise progressively with each increase of both systolic and diastolic blood pressure.

3. At all ages and blood pressures, the annual incidence of events is somewhat higher for men than for women, although the gradient of risk according to blood pressure is identical for both sexes at all ages.

By consulting the Framingham data, a physician can appreciate the degree of risk for an individual patient. For example, for a man 55 to 64 years old with a blood pressure ≥ 160/95, the risk that a stroke, myocardial infarction, or congestive heart failure will occur during the ensuing 18 years is approximately 80%.

Findings in the *placebo-treated subjects in the Veterans Administration (VA) Therapeutic Trial* and other placebo trials have added to the Framingham findings more concrete information about the risks attending untreated diastolic hypertension, albeit in subjects *selected* for a study. Table 62.2, for example, summarizes the attack rates in the VA trial for placebo-treated patients with entry diastolic pressures in two ranges (90 to 104 mm Hg and 105 to 114 mm Hg) and shows the impact of two associated characteristics (age and presence/absence of established cardiovascular or renal morbidity at entry) upon these risks. Based on these data, for example,

the 3-year risk of major morbidity in an untreated man with left ventricular hypertrophy on electrocardiogram and a usual diastolic blood pressure of 100 mm Hg would be approximately 35%.

Although hypertension, especially severe hypertension, almost always alarms physicians and patients, it is important to recognize that other treatable risk factors can be just as ominous. This is illustrated by the fact that the following two hypothetical male patients, one with mild and the other with severe hypertension, have similar long term risks:

Age	Cigarettes/ Day	Total Cholesterol	Diastolic Blood Pressure
50	0	220 mg/100 ml	125 mm Hg
50	30	250 mg/100 ml	96 mm Hg

Risk Reduction

Severe and Moderate Hypertension

The Veterans Administration Trial confirmed the benefit of treatment in patients with severe and moderate hypertension. Treatment reduced by more than 90% the morbidity in patients with entry diastolic pressures of 115 to 129 mm Hg (severe hypertension) (46) and by 50% or more the morbidity in

Table 62.2.
Placebo-Treated Subjects, Veterans Administration Trial: Impact of Blood Pressure, Age, and Cardiovascular Abnormalities on Attack Rate[a]

Risk Factor at Entry	Number Randomized	Attack Rate[b]
CARDIOVASCULAR AND RENAL ABNORMALITIES[c] AND DIASTOLIC BLOOD PRESSURE (mm Hg):		
Without abnormality		
90–104	36	0.145
105–114	51	0.173
With abnormality		
90–104	48	0.352
105–114	50	0.426
AGE AND DIASTOLIC BLOOD PRESSURE (mm Hg):		
<50 years		
90–104	43	0.121
105–114	56	0.413
50+ years		
90–104	41	0.413
104–114	54	0.459

[a] Adapted from Veterans Administration Cooperative Study Group on Antihypertensive Agents: Effects of treatment on morbidity in hypertension. III. Influence of age, diastolic pressure, and prior cardiovascular disease; further analysis of side effects. *Circulation 45:*991, 1972.
[b] Rate observed during 3 years.
[c] Presence of any of the following: grade 2 or greater hypertensive retinopathy, cardiomegaly on chest X-ray, left ventricular hypertrophy on ECG, evidence of renal damage, myocardial infarction, congestive heart failure, cerebrovascular accident.

both the subgroup with diastolic blood pressure 105 to 114 mm Hg (moderate hypertension) and in those subgroups with diastolic 90 to 104 mm Hg (mild hypertension) who either were over 50 or had one or more cardiovascular-renal abnormalities at entry to the study (Fig. 62.3) (47, 48). Specifically, the risk of congestive heart failure, cerebrovascular accident, or accelerated hypertension (*i.e.*, new retinal hemorrhages or progressive renal insufficiency) was almost entirely eliminated, while there was no significant reduction in the risk of myocardial infarction.

Mild Hypertension

The results of treatment for mild hypertension (diastolic 90 to 104 mm Hg) have been reported from five controlled trials (3, 17, 19, 32, 43, 46), most recently the British Medical Research Council (MRC) trial (24a). Table 62.3 summarizes the following aspects of these trials: number of subjects, sex of participants, entering blood pressures, design, drugs utilized in treated subjects, percentage of reduction in complications, and number of assessable events. On balance, these studies have confirmed that there is a statistically significant benefit from active treatment for mild hypertension. However, the benefit for individual subjects who were treated in these

trials was quite small, since the vast majority of both control and treatment subjects had *no* morbidity during 3 to 7 years. For example, the 5-year all-cause mortality rate in the Hypertension Detection and Follow-up Program was 7.7% for control subjects (Referred Care) and 6.4% for Stepped Care subjects, a reduction *by* 20% (from 7.7% to 6.4%) but a real reduction in expected mortality *of* only 1.3% (Fig. 62.4). In this study, reported in 1979 (19, 20), systematic treatment and follow-up ("stepped care") were compared with usual care for hypertension in the community ("referred care"). Because stepped care may have included better overall care than referred care, some critics do not regard the modest benefit shown for patients with mild hypertension as incontrovertible evidence that control of blood pressure accounted for the benefit, even though patients in the treatment group did have better blood pressure control during the 5-year period of the study.

In addition to the small size of the benefit of treatment shown in completed trials, there is evidence from the Multiple Risk Factor Intervention Trial (MRFIT) that treatment of mild hypertension with diuretics may actually increase mortality in those subjects with entry diastolic pressures of 90 to 95 mm Hg, particularly if the electrocardiogram at entry is abnormal (28).

It has been pointed out that several methodological differences and shortcomings in the completed trials make it difficult to base standard recommendations for mild hypertension upon the individual

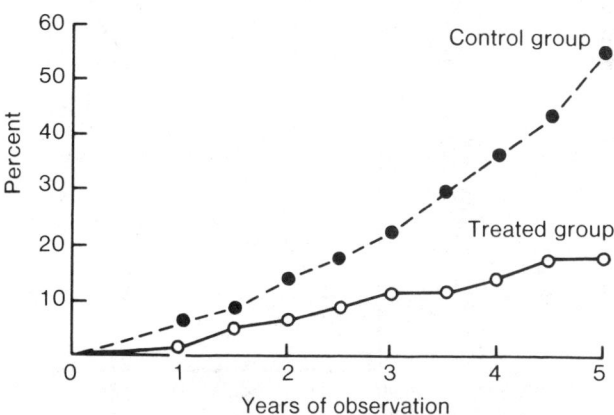

Figure 62.3. Life table analysis comparing percentage of incidence of cardiovascular complications over a 5-year period in control *versus* treated patients with initial diastolic blood pressure in the range of 90 through 114 mm Hg. (From Veterans Administration Cooperative Study Group on Antihypertensive Agents: II. Effects of treatment on morbidity in hypertension: results in patients with diastolic blood pressures averaging 90 through 114 mm Hg. *JAMA* 213:1143, 1970. © American Medical Association.)

Table 62.3.
Characteristics of Completed Controlled Trials of Treatment for Mild Hypertension

Study (Report Year)	No. of Patients Randomized	% Male	Entry Diastolic BP Range	Design		Drugs for Active[a] (Step No.)	% Reduction in Complications	No. Assessable Events	
				Control	Active			Control	Active
Veterans Administration, 1970[b]	170	100	90–104	Placebo	Stepped care	TZ (1)	35	21	14
Hypertension and Detection Follow-up Program, 1979[c]	7,825	54	90–104	Referred care	Stepped care	TZ, K-S (1) R, M (2) H (3) G (4) OTH (5)	20	287	231
Australian, 1980[b]	3,427	63	95–109	Placebo	Stepped care	TZ (1) BB, (M) (2) H, C (3)	30	127	91
Oslo, 1980[b]	785	100	90–109	No therapy	Stepped care	TZ (1) BB, M (2)	25	37	28
MRC, 1985[b]	17,354	52	90–109	Placebo	Stepped care	TZ (1) BB, M (2) or BB (1) TZ or G (2)	19	352	286

[a] TZ, thiazide or thiazide-like diuretic; R, reserpine; H, hydralazine; K-S, potassium-sparing diuretic; M, methyldopa; BB, β-blocker; C, clonidine; G, guanethidine; OTH, other drugs.
[b] Principal end points: cardiovascular morbidity and mortality.
[c] Principal end points: all-cause mortality.

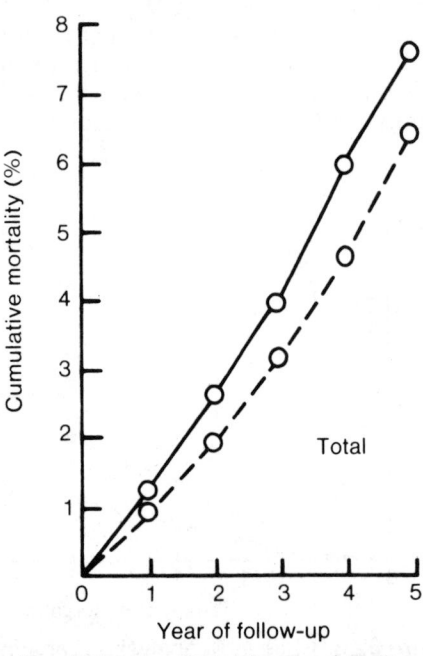
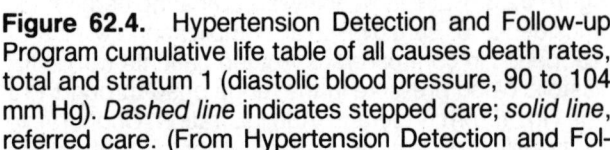
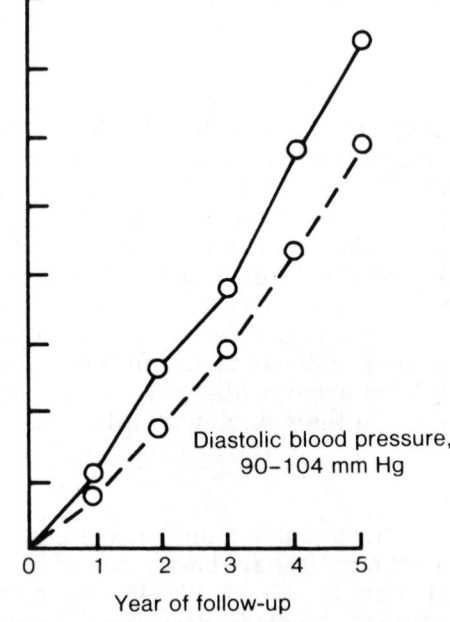

Figure 62.4. Hypertension Detection and Follow-up Program cumulative life table of all causes death rates, total and stratum 1 (diastolic blood pressure, 90 to 104 mm Hg). *Dashed line* indicates stepped care; *solid line*, referred care. (From Hypertension Detection and Follow-up Program Cooperative Group: Five-year findings of the hypertension detection and follow-up program. I. Reduction in mortality of persons with high blood pressure, including mild hypertension. *JAMA* 242:2562, 1979. © American Medical Association.)

and collective findings of these trials (40). The MRC trial (24a) provided the most extensive information, as (*a*) it included large numbers of men and women (in both sexes, treatment significantly reduced strokes but not coronary events; all-cause mortality was lower in treated men and higher in treated women, due to excess noncardiovascular deaths); and (*b*) it compared the risks/benefits of β-blocker (propranolol) monotherapy to diuretic (bendrofluazide) monotherapy (there were no differences in the impact upon overall cardiovascular morbidity or mortality except that coronary events were reduced significantly in one subgroup—propranolol-treated nonsmokers—and strokes were not reduced in propranolol-treated smokers while strokes were reduced in both smokers and nonsmokers taking bendrofluazide).

Based upon what is known, drug treatment of mild hypertension has been advocated for most patients with diastolic pressures of ≥ 100 mm Hg by the World Health Organization (15) and ≥ 95 mm Hg by the Joint National Committee on Detection, Evaluation, and Treatment of High Blood Pressure in the United States (21). Both expert groups suggest individualized treatment decisions for patients below these cut-off levels. The presence of other cardiovascular risk factors (smoking, hypercholesterolemia, overweight, diabetes), a strong family history of cardiovascular morbidity, end organ effects of hypertension (left ventricular hypertrophy on the electrocardiogram, renal insufficiency, history of cerebrovascular disease), and coexisting high systolic pressures are features which favor drug treatment for these patients if nonpharmacological treatment (see page 815) does not control the blood pressure within 2 or 3 months. For patients below the above cut-off levels, who do not have these associated risk factors, nonpharmacological treatment is advocated as the principal approach.

Other Groups of Hypertensives

Risk reduction and practical approaches to *isolated systolic hypertension* and to *hypertension in young and elderly* subjects are discussed in subsequent sections of this chapter.

PATHOPHYSIOLOGY OF ESSENTIAL HYPERTENSION

It is estimated that 95 to 99% of hypertensives do not have an identifiable etiology for their hypertension. Their problem has, therefore, been designated "essential hypertension." Nevertheless, a number of abnormal physiological characteristics have been demonstrated in essential hypertension; these provide a conceptual basis for understanding the clinical consequences of hypertension and the mechanisms of action of antihypertensive drugs.

As indicated in Figure 62.5, the patient with established essential hypertension has an increase in peripheral arterial resistance; this is hypothesized to be the final consequence of either or both of two mechanisms: inappropriate renal retention of salt and water or increased endogenous pressor activity. Serial studies on small numbers of subjects have suggested that a stage of increased cardiac output

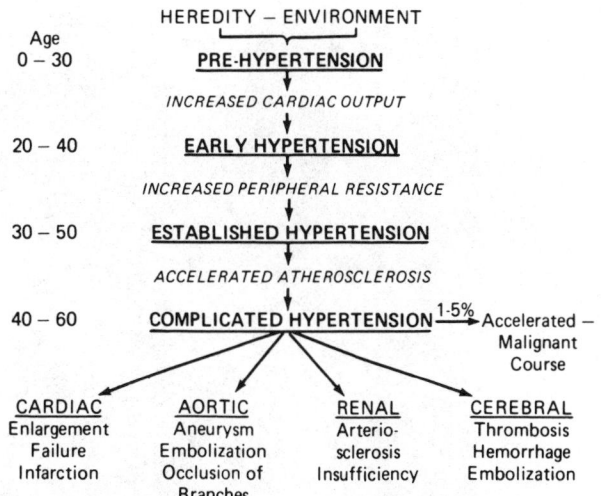

Figure 62.5. A representation of the natural history of untreated essential hypertension. (From Kaplan N: *Clinical Hypertension.* Baltimore, Williams & Wilkins, 1978.)

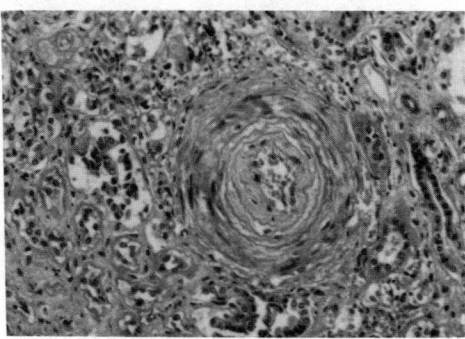

Figure 62.6. Hyperplastic arteriosclerosis in renal tissue from a patient with essential hypertension.

may precede the stage of increased peripheral resistance (5). Clinically, this earlier stage may be manifest in some young hypertensives as a high resting heart rate. In general, however, the evaluation of the individual patient with essential hypertension will not yield much information about the dominant mechanism contributing to that patient's hypertension.

The major complications of untreated hypertension are named in Figure 62.5. These complications can be seen as the clinical manifestations of two pathophysiological processes which are operating during the many "silent years" of increased peripheral resistance: (*a*) trauma to the vessels in the arterial circulation, leading to accelerated atherosclerosis in large vessels and to obliterative changes (see Fig. 62.6) or thinning and rupture (see Fig. 62.7) in small vessels; and (*b*) increase in the work load of the heart, leading to congestive heart failure and/or angina pectoris.

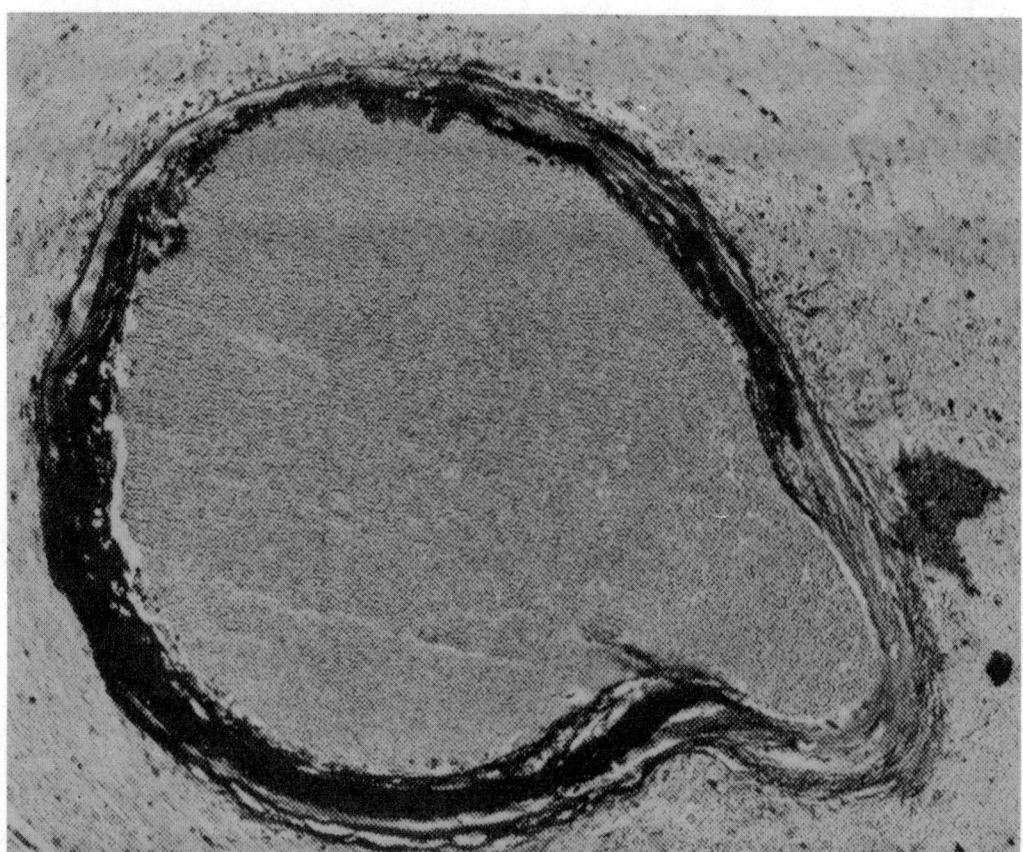

Figure 62.7.   A cross-section of a microaneurysm in a small intracerebral artery from a hypertensive patient. (From Russell RW: How does blood pressure cause stroke? *Lancet* 2:1283, 1975.)

As noted above, blood pressure reduction markedly diminishes the risk of the vascular complications due to hypertension. Although this benefit has only been assessed for drug treatment of hypertension, it is reasonable to assume that nonpharmacological measures for blood pressure reduction are at least as effective.

EVALUATION OF THE PATIENT

In this discussion, hypertension is defined as a diastolic pressure of 90 mm Hg or greater and the approaches recommended are based upon the general guidelines of the 1984 Report of the Joint National Committee on Detection, Evaluation, and Treatment of High Blood Pressure (21).

Measuring the Blood Pressure

In obtaining blood pressures, the following standard practices should be followed:

1. *Cuff selection:* Ideally, the rubber bladder in the cuff should be about 20% wider than the diameter of the arm and should encircle the arm without a significant gap or overlap. When bladder dimensions are too small for the patient's arm, the indirect blood pressure obtained may be higher than the actual blood pressure (see Fig. 62.8). The dimensions of the bladders in available cuffs are: 13 × 24 cm (standard), 17 × 32 cm (large adult), 20 × 42 cm (thigh cuff).

2. Take the initial blood pressure after *the patient has relaxed* for a few minutes in the sitting position. Measure the pressure in each arm, with the arm held across the chest and not dangling in a dependent position. If a difference between arms is noted and confirmed on repeat measurement, take all subsequent blood pressures in the arm with the higher pressure.

3. Use the first Korotkoff sound for systolic pressure. The cuff pressure should be high enough to obliterate the radial pulse; by assuring that this occurs, one will avoid reading a falsely low systolic pressure due to the silent *"auscultatory gap"* that occasionally occurs between the first and second Korotkoff sounds.

4. *Use the fifth Korotkoff sound* (disappearance) for diastolic pressure.

5. Before initiating antihypertensive treatment, take the blood pressure *when the patient is standing* in order to detect significant baseline orthostatic hypotension.

6. *After starting or increasing antihypertensive*

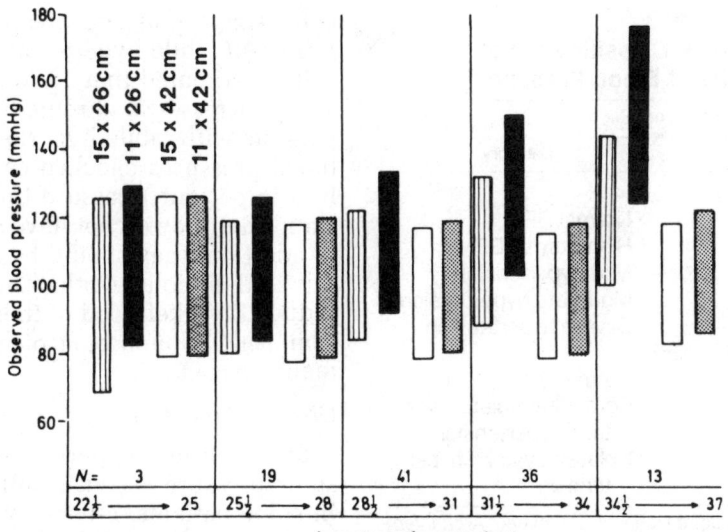

Figure 62.8. Mean blood pressure readings obtained with varying sized cuffs in normal sujects with increasing arm circumference. *N*, number of subjects. The *vertically hatched bar* is for a 15 × 26-cm cuff; the *solid* *bar* is for an 11 × 26-cm cuff; the *open bar* is for a 15 × 45-cm cuff; the *stippled bar* is for an 11 × 42-cm cuff. (From King GE: Errors in clinical measurement of blood pressure in obesity. *Clin Sci* 32:323, 1967.)

drugs, again check the blood pressure with the patient resting and with the patient standing, preferably after a standard exercise (e.g., 10 steps on a footstool or walking a fixed distance), because the orthostatic effects of drugs is often most pronounced after exercise.

7. In addition to blood pressure and heart rate, *record position, arm, and cuff size* (if large cuff used), thereby assuring that these conditions are duplicated when blood pressures are measured at subsequent visits.

Blood Pressure Variability

There are a number of psychological, biological, and pharmacological causes of blood pressure variability. These factors should be considered, in addition to following a systematic approach to measuring the blood pressure, when deciding what the measured blood pressure means in an individual patient.

In a 24-hour period, the average person's resting blood pressures fluctuate in the following ranges: systolic 20 to 40 mm Hg, diastolic 10 to 20 mm Hg. These ranges occur in patients with normal blood pressure and in hypertensive persons who are or are not taking antihypertensive drugs. During and following vigorous exercise, normotensive and hypertensive persons who are not taking antihypertensive drugs show systolic increases of as much as 60 mm Hg and sometimes a modest decrease in their diastolic pressures.

Common factors that may cause *transient or short term blood pressure elevations* are (*a*) physicians taking blood pressures, especially if the patient has

not had time to relax, (*b*) mental stress, both intellectual and psychological, (*c*) sympathomimetic decongestants (29), (*d*) nicotine use (11), (*e*) caffeine use (11), and (*f*) alcohol or sedative-hypnotic withdrawal.

Common factors that may cause a *short term decrease in a patient's blood pressure* are (*a*) intercurrent illness causing volume contraction due to fluid losses or reduced intake, (*b*) bed rest for several days, and (*c*) hospitalization without strict bed rest (18).

Clinical Classification

Evaluating hypertension in an individual patient consists of deciding with which of *four clinical presentations* one is dealing (labile, chronic, accelerated, or emergency hypertension), and, for the patient with sustained hypertension, determining in which *Joint National Committee class* the patient belongs (Table 62.4) and completing a *baseline evaluation* (see below). The classification of the patient should be accomplished carefully, for it provides the patient with a specific label (and notions) which will have a significant effect on his and his physician's future behavior. Two findings underline this point. First, almost half of those people who are found to be hypertensive in screening programs do not have sustained hypertension (8). Second, being labeled hypertensive may have significant "side effects," such as increased sick days, increased life insurance premiums, or certain employment restrictions (16).

On their initial visits, many patients will state that they have hypertension. For some of these, recorded blood pressures from other sources will be available.

Table 62.4.
Joint National Committee's Classification of Hypertension by Severity of Blood Pressure[a]

Classification of BP	
Range, mm Hg	Category[b]
Diastolic	
<85	Normal BP
85–89	High normal BP
90–104	Mild hypertension
105–114	Moderate hypertension
≥115	Severe hypertension
Systolic, when diastolic BP is <90	
<140	Normal BP
140–159	Borderline isolated systolic hypertension
≥160	Isolated systolic hypertension

[a] From The 1984 Report of the Joint National Committee: *Arch Intern Med* 144:1045, 1984.
[b] A classification of borderline isolated systolic hypertension (systolic BP, 140 to 159 mm Hg) or isolated systolic hypertension (systolic BP, >160 mm Hg) takes precedence over a classification of high normal BP (diastolic BP, 85 to 89 mm Hg) when both occur in the same person. A classification of high normal BP (diastolic BP, 85 to 89 mm Hg) takes precedence over a classification of normal BP (systolic BP, <140 mm Hg) when both occur in the same person.

Some will be taking antihypertensive drugs, presumably for sustained hypertension. Based upon this information and upon blood pressure recordings made at the initial and follow-up visits, the patient's physician should decide independently with which clinical presentation of hypertension he is dealing.

Labile Hypertension

By definition, labile hypertension is present in any individual who has a recorded diastolic blood pressure of 90 mm Hg or above, but has a usual diastolic pressure of less than 90 mm Hg. A labile rise in blood pressure can be produced in almost anyone by stresses (including visits to physicians) that provoke increased sympathetic nervous system activity. Therefore, it is no surprise that a high prevalence of labile hypertension has been found in community studies of hypertension. The best example is the Charlottesville community study (8) in which all adults having an elevated initial blood pressure were re-examined. Re-examination showed that the majority of adolescents and young adults (15 to 44 years old), half of those 45 to 55 years old, and a minority of those 55 or older had labile hypertension.

In practice, patients found to have a diastolic pressure of ≥ 90 mm Hg should have their blood pressure remeasured within 2 weeks to determine whether they have labile or sustained (i.e., chronic) hypertension. If the diastolic pressure at the first visit is relatively high (e.g., ≥ 115 mm Hg), the repeat blood pressures should be obtained within 1 week;

even single diastolic pressures in this range may represent labile hypertension.

It is estimated that 10 to 25% of labile hypertension progresses to chronic hypertension. Therefore, patients with labile hypertension should have their blood pressures checked carefully once each year. It is important to assure that such patients understand that they do not have sustained hypertension. In addition, they should be advised to avoid excess salt and to follow other healthy practices which reduce the likelihood of their developing hypertension (see "Nonpharmacological Aspects of Treatment," page 815).

Chronic Hypertension

By definition, hypertension is chronic if the diastolic pressure is consistently 90 mm Hg or greater. In some patients, especially those with high initial pressures, electrocardiographic or X-ray evidence of left ventricular hypertrophy is adequate to confirm the suspicion of chronic hypertension at the first visit. Eye ground findings indicative of arteriolosclerosis (grade 1, narrowing of arteriolar lumen; grade 2, arteriovenous crossing changes) are less reliable and less specific indicators of chronic hypertension and should not be substituted for blood pressure measurements on separate occasions.

The prognosis in untreated chronic hypertension and the benefits of treatment are summarized above ("Risks," page 789, and "Risk Reduction," page 790).

Accelerated Hypertension

By definition, hypertension is in the accelerated or malignant stage if the diastolic pressure is relatively high (usually ≥ 115 mm Hg) and there is clinical evidence of severe arteriolosclerosis, meaning either grade 3 or 4 hypertensive retinopathy (grade 3, hemorrhages and/or fresh exudates; grade 4, papilledema; see Fig. 62.9) or renal insufficiency for which there is no apparent cause except the hypertension.

The prognosis in *untreated* accelerated hypertension is poor: approximately 95% of subjects die of cardiac, renal, or central nervous system complications within 5 years of initial evaluation. Control of blood pressure and dialysis have dramatically improved the prognosis in these individuals.

Hypertensive Emergency

By definition, a hypertensive emergency exists when severe elevation of the blood pressure will cause a catastrophic outcome within hours or days. Patients with two types of hypertensive emergency—hypertensive encephalopathy and dissecting aneurysm of the thoracic aorta—may present initially in an office setting. When either of these diagnoses is suspected, the patient should be transported immediately to a hospital emergency room for definitive evaluation and treatment.

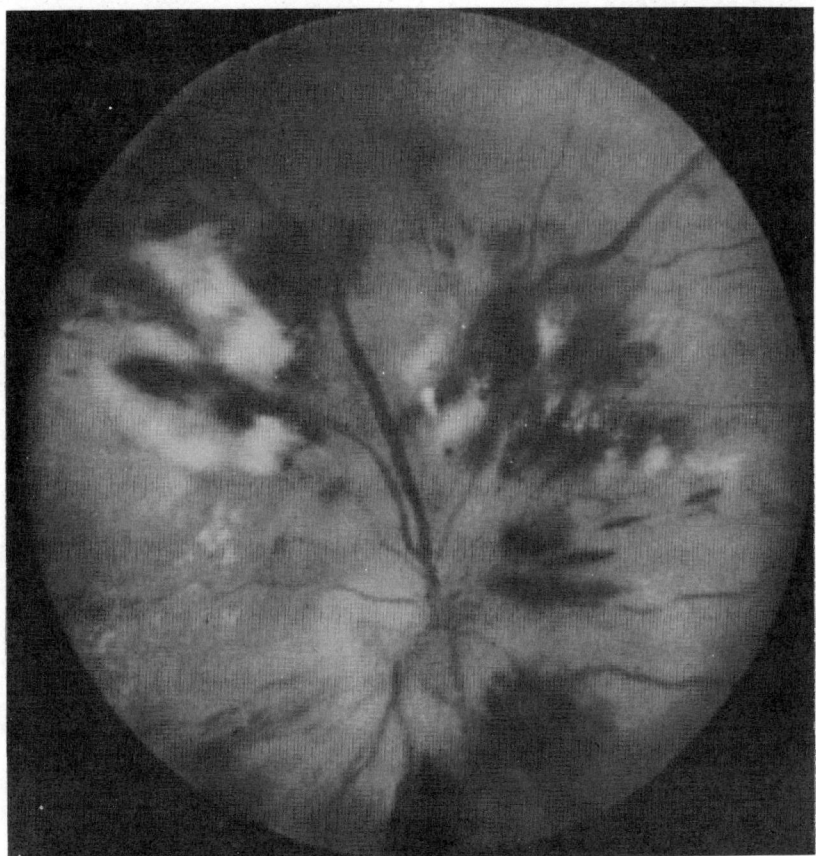

Figure 62.9.   Grade 4 Keith-Wagener retinopathy.

Hypertensive encephalopathy is the result of cerebral edema that develops gradually over 1 or more days in a patient with severe diastolic hypertension. In such a patient, global cerebral symptoms, such as headache, confusion, and irritability, have usually been present and progressive for hours or days. Papilledema may be present. Hypertensive encephalopathy is a clinical diagnosis that should be made only when intracerebral hemorrhage, which may also present with hypertension, has been excluded.

Thoracic aortic dissection results from an expanding hematoma in the wall of the aorta; in the patient who is dissecting, hypertension may promote perforation of the intima overlying the softened wall of the aorta. The patient with acute dissection will usually have a history of known hypertension and will present with a story of sudden "ripping" pain in the back. Computerized tomography and contrast aortography are both very sensitive and specific diagnostic tests for dissection. By definition, a *proximal* dissection involves the aorta between the aortic root and the left subclavian artery (pulses may be absent or decreased in the right arm and neck; there may be a murmur of aortic regurgitation) and a *distal* dissection involves only that part of the aorta distal to the left subclavian artery.

The prognosis in encephalopathy and aortic dissection, when either condition is diagnosed before there has been irreversible damage, depends upon prompt, carefully monitored blood pressure control in an intensive care setting. Despite the overwhelming threat to life without treatment, excellent outcomes can be achieved with appropriate intervention.

Baseline Evaluation: Overview

The baseline evaluation of the patient with sustained hypertension should accomplish five objectives:

1. Indicate the status of end organs affected by hypertension;

2. Identify clues to the presence of a treatable etiology for the hypertension;

3. Guide the selection of initial treatment;

4. Establish the pretreatment status of parameters commonly affected by antihypertensive drugs;

5. Detect the presence of additional cardiovascular risk factors.

Table 62.5 lists by source the information that should be obtained in the baseline evaluation to accomplish these five objectives.

Table 62.5.
Baseline Evaluation of the Patient with Sustained Hypertension

Information	Reason for Obtaining Information				
	End Organ Status	Etiology Screening	Selecting Treatment	Factors Modified by Treatment	Additional Cardiovascular Risk Factors
INTERVIEW, OLD RECORDS					
Age and race		X	X		
Blood pressure levels		X	X	X	
Hypertension treatment, results		X	X		
Family history		X	X		X
Congestive heart failure	X		X		
Angina	X		X		
Transient ischemic attack or cerebrovascular accident	X				
Renal disease	X	X	X		
Comprehension of hypertension			X	X	
Diet (Na, K, fats)		X	X	X	X
Exercise habits					X
Current drugs[a]		X	X	X	X
Alcohol use		X	X		
Tobacco use					X
Current life stresses		X	X		X
Coexisting conditions[b]		X	X		
Periodic sympathetic symptoms		X			
PHYSICAL EXAMINATION					
Weight		X	X	X	
Blood pressure (right, left, resting, standing)		X	X	X	
Heart rate		X	X	X	
Eye grounds	X		X		
Peripheral pulses	X	X	X		
Heart	X				
Lungs			X		
Abdomen (mass, bruit)		X			
Neurological	X				
LABORATORY					
Creatinine	X	X	X	X	
Potassium		X	X	X	
Sodium			X		
Fasting glucose			X	X	
Cholesterol (total, high density lipoprotein)				X	X
Uric acid			X	X	
Urinalysis		X		X	
ECG	X				

[a] Identify drugs that may cause hypertension or may interfere with antihypertensive drugs (*i.e.*, oral contraceptives, tricyclic antidepressants, sympathomimetic decongestants, appetite suppressants, corticosteroids, nonsteroidal anti-inflammatory drugs).
[b] See Table 62.7.

End Organ Status

At baseline evaluation, most patients with chronic hypertension and many of those with accelerated hypertension have no symptoms attributable to their hypertension. In the past, it was thought that headache, tinnitus, epistaxis, and dizziness were common symptoms of hypertension, but community-based studies have demonstrated that these symptoms are not more prevalent in hypertensives than in normotensives. A minority of patients do have genuine hypertensive headaches, which are occipital in location, are worse in the morning, and resolve with lowering of the blood pressure.

Heart

A history of symptoms due to congestive heart failure or to coronary artery disease will occasionally be obtained at baseline evaluation. Auscultation of the heart commonly reveals accentuation of the aortic second sound and a systolic ejection murmur.

Infrequent auscultatory findings include a systolic ejection sound at the base of the heart, paradoxical splitting of the second heart sound, or a short high pitched diastolic murmur at the base. Objective evidence of cardiac hypertrophy is frequently found at baseline evaluation, either on physical examination (left ventricular heave or fourth heart sound) or on the electrocardiogram. Evidence of left atrial abnormality is the earliest change on the electrocardiogram, reflecting atrial contraction against a left ventricle with decreased compliance. The electrocardiographic criteria for left ventricular hypertrophy (LVH) are summarized elsewhere (Table 60.3, Chapter 60). The concentric hypertrophy typical of hypertension causes only a modest increase in the left ventricular silhouette on the chest X-ray, and the plain film of the chest is much less sensitive than the electrocardiogram in identifying changes due to LVH.

The functional derangements associated with LVH have been the subject of intense study in recent years (see Messerli and Schlant, "General References"). In some asymptomatic patients, the resting ejection fraction (measured by echocardiogram) is normal but the ejection fraction shows a subnormal increase during exercise. In hypertensive patients with symptoms of left ventricular failure, echocardiographic studies have revealed that some have global left ventricular dysfunction; some have functional subaortic stenosis; some have a hyperkinetic left ventricle with a normal or high ejection fraction and with diminished relaxation during diastole; and some in the latter group (usually older patients) have "cavity obliteration" during diastole (39). Because appropriate drug therapy for patients in these groups differs in important ways (see Table 62.7 below), it is recommended that hypertensive patients with signs and symptoms of heart failure should have echocardiograms to assure that the drugs prescribed for them improve rather than worsen the heart failure.

Eye

Traditionally, examination of the retina has been emphasized in the evaluation of hypertensive patients because it offers direct inspection of blood vessels affected by hypertension. Ophthalmic symptoms attributed to hypertension (decreased acuity due to retinal hemorrhages or retinal detachment) are very uncommon, however. Most patients with chronic hypertension have evidence of arteriolosclerosis (grades 1 and 2 hypertensive retinopathy), but these findings have little practical value as they are not specific for hypertension, and there is significant interobserver and intraobserver variability in detecting them. On the other hand, grades 3 or 4 retinopathy (see Fig. 62.9) should be sought in any patient with a high diastolic pressure, for these changes signify accelerated hypertension.

Kidney

Simple tests of kidney status (urinalysis of serum creatinine level) are normal in the majority of hypertensives at baseline. In the patient with a high diastolic pressure, either an elevated creatinine concentration, proteinuria (sometimes more than 1 g/24 hours), or microscopic hematuria may be found as evidence for accelerated hypertension; other forms of urogenital disease should be excluded in such patients before these findings are attributed to hypertension.

Central Nervous System

A history of stroke—lacunar or major vessel syndromes—or transient ischemic attacks (see Chapter 83), an asymptomatic carotid bruit, or neurological findings of a remote stroke may be present at baseline evaluation, but the majority of patients will have no evidence of cerebrovascular disease when first evaluated.

Evaluation for Secondary Hypertension

Information in the baseline evaluation will identify those patients who *may* have hypertension secondary to a treatable condition. The rarity of surgically curable hypertension is indicated by the reports from referral centers in which only 1 to 3% of referred (i.e., selected) patients have had these forms of hypertension (12, 41).

Current Use of an Oral Contraceptive

This cause of hypertension should be considered in any patient currently using an oral contraceptive hormone. To confirm this etiology, there should be evidence for a normal blood pressure before oral contraceptive use; and the patient's blood pressure should become normal within 6 months of discontinuing oral contraceptives (see additional details, page 830).

Chronic Alcoholism

In some individuals, heavy, chronic alcohol use is probably the cause of sustained hypertension. For patients found to have both hypertension and alcoholism at the baseline evaluation, blood pressure control should be attempted initially through detoxification and treatment of the alcoholism (see Chapter 21). The blood pressure becomes normal in those with alcohol-induced hypertension within about 1 week of alcohol cessation (34).

Renovascular Hypertension (RVH)

A number of findings in the baseline evaluation increase somewhat the prior probability that the patient has RVH: the presence of an abdominal bruit radiating to the flank (with both systolic and diastolic components); a recent change from normal blood pressure to moderate or severe hypertension; a very high diastolic pressure (e.g., ≥ 115 mm Hg) in a person under 30 years of age; or evidence of accelerated hypertension (*i.e.*, grade 3 or 4 hypertensive retinopathy or renal insufficiency due to hypertension).

If a patient has one or more of these findings and is a candidate for surgery, the physician has three choices.

1. Attempt to control the hypertension with drugs. This choice is supported by the findings that RVH generally responds to medical therapy and that many patients with RVH due to atherosclerosis (the commonest cause of RVH) need to resume drug treatment within 1 or more years of surgery (51).

2. Screen the patient with either a hypertensive intravenous pyelogram (IVP, see "Patient Experience," below), a saralasin infusion test (saralasin, an angiotensin antagonist, is infused intravenously under standardized conditions; a positive test is a fall in blood pressure of 10/8 mm Hg during the infusion), or assay of peripheral renin activity (see protocol for renin stimulation, Table 45.7). None of these tests, when positive, enhances enough the confidence that RVH will be found on arteriography to make it a very useful screening test (14). Furthermore, because RVH is so uncommon, a normal result with any of these screening tests only increases marginally one's confidence that the patient does not have RVH. For example, a negative IVP provides the following increase in confidence in groups of patients with 1%, 5%, or 10% prevalence of RVH:

RVH Prevalence	Confidence Patient Does Not Have RVH before IVP	Confidence Patient Does Not Have RVH after Negative IVP
1%	99%	99.8%
5%	95%	98.7%
10%	90%	97.6%

3. For selected patients, proceed directly to bilateral renal arteriography and renal vein renin sampling. If unilateral renal artery stenosis with lateralizing high renal vein renin activity is found and the patient has fibromuscular hyperplasia, percutaneous transluminal angioplasty (PTA) may yield results equal to surgical correction of the RVH (36). Neither PTA nor surgery has produced very satisfactory long term results if RVH due to atherosclerosis is present. However, in some patients with the combination of hypertension resistant to medical therapy, renal insufficiency, and either bilateral renal artery stenosis or renal artery stenosis in a single functioning kidney, surgery or PTA may control the hypertension and stabilize or improve the renal function (53).

Patient experience. The patient can expect the following experience when undergoing radiological evaluation for RVH:

Hypertensive IVP: the patient takes nothing by mouth for at least 12 hours and takes a laxative the night before. Contrast material is injected as rapidly as possible by the radiologist. Mild nausea is common during injection. The patient lies supine on the X-ray table for 15 minutes while X-rays are taken at 1, 2, 3, 4, 5, 10, and 15 minutes after dye injection. Total time in the radiology suite is 20 to 30 minutes.

Renal arteriography and renal vein renin sampling: the patient is hospitalized, given nothing by mouth, and given a laxative the evening before these studies. After local anesthesia, catheter-containing needles are inserted percutaneously into a femoral vein and a femoral artery. Substantial time is devoted to positioning of catheters, under fluoroscopic guidance. When dye is injected, the patient feels intense warmth in the abdomen for a few seconds. The patient is supine throughout the procedure. Total time in the radiology suite is usually 1 ½ to 2 hours. The patient is instructed to remain at bed rest for 12 hours to allow clot formation at the site of the arterial puncture. The risks associated with angiography are hematoma formation or oozing at the arterial puncture site, and, rarely, anaphylactoid reactions or distal emboli (especially in patients with extensive atherosclerosis).

Kidney Disease

This should be suspected as a possible cause of hypertension in patients with a history of hematuria, stones, or recurrent pyelonephritis; or in patients in whom large kidneys (e.g., due to obstruction or to polycystic disease) or a large bladder are palpated; or when the urinalysis suggests acute or chronic glomerulonephritis (i.e., marked proteinuria and/or red cell casts). If obstructive uropathy is suspected, a sonogram should be obtained to check for hydronephrosis. In patients with established chronic renal failure and small kidneys, it is often difficult to determine whether the hypertension or the renal disease was the initial problem.

Primary Hyperaldosteronism

The commonest clue to this etiology is a baseline potassium level significantly below normal for which there is no explanation, such as diuretic use or gastrointestinal fluid loss. Such patients should be asked about excess consumption of licorice, which contains glycyrrhizinic acid, a moiety with mineralocorticoid-like activity. The ambulatory evaluation of the patient with suspected primary hyperaldosteronism is discussed in detail in Chapter 45, Hypokalemia.

Pheochromocytoma (6)

Clues to the possible presence of pheochromocytoma are a history of a hypermetabolic state (which may resemble hyperthyroidism) and of periodic clusters of symptoms of sympathetic nervous system hyperactivity (tachycardia, diaphoresis, palpitations, with headaches and orthostatic hypotension), especially when these are not provoked by psychological stress and when there is no evidence for reactive hypoglycemia (see Chapter 74). The absence of such symptom clusters virtually excludes the presence of pheochromocytoma. Additional symptoms that should raise concern about pheochromocytoma are (a) a marked change in blood pressure or heart rate in response to minor injury, parturition, or general anesthesia; (b) a neurocutaneous syndrome (von Recklinghausen's or von Hippel-Landau syndrome); (c) a blood relative with a pheochromocytoma; (d) possible type II multiple endocrine neoplasia (medullary carcinoma of the thyroid or parathyroid adenoma, or both, with symptoms suggesting pheochromocytoma).

Table 62.6 summarizes the sensitivity and specificity of various screening tests for pheochromocytoma. These data are based on evaluation of modest-sized groups of patients with proven pheochromocytomas and without pheochromocytoma. The best test appears to be the clonidine suppression test (sensitivity 97% and specificity 99%). In this test, 0.3 mg of clonidine is given orally and plasma catecholamine concentration is measured after 2 or 3 hours; in a positive test, the concentration remains above 500 pg/ml. The usefulness of this test depends upon access to a laboratory that measures plasma catecholamines reliably. Twenty-four-hour urine tests are also useful for screening pheochromocytoma suspects, and they can be used easily in the office setting. The patient is given a plastic container, which is acidified (contains a fixed amount of a strong acid), and instructed to collect a 24-hour specimen. One specimen can be used to screen for catecholamines, metanephrines, and vanillylmandelic acid. With modern assay techniques, no foodstuffs and only a small number of drugs interfere with test results (*catecholamines*, increased by methyldopa and L-dopa, theophylline, hypoglycemia, Isuprel, Prochlorperazine; *metanephrines*, increased by monamine oxidase inhibitors, clonidine withdrawal, occasionally methyldopa; *vanillylmandelic acid*, decreased by monoamine oxidase inhib-

itors and clofibrate, increased by nalidixic acid). In the rare patient who has a normal blood pressure between paroxysms of hypertension, the urine specimen should be taken when the patient is hypertensive. Patients with positive screening tests, ideally on more than one occasion, should be hospitalized for radiological localization of a tumor. For patients with suspected pheochromocytoma and normal office screening tests, hospital admission for provocative tests (histamine, glucagon, tyramine) should be considered, in consultation with an endocrinologist.

Coarctation of the Aorta

Clues to the presence of this condition are hypertension in a relatively young patient (most will be recognized in the pediatric age group); decreased blood pressure in the lower extremities, suggested by diminished or absent femoral pulses and corroborated by blood pressures auscultated over the popliteal artery, using a large cuff; and evidence of poststenotic dilatation of the aorta (Fig. 62.10) or collateral arterial vessels either on inspection of the trunk or on the plain chest X-ray (Fig. 62.10). In a minority of patients, the coarctation occurs proximal to the left subclavian artery, and the blood pressure will be high only in the right arm. To confirm the presence of a coarctation, the patient must be hospitalized for aortography.

Baseline Status of Factors Modified by Treatment

Table 62.5 lists a number of factors that should be documented at the baseline evaluation because of the likelihood or possibility that they will be modified as part of treatment or as a consequence of treatment. These include information obtained in the history (baseline understanding of hypertension, usual diet, alcohol consumption, current medications), in the physical examination (weight, blood pressure, heart rate and rhythm), and in the laboratory examination (creatinine, electrolytes, fasting glucose, complete blood count, uric acid, cholesterol, and urinalysis).

Table 62.6.
Sensitivity and Specificity of Various Tests for Pheochromocytoma[a, b]

Test	Referent Values	Sensitivity[e]	Specificity[f]
Plasma NE+E (after clonidine)	>500 pg/ml[c]	0.97 (31/32)	0.99 (69/70)
Plasma NE+E	>950 pg/ml[d]	0.94 (60/64)	0.97 (68/70)
Urinary MN	>1.8 mg/24 hr[d]	0.79 (34/43)	0.93 (28/30)
Urinary VMA	>11 mg/24 hr[d]	0.42 (18/43)	1.00 (30/30)

[a] From Bravo EL, Gifford RW Jr: Pheochromocytoma: diagnosis, localization and management. *N Engl J Med* 311:1298, 1984.
[b] NE+E, norepinephrine plus epinephrine; MN, metanephrines; VMA, vanillylmandelic acid. Numbers of patients are shown in parentheses. To convert values for MN and VMA to micromoles per liter, multiply by 5.265 and 5.046, respectively; to convert NE+E values to nanomoles per liter, convert to micrograms per liter and multiply by 5.911.
[c] Upper 95% confidence limits of basal values in 47 normotensive controls.
[d] Upper 95% confidence limits of basal values in 70 patients with essential hypertension.
[e] Shows number of pheochromocytoma patients with abnormal results over total number studied, in parentheses.
[f] Shows number of patients without pheochromocytoma who had normal results over total number studied.

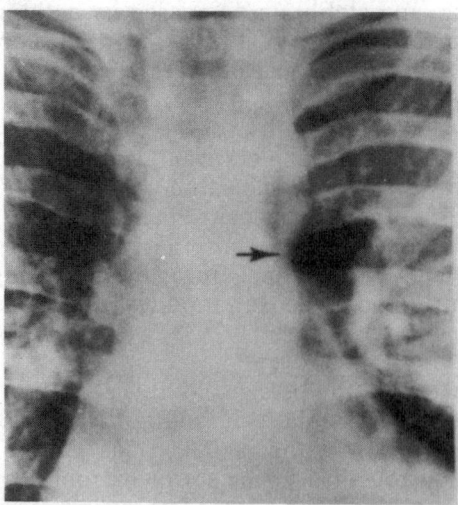 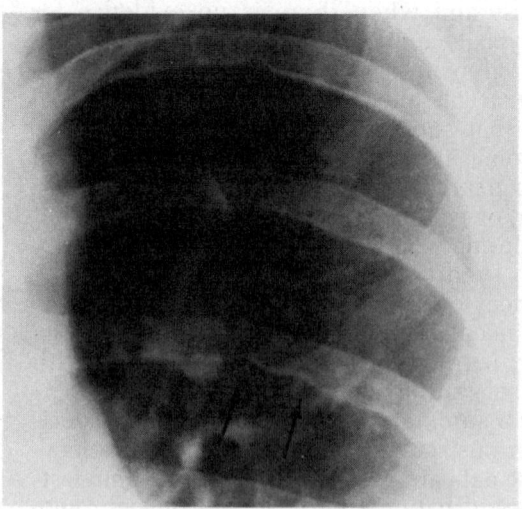

Figure 62.10. Chest X-ray features of coarctation. *Left.* The "3 sign" at the left parasternal border of the descending aorta. *Right.* Notching of the ribs from enlarged collateral vessels. (From Smith PT, Edwards JE: Pseudocoarctation, kinking, or buckling of the aorta. *Circulation* 46:1027, 1972. By permission of the American Heart Association, Inc.)

Other Cardiovascular Risk Factors (Table 62.5)

The baseline evaluation of a hypertensive patient should include checking for other factors that may increase cardiovascular risk, and these factors should be considered in planning the overall management of the patient. These include family history of premature cardiovascular disease, high cholesterol diet, sedentary living, tobacco use, stressful life style, overweight, diabetes mellitus, and hypercholesterolemia.

TREATMENT

Goals of Treatment

When sustained hypertension has been diagnosed, the initial goal of treatment is a normal blood pressure, defined as a diastolic pressure under 90 mm Hg. An appropriate long term goal is the lowest diastolic pressure that can be attained safely (for practical purposes 70 mm Hg should be the lower limit). Partial reduction of blood pressure is an acceptable goal for patients in whom it is impossible to achieve a diastolic pressure of < 90 mm Hg (38).

In most patients, satisfactory blood pressure control can be achieved within 1 to 3 months. In deciding whether treatment has altered the patient's blood pressure, it should be remembered that *a reduction of less than 10 mm Hg diastolic is not meaningful* (44). This is particularly important in deciding whether there has been a real response in the patient with mild hypertension. For example, evidence of a significant response in a patient with an average diastolic pressure of 95 mm Hg before treatment is a diastolic pressure 85 mm Hg or less after treatment.

Promoting Compliance with Treatment

Compliance with treatment as a generic feature of ambulatory care is discussed in detail in Chapter 4. Because poor compliance is so common in hypertensive patients, the problem has been studied extensively in recent years; a number of strategies in patient care have been shown to improve compliance with antihypertensive treatment (24, 33). Some of these strategies should be used routinely. More intensive strategies should be used for those patients who appear to be especially noncompliant.

The following strategies should be used routinely from the outset of treatment:

1. Assuring that the patient knows several critical facts about hypertension: that it increases the risk of grave illness later in life; that it is usually asymptomatic when initially found; that treatment reduces the risk of grave illness; and that treatment is continuous for life. This information is covered well in patient information pamphlets available from the American Heart Association and from a number of companies that manufacture antihypertensive drugs. One of these pamphlets should be given to each hypertensive patient *as an adjunct* to a verbal summary of this information by the physician or nurse, and the patient's comprehension of the fundamentals of hypertension should be ascertained periodically. (For further information on patient education, see Chapter 3.)

2. Prescribing drugs that can be taken once or twice daily (see Tables 62.9 and 62.10 below).

3. Having the patient state how he is taking his medication at each visit (including what he has taken "today" and, for drugs with a duration of action under 12 hours, when the last dose was

taken). Patients taking multiple drugs should be encouraged to bring their bottles of medicine.

4. Assuring that supervision is provided frequently enough. During the first year of treatment, this should be at least every 2 to 3 months, at scheduled visits.

5. Assuring that the practice is planned to maximize convenience for the patient, meaning that waiting time is brief, that telephone access to the practice is easy, that appointment changes are accommodated, and that prescription renewals are easy to obtain.

For patients who admit poor compliance, the reason should be explored and addressed (see practical approaches, Chapter 4).

For patients with uncontrolled hypertension in whom poor compliance is suspected but not admitted, the following strategies have been shown to help:

1. Having the adult with whom the patient has the most contact (usually the spouse) become an active participant in promoting compliance. This other adult should know in detail the treatment regimen and should be asked to provide specific reinforcement for medication taking. Sometimes it is helpful to have a visiting nurse provide initial education and check blood pressures in the patient's home.

2. Having the patient or another person take home blood pressures and bring the record to office visits. When this is done, the patient's blood pressure measurement technique should be checked periodically.

3. Observing the patient's response when his prescribed medications are given under supervision in the office (see case example in Fig. 62.12, page 822).

4. Having the patient participate in group meetings with other hypertensive patients, coordinated by someone skilled in promoting group support mechanisms.

Several additional findings have been noted in studies of compliance in hypertension:

1. Compliance-promoting strategies are additive.

2. Compliance decays in many patients who initially do well and in those noncompliers who improve after short term intensive interventions, such as home visits. Because of the problem of compliance decay, it is important to maintain some compliance-promoting strategies continuously in the long term care of hypertensive patients.

3. The cost of drugs and side effects from drugs explain only a small proportion of noncompliance in the treatment of hypertension.

Pharmacological Treatment: Stepped Care Method

For patients with moderate or severe hypertension (see criteria, Table 62.4), antihypertensive drugs are always indicated. For patients with mild hypertension (especially diastolic under 100 mm Hg), an initial trial of nonpharmacological management of hypertension is often appropriate. Nonpharmacological measures (sodium restriction, limiting alcohol use, weight reduction, regular exercise, *etc*) should always be recommended as adjuncts to drug treatment. These measures are discussed below (page 815).

In the future, objective methods may be available for selecting the most appropriate antihypertensive drug for an individual patient. The methods introduced so far, such as renin profiling and saralasin infusions, have not proven to be sufficiently reliable or practical. Therefore, drug treatment for most patients should be initiated and modified using the stepped care strategies recommended by the Joint National Committee (see Fig. 62.11). As discussed below, there *are* a number of considerations in individual patients which are important when selecting drugs in stepped care.

Step 1 in the strategy outlined in Figure 62.11 differs importantly from previous recommendations. Either a diuretic *or* a β-blocker (or another adrenergic inhibitor) is now recommended as the step 1 drug; previously, diuretic therapy was recommended as step 1 for all patients. In addition, the recommended starting and maximum doses for diuretics have been reduced to the equivalent of 25 mg and 50 mg of hydrochlorothiazide. In most patients, the principal antihypertensive effect of thiazides is realized at these doses, and higher doses may increase the likelihood of hypokalemia and other metabolic consequences of diuretics. Additional considerations related to diuretics and β-blockers are summarized below ("Properties of Individual Drugs").

More than 50% of patients can be controlled with a step 1 drug alone. *Step 2* (adding an adrenergic inhibitor to a step 1 diuretic or a diuretic to a nondiuretic step 1 drug) and *step 3* (adding a vasodilator to the step 2 regimen or utilizing captopril or a calcium channel blocker) are sequential strategies which will lead to control in most patients who do not respond to step 1.

The *step 4* drugs, guanethidine and guanadrel, are potent peripheral adrenergic inhibitors. Both cause orthostatic hypotension, often severe, at the doses needed to control the sitting or recumbent blood pressure. With judicious trials of step 3 regimens (in particular, β-blocker/hydralazine, β-blocker/minoxidil, β-blocker/nifedipine, or captopril) these unsatisfactory step 4 drugs can virtually always be avoided.

For most patients, it is reasonable to initiate a step 1 drug and assess the response after 1 to 2 weeks. In general, the patient's baseline blood pressure is not a reliable predictor of the amount or kind of drug the patient will need. However, patients with severe hypertension should be started on a step 2 regimen and should be evaluated weekly or more frequently until their blood pressure is controlled. This is feasible since the major antihypertensive effect of most

STEP 1	*STEP 2*	*STEP 3*	*STEP 4*
Initiate	*Add[a]*	*Use Combination[a]*	*Add[a]*
Thiazide diuretic	Adrenergic inhibitor (except gunadrel or guanethidine)	Add vasodilator	Guanadrel or guanethidine
or	or	or	
β-Blocker (or monotherapy with another adrenergic inhibitor, in selcted patients)	Diuretic	Try 2 adrenergic inhibitors with different actions	
		or	
		Add/substitute: angiotensin converting enzyme inhibitor	
		or	
		Add/substitute calcium channel blocker	

[a] Angiotensin converting enyzme inhibitor or calcium channel blocker may be substituted at steps 2 to 4 if side effects limit the use of other nondiuretic agents or if other agents are ineffective. For patients in whom excess total body sodium is suspected, a loop diuretic should be tried instead of large doses of step 2 and step 3 drugs.

Figure 62.11. Stepped care approach to drug therapy. (See available strengths, dose ranges, and schedules for all drugs in Tables 62.9 and 62.10.) (Adapted from The Joint National Committee on Detection, Evaluation and Treatment of High Blood Pressure: The 1984 Report of the Joint National Committee on Detection, Evaluation, and Treatment of High Blood Pressure. *Arch Intern Med* 144:1045, 1984.)

nondiuretic drugs is apparent within 1 to 2 days (see below, Table 69.10).

In stepped treatment, *diuretic therapy should always be maintained*, even in the patient whose blood pressure shows little or no response to a maximum dose of diuretic alone. This is because step 2 to 4 drugs promote renal sodium retention as a response to blood pressure lowering, attenuating the antihypertensive effect of the drug. This problem is overcome by maintaining sufficient diuretic treatment to prevent sodium retention; large doses of loop diuretics and/or the addition of diuretics which act on the distal tubule (potassium-conserving diuretics) may be needed to accomplish this in some patients, as discussed below.

Two or more of some antihypertensive drugs are available in *fixed-dose combination tablets* and more will probably be available in the future. The appropriate combination may provide additional convenience at no additional cost.

Individualizing Drug Selection

There are a variety of diuretic regimens and approximately 20 nondiuretic drugs to choose from in prescribing for hypertension. In addition to the stepped care strategy, a number of factors may be helpful in choosing drugs for individual patients.

The baseline evaluation (see Table 62.5) often discloses useful information. The patient's *previous experience with specific drugs* may be important

(e.g., a history of side effects, nonresponse, or good response). The patient's *race and age* should be considered. In general, black subjects respond less often than whites to β-blockers and more often than whites to diuretics alone (45); special considerations in managing young and elderly hypertensives are discussed in later sections of this chapter. *Coexisting medical conditions* should always be considered in selecting antihypertensive drugs. Table 62.7 summarizes considerations in patients with a number of cardiovascular conditions, obstructive airways disease, diabetes, chronic renal and liver disease, and other common conditions. New illness occurring during longitudinal care of hypertension may also affect management (see "Co-morbidity," page 824).

Drug Side Effects: Overview

Modification of the regimen may be needed when drugs control the hypertension but cause significant drug side effects. After drugs have been initiated, the patient should be encouraged to discuss any drug-associated disturbances, such as reduced mental alertness, mood change, or impairment in physical exercise or sexual activity. It should be remembered that from 5 to 15% of subjects discontinue therapy in the trials of most antihypertensive drugs because of such side effects and that many more subjects notice minor side effects as long as they are taking antihypertensive drugs. On the other hand, learning that one has hypertension may cause some

Table 62.7.
Considerations for Selecting Antihypertensive Drugs in Patients with Coexisting Medical Conditions

Coexisting Condition	Drugs Which May Be Contraindicated or Disadvantageous	Drugs Which May Have Special Advantages
Obstructive airways disease	β-blockers	None
Peripheral arterial insufficiency or Raynaud's phenomenon	β-blockers	Calcium channel blockers
Congestive heart failure		
Dilated hypokinetic heart	β-blockers	Captopril Vasodilators
Hyperkinetic heart with diminished diastolic relaxation	Vasodilators Diuretics	β-blockers Calcium channel blockers
Angina pectoris	Vasodilators	β-blockers Calcium channel blockers
Atrioventricular nodal disease	β-blockers Verapamil	None
Sinus bradycardia	β-blockers	
Vascular headaches	Vasodilators	β-blockers Calcium channel blockers
Possible renal artery stenosis (abdominal bruits, widespread atherosclerosis)	Angiotensin converting enzyme inhibitors	None
Diabetes		
On insulin	β-blockers	None
Diet controlled	Thiazide and loop diuretics β-blockers	None
Depressed mood	Central adrenergic inhibitors Reserpine Lipophilic β-blockers	None
Chronic liver disease[a]	Methyldopa	None
Chronic renal disease[a]	None	High dose loop diuretics
Chronic diarrhea (e.g., irritable bowel syndrome)	Methyldopa, guanethidine, hydralazine	None
Allergic or perennial rhinitis	Reserpine	None

[a] See Table 62.10 for principal routes of excretion for nondiuretic antihypertensives.

Table 62.8.
Prevalence of Symptoms at 12 Weeks and at 2 Years after Entry, British Medical Research Council Trial[a]

Complaint[b]	Men—percentage of affirmative answers (N = 1130)						Women—percentage of affirmative answers (N = 958)					
	Bendrofluazide		Propranolol		Placebos		Bendrofluazide		Propranolol		Placebos	
	12 Wk	2 Yr	12 Wk	2 Yr	12 Wk	2 Yr	12 Wk	2 Yr	12 Wk	2 Yr	12 Wk	2 Yr
Dizziness	13.7[c]	9.3	6.9	9.0	5.9	8.4	25.3[d]	19.4	18.1	17.8	16.8	16.1
Muscle pain	13.5	22.2	15.7	14.1	14.6	16.8	25.2	14.6[d]	21.6	17.2	22.5	26.8
Slowed walking	2.6	9.9	7.9	11.0	6.6	7.6	10.0	7.1	12.6[d]	10.6	6.2	6.9
Exertional dyspnea	16.1	23.8	19.4	27.9[d]	14.0	16.4	20.9	25.8	18.4	26.1	21.0	21.1
Headaches	19.6	16.5	21.9	19.7	27.1	26.2	31.9[d]	36.0	33.1	29.8	42.4	37.8
Cold/numb digits	8.4	15.8	14.2	12.6	11.5	10.7	18.8	16.1	18.3	29.3[d]	16.3	15.6
Paresthesias	11.6	14.9	14.7	14.3	14.7	11.2	28.9[d]	28.9	19.7	25.0	18.4	17.5
Dry mouth	13.7	12.4	11.2	7.5	7.7	7.7	26.6	28.1[d]	18.8	18.2	21.3	13.6
Blocked or runny nose	13.7	14.7	23.2[c]	26.8	12.5	18.2	11.5	18.3	20.1	22.6	19.2	12.9
Vomiting/nausea	3.9	5.0	7.9[c]	3.7	3.2	4.5	13.4	5.1	6.3	4.3	8.2	10.3
Impotence	16.2[d]	22.6[d]	13.8	13.2	8.9	10.1						

[a] From Report of Medical Research Council Working Party on Mild to Moderate Hypertension: Adverse reactions to bendrofluazide and propranol for the treatment of mild hypertension. *Lancet* 1:8246, 1981.
[b] Reported in questionnaire.
[c] $p < 0.01$.
[d] $p < 0.05$. Significance levels refer to prevalence rates for each active drug separately compared with those for all control patients. The figures do not indicate comparisons between the two active drugs.

apparent "side effects." For example, sexual impotence may be associated with all antihypertensive drugs, including diuretics, and with placebos given for hypertension. These points are illustrated in

Table 62.8, which displays the frequency of a number of side effects reported by subjects taking active step 1 drugs or placebos in the British MRC Trial.

Because *orthostatic exaggeration of the hypoten-*

sive effect can occur with any antihypertensive drug, patients should be asked about orthostatic symptoms and should have a standing blood pressure measured after every change in the regimen. For those with a systolic fall of more than 15 mm Hg, a standing blood pressure should also be measured following exercise (e.g., 10 steps on a footstool or walking a fixed distance), as exercise may exacerbate drug-induced orthostatic hypotension. For patients reporting transient orthostatic symptoms shortly after taking their daily medication, direct observation of their blood pressure response may be useful (see example case in Fig. 62.14, page 824).

Properties of Individual Drugs: Overview

The diuretics used for hypertension are listed by class in Table 69.9, which also lists available strengths and recommended dose ranges. For each nondiuretic antihypertensive, the following properties are summarized in Table 62.10: generic and proprietary names, available strengths, recommended dose range, schedule (and alternate schedule for some), onset time and duration of principal action, and principal route(s) of metabolism and elimination.

Diuretics (See Also Table 62.7)

Mechanism. Diuretics probably lower blood pressure by decreasing modestly the circulating volume and by decreasing peripheral resistance. A chronic increase in plasma renin activity has been demonstrated in diuretic-treated patients; this provides indirect evidence that the decrease in circulating volume persists as long as the patient is taking the diuretic.

Thiazide and Loop Diuretics

Doses and schedules. For step 1 or step 2 diuretic therapy, a once daily schedule, using the dose ranges listed in Table 69.9, is satisfactory, and the patient can select the time of day that is most convenient (e.g., after rather than before work because of the modest diuresis). The major antihypertensive response is seen within 1 to 2 weeks of initiating or increasing a diuretic. Full resolution of antihypertensive effect occurs within 1 week of discontinuing the drug.

Relatively high doses of *loop diuretics* (furosemide, ethacrynic acid, bumetanide) may be necessary in some patients who require large doses of steps 2 and 3 drugs (most of which promote sodium

Table 62.9.
Diuretic Drugs Utilized for Hypertension

Class/Name of Drugs[a]	Available Strengths (mg)	Dose Range for Hypertension (mg/day)
THIAZIDES AND RELATED SULFONAMIDE DIURETICS		
Bendroflumethiazide (Naturetin)	2.5, 5, 10	2.5–5
Benzthiazide	25, 50	25–50
Chlorothiazide sodium (Diuril)[b]	250, 500	250–500
Chlorthalidone (Hygroton)[b]	25, 50, 100	25–50
Cyclothiazide (Anhydron, Fluidil)	2	1–2
Hydrochlorothiazide[b]	25, 50	25–50
Hydroflumethiazide (Diucardin, Saluron)[b]	50	25–50
Indapamide (Lozol)	2.5	2.5–5
Methyclothiazide[b]	5	2.5–5
Metolazone (Diulo, Zaroxolyn)	2.5, 5, 10	2.5–5
Polythiazide (Renese)	1, 2, 4	2–4
Quinethazone (Hydromox)	50	50–100
Trichlormethiazide (Metahydrin, Naqua)[b]	2, 4	2–4
LOOP DIURETICS		
Bumetanide (Bumex)	0.5, 1	0.5–10
Ethacrynic acid (Edecrin)	50	50–200
Furosemide (Lasix)[b]	20, 40, 80	20–480
POTASSIUM-SPARING DIURETICS		
Amiloride hydrochloride (Midamor)[c]	5	5–10
Spironolactone (Aldactone)[b,d]	25, 50, 100	50–100
Triamterene (Dyrenium)[e]	50, 100	50–100

[a] If more than two proprietary formulations are available, names are not listed.
[b] Generic is available.
[c] Combination form (Moduretic): Amiloride/hydrochlorothiazide 5 mg/50 mg.
[d] Combination forms (Aldactazide and generic): spironolactone/hydrochlorothiazide 25 mg/25 mg and 50 mg/50 mg.
[e] Combination forms (Dyazide: triamterene/hydrochlorothiazide 50 mg/25 mg, and Maxzide: triamterene/hydrochlorothiazide 75 mg/50 mg).

Table 62.10.
Pharmacological Characteristics of Nondiuretic Antihypertensive Drugs

Class/Name of Drug	General Use Began	Available Strengths (mg)	Dose Range (mg/day)	Schedule (Alternative)	Major Action Onset/ Duration (Hours)	Metabolism and Elimination[a]
ADRENERGIC INHIBITORS						
β-Blockers						
Acebutolol (Sectral)[b,c]	1985	200, 400	200–1200	Once daily (twice daily)	3–8/≤24[e]	L, K
Atenolol (Tenormin)[b]	1981	50, 100	25–100	Once daily	2–4/24–48[e]	K
Metoprolol (Lopressor)[b]	1978	50, 100	50–300	Once daily (twice daily)	2–4/24–48[e]	L
Nadolol (Corgard)	1980	40, 80, 120	20–120	Once daily	2–4/24–48[e]	K
Pindolol (Visken)[c]	1982	5, 10	20–60	Twice daily	?	L
Propranolol (Inderal)[d]	1976	10, 20, 40, 60, 80	40–≥480	Twice daily	2–4/24–48[e]	L
Propranolol long acting (Inderal LA)	1984	80, 120, 160	80–≥480	Once daily	?	L
Timolol (Blocadren)	1983	5, 10, 20	20–60	Twice daily	?	L
Central acting sympatholytics						
Clonidine (Catapres)	1975	0.1, 0.2, 0.3	0.2–2.4	Twice daily	1–2/12–24	
Guanabenz (Wytensin)	1983	4, 8	8–32	Twice daily	2–4/12	
Methyldopa (Aldomet)[d]	1962	250, 500	250–3000	Twice daily (once at bedtime)	4–6/24–48	K
α-Blocker						
Prazosin (Minipress)	1976	1, 2, 5	2–≥20	Twice daily (3 times daily)	1–2/12–24	
α-β-Blocker						
Labetalol (Trandate, Normodyne)	1984	200, 300	200–≥1200	Twice daily (3 times daily)	1–3/8–24	L, K
Peripheral acting sympatholytics						
Guanadrel (Hylorel)	1984	10, 25	20–75	Twice daily	2–6/?	K
Guanethidine (Ismelin)	1959	10, 25	10–200	Every day	3–5 days/≥1 wk	K
Reserpine[d]	1952	0.1, 0.25	0.1–0.25	Once daily	1–2 wk/≥1 wk	K
VASODILATORS						
Hydralazine (Apresoline)[d]	1951	10, 25, 75, 100	20–≥300	Twice daily (3 times daily)	1–4/12–24	K
Minoxidil (Loniten)	1980	2.5, 10	5–≥40	Once daily (twice daily)	1–3/24–48	
ANGIOTENSIN-CONVERTING ENZYME INHIBITORS						
Captopril (Capoten)	1981	25, 50, 100	37.5–450	3 times daily	1–3/8–12	K
Enalapril[f]			10–40			
CALCIUM CHANNEL BLOCKERS						
Diltiazem (Cardizem)	1983	30, 60[g]	120–240	3 times daily (4 times daily)	1–3/8–12	L, K
Nifedipine (Procardia)	1983	10, 20	30–180	3 times daily	1–3/8–12	K
Verapamil (Calan, Isoptin)	1983	80, 120	240–480	3 times daily (4 times daily)	1–3/8–12	L, K

[a] L, liver; K, kidney.
[b] Cardioselective β-blockade.
[c] Has intrinsic sympathomimetic activity.
[d] Generic is available.
[e] Refers to cardioinhibitory action (principal antihypertensive effect may be delayed 1 to 7 days).
[f] Not yet released for use in USA.
[g] Twenty-milligram strength scheduled for release in 1986.

retention). These diuretics may also be needed to control hypertension in patients who will not restrict salt use and have edema that does not respond to thiazides; the serum potassium concentration should be monitored closely in such patients (e.g., within 1 or 2 weeks of adding or increasing a loop diuretic) since precipitous potassium depletion may occur.

Precautions. Mild side effects, such as increased urination and transient orthostatic symptoms, are common when diuretics are initiated. Sexual impotence is an important, though infrequent, side effect of diuretics (see Table 62.8). Of the other side effects, those seen most commonly are hypokalemia, gout related to hyperuricemia, impaired glucose tolerance, and an increase in low density lipoprotein cholesterol and triglyceride levels (thiazides and chlorthalidone). A modest reduction in total body potassium occurs in most patients, and frank *hypokalemia* (less than 3.5 mEq/liter) in some. In nonedematous patients taking thiazide diuretics, restriction of sodium intake (see below) and the use of the equivalent of 50 mg of hydrochlorothiazide or less will prevent most hypokalemia. Because ventricular ectopy may be precipitated by hypokalemia, patients should be monitored for hypokalemia (at 3 to 4 weeks; if greater than 3.5 mEq/liter, twice yearly) and the hypokalemia should be treated whenever it is detected. In nonedematous patients with hypokalemia, potassium supplements do not restore a normal potassium level as reliably as potassium-sparing diuretics (see the next section). If *diabetes* is found at the baseline evaluation or if symptomatic diabetes is provoked in the course of long term diuretic therapy, strict calorie and sodium restriction should be prescribed instead of diuretic therapy, and nondiuretic antihypertensives should be added if the patient does not adhere to a diet prescription or if dietary modification fails to control the blood pressure. With these measures, glucose tolerance does not deteriorate (or returns to normal) in many patients. Diuretic-induced *increases in plasma lipid levels* can be prevented by adherence to a diet low in saturated fat and cholesterol; therefore, it is appropriate to recommend this to all patients when thiazide diuretic treatment is started. These metabolic abnormalities are discussed in detail in Chapters 45 (hypokalemia), 69 (gout), 72 (diabetes), and 75 (hyperlipidemia).

Apart from allergy and a number of *uncommon* coexisting conditions (e.g., psychogenic polydipsia, hypercalcemia, history of hyponatremia due to inappropriate antidiuretic hormone excretion), there are no absolute contraindications for diuretics in hypertension. Because thiazide-treated patients with abnormal electrocardiograms* in the MRFIT trial had an increased mortality rate (28), some authorities caution against the use of thiazides as initial treatment in such patients.

---

* Abnormalities included high R waves in the precordial leads, negative T waves; R-R′ pattern; ectopic ventricular premature beats; left axis deviation ≤ −30°; ST depression; ST elevation; major Q waves; short P-R; first degree atrioventricular block; supraventricular tachycardia; right axis deviation ≥ +120°; and other rare conditions.

Potassium-Sparing Diuretics

The potassium-sparing diuretics (amiloride, spironolactone, and triamterene) have modest antihypertensive effects when used alone in some patients with essential hypertension. They are useful *in combination with other diuretics*, chiefly to avoid or reverse hypokalemia (see Chapter 42). They may also be used to enhance diuretic action in the occasional patient who retains sodium while taking diuretics and potent nondiuretic antihypertensives, especially the vasodilator minoxidil. In such patients blood pressure control may improve dramatically when potassium-conserving drugs are added.

To avoid iatrogenic hyperkalemia, potassium-sparing diuretics should not be given concurrently with potassium supplements or with captopril (see below) and should be used with caution in diabetic patients because some diabetics have an increased risk of developing hyperkalemia when they take these diuretics. Spironolactone has a number of undesirable endocrine side effects (especially gynecomastia and, occasionally, impotence). Therefore, amiloride or triamterene is preferable to spironolactone in male subjects. The compositions of the principal thiazide/potassium-sparing combinations are listed in the footnotes to Table 62.9.

Adrenergic Inhibitors

β-Blocking Drugs (See Also Tables 62.7 and 62.10)

The β-blocking drugs are listed in Table 62.10.

Mechanism. One or more of the following mechanisms probably accounts for the major antihypertensive effect in patients who respond to β-blocking agents: blockade of cardiac β-receptors causing decreased cardiac output, blockade of renal β-receptors causing inhibition of renin release, blockade of central nervous system β-receptors causing decreased sympathetic outflow, or blockade of presynaptic β-receptors causing decreased release of catecholamines. Evidence of some cardiac β-receptor blockade (heart rate of 64 beats or less/minute at rest and less than 80/minute after brief exercise in the office) is present in most patients whose hypertension responds to these drugs. However, there is no clinically useful way to determine which blocking mechanism is dominant in responders.

Special properties. Pindolol, propranolol, nadolol, and timolol are *nonselective* β-blockers, while metaprolol and atenolol are *cardioselective*. The major theoretic advantage of a cardioselective β-blocker is the relative lack of β_2-receptor blockade. β_2-receptors mediate bronchodilation, dilation of resistance vessels, and the sympathetic response to hypoglycemia (tachycardia, sweating). One β-blocker, pindolol, has *intrinsic β-sympathetic activity*, which may be reflected clinically by less tendency to produce bradycardia or to precipitate bronchospasm or heart failure in patients whose baseline respiratory or cardiac function is partly dependent on β-sympathetic stimulation.

Atenolol and nadolol are *less lipid soluble* and more water soluble than other β-blockers. This has two consequences that may affect clinical decisions: (a) These drugs are dependent on renal excretion and dose intervals may be longer in patients with kidney disease; (b) they enter brain tissue less readily than do other β-blockers and may cause fewer central nervous system side effects (e.g., depression, insomnia, nightmares).

Most β-blockers may be useful over a *broad dose range* (see Table 62.10). Atenolol, however, produces little or no additional blood pressure reduction when the daily dose exceeds 100 mg.

For all of the β-blocking drugs, slowing of heart rate (except pindolol) and some blood pressure response occur within 2 to 4 hours of taking an initial dose, but the full antihypertensive effect may not be seen until the patient has taken the drug for 1 week. The principal antihypertensive effect of these drugs resolves within 1 to 2 days of discontinuing the drug.

For the subset of hypertensive patients who have left ventricular heart failure, good left ventricular function, and a small left ventricular cavity due to poor diastolic phase relaxation, β-blockers, like calcium channel blockers (see below), may both reverse the diastolic stiffness and lower the blood pressure (39). This form of hypertensive cardiomyopathy has been described chiefly in older hypertensive patients.

Precautions. Whenever a β-blocking agent is being *discontinued* after prolonged use, it should be tapered over 1 to 2 weeks rather than abruptly stopped, because of the possibility of precipitating angina, acute rebound to pretreatment blood pressure levels, or a number of other withdrawal symptoms (e.g., anxiety, tachycardia, palpitations, tremor, perspiration, or increase in headaches in patients with migraine).

Switching from other β-blockers to atenolol or pindolol may be desirable in patients having central nervous system side effects or patients who might benefit from intrinsic sympathetic activity, respectively. In these instances, it is reasonable to substitute 50 mg of atenolol daily or 10 mg of pindolol twice daily for the current β-blocker.

The most common *side effects* are nausea, abdominal cramps, diarrhea, mild sedation, fatigue, nightmares, cool extremities, and asymptomatic bradycardia. Sexual impotence has been reported occasionally. Of note is the fact that hypertensive athletes tolerate β-blocking agents well.

With certain *coexisting conditions,* the β-blocking properties of these drugs may cause serious side effects. Absolute contraindications to the use of β-blockers are baseline marked bradycardia (heart rate less than 50), low cardiac output, high degree heart block, symptomatic asthma or chronic obstructive pulmonary disease, and severe peripheral vascular disease (e.g., gangrene, skin necrosis, severe or worsening claudication). For patients with mild asthma or chronic obstructive pulmonary disease, stable peripheral vascular disease, or stable insulin-requiring diabetes, low doses of the cardioselective agents, metaprolol and atenolol, or of pindolol (intrinsic sympathetic activity), may be tried if other antihypertensive regimens have been unsuccessful. It is recommended that a selective β_2-bronchodilator (see Chapter 55) be used concurrently whenever a β-blocking agent must be prescribed for a patient with asthma or chronic obstructive pulmonary disease.

Modest decreases in glucose tolerance and in high density lipoprotein-cholesterol may accompany long term use of propranolol and perhaps other β-blockers. The significance of these changes has not been established.

Drug interactions. In diabetic patients taking insulin or sulfonylureas, β-blockers may potentiate acute hypoglycemia and may mask the peripheral signs of hypoglycemia. In combination with digitalis, β-blockers may produce additional suppression of atrioventricular nodal conduction; they may also partly blunt the inotropic effect of digitalis. Cimetidine, because it decreases hepatic blood flow, may decrease the first pass extraction of the lipid-soluble β-blockers (*i.e.,* all β-blockers except atenolol and nadolol), thereby enhancing their antihypertensive and other effects. β-blockers should also be used cautiously if at all with the calcium channel blockers that have cardiodepressive effects (verapamil and diltiazem).

Combination with other antihypertensives. The addition of a diuretic usually enhances the antihypertensive effect of β-blocker therapy. The further addition of a vasodilator or the calcium channel blocker nifedipine (step 3 therapy) is usually very effective in patients not controlled with a β-blocker and a diuretic. Any other adrenergic inhibitor, or captopril, may also be synergistic with a β-blocker.

Central Acting α-Adrenergic Agonists: Clonidine and Guanabenz (See Also Tables 62.7 and 62.10)

Mechanism. These drugs are thought to act as α-adrenergic agonists, decreasing sympathetic activity in the medulla oblongata and thus diminishing sympathetic outflow to the peripheral vasculature. They suppress renin release, but a relationship between this property and the antihypertensive effect of these drugs has not been established.

Special properties. Clonidine has been used extensively since it was introduced in 1975. Its properties are therefore well known, and it is prudent to use it instead of guanabenz when selecting an α-agonist. The major antihypertensive response to clonidine occurs within 1 hour and remits after 8 to 16 hours. Because of the rapid onset of action, oral clonidine can be given hourly in doses of 0.1 or 0.2 mg in order to determine rapidly the dose needed to treat an individual patient. This property may be of value in the symptom-free patient with a very high pressure if blood pressure lowering within a few hours is desired; however, apart from hypertensive emergencies requiring hospitalization and parenteral treatment (see above), there are no absolute indications for such rapid lowering of the blood pressure.

A sustained-release clonidine patch (the Catapres Transdermal Therapeutic System, TTS), which lasts 7 days, has been released recently. In addition to the advantage of once a week application, the TTS delivers a smaller dose of the drug and may therefore cause less side effects; also blood levels subside slowly at the end of a week, eliminating the risk of rebound hypertension due to abrupt termination of clonidine. The patch is available in three sizes, (3.5 cm^2, 7.0 cm^2, and 10.5 cm^2, delivering, respectively 0.1 mg, 0.2 mg, and 0.3 mg/day). In preliminary trials about two-thirds of patients with mild hypertension have been well controlled; however, up to 20% of patients have had to discontinue the clonidine TTS because of a rash. The role of the TTS in managing a broad spectrum of hypertensive patients has not yet been established.

Guanabenz lowers total serum cholesterol by about 20%, a unique property among antihypertensive drugs.

Precautions. Rapid *rebound to pretreatment blood pressure* with accompanying symptoms of increased sympathetic nervous system activity (tachycardia, perspiration, headache, palpitations) may follow abrupt discontinuation of clonidine or guanabenz. Treatment for this problem is reinstitution of the drug. As there is no way to recognize prospectively the few patients in danger of this severe reaction, all patients must be regarded as at risk. In selecting antihypertensive drugs, patients known to be erratic in medication taking should thus not receive these drugs, and all patients for whom they are prescribed should be warned explicitly of the risk of discontinuing the drug.

The most common *side effects* are sedation, dry mouth, constipation, and orthostatic symptoms. Impotence has been reported. There are no absolute contraindications to the use of clonidine or guanabenz.

Drug interactions. Tricyclic antidepressants may diminish the blood pressure-lowering effect of clonidine; excessive sedation may occur when clonidine or guanabenz is taken concurrently with any drug having central nervous system depressant effects, including alcohol.

Combination with other antihypertensive drugs.

Clonidine has been used with hydralazine to prevent the reflex sympathetic response to hydralazine (see below). This combination is useful in patients needing step 3 drugs who cannot take the more widely studied combination of β-blocking drugs and hydralazine, such as patients with a history of bronchospasm. Synergy between clonidine and prazosin has also been demonstrated.

Other Central-Acting Adrenergic Inhibitors: Methyldopa (See Also Tables 62.7 and 62.10)

Mechanism. There is evidence that the derivative of methyldopa, methylnorepinephrine, displaces norepinephrine in the central nervous system and that the hypotensive effect of methyldopa is related to this process. Methyldopa suppresses renin release, but a relationship of this property to its antihypertensive action has not been clearly established.

Special properties. Although 250 to 3000 mg is the daily dose range publicized frequently, an additional hypotensive response is rarely attained with doses greater than 2000 mg. Over long intervals of continuous treatment (e.g., 10 years), most patients require a gradual increase in their daily dose of methyldopa to maintain satisfactory blood pressure control.

In studies of small numbers of patients, it has been shown that hypertension is controlled for 24 hours regardless of whether the same total daily dose is given on a four times daily, three times daily, twice daily, or once daily schedule. For patients who comply poorly or who experience sedation after daytime doses of methyldopa, a single dose at bedtime can be tried in place of the usual twice daily schedule. The major antihypertensive effect of methyldopa occurs within 4 to 6 hours of oral administration, and the hypotensive response remits within 1 to 2 days.

Precautions. Rapid rebound to pretreatment pressures, with or without symptoms, has been reported in a few patients after abrupt discontinuation of methyldopa. The most common side effects are orthostatic symptoms, sedation, mood alteration, impotence, and diarrhea (soft stools, two to four times daily). After 6 to 12 months, about 10% of patients taking methyldopa develop a positive direct Coombs' test, and rarely there is associated hemolysis. Because methyldopa may cause hepatitis, it is contraindicated in patients with active liver disease.

Drug interactions. Tricyclic antidepressants may diminish the blood pressure-lowering effect of methyldopa; chronically coadministered phenobarbital may reduce the effect of methyldopa due to induction of hepatic microsomal enzymes. When methyldopa is given with L-dopa, the hypotensive effect of the former may be potentiated and the antiparkinsonian effect of the latter may be reduced. Finally toxicity from lithium and from haloperidol may be increased when methyldopa is taken concurrently.

Combination with other antihypertensive drugs.

The combination of methyldopa and a β-blocker is more effective than either drug alone. In patients who show a partial response to one of these drugs, adding a small amount of the other may at times be more practical than starting a different drug. This is especially true in the patient who may have failed to respond to two or more step 2 drugs. Synergy with prazosin and with hydralazine has also been demonstrated.

α-Adrenergic Blocker: Prazosin (See Also Tables 62.7 and 62.10)

Mechanism. Prazosin blocks postsynaptic α-receptors in arterioles and venules, presumably decreasing blood pressure by impairing sympathetic tone at both sites. Prazosin does not block presynaptic α-receptors. This may explain why prazosin does not predictably cause tachycardia and renin release, as both of these adaptive responses to blood pressure lowering are inhibited by activation of the presynaptic α-receptors.

Selected properties. Although the recommended upper limit for hypertension is 30 mg/day, an additional antihypertensive effect may be attained at higher doses (up to 80 mg daily); in the patient with hypertension refractory to other drugs, a trial of high dose prazosin is therefore worthwhile. Because of the broad range of doses which may be needed to control blood pressure in different patients (e.g., from 1 mg to 25 mg two or three times daily), prazosin requires more dosage changes than most antihypertensive drugs in patients who do not respond to an initial low dose.

The usual schedule is twice daily. Clinical studies have shown that some patients may have to follow a three times daily schedule, while others may be able to take prazosin once a day. It is helpful to check the blood pressure just before the next scheduled dose in order to determine the most appropriate schedule for prazosin. The major antihypertensive response to a dose of prazosin occurs within 1 to 2 hours and remits entirely after 24 hours.

Prazosin has the effect of lowering serum low density lipoprotein-cholesterol; when added to diuretics or β-blockers, it may counterbalance the unfavorable effects of these drugs on serum lipids.

Doxazosin, a sustained-release form of prazosin, offers the advantage of once daily administration. This drug is presently being tested for release in the United States.

Precautions. The most common side effects are postural hypotension, headache, drowsiness, dry mouth, and palpitations. Sexual impotence is very uncommon. Postural hypotension, usually without tachycardia and at times asymptomatic, occurs as a transient problem in up to half of patients during the first few days they take prazosin. Syncope occurring within ½ hour after the initial dose of prazosin is a very rare, but severe, side effect. It may occur after taking a 1-mg dose. Clearly, warning and reassurance about postural symptoms (for the first few days) are important whenever this drug is prescribed. In addition, patients should either take their first dose in the office (and be observed for about 1 hour) or they should be instructed to take it at bedtime, so that they will be recumbent during the initial adjustment to the drug.

There are no absolute contraindications to the use of prazosin.

Drug interactions. Apart from the risk of additive orthostatic hypotension when it is given with drugs that can cause this problem, there are no important interactions with drugs that might be administered with prazosin.

Combination with other antihypertensive drugs. The combination of prazosin and a β-blocker is frequently effective in patients with moderate or severe hypertension that does not respond to either drug alone. Synergism has also been reported with clonidine, methyldopa, and hydralazine.

The use of prazosin in the ambulatory management of congestive heart failure is discussed in Chapter 61.

α-β-Blocker: Labetalol (See Also Tables 62.7 and 62.10)

Mechanism. Labetalol combines three actions that can lower blood pressure: nonselective β-blockade, α_1-blockade (vasodilating activity), and β_2-stimulation (vasodilating activity). During labetalol treatment, control of hypertension is usually accompanied by a modest reduction in resting and postexercise heart rate. The cardiac index and peripheral resistance are reduced during the first year of treatment, but after several years cardiac index returns to normal while total peripheral resistance remains lower.

Special properties. Based upon early experience, labetalol is effective as step 1 or step 2 therapy in somewhat more than 50% of patients with mild or moderate hypertension and about one-third of patients with severe hypertension. It seems to be equally effective in black and white subjects.

The dose range is large (200 to ≥1200 mg/day). Because the full impact of a dose occurs within 1 to 3 hours, the dose can be titrated up rapidly. Most responders are controlled with daily doses of 400 to 800 mg. Abrupt discontinuation does not appear to cause a withdrawal state similar to that observed occasionally with the β-blockers.

Precautions. The most frequent side effects seen with labetalol are fatigue, nausea, dyspepsia, dizziness, nasal stuffiness, and pruritic rash. Impotence has been the commonest reason for early termination of labetalol.

Because of its β_2-activity, labetalol may be somewhat safer than pure β-blockers in patients with obstructive airways disease; however, it has been associated with a modest fall in 1-second forced expiratory volume when given chronically to patients with mild obstructive airways disease. Labetalol is contraindicated in patients with greater than first degree heart block.

Drug interactions. Because the experience with labetalol is limited, the risk of adverse drug interactions is not yet well established. However, apart from an enhancement of the bioavailability and action of labetalol when it is taken concurrently with cimetidine, interactions with commonly prescribed drugs have not been described.

Combination with other antihypertensive drugs. To date, there have been no sizable trials of labetalol in combination with other antihypertensive drugs apart from diuretics. As is true of all antihypertensives, diuretics may enhance the effect of labetalol on blood pressure.

Peripheral Acting Sympatholytics: Guanadrel and Guanethidine (*See Also Tables 62.7 and 62.10*)

Mechanism. These drugs prevent release of and deplete stores of norepinephrine in peripheral tissues but not in the central nervous system. Their hypotensive action is ascribed to the loss of sympathetic regulation of vessel tone in the venous and arterial circulation. Because their hypotensive effect depends predominantly upon impaired venous tone, the effects of guanethidine and guanadrel are always more pronounced when patients are standing, particularly after exercise.

Special properties. The major antihypertensive effect of guanadrel occurs within 4 to 6 hours of the first dose and lasts 12 to 24 hours. The major effect of guanethidine is seen after 3 to 5 days of initiating treatment and remits within 1 to 2 weeks of discontinuing the drug.

Precautions. Orthostatic exaggeration of the hypotensive response severely limits the usefulness of these drugs. As shown in Table 62.11, most guanethidine-treated patients show one of two unsatisfactory patterns: a high resting pressure and an unacceptably low pressure after exercise, or a high resting pressure and a normal pressure after exercise. In addition, sexual dysfunction in male patients (impairment of ejaculation and/or erection) and diarrhea are quite common. Because of the frequency of orthostatic hypotension and because of the availability of minoxidil, captopril, and nifedipine, the initiation of guanethidine or guanadrel (step 4 therapy) can almost always be avoided in the management of hypertension. Patients who currently take either of these drugs should be monitored carefully, and an alternative drug should be considered whenever there is any suggestion that the exaggerated orthostasis is producing symptoms.

Drug interactions. Tricyclic antidepressants and sympathomimetic decongestants may reverse the antihypertensive effect of guanethidine. Presumably the same may occur with guanadrel.

Table 62.11.
Blood Pressures of 16 Consecutive Patients Receiving Guanethidine, at Their Most Recent Visit[a]

Patient	Resting	Standing	Standing after Exercise	Guanethidine Dose[b] (mg)
1	190/120	140/114	124/94	50
2	210/132	134/100	100/84	50
3	170/120	170s/100	130/80	50
4	160/100	150/100	130/84	10
5	208/110	126/90	100/70	50
6	142/100	120/90	114/84	50
7	190/108	160/110	160/104	75
8	180/92	120/80	110/60	100
9	156/108	160/108	150/96	75
10	164/100	154/94	150/82	75
11	240/100	220/88	170/70	60
12	150/110	140/105	140/100	50
13	140/100	130/96	125/85	37.5
14	170/105	140/110	130/100	25
15	170/120	140/110	150/100	20
16	194/120	168/116	144/112	150
Mean	177/109	148/104	133/88	55

[a] From Barker LR: Guanethidine, exercise, and hypotension. *Lancet* 2:1297, 1976.
[b] All patients also on a diuretic.

Combinations and interactions. Guanethidine has been used effectively as a sympatholytic drug in conjunction with hydralazine. Because of its undesirable side effects, it provides no advantage over the other sympatholytic drugs that have been tested with hydralazine (β-blockers, clonidine, reserpine).

Peripheral/Central Sympatholytic: Reserpine (*See Also Tables 62.7 and 62.10*)

Mechanism. Chronic administration of reserpine depletes the stores of catecholamines in many tissues, probably by impairing the uptake of essential precursors. The antihypertensive effect is attributed to impaired uptake centrally and peripherally of dopamine, a precursor for the intracellular synthesis of norepinephrine.

Special properties. The major antihypertensive effect occurs 1 to 2 weeks after initiating treatment and remits within 1 to 2 weeks of stopping the drug. The principal advantages of reserpine are the once a day schedule and low cost.

Precautions. Frank depression occurs in some patients, and slight decrease in mental alertness is common. Both are dose related and occur chiefly at doses higher than the recommended range (0.1 to 0.25 mg) (13). Nasal and gastric hypersecretion occurs at therapeutic doses and may produce nasal stuffiness or dyspepsia. An association between reserpine and breast carcinoma, reported in 1974, was not confirmed by carefully controlled observations. Because of side effects and the availability of other step 2 drugs, reserpine has not been recommended prominently in recent years. Two definite contraindications are active peptic ulcer or a history of depression.

Drug interactions. Reserpine may interact unfavorably with a number of drugs. Because it releases stored norepinephrine, a hypertensive crisis may occur if it is given with a monoamine oxidase inhibitor. Reserpine plus digitalis may cause cardiac arrhythmias (ventricular ectopy and atrial arrhythmias, similar to those caused by digitalis toxicity). Tricyclic antidepressants can reduce the blood pressure-lowering effect of reserpine. The central nervous system depressant effects of many drugs may be increased by reserpine. Finally reserpine antagonizes the antiparkinsonian effect of L-dopa.

Combination with other drugs. In the Veterans Administration controlled trial (see above, page 790), the combination of reserpine, hydralazine, and hydrochlorothiazide was shown to be highly effective. These three drugs are available in a fixed-dose combination tablet (the CIBA product Ser-Ap-Es and generic) which contains 0.10 mg of reserpine, 25 mg of hydralazine, and 15 mg of hydrochlorothiazide.

Vasodilators

Hydralazine (See Also Tables 62.7 and 62.10)

Mechanism. Hydralazine directly relaxes smooth muscle in resistance vessels (arterioles and small arteries); it has a similar but lesser effect on capacitance vessels (venules and small veins). Secondary effects are stimulation of renin release and reflex increase in activity of the sympathetic nervous system that may cause tachycardia, palpitations, headache, or increased angina. Because of this latter effect, hydralazine is recommended as a step 3 drug to be added to a regimen containing an adrenergic inhibitor.

Special properties. The daily dose range is 20 to 400 mg. An upper limit of 200 mg is sometimes recommended because of the increased risk of hydralazine-induced lupus at higher doses. However, 400 mg or more may be effective and appropriate in patients with severe hypertension who are difficult to control and who do not tolerate other drugs.

Hydralazine can be taken twice daily. The major antihypertensive response occurs within 2 to 4 hours and remits within 12 to 24 hours. If there is evidence that an individual patient's response does not persist for 12 hours, a three times daily schedule may be required. Hydralazine should be taken with meals, as absorption is maximal with food and blood pressure response may be erratic if the drug is taken irregularly with respect to eating.

Precautions. The most common side effects (headache, palpitations, tachycardia) occur when hydralazine is given without an adrenergic inhibitor. The uncommon but widely publicized lupus-like hydralazine syndrome has the following features in most affected subjects: occurs after 6 or more months of exposure to 200 mg or more daily, begins as new

arthritis or arthralgia, rarely affects the kidneys, stimulates the production of antinuclear antibodies, and remits entirely within 6 months of discontinuing hydralazine (a few patients have had persistence of rheumatological symptoms or antinuclear antibodies long after discontinuation of hydralazine). Another uncommon, reversible side effect is peripheral sensory neuropathy presenting as paresthesias and numbness and responding to pyridoxine, 50 mg daily, or to discontinuation of the drug. There are other uncommon toxic reactions to hydralazine, but when used as a step 3 drug, hydralazine is generally well tolerated.

Except for a history of systemic lupus erythematosus, there are no absolute contraindications to hydralazine when used in combination with an adrenergic inhibitor.

Interactions with other drugs. There are no significant unwanted interactions between hydralazine and other commonly used drugs.

Combination with other drugs. When hydralazine is added to any adrenergic inhibitor, the hypertension responds well in the majority of patients who are not controlled with the adrenergic inhibitor alone. The addition of hydralazine to a β-blocking agent is widely practiced, both because of the effectiveness of this combination and the protection against reflex sympathetic activity that the β-blockers provide.

Minoxidil (See Also Tables 62.7 and 62.10)

Mechanism. Minoxidil relaxes arteriolar smooth muscle and is thus a peripheral vasodilator. Like hydralazine, it stimulates renin release and induces reflex hyperactivity of the sympathetic nervous system. Therefore, the patient should always be on an adequate dose of an adrenergic inhibitor (usually a β-blocker) before minoxidil is initiated.

Special properties. The daily dose range is 5 to 40 mg. Daily doses greater than 40 mg (up to 100 mg) may be effective. Because of its extraordinary potency, minoxidil should be initiated at a trial dose of 2.5 mg; dose increases can be made daily until a response occurs. The major antihypertensive effect occurs within 1 to 3 hours and remits within 1 to 2 days.

Minoxidil can be given once or twice daily. When minoxidil is being substituted for another drug (hydralazine, for example), this drug should be continued until a response to minoxidil occurs; then the other drug should be gradually discontinued while the minoxidil dose is increased if necessary.

Precautions. Fluid retention, often marked, occurs in most patients as a consequence of the hypotensive action of the drug; furosemide or another potent loop diuretic should be given in a dose adequate to eliminate the problem. Most patients also develop hirsutism within 1 month of starting minoxidil, limiting severely the acceptance of this drug by women. There are no other common side effects. A minority of patients (estimated at 3% of those not on dialysis) develop a pericardial effusion (transudate) after prolonged use of minoxidil; rarely tampanode occurs. The effusion usually resolves or decreases with added diuretic treatment; it resolves entirely if minoxidil is discontinued. The development of anasarca, which remits when the drug is stopped, has been seen in an occasional patient taking minoxidil.

Interactions with other drugs. Like hydralazine, there are no significant interactions between minoxidil and other commonly used drugs.

Combination with other drugs. Minoxidil should always be used in conjunction with an adrenergic inhibitor. All minoxidil studies to date have utilized β-blockers. Presumably the other sympatholytics are also effective with minoxidil.

For patients with severe hypertension, a once daily regimen of minoxidil, a long acting β-blocker, and a diuretic is highly effective and increases the likelihood that the patient will not forget a dose.

Angiotensin Converting Enzyme Inhibitors (See also Tables 62.7 and 62.10)

Captopril

Mechanism. Angiotensin I is the product of the interaction between the proteolytic enzyme renin and an α_2-globulin, renin substrate. Captopril inhibits the enzymatic conversion of angiotensin I to the potent vasodilator angiotensin II; its antihypertensive effect has been attributed to this action. Because captopril lowers the blood pressure in patients with low and normal peripheral renin activity as well as those with high peripheral renin activity, and because it also may inhibit the enzymatic degradation of the potent vasodilator bradykinin, there is controversy regarding its mechanism of action. The drug does not cross the blood-brain barrier, and its antihypertensive action is therefore strictly a peripheral effect.

Special properties. The daily dose range is 37.5 to 450 mg. The drug should be initiated in a trial dose of 12.5 mg, three times daily. When it is being substituted for other drugs, these should either be discontinued or gradually tapered while captopril is being introduced. Because a profound fall in blood pressure (and occasional syncope) may follow the first dose, this dose should be given and sitting and standing blood pressure should be measured for 1 to 2 hours in the office whenever possible.

Patients should be instructed to take captopril at least 1 hour before meals since absorption is impaired when the drug is taken with meals.

The major antihypertensive effect occurs within a few hours of a dose and remits within 12 hours. The full impact of a dose is seen after 1 to 2 weeks at that dose. After prolonged use of captopril, the antihypertensive effect may diminish in occasional patients with severe hypertension, and a larger dose may be required. Black individuals seem to be less responsive to captopril than are whites.

Precautions. The commonest side effects of captopril are maculopapular rash and dysgeusia (decreased, totally lost, or unpleasant taste). Both effects occur in 5 to 10% of persons within the first 1 to 2 months of use; both remit with either a temporary decrease in dose or discontinuation of the drug. The most series adverse reactions are proteinuria and neutropenia. Proteinuria (1 or more g/24 hours) occurs in 1 to 2% of patients during the first year of treatment. In most cases, proteinuria subsides or resolves within 6 months even if captopril is continued; in a small number of patients, however, the nephrotic syndrome has occurred. Patients should be monitored for proteinuria before treatment and monthly for the first year of treatment; if new proteinuria develops, it is prudent to change to another drug. Neutropenia occurs in less than 1% of patients, within 12 weeks of starting the drug; it remits promptly with discontinuation. The neutropenia develops gradually; therefore, it is prudent to obtain a white blood cell count every 2 weeks for the first 3 months of treatment. Patients should be warned to report any signs of infection during this period. Captopril may cause acute renal failure in patients with bilateral renal artery stenosis, unilateral renal artery stenosis, or in renal transplant patients with stenosis of the transplanted renal artery. The type of patients most likely to have the former two problems are those with widespread atherosclerosis, manifested by multiple bruits and diminished peripheral pulses. The renal deterioration remits after captopril is discontinued.

Drug interactions. In some patients, indomethacin reduces the antihypertensive action of captopril. This property may be related to the inhibition of the synthesis of vasodilating prostaglandins, which may mediate the captopril response in some patients. The other important drug interactions are those between captopril and other drugs used in managing hypertension.

Combination with other drugs. Like other antihypertensive drugs, the action of captopril is enhanced by concurrent use of a diuretic. Captopril prevents secondary hyperaldosteronism, which is dependent upon angiotensin II. This has two important implications regarding diuretics: (a) the development of diuretic-induced hypokalemia, a problem due largely to secondary hyperaldosteronism, is less likely during concurrent treatment with thiazide or loop diuretics, and potassium supplements should be given only for well documented hypokalemia, with careful monitoring to avoid hyperkalemia; and (b) potassium-sparing diuretics should not be utilized in conjunction with captopril, as this combination increases the risk of hyperkalemia. Captopril should be used cautiously with agents that affect sympathetic activity, as the sympathetic nervous system may be especially important in supporting the blood pressure in the event of acute hypotension. Despite this concern, β-blockers have been used in conjunction with captopril in patients whose blood pressure did not respond to captopril alone. Theoretically, captopril may add to the antihypertensive effect of vasodilators (hydralazine and minoxidil) or calcium channel blockers, and such combinations may be reasonable for an occasional patient with very resistant hypertension.

Enalapril

Enalapril (not yet released for general use) is an angiotensin converting enzyme inhibitor that has the advantages over captopril of once or twice daily dosing and a lower incidence of side effects. The drug is manufactured in two strengths, 10 mg and 20 mg. The initial dose is 10 mg daily, and the maximum recommended daily dose is 40 mg. Because there has not yet been extensive experience with enalapril, its advantages and risks are not yet well established.

Calcium Channel Blockers (See Also Tables 62.7 and 62.10)

Mechanism. Although none had been approved formally in 1985 for use in hypertension, calcium channel blocking drugs are very effective antihypertensives. They block or alter cell membrane calcium flux, thereby reducing blood pressure through one or more of the following mechanisms: decreased vascular smooth muscle contractibility in both the arterial and venous circulation, negative inotropic and chronotropic effects (slows atrioventricular nodal conduction) on the heart, and inhibition of secretion of catecholamines. Nifedipine (and related agents) lowers blood pressure chiefly *via* arteriolar and venous vasodilatation, and it has little cardiodepressive effect. Verapamil (and related agents) and diltiazem probably lower blood pressure *via* combined peripheral vasodilatation and a negative inotropic effect. These differences in mechanism may be important in drug selection as noted below.

Special properties. Both nifedipine and verapamil have been shown to be effective step 1 or step 2 drugs. Nifedipine is also an effective step 3 drug (added to a diuretic/β-blocker regimen); when used with a β-blocker, one of the common side effects of nifedipine, sinus tachycardia, does not occur. All of the calcium channel blockers must be taken three times daily. Long acting preparations will probably be available for general use in the near future. Because the full impact of a dose occurs within 1 to 2 hours, the response to a calcium channel blocking agent can be evaluated rapidly. The liquid contents of a 10-mg nifedipine capsule can be given sublingually if there is need to lower blood pressure rapidly; however, this is rarely necessary in an ambulatory setting. The heart rate and the cardiac output

may increase during nifedipine treatment, while verapamil causes a fall in heart rate that may persist chronically.

Precautions. Side effects commonly reported with nifedipine are nausea, flushing, headache, and tachycardia. Vasodilator effects (flushing and headache) are not common with verapamil and diltiazem. All of these drugs may cause orthostatic symptoms, ankle edema (not due to salt retention), and palpitations. Verapamil causes constipation, especially when large doses are used, and nifedipine occasionally causes diarrhea. Of the three calcium channel blockers, nifedipine causes side effects leading to discontinuation most frequently and diltiazem least frequently.

Because of their effects on the heart, diltiazem and verapamil are contraindicated in patients with bradycardia, atrioventricular conduction disturbances, or uncontrolled heart failure. Because the cardiodepressive effects of these two drugs may be additive to the cardiodepressor effects of β-blocking drugs, such combinations should be avoided in hypertensive patients. Nifedipine may be particularly effective in treating left ventricular failure in patients with severe hypertension and well preserved cardiac function, whose heart failure is due to the diastolic stiffness associated with left ventricular hypertrophy (39). There are no absolute contraindications for nifedipine.

Drug interactions. The serum digoxin level increases after nifedipine or verapamil, and the potassium level may fall during nifedipine treatment. Because of the latter property, a potassium-sparing agent should be considered when nifedipine is used with a thiazide or loop diuretic.

Combinations with other drugs. The combination of nifedipine and a β-blocker has been shown to be an excellent step 3 regimen in patients with severe hypertension. Nifedipine has also been shown to be additive when combined with methyldopa. Additional combinations of nondiuretic drugs with calcium channel blockers have not been reported for the control of hypertension.

Nonpharmacological Aspects of Treatment (See Kaplan, 1985, "General References")

Four nonpharmacological modalities may promote lowering of blood pressure: sodium restriction, weight reduction, physical exercise (sufficient to achieve the conditioning effect—see Chapter 58), and various techniques combining psychological and physical relaxation. All four have been shown to enhance the blood pressure-lowering effect of antihypertensive drugs. Systematic trials of initial management with nonpharmacological therapies are in progress; it is hoped that such trials will indicate how often the blood pressure can be controlled plus the impact of these means of blood pressure control upon hypertension-associated mor-

Table 62.12.
Information for Patients Who are Advised to Follow a 2-g Sodium Diet[a]

Americans eat about **20 times more sodium** than they need, most of which comes from salt, which is one source of sodium.

Sodium is:

found naturally in foods, even those that do not taste salty.

added to food by manufacturers in food processing.

added in cooking in the form of salt, baking powder, baking soda, or seasonings such as monosodium glutamate (MSG).

added as salt to food at the table.

In the body, sodium acts like a sponge to hold water in the body tissues. Sometimes the body cannot get rid of enough of the sodium. High blood pressure may result. If not controlled, high blood pressure leads to stroke, kidney failure and heart disease.

Using no salt in cooking or at the table and eliminating highly salted food cuts down the sodium level of the food you eat to about **2000 mg a day.**

ADD NEW FLAVORS TO YOUR FOOD!

☐ Herbs and spices can give new zest to your unsalted cooking.

☐ A little herb goes a long way. If you are making your own substitution without the benefit of a recipe, try 1/4 teaspoon of dried herb or spice to:

a recipe for 4 servings,

a pound of meat, poultry, fish, or vegetable or 2 cups of sauce.

If you are using red pepper or garlic powder start with only 1/8 teaspoon. Taste and add a little more depending on your preference.

☐ If you use fresh herbs use 4 times the amound of dried herb. Instead of 1/4 teaspoon of dried herb use 1 full teaspoon of fresh herb.

☐ Add dried herbs to soups and stews during the last hour of cooking.

☐ Use whole spices in slow cooking dishes and add them at the beginning of the cooking period.

☐ When using ground spices add them 15 minutes before the end of the cooking period. If adding them to uncooked dishes, add them several hours before serving. As a start, try one or a combination of the following popular herbs:

Basil	Rosemary
Celery seed	Sage
Marjoram	Savory
Mint	Thyme

BEWARE OF HIDDEN SODIUM!

Processed Foods

Salt is added to many packaged, convenience, "fast," and canned foods. Examples are: packaged dinners (such as macaroni and cheese), packaged coatings and "helpers," combination dinners (such as frozen meals and casserole dishes), canned soups, dried soups, canned vegetables, and frozen vegetables with sauces.

"Fast Foods"

Generally, meals served at "fast food" places are high in sodium. A typical meal of a hamburger, french fries, and a vanilla shake can total over 1000 mg of sodium—more than half of your total daily allowance. Remember pizza, hot dogs, burgers, fried chicken, fried fish, omelettes, and tacos served at "fast food" places are usually high in sodium. Just one whole dill pickle contains 1900 mg of sodium, almost the total allowed in this diet.

Read labels carefully. Foods which list salt or sodium as ingredients should be avoided. Compare different brands of the same product. It's unnecesary to purchase special dietetic foods. Many dietetic foods contain sodium or salt, **so read the labels carefully.**

SOME TIPS ON EATING OUT!

☐ Select restaurants that offer à la carte service.

☐ For breakfast, order from the allowed cereals. Poached or boiled eggs with toast may be ordered at most restaurants.

Additives

Sodium may be added to food as a preservative; for quick cooking; to soften or loosen skins of fruits and vegetables; to cure meats, fish, sausage; to stop growth of molds. Additives which contain sodium include:

Monosodium glutamate (MSG)

Baking soda

Disodium phosphate

Sodium alginate

Sodium benzoate

Sodium hydroxide

Sodium nitrate

Sodium propionate

Sodium sulfite

☐ In ordering rice, ask if it has been cooked in salted water. Some restaurants cook rice without salt. Rice pilaf is usually prepared with salt.

☐ You can count on baked potato. For toppings use butter, margarine or sour cream.

Table 62.12.—*Continued*

☐ For lunch, try fruit or tossed salads; roast beef, sliced chicken or turkey breast sandwich; and fruit for dessert.

☐ At dinner, try fruit (fresh, canned, or frozen), fruit juice, or fruit cup as an appetizer.

☐ If you select broiled meats, fresh fish, or chicken, you may request that no salt or other condiments like garlic salt or onion salt be added before or after broiling.

☐ Inside cuts of roast beef, lamb, pork, veal, chicken and turkey have less sodium than outside cuts. Trim off the edges that would have been salted. Ask that it be served without gravy or sauce.

TO SUM IT UP!

☐ Using less salt is advisable for almost everyone, even children, so let the whole family join in.

☐ Avoid shaking salt on your food. Substitute a blend of herbs for your salt shaker.

☐ Cook without salt. Try leaving it out of recipes.

☐ Experiment with new flavors by using herbs and spices. Fine restaurants rely on herbs, spices, and the natural flavor of food, *not salt*, for good taste.

☐ Avoid "fast foods" and other processed foods high in sodium.

☐ Read the labels of foods and medicines to find "hidden" sodium.
  Look for the symbol: Na$^+$;
      the words: salt, sodium, soda, brine

☐ Become familiar with foods high in sodium.

☐ If in doubt about cooked vegetables, order sliced tomatoes or a salad such as tossed salad, lettuce wedge or fruit salad. Try lemon or oil and vinegar for the dressing. Ask the waiter to leave off the croutons!

☐ Help yourself to the bread basket, but avoid salted breadsticks and crackers with salted tops.

☐ For dessert select fruit, sherbet, ice cream, or plain yogurt.

☐ Most airlines provide "special meals." A low sodium meal may be ordered at no extra cost when you make your flight reservation.

☐ "Fast food" menu items (except for the salad bar where you can select low sodium items) have usually been salted. If food can be prepared to order, request that no salted seasonings be added.

☐ Low sodium salt, such as "Lite Salt," is a combination of sodium and potassium. Do not be misled that it is free of sodium. It has about half the sodium content of regular salt.
  Use of low sodium salt and salt substitutes can be dangerous because of their very high potassium content. It is **essential** that you ask your doctor if you may use them. Also ask **how much** you may use each day.

[a] From "Health Is In—Salt is Out," courtesy of The Maryland High Blood Pressure Coordinating Council.

bidity and mortality. So far, only weight reduction in obese subjects (31) and marked sodium restriction (meaning less than 1 g of sodium daily) (26) have been shown to control chronic hypertension.

In one preliminary trial (23), subjects whose hypertension had been controlled on medication for 5 years in the Hypertension Detection and Follow-up Program (HDFP) (see description, page 791) were randomly allocated to a no-medication control group, a weight reduction group (obese subjects), or a sodium restriction group (70 mEq, or 2 g, or less/day). Participating subjects agreed to discontinue their medications at the outset; medications were resumed if the diastolic pressure rose above 95 mm Hg. The dietary interventions consisted of frequent group therapy sessions. The end point, blood pressure control without resuming medication, was attained and maintained for the duration of the study (up to 56 weeks) by over 70% of those subjects in both the sodium restriction and weight reduction groups and also by over 50% of the control subjects who received *no* dietary intervention.

Because nonpharmacological measures require significant changes in life style, it is generally more difficult to achieve long term adherence to them than to drug treatment. Nevertheless, in initiating

care for the individual patient, one or more of these modalities should be recommended as an adjunct to drug treatment. For motivated patients with mild or moderate hypertension, one or more of these can be tried as primary treatment.

Weight Reduction and Sodium Restriction

In 1979, the National High Blood Pressure Coordinating Committee published the following practical recommendations for weight reduction and sodium restriction in the care of and prevention of hypertension. These recommendations, with modifications made in the 1984 report (21), are as follows:

Weight reduction:

1. Weight reduction should be considered routinely in the treatment of overweight borderline hypertensives, both for its potential in lowering blood pressure and for its general health benefits.

2. Practitioners should encourage weight reduction for the obese hypertensive patient, and if blood pressure is reduced to and maintained at normal levels, it should be used as definitive therapy.

3. For overweight patients who experience significant side effects from drugs, weight reduction should be considered as adjunctive therapy to help reduce drug dosages.

Table 62.13
Food List for Patients Who Are Advised to Follow a 2-g Sodium Diet (Shows What to Eat and What Not to Eat)[a,b]

What to Eat	What Not to Eat	What to Eat	What Not to Eat
Vegetables			
Fresh and most frozen vegetables	Canned vegetables	Cracked wheat	Danish pastries
Artichoke	Canned tomato juice	French	Muffins
Asparagus	Canned vegetable juice	Hamburger roll	Pancakes
Avocado	Frozen peas	Hot dog roll	Pizza
Bamboo shoots	Frozen lima beans	Italian	Spoonbread
Bean sprouts	Frozen vegetables with seasoned sauce	Raisin	Stuffing mix
Beets	Olives	Rye	Sweet rolls
Broccoli	Pickled vegetables	Vienna	Waffles
Brussels sprouts	Pickles	White, enriched	
Cabbage	Sauerkraut	Whole wheat	**Crackers/Snack Foods***
Carrots	Seaweed	**Cereals**	Crackers with salted tops
Cauliflower		Barley	Pretzels
Celery		Cream of Wheat, regular	Soda crackers
Chicory		Cornmeal	*Consider crackers, chips, pretzels to be high in sodium unless labeled as "unsalted"
Collards		Granola	
Corn		Grits, regular	**Cereals**
Cucumber		Oatmeal, regular	Dry cereals, except those listed under "What to Eat"
Dried beans		Petitjohns	Instant grits
Dried peas		Popcorn, unsalted	Instant hot cereals
Eggplant		Puffed Rice	Salted popcorn
Endive		Puffed Wheat	**Pastas**
Escarole		Ralston	Chow mein noodles
Green beans		Rice	Prepackaged meals, such as macaroni, noodle, or spaghetti dinners
Kale		Shredded Wheat	
Kohlrabi		Special K	
Leeks		Tapioca	
Lettuce		Wheatena	
Lima beans		**Pastas, Cooked without Salt**	
Mixed vegetables		Macaroni	
Mushrooms		Noodles	
Mustard greens		Spaghetti	
Okra			
Onion		*Fruits*	
Parsley		**Fresh, frozen, canned or dried fruit**	Dried fruits that contain sodium preservative
Parsnips		Apple	
Peas		Apple juice	
Peppers		Applesauce	
Potato, sweet white		Apricots	
Pumpkin		Banana	
Radishes		Berries	
Rutabaga		*Cantaloupe	
Scallions		Cherries	
Soybeans		Cranberries	
Spinach		Dates	
Squash, summer acorn winter		Figs	
Tomato		*Grapefruit	
Tomato juice, low sodium		*Grapefruit juice	
Turnip		*Lemon	
V-8 Juice, low sodium		Nectarine	
Water chestnuts		*Orange	
Watercress		*Orange juice	
Wax beans		Peach	
Yams		Pear	
Note: Low sodium canned vegetables may be used.		Pineapple	
		Pineapple juice	
Protein Foods		Plums	
Lean fresh meat	Bacon	Prunes	
Beef	Canned meats	Prune juice	
Lamb	Corned beef	Raisins	
Liver	Dried chipped beef	Raspberries	
Pork	Ham, cured or "low salt"	Rhubarb	
Veal	Mean extenders and "helpers"		
	Hot dogs		
	Luncheon meats		
	Salt pork		
	Sausage		
	Scrapple		
	Smoked meats		
	Salted or pickled meats		
	TV and frozen meat dinners		
	"Fast food" meats		

Fresh fish
Bass
Bluefish
Carp
Cod
Flounder
Haddock
Hake
Halibut
Ocean perch
Pike
Pollack
Pompano
Porgy
Red snapper
Rockfish
Salmon
Shad
Sole
Swordfish
Trout
Tuna
Whitefish

Anchovy
Canned fish
Commercially frozen fish
"Fast food" fish
Herring
Salted fish
Sardines
Smoked or pickled fish
TV and frozen fish dinners

Fresh Shellfish
Crab
Lobster
Oysters*
Shrimp

Crabs, prepared with salty seasoning
Mussels
Scallops

* If from saltwater bed, rinse saltwater out with fresh water.

Peanut butter

Dried beans, cooked without salt, salt pork, or ham

Canned beans

Lean fresh poultry
Capon
Chicken
Cornish hen
Duck
Goose
Turkey

Canned chicken
Canned turkey
Commercial fried chicken
TV dinners
Turkey roll
Frozen turkey or chicken casseroles/pies
Frozen omelet
Frozen souffle
Frozen quiche

Beverages

Alcoholic beverages, in moderation
Club soda
Cocoa
Coffee—ground, instant, decaffeinated
Soft drinks
Sugar-free beverages, in moderation
Tea—loose, teabags, instant
Tonic water
Wine

Breads, Crackers, Cereals, Grains

Breads
Cinnamon
Corn and molasses

Crackers
Any crackers with unsalted tops

Breads
Biscuits
Cornbread
Croutons, packaged

Desserts

Grapes
Grape juice
Honeydew
*Strawberries
*Tangerine
Watermelon

Custard, homemade
Fruit
Fruit cake
Fruit cobbler
Gelatin desserts, all flavors
Ice cream
Ice milk
Lady fingers
Sherbert
Sponge cake, homemade
Yogurt, plain

Commercially prepared:
Cake
Cookies
Donuts
Pie
Pudding mixes
Sweet rolls

Seasonings

Garlic, fresh or powdered
Herbs and spices
Horseradish, fresh or prepared
Lemon, juice and peel
Onion, fresh, powered, flaked
Pepper
Tabasco sauce
Vanilla extract
Vinegar
Wine
Worchestershire sauce (used sparingly)

Barbeque sauce
Catsup
Celery salt
Chili sauce
Cooking wine (has salt added)
Garlic salt
Lemon pepper seasoning
Meat tenderizers
Monosodium glutamate (MSG)
Onion salt
Pickle relish
Prepared mustard
Salt, seasoned or plain
Sea salt
Soy sauce
Steak sauce

Dairy Products

Skim
Dry
Evaporated
Yogurt, plain
Brie
Chedder
Colby
Cottage
Gruyere
Monterey
Mozzarella
Muenster
Natural swiss
Neufchatel
Port du Salut
Ricotta
Cheese labeled "low sodium" or "unsalted"

Buttermilk (commercial)
Condensed milk
"Fast food" shakes
Blue
Camembert
Cheezola
Edam
Feta
Gouda
Limburger
Parmesan
Processed Cheese, American and Swiss
Processed cheese foods
Processed cheese spreads
Provolone
Roquefort
Romano
Slim Line cheese
Tilsit

ª Adapted from "Health Is In—Salt Is Out," courtesy of The Maryland High Blood Pressure Coordinating Council.
ᵇ Useful conversions: 100 mg of sodium = 4.35 mEq of sodium.
100 mg of sodium = 250 mg of salt.
1 teaspoon of salt = 6 g of sodium.

4. Persons with a family history of hypertension should avoid excessive weight gain and should reduce if overweight.

5. Prevention or control of obesity in the young should be regarded as having positive health benefits and as a possible preventive step for hypertension.

Chapter 76 contains a full discussion of obesity and its treatment.

Sodium restriction:

1. Moderate sodium restriction (70 to 90 mEq daily, approximately 2 g of elemental sodium or 5 g of salt) should be routinely prescribed and if blood pressure is reduced to and maintained at normal levels, it should be used as definitive therapy.

2. For patients who experience significant side effects from drugs, sodium restriction should be considered as adjunctive therapy to help reduce drug dosages or increase drug efficacy.

3. Persons with a family history of hypertension should be encouraged to restrict sodium intake even though they may not be hypertensive.

4. Practitioners recommending sodium restriction should indicate specific diets appropriate to each patient's condition and life style and should ensure that the diet is explained satisfactorily.

Tables 62.12 and 62.13 summarize what the patient should know in order to follow a low salt diet.

As pointed out above (page 808), when a patient continues to ingest substantial salt while taking diuretics, potassium wasting is increased. Therefore, salt restriction may both prevent excessive potassium loss and facilitate blood pressure reduction in patients taking diuretics. Some investigators even suggest that the blood pressure reduction due to salt restriction is caused in part by the increased potassium consumed in many low sodium foods.

Muscle Relaxation and Biofeedback

The 1984 Joint National Committee (JNC) on Detection, Evaluation and Treatment of High Blood Pressure report (21) points out that muscle relaxation and biofeedback techniques have been shown to produce sustained modest blood pressure reduction, both in patients who are poorly controlled on drug therapy and in patients who are not on drug therapy. These techniques can therefore be recommended to motivated patients. Muscle relaxation techniques are described in Chapter 13. Biofeedback techniques and "doses" vary and require the involvement of therapists experienced with the method (4).

Physical Exercise

The 1984 JNC report (21) strongly recommends advising motivated patients to engage in conditioning level isotonic exercises. There is suggestive evidence that such exercise may produce sustained blood pressure reduction and/or a need for less antihypertensive medication to control blood pressure. Chapter 58 provides details regarding the exercise needed to achieve cardiovascular conditioning.

Although physical conditioning may be recommended as part of the initial treatment for selected patients, all patients should be informed about the *implications of hypertension and antihypertensive drug therapy for ordinary physical activity.* Studies have shown that subjects with untreated hypertension have the same patterns of blood pressure fluctuation during exercise as normotensive subjects, only at higher pressures: with vigorous exercise, the systolic pressure rises (as much as 60 mm Hg) while the diastolic pressure may rise or fall slightly. Similar patterns are found in patients treated for hypertension with β-blockers alone (49) and in combination with hydralazine (22). The impact of a number of antihypertensives and other cardiovascular drugs on blood pressure during exercise is summarized in Chapter 58, Table 58.9. Overall, it is reasonable for the physician to inform his patient that hypertension does not make a person "different" and to reassure each patient that he can engage in all of his usual activities after beginning treatment for hypertension.

Other Nonpharmacological Measures

A number of other measures may promote blood pressure reduction and should be recommended to hypertensive patients. These are:

1. Limiting *alcohol* intake to 2 ounces/day in social drinkers and treating alcoholism as a primary mode of treatment for hypertension in alcoholics (see Chapter 21).

2. Consuming a diet with substantial *potassium* content. This often occurs as a consequence of changing to a low sodium diet, which tends to contain more potassium-rich natural foods in place of processed food (Chapter 45, Table 45.2 contains an extensive list of potassium-rich foods).

3. Reducing dietary *saturated fats.*

Recently, there has been enthusiasm for supplementing the diet of hypertensive patients with *calcium and magnesium.* To date, there is insufficient evidence to suggest this as part of the nonpharmacological approach to hypertension.

Life Style and Primary Prevention of Hypertension

In addition to the role they may have in the management of established hypertension, the nonpharmacological measures discussed above have important implications for *preventing* hypertension. Although there has not been a prospective "therapeutic trial" to confirm that primary prevention of hypertension is possible, there is abundant epidemiological evidence that suggests that avoiding weight gain, avoiding excessive salt and alcohol intake, maintaining physical fitness, avoiding excessive stress, and engaging in relaxation techniques may forestall or prevent blood pressure increase. Measures such as these and other measures known to protect cardiovascular health (e.g., not smoking, avoiding a diet high in saturated fats) should be recommended to anyone who is motivated to follow a healthy life style and especially to those who have a family history of hypertension or have high normal blood pressures.

Problems in the Course of Treatment

There are three problems which will occur during the long term treatment of most patients with hypertension: the need for adjustment of the antihypertensive regimen, instability in blood pressure control, and intercurrent or concurrent morbidity.

Medication Adjustment

Within 2 to 3 months of initiating treatment, the average patient should have satisfactory blood pressure control. In the ensuing months and years, minor or major changes in the medical regimen will be needed for many patients. Each medication change requires the patient to learn a new habit and contains the potential for medication error. Therefore, whenever a medication adjustment is contemplated, the reason should be well established. If the reason is loss of blood pressure control, this should be confirmed at more than one visit; if the reason is a possible drug side effect, this should also be confirmed at serial visits in some instances. When the adjustment involves a drug the patient is already taking, it is critical to *write down the change* for the patient, to avoid confusion with instructions on the current medication bottle.

Instability in Blood Pressure Control

Most patients have inadequate blood pressure control at an occasional visit during long term follow-up. At those visits, the physician can usually identify the probable cause and design a plan to restore blood pressure control. A prompt follow-up visit should always be part of this plan. In assessing loss of blood pressure control for which the cause is not clear, it is always useful to look at the information recorded at the most recent visit where the blood pressure was controlled and ask the question: "What is different today?" The differential diagnosis of instability in blood pressure control is summarized in Table 62.14, divided into common and uncommon causes.

Noncompliance

Noncompliance can be identified by review of medication taking. Effective ways to approach this are illustrated in Chapter 4, Patient Compliance with Medical Advice.

At certain times, the patient will simply omit the medication on the day of the visit. On the other

Table 62.14.
Differential Diagnosis of Instability in Blood Pressure Control

COMMON CAUSES:
Noncompliance
Increased salt consumption
Psychological stress
UNCOMMON CAUSES:
Concurrent medications[a]
Tolerance
Refractory hypertension

[a] See Table 62.15.

hand, the patient may be taking medication faithfully but incorrectly. Because this may be due to an error in dispensing of medication, the patient's medication bottles should be checked.

History taking is obviously important. If the patient has deliberately discontinued a medication, he will often explain his reasons.

If the patient denies noncompliance, this can be further evaluated by having the patient take his medicine under supervision in the office and then measuring his blood pressure response for several hours (see example case, Fig. 62.12).

Increased Salt Consumption

A significant increase in salt consumption may lead to a positive sodium balance, which can blunt the effects of antihypertensive drugs. This problem is not uncommon in the summer months. It should be expected whenever loss of blood pressure control is associated with a weight gain of 2 to 3 lb (1 kg) or more, with or without edema. Brief review of the patient's current diet will often help to support this hypothesis. Management consists of having the patient resume moderate sodium restriction or substituting more potent diuretic treatment. Temporary use of furosemide (40 to 80 mg daily for 1 or more weeks) to eliminate excess sodium is often useful in this situation. For patients in whom sodium overload is a recurrent problem, furosemide in doses adjusted to maintain a stable weight is very effective (27).

Psychological Stress

In the patient who is adhering faithfully to treatment, psychological stress may explain his failure to respond as usual to antihypertensive drugs. This is probably because increase in sympathetic nervous system activity is often present during psychological stress.

Stress may be associated only with visits to a physician's office and the rise in blood pressure may be strictly transient. This problem can be minimized by assuring that the patient is at ease before taking the blood pressure and by repeating the measurement later in the visit if the initial pressure is high. When stress is suspected as the reason for erratic office blood pressures, blood pressure measurements

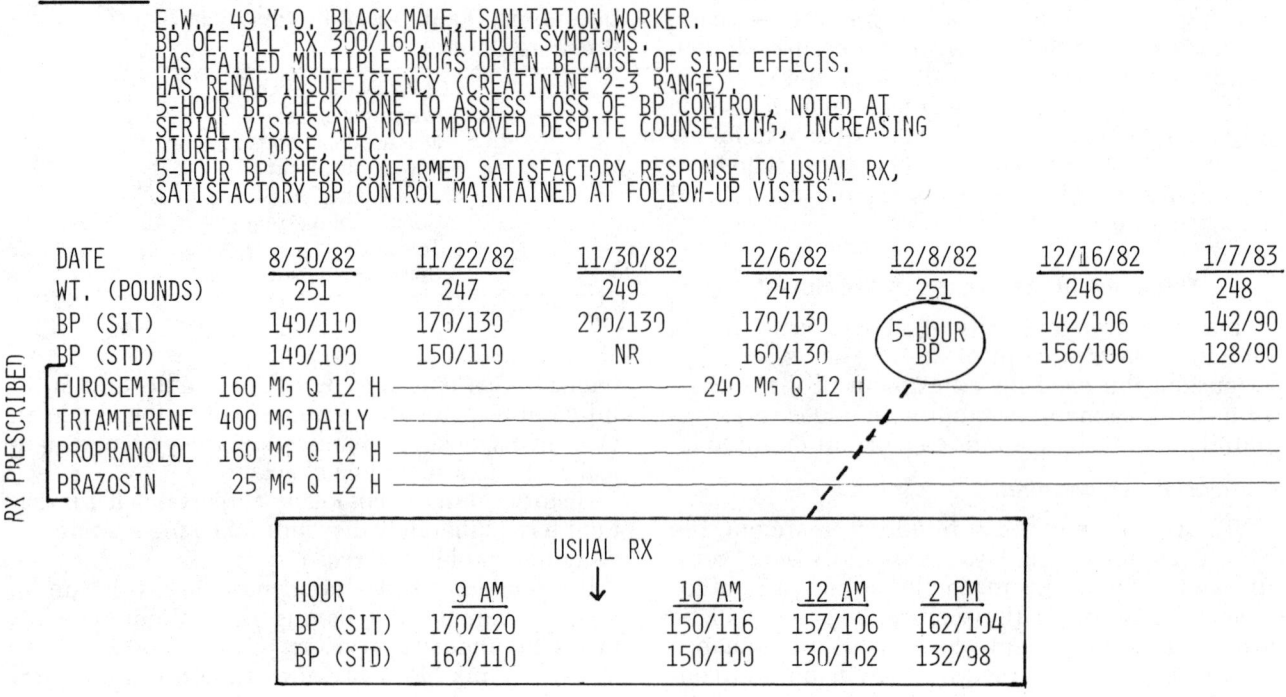

SUMMARY

E.W., 49 Y.O. BLACK MALE, SANITATION WORKER.
BP OFF ALL RX 300/160, WITHOUT SYMPTOMS.
HAS FAILED MULTIPLE DRUGS OFTEN BECAUSE OF SIDE EFFECTS.
HAS RENAL INSUFFICIENCY (CREATININE 2-3 RANGE).
5-HOUR BP CHECK DONE TO ASSESS LOSS OF BP CONTROL, NOTED AT
SERIAL VISITS AND NOT IMPROVED DESPITE COUNSELLING, INCREASING
DIURETIC DOSE, ETC.
5-HOUR BP CHECK CONFIRMED SATISFACTORY RESPONSE TO USUAL RX,
SATISFACTORY BP CONTROL MAINTAINED AT FOLLOW-UP VISITS.

DATE		8/30/82	11/22/82	11/30/82	12/6/82	12/8/82	12/16/82	1/7/83
WT. (POUNDS)		251	247	249	247	251	246	248
BP (SIT)		140/110	170/130	200/130	170/130	5-HOUR BP	142/106	142/90
BP (STD)		140/100	150/110	NR	160/130		156/106	128/90
FUROSEMIDE	160 MG Q 12 H				240 MG Q 12 H			
TRIAMTERENE	400 MG DAILY							
PROPRANOLOL	160 MG Q 12 H							
PRAZOSIN	25 MG Q 12 H							

RX PRESCRIBED

USUAL RX

HOUR	9 AM	↓	10 AM	12 AM	2 PM
BP (SIT)	170/120		150/116	157/106	162/104
BP (STD)	160/110		150/100	130/102	132/98

Figure 62.12. Five-hour office observation of response to usual antihypertensive regimen to determine whether "refractory hypertension" is due to tolerance or noncompliance.

taken at home by the patient or another responsible person may provide better information for judging the effectiveness of treatment and may spare patients from inappropriate increases in antihypertensive drugs and the associated side effects.

Psychological stress may also be due to serious job- or family-related crisis. Brief inquiry may reveal additional stress-related symptoms, such as headache, dyspepsia, sleeplessness, irritability, *etc.* In such patients, managment consists of supportive counseling (see Chapter 11) and, at times, short term prescription of minor tranquilizers (see Chapter 13). This is the one situation in which minor tranquilizers may contribute to blood pressure control.

Concurrent Medications

A number of commonly prescribed and over-the-counter medications (Table 62.15) may attenuate the response to antihypertensive drugs. Therefore, inquiry about concurrent medications is always important in assessing unstable blood pressure control. Hypertensive patients should be told which common drugs are contraindicated and that chronic use of such drugs as nonsteroidal anti-inflammatory agents and over-the-counter decongestants requires careful supervision of blood pressure.

Tolerance

With the possible exception of methyldopa, the development of tolerance to antihypertensive drugs

Table 62.15.
Medications That May Attenuate Response to Antihypertensive Drugs

PROMOTES POSITIVE SODIUM BALANCE:
  Nonsteroidal anti-inflammatory drugs (not aspirin)
  Corticosteroids
  Estrogens
  Sodium-containing antacids
SYMPATHOMIMETIC:
  Decongestants (oral)
  Amphetamine
  Bronchodilators
MECHANISM NOT ESTABLISHED
  Tricyclic antidepressants
  Phenothiazines
  Monoamine oxidase inhibitors
  Oral contraceptives

has not been demonstrated. Therefore, whenever a patient appears to become "tolerant" to a drug which worked well initially, other causes of unstable blood pressure control should be sought.

After a number of years of taking methyldopa, many patients require larger amounts of the drug to maintain adequate blood pressure control. This finding may signify the development of true tolerance, or it may signify progressive hypertension. If the latter explanation is correct, a similar need for higher doses may be found with other drugs after they have been in general use for 10 or more years.

In evaluating apparent tolerance to a previously effective drug or combination of drugs, office observation of a patient's response to his usual regimen can be quite helpful (see case example, Fig. 62.12).

Refractory Hypertension

Rarely, a patient's blood pressure may become refractory to previously effective drugs, and none of the above causes will be found. In such patients, two questions must be answered:

1. *Is the hypertension really refractory to the patient's usual medication?* This question can be answered best by a brief hospital admission to ensure that the patient receives his medications correctly; because of the blood pressure-lowering effect of bed rest, patients should be encouraged to remain active while in the hospital. Alternatively, supervision of medication taking and blood pressure response in the office or at home by a nurse may suffice. It is usually found that these patients were not taking their medication correctly (see Fig. 62.12) and that, under supervision, they respond appropriately. Some patients, however, do not respond at all to previously effective drugs.

2. *What is the reason* (for the occasional patient whose refractory hypertension is confirmed)? Confirmed refractory hypertension in a previously responding patient suggests that one of the causes of secondary hypertension may be present, especially RVH. Evaluation for RVH or a trial of a different

drug regimen is appropriate at this juncture. For those patients without surgically treatable hypertension, an effective drug regimen can almost always be found.

Occasionally, a newly diagnosed patient fails to respond to a variety of drugs and doses. This apparent primary refractoriness to antihypertensive drugs should also be evaluated by hospital or office supervision of the blood pressure response to drugs (see example case, Fig. 62.13).

Regimens which may be particularly effective in controlling refractory hypertension are:

1. Minoxidil or nifedipine with a β-blocker;
2. Captopril;
3. High dose furosemide in conjunction with a step 2 or step 3 regimen;
4. High dose prazosin.

Orthostatic Symptoms

Many patients describe occasional orthostatic symptoms, particularly when they first stand up in the morning. Advice to sit for a few minutes before standing or a modest reduction in drug dose will usually alleviate the problem.

At times a patient who has satisfactory blood pressures at office visits will describe orthostatic symptoms lasting an hour or more after taking medicine. In this situation, it is important to try reducing or discontinuing the medication promptly. In such a patient who has severe hypertension off of medi-

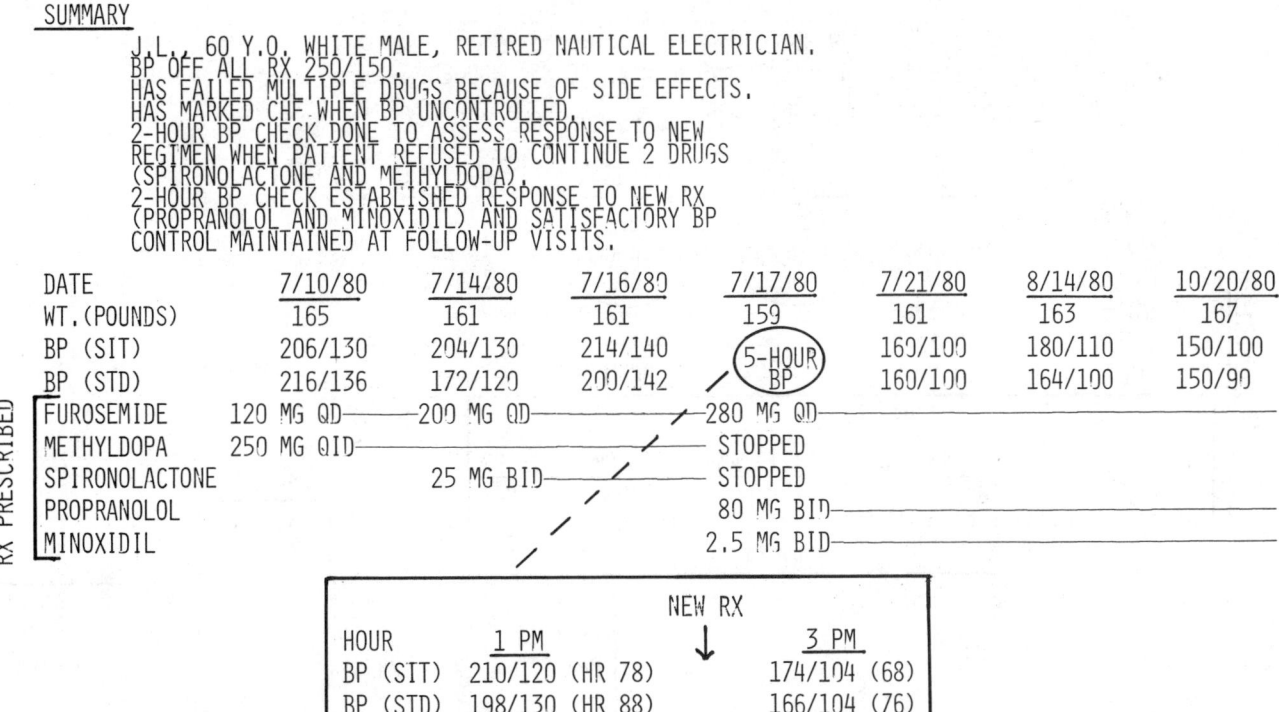

SUMMARY

J.L., 60 Y.O. WHITE MALE, RETIRED NAUTICAL ELECTRICIAN.
BP OFF ALL RX 250/150.
HAS FAILED MULTIPLE DRUGS BECAUSE OF SIDE EFFECTS.
HAS MARKED CHF WHEN BP UNCONTROLLED.
2-HOUR BP CHECK DONE TO ASSESS RESPONSE TO NEW
REGIMEN WHEN PATIENT REFUSED TO CONTINUE 2 DRUGS
(SPIRONOLACTONE AND METHYLDOPA).
2-HOUR BP CHECK ESTABLISHED RESPONSE TO NEW RX
(PROPRANOLOL AND MINOXIDIL) AND SATISFACTORY BP
CONTROL MAINTAINED AT FOLLOW-UP VISITS.

DATE	7/10/80	7/14/80	7/16/80	7/17/80	7/21/80	8/14/80	10/20/80
WT.(POUNDS)	165	161	161	159	161	163	167
BP (SIT)	206/130	204/130	214/140	(5-HOUR BP)	160/100	180/110	150/100
BP (STD)	216/136	172/120	200/142		160/100	164/100	150/90

RX PRESCRIBED

FUROSEMIDE   120 MG QD———200 MG QD———280 MG QD————————————
METHYLDOPA   250 MG QID—————————————— STOPPED
SPIRONOLACTONE   25 MG BID——————— STOPPED
PROPRANOLOL   80 MG BID———————————
MINOXIDIL   2.5 MG BID—————————————

NEW RX		
HOUR	1 PM	3 PM
BP (SIT)	210/120 (HR 78)	174/104 (68)
BP (STD)	198/130 (HR 88)	166/104 (76)

Figure 62.13. Two-hour office observation of response to new regimen in a patient being changed to a more potent antihypertensive drug (minoxidil).

cine, it is important to evaluate objectively the orthostatic symptoms before reducing medications (see case example, Fig. 62.14).

Rarely, an older patient who has atherosclerosis of his cerebral arteries may describe orthostatic symptoms related to medications, even when he has normal standing blood pressures (25). When such positional cerebral ischemia appears to be present, a trial of less (or no) antihypertensive drugs is appropriate.

Co-morbidity

During long term treatment, most hypertensive patients will develop acute or chronic conditions that require adjustment of their antihypertensive drugs. One of the commonest situations in which less medication may be needed to control hypertension is hospitalization for any reason (18). For patients with selected chronic conditions, one or more antihypertensive drugs may be inappropriate, as summarized in Table 62.7. There are a number of conditions that require extra caution with *any* antihypertensive drug regimen.

Acute Illness

From time to time, each patient with hypertension will have an intercurrent acute illness. The following factors, which increase a person's sensitivity to antihypertensive drugs, may accompany some of those intercurrent illnesses:

1. Reduced intake of food, including salt.
2. Bed rest for several days to several weeks. In previously healthy individuals, it has been demonstrated that bed rest for more than a few days produces a modest reduction in recumbent blood pressures and a marked reduction in standing blood pressure.
3. Vomiting or diarrhea, leading to fluid and electrolyte deficits.
4. Hypotension, presumably due to vasodilation, during febrile illnesses.

Short term decrease or withholding of antihypertensive drugs will protect such patients from the additional morbidity brought by hypotension or electrolyte depletion. The patient's usual antihypertensive regimen should be resumed gradually as the blood pressure returns to hypertensive levels. In

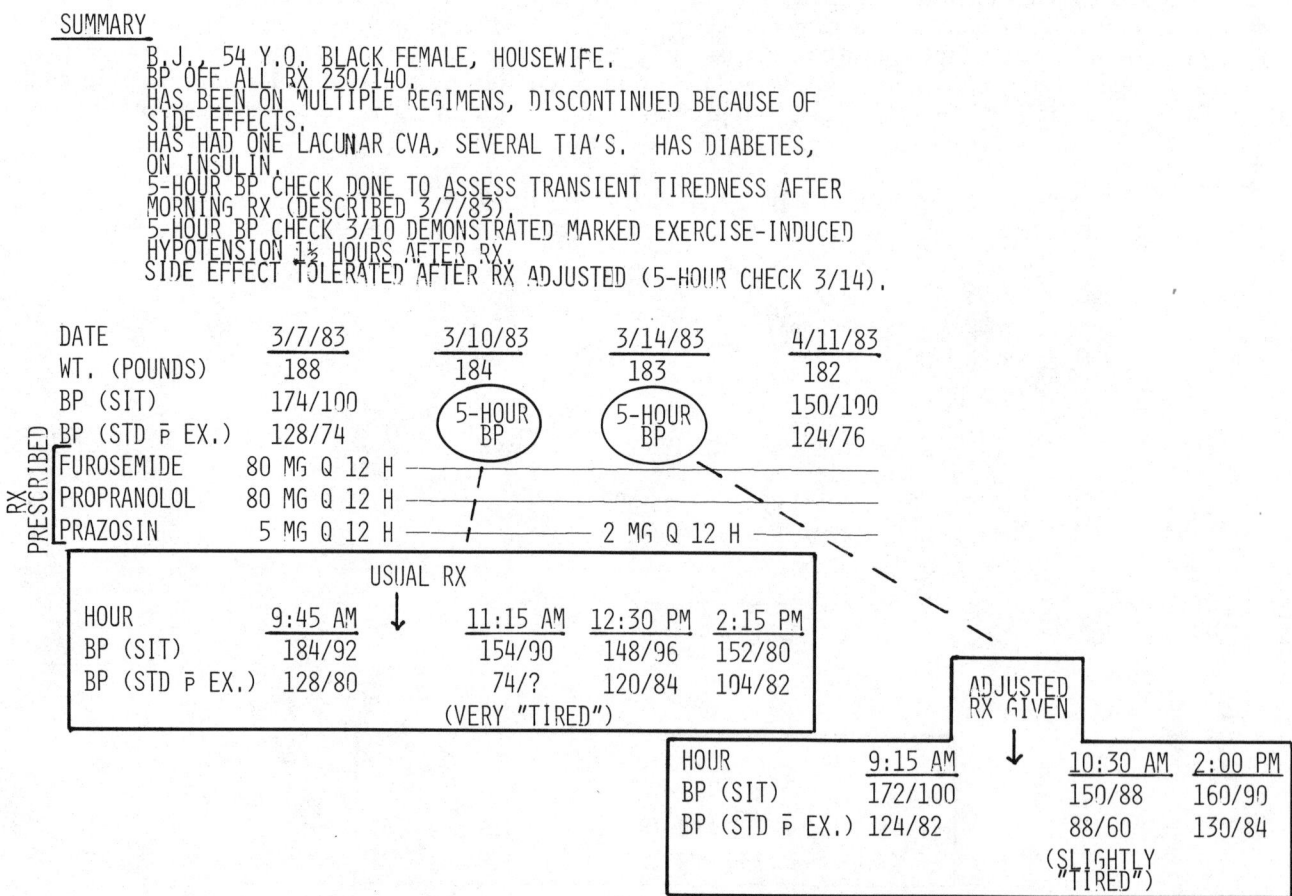

Figure 62.14. Five-hour observation of response to usual medication in a patient who described transient symptoms after medication every day but had satisfactory pressures at office visits.

some situations, for example, following major surgery, the previous regimen may not be needed for 1 or more months.

Concurrent Chronic Illness

CEREBROVASCULAR DISEASE. Hypertensive patients with suspected or known cerebral atherosclerosis should have their blood pressure lowered carefully to avoid hypoperfusion of an already compromised vascular network. Patients who develop typical orthostatic symptoms despite standing blood pressures in the "normal" range should have a trial of lower dose treatment or no treatment to determine whether positional cerebral ischemia is present.

In patients with completed strokes, controlled studies of antihypertensive treatment have shown both a reduction or no reduction in the occurrence of second strokes; these studies have not reported the incidence of other hypertensive morbidity in poststroke patients, particularly congestive heart failure, which should be reduced by antihypertensive treatment. Therefore, patients who remain hypertensive after their neurological status has stabilized should be treated.

CORONARY ARTERY DISEASE. In the hypertensive patient with angina pectoris, management of the angina always includes adequate blood pressure control.

The hypertensive patient who has a myocardial infarction may have a normal blood pressure or less severe hypertension during convalescence. Because this may be transient, the blood pressure should be evaluated at least monthly in the first 3 to 4 months after discharge.

DIABETES. In the patient with coexisting diabetes, consistent control of hyperglycemia will prevent erratic responses to antihypertensive drugs; the diabetic patient who periodically develops volume deficits from osmotic diuresis risks symptomatic hypotension. In the sizable subgroup of diabetics who have postural hypotension due to diabetic neuropathy, the risk of exaggerated hypotension accompanies any antihypertensive regimen; the orthostatic pressure and not the recumbent pressure should be monitored to determine the response to therapy in these and other patients with baseline orthostasis.

ASTHMA. In the hypertensive patient with coexisting asthma, blood pressure elevation may accompany episodes of increased bronchospasm. This may occur in untreated hypertensives as well as in those whose blood pressures are usually controlled on antihypertensive drugs. In treated patients, restoration of blood pressure control depends upon improvement in the asthma and not upon increased antihypertensive medications. As noted in Table 62.9, hypertensive patients with a history of bronchospasm should not receive β-adrenergic blocking agents.

Preplanned Surgery (See Chapter 86)

HYPERTENSION IN ADOLESCENTS AND YOUNG ADULTS

Adolescents and young adults have not been included in the major studies of the epidemiology and treatment of hypertension. In recent years; preliminary findings about the natural history of hypertension in this age group and recommendations for management have been published. (See symposium on high blood pressure in the young (Kotchen and Havlik in "General References").

Epidemiology

A single longitudinal study, in Evans County, Georgia, has provided information about the prevalence of hypertension and the incidence of new hypertension in adolescents and young adults (42). The study utilized a probability sample of the population between the ages of 15 and 24 at entry. Hypertension was defined as an average of three diastolic blood pressure readings of 90 mm Hg or greater. At entry in 1960, the overall *prevalence of hypertension* was 14.6% (3.0% for subjects 15 through 19 years of age and 20.6% for subjects 20 through 24 years of age). The follow-up study in 1976, when all subjects were in their third or fourth decade, showed an overall prevalence of hypertension of 26.4%; during 16 years there was a 26% *incidence of new hypertension* for those 15 to 19 years old at entry and a 12% incidence for those 20 to 24 years old at entry. Overweight status and the development of obesity correlated highly with prevalence and incidence of hypertension, respectively. A small percentage of those hypertensive at entry had a normal blood pressure at follow-up; presumably they had labile hypertension when first examined.

In addition to prevalence and incidence rates, this study has yielded preliminary data on *long term morbidity* in the young adult with hypertension. During the first 10 years of follow-up (before the publication of the Veterans Administration study results) none of the hypertensive subjects was treated. An interim study in 1968 disclosed that a number of those hypertensive at entry had developed cardiovascular events attributable to hypertension. The 16-year follow-up in 1976 disclosed a much higher incidence of electrocardiographic abnormalities in those hypertensive at entry compared to those normotensive at entry.

Other epidemiological studies of hypertension in young adults have indicated that labile hypertension may be more common than sustained hypertension in teenagers; that there is a striking incidence of sustained new hypertension between the ages of 15 and 25; and that most young adults with sustained

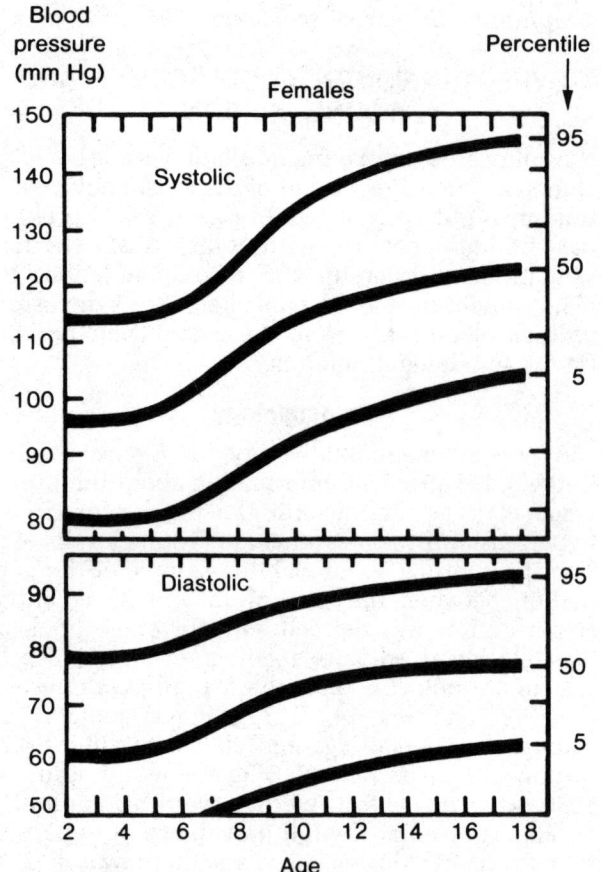

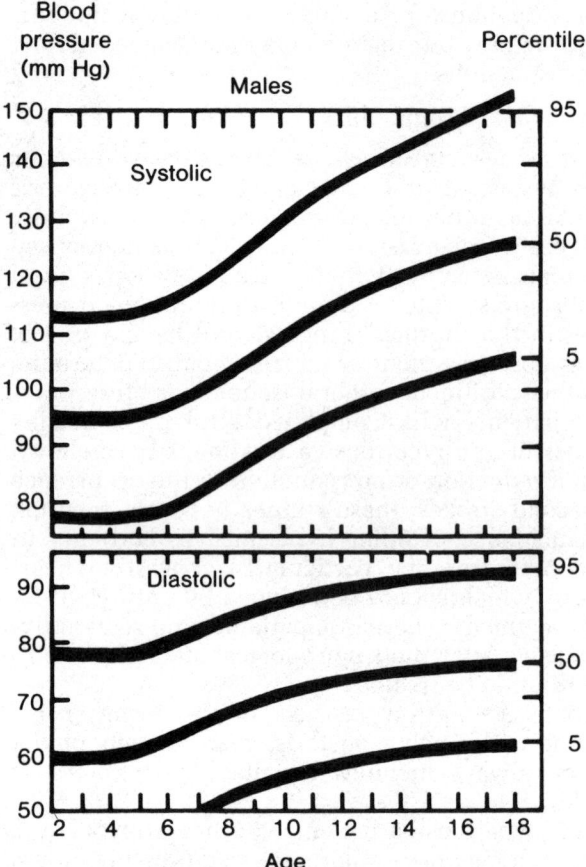

Figure 62.15. Percentiles of blood pressure measurement (right arm, seated) in children and adolescents.

(From Report of the Task Force on Blood Pressure Control in Children. *Pediatrics* 59 (suppl):803, 1977.)

hypertension have essential hypertension. The guidelines for baseline evaluation and for suspecting secondary hypertension are therefore the same as those summarized earlier (pages 799 to 801). Oral contraceptive treatment is a particularly important etiology to consider in the baseline evaluation of all young women with hypertension (see below, page 830).

Recommendations

In 1977, the National High Blood Pressure Coordinating Committee made the following recommendations for managing adolescent hypertension:

All adolescents with blood pressure levels above the 95th percentile (see Fig. 62.15) and a diastolic pressure of less than 100 mm Hg should receive the following surveillance and counseling.

1. Periodic blood pressure determination.
2. Advice on weight reduction, if needed.
3. Avoidance of salt abuse (placement on a moderate salt-restricted diet—5 g/day for teenagers, less for younger children).
4. Encouragement to be physically active.
5. Encouragement to discontinue smoking ciga-

rettes (nonsmokers should be discouraged from starting the habit).

6. Examination for other risk factors (i.e., serum lipids, glucose, etc).

All patients with sustained diastolic pressures of 100 mm Hg or greater should receive drug treatment by the stepped method. Methyldopa and β-blocking agents are recommended as step 2 drugs.

For those patients whose diastolic pressure remains in the range 90 to 100 mm Hg after 1 year of nonpharmacological management, drug treatment should be strongly considered.

Because of the psychological and social stresses associated with adolescence, the care of a chronic condition such as hypertension requires special considerations in this age group (see Chapter 5).

HYPERTENSION IN OLDER PATIENTS

Physicians frequently find sustained hypertension in their older patients. This is not surprising in light of the prevalence data summarized above in Figure 62.1. In 1979, the National High Blood Pressure Coordinating Committee announced recommendations for the treatment of two subgroups of older patients with hypertension: those with systolic-diastolic hypertension; and those with isolated systolic hypertension (considered in the following section).

Recommendations

The 1979 recommendations for older patients were modified somewhat in the 1984 report of the JNC (21), on the basis of the results of the HDFP (20), which showed a modest benefit in patients 60 to 69 years of age whose hypertension was controlled (stepped care) as compared to those with inadequately controlled hypertension (referred care). For older individuals with sustained diastolic pressures of 90 mm Hg or greater (105 mm Hg or greater in the 1979 report), reduction of the pressure to less than 90 mm Hg is now recommended. In addition to the HDFP results, this recommendation is supported by (a) the earlier results of treatment in the subgroup of men with diastolic pressures of 90 to 114 mm Hg who were 60 years of age and older at entry to the Veterans Administration (VA) study (see description of study, page 790, and Table 62.16) and (b) the recently completed study of the European Working Party or High Blood Pressure in the Elderly (EWPHE)(2). EWPHE utilized a placebo trial similar to the VA trial but designed specifically to assess the effectiveness of treatment in older (average age 71 years at entry) hypertensives, both men and women. In the trial, it was shown that both systolic and diastolic pressures could be reduced effectively and safely (by about 30 to 50%) by the drugs used in the study: hydrochlorothiazide, triamterene, and methyldopa. Both mortality and morbidity due to cardiovascular and cerebrovascular disease were reduced

Table 62.16.
Veterans Administration Trial Results in Patients 60 Years Old and Older, Diastolic 90 to 114 mm Hg[a]

	Placebo	Treated
NUMBER OF SUBJECTS	43	38
INCIDENCE OF MORBID EVENTS (%)	62.8	28.9
TYPE OF MORBID EVENT (NO.):		
Cerebrovascular accident	10	3
Congestive heart failure	9	0
Accelerated hypertension	0	0
Coronary artery disease	5	5
Atrial fibrillation	2	0
Dissecting aneurysm	1	0
Other	0	3
Diastolic > 124 mm Hg	2	0
TOTAL	29	11

[a] Adapted from Veterans Administration Cooperative Study Group on Antihypertensive Agents: Effects of treatment on morbidity in hypertension. III. Influence of age, diastolic pressure, and prior cardiovascular disease; further analysis of side effects. *Circulation* 45:991, 1972 (48).

significantly in treated subjects, although their overall mortality during the study period was not significantly reduced.

In addition to reducing the cut-off level for treatment from 105 to 90 mm Hg, the JNC now strongly recommends trying nonpharmacological measures before drugs in older patients with mild hypertension and has issued a number of caveats about drug treatment of older persons with hypertension.

Caveats

Several special characteristics of older persons should be considered in deciding how to treat their hypertension.

Orthostatic hypotension unrelated to drugs is common in elderly subjects. Approximately one-fourth of those living at home have a 20 mm Hg or greater fall in systolic pressure upon standing (7). A combination of incresae in sedentary activity and blunting of autonomic reflexes probably explains this. Thus it is particularly important to obtain baseline and follow-up standing blood pressure (including standing after walking) in older patients taking antihypertensive drugs. When drug treatment is selected for an older person, it is prudent not to select the step 2 adrenergic inhibitor, prazosin, because of its tendency to produce marked orthostasis at low doses in some patients.

Other characteristics of older subjects that increase the risk of chronic antihypertensive drugs include:

1. Salt and fluid intake may vary significantly from week to week.

2. Concomitant large vessel atherosclerosis (kidneys, brain, heart) may increase the risk of ischemic damage resulting from accidental drug-induced hypotension.

3. Medication-taking errors may be increased.

4. Drug excretion rates are generally reduced as a function of aging.

Three precautions will minimize the risks of antihypertensive drugs in older patients: using the smallest recommended dose and increasing the dose very slowly; keeping the drug schedule simple; and promptly decreasing or discontinuing drugs if there are signs or symptoms of significant orthostatic hypotension or annoying side effects.

ISOLATED SYSTOLIC HYPERTENSION

Sustained isolated systolic hypertension (defined as a blood pressure ≥ 160/< 90 mm Hg) is quite common in older patients and may be seen in any age group. The Framingham data and other studies have confirmed that systolic hypertension is an independent and powerful risk factor for cardiovascular morbidity. To date, there has been no formal study of the health impact of treatment for isolated systolic hypertension. However, in 1981 a multicenter controlled trial of treatment of isolated systolic hypertension in patients over 60 was initiated in the United States (the Systolic Hypertension in the Elderly Program). In recent years, the physiological basis for isolated systolic hypertension has been studied and practical recommendations for long term management have been published.

Pathophysiology (1, 35)

Isolated systolic hypertension (ISH) may be found in patients at any age who have conditions associated with an increased cardiac output (arteriovenous fistula, patent ductus arteriosus, severe anemia, erythroderma, thyrotoxicosis, Paget's disease of the bone, *etc*). However, in individuals without one of these conditions, the mechanisms for isolated systolic hypertension appear to be different in young and old subjects. In younger subjects, there is a usually hyperkinetic circulation (increased heart rate, increased left ventricular ejection rate and cardiac indices, and normal peripheral resistance) and the hypertension responds to β-blocking agents. Older subjects with ISH usually have a normal heart rate, decreased left ventricular ejection rate and cardiac indices, and increased peripheral resistance; and the hypertension responds to vasodilator treatment.

Recommendations

In its 1979 statement of hypertension in the elderly, the National High Blood Pressure Coordinating Committee gave no definitive recommendations for ISH but stated that for the individual patient the goal should be an acceptable range (140 to 160 mm Hg) rather than a normal blood pressure (< 140 mm Hg). The 1984 JNC report reiterated this position (21) and indicated that in the preliminary part of the Systolic Hypertension in the Elderly Program it was established that diuretic therapy alone was effective in a substantial proportion of patients, that clonidine and methyldopa seem to be more effective than β-blockers as step 2 drugs, and that hydralazine may be added as step 3 drug if needed.

Treatment of isolated systolic hypertension should be strongly recommended for the following patients: those with left ventricular failure, those with poorly controlled angina, and those with consistently very high systolic pressure (i.e., ≥ 200 mm Hg). In each of these situations, reduction of the actual or potential increase in cardiac work due to systolic hypertension is the rationale for treatment. The stepped method for drug selection discussed earlier is appropriate.

A subset of older hypertensive patients develop heart failure because of left ventricular cavity obliteration, due to inappropriate "stiffness" of the myocardium during diastole (39). This problem has been reported chiefly in patients with diastolic hypertension; however, in a patient with ISH whose heart failure does not respond to empiric treatment, an echocardiogram should be obtained to look for this problem; the most effective treatment is with nifedipine or a β-blocker (see above).

HYPERTENSION IN PREGNANCY

Normally, the blood pressure falls slightly during the first and second trimesters of pregnancy and reverts to prepregnancy level in the third trimester. The fall in blood pressure is probably due to the general vasodilation which accompanies pregnancy. An increase in renin and aldosterone levels also occurs in normal pregnancy.

Based on previous records or history from the patient, it should be possible at the first prepartum visit to decide for most women whether they are usually normotensive or have chronic hypertension. This decision is very helpful in managing the sevral patterns of hypertension that may be associated with pregnancy. These are pregnancy-induced hypertension (pre-eclampsia and eclampsia), chronic hypertension, and new postpartum hypertension. Management of the last-mentioned form of hypertension will usually be the task of the patient's primary physician, while management of the first two is the province of the physician supervising the pregnancy.

Depending upon the population and the criteria for hypertension, the reported incidence of hypertension during pregnancy varies from 5 to 30%. The hypertension is pregnancy induced in about 75% of patients and chronic in the remaining 25%.

Pregnancy-Induced Hypertension

Pregnancy-induced hypertension (PIH), or pre-eclampsia, is a syndrome in which the clinical data must be carefully considered before making the diagnosis, in particular to distinguish it from pre-existing chronic hypertension. Untreated PIH is associated with a high incidence of fetal mortality and maternal morbidity. The major pathophysiological derangements are placental hypoperfusion, generalized vasospasm, and decreased glomerular filtration rate. The clinical manifestations which permit the firm diagnosis of PIH are:

1. New development of hypertension during the last trimester. The definition for hypertension in this instance is an absolute blood pressure exceeding 140/90 (on two occasions at least 6 hours apart) or a rise, between visits, of 30 mm Hg systolic or 15 mm Hg diastolic.

2. The development of *new* proteinuria during the last trimester.

3. The development of *new*, generalized edema during the last trimester (dependent edema alone is not a predictor of pre-eclampsia; it is seen in approximately one-third of pregnant women whose blood pressure remains normal).

In the patient who lacks the full clinical triad of findings, the following considerations may help to decide whether to treat her as if she is pre-eclamptic:

1. Does she have one of the known risk factors for PIH? The majority of affected women are primigravidas at the extremes of the childbearing age range. A primigravida whose mother or a sister had eclampsia is at particularly high risk. These and other risk factors are summarized in Table 62.17.

2. Was the same degree of hypertension in fact present before the twentieth week of gestation (i.e., chronic hypertension)?

Fortunately most PIH develops late in the third trimester when the fetus is mature and delivery can be planned promptly. The management for PIH that develops before the fetus is mature is hospital admission, modified bed rest, frequent monitoring of maternal blood pressure and fetal status, and antihypertensive drugs when the diastolic pressure exceeds 110 mm Hg. These measures are effective in resolving the manifestations of pre-eclampsia and ensuring a successful outcome of the pregnancy in almost all patients. If despite treatment pre-eclampsia remains severe or worsens, the treatment is delivery regardless of the maturity of the fetus.

PIH resolves within 6 weeks of delivery. About 25% of primigravidas with PIH will develop PIH during a future pregnancy. Epidemiological studies have shown, however, that women with a history of PIH do not have an increased risk of developing chronic hypertension (9). This finding is consistent with the concept that PIH is a specific and self-limited complication of pregnancy.

Chronic Hypertension in Pregnancy

Chronic hypertension will be seen more commonly in pregnant women who are in their thirties because the prevalence of hypertension increases with age (Fig. 62.1). Because of the fall in blood pressure which occurs during the first two trimesters, a sustained blood pressure of 130/80 or above is the geneally accepted criterion for chronic hypertension during these trimesters, and 140/90 is regarded as hypertension in the last trimester.

There are two important questions to consider in patients with chronic hypertension:

Table 62.17.
Risk Factors for Pregnancy-Induced Hypertension

Primagravida
Familial history of pre-eclampsia/eclampsia
Diabetes
Multiple gestation
Extremes of age
Pre-existing hypertensive vascular or renal disease
Hydatidiform mole
Fetal hydrops, but not isoimmunization *per se*
Previous history of pre-eclampsia/eclampsia

1. *Should a woman with chronic hypertension avoid pregnancy?* In the woman with mild to moderate hypertension, there is little or no increased risk to the mother or the infant. However, in a woman with evidence for major end organ damage (significant cardiomegaly, renal impairment, or eye ground changes of accelerated hypertension), infant mortality is greatly increased. Such women should be advised to avoid pregnancy.

2. *How should chronic hypertension be treated during pregnancy?* In general, a patient who becomes pregnant while taking antihypertensive medication should remain on her usual medication unless she becomes hypotensive during the pregnancy. In these patients, it is important to confirm that chronic hypertension was documented adequately before drug treatment. For patients not taking antihypertensives whose chronic hypertension is discovered during the first or second trimester, the hypertension should be treated. This recommendation is based on the finding of improved fetal survival in a controlled trial of methyldopa treatment (without diuretics) for women with chronic hypertension, defined as a blood pressure exceeding 140/90 on at least three separate occasions (30).

Management of Hypertension during Lactation

Because there has been widespread recommendation for an increase in breast-feeding in the past decade, some women who need antihypertensive drugs will want advice regarding the risks and benefits of breast-feeding. Most antihypertensive drugs appear in breast milk, and their impact upon suckling infants has not been well delineated. Based on what is known, the following guidelines have been suggested by White (52): The use of diuretics should probably be avoided during lactation because diuretics may significantly reduce milk volume. If a β-blocking agent is indicated, propranolol should be used because it has the lowest ratio of milk to plasma concentration among β-blockers; suckling infants of mothers taking propranolol, and other β-blockers, have not had adverse effects. Because there is too little information about other adrenergic inhibitors, vasodilators, or calcium channel blockers, the drugs should probably be avoided when more potent drugs are needed. Captopril yields a very low concentration in milk relative to plasma, and it can be recommended in a breast-feeding woman who needs a more potent antihypertensive drug.

New Postpartum Hypertension

New hypertension is detected occasionally at the sixth week postpartum visit. At the end of 1 year, some of these patients remain hypertensive, while most revert to a normal blood pressure (37). When the hypertension is first detected at the sixth-week visit, a urinalysis is critical in order to exclude the rare syndrome of postpartum nephrosclerosis.

Women with diastolic blood pressures repeatedly 100 mm Hg or greater should be treated according to the stepped care strategy discussed earlier (page 803). For women with milder hypertension (diastolic always under 100 mm Hg or less) and a normal urinalysis, nonpharmacological measures (see above, page 815) and regular follow-up are appropriate for the first 6 months to 1 year. A small proportion of these women remain hypertensive after this interval, and they should be treated for chronic hypertension.

ORAL CONTRACEPTIVES AND HYPERTENSION

Epidemiology

Longitudinal studies of women taking oral contraceptive pills (OCP) have shown the following:

1. *A mild increase in blood pressure* (systolic 5 to 6 mm Hg and diastolic 1 to 2 mm Hg) occurs shortly after initiating OCP in most women (50).

2. During the first 5 years of OCP use, there is a progressive rise in the blood pressure (mean 14 mm Hg systolic and 8 mm Hg diastolic) (50).

3. The reported incidence of *new hypertension* has varied from 3 to 6/1000 OCP users after 3 years of use. These rates were 2 to 3 times higher than the rates in comparable nonusers (10).

Population studies in recent years have shown that OCP use does increase the risk of death from cerebrovascular and cardiovascular diseases. The absolute number of women affected is very small, but physicians must be aware of the potential hazards of this form of contraception.

The physiological basis for the modest increase in blood pressure accompanying OCP use may be volume expansion. After 3 weeks, it has been found that most individuals show a 100 to 200 mEq increase in total body sodium. In addition, increased renin and aldosterone activities are found. There is no difference in the degree of these changes between those women who remain normotensive and those who develop hypertension. A history of pregnancy-induced hypertension does not increase the risk of OCP-induced hypertension and is not a contraindication to OCP use. Furthermore, there are no contraindications to OCP use in the patient with well controlled chronic hypertension who may wish to use this kind of contraception.

Approach to the Patient

The use of oral contraceptives has played a major role in the reduction of unwanted pregnancy during the past 20 years (see Chapter 93). Most physicians will find that a substantial proportion of women in the childbearing age range are OCP users or will select OCP prophylaxis. Therefore, it is important to have an approach to the occasional woman who may develop hypertension while taking oral contraceptives. The following approach is recommended:

1. Assure that a baseline blood pressure is obtained before OCP use.

2. Dispense no more than a 6-month supply at one time.

3. Measure the blood pressure at least every 6 months. If the patient develops hypertension or if the blood pressure rises significantly (though remaining below 140/90), the patient should be advised to select another form of contraception, and when this has been done OCP should be discontinued.

4. Approximately one-half of women developing hypertension during OCP use will revert to normal blood pressure within 3 months of discontinuation of OCP use. If the blood pressure does not revert to normal, the patient should be managed for chronic hypertension as described earlier in this chapter.

5. In the OCP user who develops hypertension and must continue OCP use, treatment for sustained hypertension as outlined earlier is appropriate.

General References

Chesley LC: *Hypertensive Disorders in Pregnancy.* New York, Appleton-Century-Crofts, 1978.
> Monograph covering many aspects of hypertension in pregnancy.

Kaplan NM: *Clinical Hypertension.* Baltimore, Williams & Wilkins, 1982 (new edition scheduled 1986).
> Monograph covering in detail what the clinician needs to know about essential and secondary hypertension.

Kaplan NM: Nondrug treatment of hypertension. *Ann Intern Med* 102:359, 1985.
> Thoroughly referenced review of this subject.

Kotchen T, Havlik R (eds): High blood pressure in the young. *Hypertension* 2: I-1, 1980.
> Entire issue devoted to papers presented at a 1979 symposium.

McMahon FG: *Management of Essential Hypertension.* Mt Kisco, NY, Futura, 1984.
> Monograph providing a systematic account of each available antihypertensive drug, particularly useful for compilation of reported side effects. Extensive referencing is provided.

Messerli FH, Schlant, RC: Left ventricular hypertrophy in essential hypertension: mechanisms and therapy. *Am J Med,* September 26, 1983 (special issue).
> A large collection of papers on the subject.

Paul O: *Epidemiology and Control of Hypertension.* New York, Stratton Intercontinental, 1975.
> Multicontributor symposium covering all significant information about epidemiology of hypertension prior to 1975.

The 1984 Report of the Joint National Committee on Detection, Evaluation, and Treatment of High Blood Pressure. *Arch Intern Med* 144:1045, 1984.
> Specific recommendations based on the consensus of a national panel of experts.

Specific References

1. Adamopoulos PN, Chrysanthakopoulis SG, Frohlich ED: Systolic hypertension: nonhomogeneous diseases. *J Cardiol* 36:697, 1975.
2. Amery A, Birkenhäger W, Brixko P, et al: Mortality and morbidity results from the European Working Party on High Blood Pressure in the Elderly trial. *Lancet* 1:1349, 1985.
3. The Australian therapeutic trial in mild hypertension (editorial). *Lancet* 1:1261, 1980.
4. Biofeedback for Hypertension. Health and Public Policy Committee, American College of Physicians; Philadelphia, Pa. *Ann Intern Med* 102:709, 1985.

5. Birkenhager WH, Krauss XH, Schalekamp MADH, Kolsters G: Consecutive haemodynamic patterns in essential hypertension. *Lancet* 1:560, 1972.

6. Bravo EL, Gifford RW Jr: Pheochromocytoma: diagnosis, localization and management. *New Engl J Med* 311:1298, 1984.

7. Caird FI, Andrews GR, Kennedy RD: Effect of posture on blood pressure in the eldery. *Br Heart J* 35:527, 1973.

8. Carey RM, Reid RA, Ayers CR, et al: The Charlottesville blood-pressure survey. Value of repeated blood-pressure measurements. *JAMA* 236:847, 1976.

9. Chelsey LC, Annitto JE, Cosgrove RA: The remote prognosis of eclamptic women: sixth periodic report. *Obstetrics* 124:446, 1976.

10. Fisch IR, Frank J: Oral contraceptives and blood pressure. *JAMA* 237:2499, 1977.

11. Freestone S, Ramsay LE: Pressor effect of coffee and cigarette smoking in hypertensive patients. *Clin Sci* 63:403s, 1982.

12. Gifford RW Jr: Evaluation of the hypertensive patient. *Chest* 64:336, 1973.

13. Goodwin FK, Bunney WE, Jr: Depression following reserpine: a reevaluation. *Semin Psychiatry* 3:435, 1971.

14. Grim CE: Evaluation of patients with renovascular hypertension: another view. *Hypertension* 6:591, 1984.

15. Guidelines for the treatment of mild hypertension: memorandum from a W.H.O./I.S.H. Meeting. *Lancet* 1:457, 1983.

16. Haynes RB, Sackett DL, Taylor DW, et al: Increased absenteeism from work after detection and labeling of hypertensive patients. *N Engl J Med* 299:741, 1978.

17. Helgeland A: Treatment of mild hypertension: a five-year controlled drug trial. The Oslo study. *Am J Med* 69:725, 1980.

18. Hossmann V, Fitzgerald GA, Dollery CT: Influence of hospitalization and placebo therapy on blood pressure and sympathetic function in essential hypertension. *Hypertension* 3:113, 1981.

19. Hypertension Detection and Follow-up Program Cooperative Group: Five-year findings of the hypertension detection and follow-up program. I. Reduction in mortality of persons with high blood pressure, including mild hypertension. *JAMA* 242:2562, 1979.

20. Hypertension Detection and Follow-Up Program Cooperative Group: Five-year findings of the hypertension detection and follow-up program. II. Mortality by race, sex, and age. *JAMA* 242:2572, 1979.

21. The Joint National Committee on Detection, Evaluation, and Treatment of High Blood Pressure: The 1984 Report of the Joint National Committee on Detection, Evaluation, and Treatment of High Blood Pressure. *Arch Intern Med* 144:1045, 1984.

22. Koch G: Haemodynamic adaptation at rest and during exercise to long-term antihypertensive treatment with combination of β-receptor blocking and vasodilator agent. *Br Heart J* 38:1240, 1976.

23. Langford HG, Blaufox MD, Oberman A, et al: Dietary therapy slows the return of hypertension after stopping prolonged medication. *JAMA* 253:657, 1985.

24. Levine DM, Green LW, Deeds SG, et al: Health education for hypertensive patients. *JAMA* 241:1700, 1979.

24a. MRC Trial of Treatment of Mild Hypertension: Principal results. *Br Med J* 291:97, 1985.

25. Meyer JS, Leiderman H, Denny-Brown, D: Electroencephalographic study of insufficiency of the basilar and carotid arteries in man. *Neurology (Minneap)* 6:455, 1956.

26. Morgan T, Gillies A, Morgan G, et al: Hypertension treated by salt restriction. *Lancet* 1:227, 1978.

27. Mroczek WJ, Davidov M, Finnerty FA Jr: Large dose furosemide therapy for hypertension: long-term use in 22 patients. *Cardiology* 33:546, 1974.

28. Multiple Risk Factor Intervention Trial Research Group: Multiple risk factor intervention trial: risk factor changes and mortality results. *JAMA* 248:1465, 1982.

29. Pentel P: Toxicity of over-the-counter stimulants. *JAMA* 252:1898, 1984.

30. Redman CWG, Beilin LJ, Bonnar J, Ounsted MK: Fetal outcome in trial of antihypertensive treatment in pregnancy. *Lancet* 2:753, 1976.

31. Reisin E, Abel R, Modan M, et al: Effect of weight loss without salt restriction on the reduction of blood pressure in overweight hypertensive patients. *N Engl J Med* 298:1, 1978.

32. Report of Medical Research Council Working Party of Mild to Moderate Hypertension: Randomized controlled trial of treatment for mild hypertension: design and pilot trial. *Br Med J* 1:1437, 1977.

33. Sackett DL: The hypertensive patient; 5. Compliance with therapy (editorial). *Can Med Assoc J* 121:259, 1979.

34. Saunders JB, Beevers DG, Paton A: Alcohol-induced hypertension. *Lancet* 2:653, 1981.

35. Simon AC, Safar MA, Levenson JA, et al: Systolic hypertension: hemodynamic mechanism and choice of antihypertensive treatment. *Am J Cardiol* 44:505, 1979.

36. Sos TA, Pickering TG, Phil D, et al: Percutaneous transluminal renal angioplasty in renovascular hypertension due to atheroma or fibromuscular dysplasia. *N Engl J Med* 309:274, 1983.

37. Stout ML: Hypertension six weeks postpartum in apparently normal patients. *Am J Obstet Gynecol* 27:730, 1934.

38. Taguchi J, Freis ED: Partial reduction of blood pressure and prevention of complications in hypertension. *N Engl J Med* 291:329, 1974.

39. Topol EJ, Traill TA, Fortuin NJ: Hypertensive hypertrophic cardiomyopathy of the elderly. *New Engl J of Med* 312:277, 1985.

40. Toth PJ, Horwitz RI: Conflicting clinical trials and the uncertainty of treating mild hypertension. *Am J Med* 75:482, 1983.

41. Tucker RM, Labarthe DR: Frequency of surgical treatment for hypertension in adults at the Mayo Clinic from 1973 through 1975. *Mayo Clin Proc* 52:549, 1977.

42. Tyroler HA, Heyden S, Sneiderman C, et al: A 16-year follow-up of blood pressure in young adult residents of Evans County. *Medical Horizon Symposium: Hypertension in Childhood and Adolescents*, Pittsburgh, September 1976.

43. US Public Health Service Hospitals Cooperative Study Group (Smith WM): Treatment of mild hypertension: results of a ten-year intervention trial. *Circ Res* 40 (suppl I):98, 1977.

44. Varady PD, Maxwell MH: Assessment of statistically significant changes in diastolic blood pressures. *JAMA* 221:365, 1972.

45. Veterans Administration Cooperative Study Group on Antihypertensive Agents: Comparison of propranolol and hydrochlorothiazide for the initial treatment of hypertension. II. Results of long-term therapy. *JAMA* 248:2004, 1982.

46. Veterans Administration Cooperative Study Group on Antihypertensive Agents: Effects of treatment on morbidity in hypertension: results in patients with diastolic blood pressures averaging 115 through 129 mm Hg. *JAMA* 202:116, 1967.

47. Veterans Administration Cooperative Study Group on Antihypertension Agents: II. Effects of treatment on morbidity in hypertension: results in patients with diastolic blood pressures averaging 90 through 114 mm Hg. *JAMA* 212:1143, 1970.

48. Veterans Administration Cooperative Study Group on Antihypertensive Agents: Effects of treatment on morbidity in hypertension. III. Influence of age, diastolic pressure, and prior cardiovascular disease; further analysis of side effects. *Circulation* 45:991, 1972.

49. Watson RDS, Stallard TJ, Littler WA: Influence of once-daily administration of β-adrenoceptor antagonists on arterial pressure and its variability. *Lancet* 1:1210, 1979.

50. Weir RJ, Briggs E, Mack A, et al: Blood pressure in women taking oral contraceptives. *Br Med J* 1:533, 1974.

51. Whelton PK, Harris AP, Russell RP, et al: Renovascular hypertension: results of medical and surgical therapy. *Johns Hopkins Med J* 149:213, 1981.

52. White WB: Management of hypertension during lactation. *Hypertension* 6:297, 1984.

53. Ying CY, Tifft CP, Gavras H, Chobanian AV: Renal revascularization in the azotemic hypertensive patient resistant to therapy. *N Engl J Med* 311:1070, 1984.

SECTION 9

Musculoskeletal Problems

CHAPTER SIXTY-THREE

Shoulder Pain

NOBLE M. HANSEN, M.D., AND JOHN R. BURTON, M.D.

Shoulder pain is a common complaint in ambulatory practice. Most often the general physician can establish the correct diagnosis and can direct therapy without an orthopaedic or rheumatologic consultation. This chapter will review the major causes of shoulder pain and provide a basis for treatment of these conditions. Two problems often associated with shoulder pain are discussed in other chapters: shoulder-hand syndrome in Chapter 83 and polymyalgia rheumatica in Chapter 79.

REFERRED PAIN (Table 63.1)

When a patient complains of shoulder pain, the physician should consider first that the pain might be referred from another region of the body. Unlike a primary disorder of the shoulder, referred pain is not made worse when the patient actively moves just his shoulders.

Shoulder Pain Referred from Cervical Spine or Thoracic Outlet

Problems arising in the *cervical spine* (see Chapter 64) often produce shoulder pain as a major manifestation; but on closer questioning, the patient usually will have some pain in the neck as well. In addition, the pain will be exacerbated by motion of the neck. It is important to evaluate this possibility by having the patient extend, flex, and rotate his neck. This will increase or elicit pain due to cervical disc dis-

ease, degenerative joint disease, or other cervical problems. Pain arising from a problem within the cervical spine will often extend beyond the shoulder to below the elbow.

The *thoracic outlet syndrome* is a less common cause of shoulder pain and results from compression of vascular and neural structures between the 1st rib and the clavicle or between the anterior and middle scalene muscles (Fig. 63.1). The thoracic outlet syndrome may be caused by a variety of structural disorders such as an unusual insertion of the anterior scalene muscle or the presence of a cervical rib (usually arising from the 7th cervical vertebra). Most often the symptoms are weakness, numbness, and pain along the medial aspect of the arm and in the forearm along the distribution of the ulnar nerve (see Table 84.6, Chapter 84). These symptoms can often be exacerbated by asking the patient to assume an exaggerated military position with the shoulders held backward and downward. The symptoms may also be elicited and the radial pulse may weaken or disappear when the patient compresses the neurovascular bundle by extending the neck and rotating it toward the examined side just after a deep inspiration. There are usually no objective neurological findings on examination of the patient when he is not having symptoms. When the thoracic outlet syndrome is diagnosed, it is especially important to explain to the patient the mechanism and to reassure him that he does not have a serious or crippling disease. Specific exercises that strengthen the muscles around the shoulder and avoidance of certain activities may be helpful in preventing symptoms. A physical therapist should be consulted to teach the patient about these exercises and activities.

Shoulder Pain Referred from Other Regions of the Body

Diseases of various viscera may cause pain to be referred to the shoulder, sometimes without any other evidence that a problem exists. Ischemic heart disease, pericarditis, carcinoma of the lung, and gallbladder disease are especially common processes that should be considered when the clinical presentation suggests that shoulder pain is referred (i.e., pain not exacerbated by pressure on or movement of the shoulder joint).

ANATOMY, FUNCTION, AND PATHOPHYSIOLOGY OF THE SHOULDER

For the physician to diagnose and treat disorders of the shoulder joint (also called the glenohumeral or scapulohumeral joint) properly, he should understand several aspects of shoulder anatomy (see Fig. 63.2) and function. Movement of the humeral head upon the glenoid fossa of the scapula is intricate, in that the humeral head is actually larger than the fossa and thus does not fit into it: the shoulder joint is not a snug ball-and-socket joint. During humeral motion, the humeral head *glides* into different relationships with the fossa. The muscles of the shoulder girdle are especially important in maintaining the stability of the joint in addition to governing its wide variety of motions.

At the superior aspect of the shoulder, just lateral to the acromial process of the scapula, are the tendons of the supraspinatus and the infraspinatus muscles; these tendons comprise what is called the *rotator cuff*. These muscles arise from the supraspinatus and infraspinatus fossae of the scapula, sweep under the rigid arch formed by the acromion and the acromiocoracoid ligament, and insert into the lateral aspect of the head of the humerus. These

Table 63.1.
Causes of Referred Shoulder Pain

CERVICAL SPINE DISEASE AND THORACIC OUTLET
  SYNDROME
DISORDERS IN OTHER PARTS OF THE BODY:
  Cardiac or pericardial disease
  Pleural disease—*e.g.*, carcinoma of the superior parts of
    the lung
  Diaphragmatic irritation—*e.g.*, subphrenic abscess
  Gallbladder disease

muscles function to initiate elevation of the arm through the first 20° of abduction.

The long head of the biceps (*biceps tendon*) originates in the glenoid portion of the scapula and runs through a bony groove in the head of the humerus. The short head of the biceps arises from the coracoid process of the scapula and converges upon the muscle body, with the long head. The biceps muscle

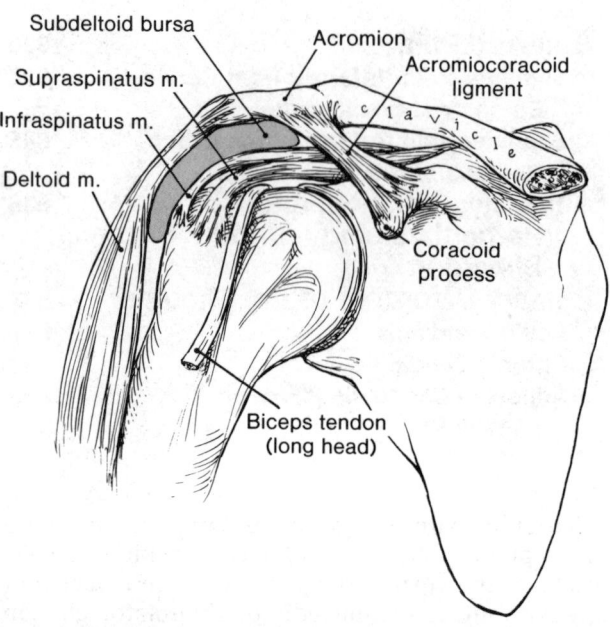

Figure 63.2. Coronal section of shoulder anatomy. Note the relationship of the subdeltoid bursa lying next to the supraspinatus tendon, but separate from the shoulder joint. Note the acromion, which is in a position to impinge the supraspinatus tendon on abduction of the arm.

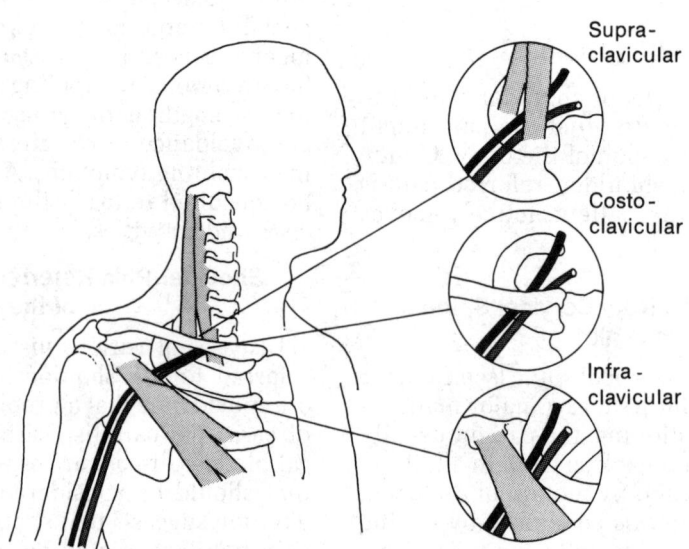

Figure 63.1. Points of neurovascular compression in the thoracic outlet syndrome. (From Ramamurti CP: *Orthopaedics in Primary Care.* Tinker RV (ed). Baltimore, Williams & Wilkins, 1979.)

inserts, as a single tendon, into the inner aspect of the radius. The biceps aids in movement of the arm directly forward from the body; during this motion the biceps tendon actually remains fixed, and the head of the humerus glides under the tendon. The second function of the biceps muscle is to flex the arm at the elbow.

The *deltoid muscle* arises anteriorly from the clavicle, laterally from the acromion, and posteriorly from the spine of the scapula, and passes down in front of, lateral to, and behind the shoulder joint; it attaches distally to the anterior-lateral area of the middle third of the humerus. Deltoid muscle contraction causes elevation of the humerus and tends to force the humeral head up against the acromio-coracoid ligament.

Problems of the tendinous portions of the shoulder will account for the vast majority of complaints of shoulder pain seen in an ambulatory practice. As the shoulder is abducted actively, the rotator cuff tendons become impinged against the bony arch and the humeral head (Fig. 63.2). During this impingement, the blood flow to the rotator cuff tendons is markedly decreased and may be totally obliterated as the arm is abducted (4). In this region of intermittently decreased blood flow, progressive degenerative changes in the rotator cuff occur frequently after the age of 30. Inflammation in the rotator cuff tendons and/or the biceps tendon may accompany this degenerative process, and pain is characteristically brought on as the inflamed tendon is compressed or impinged against the rigid acromial arch. These aspects of the anatomy and pathophysiology of the tendons of the shoulder joint explain two important clinical observations: First, the patient with pain related to a tendon injury usually gives a history of recurrent exacerbations of symptoms from the underlying degenerative process. Second, the symptoms are related to activity. Therefore, it is extremely important to consider recreational or occupational demands on the shoulder joint when managing these patients.

With the functional anatomy in mind, the physician should *examine the shoulder*. The shoulders should be compared visually with the arms hanging straight down in the position of rest. This will permit the identification of deformity or of erythema. The joint should then be moved actively through the full range of motion first with no force and then, if no abnormality is identified, repeated with the physician applying resistance in order to detect subtler degrees of inflammation or injury. The full range of motion of both shoulders is easily assessed and compared by having the patient sit or stand facing the physician and performing the following movements:

With the arms hanging loosely at the side, the elbows should be flexed; the arms may then be flexed anteriorly, posteriorly and abducted; the arms should then be externally rotated 90° and abducted again attempting to place the hands on the head. (This latter movement will aid in the diagnosis of rotator cuff problems since it permits the greater tuberosity of the humerus to pass under the cora-coacromial process and impinge on structures more medially located.)

"False abduction" of the shoulder can be prevented by the physician holding the patient's shoulder downward, thereby preventing the patient from swinging the scapula laterally to accomplish abduction. Pain persisting with passive movements of the shoulder may help to localize the problem in the joint itself as opposed to the supportive muscles and tendons. This distinction is not always precise, however.

The shoulder should be carefully palpated since a localized area of tenderness (e.g., along the bicipital tendon) will localize the problem.

PRIMARY DISORDERS OF THE SHOULDER

A history of trauma is most important in the assessment of primary shoulder problems. Significant trauma indicates the need for an X-ray of the shoulder joint to rule out the possibility of a nondisplaced fracture or of dislocation. The majority of patients with shoulder pain will give a history of trauma, such as repetitive actions during work or sports, and they will have a problem located in the tendinous portion of the shoulder joint. The three major problems are acute tendinitis, chronic tendinitis, and adhesive capsulitis. An X-ray of the shoulder is not needed when these problems are suspected; it should be obtained, however, if pain persists or worsens in spite of conservative therapy (see below). For this reason the patient should be followed up in 1 to 2 weeks by either telephone or an office visit. This encounter will also permit the physician to educate the patient about exercises and activities that may help to prevent recurrences (see below).

Acute Tendinitis

Diagnosis

Acute tendinitis of the shoulder is a dramatic illness. The rapid onset of severe pain is characteristic, and the pain can be incapacitating. The patient complains of pain over the anterior or lateral aspect of the shoulder resulting in the characteristic "deltoid ache." The pain frequently will radiate down to the elbow, but should not involve the forearm or neck, as referred pain sometimes does (see above). Motion of the shoulder, especially arm abduction (compression of the rotator cuff), is very painful. The most characteristic physical finding is localized tenderness over one of the rotator cuff tendons or the biceps tendon. Tenderness directly at the superior aspect of the shoulder just lateral to the acromion is in the region of the supraspinatus tendon, and tenderness just posterior to this is in the region of the infraspinatus tendon. If the arm is externally rotated and the anterior aspect of the humeral head is palpated, the biceps tendon in its groove can be felt; commonly tenderness will be localized at this point. When the biceps tendon is inflamed, active external rotation and then elevation of the arm will give maximum discomfort. While an X-ray of the shoulder is not necessary for the diagnosis of tendinitis, if obtained, it may show calcium within the rotator cuff just superior and lateral to the humeral head. Deposits of calcium begin within the rotator cuff tendon itself but occasionally extend into the subdeltoid bursa. These deposits can form within 24 to 48 hours, and they frequently resolve as the symptoms subside. Occasionally, the calcium may persist long after symptoms have disappeared, and in this case its presence is of no concern. It is important to understand that the primary inflammatory process is occurring within the rotator cuff tendon itself and that the subdeltoid bursa becomes inflamed secondarily. The terms *subacromial bursitis, subdeltoid bursitis,* or "bursitis" of the shoulder are commonly used interchangeably and have led to the erroneous idea that the primary inflammatory response is within the bursa.

Treatment

In considering treatment, it should be emphasized that acute tendinitis is generally a self-limited illness lasting up to 2 weeks. The most important complication, in those who do not initially respond, is adhesive capsulitis (see below).

The initial aim of treatment of acute tendinitis is to relieve pain. In mild cases, the shoulder should be rested in a sling and the patient should be given a rapidly acting oral anti-inflammatory agent such as piroxicam (Feldene), 20 mg once a day. Alternative nonsteroidal anti-inflammatory agents may be used (see Chapter 70, Rheumatoid Arthritis, Table 70.11). If the patient is having very severe pain, an analgesic such as codeine, 30 to 60 mg every 4 to 6 hours, for several days may be helpful. Also, the application of moist or dry heat for 20 to 30 minutes two or three times/day may provide comfort and muscle relaxation.

If the response to this treatment after 2 weeks is not adequate, local injections of a glucocorticoid suspension into the region of maximum tenderness may give immediate dramatic relief. This procedure may be performed by the general physician using a 22 gauge needle; the corticosteroid is injected in a dose of 1 ml of Aristospan, Celestone, or Kenalog diluted with 3 ml of 1% Xylocaine (see Chapter 66, page 866 for further details regarding injection of glucocorticoid suspension). An occasional patient will not respond to initial treatment, and an X-ray may show a significant calcium deposit in the tendon; aspiration of the calcium with a 16 gauge

needle, usually by an orthopaedist or rheumatologist, may provide immediate relief to such patients.

As the pain of acute tendinitis subsides following initial treatment, the patient should begin gentle range of motion exercises (Fig. 63.3) to prevent the development of adhesive capsulitis (see below). The physician may teach the exercise to the patient. It is best that the patient perform circumduction exercises by bending forward 90° at the waist and dangling the arm straight down and then swinging the elbow in a circular fashion. This will allow the shoulder to move without the patient actively using the rotator cuff tendons to elevate the arm. Another home exercise is to have the patient stand facing a wall and to flex the shoulders forward until the fingers touch the wall; then the fingers are "walked" up the wall, carrying the arm and shoulder into full forward flexion. Either or both of these exercises can be done for 10 minutes twice a day.

Quite often attacks of acute tendinitis are recurrent; thus, a change in recreational or occupational activity may be necessary. If the patient is not able to regain full range of motion of the shoulder within

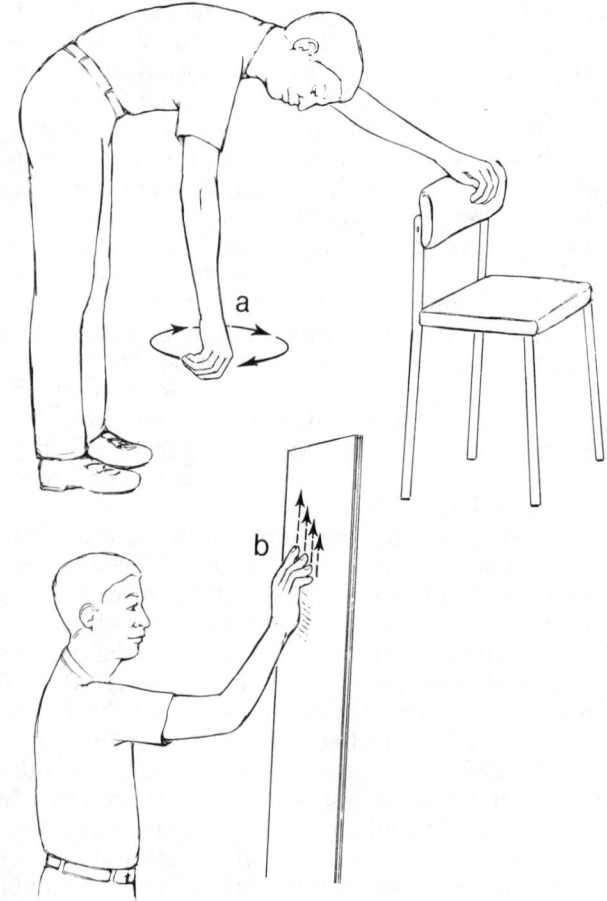

Figure 63.3. Range of motion exercises of the shoulder. Circumduction exercises of the shoulder (*a*) and the wall-climbing exercises for the shoulder (*b*) as described in the text.

2 to 4 weeks, a physical therapy consultation should be requested. The therapist can supervise the exercises and encourage the patient to do them. If there is still a poor response or continuing pain after a period of 2 weeks, a consultation by an orthopaedist or rheumatologist is appropriate. However, there is, in general, no place for surgery in the treatment of acute tendinitis of the shoulder.

Chronic Tendinitis

Diagnosis

Chronic tendinitis of the shoulder has the same basic etiology as acute tendinitis. It is, however, a milder but more persistent problem. The patient most often develops activity-related pain over the lateral or anterior aspect of the shoulder and upper arm. The patient often recognizes a particular motion or activity that makes the pain worse. Active elevation of the arm almost always causes the pain to worsen because of impingement of the tendons; however, passive range of motion is normal. There is mild tenderness over the rotator cuff or biceps tendon.

Treatment

Treatment consists of the application of dry or moist heat, gentle circumduction exercises, and anti-inflammatory agents with a rapid onset of action, such as piroxicam (Feldene), 20 mg once a day. Alternative nonsteroidal anti-inflammatory agents may be used (see Chapter 70, Rheumatoid Arthritis, Table 70.11). If the tenderness is particularly severe and localized, injection of a glucocorticoid suspension as described above can give significant relief; this is especially effective when the biceps tendon is involved. The patient should be instructed to avoid any aggravating activities.

If the patient does not respond to conservative therapy in several months or if there are repeated episodes of protracted pain, an orthopaedic consultation is indicated. The consultant should obtain or review an X-ray of the shoulder and should search for *aggravating mechanical factors,* such as spur formation along the acromion that has led to increased impingement. There are several surgical procedures designed to remove parts of the coracoacromial arch to decrease impingement of the inflamed rotator cuff, but these all require general anesthesia and hospitalization may be necessary (2). In addition, if there is biceps tendinitis, this tendon may be removed from its groove in the humeral head and attached more distally to the shaft of the humerus.

Finally, in the patient with chronic pain not helped by conservative therapy, the consultant will need to consider the less common complication of a *tear of the rotator cuff* (3). This diagnosis should be considered when the physical examination reveals weakness in elevation of the arm and atrophy of the deltoid, supraspinatus, and infraspinatus muscles.

Occasionally, there is a palpable cleft in the rotator cuff tendon. In suspected cases the consultant will suggest an *arthrogram of the shoulder.* This requires an injection into the articular cavity of approximately 15 ml of Renograffin mixed with air, followed by X-rays to see if the dye remains within the joint or flows through a tear of the rotator cuff into the subdeltoid bursa as shown in Figure 63.4. Ordinarily, the subdeltoid bursa does not connect with the articular cavity. In individuals who are over the age of 40, the rotator cuff usually tears because of attrition. In these patients there are no sudden symptoms, and often surgical repair of the tear is quite difficult. Frequently, the best result that can be obtained from surgery of a tear of a rotator cuff in patients in this group is some decrease in the pain, but residual loss of motion persists. In some older individuals rotator cuff tears are associated with hydroxyapatite crystal deposition (see "Milwaukee Shoulder," in Chapter 69). In younger individuals, there is more often a history of trauma, such as from swinging on a rope or a throwing injury, leading to sudden tear of the rotator cuff, and in this instance early surgical repair may give much better results.

Adhesive Capsulitis ("Frozen Shoulder")

Diagnosis

This problem results from inflammation and fibrous band formation of the capsule of the shoulder

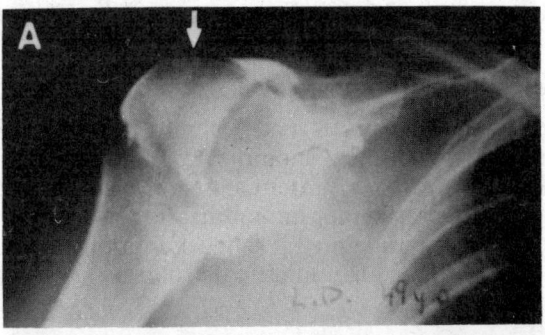
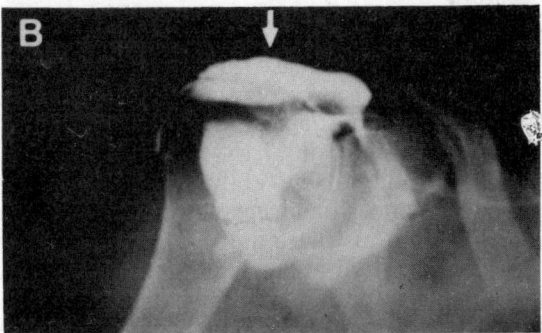

Figure 63.4. *A.* Normal shoulder arthrogram. The superior aspect of the joint should be smooth with a fine layer of contrast material. *B.* Rotator cuff tear. Note extravasation of the dye from the glenohumeral joint into the subdeltoid bursa, indicating a large tear of the rotator cuff tendon.

joint and is characteristically seen in patients who are between the ages of 40 and 70 years. It is more common in women and is usually preceded by a period of inactivity of the shoulder (for example, following a stroke, a shoulder injury, or an exacerbation of chronic tendinitis). The patient presents with slowly progressive stiffness of the shoulder that is usually painless or is associated with mild discomfort in the anterior and lateral aspect of the shoulder. The patient may also complain that he is unable to bring his hand to his mouth when he eats or that he has difficulty in combing his hair. On physical examination marked reduced passive range of motion of the glenohumeral joint will be demonstrated; but the shoulder is usually not tender. The examiner should put a hand on the top of the shoulder to prevent elevation of the scapula (which could mask loss of glenohumeral motion) and should then passively abduct the arm. The maximum angle between the humerus and the side of the chest with the scapula fixed is a measure of motion between the glenoid and humerus; normally the angle is at least 90°.

Natural History

Adhesive capsulitis may last as long as 1 to 2 years. Generally, the patient's range of motion slowly improves, although a complete return to full range of motion is very unlikely. Most often a satisfactory range of motion is achieved that permits the patient to raise his hand to the back of the head, the mouth, and the low back.

Prevention

Adhesive capsulitis is a potential complication whenever a patient's shoulder is immobilized, and eventually it may represent a greater disability than the primary reason for immobilization. This complication can be prevented if range of motion exercises of the shoulder are initiated as soon as acute pain subsides.

Treatment

The primary aim of treatment of adhesive capsulitis is gradually to increase the activity of the shoulder. A specific exercise program in passive (someone in the patient's household should be trained to do this) and active motion of the shoulder should include forward flexion and abduction and rotation of the shoulder and should be performed for a minimum of 10 minutes twice daily. Circumduction exercises and wall-climbing exercises are excellent (Fig. 63.3). It is important that the patient understand (a) that improvement is expected over the course of months, not days or weeks, and (b) that the range of motion achieved may not be entirely normal but, it is to be hoped, will permit him to reach his hand to his head, mouth, and back. Long term use of anti-inflammatory medications usually has no place in

the treatment of adhesive capsulitis; but a 2-week course of an anti-inflammatory medication (see above) during the initiation of treatment may be helpful if pain is exacerbated. Occasionally injection of a glucocorticoid suspension (see above) into the region of the shoulder joint at the initiation of therapy is useful if discomfort prevents adequate exercising. Prescribing an analgesic medication to allow physical therapy is important. Most patients are adequately treated by the primary physician after an initial physical therapy consultation, which will aid the patient in understanding the exercise program. If the patient fails to improve the range of motion of his shoulder after several months of therapy, consultation with an orthopaedic surgeon is indicated. Very occasionally, manipulation of the shoulder under local anesthesia and simultaneous glucocorticoid suspension injection into the shoulder joint may improve the patient's range of motion (1), which then can be maintained by further physical therapy.

General References

Bateman JE: *The Shoulder and Neck*, ed 2. Philadelphia, WB Saunders, 1978.
> Comprehensive book on the shoulder containing a complete differential diagnosis. Excellent discussion of anatomy and biomechanics of the shoulder joint.

Calliett R: *Shoulder Pain*, ed 2. Philadelphia, FA Davis, 1981.
> A concise and well illustrated manual with much practical information.

Halbach JW, Tank RT: The shoulder. In Gould JA, Davies GJ (eds): *Orthopaedic and Sports Physical Therapy*. St Louis, CV Mosby, 1985.
> A well illustrated, useful resource for understanding the mechanism of injury and the techniques of evaluation and rehabilitation of shoulder problems.

Post M (guest ed): The painful shoulder. *Clin Orthop* 173:March, 1983.
> A comprehensive monograph covering all aspects of shoulder pain problems.

Ramamurti CP: *Orthopaedics in Primary Care*. Tinker RV (ed.) Baltimore, Williams & Wilkins, 1979.
> A very practical and well illustrated text with chapters on the thoracic outlet syndrome and the shoulder.

Thornhill TS: The painful shoulder. In Kelley WM, Harris ED, Ruddy S, Sledge CB (eds): *Textbook of Rheumatology*, ed 2. Philadelphia, WB Saunders, 1985.
> An excellent chapter in a comprehensive textbook.

Wilgis EFS: *Vascular Injuries and Diseases of the Upper Limb*. Boston, Little, Brown, and Co, 1983.
> A well illustrated monograph with a good chapter on compression syndromes of the shoulder, girdle and arm.

Specific References

1. Lloyd JA, Lloyd HM: Adhesive capsulitis of the shoulder. *South Med J* 76:879, 1983.
2. Neer CS II: Anterior acromioplasty for the chronic impingement syndrome in the shoulder. *J Bone Joint Surg* 54A:41, 1972.
3. Neviaser JS: Ruptures of the rotator cuff of the shoulder. New concepts in the diagnosis and operative treatment of chronic ruptures. *Arch Surg* 102:483, 1971.
4. Rathbun JB, Macnab I: The microvascular pattern of the rotator cuff. *J Bone Joint Surg* 52B:540, 1970.

CHAPTER SIXTY-FOUR

Neck Pain

NOBLE M. HANSEN, M.D., AND JOHN R. BURTON, M.D.

Neck pain is a common problem. Nearly 50% of individuals over 50 years of age experience neck pain at some time. Since there are many structures in the neck that, when diseased, may cause pain, as well as multiple sources of referred pain, the physician must systematically evaluate patients who complain of neck pain that is new or persistent. This chapter provides a review of the skeletal structures of the neck; the method of evaluation for complaints of neck pain; a description of common problems and their treatment; and guidance for referral of selected patients with neck pain.

ANATOMY AND SOURCES OF PAIN
(Fig. 64.1)

The cervical spine consists of seven vertebral bodies connected by an *anterior and a posterior longitudinal ligament*. These ligaments provide stability when the neck is flexed and extended. The vertebral bodies are joined by *intervertebral discs* composed of a gel-like material (the *nucleus pulposus*) which absorbs increased pressure applied to the spine. The nucleus pulposus is contained within an *annulus fibrosus*, a fibrous structure ringing the outer margin of the disc. During the fourth decade of life, both the nucleus pulposus and the annulus fibrosus undergo progressive degeneration, seen microscopically as a loss of the fibrous pattern and of the collagen alignment. As a result, the ability of the disc to absorb shocks is reduced. There are *facet joints* found between vertebral elements posteriorly, one on each side of the spine; they are apophyseal (projecting) joints with a synovium-lined capsule. It

is within these small joints in the posterior spine that osteoarthritis can occur—osteoarthritis being a breakdown of the articular cartilage within the joints. The *intervertebral neural foramina*, located laterally on either side of the vertebral bodies, are the canals through which the individual nerve roots emerge from the spinal canal. The spinal canal and the foramina can be encroached upon by a bulging intervertebral disc or an osseous proliferation (bony spur) originating in a vertebral body, a facet joint, or from the bony margin of a neural foramen (Fig. 64.1). When the encroachment involves a nerve root, pain in the distribution of that root (radicular pain) may occur. The facet joint capsules and the intervertebral disc are innervated by fine unmyelinated nerves (called C fibers) which have simple nerve endings. When these nerve endings are stimulated by degenerative disease within the disc or joint capsules, the patient may experience pain, which is referred to the posterior aspect of the neck at any level. The pain felt in the neck may not be at the cervical level from which the nerve is arising. In addition, C fiber stimulation can cause pain to be referred to the interscapular area, superiorly and laterally over the shoulders, and in the lower arm and the hand. C fiber stimulation occasionally causes a decrease in sensation in the lower arm and in the hand. Spasm of any of the many muscles of the neck region is also a common source of pain.

EVALUATION OF THE PATIENT
History

The date of onset of the patient's symptoms and of any associated trauma should be ascertained. A history of trauma is an indication for a complete set of cervical spine x-rays (see below). Often, knowledge of the specific activity the patient was performing at the onset of pain will be quite helpful in establishing the cause of the pain. Prolonged extension of the neck, such as occurs in people doing overhead work, is a common occupational situation that can give rise to pain in the cervical region. It is quite common that a patient sustains a minor twisting injury or trauma to the neck and does not experience neck pain within the first 24 hours. The patient's first pain may then begin to appear and may progress. Reproduction or increase of pain by neck motion is very helpful in localizing the problem

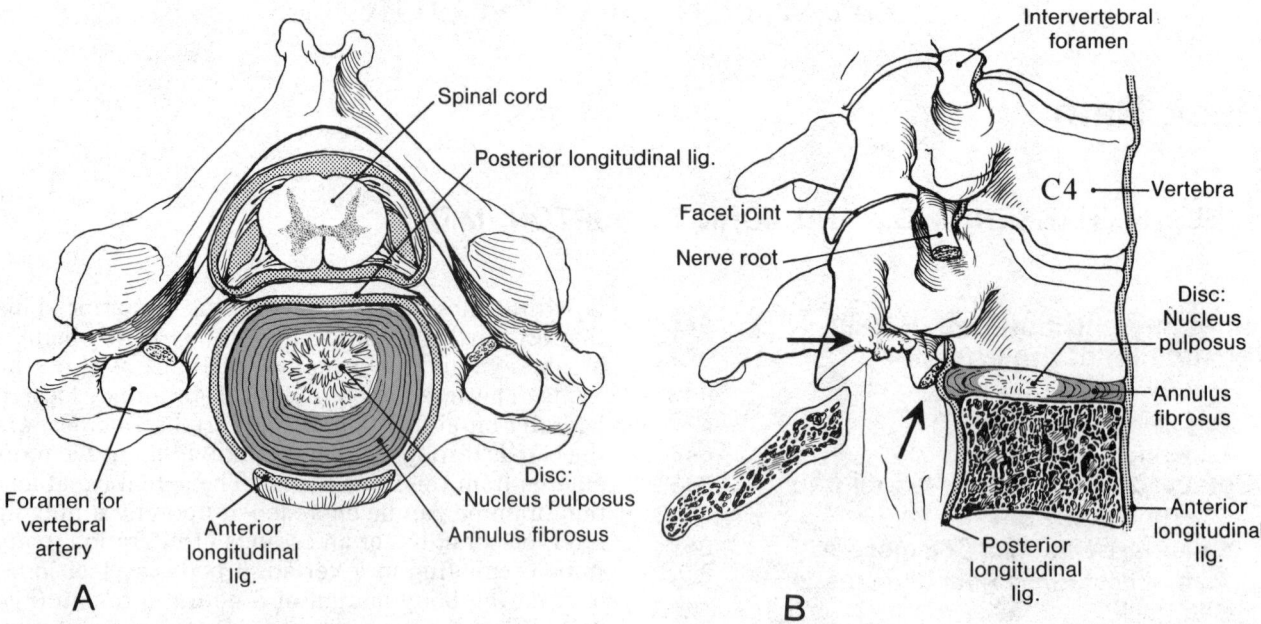

Figure 64.1. Anatomy of disc and ligaments of the cervical spine. *A.* Superior view. Note relationship of anterior and posterior longitudinal ligament to the intervertebral disc. *B.* Lateral view. Note relationship of intervertebral foramen to the intervertebral disc and facet joint. Bulging of the intervertebral disc or bone spurs forming from the facet joint may cause compression of the nerve root within the intervertebral foramen (*arrows*).

Table 64.1.
Sources of Referred Pain in the Neck

The clue to referred pain is the absence of any tenderness in the neck or of exacerbation of symptoms with manipulation of the neck.

DISORDERS OF THE HEAD:

Migraine or tension headache—pain anterior or posterior.

Sinus infection—most often the pain is anterior but occasionally posterior, especially when muscle spasm is present.

Temporomandibular joint problem—usually pain is anterolateral.

DISTANT LESIONS:

Irritation of the surface of the diaphragm innervated by the phrenic nerve (C3, 4, and 5)—frequently shoulder as well as low neck pain, but more medial diaphragmatic lesion may be associated with just neck pain. An example is gastric ulcer.

to the cervical spine rather than to a referred source (Table 64.1). It is also important to know if the pain is felt outside the neck as well, such as in the head, posteriorly between the scapulae, about the shoulder, down the arm, or in the hand. The patient should be asked about decreased sensation in his hands and, if he is able, to say specifically which fingers are involved. If the pain and numbness are felt in a dermatome distribution, this indicates nerve compression (Table 64.2). Pain associated with motion of the shoulder is not characteristic of cervical spine disease and suggests that the problem is within the shoulder joint (see Chapter 63). Symptoms such as dizziness, visual changes, and ataxia are not usually associated with cervical problems arising from simple nerve root compression or degenerative disc disease, but may be found when bony spurs encroach on the vertebral foramina (see Fig. 81.2, Chapter 81) and compress the vertebral arteries. These relatively rare symptoms usually occur when the neck is in a certain position, and they are usually of short duration.

Physical Examination

In the physical examination, the patient should be asked to demonstrate active range of motion of the neck, including flexion, extension, rotation, and lateral bending. Normally, the chin can be placed easily upon the anterior chest and the neck can be extended so that the patient is looking directly above. Normally, there is almost 90° of rotation of the neck to both sides. Simple hyperextension of the neck commonly exacerbates the pain caused by cervical disc degeneration. The patient should be asked to extend his neck and maintain this position for a period of 30 seconds to determine whether the pain is made worse. Putting direct compression on top of the head also may produce or exacerbate pain in the patient with degenerative disc disease, especially if the head is compressed while the neck is extended. The posterior neck muscles are palpated for muscle spasm, which may be asymmetric and may give the patient the appearance of torticollis (wry neck). Next, the shoulder should be subjected to a range of motion to see if this elicits pain within the shoulder itself.

Selected neurological tests (see Fig. 78.2, Chapter 78 and Table 84.6, Chapter 84) are important in the evaluation of the patient with neck pain whenever there is any suggestion of nerve root involvement or cord compression. These tests include reflex testing of the upper and lower extremities; muscle strength testing of the upper extremities; and sensory testing of the upper extremities. The reflex testing should include the biceps, triceps, brachioradial, quadriceps, and gastrocnemius tendons, and the Babinski test. Muscle strength in the upper extremities should include the biceps (flexion of elbow), triceps (extension of elbow), wrist extensors and flexors, hand and finger flexors, and intrinsic muscles of the hand. The intrinsic muscles of the hand are tested by having the patient hold the fingers tightly together while the examiner tries to separate them. A sensory examination is then performed. An objective sensory deficit is one which conforms to a dermatome distribution (see Fig. 78.2, Chapter 78 and Table 84.6, Chapter 84).

Occasionally, cervical spine problems can cause cervical myelopathy when a bone spur forms posteriorly at the margin of an intervertebral disc and then impinges on the spinal cord, producing signs of cord compression: increased reflexes in the lower extremities with a positive Babinski sign. A spinal cord tumor at this level could give similar findings.

Laboratory Assessment

If the history reveals an episode of recent trauma or if the neurologic examination reveals abnormalities, a complete set of cervical spine X-rays should be obtained. These films should include an assessment of levels C1 through C7 with oblique and openmouth odontoid views. These X-rays will help the physician to rule out fracture or metastatic disease. There is not, however, a good correlation between clinical symptoms or signs and degenerative abnormalities on X-ray. In fact in asymptomatic individuals after the age of 40, cervical degenerative changes (spondylosis) are common and after the age of 50 are evident in over 90% of individuals (1). On the other hand, there may be serious cervical disease with minimal or no changes on X-ray. If there is no history of trauma and if the neurological examination is normal, initial X-rays are not necessary, but should be obtained if there is an inadequate response after 1 or 2 weeks of therapy.

Computerized tomography is also useful in the evaluation of problems of the upper cervical spine (2), especially after significant trauma when X-ray studies reveal no abnormality or if the positioning necessary for regular X-rays is difficult. Bone scans using radionuclides may be helpful when neoplastic disease is suspected; however, arthritis or positioning artifacts may confuse interpretation (4).

SELECTED SYNDROMES ASSOCIATED WITH NECK PAIN

Many problems of the neck may result in neck pain (Table 64.3). Because the most common problems—cervical disc disease and cervical spondylosis (degenerative changes)—may have similar manifestations, they are discussed together based on the presence or absence of neurological findings (see below); and two other common problems, stiff neck and whiplash injury, are discussed separately.

Pain with Nerve Root Compression

Diagnosis

The objective signs of nerve root compression are muscle weakness, a decreased reflex, and decreased sensation in a dermatome distribution.

Table 64.2.
Characteristic Findings at Individual Cervical Nerve Root Levels

Nerve Root	Disc Level	History	Examination[a]
C3	(C2–3)	Pain into the back of the neck and around the mastoid process	No reflex changes
C4	(C3–4)	Pain into the back of the neck to the levator scapulae to anterior chest	No reflex changes
C5	(C4–5)	Pain into side of neck to the superior lateral shoulder, numbness over the deltoid muscle	Deltoid muscle atrophy and weakness of shoulder abduction
C6	(C5–6)	Pain to the lateral aspects of the arm and forearm and into the thumb and index finger with numbness of thumb and dorsum of hand	Weak biceps and brachioradial muscles and decreased biceps and brachioradial tendon reflexes
C7	(C6–7)	Pain into the midforearm to middle and ring fingers	Triceps muscle weakness with decreased triceps muscle reflex
C8	(C7–T1)	Pain to the medial aspect of the forearm into the ring and small fingers with numbness of the ulnar border and small finger	Triceps weakness with weakness of intrinsic muscles of the hand

[a] Sensory testing will usually show abnormalities in dermatome of the affected nerve root (see Fig. 78.2).

Table 64.3.
Selected Problems of the Neck Which May Result in Neck Pain

Problem	Comment
Arthritis	Especially rheumatoid (see Chapter 70) and degenerative joint disease (see the text and Chapter 68).
Disc disease	See the text.
Fibrositis	See Chapter 66.
Infection	Osteomyelitis or soft tissue infection—look for point tenderness.
Neoplasia	Myeloma or metastatic disease is associated with point tenderness and X-ray abnormalities.
Neuritis	Any nerve may be involved. A relatively common one is the spinal accessory nerve. Look for tenderness over the nerve—lateral aspect of upper one-third of sternomastoid muscle.
Platybasia	A congenital disorder which may not manifest symptoms before age 40 or from Paget's disease, X-rays show characteristic changes (*i.e.*, invagination of the base of the skull).
Sprain	Whiplash (see the text).
Structures in neck	Any organ or structure located in the neck may become a source of neck pain. Careful examination will detect abnormalities such as thyroiditis, lymphadenitis, pharnygitis, sialadenitis, or tender carotid artery (carotodynia).
Tendinitis	Any tendon may be involved but occipital and sternomastoid are particularly common. Local tenderness is a clue.
Torticollis (wry neck)	Diagnosis is usually obvious by observation. An underlying structural problem could produce reflex muscle spasm; therefore, with an initial episode an underlying problem (such as tumor or infection) should be considered.
Trauma	Because of the danger of cord injury, trauma associated with neck pain should be carefully evaluated.
Vascular	Arteritis or dissection may cause neck pain.

Patients with nerve root compression present with the acute or gradual onset of posterior neck pain that radiates to the shoulder and down one arm into the lower arm and often into the hand itself. The pain will occasionally radiate into a finger that corresponds to the dermatome of the nerve root involved. The pain is made worse by movement of the neck and by extreme neck positions. The patient may, in addition, complain of decreased sensation in the arm and of paresthesia in the hand. The physician should bear in mind that a patient may have nerve root compression from the cervical spine but have little or no neck and arm pain, and instead have arm weakness and loss of sensation. Nerve root compression can be caused by impingement of the nerve by a cervical disc—most common in younger individuals—or by osseous proliferation that can impinge upon the nerve as it exits through its foramen—most common in patients over 50. Also, the thoracic outlet syndrome may be confused with cervical disease associated with neurological findings, and this syndrome should be ruled out (see Chapter 63).

Management

Patients with neurological findings are probably best referred to an orthopaedist or to a neurosurgeon for more complete examination and follow-up. If muscle weakness and sensory impairment are of such a degree that they would be unacceptable if permanent, immediate surgical decompression should be considered. The orthopaedist or neurosurgeon will evaluate these patients further with computerized tomography and/or myelography.

In mild cases of nerve root compression, treatment consists first of immobilization of the neck by use of a *soft cervical collar* which should allow slight flexion of the neck. If the collar forces the neck into some extension, it may exacerbate the symptoms. A soft cervical collar, made of foam rubber and stockinette and fastened behind the neck, serves more as a reminder to a patient to restrict his neck motion, as it will actually only restrict approximately 25% of flexion-extension and approximately 20 and 10% of rotational and lateral motion, respectively (3). These collars are well tolerated, inexpensive, and easily accessible (made in the office or available in pharmacies). Cervical collars that more fully restrict neck movements (such as the Philadelphia collar, Somibrace, four-poster brace, or cervicothoracic brace) are difficult to use, more expensive, and should be recommended only after consultation with an orthopaedist or neurosurgeon.

If the pain is severe, *bed rest* may be necessary. It is helpful to place a small pillow under the nape of the neck to provide proper positioning. If muscle spasm is present, moist or dry *heat* applied to the neck may give symptomatic relief. *Analgesia* using aspirin or acetaminophen may help. If a stronger analgesic becomes necessary, the addition of codeine, 30 to 60 mg orally three or four times daily, may be used. While not a first line agent, a muscle relaxant may be helpful (see Chapter 65, Low Back Pain) if symptoms persist after 3 or 4 days.

The acute phase usually lasts only 1 or 2 weeks.

When symptoms have been recurrent, intermittent *cervical traction* may provide relief and, although not studied in a controlled fashion, could be tried after the exacerbation subsides. This is performed initially by a physical therapist. For a period of 30 minutes, 15 to 20 lb of chin halter traction are applied to the neck. The neck must be positioned in slight flexion; extension, which could worsen symptoms, must be avoided. After several sessions, the patient can be instructed in the use of a home cervical traction unit, which then can be applied for 30 minutes at a time, up to three times/day, for several months. Should the acute symptom not subside or if new signs develop, referral to an orthopaedist or a neurosurgeon is necessary for confirmation of the diagnosis and for consideration of the use of a complex brace and possible surgery (usually discectomy and anterior interbody fusion).

Even when symptoms and signs subside there is, unfortunately, a relatively high rate of recurrence of symptoms. It is therefore important for the physician to educate the patient in activities or positions that should be avoided and in exercises that may help to relieve muscle spasm (Fig. 64.2 and 64.3).

Pain without Nerve Root Compression

Diagnosis

The majority of patients who present with neck pain have no objective neurological findings. Changes in sensation in the lower arm or hand can occur from C fiber i.e., those fibers innervating the disc and surrounding tissue) irritation from degenerative disc disease or from degeneration of the facet joints within the neck and, therefore, may be present without true nerve root compression. The patient may present either with an *acute onset* of pain (most of the time a disc herniation) or with a *slowly progressive* discomfort (most often from degenerative joint disease) that has been building over several months. In the acute disc herniation syndrome, the patient presents with the rather sudden onset of neck pain that is associated with decreased range of motion of the cervical spine, bilateral muscle spasm, or occasionally asymmetric muscle spasm, which produces torticollis (wry neck). The patient may have pain in the shoulder or arm but have no objective weakness or sensory findings on examination. X-rays of the cervical spine may be entirely normal.

Treatment

Initial treatment is basically the same as that outlined above for patients with nerve root compression. The neck is "immobilized" with a soft cervical collar; local heat and analgesics also may give symptomatic relief. Muscle relaxants (see Chapter 65, Low Back Pain) may be tried if symptoms persist after 3 or 4 days of initial treatment. When the pain has subsided, the patient may benefit from intermittent cervical traction. In patients who have a chronic, more insidious onset of pain, it is helpful to examine the patient's occupational situation more closely to see if there are exacerbating circumstances. Any activity that creates prolonged extension of the neck, such as overhead work (*e.g.*, painting) may aggravate a pre-existing problem. If after initial treatment pain lasts more than 2 or 3 weeks, X-rays of the cervical spine should be obtained to look for a possible vertebral collapse, metastatic disease, or foraminal encroachment by bone. The treatment is based on the severity of the symptoms. An oral, rapid acting anti-inflammatory agent, such as piroxicam (Feldene), 20 mg once a day, may be tried over a course of 2 or 3 weeks. (Alternative nonsteroidal anti-inflammatory agents, including aspirin, may be tried also; see Chapter 70, Table 70.11). When cost is a factor, aspirin is preferred; however, a daily dose of 3 to 6 g is needed for 7 to 10 days to achieve an anti-inflammatory effect. Shorter courses and lower doses of aspirin do provide some analgesic benefit, however. The patient should be informed that his symptoms often may be chronic or recurrent, and he should be advised about how to avoid recurrences (Fig. 64.2).

If an acute severe episode of neck pain in this situation does not respond to treatment within the first week or two, the patient should be referred. When the symptoms are more mild and chronic, a trial of treatment for several months would be reasonable before referral. Further evaluation by an orthopaedic surgeon or a neurosurgeon will include a complete cervical spine X-ray and a computerized cervical tomogram or myelogram to identify the problem and its location. If a herniated disc is identified, consideration can be given to its removal with anterior interbody fusion. This operation can give excellent relief of pain if the correct level of involvement has been identified (5).

Stiff Neck

Stiff neck is very common and is not a diagnosis, but rather a description of a symptom. Strain of the muscles or ligaments, of the neck, cold-induced muscular spasm, fibrositis, and neuritis are all possible causes. The problem is characterized by posterior cervical muscular spasm on one or both sides. The spasm usually lasts only 1 to 4 days and is relieved by the application of heat and by mild analgesics, such as aspirin or acetaminophen. The patient should receive advice about relieving muscle spasm and preventing recurrences (Figs. 64.2 and 64.3). Should the discomfort last beyond a week, an underlying disorder should be considered (*e.g.*, disc disease), and an evaluation should be initiated.

Whiplash

Mechanism

Whiplash is a term given to acute injuries of the neck caused by sudden extension of the cervical

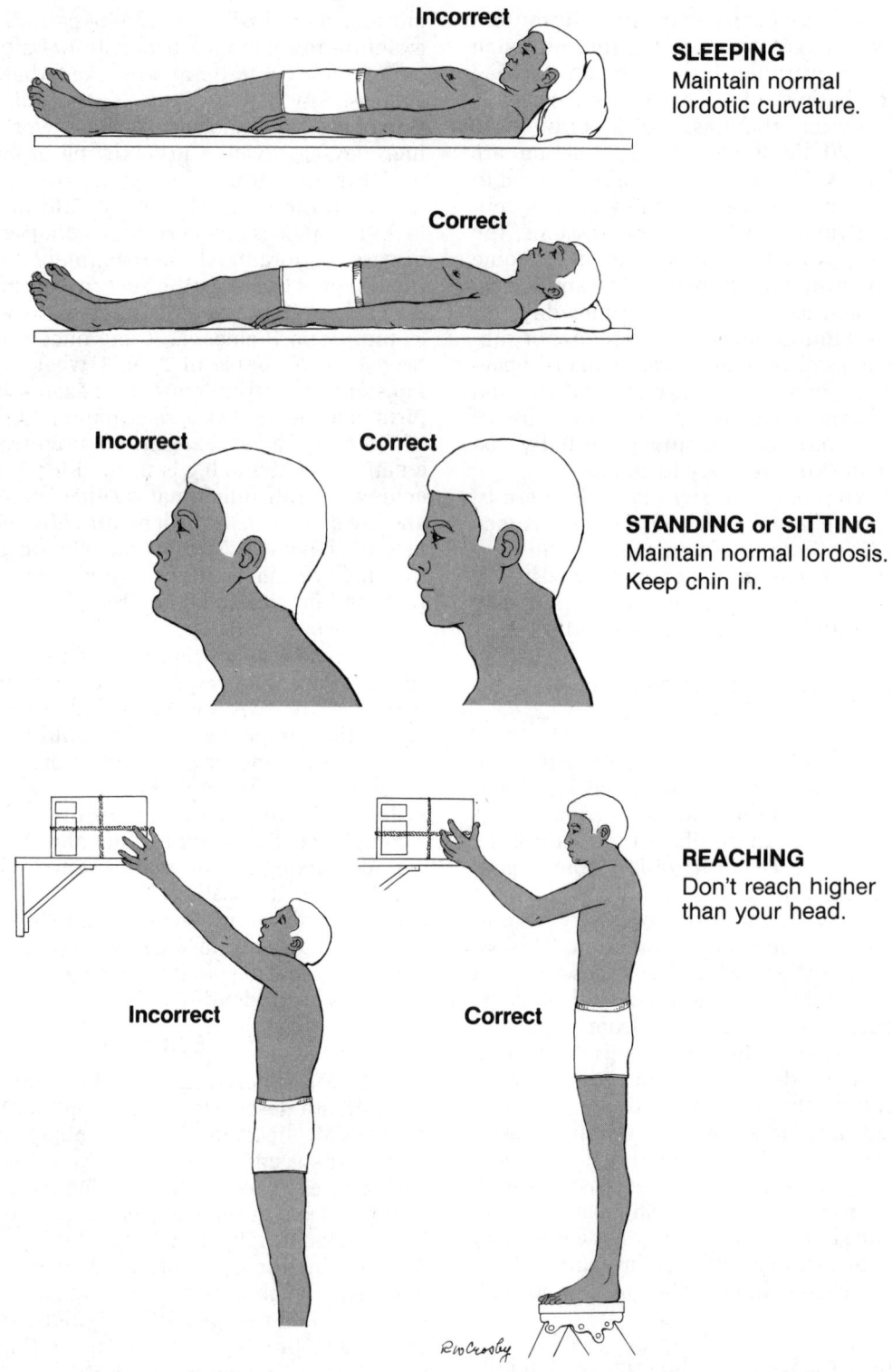

SLEEPING
Maintain normal
lordotic curvature.

STANDING or SITTING
Maintain normal lordosis.
Keep chin in.

REACHING
Don't reach higher
than your head.

Figure 64.2.   Position to prevent recurrence of neck pain.

spine. In this country, the most common cause is a
rear-end automobile collision. Patients with whiplash are frequently involved in litigation and compensation situations, which makes physicians skeptical of their complaints; it is however, well documented experimentally that significant injury can
occur by this mechanism. In cadaver studies, it has
been shown that when the neck is suddenly and

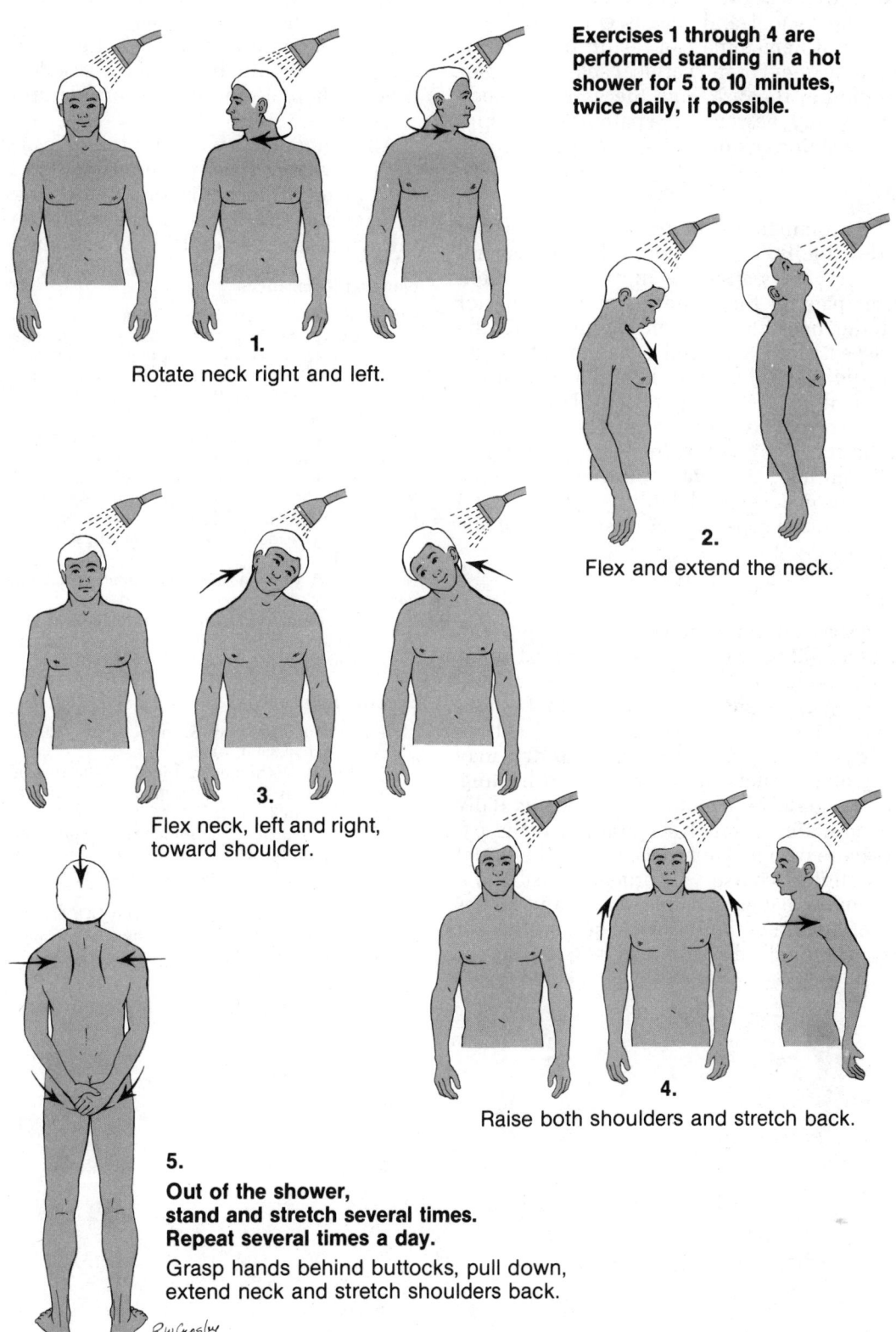

Exercises 1 through 4 are performed standing in a hot shower for 5 to 10 minutes, twice daily, if possible.

1.
Rotate neck right and left.

2.
Flex and extend the neck.

3.
Flex neck, left and right, toward shoulder.

4.
Raise both shoulders and stretch back.

5.

Out of the shower, stand and stretch several times. Repeat several times a day.

Grasp hands behind buttocks, pull down, extend neck and stretch shoulders back.

Figure 64.3. Exercises to rehabilitate the neck.

forcefully hyperextended, the muscles of the anterior aspect of the neck are stretched or torn, including the sternomastoid and longus coli muscles; a retropharyngeal hematoma can result; the anterior longitudinal ligament of the cervical spine may tear; and separation of the disc from the vertebral body can occur. Usually, however, the patient with whiplash injury sustains less intensive damage.

Diagnosis

It is not uncommon for the patient to be without discomfort initially. Pain usually begins several hours to 1 or 2 days after the injury. The patient experiences pain in the posterior and/or anterior region of the neck. It commonly radiates to the occipital aspect of the head and it may radiate to the shoulders and down the upper lateral aspect of the arms. Occipital headaches often occur. Disc herniation and nerve root compression rarely occur from whiplash injury. X-rays following whiplash injuries are usually normal. However, there may be some loss of the normal cervical lordosis, which is an indication of muscle spasm and of splinting of the neck.

Treatment

If muscle spasm or limitation of motion is present, the patient should be placed in a soft cervical collar (see above). Analgesics, in adequate doses, should be given. The patient should be warned that extension of the neck will exacerbate his pain. Heat applied to the cervical spine, either moist or dry, may give symptomatic relief but does not speed healing. The patient should be encouraged to do his daily work and activities as much as possible. If the patient has severe pain and muscle spasm at the initial injury, his clinical course will probably last 4 to 6 weeks. When the patient's pain subsides and he has full range of motion without muscle spasm, the soft collar can be gradually discontinued, and the patient should also be advised of the methods of relieving muscle spasm and preventing recurrent symptoms (Fig. 64.2 and 64.3). If there are no symptoms of nerve root compression, the patient with persistent symptoms should be treated for a long period of time, perhaps a year, before consideration of further workup.

All patients with whiplash injury, especially those with nerve root signs, are probably best seen at least once by an orthopaedist or a neurosurgeon for confirmation of the diagnosis and for follow-up should the symptoms not resolve in a reasonable time.

General References

Cailliet R: *Neck and Arm Pain*. Philadelphia, FA Davis, 1981.
> A very practical, concise, and well illustrated manual covering the common causes of neck pain.

Nakano, KK: Neck pain. In Kelley WN, Harris ED, Ruddy S, Sledge CB (eds): *Textbook of Rheumatology*, ed 2. Philadelphia, WB Saunders, 1985.
> An excellent discussion of the anatomy and biomechanisms and of the diagnosis, treatment, and differential diagnosis of common cervical spine problems.

Ramamurti CP: *Orthopaedics in Primary Care*. Tinker RV (ed). Baltimore, Williams & Wilkins, 1979.
> A very readable book with practical information relevant to the neck.

Rothman RH, Simeone FA: *The Spine*. Philadelphia, WB Saunders, 1975.
> An exhaustive textbook with excellent chapters covering anatomy, differential diagnosis, cervical disc disease, and arthritis of the spine.

Specific References

1. Elias F: Roentgen findings in the asymptomatic cervical spine. *NY J Med* 58:3300, 1958.
2. Geehr RB, Rothman SL, Kier EL: The role of computed tomography in the evaluation of upper cervical spine pathology. *Comput Tomogr* 2:79, 1978.
3. Johnson RM, Hart DL, Simmons EF, *et al*: Cervical orthoses. *J Bone Joint Surg* 59:332, 1977.
4. Oppenheim BE, Cantez S: What causes lower neck uptake in bone scans? *Radiology* 124:749, 1977.
5. Robinson RA, Walker AE, Ferlic DC, *et al*: The results of anterior interbody fusion of the cervical spine. *J Bone Joint Surg* 44A:1569, 1962.

CHAPTER SIXTY-FIVE

Low Back Pain

ANDREW F. BROOKER, Jr., M.D., DAVID T. SOWA, M.D., AND
JOHN R. BURTON, M.D.

As many as 65 to 80% of the population experience low back pain at some time in their lives, and this problem is a major cause of time lost from work (5, 8). While perhaps as many as one-third of these patients do not seek the advice of a physician (11), the remainder do so; therefore, most physicians often will need to evaluate patients with this problem. This chapter reviews the patterns of back pain most frequently described by patients, outlines the process of evaluating these patients, and recommends acute and intercritical treatment.

Symptoms of low back pain most often begin in the third and fourth decades of life, and approximately 60 to 65% are not associated with acute trauma, lifting, or strain (10). The back is a complex anatomical and functional region that is not easily analyzed. Therefore, it is often very difficult precisely to diagnose patients complaining of back pain. Physicians must use considerable judgment in deciding how best to evaluate and manage these patients. Most important, serial observation is a critical component in the care of patients with low back pain.

ANATOMY AND BIOMECHANICS OF THE LUMBAR AREA

Figure 65.1 emphasizes the anatomical complexity of the lumbar region and illustrates the important structures in the region.

The lumbar vertebrae are exposed to tremendous forces. This is due principally to the magnification of stresses that result from the lever effect of the arm in lifting and to vertical forces associated with man's upright position. Figure 65.2 demonstrates how lifting an object away from the body introduces the lever magnification phenomenon, resulting in a marked increase in forces on the vertebral bodies and discs. Because each intervertebral disc is a fluid system, there is a hydraulic pressure created whenever a load is placed on the axial skeleton. This hydraulic pressure magnifies 3 to 5 times the force that occurs on the annulus fibrosus. This force is akin to the hoop stress which occurs in a barrel when pressure is applied to its liquid content. The ability of the annulus fibrosus to withstand stress decreases significantly with age, and by 60 years many individuals have only 50% of the strength in these fibers that they had at age 30.

The lumbar spine, however, is not just an isolated structure. Much support is obtained by the muscles and ligaments of the spine and by the muscles of the thoracic and abdominal cavities. These latter structures act as a sort of muscular cylinder that helps to decrease the load on the axial skeleton by as much as 30% in the lumbar area and 50% in the thoracic spine (17).

ASSESSMENT OF PATIENTS WITH LOW BACK PAIN

Important information will always be obtained from the history and physical examination in the patient with low back pain.

History

The history may provide a clue that the cause of low back pain may not be a regional problem. The patient's *age* is the first important factor. Older individuals, especially those over 60 years of age, who are seen with new back pain are more likely to have referred pain or a less common cause of back pain than are younger individuals. Further, any

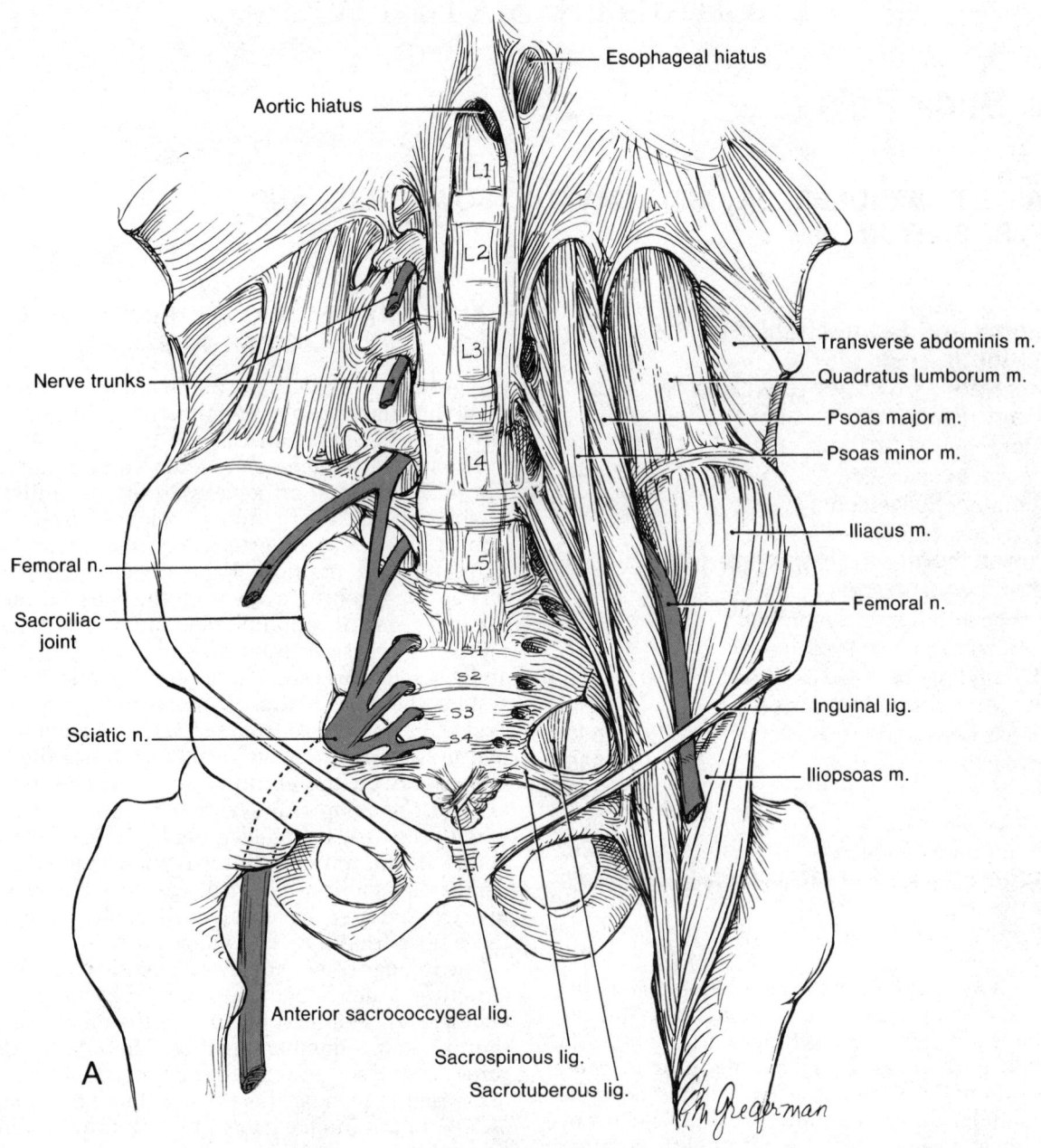

Figure 65.1. *A.* Normal anatomy: anterior view.

history of *systemic illness*—such as fever, weight loss, arthritis, gastrointestinal or genitourinary symptoms—should suggest a less common cause of the back pain (see below).

The *occupational* and *recreational history* will provide information about predisposing factors, including features of the patient's life which may need to be modified should the problem become chronic.

A thorough assessment of the *chronological development* of the pain and of the factors which aggravate and alleviate the pain will guide the physician in directing the evaluation and management of the patient. The pain should be characterized with re-

spect to its severity, quality, localization, and duration to aid determination of the etiology as well as the anatomical localization of the problem. Historical evidence of motor or sensory nerve root irritation or of sexual or sphincter dysfunction (bladder or bowel incontinence) should be sought.

Physical Examination

The examination of the back should receive special emphasis, but a general physical examination should also be done in those patients in whom referred pain or a less common cause of back pain is suspected.

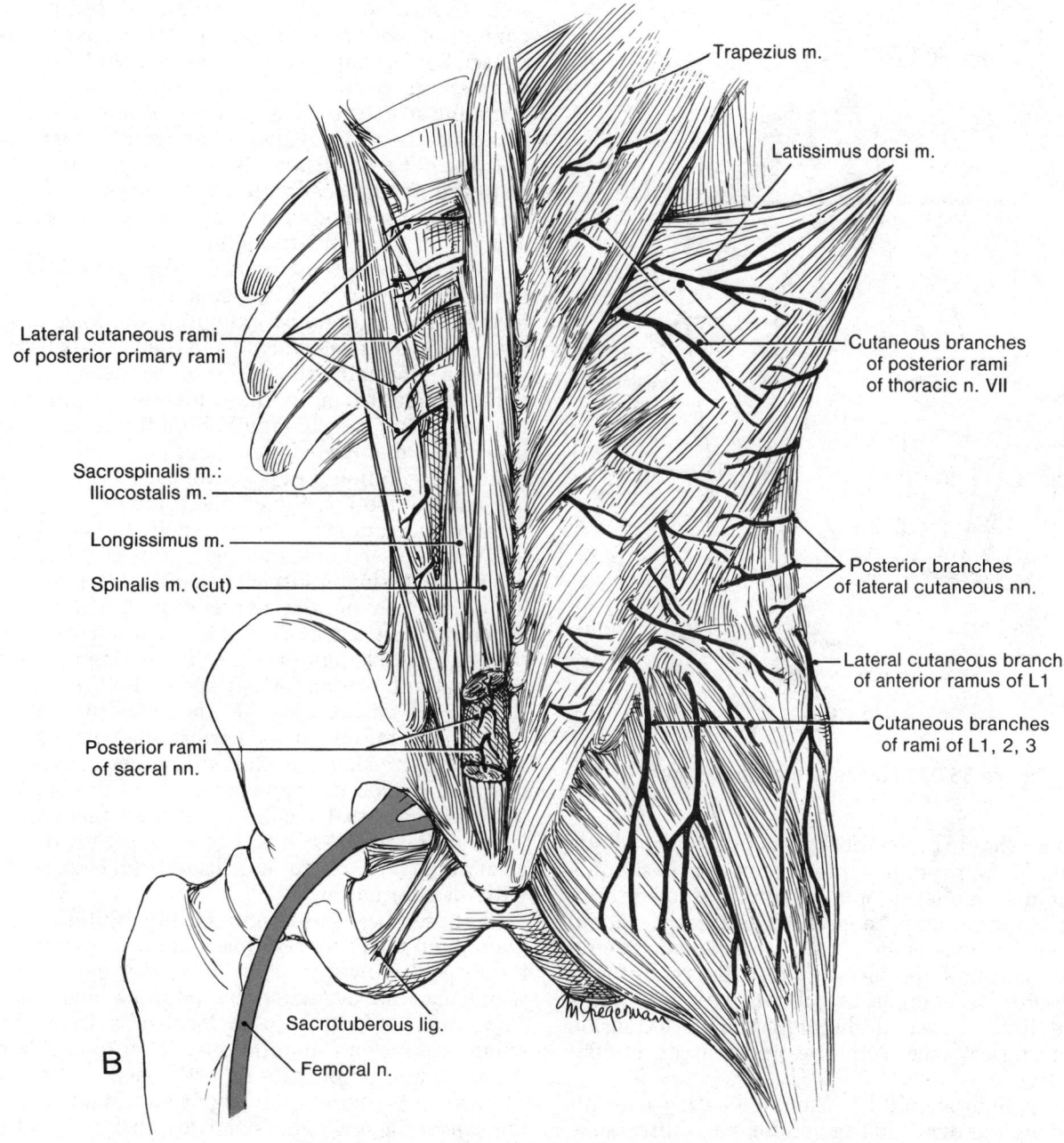

Trapezius m.

Latissimus dorsi m.

Lateral cutaneous rami
of posterior primary rami

Cutaneous branches
of posterior rami
of thoracic n. VII

Sacrospinalis m.:
Iliocostalis m.

Longissimus m.

Spinalis m. (cut)

Posterior branches
of lateral cutaneous nn.

Lateral cutaneous branch
of anterior ramus of L1

Cutaneous branches
of rami of L1, 2, 3

Posterior rami
of sacral nn.

Sacrotuberous lig.

Femoral n.

B

Figure 65.1. *B.* Normal anatomy: posterior view.

Examination of the Back and Associated Musculoskeletal Areas

The patient should wear only a gown that opens in the back and should be barefoot.

First, the patient should be examined while he is *standing.* The spinal column should be checked for kyphosis, lordosis, or scoliosis. Kyphosis and lordosis are readily apparent. The presence of scoliosis can best be determined by having the patient flex at the waist with arms extended in front. The asymmetry of even subtle curves can be appreciated. Any de-

viation of a spinous process from the midline should be noted. Firm palpation of the paravertebral muscles and of each vertebral spine should be performed. Isolated tenderness of one or two spinous processes suggests a local problem, such as compression fracture, abscess, or tumor. Hardened paravertebral muscles result from spasm secondary to pain or guarding.

Mobility of the spine should then be assessed. The patient should bend forward and attempt to touch his toes. Range of flexion can be quantitated by noting the distance of fingertips from the floor or the angle between trunk and legs. During this proc-

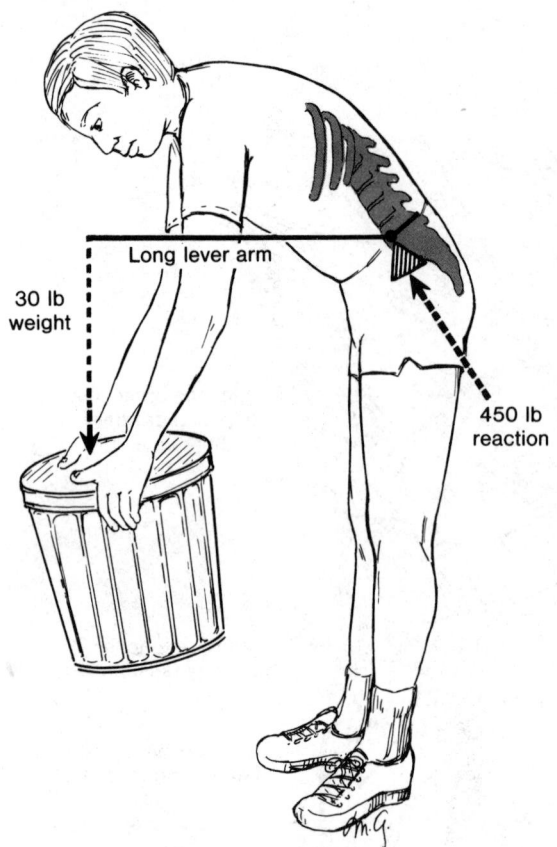

Figure 65.2. Forces in the lumbar area.

ess there should be a normally smooth rhythm down and up. If the rhythm is interrupted or is hesitant, a problem with a facet joint or significant lower back muscle spasm may be present. Similarly, lateral flexion and extension should be assessed. Lateral flexion is usually preserved in disc disease but may be absent, for example, in patients with ankylosing spondylitis. Increased discomfort with extension might suggest facet joint involvement or lumbar stenosis.

The patient should be examined *sitting with his legs dangling* over the edge of the examining table. The deep tendon reflexes of the knees and ankles should be tested. They assess the reflex arcs involving the nerve roots, L4, and S1, respectively. An absent reflex may signify nerve root irritation due to a herniated intervertebral disc. While the patient remains seated, the physician should perform a *"distracted" straight leg* raising examination by extending the patient's knee. Flexion of the hip and extension of the knee stretch the lumbar nerve roots; if radicular pain (down the leg and not limited to the back) is produced by this maneuver, nerve root irritation is present. The irritation can be confirmed by lowering the leg just to the point where the pain disappears and then dorsiflexing the foot, which again stretches the nerves and reproduces pain. This

sign, if positive, suggests a herniated disc or, less commonly, bony impingement of a nerve root caused by degenerative disease of a facet joint, lumbar stenosis, or, rarely, a tumor of the cord or surrounding structures. The absence of radicular pain, especially in an individual over age 30 years, does not rule out a herniated disc that may be too small or in the wrong location to irritate the nerve roots. This variant method of straight leg testing serves as a check on the standard method.

Next, the patient assumes the supine position, so that a *standard straight leg raising test* can be performed. This is done by extending the knee of the side expected to be involved and then slowly flexing the hip. Normally the hip can be flexed to 80° without pain, except perhaps for some tightness in the hamstring muscles and behind the knee. A positive test is manifested by pain or paresthesia in the sciatic distribution (*i.e.,* posterior aspect of the thigh, leg, and the foot) on the affected side or bilaterally. It is an indication of nerve root irritation. During this test, reported radicular pain present at less than 30° of hip flexion is suspect because of the mechanics of traction on the nerve root. In addition, a differentiation must be made between radicular pain and muscle tightness (*i.e.,* hamstring tightness) that patients often experience. Following the straight leg raising test, the unaffected or well leg should be raised, thus performing the *crossed straight leg raising test*. This procedure causes tension and stretch of the nerve roots of the opposite (affected) side and results in pain in the affected lower extremity. When this test is positive, there is a very high (7, 9, 24) but not absolute (22) correlation with disc herniation.

Next, *sensory assessment* of the buttock, perineum, and lower extremities can be accomplished. Figure 65.3 shows the relevant sensory dermatomes which can be evaluated by pinprick and touch. Abnormalities will help to localize a lesion and when present will help the physician to decide on the need and urgency of an orthopaedic or neurosurgical consultation. An important component of the sensory assessment is the search for signs that would suggest the presence of a *cauda equina syndrome* (compression of the lower portion of the spinal cord and its nerve roots, often secondary to a central disc herniation). This syndrome, if present, is an indication for immediate hospitalization and neurosurgical or orthopaedic consultation. The signs of compression of the lower end of the spinal cord are saddle anesthesia, loss of anal sphincter tone (assessed by rectal examination) and cremasteric reflexes, as well as historical evidence of bowel, bladder, or sexual dysfunction.

A *detailed assessment of motor function* in the legs will also help to localize a lesion in the patient in whom neurological involvement is suspected (Chapter 84, Table 84.7). This assessment should include,

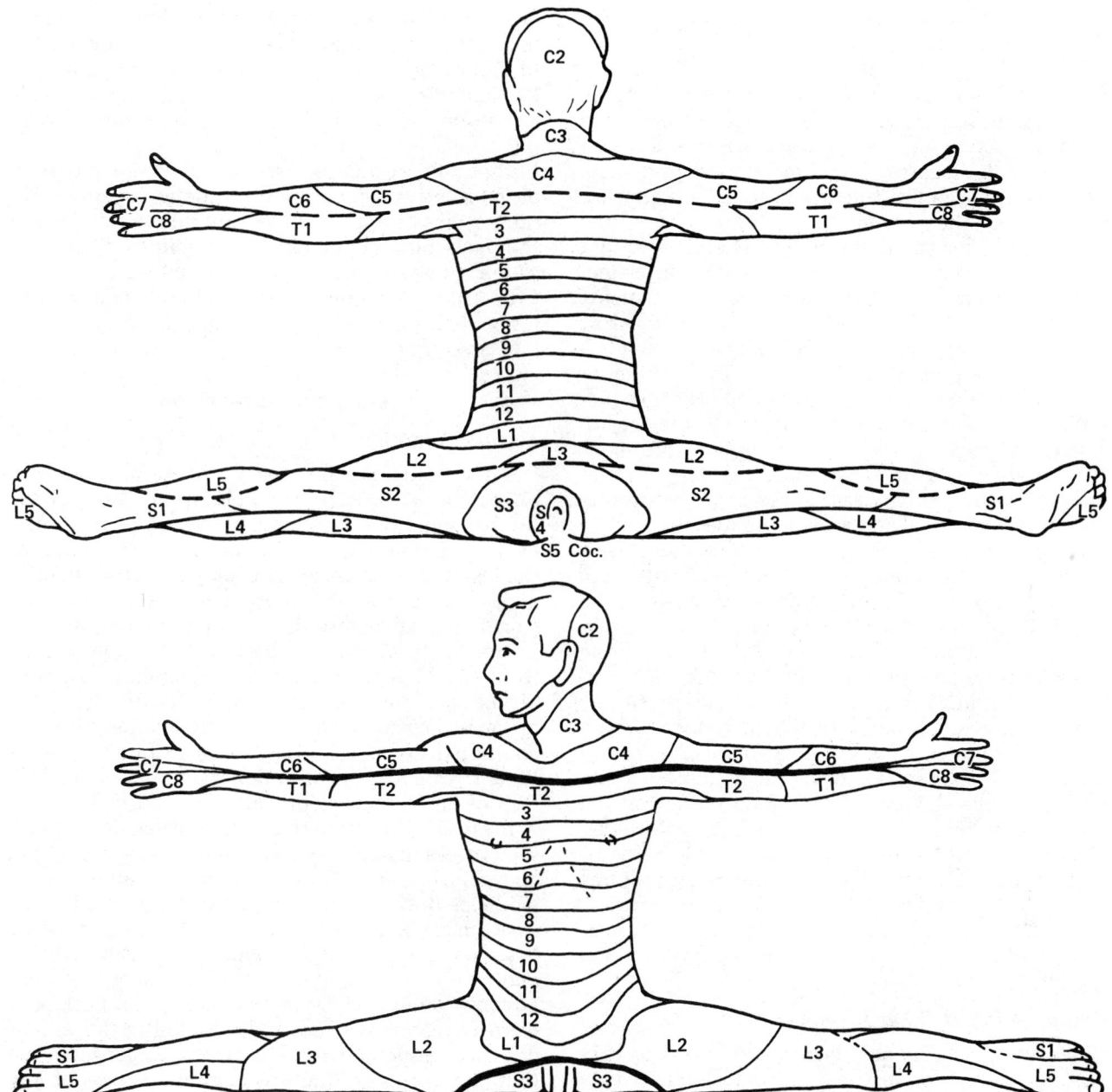

Figure 65.3. Sensory dermatomes. The numbers correspond to the spinal cord level of the dermatome. *C*, cervical; *T*, thoracic; *L*, lumbar; *S*, sacral. (From Haymaker W, Woodhall B: *Peripheral Nerve Injuries*, ed 2. Philadelphia, WB Saunders, 1962.)

while the patient is sitting, the knee extensors (L2-4), the dorsiflexors of the foot (L4-5), and the plantar flexors of the foot (S1-2). In order to demonstrate subtle weakness, the patient should stand and walk normally as well as on toe (gastrocnemius muscle group—S1-2) and heel (tibialis anterior muscle—L4-5). The symmetry of the buttock also can be assessed at this time (gluteus maximus—L5, S1-2).

As an adjunct to the routine evaluation of back pain in the difficult patient when there is suspicion of "malingering" or the presence of a psychogenic

component, it is useful to attempt to elicit the five *nonorganic physical signs of Waddell* (23): First, overreaction during examination was found to be the single most important nonorganic sign. This may take the form of collapsing, sweating, tremor, muscle tension, facial expression, or disproportionate verbalization. Second, simulation testing may be used to elicit nonorganic pain. Two useful examples are axial loading and rotation. In the first test, low back pain is reported on vertical loading by the examiner's hands on the patient's head. Neck pain is common and does not constitute a positive sign. In the rotation test, the patient stands with feet together and arms fixed firmly to his sides. The shoulders and pelvis are then passively rotated in the same plane. Reports of low back pain constitute a positive nonorganic sign. However, in the presence of true radiculopathy, leg pain may be produced. Third is the use of distraction testing. This consists of observing the patient during the course of the examination for variable findings when the patient is unaware that he is being observed or tested. Specific tests include "distracted" straight leg raising (see above). Fourth, superficial, nonanatomical or variable tenderness is also a nonorganic sign. A useful technique is *Magnuson's test* in which tender areas are marked and later examined for reproducibility. Fifth, nonanatomical motor or sensory regional disturbances are important nonorganic signs. "Giving way" and nonanatomical sensory changes often affect the same area and may be associated with nonanatomical and regional tenderness.

An assessment of the *hip, sacroiliac, and knee joints* should be done, as abnormalities in these joints may cause back or leg pain and mislead the physician into assuming that a primary lumbar problem is present. The hip and knee joints should be assessed by moving these joints through a normal range of motion. This is done with the patient supine in order to exclude nonarticular discomfort which may be generated by active movement. The sacroiliac joint is best assessed when the patient is supine with the knee flexed and the ankle placed on the opposite straight leg at the knee. The physician places his hands on the flexed knee and the ipsilateral anterior superior iliac spine, and, by pressing down, the sacroiliac joint on that side is stressed. When the patient is not supine, firm pressure over the sacroiliac joints will also elicit discomfort when sacroiliitis is present.

Examination of Other Regions

Because pain may be referred to the back or may be due to changes in the back that are part of a systemic process (see above), a selective general examination is important in some patients, particularly if (*a*) the patient is over 50 years of age, (*b*) there is fever, (*c*) historical clues suggest a systemic process, (*d*) the assessment of the back is normal, or (*e*) the back discomfort persists or progresses in spite of conservative therapy.

Metastatic cancer of the spine is especially common from primary tumors of the breast, lung, prostate, thyroid, kidney, and rectum. These regions should therefore be examined carefully. Further, an abdominal examination and, in women, a pelvic examination are necessary. Referred pain from cancer may also be felt in the back. For example, pancreatic lesions may cause pain to be referred to the high lumbar or low thoracic vertebral region. Bowel or urinary tract lesions may cause pain to be referred to the mid or low lumbar region, and disease located in the pelvis may cause lower lumbar or sacral pain. Particular attention to the lymph nodes may provide a clue to the presence of an intra-abdominal lymphoma.

Important also is the assessment of the adequacy of the arteries emanating from the lower aorta. Abnormalities here may cause pain due to ischemia in the back, buttock, or lower extremities during exertion. In addition to diminished pulses and bruits over arteries, cutaneous signs of ischemia (ulcers, loss of hair or nails) should be sought in the legs or feet (see also Chapter 87).

Laboratory Evaluation

X-ray Evaluation

It is usually not necessary, in the absence of a history of major trauma, to obtain an X-ray of the lumbar spine when patients with back pain are first evaluated. The study is important in checking for the less common causes of back pain rather than in diagnosing the more common problems—acute or subacute lumbar disc disease or muscular strain—in which the X-ray will be normal or nonspecific. By age 50, 67% of normal individuals show evidence of "disc disease" characterized by narrowing of one or more disc spaces and disc calcifications; and an additional 20% of individuals are found to have lumbar osteophyte formations alone, so that only 13% of individuals at this age have normal lumbar X-rays. On the other hand, abnormal X-rays are seen in less than 5% of individuals who are less than 20 years of age (10). Two-thirds of patients with evidence on X-ray of lumbar degenerative disc disease are asymptomatic. Also, there is no correlation between the presence of facet joint osteoarthritis and symptoms (15). Lumbar X-rays should be obtained whenever there is a suspicion that back pain has a less common cause and especially if the patient does not respond within 3 weeks to conservative therapy. In this setting less common causes of low back pain, such as a collapsed vertebra, osteomyelitis, osteoblastic or osteolytic lesions, may be detected by the X-ray. It is often useful to obtain an anteroposterior pelvis X-ray at the time of lumbar X-ray to rule out hip diseases as a source of back pain (16).

Other Laboratory Tests

Certain tests should be performed when back pain is suspected to be due to a less common cause. While the evaluation may be quite varied, several screening tests are particularly helpful: urinalysis (renal disease), stool occult blood (intestinal cancer), complete blood count with differential and erythrocyte sedimentation rate (inflammatory or neoplastic disease), serum calcium and alkaline phosphatase levels (diffuse bone disease), and, in males, acid phosphatase level (metastatic prostatic cancer). Other tests may be indicated based on the suspicion of the diagnostic possibilities.

Serial Observation

It is most important when first evaluating a patient with back pain, to establish rapport and to ensure follow-up of the patient either by telephone or by a subsequent office visit, since a diagnosis of the specific cause of back pain is often impossible at the initial visit. Even when there is a history of trauma, the diagnosis is not certain since, for example, 10% of patients with neoplasia as a cause of back pain give a history of trauma (8). Even when there is no initial clue in the history or in the physical examination, a serious or less common disorder is not ruled out.

If on reassessment there are symptoms or signs of progression or if there is an incomplete response to treatment, evaluation for an alternative diagnosis is necessary. After conservative management for an episode of back pain, 40% of patients will be symptom free in 1 week, and symptoms will have remitted in 75% by 3 weeks (6). Regardless of the initial problem formulation, follow-up contact with the patient within 3 weeks is mandatory. By following this approach routinely, considerable initial laboratory testing can be avoided, and clues to the presence of an underlying less common and potentially serious disorder will not be missed. A follow-up visit also provides an opportunity for education regarding recurrent symptoms (very common) and for advice regarding prophylactic measures (see below).

COMMON REGIONAL (NONSYSTEMIC) BACK SYNDROMES

Three problems account for the majority of complaints of low back pain: lumbosacral strain, acute and subacute disc disease.

Lumbosacral Strain Syndrome

Lumbosacral strain is the most common back problem encountered in practice. It is caused by an exertional or stress injury to the lumbosacral muscles or to the facet joints. This problem can occur at any age but is most common between the ages of 25 and 50. Predisposing factors include obesity, chronic occupational strain requiring bending and lifting, abnormal forward pelvic tilt (accentuated lordosis), leg length discrepancy, or X-ray evidence of vertically oriented lumbar facets (20).

Diagnosis

The patient complains of pain that may be severe in the back, buttock, or in one or both lower extremities. Usually symptoms follow a recent increase in physical activity for that individual, such as gardening, lifting, or an infrequently played sport. Usually the patient experiences no (or only minimal) discomfort during or immediately after the activity. Within the next 12 to 36 hours, however, pain develops and is associated with a feeling of muscular stiffness.

Examination of the back (see above) may show nonspecific signs of muscle spasm and of loss of lumbar lordosis, but characteristically there is no evidence of nerve root irritation.

Management

The patient should be advised to adhere to strict bed rest for a minimum of 3 to 4 days. To minimize back motion, he should either have a bed board cut to size from 5/8-inch particle board (plywood is usually much more expensive and unnecessary) placed under his mattress or have the mattress moved to the floor. He should position a small pillow beneath his head and knees, as shown in Figure 65.4. This relaxes the muscles and relieves stretch on the nerve roots. An equally comfortable position is the semifetal position (lying with the back slightly flexed). The patient should be out of bed only for bathroom use. The application of *dry heat* by a heating pad for 20 to 30 minutes several times a day (on low or medium setting with a protective towel between skin and pad to prevent burns) will often relieve muscular spasm and thereby provide comfort. Occasionally a patient will feel that heat worsens symptoms, in which case heat application

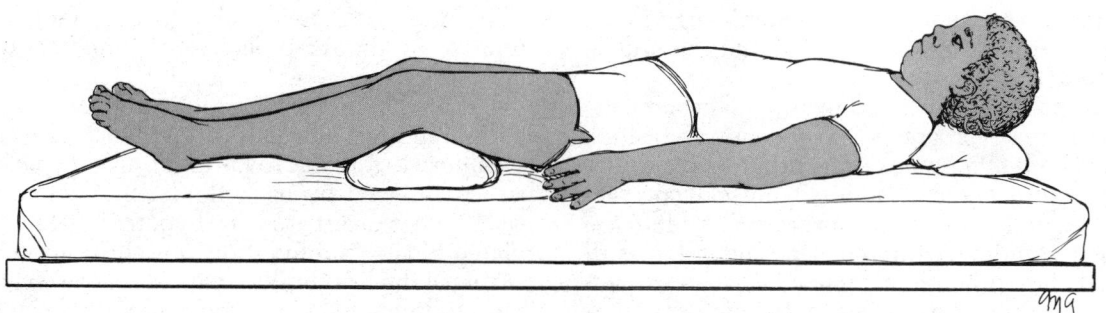

Figure 65.4. Recumbent position.

should be discontinued. Application of *moist heat* also may be used (and is preferred by some patients) for symptomatic relief of back pain. Moist heat may be accomplished by using hot towels, or a heat pack which produces sustained heat for up to ½ hour (available at pharmacies). *Analgesics*, such as codeine, 30 to 60 mg, in combination with aspirin or acetaminophen, every 4 to 6 hours may be necessary for the first several days. Subsequently, acetaminophen or aspirin alone is usually sufficient to control pain. An *anti-inflammatory agent* with rapid onset of action, such as naproxen (Naprosyn), 250 mg two times a day, or piroxicam (Feldene), 20 mg once a day, is an important adjuvant to bed rest. *Muscle relaxants* are not first line therapeutic agents, but they may be used in the occasional patient who has not responded in a day or two to the above treatments. Carisoprodol (Soma), 350 mg four times a day, has been found in controlled studies to be more effective than placebo in relieving discomfort in patients with low back pain (1). Cyclobenzaprine (Flexeril), 10 to 20 mg three times a day, has also been shown to be more efficacious than placebo in the treatment of intractable pain syndromes with muscle spasm, but it is associated frequently with a dry mouth, drowsiness, and dizziness (2). Diazepam (Valium), 5 mg two to three times a day, promoted as a muscle relaxant, has been variably shown to be no more effective to slightly more effective than placebo (18). Its sedating properties, however, may be useful in the patient who finds adherence to bed rest difficult. Only a 3- to 7-day supply should be given because of its potential for abuse.

When improvement occurs after 3 to 4 days, the patient may be permitted out of bed for short leisurely walks. Sitting should be avoided as it will tend to increase low back stresses and may cause a recurrence of pain. Over a period of 1 to 2 weeks, ambulation is increased with a gradual decrease of the dose of analgesic until the patient can return to his usual activities without medication. During this recovery period it is especially important to advise the patient to avoid activities that greatly increase the forces applied to the lower spine (e.g., lifting, pushing, force on outstretched upper extremity as in making beds or vacuuming, lurching, or bending). Should the patient fail to respond or should there be a recurrence, he should be re-examined and an orthopaedic or neurosurgical consultation should be considered.

For the patient who is recovering satisfactorily, various exercise programs have been advocated. One simple but effective *exercise program* combines isometric gluteal and abdominal muscle contractions and pelvic tilt. These exercises, which are performed standing with the back against a wall (Fig. 65.5) should be recommended as soon as pain subsides. Additional exercises that *stretch* the lum-

bosacral muscles (Fig. 65.6) also may provide comfort. The exercises should be performed for a few minutes four to six times a day. Exercises that are designed to strengthen the abdominal musculature, such as sit-ups with the knees flexed or straight leg raising, have been shown to magnify markedly the lower lumbar forces, could exacerbate symptoms, and are not recommended.

With continued healing the discomfort should resolve entirely, and the patient then can be advised about prophylactic measures (see below).

Physical therapy is usually not necessary in managing these patients; in particular, active exercise programs may intensify symptoms and should be avoided. Therapy such as ultrasound, shortwave, diathermy, heat or cold packs may provide short term relief, but there is no evidence that there is any effect on the disc lesion or any long term effect on symptoms. Also, such therapy is often quite inconvenient for patients and therefore may detract from overall compliance. Lumbar traction has not been shown to be more effective than bed rest in the treatment of lumbar disc disease (5).

In addition, once the patient is ambulating he may benefit from the use of a *lumbosacral support*. While these devices have not been evaluated in a controlled study, theroretically they can help by increasing intra-abdominal pressure, which will provide support to the vertebral column, and by limiting (or reminding the patient to limit) spinal motion (clearly the spine is not immobilized, however). A lumbosacral support is prescribed by the physician and is fitted by an orthotist (brace maker) at an orthopaedic appliance shop. The most practical and most common device is a cloth corset fitted with metal stays posteriorly. The patient should use the support when ambulating and then, as healing occurs, should gradually be weaned from it over a period of 2 to 3 weeks until usual activities are resumed. It is important for this group of patients to return gradually to full activity because an abrupt return may cause a recurrence of low back pain. As in the other syndromes associated with back pain (see below), the physician should establish rapport at the first visit and ensure follow-up since a less common cause of back pain could present with the symptoms and signs of muscle strain. Prompt re-evaluation is necessary should the symptoms not improve or should progressive symptoms or signs develop.

Chronic lumbosacral strain (facet syndrome) may follow repeated episodes of low back pain that are secondary to forceful hyperextension. Typically, the pain is relieved by back flexion (i.e., bending forward) and exacerbated by hyperextension. This is related to facet subluxation caused by stretching or tearing of the ligamentous capsule of the facet joints. The syndrome may be associated with degenerative

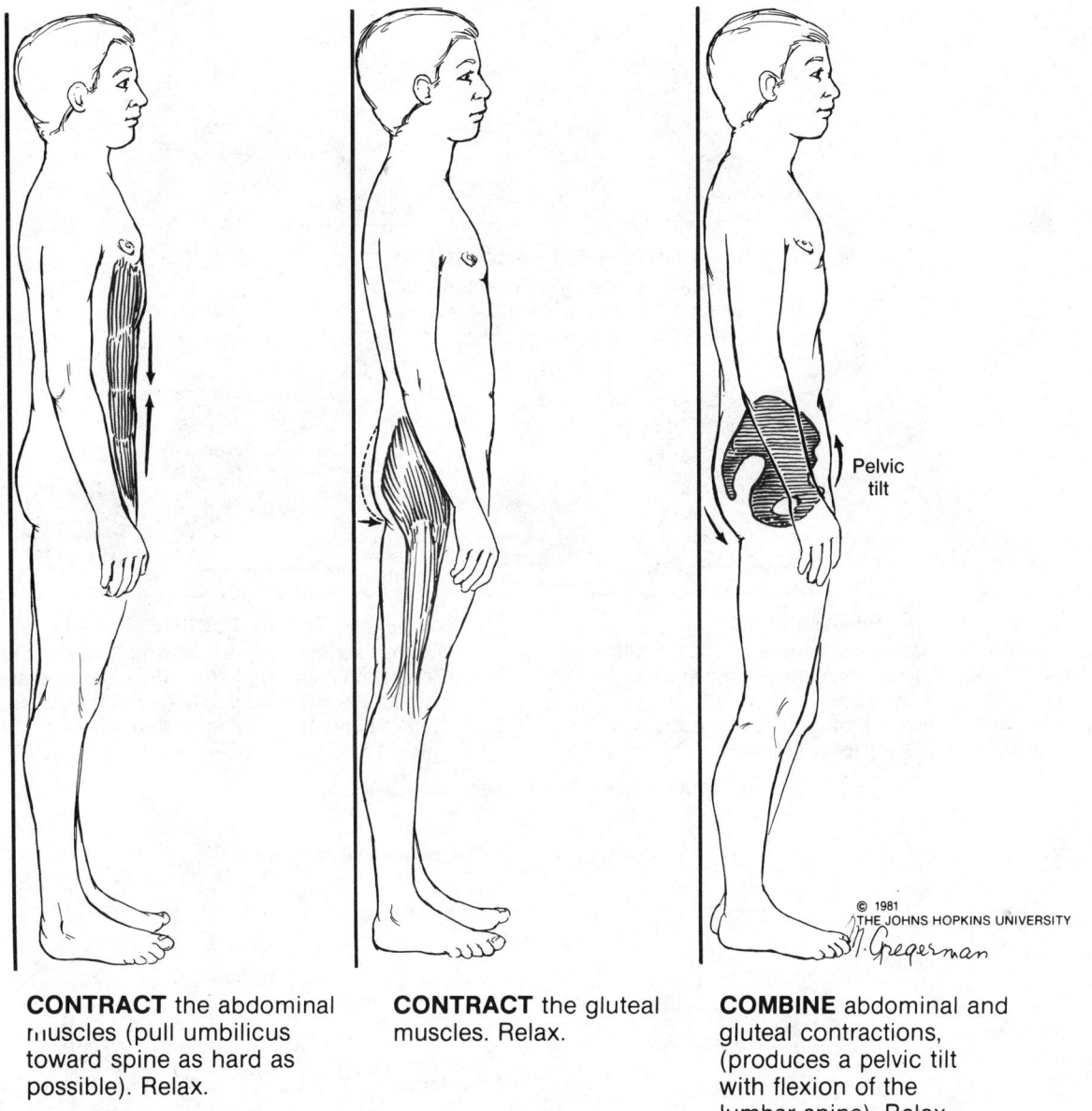

CONTRACT the abdominal muscles (pull umbilicus toward spine as hard as possible). Relax.

CONTRACT the gluteal muscles. Relax.

COMBINE abdominal and gluteal contractions, (produces a pelvic tilt with flexion of the lumbar spine). Relax.

Pelvic tilt

© 1981
THE JOHNS HOPKINS UNIVERSITY

Figure 65.5.   Exercises—abdominal muscles and pelvic tilt.

arthritis involving the intervertebral joints. Treatment is initiated to decrease back hyperextension by strengthening abdominal muscles.

Acute Lumbar Disc Disease

The annulus fibrosus degenerates with time, which predisposes to disc rupture and to herniation of the nucleus pulposus (Fig. 65.7), resulting in the acute lumbar disc syndrome. There may be mild transient episodes of low back pain associated with this degenerative process, but it is herniation that produces the sudden severe discomfort. A sudden increase in the pressure in the lumbar spine which might occur with a flexion injury: e.g., bending over to lift a heavy object, lifting with the arms extended away from the body (the lever magnification of stresses, illustrated in Fig. 65.2), a sudden lurch, or even a sneeze or cough can precipitate the rupture. However, many patients who have a ruptured disc will not give a history of injury or of a sudden increase in pressure. Lumbar disc disease is most common at the L4-5 level and at the L5-S1 level and is less common between the other vertebral bodies. Acute lumbar disc disease is less common than subacute disc disease or lumbosacral strain syndrome.

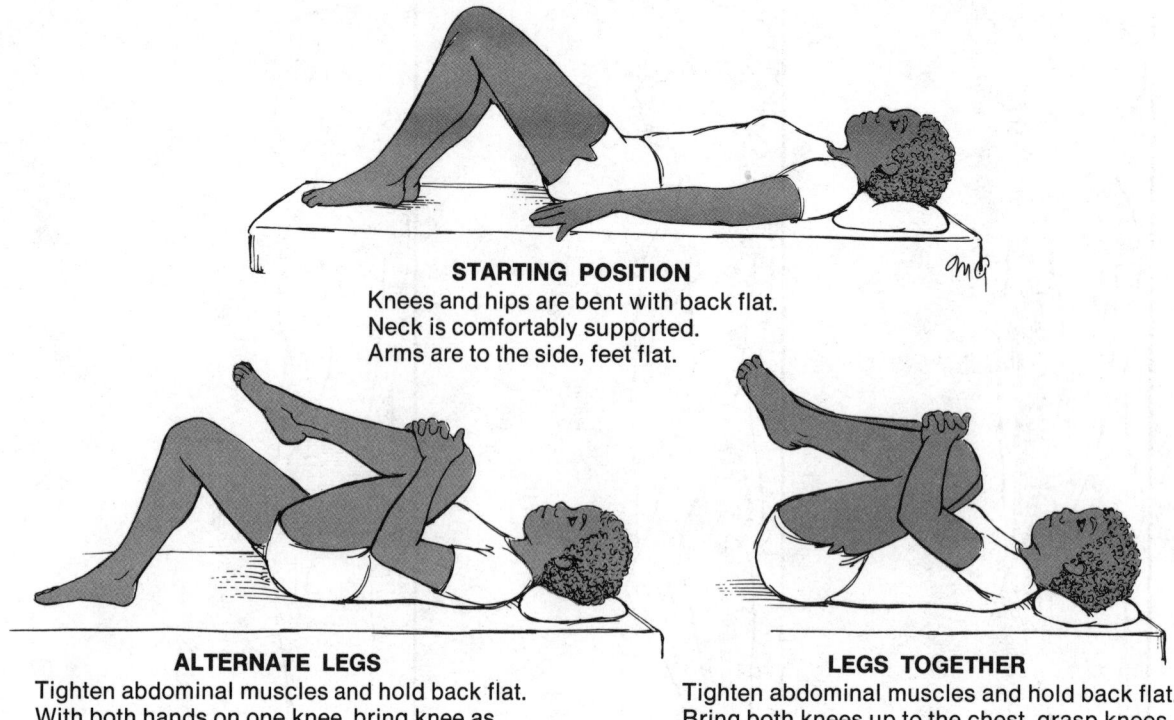

STARTING POSITION
Knees and hips are bent with back flat.
Neck is comfortably supported.
Arms are to the side, feet flat.

ALTERNATE LEGS
Tighten abdominal muscles and hold back flat.
With both hands on one knee, bring knee as
near chest as possible.
Return slowly to starting position. Relax.
Repeat, alternating legs, 10 times.

LEGS TOGETHER
Tighten abdominal muscles and hold back flat.
Bring both knees up to the chest, grasp knees
with hands and hold position for 30 seconds.
Return slowly to starting position. Relax.
Repeat 5 times.

Figure 65.6.   Knee-chest exercises.

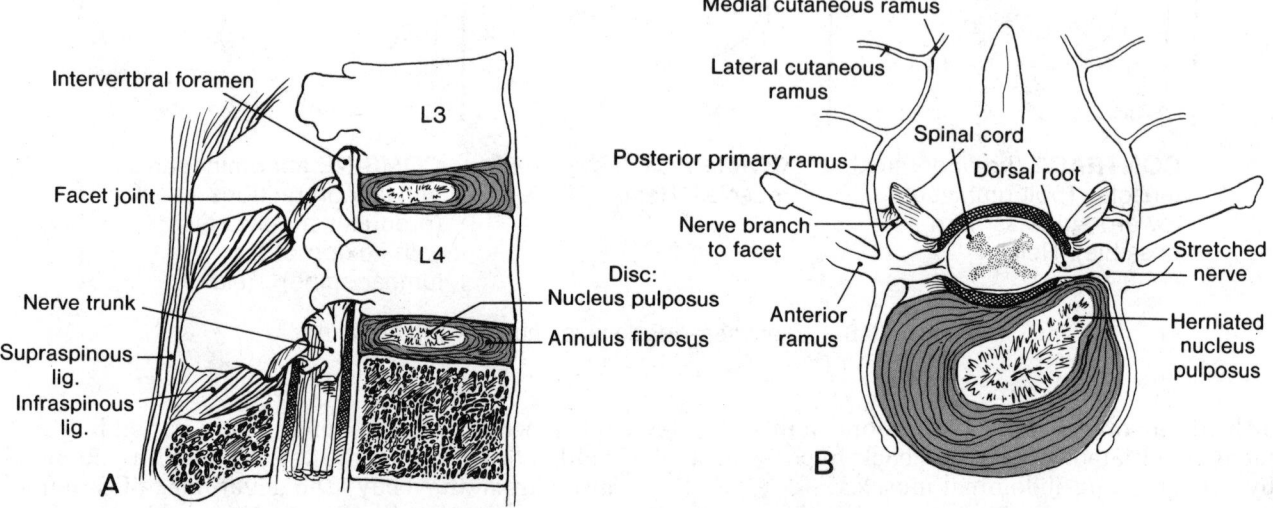

Figure 65.7.   *A.* Normal disc. *B.* Herniated disc.

Diagnosis

Patients with this problem describe severe back, buttock, and/or leg pain which is either unilateral or bilateral. The pain may be so severe that the patient resists examination and splints the back in an awkward position of lateral lumbar flexion and hip flexion. The patient is still or else moves very slowly. Any suggestion of restlessness or pain worsened by quiet rest in bed suggests the dangerous cauda equina syndrome (see above). The diagnosis of acute lumbar disc herniation is most likely when examination (see above) reveals signs of nerve root irritation with either a loss of motor function, loss of deep tendon reflexes, and/or a localized sensory deficit. Specific disc herniations may result in well defined motor, sensory, and reflex deficits that aid in their diagnosis (Table 65.1).

Management

If the patient has a neurological defect or has extreme pain, immediate hospitalization and urgent orthopaedic or neurosurgical consultation are necessary. After hospital admission a decision must be made about further confirmation of a neurological deficit (occasionally necessary by electromyography, which may show denervation of leg muscles) or about myelography or computerized axial tomography (CT) of the lumbar region. Before the advent of CT, myelography was the mainstay of diagnosis in lumbar disc herniation. Today, they are complementary procedures with performance of a standard lumbar myelogram followed the same day by CT scanning (3, 13).

Patient experience. Myelography is generally performed as an inpatient procedure. Cerebrospinal fluid is withdrawn for routine diagnostic tests, and the contrast agent is introduced intrathecally. The patient often experiences a warm or burning sensation, but severe pain is rarely experienced.

Routine X-ray views are taken and flow of the contrast is enhanced by use of the tilt table. CT scanning is then performed a few hours later. The CT scan can demonstrate a disc that has ruptured but has not impinged the dural sac. It is also effective in demonstrating spinal stenosis, facet lesions, extradural tumors, or vertebral body destruction (3).

After a metrizamide myelogram (water-soluble contrast) the patient is returned to his room and typically is instructed to remain supine with the head of the bed elevated to 20°. After a myelogram, the patient may experience a headache, but the chances of its development are lessened by adequate pre- and postprocedure hydration, by the use of the small spinal needles, and by keeping the patient in bed 12 hours after the procedure. Nausea may also develop after a myelogram but should not be treated with phenothiazines, which lower the seizure threshold.

Depending on the patient's response to initial treatment and on the above studies, surgery may be considered. Most patients, however, will respond to conservative therapy. When followed for several years, similar patients who have been treated surgically or conservatively have the same fitness for work. Also, approximately 60% of those who had surgery and approximately 40% who were treated conservatively will be symptom free when studied 8 years after hospitalization (18). Those with conservative therapy, however, may have more symptoms in the earlier posthospitalization period. In cases of spontaneous remission of an acute disc herniation, actual reduction of the disc is unlikely. It is more likely that the annulus and posterior longitudinal ligament "adjust" to the presence of the herniated fragment with the resolution of edema, inflammation, back pain, and leg pain. Also desiccation of the fragment may play a role in resolution of symptoms (21).

Should the patient not be hospitalized initially, very close surveillance is necessary with immediate hospitalization should signs progress or should the pain not remit promptly. The conservative management of patients with this problem is discussed under "Subacute Lumbar Disc Disease," as patients

Table 65.1.
Common Findings in Lumbar Disc Herniations[a]

Level of Disc Herniation	Nerve Root Compressed	Pain	Numbness (See Fig. 65.3)	Weakness	Reflexes (Decreased or Absent)
L3-L4	L4	Sacroiliac joint, hip, posterolateral thigh, anterior aspect of leg	L4 dermatome	Extension of knee (quadriceps)	Knee jerk
L4-L5	L5	Sacroiliac joint, hip	L5 dermatome (includes great toe)	Dorsiflexion of great toe (extensor hallucis longus)	
L5-S1	S1	Lateral aspect of leg and foot	S1 dermatome (includes lateral toes)	Unusual (plantar flexion of foot)	Ankle jerk
Massive midline lumbar disc herniation Cauda equina syndrome (usually L4 or L5)	Multiple roots in dural sac	Midline of back, posterior aspect of both thighs and legs	Perineum, posterior thighs, plantar aspect of feet	Paralysis of feet and sphincters	Absent ankle jerk

[a] Adapted from Vanden Briuk KD, Edmonson AS: The spine. In Edmonson AS, Crenshaw AH (eds): *Campbell's Operative Orthopaedics.* St Louis, CV Mosby, 1980.

with this latter syndrome are more frequently managed at home (see below).

Subacute Lumbar Disc Disease

This problem is similar to acute lumbar disc disease, but the onset is not sudden nor is the condition totally incapacitating. Frequently, the history is of several weeks' or even years' duration. The disease is caused either by a herniated disc or by an osteophyte (bony spur) impinging on a nerve root.

Diagnosis

The patient with this problem describes back, buttock, or lower extremity pain (usually radiating below the knee) that is most commonly unilateral. Examination usually reveals evidence of irritation of a specific nerve root resulting in loss of a localized motor or sensory neurological function or of an absent deep tendon reflex (L5-S1 disc, ankle; or L3-4 disc, knee). The straight (or crossed straight) leg raising test is often positive. In this situation, conservative management at home is most appropriate. However, a re-evaluation and/or consultation is mandatory should neurological symptoms or signs progress or if a prompt remission of symptoms does not occur. Of some concern is the fact that tumors of the spinal cord, especially those about the conus and cauda equina, may cause symptoms simulating disc herniation.

Management

The management of this problem is identical to that described for lumbosacral strain syndrome (see above).

LESS COMMON SYNDROMES

There are other regional and systemic disorders which are manifest by complaints of low back pain.

Lumbar Stenosis

Some people have a congenitally narrow spinal canal which fails to produce symptoms until adult life. Characteristically, the diagnostic clue is a story suggesting irritation of multiple nerve roots at different levels on both sides. More commonly, however, lumbar stenosis develops in patients with no congenital narrowing who develop a progressive stenosis as a result of hypertrophic degenerative arthritis or repetitive or chronic trauma. This syndrome presents in the fifth to seventh decade and is more common in males than females (21). Typically, these patients complain of chronic low backache with unilateral or bilateral lower extremity discomfort and may develop frank hypesthesia or dysesthesia. There may be a history of prior disc surgery. In 30 to 40% of patients with lumbar stenosis the characteristic syndrome of "neurogenic claudication" may develop (12). These patients develop lower extremity claudication with standing, walking, or hyperextension of the spine in the absence of any evidence of peripheral vascular disease. Painful paresthesias are present in the feet or legs and may progress to the hip girdle or lower trunk. If there is no alteration in activity, this may progress to lower extremity numbness and weakness, and the patient may experience frequent falls. These symptoms are relieved by rest or flexion of the spine (the patient may report that he regularly gets relief by bending forward as if to tie his shoes). Physical examination may show no abnormalities until the patient becomes active when motor or sensory deficits may appear. Plain X-rays show degenerative changes in the facet joints and decreased anteroposterior canal diameter. Plain myelography is rarely helpful. The major diagnostic test in suspected lumbar stenosis is CT, which shows the narrowed canal and/or the impingement of osteophytes upon the intervertebral foramina.

When the diagnosis of lumbar stenosis is considered, orthopaedic or neurosurgical consultation should be obtained. Conservative management is rarely beneficial. Laminectomy gives very satisfying results, whereas conservative therapy may be associated with progressive neurological dysfunction in the lower extremities.

Sacroiliitis

Pain from an inflammatory process of the sacroiliac joint is not uncommon. Frequently the process is manifest as leg or buttock pain rather than as back pain. It may be the first symptom of ankylosing spondylitis when it is identified in a young man. Sacroiliitis may also be seen in older men and women because of a nonspecific inflammatory process in this joint. A clue to the presence of sacroiliitis is tenderness when the joint is stressed while the patient is in the prone or in the supine position (see above). Conditions affecting the sacroiliac joint are discussed in Chapter 71.

Discitis

Although rare, discitis must be considered in any patient with back pain. Discitis is a closed space infection of the intervertebral disc with peridiscal osteomyelitis of the vertebral body. Symptoms include the onset over several days of severe back pain, often with radiation to the extremities, flanks, lower extremities, or inguinal area. The pain is usually well localized. Patients tend to avoid motion of the back and prefer to lie still in bed. There are usually few local or systemic signs of infection, but many patients are febrile. The most common physical finding is paravertebral muscle spasm, which may be associated with a positive straight leg raising test. Typically, the leukocyte count is normal, but the erythrocyte sedimentation rate is elevated. These laboratory tests should be obtained in patients with severe, well localized back pain that does not respond to conservative measures. Roentgenographic changes in discitis may not be present for months, but a bone scan will show increased radiotracer uptake at the infection site (although this abnormality is not specific). Because discitis may progress to frank vertebral osteomyelitis (see Chapter 31), it is important to identify the pathogen so that appropriate antimicrobial therapy can be initiated. If blood cultures fail to yield the organism, the patient should be referred to an orthopaedist for admission to hospital and the performance of a needle biopsy under fluoroscopic or CT guidance. While awaiting culture results, the patient should be hospitalized and treated with an aminoglycoside and a penicillinase-resistant penicillin. Cephalosporins are not used because of poor disc penetration. *Staphylococcus aureus* is the most common organism, but Gram-negative discitis may occur. The antibiotic should be modified when culture results are available and should be continued for a minimum of 6 weeks. Early mobilization is encouraged. Erythrocyte sedimentation rates should be followed and expected to decrease with appropriate therapy (14).

Vertebral Fractures

Vertebral compression fractures are common and usually the result of a flexion injury when the spine is abruptly and violently flexed as it is, for example, during jumping. The force needed to compress a vertebral body in healthy bone is considerable. However, when the bone is diseased, as, for example, in osteoporosis, multiple myeloma, metastatic cancer, or hyperparathyroidism, the injury may be relatively insignificant. Pain is usually localized and immediate, although it may be delayed for several days following the fracture. Often tenderness over a single vertebra indicates the presence of this problem, but an X-ray is necessary to confirm the diagnosis.

In the presence of neurological deficit, CT and myelography are indicated since neurological deficit usually suggests that there is more damage than a single compression fracture of the vertebral body. A bone scan is often useful in demonstrating whether the process is isolated. It is important in the evaluation to consider a process (such as multiple myeloma) that may have weakened the bone and predisposed it to fracture. With lumbar or thoracic vertebral compression fractures, management includes rest, adequate analgesia, and gradual ambulation when the patient is pain free. A lumbosacral support or, for the patient with a thoracic vertebral fracture, a chair-back or hyperextension brace may be helpful in alleviating pain. These may be obtained by prescription from an orthopaedic appliance shop.

Other Causes

Many other regional or systemic problems may cause patients to come to physicians with complaints of back pain (see Table 65.2).

MANAGEMENT OF THE INTERCRITICAL PERIOD

While most patients with low back pain have a complete remission of symptoms within 3 weeks (6), many patients will experience recurrence. For this reason the physician should discuss with the patient ways to prevent recurrence. The important subjects of posture, weight control, exercise, and activities will need to be discussed.

Figure 65.8 shows some correct and incorrect postures and practical advice which may be useful to give to patients who have had low back pain. Weight reduction is desirable in the obese patient, as excessive weight directly increases the load on the lower vertebral column and its supporting structures. Exercises designed to strengthen the muscles of support are frequently prescribed, although they have not been shown to be preventive. However, weakness of muscles regularly occurs with bed rest and with modified activity that is part of the treatment of patients with acute back pain syndromes. Also, it has been demonstrated that sudden loading of the spine when the back is flexed and when the knees are straight markedly increases lumbar forces compared to when the knees are bent and the back is straight. Exercises which strengthen the quadriceps

Table 65.2.
Some Less Common Causes of Low Back Pain[a]

REFERRED PAIN (A clue that the pain is referred is the absence of any tenderness, limitation of motion, or aggravation of pain or spasm during the physical examination of the back.)
Sacral pain—from a pelvic problem (*e.g.*, endometriosis or metastatic cancer)
Lower lumbar pain—from a lower abdominal disease process (*e.g.*, aortic aneurysm)
Lower thoracic and upper lumbar pain—from an upper abdominal disease process (*e.g.*, pancreatic tumor).
SYSTEMIC OR REGIONAL DISEASE SOMETIMES ASSOCIATED WITH MUSCULOSKELETAL BACK PAIN
Infection—tuberculosis, osteomyelitis, spinal or epidural abscess, herpes zoster
Neoplastic diseases—myeloma, lymphoma, retroperitoneal sarcoma, neural tumor, or metatastic disease
Metabolic disease—osteoporosis, osteomalacia, Paget's disease, ankylosing spondylitis, Reiter's syndrome
Postural back pain (increased lordosis, as with high heel use)
PSYCHIATRIC CAUSES OF BACK PAIN, *e.g.*, depression

[a] These causes should be considered when the patient fails to respond to conservative treatment or if there is suspicion on initial evaluation.

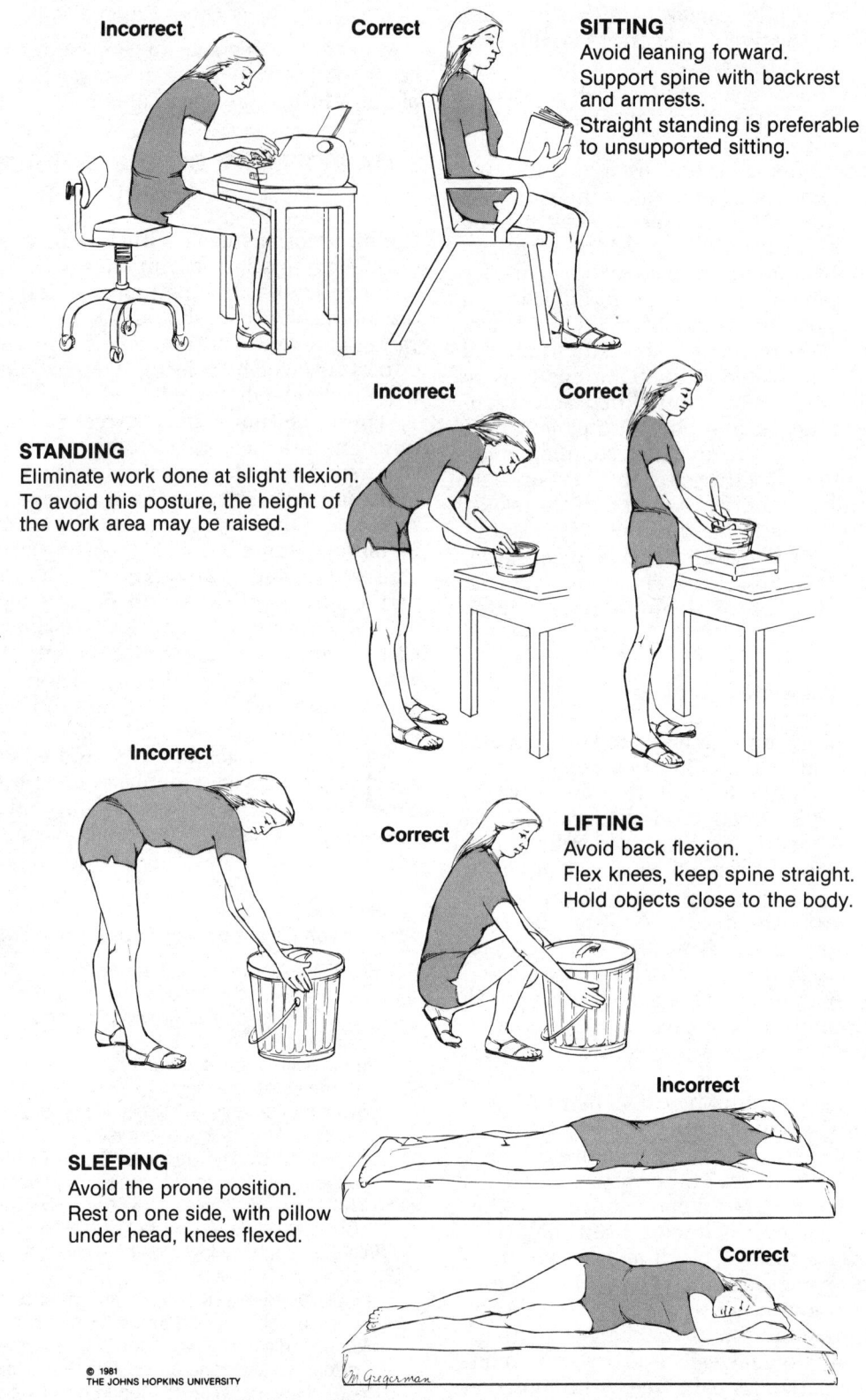

SITTING
Avoid leaning forward.
Support spine with backrest and armrests.
Straight standing is preferable to unsupported sitting.

STANDING
Eliminate work done at slight flexion.
To avoid this posture, the height of the work area may be raised.

LIFTING
Avoid back flexion.
Flex knees, keep spine straight.
Hold objects close to the body.

SLEEPING
Avoid the prone position.
Rest on one side, with pillow under head, knees flexed.

© 1981
THE JOHNS HOPKINS UNIVERSITY

Figure 65.8. Postural attitudes—correct/incorrect.

(extend knees) are theoretically sound and include swimming, cycling, or jogging on a flat surface. The patient should be advised to exercise only if it does not initiate or increase back pain. In addition, because the abdominal musculature is important in supporting the spine when a weight is brought to bear on it (see above), exercises that strengthen the abdominal musculature (Fig. 65.5) are important. More complex exercise programs are likely to be followed by only an occasional patient and therefore are not recommended.

Work or athletic activities may need to be modified, although there is no convincing support for the concept that heavy labor or lifting predisposes to the development of low back pain (19). Several points are, however, worth emphasis: (a) improper technique in lifting produces backache, (b) there is a high incidence of low back pain in those people who either sit for prolonged periods or who are unable to sit at all during the workday, (c), sudden maximal physical activity (e.g., participation in an occasional vigorous game without conditioning) results in a high incidence of back pain. Further, there is evidence that back pain occurs more frequently in individuals who consider their occupation to be physically hard and in those who feel that the work they perform is particularly stressful to the spine (4). These observations are important for the physician to bear in mind as he educates the patient about recurrences of back pain after the acute episode has resolved.

General References

Helfet AJ, Gruebel-Lee DM: *Disorders of the Lumbar Spine.* Philadelphia, JB Lippincott, 1978.
>A readable well illustrated monograph on low back pain.

Macnab I: *Backache.* Baltimore, Williams & Wilkins, 1977.
>A very well organized, practical text with many helpful schematic illustrations covering all aspects of low back pain.

Rothman RH, Simeone FA: *The Spine.* Philadelphia, WB Saunders, 1982.
>A textbook of spinal disorders and their treatment.

Ramamurti CP: *Orthopaedics in Primary Care.* Tinker RV (ed). Baltimore, Williams & Wilkins, 1979.
>A well illustrated and practical book.

Specific References

1. Baratta RR: A double-blind comparative study of carisoprodol, propoxyphene, and placebo in the management of low back syndrome. *Curr Ther Res* 20:233, 1976.
2. Brown BR Jr, Womble J: Cyclobenzaprine in intractable pain syndromes with muscle spasm. *JAMA* 240:1151, 1978.
3. Carrera GF, Williams AL, Houghton VM: Computed tomography in sciatica. *Radiology* 137:433, 1980.
4. Dehlin O, Hedenrud B, Horal J: Back symptoms in nursing aides in a geriatric hospital. *Scand J Rehabil Med* 8:47, 1976.
5. Deyo RA: Conservative therapy for low back pain. Distinguishing useful from useless therapy. *JAMA* 250:1057, 1983.
6. Dillane JB, Fry J, Kalton G: Acute back syndrome—a study from general practice. *Br Med J* 3:82, 1966.
7. Hakelius A, Hindmarsh J: The significance of neurological signs and myelographic findings in the diagnosis of lumbar root compression. *Acta Orthop Scand* 43:239, 1972.
8. Horal J: The clinical appearance of low back disorders in the city of Gothenburg, Sweden. *Acta Orthop Scand Suppl* 118:1, 1969.
9. Hudgins WR: The predictive value of myelography in the diagnosis of ruptured lumbar discs. *J Neurosurg* 32:152, 1970.
10. Hult L: Cervical, dorsal and lumbar spinal syndromes. *Acta Orthop Scand Suppl* 17:1, 1954.
11. Kane RL, Leymaster C, Olsen D, et al: Manipulating the patient. A comparison of the effectiveness of physician and chiropractor care. *Lancet* 1:1333, 1974.
12. Karayannacos PE, Yashon D, Vasko JS: Narrow lumbar spinal canal with "vascular" syndromes. *Arch Surg* 111:803, 1976.
13. Kieffer SA, Cacayorin ED, Sherry RG: The radiological diagnosis of herniated lumbar intervertebral disk. *JAMA* 251:1192, 1984.
14. Kornberg M, Eismont FJ: Discitis: an elusive infection. *Infect Surg* 2:818, 1983.
15. Lawrence JS, Bremner JM, Bier F: Osteo-arthrosis. Prevalence in the population and relationship between symptoms and X-ray changes. *Ann Rheum Dis* 25:1, 1966.
16. Mooney V: Evaluating low back disorders in the primary care office. *J Musculoskeletal Med* 1 (2):16, 1984.
17. Morris JM, Lucas DB, Bresler B: Role of the trunk in stability of the spine. *J Bone Joint Surg* 43A:327, 1961.
18. Quinet RJ, Hadler NM: Diagnosis and treatment of backache. *Semin Arthritis Rheum* 8:261, 1979.
19. Rowe ML: Low back pain in industry. *J Occup Med* 11:161, 1969.
20. Turek SL: *Orthopaedics: Principles and Their Application,* Philadelphia, JB Lippincott, 1984, pp 1483–1656.
21. Vanden Briuk KD, Edmonson AS: The spine. In Edmonson AS, Crenshaw AH (eds): *Campbell's Operative Orthopaedics.* St Louis, CV Mosby, 1980.
22. Vaz M, Wadia RS, Gokhale SD: Another cause of positive crossed-straight-leg-raising-test. *N Engl J Med* 295:779, 1978.
23. Waddell G, McCulloch JA, Kummel E, et al: Nonorganic physical signs in low-back pain. *Spine* 5:117, 1980.
24. Woodhall B, Hayes GJ: The well-leg raising test of Fajersztajn in the diagnosis of ruptured lumbar intervertebral disc. *J Bone Joint Surg* 32A:786, 1950.

CHAPTER SIXTY-SIX

Nonarticular Rheumatism: Bursitis, Tenosynovitis, Trigger Finger, Dupuytren's Contracture, Raynaud's Phenomenon, and Fibrositis

RAYMOND L. MALAMET, M.D., AND GREGORY B. KELLY, M.D.

BURSITIS

General Considerations

Definition

Bursitis, the inflammation of a bursal sac, is a very common problem. Bursal sacs are structures lined with synovial membrane that secretes and absorbs liquid. The bursae provide, thereby, a lubricating mechanism between structures such as bones, ligaments, tendons, muscles, and skin. Although usually isolated, occasionally they are in communication with a joint space. There are over 150 such structures in the body, but the number is not fixed and a new bursa may appear whenever there is friction between structures (2).

Most instances of bursitis can be diagnosed properly and treated in the office by the general physician; however, occasionally, because of the location of the bursa, the uncertainty of the diagnosis, or frequent recurrences of the problem, referral to an orthopaedist or rheumatologist may be necessary.

Etiology

The most common cause of bursitis is trauma; less often, a systemic process, such as rheumatoid arthritis or gout, causes the inflammation. Septic bursitis following trauma is especially a concern in patients with superficial bursitis (such as olecranon or prepatellar bursitis) (10). When a bursa has become inflamed from any cause it may be associated with amorphous deposits of calcium.

Manifestations

Bursitis is particularly common in middle-aged and older individuals of either sex, but the reason for this age distribution is not known. Patients with acute bursitis usually describe the abrupt onset of localized pain and discomfort that is worsened by any movement of the structures adjacent to the bursa. Frequently, there is a history of trauma or of repetitively performed activity. Fever is occasionally present.

When the inflamed bursa is superficial, an obvious swelling may be present, which is often erythematous and tender. On the other hand, inflammation in deep bursae may be manifest only by regional tenderness and by some limitation of motion.

Aspiration of Bursae

When there is identifiable swelling that is fluctuant, especially accompanied by fever or evidence of surrounding cellulitis, it is important to aspirate fluid from the bursa. Examination of the fluid will differentiate between septic and nonseptic bursitis. Aspiration may be easily accomplished by the general physician when the bursa is superficial (Table 66.1). The appearance of the fluid varies, depending on the cause. It should be analyzed routinely (Table 66.1) in order to establish the diagnosis (Table 66.2). Septic bursal fluid manifests a significant leukocytosis with polymorphonuclear cell predominance (Table 66.2). Confirmation of sepsis occurs with culture proof of infection. The vast majority of septic bursae are caused by *Staphylococcus aureus*.

Therapy

If a septic bursitis is identified, the patient should be hospitalized to receive parenteral antibiotics and repeated aspiration of the bursa. Gout, pseudogout, or rheumatoid arthritis should be treated with antiinflammatory agents (see Chapter 69).

Usually traumatic bursitis will heal spontaneously if the area of inflammation is rested. The spontaneous healing, however, requires several weeks and therapy shortens this period considerably. Therefore, if sepsis and crystalline disease are ruled out, the treatment outlined in Table 66.3 is indicated.

If there is no initial response to treatment, then the patient should be treated by an *injection* into the inflamed bursa of a mixture of Xylocaine and depo-steroid (Table 66.4).

Usually, injection of an inflamed bursa with Xylocaine results in an immediate and dramatic relief of pain, and this response indicates that the proper site has been injected. The anti-inflammatory effect of the steroid injection is seen in approximately 72 hours. If a satisfactory response has not occurred,

the bursa may be reinjected in approximately 2 weeks. Waiting for 2 weeks before reinjection provides ample time to rule out iatrogenic sepsis, which occasionally occurs after a steroid injection. If a bursitis does not respond to two steroid injections, orthopaedic consultation is necessary, as rarely definitive treatment by *surgical excision* of the bursa may be necessary.

Specific Forms

Several forms of bursitis are particularly common; their unique aspects are described here.

Olecranon Bursitis

This common form of bursitis—also called student's or miner's elbow—is easily recognized by its location just behind the olecranon process of the ulna. Its special features are: (*a*) it is frequently

Table 66.1.
Technique for Aspiration of Superficial Bursae (or Joints) and of Analysis of Bursal (or Synovial) Fluid

1. Determine by palpation the area of maximum tenderness and/or fluctuance and outline with indelible pen.
2. Determine and outline with an indelible pen any structures to be avoided.
3. Clean the skin with iodine solution such as povidone (Betadine).
4. Anesthetize the skin with Xylocaine in the area of planned aspiration.
5. An 18 gauge needle should be used to aspirate.
6. The fluid should be grossly inspected by the physician and analyzed for the following:
   a. Cell count and differential—fluid needs to be in a tube containing heparin.
   b. Glucose and total protein—fluid needs to be placed in a tube without anticoagulant.
   c. Type of crystals (see Chapter 69).
   d. Gram stain and culture using transport media (even in the absence of a high white cell count).
   e. Mucin clot analysis.
      (1) Add 1 to 2 drops of bursal fluid to 1 ml of 2–5% acetic acid in a test tube.
      (2) Shake the mixture a few moments and observe the clot (good, if clot remains intact and this is normal or a noninflammatory state; poor, if clot disintegrates and this represents inflammatory disease states) (see Table 66.2).

Table 66.3.
Treatment of Bursitis

1. Splint where feasible (especially effective in the hand and fingers).
2. Application of heat for 20–30 minutes several times a day; *i.e.*, heating pad at low heat and wrapped in a towel to prevent burning.
3. Anti-inflammatory agents: A nonsteroidal anti-inflammatory agent with a rapid onset of action is preferred if cost is not a restriction: naproxen (Naprosyn), 375–500 mg two times a day, or piroxicam (Feldene), 20 mg once a day, are two agents that have a rapidly achieved effect. (Other nonsteroidal anti-inflammatory agents, including aspirin, may be used and are discussed in Chapter 70. If cost is a factor, aspirin is recommended, although it takes 7–10 days at a dose of 3–4 g/day to achieve an anti-inflammatory effect (as opposed to its analgesic effect which is achieved at a lower dose.)
4. Improvement is usual in several days, but the anti-inflammatory agent should be continued an additional 4–5 days to prevent recurrence.
5. If no signifcant response is noted in 5–7 days and if sepsis has been ruled out, the bursa may be injected with Xylocaine and/or a steroid preparation (see Table 66.4).

Table 66.2.
Patterns on Bursal (or Joint) Fluid Findings in Common Problems

	Normal	Trauma	Sepsis	Rheumatoid Inflammation	Microcrystalline Inflammation
Color of fluid	Clear yellow	Bloody, xanthochromic	Yellow to cloudy	Clear yellow to cloudy	Clear yellow to cloudy
WBC/RBC	0–200/0	< 1200/many	10,000–200,000/few	1000–20,000[a]/few	1000–20,000[a]/few
Protein	Low	Low	Slightly increased	Slightly increased	Slightly increased
Glucose	Same as plasma	Normal	Decreased	Slightly decreased	Variable
Crystals	–	—	—	—	+[b]
Mucin clot	Good	Good to intermediate	Poor	Poor	Poor
Culture	–	—	+	—	—

[a] Cell count in noninfected inflammatory fluid may sometimes be as high as it is with sepsis; thus the need for culture.

[b] Gout: negatively birefringent sodium urate (see Chapter 69). Pseudogout: positively birefringent sodium pyrophosphate (see Chapter 69).

Table 66.4.

Methods of Injection of Bursae or Joints with Xylocaine and/or Depo-glucocorticoid Preparations[a]

1. Be certain sepsis has been ruled out (Tables 66.1 and 66.2).
2. Outline with an indelible pen both area of injection and surrounding structures that should be avoided.
3. Prepare the skin carefully with an iodine-containing solution such as povodine (Betadine).
4. Anesthetize the skin with intradermal Xylocaine.
5. Mix 2–3 ml of 1–2% Xylocaine with 20–40 mg of a depoglucocorticoid (such as Aristocort or Kenalog) being sure that the corticosteroid is well suspended and inject the bursa with 1–3 ml of this mixture using a 20–22 gauge needle.

[a] *Notes of caution:* (a) injection into the skin will cause atrophy and thus should be avoided; the patient should understand that there is a possibility of this complication; and (b) injection into tendons themselves may cause degeneration and, in time, rupture and these structures should be avoided by careful palpation.

associated with *systemic disease*, such as rheumatoid arthritis or gout; (b) symptoms frequently are *chronic*, in that they have been present for 2 or 3 weeks before a patient sees a physician; and (c) it is a common site for *septic bursitis* following trauma and may be associated with surrounding cellulitis (6, 10). If rheumatoid arthritis or gout is present, it is important to realize that sepsis sometimes coexists. Traumatic olecranon bursitis is usually hemorrhagic, although xanthochromic fluid may be present.

Swelling in the area of the olecranon bursa should always be aspirated (see Tables 66.1 and 66.2) and a stain, culture, white blood cell count, and crystal identification with polarizing microscopy should always be obtained.

Therapy. Therapy depends on the characteristics of the fluid. If gout is present, specific therapy is indicated (see Chapter 69). Traumatic bursitis responds to simple removal of fluid; but if the fluid reaccumulates, a steroid injection (Table 66.4) should be given. If sepsis is identified, the patient should be hospitalized for parenteral antimicrobials and frequent aspiration and an X-ray of the elbow should be obtained to rule out osteomyelitis if the process has been present for more than 2 weeks.

Prepatellar Bursitis

Prepatellar bursitis (housemaid's or carpenter's knee) is a very common form of bursitis, easily recognized by its location in front of the patella. It is particularly common in carpet layers, plumbers, and carpenters. It is most often caused by trauma from kneeling, but it may also be a site of sepsis, and the bursa, for this reason, should always be aspirated even if it feels dry (6).

Anserine Bursitis

The anserine bursa is fan shaped and lies between the confluence of tendons and the tibia bone at the anterior medial aspect of the knee just below the joint space. Anserine bursitis is most often seen in individuals with arthritis, such as degenerative joint disease, and is recognized by its location; the pain is typically produced when the knee is flexed and is particularly troublesome at night. The patient often seeks comfort by sleeping with a pillow between his thighs.

If there is surrounding erythema or if the patient is febrile, aspiration should be attempted because sepsis, although uncommon, may be present. Therapy depends on the findings (see Tables 66.2 and 66.3). When injection therapy is used, the solution should be injected in a fan-shaped pattern so that the entire bursa is treated.

Ischial Bursitis (13)

The ischial bursa is located over the ischial tuberosity, close to the sciatic nerve. When a person is sitting, the ischial bursae are covered only with subcutaneous tissue and skin; when a person is erect, the gluteus maximus also covers the bursa.

The most common reason for inflammation of this bursa is trauma, such as may occur in bicycling. It also may be a site of hemorrhage after minor trauma, especially in patients who have been taking anticoagulants. It is rarely a site of sepsis.

Usually the inflammation results in an abrupt onset of pain, but occasionally the onset is more insidious. The patient often has exquisite pain when sitting or lying. Because of the close proximity of the sciatic nerve to the bursa, there may be an associated neuritis resulting from pressure on the nerve, which causes pain to radiate into the leg. Direct pressure over the ischial tuberosity will cause sharp pain. In addition, the pain is intensified when the patient is supine and his hip is passively flexed.

The differential diagnosis of ischial bursitis includes lumbar spine disease and thrombophlebitis. Similar pain may also be seen in association with ankylosing spondylitis or Reiter's syndrome (see Chapter 71). Localization of the pain over the ischial tuberosity and the finding of induration near the ischial tuberosity on rectal examination establish the diagnosis of ischial bursitis.

Aspiration of the bursa, even when it is inflamed, is not recommended because it is often difficult to localize, and the surrounding structures, especially the sciatic nerve, may be injured. If aspiration is indicated because there is associated fever and, therefore, the possibility of septic bursitis, the patient should be referred to a rheumatologist or an orthopaedist for immediate evaluation.

Standard therapy (Table 66.3) usually provides dramatic improvement within 2 to 3 days; but if there has been associated leg pain or weakness from sciatic nerve inflammation, those symptoms may persist for several months.

Ultrasound, administered by a physical therapist, is effective, especially when symptoms are chronic, and it should be considered if initial therapy has not relieved the symptoms within several days.

If the diagnosis is unclear, if there is a question of sepsis, and if the patient does not respond within a week to therapy, consultation with a rheumatologist or orthopaedist is recommended. If the diagnosis is confirmed, the consultant may aspirate the bursa and, if sepsis is ruled out, inject it with Xylocaine and depo-corticosteroids, which often results in dramatic improvement.

Semimembranosus-Gastrocnemius Bursitis (Baker's Cyst) (5)

The semimembranosus-gastrocnemius bursa—commonly called a cyst—lies in the posterior medial aspect of the knee behind the femoral condyle and in 50% of individuals is continuous with the knee joint. Inflammation of this bursa is commonly associated with other knee problems such as internal derangements, rheumatoid arthritis, or degenerative arthritis. The bursa is rarely traumatized or infected. When the bursa is inflamed, pain is the major manifestation, especially during activities that require movement of the knee, and often it is relieved by rest. Contraction of the quadriceps (knee extension) compresses the supratellar bursa (which communicates often with the knee joint), causing fluid in the knee joint to flow directly into the semimembranosus-gastrocnemius bursa, thereby causing pain. A Baker's cyst can also be associated with calf swelling and tightness (the bursa descending several centimeters into the leg). Tenderness is present over the bursa, and often the patient complains of pain when the gastrocnemius muscle group is stretched—a positive Homan's sign. The location of the swelling often leads to confusion with thrombophlebitis or with a popliteal aneurysm. For this reason, careful examination, including palpation of the venous and arterial systems, is necessary. When there is any doubt about the diagnosis, special diagnostic studies and appropriate consultation as outlined in Chapters 70 (Rheumatoid Arthritis) and 87 (Peripheral Vascular Disease), respectively, may be indicated. Occasionally a Baker's cyst ruptures spontaneously, resulting in swelling, heat, and diffuse tenderness of the calf. These features can mimic an acute deep vein thrombophlebitis (see Chapter 51). In those patients in whom the diagnosis is unclear, venography should be performed to exclude phlebitis.

Management of a patient with an uncomplicated Baker's cyst includes aspiration of the cyst (and of the knee if synovitis is present) by an orthopaedist or rheumatologist and instillation of a corticosteroid-anesthetic mixture into the cyst and joint cavity. Because of the important structures in the popliteal fossa (artery, nerve, and vein), aspiration of the bursa by the general physician is not recommended unless he has received training in this technique. Weight bearing should be minimized for several days or weeks. The response to this therapy is usually excellent. Management of a ruptured cyst consists of bed rest, heat, and elevation. Instillation of corticosteroids into the joint that has an effusion may be helpful. Nonsteroidal anti-inflammatory agents may also be of assistance; after symptoms have begun to abate, ambulation can slowly be increased.

Iliopectineal Bursitis

The iliopectineal bursa lies anterior to the hip joint with which it communicates in approximately 15% of individuals. It lies between the inguinal ligament and the iliopsoas muscle just lateral to the femoral artery. Pain in the anterior pelvis, groin, and thigh is the most frequent manifestation of iliopectineal bursitis; swelling may result in a bulge resembling a femoral hernia (see Chapter 91) below the inguinal ligament. Bursitis may result from intrinsic joint disease, such as rheumatoid arthritis. Extension of the hip (for example, during walking) intensifies the pain so that the patient often limits the stride of the affected side. The anterior crural nerve (the largest branch of the lumbar plexus) lies just below the bursa and it may be irritated from bursal inflammation; resulting neuritis causes pain in the thigh, which often is also intensified by walking, and there may also be weakness of anterior muscles of the thigh. When a bursa is quite enlarged it may compress the femoral vein, resulting in edema in the affected leg.

If a hernia can be ruled out (see Chapter 91), the bursa should be aspirated by a rheumatologist or orthopaedist. Aspiration and injection with Xylocaine and usually a corticosteroid results in lasting improvement.

Trochanteric Bursitis (12)

The trochanteric bursa lies in the lateral aspect of the thigh over the greater trochanter of the femur and is closely associated with tendons of the glutei muscles. The problem primarily affects older individuals. Most cases are of unknown etiology, although many are thought to result from osteoarthritis. Trauma accounts for approximately 20% of cases and sepsis is rare. The onset of abrupt pain, frequently with radiation to the knee or even to the groin, is most common. Discomfort is intensified by movement from the sitting to the standing position, going up and down stairs, or sleeping on the affected side.

On examination there is point tenderness over the bursa with reproduction of the pain. An X-ray of this area is indicated, as frequently calcium is identified and its presence supports the diagnosis. Also, an X-ray may identify a problem in the hip joint that is causing referred pain, which may simulate trochanteric bursitis.

Therapy, as outlined in Table 66.3, is usually quite effective. If calcium has been identified on X-ray, it is usually in the area of the inflammatory process, and for this reason steroid injections should be aimed at the calcium. Additionally, it is important for the patient to sleep with a small pillow under the involved buttock to keep weight shifted off the bursa.

TENOSYNOVITIS

As with bursae there are many sites of potential tenosynovial inflammation. Tendinitis and tenosynovitis generally occur simultaneously. The synovial-lined tendon sheath is usually the site of maximal inflammation.

Inflammation of a sheath of a tendon is a relatively common problem. For the most part, only long tendons have sheaths. Tenosynovitis most often occurs from exercise, especially when a tendon has been used repetitively when the individual is not properly conditioned (see Chapter 67). Tenosynovitis also may be part of a generalized inflammatory process, such as rheumatoid arthritis, systemic lupus erythematosus, systemic sclerosis, gout, Reiter's syndrome, sarcoidosis, type II hyperlipoproteinemia, and gonococcal infections. Sometimes, tenosynovitis is the first manifestation of one of these diseases.

Tenosynovitis often affects the dorsal extensor tendons of the wrist. It is manifest most commonly by pain that is intensified with hand extension. In the acute stage, swelling and pain over the dorsal aspect of the wrist or over the dorsal radioulnar joint may occur. Occasionally, a friction rub is felt and/or heard when the appropriate muscle is contracted.

When tenosynovitis is identified in the absence of trauma, a systemic disease should be suspected, and if present, therapy for that disease is obviously important. Gonorrhea, especially, should be suspected in sexually active individuals, if inflammation involves the tendons of the ankle or wrist. This should be suspected in the setting of a monoarthritis, fever, and skin rash. Using Transgrow media, culture of the endocervical canal and rectum in women and of the urethra in men is indicated (see Chapters 27 and 94).

If the tenosynovitis has developed because of trauma, such as exercise, or because of unknown reasons, nonspecific therapy, as for bursitis (Table 66.3), is appropriate. The fingers should be splinted in the position of function (see Chapter 67, Figure 67.17). If symptoms persist after 3 or 4 days of conservative therapy, the peritenon (loose tissue surrounding the tendon) should be injected with Xy-locaine and a corticosteroid (such as Aristocort or Kenalog) after the tendon is outlined with an indelible pen (Table 66.4). Occasionally, symptoms are recurrent, in which case referral to a rheumatologist or orthopaedist is indicated.

Tenosynovitis and tendinitis are also discussed in Chapters 63 (Shoulder Pain), 67 (Exercise-Related Musculoskeletal Problems) and 102 (Common Problems of the Feet).

STENOSING TENOSYNOVITIS

Stenosing tenosynovitis is not a complication of tenosynovitis; rather, it occurs primarily when trauma is severe and localized. In stenosing tenosynovitis either a nodule forms on a tendon or an actual stenosis of a tendon sheath of a long tendon develops. This results in the affected part "sticking" in a position. The patient is unable to flex a digit fully or else, once it is flexed, the digit locks and literally must be straightened by external force until it suddenly snaps free. When stenosing tenosynovitis is present in the abductor or extensor tendon of the thumb, it is called De Quervain's disease, the most common form of stenosing tenosynovitis. Stenosing tenosynovitis is caused by repeated trauma, but it is occasionally seen in association with rheumatoid arthritis, amyloidosis, pregnancy, and myxedema.

The treatment is identical to that of bursitis as outlined in Tables 66.3 and 66.4. If the patient resists several weeks of conservative therapy, surgical release may be necessary. When a nodule is palpated, it should be injected with a small amount of corticosteroid (such as 10 to 20 mg of Aristocort or Kenalog) with a small amount of Xylocaine and, frequently, it will resolve in several weeks (15).

TRIGGER FINGER

Repeated trauma of the flexor tendon (or its sheath), especially of the middle or ring finger or thumb, results in thickening and nodule formation. This results in the impediment of movement of the tendon through its sheath. Most often this impingement is near the metacarpal head and results in the tendon snapping and even locking as it flexes. If patient function is interfered with, corticosteroid injection (see Table 66.4) into the tendon sheath may relieve the problem. If injection therapy is not successful, or if the physician is unfamiliar with the technique, the patient should be referred to an orthopaedic surgeon. Surgical release of the tendon sheath may be necessary.

DUPUYTREN'S CONTRACTURE

The palmar fascia may undergo nodular, hypertrophic degeneration of unknown cause. This results over many years in the ultimate development of a flexion contracture (Dupuytren's contracture). The process causes the skin to be fixed to the underlying fascia by adhesive bands, resulting in a fixed, puckered appearance. A Dupuytren's contracture is almost always painless but may result in significant functional disability. Although all digits may be involved, the little and ring fingers are affected most commonly. The condition primarily affects middle-aged or older men and, in nearly 40%, it is bilateral. Once the condition is present, passive extension of the fingers does not retard the process; in fact, it may accelerate it. If functional disability is present, the patient should be referred to an orthopaedic surgeon for consideration for injection therapy or surgery. Oral anti-inflammatory agents are not effective in retarding the process.

FIBROSITIS

Fibrositis is a form of nonarticular rheumatism characterized by chronic aches, pain, and stiffness in muscles, ligaments, tendon insertions, and subcutaneous tissues accompanied by increased tenderness at specific anatomic sites known as *tender points*. It is a clinical and not a pathological diagnosis. The recognition and management of fibrositis as a distinct entity is important because of its high prevalence (20 to 30% of patients referred to a rheumatologist) (16) and because of the conditions with which it may be confused. The syndrome is considered *primary* when no known cause or associated disorder is present. *Secondary* fibrositis includes rheumatic and nonrheumatic conditions that have some of the same clinical features seen in the primary group. Some of the secondary forms include osteoarthritis, rheumatoid arthritis, various connective tissue diseases (polymyositis, polymyalgia rheumatica, systemic lupus erythematosus) and nonrheumatic disorders, such as chronic infections, hypothyroidism, and malignancy (Table 66.5).

Manifestations

The cardinal features of fibrositis are widespread soft tissue aching and stiffness in the cervical and lumbar spine of more than 3 months' duration that is aggravated by fatigue, tension, excessive work activity, immobilization, and changes in the weather. The condition primarily affects young and middle-age-women. The stiffness occurs more diffusely than in specific joint areas, which differs from the pattern of morning stiffness in rheumatoid arthritis. Essential to the diagnosis of fibrositis are the presence of at least *four tender points*, defined as areas of permanent localized tenderness elicited on firm palpation of specific anatomical sites (11). The most common sites of tender points are shown in Figure 66.1. They are the midpoint of the upper fold in the trapezius muscle, the second costochondral junction, lateral epicondyles, supraspinatus muscle

Table 66.5.
Causes of Secondary Fibrositis[a]

CONNECTIVE TISSUE DISEASE
  Any may be associated with this syndrome but is more common with rheumatoid arthritis
SKIN DISEASE
  Erythema nodosum, psoriasis
INFECTION
  Syphilis, tuberculosis, brucellosis, streptococcal infections, bacterial endocarditis, gonorrhea, rubella, and viral hepatitis
ENDOCRINE
  Hypothyroidism, hyperparathyroidism
MALIGNANT DISEASE
DRUG REACTION
  Hypersensitivity vasculitis and drug-induced lupus
INFLAMMATORY BOWEL DISEASE
SARCOIDOSIS

[a] Adapted from Beetham WP: Diagnosis and management of fibrositis syndrome and psychogenic rheumatism. *Med Clin North Am* 63:422, 1979.

near the medial border, over the lower cervical and lower lumbar spine, and the medial fat pad proximal to the joint line overlying the collateral ligament of the knee. Patients often complain of swelling in the hands and fingers, although there is no objective evidence noted by the physician. Patients may also complain of numbness, usually in a nonradicular distribution and in the setting of a normal neurological examination. A frequent finding in these patients is sleep disturbance. Characteristically the patient feels more tired in the morning than prior to going to bed the night before. It has been noted that nonrapid eye movement sleep is disturbed and that deep sleep (stage 4 sleep) is never entered (7). Other findings in these patients are headaches, symptoms of irritable bowel syndrome, and anxiety. Symptoms generally persist for years unless treatment is given (see below).

A complete physical examination should be performed, as other conditions must be excluded before the diagnosis of fibrositis is made. Careful examination of the joints, blood vessels, and muscles should be done to exclude inflammatory diseases such as rheumatoid arthritis and polymyositis. Other conditions such as osteoarthritis, polymyalgia rheumatica, hypothyroidism, malignancy, and infections (viral, and endocarditis, toxoplasmosis) should be carefully considered (see above). It should be emphasized that tender points are always tender in patients with fibrositis, even during periods of remission. Therefore, the physician must be experienced in evaluating the degree of tenderness at characteristic sites using palpation in individuals without musculoskeletal symptoms. Palpation of the tender points may elicit the characteristic *jump sign*, which is the recoil of the patient out of proportion to the amount of pressure exerted by the physician.

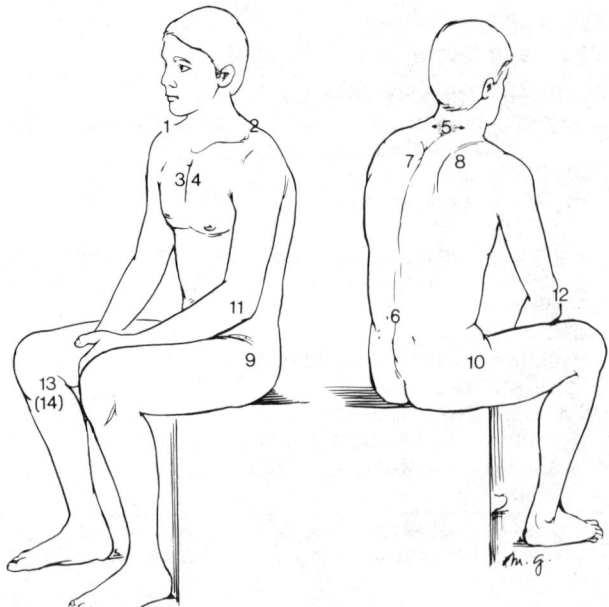

Figure 66.1. The more common tender points of fibrositis. *1, 2,* midpoint of upper fold of trapezius muscle; *3, 4,* second costochondral junction most often on the superior surface (occasionally there is also tenderness of more inferior costochondral junctions); *5,* area immediately anterior to the trapezius muscle, on the right and left sides; *6,* along the L4-S1 interspinous ligaments; *7, 8,* at the origin of the supraspinatus muscle near the medial border of the scapula; *9, 10,* in the upper and outer quadrant of the buttocks; *11, 12,* the tennis elbow site at the lateral epicondyle just distal to the radial head; *13, 14,* over the medial collateral ligament of the knee, proximal to the joint line and anterior to the semimembranosus and semitendinosus tendons; the medial fat pad.

The physician should note: (a) It is important to apply deep firm pressure when examining these trigger sites; (b) these areas, except site 6, are often somewhat tender to deep firm pressure in normal individuals; the discomfort is extreme in patients with fibrositis; and (c) the areas of tenderness are reproducible and very defined; pressure applied 1 or 2 cm away, except at site 5, does not produce discomfort. (Adapted from Smythe HA, Moldofsky H: Two contributions to understanding of the fibrositis syndrome. *Bull Rheum Dis* 28:928, 1977.)

Laboratory tests that should be performed include complete blood counts and measurement of erythrocyte sedimentation rate, serum proteins, muscle enzymes, and antinuclear and rheumatoid factor determinations. Thyroid function tests are appropriate if there is a suspicion of hypothyroidism (see Chapter 73). By definition, these studies are normal in patients with fibrositis, and therefore any abnormalities should warrant a further search for an underlying disease.

Treatment should begin with reassurance and a clear explanation of the nature of illness. Proper support for the neck (see Chapter 64) and back areas helps to reduce the pain these patients experience. Physical therapy with mobilizing exercises as prescribed by a physical therapist should be part of the regimen of every patient with fibrositis. Local heat and ultrasound are also useful. Stretching exercises (see Chapter 67) are advised to keep the muscles supple as well as for posture correction and abdominal support. Although rest and relaxation are important for many of these patients to relieve tension, it is equally important for the patient to be mentally and physically active to avoid fixation on his symptoms.

Amitriptyline (Elavil) or Doxepin (Sinequan) at bedtime is helpful for the sleep disorder. The dosage may be gradually increased from 25 to 100 mg until restful sleep is achieved. These drugs act slowly and are best taken in the early evening rather than at bedtime to give effects lasting throughout the night.

Aspirin may be useful to control symptoms when prescribed in anti-inflammatory doses (see Chapter 70, Rheumatoid Arthritis). Other nonsteroidal anti-inflammatory drugs, such as Motrin, Naprosyn, Indocin, and Clinoril, are useful and should be tried if adequate doses of aspirin are not taken or, if taken, fail to provide sufficient relief or are not well tolerated. Injection of tender points with a local anesthetic, such as Xylocaine, and with corticosteroids often will provide temporary relief, but a rheumatologist should be consulted about this as one injection may lead to the request by the patient for frequent injections. The efficacy of systemic corticosteroids has not been studied in a controlled fashion, and therefore these drugs are not recommended (1).

RAYNAUD'S PHENOMENON

Raynaud's phenomenon is a syndrome characterized by episodic vasospasm of the digital vessels in response to cold or emotional stress. Classically, a triphasic response occurs: first cutaneous pallor, extending from the fingertips to the midfingers; then mottling of the skin and cyanosis rapidly follows as a consequence of venous blood refluxing back into an empty cutaneous capillary bed (this pallor and/or cyanosis persists until rewarming of the digits); finally the recovery phase occurs over 15 to 20 minutes, resulting in intense hyperemia. Vasospasm is usually triggered by an abrupt change of environmental temperature, and, therefore, it may occur even in the summer months when a patient moves into air-conditioned or refrigerated areas. One or two digits may have more intense vasospasm, but generally the episodes are bilateral and symmetrical. Also, the feet and other acral parts (such as the ears or nose) may be involved. Patients often do not describe spontaneously the classical phases of Raynaud's phenomenon, but do commonly note deep cyanosis associated with numbness, a pins and needles sensation, or frank pain on cold exposure.

Raynaud's phenomenon may occur secondary to a defined vascular abnormality or in association with a specific disease process (Table 66.6). It occurs most commonly in an idiopathic or primary form, *Raynaud's disease*, in which no underlying abnormality can be defined. Primary Raynaud's phenomenon is thought to be quite common, occurring principally in women age 20 to 30 years. The true prevalence of Raynaud's phenomenon is unknown, but it has been estimated to be 6% of the general population and up to 20% of the selective population of young women (8). Patients with primary Raynaud's phenomenon are otherwise healthy, generally have relatively infrequent attacks (one to four episodes weekly), and rarely develop local cutaneous complications, such as digital pitting, ulcerations, or loss of hand function. Patients with primary Raynaud's phenomenon usually have an uncomplicated course

Table 66.6.
Classification of Raynaud's Phenomenon

		Percentage of Patients with Stated Disorder Who Also Have Raynaud's Phenomenon
A. Primary: Idiopathic Raynaud's, Raynaud's disease		
B. Secondary: Disorders associated with Raynaud's phenomenon		
1. *Connective tissue diseases*		
a. Systemic sclerosis		90
b. Systemic lupus erythematosus		20
c. "Mixed" connective tissue disease"		75
d. Dermatomyositis/polymyositis		20
e. Rheumatoid arthritis		10
2. *Neurovascular compression*		
a. Thoracic outlet syndrome (*e.g.*, cervical ribs, scalenus anticus syndrome)		
b. Carpal tunnel syndrome		
3. *Arterial disease*		
a. Arteriosclerosis		
b. Arteritis (thromboangiitis obliterans)		
4. *Hematological Disorders*		
a. Paraproteinemia		
b. Cryoglobulinemia		
c. Polycythemia		
d. Hyperviscosity syndrome		
5. *Occupational*		
a. Vibratory tools (white finger syntrome)		
b. Polyvinyl chloride exposure		
6. *Drugs*		
a. Ergot-containing drugs (such as ergotamine)		
b. β-Adrenergic blockers		
c. Sympathomimetic agents (such as Actifed)		
d. Methysergide (Sansert)		
7. *Miscellaneous*		
a. Primary pulmonary hypertension		30
b. Migraine headache		10

with gradual improvement over a number of years in the frequency of episodes. Estimates suggest that 8 to 13% of patients felt initially to have the primary form will in time develop a defined secondary form (usually a connective tissue disease) (14).

When patients present with Raynaud's phenomenon to a general physician, approximately 40% will have a defined secondary cause, the most common being a connective tissue disease (Table 66.6). Raynaud's phenomenon occurs in greater than 90% of patients with *systemic sclerosis* and may be the initial symptom, preceding the other features of the disease by years. Approximately 40% of patients with *systemic lupus erythematosus* and 20% of patients with *rheumatoid arthritis* may also have associated Raynaud's phenomenon. Raynaud's phenomenon may be a presenting feature in patients who have a *systemic vasculitis*. Disturbances of the axillary or cervical neurovascular bundle also can lead to Raynaud's phenomenon. Approximately 20% of patients with *neurovascular compression syndromes* (cervical rib, scalenus anticus syndrome) and *proximal vascular lesions* (atherosclerosis) may present with unilateral Raynaud's phenomenon. *Hematological abnormalities*, such as cryoglobulinemia, paraproteinemia, or cold hemagglutinins, may present as typical Raynaud's phenomenon. Ergot-containing *drugs*, such as ergotamine, and β-blocking agents may be causative or potentiating agents. *Occupational injury* (vibration white finger syndrome) occurs in a high proportion of workers operating vibratory tools (such as lumberjacks, shipyard workers, or meat cutters).

It may be difficult to determine if a patient has a primary or secondary form of Raynaud's phenomenon when he initially presents to a physician; however, there are certain clues which should suggest a secondary form. Raynaud's phenomenon in children, males, or in women over age 30 is more likely to be a secondary form. Likewise, involvement limited to a single digit, vasospasm extending past the proximal interphalangeal joint, or unilateral Raynaud's are more commonly associated with a secondary defined vascular occlusive lesion. Patients with signs or symptoms of another disease are likely to have a secondary form of Raynaud's phenomenon, especially if symptoms of a connective disease are present, such a myalgia, arthralgia, or unexplained fever.

Every patient presenting with Raynaud's phenomenon should have a complete history (including a drug review) and physical examination looking for underlying disease. An extension of the examination, evaluation of the nailbed with an ophthalmoscope, may reveal small telangiectasia or abnormal cutaneous capillary loops; these small vessel changes may be the earliest findings in an associated underlying connective tissue disease, primarily scleroderma. The presence of ulcers on the digits should alert the physician that the Raynaud's is very severe and that the patient is very likely to have a secondary form of Raynaud's phenomenon. Patients with unilateral Raynaud's phenomenon should be carefully evaluated for a local vascular lesion, including bilateral blood pressure determination, auscultation over major vessels to determine the presence or absence or vascular bruits, and assessment of the peripheral pulses. Special testing for possible neurovascular compression syndrome (see Chapter 63) and consideration for chest X-ray and a noninvasive evaluation of the peripheral circulation (Doppler studies or digital plethysmography studies) is appropriate. Angiography may be necessary in cases in which a correctable occlusive vascular lesion is strongly suspected. Carpal tunnel syndrome has been implicated both in unilateral and bilateral Raynaud's phenomenon, and nerve conduction studies may be appropriate when a nerve compression syndrome is suspected (see Chapter 84).

Patients with typical symmetrical Raynaud's phenomenon should have, even in the absence of a suspicion of an underlying disorder, a complete blood count, Westergren sedimentation rate, urinalysis, antinuclear antibody (ANA) screen, cryoglobulins, and serum protein determination. Other studies may be initiated on an individual basis depending on the history, the physical findings, or the results of the screening studies (see above). Patients with a positive ANA are more likely to develop a clinically active connective tissue disease. Even when an associated illness is not identified, the patient should be followed carefully because an underlying illness might not manifest fully for 5 to 10 years (see above).

The principal mode of *treatment* in those cases in which a correctable cause cannot be found is *avoidance of the cold*. This includes protection of the hands and feet with mittens or gloves and avoiding a general chill of the body by wearing a hat and loose-fitting warm clothing in winter months. *Smoking* has been shown to aggravate Raynaud's phenomenon and should be stopped (4). *Emotional stress* should be assessed and controlled by appropriate measures (see Chapter 13). Patients with mild Raynaud's phenomenon often improve with education as to the cause and nature of these episodes. *Biofeedback* therapy usually offered by behavioral psychologists is available in some communities and may provide partial benefit in patients with mild primary Raynaud's phenomenon. The nonpharmacological management of patients with Raynaud's phenomenon is summarized in Table 66.7. The majority of patients, particularly those with primary Raynaud's phenomenon, do not need and should not be treated with drugs. Rather, pharmacological treatment should be limited to patients with repeated attacks which either limit their daily activities or have significant loss of nutritional blood flow such that

Table 66.7.
Management of Patients with Raynaud's Phenomenon

Education and reassurance
  Establish precipitating factors (such as refrigerator/freezer, air conditioning, emotional stress).
  Provide emotional support, *e.g.*, assurance of the mild nature of the disease in most patients may reduce some of stress that can precipitate attacks.
Avoidance of precipitating factors
  Wear gloves before reaching into refrigerator or freezer.
  Warm body clothing to avoid cold exposure when dressing.
  Keep head covered to avoid heat loss.
  Keep extremities warm and body well covered in cool weather or in air-conditioned environments.
  Be aware that stress can cause Raynaud's attacks.
  Move to a warmer climate (when feasible).
Avoidance of certain drugs which precipitate attacks
  β-Blockers (such as propranolol)
  Ergot-containing drugs (*i.e.*, ergotamine)
  Sympathomimetric agents (such as isoproterenol, Actifed, or other cold remedies)
  Nicotine (smoking)
  Oral contraceptives

skin breakdown or ulceration may occur. There is no evidence that decreasing the number of episodes of Raynaud's phenomenon will alter the progressive changes that may occur in patients with scleroderma or another connective tissue disease.

A wide variety of vasoactive agents have been used in patients with Raynaud's phenomenon, but few agents have been proven of definite benefit. The physician should remember that many of these patients are young women who have the potential of childbearing; therefore, unproven treatment which may have a teratogenic effect should be avoided.

The calcium channel blockers, nifedipine and diltiazem, but not verapamil, have been demonstrated to be effective in several prospective, controlled, and double-blind studies (9). These agents relax smooth muscle, reduce peripheral vascular resistance, and increase peripheral blood flow. Patients with primary Raynaud's tend to respond better than do patients with Raynaud's phenomenon secondary to a connective tissue disease, especially scleroderma. The major side effects of these agents are secondary to their vasodilatory activity and include hypotension, dizziness, headache, and peripheral edema. Approximately 40 to 50% of patients will experience some light-headedness and flushing on initiation of the calcium channel blockers; however, these side effects are usually transient, lasting 1 to 2 days, and do not require the discontinuation of the medication. Calcium channel blockers should never be used during pregnancy or in a patient planning to become pregnant, because they have been shown in animal models to be teratogenic.

The calcium channel blocker that has been more

extensively studied and the drug of first choice is nifedipine (Procardia, 10-mg capsules). The initial dose should be 10 mg orally given while the patient is in the physician's office. Sitting and standing blood pressures and pulse should be monitored in 15-minute intervals for 30 to 45 minutes. If the patient does not experience any significant adverse effects (a decrease in systolic pressure of 20 mm or greater below baseline, or a fall below 90 mm Hg) then Procardia may be prescribed at a dose of 10 mg orally three times daily. The patient should be encouraged to assume his usual activities and to keep a diary of the number and intensity of his Raynaud's phenomenon. The dose then may be increased every 3 to 4 days by 10 mg to a maximum of 30 mg three times daily or until good control is achieved. Once an effective dose has been achieved, monitoring every 2 to 4 months is important since the initial response may be transient and side effects may limit the usefulness of the drug. If nifedipine fails or is not tolerated, diltiazem (Cardizem, 30- and 60-mg tablets) at a dose of 30 mg four times a day may be tried as an alternative calcium channel blocker. The dose may be advanced by 30 mg/day every 3 to 4 days until the symptoms improve or a maximum of 60 mg four times a day is reached. Patients generally have resolution or a dramatic reduction in the intensity and number of episodes of Raynaud's phenomenon in the summer months. For this reason, medication should be discontinued unless repeated cold exposure or active Raynaud's phenomenon is documented.

Other drugs which are used for the treatment of Raynaud's are prazosin (Minipress), reserpine, phenoxybenzamine (Dibenzyline), and guanethidine (Ismelin). These agents have been generally disappointing with both unproven long term control and intolerable side effects (orthostatic hypotension, reflex tachycardia, impotency, lassitude), and therefore they are not recommended. Topical nitroglycerin paste applied to the digits has been used with some success, but its indications are not established and consultation with a rheumatologist is suggested before prescribing it. Research is now active in determining whether prostaglandins (PGE, prostacyclin) or a serotonin inhibitor (Kentaserin) are helpful in the treatment of Raynaud's phenomenon.

Surgical sympathectomy was once popular for the treatment of Raynaud's phenomenon but is now infrequently performed, primarily because of the high relapse rate (40 to 50%) and frequency of significant posturdal hypotension (3). Selective digital sympathectomy may be done in centers where microsurgery is available; however, long term controlled studies of this procedure are lacking. Sympathectomy should only be considered for short term relief from an intractable course complicated by digital ulceration which has failed medical treatment. All patients who have had such a severe course or who have ulcers on their digits should be seen in consultation by a vascular surgeon and/or a rheumatologist. Local digital block performed by a vascular surgeon or rheumatologist has been used for temporary treatment of patients with significant digital tissue compromise; also a good response may predict which patient may have a good effect from digital or cervical sympathectomy. A patient who has severe disease with digital ulcers is susceptible to developing secondary soft tissue infection. Local debridement and antimicrobial treatment may be necessary if ischemic ulcerations become infected. Whirlpool treatment is the most effective method of ulcer debridement. In instances of secondary complications, consultation with a vascular surgeon and/or a rheumatologist is advised.

General References

Coffman J, Davies WT: Vasospastic disease: a review. *Prog Cardiovasc Dis* 18:123, 1975.
    A review of all nonspastic diseases including Raynaud's phenomenon.
Owen DS Jr: Aspiration on injection of joint and soft Tissues In Kelley WN, Harris EDD, Ruddy S, Sledge CB (eds): *Textbook of Rheumatology*, ed 2. Philadelphia, WB Saunders, 1985.
Schumacher HR: Synovial fluid analysis In Kelley WN, Harris EDD, Ruddy S, Sledge CB (eds): *Textbook of Rheumatology*, ed 2. Philadelphia, WB Saunders, 1985.
    These three chapters provide a comprehensive review of these important subjects.
Smythe H: Fibrositis and other diffuse musculoskeletal syndromes In Kelley WN, Harris EDD, Ruddy S, Sledge CB (eds): *Textbook of Rheumatology*, ed 2. Philadelphia, WB Saunders, 1985.
Spencer-Green G. Raynaud's phenomenon. *Bull Rheum Dis* 33:1, 1983.
    A well referenced review.

Specific References

1. Beetham WP: Diagnosis and management of fibrositis syndrome and psychogenic rheumatism. *Med Clin North Am* 63:433, 1979.
2. Bywaters EGL: Tendinitis and bursitis. *Clin Rheum Dis* 5:883, 1979.
3. Buddeley RM: The place of upper dorsal sympathectomy in the treatment of primary Raynaud's disease. *Br J Surg* 52:426, 1965.
4. Coffman JD: The attenuation by reserpine or guanethidine of the cutaneous vasoconstriction caused by tobacco smoking. *Am Heart J* 74:229, 1967.
5. Doppman JL: Baker's cyst and normal gastrocnemius-semimembranosus bursa. *AJR* 94:646, 1965.
6. Ho G, Tice AD, Kaplan SR: Septic bursitis. *Ann Intern Med* 89:21, 1978.
7. Moldofsky H, Searisfrick P, England R, *et al*: Musculoskeletal symptoms and non-REM sleep disturbance in patients with "fibrositic" syndromes and healthy subjects. *Psychosom Med* 37:341, 1975.
8. Olsen N, Nielsen SL: Prevalence of primary Raynaud's phenomenon in young females. *Scan J Clin Lab Invest* 37:761, 1978.
9. Rodeheffer RJ, Rammer JA, Wigley F, Smith CR: Controlled double-blind trial of nifedipine in the treatment of Raynaud's phenomenon. *N Engl J Med* 303:880, 1983.
10. Simonelli C, Zoschke D, Bakhurst A, Messner R: Septic bursitis. *Ann Intern Med* 98:975, 1978.
11. Smythe HA, Moldofsky H: Two contributions to understanding of the fibrostis syndrome. *Bull Rheum Dis* 28:928, 1977.

12. Spear IM, Lipscomb PR: Noninfectious trochanteric bursitis and peritendinitis. *Surg Clin North Am* 32:1217, 1952.

13. Swarbout R, Compere E: Ischiogluteal bursitis—the pain in the arse. *JAMA* 227:551, 1974.

14. Velogos E, Robinson H, Porcluncula F, Masi A: Clinical correlation analysis of 137 patients with Raynaud's phenome-

non. *Am J Med Sci* 262:347, 1971.

15. Younghusland DZ, Black JD: De Quervain disease. *Can Med Assoc J* 89:508, 1963.

16. Yunus M, Masi A, Calabro J, *et al*: Primary fibromyalgia (fibrositis): clinical study of 50 patients with matched normal controls. *Semin Arthritis Rheum* 11:151, 1981.

CHAPTER SIXTY-SEVEN

Exercise-Related Musculoskeletal Problems

RONALD P. BYANK, M.D.

Activities such as jogging, marathon running, golf, tennis, softball, bowling, and many others are an integral part of the lives of millions of Americans.* Consequently, physicians are contacted frequently by patients with exercise-related problems. This chapter describes for a number of common exercise-related syndromes the mechanism of injury, the usual signs and symptoms, the treatment, the indications for referral, and the methods of preventing recurrences of the problem. Most of the injuries associated with exercise may also occur in nonexercising individuals who suffer mechanical stress due to falls, missteps into depressions, *etc.* Evaluation and management are similar for exercising and nonexercising persons with these injuries.

KNEE STRUCTURE AND FUNCTION
(Fig. 67.1, *A* and *B*)

The knee is the largest joint in the body. It has both hinge-like motion and rotatory motion (of the tibia on the femur) during flexion and extension. The principal components of the knee and their functions are the following:

1. *Three articulations* which have a common articular cavity: The lateral and medial tibiofemoral articulations each of which has an important cartilaginous buffer, the lateral and medial *menisci*, and the patellofemoral articulation.

2. *The muscles* which control the motion of the

---

* See Chapter 58 for a discussion of physical conditioning from the standpoint of the cardiovascular system.

knee: *Flexors*—the hamstring muscles, which arise from the ischium and the gastrocnemius, which arises from the femur and diverge to form tendons which insert into the tibia and the fibula; and *extensors*—the quadriceps muscles, which originate at the ilium and the femur and converge distally as the common quadriceps tendon which attaches to the superior aspect of the patella.

3. *The external ligaments:* The patellar tendon, a continuation of the common tendon of the quadriceps that joins the patella to the tibial tuberosity and makes possible extension of the knee joint; and the collateral ligaments which gave stability to the joint—the lateral connects the lateral femoral condyle to the fibula, and the medial connects the medial femoral condyle to the medial condyle and surface of the tibia.

4. *The cruciate ligaments*, which are located inside the joint and stabilize the joint in the anteroposterior plane: the anterior cruciate ligament, which is attached anteriorly to the intercondylar eminence of the tibia and posterosuperiorly to the lateral femoral condyle; and the posterior cruciate ligament, which is attached posteriorly to the posterior intercondylar fossa of the tibia and to the lateral meniscus and anterosuperiorly to the medial femoral condyle.

5. *The bursae of the knee*, which provide lubrication between the many dynamic components of the knee.

KNEE INJURIES: GENERAL EVALUATION

Traumatic knee injury may be caused by a single event in which the knee is suddenly stressed or by chronic, repetitive stress. When there is no history of sudden trauma, two features are especially helpful in evaluating knee pain: (a) identification of any recently initiated physical activities; and (b) identification of problems elsewhere in the lower extremity which may cause inappropriate stresses upon the structure of the knee (e.g., excessive pronation of the feet, see Chapter 102). When there is no clear-cut history of trauma and physical examination does not indicate injury to one or more anatomical structures, conditions which may cause spontaneous knee pain should be considered (see Chapter 66, Nonarticular Rheumatism; Chapter 68, Degenerative Joint Disease; Chapter 69, Crystal-Induced Arthritis; Chapter 70, Rheumatoid Arthritis).

Knee pain may be due to injury to any one of the structures described above. Except when there is a large effusion, the structure(s) accounting for pain can usually be identified by systematic examination. Focal tenderness to palpation is present when pain is due to bursitis or to ligament, meniscus, or muscle injury. Specific tests for meniscal injury, ligament injury, and patellofemoral arthralgia are described below.

Examination for a small or moderate *knee joint effusion* is done in one of two ways:

1. By inspection, with the patient seated and both knees flexed 90°; if there is an effusion in the symptomatic knee, there will be a bulge on either side of the patellar ligament which is not seen in the normal knee.

2. By ballottement (Figure 67.2), with the patient supine and the knee fully extended; the knee is compressed above and on either side of the patella, in order to localize any fluid under the patella, then the patella is compressed with an examining finger to determine whether it is ballotable.

PROBLEMS OF THE KNEE

Meniscal and Ligament Injuries

Definition and Mechanism of Injury

Tears of the medial or lateral meniscus (a disc-shaped fibrous cartilage) of the knee are common. When a rotary force is applied to the flexed knee joint, the meniscus is trapped between the femur and the tibia; then when the knee is extended, the cartilage may be torn (5). Tears of the medial meniscus are about 10 times as common as those of the lateral meniscus. This problem is encountered, especially, in individuals who play football, basketball, and lacrosse as well as in persons who are bowlers, golfers, or baseball players.

Sprains or tears of the collateral ligaments and the cruciate ligaments are caused by a combination of angulating forces at the knee with rotational forces which cause rotation of the leg at the knee. Those forces which most frequently cause ligament injuries are forces which produce abduction of the leg at the knee (e.g., a direct blow to the lateral aspect of the leg on the playing field). In these injuries, the order of vulnerability to damage is as follows: medial collateral ligament, anterior cruciate ligament, posterior cruciate ligament, and lateral collateral ligament.

Symptoms and Signs

Meniscus injury. The patient with a meniscus injury usually describes a twisting flexion injury of the knee followed by pain, and inability to flex the knee fully or to bear weight. Examination usually reveals knee joint effusion and tenderness over the joint line, either medially (medial meniscus injury) or laterally (lateral meniscus injury). Sometimes the onset is insidious and the patient notes episodes of knee effusion or of clicking or locking of the knee (which may last for several minutes or several hours). Examination of patients who suffer from this more chronic condition often reveals only minimal joint line tenderness. Certain maneuvers are helpful in the diagnosis of meniscal injury; they are more likely to be diagnostic in patients with acute symp-

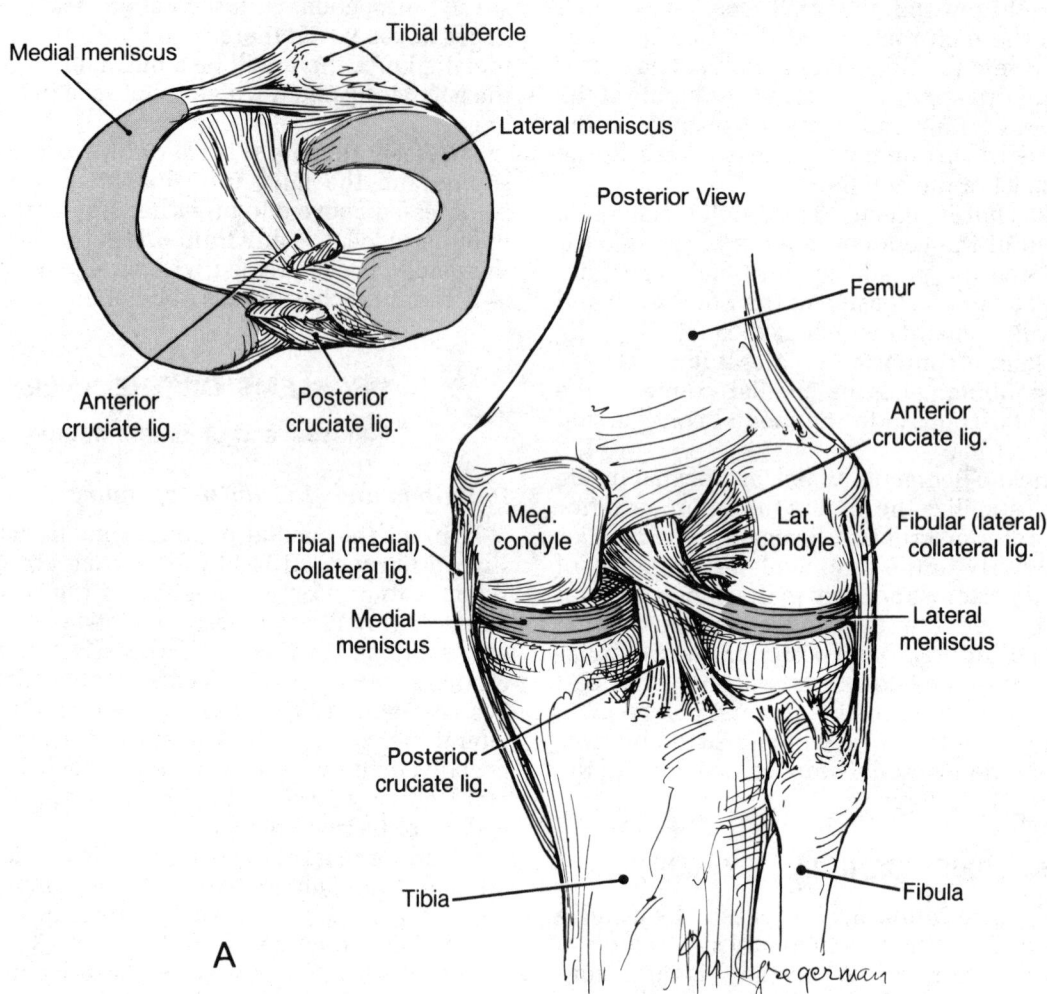

Superior View

Medial meniscus

Tibial tubercle

Lateral meniscus

Posterior View

Anterior
cruciate lig.

Posterior
cruciate lig.

Femur

Anterior
cruciate lig.

Med.
condyle

Lat.
condyle

Fibular (lateral)
collateral lig.

Tibial (medial)
collateral lig.

Medial
meniscus

Lateral
meniscus

Posterior
cruciate lig.

Tibia

Fibula

A

Figure 67.1.   *A.* Important structures of the knee.

toms than in patients with chronic symptoms. The *McMurray test* is performed with the patient lying supine with the hip and knee fully flexed and the foot rotated outward to its full capacity to test the medial meniscus and inward to test the lateral meniscus (Fig. 67.3A). The knee is extended with the foot at first rotated out and again with it rotated in and a painful click in the knee indicates a positive test. Not all meniscal tears will result in a positive test. The *Apley* or grinding test is performed by flexing the knee 90° when the patient is in the prone position, and then rotating the tibia internally and externally on the femur while compressing the leg against the femur, and then repeating the rotation while pulling the leg away from the femur (Fig. 67.3B). Pain during compression may be due to a meniscal tear, and pain while pulling the leg is likely from a ligamentous injury.

Ligament Injuries

With a sprain of a ligament (usually the medial collateral ligament), the patient will describe pain at the time of injury and there will be stiffness of the knee in addition to pain, tenderness, and often fullness, over the ligament. Occasionally, there will be a serous joint effusion.

When injury to a ligament of the knee joint is suspected, the joint should be carefully evaluated for ligament instability, as illustrated in Figure 67.4. The laxity of ligaments varies tremendously between individuals; therefore, assessment of the normal knee first is important in evaluating an injured knee. The stability of the collateral ligaments should be tested with the patient supine and the knee in about 20° of flexion. Force is applied, as shown in Figure 67.4, *D* and *E*. If there is a sprain, the affected

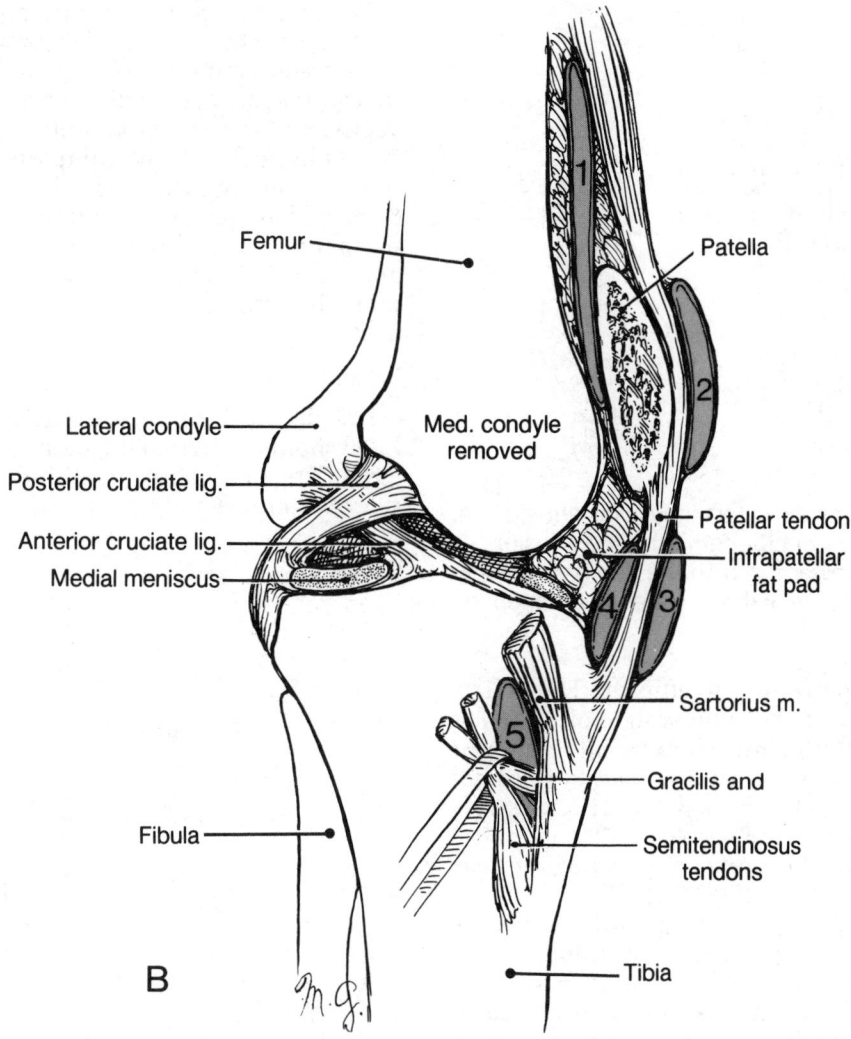

Femur

Patella

Lateral condyle

Med. condyle removed

Posterior cruciate lig.

Anterior cruciate lig.

Medial meniscus

Patellar tendon

Infrapatellar fat pad

Sartorius m.

Gracilis and

Fibula

Semitendinosus tendons

B

Tibia

Figure 67.1. *B*. Five bursae of the knee: *1*, suprapatellar; *2*, prepatellar; *3*, superficial patellar tendon; *4*, retropatellar tendon; *5*, pes anserinus.

ligament will be painful and tender, but there will be no excessive laxity to indicate that the ligament has been ruptured. The integrity of the anterior and posterior cruciate ligaments is tested with the knee flexed to 90° (see Fig. 67.4, *B* and *C*). Grasping the leg, the examiner exerts pressure posteriorly to test the posterior cruciate and then anteriorly to test the anterior cruciate. Laxity in the direction of pressure indicates a tear of the cruciate ligament being tested.

Additional Evaluation

X-rays of the knee should always be obtained to exclude other problems, such as loose bodies within the knee, osteochrondritis dissecans, fractures, or arthritis. If a large effusion is present, it should be aspirated for two reasons: first, removal of the fluid will result in relief of discomfort; and second, if a

hemarthrosis is present, it may indicate a serious injury and the patient should be referred to an orthopaedist. If referral cannot be accomplished for several days, the knee should be splinted with a knee immobilizer (see below). Aspiration of the knee joint is easily accomplished after preparing the skin with an iodine-containing solution (such as Betadine) and anesthetizing it with Xylocaine. Generally the easiest approach to aspiration is medially at the patellofemoral joint.

Treatment and Prognosis

Meniscus injuries. When a meniscus injury is diagnosed or suspected, the initial treatment consists of immobilization of the injured knee with a knee immobilizer (a rigid support available from large pharmacies or orthopaedic appliance stores). An Ace bandage is not sufficient to provide stability, al-

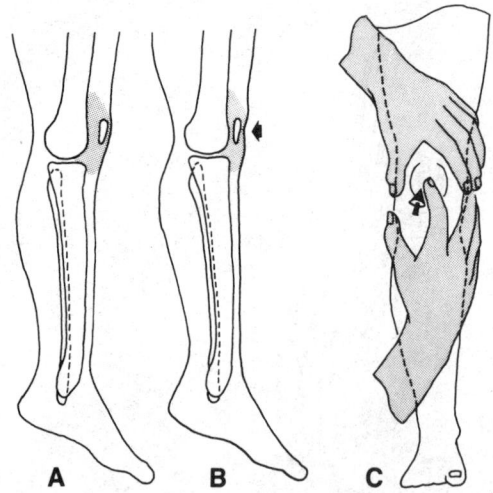

Figure 67.2. Examination for knee joint effusion. *A.* Patella forced away from the femur by the effusion. *B.* Patella forced downward into the femor ballottement maneuver. *C.* Illustration of the ballottement maneuver.

though it may help to diminish effusion. The patient should use crutches to keep his weight off the knee and should elevate the injured extremity when he lies down. Ice packs should be applied to the knee for 15 minutes several times a day to reduce swelling. Isometric quadriceps-strengthening exercises should be recommended as soon as the patient can do these comfortably (see Fig. 67.5).

Most often symptoms subside within 14 days; if symptoms resolve, the prognosis is variable. In the instance of a small tear, complete healing may occur without subsequent symptoms. On the other hand, a larger tear may result in recurrent symptoms after initial improvement. Therefore, if symptoms persist beyond 2 weeks with conservative treatment or if they recur following return to normal activity, an orthopaedic referral is indicated for consideration of an arthrogram and/or arthroscopy to establish the diagnosis. An *arthrogram* is an X-ray of the joint and requires the injection of iodinated contrast material and air into the joint space. This is done by a radiologist or orthopaedist after administration of local anesthesia. After the procedure, which generally is well tolerated, crutches should be used for 1 to 2 days, during which time only mild analgesics are usually needed. *Arthroscopy*, which may be accomplished in 30 to 45 minutes by the orthopaedist using local or general anaesthesia, involves the insertion of the arthroscope (a 2- to 4-mm diameter instrument) through a stab wound in the anterior lateral aspect of the knee. The patient usually requires crutches for 2 to 3 days and mild analgesics. If the diagnosis is confirmed, surgical excision of the torn portion of the meniscus or of the entire meniscus may be necessary and may be performed either by arthroscopic surgery or through arthrotomy.

Following surgery for a torn meniscus, the patient is often able to return to light sports activity within 6 to 8 weeks, but it may be 3 months or longer before he can resume such activities as running or tennis. A proper postoperative conditioning period of supervised physical therapy is important and will consist of strengthening the quadriceps muscles (see Fig. 67.5) and of range of motion exercises to ensure normal mobility of the knee. Joint space narrowing and arthritic change almost always follow meniscectomy, but may not limit a patient's activity significantly.

Ligament Injuries

If a ligament rupture is suspected, the patient's knee should be immobilized in a posterior splint or a rigid knee immobilizer, and the patient should be referred immediately to an orthopaedist.

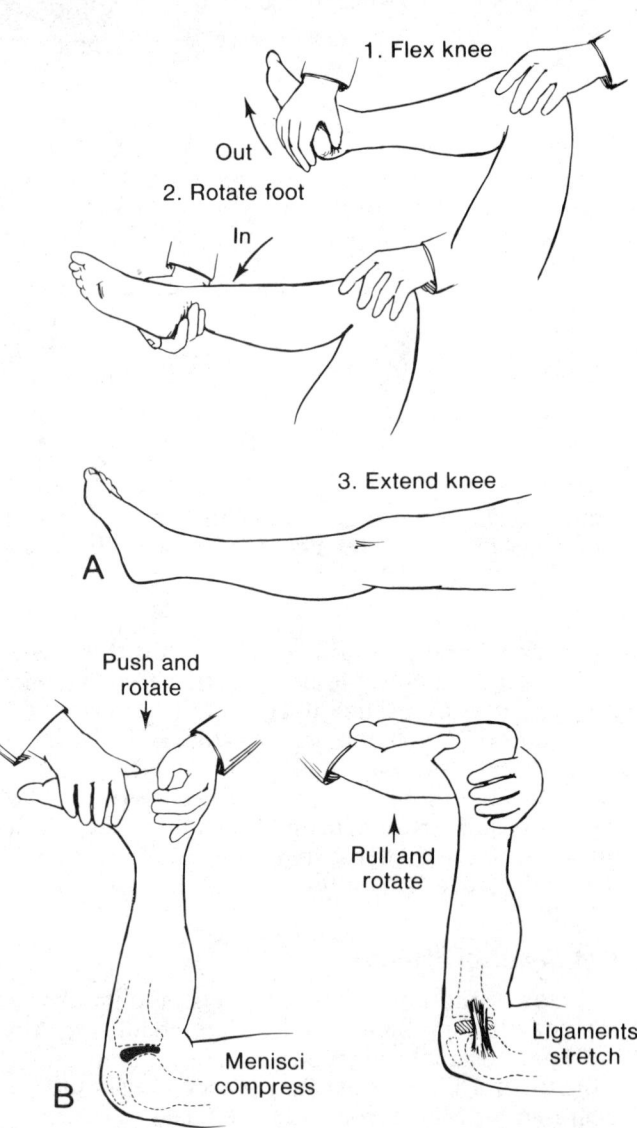

Figure 67.3. *A.* McMurray test. *B.* Apley test.

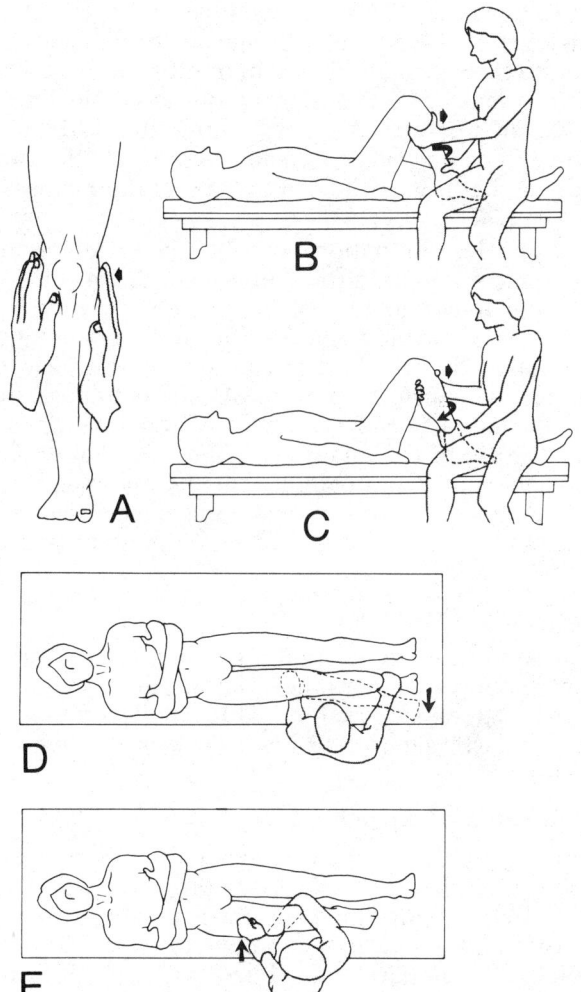

Figure 67.4. Examination for collateral and cruciate ligament injuries. *A.* Palpation for tenderness. *B.* Manipulation for laxity of posterior cruciate and posterolateral capsule. *C.* Manipulation for laxity of anterior cruciate. *D.* Manipulation for laxity of anterior cruciate and medial collateral ligament tear. *E.* Manipulation for laxity of medial collateral ligament alone. (From Ramamurti CP: *Orthopaedics in Primary Care.* Tinker RV (ed). Baltimore, Williams & Wilkins, 1979.)

If a collateral ligament sprain is diagnosed, a patient with minor symptoms can be permitted to increase his activity gradually over the succeeding 1 to 2 weeks. For more pronounced symptoms, the knee should be immobilized with a knee immobilizer, and the patient should use crutches for 5 to 10 days. Ice packs and isometric quadriceps-tensing exercises should be recommended, as for meniscus injuries. When the knee brace is removed, the patient can progressively increase his activity and should begin isotonic quadriceps exercises (see Fig. 67.5) and range of motion exercises.

Prevention

Acute meniscus injury occurs by chance when a rotational force is applied to the knee when it is in the flexed position; it cannot be prevented by conditioning. Ligamentous injuries can be prevented to some degree by proper conditioning.

Patellofemoral Arthralgia (Chondromalacia (1, 2))

Definition and Mechanism of Injury

Patellofemoral arthralgia refers to pain originating from the patellofemoral joint associated with changes in the articular cartilage of the patella. The patellar cartilage shows softening (chondromalacia), which is caused by lateral subluxation or hypermobility of the patella, usually due to an increased angle (Q-angle) between the quadriceps and patellar tendon, and by patella alta. The normal *Q-angle* is up to 20°; if it is greater than this, increased lateral displacement of the patella results (Fig. 67.6). An abnormal Q-angle is sometimes associated with excessive pronation of the feet (flat feet, see Chapter 102). *Patella alta* is an anatomical variant in which the patella rides more proximally than usual, so that

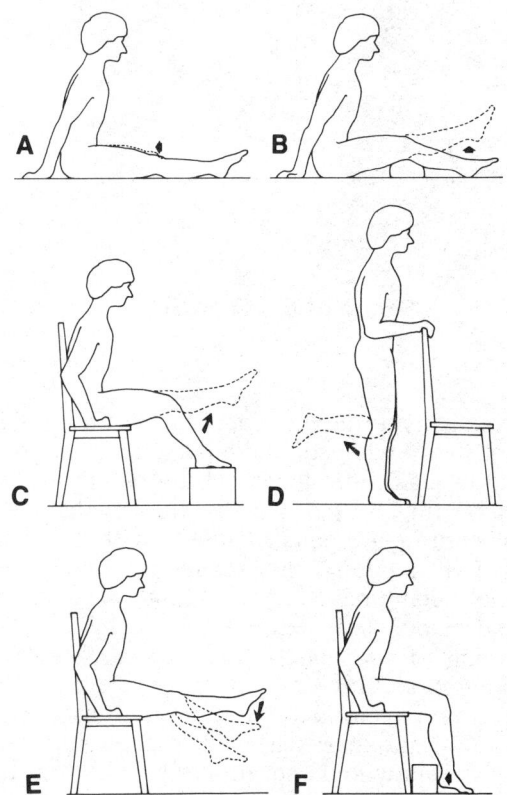

Figure 67.5. Restorative knee exercises. *A.* Isometric quadriceps exercise. *B* and *C.* Isotonic quadriceps exercises. *D,* Gravity-resisted isotonic flexion exercise. *E.* Gravity-assisted isotonic flexion exercise. *F.* Isometric flexion exercise.

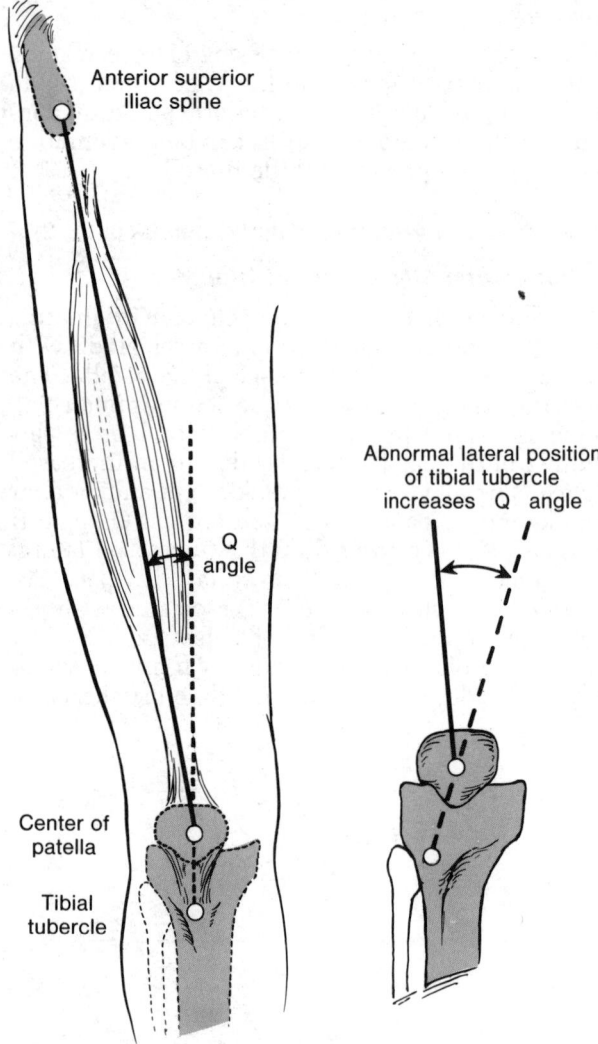

Anterior superior
iliac spine

Q
angle

Abnormal lateral position
of tibial tubercle
increases Q angle

Center of
patella

Tibial
tubercle

Figure 67.6. Q angle.

it becomes hypermobile. Patella alta can be identified on X-ray when the patellar tendon length exceeds the maximum length of the patella by more than 1 cm (Fig. 67.7). Normally, the lengths of these two structures are equal. Patients with a variation in hip joint anatomy that results in compensatory external tibial torsion (external rotation of lower leg in axial plane, slew foot) will also have lateral displacement of the patella and excess wear of the patellofemoral joint.

Chondromalacia is a very common disorder, especially in inexperienced adolescent and young adult runners who do not properly condition themselves, but accelerate their activities too rapidly.

Symptoms and Signs

Pain, usually described as a soreness or aching around or under the patella, is the hallmark of this problem. The discomfort is aggravated by running

up hills, climbing stairs, kneeling, or hyperflexing the knee. Pain frequently disappears during activity only to recur just at the end of or after activity. The patient may also complain of the knee "locking"; however, upon careful questioning, this locking is found to be only very transient and is not the true locking that is experienced in tears of the meniscus (see above).

Physical examination reveals any or all of the anatomical abnormalities described above. Patella alta and hypermobility of the patella are very frequent. Pain and/or crepitus with patellofemoral manipulation or palpation of the articular surface of the patella is usually present. Attempts to push the patella laterally may cause pain and involuntary contracture of the quadriceps, the so-called *apprehension sign*. If the patient extends his knee from 30° of flexion to full extension against resistance, pain will result. A knee effusion is frequently present.

Additional Evaluation

X-rays of the knees should be obtained routinely and should include a tangential or sunrise view to look for lateral subluxation of the patella, often with a hypoplastic lateral trochlear facet of the femoral sulcus.

Differential Diagnosis

Other problems which occasionally may be confused with chondromalacia are prepatellar bursitis (Fig. 67.1B) (pain and tenderness localized to the prepatellar bursa, see Chapter 66), retropatellar (also called infrapatellar) tendon bursitis (Fig. 67.1B) (pain and tenderness localized to the area below the patella and behind the tendon), pes anserinus bursitis (Fig. 67.1B) (pain and tenderness in the bursa that lies deep to the combined insertion of the sartorius, gracilis, and semitendinosus tendons into the prox-

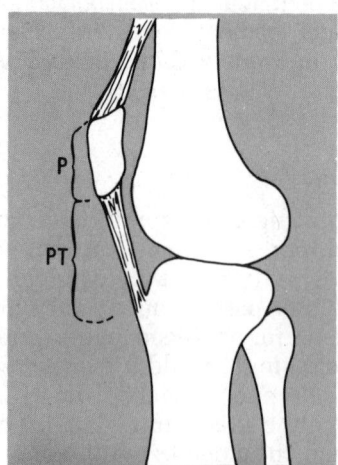

P

PT

Figure 67.7. Patella alta. *P*, patella; *PT*, patellar tendon.

imal medial tibial metaphysis), fat pad syndrome (trauma-related inflammation of the infrapatellar fat pad) (Fig. 67.1*B*), meniscal injury (see above), ligamentous instability of the knee (see above), arthritis, and osteochrondritis dissecans (necrosis within the condylar epiphysis characterized by insidious onset of knee ache at rest, worsened by weight bearing and confirmed by X-ray). Hip or pelvic disease is associated with referred pain from sciatic nerve root irritation. These problems can be differentiated by careful physical and radiological examination; if there is any doubt, referral to an orthopaedic surgeon is appropriate.

Treatment and Prognosis

Therapy is initiated as soon as possible after the appearance of symptoms. The use of crutches for up to 7 days to rest the knee is important; and the application of ice to the knee for approximately 15 minutes several times a day will help to decrease swelling. In addition, analgesic medications should be prescribed, such as aspirin, 600 mg four times a day, or Tylenol, 650 mg four times a day.

After the initial 24 hours, the application of ice may be discontinued and heat may be applied for 15 to 20 minutes several times a day. The patient should avoid vigorous sports activities until symptoms subside, which often takes several weeks. Progressive resistance exercises of the quadriceps should be supervised by a physical therapist (especially one experienced in sports medicine) to maximize quadriceps strength and stability (see Fig. 67.5). The course of patients with this problem is unpredictable. Orthopaedic referral is usually necessary if the patient has been forced to abandon his major sport for more than a few weeks, or if the problem recurs. Intra-articular corticosteroid injections by the orthopaedist may alleviate symptoms, but this treatment must be restricted, as it will increase cartilage deterioration if done to excess. Correction of the tracking problem in the patellofemoral joint may require the use of an orthotic to correct excess pronation of the foot (see chapter 102) or the use of a cartilage knee brace (a heavy elastic brace containing a horseshoe-shaped pad to stabilize the patella—available from large pharmacies or orthopaedic appliance stores without prescription). Occasionally, surgical treatment of chondromalacia is necessary if conservative treatment fails. Surgery is designed to prevent subluxation of the patella. Results are variable depending on the extent of the problem and the type of surgery but, occasionally, the patient may not be able to return to sports which place stress on the knee.

Prevention

Prevention of chondromalacia requires the use of proper foot gear (see Chapter 102), often including the use of orthotics, and "proper conditioning" of the athlete by gradually increasing his level of activity and by the performance of stretching exercises (see below).

PROBLEMS OF THE LEG

Apophysitis of the Tibial Tubercle (Osgood-Schlatter's Disease)

This is a relatively common cause of knee pain in adolescents. It is thought to be due to repetitive avulsions or stress fractures due to traction of the patellar ligament upon the growth plate of the tibial tubercles.

The patient describes the insidious onset of pain of the tibial tubercle with activity. On examination there is enlargement and tenderness of the tubercle. There may be quadriceps atrophy from decreased activity, which frequently occurs because of use pain.

The adolescent with Osgood-Schlatter's disease should be instructed to avoid activities which entail resisted knee extension, such as climbing, running, and kicking until pain has resolved (usually 6 to 8 weeks). If pain persists after ossification is complete, surgical excision of heterotopic bone at the tibial tubercle and reattachment of the patellar ligament are sometimes necessary.

Shin Splints (4)

Definition and Mechanism of Injury

Shin splints are the occurrence of pain over the anteriomedial aspect of the mid to distal portion of the lower leg (Fig. 67.8, site A). They are caused by overuse of the muscles of this region as may occur with running, jogging, or sustained walking. The pain is though to result from tendinitis of the posterior tibial tendon and by periostitis from the pulling of this muscle from its bony attachment along the medial aspect of the tibia, the interosseous membrane, and the fibula.

Shin splints develop most often in individuals who (*a*) are not properly conditioned, (*b*) do not warm up properly, (*c*) run on hard or uneven surfaces, (*d*) wear improper foot gear, or (*e*) have anatomical abnormalities such as variation in the anatomy of their hip joint with resultant excessive tibial torsion (external rotation of tibia in the axial plane, slew feet) and hyperpronation of the feet (flat feet).

Symptoms and Signs

Shin splints are characterized by pain, usually gradual but occasionally abrupt in onset, which occurs during or just after exercise. Frequently, athletes continue to exercise in spite of the discomfort; but occasionally the pain is so severe that the exercise must be stopped. Examination reveals only the presence of tenderness along the medial aspect of the tibia.

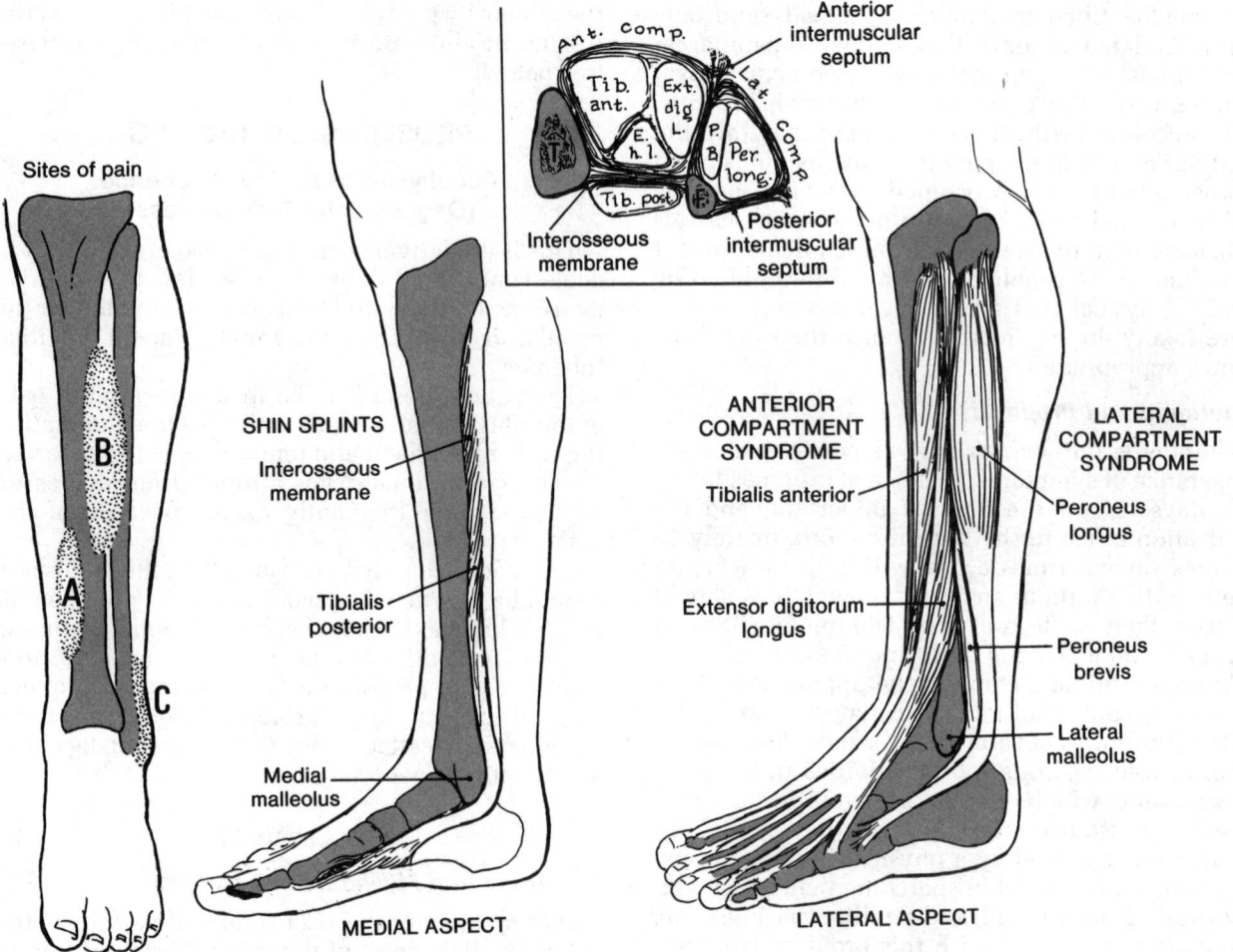

Figure 67.8. Sites of pain and relevant anatomy of (*A*) shin splints, (*B*) anterior compartment syndrome, and (*C*) lateral compartment syndrome.

Differential Diagnosis

If the area of tenderness is localized, a stress fracture may have occurred, although it is quite unusual in the tibia or fibula (see below). A compartment syndrome is similar but the location of pain and tenderness is different (see below). Occasionally fascial hernias, tenosynovitis, or tears of the interosseous membrane may produce symptoms suggesting shin splints; and, for this reason, an orthopaedic consultation should be requested if there is persistence of the symptoms after 3 weeks of therapy (see below) or if there is recurrence of symptoms. The orthopaedist will confirm the diagnosis and will look for anatomical abnormalities that predispose to this condition (see below). Also, an X-ray (indicated when symptoms are prolonged or recurrent) of the leg in the case of shin splints will occasionally show irregular bone formation of the tibia or fibula as a result of periostitis. A radionuclide bone scan is more sensitive than an X-ray in the diagnosis of shin splints and may be necessary if the

diagnosis is uncertain. A positive bone scan shows increased uptake of radionuclide by the tibia, fibula, or interosseous membrane.

Treatment and Prognosis

Ice packs should be applied several times a day for 15 minutes at a time in order to reduce swelling and inflammation. In severe cases, the patient should avoid, for several weeks, the exercise which has precipitated the problem. The use of an elastic wrap on the lower leg provides some comfort and the prescription of analgesic agents, such as aspirin, 600 mg four times a day, or Tylenol, 650 mg four times a day, will help to control the discomfort.

Acute shin splints should resolve in 3 weeks; and, after this, conditioning is necessary before the patient can return to his sport. The syndrome rarely recurs if conditioning has been correct.

Prevention

Prevention of this problem requires stretching exercises before physical activity (see below), running or walking on soft level surfaces, and use of proper shoes (Chapter 102). An orthotic device may also be prescribed by an orthopaedist or podiatrist if hyperpronation of the feet or excessive tibial rotation is present. These also will be helpful in preventing recurrences.

Compartment Syndromes

Definition and Mechanism of Injury

There are two compartments in the leg which are prone to injury and subsequent swelling: the anterior (tibial) compartment and the lateral (peroneal) compartment. The anterior compartment syndrome is also called lateral shin splints and occurs when an athlete runs to excess on his toes or on a hill, or runs with shoes that have a sole which is too flexible.

Compartment syndromes are usually seen in competitive runners and they are much less common than shin splints.

Symptoms and Signs

Anterior Compartment Syndrome

The patient notices pain in the extensor muscles of the leg and in the lower leg, ankle, and foot. Discomfort usually occurs during or just after exercise. Examination reveals tenderness and often swelling of the anterior compartment, which is located over the midlateral aspect of the lower leg (Fig. 67.8, site *B*).

Lateral Compartment Syndrome

In this situation the pain is located in the posterolateral aspect of the ankle above and behind the lateral malleolus (Fig. 67.8, site *C*); this is the area where the peroneal tendons are located. Frequently the patient feels as if his ankle has "given out." This syndrome is caused by excessive pronation of the foot (flat foot) and ankle (eversion) in runners with hypermobile ankles (weak ankles).

Treatment and Prognosis

Initially, ice should be applied for 15 minutes several times a day, and the patient must rest from exercise for 3 to 4 weeks. Anti-inflammatory agents are very helpful in controlling the inflammatory response. An anti-inflammatory agent with a rapid onset of action is suggested if cost is not a restriction: naproxen (Naprosyn), 375 to 500 mg two times a day, and piroxicam (Feldene), 20 mg once a day, are both effective. If cost is a factor, aspirin is recommended, although it takes 7 to 10 days at a dose of 3 to 4 g/day to achieve an anti-inflammatory effect. Once symptoms subside, the patient should condition himself before returning to full exercise. This conditioning requires pre-exercise stretching (see below), especially of the muscles that are involved, and then gradual return to running. The patient

should have well designed running shoes (see Chapter 102), should avoid toe running, and should always run on a level surface.

In the management of the lateral compartment syndrome an orthopaedist or podiatrist should be consulted to evaluate the use of an orthotic device or heel wedge to prevent hyperpronation, which predisposes to recurrence of the problem.

The prognosis for patients with either of these compartment syndromes is excellent provided the patient is properly conditioned.

Differential Diagnosis

Should symptoms not respond within a 7- to 10-day period, an X-ray of the area should be obtained to rule out other causes, such as a stress fracture or osteoid osteoma. A compartment syndrome also can be confused initially with thrombophlebitis, cellulitis, or vascular insufficiency and these should all be investigated by means of serial observations and appropriate specific tests when indicated.

Prevention

Prevention of compartment syndromes requires stretching exercises (see below) before running, especially of the musculature involved in each of the compartments, and the use of good quality running gear, often including orthotics.

PROBLEMS OF THE ANKLE AND FOOT

Injuries of the Ankle Joints

Ankle Structure and Function

The ankle joint consists of articulations between the distal tibia and fibula, which form an arch, or mortice, and the talus, which fits into the mortice (see Fig. 67.9). The talus fits tightly into the mortice during dorsiflexion of the foot and is relatively mobile during plantar flexion. The stability of the ankle is provided by the various ligaments shown schematically in Figure 67.9.

Mechanism of Injury

Ankle injuries occur when there is sudden stress on one or more of the supporting ligaments. Such injuries may occur during vigorous activity or as a consequence of inadvertently stepping onto an uneven surface or off of an unnoticed curb's edge, *etc.* Figures 67.10 and 67.11 illustrate schematically the spectrum of ankle ligament injuries and the stresses which cause them. A ligament injury may be a *strain*—stretching without actual disruption of tissue—or a *sprain*—partial or complete disruption of tissues.

Signs and Symptoms

The patient usually can recall the position of the foot and whether there was a sensation or sound of

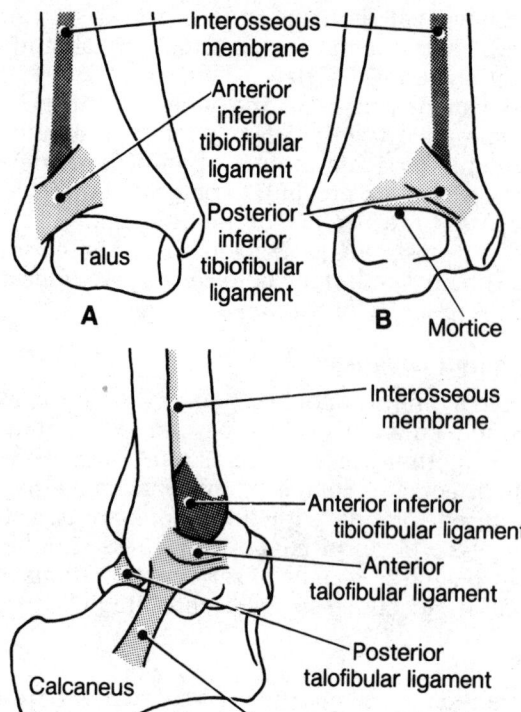

Figure 67.9. Distal tibiofibular joint and tibiotalar joint. *A.* Anterior view. *B.* Posterior view. *C.* Lateral view. (From Ramamurti CP: *Orthopaedics in Primary Care.* Tinker RV (ed). Baltimore, Williams & Wilkins, 1979.)

tearing at the ankle. Immediate pain is noted, and if there has been a sprain the patient will be aware of instability with weight bearing. Swelling over the injured ligament occurs within 1 hour of the injury, and it may be followed later by diffuse swelling of the foot and by an ecchymosis if there has been a significant ligament tear.

Examination of the strained or sprained ankle reveals marked tenderness over the injured ligament(s), made worse by replicating the stress which led to the injury (most commonly inversion of the foot). If there is not tense swelling, joint instability (e.g., obvious looseness or tilting of the talus with inversion of the foot) can be demonstrated when there has been a significant ligament tear. When the ankle cannot be easily manipulated to test for instability, a stress X-ray, under block anesthesia if needed, provides definitive diagnosis of severe sprain (see example, Fig. 67.12).

Treatment, Prognosis, and Prevention

Promptly following injury, the ankle should be immobilized (no walking, elastic bandage), ice packs (or ice water immersion) should be used for 10 to 15 minutes, and the leg should be elevated. If examination suggests that the injury represents a strain or

minor sprain (i.e., only modest pain, tenderness, and swelling, and no obvious instability), the ankle can be managed with an elastic bandage (used for 1 to 3 weeks), rest and elevation whenever possible, use of a cane for partial weight bearing, and gradual return to normal activities over 2 to 4 weeks. The technique and instructions for wrapping the ankle with an elastic bandage are shown in Figure 67.13.

If there is marked pain, swelling, or instability, it is likely that the patient has a significant sprain of one or more ligaments, or, in the case of an eversion injury, an avulsion fracture (see Fig. 67.11). Referral to an emergency room or an orthopaedic surgeon's office for definitive diagnosis and management is indicated. For these patients, treatment consists of immobilization with a rigid ankle splint for 3 to 6 weeks and no weight bearing (i.e., use of a crutch) for 2 weeks, followed by progressive return to weight bearing. In order to assure optimum long term outcome, convalescence from a significant ankle sprain should be planned and supervised by an orthopaedic surgeon. For severe injuries and for instability which does not improve with conservative management, surgical realignment or repair may be necessary.

Prevention

Recurrent ankle sprain is common. The optimal method for preventing recurrent injury, especially for an athlete with lax ankle joint(s), is to tape the ankle before engaging in exercise involving running. Alternatively, the patient can use a commercially available elastic ankle support whenever he exercises; these supports permit full range of motion but prevent the foot from falling into excessive inversion when it is not touching the ground.

Achilles Tendinitis

Definition and Mechanism of Injury

Achilles tendinitis is inflammation of the heel tendon and surrounding tissue and is due to overuse. The problem is most often caused by repetitive stretching of the tendon when the athlete is not properly conditioned. However, even with good conditioning it occurs in athletes who run on hills or who wear shoes with rigid soles. Furthermore, structural abnormalities such as tibia vara (bowlegged deformity), tight hamstring and calf muscles, a cavus foot (high arched foot often with claw toes), and a varus (inverted) heel deformity predispose to Achilles tendinitis. Initially, the peritenon (loose soft connective tissue surrounding the tendon) is inflamed, but in chronic cases the tendon itself undergoes mucoid degeneration with the formation of longitudinal fissures and often nodule formation in the degenerate tendon.

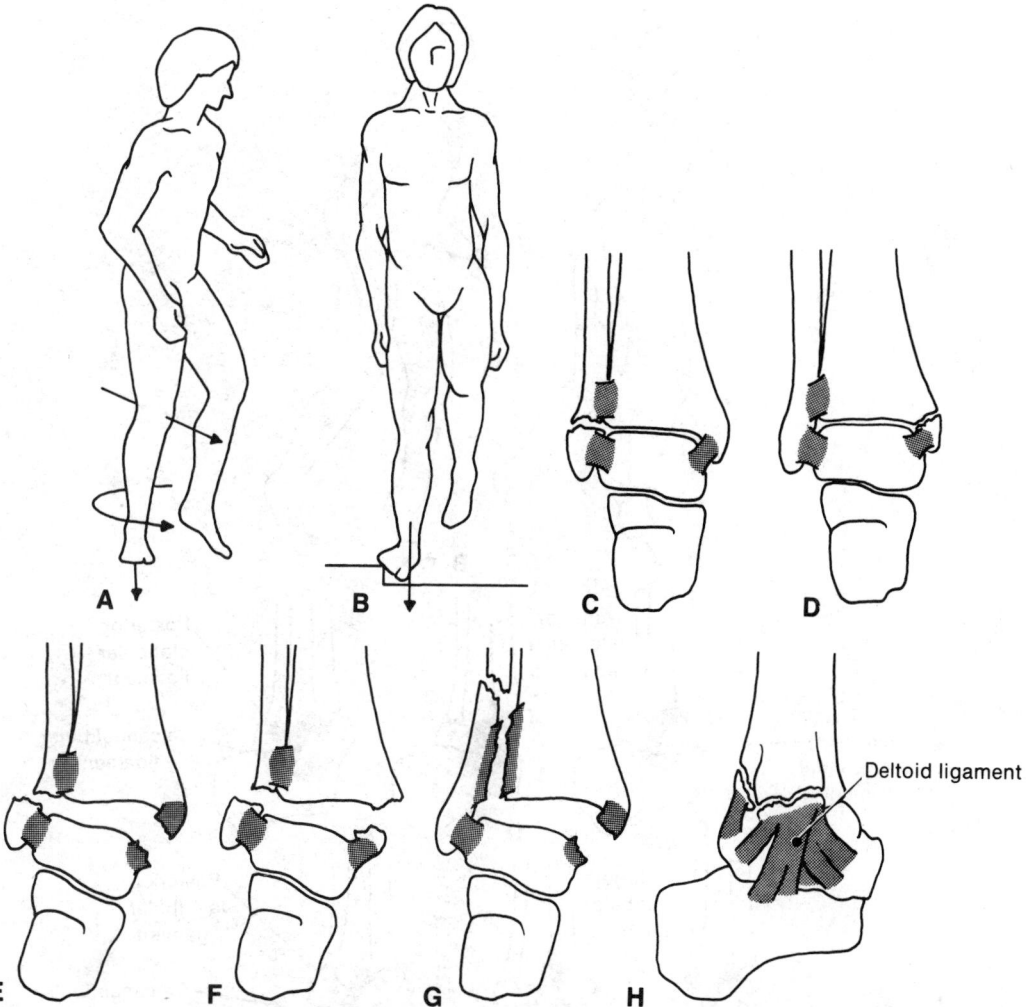

Figure 67.10. Pronation injuries of the ankle. *A* and *B.* Modes of injury. *A.* Extremity rotates internally on the fixed foot. *B.* The foot is forced into pronation by weight taken on the lateral aspect of the forefoot. *C* and *D.* Brief forces of lesser severity may fracture a malleolus without tearing a ligament. *E* through *G.*

Forces of greater severity will destroy the mortice in one of three ways. *H.* When forward displacement of the tibia accompanies severe pronation forces, the posterior margin of the tibial articular surface may be fractured as well.

This problem is commonly seen in recreational athletes, as well as in more serious runners.

Symptoms and Signs

The athlete with this problem notices a burning sensation in the heel, usually early during a run, which then lessens or disappears completely as running progresses. The discomfort often recurs upon completion of the run, in which case it is often more severe. Occasionally, a runner may note heel pain soon after awakening from sleep, which then subsides with daily activities.

On examination there is local or diffuse tenderness in the Achilles tendon; and, when the condition is chronic, there may be a tender nodule in the tendon, crepitus, and swelling.

Treatment and Prognosis

The application of an ice pack to the area for 15 minutes several times a day will provide comfort and reduce swelling. Analgesic agents, such as aspirin, 600 mg four times a day, or Tylenol, 650 mg four times a day, for several days will help to control the discomfort. The runner should rest for several days, then reduce his running mileage and avoid hills until symptoms have been absent for 10 to 14 days. Exercises that gently stretch the tendon are important to condition the runner (see below) and to prevent recurrences. If symptoms persist, a rest from exercise for a period of 3 to 4 weeks or longer may be necessary to permit healing. Local injection of corticosteroids into the Achilles tendon must be

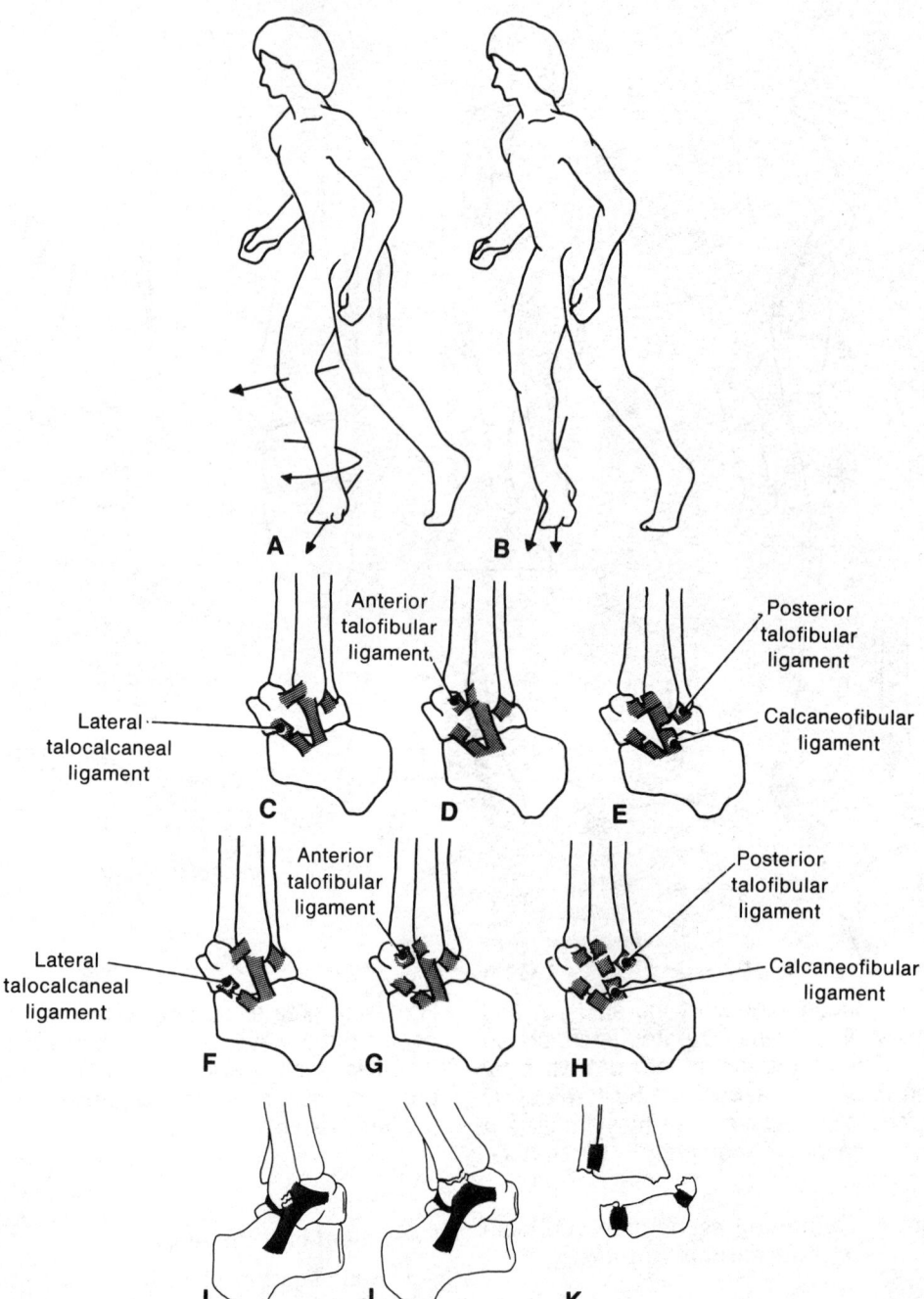

Figure 67.11.   Supination injuries to the ankle. *A* and *B*. Modes of injury. *A*. Extremity rotates externally on the fixed foot. *B*. Plantar-flexed foot is forced into supination. *C* through *E*. Sequence of injuries. Lateral talocalcaneal ligament (*C*) is injured before the anterior talofibular (*D*), which is injured before the calcaneofibular (*E*). *F* through *H*. When the injuring force is sufficient, the ligaments will tear completely and in the same sequence. *I* through *K*. Rather than tear the lateral ligaments, the injuring force may avulse a flake of fibula (*I*), or fracture off the end of the fibula (*J*), or fracture off both the end of the fibula and the medial malleolus (*K*).

avoided as this can weaken the tendon and cause a rupture. (Achilles tendinitis, if chronic, may lead to increased risk of rupture.)

In resistant cases, physical therapy, especially ultrasound, is helpful. In addition, when the syndrome is severe, splinting or casting of the ankle joint and the use of crutches are necessary to immobilize the Achilles tendon. In mild cases, with initial treatment and then proper conditioning, the prognosis is excellent. If the condition does not respond to therapy

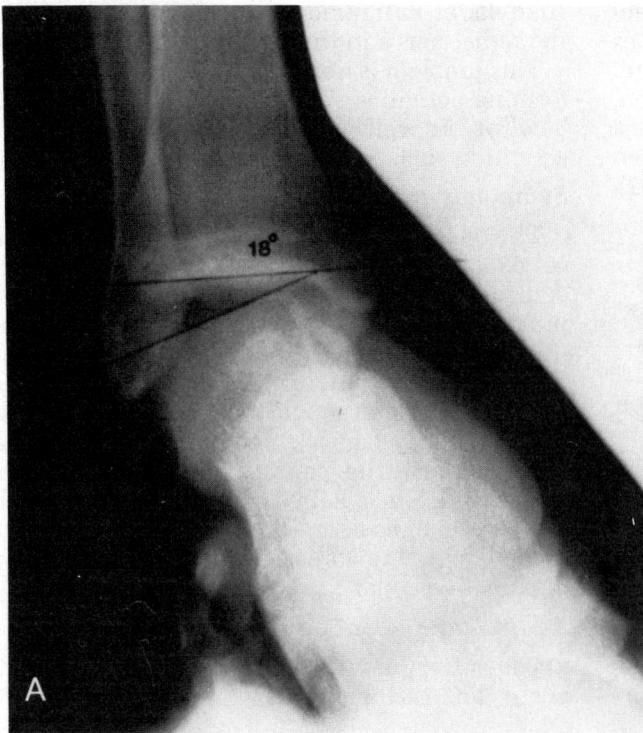

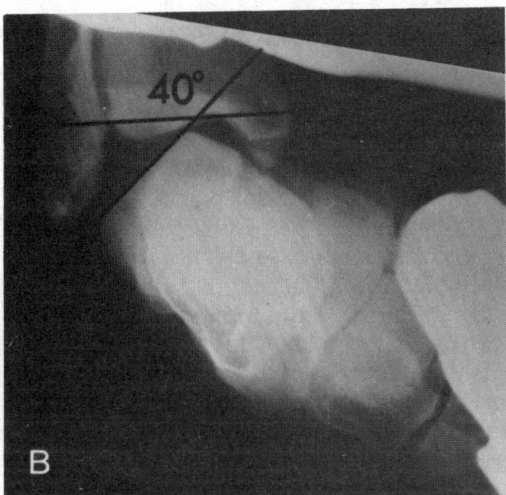

Figure 67.12. Examples of talar tilt. *A.* 15 to 20°. Complete single ligament tear with partial or complete injury to second ligament. *B.* Greater than 25°. Double ligament injury requiring more intensive treatment.

(From Scott NW, Nisonson B, Nicholas JA (eds): *Principles of Sports Medicine.* Baltimore, Williams & Wilkins, 1984.)

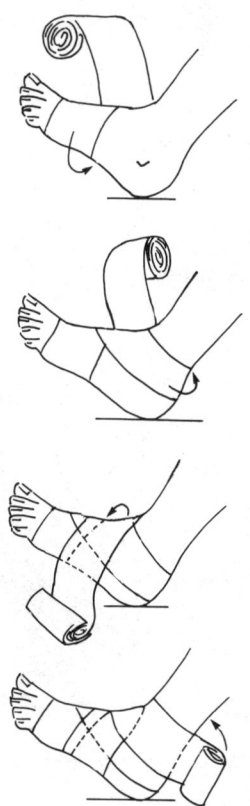

Figure 67.13. Technique for wrapping the ankle.

within 1 to 2 weeks, an orthopaedic consultation should be obtained since occasionally surgery is necessary. If surgery must be performed, it is unlikely that the athlete will be able to return to running, although other exercises, such as swimming or cycling, may be readily performed.

Prevention

Prevention of this problem requires the use of good running shoes (see Chapter 102) with flexible soles, a well molded Achilles pad, and a rigid heel wedge. If the runner has a cavus foot (see above) an orthopaedist or a podiatrist should be consulted about the use of an orthotic device.

Plantar Fasciitis (Heel Spur)

Plantar fasciitis or "heel spur syndrome" is the most common cause of heel pain; it occurs most often in people who hike or run, but it may also occur in individuals who are not athletic. The name "heel spur syndrome" derives from the finding of a bone spur on X-ray of the calcaneus, but it is unlikely that this spur causes the symptoms in most patients. This problem is fully discussed in Chapter 102.

Retrocalcaneal Bursitis

Inflammation of the bursae which overlie the calcaneus (heel bone) may produce symptoms similar to those of Achilles tendinitis. Bursitis of the heel affects runners, but it may also occur, at the upper border of the calcaneus, when tight-fitting shoes rub the heel with ordinary walking. On examination, there is focal tenderness confined to the calcaneus. Heel bursitis is managed with rest, properly fitted shoes, and, in runners, a heel pad (see Chapter 102).

PROBLEMS OF THE ELBOW (Fig. 67.14)

Lateral Epicondylitis (Tennis Elbow)

Definition and Mechanism of Injury

The term "tennis elbow" refers to inflammation in the region of the lateral epicondyle of the humerus at the origin of the common extensor muscles; it is a common exercise-related syndrome. It is caused by activities that combine excessive pronation and supination of the forearm with an extended wrist. Although the mechanism by which tennis elbow is produced is not known, the actual cause of pain may be due to radiohumeral synovitis or bursitis, tendinitis of the common extensor origin, traumatic epicondylitis or periostitis of the lateral epi-

condyle, or entrapment by scarring of a branch of the radial nerve in this region.

This problem is quite common in individuals performing activities such as tennis, badminton, and bowling, as well as with many non-sports-related activities, such as using a screwdriver or a wrench.

Symptoms and Signs

The onset of symptoms is usually gradual. Physical examination reveals tenderness over the lateral epicondyle or over the radiohumeral joint. The proximal common extensor muscle is often tender to palpation and, on occasion, there is swelling in this area. The elbow usually has a normal flexion and extension, although the latter may sometimes be temporarily painful. Supination and, especially, pronation may be painful if they are performed against resistance. Pain can be elicited by stretching the wrist extensors by holding the elbow fully extended with the forearm pronated and the wrist maximally palmar flexed (Fig. 67.15).

Additional Evaluation

The history and physical examination are diagnostic, and further studies are not indicated unless

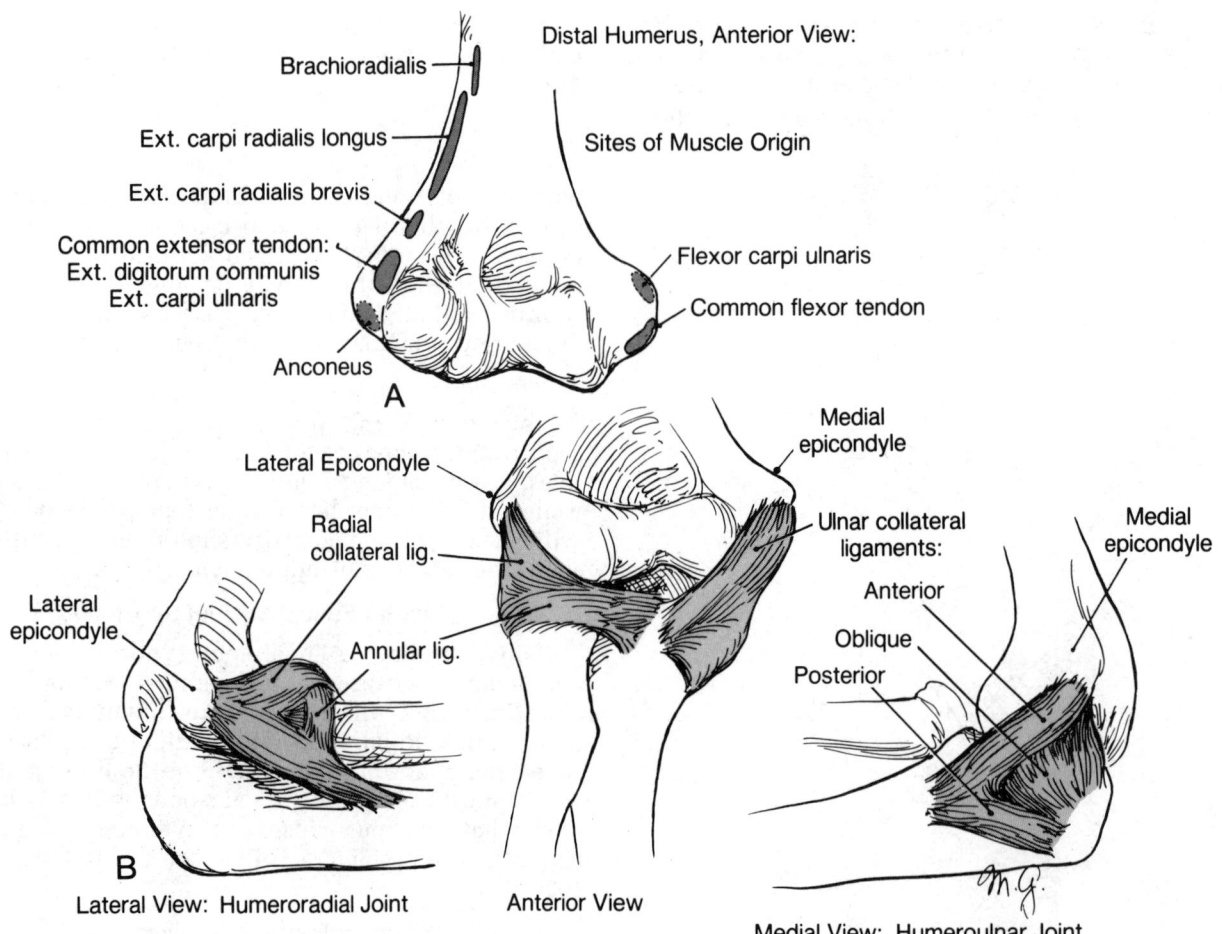

Figure 67.14. Important structures of the elbow.

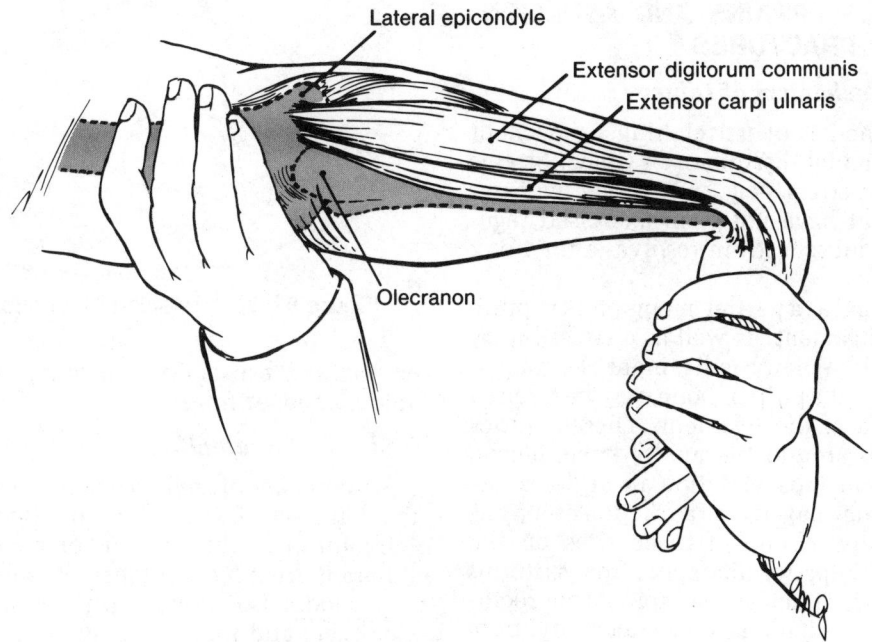

Lateral epicondyle

Extensor digitorum communis

Extensor carpi ulnaris

Olecranon

Figure 67.15. Tennis elbow.

symptoms fail to improve with treatment. In that case, an X-ray of the elbow should be obtained; on occasion, there may be calcium deposits noted at the lateral epicondyle of the humerus.

Treatment and Prognosis

The painful arm should initially be immobilized in a sling or, if symptoms are severe, immobilized in a long arm splint with the wrist held in dorsiflexion to rest the extensor tendons. Aspirin or Tylenol or other analgesic agents will help to control symptoms. If mild analgesics are inadequate, a rapid acting anti-inflammatory agent such as naproxen (Naprosyn) or piroxicam (Feldene) as described above (page 883) may be prescribed. The injection of the area at the point of tenderness with a mixture of 3 ml of 1 to 2% Xylocaine and 1 ml of glucocorticoid suspension (such as Aristocort or Kenalog) followed by the use of a sling for 1 or 2 weeks often provides dramatic relief of pain. A second injection may be repeated in approximately 3 weeks if symptoms fail to improve or if they recur during this period.

The prognosis is quite variable and depends to a large extent on the patient's activities. Tennis elbow may recur even in patients who are conscientious about their activity. If symptoms recur or if they fail to respond promptly to treatment, an orthopaedic consultation is indicated. Surgery may occasionally be required. The type of surgery depends on the problem and occasionally a return to the vigorous activity that precipitated the problems may not be possible.

Prevention

Prevention of this problem requires conditioning of the muscle groups in the forearm and wrist through an exercise program. This program often needs to be specialized, and a physical therapist should be consulted. Often the use of a tennis elbow strap (available at sports stores) in the area of the muscle mass of the proximal portion of the forearm is helpful since it decreases strain of the common extensor origin at the lateral epicondyle.

Medial Epicondylitis (Golfer's Elbow)

Definition and Mechanism of Injury

Medial epicondylitis of the elbow is due to inflammation of the tissues in the area of the medial epicondyle where the muscles that flex and pronate the wrist originate. It is caused by overuse of these muscles.

This problem is less common than tennis elbow and is seen in individuals performing repetitive pronation exercises, such as occur in golf.

Symptoms and Signs

The manifestations of this problem are very similar to those of tennis elbow except that the location is in the area of the medial, rather than the lateral, epicondyle.

Treatment, Prognosis, and Prevention

These aspects are similar to those of tennis elbow.

MISCELLANEOUS SPRAINS AND AVULSION FRACTURES

Definition and Mechanism of Injury

A *strain* is defined as overstretching a muscle or tendon, without actual disruption of tissue. Strains occur during mild stress—e.g., when one overuses muscle groups that have not been exercised regularly. The pain of muscle strain resolves after 1 or 2 days.

A *sprain* is defined as a partial or complete rupture of the fibers of a ligament, as well as a stress injury to the joint capsule. When the ligament is strong, it does not rupture, but a chip of bone may be *avulsed* from the insertion of the ligament. These injuries are most common around the ankle, knee, elbow, and fingers. Violent muscle action in athletes, especially adolescents, may avulse a traction epiphysis (apophysis), usually at one of three sites on the pelvis: (*a*) anterior superior iliac spine from sartorius avulsion, (*b*) anterior inferior iliac spine from rectus femoris avulsion, and (*c*) ischial tuberosity from avulsion of the hamstring (Fig. 67.16). Also, injuries to the joint capsules and ligaments of the fingers are particularly common.

Sprains and related injuries of the ligaments of the knees and ankles are discussed above.

Sprains and avulsion fractures result from sudden forceful muscle contraction and are very common in athletes.

Symptoms and Signs

The hallmark of a sprain or an avulsion fracture is pain in the area of the injury. Physical examination reveals swelling and stiffness of the involved joint with increased pain as the patient attempts to use it. The joint may be unstable if the ligament rupture is complete. Maximal swelling and tenderness are usually localized at the area of the sprain

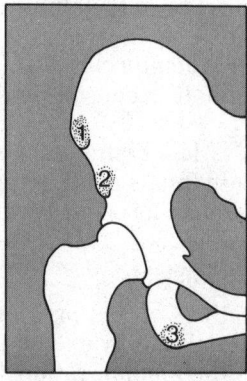

Figure 67.16.   Common sites of avulsion fracture: (*1*) anterior superior iliac spine, (*2*) anterior inferior iliac spine, and (*3*) ischial tuberosity.

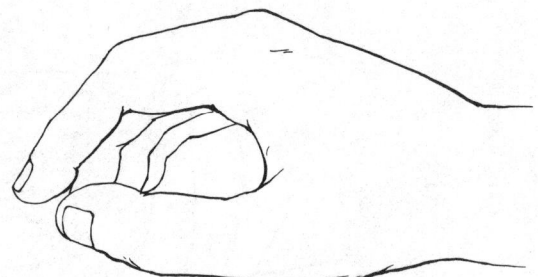

Figure 67.17.   Position of function of fingers.

or fracture, especially if it is superficial as in the ankle, knee, or finger.

Additional Evaluation

X-rays of an injured area must be done to establish the diagnosis of an avulsion fracture.

If joint instability is found on examination, a consultation from an orthopaedic surgeon should be requested. Also, stress X-rays, especially of the ankle, knee, and finger, are often done by the orthopaedic surgeon either under local or general anesthesia to evaluate the degree of instability of the joints.

Surgical intervention by the orthopaedic surgeon to repair joint instability is occasionally necessary, especially in injuries in the area of the ankle and knee; even after surgery, an athlete will often not be able to return to the activity that resulted in the injury.

Treatment and Prognosis

The initial treatment of sprains and/or avulsion fractures consists of immobilization of the area with a splint, elevation, and application of ice for approximately 15 minutes several times a day to decrease swelling, and the prescription of analgesics such as aspirin or Tylenol alone or in combination with codeine, 30 to 60 mg every 4 to 6 hours. If the injury is in the area of the ankle or knee, the patient must keep his weight off the injured joint by the use of crutches (see above). It is important to immobilize a finger for no more than 3 weeks and then only in the *position of function*, in order to avoid permanent stiffness of the joint (Fig. 67.17).

The prognosis for sprains and avulsion fractures is quite variable and depends to a large extent on the location of the injury; but with proper treatment and with subsequent conditioning of the patient, the prognosis is generally good.

Prevention

The prevention of sprains and avulsion fractures requires proper conditioning, especially by the performance of stretching exercises (see below) before exertion, and the use of proper foot gear and protective equipment.

STRESS FRACTURES (3, 6)

Definition and Mechanism of Injury

A stress fracture is a crack, which is sometimes minute, that can occur in almost any bone that has been repetitively subjected to impact. The most common sites of stress fractures are the metatarsal shafts, especially the second and third metatarsals, the distal fibula, the proximal tibia, and the symphysis pubis. Stress fractures may, however, occur in other bones, such as the lumbar vertebrae, the sacroiliac joint, the distal femur, the distal aspect of the tibia, and the lateral malleolus.

Stress fractures occur most commonly from walking or running, usually when an athlete has tried to do too much too fast, has used improper shoes, or has exercised on hard surfaces. Stress fractures occur in both poorly conditioned individuals and in highly conditioned athletes.

Symptoms and Signs

A patient who has sustained a stress fracture notices the gradual onset of aching of the affected bone during or just after exercising. Examination reveals localized tenderness and occasional swelling.

Additional Evaluation

The diagnosis depends on the symptoms and signs since X-rays of the affected area are usually normal at first; only after 2 to 4 weeks (sometimes longer) they may show bone resorption at the fracture site and/or the formation of callus (new bone). A radionuclide bone scan is positive, however, before the fracture can be identified on X-ray, and the scan may remain positive for up to 2 years after the injury. Therefore, a bone scan is indicated if symptoms persist for more than a few weeks and X-rays are negative.

Differential Diagnosis

Tibial stress fractures may be confused with pes anserinus bursitis, shin splints, and bone tumors, especially osteoid osteoma. If there is uncertainty about the correct diagnosis, a consultation should be requested from an orthopaedist.

Treatment and Prognosis

The treatment of stress fractures involves complete immobilization of the injured part in a splint. If the injury is in a lower extremity, the patient should not bear weight on it. The injured part should also be elevated, and ice should be applied initially for approximately 15 minutes several times a day until the swelling subsides, which usually occurs in 24 to 36 hours. After the swelling has subsided, heat may be applied for 15 minutes several times a day; but this should be discontinued if the discomfort is made more severe, which occasionally occurs. Pain should be controlled with aspirin or Tylenol alone or combined with codeine, 30 to 60 mg every 4 to 6 hours as needed.

Metatarsal stress fractures should be treated initially with a cast, which should be left on 4 to 8 weeks. (If the physician is unfamiliar with the application of a short leg cast, referral to an orthopaedist is indicated.) Stress fractures of the tibia and fibula require more prolonged periods of immobilization and may require a cast for up to 12 weeks or longer. All patients with suspected stress fractures of the tibia or fibula should be seen by an orthopaedist.

With proper treatment and then appropriate conditioning, the prognosis is excellent and most patients will be able to return to normal sports activities.

Prevention

Prevention of stress fractures requires proper conditioning with pre-exercise stretching exercises, proper footwear, and avoidance of hard surfaces and of too rapid an acceleration of physical activity.

STRETCHING EXERCISES

It has been pointed out that the occurrence (and recurrence) of some of the problems described in this chapter can be prevented by several measures—that is, selecting good shoes (see Chapter 102 for a description and illustration), not increasing the amount of stress on the musculoskeletal system too rapidly, and stretching the major muscle groups of the lower extremity before participating in sports. The four stretching exercises which should be practiced routinely are illustrated in Figure 67.18. Each exercise should be done for both sides for 15 to 30 seconds at a time for a total of 10 to 15 minutes before engaging in sports activities.

ARTHROSCOPY

Arthroscopy can be used in the evaluation and treatment of various joint injuries and conditions. The most commonly arthroscoped joint is the knee, but the shoulder, ankle, and other joints also can be examined by this method. Tears of menisci in the knee can be excised or repaired by utilizing the arthroscope. Cruciate ligament injuries in the knee can be diagnosed and sometimes repaired. Loose bodies and articular cartilage defects can also be diagnosed and treated by removal or debridement using this method. Arthroscopy can be done under general or local anesthesia and, usually, without the need for hospitalization. Treatments performed arthroscopically generally need less time to heal than those done by arthrotomy, and there is a lower incidence of morbidity. Complications are rare, but

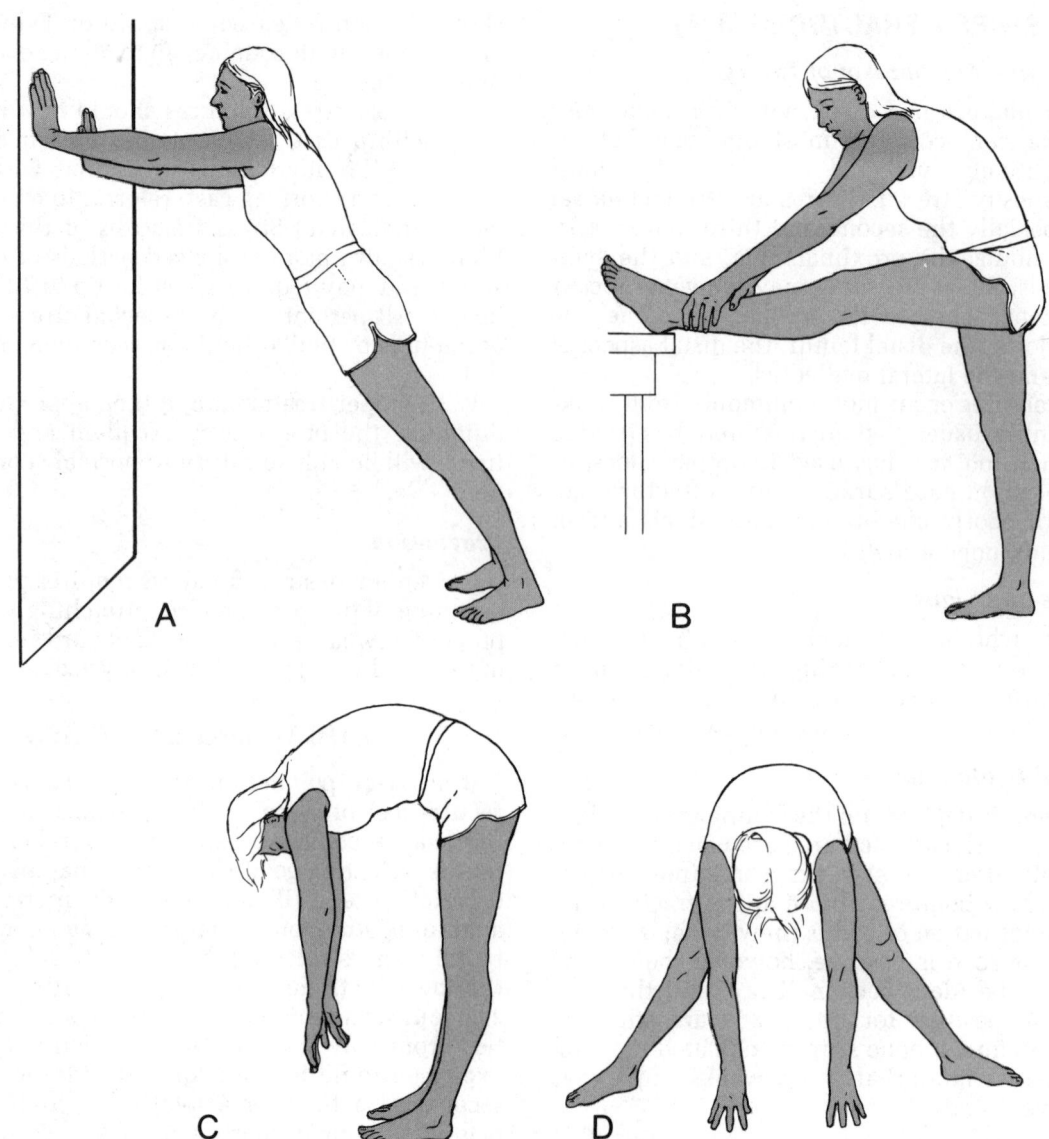

Figure 67.18. *A.* Stretch the Achilles tendon by leaning forward with the feet flat and placed at least 4 feet from the wall. *B.* Stretch the hamstring and gastrocnemius muscle groups by elevating the leg and bending forward as far as possible. *C.* Stretch the hamstring and back muscles by touching the toes slowly; bouncing should be avoided. *D.* Stretch the adductor muscle by gradually spreading the legs as far apart as possible; place the fingers on the floor for support.

do include infection, synovitis, phlebitis, neuropraxia, and compartment syndromes.

General References

Brody DM: Running injuries. *Ciba Clin Symp 32:* Nov 4, 1980.
    An excellent review of running injuries, including superb anatomical illustrations and a description of specific stretching exercises.
Mirkin G, Hoffman M: *The Sports Medicine Book.* Boston, Little, Brown, and Co, 1978.
    An excellent general reference book, which contains descriptions of stretching exercises.
Ramamurti CP: *Orthopaedics in Primary Care,* Tinker RV (ed): Baltimore, Williams & Wilkins, 1979.
    A practical and well illustrated text.
Scott WN, Nisonson B, Nicholas JA (eds): *Principles of Sports Medicine.* Baltimore, Williams & Wilkins, 1984.
    An excellent reference book with detailed information about the prevention, diagnosis, and management of athletic injuries; the book contains a good section on the use of arthroscopy.

Specific References

1. Ficat RP, Hungerford DS: *Disorders of the Patello-Femoral Joint.* Baltimore, Williams & Wilkins, 1977.
2. Insall J: Chondromalacia patellae. *J Bone Joint Surg* 58A:1, 1976.
3. Pavlov H, Nelson TL, Warren RF, *et al*: Stress fractures of the pubic ramus. *J Bone Joint Surg* 64A:1020, 1982.
4. Slocum DB: The shin splint syndrome—medical aspects and differential diagnosis. *Am J Surg* 114:875, 1967.
5. Slocum DB, Larson RL: Rotatory instability of the knee. *J Bone Joint Surg* 50A:211, 1968.
6. Torg JS, Pavlov H, Cooley LH, *et al*: Stress fractures of the tarsal navicular. *J Bone Joint Surg* 64A:700, 1982.

CHAPTER SIXTY-EIGHT

Degenerative Joint Disease

ALEXANDER S. TOWNES, M.D.

The common occurrence, the chronic and often benign course, and the lack of definitive treatment of degenerative joint disease or osteoarthritis have generated a general apathy and disinterest on the part of many physicians about this disease. A common attitude also among patients is that this form of arthritis is an inevitable consequence of aging and must be accepted as such. Advances in understanding of the pathophysiology of degenerative joint disease, especially in the past decade, have accomplished a great deal in dispelling these undeserved attitudes. As a result a better perspective of the multiple etiological factors potentially involved in this disease, and a better understanding of the clinical problems presented by patients with this disorder have developed.

Degenerative joint disease is particularly important to the general physician who sees ambulatory adult patients. Estimates indicate that approximately half of all visits to physicians for joint disease are for this diagnosis. Degenerative joint disease is the most common arthritis diagnosed in a general practice (10).

PREVALENCE

Prevalence of degenerative joint disease increases with advancing age, beginning perhaps as early as the third decade of life and being almost ubiquitous as detected by radiography or by biochemical changes in articular cartilage in the seventh and eighth decades and beyond. It is fortunate and important, however, that clinical symptoms are not necessarily associated with structural changes, so that estimates of prevalence based on these findings exceed the magnitude of the clinical problem. Thus, symptoms and clinical findings of degenerative joint disease are not an inevitable accompaniment of aging. However, symptoms and findings are uncommon below age 35 and are more frequent above age 65, with perhaps as much as 30 to 40% of the population age 65 and above having some symptoms related to this diagnosis.

PATHOPHYSIOLOGY

The pathogenesis of degenerative joint disease is probably multifactorial; however, the final common pathway is believed to be *injury to articular cartilage*, which then undergoes a sequence of changes resulting eventually in loss of its proteoglycan matrix, cellular proliferation in attempted repair, release of enzymes with more destruction of all cartilage elements, and proliferation of subchondral bone. Changes are most severe in or may be confined entirely to areas of maximal stress on the articular cartilage, most striking in weight-bearing areas of the large joints. Although one hypothesis suggests a primary synovial lesion (4), most observers have concluded that the chronic synovitis that is found in more advanced cases of degenerative joint disease is probably secondary to cartilage degeneration with reaction to detritus shed into the joint cavity from this process. A possible role for immune response to cartilage antigen has been suggested by the demonstration of antibodies to collagen in eluates of articular cartilage from patients with osteoarthritis (7a). An important role of crystalline deposits of calcium pyrophosphate or hydroxyapatite in the synovial inflammatory response in certain patients, especially those with more advanced osteoarthritis, has been demonstrated (7) (see also Chapter 69). Remodeling and microfractures of subchondral bone with hardening and loss of ability to absorb stress as primary mechanisms in production of osteoarthritis have also been suggested (14).

Since there are no nerve fibers in articular cartilage, there are no symptoms due to early changes in the joints. There are multiple sources of pain, however, as the disease progresses. Periosteal irritation as a result of proliferating bone, denuded bone, microfractures of subchondral bone, stress on ligaments as a result of loss of cartilage and joint incongruity, low grade synovitis, effusion, and spasm of surrounding muscles are all potential sources of pain in osteoarthritis.

ETIOLOGY AND PREDISPOSING FACTORS

The cause of degenerative joint disease is not known. It is quite likely that there are multiple causes and many factors that may influence disease expression, some of which are listed in Table 68.1.

Because of multiple etiological mechanisms in the pathogenesis of osteoarthritis, the history should

Table 68.1.
Factors Contributing to Development of Osteoarthritis

AGING
    Diminished proteoglycan aggregation
    Diminished resistance of cartilage to fatigue fracture
        (? defective collagen network)
    Decreased resiliency of soft tissues
    Loss of normal anatomical relationship (hip)
HEREDITY
    Heberden's nodes
    Primary generalized osteoarthritis
    Postural or developmental defects (*e.g.*, scoliosis, slipped
        capital femoral epiphyses, Legg-Calvé-Perthes disease,
        etc
    Metabolic defects (ochronosis, Wilson's disease)
ABNORMAL DISTRIBUTION OF MECHANICAL STRESS
    Postural or developmental defects
    Joint instability or hypermobility
    Local incongruity of joint surfaces post-traumatic, after
        meniscectomy, prolonged immobilization
    Obesity (abnormal stress on knees due to adiposity)
EXCESSIVE REPETITIVE STRESS
    Occupational
    Sports related
    Associated with neuropathy
CRYSTALLINE DEPOSIT DISEASE
    Calcium pyrophosphate
    Hydroxyapatite
PREVIOUS INFLAMMATORY JOINT DISEASE
METABOLIC ABNORMALITIES
    Ochronosis
    Wilson's disease
    Acromegaly
    ? Diabetes mellitus

seek to determine specific factors that may be implicated in each patient. *Heredity* may be important, especially in development of Heberden's nodes (19) (see below). A family history may also draw attention of the patient to the benign occurrence of these bony enlargements in elderly family members and serve to reassure them regarding their course.

Obesity is perhaps an obvious factor, but its extent and duration are important in assessing potential damage to weight-bearing joints, especially the knees. *Preceding trauma* may be important in subsequent development of degenerative arthritis in a joint damaged by ligamentous instability, meniscal tear in the knee joint, *etc.* Traumatic episodes with sufficient damage to induce these abnormalities are likely to be severe enough to be recalled, for example, as severe "sprains" with swelling lasting several days or longer following a sports-related or other injury. Jogging is not known to predispose to degenerative joint disease unless an injury has been sustained, or pain, emanating from a joint, regularly results from the exercise. *Prior joint surgery* with removal of a torn meniscus in the knee is also a predisposing factor to osteoarthritis of the knee. *Repetitive stress* of minor trauma may also predispose to development of osteoarthritis (for example, in knees of basketball players) and may account for osteoarthritis in joints not commonly affected (e.g., elbows of baseball pitchers and elbows as well as shoulders of air hammer operators). Lifelong postural or mechanical defects also predispose to degenerative changes as the result of abnormal distribution of stress to the joint when force is applied. Since abnormalities such as varus or valgus deformities of the knees may also occur as a result of osteoarthritic damage to the joint, the history is important in determining which came first.

Degenerative joint disease may also be associated with other disease states: preceding inflammatory arthritis; metabolic diseases, such as ochronosis, with deposition of metabolites in cartilage; diseases predisposing to chondrocalcinosis such as hemochromatosis and hyperparathyroidism; and acromegaly. Diabetes mellitus may also predispose to osteoarthritis, although this association is less well documented.

GENERAL CLINICAL FEATURES

History

Characteristically there is involvement of only one or a few joints in osteoarthritis. Joints commonly affected and those usually spared are shown in Table 68.2. Since the presentations of patients may differ, depending upon the pattern of joints involved and predisposing factors, some of these presenting symptoms will be highlighted separately after a general discussion of the symptoms and findings in this disease.

Table 68.2.
Distribution of Joint Involvement in Osteoarthritis

COMMONLY AFFECTED
  Hands:
    Distal interphalangeal (Heberden's nodes)
    Proximal interphalangeal (Bouchard's nodes)
    Carpometacarpal of the thumb (joints between first metacarpal and greater multangular and between greater multangular and navicular)
  Knees
  Hips
  Spine:
    Cervical
    Lumbar
    Thoracic
  Feet:
    Metatarsophalangeal (especially first)
USUALLY SPARED
  Hands:
    Metacarpophalangeal
    Carpometacarpal (except first)
  Wrists
  Elbows
  Shoulders

Degenerative joint disease usually begins insidiously and progresses slowly. Aching discomfort early in the course characteristically increases in severity with use of the joint; therefore it tends to reach a peak after the day's activity and is relieved by rest. Pain is often aching in character and may be difficult for the patient to localize precisely. It is usually felt in the areas surrounding the involved joint. However, it is important to remember that hip pain may be referred to the medial aspect of the thigh, the lateral portion of the buttock, or to the knee. Morning stiffness and stiffness after rest may be absent, or if present, last only 15 to 20 minutes or less, in contrast to a longer duration in inflammatory joint disease, such as rheumatoid arthritis. However, in advanced disease stiffness may be more profound, and pain may occur at rest. When joint destruction is marked, the patient may be kept awake at night by the pain.

As the disease progresses, large pieces of degenerated cartilage may shed into the joint, producing loose bodies which may cause locking or giving away of the joint in addition to pain.

There are no systemic symptoms in osteoarthritis. This is an important negative feature of the history that helps to differentiate this disease from other forms of arthritis.

Physical Findings

Early in the disease there may be no physical findings. Most patients who present with symptoms will have some pain on passive motion of the involved joints or on motion against resistance. This is frequently a sense of crackling or crepitus as the joint is moved, probably due to joint surface incon-gruities and irregularities of opposing cartilaginous surfaces. Crepitus may be exaggerated by movement with weight bearing or by manual compression of the joint during movement (for example, compression of the patella against the condyle of the femur when patellofemoral arthritis is present). In more advanced disease, joint motion may be limited and gross deformities may develop. Tenderness along the joint line is common, but may be mild or absent. In contrast to most inflammatory joint diseases, soft tissue swelling is usually absent or minimal in osteoarthritis except in its most advanced stages. Bony enlargement and irregularity are common, especially in the hands at the distal interphalangeal joints (Heberden's nodes) and less commonly in the proximal interphalangeal joints (Bouchard's nodes). Joint effusions are relatively infrequent compared to more inflammatory forms of joint disease. However, they may occur, especially in the knees. There is usually no detectable heat or redness over involved joints, although some warmth may be present as the disease progresses and chronic synovitis develops.

Physical examination of the patient with osteoarthritis should always include a careful evaluation of the neurological system and peripheral vascular system since disease in these systems may produce pain or limited motion in an extremity which may be erroneously attributed to degenerative joint disease (see "Diagnosis and Differential Diagnosis").

Laboratory Findings

Degenerative joint disease is characterized by normal laboratory tests unless it is associated with some other disease process. In particular the erythrocyte sedimentation rate (ESR) is characteristically normal, in contrast to the inflammatory arthritides. Mild and transient elevation of ESR may occasionally be associated with the acute inflammatory events described below, or may be due to intercurrent disease elsewhere.

Examination of synovial fluid is helpful when effusion is present in a large joint. Synovial fluid in osteoarthritis is usually of the noninflammatory type, i.e., with good viscosity, white blood cells < 2000/mm³, protein content < 4 g/dl, glucose concentration approximately equal to a simultaneous serum glucose concentration, and a good mucin clot when mixed with acetic acid. When crystals of calcium pyrophosphate or hydroxyapatite are present (see Fig. 69.1 and Table 69.1 in Chapter 69) the white cell count of the fluid may be elevated and the protein content increased.

X-ray Findings

Radiographic findings are important in the diagnosis and differential diagnosis of degenerative joint disease since certain abnormalities are characteristic of this disorder. Therefore X-ray examination of the affected joints is indicated in the evaluation of

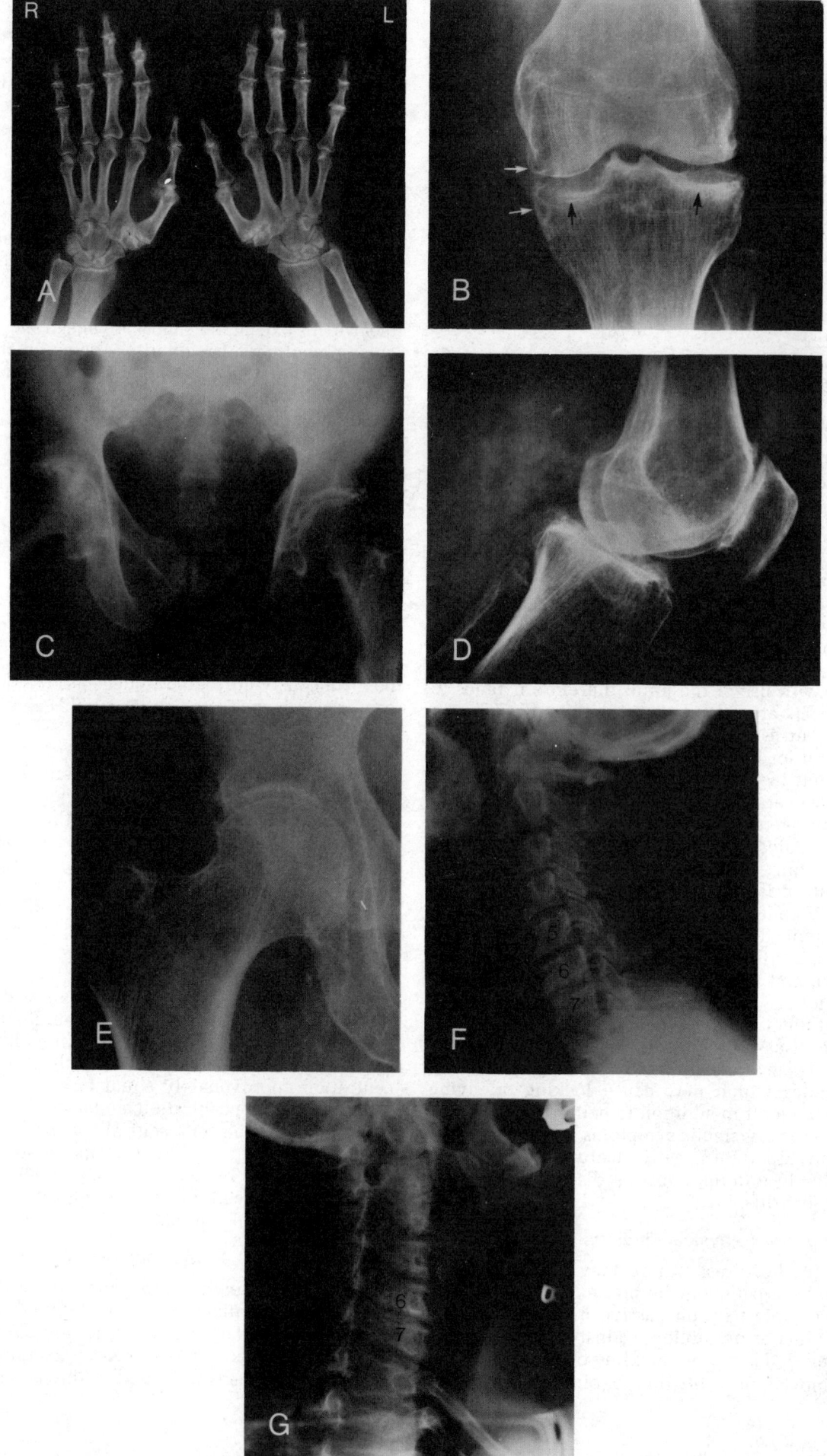

Table 68.3.
X-Ray Findings in Osteoarthritis

EARLIEST:
  No abnormality
EARLY:
  Slight loss of articular cartilage thickness (narrowing of
    radiological joint space)
MODERATE:
  Marginal osteophyte formation
LATE:
  Loss of cartilage space (often focal in weight-bearing joints)
  Sclerosis of subchondral bone
  Subchondral cyst formation
  Loose bodies
  Subluxation or deformity

most patients to confirm the diagnosis and to determine the extent of abnormalities present. However, it is important to point out that in early disease X-rays may be normal, and even with characteristic findings of joint narrowing and proliferation of subchondral bone with spur formation, symptoms may be absent. Hence, the importance of relating radiographic findings to the history and physical examination cannot be overemphasized. In general the more severe the radiographic changes, the more likely the patient is to have symptoms and findings of osteoarthritis. Radiographic findings from the earliest to the most advanced changes are listed in Table 68.3 and examples of X-rays are shown in Figure 68.1.

For evaluation of *hands* a single anteroposterior (AP) view of both hands is sufficient in most cases. Both *hips* can be visualized on a single AP film of the pelvis; more specific films may be required if an abnormality is detected or if findings do not correlate with the clinical picture. AP and lateral films are required for adequate evaluation of the *knee* joint. Special views of the patella ("skyline" view) may also be required to demonstrate the extent of patellofemoral arthritis. In evaluating the *spine*, AP, lateral, and oblique views are needed, the latter to visualize the neural foramina and the localization of nerve root compression by bony spurs.

In patients with degenerative disease of the spine, computerized tomography (CT) scans may demonstrate encroachment of osteophytes or of disc material on nerve roots. However, abnormal findings on CT scan in the absence of symptoms, or negative findings despite significant symptoms and signs are not infrequent. In the cervical spine, false positive and false negative CT scan readings approximate 30% (1). Thus, as with plain radiographs, careful correlation of findings with clinical symptoms is imperative. In general, CT scans are reserved for patients in whom conservative management has failed and in whom surgery or alternative causes of radiculopathy are being strongly considered.

CLINICAL PATTERNS OF OSTEOARTHRITIS

Heberden's Nodes

These bony enlargements of the distal interphalangeal joints are more frequent in women and commonly begin to appear in the fifth or sixth decade of life. They are often asymptomatic but a source of concern on the part of many patients who may view them as an outward sign of aging or as the beginning of a more serious and disabling arthritic disorder. Thus the physician must be aware of and be prepared to deal with the emotional investment of the patient that may focus concerns about declining functions (including menopause) upon an obvious change in physical appearance such as Heberden's nodes. With a curt dismissal, no explanation of the true significance of this abnormality, and no opportunity for the patient to ventilate her concerns, the physician will miss an important therapeutic opportunity.

Primary Generalized Osteoarthritis

This term was applied by Kellgren and Moore (8) to a group of patients whom they characterized as having osteoarthritis involving the distal and prox-

Figure 68.1. *A. Hands of patient* with degenerative joint disease. Note the following characteristics: soft tissue enlargement on right over the second distal interphalangeal joint (Heberden's node); the loss of joint space and bony proliferation of all distal interphalangeal joints, especially 2 and 3 in the right hand and 3 in the left hand; involvement of carpometacarpal joint of both thumbs with narrowing and increased density of subchondral bone; and normal metacarpophalangeal joints and wrist joints. *B. X-ray of knee* showing degenerative joint disease with loss of joint space (cartilage) especially in medial compartment, sclerotic subchondral bone, subchondral cysts, and early marginal spurs especially on lateral side. *C. Pelvic film* of a patient with advanced degenerative joint disease in the right hip.

Notice the joint space narrowing and proliferation of subchondral bone. The left hip shows the minimal change of marginal sclerosis. *D. Lateral X-ray of same knee* (in *B*) illustrating involvement of patellofemoral joint with narrowing and spur formation superiorly. *E. X-ray of a hip* showing relatively early degenerative joint disease. Notice the narrowed joint space and spur formation of femoral head at upper margin of acetabulum. *F. X-ray of the lateral cervical spine* showing degenerative joint disease. Note narrowing of C5-6, and especially C6-7 interspace with anterior lipping and spur formation. *G. Oblique X-ray view of cervical spine* of same patient (*F*) showing osteophytes encroaching on neural foramina C5-6, C6-7.

imal interphalangeal joints and the carpometacarpal joint of the thumb in addition to involvement of multiple other joints (hips, knees, metatarsophalangeal, and spine). This pattern of osteoarthritis affects mostly middle-aged women who have a positive family history of a similar disorder. It is an uncommon pattern of osteoarthritis. Occasionally in early phases they will have had some inflammatory symptoms with an elevated ESR and an episodic course. It is suggested that these patients constitute a subgroup of patients with a heritable form of osteoarthritis that involves multiple joints and that perhaps has some distinctive radiological features. However, the nature of the proposed heritable factor has not been determined. It is important to recognize the syndrome clinically, primarily in order to differentiate it from rheumatoid arthritis and other polyarticular diseases. Recent studies have suggested that primary osteoarthritis involving the hands and other joints may also predispose to the development of secondary osteoarthritis such as that following meniscectomy (2).

Erosive Osteoarthritis of Hands

This term has been applied to patients with severe osteoarthritis of the hands (distal interphalangeal (DIP) and proximal interphalangeal (PIP) joints) in which extensive erosion of subchondral bone occurs with eventual deformity and significant limitation of motion of the finger joints (13). These patients also may have episodes of acute inflammation in these joints and their surrounding tissues. X-rays reveal the extensive bony erosion and subchondral cyst formation that may be interpreted incorrectly as rheumatoid or gouty erosions. The distribution of involvement in DIP and first carpometacarpal joints, sparing the metacarpophalangeal and wrists, should easily establish the true nature of the process. From the clinical point of view this syndrome is important because of the severity of symptoms and physical findings, which are not common in milder forms of osteoarthritis of the hands.

Hip

Hip involvement is potentially the most painful and disabling joint abnormality in osteoarthritis (see also Chapter 67). It is more often unilateral. Developmental defects in the structure of the hip, including congenital hip dysplasia, slipped capital femoral epiphysis, or unrecognized avascular necrosis, may have gone undetected but have predisposed the patient to develop osteoarthritis; with age, disturbance of the normal anatomical relationship between femoral head and acetabulum may also predispose to osteoarthritis. In contrast to osteoarthritis of the knee, obesity is not a major causal factor in osteoarthritis of the hip.

Pain, which early in the disease is associated with weight bearing and movement, may become severe even at rest, and night pain is common in advanced disease. Patients may walk with a limp or with an abnormal gait. Pain and limitation of motion during internal rotation and extension are early physical signs, and subsequently all motions may be painful and restricted. Clear identification of pain on motion of the hip is important in differentiating hip disease from other causes of pelvic pain. Flexion and adduction contracture and shortening may occur as disability progresses. Most patients who are symptomatic will have characteristic changes of osteoarthritis on X-rays of the hip. Progression of disease is variable but perhaps more likely to occur rapidly in the hip than in other joints.

Knee

The knee is the most common symptomatic joint in osteoarthritis (see also Chapter 67). There is a definite relationship to obesity, and the weight bearing areas of the medial compartment are most often involved. Patellofemoral joint involvement is also common.

Chondromalacia patellae (see also Chapter 67, Exercise-Related Musculoskeletal Problems) is a syndrome occurring usually in younger individuals (second, third, and fourth decades), probably resulting from trauma and shearing forces against the patella as it contacts the femur in midflexion. Knee effusion is frequently associated with this syndrome. In younger patients with knee effusion who do not respond to rest or palliative aspiration (see Chapter 66), then arthroscopy may be indicated and will show characteristic changes. In this instance, surgery may be indicated (see below). The relationship of this rather common syndrome to osteoarthritis is not entirely clear, although a distinct etiological mechanism and pathology have been suggested.

Spinal Syndromes

Degenerative joint disease can result in neck or back pain that may be acute or chronic (see Chapters 64 and 65). Particularly in cervical spine involvement, symptoms may be more related to referred pain than to neck pain. These syndromes can also result in pain without obvious nerve root compression or neurological abnormalities. Low cervical spine involvement can cause pain that is usually aching or burning in quality referred to the upper anterior chest, to the lower border of the scapula, and radiating down the arm to the elbow. Confusion with anginal pain may occur, but the history usually makes it clear that pain is localized to one side and occurs at rest, particularly during the night or in the early morning after sleep (probably due to positioning of the head during sleep). Although it may also be exacerbated by activity during the day, pain related to cervical arthritis does not subside rapidly with rest and is not related to specific exertion. Physical examination usually can reproduce the

Table 68.4.
X-Ray Abnormalities in Diffuse Idiopathic Skeletal Hyperostosis[a]

SPINAL

Laminated calcification and ossification along the anterior lateral aspect of the vertebral bodies continuing across the disc spaces and varying in thickness from 1 to 20 mm (see Fig. 68.2A, *arrows*)

Bumpy spinal contour appearance from increased bone deposition located at the anterior disc space margins (see Fig. 68.2A)

Radiolucent disc extension (*i.e.*, L-, F-, or Y-shaped lucencies within the bone deposition along the anterior disc margin) (see Fig. 68.2B, *arrow*)

Radiolucency beneath deposited bone linearly located between the anterolateral calcification and the vertebral bodies (see Fig. 68.2A, *arrows*)

EXTRASPINAL

(Frequent and distinctive features which permit a diagnosis even without spinal X-rays)

Bony proliferation

Ligament calcification, ossification

Para-articular osteophytes

(These changes are always present in the pelvis and in approximately 75% of cases in the heel and foot and less commonly in the elbows, knees, shoulders, humerus, wrist, and hands.)

[a] Adapted from Resnick D, Shapiro RF, Wiesner KB, *et al.*: Diffuse idiopathic skeletal hyperostosis (DISH) (ankylosing hyperostosis of Forestier and Rotes-Querol). *Semin Arthritis Rheum* 7:153, 1978.

pain on extremes of movement of the neck or with manual compression of the cervical segments in hyperextension, rotation, or lateral flexion. Degenerative arthritis of the thoracic spine can also cause radicular pain in the thoracic area, but this is surprisingly uncommon in contrast to frequent radiological findings of spur formation in the thoracic spine, probably because of the anterior position of most of these bony abnormalities.

Another spinal syndrome, the relationship of which to osteoarthritis is not clear, is diffuse idiopathic skeletal hyperostosis (DISH). Table 68.4 lists the radiological criteria for this diagnosis (15). Despite extensive hyperostosis and bony bridging between the vertebral bodies, motion and function are usually maintained since the apophyseal joints are usually spared. This syndrome is chiefly important because of its impressive radiographic appearance (Fig. 68.2), the diffuse bony changes with hyperostosis, and the importance of distinguishing it from ankylosing spondylitis (see Chapter 71).

"Acute" Exacerbations of Osteoarthritis

Patients with degenerative joint disease may present occasionally with acute or subacute painful episodes with swelling of the affected joint. These episodes are usually superimposed upon more typical preceding symptoms and signs of osteoarthritis,

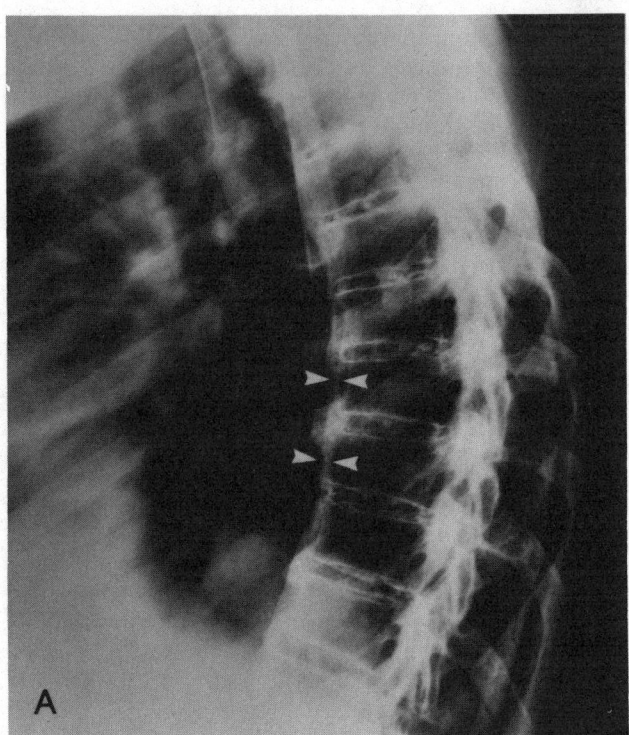

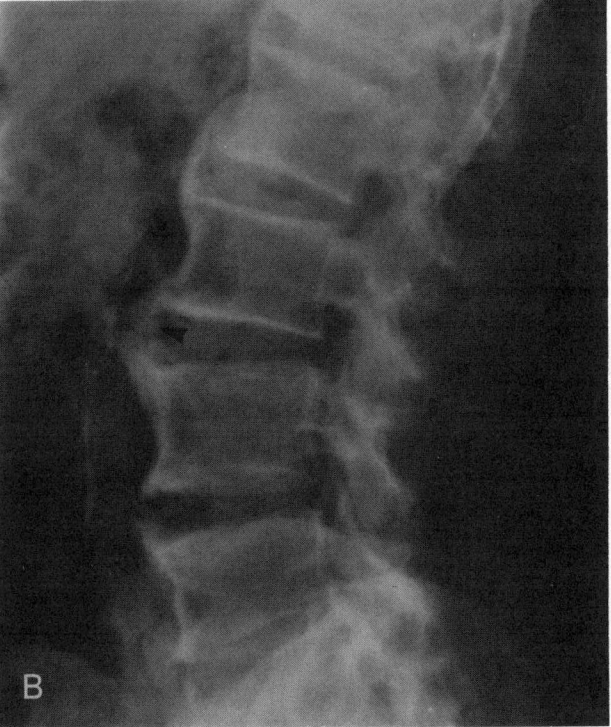

Figure 68.2. *A.* Lateral X-ray of thoracic spine of patient with diffuse idiopathic skeletal hyperostosis. *B.* Lateral X-ray of lumbar spine of patient with diffuse idiopathic skeletal hyperostosis. Prominent bony fusion and lipping anteriorly are seen.

but may be the event precipitating an initial visit to the physician. In these patients there may be evidence of inflammation with pain, swelling, warmth, and some erythema on occasion. When the knee is involved, there may be a joint effusion. The episodes, which may be precipitated by minor trauma, probably are caused by sudden release into the joint of large amounts of cartilaginous debris and/or microcrystalline deposits contained therein, and very rarely by complicating sepsis. In a study by Huskisson et al (7) either calcium pyrophosphate or hydroxyapatite crystals or both were found in a high proportion of knee effusions of patients with such episodes, but, in addition, in a significant proportion of unselected patients with osteoarthritis of the knee with effusion. Thus the concurrence of crystalline deposit disease and osteoarthritis seems to be well established, although the relationship of cause and effect is not yet clear. From the clinical point of view, however, this interrelationship provides a better understanding of these acute inflammatory episodes which punctuate the course of otherwise typical osteoarthritis (see also Chapter 69, Crystal-Induced Arthritis). Sepsis may occasionally complicate an osteoarthritic joint, but it is a much less common event than occurs in a rheumatoid arthritic joint.

For these reasons a patient with established osteoarthritis who develops an acutely swollen, painful, hot joint should have the joint aspirated and the fluid analyzed because of the possibility of there being either a complicating microcrystalline-induced or a septic arthritis.

DIAGNOSIS AND DIFFERENTIAL DIAGNOSIS

The diagnosis of degenerative joint disease is based upon the history and physical findings related to the joints, the absence of systemic signs, and typical radiological findings. Differentiation from other forms of arthritis is usually not difficult, with the possible exception of some of the more unusual diffuse or inflammatory patterns of involvement described above. Consideration of the age of the patient, the distribution of the joints involved, and the radiological findings will usually lead to the correct diagnosis.

The most common errors in differential diagnosis occur in attributing symptoms of pain or restricted movement to degenerative joint disease when the problem is not the joints. This is a common mistake in the evaluation of shoulder pain particularly (see Chapter 63). Since X-rays may demonstrate changes of degenerative joint disease in asymptomatic or mildly symptomatic patients, the physician must rely upon a careful history and physical examination to localize the disease to the joints. Table 68.5 lists other disorders, also common in older age groups, which often give rise to pain and to painful

Table 68.5.
Differential Diagnosis of Osteoarthritis: Extra-articular Causes of Pain or Restricted Movement

BONE DISEASE
   Osteopenia or osteoporosis (see Chapter 74)
   Malignancy: myeloma, metastatic
   Paget's disease
   Osteomyelitis (see Chapter 31)
PERIARTICULAR SOFT TISSUE ABNORMALITIES
   Soft tissue contractures (Dupuytren's, postcerebrovascular accident, or debilitating disease with disuse)
   Tendinitis or bursitis (see Chapters 63 and 66)
   Reflex sympathetic dystrophy
NEUROMUSCULAR DISEASES
   Neuropathy (diabetic, alcoholism, B_{12} deficiency) (see Chapter 84)
   Parkinsonism (see Chapter 82)
   Tardive dyskinesias (see Chapters 16 and 82)
   Senile dementia with rigidity (see Chapters 17 and 82)
VASCULAR DISEASES (see Chapter 87)
   Atherosclerotic
   Diabetic
   Vasculitic

or restricted movement and which may be erroneously attributed to degenerative "arthritis" unless a careful examination is done.

MANAGEMENT

There is no cure for degenerative joint disease and no therapy that can be directed toward the specific pathophysiology of cartilage degeneration. However, much can be done to relieve symptoms, to minimize disability, and perhaps to delay progression of the disease. Certainly a nihilistic approach to therapy, e.g., "take aspirin and accept the fact you are getting older," which has been common advice in the past, is not justified. The criteria for the determination of medical disability under Social Security are listed in Table 9.5 on page 121.

General Measures

Patient Education

Explaining to the patient the nature of the disease, that other joints are not likely to be involved, that progression of disease is slow, and that preservation of function is likely will reassure most patients. For the patient with Heberden's nodes or mild disease in other joints, this reassurance and understanding will be the most important therapeutic step in management. The physician should suggest some reading material for the patient such as *Learning to Live with Osteoarthritis* published in 1984 by Medicine in the Public Interest, Inc (Suite 720, 600 New Hampshire Ave NW, Washington, DC 20037.)

Rest

Pain and discomfort of degenerative joint disease are frequently exacerbated by use, especially continuous use or weight bearing. Further, excessive use of joints already damaged by osteoarthritis may accelerate cartilage degeneration. Therefore, rest is an important modality of treatment for osteoarthritis. Short periods of rest through the day are usually more effective than are less frequent longer periods. With weight-bearing joints, rest is particularly important. Many patients, especially elderly ones, have the notion that use of a joint becomes limited if it is rested too much, so that needless overuse is common. When an understanding of the value of rest and reassurance about function are given, patients will often quickly learn to live within their own limitations without undue restrictions of activity and with improvement in symptoms.

Use of Canes, Crutches, and Walkers

In more severe disease, rest from weight bearing and stability when walking may be partially achieved by the use of a crutch, a cane, or a walker. The patient's attitude about the use of such assistive devices is an important consideration here since some will interpret their cane as a sign of infirmity and fail to use it, while others may carry it proudly as a badge of dependency even when it is not needed. Instruction in proper use of a cane, a crutch, or a walker should be given by the physician or a physical therapist. It should be remembered that the object is to take weight off the affected limb; thus a cane or a crutch should always be used on the opposite side and used simultaneously with the affected limb for weight bearing. Also, a cane should be held tightly and close to the body. Proper use is assured by pressing the handle against the good hip. A walker does not provide this type of unilateral support, but it may be needed in patients with bilateral knee pain or in patients whose instability requires more support than that provided by a cane or a crutch.

Correction of Postural or Mechanical Strain

This is an important consideration in patients with poor body mechanics. Thus the patient with pronated feet (see Chapter 102, Common Problems of the Feet) will have excessive stress on the knees and low back. Genu varus or valgum will stress the lateral or medial compartment excessively. Instruction in proper lifting and avoidance of unnecessary strain on certain joints or muscles by occupational or other activities may also need attention—for example, use of a cervical pillow in the patient with neck involvement (see also Chapters 64, Neck Pain, and 65, Low Back Pain).

Physical Therapy

Simple measures can be prescribed for home use without the need for referral to a physical therapist in patients with mild disease. However, the physician must be sure that the patient understands directions. Reinforcement on subsequent visits is also important to ensure compliance. Patients with more advanced disease should be referred to a physical or occupational therapist for more extensive instruction in an exercise program, joint protection maneuvers, use of assistive devices, gait training, and the like.

Heat

Application of heat often provides symptomatic relief of pain, reduces muscle spasm, and facilitates subsequent performance of an exercise program. Most patients prefer moist heat, which can be applied for 15 to 20 minutes *via* bathtub, hot towels, or commercially manufactured packs. Electric heating pads may also be used. Paraffin wax baths (available from large pharmacies) may be useful in patients with extensive hand involvement. With all modalities of heat therapy, temperatures that are very hot (above 110°F (43°C)) and prolonged or uninterrupted use should be avoided, to prevent skin damage. Use of diathermy, ultrasound, heat cabinets, and the like offers little advantage in most cases and requires a physical therapist.

Exercise

Goals of an exercise program are to maintain or improve function by preserving range of motion and improving muscle strength. The latter is important to help stabilize the joint and, by maintaining soft tissue cushioning of stress, to reduce the stress applied to the joint. Gradual conditioning is important so that muscle pain and soreness are not aggravated. Exercise should be graded according to the ability of the individual patient and carried out at least three times/day for optimal effect. In general, if muscle soreness or joint pain is worse after exercise, the intensity of the exercise should be reduced or progression halted until symptoms subside. Swimming is also a valuable means of exercise that does not involve weight-bearing stress. Bicycling also provides exercise with less weight-bearing stress than does walking.

Maintenance of quadriceps strength is particularly important in osteoarthritis of the knee. This can be accomplished by beginning with slow full extension of the knee against gravity, and then, as symptoms and progress allow, by extension with progressively increasing weight attached to the lower leg (an old pocketbook or bag with a strap to which are added canned goods of specific weight from the pantry shelf will suffice). In patients whose pain prevents active quadriceps strengthening, isometric exercises are useful. With the knee extended the patient is instructed to tighten the quadriceps maximally so that the patella becomes fixed, hold for 10 to 15 seconds by count, release, and repeat.

Other Measures

For cervical spine disease gentle overhead traction may improve symptoms. This can be accomplished at home with a halter device and pulley and may be combined with the use of a soft cervical collar (see Chapter 64).

Many patients report remission of stiffness and pain and a sense of joint protection through the use of elastic supports around the joint. Such devices used at the knee, however, often obstruct venous circulation in the leg and cause edema, so that their use is not generally recommended. Wearing nylon stretch gloves (such as Iso-Toner gloves, available in department stores) may provide relief for some patients with extensive hand involvement (3).

Diet

Control of obesity (Chapter 76) is important in osteoarthritis of the knees, hips, and metatarsophalangeal joints. Otherwise there is no dietary imperative either to omit or to eat any specific foods, vitamins, or nutrients. Niacin, promoted by some as effective in controlling arthritis, has not been demonstrated scientifically as beneficial in the treatment or prevention of degenerative joint disease. Patients should be cautioned against food fads and unwarranted claims of relationship of diet and osteoarthritis.

Drug Therapy

Nonsteroidal Anti-inflammatory Drugs

Nonsteroidal anti-inflammatory drugs (NSAIDs) and analgesic agents are the mainstay of drug treatment of osteoarthritis. For patients with mild disease, pain is usually related to mechanical factors rather than to inflammation. Thus, analgesic doses are all that is required. Aspirin is an effective analgesic and usually is well tolerated in divided doses of 1.2 to 2.4 g/day. Tylenol is equally effective as an analgesic in patients unable to take aspirin.

Although mild by comparison to that of rheumatoid arthritis, the inflammatory component of osteoarthritis becomes more evident as the disease progresses and may warrant the use of anti-inflammatory doses of salicylates or other NSAIDs. The average dose of aspirin required may vary from 3.6 to 4.8 g/day for anti-inflammatory effect. At this dose gastrointestinal side effects of aspirin, including gastric ulceration and increased blood loss in the stool, are common. This may be largely obviated by the use of enteric coated aspirin, but erratic absorption in some patients requires a measure of blood salicylate level after several days of therapy to ensure an optimum level of 15 to 25 mg/dl. Other salicylate preparations such as choline salicylate (Arthropan liquid, 870 mg/5 ml, available without prescription), choline magnesium salicylate (Trilisate, 1500 mg), and salicylsalicylic acid (Disalcid, 500 mg) (both requiring a prescription) are also effective and have better gastrointestinal tolerance than aspirin, but are also significantly more expensive—about equal in cost to other nonsteroidal anti-inflammatory drugs.

A large number of NSAIDs (18) in addition to salicylates are now available and more are being developed. It is probable that the efficacy and side effects of aspirin and the nonsteroidal anti-inflammatory agents are mediated, at least in part through the ubiquitous prostaglandin system by inhibition of cyclo-oxygenase enzymes which are involved in the synthesis of prostaglandins from fatty acids of the cell membrane, principally arachidonic acid. The anti-inflammatory potency, duration of action, and side effects of each agent are somewhat variable because of the differences in tissue distribution and metabolism of the various drugs. For example indomethacin (Indocin) is a potent NSAID which penetrates most tissues, including the central nervous system. Tolmetin (Tolectin) has a somewhat similar molecular structure and efficacy, but because it is largely excluded by the blood-brain barrier, has fewer central nervous system side effects, such as headache and psychic disturbances. Sulindac (Clinoril) is converted to an active metabolite after absorption so that it bypasses and does not inhibit the local gastro-protective effect of prostaglandins in the gastric mucosa. It also has little effect on renal function, perhaps because of tissue distribution of active metabolites in the kidney. Naproxen (Naprosyn) and piroxicam (Feldene) have a long half-life in the plasma, so that intervals between doses can be increased.

In controlled clinical trials none of the NSAIDs has been shown to differ significantly from aspirin in efficacy in the treatment of osteoarthritis or other forms of arthritis, although the frequency of side effects has been lower with some of these drugs than with regular aspirin. Also, any one agent may be unaccountably more effective than another, so that a serial trial approach is often warranted. NSAIDs have been shown to have variable effects on cartilage metabolism, including decrease of proteoglycan synthesis (11), and in experimental models of osteoarthritis may accelerate cartilage loss (12). Whether or not these observations are relevant to human disease or to the choice of a particular NSAID is not known. Adverse effects on progression of hip osteoarthritis by indomethacin have been suggested (17). However, until more specific therapy is available, NSAIDs will continue to be the principal drug treatment for symptomatic relief of osteoarthritis.

Although use of combinations of NSAIDs is fairly common practice, there is no convincing evidence that this practice is beneficial. Interference with absorption of indomethacin by aspirin, displacement from protein binding, and other potential interactions of NSAIDs would seem to indicate that the prudent choice is to use a single agent to its maximal effect. This may require increasing dosage over a period of 2 to 6 weeks until symptoms are relieved, side effects occur, or lack of efficacy is established before switching to an alternative agent.

Since many patients with osteoarthritis have other medical conditions for which they are receiving therapeutic drugs, one must be alert to problems of interactions with NSAIDs. For example, NSAIDs may mitigate the therapeutic effect of agents that depend on prostaglandins to mediate a response, such as the naturetic and antihypertensive effects of furosemide, thiazides, or captopril (16).

Some of the factors in choice of an NSAID include cost (18), frequency of administration required (a major factor in compliance), and side effects, which may be variably tolerated by different patients (see Table 70.11, page 930 for list of side effects and dosage). Aspirin is clearly the cheapest and generally the drug of first choice in treatment of osteoarthritis. Ibuprofen (Motrin) is now available without prescription (as Advil or Nuprin) but costs more than regular or enteric coated aspirin.

Corticosteroids

Intra-articular injection of suspensions of corticosteroids (see Table 66.4, page 866) has been shown to be useful in the management of osteoarthritis, when associated with effusions in large joints such as the knee (6). The removal of joint fluid (without corticosteroid injection) when an effusion is present in degenerative arthritis usually does not improve symptoms unless a microcrystalline arthritis is superimposed (see Chapter 69). If prolonged relief lasting several months is not achieved with one or two injections, this therapy should not be continued. The risk of serious side effects including enhanced destruction of the joint and infection may follow repeated injections, which should therefore be avoided.

There is absolutely no indication for systemic administration of corticosteroids in the management of osteoarthritis.

Orthopaedic Surgery

The orthopaedist should be consulted in management of patients with osteoarthritis who have a problem of malalignment or major instability in weight-bearing joints, for symptoms or findings of loose bodies in the joint, and for intractable pain with advanced disease of the hips or knees. Osteotomy may correct malalignment. Arthroplasty to improve instability and remove loose bodies, meniscal fragments, and perhaps large spurs may be useful in some patients. When pain or disability is refractory

to treatment and joint destruction of a hip or a knee is advanced, consideration should be given to total joint replacement (5). Disabling pain is the principal indication for this procedure. Contraindications include neuromuscular or sensory deficits, severe peripheral vascular disease, marked obesity, dementia, and lack of motivation or inability to cooperate with a postoperative rehabilitation program. Results of joint replacement in osteoarthritis of the hip are generally excellent. Knee replacement has been somewhat less successful, but results have improved with new prostheses and in the hands of experienced surgeons; relief of pain approximates 90% but functional improvement is less certain. Arthrodesis (i.e., surgical fusion of the joint) is still useful in patients with unilateral, intractable, and severe knee involvement and may also be done when joint replacement has failed. Major complications of joint replacement are postoperative thrombophlebitis and infection. Elimination of potential foci of infection is important preoperatively, and prophylactic antibiotics are indicated after joint replacement surgery during dental or urinary tract procedures which might produce bacteremia (9). Although the continued improvement in synthetic materials and surgical techniques has prolonged the durability of an artificial joint, still most rheumatologists do not refer patients with hip or knee arthritis for surgery until symptoms are pronounced and functional impairment is considerable.

Recurrent symptoms of chondromalacia patellae may also be an indication for orthopaedic referral. Arthroscopy can confirm the diagnosis, and surgery may be indicated in some patients, although there is not uniform agreement on the procedure or its outcome.

PREVENTION

Since the etiology of degenerative joint disease is uncertain, so is its prevention. However, recognition of predisposing factors and elucidation of normal physiology of articular cartilage suggest certain prudent steps which can be recommended.

Immobilization with avoidance of joint stress gives rise to biochemical changes in cartilage similar to early lesions in osteoarthritis. Thus normal stress and functioning of joints are important in maintenance of normal cartilage physiology. Perhaps one can abstract from this that a sedentary and inactive life is not good for the integrity of articular cartilage. Further, since strong periarticular muscles lend stability and help to absorb stress applied to joints, it seems logical that physical conditioning to maintain muscle strength and a lean habitus may be important in prevention of degenerative joint disease. Soft tissues tend to lose mobility with advancing age and such changes have been shown to increase impact stress of joints. Physical activity may retard this loss of mobility and therefore should be encouraged in aging individuals.

At the same time it is evident that repetitive stress, especially when abnormally applied, is a strong predisposing factor to osteoarthritis. Thus correction of abnormal mechanical forces from developmental or postural defects, avoidance of unusual occupational stress, and avoidance of traumatic injury to joints are important in prevention of osteoarthritis.

General References

Brandt KD: Pathogenesis of osteoarthritis. In Kelley WN, Harris CD, Ruddy S, Sledge CB (eds): *Textbook of Rheumatology.* Philadelphia, WB Saunders, 1985, vol 2.

    This chapter provides an in-depth review of the pathogenesis of osteoarthritis.

Bland JH, Stalberg SD: Osteoarthritis: pathology and clinical patterns. In Kelley WN, Harris CD, Ruddy S, Sledge CB (eds): *Textbook of Rheumatology.* Philadelphia, WB Saunders, 1985, vol 2.

    This chapter provides an in-depth review of the pathology and patterns of osteoarthritis.

Gardner PL: The nature and causes of osteoarthritis. *Br Med J* 286:418, 1985.

    Provides a good review of mechanisms involved in pathogenesis of this disease.

Miskowitz RW, Howell DS, Goldberg VM, Mankin HJ (eds): *Osteoarthritis, Diagnosis and Management.* Philadelphia, WB Saunders, 1984.

    A multiauthored text providing extensive basic and clinical information on the subject.

Radin EC: Chondromalacia of the patella. *Bull Rheum Dis* 34:1, 1982.

    An excellent review of chondromalacia patellae.

Robertson WD: Management of degenerative disease. In Kelley WN, Harris CD, Ruddy S, Sledge CB (eds): *Textbook of Rheumatology.* Philadelphia, WB Saunders, 1985, vol 2.

    This chapter provides an in-depth review of the management of osteoarthritis.

Specific References

1. Daniels DC, Grogan JP, Johansen JG, et al: Cervical radiculopathy: computed tomography and myelography compared. *Radiology* 151:109, 1984.
2. Doherty M, Watt I, Dieppe P: Influence of primary generalized osteoarthritis on development of secondary osteoarthritis. *Lancet* 2:8, 1983.
3. Ehrlich GE, DiPiero AM: Stretch gloves: nocturnal use to ameliorate morning stiffness in arthritic hands. *Arch Phys Med Rehabil* 52:479, 1971.
4. Glynn LE: Primary lesion in osteoarthritis. *Lancet* 1:574, 1977.
5. Harris WH: Total joint replacement. *N Engl J Med* 297:650, 1977.
6. Hollander JL: Treatment of osteoarthritis of the knees. *Arthritis Rheum* 3:564, 1960.
7. Huskisson EC, Dieppe PA, Tucker AK, Channel LB: Another look at osteoarthritis. *Ann Rheum Dis* 38:423, 1979.
7a. Jasin HE: Autoantibody specificities of immune complexes sequestered in articular cartilage of patients with rheumatoid arthritis and osteoarthritis. *Arthritis Rheum* 28:241, 1985.
8. Kellgren JH, Moore R: Generalized osteoarthritis and Heberden's nodes. *Br Med J* 1:181, 1952.
9. Liang MD, Cullen KE, Poss R: Primary total hip or knee replacement: evaluation of patients. *Ann Intern Med* 97:735, 1982.
10. Marsland DW, Wood M, Mayo F: Content of family practice. I. Routine order of diagnosis by frequency. II. Diagnosis by disease category and age/sex distribution. *J Fam Pract* 8:37, 1976.
11. Palmoski MJ, Brandt KD: Effects of some nonsteroidal anti-inflammatory drugs on proteoglycan metabolism and organization in canine articular cartilage. *Arthritis Rheum* 23:1010, 1980.
12. Palmoski MJ, Brandt KD: *In vivo* effect of aspirin on canine osteoarthritic cartilage. *Arthritis Rheum* 26:994, 1983.
13. Peter JB, Pearson CM, Marmnor L: Erosive osteoarthritis of the hands. *Arthritis Rheum* 9:365, 1966.
14. Radin EL, Parker HG, Pugh JW, et al: Response of joints to impact loading. III. Relationship between trabecular microfractures and cartilage degeneration. *J Biomech* 6:51, 1973.
15. Resnick D, Shapiro RF, Wiesner KB, et al: Diffuse idiopathic skeletal hyperostosis (DISH) (ankylosing hyperostosis of Forestier and Rotes-Querol). *Semin Arthritis Rheum* 7:153, 1978.
16. Rizack MA, Hillman CDM (eds): *The Medical Letter Handbook of Drug Interactions.* New Rochelle, NY, The Medical Letter, 1983.
17. Ronnigen H, Langeland N: Indomethacin treatment in osteoarthritis of the hip joint. *Acta Orthop Scand* 50:169, 1979.
18. Simon LS, Mills JA: Non-steroidal anti-inflammatory drugs. *N Engl J Med* 302:1179, 1237, 1980.
19. Stecker RM: Heberden's nodes, heredity in hypertrophic arthritis of the finger joints. *Am J Med Sci* 201:801, 1941.

CHAPTER SIXTY-NINE

Crystal-Induced Arthritis

ALEXANDER S. TOWNES, M.D.

INTRODUCTION

Gout was the first form of arthritis that was recognized to be caused by the deposition of (urate) crystals in the joints and periarticular tissues. It is now known that other crystalline substances—most commonly calcium pyrophosphate dihydrate and hydroxipatite—also are implicated in the pathogenesis of certain kinds of arthritic disease. Although disorders associated with these various crystals differ in etiology and in specific characteristics, they have in common the deposition of crystals in and around joints, the propensity to episodes of acute inflammatory arthritis and sometimes the development of a destructive arthropathy. It is therefore appropriate to consider these varied clinical disorders together under the unifying concept of crystal-induced arthritis.

Mechanisms of Crystal-Induced Arthritis

The inflammatory properties of crystals such as sodium urate and calcium pyrophosphate dihydrate when injected into joints or soft tissues depend upon the interaction of the crystals by polymorphonuclear leukocytes (PMN). Leukocytes which have phagocytized crystals generate and release a potent low molecular weight chemotactic factor, a glycopeptide, which attracts more neutrophils and amplifies the response. During the process of phagocytosis, leukocytes also release into the surrounding tissue lysosomal enzymes which further activate mediators of inflammation. Urate crystals, by the nature of their electrostatic surface charge, also interact with other plasma proteins to activate the complement system and the kinin system, contributing further to the inflammatory response.

Although the events which trigger acute inflammation are not entirely clear, it seems likely that there is, in association with rapid changes in serum urate concentration, a sudden release of a sufficient volume of crystalline material from tissue sites into joint spaces to begin the cycle of phagocytosis and inflammation (8, 9).

The invariable association between phagocytosis of crystals and the acute inflammatory response is important clinically since demonstration of crystals within leukocytes from synovial fluid constitutes a convenient method of making a definitive diagnosis in patients with acute inflammatory crystal-induced arthritis.

Although gouty arthritis and other crystal-induced diseases are usually characterized by symptoms and signs of acute inflammation, sometimes destructive arthropathy occurs with little evidence of inflammation.

Crystal Identification

The identification of crystals in synovial fluid or in periarticular tissue is fundamental to the diagnosis and management of patients with crystal-induced arthritis. Crystals of monosodium urate are best identified by placing a drop of aspirated tissue fluid directly on a glass slide and by examining the wet preparation through a microscope under polarized light (16); the crystals are difficult to see under nonpolarized light. Although specialized equipment is ideal, crystals can be demonstrated adequately in the physician's office by placing a plastic polarizing lens (made from an old pair of sunglasses, for example) between the light source and the microscopic stage, and by placing another lens in the body or in the eyepiece of the microscope. When one lens is rotated so that the field becomes dark, the negatively birefringent urate crystals (i.e., crystals capable of bending light rays in two planes; the notation of negativity is an arbitrary term used by physicists to describe the direction of bend), dimly seen in ordinary light, stand out brightly and can be identified within the cytoplasm of polymorphonuclear leukocytes. If a red plate compensator is placed between the light source and the stage of the microscope (one can be fabricated by wrapping a glass slide longitudinally with two layers of transparent (cellophane) tape (occasionally more layers of tape are required)) (2), the crystals are even more easily identified since the field turns red and crystals parallel to the axis of the compensator will appear yellow, while those perpendicular to the axis will appear blue. Monosodium urate crystals are usually needle or rod shaped. The size varies, but some large crystals equal to or larger than the diameter of the leukocyte are usually seen. A wet slide of joint fluid prepared in this manner may be kept for several hours at room temperature; however, once the cells die and lyse, evaluation is less valid. In the event the aspirated fluid cannot be examined immediately, it may be preserved overnight by refrigeration in a plain test tube.

Monosodium urate crystals (which are usually present in abundance) are pathognomonic of gout (see Table 69.1 and Fig. 69.1). Absence of crystals is strong evidence against the diagnosis, and, especially if leukocytosis is significant, infection or another diagnosis should be considered.

Monosodium urate is usually easily distinguished from calcium pyrophosphate dihydrate (CPPD) on the basis of morphology and of characteristics of the crystals under polarized light (see Table 69.1 and Fig. 69.1). CPPD crystals vary much more in size and shape from rod-like to rhomboid and irregular forms, are usually much shorter, and are never needle-like. They are usually refractile without polarized light and do not increase appreciably in brilliance when the light is polarized. They are weakly positively birefringent and change color in the opposite direction to urate when the red plate compensator is placed between the polarizing lens (i.e., blue when parallel to the axis and yellow when perpendicular).

Because CPPD crystals are small and do not stand out in polarized light, they are overlooked more frequently by the occasional observer. Routine reports from unspecialized clinical laboratories are often falsely negative.

Other crystalline materials which may be seen include those from previously injected corticosteroids (which appear as crystals of varying and unusual configuration), and occasionally cholesterol crystals which are easily distinguished from all of the above (resembling a folded envelope). Contaminating crystalline or refractile substances, such as ethylenediaminetetraacetic acid anticoagulant, talc, *etc*, can be avoided by use of careful technique.

Table 69.1.
Identification of Crystals in Synovial Fluid

MONOSODIUM URATE
  Morphology:
    Rod or needle shaped
    Length usually approaches diameter of polymorphonuclear leukocyte (PMN)
  Polarized light:
    Stand out brightly when field is dark
    Strongly negative birefringent
  Red plate compensator:
    Yellow crystals parallel and blue crystals perpendicular to axis
CALCIUM PYROPHOSPHATE DIHYDRATE
  Morphology:
    Rhomboid, rod, or irregular rhomboid shape
    Length variable, often smaller than one lobe of a PMN nucleus
  Polarized light:
    No increase in refractile appearance when field is dark
    Weakly positively birefringent
  Red plate compensator:
    Blue crystals parallel and yellow crystals perpendicular to axis
HYDROXYAPATITE
Not usually seen with ordinary or polarized light microscopy
Stain nonspecifically with alizarin Red S (available in histology laboratories) as clusters of crystalline material. Useful as a screening test.
Requires electron microscopy, X-ray diffraction, or microprobe analysis for more definite identification.

GOUT

Pathophysiology

Gout is a syndrome that is caused by an alteration in purine metabolism, the end product of which is uric acid. This alteration results in hyperuricemia and in the deposition of urate crystals in various tissues. Periodic attacks of acute inflammatory arthritis, characteristic of gout, are due to the deposition of urate crystals in and about joints. *Primary gout* is caused by an inborn error in the production or excretion of uric acid. *Secondary gout* is caused by an increased breakdown of nucleic acids in association with one of a variety of acquired diseases or by impaired excretion of urate as a consequence of acquired renal disease (Table 69.2).

Most patients with gout (approximately 85%) have, usually for unknown reasons, an elevated renal threshold for the excretion of uric acid. The rest (approximately 15%) overproduce uric acid, although precise enzymatic defects in purine catabolism only rarely have been identified. Production and excretion of uric acid are best assessed by meas-

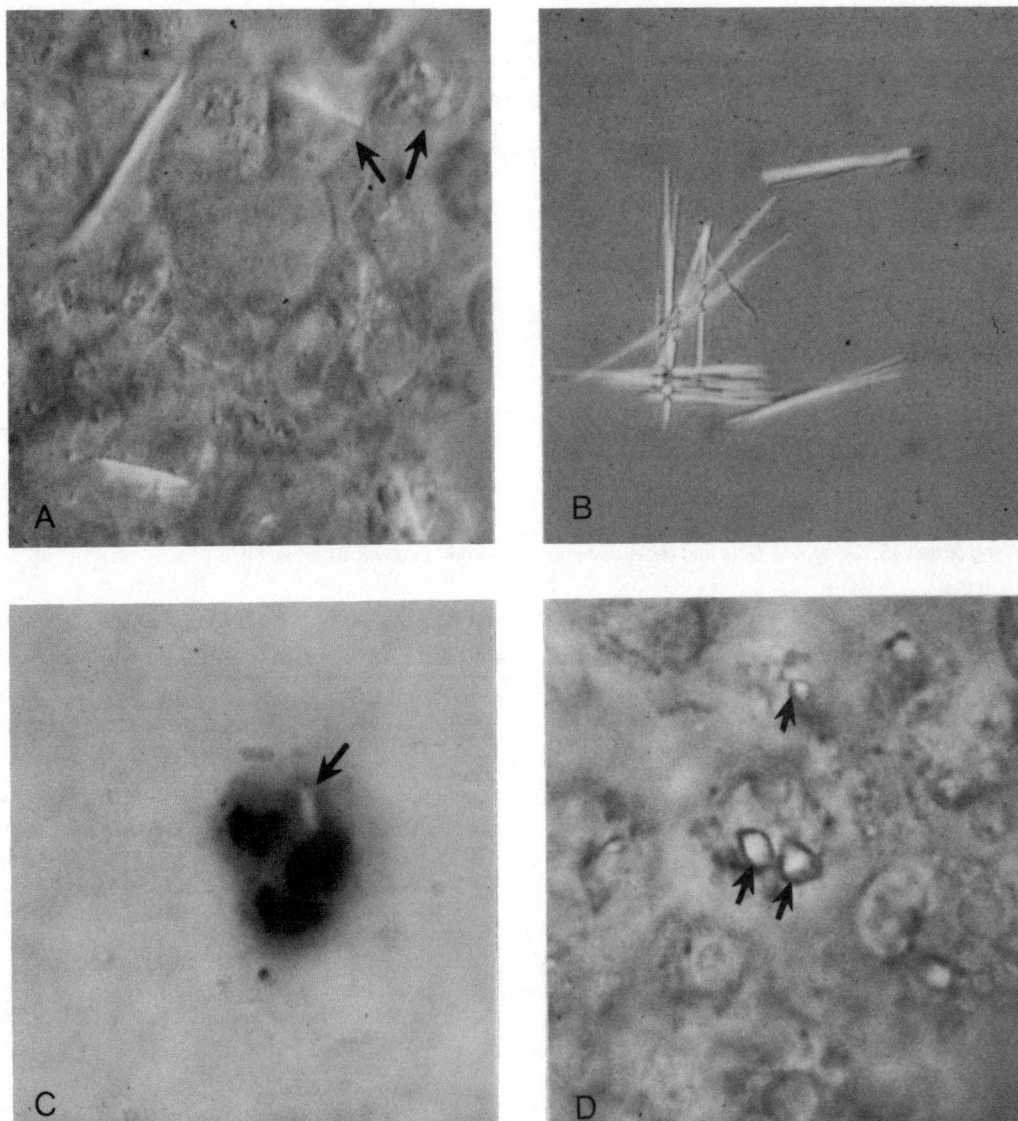

Figure 69.1. *A.* Urate crystals in synovial fluid examined by polarized light microscopy. Note the needle shape and variable size, but many have a larger diameter than white blood cells (oil immersion). *B.* Urate crystals from tophus examined by polarized light with red plate compensator (oil immersion). *C.* Calcium pyrophosphate dihydrate (CPPD) crystal in white blood cell found on Gram stain (oil immersion). Note the shape and size relative to nucleus and cytoplasm. Gram stain is not the usual method of demonstration, but it is occasionally useful. *D.* Wet preparation of synovial fluid demonstrating varied size and shape of CPPD crystal phagocytized by white blood cell (oil immersion lens, polarized light). Size and shape varies from squat rhomboid to rod shaped. Note several crystals in some cells.

urement of urate in a 24-hour sample of urine; normally less than 600 mg/day are excreted if the diet for 5 days has been free of foods that are rich in purines (fish, meat, and poultry—especially the solid organs of these food sources); while there is considerable dietary variation, an excretion of more than approximately 750 to 800 mg/day while eating a nonrestricted diet may be considered indicative of overproduction in the absence of purine gluttony (4).

Normal levels of serum urate vary widely in the population, with a range of 3 to 8 mg/dl; also, there may be spontaneous variation within individuals. The upper limit of normal for serum urate measured by the uricase method usually is considered to be 7.0 mg/dl for adult males and 6.0 mg/dl for females. Ranges may be higher by 1 mg/dl or more if automated colorimetric methods, commonly used in multiphasic screening tests, are employed.

Serum "uric acid" concentration is primarily a

Table 69.2.
Causes of Hyperuricemia[a]

With Increased Urinary Uric Acid	With Normal or Low Urinary Uric Acid
10–25% of primary gout (defect unknown)	75–90% of primary gout (defect unknown)
Specific enzyme defects with primary gout	
Secondary causes:	Secondary causes:
Myeloproliferative disease	Renal insufficiency
Lymphoproliferative disease	Lead intoxication
Hemolytic anemias	Drugs:
Obesity	Salicylates (low dose, *i.e.*, < 2.4 g/day)
Glycogen storage disease	Diuretics
Exercise	Pyrazinamide
Psoriasis	Ethambutol
	Nicotinic acid
	Alcohol
	Others
	Obesity
	Sarcoidosis
	Starvation

[a] Modified from Wyngaarden JB, Kelley WN: *Gout and Hyperuricemia*. New York, Grune & Stratton, 1976.

measurement of urate. The concentrations of urate and uric acid are related to pH: at normal blood and interstitial fluid pH of 7.40, the ratio of urate to uric acid is approximately 45:1; as the pH falls—e.g., in the urinary tubule—the relative concentration of uric acid rises (e.g., at a pH of 4.50 the urate to uric acid ratio is approximately 0.06:1).

Prevalence

Gout is estimated to occur at a lifetime frequency of 3/1000 population in the United States. It is 10 times more common in males in all of its forms and is rare in premenopausal females. Gout is infrequent below age 30 and increases in frequency to a plateau at about age 60. Age at onset is probably related to the duration and severity of preceding hyperuricemia. Gout is more common in obese or in hypertensive people, although the relationships are complex. The frequency of gout in hypertensive subjects, for example, is magnified if they are treated with thiazide diuretics (see below). Gout is also more common in patients with a chronically high alcohol intake, especially if they also are obese or have mildly impaired renal function. Associations of gout with hyperlipidemia and with atherosclerotic coronary disease have also been reported, but these relationships need further clarification.

Clinical Features (Table 69.3)

Acute Arthritic Attack

The acute arthritic attack is the hallmark of gout. It is characterized by the onset of pain, swelling, and discomfort that progress rapidly to a peak level of intensity within 24 to 36 hours after onset. The pain is often severe enough to prevent use of the affected joint or even for the patient to bear the weight of bed clothing. The metatarsophalangeal joint of the great toe is the most commonly affected joint, fol-

Table 69.3.
Clinical Features of Gout

EPIDEMIOLOGY
  Sex: Males 10 to 1; Rare in premenopausal women
  Age: Usually middle age or older (peak age 60)
ACUTE GOUT
  History:
    Acute attacks, recurrent, with disease-free intervals
    Rapid progression to peak severity within 24 hours
  Physical findings:
    Usually monoarticular with swelling, tenderness, erythema, and intense inflammation
    Big toe metatarsophalangeal joint commonly involved (podagra)
    Forefeet, heels, ankles, knees, wrists, fingers, elbows, and other joints may be affected
    Occasionally polyarticular
    Fever may occur
  Laboratory: Joint aspiration with leukocytosis and identification of urate crystals is diagnostic
INTERCRITICAL GOUT
  No symptoms or findings except hyperuricemia
CHRONIC GOUT
  Often polyarticular
  Symptoms may persist between attacks
  Tophi are common (approximately 90–95%)
  Deformities may develop

lowed by the forefoot, heel, ankle, knee, wrist, fingers, and elbow. The great toe is affected at some time during the course of perhaps 90% of gouty subjects. Usually a single joint is involved early in the course of the disease but pauciarticular arthritis (two or three joints) may occur; polyarticular (more than three joints) onset is rare. Polyarticular gout is more common is late disease associated with soft tissue tophi. Recurrent acute arthritis is more common in previously affected joints.

There are several events that may trigger an acute

attack of gout: trauma, an acute illness such as an acute myocardial infarction, dietary indiscretion, overuse of alcohol, starvation, and recent administration of drugs that lower serum urate concentration. Most of these events are associated with rapid changes in serum urate concentration, and it has been postulated that such changes cause dissolution of tissue deposits with discharge of crystalline material locally to induce the acute attack.

A family history of gout should be sought in patients with primary gout, and especially in those patients who excrete excess amounts of uric acid in whom a specific enzyme defect may be suspected. However, a positive family history is obtained in less than half of gouty subjects so that a negative history is of no differential diagnostic value.

On physical examination of the patient with acute gouty arthritis there is frequently erythema overlying or adjacent to the affected joints, especially when small joints are involved. The erythema often involves only a localized area rather than the entire joint. The intensity of the inflammatory reaction frequently results in a mistaken diagnosis of cellulitis, a diagnosis which may appear to be supported by a fever which may reach 101°F (38°C) or higher. Joint swelling usually is marked and joint effusion is also common. Tenderness on palpation or motion of the affected part also usually is marked.

The intensity and severity of these classical acute signs and symptoms may vary from one attack to another and may be less evident when a large joint such as the knee in involved, especially in elderly patients and in patients with polyarticular gout. However, the history will almost always indicate rapid progression to a peak intensity within 24 to 36 hours, an important feature in differential diagnosis.

Laboratory findings may include a mild leukocytosis and an elevated erythrocyte sedimentation rate. Serum uric acid almost always is elevated but is of limited diagnostic value because of the frequency of hyperuricemia in the absence of gout, and because the acute attack, which is related principally to the concentration of tissue urate, may occur at a time when the serum urate may be normal as a result of previous drug administration (such as high dose aspirin (>3.5 g/day) or another uricosuric agent) or of spontaneous variation. Examination of the synovial fluid provides diagnostic findings in almost all instances in which it can be obtained. There is a brisk leukocytosis in the joint fluid with polymorphonuclear leukocytes that, when examined under polarized light, can be seen to contain phagocytized urate crystals (see section on crystal identification).

The acute attack is self-limited and even without treatment will subside in several days to weeks. Once the acute attack subsides or is treated, there are no residual joint symptoms—another important point in the differential diagnosis.

Recurrent acute attacks are usual: approximately 75% of patients will have a second gouty attack within 2 years of their first and most of these will have occurred within the first year; occasionally 10 years or more may elapse between attacks (22).

Intercritical Gout

Between acute attacks of gout, patients will be totally asymptomatic with no abnormal physical findings unless tophi are present or unless the disease has progressed to the chronic phase. If the patient's first visit to the physician is at this stage, a presumptive diagnosis can be made on the basis of a history of a typical prior attack, especially if there have been multiple attacks, and on the basis of hyperuricemia. The observation that aspiration of the great toe during intercritical gout, with the demonstration of urate crystals, would establish a definitive diagnosis of gout (20) has been challenged by a subsequent report that demonstrated that urate crystals may be found in the joint spaces of patients without gout who simply have hyperuricemia (19).

Chronic Gout

This form of the disease is infrequent, especially since the advent of effective therapy to control hyperuricemia. Patients with chronic gout frequently have some persistent symptoms (such as morning stiffness) and manifest signs of synovial tissue thickening and some joint deformity. Acute exacerbations are still frequent and are often polyarticular. Tophi (soft tissue deposits of sodium urate) are present in 90 to 95% of patients. The rate of formation of tophi seems to be a direct function of the level and duration of hyperuricemia. Tophi are chalky or pinkish, gritty, usually superficial deposits that are palpable in joints or tendons, over pressure points, or in the pinnae of the ears. They are usually painless but as from palpation they may be tender. Large tophi may look like bulbous swellings of the joints or, when they are located over the extensor surface of the forearm or in the ulnar bursa, may be mistaken for rheumatoid nodules. In such circumstances, aspiration or biopsy of tophi with demonstration of urate crystals will confirm the diagnosis of chronic gout. The actual concurrence of gout and rheumatoid arthritis is extremely rare.

Extra-articular Manifestations

It has long been known that primary gout may be associated with renal disease in three forms: *chronic gouty nephropathy, nephrolithiasis, and acute uric acid nephropathy.*

Chronic gouty nephropathy develops after many years of hyperuricemia and results from the deposition in the interstitial medullary tissue of sodium urate crystals that cause, ultimately, an interstitial nephritis. The frequency of this complication, until recently, had been assumed to be high. Recent controlled studies, however, indicate that the incidence of renal insufficiency solely from gout and hyperuricemia is low and that renal dysfunction is usually mild; most often renal failure in patients with gout can be attributed to age, vascular disease, or primary renal disease (1, 3). Renal failure from primary gout and hyperuricemia is usually silent and suspected only because of the identification of a mild abnormality of the concentration of blood urea nitrogen or of serum creatinine. Some patients will have slight proteinuria; only a few will be found to have peripheral tophi. It is not known whether secondary gout is associated with the development of chronic gouty nephropathy. The evaluation and management of patients who have renal failure are discussed in Chapter 47.

Uric acid nephrolithiasis accounts for only a small number of patients who have urinary calculi (see Chapter 46). However, approximately 20% of patients with gout develop calculi, although the stones may antedate acute gouty arthritis by years. From a different perspective, about 25% of patients with uric acid calculi have an abnormal serum urate concentration. The prevalence of uric acid calculi increases proportionate to the concentration of serum urate or to the excretion of uric acid whether or not gout is present. In one study, in which a cohort of men was followed for 12 years, serum levels of urate of 7 to 8 mg/dl, 8 to 9 mg/dl, and > 9 mg/dl were associated with renal stones in 12.7%, 22%, and 40%, respectively (5). Also in gouty patients, urinary excretion rates of < 300, 300 to 700, 700 to 1100, and > 1100 mg/24 hours of uric acid were associated with a prevalence of renal stones of 11, 21, 35, and 50%, respectively (23). The development of uric acid calculi is related not only to uric acid excretion but also to urinary pH and concentration. This subject is more fully discussed in Chapter 46.

Acute uric acid nephropathy is associated with a sudden increase in urate production and a marked rise in uric acid excretion, resulting in the formation of microcrystals in the renal tubules. This most often occurs in patients with lympho- or myeloproliferative disorders, especially during treatment. Acute uric acid nephropathy is rarely encountered in ambulatory practice.

Differential Diagnosis

During the acute attack gout must be differentiated principally from acute infectious arthritis, from bursitis related to a bunion (see Chapter 102), or from other forms of crystal-induced arthritis. It is important therefore to aspirate joint fluid for smear and culture (see Chapter 66 for technique) as well as for crystal identification. Infectious arthritis is associated with a very low synovial fluid glucose, not found in gouty fluids.

X-rays (Fig. 69.2)

In the early course of gout, X-rays are normal except for acute soft tissue swelling. As the disease

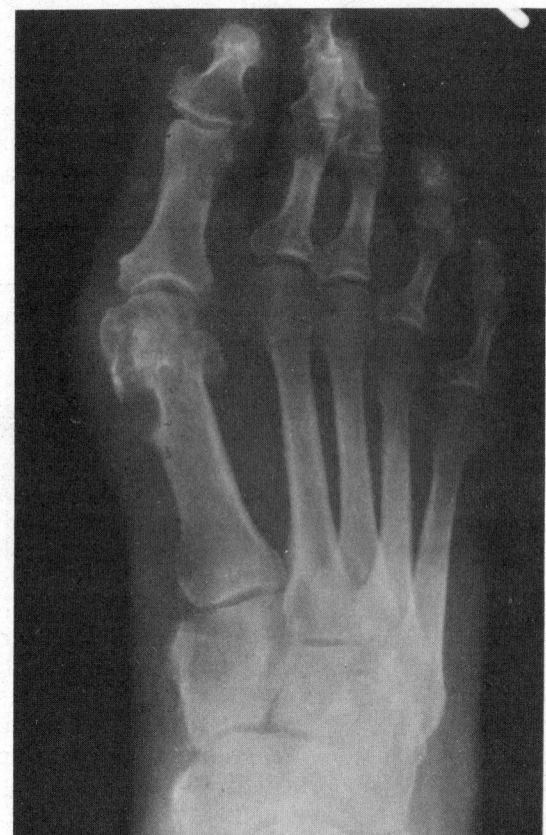

Figure 69.2. X-ray of foot in patient with gout showing soft tissue swelling over first metatarsophalangeal joint and typical gouty erosion: away from joint margin, punched out with overhanging edge and no osteoporosis.

progresses, lucent areas of urate deposits may be seen in bone adjacent to the joints. These lesions may be mistaken for the erosions that are seen in rheumatoid or other arthritides but may be distinguished from them in that osteoporosis and bony sclerosis, which are common in other erosive diseases, are not present. Overhanging margins of bone are said to be characteristic of gouty erosions but are not frequently found.

X-rays of gouty joints are thus indicated mainly to evaluate the extent of possible tophaceous deposits in patients with gout of long duration, and only occasionally are indicated as an aid to diagnosis or differential diagnosis.

Management

If the diagnosis of gout can be established with certainty by the demonstration of urate crystals, the treatment is relatively simple and straightforward. Hospitalization is seldom required unless the diagnosis is in doubt; even the most severe case can be effectively managed on an ambulatory basis. The key elements in management are control of the pain of the acute attack and patient education to assure compliance with therapy administered to reduce serum urate concentration and to prevent recurrent attacks and progression to chronic tophaceous gout.

Management of the Acute Attack

If the diagnosis of acute gout is established or if gout has been diagnosed previously by the identification of urate crystals in the affected joints, rapid relief can be obtained in almost all cases by the administration of nonsteroidal anti-inflammatory drugs in appropriate doses. Indomethacin (Indocin) 50 mg (i.e., two 25-mg capsules) every 6 hours for six to eight doses is dramatically effective. There are few side effects if the dose is then quickly reduced to 25 mg every 6 hours after the initial response and maintained until the attack is completely resolved, usually no more than 5 to 7 days. Alternatively, other nonsteroidal anti-inflammatory drugs may be used (see Table 70.11, Chapter 70). Phenylbutazone (Butazolidin), a potent anti-inflammatory agent, has been largely replaced by better tolerated and safer drugs. The plasma concentration and therapeutic effect of indomethacin (and of naproxen but apparently not of other nonsteroidal anti-inflammatory agents) are potentiated by an unknown mechanism by the simultaneous administration of probenecid (see below). While the clinical sigificance of this interaction is unclear, especially with short course therapy, the manufacturer recommends that the dose of the nonsteroidal drug be reduced in patients who also are taking probenecid.

Colchicine is the time-honored drug for treatment of acute gout; but its efficacy is limited by side effects that are almost invariable if an adequate dose is administered orally. The usual regimen is 0.6 mg every 2 hours up to 16 doses until relief is obtained or until side effects, usually diarrhea, nausea, or vomiting, develop. It is no longer necessary to subject a patient to severe diarrhea when he already has a very painful joint, so that oral colchicine has largely been replaced by nonsteroidal anti-inflammatory agents. They are at least as effective and have fewer side effects. The exception is in the well instructed patient who immediately after recognizing the onset of an acute attack of gout can institute oral colchicine and in doing so can abate the attack with a few doses and with minimal side effects.

Intravenous administration of colchicine rapidly provides a therapeutic plasma level of the drug and does not cause gastrointestinal side effects. It is particularly useful in treatment of acute gout when the patient cannot take medication by mouth and in the patient with peptic ulcer disease, or with another contradindication to the use of nonsteroidal agents. Two milligrams of colchicine (available in ampules containing 1 mg in 2 ml) diluted with isotonic saline to 20 ml and given slowly (i.e., over 10 minutes) intravenously usually provide relief within 6 to 8 hours and, if necessary, may be followed by one or two doses of 1 mg in 20 ml of isotonic saline intra-venously in 12 to 24 hours, not to exceed 4 mg in 24 hours. Reduced dosage is necessary in patients with impaired renal function. Care must be used to prevent extravasation of colchicine into the soft tissues since it may cause necrosis.

A diagnostic therapeutic trial of colchicine has limited value (except with podagra, see below) since acute gout of several days' duration may not respond to colchicine and since pseudogout due to calcium pyrophosphate dihydrate-induced arthritis often shows a dramatic response as well.

Drugs administered to lower serum urate have no place in the treatment of the acute gouty attack. In fact, these agents may cause exacerbation of acute attacks by the associated changes in plasma urate levels (see above).

Acute Podagra

Podagra is an acute inflammatory arthritis of the first metatarsophalangeal joint and is a characteristic manifestation of gout. Other acute arthritides are much less likely to involve the great toe. It is quite difficult to aspirate the first metatarsophalangeal joint when it is acutely inflamed; in fact an inexperienced physician may cause marked discomfort for the patient. For this reason, if the physician is inexperienced, he should made a presumptive diagnosis on clinical grounds, supported by the demonstration of an elevated serum urate concentration, although this finding is not always present. In this situation, the diagnosis will be further strengthened by the resolution or marked improvement of the problem within 6 to 8 hours after the administration of intravenous colchicine by the physician in his office. A response of early podagra to colchicine is more specific for gout than is a response to a nonsteroidal anti-inflammatory agent. Intravenous colchicine, therefore, is suggested when a patient is first seen and the diagnosis has not been definitively established.

Intercritical Gout

The efficacy of colchicine in doses of 0.6 mg one, two, or three times daily (dose frequency depends on control; most require two doses a day) in reducing the frequency of acute attacks of gout has been well established (22). Thus, prophylactic colchicine should be given to all patients who have had more than one episode of acute gout to prevent recurrent attacks or to reduce the frequency of those attacks. In patients without tophi (nontophaceous gout), with infrequent acute attacks and with mild hyperuricemia (i.e., < 8 to 9 mg/dl), this therapy may be all that is required. Some patients who have nontophaceous gout with infrequent attacks of arthritis (e.g., less than one or two a year) and who have relatively mild hyperuricemia (i.e., < 8 to 9 mg/dl) may as an option elect not to take regular colchicine prophylaxis; in this instance, the episodic use of a nonsteroidal anti-inflammatory drug such as indomethacin

(Indocin) (see above) is appropriate to control acute attacks. However, in most patients with gout and with persistent hyperuricemia of 9 mg/dl or higher, the serum urate concentration should be reduced to prevent recurrent gout and to reverse the accumulation of urate in the tissues. In this instance, colchicine prophylaxis should be continued until the patient has been free of attacks for at least 3 to 6 months after the concentration of serum urate has returned to normal.

Two classes of drugs that lower serum urate concentration are available: *uricosuric agents* promote urinary excretion of urate by blocking tubular urate resorption, and *allopurinol* (Xyloprim) decreases production of urate through inhibition of purine metabolism. Indications for the use of allopurinol are a history of urinary calculi or the presence of renal insufficiency, of chronic tophaceous gout, of excessive basal urinary uric acid excretion (*i.e.*, > 750 to 800 mg/24 hours), or of high levels of serum urate associated with secondary gout. Uricosuric agents are most effective in patients with nontophaceous gout with normal renal function and normal uric acid excretion (*i.e.*, < 750 to 800 mg/24 hours). Evaluation of *urinary uric acid excretion* is thus important not only as a clue to the mechanism of hyperuricemia (Table 69.2) but in the choice of therapy.

Probenecid (Benemid) is the uricosuric agent of choice because of its well established safety and its relatively long duration of effect. An initial dose of 0.5 g twice daily should be increased to 1.5 g daily or to a maximum of 2 g/day (in two or three divided doses) to achieve a serum urate concentration consistently below 6.5 mg/dl, the level required to produce a urate gradient from tissue to plasma and to prevent further deposition of urate. In order to minimize the chance of precipitating a recurrent arthritic attack, the uricosuric agent should not be initiated until at least a week after an acute attack of gout has subsided and only after colchicine prophylaxis (see above) has been initiated for 3 or 4 days. The principal side effect of probenecid is gastrointestinal distress, but there is a risk of the formation of uric acid calculi in the renal tubules in the first week of therapy (the period of negative uric acid balance), especially when there is a large basal uric acid excretion (*i.e.*, 600 to 800 mg/day); this risk can be eliminated if the patient drinks 2 to 3 liters of fluid/day and takes an alkalinizing agent such as sodium bicarbonate or citrate salt (Polycitrate) 0.5 to 1 mEq/kg of body weight in five or six doses a day to keep the urine pH above 6.0 to 6.5 for the first week of uricosuric therapy. Small doses of aspirin (2.4 g/day) block the effect of probenecid on renal excretion of urate and should be avoided.

Sulfinpyrazone (Anturane) is a more potent uricosuric agent but must be given every 4 to 6 hours (400 to 600 mg/day) for maximum effect. This agent, which is an analog of phenylbutazone, may cause gastric ulceration and platelet dysfunction. For these reasons, it should be used only when probenecid or allopurinol (see below) is not tolerated.

Allopurinol (Xyloprim) is a potent agent that reduces the concentration of serum urate, Since it blocks urate production, it is particularly useful in patients with renal dysfunction or with uric acid calculi. Serious side effects of rash, fever, leukopenia, hepatitis, and/or occasionally a generalized vasculitis occur in less than 2% of patients. These symptoms are most likely to occur within the first 2 months after initiation of therapy so that patients should be kept under close surveillance during this period. Toxicity seems to be enhanced when the drug is administered concomitantly with thiazide diuretics. Allopurinol (Xyloprim, available in 100- and 300-mg tablets) should be started at a dose of 200 mg daily and increased gradually (*i.e.*, over 2 or 3 weeks) until the serum urate is consistently below 6.5 mg/dl; no more than 300 mg should be administered as a single dose. Prolonged use of doses in excess of 300 mg twice a day increases the risk of toxicity.

Concomitant use of allopurinol and probenecid has been advocated (18). These agents seem to have an additive effect in lowering serum uric acid. However, use of a single agent is preferable if possible.

Compliance is the major factor in the effective therapy of intercritical gout. Patients feel well between attacks, and continued compliance with medications requires reinforcement in patient education and in follow-up visits to ensure maintenance of normal serum levels of urate.

Dietary advice to patients with gout should be kept simple. Because of the complexity of urate metabolism and secretion, the role of ingestion of purine in gout is of importance only in extreme situations. Patients with an excretion of urate that is greater than 1100 mg/24 hours should be advised to decrease the use of purine-rich foods if they give a history of this gluttony. Purine-rich foods, such as liver, kidney, and fish roe, are not, however, commonly used in excess. More importantly, dietary advice is to avoid alcohol debauchery and fasting beyond 24 hours as both these situations may be associated with acute increase of serum urate concentration and this change may precipitate an attack of gout.

Chronic Gout

Compliance with appropriate therapy should eliminate this phase of gout except for a few patients with severe disease who are intolerant of one or more drugs used in treatment. Prolonged use of nonsteroidal anti-inflammatory agents (including aspirin in doses greater than 3.5 g/day—a uricosuric dose) may be required in some of these patients for adequate control of inflammation and chronic symptoms. Effective reduction in serum urate for months or years will result in dissolution of tophi and in general improvement. However, very large tophi may require surgical removal.

Asymptomatic Hyperuricemia

Asymptomatic hyperuricemia (> 7 mg/dl in males and > 6 mg/dl in females) should be evaluated first by assessment of urine uric acid excretion. If urinary uric acid excretion is significantly elevated (> 600 mg/day on low purine diet or > 750 to 800 mg/day in the absence of purine gluttony), a careful search for causes of hyperuricemia (see Table 69.2) should be made and consideration should be given to allopurinol therapy in order to prevent urinary stones and chronic renal insufficiency from interstitial deposition of urate. However, in the majority of such patients urine uric acid excretion will be normal or reduced despite hyperuricemia. In this situation, some of these patients may subsequently develop gouty arthritis, but the risk of urinary stones or renal disease is much less than if the urine uric acid excretion were elevated. Fessel *et al* (3) have suggested that azotemia attributed to hyperuricemia is of no clinical significance until serum uric acid levels reach 13 mg/dl in men and 10 mg/dl in women. The expense and potential toxicity of therapy to lower serum urate, therefore, are probably not warranted since therapy can be successfully initiated if gout develops (7); this issue is controversial, however, and some would initiate therapy when serum levels are consistently > 9 mg/dl in the hope of preventing potential renal damage and acute gout (21).

Hyperuricemia Secondary to Diuretics

The renal tubular handling of uric acid is complex: there is complete glomerular filtration followed by tubular resorption. tubular secretion, and further tubular resorption. The resorption of uric acid is in part modulated by the volume of extracellular fluid (expansion increases excretion and contraction decreases excretion). Diuretics modify the renal handling of uric acid by their effect on volume and also some diuretics may directly affect urate transport. Thiazides regularly cause a dose-related rise of the serum urate level. This elevation is reversed upon withdrawal of the agent. The increase in concentration averages 1 to 2 mg/dl but occasionally may be 4 to 5 mg/dl. Furosemide also is frequently associated with a rise in concentration of serum urate; less commonly ethacrynic acid, acetazolamide, and rarely triamterene are associated with hyperuricemia. Spironolactone *per se* is not associated with hyperuricemia.

The incidence of gout after the initiation of a diuretic is a complex issue. Other factors which affect the incidence of gout—such as hypertension or obesity—are often present in diuretic-treated patients. Approximately 10% of hypertensive patients with hyperuricemia secondary to diuretic therapy actually develop gout. This risk increases in patients with known gout and those patients with diseases associated with elevation of serum urate, such as myeloproliferative disorders or psoriasis. Also in association with diuretic therapy uric acid excretion is diminished and there is no increase in the incidence of urinary calculi. The risk of developing urate nephropathy is unknown (see above). For these reasons expectant management of patients with asymptomatic hyperuricemia secondary to diuretics is appropriate.

Should acute gout develop, treatment as described above may be initiated. Intercritical gout is managed similarly to primary gout and uricosuric therapy with probenecid (if there is no renal failure) or therapy with allopurinol to decrease production of urate may be used. Stopping the diuretic is usually associated with a slight fall in the plasma urate concentration, but many patients will continue to have attacks of gout. Therefore, if a patient develops gout while taking diuretics, and the need for the diuretic continues, it is best to treat the gout as discussed above and to continue the use of the diuretic.

CALCIUM PYROPHOSPHATE DIHYDRATE (CPPD)-INDUCED ARTHRITIS

Pathophysiology

Pseudogout is a syndrome caused by the deposition of calcium pyrophosphate dihydrate in fibrocartilage and joint tissue and in ligaments and tendons with an occasional resulting inflammatory response. It most often is idiopathic but may be associated with certain other diseases (see below).

Inorganic pyrophosphate is an important metabolite in many biosynthetic reactions where it is removed from macromolecules through the action of pyrophosphatases. It is adsorbed to hydroxyapatite and is probably involved in the regulation of mineralization, both in the accretion from amorphous calcium phosphate and in the dissolution of crystalline hydroxyapatite.

Prevalence

Chondrocalcinosis increases in frequency with age; it is present in about 5% of the adult population at the time of death and in 20 to 30% of people above age 80. The exact prevalence of CPPD disease is not known. In one series of consecutive patients with newly diagnosed crystal-induced arthritis, CPPD disease accounted for about one-third of the cases (10). Males are probably affected more than females with a ratio of males to females of 1.5:1 in the largest reported series (10).

Etiology

Familial cases with an autosomal dominant inheritance have been described (17) in which chondrocalcinosis appears at an earlier age. These families are uncommon, and many of these patients will remain asymptomatic for many years; the metabolic defect has not been identified, however. Most cases of CPPD disease are sporadic and idiopathic; a few are associated with one of a variety of metabolic diseases. Many of the diseases associated with deposits of CPPD involve metabolic abnormalities in connective tissues, but the precise mechanisms of CPPD crystallization are unknown. A list of these associated diseases is presented in Table 69.4.

Clinical Features (Table 69.5)

Patients are usually middle-aged to elderly at the time of onset of arthritic symptoms. There are several possible patterns of presentation: about one-quarter present with *self-limited acute gout-like attacks* (*pseudogout*) predominantly affecting the knees and wrists, but occasionally involving other joints, including rarely the first metatarsophalangeal joint. Monoarticular attacks are the rule, but involvement of symmetrical joints and polyarthritis may occur rarely. Symptoms are often less intense than they are in gout, but the presentation is variable and some attacks may be quite severe. Systemic symptoms, including fever to 101°F (38°C) or more, may occur as in gout, and patients are frequently misdiagnosed as having infection. Attacks are often exacerbated by trauma and by acute illness. Long intervals (sometimes years) between attacks are common.

In about half the patients, and especially in women, the presentation *resembles osteoarthritis* with bilateral involvement, especially of the knees. The wrists, the metacarpophalangeal (MCP) joints, hips, shoulders, elbows, or ankles also may be affected. Acute exacerbations occur in about half of these patients with features that resemble osteoarthritis except that the disease is more progressive and destructive. Varus or valgus knee deformities are common, and extensive calcification around the patella may be seen on X-ray. Flexion contractures may occur also. The relationship to ordinary osteoarthritis is still unclear, except that the involvement of joints not usually affected in osteoarthritis (MCPs, wrists, shoulders, elbows) suggests a different pathogenesis (see also Chapter 68).

In a few patients persistent subacute inflammation with fatigue, morning stiffness, and synovial swelling in multiple joints lasting weeks or months *resembles rheumatoid arthritis*.

A few patients also have been reported with severely *destructive arthritis* resembling the Charcot joints of neuropathic arthropathy but associated with a normal neurological examination (13). CPPD

Table 69.4.
Diseases Associated with Calcium Pyrophosphate Dihydrate (CPPD) Deposition Disease

Gout
Hemochromatosis—hemosiderosis
Hyperparathyroidism
Hypomagnesemia
Hereditary hypophosphatasia
Hypothyroidism
Neurogenic arthropathy

Table 69.5.
Clinical Features of Calcium Pyrophosphate Dihydrate (CPPD) Deposit Disease

EPIDEMIOLOGY
  Age: Middle aged or elderly
SITE
  Knee and wrist most common joints involved
  Metacarpophalangeal joints, hips, shoulders, elbows, ankles may be affected
  Arthritis usually monoarticular
PATTERN
  Acute gout-like attacks with symptom-free intervals in 25%
  Osteoarthritis-like disease in 50%, with superimposed acute attacks in half of these patients
  Rheumatoid-like polyarthritis in 5%
  Neuropathic-like arthritis without neurological damage (rare)
  Asymptomatic chondrocalcinosis in 20%
LABORATORY
  Synovial fluid shows leukocytosis and characteristic CPPD crystals

disease may also be associated with a true neuropathic arthritis due to tabes dorsalis.

Laboratory Findings

Patients may have peripheral leukocytosis and an elevated erythrocyte sedimentation rate in association with acute or subacute attacks of arthritis. The synovial fluid will show polymorphonuclear leukocytosis which may exceed 50,000/mm³ in acute pseudogout, but is more commonly in the range of 15,000 to 25,000. Crystal identification is the key to diagnosis (see above). In the absence of acute or subacute inflammation, leukocyte counts may be low (< 2000/mm³) and crystals may be largely extracellular.

Because of the occasional association with other disorders (Table 69.4), the patient's serum calcium, phosphorus, alkaline phosphatase, and uric acid concentrations should be measured, although they will usually be normal (12). Because pseudogout may be the presenting manifestation of hemochromatosis and because of the importance of early diagnosis in this disorder, measurement of serum ferritin is also indicated if there is any suspicion of this diagnosis.

X-ray Findings

The typical X-ray findings of CPPD deposit disease are punctate and linear calcifications (chondrocalcinosis) seen most frequently in the fibrocartilage of the menisci of the knee, usually bilaterally (Fig. 69.3). Other fibrocartilages may show similar changes, including the disc in the distal radioulnar joint, the symphysis pubis, the lip of the acetabulum or the glenoid fossa or intervertebral discs. Hyaline cartilage may also be involved with similar punctate linear calcifications which may be identified as a dense line parallel to the subchondral bone. Calcification in the soft tissues of the joint capsule and occasionally in ligaments and tendons may also be seen but is less characteristic. In patients with the type of CPPD disease that resembles osteoarthritis, subchondral cyst formation with bony collapse may be prominent. Osteophyte formation is variable and inconsistent.

These radiographic findings may be helpful in suggesting or confirming the diagnosis of CPPD disease. However, it may not be possible to visualize the extent of deposits radiographically, and their absence does not exclude the diagnosis if typical crystals can be demonstrated in synovial fluid or in biopsy material.

Management

There is no therapy which influences the deposition or resolution of tissue deposits of CPPD. In the acute episode diagnostic aspiration of synovial fluid with removal of crystals and leukocytes may provide significant clinical improvement. Local injection of depo-corticosteroid is often effective and avoids potential side effects of systemic drug therapy (see Chapter 66, for technique). Efficacy of colchicine has been debated, and although it is sometimes effective, especilly if given intravenously, the use of indomethacin (Indocin) or other nonsteroidal anti-inflammatory agents is generally preferred as described above for acute gout (see above). Since many of these patients are elderly (and may therefore have an impaired glomerular filtration rate), caution regarding renal toxicity of these agents should be exercised (see Chapter 47, Table 47.9). In patients with only recurrent acute attacks, no therapy is indicated between attacks, but early administration of anti-inflammatory agents on exacerbation may minimize or abort attacks. Therapy for patients with more subacute inflammation or for those with osteoarthritis-like disease is similar to that described for osteoarthritis (see Chapter 68), except that anti-inflammatory levels of drugs may be required for optimal symptomatic control.

HYDROXYAPATITE-INDUCED ARTHRITIS

The capacity of hydroxyapatite crystals to induce an inflammatory response was first appreciated in some patients with acute tendinitis (15). More re-

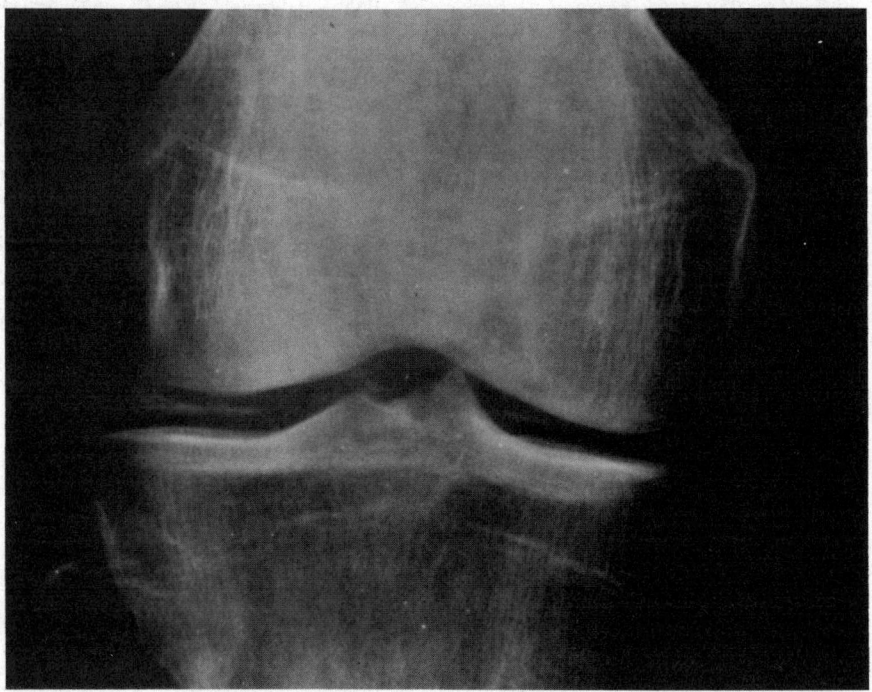

Figure 69.3. X-ray of knee of a patient with chondrocalcinosis. Stippled calcification of the medial and lateral menisci is easily identified.

cently hydroxyapatite crystals have been identified in patients with osteoarthritis, especially in association with acute inflammatory episodes (6), and in patients with destructive arthropathy of the shoulder joint (11). The latter, termed *Milwaukee shoulder* (see Chapter 63), is associated with painful limited shoulder motion, complete disruption of the rotator cuff, and extensive degenerative changes in the bone. Alizarin Red S dye (available from scientific supply houses) may be used by the physician to stain wet preparations of synovial fluid to screen for the presence of hydroxyapatite crystals, which appear with ordinary light microscopy as red-stained clumps of crystalline material (14). Since all other calcium-containing crystals and even noncrystalline calcium salts stain with this dye, specific identification of hydroxyapatite crystals will require techniques not usually available, such as electron microscopy, microprobe analysis, or X-ray diffraction. Further definition of the role of hydroxyapatite in crystal-induced arthritis and of the spectrum of its clinical manifestations will be forthcoming as identification of crystals is applied more widely. At this time the physician need only be aware of the potential inflammatory properties of this crystalline material and consider its implication in the above clinical situations.

General References

Dieppe P, Doherty M, Macfarlane D (ed): Symposium on the crystal-related arthropathies. *Ann Rheum Dis* 42 (suppl 1), London, 1983.

A collection of recent papers on this topic.

Howell DS: Diseases due to the deposition of calcium pyrophosphate and hydroxyapatite. In Kelley WN, Harris ED Jr, Ruddy S, Sledge CB (eds): *Textbook of Rheumatology*, Philadelphia, WB Saunders, 1985.

Kelley WN: Gout and related disorders of purine metabolism. In Kelley WN, Harris ED Jr, Ruddy S, Sledge CB (eds): *Textbook of Rheumatolgy*, Philadelphia, WB Saunders, 1985.

These two chapters in this comprehensive textbook provide an up-to-date review of all aspects of crystal-induced arthritis.

McCarty P: Heberden Oration, 1982. Crystals, joints and consternation. *Ann Rheum Dis* 42:243, 1983.

An update by a pioneer investigator in this field.

Steinbroker O, Neustadt PH: Aspiration and injection therapy. In *Arthritis and Musculoskeletal Disorders*. Hagerstown, MD, Harper & Row, 1972.

This is a very practical manual to aid the physician in the techniques of joint aspiration.

Specific References

1. Berger L, Yu TF: Renal function in gout. *Am J Med* 59:605, 1975.
2. Fagan TJ, Ludsky MD: Compensated polarized light microscopy using cellophane adhesive tape. *Arthritis Rheum* 17:256, 1974.
3. Fessel WJ, Siegelaub AB, Johnson ES: Correlates and consequences of asymptomatic hyperuricemia. *Arch Intern Med* 132:44, 1973.
4. Gutman AB, Yu TF: Uric acid nephrolithiasis. *Am J Med* 45:756, 1968.
5. Hall AP, Barry PE, Dawber TR, et al: Epidemiology of gout and hyperuricemia. *Am J Med* 42:27, 1967.
6. Huskisson EC, Dreppe PA, Tucker AK, Cannell LB: Another look at osteoarthritis. *Ann Rheum Dis* 38:423, 1979.
7. Liang MH, Fries JF: Asymptomatic hyperuricemia: the case for conservative management. *Ann Intern Med* 88:666, 1978.
8. Malawista SW: Gouty inflammation. *Arthritis Rheum* 20:5241, 1977.
9. McCarty DJ: The gouty toe—a multifactorial condition. *Ann Intern Med* 86:234, 1977.
10. McCarty DJ: Pseudogout and pyrophosphate metabolism. *Adv Intern Med* 25:363, 1980.
11. McCarty DJ, Halverson PB, Carrera GF, et al: "Milwaukee shoulder"—association of microspheroids containing hydroxyapatite crystals, active collagenase and neutral protease with rotator cuff defects. I. Clinical aspects. *Arthritis Rheum* 24:464, 1981.
12. McCarty DJ, Silcox DC, Coe F, et al: Diseases associated with calcium pyrophosphate dehydrate crystal deposition. A controlled study. *Am J Med* 56:704, 1974.
13. Menkes CJ, Simon F, Delrieu F, et al: Destructive arthropathy in chondrocalcinosis articulosis. *Arthritis Rheum* (suppl) 19:329, 1976.
14. Paul H, Reginato AJ, Schumacher R: Alizarin Red S staining as a screening test to detect calcium compounds in synovial fluid. *Arthritis Rheum* 26:191, 1983.
15. Pinals RS, Short CL: Calcific periarthritis involving multiple sites. *Arthritis Rheum* 7:359, 1964.
16. Phelps P, Steele AD, McCarty, DJ, Jr: Compensated polarized light microscopy. *JAMA* 203:508, 1968.
17. Reginato A, Valenzuela F, Martinez V, et al: Polyarticular and familial chondrocalcinosis. *Arthritis Rheum* 13:197, 1970.
18. Rundles RW, Metz EN, Silberman JR: Allopurinol in the treatment of gout. *Ann Intern Med* 64:229, 1966.
19. Wall B, Agudelo CA, Tesser JRP, et al: An autopsy study of the prevalence of monosodium urate and calcium pyrophosphate dihydrate crystal deposition in the first metatarsophalangeal joints. *Arthritis Rheum* 26:1522, 1983.
20. Weinberger A, Schumacher HR, Agudelo CA: Urate crystals in asymptomatic metatarsophalangeal joints. *Ann Intern Med* 91:56, 1979.
21. Wyngaarden JB, Kelley WN: *Gout and Hyperuricemia*. New York, Grune & Stratton, 1976.
22. Yu TF, Gutman AB: Efficacy of colchicine prophylaxis in gout. Prevention of recurrent gouty arthritis over a mean period of five years in 208 gouty subjects. *Ann Intern Med* 55:179, 1961.
23. Yu TF, Gutman HB: Uric acid nephrolithiasis in gout. Predisposing factors. *Ann Intern Med* 67:1133, 1967.

CHAPTER SEVENTY

Rheumatoid Arthritis

FREDRICK M. WIGLEY, M.D., AND PHILIP D. ZIEVE, M.D.

Rheumatoid arthritis is a chronic inflammatory systemic disease of unknown etiology that has a predilection for involvement of the joints. The articular inflammation has a variable course, but an additive (see below) symmetrical chronic polyarthritis associated with joint destruction, deformity, and loss of function is the primary clinical problem. Extra-articular features are recognized as an integral part of the disease and may antedate the onset of the inflammatory arthropathy by months.

In the past, patients with inflammatory arthritis were lumped under the diagnostic umbrella of either "rheumatoid arthritis" or "gout." In the last few decades it has been recognized that the spectrum of inflammatory arthritis could be separated into a number of individual disease processes. A clinician is now faced with an increasing complexity of diagnostic possibilities and, therefore, must develop a comprehensive approach that encompasses the history, physical examination, and appropriate laboratory studies.

EPIDEMIOLOGY

Population surveys have used somewhat different criteria for diagnosis of rheumatoid arthritis, but most have agreed that it has a worldwide distribution and, in white populations, a prevalence of definite classical disease of 1 to 2% (3). Important geographic and ethnic/racial variations exist. A high prevalence has been noted in North American Indians (3.5 to 5.3%) and a low prevalence has been reported in rural South African blacks and in Japanese (0.1%).

The prevalence increases with age, approaching 5% in women over age 55. The average annual incidence rate in the United States is about 70/100,000/year. Both incidence and prevalence of rheumatoid arthritis are 2 to 3 times greater in women than men. Although rheumatoid arthritis may present at any age, it most commonly affects patients in the third to sixth decades. Women tend to have a more severe articular disease, while extra-articular features are more common in men.

Seropositive rheumatoid arthritis (see below) aggregates in families, suggesting genetic and/or environmental influences on disease expression. The B cell alloantigen HLA-DR4 has been found in 70% of Caucasian seropositive patients compared to 25% of unaffected controls (14). DR4 associations have been confirmed in family studies in a variety of ethnic groups, thus defining an increased relative risk of 6 to 12 times in the DR4-positive individual.

PATHOGENESIS

Although the cause of rheumatoid arthritis is unknown, the infiltration of the synovia of affected joints by lymphocytes, plasma cells, and macrophages, associated with synovial lining cell proliferation (the so-called pannus), has suggested a cell-mediated immune process (8). Local production of rheumatoid factor-containing immune complexes that are capable of activating complement and attracting inflammatory cells also has been shown. The inflammatory process is amplified by a variety of mediators including prostaglandins and lymphokines. The subsequent release of destructive enzymes and the altered cellular function cause destruction of cartilage and bone and subsequent loss of normal joint architecture.

HISTORY

The presentation of the disease (Table 70.1) varies from situations in which the diagnosis is obvious to ones in which the presentation is so atypical that it suggests other conditions. Diagnosis may be complicated further by the fact that rheumatoid arthritis may present with signs and symptoms that mimic other musculoskeletal disorders, such as gout or pseudogout (Chapter 69), polymyalgia rheumatica (Chapter 79), and fibrositis (Chapter 66).

The typical case of rheumatoid arthritis begins insidiously with the slowly progressive development of symptoms and signs over a period of weeks to months. Occasionally, however, patients will experience an acute onset, usually polyarticular, within 24 to 48 hours; sometimes an acute presentation appears to be associated with either emotional or physical stress (for example, loss of a loved one or a recent injury).

Nonspecific systemic symptoms, primarily fatigue, malaise, and depression, are common but not invariable, and may precede other symptoms of the disease by weeks to months. Usually the patient does not feel tired upon awakening but complains of rather severe fatigue 4 to 6 hours later. Fever occurs occasionally and is almost always low grade (37 to 38°C; 99 to 100°F); a higher fever suggests another illness, such as infection.

Arthritic symptoms (and signs) provide the definitive clues by which a specific diagnosis is made. Often the patient first notices stiffness (see below) in one or more joints, usually accompanied by pain on movement and by tenderness in the joint. Unlike a patient with gout (Chapter 69), a patient with rheumatoid arthritis can bear weight and can move the inflamed joint but has a persistent, deep, gnawing discomfort. In fact, severe pain in a patient with

established rheumatoid arthritis should suggest a superimposed infection or an acute structural abnormality. The number of joints that are involved is highly variable, but almost always the process is eventually polyarticular (involvement of five or more joints). Rheumatoid arthritis is called an "additive" polyarthritis (there tends to be sequential involvement of joints) in contrast to the migratory or evanescent arthritis that can be seen in systemic lupus erythematosus or in the episodic arthritis of gout. The American Rheumatism Association, in its criteria for the diagnosis of rheumatoid arthritis (11), has emphasized the importance of persistent swelling of the joints for greater than 6 weeks, stating that persistent soft tissue swelling of (or increased fluid in) a joint, followed by swelling of symmetrical joints, is characteristic of the disease. Any joints may be involved; but there is a predilection for peripheral joints with a relative sparing of the axial skeletal; the joints involved most often are the proximal interphalangeal (PIP) and metacarpophalangeal (MCP) joints of the hands, the wrists (particularly at the ulnar-styloid articulation), knees, elbows, temporomandibular joints, hips, ankles, and metatarsophalangeal (MTP) joints.

Morning stiffness may be a feature of any inflammatory arthritis but is especially characteristic of rheumatoid arthritis (almost all patients complain of it) and, in fact, is a useful gauge to measure the activity of the disease. The symptom is defined as stiffness, predominantly over joints, which persists at least for several hours (the average is 3 to 4 hours), thus distinguishing it from the transient gelation phenomenon of degenerative arthritis which lasts but a few minutes (see Chapter 68). Similar stiffness may, of course, occur after any prolonged period of inactivity.

It is typical of patients with rheumatoid arthritis that their symptoms wax and wane, especially at the beginning of the illness. Because of this and because objective signs may not be present at first, it is not unusual that the diagnosis is delayed for months. During this time the physician can best serve the patient by reassurance, careful interval history and periodic physical examination (see below), and, if appropriate, selected screening tests (page 920). Symptomatic treatment with anti-inflam-

Table 70.1.
Symptoms and Signs of Rheumatoid Arthritis

Symptoms		Signs	
Extra-articular	Articular[a]	Extra-articular	Articular
Fatigue	Morning stiffness	Rheumatoid nodules	Pain on passive motion
Depression	Pain and tenderness	Lymphadenopathy	Tenderness
Malaise	Swelling	Splenomegaly	Swelling
Anorexia		Ocular disease	Heat
		Entrapment neuropathies	Typical deformity

[a] Persistence (6 weeks or more) and symmetrical nature of signs and symptoms are important, but not invariable, diagnostic features.

matory drugs may be instituted during this period (page 930).

PHYSICAL EXAMINATION

A complete physical examination initially and then a limited examination every 3 to 6 months are important in patients with suspected rheumatoid arthritis, not only to make the diagnosis but to establish a baseline against which to assess the possible later development of both articular and extra-articular disease.

However, the primary focus of examinations in the physician's office will be the joints—repeated examinations and careful records of the status of affected joints, determined by history and previous examinations.

Joints

Swelling is the most measurable change that occurs in a joint that is affected by rheumatoid arthri-

tis. The first change in involved joints is usually soft tissue swelling; eventually increased amounts of fluid within the joint space produce more readily recognizable (and, often, persistent) changes. In the hands, where the disease is often first manifest, typical fusiform swelling of the PIP joints commonly occurs (Fig. 70.1); the distal interphalangeal joints are less often involved. The MCP joints and the wrists are swollen even more often than are the PIP joints. The elbows, knees, ankles, and MTP joints are other common sites of disease where swelling may be readily apparent. Swelling of symmetrical joints, although not invariable, is characteristic of rheumatoid arthritis.

In contrast to gout (see Chapter 69) or to septic arthritis, redness of affected joints is not a prominent feature of rheumatoid arthritis.

Tenderness and pain on passive motion, although not specific for rheumatoid arthritis, are the most sensitive indices of inflammation of a joint. It is

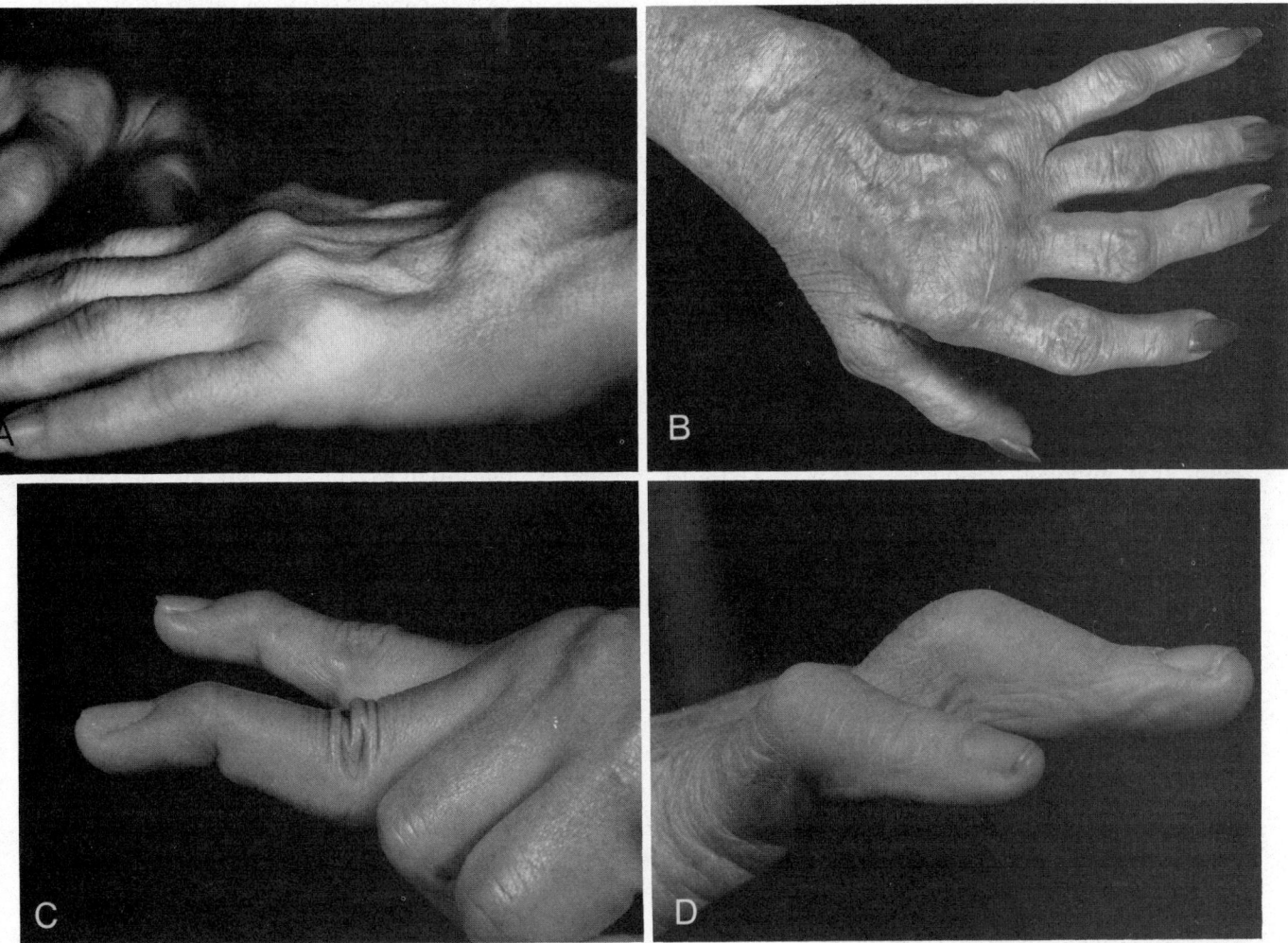

Figure 70.1. Hand deformities in rheumatoid arthritis. *A.* Typical fusiform swelling of the PIP joints; note also the synovial swelling of the wrist and MCP joints. *B.* Ulnar deviation of the fingers. *C.* Swan-neck deformity (hyperextension of PIP joint). *D.* Boutonnière deformity (flexion contracture of PIP joint).

important for the physician to apply gentle but firm pressure when examining a joint so that tenderness due to inflammation will be elicited, but not so much pressure that a normal joint will be inappropriately symptomatic. Inflamed joints are also usually warmer than normal joints; the examiner may assess this best by feeling them with the back of his fingers.

The range of motion of the joint may be limited by inflammation and/or structural deformity, and it is important to determine which of these processes is playing the major role in this regard so that appropriate therapy (see below) can be prescribed.

Weakness is a common feature of patients with rheumatoid arthritis; but, like range of motion, it is not easy to assess. The fatigue produced by the illness (see above) may contribute to an overall sense of weakness; but weakness of one or more limbs or parts of limbs may be caused by muscle atrophy, a result of joint deformity and of disuse. However, weakness may only seem to be present at times when, because of pain, the patient is unwilling to apply his full strength.

Permanent deformity may be an end stage of the inflammatory process that is first apparent as joint swelling. Persistent tenosynovitis and synovitis may lead to the formation of synovial cysts, which sometimes rupture (see below), to displaced tendons, and to compression by synovial fluid of the normal supporting structures of the joint (leading, for example, to muscle atrophy). These anatomical changes result in flexion contractures and subluxation (incomplete dislocation) of articulating bones. Typical visible changes (Fig. 70.1) include ulnar deviation of the fingers at the MCP joints, hyperextension or hyperflexion of the joints of the fingers, and, occasionally, ankylosis of the carpal and tarsal joints. Ankylosis of other joints is rare and may be a distinguishing feature when comparing rheumatoid arthritis to diseases that mimic it. Displaced toes ("cocked-up") with hallux valgus formation (angulation of the great toe laterally) are also common.

Synovial cysts are common in patients with rheumatoid arthritis and can be readily seen and palpated overlying the joints with which they communicate. Synovial cysts of the popliteal space (Baker's cysts) may develop in patients with a variety of disorders of the knee but seem to be especially prevalent in patients with rheumatoid disease. If popliteal cysts rupture, the signs and symptoms resemble closely those of acute thrombophlebitis (calf swelling and tenderness—even a positive Homans' sign). Proper therapy depends on the physician's ability to make the right diagnosis. An arthrogram (performed by injection of a radiopaque dye into the joint, followed by an X-ray of the knee) often will show the cyst and its connection with the joint space (Fig. 70.2). Decompression of the cyst by aspiration of synovial fluid from either the joint or the cyst and injection of a croticosteroid into the joint (see

below, page 932) usually effectively relieve the symptoms of the condition.

LABORATORY TESTS

Baseline laboratory information in patients with suspected rheumatoid arthritis should include a hematocrit value, white blood cell count and differential count, erythrocyte sedimentation rate, urinalysis, and rheumatoid factor titer. In selected patients, synovial fluid analysis, additional serological studies, and appropriate X-rays may also be important (see below).

Hematology

A mild anemia with hematocrit values in the range of 30 to 34% occurs in approximately 25 to 35% of patients with rheumatoid arthritis. In most cases the reduced red cell mass is due to the so-called anemia of chronic disease (see Chapter 49) and is a normocytic-normochromic process characterized by a low concentration of serum iron, a low serum iron-binding capacity, and a normal or increased serum ferritin concentration. However, occasionally true iron deficiency anemia develops because of intercurrent stress ulceration and/or because of the irritative effects of aspirin (see below, page 933) on the gastric mucosa.

The white cell count is usually normal in patients with rheumatoid arthritis, but occasionally it is elevated in patients with a great deal of inflammatory disease and rarely is depressed (especially in association with Felty's syndrome, see page 926). Similarly the platelet count is usually normal but also may be elevated in association with the inflammatory process and may be reduced in patients with Felty's syndrome.

The erythrocyte sedimentation rate (ESR), most reliably measured by the Westergren method, is usually elevated in patients with rheumatoid arthritis and is an excellent way to follow the activity of the disease (see below).

Serology

Rheumatoid Factors

These are antibodies that react with the Fc fragment (a part of the molecule that can be produced in the laboratory by enzymatic cleavage of immunoglobulin G (IgG)). Although they may belong to any of the three major classes of immunoglobulins—IgG, IgM, and IgA—rheumatoid factors, as measured for clinical purposes, are IgM antibodies. The antibodies are by no means pathognomonic of rheumatoid arthritis, nor do they seem to be involved in its pathogenesis, but they are detectable in the serum of 70 to 80% of patients with the disease (13). A significant titer of rheumatoid factor is 1:80 or greater. The titer does not correlate with the activity

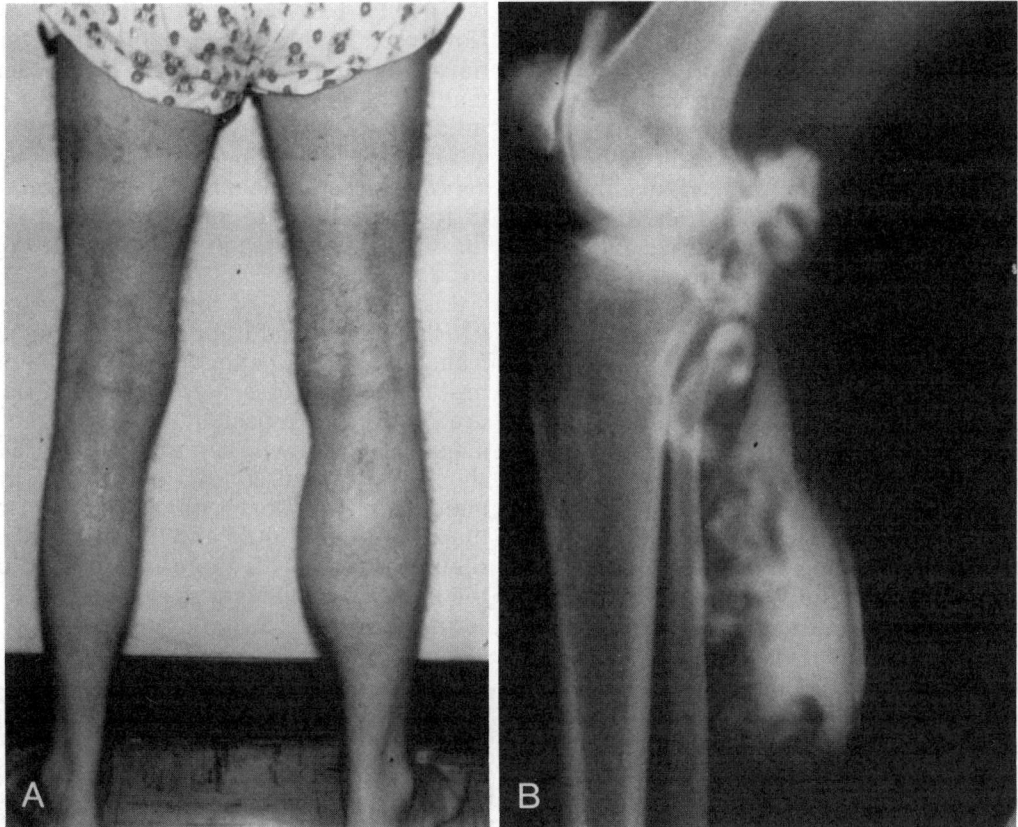

Figure 70.2. Baker's cyst. *A.* Swelling of the calf secondary to dissection of the cyst. *B.* Arthrogram of the knee, demonstrating the cyst.

of disease, but it does appear that patients with very severe erosive arthritis or with extensive extra-articular disease are likely to have relatively high titers.

Rheumatoid factor is also detectable in the serum of many patients without rheumatoid arthritis; most of these patients have had demonstrated or presumed chronic antigenic stimulation, such as prolonged infection (bacterial endocarditis, tuberculosis, viral hepatitis), collagen vascular disease, chronic lung disease (pulmonary fibrosis, asthma), and dysproteinemia (myeloma, macroglobulinemia, mixed cryoglobulinemia). Also, transient appearance of rheumatoid factor may occur in patients who have been recently vaccinated or who have had a self-limited viral infection. Finally, rheumatoid factor may be detected in the serum of apparently normal people, especially people over the age of 50, where its prevalence is anywhere from 10 to 25%, depending on the assay.

All of the clinical tests for rheumatoid factor depend on the agglutination, by serum which contains it, of particles (sheep red cells, latex, bentonite) coated with aggregated human or animal IgG. There is some variation in sensitivity of detection of rheumatoid factor according to which technique is used, so that the clinician should be familiar with the procedure used by his reference laboratory. The tests that employ latex or bentonite are more sensitive but less specific than tests that employ sheep red cells (1).

Antinuclear Antibodies

Antinuclear antibodies (ANA), measured by immunofluorescent techniques, are present in approximately 20 to 30% of patients with rheumatoid arthritis. ANA are more common in patients with extra-articular manifestations of disease and in patients with a high titer of rheumatoid factor. In comparison to systemic lupus erythematosus (SLE) the titer of antinuclear antibodies is ordinarily low in patients with rheumatoid disease, and antibodies to native DNA are unusual. The test is most useful as a predictor of extra-articular disease.

Serum Complement

Serum hemolytic complement (C′H50), C_3 or C_4, is generally normal or increased in patients with rheumatoid arthritis; it may be low in an occasional patient with severe disease or with systemic vasculitis. The test is most useful in helping to distinguish the patient with early rheumatoid arthritis from patients with early SLE in whom it is often markedly decreased.

Synovial Fluid (Table 70.2)

Synovial fluid should be analyzed in a patient with monarticular arthritis, with polyarticular arthritis and fever, or in any patient with a joint effusion in whom the diagnosis is in doubt. Also patients with known rheumatoid arthritis who develop disproportionate discomfort and swelling of one joint should have fluid aspirated from that joint to rule out infection. If the primary physician is not familiar with the technique of arthrocentesis (see Table 66.1, page 865) or if he does not feel comfortable about tapping the joint in which there is an effusion, the patient should be referred to a rheumatologist or to an orthopaedic surgeon. The patient should be told that the overlying skin will be anesthetized before the aspiration and that he will experience minimal discomfort during the procedure.

Early in the course of rheumatoid arthritis, joint fluid may not show the characteristic inflammatory changes that ultimately develop. Thereafter, however, the normally clear fluid becomes yellowish-white and turbid and, because of the degradation of hyaluronic acid by lysosomal enzymes, the viscosity of the fluid falls considerably and the so-called mucin clot becomes poor. (A simple method of testing the mucin clot is to add 1 ml of joint fluid to 4 ml of 2% acetic acid (Fig. 70.3).) Fluid aspirated from an inflamed joint also often clots spontaneously, another feature distinguishing it from normal. There is considerable variation in the total white cell count and the neutrophil count in synovial fluid of rheumatoid joints, but in general many more leukocytes (predominantly neutrophils) are present than are seen in the fluid of either normal joints or joints that are arthritic but are not acutely inflamed. Cell counts can be done in the office with normal saline as a diluent. At the same time, a smear can be made and stained for differential counting of white cells. If the physician is unable to perform these counts, the fluid should be transported to an appropriate laboratory, in which case the fluid should be added to a tube containing ethylenediaminetetraacetic acid to prevent clot formation. The cells will not lyse even if 4 to 6 hours pass before they are counted. However, rapid transport to the laboratory is essential so that an accurate glucose measurement can be made. The concentration of glucose in the fluid of inflamed joints, though usually normal, is occasionally moderately reduced; if it is less than half the serum glucose concentration, it suggests septic arthritis. The protein concentration in the synovial fluid is usually greater than 3 g/dl, typical of an exudative process.

A measurement of total hemolytic complement (C′H50) in synovial fluid can be of diagnostic significance when the patient with rheumatoid arthritis has an atypical presentation. It need not be measured routinely, especially in patients in whom the diagnosis is known. If measured, C′H50 in serum should be measured simultaneously. In nonrheumatoid inflammatory arthritis, the titer of C′H50 is the same in joint fluid and in serum. In seropositive rheumatoid arthritis there is a marked decrease in the titer of complement in synovial fluid (but not in serum). However, a similar decrease may be seen in

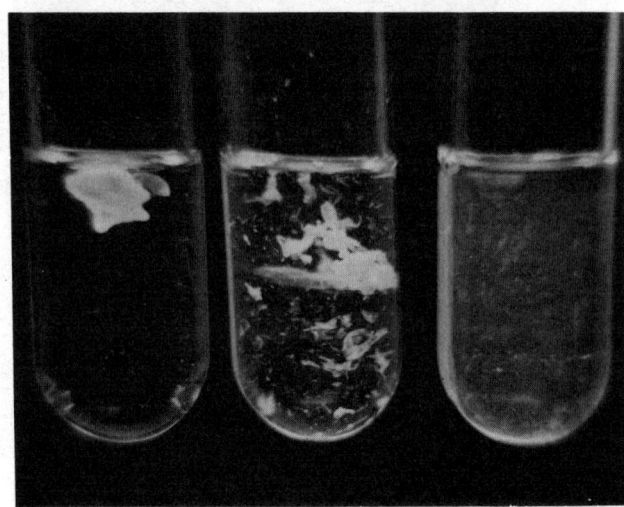

Figure 70.3. Mucin clot demonstrating (left to right) good, intermediate, and poor mucin clots.

Table 70.2.

Synovial Fluid	Normal	Rheumatoid Arthritis	Noninflammatory Arthritis	Septic Arthritis
Color	Clear	Yellow	Clear-yellow	Variable
Clarity	Transparent	Turbid	Transparent	Opaque
Viscosity	High	Low	High	Low
Mucin clot	Good	Fair to poor	Fair to good	Poor
White cells (per mm³)	< 150	3,500–50,000	< 3000	50,000 → 100,000
Polymorphonuclear leukocytes (%)	< 25	> 70	< 25	> 75
Serum-synovial fluid glucose difference	0	≥ 30	≤ 5	≥ 30
Protein (g/dl)	1.8	4.2	3.0	4.9
C′H50: protein[a]	> 2.5	< 2.5	> 2.5	Variable

[a] This ratio is low in synovial fluid of patients with arthritis associated with local immune complex formation (rheumatoid arthritis, SLE); it can be low in states associated with local consumption of complement (gout, infection), but it is frequently high or normal in other forms of arthritis.

microcrystalline arthritis and in septic arthritis. For complement determination the joint fluid and serum should be packed in ice and transported to the laboratory within hours of collection. If that is not possible, the specimens may be stored at −20°C (the usual temperature of a freezer in a refrigerator) for up to 1 week.

Radiology (Fig. 70.4)

Roentgenograms are rarely necessary in the diagnosis of rheumatoid arthritis but are useful in following the progression of the erosive process. Furthermore, X-ray changes lag behind and require sufficient time (months) to evolve in a characteristic manner, limiting their usefulness early in the course of the disease.

Radiological findings vary in rheumatoid arthritis depending on the duration and severity of the illness. Early in the disease X-rays may show nothing other than soft tissue swelling. Thereafter periarticular osteoporosis may develop, and it is usually most noticeable in the small joints of the hands, wrists, and feet. With progression of the disease, narrowing of the joint space occurs due to loss of cartilage, and juxta-articular erosions appear, generally at the point of attachment of the joint capsule. In end-stage disease, large cystic erosions of bone may be seen, bony proliferation may occur because of degenerative changes that follow inflammation, and the marked deformities that are visible to the naked eye (see above, page 919) are also visible radiologically. These changes are in contrast to the bony hypertrophy and fusion seen in patients with osteoarthritis (Chapter 68).

In general serial X-rays are not necessary in the management of patients with rheumatoid arthritis; they should be obtained if there is a suspicion of structural damage of a joint.

Special radiological studies are helpful in certain situations. *Arthrography* can be used to define possible internal joint derangement or injury to a supporting structure, such as a torn rotator cuff of the shoulder; and *bone scan* can be helpful in establishing the diagnosis of aseptic necrosis.

Biopsies

Although the histology of rheumatoid arthritis is characteristic (see above, page 917), synovial biopsy is rarely necessary in the diagnosis of the disease. Similarly, biopsy of a nodule is only indicated to distinguish it from another process (e.g., a tumor); occasionally a nodule is excised because it is unsightly or because it has ulcerated or has eroded into an adjacent structure.

EXTRA-ARTICULAR DISEASE (4)

Rheumatoid arthritis is a chronic inflammatory *systemic* disease. Although the joints are almost always the principal focus of the illness, other organ systems may also be involved, either because of rheumatoid granuloma formation or because of a generalized vasculitis. Usually, extra-articular manifestations of rheumatoid arthritis occur in patients with relatively more severe disease. In contrast to the predilection of classic rheumatoid arthritis for women, extra-articular manifestations of the disease (Table 70.3) are more common in men.

Rheumatoid Nodules

Although not specific for rheumatoid arthritis (similar nodules may be seen in patients with SLE or with rheumatic fever) the subcutaneous nodule is the most characteristic extra-articular lesion of the disease (Fig. 70.5). Nodules occur in 20 to 30% of cases, almost exclusively in seropositive patients. They vary in size from a few millimeters to several centimeters and may be either fixed to surrounding tissue or be freely movable beneath the skin. They are located most commonly on the extensor surfaces of the arms and elbows, but are prone to develop also at pressure or contact points on the feet, the knees, and, rarely, the scapulae, the back of the head, the ischial tuberosities, and the base of the spine. Occasionally subcutaneous nodules may become painful, erode underlying bone, or ulcerate, but usually they are asymptomatic. Rheumatoid nodules may arise within tendons or ligaments and can result in joint dysfunction or tendon rupture. Rarely nodules may arise in visceral organs, such as the lungs, the heart, or the sclera of the eye. Wherever their location, nodules usually persist but occasionally regress when there is a remission of activity of the disease.

Pleuropulmonary Disease

There are several pulmonary manifestations of rheumatoid arthritis including pleurisy with or without effusion, intrapulmonary nodules, rheumatoid pneumoconiosis (Caplan's syndrome), diffuse interstitial fibrosis, and, rarely, bronchiolitis obliterans, pneumothorax, or pulmonary arteritis (7). Severe lung involvement is more common in males and tends to occur in patients with high titer rheumatoid factor in the presence of other manifestations of rheumatoid arthritis. Commonly, there is a restrictive ventilatory defect with reduced lung volumes and a decreased diffusing capacity for carbon monoxide. Although the issue is controversial, most rheumatologists believe that rheumatoid arthritis does not cause intrathoracic obstructive airway disease. Extrathoracic airway obstruction may occur secondary to involvement of the cricoarytenoid joints of the larynx.

Pulmonary involvement may precede by months the onset of arthritis. Pleurisy, the most common problem, is clinically apparent in 5% of patients, but at autopsy is found 50% of the time, manifest by

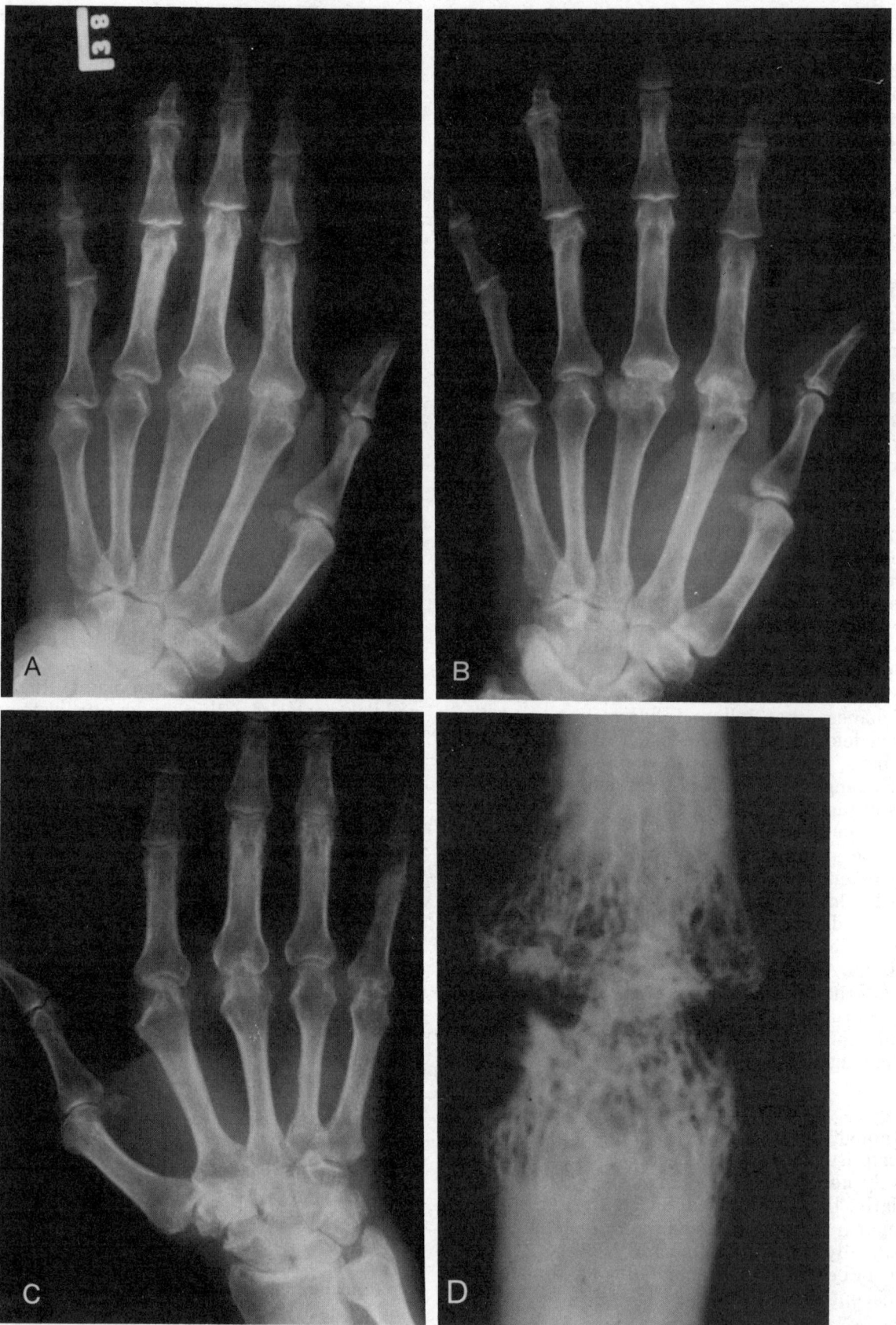

Figure 70.4. Radiological changes in rheumatoid arthritis. *A.* Early joint space narrowing in second and third MCP joints. *B.* Cystic changes, erosions, and further bony proliferation in second and third MCP joints. *C.* Periarticular osteoporosis, most noticeable in the interphalangeal joints, and numerous marginal erosions and cysts in the carpal bones and metacarpal heads. *D.* Juxta-articular erosions in a PIP joint.

Table 70.3.
Systemic Manifestations of Rheumatoid Arthritis (Rheumatoid Disease)

I. General
  A. Fever
  B. Fatigue, malaise, diffuse stiffness
  C. Adenopathy
  D. Splenomegaly
II. Pulmonary
  A. Pleuritis (± effusion)
  B. Intrapulmonary nodules
  C. Interstitial pneumonitis
  D. Rheumatoid
     pneumoconiosis (Caplan's syndrome)
  E. Pulmonary fibrosis
  F. Arteritis (rare)
III. Cardiovascular
  (1) Heart
  A. Pericarditis, effusion, tamponade, constriction
  B. Myocarditis
  C. Endocarditis, including valvulitis
  D. Rheumatoid nodule (conduction defects)
  (2) Peripheral
  A. Vasculitis or arteritis
IV. Nervous system
  A. Peripheral neuropathy (mononeuritis multiplex) (sensory, motor, or both)
  B. Central nervous system
     1. Spinal cord lesion
        a. Vascular thrombosis
        b. Rheumatoid nodule
     2. Intracranial
        a. Arteritis (rare)
        b. Rheumatoid nodule (rare)
V. Ocular
  A. Keratoconjunctivitis (Sjögren's syndrome)
  B. Episcleritis (simple or nodular)
  C. Scleritis
     1. Diffuse
     2. Nodular (scleromalacia perforans)
     3. Necrotizing
VI. Hematological
  A. Anemia (chronic disease)
  B. Neutropenia (Felty's syndrome)
  C. Thrombocytosis
  D. Eosinophilia
VII. Skin
  A. Palmar erythema
  B. Nodules
  C. Vasculitic lesions
  D. Leg ulcers (Felty's syndrome)
VIII. Others
  A. Sjögren's syndrome
  B. Osteoporosis
  C. Hyperviscosity
  D. Lymphoma (Sjögren's syndrome)
  E. Secondary amyloidosis (controversial)

pleural thickening and inflammation. Pleural effusions, either unilateral or bilateral, are usually exudates (high lactate dehydrogenase activity and a protein concentration greater than 3 g/dl), but even in transudates the glucose concentration of the fluid is usually low (less than 30 mg/100 ml). A logical first approach to the management of a pleural effusion includes a diagnostic aspiration and/or pleural biopsy to exclude infection or malignancy.

Rheumatoid nodules in the lung are usually asymptomatic, but cavitation simulating cancer or infection may occur. Therefore, appropriate diagnostic steps should be taken to assure that an isolated pleural or pulmonary nodule is in fact rheumatoid in origin and not due to a complicating, intercurrent process.

Interstitial pneumonitis may precede a progressive pulmonary fibrosis, the most severe form of rheumatoid lung disease. This process is more common among patients who smoke.

To date no regression of rheumatoid lung disease has been shown with conventional modes of treatment. Patients with symptomatic pleural or pulmonary manifestations of rheumatoid arthritis should be followed in consultation with a rheumatologist and/or a pulmonologist.

Cardiac Disease (9)

Pericarditis is the most common cardiac manifestation of rheumatoid arthritis. Echocardiographic studies have demonstrated pericardial effusion in 55% of patients with subcutaneous nodules and in 15% of patients who do not have nodules. Symptomatic pericarditis usually presents with fever, chest pain, and a pericardial rub that resolve spontaneously. Recurrent or persistent pericardial disease, complicated by tamponade or constriction, is unusual. Myocarditis and conduction abnormalities secondary to nodule formation in the heart have been reported rarely. The treatment of patients with

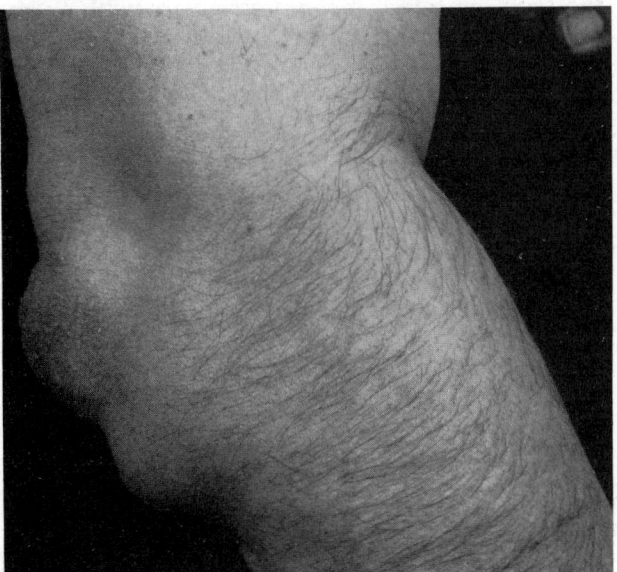

Figure 70.5. Rheumatoid nodules along the extensor surface of the forearm.

symptomatic cardiac disease should be planned in consultation with a rheumatologist.

Ocular Disease

The most common ocular manifestation of rheumatoid arthritis is the keratoconjunctivitis of Sjögren's syndrome (see below). *Episcleritis*, ordinarily a self-limited process of a few weeks' duration, occurs occasionally. It is manifest by discomfort, mild pain, and intense redness of the affected eye. *Scleritis* is a rarer but more serious problem. Unlike episcleritis it is a slowly progressive, frequently bilateral process; it is characterized by nodularity, intense redness, and often severe pain; and it may lead to perforation and/or loss of vision. The distinction between episcleritis and scleritis is difficult, and all patients with suspected scleritis should be referred to an opthalmologist.

Neurological Disease

The most common neurological manifestation of rheumatoid arthritis is a mild, primarily sensory, *peripheral neuropathy*, usually more marked in the lower extremities. Entrapment neuropathies (for example, the carpal tunnel syndrome) sometimes occur in patients with rheumatoid arthritis because of compression of a peripheral nerve by inflamed edematous tissue. This problem is discussed in Chapter 84. Cervical myelopathy, secondary to arthritis of the cervical spine, is a particularly worrisome, although uncommon, complication; if caused by atlantoaxial subluxation, permanent—even fatal—neurological damage may ensue. Thirty percent of patients with rheumatoid arthritis have atlantoaxial subluxation without symptoms, and very few of them develop neurological dysfunction. However, neurosurgical consultation should be sought at the first sign of cord compression (radicular pain, difficulty voiding, focal weakness).

Lymphoid Hyperplasia

Lymphadenopathy, either local or generalized, occurs in 25% or more of patients with rheumatoid arthritis and is probably more common than that in seropositive patients. The nodes are nontender, firm, and freely movable; and, although the diagnosis of lymphoma sometimes is considered, the process almost always proves to be benign. When examined by biopsy, the nodes show a proliferation of normal plasma cells, consistent with the immunological reactivity of the disease. *Splenomegaly* occurs more rarely (5 to 10% of patients), usually in association with lymphadenopathy.

Felty's Syndrome (12)

Felty's syndrome is characterized by rheumatoid arthritis, splenomegaly, and leukopenia—predominantly granulocytopenia. Patients with the syndrome usually are older, have a high titer of rheumatoid factor, and have relatively severe arthritis, often with other extra-articular manifestations of the disease. Recurrent bacterial infections and chronic refractory leg ulcers are the major complications, and splenectomy may benefit patients whose infections are severe.

Rheumatoid Vasculitis

Vascular inflammation is found in 10 to 25% of patients with rheumatoid arthritis on whom autopsies are performed. The most common *clinical* manifestations of vasculitis are small digital infarcts along the nailbeds. In a very small proportion of patients (less than 1%) a syndrome of accelerated vasculitis is seen, characterized by distal cutaneous ulcerations and gangrene, peripheral polyneuropathy, and visceral (intestinal, renal, cardiac, cerebral) ischemia. There does not appear to be a positive correlation, as was once thought, between the long term administration of corticosteroids and the severity of this process. The syndrome ordinarily emerges after years of seropositive, persistently active, rheumatoid arthritis. Immediate consultation with a rheumatologist and, usually, hospitalization are indicated.

Sjögren's Syndrome

About 10 to 15% of patients with rheumatoid arthritis (most of them women) have Sjögren's syndrome, a chronic inflammatory disorder characterized by lymphocytic infiltration of lacrimal and salivary glands with impaired secretion of saliva and tears that results in the *sicca complex*, dry mouth (xerostomia) and dry eyes (keratoconjunctivitis sicca) (10). Variably, other exocrine glands are affected as well. There is also commonly a lymphoproliferative reaction, characterized by lymphadenopathy and sometimes, splenomegaly that may mimic or, rarely, actually transform into a malignant lymphoma. The syndrome may also be associated with a number of other systemic manifestations, including vasculitis, peripheral neuropathy, and thyroiditis, and with diffuse hypergammaglobulinemia (sometimes in association with renal tubular acidosis), cryoglobulinemia, an elevated titer of antinuclear antibodies, and a number of tissue-directed autoantibodies.

COURSE

Rheumatoid arthritis is a variable illness, and its course cannot be predicted precisely in a given patient. Several different patterns of activity can be described: *Spontaneous remission* may occur, particularly in the seronegative patient. *Recurrent explosive attacks* followed by periods of quiescence can be seen in the early phases, but activity usually is *persistent and unpredictably waxes and wanes* in intensity. Rarely, the inflammatory process is *rapidly destructive*, leading to early loss of function and to joint deformity. The degree of disability is probably directly proportionate to the severity and the duration of the inflammatory process. Although treatment can alter the course of the illness, complete remission is unlikely in people who have had symptomatic rheumatoid arthritis for a year or more. There is no clear-cut way to predict which patients will develop significant deformities (subluxation, ankylosis, *etc*; see above, page 920); most will not. On the other hand, a recent study has shown that 60% of patients with rheumatoid arthritis are unable to work 10 years after onset of their illness (15). A minority of patients (approximately 25%) will have a course characterized by remissions and exacerbations—often with months or even years during which they are asymptomatic; a few have permanent remissions. Such patients often have an abrupt onset of their disease, which paradoxically may herald a better prognosis. Some patients who at first have episodic attacks of arthritis ultimately develop a more typical sustained progressive course. Patients who have a high titer of rheumatoid factor and nodules, particularly men, tend to have more severe disease and, conversely, seronegative patients are more likely to have spontaneous remissions and/or less severe disease.

DIFFERENTIAL DIAGNOSIS

The difficulty of diagnosing early rheumatoid arthritis emphasizes the importance of a systematic approach to patients with arthritis (Table 70.4). Epidermiological studies have clarified that the age, sex, and genetic matrix of the patient influence disease expression. Therefore, a clear definition of host features will form a framework to begin the evaluation of a patient with arthritis. Table 70.5 outlines examples of the differential diagnosis of polyarthritis based on prevalence of disease expression defined by age and sex. Other important factors

Table 70.4.
Outline of Diagnostic Approach to Polyarthritis

A. Define the host features
  1. Age, sex, and ethnic background
  2. Genetic matrix
  3. Environmental factors
B. Describe the joint involvement
  1. Number
  2. Patterns
  3. Specific joints
  4. Intensity of pain
  5. Course
C. Characteristics of extra-articular features
D. Supporting laboratory studies
E. Response to therapeutic trial

Table 70.5.
Differential Diagnosis of Polyarthritis Based on Age and Sex

	Male	Both Sexes	Female
Childhood (1–15)	Juvenile ankylosing spondylitis (Chapter 71)	Juvenile rheumatoid arthritis—systemic onset (Still's disease)[a]	Juvenile rheumatoid arthritis[a]
	Kawasaki's syndrome[a]	Rheumatic fever[a]	Pauciarticular arthritis[a]
	Hemophilia (Chapter 50)	Leukemia[a]	Juvenile rheumatoid arthritis—polyarthritis onset[a]
Young adult (15–30)	Ankylosing spondylitis (Chapter 71)	Psoriatic arthritis (Chapter 100)	Systemic lupus erythematosus[a]
	Reiter's syndrome (Chapter 71)	Lyme disease[a]	Gonococcal arthritis (Chapter 27)
	"Reactive" arthritis[a] Behcet's syndrome[a]	Inflammatory bowel disease (Chapter 38)	Scleroderma[a]
Middle years (30–60)	Gout (Chapter 69)	Seronegative polyarthritis (Chapter 70)	Rheumatoid arthritis Sjögren's syndrome
	Palindromic rheumatism[a]	Hypersensitivity reactions (Chapter 23)	Sarcoidosis[a] Polymyositis[a]
	Whipple's disease[a]	Vasculitic syndromes[a] Relapsing polychondritis[a]	Erosive osteoarthritis (Chapter 68)
Elderly (60+)	Diffuse idiopathic skeletal hyperostosis (DISH) (Chapter 68)	Pseudogout (Chapter 69)	Primary generalized osteoarthritis (Chapter 68)
	Hypertrophic pulmonary osteoarthropathy (HPO)[a]	Tumor-related syndromes Secondary osteoarthritis (Chapter 68) Metabolic disorders	Polymyalgia rheumatica (Chapter 79)

[a] These conditions are not discussed in this book. Information about them is contained in any of the general references at the end of this chapter.

include the patient's occupation, habits, drug usage, and past medical history (Table 70.6). Finally, the characteristics of the arthritis itself provide important information in approaching the differential diagnosis (Tables 70.7 and 70.8).

MANAGEMENT

General Principles

Rheumatoid arthritis is a chronic disorder for which there is no known cure. It therefore requires a comprehensive program that combines medical, social, and emotional support for the patient. An understanding of each patient's specific problems is essential. Serial observations (Table 70.9) and in-depth investigation of the impact of the disease on both the patient and his family provide the basis for effective management.

The major goals of treatment of the arthritis are (a) to reduce pain and discomfort, (b) to prevent deformities and loss of normal joint function, and (c) to maintain a productive and active life. To achieve these goals an understanding of the cause of pain is important. In rheumatoid arthritis pain and dysfunction are caused by (a) acute inflammation, (b) chronic proliferative synovitis, and (c) subsequent mechanical and structural abnormalities. Each of these processes warrants a different therapeutic approach. Often all three are present at once, although, depending on the stage of disease, one process may be predominant. Acute inflammation is always the major problem in early disease, while mechanical and structural abnormalities do not ordinarily develop until several years after onset.

Management begins with effective communication between physician and patient. It is essential that the patient and his family be educated about the nature and course of the disease—the specific causes of the discomfort and the goals, problems, and expectations of treatment. Chronic arthritis is a major emotional, as well as physical, stress that often requires a major change in life style. A misunderstanding about the disease and the setting of inappropriate goals will lead to frustration, depression, and withdrawal from social activity and from medical support.

Treatment options include (a) reduction of joint stress, (b) physical and occupational therapy, (c) drug therapy, and (d) surgical intervention.

Reduction of joint stress is accomplished by a number of practical measures, which do not depend on the use of drugs. Because of the stress of obesity on the musculoskeletal system, an ideal body weight should be maintained. Rest, in general, is an important feature of management; 8 to 9 hours' sleep at night and a 2-hour rest period in the middle of the day are reasonable recommendations for everyone with active disease. Also, vigorous activity (heavy work, brisk exercise) should be avoided because of the danger of intensifying joint inflammation. On the other hand, patients should be urged to maintain a modest level of activity to prevent joint laxity and muscular atrophy. Splinting of acutely inflamed joints, walking aids (canes, walkers), and specially designed furniture and household utensils are all effective means of reducing stress on specific joints; such aids are provided, on recommendation of the consultant rheumatologist, by an orthopaedist, a physiatrist or physical therapist, or an orthotics appliance store.

The *physical and the occupational therapist* should be consulted early in the course of a patient with rheumatoid arthritis. The therapist can effectively design a program of balanced rest and activity that is appropriate for the stage of the disease. Passive exercise (moving the joints through a full range of motion) is used when inflammation is active and poorly controlled; an active exercise program, when tolerated, can be designed to prevent contractures and muscular atrophy. Local heat, education in the use of various supporting aids and in joint protec-

Table 70.6.
Examples of Environmental Factors in Diagnosis of Arthritis

Occupation	Disease
Bartender, lead exposure	Gout (Chapter 69)
Health workers	Hepatitis (Chapter 42)
Sports	Secondary osteoarthritis (Chapter 68)
Outdoorsman	Lyme disease[a]
Gardener	Sporotrichosis[a]
Deep sea diver	Aseptic necrosis of bone[a]
Habits	
Alcohol abuse	Gout (Chapter 69), aseptic necrosis[a]
"Moonshine" ingestion	Saturnine gout (Chapter 69)
Smoking	Hypertrophic osteoarthropathy[a]
Intravenous drug abuse	Septic arthritis,[a] hepatitis, vasculitis
Sexual promiscuity	Gonococcal arthritis (Chapter 27), hepatitis (Chapter 42), Reiter's syndrome (Chapter 71)
Drugs	
Diuretics	Gout (Chapter 69)
Corticosteroids	Aseptic necrosis[a]
Hydralazine, procainamide	Systemic lupus erythematosus[a]
Any drug	Hypersensitivity reactions (Chapter 23)

[a] These conditions are not discussed in this book. Information about them is contained in any of the general references at the end of this chapter.

Table 70.7.
Assessment of Joint Involvement

A. Number:

Monarthritis	Oligoarthritis (2–4)	Polyarthritis ($\geqslant$ 5)
Septic arthritis[a]	Reiter's syndrome	Rheumatoid arthritis
Gout	Inflammatory bowel disease	Systemic lupus erythematosus[a]
Pseudogout	Psoriatic arthritis	Serum sickness
Other crystals	Rheumatic fever[a]	Psoriatic arthritis
Local tumor[a]	Juvenile rheumatoid arthritis[a]	Tophaceous gout

B. Patterns:

Symmetrical	Asymmetrical
Rheumatoid arthritis	Psoriatic arthritis
Serum sickness	Reiter's syndrome
Systemic lupus erythematosus[a]	Gout, pseudogout

C. Intensity of pain:

Severe	Moderate
Septic arthritis[a]	All others including rheumatoid arthritis
Microcrystalline arthritis	

D. Course:

Acute	Infection, gout, pseudogout
Chronic	Psoriatic arthritis, rheumatoid arthritis, ankylosing spondylitis
Additive	Rheumatoid arthritis
Migratory	Rheumatic fever,[a] systemic lupus erythematosus[a]
Evanescent	Systemic lupus erythematosus,[a] viral[a]
Episodic	Gout, pseudogout, palindromic rheumatism[a]

[a] These conditions are not discussed in this book. Information about them is contained in any of the general references at the end of this chapter.

Table 70.8.
Diagnostic Clues Provided by Involvement of Specific Joints

First metatarsal (podagra)	Gout
Knee (acute, episodic)	Pseudogout
Distal interphalangeal	Psoriatic arthritis
	Osteoarthritis
Metacarpals, wrists, metatarsals	Rheumatoid arthritis
Sausaged digits	Reiter's syndrome
	Psoriatic arthritis
	Sarcoidosis
Sacroiliac	Ankylosing spondylitis
	Reiter's syndrome
	Psoriatic arthritis
	Inflammatory bowel disease
Sternoclavicular	Septic arthritis
	Polymyalgia rheumatica
Heel/ankle	Reiter's syndrome

Table 70.9.
Measurements to Be Made Serially in Patients with Rheumatoid Arthritis[a]

Duration of morning stiffness
Time of onset of fatigue
Aspirin need/day
Grip strength
Number of joints that are tender or are painful on passive motion
Degree of swelling of affected joints
Erythrocyte sedimentation rate (Westergren)

[a] Adapted from McCarty DJ: Clinical assessment of arthritis. In McCarty DJ (ed): *Arthritis and Allied Conditions*, ed 9. Philadelphia, Lea & Febiger, 1979.

tion, and maintenance of good joint function are all part of the therapist's role.

Either wet or dry local heat gives transient symptomatic relief of pain and stiffness, particularly to patients with chronic synovitis. A hot shower in the morning, coupled with passive "warming up" exercises, may relieve stiffness and help the patient to get the day started.

During periods when the inflammatory process is particularly intense, especially if they occur at the onset of the illness, *hospitalization* is helpful in removing the patient from the stresses of his everyday life, in beginning a structured rehabilitation program, and in evaluating the effect of drugs (see below) on the illness.

There is increased susceptibility of the rheumatoid joint to infection, usually by Gram-positive organisms. Whenever a single joint flares up or is accompanied by increased body temperature or follows a recent procedure (e.g., dental), infection should be ruled out by means of synovial fluid examination (see page 922).

Drug Treatment (5)

A general discussion of the pharmacological approach to rheumatoid arthritis is followed by a description of the characteristics of individual drugs.

Anti-Inflammatory Drugs

In the presence of acute and/or chronic inflammation, it is appropriate first to prescribe aspirin or another nonsteroidal anti-inflammatory drug (NSAID). They should always be used in conjunction with the general modalities of rest, heat, *etc* discussed above. The major effect of these agents is to reduce acute inflammation and thereby to decrease pain, improve function, and, it is hoped, prevent joint destruction. Recent studies have suggested that NSAIDs also may have more than an anti-inflammatory effect—i.e., they may alter cell function and, subsequently, the immune and/or inflammatory process, but the issue is controversial. All of these drugs also have mild to moderate analgesic properties independent of their anti-inflammatory effect.

Aspirin is usually the drug of first choice because of long familiarity with its use and because of its low cost. Aspirin is the generic name of acetylsalicylic acid. Several different preparations exist, including regular aspirin, aspirin buffered with antacids, and enteric coated aspirin (Table 70.10). Nonacetylated salicylates are mainly analgesic agents with only mild anti-inflammatory activity. The main disadvantages of aspirin are the high incidence of gastrointestinal intolerance, the inconvenience of taking multiple doses, and the relatively long interval (4 to 7 days) before a full anti-inflammatory effect is reached. Gastrointestinal symptoms can be reduced by the use of various enteric coated preparations. A trial of aspirin is usually continued for 4 to 6 weeks; if tolerated, 70 to 80% of patients can be expected to respond during this time. A lack of response may be due to noncompliance or to an inadequate dosage, so that a salicylate level should

Table 70.10.
Salicylates

		Available Strength (mg)
Acetylated preparations		
Regular aspirin	Multiple brands	300–800
Buffered aspirin	Multiple brands	300–650
Enteric coated aspirin	Ecotrin, Encaprin	325–500
	Cosprin	325–650
	APF	500
	Easprin	950
Nonacetylated preparations		
Sodium salicylate	Pabalate	300
Salicylsalicyclic acid	Disalcid	500, 750
Choline-magnesium trisalicylate	Trilisate	500, 750
Salicylate derivative		
Diflunisal	Dolobid	250–500

Table 70.11.
Nonsteroidal Anti-inflammatory Drugs

		Available Strengths (mg)	Recommended Dosage	Maximum Daily Dosage (mg/day)
Propionic acid derivatives				
Ibuprofen	Motrin, Rufen	300, 400, 600, 800	600 mg 3 to 4 times a day	3200
	Nuprin,[a] Advil[a]	200		
Naproxen	Naprosyn	250, 375, 500	500 mg twice a day	1000
	Anaprox	275		
Fenoprofen	Nalfon, Fenopron	200, 300, 600	600 mg 3 times a day	2400
Pyroxicams				
Piroxicam	Feldene	10, 20	20 mg a day	20
Indoles				
Indomethacin	Indocin	25, 50	50 mg 3 to 4 times a day	150–200
		75 (slow release)	1–2 times a day	
Sulindac	Clinoril	150, 200	200 mg twice a day	400
Tolmetin	Tolectin	200, 400	400 mg 3 to 4 times a day	2000
Fenamates				
Meclofenamate	Meclomen	50, 100	50–100 mg 3 to 4 times a day	400
Pyrazoles				
Phenylbutazone	Butazolidin	100	100 mg 3 times a day	300 for no more than 7 days

[a] Over-the-counter.

be measured before changing medications. If aspirin is not tolerated or if there is a lack of response at ideal drug levels (see details below), another NSAID should be prescribed.

There are now a large number of NSAIDs from which to choose (Table 70.11), but at full dosage all are potentially equally effective. In general, the NSAIDs have a more rapid onset of action, have a simpler dosage schedule, and are often better tolerated than aspirin. However, there is a great deal of individual variation in patient tolerance and response to a particular NSAID. Therefore, a trial of approximately 4 weeks with one of these agents as a second choice to aspirin is indicated. Failure of response or intolerance can be followed by a new trial with another NSAID, usually of a different chemical class (Fig. 70.6). (Combinations of two NSAIDs should be avoided.) If the second trial is also a failure, it is best to consider another approach.

Corticosteroids

Corticosteroids have both anti-inflammatory and immunoregulatory activity. Whether or not they can induce actual remission of rheumatoid arthritis is controversial. They can be taken systemically or can be injected intra-articularly depending on the clinical situation. If good control of active inflammation is not achieved with aspirin or another NSAID, a *low* dose (5 to 15 mg by mouth once a day) can be added, but the clinician should understand that, once started, corticosteroid therapy is very difficult to discontinue. Higher doses are rarely necessary unless there is a life-threatening systemic disease and, if used for prolonged periods, will lead to steroid toxicity. Although it is reasonable to initiate therapy with an every-other-day regimen, most patients will require corticosteroids daily. Repetitive short courses of high dose corticosteroids, intermittent intramuscular injections, adrenocorticotropic hormone injections, and the use of corticosteroids as the sole therapeutic agent are all to be avoided. The recent use of "pulse therapy" (1 g of intravenous methylprednisolone once a month for 2 months) for management of very difficult cases is controversial and should be initiated only in conjunction with a rheumatologist.

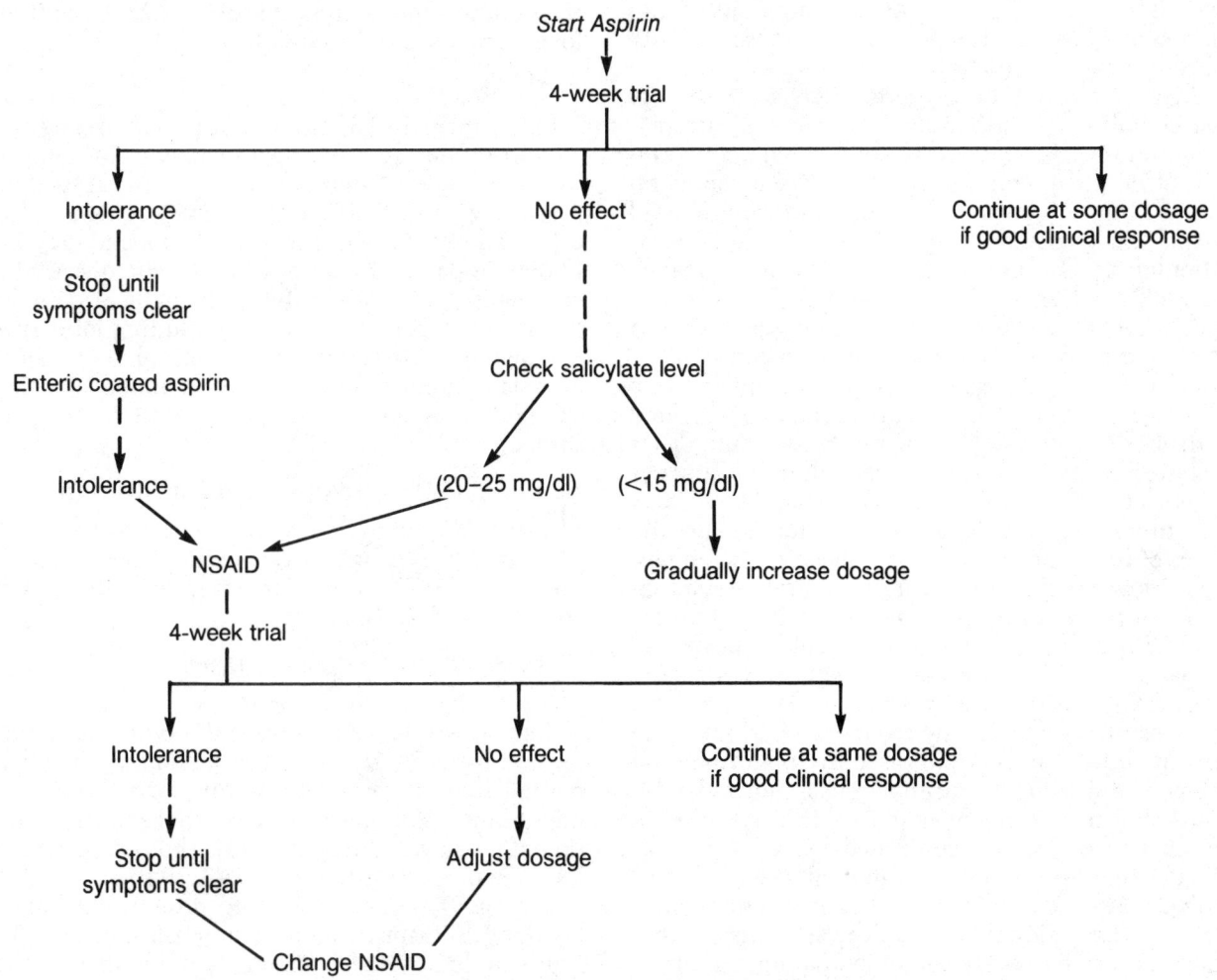

Figure 70.6. Pharmacological approach to patients with rheumatoid arthritis.

Intra-articular corticosteroids (e.g., 40 mg of triamcinolone in a knee, 20 mg in a shoulder, or 2 mg in a finger) are an effective means of controlling a local flare in one or two joints without changing the overall drug regimen (see Chapter 66 for details about the technique of injection). Joint fluid should always be obtained, studied, and cultured to be certain that a complicating infection has not developed. The injection should be administered by a rheumatologist or an orthopaedist if the primary physician is inexperienced with the techniques. Many rheumatologists think that the same joint should not be injected more than twice a year because of possible deterioration of intra-articular cartilage.

Remission-Inducing Agents (Agents with Delayed Onset of Action)

While NSAIDs control the symptoms of active rheumatoid arthritis, remission-inducing agents theoretically alter the disease process itself—although whether or not that is so is still being debated. In any case they do have an effect upon rheumatoid arthritis that is different and more delayed in onset than is the effect of the anti-inflammatory drugs discussed above. Once persistent disease activity (chronic synovitis) is established, a remission-inducing agent should be considered. Persistent disease can be defined as either continued activity despite an optimum trial of an anti-inflammatory program (2 to 3 months) or the development of erosions on X-rays of the involved joints. High titer rheumatoid factor, the presence of nodules or of other extra-articular features of rheumatoid arthritis, or aggressive joint activity all predict progressive disease, and, therefore, a remission-inducing agent should be started early in such cases. The decision to use a remission-inducing agent is complicated by the time commitment, expense, and potential toxicity related to drugs of this class. The currently available drugs include antimalarials, gold, D-penicillamine, and cytotoxic agents.

Antimalarials or *gold salts* (chrysotherapy) are the drugs of first choice. Antimalarials have the advantage of low toxicity. However, in general, they probably are better utilized in patients with relatively mild, although persistent, disease; gold is best used in patients with more active, aggressive disease. Consultation with a rheumatologist will be helpful in choosing the appropriate regimen. Approximately 60% of patients have some response to antimalarial drugs. The response to antimalarials is delayed, with increasing improvement noted up to 6 months; in patients who respond, continued use of the drugs dictates that the patient be examined by an ophthalmologist every 6 months so that early signs of ocular toxicity, the major side effect, can be detected (see below). Fifty to seventy percent of patients improve after 2 to 4 months of chrysotherapy. If no response

has occurred within 6 months or if toxicity is observed (see below), the drug is discontinued. If there is a good response, gold is given in a reduced dosage indefinitely.

If there is an inadequate or toxic response to gold and/or to antimalarial drugs, the next step in the treatment of rheumatoid arthritis is the use of D-penicillamine. In fact, some rheumatologists prefer this drug to gold or antimalarials and use it as their first choice when a remitting agent is indicated. Approximately 80% of patients will respond to this drug after it is given for 3 or 4 months. The use of D-penicillamine is often limited by its toxic effects (see below); and again, it should not be given without the advice of a rheumatologist. In patients who respond favorably, the drug can be administered indefinitely at a relatively low maintenance dose (see below).

Cytotoxic drugs have a very limited role in the treatment of rheumatoid arthritis. They should be reserved for the relatively small number of patients with progressive, otherwise uncontrollable or life-threatening disease and should be used only in consultation with a rheumatologist and then only after the patient understands the risks of both short and long term toxicity (see below).

Analgesic Drugs

Pain caused by inflammation is best treated with an anti-inflammatory drug (see above), although occasionally acetaminophen may be prescribed, together with an NSAID, for temporary analgesia. Narcotics should not be prescribed; dependency is a hazard in patients who have a chronic disease that may cause pain indefinitely. Mechanical pain secondary to structural changes, including joint space narrowing, subluxation, muscle atrophy, and weakness, is best approached through nonpharmacological modalities, such as splints, joint protection, surgery, etc.

Approach to Drug Treatment of Patients with Rheumatoid Arthritis

Figure 70.7 outlines a recommended sequence of therapeutic trials in the treatment of patients with rheumatoid arthritis.

Characteristics of Individual Drugs

Aspirin (acetylsalicylic acid).

MECHANISM. Aspirin inhibits the synthesis of prostaglandins, a family of potent mediators of inflammation that is derived from fatty acids within cell membranes. While aspirin has other effects, inhibition of prostaglandin synthesis is thought to account for its major anti-inflammatory activity.

DOSAGE. The usual starting dose is 900 mg (3 regular USP aspirin tablets) four times a day. The drug should be taken with meals and with a bedtime snack to minimize gastrointestinal side effects. If

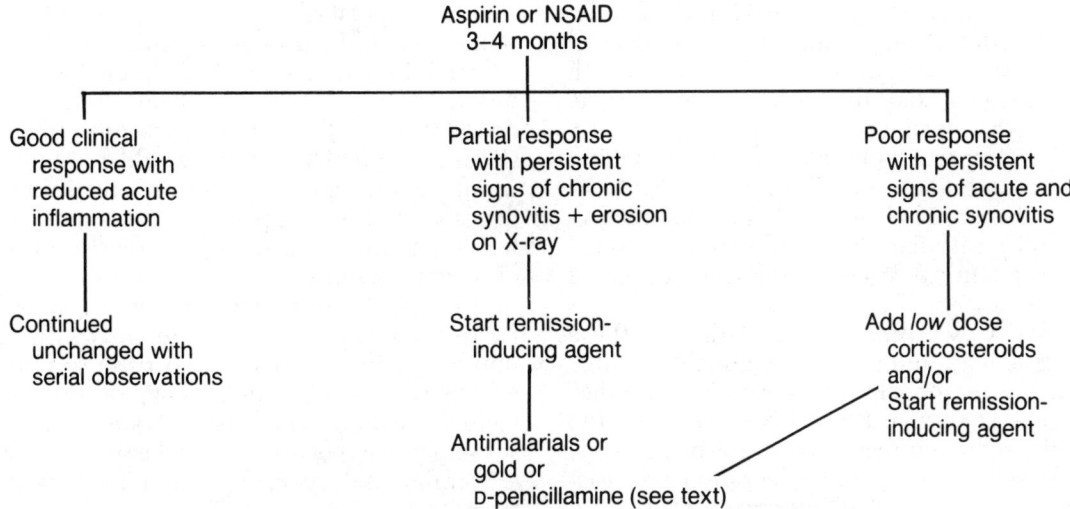

Figure 70.7. Suggested approach to anti-inflammatory drug treatment in rheumatoid arthritis.

side effects do develop, dropping to a lower dosage (6 tablets/day) and increasing by 1 tablet a day back to full dosage schedule may improve tolerance. Elderly patients are predictably less tolerant, and, therefore, a reduced dosage is advised at onset of treatment (8 to 10 tablets daily). A random serum salicylate level should be obtained approximately 7 to 10 days after beginning full dosage. A therapeutic level is 20 to 25 mg/dl, but elderly patients may be maintained between 15 to 20 mg/dl. If this level is not achieved on the initial schedule, and if the patient is believed to be compliant (see Chapter 4), the dose should be increased by 1 or 2 tablets a day until the desired anti-inflammatory level of salicylate is reached. There is a narrow margin between a good therapeutic level and toxicity. The earliest manifestation of toxicity is tinnitus or mild deafness. Should these symptoms occur, aspirin should be stopped until they abate and then restarted at a lower total dose that has been reduced by 1 or 2 tablets. After each change of dosage, it may take a week for a new steady state to be achieved. Younger patients can tolerate higher salicylate levels and do not usually have tinnitus or deafness until 30 to 35 mg of salicylate /dl.

Usual time to maximal effect. The maximum anti-inflammatory effect of aspirin is achieved in 10 to 14 days if therapeutic levels are reached. Patients should be told of the importance of taking the medicine exactly as prescribed in order for the therapeutic effect to be achieved.

SIDE EFFECTS. Tinnitus (see above) and dyspepsia (nausea, heartburn, anorexia) are common side effects of aspirin therapy; both can be controlled: tinnitus, by reducing the dosage; dyspepsia, by taking the aspirin with food. Enteric coated aspirin reduces the incidence of dyspeptic symptoms, and, although absorption is somewhat reduced, an effec-

tive dosage can usually be achieved by appropriate monitoring of salicylate levels. Buffered aspirins are more expensive than, and have no clear-cut advantage over, the standard preparation.

The most troublesome side effects are gastrointestinal bleeding and peptic ulceration, due primarily to the effect of the drug on the gastric mucosa. These problems occur in less than 5% of patients and are reasons to substitute another drug after symptoms have abated. Because of the inhibition of platelet function by aspirin (see Chapter 51), it should never be prescribed to a patient with an underlying bleeding tendency (including patients taking anticoagulant drugs).

Nonsteroidal anti-inflammatory drugs (NSAIDs).

MECHANISM. Although chemically dissimilar, these agents, like aspirin, inhibit the synthesis of prostaglandins, currently their only well defined anti-inflammatory effect.

DOSAGE. NSAIDs have an advantage over aspirin in that the dose schedule is simpler and peak levels are achieved within hours of the first dose. Some preparations can be given once a day or twice a day, a schedule that maintains drug levels equivalent in effect to full doses of aspirin and that is particularly important in the treatment of elderly or less compliant patients.

If there is active inflammation, a full dosage of a NSAID should be prescribed (see Table 70.11); a lower dosage can be started if inflammation is mild, if mechanical pain is the major problem, if the patient is elderly, or if he is at added risk for toxicity (see below). Ibuprofen, naproxen, piroxicam, and tolmetin are the agents used most frequently in rheumatoid arthritis. If a particular preparation is ineffective or is not tolerated, then following resolution of symptoms of toxicity a trial for 4 weeks of another NSAID can be initiated. It has been demonstrated that a single dose (50 to 75 mg) of indomethacin at bedtime can be added to full doses of aspirin with good effect, particularly in patients with active disease who continue to have considerable discomfort in the morning (6).

There is an unpredictable and varied individual response in both tolerance and response to NSAIDs. In addition, assays of blood levels are not readily available, so that unlike aspirin, the clinician must depend on the clinical response to a trial of a given NSAID.

USUAL TIME TO MAXIMAL EFFECT. Although these agents have a maximum anti-inflammatory effect within hours, a reasonable trial period is 1 month.

SIDE EFFECTS (TABLE 70.12). All NSAIDs have the potential of producing dyspepsia (15% of patients) and, to a lesser extent, peptic ulceration and gastrointestinal bleeding. Meclofenamate frequently causes diarrhea and therefore should not be the first choice as an NSAID in the treatment of rheumatoid arthritis.

Table 70.12.
Side Effects of Nonsteroidal Anti-inflammatory Drugs

	Approximate Prevalence
Gastrointestinal	10–20%
Epigastric pain, nausea	
Anorexia, dyspepsia, peptic ulceration	
Overt or occult bleeding	
Hypersensitivity reactions	1–5%
Rashes, rarely Stevens-Johnson syndrome	
Very rarely, anaphylactoid reactions	
Aggravation of allergic rhinitis or asthma	10% of sufferers
Renal effects	> 5%
Transient renal failure	
Water and salt retention	
Hypokalemia, inhibit diuretic action	
Interstitial nephritis, nephrotic syndrome	< 1%
Hepatic effects	5–15%
Cholestatic hepatitis	
Central nervous system	> 5%
Tinnitus/deafness	Primarily aspirin
Headache, vertigo, confusion	Higher with indomethacin
Others	
Agranulocytosis, aplastic anemia	< 1% (phenylbutazone)
Diarrhea	10–15% (mefenamic acid, other fenamates)
Aggravation of congestive heart failure, angina	> 1%
Parotitis	< 1% (phenylbutazone)
Toxic amblyopia	< 1% (ibuprofen)

Because prostaglandins play a role in the regulation of renal blood flow, NSAIDs may impair renal function in patients whose fluid balance is compromised (e.g., patients with heart failure, cirrhosis, dehydration (2)). If NSAIDs are prescribed in such situations, renal function should be monitored by serial measurements of serum creatinine and the drugs should be stopped if there is evidence of deterioration (increased edema or rise in concentration of serum creatinine).

Less than 5% of patients develop a hypersensitivity reaction, usually a rash, to an NSAID; the reaction is specific to a particular drug so that another NSAID can be substituted. Very rarely, an anaphylactoid reaction occurs (see Chapter 23) and, if so, subsequent exposure to all classes of nonsteroidal anti-inflammatory agents (including aspirin) is contraindicated.

Some side effects are more common for a particular NSAID. Phenylbutazone imposes an uncommon but important risk of producing aplastic anemia and, given the availability of many equally effective agents, should not be used in the treatment of rheumatoid arthritis. Indomethacin is more commonly associated than are other NSAIDs with gastrointestinal side effects and with neurological symptoms including severe frontal headache, dizziness, vertigo, light-headedness, and mental confusion. Its long term usefulness is therefore limited, particularly in elderly patients. The propionic acid derivatives (ibuprofen, naproxen, fenoprofen) are generally well tolerated (Table 70.14), although fenoprofen has been more frequently reported to cause acute interstitial nephrtis than has other NSAIDs.

Significant drug interactions can occur with any of the nonsteroidal anti-inflammatory drugs (Table 70.13) and must be anticipated.

Gold. Gold is effective in the treatment of rheumatoid arthritis when it is given intramuscularly as a water-soluble thiosalt (gold sodium thiomalate (Myochysine) or gold thioglucose (Solganol)). A new oral gold compound (auranofin) is now available. Initial studies have demonstrated that it is as effective as intramuscular gold.

MECHANISM. A number of mechanisms have been postulated, but none has been proved to explain the effect of gold in patients with rheumatoid arthritis.

DOSAGE. Myochrysine or Solganol therapy should be initiated at 10 mg intramuscularly; if this is tolerated, 25 mg intramuscularly should be given the second week; and if that is tolerated, 50 mg intramuscularly should be given weekly until a response has occurred or until a total of 1 g has been given. If there is a favorable response, therapy should be maintained with 50 mg intramuscularly each month indefinitely.

Auranofin (oral gold) is now preferred by many rheumatologists because of ease of administration and, potentially, a lower incidence of serious toxic-

Table 70.13.
Nonsteroidal Anti-inflammatory Drug: Drug Interactions

Antacids	Reduce rate and extent of absorption of NSAIDs; variable effect.
Anticoagulants	Phenylbutazone and oxyphenbutazone enhance the activity of warfarin. Aspirin, and potentially all NSAIDs, increases the risk of bleeding of an anticoagulated patient.
Oral hypoglycemic drugs	Aspirin, phenylbutazone, and oxyphenbutazone may potentiate the activity of sulphonylurea drugs. Other NSAIDs do not.
Antihypertensive/diuretics	NSAIDs may attenuate the effect of diuretics, β-blockers, and hydralazine.
Methotrexate	Salicylate inhibits the renal clearance of methotrexate, and toxic levels may occur.
Phenytoin	Phenylbutazone inhibits the metabolism of phenytoin. Salicylates displace phenytoin from albumin and increase the concentration of free drug.
Probenecid	Inhibits renal clearance of several NSAIDs.
Combinations of NSAIDs	Should be avoided.

ity. The dosage is either 6 mg once a day or 3 mg twice a day.

USUAL TIME TO MAXIMAL EFFECT. Maximal effect is achieved within 4 to 6 months or after administration of 1 g of gold.

SIDE EFFECTS. Chrysotherapy is associated commonly with side effects. Thirty percent of patients develop a rash, which can vary from a simple pruritic erythematous patch to a severe exfoliative dermatitis. Ulcerations and/or inflammation of the mouth, tongue, and pharynx occur occasionally as well. Up to 10% of patients have proteinuria, which is usually mild but rarely may be in the nephrotic range. Hematological reactions—immune thrombocytopenia, granulocytopenia, and aplastic anemia—occur rarely. Myochrysine, and less often Solganol, may produce a "nitritoid" reaction (flushing, dizziness, or fainting). Rarely, there is a paradoxical aggravation of musculoskeletal symptoms that requires discontinuation of treatment.

Patients receiving gold should have complete blood counts, including platelet counts, and have their urine tested for protein before each dose. Any evidence of hematogical or renal toxicity warrants stopping treatment permanently. If a mild mucocutaneous eruption occurs, crysotherapy should be interrupted, but if the eruption abates, therapy may be restarted at a dose of 10 to 15 mg a week (and then increased by 5 to 10 mg every few weeks up to 50 mg a week again).

Oral gold (see above) is more likely to cause cutaneous eruptions or diarrhea than is intramuscular gold but is less likely to cause serious hematological or renal toxicity.

Antimalarials. Antimalarials are rapidly absorbed, relatively safe, inexpensive, and often effective, remitting agents in the treatment of rheumatoid arthritis.

MECHANISM. As is the case with gold, the mechanism of action of antimalarials in the treatment of patients with rheumatoid arthritis is unknown.

DOSAGE. Hydroxychloroquine (Plaquenil) is the drug of choice among antimalarials (chloroquine is no longer recommended because of its greater ocular toxicity). The daily dose should not exceed 400 mg/

day (6 mg/kg); normally it is prescribed as a nighttime dosage to avoid gastrointestinal symptoms. The initial dosage of 6 mg/kg can be continued for 2 to 3 months, or until a good clinical response is noted, and then lowered to a maintenance dose of 200 mg/day.

USUAL TIME TO MAXIMUM EFFECT. A period of 3 to 6 months is usual. A 6-month period without clinical effect should be considered as drug failure.

SIDE EFFECTS. The most important toxicities are ocular: loss of the corneal reflex, extraocular muscular weakness, loss of accommodation, and an irreversible retinopathy that may progress to visual loss. At the dosage recommended these toxicities are rare, but a baseline ophthalmological examination and a follow-up examination every 6 months are mandatory during the period of treatment. Gastrointestinal upset, pigmentation changes, leukopenia, and a variety of neurological side effects can rarely be seen also.

D-Penicillamine. Dimethylcysteine, a product of hydrolysis of penicillin, is named penicillamine. It has remitting effects in the treatment of rheumatoid arthritis similar to those of gold.

MECHANISM. Penicillamine chelates metals, interferes with cross-linking of collagen fibrils, and disrupts sulfhydryl-disulfide bonds; but whether any of these actions explains the effects of the drug in patients with rheumatoid arthritis is unknown.

DOSAGE. Penicillamine (Cuprimine, Depen) is available in 125- and 250-mg capsules. Toxicity is reduced by starting at a low dosage (250 mg taken without other medications 1 to 1½ hours after a meal once a day) and increasing the dose slowly (125 to 250 mg a day/every 3 months) until clinical benefit is observed or maximal dosage (750 to 1000 mg a day) is reached. Occasionally a slight reduction in dose (125 to 250 mg a day) may cause a dose-dependent side effect to abate (see below).

USUAL TIME TO MAXIMAL EFFECT. Maximal effect is noted within 4 to 6 months. The earliest response to therapy takes 8 to 12 weeks, and each time the dose is increased, another 8 to 12 weeks must pass before a response can be expected. If after 6 to 9 months of treatment, during which time the maximum dosage has been given for at least the last 8 to 12 weeks, a good clinical response has not been effected, the treatment should be stopped.

SIDE EFFECTS. Like gold, D-penicillamine treatment requires careful periodic monitoring of blood and urine, first on a weekly basis and then monthly once a stable dosage schedule is attained. The major early toxicities include skin rash, loss of taste, and gastrointestinal upset. These early side effects may be dose dependent and transient. After 3 to 4 months of treatment mouth ulcers, thrombocytopenia, renal toxicity (proteinuria, nephrotic syndrome) and skin eruptions are more likely to occur. Patients who have a history of gold-induced nephrotoxicity are more likely to have a nephrotoxic reaction to D-penicillamine. There is an increasing number of cases reported of unusual autoimmune syndromes secondary to penicillamine, including Goodpasture's syndrome, SLE, myasthenia gravis, polymyositis, and pemphigus. One or more of these side effects may occur in up to 30% of patients taking the drug, in which case treatment must be stopped.

Cytotoxic agents. The most commonly used drugs are methotrexate and azathioprine (Imuran). (Cyclophosphamide-Cytoxan, another popular cytotoxic agent, is not often used in the treatment of rheumatoid arthritis because of a somewhat higher incidence of toxic reactions.)

MECHANISMS. These drugs interfere with the synthesis of nucleic acids; one of the consequences of that interference is suppression of the immune response. The explanation for the effect of cytotoxic agents in patients with rheumatoid arthritis is unknown but presumably relates to these basic mechanisms.

DOSAGE. Methotrexate (available as a 2.5-mg tablet) is prescribed in an initial dosage of 2.5 mg every 12 hours for three doses (total 7.5 mg) once a week. If there is no effect in 6 weeks, the dose can be increased to 5 mg every 12 hours for three doses once a week. Azathioprine (available as a 50-mg tablet) is used as a dosage of 1.0 to 2.5 mg/kg/day (100 to 200 mg), starting with the lower dosage and increasing it if necessary after 12 weeks of therapy.

USUAL TIME TO MAXIMAL EFFECT. Maximal response to therapy is seen in 2 to 6 months.

SIDE EFFECTS. Probably the most common side effect, in the first few months in this dose range, is a slowly falling blood cell count secondary to dose-related marrow depression; this effect is reversible if the drugs are withdrawn. The most serious side effect is the increased incidence, over a period of years, of malignant neoplasma (bladder cancer and lymphoproliferative and myeloproliferative neoplasms); however, this risk has been associated primarily with the use of cyclophosphamide. Less serious, but still important, complications of cytotoxic drugs are increased susceptibility to infection, dys-

pepsia (azathioprine) and hepatic toxicity (methotrexate). Thus, these agents should be strictly reserved for life-threatening complications of the rheumatoid process (e.g., vasculitis) or for patients with intolerable progressive disease despite conventional treatment.

Experimental Treatment Modalities

A number of experimental approaches to the treatment of rheumatoid arthritis have been devised but are not generally available. Levamisole is another new immunoregulatory drug that has been shown to be effective in rheumatoid arthritis, but it has unacceptable side effects. Plasmapheresis, lymphopheresis, and total nodal irradiation have all also been studied but, because of lack of controlled trials and of long term follow-up, are not recommended.

Surgery

While rheumatoid arthritis is generally an inflammatory process of the synovium, structural or mechanical derangement is a frequent cause of pain or

Table 70.14.

Indications for Hospitalization of Patients with Rheumatoid Arthritis

Early in the course for assessment of the extent of the disease and for institution of a therapeutic regimen

At the time of acute painful flareups of arthritis

For assessment and treatment of severe manifestations of extra-articular disease (page 923)

Table 70.15.

Indications for Referral of Patients with Rheumatoid Arthritis for Consultation

TO A RHEUMATOLOGIST:
1. If there is any question about the validity of the diagnosis.
2. If a synovial tap is indicated and the primary physician is not comfortable in performing the procedure (an orthopaedist can also do this procedure).
3. For advice about splinting (an orthopaedist can also provide this advice).
4. If the therapeutic regimen requires the use of remitting agents (see the text), at least telephone contact should be made.
5. If there is any consideration of corrective surgery (an orthopaedist can also provide this advice).
6. If there are severe manifestations of extra-articular disease.

TO AN ORTHOPAEDIST:
1. For advice about splinting.
2. If there is any consideration of corrective surgery.

TO A PHYSICAL THERAPIST:
1. Soon after diagnosis to advise and institute appropriate physical therapy.

loss of joint function and may be improved by a surgical procedure. The patient, the primary physician, the rheumatologist, and the orthopaedist should participate in the consideration of such operations. The decision to have surgery is a complex one that must consider the motivation and goals of the patient, his ability to undergo rehabilitation, and his general medical status.

Synovectomy is ordinarily not recommended to patients with rheumatoid arthritis, primarily because relief is only transient. However, synovectomy of the wrist is an exception and is recommended if intense synovitis is persistent despite medical treatment (6 to 12 months) in order to prevent extensor tendon sheath rupture.

Total joint arthroplasties, particularly of the knee, hip, wrist, and elbow, are highly successful. Arthroplasty of the MCP joints also can reduce pain and improve function. Other operations include release of nerve entrapments (e.g., carpal tunnel syndrome), arthroscopic procedures, and, occasionally, removal of a symptomatic rheumatoid nodule.

Summary of Indications for Hospitalization or Referral

See Tables 70.14 and 70.15.

General References

Kelly WN, Harris ED Jr, Ruddy S, Sledge CB (eds): *Textbook of Rheumatology*, ed 2. Philadelphia, WB Saunders, 1985.
> A comprehensive, extensively referenced, especially well illustrated text.

McCarthy DJ (ed): *Arthritis and Allied Conditions*, ed 10. Philadelphia, Lea & Febiger, 1985
> A comprehensive extensively referenced text: the information about rheumatoid arthritis is scattered among a number of chapters.

Rodnan GP, Schumacher HR, Zvaifler NJ: *Primer on the Rheumatic Diseases*, ed 8. Atlanta, Arthritis Foundation, 1983.
> An overview of the rheumatic diseases.

Specific References

1. Cathcart ES: Rheumatoid factor B. Serologic techniques and *in vitro* assays of humoral and cellular immune function. In Cohen AS (ed): *Laboratory Diagnostic Procedures in the Rheumatic Diseases*, ed 2. Boston, Little, Brown, and Co, 1975, p 107.
2. Garella S, Matarese RA: Renal effects of prostaglandins and clinical adverse effects of nonsteroidal anti-inflammatory agents. *Medicine* 63:165, 1984.
3. Hochberg MC: Adult and juvenile rheumatoid arthritis: current epidemiologic concepts. *Epidemiol* Rev 3:27, 1981
4. Hund ER: Extraarticular manifestations of rheumatoid arthritis. *Semin Arthritis Rheum* 8:151, 1979.
5. Huskisson E: *Antirheumatic drugs in Clinical Pharmacology and Therapeutics Series*, New York, Praeger Scientific, 1983, vol. 3
6. Huskisson EC, Taylor RT, Burston D, et al: Evening indomethacin in the treatment of rheumatoid arthritis. *Ann Rheum Dis* 29:396, 1970.
7. Hyland RH, Gordon DA, Broden I, et al: A systematic controlled study of pulmonary abnormalities in rheumatoid arthritis. *J Rheum* 10:395, 1984.
8. Krane SM: Aspects of the cell biology of the rheumatoid synovial lesion. *Ann Rehum Dis* 40:433, 1981.
9. Lebowitz WB: The heart in rheumatoid arthritis (rheumatoid disease). A clinical and pathological study of sixty-two cases. *Ann Intern Med* 58:102, 1963
10. Mason AM, Grumpel JM, Golding PL: Sjögren's syndrome—a clinical review. *Semin Arthritis Rheum* 2:301, 1973.
11. Ropes MW, Bennett GA, Cobb S, et al: 1958 Revision of diagnostic criteria for rheumatoid arthritis. *Arthritis Rheum* 2:16, 1959.
12. Spivak JL: Felty's syndrome: an analytical review. *Johns Hopkins Med J* 141:156, 1977.
13. Stage DE, Mannik M: Rheumatoid factors in rheumatoid arthritis. *Bull Rheum Dis* 23:720, 1973.
14. Stastny P: Association of the B-cell alloantigen DRW4 with rheumatoid arthritis. *N Engl J Med.* 298:869, 1978.
15. Yelin E, Meenan R, Nevitt M, Epstein W: Work disability in rheumatoid arthritis: effects of disease, social, and work factors. *Ann Intern Med* 93:551, 1980.

CHAPTER SEVENTY-ONE

Sacroiliitis, Ankylosing Spondylitis, and Reiter's Syndrome

FRANK C. ARNETT, JR., M.D.

SACROILIITIS

Chronic inflammation of the sacroiliac joints, *sacroiliitis*, may occur as an isolated clinical syndrome or as a component feature of several other chronic rheumatic disorders. Sacroiliitis is considered the *sine qua non* for early *primary ankylosing spondylitis*; however, this latter diagnosis should only be applied when symptoms or signs indicate ascension of inflammation into additional segments of the axial skeleton. *Secondary forms of sacroiliitis* or spondylitis may complicate the clinical course in 10% of patients with inflammatory bowel disease (ulcerative colitis and Crohn's disease), 5 to 10% of those with psoriatic arthritis, and nearly one-third of those with Reiter's syndrome. The dominant clinical problems which bring the patient with primary spondylitis to a physician and require careful management over many years relate to pain, limitation of motion, and deformity of the spine. In secondary spondylitis the same principles of diagnosis and management of the axial problem apply but must be accompanied by attention to the cutaneous, gastrointestinal, genitourinary, and peripheral articular manifestations of the primary disorders.

The pathogenesis of axial inflammation is unknown; however, there is a strong hereditary component marked by the histocompatibility antigen, HLA-B27. This genetic marker is strongly associated with sacroiliitis and spondylitis regardless of clinical setting (Table 71.1). Approximately 90% of patients with primary ankylosing spondylitis have HLA-B27. Conversely, if "normal" individuals with HLA-B27 are carefully assessed, clinical and/or radiographic evidence of disease can be found in nearly 20% (3). In addition to this genetic predisposition, certain environmental agents appear to be associated with these diseases in the B27-positive host. There is increasing evidence that certain *Klebsiella* species in the gastrointestinal tract may be implicated in the pathogenesis of primary ankylosing spondylitis (4). A secondary spondylitis may occur in the setting of Reiter's syndrome which has been triggered by certain gastrointestinal or genitourinary infections (see "Reiter's Syndrome").

ANKYLOSING SPONDYLITIS

Prevalence

The prevalence of spondylitis parallels the frequency of HLA-B27 in different populations in the United States and other regions of the world. This tissue type occurs in 8 to 10% of Caucasian Americans and the disease occurs in 1 to 2% of the white population (Table 71.1). Black Americans have a much lower frequency of both disease and the HLA-B27 antigen (13). On the other hand, there is a high frequency of spondylitic disease and of HLA-B27 in American Indians (7). In other parts of the world, ankylosing spondylitis is common in Europeans but is found rarely in African Blacks or Orientals, again reflecting the relative frequency of the B27 marker.

Histopathology

The spondylitic diseases are characterized by chronic inflammation involving *synovial joints*, especially those in the axial skeleton, *fibrous joints* such as sacroiliacs and symphysis pubis, and nonarticular bony areas where tendons and fascia have their *insertions* (*enthesopathy*). The chronic inflammatory infiltrates are nonspecific and histologically indistinguishable from those of rheumatoid arthritis. On the other hand, unlike the rheumatoid process where there is cartilaginous and bony destruction, this inflammatory process tends to promote new bone formation and fusion across previous articula-

Table 71.1.
Classification of Spondylitis and Frequency of HLA-B27[a]

Classification	HLA-B27 Positive
PRIMARY	
Isolated sacroiliitis[b]	70–90%
Ankylosing spondylitis	90%
SECONDARY	
Spondylitis of inflammatory bowel disease	50%
Psoriatic spondylitis	50%
Reiter's disease with spondylitis	90%
INFECTIOUS	
Sacroiliitis	Not increased
Discitis	Not increased
Osteomyelitis	Not increased
Degenerative spondylosis	Not increased

[a] Found in 8 to 10% of normal white and 2 to 4% of black Americans.
[b] May be the mildest form of ankylosing spondylitis.

Table 71.2.
Clues to Early Ankylosing Spondylitis

A young man
Pain/stiffness in buttocks, low back, chest wall
 Worse with rest
 Better with exercise
Sciatic-like pains
Family history of spondylitis
History of iritis

tions. This ossification and calcification of the articular and ligamentous structures of the spine results in eventual fusion, and gives rise to the characteristic radiographic findings.

History

The typical patient with sacroiliitis or ankylosing spondylitis is a young white man under the age of 40 years (Table 71.2). Women appear to be affected less often than men; however, this may be due to underrecognition of the disease in females. The initial symptoms of the disorder in women may be peripheral or cervical arthritis, and low back involvement may be absent or overshadowed by these complaints. Many are misdiagnosed and labeled seronegative rheumatoid arthritis (see Chapter 70). Therefore, the physician must be mindful of these differences between men and women and consider an emerging sondylitic process in young women presenting with a seronegative arthritis. Similarly, children are also more likely to develop a peripheral oligoarticular lower extremity arthropathy, and symptoms in the axial skeleton may not develop for many years, if ever. Their illness is often labeled juvenile rheumatoid arthritis (1).

The usual presenting symptoms of sacroiliitis or ankylosing spondylitis are those of pain and stiffness in the low back or buttocks. These symptoms begin insidiously, and the patient has usually noticed them for at least 3 months before seeking medical advice. Unlike mechanical low back syndromes, the pain and stiffness of inflammatory disease are usually worsened by rest and improved by exercise. The patient is unable to rest at night or sit for prolonged periods and must arise and walk in order to obtain relief. Like discogenic disease, however, symptoms of shooting pains into the buttocks and down the posterior or lateral thighs may mimic

sciatica. These pains are usually transient and not associated with any demonstrable neurological deficits. Frequently, patients will already have been evaluated myelographically and/or treated conservatively or surgically for presumed disc disease.

With time the disease progresses into the lumbar and thoracic regions. Chest wall radicular pain occurs frequently and may mimic pleuritic, pericardial, or anginal pain syndromes. Progressive limitation of spinal movements ensues, and patients may note more difficulty in bending forward, the development of a stooped posture, and actual loss of height. Finally, the disease process reaches the cervical spine, and if appropriate preventive measures are not taken, the neck may become fused in a kyphotic position. Although other peripheral joints are uncommonly affected, the root joints (hips and shoulders) eventually become involved in 50% of patients. Occasionally fusion of the back may be entirely asymptomatic, and the patient will develop complaints only when the disease reaches the cervical spine, hips, or shoulders (11).

Additional important historical facts should be sought in the assessment of the patient. The family history will be positive for a first degree relative with spondylitis in 16% of patients (10). The past history should seek out prior episodes of peripheral arthritis, perhaps beginning in childhood, or even an episode of Reiter's syndrome. Acute anterior uveitis (iritis) may have been a harbinger of the articular syndrome, and at least 25% of patients will have iritis at sometime before or during their course of illness. The review of systems as well as the family history should seek out symptoms or diagnoses of psoriasis or inflammatory bowel disease in the patient or his family members. The patient with spondylitis may have relatives with psoriasis or inflammatory bowel disease but never manifest these disorders himself (5).

Physical Examination

A complete physical examination initially and every 4 to 6 months is important in patients with suspected inflammatory back disease. This practice ensures the diagnosis and provides the baseline with which the physician can assess future articular or extra-articular complications or the superimposition of unrelated systemic or musculoskeletal disorders.

It must be emphasized that ankylosing spondylitis is a disease where the patient requires management over decades, and each new complaint cannot necessarily be ascribed to the basic disease process. Thus, while the primary focus of examinations will be the musculoskeletal system, especially the axial skeleton, shoulders, hips, and peripheral joints, additional attention must be directed toward the eyes, heart, skin, and gastrointestinal tract.

Articular Features (Table 71.3)

There are few measurable abnormalities in early spondylitis. In fact the patient with *sacroiliitis*, despite significant symptoms of pain and stiffness in the low back region, may have an entirely normal physical examination. At most, there may be tenderness on direct palpation of these joints in the buttocks or upon compression of the pelvis. Stressing the sacroiliac joint to elicit pain (see Chapter 65, Low Back Pain) may also be useful.

Those abnormalities which eventually appear in the patient who has progressive disease relate to loss of range of motion and deformity in mobile structures. After evaluation of the sacroiliac regions the physician should next direct his attention to the *lumbar spine*. The patient with lumbar involvement has often lost the normal lordosis, and there is flattening of that segment of the back. In addition, there is loss in range of motion when the patient attempts to bend forward and touch his toes. It should be recalled that hip motion accounts for 90° of the flexion of trunk on the lower extremities and that the lumbar spine provides the remaining stretch by reversing its lordosis and becoming kyphotic. It is important to obtain serial measurements of the distance between the patient's fingertips and the floor with maximal forward bending. Another objective measurement of lumbar motion is the *Schober test*.

Table 71.3.
Physical Examination in Ankylosing Spondylitis

SACROILIAC JOINTS	THORACIC SPINE
Tenderness	Increased kyphosis
Pain with compression/ stress	Tenderness
LUMBAR SPINE	Pain with rib cage compression
Tenderness	Decreased chest expansion (< 3 cm)
Paravertebral muscle spasm	CERVICAL SPINE
Loss of lordosis	Tenderness
Decreased flexion:	Pain on motion
Schober test (< 5 cm) (see the text)	Muscle spasm
Abnormal finger-floor	Decreased motion
Decreased lateral motion and extension	Kyphosis, decreased lordosis
HIPS, SHOULDERS	Occiput to wall movement (see the text)
Pain on motion	
Decreased range	

With the patient standing erect, a horizontal line is drawn at the L5-S1 region and another line 10 cm above that. With forward flexion the distance between these two points should increase to 15 cm in the normal lumbar spine. This test is best applied and interpreted in the young patient since lumbar motion normally decreases with age. Lateral bending of the lumbar spine should also be assessed at the same time.

Involvement of the *thoracic spine* is determined subjectively by the patient's complaints of pain or stiffness in that region and by demonstrable tenderness along the vertebral column and paravertebral muscles. Compression of the rib cage laterally and over the sternum may also elicit pain. Objective determination of fusion of the costovertebral joints is obtained by measuring the chest expansion. A tape measure is placed around the patient's chest wall at the nipple line, and the change in circumference from full expiration to full inspiration is measured. Less than 3 cm is considered abnormal.

The range of motion of the cervical spine should be determined for extension, right and left rotation, lateral flexion, and forward flexion. Loss of extension is usually the earliest abnormality, and as the disease progresses there is a tendency for the patient to develop fixed deformity in the forward flexed position. Therefore, another rough estimate of developing cervical kyphosis is the occiput-to-wall measurement. This is obtained with the patient placing his heels against the base of the wall and attempting to extend his neck fully to touch the wall with the back of his head. This is normally readily accomplished.

Examination of the range of motion and elicitation of any pain on motion of both shoulders and hips is important since from one-third to one-half of patients will develop involvement of these root joints at sometime during the course of the disease. Less often, peripheral joints become inflamed, but usually only transiently. The joints most commonly involved are the knees, ankles, and wrists. Approximately 10% of patients with ankylosing spondylitis will complain of pain in the heels either at the Achilles tendon insertion or over the attachment of the plantar aponeurosis in the sole of the foot. Swelling is usually not apparent in these areas, but tenderness to direct palpation is found.

Extra-articular Features (Table 71.4)

Cardiac abnormalities occur in less than 5% of patients with ankylosing spondylitis. The most common, first degree atrioventricular (AV) block, can be determined only electrocardiographically. A history of palpitations or syncope and the finding of a slow or irregular pulse on examination should alert the physician to higher degrees of AV block. At times a cardiac pacemaker is required for serious arrhythmias or complete AV dissociation. Aortic regurgita-

Table 71.4.
Extra-articular Manifestations and Complications of Ankylosing Spondylitis

CARDIAC	5%
First degree atrioventricular block	
Second and third degree atrioventricular block	
Aortic regurgitation	
OCULAR	25%
Acute iritis	
Chronic iritis	
NEUROLOGICAL	Rare
Cauda equina syndrome	
Cord injury due to fractures	
AMYLOIDOSIS	4%
PULMONARY FIBROSIS	Rare

tion due to inflammatory thickening of the aortic valve and root is another serious cardiac complication. Once the diastolic murmur becomes apparent there is usually cardiac decompensation requiring valve replacement in 1 to 2 years.

Iritis occurs in approximately 25% of patients with ankylosing spondylitis and does not necessarily parallel the course of the articular disease. It may occasionally be the sentinel symptom. Its onset is usually abrupt and unilateral with intense pain, redness, and photophobia as the cardinal symptoms. Immediate ophthalmological attention is required to prevent serious damage to the anterior chamber of the eye. Local corticosteroids are usually successful in abating an acute episode; however, frequent slit-lamp examinations determine the response and help to dictate whether systemic steroids are required.

The cauda equina syndrome is a rare but serious neurological complication of spondylitis (see also Chapter 65). It is believed to be related to entrapment of exiting lumbar and sacral nerves through the inflamed spinal column; however, compressive inflammatory lesions within the spinal column may be found in some cases and are surgically remediable. Patients with ankylosing spondylitis should be questioned regularly about paresthesias and pain or weakness in the legs, as well as symptoms of bladder and/or bowel sphincter dysfunction. *Other neurological sequelae* of the disorder include injuries to the spinal cord from fracture dislocation of a rigid and brittle spine. The neck is especially prone to fracture, and paraplegia or quadriplegia may result.

Secondary amyloidosis can be found in approximately 4% of patients with ankylosing spondylitis, usually after many decades of persistent inflammatory disease. Proteinuria and nephrotic syndrome indicate renal involvement, which is usually the most serious organ manifestation of amyloid.

Apical pulmonary fibrosis, sometimes with cavity formation, is rare and usually is of no clinical consequence. This radiographic abnormality may mimic tuberculosis, and *vice versa*.

Laboratory Tests

Radiographic evaluation of the sacroiliac joints provides the single most specific test for this disorder. Although a diagnosis of sacroiliitis/spondylitis can be suspected based on the history and physical examination, definitive diagnosis cannot be established without radiographic findings. A single anteroposterior view of the pelvis is usually adequate to define sacroiliitis; however, at times special views such as Ferguson's or oblique views are necessary to evaluate fully the integrity of the sacroiliac joints. The earliest radiographic change is usually bony sclerosis on both sides of the joint margins. Shortly thereafter bony erosions occur (Fig. 71.1). There is eventual fusion across the joint space with subsequent loss of the early sclerotic changes (Fig. 71.2). Sacroiliitis is not infrequently confused with the radiographic anomaly, *osteitis condensens ilii*, where there is symmetrical sclerosis on the iliac side of each sacroiliac joint without any erosions. This finding is most common in young women who have borne children.

If the inflammatory disease has progressed beyond the pelvis, an early radiographic finding on lateral lumbar spine films is "squaring" of the vertebral bodies. This phenomenon may also be seen in the thoracic and cervical regions. The apophyseal joints of the spine become fused and, presumably due to immobility, diffuse osteoporosis ensues. Calcification and ossification of the ligamentous structures between vertebral bodies result in the characteristic syndesmophytes seen on X-ray, *i.e.*, the bamboo spine (Fig. 71.2).

Radionuclide scanning (scintigraphy) of the sacroiliac joints has recently been advocated as a sensitive test in early disease, before radiographic changes are observed. Unfortunately, there are wide ranges of tracer uptake in normal sacroiliac joints, and there is a great deal of controversy regarding their specificity. They may be useful in detecting unilateral sacroiliitis and are probably of most value in localizing pyogenic infections in the sacroiliac joints and other spinal structures (8, 9).

Hematological studies are usually normal. In patients with severe disease, however, there may be a mild normocytic-normochromic anemia reflective of chronic disease. The white blood cell count is usually normal as is the platelet count, although again those with highly inflammatory disease may demonstrate mild thrombocytosis. The erythrocyte sedimentation rate is usually elevated. *Serological studies* are characteristically negative for rheumatoid factor and antinuclear antibodies, and serum complement levels are normal.

Tissue typing. HLA-B27 occurs in 90% of patients with sacroiliitis or spondylitis. This genetically determined tissue type occurs in approximately 8% of the normal white American population. Recently,

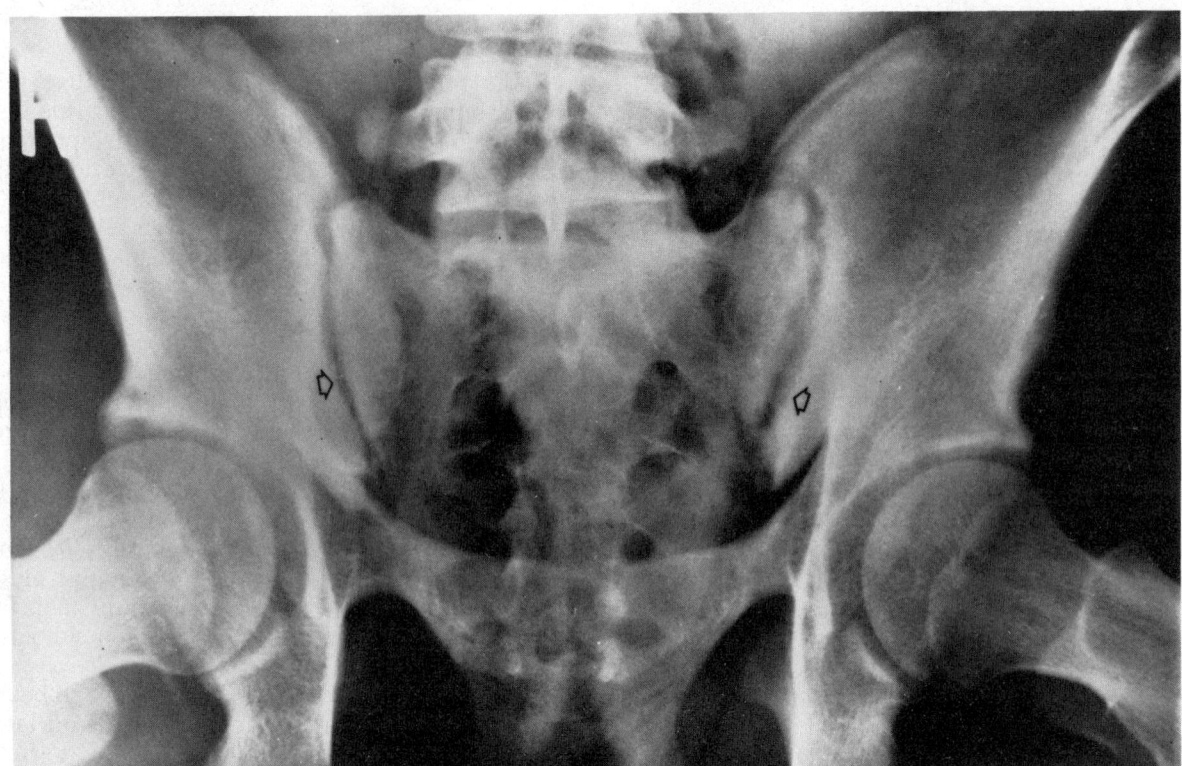

Figure 71.1. Relatively early X-ray changes of sacroiliitis showing bony sclerosis on both sides of the joint margins (see *arrows*). Joint space erosions, a later manifestation of the disease, are present on both sides also.

HLA typing by many commercial laboratories has become available to practicing physicians and when properly used may be a helpful diagnostic aid in the assessment of a patient with low back symptoms or seronegative peripheral arthritis (12). It must be emphasized, however, that indiscriminate HLA typing cannot be substituted for a thorough clinical and radiographic evaluation of the patient. In fact, determination of B27 is rarely needed in making the diagnosis of spondylitis. There are unusual circumstances, however, where the patient gives a strong history suggestive of inflammatory back disease but in whom the radiographs are not yet diagnostic of sacroiliitis. It is in such situations that HLA typing may be helpful, most especially for children and women with early or atypical disease. Even then a positive B27 *does not confirm* a diagnosis of sacroiliitis, but provides supporting data for the diagnosis when the most specific finding (radiographic sacroiliitis) is not present.

Many patients will already know their tissue type or wish to have the test performed because of the hereditary impact of disease on their family. In these circumstances the physician must offer proper genetic counseling. The facts should be simply presented to the patient as they are currently known.

It should be emphasized that spondylitis is not usually a life-threatening or crippling disorder and that symptoms can be controlled medically in the majority of patients. The likelihood that a family member will develop inflammatory back disease is low. Since HLA antigens, including B27, are inherited in a Mendelian dominant fashion, the risk of inheriting this tissue type would be 50% for each of a patient's children (this assumes that the opposite parent is negative for B27). Even if a child inherits this tissue type, his likelihood of developing arthritis is only 20% (see above). Therefore, without any knowledge of HLA status, every child of a patient with B27-positive spondylitis has roughly a 10% (50% times 20%) chance of developing spondylitis.

The 90% probability of never developing this form of arthritis needs to be emphasized to patients concerned about this hereditary factor.

Diagnostic Criteria

The diagnostic criteria for ankylosing spondylitis are summarized in Table 71.5.

Course

It is impossible to predict the ultimate course of any patient presenting with sacroiliitis. The inflam-

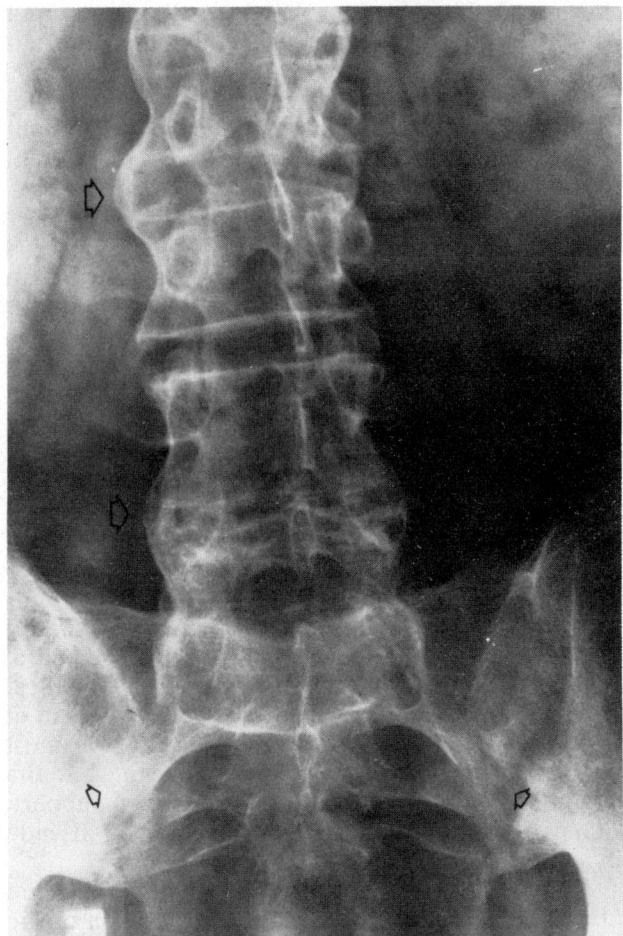

Figure 71.2. Late X-ray changes of sacroiliitis showing complete fusion of the joint space and loss of the early sclerotic change (*small arrows*). Bridging syndesmophytes are also present in the lumbar spine (*large arrows*).

Table 71.5.
New York Diagnostic Criteria for Ankylosing Spondylitis[a, b]

CLINICAL
1. Limitation of motion of the lumbar spine in all three planes—anterior flexion, lateral flexion, and extension.
2. History or presence of pain at the dorsolumbar junction *or* in the lumbar spine.
3. Limitation of chest expansion to 2.5 cm (1 inch) or less, measured at the level of the fourth intercostal space.
RADIOGRAPHIC
1. Sacroiliitis: grade 3 (sclerosis and erosions of the joint margins) or grade 4 (fusion across the joint).

[a] From Bennet PH, Burch TA: New York Symposium on population studies in the rheumatic diseases: new diagnostic criteria. *Bull Rheum Dis* 17:453, 1967.
[b] Definite ankylosing spondylitis = grade 3 or 4 bilateral sacroiliitis with at least one clinical criterion *or* unilateral grade 3 or 4 or bilateral grade 2 (sclerosis of joint margins) sacroiliitis with clinical criterion 1 *or* with both clinical criteria 2 and 3.

Table 71.6.
Principles of Management in Ankylosing Spondylitis

Ensure patient understanding of disease process and objectives in management
Alleviation of pain and stiffness with anti-inflammatory drugs
Physical measures to maintain posture and range of motion in affected areas

matory process may remain confined to these isolated joints or it may progressively ascend into the lumbar, thoracic, and cervical spinal segments. Likewise, the duration of time from onset of symptoms to fusion of higher spinal segments is highly variable. Thus, each patient should understand the nature of this illness and the need for *continued medical surveillance*, as well as the principles of physical and pharmacological management of the disorder (Table 71.6).

Management

Pharmacological

Anti-inflammatory drugs are used to relieve the pain and stiffness of the disease and to promote the patient's ability to perform the physical exercises so important to maintaining a good posture. It is unclear whether these drugs actually affect the natural history of the disease since no long term controlled studies are available. It seems likely, however, that they do alter and improve the overall functional capacity of the patient. Most often their use is required throughout the person's life; but, occasionally when symptoms completely remit, the anti-inflammatory agent may be tapered over several weeks and reinstituted if symptoms recur. Silent progress of the disease may occur; therefore, the physician should closely monitor these patients even when they are not on medication.

Salicylates (aspirin) may be tried as the initial anti-inflammatory drug. An initial dose of 3 tablets four times/day is usually sufficient to attain blood salicylate levels that are anti-inflammatory (15 to 25 mg/dl). Blood salicylate levels should be measured and the dosage adjusted to attain these levels. The majority of patients with ankylosing spondylitis will not have a dramatic response to salicylates; however, a trial of these inexpensive agents is often warranted before consideration is given to more potent and expensive nonsteroidal anti-inflammatory drugs.

Indomethacin (Indocin) is effective therapy in many patients in dosages up to 75 to 150 mg/day. Although hematological reactions are far less common with this drug compared with phenylbutazone (see below), gastrointestinal intolerance and peptic ulcer disease, as well as the central nervous system effects of severe morning frontal headache, vertigo, depression, psychosis, hallucinations, and feelings of dissociation, may limit its usefulness. Additional *newer nonsteroidal anti-inflammatory agents* are now available including tolmetin (Tolectin), sulindac (Clinoril), naproxen (Naprosyn), piroxicam (Feldene), and others which may prove more useful in individual patients or in those intolerant of indomethacin (see Chapter 70).

Phenylbutazone (Butazolidin, Azolid) appears to be the most effective agent in the majority of patients with spondylitic disease. Its long term use is indicated in patients with very active disease unresponsive to other anti-inflammatory agents; however, because of its potential serious side effects (see below), its prolonged use is not recommended without a thorough understanding by the patient of these risks (see below) and without consultation with a rheumatologist. The dosage varies from 200 to 400 mg/day with occasional patients requiring 600 mg for several days in order to suppress highly aggressive disease. Phenylbutazone has a long serum half-life (approximately 80 hours) and a single daily dose may be possible in some patients. The majority, however, will require divided doses usually two to three times/day. Lower doses should be used in older patients and in those with hepatic and renal disease. There are multiple interactions of this drug with other pharmacological agents, such as sulfa drugs (increased sulfonamide effect), anticoagulants (increased anticoagulant effect), oral hypoglycemics (increased effects of sulfonylureas), and phenytoin (increased phenytoin toxicity), and the physician should make himself aware of interactions with any other drug his patient is currently taking. The most serious potential side effect of phenylbutazone therapy relates to bone marrow suppression. Aplastic anemia, pancytopenia, granulocytopenia, or thrombocytopenia, developing within the first few months of exposure, occurs approximately 2 to 10 times for each 1 million prescriptions filled. Gastrointestinal effects include nausea, vomiting, peptic ulcer disease, and gastrointestinal bleeding. The drug should be used cautiously in patients with compromised cardiovascular status since fluid retention can result in congestive heart failure or pulmonary edema. Reduction of salt intake, especially in older patients, may reduce edema and the likelihood of fluid overload. Other side effects include skin rashes, hepatotoxicity, myocarditis, acute parotitis, vertigo, and anaphylaxis. Thus each patient should be informed of the potential side effects of phenylbutazone use, especially the hematological ones, and should consent to this avenue of therapy. Furthermore, complete blood counts should be obtained every 1 to 2 weeks during the first 3 months of therapy and usually at 4- to 6-month intervals thereafter; however, once a fall in the blood count occurs from aplasia, stopping the drug usually will not reverse the process. If the patient is noncompliant or cannot obtain adequate hematological follow-up, alternative agents should be used.

Radiation therapy to the spine was once an effective means of relieving pain. This form of treatment is no longer recommended because of the risk of subsequent leukemia.

Physical Measures

While anti-inflammatory agents relieve the pain and stiffness of spondylitis, an equally important function is their promotion of the patient's ability to perform the physical therapy necessary to prevent spinal deformity and loss of motion in the joints. In fact, such a program can usually not be instituted until symptoms have been brought under control. The natural history of the disease should be explained so that the patient understands the rationale for the exercise program which he must follow (and which the physician will need to reinforce) over many years. An erect posture when sitting or standing should be encouraged. The patient's bed should be quite firm or should be supported by a bed board. Use of a pillow should be avoided, or the smallest possible pillow should be used to prevent flexion of the neck. Sleeping in the prone position is most efficacious in promoting spinal extension, but the supine position is adequate if there is good support. The patient should refrain from sleeping on his side in a curled up posture.

An active exercise program, to promote extension of the back, and to increase range of motion of the axial and peripheral joints, as well as breathing exercises to maintain chest expansion should be instituted and executed two to three times/day. Referral to a physical therapist to provide specific instructions and to determine that the patient is performing well is a good investment. Swimming is an excellent exercise for the patient with ankylosing spondylitis.

If spinal structures undergo complete ankylosis, the danger of spinal fracture after even minor trauma is increased. This is especially true in the neck, where whiplash types of injury occur. Thus, the spondylitic patient should take special precautions to prevent injury, including the use of a soft cervical collar when automobile riding or when walking on slippery surfaces.

Prognosis

The prognosis for ankylosing spondylitis is excellent. The majority of patients can be managed successfully by pharmacological and physical means. Most continue to lead productive lives and change in vocational plans is usually not indicated. The morbidity from articular and extra-articular complications is low, and life span is not reduced significantly, if at all. In many instances pain in an affected area of the spine disappears after that segment has fused and often disease halts at a particular segment and does not proceed to others. While these facts should be optimistically presented to the patient, they are not cause for laxity in following the postural and exercise program and in maintaining close medical surveillance.

REITER'S SYNDROME

Definition

Unlike ankylosing spondylitis, Reiter's syndrome is primarily a peripheral arthritis. However, it shares with ankylosing spondylitis a predisposition to affect young white men and a tendency for sacroiliitis or spondylitis, inflammation of tendon and fascial attachments, uveitis, the same cardiac complications, and a strong association with HLA-B27 (75% positive). Although classically defined as the triad of nongonococcal urethritis, conjunctivitis, and arthritis, it has recently been found that the majority of patients do not express the classical triad, and that approximately 40% of patients will have arthritis as the only feature of the triad. This latter group has been termed "incomplete Reiter's syndrome," and diagnosis depends upon recognition of the typical pattern of arthritis, the presence of mucocutaneous lesions, and other features that are discriminating (2). Reiter's syndrome may, in fact, be the most common cause of arthritis in young men, even exceeding the prevalence of ankylosing spondylitis. Women are less often affected and comprise only 10 to 15% of most series. The diagnosis and management of the disease focus primarily on symptoms and signs referable to the joints and nonarticular musculoskeletal structures. The diagnosis is made on clinical grounds based upon a constellation of symptoms and signs. Typing for HLA-B27 may be a useful diagnostic aid in the incomplete or atypical case.

History and Examination

The principal clues to the diagnosis of Reiter's syndrome are summarized in Table 71.7. The patient presenting with Reiter's syndrome is usually a young white male between puberty and age 40. Blacks and Orientals are affected far less commonly, presumably due to the relatively low frequency of

Table 71.7.
Clues to the Diagnosis of Reiter's Sydrome

A young man with arthritis
Preceding diarrhea, urethritis, or conjunctivitis
Lower extremity oligoarthritis (knee, ankle, foot)
Heel pain and/or sausaging of digits
Rash on soles, penis; painless oral ulcers; dystrophic nails
Fever, weight loss, leukocytosis

HLA-B27 antigen

HLA-B27 in these groups. The reason so few females are affected is unclear.

The disorder occurs in two settings. First, the disease may follow an episode of diarrhea caused by *Shigella, Salmonella, Yersinia,* or *Campylobacter* (see Chapter 26). This postdysenteric form constitutes approximately 15% of most series in the United States. Second, the endemic form is believed by some to result from venereal exposure to unknown pathogens, and *Chlamydia trachomatis* (see Chapters 27 and 94) may be a causative agent. Much of the evidence supporting this notion is debatable and clearly there are a large number of patients with Reiter's disease where no antecedent diarrheal or venereal event can be ascertained.

In the classical form, *urethritis*, usually painless or with mild dysuria and a mucopurulent discharge, is usually the first symptom. Also, the prostate gland may be tender, although symptomatic prostatitis is not common. It generally lasts only 1 to 2 weeks. *Conjunctivitis* usually follows shortly. This is most often mild with redness, weeping, and morning crusting. Photophobia is unusual, and its presence suggests uveitis (see below). *Arthritis* is usually the last feature of the triad to appear, usually from several days up to 1 month following the onset of urethritis. The arthritis is typically in the lower extremities, involving only one to four joints, most commonly the knees, ankles, and small joints of the feet. The patient notes pain, swelling, heat, and erythema over the joints in the majority of cases of this highly inflammatory disease. In addition to frank arthritis, over 50% of patients will have *nonarticular musculoskeletal pain*. Heel pain due to inflammation of the plantar aponeurosis or of the Achilles tendon insertion is one of the most prominent symptoms of the disease and may be one of the most disabling. Diffuse swelling of digits (sausaging), especially the toes, also occurs in over 50% of patients and is indicative of involvement not only of the joints but of tendons and periosteal structures.

The *mucocutaneous features* of Reiter's syndrome are often asymptomatic and must be sought on physical examination. These include (a) painless shallow oral ulcers, usually on the tongue and palate, (b) circinate balanitis (see Fig. 71.3) manifested by shallow moist painless ulcers on the glans penis in uncircumcised men or a dry scaling eruption on the glans in the circumcised, (c) hyperkeratosis and crumbling of nails (see Fig. 71.4), and (d) keratoderma blennorrhagica (see Fig. 71.5), a papulosquamous skin eruption usually beginning on the palms and soles which closely resembles pustular psoriasis.

Additional features include fever in approximately one-third of patients, weight loss, and uveitis. The disease may begin abruptly and run a toxic course, or begin very insidiously and pursue an indolent one. Not infrequently heel pain (see Chapter 102) is the first symptom, and this complaint in

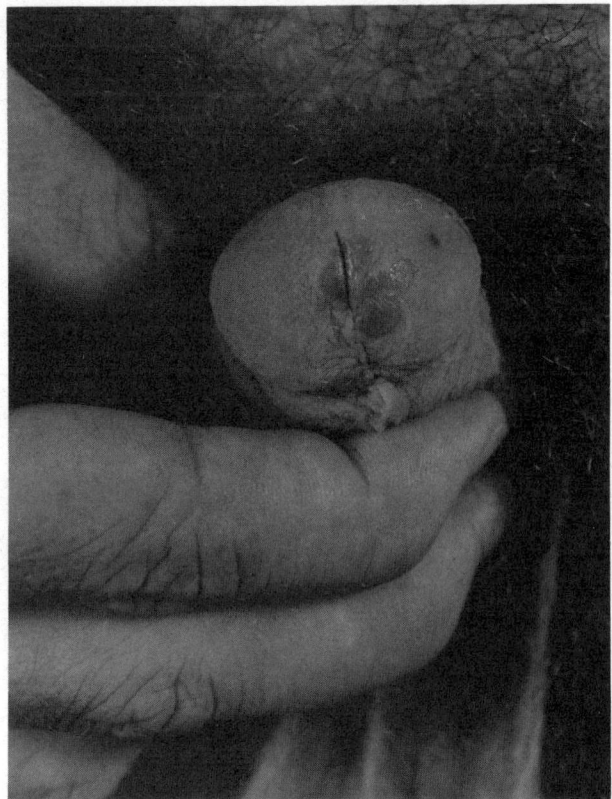

Figure 71.3. Moist, shallow circular lesions on the glans penis characteristic of circinate balanitis.

a young man should raise the question of emerging Reiter's syndrome.

Laboratory Tests

Hematological studies will usually demonstrate a mild normocytic normochromic anemia characteristic of chronic disease. The hematocrit value rarely falls below 30%. A modest leukocytosis in the range of 10,000 to 15,000/mm³ with a mild shift to the left occurs frequently in those with an acute toxic presentation. Thrombocytosis with platelet counts in the range of 400,000 to 600,000/mm³ is found in approximately one-third. The erythrocyte sedimentation rate is usually elevated.

Serological studies for rheumatoid factor and antinuclear antibodies are negative. Serum complement is typically normal or elevated as an acute phase reactant. *HLA typing* will reveal the B27 antigen in 75% of cases, but is rarely required in diagnosing the disease. *Radiographs* are typically normal early in the course of the disease; however, over time periostitis may be seen involving the calcaneus or along the shafts of swollen digits. Should sacroiliitis appear (it does in about 20% of cases), it is more likely to be unilateral in this disease than in ankylosing spondylitis. This may be detected by examination (see above) and confirmed by X-ray if there

is doubt. In severe disease cartilage may be lost in joint spaces and bony ankylosis may ensue.

Synovial fluid has the characteristics of a moderate inflammatory process with a poor mucin clot, white blood cell counts ranging from 5,000 to 50,000/

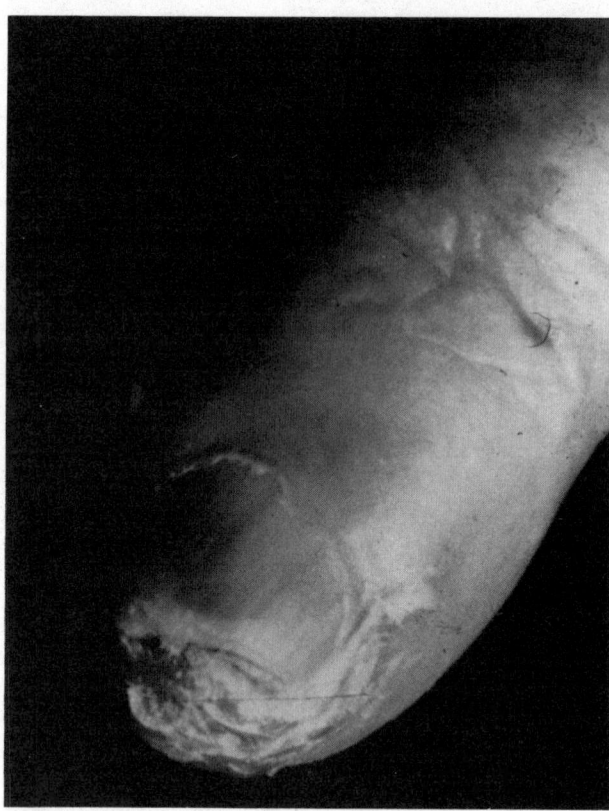

Figure 71.4. Opacification and onychodystrophy of fingernails in Reiter's syndrome. (Taken with permission from Arnett FC: Reiter's syndrome. In Fitzpatrick TB, Eisen AZ, Wolf K, *et al* (eds): *Dermatology in General Medicine*, ed 3. New York, McGraw-Hill, 1985.)

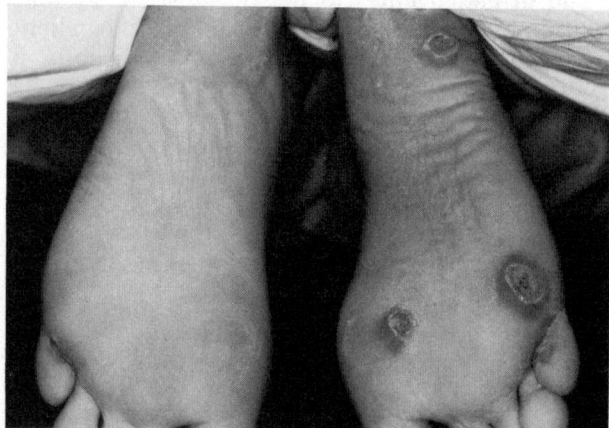

Figure 71.5. Typical keratoderma blennorrhagica involving the sole.

mm³, elevated protein, normal glucose, and a high complement (in contradistinction to the synovial fluid hypocomplementemia of rheumatoid arthritis). Culture shows that the synovial fluid is sterile. *Synovial biopsy* demonstrates an acute and chronic inflammatory process which is nonspecific and indistinguishable from that of many other inflammatory synovitides, and therefore it is not usually necessary. A urinalysis performed on the first voided specimen in the morning is a useful way to identify asymptomatic urethritis. *Urethral stains and cultures are* negative for gonococci in the majority, although the concurrence of gonococcal urethritis with Reiter's syndrome has been documented. Therefore, this culture should not be overlooked.

Course and Prognosis

Reiter's syndrome follows a self-limited course and completely resolves in 3 months to 1 year in approximately one-third of patients. Another 30 to 40% of patients will have relapses after months or years of quiescence. It has been estimated that a patient with this disease has a 15% chance of having another episode each year for as long as 30 years. Less commonly, a chronic progressive course ensues, resulting in articular destruction and fusion of peripheral, and usually axial skeletal joints. Disability results primarily from severe heel pain, deformities of the feet, visual loss due to uveitis, and, less commonly, cardiac complications. Approximately 10% of patients will become permanently disabled and unable to work (6).

Management

Treatment is directed toward suppressing the inflammatory process in joints and tendon insertions and preventing deformity of the peripheral and axial skeleton. Urethritis does not require specific therapy, but the patient should be advised to use a condom during sexual intercourse. Rarely an urgent circumcision is indicated if balanitis is extreme, but usually a protective dressing (e.g., petroleum gauze) is all that is needed to control discomfort. Conjunctivitis responds to compresses or astringent drops (see Chapter 99). Uveal tract involvement, if present, requires close follow-up and treatment by an ophthalmologist in order to prevent permanent visual loss. Phenylbutazone and indomethacin have been found to be most effective in suppressing the articular inflammation in this disease. Salicylates are helpful in a minority of patients but may be worthy of trial. Dosage recommendations and adverse side effects are similar to those for ankylosing spondylitis. Systemic corticosteroids may be necessary to treat severe uveitis or inflamed joints which have been unresponsive to phenylbutazone or other nonsteroidal anti-inflammatory drugs, and in these instances consultation with a rheumatologist is suggested. At times, intra-articular corticosteroid injection (usually performed by a rheumatologist) may be useful when systemic therapy has not completely suppressed the inflammatory process. Only occasional patients with extensive cutaneous and articular disease will require more radical therapy (e.g., cytotoxic drugs), and consultation with a rheumatologist should be sought in these circumstances. Anti-inflammatory agents are generally continued for several months and then tapered in those whose symptoms are completely controlled. However, many patients will need continued, lifelong anti-inflammatory agents to suppress the inflammatory activity of the disease. Also, approximately 30 to 40% (see above) of those who have had symptomatic remissions will experience a relapse and require the reinstitution of anti-inflammatory medications. *Tetracycline or erythromycin* may be effective in treating the nongonococcal urethritis; however, it is unclear whether this therapy influences the subsequent emergence or course of the articular disease.

Physical measures are important adjuncts in the management of this disorder as in ankylosing spondylitis. There is a tendency for fusion of affected peripheral and axial joints. During acute inflammatory episodes, rest is important, and severely inflamed joints should be splinted to ensure comfort for the patient. As soon as inflammation can be brought under control with drugs, it is important that affected joints be exercised to maintain their ranges of motion. At first passive range of motion should be encouraged in all affected joints. Later, more active range of motion and strengthening exercises should be prescribed as the patient improves.

Painful feet, especially heels, may be helped by shoe inserts which shift weight bearing to nonaffected areas (see also Chapter 102).

General References

Calin A (ed): *Spondylarthropathies.* New York, Grune & Stratton, 1983.
> An authoritative text on all aspects of the spondylarthropathies.

Sharp JT: Reiter's syndrome. In McCarty DJ (ed): *Arthritis and Allied Conditions,* ed 10, Philadelphia, Lea & Febiger, 1985.
> This chapter provides a comprehensive review of this common form of sacroiliitis.

Specific References

1. Arnett FC, Bias WB, Stevens MB: Juvenile-onset chronic arthritis: clinical and roentgenographic features of a unique HLA-B27 subset. *Am J Med* 69:369, 1980.
2. Arnett FC, McClusky OE, Schacter BZ, Lordon RE: Incomplete Reiter's syndrome: discriminating features and HL-A W27 in diagnosis. *Ann Intern Med* 84:8, 1976.
3. Calin A, Fries JF: Striking prevalence of ankylosing spondylitis in "healthy" W27 positive males and females. *N Engl J Med* 293:835, 1975.
4. Edmonds J, Macauley D, Tyndall A, *et al*: Lymphocytotoxicity of anti-Klebsiella antisera in ankylosing spondylitis and related arthropathies. *Arthritis Rheum* 24:1, 1981.

5. Enlow RW, Bias WB, Arnett FC: The spondylitis of inflammatory bowel disease. *Arthritis Rheum* 23:1359, 1980.

6. Fox R, Calin A, Gerber RC, Gibson D: The chronicity of symptoms and disability in Reiter's syndrome. *Ann Intern Med* 91:190, 1979.

7. Gofton JP, Chalmers A, Price GE, Reeve CE: HL-A27 and ankylosing spondylitis in B.C. Indians. *J Rheumatol* 2:314, 1975.

8. Gordon G, Kabins SA: Pyogenic sacroiliitis. *Am J Med* 69:50, 1980.

9. Greyson ND: Radionuclide bone and joint imaging in rheumatology. *Bull Rheum Dis* 30:1034, 1980.

10. Hochberg MC, Bias WB, Arnett FC: Family studies in HLA-B27 associated arthritis. *Medicine* 57:463, 1978.

11. Hochberg MC, Borenstein DG, Arnett FC: The absence of back pain in classical ankylosing spondylitis. *Johns Hopkins Med J* 143:181, 1978.

12. Khan MA: Clinical application of the HLA-B27 test in rheumatic disease. *Arch Intern Med* 140:177, 1980.

13. Khan MA, Braun WE, Kushner I, et al: HLA-B27 in ankylosing spondylitis: differences in frequency and relative risk in American blacks and Caucasians. *J Rheumatol* 3:39, 1977.

Metabolic and Endocrinological Problems

CHAPTER SEVENTY-TWO

Diabetes Mellitus

ROBERT I. GREGERMAN, M.D.

DEFINITION AND CLASSIFICATION

Diabetes mellitus is a condition characterized by an abnormality of glucose utilization and associated with elevation of blood glucose concentration. Approximately 10 million people in the United States are diabetic by this definition. Diabetes mellitus is not a single distinct disease entity. The commonest varieties of diabetes mellitus are known to be associated with abnormalities of insulin secretion and concentration, with cellular resistance to insulin action, and with vascular abnormalities such as basement membrane thickening. Nonetheless, diagnosis is based on the finding of persistently abnormal blood glucose concentrations at some time in life.

Until recently there has been no general agreement on the classification of diabetes mellitus, based either on etiology or manifestations. A new terminology has recently been proposed by the National Diabetes Data Group of the National Institutes of Health (9). This classification is followed in this chapter; it has the endorsement of at least the majorities of the American Diabetes Association and of many diabetologists in the United States, the United Kingdom, and elsewhere (Table 72.1)

Table 72.1.
Classification of Diabetes Mellitus and Other States of Glucose Intolerance

Type of Diabetes	Former Terminology	Clinical Characteristics
INSULIN-DEPENDENT TYPE (IDDM, TYPE I)	Juvenile diabetes Juvenile onset type diabetes Ketosis-prone diabetes Brittle diabetes	Onset usually in youth but occurs at any age. Insulin deficiency requires exogenous insulin to prevent ketosis-acidosis. Non-insulin-dependent phases may occur during natural history. 10–12% of all cases.

NON-INSULIN-DEPENDENT TYPES (NIDDM, TYPE II):
  Nonobese NIDDM
  Obese NIDDM
	Adult onset diabetes, maturity onset diabetes (MOD), stable diabetes, nonketosis-prone diabetes; in young people was called maturity onset diabetes of youth (MODY)	Onset generally after age 40, but may occur in young; not insulin dependent or ketosis prone, but may need insulin for control of persistent hyperglycemia; periods of ketosis-acidosis may occur during stress of illness; weight control of obese subtype may ameliorate disease. 80% of all cases.

OTHER TYPES:
  Diabetes mellitus associated with
    Pancreatic disease
    Hormone excess due to endocrine disease or hormone treatment (steroids of glucocorticoid type)
    Drug use
    Insulin receptor abnormalities
	Secondary diabetes	Diagnosis demands usual abnormalities of glucose handling and documentation of associated condition.

Impaired glucose tolerance (IGT)
    Nonobese IGT
    Obese IGT
    IGT associated with certain conditions and syndromes
    Drug (chemical) induced
    Insulin receptor abnormalities
    Genetic syndromes
	Asymptomatic diabetes; chemical diabetes; subclinical diabetes; borderline diabetes; latent diabetes	Diabetes is based on abnormality of glucose handling: may represent a stage of development of diabetes, although most remain in this class for years or revert to normal glucose tolerance.

Gestational diabetes mellitus (GDM)	Gestational diabetes	Glucose intolerance has *onset* during pregnancy; does not include diabetic who becomes pregnant: increased risk of perinatal complications and future diabetes.

Non-Insulin-Dependent Diabetes Mellitus (NIDDM: Type II)

This is the commonest form of diabetes mellitus and accounts for about 90% of patients presenting with an abnormality of glucose metabolism. About 9 to 10 million people in the United States are affected. The majority of patients are obese. Patients with NIDDM are neither absolutely dependent on treatment with insulin nor ketosis prone. Nonetheless, treatment within insulin may be necessary in the short term in order to control hyperglycemia, which leads to symptoms through osmotic diuresis or infection. Treatment with insulin may also be undertaken in an effort to prevent vascular complications, now believed by many to be a direct consequence of hyperglycemia. Furthermore, such patients do sometimes develop insulin dependence as the result of stress (severe infections, trauma).

NIDDM is very likely a heterogeneous disorder. Although most patients are over age 40 at the time of diagnosis, this type of disease is also seen in young persons, and it is for this reason that older terms such as "maturity onset type diabetes" should be abandoned.

NIDDM has a much more obvious familial pattern of expression than does insulin-dependent diabetes mellitus (IDDM, see below). Included in the group of NIDDM are patients who develop the disease before they reach adulthood (formerly known as "maturity onset diabetes of the young" or MODY). Behavioral and possibly environmental factors appear to be involved in the onset of NIDDM. Especially prominent is the role of excessive caloric intake and subsequent obesity in 60 to 90% of cases. In this type of diabetes, association with certain histocompatibility antigen (HLA) subtypes and antibodies to islet cells has not been found. Blood insulin levels are variable and may be normal, subnormal, or even supranormal; insulin resistance is common. However, measurement of insulin concentration has no diagnostic usefulness.

Insulin-Dependent Diabetes Mellitus (IDDM: Type I)

This type of diabetes—which accounts for about 5 to 10% of cases—*generally* has its onset in childhood or in early adulthood, hence the former name "juvenile onset diabetes mellitus." However, that designation was misleading, since this type of diabetes can occur at any time of life. Moreover, its essential characteristic is that insulin dependence is absolute; without insulin therapy, ketosis-acidosis usually ensues rapidly. Although the disease is probably heterogeneous, genetic determinants are important in most of these patients (see below). Rare cases may have a viral basis, but even in these, genetic predisposition may be important. A minority of siblings of patients with IDDM develop diabetes; when tested initially, these individuals may show only impaired glucose tolerance but eventually develop overt IDDM. Increased or decreased frequency of certain histocompatibility antigens, abnormal immune responses and autoimmunity, and antibodies to islet cells have been demonstrated in IDDM. None of these findings is currently useful in a diagnostic sense.

Recent studies have focused on IDDM as an autoimmune disease. When immunosuppressive therapy has been given within a few weeks after onset, remissions have been induced. Such therapy is experimental. Viruses have also been linked to the onset of IDDM, but their precise role in the causation of the disease is unclear.

Inheritance and Genetic Counseling

The genetics of IDDM (formerly juvenile) and NIDDM (formerly adult onset) are different; surprisingly, familial expression is greater in the latter group. The precise genetics, however, is not clear, and prediction of the occurrence of diabetes in offspring of diabetic parents is not possible; even statistical estimates are crude (7). The prevalance of overt diabetes in offspring of conjugal diabetic parents is remarkably low, ranging from 3 to 12% in most reports. Contributing to the difficulty of prediction are the criteria for detection of diabetes (overt diabetes *versus* diabetes detected by glucose tolerance testing; see pages 955–957) and age of onset.

The conclusion that hereditary factors are more important in NIDDM than in IDDM comes from studies of twins. If expression of diabetes were based entirely on genetic grounds, one would expect 100% concordance for diabetes in monozygotic twins; but this is not the case for patients diagnosed when young (before age 40). Both members of pairs become diabetic only about 50% of the time. Only in twins in whom diagnosis is made later in life is 100%

concordance approached. Thus, environmental factors must be important in younger diabetics.

Studies of ethnic groups show distinctive patterns of diabetes and superimposed geographic (environmental) effects upon these patterns. The most easily apparent determinant is obesity. Certain American Indian tribes show a remarkably high prevalence of diabetes (Pima, Navajo); obesity appears to be the major factor in expression of the disease in these people. In terms of the patterns of disease, in South Africa, black and Indian populations have similar environments and diets, but only the black diabetics are ketosis prone. In contrast, the Indians have more frequent vascular disease. In non-Indian populations in the United States, no such distinctive ethnic or racial patterns have been recognized to date.

Parents who have produced an insulin-dependent diabetic offspring often wish to know the risk to future offspring. Prenatal HLA typing of fetal cells obtained at amniocentesis could be compared to that of the diabetic sibling; a fetus with the same HLA identity would increase the risk, but the accuracy of the prediction would still be only about 50%. The imprecise nature of this assessment is in contrast to the nearly 100% certainty of predicting Tay-Sachs disease or Down's syndrome. Thus, even with an accurate family history and pedigree, together with chemical assessment of diabetes (glucose tolerance testing), only crude predictions can be made for a couple who wish to know their own chances of developing diabetes and the risk for their offspring (7).

At this point, only a few generalities seem safe. Prospective parents should not be told to avoid procreation merely because one parent is diabetic. Even when both parents are diabetic, the risk seems relatively low. If avoidance of pregnancy is decided upon, a diabetic mother may be at increased risk from several commonly used contraceptive measures, although the evidence for this increased risk is not firm. Estrogen-based contraceptives may be unwise because of possibly increased risk in the diabetic of vascular thrombosis and hyperlipidemia. Intrauterine devices may possibly produce infection more often in a diabetic. Thus, mechanical means of contraception such as diaphragm or condom would seem to be the safest methods (see Chapter 93).

Other Types of Diabetes

Sometimes diabetes is associated with another condition or disease; usually the association is infrequent but more common than in the general population (Table 72.2). This heterogeneous group includes some disorders in which there is a clear relationship between the associated disease and the diabetes and others in which an association has been noted but is not well understood. For example, in pancreatic insufficiency due to pancreatitis, insuf-

Table 72.2.
Diseases Associated with Diabetes Mellitus or Abnormal Glucose Tolerance

ENDOCRINE DISORDERS
  Acromegaly
  Aldosteronism
  Glucocorticoid excess (Cushing's syndrome; iatrogenic)
  Hyperthyroidism
  Pheochromocytoma
AUTOIMMUNE DISORDERS
  Adrenal insufficiency (Addison's disease)
  Hashimoto's disease
  Hypoparathyroidism
  Myasthenia gravis
  Pernicious anemia
  Polyglandular failure (adrenals/gonads/thyroid)
  Primary hypothyroidism
OTHER DISORDERS
  Chronic pancreatitis
  Hemochromatosis

ficient insulin may be produced and insulin-dependent diabetes mellitus ensues. At the opposite extreme, an association between aldosterone excess in primary aldosteronism and diabetes mellitus has been observed, but the mechanism is not clear. Glucocorticoid excess, as in Cushing's syndrome or steroid therapy, may produce diabetes mellitus. Recently, rare cases of diabetes associated with antibodies to insulin receptors have been described.

Problems in Classification of Individual Patients

On occasion, classification may be difficult. For example, an adult presenting with ketoacidosis may be erroneously classified as IDDM when in fact the individual's diabetes is of the NIDDM type, with insulin dependence having been precipitated by the stress of infection. Similarly, the process of distinguishing between a patient with IDDM and a thin NIDDM patient for whom insulin has merely been prescribed may require discontinuation of the insulin therapy, a procedure which may be impractical. Diagnostic procedures necessary to exclude the possibility that the diabetes is one of the other types (e.g., Cushing's syndrome, hemochromatosis, etc) may not have been performed. In addition, for those patients in whom diagnosis was based on an abnormality of glucose tolerance, diagnostic criteria may not have been met or may have been equivocal (see page 955). In these situations, classification should be considered tentative.

CLINICAL PRESENTATION

Most diagnoses of diabetes mellitus are now made at an asymptomatic stage of the disease as a result of routine blood tests which reveal elevation of blood glucose concentration. In some institutions where the diagnosis is actively sought, glucose tolerance

tests reveal many cases. Of those patients who are symptomatic at time of diagnosis, most will complain of increased frequency of urination (polyuria), excessive thirst with increased fluid intake (polydipsia), and, if the disease is very severe, increased appetite and increased food consumption (polyphagia) associated with weight loss. All of these symptoms are manifestations of excessive blood sugar and of secondary glucosuria. Other symptomatic manifestations include blurred vision, vaginitis (usually due to monilial infection), and skin infections. Furuncles and carbuncles, once common, are now rarely seen, but intertriginous moniliasis is common in the obese. Oral moniliasis is uncommon.

Usually, these symptoms are present for weeks or months before medical attention is sought. The onset of symptoms is often insidious and may be attributed by the patient, or even by the physician, to emotional factors or to a common problem such as a urinary tract infection. Indeed, the diagnosis may be missed for a time because the physican "knows" that the patient is not a diabetic on the basis of previous evaluation.

Some patients present with absent or minimal diabetic, i.e., glucosuria-related, symptoms but have already developed complications of the diabetic state such as neuropathy or, more commonly, vascular disease. However, only rarely will a patient be unaware of diabetes and yet present with severe complications of the disease such as diabetic retinopathy or nephropathy.

DIAGNOSIS

Elevation of blood sugar concentration is the hallmark of diabetes mellitus. Glucosuria alone is not a diagnostic finding, however, since rare individuals may have a renal tubular glucose "leak" (renal glucosuria) at normal concentrations of blood sugar. Only infrequently will individuals show diagnostically elevated blood sugar levels before glucosuria develops ("elevated renal threshold").

Criteria for Diagnosis of Diabetes Mellitus

Criteria have been suggested as follows (Tables 72.3 and 72.4) (9): (a) unequivocal elevation of plasma glucose (PG) concentrations associated with classic symptoms of diabetes mellitus, or (b) elevation of fasting plasma glucose (FPG) on more than one occasion, or (c) elevation of PG following an oral glucose challenge on more than one occasion. A single elevated FPG or a single oral glucose tolerance test never establishes the diagnosis.

In most modern laboratories glucose is determined in plasma or serum. Plasma and serum values are identical, but both are 5 to 15% higher than are obtained using whole blood. The physician should be aware of the laboratory's procedure, lest inappro-

Table 72.3.
Normal Plasma Glucose Concentrations[a]

Fasting state (10–16 hours postprandial)

Venous plasma	< 115 mg/dl
Venous whole blood	< 100 mg/dl
Capillary whole blood	< 100 mg/dl

2-Hour oral glucose tolerance test (OGTT)

Venous plasma	< 140 mg/dl
Venous whole blood	< 120 mg/dl
Capillary whole blood	< 140 mg/dl

Values between those which are diagnostic (see Table 72.4) and those which are normal should be considered *nondiagnostic*. Impaired glucose tolerance (IGT) is considered present when three criteria are met: (*a*) fasting level is below diagnostic (*b*) 2-hour value is intermediate, and (*c*) some other value (½, 1, 1½) must be elevated to:

Venous plasma	> 200 mg/dl
Venous whole blood	> 180 mg/dl
Capillary whole blood	> 200 mg/dl

[a] To express values as millimoles per liter, multiply glucose in milligrams per deciliter × 0.056. Serum and plasma values are the same.

priate diagnosis is made because of methodological differences.

Impaired Glucose Tolerance (IGT) *versus* Diabetes Mellitus

The standards promulgated in Tables 72.3 and 72.4 are not arbitrary, but have been derived from many studies and numerous considerations, including prospective studies conducted in the United States and Britain over the past 15 years. These standards, first published in 1979, supersede those in general use for many years. The older standards for the oral glucose tolerance test (OGTT) were clearly set at levels of blood sugar that were too low and reduced the specificity of the test (high number of false positive results). Perhaps most widely used in the past were the criteria of Fajans and Conn and standards promoted by the US Public Health Service, World Health Organization, *etc.* In general, the upper limits of normal at 1 hour had been set at between 180 and 195 mg/dl; and for 2 hours, at 140 to 160 mg/dl.

Although some disagreement will inevitably exist on all standards, perhaps the most important point for the clinician to recall is that no single value of fasting glucose or combination of values in glucose tolerance tests sharply divides diabetics from nondiabetics. Most populations exhibit a continuous unimodal distribution of values, usually skewed to the higher end. (An exception is the Pima Indian population in which bimodal distribution of both fasting and 2-hour postglucose values is seen (12)). The Fajans and Conn criteria were simply statistically based, *i.e.*, individuals were deemed diabetic if their 1-, 1½-, and 2-hour values were greater than 2 standard deviations above the mean for a group of healthy adults who were less than 50 years old. In

contrast, the new criteria are derived from prospective observations of the fate of individuals whose glucose concentrations fall within certain ranges. The conclusions from such studies are as follows:

1. Individuals whose plasma glucose levels during the OGTT fall between normal (1 hour < 160 mg/dl; 2 hours < 140 mg/dl) and diabetic should be clearly classified into a group (impaired glucose tolerance, IGT) separate from those with overt glucose intolerance.

2. In this IGT group, one can expect 1 to 5%/year to develop symptomatic diabetes mellitus or diagnostically abnormal glucose tolerance. On the other hand, many such individuals eventually show normalization of glucose tolerance, while still others remain in the IGT range. The higher the blood sugar within the range of IGT, the greater the tendency for tolerance to deteriorate.

Perhaps the most convincing evidence on IGT progression has come from a long term study of Pima Indians (3, 9, 12). The risk of progression to overt diabetes in this group was clearly related to the level of glucose within the range of 160 to 200 mg at 2

Table 72.4.
Diagnosis of Diabetes: Diagnostic Concentrations of Glucose

Fasting state (10–16 hours postprandial)

Venous plasma[a]	> 140 mg/dl
Venous whole blood	> 120 mg/dl
Capillary whole blood	> 140 mg/dl

Oral glucose tolerance test (OGTT) *preparation*: fasting 10–16 hours during which no caffeine-containing drinks or smoking is permitted.

75-g glucose (40 g/m^2)

Use in nonpregnant adults: (1.75 g/kg for children. Up to 75 g maximum). Dosage form: flavored water, 25 g of glucose/100 dl. Drink over 5 minutes. Obtain blood samples at 0, ½, 1, 1½, 2 hours.

Test positive for diabetes mellitus: *both* the 2-hour sample *and* at least one other sample must meet following criteria:

Venous plasma	> 200 mg/dl
Venous whole blood	> 180 mg/dl
Capillary whole blood	> 200 mg/dl

100-g glucose

Use only in pregnant adults: obtain blood samples at 0, 1, 2, 3 hours.

Test positive for diabetes mellitus: *two* or more of the following values must be met or exceeded:

	Venous plasma (mg/dl)	Venous Whole Blood (mg/dl)	Capillary Whole Blood (mg/dl)
Fasting	105 mg/dl	90	90
1 hour	190	170	170
2 hours	165	145	145
3 hours	145	125	125

[a] Serum and plasma values are the same.

hours (3 times that of persons with lower values). In this group, however, the rate of decompensation to overt diabetes was still only 3%/year.

3. Treatment of the IGT group with oral antidiabetic (hypoglycemic) agents had no effect on the eventual development of diabetes.

4. Diabetic microvascular complications (retinopathy or nephropathy) do *not* develop in individuals with IGT. On the other hand, in the study of Pima Indians, values > 240 mg/dl were associated with such changes.

Significance of Impairment of Glucose Tolerance for Development of Cardiovascular Disease

Although morbidity and mortality from cardiovascular disease are unequivocally increased in patients with clinical diabetes mellitus, the issue of the impact of IGT on such events is unsettled. The National Diabetes Data Group Study concluded that morbidity and mortality from arteriosclerotic disease appeared to be significantly increased in patients with IGT, although to a lesser degree than the 2- to 3-fold increase seen in overt diabetes (9). On the other hand, no such conclusion could be drawn from later studies in 15 populations of the impact of IGT on development of coronary artery disease (14). In some of these studies, a strong relationship was found between IGT and coronary heart disease death rates, but in others no such relationship was evident. No satisfactory explanation is available to explain these discrepancies. At this time, IGT cannot be designated as an established risk factor for coronary heart disease or other cardiovascular diseases.

Fasting Plasma Glucose (FPG)

Elevation of FPG should be followed up by several repeat measurements of the FPG on different days. Since over 90% of individuals with repeated elevations of FPG will have an abnormal glucose tolerance test (OGTT), little is gained by proceeding directly to such a test. FPG may be elevated by stress and illness, but is actually less subject to this change than is the OGTT. When an illness results in elevation of FPG (or an abnormal OGTT) only to revert to normal with recovery, the question which arises is whether a "diabetic" state has been unmasked or whether the transient elevation is simply the result of disturbed carbohydrate metabolism associated with the illness. Only long term follow-up may sometimes provide an answer. In the interim, the individual may be deemed to have IGT (see above). Such terms as subclinical, preclinical, chemical, latent, and borderline diabetes should be avoided, both because of their uncertain meaning and because of the psychological trauma and economic penalties (e.g., insurance ratings, job qualifications) that are often needlessly created.

The 2-Hour Postprandial Blood Sugar as a Screening Test

This frequently used procedure should be abandoned. Only infrequently will a gross elevation of postprandial sugar be seen when the FPG is normal. Initially nondiagnostic but abnormal elevations (e.g., 140 to 200 mg/dl) are often not observed on follow-up testing with an OGTT. Even a normal glucose concentration 2 hours postprandially has no established value for predicting that an OGTT would be normal. The 2-hour postprandial blood sugar with glucose added to the meal is similarly to be avoided.

Use of the Oral Glucose Tolerance Test

Diagnostic criteria for the OGTT are listed in Tables 72.3 and 72.4; Table 72.4 also shows how the test is performed. The OGTT is not necessary if there is unequivocal elevation of plasma glucose in a patient who has classic symptoms of diabetes or if the FPG is elevated on more than one occasion (see page 955). Indeed, in the absence of signs and symptoms of diabetes, relatively few clinical indications exist for attempted establishment of a diagnosis of diabetes mellitus solely by use of the OGTT.

Indications

The physician may wish to perform the test because of a positive family history. Occasionally, he may wish to prognosticate for a sibling of a diabetic. The OGTT does have a place in diagnosis during pregnancy (see below). The test is also sometimes performed in an individual who manifests premature atherosclerosis or has unexplained neuropathy or retinopathy. However, under such conditions a positive OGTT is ordinarily, at most, no more than suggestive of a cause of the disorder at hand. For example, premature atherosclerosis certainly occurs in nondiabetics and in the face of normal glucose tolerance. Perhaps a greater constraint on the use of the OGTT for early diagnosis is the realization that, given the limitations of currently available therapeutic measures, the physician does not—except in obese individuals—undertake therapy directed at improvement of an abnormal OGTT. In many patients, therefore, no immediate therapeutic benefit is likely to result from uncovering an abnormal OGTT. Moreover, the "labeling effect" associated with an abnormal OGTT may create unnecessary morbidity in a previously healthy person.

Limitations

A number of other considerations impose limitations on the usefulness of the OGTT. A variety of illnesses, both acute and chronic, produce abnormalities of the OGTT. Infection, trauma, drugs, and even physical inactivity may produce a "diabetic" OGTT (Table 72.4). Following myocardial infarction, many weeks may be required before normal glucose tolerance is again seen, and at least 2 weeks may be required after a febrile illness. Testing with OGTT should certainly be postponed under these circumstances. Reduced food intake with less than 150 g of carbohydrate/day can also produce an abnormal test within a few days as can fasting beyond 16 hours. Even performance of the test in the afternoon rather than in the morning may produce elevated levels of blood sugar. Smoking immediately before or during the test can produce an abnormal result, as may the ingestion of caffeine-containing drinks (coffee, tea) in the period of fasting. If nausea, vomiting, or diaphoresis occurs during the test, the results are invalid and the test should be terminated. A repeat test may not necessarily provoke these symptoms. Beyond all of these caveats, great variability in any patient's OGTT response is well established, so that a diagnosis of diabetes *cannot* be established on the basis of a single abnormal test.

Drug Effects on Glucose Tolerance

Table 72.5 gives a list of drugs and related substances which have been reported to be associated with decreased glucose tolerance and even with the development of symptomatic diabetes mellitus. The

Table 72.5
Drugs Associated with Abnormal Glucose Tolerance or Diabetes Mellitus

HORMONES AND RELATED AGENTS
  ACTH
  Catecholamines (epinephrine, isoproterenol, levodopa)
  Dextrothyroxine
  Estrogens (oral contraceptives)
  Glucocorticoids (cortisone and derivatives)
  Thyroxine and triiodothyronine (toxic doses)
DIURETICS AND ANTIHYPERTENSIVE DRUGS
  Chlorthalidone (Hygroton, Combipres, Regroton)
  Clonidine (Catapres, Combipres)
  Ethacrynic acid (Edecrin)
  Furosemide (Lasix)
  Thiazides (Diuril, Hydrodiuril, etc)
PSYCHOACTIVE AGENTS
  Chlorprothixene (Taractan)
  Haloperidol (Haldol)
  Lithium (Lithane, Eskalith)
  Phenothiazines (Thorazine, Trilafon, Etrafron, Triavil, *etc*)
  Tricyclic antidepressants
    Amitriptyline (Elavil, Endep, Triavil, *etc*)
    Desipramine (Norpramin, Pertofrane)
    Doxepin (Adapin, Sinequan)
    Imipramine (Presamine, Tofranil)
    Nortriptyline (Aventyl)
MISCELLANEOUS
  Antineoplastic drugs (L-asparaginase, streptozotocin)
  Indomethacin
  Isoniazid (INH)
  Nicotinic acid

agents most often responsible are glucocorticoids (cortisone, prednisone, *etc*) and the diuretics used in the long term therapy of hypertension. Potassium depletion—which can be present even when serum potassium is normal—is one mechanism by which diuretics can produce glucose intolerance. Other drugs also affect glucose tolerance, but do so much less often. Despite their tendency to decrease glucose tolerance, these drugs should not be withheld when their use is indicated. A common error is to fail to use a diuretic in a diabetic hypertensive patient for fear of exacerbating glucose intolerance. Although blood pressure control may be attempted by using nondiuretic agents (see Chapter 62), failure to achieve satisfactory blood pressure control should prompt the physician to proceed with use of a diuretic. If glucose tolerance worsens, therapy with the usual modalities for control of blood sugar should then be instituted. If the patient is already receiving insulin, an increase of insulin dose may be all that is needed. Similar considerations pertain to the use of glucocorticoids. The course of diabetes provoked by the administration of corticosteroids or diuretics, once these agents have been discontinued, is variable.

Other Aspects of the Glucose Tolerance Test Including Effect of Age

Previous schemes for interpretation of the OGTT include summation of the fasting and 2-hour glucose levels, *etc*. These approaches are usually arbitrary and should be abandoned.

The effect of age on glucose tolerance is a special circumstance. Although age has no effect on FPG, the values in the OGTT tend to increase with age. One method for dealing with this phenomenon was to report any given value as a percentile rank. Although this was a reasonble approach, the diagnostic criteria of the National Diabetes Data Group, as proposed above, take into account this effect of age (9). By this approach, aging merely results in IGT and is associated with the corollaries of this state, *viz*, the possibility of higher risk for development of atherosclerotic disease and overt diabetes.

Gestational Diabetes

The term gestational diabetes (GDM) refers only to women who become overtly diabetic during pregnancy. Women who are known to have diabetes and become pregnant are not included. The majority of gestational diabetics return to a state of normal glucose tolerance postpartum. GDM occurs in some 1 to 2% of all pregnancies. Such patients are at increased risk (about 30%) for developing diabetes within 5 to 10 years after parturition.

Proper management of the patient with GDM is important, since the increased morbidity and mortality of poorly controlled diabetes can be greatly reduced. Indications for detection of such patients using the OGTT include recognition of glucosuria, family history of diabetes, a history of stillbirth or fetal malformations, spontaneous abortions, and an earlier heavy baby (see page 985).

Previous (PrevAGT) and Potential (PotAGT) Abnormalities of Glucose Tolerance

Persons with a normal OGTT who previously showed either IGT or overt diabetic hyperglycemia should be classified as PrevAGT. These individuals are not to be considered diabetic and should not be labeled, as in the recent past, with the terms prediabetes or latent diabetes. The economic and psychosocial stigmata of such labels are not justified. Furthermore, if, following development of glucose intolerance during pregnancy or some other occasion, an individual reverts to normal OGTT, reclassification to PrevAGT is warranted. The stress associated with trauma, burns, surgery, and infection may also result in hyperglycemia or abnormalities of OGTT which revert to normal and warrant classification as PrevAGT.

The term potential abnormality of glucose tolerance (PotAGT) should never be used as a diagnostic label for any person. The term is useful only in research.

TREATMENT OF DIABETES MELLITUS

Education of the Patient

Of those chronic conditions which are common in ambulatory practice, diabetes stands apart because of the broad scope and the critical importance of patient education and long term management. For *all* diabetics, the following factors are important: the impact of diet on diabetes; the implications of diabetes for ordinary activities; recognition of the signs of worsening diabetes; the importance of proper care of the feet; and the clarification of misconceptions about diabetes. For patients receiving insulin, the following additional factors are important: correct administration of insulin, the unique constraints which insulin therapy places on dietary management and changes of activity, the recognition of the symptoms of hypoglycemia, and the adjustment of insulin dose during intercurrent illness.

The patient's response to being informed of a diagnosis of diabetes varies widely. Many patients have already suspected the diagnosis as the result of previous observations of similar symptoms in family members. These individuals are often also aware of the complications of the disease (loss of vision, amputations) and the use of "the needle" (insulin, self-administration). Transient anxiety or depression occurs frequently and should be anticipated by the physician. Management of these minor mood disturbances is described in Chapter 13.

Many patients are reluctant to accept the need for self-injection of insulin, and many physicians are unwilling to press the issue. The result is poor control, inappropriate use of oral hypoglycemic drugs, or both. Reluctance of both patient and physician may stem from unfamiliarity with the techniques. In point of fact, insulin injection is simple and almost without discomfort. A firm attitude on the part of the physician will overcome patient reluctance in almost all cases. The use of disposable syringes has eliminated the inconvenience of sterilization while the modern thin, very sharp, plastic-hubbed or syringe-attached needles render the injections practically painless. Aspects of technique are described below (page 966).

A substantial proportion of "new" diabetics will quickly reveal a noncompliant pattern of handling their particular chronic illness. These patterns are usually difficult to alter. Perhaps the best way to prevent the development of poor compliance is to educate the patient and other members of the patient's household from the outset (see Chapter 4 for a detailed discussion of compliance-promoting strategies).

Educational Process

The educational process should be as frank and as authoritative as possible, since much misinformation is apt to deluge the patient. Misconceptions should be explained and countered. The physician is not able to undertake and continue this process in the detail it deserves; therefore, a nurse or other trained individual should be available whenever possible to instruct the new diabetic and to continue the educational process as necessary. Excellent booklets are available from the American Diabetes Association and pharmaceutical manufacturers as adjuncts to personal instruction, as are a variety of teaching films and newsletters dealing with all aspects of diabetic care (6). In all aspects of management the need for reinforcement and continuing patient education must be stressed. Even the most intelligent patient often needs reiteration of treatment principles and procedures.

The goal of such instruction is correct patient self-care. Even such procedures as altering the dose of insulin to conform to changing needs should, whenever possible, be taught. Successful management is never possible without such education. On the other hand, all patients will need assistance from time to time. Telephone contact with the physician should be available and encouraged. Many problems of adjustment of insulin dosage, *etc*, can and should be handled by telephone in order to avoid excessive use of office time and unnecessary expense and loss of work time for the patient. Finally, the need for education of key members of the patient's family should not be forgotten. Alterations of diet and of eating patterns are not often made easily and may not be made at all if a spouse is unaware, for example, that punctual meals are essential for the patient receiving "conventional" insulin therapy. The distinctions between conventional, intensive conventional, and insulin therapy utilizing pumps are described below ("Insulin Therapy," page 966). The various programs impose different demands on the therapeutic process; conventional therapy is the most demanding in terms of the need for punctual meals.

Diet Therapy

Different diet strategies guide therapy for diabetes, depending on whether one is dealing with an obese, non-insulin-dependent (NIDDM) patient or an individual of appropriate weight who has insulin-dependent disease (Table 72.6). For the obese NIDDM diabetic, the immediate and long term goals are *weight reduction*, and almost any weight reduction scheme (diet plan) will suffice (see Chapter 76). Ideally, diet composition should approximate that shown in Table 72.7. Most obese diabetics are not symptomatic and do not require therapy with insulin or oral hypoglycemic agents for control of symptoms. The latter, if used, have the advantage that

they do not complicate a low calorie diet. Simultaneous institution of a weight reduction program and treatment with insulin, if prescribed, often lead to hypoglycemia and must be approached cautiously. The short term goal of insulin therapy under these conditions is the relief of symptoms due to hyperglycemia. No attempt at "tight" control should be made at this time; such efforts should be deferred until efforts at weight loss have ended.

The importance of weight reduction for the obese diabetic cannot be overstated. Population studies indicate that most diabetes is either made manifest by obesity in genetically predisposed persons or is actually caused by obesity. Hence, most overt diabetes in obese patients is potentially either preventable or "curable" by weight reduction provided that the diabetes has not been present for more than a few years. However, most patients are unable to achieve and/or maintain a weight that will reverse overt diabetes, even though they are made aware of the necessity for doing so. Chapter 76 on obesity, Chapter 3 on patient education, and Chapter 4 on compliance deal with this problem in greater detail.

The second goal of diet therapy is prevention of atherosclerotic disease. The evidence that this major problem of the diabetic *may* be preventable is to a large degree based on comparisons of the prevalence of atherosclerotic disease in different populations with widely varying diets. A detailed discussion of the evidence bearing on this issue can be found elsewhere (16, 17). In any case, the diabetics in this country who have followed conventional diabetic diets—at least until about 1970—have had the highest rate of coronary disease seen anywhere in the world (3 times the rate of the general population in this country). Because of this and the evidence from population studies, the American Diabetes Association recommended in 1971 that its old standard diabetic diets be abandoned. Unfortunately, the new diets, high in starch and low in saturated fats, have not been widely accepted by either physicians or patients, perhaps because of the long held notion that carbohydrate is harmful to the diabetic (Table

Table 72.6.
Dietary Strategies for Diabetics[a]

Strategy	Obese, Non-insulin-requiring[b]	Lean, Insulin-requiring
Reduce caloric intake	Yes	No
Improve pancreatic β cell function (disease reversal)	Weight reduction effective	Not possible
Day-to-day dietary constancy	Not critical	Yes—essential[c]
Extra feedings	No	Yes[c]
Consistent timing of meals	No	Yes—essential
Extra food for exercise	No	Usually
Frequent small feedings during intercurrent illness	No	Yes

[a] Modified from West KM: Diet therapy of diabetes: an analysis of failure. *Ann Intern Med* 79:425, 1973.
[b] Includes patients on oral hypoglycemics.
[c] Patients using intensive conventional therapy or insulin pumps have greater freedom to deviate from these rules.

Table 72.7.
Distribution of Major Nutrients in Normal and Diabetic Diets (United States)[a]

Diet	Nutrients (Percentage of Total Calories)						
	Starch and other polysaccharides	Sugars and dextrins	Total carbohydrate	Fat		Protein	Alcohol
				Total	% Polyunsaturated		
"Typical" diet	25–35	20–30	45–50	35–45	30	12–20	0–10
Traditional diabetic diet	25–30	10–15	35–40	40–45	30	15–20	0
Newer diabetic diets	30–45[b]	5–15	45–55	25–35[b]	50	12–25	0–6

[a] Modified from West KM: Diet therapy of diabetes: an analysis of failure. *Ann Intern Med* 79:425, 1973.
[b] Even higher levels of starch and lower levels of fat would be desirable, but are seldom possible in Western societies because they differ too much from the traditional diets of these cultures.

72.7). In fact, the new relatively high carbohydrate diets do not result in higher blood glucose levels. Similarly, the notion that high carbohydrate diets increase hyperlipidemia is not corroborated by observations in diabetic patients. Another problem in instituting the new dietary approach is the lack of standardized diets to replace the old ones. The American Diabetes Association has taken the view that diets should be individualized. Such individualization may be logical but seems to be beyond the capacity of all but the most sophisticated centers, even though in theory any dietitian could construct such a diet.

A guiding principle of individualization of diabetic diets should be the recognition that individual food preferences must be respected whenever possible. The dietician should obtain the patient's *preferred* dietary history and then attempt to construct the diet around these preferences. Such an approach is demanding for the dietitian, but the issuance of a standardized "American" diet to a diabetic from an ethnic minority simply guarantees noncompliance.

In the past few years, diets containing large quantities of nonabsorbable plant fibers have been explored for use in diabetics. Fiber-rich foods decrease blood glucose following glucose loads or meals in both normal persons and in patients with NIDDM, while chronic ingestion of high fiber, high carbohydrate diets decreases fasting blood glucose and may permit decreased doses of oral hypoglycemic drugs or lower insulin requirements. The mechanisms of these effects are not fully understood. Although delayed carbohydrate absorption probably accounts for most of the acute effect, increased sensitivity to insulin seems also to be involved. Abnormalities of blood lipids often improve. However, a role for high fiber diets in routine therapy has not been established. In many patients these diets produce a variety of unpleasant side effects, including increased frequency of stools, diarrhea, abdominal pain, and flatulence. The formulation of fiber-rich diets is difficult, and most patients do not accept the major alterations of diet that are necessary to produce the desired effects on blood glucose levels.

Diet during Conventional Insulin Therapy

Any patient receiving insulin faces a special problem with diet, one that for the insulin-dependent patient is usually even more difficult than for the individual with NIDDM. Unlike patients who are not receiving insulin—who require no special timing of meals and whose total intake can vary from day to day—the pattern of food intake for the individual receiving conventional therapy with insulin must be quite rigid; greater flexibility is possible with intensive conventional therapy (see page 968). Total caloric intake must be distributed among the meals of the day, which usually include midafternoon and bedtime snacks as well, so that insulin

dose can be adjusted according to the patient's needs. The reverse procedure, selection of an insulin dose and adjustment of total caloric intake to this dose, is unphysiological and should never be used. Occasional patients strive to reduce insulin dosage by senseless starvation, incorrectly assuming that insulin dose has some relationship to "severity" of their disease. Needless to say, patients must be dissuaded from such practices.

The exact composition of the diet for the IDDM patient is less important—from the point of view of blood sugar control—than is the constancy of distribution of the amount of food at each meal from day to day. Insulin effect (duration, intensity), even for a particular type of insulin, varies from patient to patient. Accordingly, avoidance of extremes of blood sugar concentration (hypo- and hyperglycemia) requires some adjustment of food apportionment for each individual. However, one should attempt to simulate as closely as possible the patient's usual and preferred pattern of food intake. The main modification is usually to add between-meal snacks. Once an acceptable food pattern has been established and insulin dose adjusted to that pattern, the patient must adhere to the program if extremes of blood sugar are to be avoided. Patients learn by trial and error how much latitude they can tolerate. Problems, not easily solved, are encountered in individuals who engage in strenuous sports or work which varies from day to day. Such persons may have to eat more on some days than others or make frequent adjustments of their insulin dose. Rigid control of blood sugar by use of conventional insulin therapy is not possible in such cases. Intensive conventional therapy (page 968) allows for better control of blood sugar and for greater variation in the level of physical activity.

The major adaptive problem with diet in patients treated with conventional insulin therapy (see page 966) is the need for most of them to eat in a programmed fashion, i.e., by the clock. No longer can the individual wait for hunger to prompt a meal; nor can he approach dining out at a restaurant with indifference to the time the meal will be served. To do so is to court a major hypoglycemic episode. However, delay of a meal may be unavoidable. In order to prevent hypoglycemia in this circumstance, about 10 g of carbohydrate/½ hour should be ingested. This can be provided by 4 to 6 oz (180 ml) of a sugar-containing soda ("soft drink") or 4 oz of orange juice, palatable premeal alternatives to a candy bar (see "Hypoglycemia during Insulin Therapy," page 972).

Estimation of Caloric Needs

Caloric requirements for maintenance of weight vary somewhat from individual to individual but are mainly determined by activity level. Required calories are *approximately* 40 kcal/kg or 20 kcal/lb/

day for an adult with "normal" activity. Thus an individual of 70 kg may require 2800 kcal, although some lean men performing ordinary activities may require as much as 3000 to 3500 kcal/day. Individuals who perform manual labor may need 4000 or more kcal, while sedentary persons may need only 2000 kcal or less.

In prescribing diets caloric requirements are often underestimated. Physicians commonly prescribe an 1800-kcal diet for maintenance even if it is grossly inadequate for a particular patient's caloric needs. Prescription of such a diet leads to frustration and noncompliance. Overzealous decreases of calories for weight reduction may be equally defeating. When maintenance of weight is the goal, a careful dietary history by a skilled dietician may give a good starting point for establishment of an individual's needs; the prescribed diet should then become simply a modification of that patient's ordinary pattern.

Other Aspects of Diet and Insulin Therapy

After a dietitian estimates the constituents that will be acceptable to a patient, joint discussion should be held with the spouse or other involved family members. Cooperation and participation of a spouse in the process may be essential for successful adaptation, which, for practical reasons, may require that both partners participate in the diet modifications.

The intelligent use of diet exchange lists (food equivalents) is necessary for most IDDM patients. Such lists are available from the American Diabetes Association, the American Dietetic Association, and most hospital dietetic units. There is no necessity for such exchanges in NIDDM.

Special "diabetic" or "dietetic" foods are expensive and usually are unnecessary. Some such foods do contain less free sugar than is ordinarily the case, but the patient must read the labels carefully to avoid self-deception.

Exercise during insulin therapy. The patient must be instructed on dietary self-management in several situations. Modest exercise (walking briskly) requires about 10 g of extra carbohydrate/hour. Vigorous exercise (basketball playing) requires about an extra 20 to 30 g/hour (e.g., 12 oz of soda or orange juice). To some extent the hypoglycemic effect of exercise may be greater if the insulin has been injected into an extremity being exercised. Many patients prefer to inject insulin into the thigh, but persons who engage in vigorous exercise (jogging, other sports, manual labor) may have to use abdominal or arm injection sites to avoid excessive insulin effect due to exercise-induced rapid absorption.

Effect of anorexia. When a patient with IDDM develops anorexia because of mild short term illness ("cold," "flu," gastroenteritis), insulin should not be discontinued, but a reduction of the normal dose by one-third to one-half may be needed. More severe illness (e.g., a marked febrile state) may require continuation of the usual dose or even an increase in the dose. Every effort should be made to ensure intake of 50 g of carbohydrate in every 8-hour period to avoid both starvation ketosis and hypoglycemia. Careful monitoring of urine ketones (and glucose) during such periods and prompt adjustment of insulin dose if necessary may prevent a hospitalization for ketoacidosis.

Selection of Patients for Oral Hypoglycemic Drugs or Insulin Therapy

Non-Insulin-Dependent Diabetes

As previously noted, the initial approach to the obese non-insulin-dependent (NIDDM) patient is weight reduction. Such therapy—if followed—can be expected to reduce blood sugar within a few weeks. If FPG is less than 200 to 300 mg/dl, glucosuria will not ordinarily produce enough symptoms to be troublesome during this period and no additional drug therapy (oral hypoglycemics or insulin) is needed. Even a FPG of 300 to 400 mg/dl is ordinarily well tolerated. These patients are not ketosis prone; no urgency exists for instituting drug therapy. On the other hand, symptomatic glucosuria, persisting for weeks despite efforts at (or actual) weight loss, should not be ignored. In this case, drug therapy is indicated for symptomatic relief and can be discontinued if weight reduction is successful.

In the past, many NIDDM patients with symptomatic disease have been treated with oral hypoglycemic drugs (see page 973). However, even asymptomatic patients have also been treated for only modest elevations of FGP or even for abnormal glucose tolerance. Such treatment may improve or normalize glucose tolerance. Extrapolation of results from patient surveys relating abnormalities of glucose tolerance to development of complications of diabetes would suggest that such treatment might be beneficial. However, no evidence exists to support this possibility. In fact, a study of long term use of tolbutamide—although controversial—suggests that the drug itself may increase the frequency of occurrence of cardiovascular problems. (see discussion of the UGDP study, page 973). Thus, at present, drug therapy of modest elevations of FPG or OGTT abnormalities is not routinely recommended.

The official recommendation of the American Diabetes Association, the AMA Council on Drugs, and the Food and Drug Administration is that sulfonylureas be limited to patients with symptomatic NIDDM who cannot be controlled by diet and in whom addition of insulin is impractical and/or unacceptable. This stand may be inappropriately conservative.

The indications for use of insulin in patients with *asymptomatic* NIDDM are unclear. Although evidence is accumulating that modest elevations of blood sugar do indeed relate to at least some of the complications of diabetes (3), no prospective studies are available to demonstrate that insulin therapy of patients with asymptomatic hyperglycemia (FPG or OGTT) is beneficial. Insulin therapy is certainly indicated for control of *symptomatic* diabetes (see above, page 954) in NIDDM that cannot be controlled with diet.

Determination of hemoglobin A_{1c} under these circumstances can serve as a guide to the physician (see page 971). A normal value would deter a recommendation for drug or insulin therapy, whereas an elevated value would suggest that long term benefit might outweigh the possible risks or inconvenience. Recommendations for or against therapy under these circumstances are presently determined not only by the clinical circumstances, but by the physician's convictions concerning the long term deleterious effect of hyperglycemia (see "Normoglycemia as a Goal of Insulin Therapy," below).

Insulin-Dependent Diabetes

The IDDM patient should be started on insulin therapy as soon as insulin need is apparent. Ordinarily these patients have been hospitalized for treatment of ketoacidosis and have been switched from short acting insulin, used in the treatment of the acute phase, to an intermediate or long acting preparation. The insulin dependence has been established by the occurrence of the acute episode. Unless this acute event was precipitated by stress in an otherwise NIDDM patient, insulin dependence is usually absolute and permanent. Occasionally in adults (more often in children), insulin requirement may decrease or even disappear over several months; relapse is the rule in such cases.

Other Circumstances Requiring Insulin Therapy

Some patients who are not, strictly speaking, insulin dependent also need insulin therapy. Patients with NIDDM may be prescribed hypoglycemic drugs to control blood glucose but may be unresponsive with an initial attempt ("primary failures"). Others, adequately controlled by hypoglycemic drugs for a time, may become unresponsive to these agents ("secondary failures"). Insulin therapy may become essential in such cases. Other patients with NIDDM may develop grossly uncontrolled hyperglycemia during stress (trauma, infection, surgery). Whether or not ketosis ensues, the gross hyperglycemia may produce severe osmotic diuresis and its sequelae. Obviously, such patients require control of hyperglycemia with insulin therapy which may be discontinued as soon as the situation warrants. Most young people of normal weight who develop diabetes will require insulin, even though they are not ketosis prone. The group of children or young adults recently described and termed MODY are also candidates for insulin, although many may be managed on diet alone.

Occasional adults, usually thin and not necessarily exhibiting much glucosuria, may exhibit unexplained weight loss and lack of well-being. Such patients may show dramatic improvement with insulin.

Some patients will be encountered who are receiving insulin therapy needlessly. Typically these are elderly individuals with NIDDM who have already developed an array of medical problems, usually cardiovascular. The degree of blood sugar control with large amounts of insulin (50 to 100 units) is poor. Although aggressive use of insulin will certainly normalize blood glucose, the development of hypoglycemia is risky in such persons. On the other hand, abrupt discontinuation of insulin in these patients often results in no worsening of diabetic control and reveals that, in fact, no significant insulin effect had been manifest at the prescribed dosage. Adherence to a proper diet and to weight reduction may suffice in such cases and will actually control hyperglycemia to a greater degree than does the use of insulin at an ineffective dosage.

Normoglycemia as a Goal of Insulin Therapy

In view of the growing evidence that control of hyperglycemia may prevent development of the microvascular complications of diabetes (3), no one would argue that normalization of blood sugar with insulin is undesirable, but this goal is not usually achievable using single dose or even two-dose insulin schemes without incurring the risk of unacceptable episodes of hypoglycemia. In which patients should the effort be vigorously promoted, and when in the history of the disease should such a program be undertaken?

Young patients with IDDM in the early years of their disease, at least in theory, stand to gain the most from "tight control," since prevention of complications is the goal. Patients with IDDM who already have advanced complications of diabetes may not benefit at all, since no evidence is available that such complications are reversible or can even be stabilized. Nonetheless, the patient's hopes must be considered under these circumstances while the physician remains as supportive as possible.

For those patients with NIDDM, prevention of vascular complications is also the most important rationale for tight control. Relatively young or even middle-age patients with NIDDM may stand to gain as much as young patients with IDDM. In the elderly, whose life expectancy is limited by age, complications of diabetes, or concurrent disease, the problems associated with tight control should strongly influence the physician to avoid this approach, since the prevention of complications is not an issue.

After an initial period of conventional therapy the

issue of tight control should be considered and discussed with patients who are suitable candidates. In those to whom tight control is suggested, it is the physician's obligation to explain the current view that maintained normoglycemia may prevent the long term complications of diabetes mellitus. The magnitude of the effort that is necessary to maintain normoglycemia must be explained, including the need for home blood glucose monitoring. One of the frequent-dose, intensified conventional insulin therapy schemes or its alternative, infusion pump delivery of insulin, must also be presented (see page 968). If the patient understands and accepts the problems and effort required, the physician may consider a program of tight control. However, serious consideration should be given to referral of the patient to an endocrinologist familiar with such a program since the process is difficult, very demanding of the physician's time, and usually requires a team approach utilizing a specially trained physician's assistant or nurse practitioner. The demands on the patient and the physician are greatest at onset of tight control therapy. The effort should always be made only when the schedules of all parties permit the undertaking.

When should an effort be made using conventional therapy to achieve *near* normalization—as opposed to tight control—of blood sugar? Individuals with NIDDM tend to have relatively stable blood sugars and predictable responses to insulin, and an attempt to achieve near normalization can be made in such patients. In many, at least the fasting blood glucose can be normalized (see Table 72.3) without great difficulty using one or two doses of intermediate acting insulin. Patients with IDDM are much more difficult to control, and even this degree of control is usually not possible using conventional therapy. Many physicians nonetheless still go through an agonizing trial of conventional therapy with such patients, only to have the effort end in failure and frustration for all involved. Usually several types and mixtures of insulin are tried along with both single and two-dose schedules. At this point, a simplified treatment scheme that avoids excessive glucosuria with resultant symptoms and prevents development of ketoacidosis should be accepted. Reconsideration of institution of intensive conventional therapy may be appropriate at this stage.

Types of Insulin

Most of the preparations now in use are suspensions of insulin which have been chemically or physically modified to prolong their action following subcutaneous injection. The characteristics of these insulins are summarized below and in Table 72.8.

Crystalline Zinc Insulin (CZI; Regular Insulin)

This unmodified insulin is a completely dissolved ("clear") preparation, the main use of which is for acute therapy of ketoacidosis in hospitalized patients. In the ordinary treatment of ambulatory patients, regular insulin is not used alone, but rather used in conjunction with other insulins. The onset of action of subcutaneously injected regular insulin is 30 to 60 minutes; peak action is at 2 to 4 hours; and the duration of action 6 to 8 hours. In occasional patients receiving one dose of intermediate acting insulin daily, regular insulin may be given as the second dose. This preparation is the only one now being used for continuous subcutaneous injection with portable infusion pumps. It is also increasingly used in combination with Ultralente insulin in tight control schemes; the long acting preparation provides the equivalent of background activity provided by the basal infusion rate of a pump, while superimposed injections before meals are equal to bolus injections of the pump (see page 968).

Protamine Zinc Insulin (PZI)

This preparation, a loose chemical combination of insulin with the carrier protein, protamine, was the first long acting insulin. Until recently, PZI was

Table 72.8.
Characteristics of Commonly Used Insulin Preparations

Type	Physical State	Modifying Protein	Peak Action (hr)	Duration of Effect (hr)
SHORT ACTING (RAPID ONSET)				
Regular (CZI)	Clear solution	None	1–2	6–8
Semilente	Suspension (turbid)	None	2–4	8–14
INTERMEDIATE ACTING				
NPH	Suspension (turbid)	Protamine	3–8	18–36
Lente	Suspension (turbid)	None	3–8	18–36
LONG ACTING				
Protamine zinc (PZI)	Suspension (turbid)	Protamine	8–12	18–36
Ultralente	Suspension (turbid)	None	8–12	18–36

amorphous material containing an excess of protamine which precluded addition of regular insulin. However, all PZI now available is crystalline, contains no excess protamine, and can be mixed with regular insulin. Indeed, the commonly used NPH insulin approximates such a mixture (see below). PZI has a duration of action exceeding 24 hours.

PZI is rarely used by itself. Exceptions include diabetics who are not eating because of intercurrent acute or chronic illness. Other patients who may benefit from PZI are those who experience unacceptably frequent episodes of insulin-induced hypoglycemia when the "intermediate" insulins are used. When a long acting form is to be used as sole therapy, some authorities have preferred—because of its allegedly more predictable effect—Ultralente insulin to PZI. For practical purposes, the two forms have identical uses and effects.

Neutral Protamine Hagedorn Insulin (NPH; Isophane Insulin)

This preparation is a standardized crystalline suspension prepared from regular insulin and protamine. Often termed "intermediate acting," NPH in fact exhibits rather rapid onset of action and a duration of action usually over 24 hours. Ideally, with a single injection of NPH, the short acting component provides insulin effect during the day when meals are elevating the blood glucose, while the long acting portion of PZI provides insulin effect through the night. For many patients the achieved ratio of insulin effects is satisfactory. However, if NPH is not satisfactory, other mixtures of insulins can be prepared as needed (see below). NPH insulin is always given subcutaneously in either one or two injections daily.

The Lente Insulin Series

This group of insulins was devised at a time when PZI contained excess protamine, thus precluding the preparation of mixtures of short acting regular with long acting PZI. Controlled addition of zinc was used to prepare a microcrystalline, rapidly absorbed, and rapidly acting material (Semilente insulin) and another crystalline product with much slower absorption and longer action, Ultralente insulin. These insulins avoided the use of a foreign protein, protamine, and could be mixed in varying proportions. In some geographic areas, in both the United States and abroad, the Lente insulins are used almost exclusively.

Semilente insulin. This preparation is similar to regular insulin in onset and duration of action, although its effects are somewhat slower in onset and more prolonged. Semilente is always given subcutaneously. The chief use of Semilente is in mixtures with Ultralente or as a supplementary dose in conventional therapy schemes.

Ultralente insulin. This preparation has a duration of action exceeding 24 hours and is indistinguishable from PZI. Ultralente may, like PZI, occasionally be used alone (see PZI). However, the main use of Ultralente is as the long acting component in the mixture that is known as Lente insulin. Recently, Ultralente insulin has become the backbone of "intensified conventional therapy." The prolonged effect of this preparation provides the background activity equivalent to the basal infusion rate of an insulin pump (see page 968).

Mixtures of Insulins

The usual goal of conventional insulin therapy is a single injection once daily. If this goal is to be reached, insulin effect must be prolonged sufficiently to produce normoglycemia in the morning and at the same time provide adequate daytime control of the increases of blood glucose that occur postprandially. While the use of NPH or Lente insulin is often successful, the patterns of effect that these insulins provide are not always satisfactory. Either one of two scenarios is observed. In the first, the excessive daytime hyperglycemia and glucosuria dictates the need for additional rapidly acting insulin. Thus, regular insulin is added to NPH or Lente; or Semilente is added to Lente. The second and opposite situation is seen when a single injection of NPH or Lente controls daytime hyperglycemia and glucosuria, but the total duration of action is inadequate, resulting in hyperglycemia at the beginning of the next day. Under these circumstances, additional long acting component is needed. Ultralente can be added to Lente, or a mixture of Semilente and Ultralente can be used with a ratio of 20:80 or 10:90. In this situation many diabetologists, rather than attempt to control fasting (overnight) hyperglycemia by addition of more long acting insulin to a single injection, prefer to give a second small dose of NPH or Lente insulin. The A.M. dose may have to be reduced somewhat, resulting in a "split dose" program (see below, "Insulin Therapy"). Such regimens are often necessary in patients with IDDM who are being treated with conventional therapy, in some persons with NIDDM who have been receiving insulin for many years and in whom the duration of insulin effect seems to lessen, in persons with either type of diabetes requiring relatively large doses of insulin (greater than 60 units daily), and during pregnancy.

Commercial Insulin Preparations

New Insulin Preparations of Increased Purity

Until the last few years, all available preparations regardless of type were of essentially the same purity. With the realization that the commercial products did contain small amounts of other related and unrelated proteins (proinsulin, insulin degradation products, *etc*) and that these impurities might possibly contribute to "insulin allergy," antibody formation, *etc*, further purification procedures were introduced. The ordinary insulins (Lilly, Squibb) now in greatest use are > 98% pure. Beginning in 1972 these materials were unofficially designated "single peak" insulins, because they are pure enough to appear as such on gel chromatography. Still more highly purified material was introduced a few years ago into the US market by several European manufacturers (Novo; Nordisk) and is unofficially termed "monocomponent" insulin. Similar preparations were made available by Lilly, the major US manufacturer, and in 1980 the preparation became commercially available. The unofficial term for this was "single component" insulin. Henceforth, this material will be known simply as purified pork insulin (Iletin II, pork; Lilly).

Although the highly purified insulins are currently being aggressively marketed in the United States by their European manufacturers, no proof is available that they offer the patient or physician any advantage. They do offer a considerable (severalfold) increase in cost. Most of the problems encountered with insulin in the past disappeared with introduction of the relatively pure "single peak" insulins after 1972. Allergic reactions and lipoatrophy were the two most troublesome events; both do appear to have been related to impurities.

Allergy to insulin is most commonly a local reaction at the site of injection. Local redness, swelling, heat, and itching occur within minutes to an hour after injection and persist for a few hours to a day, often with formation of an area of induration. Such reactions, no longer common, occur during the first few weeks of therapy and usually disappear as therapy is continued. Rarely, similar reactions develop many hours or up to a day after injection (delayed hypersensitivity).

Systemic allergic reactions, with or without a local reaction, are rare; they are manifest by urticaria, angioedema, and even anaphylactic shock (IgE-mediated; see Chapter 23). Such reactions seem to occur most often in persons who have previously received insulin and appear during reinstitution of therapy after a lapse of months or years. Local reactions may progress to systemic ones; if this seems to be occurring, one should treat the patient before anaphylaxis occurs. The first maneuver involves a trial of highly purified insulin. If this approach fails, drugs such as antihistamines and glucocorticoids are helpful, but persistent insulin allergy is best treated by desensitization. With the patient receiving no antihistamines or steroids and no insulin in the preceding 12 to 24 hours, the procedure involves injection of 0.1-ml volumes of insulin that have been diluted 1:100 in 0.1% human serum albumin to prevent adsorption losses onto glass. An initial dose (0.001 unit) is given intradermally. Subsequent doses of 0.1 ml contain doubling amounts (units). After several in-

tradermal injections at 30-minute intervals, the subcutaneous route is used. If a reaction occurs, epinephrine may be administered; the dose of insulin is reduced, but the process is continued. This procedure requires a series of solutions of insulin. These may be prepared by the physician or pharmacist, but are also available in kit form by telephone request to Dr. John Galloway, Eli Lilly Co., Indianapolis, Indiana. Special kits and instructions for desensitizing patients who have delayed hypersensitivity reactions are also available from the same source.

Insulin lipoatrophy is now an uncommon event. Harmless but disfiguring localized atrophy of subcutaneous fatty tissue occurs around the site of insulin injections and is sometimes seen simultaneously with insulin allergy. The process may be related to impurities in insulin preparations rather than to insulin itself, since newer preparations ("single peak") are much less likely to produce this problem. In addition, the injection of highly purified "monocomponent" or "single component" insulins into the atrophied areas has sometimes resulted in disappearance of the atrophy

Insulin lipohypertrophy is even less common than insulin atrophy. This phenomenon is probably due to an intrinsic action of insulin and has not been improved by use of purer insulins. Repeated injections into the same area do appear to predispose to lipohypertrophy.

Trade Names, Unit Designations, and Syringes

Lilly designates all of its insulin as Iletin. The newest, most highly purified material is Iletin II. Squibb uses no trade name, while foreign manufacturers have regrettably introduced a bewildering array of designations.

All insulin, regardless of type or source, is standardized at a specific concentration per milliliter. The symbol U refers to the insulin concentration in units per milliliter. Until 1973 when U-100 was introduced into use in the United States, the standard forms were U-80 and U-40. The shift to U-100 was made in the expectation of phasing out the old strengths and with the hope of reducing confusion by patients. By 1980 about 90% of the insulins in use were U-100, and U-80 was no longer being manufactured by Lilly. Within the next few years U-40 insulin will probably be withdrawn from the US market.

Several sizes of syringe are available for use with U-100. A 1-ml syringe can be used for all doses up to 100 units, but most accurate dispensing of less than 30 units is made when syringes of 0.5-ml capacity are used. The bores of these syringes are smaller and the scales are consequently expanded. Occasional patients require more than 100 units/single injection. For such use 2-ml syringes (200-unit capacity) are manufactured, but these are in short supply and are difficult to obtain. The use of disposable plastic syringes with attached needles has greaty simplified use of insulin and is preferred by almost all patients (Becton-Dickinson: B-D, or equivalent). Reusable glass syringes requiring detachable needles are also available. Special syringes are available for use by patients with severe impairment of vision that prevents them from accurately measuring their insulin dose. However, a simple solution to this problem is often possible. Disposable syringes can be prefilled with ordinary sterile precautions by an able person (relative, friend) and safely stored in a refrigerator for at least a week.

Insulin Injection Technique

Following initial instruction the patient should be observed during self-administration of insulin to be certain that the correct volume is being drawn into the syringe and that the technique of injection is proper. Sterilization of the skin with an alcohol wipe is not necessary, although the injection site should be clean. If the injection is made through skin that is wet with alcohol, unnecessary burning discomfort will be produced.

For use in ambulatory patients insulin preparations should always be given subcutaneously. Most needles in present use are ½ inch in length. Unless the individual is very thin, the best technique involves insertion of the needle at 90° to the skin surface. If the patient is very thin, or the needle is ⅝ inch in length, or the site is covered by thin skin, the needle may be inserted at up to 45°. The objective is subcutaneous rather than intradermal or intramuscular injection. Following injection, the area should not be massaged, since that may accelerate absorption.

The choice of injection site is important, since the rate of insulin absorption—and hence the duration and magnitude of insulin effect—varies considerably between anatomical locations. Absorption is slowest from the thigh, fastest from the anterior abdominal wall, and intermediate from the arm. In addition, absorption from an exercising extremity is accelerated (page 961). The long used technique of rotation of sites is perhaps unwise and may contribute to erratic control. On the other hand, the repeated use of precisely the same spot within a site should be avoided.

Beef, Pork, and Human Insulins

Most of the insulin sold in the United States is derived from beef or pork pancreas. Most ordinary preparations marketed by Lilly are a variable mixture of beef (bovine) and pork (porcine) insulins with the beef-derived component predominating (about 80%), but the precise proportions vary with available supply. The products marketed by Squibb are derived entirely from beef. Lilly's most highly purified material (Iletin II) is exclusively prepared from pork sources. Porcine insulin differs from the human

form by only a single amino acid, while the beef material has several additional amino acid substitutions. As a result, pork insulin is, in some persons, less allergenic than the beef material. Clinically, this is of significance in occasional cases of insulin allergy and may affect insulin requirements. Switching a patient with allergy to beef insulin from beef-pork or all-beef preparation to an all-pork material will double cost and may result in reduction of 30% in the number of units needed. Such a maneuver is hardly cost effective. On the other hand, an inadvertent shift of preparations may result in loss of blood sugar control or hypoglycemia.

Insulin identical to that of the human hormone (human insulin) has recently become available for general clinical use. Such material is produced by bacterial recombinant DNA techniques (Humulin, Lilly) or is partially synthetic (Squibb/Novo). Whether human insulin will offer any advantages over other insulins remains to be established. Human insulin is definitely antigenic when given subcutaneously. The dose required is comparable to that of other insulins. Cost is comparable to that of the highly purified insulins of animal origin.

Insulin Therapy

Strategy of "Conventional" Insulin Therapy: Initiation of Therapy

"Conventional" therapy with insulin is the term applied to the type of insulin administration schedule most commonly used. The goal of such therapy is near normalization of blood sugar, discussed elsewhere ("Normoglycemia as a Goal of Insulin Therapy," page 962). Insulin is given as one or two doses of an intermediate acting preparation (NPH or Lente), sometimes mixed with shorter acting regular or Semilente insulin. Ordinarily, the degree of control is such that modest hyperglycemia exists at least part of the day but hypoglycemia is usually avoided. In some cases near normalization of blood sugar can be achieved. However, true normalization can only be accomplished by "intensive conventional therapy" or with an insulin pump. Both of the latter procedures require home blood glucose monitoring and are discussed separately (page 968).

The fundamental information which the patient should understand when insulin therapy is initiated is reviewed in Table 72.6. Institution of insulin therapy coincides with or follows the establishment of a diet (see above). As pointed out earlier, relative constancy of food intake is essential. If such dietary compliance cannot be assured, the goal of insulin therapy should be modest, i.e., the avoidance of symptomatic hyperglycemia and ketoacidosis. Attempts to manipulate insulin dose while diet is varying widely will unquestionably result in hypoglycemic episodes. In any case, insulin therapy cannot possibly achieve even a near approach to normoglycemia when diet is varying.

First attempts at blood sugar control in almost all ambulatory patients treated by the conventional approach should be done with an intermediate acting insulin (NPH or Lente). A safe initial dose for a non-insulin-dependent patient who has not received previous insulin therapy is 20 units for a nonobese individual and 30 units for an obese patient.

Previously treated patients often require higher initial doses. Insulin-dependent patients will ordinarily have been started on insulin therapy while in the hospital, but the scheme below can be used for further adjustment of dose for both types of patient.

The dose of insulin can be increased by 5 units every 3 days until satisfactory control is approached. Usually, such a program will bring the patient under control within a few weeks. Increments of 10 units every 3 days are also safe if the patient is markedly symptomatic or if no effect is apparent within a week. During this time the patient should be monitoring urine glucose (see "Monitoring Conventional Insulin Therapy"). A telephone call to the physician can be made every week or 10 days, but the patient should be encouraged to proceed with the adjustments of dose as planned and should not require or expect a physician's instructions at each dose increment. Unnecessary dependence is thus discouraged, and the patient's involvement in management is enhanced.

When glucosuria begins to subside, almost always first apparent as decreased glucosuria or aglucosuria in the first A.M. specimen, the dose of insulin should be held constant until such time as FPG can be obtained. Sometimes glucosuria first subsides during the day rather than in the A.M. If this pattern develops, the dose of insulin should be held constant until both FPG and the PG at the aglucosuric time are measured. At the time the PG is measured, a double voided urine sample should be obtained and glucosuria should be measured simultaneously. A few such determinations allow an estimate of the patient's renal threshold; thereafter the physician can approximate the PG for that particular individual from the glucosuria. From the point of development of aglucosuria during some portion of the day to eventual "control" requires continued adjustment of insulin dosage, almost always upward, and adjustment of the patient to the diet and the routine of monitoring. During this time the patient often needs reassurance that the period of close dependency on the physician will soon come to an end. Every effort must also be made to avoid rigidly scheduled visits to the physician's office or the clinical laboratory that interfere with the patient's livelihood or important personal affairs. Such intrusions will only discourage the patient and promote future noncompliance. On the other hand, achievement of reasonable control should not be prolonged and should be possible within a few weeks. When months pass and the patient's control remains irregular, seems to follow no pattern, or is marked by many hypoglycemic episodes, the problem is either noncompliance (see Chapter 4), usually dietary, or improper prescription of insulin. Noncompliance in the use of insulin can sometimes be ascertained by comparison of frequency of insulin purchase with the volume predicted by prescribed therapy. For example, a 10-ml vial of U-100 insulin contains 1000 units; if the patient received 50 units daily, a vial should last 20 days (1000/50).

Many patients will not be controlled with a single dose of intermediate acting insulin (NPH or Lente; see "Mixtures of Insulin" above). In these individuals hyperglycemia and glucosuria improve; the late A.M. or afternoon glucose measurements are the first to show a tendency to normalize. However, the long acting component of the insulin preparation is insufficient to ensure normoglycemia in the fasting state, i.e., in the early morning. Two maneuvers can be tried. Usually, a predinner dose of the same intermediate acting insulin can be added, sometimes requiring a concomitant reduction of the A.M. dose. For example, if such a patient is receiving 60 units daily, up to 15 units may be given in the evening—usually before the dinner meal—and the A.M. dose can be reduced to 50 units. Additional increments of 5 units may then be made to either dose, depending on whether the fasting or postprandial glucose needs lowering. Patients requiring a "split dose" schedule, as this is sometimes called, usually are receiving 60 units or more daily. To avoid a two-dose schedule the alternate approach of increasing the long acting component can be instituted. In this case, the Lente insulins are best employed (see "Types of Insulin"). If the patient is already receiving NPH, a switch to the same dose of Lente is made. Ultralente insulin may then be mixed with Lente in daily increments of 5 to 10 units. Since Lente insulin is already a mixture of Semilente and Untralente in a proportion of 30:70, addition of Ultralente merely alters this ratio in favor of the longer acting component, thus providing a greater likelihood that early A.M. PG will be controlled without producing midday hypoglycemia. To some extent, addition of more long acting component does, however, effect a lowering of glucose even during the day. In any case, some patients can be controlled on a single dose of insulin in this way. For the patient who does not want a second daily injection, this approach may be worthwhile.

Many patients given an intermediate acting insulin readily achieve normoglycemia in the fasting state, but have heavy glucosuria during the day, i.e., postprandially. In such individuals, addition of Semilente insulin to Lente provides additional short acting effect during the period when hyperglycemia needs control. For this purpose one may also add regular insulin to NPH or to Lente.

Much effort can be expended in such "fine tuning." Once the FPG is normalized, efforts to achieve "tight control" during the day can sometimes be made successfully, but often result in unacceptable hypoglycemic episodes. In the absence of evidence that normalization of blood sugar is ordinarily possible by the schemes described, one may properly question the desirabililty of extreme machinations of this type in the ordinary case. This point is *not* in conflict with the evidence that hyperglycemia *may* be important as a cause of increased cardiovascular disease. The point is simply that "tight control" is usually unachievable in most diabetics treated with conventional therapy.

Intensive Therapy with Insulin: Multiple Dose Insulin Programs and Continuous Infusion Pumps for Administration of Insulin

Normalization of blood glucose is not possible in IDDM with one daily dose of insulin or with mixtures of insulin; only rarely is normalization possible with two doses. However, two approaches now make it possible to achieve a state closely approaching normalization in many such patients. Diet must be optimized and home monitoring practiced before initiating any program of intensive therapy with insulin.

Continuous subcutaneous insulin infusion (CSII) using a pump was first reported in 1978. In the past few years, many efforts attest to the efficacy and advantages of this approach and have defined the complications and risks of this method of therapy. Not as generally appreciated is the demonstration during the past few years that identical success at normalization can be achieved by multiple dose programs that do not use a pump but do use utilize a similar principle, viz., delivery of insulin continuously from a subcutaneous depot site with additional doses of short acting insulin given in bolus form (Fig. 72.1). Background insulin activity is provided not by the basal delivery rate of a pump but by absorption from the depot of long acting insulin (usually Ultralente, sometimes NPH). The boluses are given prior to meals as individual injections of regular insulin. Approximately 50 to 60% of the total daily dose of insulin is given as a long acting depot injection in the morning; the remainder is divided and given prior to meals as bolus injections of regular insulin. Regular insulin can be mixed with the long acting form prior to breakfast, but two or three later injections are necessary. This approach has received several names, the most commonly used of which may be "intensive conventional therapy" (ICT).

If a physician decides to institute therapy with a pump, referral to a specialist familiar with one of these devices is usually necessary. Selection of a suitable current model of pump (cost $1500 to $3000) and initiation of therapy are best made by a team active in this specialized field, although if necessary

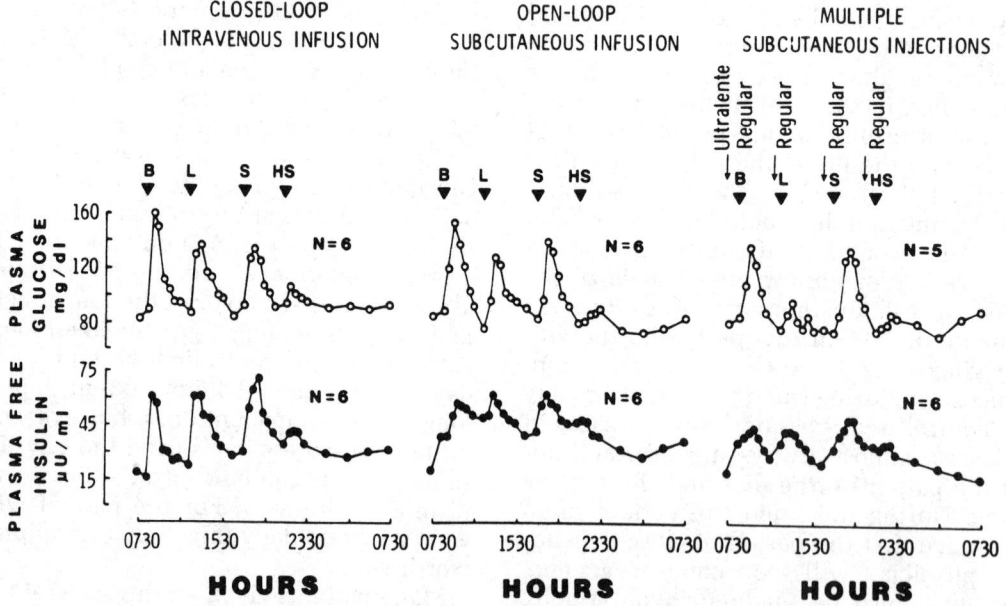

Figure 72.1.   Plasma glucose and free insulin levels in patients with IDDM treated by three methods: closed-loop intravenous infusion (plasma glucose sensor controlled apparatus); open-loop subcutaneous infusion (insulin pump); and multiple subcutaneous injections (intensive conventional therapy). *B*, breakfast; *L*, lunch; *S*, supper; *HS*, bedtime snacks. Note that the results are essentially the same with all methods used. (Modified from Rizza *et al* (11) by Schade *et al* (13).)

the continuation of therapy can thereafter be supervised by the general physician following the instructions available in published material (13).

Pumps are in a state of technological evolution. New models include fail-safe devices and alarms to guard against runaway pump action, power (battery) failure, empty insulin reservoir, and inadvertent turn-off. The insulin is administered through a 25 gauge scalp-vein needle attached to the pump *via* a piece of plastic tubing and inserted into the subcutaneous tissue of the abdomen. The needle is replaced every day or two. Insulin reservoirs vary greatly in size and can accommodate one to several days' supply. Pumps must be worn almost continuously, being removed for only short periods of up to 15 minutes to allow showering, bathing, or swimming. Other physical activities, including sports, are performed with the pump in operation.

Initiation of therapy can be expected to take about 2 weeks, generally during a hospitalization in which the patient becomes familiar with pump operation and the dosage schedule is adjusted. Despite the apparent inconvenience of wearing the device, acceptance of the pump is remarkable. Most patients continue therapy for prolonged periods, and some have now used pumps for several years. Many patients, observing the improved blood glucose levels, are gratified by a sense of control of their destinies. In addition, they experience a normalization of activities by being freed from the tyranny of a clock-oriented existence, since meals no longer need be taken at fixed times but can be taken at will without great concern over the possible development of hypoglycemia. (However, hypoglycemia does occur occasionally even in the best managed cases.) The concentrations of lipids and lipoproteins, invariably abnormal in diabetics with even modest elevations of blood sugar, return to normal, in theory decreasing the increased risk of atherosclerosis of conventionally treated patients.

These forms of therapy have been in use for only a few years, and it is not surprising that information on prevention of complications of diabetes is not yet available. Amelioration of minor degrees of proteinuria has been claimed, possibly a result of membrane permeability changes, but renal insufficiency and major proteinuria are not reversed. Established retinopathy does not appear to be improved. Neuropathy is not clinically improved, although nerve conduction may improve.

A number of problems with pump therapy have become obvious. Pump failure, due to failure of the pump itself or to clogging of its infusion line, sometimes occurs. Diabetic ketoacidosis (DKA) rapidly ensues, often overnight, when the insulin infusion is interrupted. Local infection at the needle site also predisposes to ketoacidosis due to poor absorption of insulin, and may be severe enough to require antibiotic therapy and hospitalization. The approximate frequency of DKA has been estimated at 1 episode/100 patient months; infection, at 1/40 patient months; and severe hypoglycemia, at 1/130 patient months.

Intensified conventional insulin therapy has the advantage over the pump approach of lower cost and freedom from the hazards of DKA and local infection, but the disadvantage of requiring multiple injections. In crossover studies, an equal number of patients prefer one or the other form of therapy.

Monitoring Conventional Insulin Therapy

Efficacy of treatment in the conventionally treated ambulatory patient should be monitored by measuring FPG and urine glucose. Normalization of FPG—more reproducible than postprandial sugars—represents the basic or "coarse" adjustment of insulin dose, while postprandial normalization can be viewed as the "fine" adjustment. No useful purpose is served by attempts to adjust postprandial PG before normalization of the FPG is achieved; only thereafter should PG be monitored at midafternoon or before the evening meal. *Urine* glucose monitoring before meals and before bedtime is also important and too often neglected (Table 72.9). Double voiding technique should be used whenever possible, especially for the first morning specimen, if the patient has not voided during the night. While heavy daytime glucosuria is still present, no useful purpose is served by additional frequent monitoring of PG. On the other hand, when afternoon (before dinner) glucosuria has cleared, PG determination—like that of FPG—becomes essential to determine whether the PG has reached, or is approaching, hypoglycemic levels. The development of such episodes is, of course, an indication of need for adjustment of the treatment program, usually reduction in insulin dose.

In ketosis-prone patients, the urine should also be monitored for ketonuria. This can be accomplished using Acetest tablets or one of the combination "stix" (Table 72.9). Ordinarily, monitoring for ketones is not necessary as a routine procedure.

The optimal frequency of monitoring of FPG and/or of urinary glucose must be determined for each patient. During initiation of therapy, determination of glucosuria four times daily (first voided A.M. specimen, prelunch, predinner, and at bedtime) is essential if insulin is to be varied (increased) as described above. Typically, FPG must be determined every week or two while insulin dose is being adjusted, and thereafter less often—perhaps monthly or even every 2 to 3 months. The required frequency depends on the degree of control which is being sought. For most patients the *practical* goal will be avoidance of fasting and postprandial hyperglycemia and the prevention of heavy glucosuria. It is for such patients that the monitoring schedule has been described above. If "tight control" is the goal,

Table 72.9.
Monitoring of Urine Glucose[a]

Diagnostic Method	Glucosuria (g/100 ml)						
	0	0.1	0.25	0.5	0.75	1	2
Clinitest	Blue	—	Blue-green trace	Green (+)	Green-brown (++)	Brown-orange (+++)	Orange (++++)
Testape	Yellow	Green-yellow (+)	Green (dark) (+++)	Green-blue (+++)			Black (++++)
Clinistix	Pink		Pink (+)	++	Purple (+++)	Nonquantitative	
Diastix	Aqua	Light green trace	Green (+)	Green-brown (++)		Yellow-brown (+++)	Brown (++++)

[a] Note that the colors in the different methods do not indicate comparable degrees of glucosuria. All colors should be matched against the chart supplied by the manufacturer. Clinitest will indicate up to 4–5% glucosuria, provided that 2 drops of urine rather than 5 drops are used. A number of products are availble to test for ketones, including Acetest tablets and strips, such as Ketostix. The cost of these materials varies widely. Materials that test for both glucose and ketones (*e.g.*, Keto-Diastix) are much more expensive than those which test for glucose alone. Attention should be given to the shelf stability of these preparations. Storage under improper conditions of temperature and/or humidity will lead to inaccuracies of testing.

a much more frequent schedule is necessary. In the patient with NIDDM, complete absence of glucosuria can sometimes be achieved without the need for frequent determinations of FPG, but in patients with IDDM monitoring is more difficult. As mentioned earlier ("Normoglycemia as a Goal of Insulin Therapy," page 962), tight control of IDDM using conventional therapy with insulin is not possible; nonetheless, even the conventional approach is greatly aided by home blood glucose monitoring (see below).

Home Blood Glucose Monitoring (HBGM)

The principle indication for home (self) blood glucose monitoring (HBGM) is to permit normalization of blood glucose—tight control—by intensive conventional therapy or by insulin pump. However, other indications include patients with unusually low or high renal threshold for glucose, many patients with IDDM treated conventionally, all patients prone to hypoglycemic episodes, pregnant patients, and some patients with IDDM who, despite an inability to master effective therapy, seem to find HBGM more satisfying than the simpler and less expensive procedures of testing urine.

The process of HBGM should be initiated as a prelude to tight control since, unless the patient shows an ability to master the technique and accept it as an ongoing necessity, the effort at tight control will fail. HBGM does not eliminate the need for dietary compliance. Recent studies indicate that, within the wide range of normal, neither intelligence, socioeconomic status, nor personality type has any predictive value for success with HBGM. Patients of limited financial means may drop out of such a program because of its high cost.

With tight control programs initial frequency of monitoring may be up to seven times daily: 1 hour before and after breakfast, lunch, and dinner, and before bedtime. Testing may be reduced to two to four times daily once a pattern of normalization is achieved. Patients who monitor less than four times

daily are unlikely to maintain normalization of blood glucose.

The basis for all HBGM methods is a paper strip inpregnated with an enzyme reagent (glucose oxidase) and suitable dyes. When placed in contact with a drop of capillary blood, the change of color intensity indicates the glucose concentration. Some strips are read only visually, others either visually or with a reflectance photometer. The characteristics of the commonly used strips are presented in Table 72.10. Remarkably, accuracy of strips properly examined visually is excellent. For most patients a meter is not a necessity, but many feel more secure with machine readings. In the US two meters are presently in wide use (13). The Dextrometer (Ames) is used with Dextrostix strips; the Accu-Chek bG is used for Chemstrip bG. Both machines are reliable, portable, battery operated, and cost about $150 to $300. The characteristics of these and other machines are given elsewhere (13).

The retail cost of the strips varies widely but approximates $0.55/strip. Chemstrips bG read visually can be split linearly to reduce the cost by one-half. For frequency of measurements from two to four times daily, cost for strips alone will range from $30 to $60/month.

Capillary blood is most commonly obtained from the tip of the finger, although some patients prefer the earlobe. The required drop of blood is obtained almost painlessly using a spring-triggered device termed an Autolet. Disposable Monolet lances are used to produce the puncture. Some patients use the Monolet lance without the Autolet, and others use an ordinary 25, 26, or 27 gauge, ⅝-inch disposable needle. A spring-triggered device is also available for use with these needles (13). At a current cost of $0.06 per Monolet, the monthly cost approximates $10.

Blood flow from the finger can be enhanced prior to puncture by holding the hand in warm (not hot) water for 30 seconds. The skin should be quickly

Table 72.10.
Types of Reagent Strips for Home Blood Glucose Monitoring

Strip	Reading by		Blood Removed by	
	Meter	Visually	Wash	Blot Dry[a]
Dextrostix	+		+	
Chemstrip bG	+	+		+
Visidex		+	+	
Stat-Tek	+			+
Glucoscan	+			+

[a] Strips that are blotted dry before reading are simpler to use.

dried. Puncturing the thumb is least painful, but the ring finger has the best blood supply. Puncturing the lateral aspect of the fingertip (distal phalanx) is less painful than puncturing the ball. Pain is also less when sufficient pressure to produce erythema is applied to the palmar surface (ball) of the distal phalanx; an opposing digit of the same hand is used to apply the pressure. The first drop of blood produced suffices; the presence of extravascular fluid does not affect the result. An ideal puncture produces a ±5-mm drop. The finger is inverted and the drop is allowed to fall to the strip; timing is begun. The strip is blotted or the blood is otherwise removed, following directions of the supplier, and the glucose level is read. If the earlobe is used, a second or third sample can subsequently be obtained without repuncture if the site is rubbed with an alcohol wipe, allowed to dry, and the earlobe is flipped with the finger. This procedure is preferred by some patients.

Glycosylated Hemoglobins

Long term monitoring of overall blood sugar control by measurement of one of the chronic *effects* of hyperglycemia provides clinically useful information. Glucose reacts nonenzymatically in a concentration-dependent manner with the amino groups in proteins to produce glycosylated derivatives.

Chronic elevation of blood glucose results in an increase in the concentration of glycosylated hemoglobins, a major component of which is hemoglobin A_{1c} (Hgb A_{1c}). Determination of the level of either the total glycosylated hemoglobin or Hgb A_{1c} gives essentially the same information, an integrated *estimate* of the degree of hyperglycemia over a period of weeks to months. The normal range of Hgb A_{1c} is 4 to 8% of total hemoglobin and may rise to 15% with chronic hyperglycemia. Glycosylated hemoglobin levels fall slowly with reduction of mean glucose, since circulating red blood cells containing high levels of glycosylated hemoglobin disappear normally in approximately 120 days. If euglycemia is established, glycosylated hemoglobins subsequently normalize in 4 to 6 weeks. Conversely, persistent hyperglycemia must be present for 1 to 4 weeks before elevated levels of glycosylated hemo-

globins are seen. Short periods of hyperglycemia (6 to 24 hours' duration) may result in disproportionate elevations, since some methods include measurement of unstable glycosylated derivatives. Other conditions render interpretations of glycosylated hemoglobin values uncertain, including any in which red cell life span is low (bleeding; hemolysis) or in which hemoglobin F is increased (some thalassemia disorders).

The measurement of glycosylated hemoglobins is a useful clinical adjunct in the assessment of the efficacy of control of hyperglycemia. However, proteins other than hemoglobin that also undergo glycosylation exist in nerve, ocular lens, kidney, cell membranes, and plasma. Of great importance is the realization that glucose is not an inert substance but one that can produce postsynthetic modification of many proteins. Some of these alterations may be harmful and provide for the first time a possible biochemical mechanism by which hyperglycemia, *per se*, may result in deleterious alterations of tissue structure and function and produce long term complications of the diabetic state.

Factors Affecting Insulin Requirement during Chronic Therapy

Insulin resistance. Classically, the term insulin resistance refers to a state in which the requirement for insulin exceeds 200 units daily. This extreme type of insulin resistance is usually due to the development of antibodies to insulin (see below). However, resistance to insulin occurs even in the absence of antibodies to insulin. This resistance—or decreased sensitivity to insulin—is most apparent in the diabetes that is associated with obesity and the state now termed non-insulin-dependent diabetes mellitus. Even nondiabetic obese individuals who maintain *normal* levels of blood sugar do so by secreting supranormal amounts of insulin.

Although obese diabetics are insulin resistant in terms of their glucose homeostasis and certain aspects of lipoprotein metabolism, their metabolic state is not so deranged as to allow development of ketoacidosis. In the majority of insulin-resistant diabetics, weight reduction will reverse the insulin resistance. Glucose tolerance often improves to (or toward) normal, and the need for insulin to control hyperglycemia may decrease or disappear. In contrast, some nonobese patients with NIDDM have lower than normal levels of plasma insulin. Such patients comprise a spectrum of combinations of insulin resistance and insulin deficiency.

Recent evidence suggests that sulfonylurea compounds, in addition to their action in facilitating insulin release, may act by returning insulin sensitivity toward normal, perhaps by increasing insulin receptors. The use of these drugs is dictated, however, by other considerations.

Increases of insulin requirement. The stress of infection or trauma may increase insulin requirements quickly. Usually the site of any infection that is severe enough to produce this effect is obvious, or at least there is good evidence of an infectious process (fever, leukocytosis). Only rarely will a search for a hidden focus provide an explanation for changing insulin requirements or even for the development of ketoacidosis. Most episodes of ketoacidosis that are not related to stress are not caused by an increased insulin requirement. Rather, such episodes are usually related to noncompliance, although this may be unintentional, as when the patient mistakenly omits insulin because of intercurrent viral illness. In the past a common cause of an *apparent* increase in insulin requirement was use of the wrong insulin concentration (U-40 for U-80). Insulin requirement tends to increase after the end of the first trimester of pregnancy (see below).

A slow increase of insulin requirement (for the commonly used insulin of beef-pork origin) occurring over months may be related to development of insulin antibodies of the IgG type. Usually the patient may be stabilized at a new, higher dose level. Under these circumstances, the duration of action of short acting insulin is often prolonged, while intermediate or long acting insulins may not carry a 24-hour effect. Insulin requirement may exceed 200 units/day and administration may become a problem. A switch to purified pork insulin may result in up to a 30% decrease in requirement. Occasionally, a short course of glucocorticoid therapy is necessary to effect a dose reduction. Prednisone (40 to 60 mg daily), rather than increase insulin requirement, will usually produce a dramatic fall in insulin requirement beginning at 7 to 10 days. Hospitalization should be considered after the first 5 days of such therapy in anticipation of rapid decrease of insulin requirement. When the decrease occurs, glucocorticoid therapy can be abruptly discontinued. Recurrence of the resistant state is infrequent and may not occur for months or years.

Still another type of insulin "resistance" has been recently recognized. It has long been appreciated that in most patients a modest proportion of the insulin injected subcutaneously undergoes local destruction by tissue proteinases. However, in rare patients very large amounts may be destroyed in this way leading to massive *apparent* resistance. In these individuals, when insulin is injected subcutaneously together with a proteinase inhibitor, required insulin dose is greatly reduced. This phenomenon may explain the large difference frequently observed between insulin dose required by intravenous route and that given subcutaneously. At present no insulin additive is approved that obviates this problem, and one can only inject as much insulin as seems to be required.

Decreases of insulin requirement. Vigorous exercise reduces blood glucose and, in anticipation of such activity, the dose of insulin may need to be reduced (see page 961).

During pregnancy, insulin requirement drops during the first trimester, rises and may double during the second and third trimesters, and falls suddenly at delivery (see below). Diabetics who develop nephropathy often show a decreased insulin requirement. A tendency to normoglycemia or even to hypoglycemia develops occasionally in patients previously requiring insulin who develop chronic congestive heart failure. Development of adrenal or pituitary insufficiency will also result in a decreased insulin requirement, but these are rare events and not specifically related to diabetes mellitus.

Hypoglycemia during Insulin Therapy: Recognition, Prevention, and Treatment

Hypoglycemia is, of course, an inevitable effect of an excessive insulin dose. Especially when severe, hypoglycemia causes central nervous system symptoms ranging from headache, confusion, and visual disturbances to personality change, seizures, unconsciousness, and transient hemiparesis. When hypoglycemia occurs during waking hours and is accompanied by the usual symptoms of epinephrine release (tremor, sweating, tachycardia, and palpitations), there is no problem in recognizing the condition. However, in diabetics, as in some other persons, even mild reductions of blood glucose to levels (50 to 70 mg/100 ml) not clearly identifiable as hypoglycemia can sometimes produce epinephrine release with its resulting symptoms (2) (see also Chapter 74). Under these circumstances, documentable hypoglycemia is not present and the clinical situation may be confusing.

By far the most frequent cause of hypoglycemia in the diabetic receiving insulin therapy is failure of the patient to eat at normal times. Despite repeated warnings many patients not only miss meals, but obfuscate the treatment program further by lying to the physician about food intake. The physician must be ever on guard but tactful in constantly considering this possibility.

Diabetics may develop defects in mechanisms that normally counterregulate hypoglycemia (2). This pathophysiological state may occur within a few years of onset of the disease. Deficiencies of glucagon secretion are common in IDDM and sometimes occur in NIDDM. Defective counterregulation due to impaired secretion of epinephrine also becomes manifest in patients with autonomic (adrenergic) neuropathy late in the course of IDDM, although it occasionally develops within a year of onset of the disease. Other patients show defective counterregulation due to impairment of epinephrine *action* as a result of treatment with β-adrenergic blocking drugs, such as propranolol. In addition, such agents may mask many of the symptoms of epinephrine excess. Regardless of their precise mechanisms, these defective counterregulatory responses undoubtedly contribute in many diabetics to their high risk of developing severe hypoglycemia during therapy with insulin, especially during intensive therapy (2).

Excessive insulin action may occur during the night or early morning hours. The hypoglycemia-induced release of epinephrine and other counterregulatory hormones (cortisol, growth hormone, glucagon) causes rebound hyperglycemia, glucosuria, and ketonuria (Somogyi phenomenon). If the physician notes an elevated blood sugar at this point and prescribes still more insulin, the result is further hypoglycemia, perpetuation of the cycle, and possible serious consequences. The physician is obliged to question the patient carefully for clues to the presence of nocturnal hypoglycemia leading to this sequence, such as nightmares, night sweats, and headache during the night or on arising. Often, but not always, the pattern of daytime glucosuria shows minimal spill. Increasing intake of carbohydrate in the late evening and/or reduction of insulin dose by 10% in IDDM and up to 30 to 40% in NIDDM will often identify and correct the situation. In the latter patients, such a brief and substantial reduction in insulin dose can be made with impunity. If the situation cannot be resolved by such maneuvers, frequent blood glucose monitoring may be necessary (see "Home Blood Glucose Monitoring," page 970).

The classical Somogyi phenomenon must be distinguished from waning of insulin effect which frequently occurs during the early morning hours ("dawn phenomenon"). Although this can occur merely as a result of inadequate dosage of insulin, recent work indicates that resistance to the action of insulin often occurs during the early morning hours and may be the result of nocturnal oversecretion or excessive action of growth hormone (2). Therapy of waning insulin effect, regardless of the cause, requires increasing the dose of insulin to provide additional effect in the preawakening hours.

The immediate therapy of hypoglycemia in a conscious patient is ingestion of food, preferably sugar. Patients should carry a ready carbohydrate source, such as candy, and must realize that a tiny piece of such material will not suffice. Five or six Lifesavers provide the necessary 10 g of carbohydrate, as will a piece of fruit. If available, 4 to 6 ounces of sweetened juice or a soft drink are most satisfactory. A tablespoon of sugar may be added to fruit juice or merely dissolved in ½ cup of water. Relief should be obtained in 10 to 20 minutes. Family members or friends should be instructed in the treatment of such an emergency and should not waste time in attempting to reach medical assistance before administering sugar. Although no objection exists to seeking emergency medical care after sugar is given, the problem is usually resolved by the time medical assistance can be obtained. If no obvious cause is apparent for the episode of hypoglycemia—such as a missed meal which is subsequently eaten—the patient should be on guard for recurrence over the next few hours, during which time repeated ingestion of sugar, at hourly intervals, may be advisable.

Most patients will never require emergency medical assistance for treatment of hypoglycemia. However, occasional individuals will be prone to this problem and sometimes cannot be treated by the simple means described. Either because of a hypoglycemia-related alteration of mental status or because of unconsciousness, such persons will not be able to take oral sugar. A safe and effective emergency therapy is administration of 1 mg of glucagon subcutaneously by a person instructed in this technique. Glucagon is readily available in single dose form (1-mg vial) and should be kept available during initiation of insulin therapy and in hypoglycemia-prone persons. About 10 to 15 minutes are required for an obvious effect on sensorium. As soon as possible, oral sugar should then be given. An effort should always be made to identify the cause of the hypoglycemic episode and to reduce dosage or take other appropriate action to prevent recurrence.

Oral Hypoglycemic Drugs (Sulfonylureas)

Mechanism of Action

Within a few years after their introduction 25 years ago, these drugs came into wide use for the treatment of NIDDM. The acute hypoglycemic effects of the sulfonylureas appear to be mediated through insulin release. However, in chronic administration, during which blood glucose has been lowered, no increase of plasma insulin is apparent. Recent studies on the mechanisms of action of these drugs show both an increase in the number of insulin receptors and a potentiation of insulin action. Numerous effects other than the desired hypoglycemic action of the sulfonylureas have been studied in connection with drug-drug interactions of these compounds (see below).

Current Place in Therapy: University Group Diabetes Program (UGDP)

Although sometimes used to good purpose for treatment of symptomatic hyperglycemia, oral hypoglycemic drugs were often administered to patients with NIDDM who could have been treated with diet (i.e., by weight reduction). Many patients with minimal fasting or postprandial hyperglycemia or other abnormalities of glucose tolerance were also given these drugs.

A multicenter long term cooperative study (University Group Diabetes Program, UGDP) attempted to assess the usefulness of these agents in asymptomatic diabetics by comparing tolbutamide with diet and insulin treatment. The study began a vitriolic controversy beginning in 1970 when it first reported that tolbutamide-treated patients fared no better than those given placebo and indeed had a higher cardiovascular (but not overall) death rate. Since that report, diabetologists have been divided concerning the usefulness (or dangers) of these agents. While the harmfulness of these agents seems now, on reanalysis of the data, to be open to serious question, the long term benefits in terms of prevention of complications of diabetes remain questionable. It is almost certain that the original UGDP study was too brief and too few patients were studied to have permitted answers to questions concerning prevention of complications. A number of other studies of this issue have now concluded that sulfonylureas do not result in harmful effects.

Therapeutic Effects versus Side Effects

No doubt exists that short term symptomatic relief of hyperglycemia and its sequelae can be obtained in most NIDDM patients treated with sulfonylureas. This result can be most gratifying in properly selected patients. For example, patients who may have difficulty in self-administering insulin because of visual or other physical handicaps may benefit symptomatically from use of sulfonylureas. On the other hand, the use of sulfonylureas is not harmless, because of their intrinsic pharmacological action in lowering blood glucose and a number of toxic effects. Hypoglycemia can occur and may be both severe and protracted, especially in the elderly or in patients with decreased renal function. Administration of certain of these agents to elderly patients, especially to patients with impaired cardiovascular function, may produce water retention and a syndrome identical to that of inappropriate secretion of antidiuretic hormone (SIADH) with severe hyponatremia and symptoms as profound as coma (15). The volume expansion that occurs may precipitate or worsen congestive heart failure. Chlorpropamide (Diabinese) is the classic offender in this regard, although tolbutamide (Orinase) has been rarely involved as well.

Candidates for Therapy with Sulfonylureas

Obese NIDDM patients who have not responded to a weight reduction diet or who, having started on a diet, need interim symptomatic relief from hyperglycemia that is producing osmotic diuresis (polyuria, polydipsia) may benefit. Typically these individuals are over age 40 and are more likely to respond if their diabetes has been present for only a few years. Other candidates are those who are unwilling to accept insulin therapy or in whom the risks of hypoglycemia seem unacceptable. The latter might include persons with occupations involving hazardous conditions (vehicle or dangerous equipment operators). Still others include nonobese individuals in whom insulin therapy is unacceptable, but for whom persistent hyperglycemia is felt by the

physician to constitute a long term risk factor for atherosclerotic and microvascular disease.

Although most physicians would currently be reluctant to change therapy to an oral agent for a patient who is managing well with insulin, such a change—if undertaken—is more likely to succeed if the diabetes has required less than about 40 units of insulin. Patients with a previous history of ketoacidosis are ordinarily not candidates for a transfer from insulin. A history of hyperosmolar nonketotic coma does not preclude a successful change from insulin. Patients with no tendency to ketosis, but whose diabetes is so severe that it has produced weight loss, may not respond to sulfonylureas given as initial therapy but may respond after hyperglycemia has been controlled for a short time with insulin.

Oral agents should not be prescribed for certain patients: individuals with a history of ketoacidosis, unless the latter has developed in relation to stress; patients with a history of severe toxic reaction to a sulfonylurea; and patients with severe hepatic or renal disease, although correct choice of an agent may make such therapy possible (see Table 72.11).

Effectiveness. In optimally selected patients about one-half can be expected to experience normalization of fasting blood sugar while about one-third will not respond. In others, some drug effect will be evident, perhaps to a degree which permits symptomatic relief. Maximal drug effect can be expected within a few days to a week. Those who do not respond during initial therapy are considered to be "primary" sulfonylurea failures. In other cases, following a month or more of good response, the drug seems to become ineffective ("secondary" sulfonylurea failure). The frequency of this response has been estimated at 3 to 10%. Many secondary failures are due to noncompliance. Only occasionally in secondary failure will a switch from a maximal dose of one agent to another be successful.

Transfer from insulin or from one sulfonylurea to another sulfonylurea. An ineffective agent may be stopped abruptly and a new one started. NIDDM patients receiving insulin can also be abruptly switched, provided that they do not need more than 40 units of insulin. A need for maximal doses of sulfonylurea can usually be anticipated in such cases. If the patient has manifested ketosis in the past, as for example during stress, but is otherwise thought to be a candidate for a switch to an oral agent, the dose of insulin may be cut in half as the drug is started. Subsequent monitoring over the next few days will show whether the oral agent can control hyperglycemia or must be abandoned.

Choice of drug. Tolbutamide is the only sulfonylurea studied in the UGDP. Although the Food and Drug Administration's admonitions concerning other oral agents extrapolate from this study of tol-

Table 72.11.
Characteristics of Hypoglycemic Drugs (Sulfonylureas)

Compound	Trade Name	Tablet Size	Daily Dose Range	Duration of action (hr)	Doses/ Day	Route of Inactivation
Tolbutamide	Orinase	0.5 g	1–3 g	12	2–3	100% in liver
Chlorpropamide	Diabinese	0.1 g 0.25 g	0.1–0.5 g	36+	1	80% excretion by kidney as intact drug; 100% excretion as intact drug *plus* metabolites, activities unknown
Acetohexamide	Dymelor	0.25 g 0.5 g	0.25–1.5 g	12–18	1–2	Partial liver metabolism; 100% kidney excretion as active metabolites plus unchanged drug
Tolazamide	Tolinase	0.1 g 0.25 g 0.5 g	0.25–1.0 g	12–18	1–2	Partial liver metabolism; partial excretion *via* kidney
Glyburide	Micronase Diabeta	1.25 mg 2.5 mg 5 mg	1.25–20 mg	24	1–2	100% metabolized to inactive compounds
Glipizide	Glucotrol	5 mg 10 mg	2.5–40 mg	16–24	1–3	100% metabolized to inactive compounds

butamide, it may be useful to remember that the related available drugs might have fared better or worse. This caveat aside, for patients with normal hepatic and renal function, there is little to lead one to choose among the available agents (Table 72.11) except that the longer acting drugs need not be taken as often. The frequency of toxicity with tolbutamide is very low, probably lower than with the other agents, even at maximal doses. Chlorpropamide should never be used at a dose greater than 500 mg/ day (above which hepatic toxicity is frequent). Because of the unique ability of chlorpropamide among the sulfonylureas to produce a syndrome of drug-induced water intoxication (SIADH) (see above), this drug should be avoided in the elderly in whom this effect has been seen almost exclusively. Acetohexamide is the least used agent, partly because it was introduced later than tolbutamide and chlorpropamide and partly because of lack of aggressive marketing. Tolazamide was introduced 20 years ago but has been marketed vigorously only within the past few years. Phenformin, a biguanide (not a sulfonylurea), was withdrawn from the market in 1977 as an "imminent hazard to the public health" *after* 18 years of general use. Fatal lactic acidosis, hypertension, and persistent tachycardia were associated with its use. The drug is available free of charge to any physician who files an application with the Food and Drug Administration, but for practical purposes use of phenformin has been abandoned by all but a few diabetologists.

For many years, "second generation" sulfonylureas have been in wide use outside the United States. Glyburide (Micronase, Diabeta) and glipizide (Glucotrol) have recently been introduced into use

in the United States and are being aggressively marketed. These drugs are safe agents and, although up to 200 times more potent than the older sulfonylureas, do not offer clear advantages over the older drugs. No long term studies of the UGDP type are available with these agents.

Comparative cost. At present, the approximate monthly retail cost of therapy with these drugs is from $10 to $50 depending on the dose and the agent used. Two of the drugs, tolbutamide and chlorpropamide, are currently available in their generic forms at one-half to one-third the price of the trade name products. The cost of insulin therapy may be significantly less than that with the oral agents, depending on the doses required.

Instruction to the Patient on Use of Sulfonylureas

The obese patient must be made to realize that diet, *i.e.*, weight reduction, is the mainstay of therapy. In order to avoid unnecessary anxiety, the current status of the UGDP controversy should be discussed with the patient and the possible risks and goals of therapy clearly outlined. Although hypoglycemia is not common with the sulfonylureas, when it does occur, it is likely to be both severe and prolonged. The symptoms of hypoglycemia should be clearly described to the patient, family, and/or friends and corrective measures outlined (see "Insulin Therapy"). The possibility of drug-drug interactions (see below) should be mentioned lest another physician prescribe a drug which potentiates or decreases the effectiveness of the sulfonylureas. Loading doses of sulfonylureas may have a place in patients under observation in hospital but should not be used in ambulatory patients.

Monitoring Therapy with Sulfonylureas

Since patients receiving sulfonylurea drugs are not ketosis prone and have fairly stable diabetes, monitoring is relatively simple. Similar considerations apply to patients being treated with diet alone. No compelling indication exists for home blood glucose monitoring in most such patients (see page 970). Patients who have FPG in or near the normal range exhibit little or no fasting glucosuria but may show glucosuria in the postprandial state. Such patients can check their overnight (early A.M.) urine samples for glucose as infrequently as once a week or even every 2 weeks. More important they should understand that appearance of glucosuria where none had been evident or the worsening of glucosuria is an indication for contact with a physician. Similarly, these patients must be taught that, should they develop symptoms and signs of uncontrolled hyperglycemia (heavy glucosuria, polyuria, polydipsia), prompt advice from a physician is absolutely necessary. Testing for urinary acetone is not necessary unless the patient has glucosuria and at some earlier time had an episode of ketoacidosis, perhaps during stress.

FPG should be determined every few months in most patients and is the best means of monitoring sulfonylurea-treated patients who respond to treatment with normalization of blood sugar. Determination of glycosylated hemoglobin is also useful (page 971). Development of hypoglycemia—which may be detected before symptoms develop—is an indication for downward adjustment of drug dosage.

Some patients relentlessly monitor their urine at very frequent intervals—perhaps daily—even though years pass without glucosuria. Such practices are to be discouraged, but certain patients persist despite advice to the contrary, perhaps out of compulsiveness or because of their constant need for reassurance.

Special Considerations in Treatment of the Geriatric Patient

Some elderly patients may best be treated with oral agents. These individuals may have special problems (*e.g.*, poor vision or manipulative skills) which make self-administration of insulin more difficult than usual. Moreover, simple symptomatic therapy may be the foremost consideration in these individuals. On the other hand, many elderly persons can manage insulin therapy, especially of the type that is not excessively aggressive, and age alone should not deter the physician from appropriate institution of insulin therapy. As noted above (page 966), insulin syringes can be prefilled and stored in the refrigerator for 1 to 2 weeks; this plan is useful for the older person who cannot accurately draw up the correct amount of insulin. The elderly are especially likely to suffer from multiple diseases and to use multiple drugs. The risk of drug-drug inter-

actions in this group is therefore greater than in younger individuals (see below). The elderly are also especially prone to development of severe and prolonged hypoglycemia with use of the sulfonylureas, which may be related, in part, to the decrease of renal function that normally accompanies aging and that may be worse in the diabetic. Decreased renal function (glomerular filtration rate, creatinine clearance) is frequently present in the elderly even when the serum creatinine is normal, since creatinine production decreases with age as muscle mass decreases. Thus, sulfonylureas which are disposed of exclusively by excretion (acetohexamide) or in part by this route (chlorpropamide, tolazamide) are more likely to produce hypoglycemia when renal function decreases. Chlorpropamide is also uniquely capable of inducing enhanced endogenous antidiuretic hormone action and of inducing a water intoxication syndrome, a phenomenon seen almost exclusively in elderly diabetics (15). Tolbutamide and tolazamide are probably the safest of the sulfonylureas for use in the elderly; the initial dose should be low and increases should be made cautiously. Loading doses should not be used in the elderly.

Drug-Drug Interactions

Various drugs enhance the hypoglycemic action of sulfonylureas, while others decrease their effect. The magnitude of the effects varies with the different sulfonylureas. Several mechanisms are involved, some of which are known. Among the more commonly used drugs, salicylates, some sulfonamides, chloramphenicol, phenylbutazone and its derivatives, and bishydroxycoumarin all enhance the hypoglycemic action of the sulfonylureas either by displacement of binding to plasma proteins or by interfering with metabolic disposal. Propranolol (Inderal) and other β-blockers may mask the hypoglycemia-induced release of epinephrine and thus prolong and intensify the hypoglycemic reactions. Propranolol, by blocking insulin release, may also precipitate hyperosmolar coma. Clonidine (Catapres) may, like propranolol, mask the signs and symptoms of hypoglycemia. Acute ingestion of alcohol can enhance hypoglycemia; chronic alcohol use accelerates metabolic disposal of sulfonylureas and antagonizes their hypoglycemic action. Sulfonylureas, especially chlorpropamide, interfere with the metabolism of alcohol and may produce a disulfiram-like (Antabuse) effect (see Chapter 21). The thiazide diuretics, chlorthalidone, furosemide, and ethacrynic acid may produce hyperglycemia even in normal persons and antagonize the sulfonylureas. Another commonly used drug, the anticonvulsant phenytoin (Dilantin), also has an antagonist action. Numerous other drugs may enhance or negate the effect of the sulfonylureas; equally important, the sulfonylureas themselves produce numerous alterations of drug action. These problems should not be overstated, but the physician should be aware of these possibilities and interactions.

Treatment of "Other Types" of Diabetes Mellitus (Secondary Diabetes)

Drug-induced diabetes (e.g., thiazides) and diabetes associated with the use of glucocorticoids are usually not ketosis prone and ordinarily resemble that of NIDDM. Treatment with sulfonylureas may be tried, but insulin is often necessary. Withdrawal of the offending agent does not always ameliorate the diabetic state. The possibility of precipitating diabetes in patients with a strong family history should not deter the physician from the judicious use of diuretics or glucocorticoids when these agents are necessary. Similarly, a diabetic who is already receiving insulin should not be denied diuretic therapy (e.g., when hypertension develops) or glucocorticoids for fear of "aggravating" the diabetes. If such aggravation occurs, usually only an increase of insulin dose is necessary to re-establish the previous state of control.

Diabetes secondary to *chronic pancreatitis or pancreatectomy* should be treated with insulin. The insulin requirement is usually 20 to 40 units/day. The patients should be instructed to follow the dietary strategy outlined for insulin-dependent diabetes in Table 72.6. Alcoholic patients with this form of diabetes are particularly difficult to manage if they continue to drink heavily and to eat erratically.

COMPLICATIONS OF DIABETES MELLITUS

Diabetes mellitus is a leading cause of death in the United States today. Most of these deaths are due to the complications of the disease—primarily those complications associated with accelerated atherosclerosis and with chronic renal failure (Fig. 72.2). The risk of both atherosclerotic heart disease and of atherosclerotic peripheral vascular disease is increased approximately 3-fold in diabetics and is proportionate to the duration of disease (in patients with both NIDDM and IDDM). Atherosclerotic disorders are discussed in Section 8 and in Chapters 83 and 87; chronic renal failure is discussed in Chapter 47.

Diabetic Neuropathy

(See Chapter 84 for a general discussion of peripheral neuropathy.)

The incidence of neurological deficit in diabetes mellitus is not known, although it is clear that in most patients the occurrence and severity of involvement are related to duration of the disease (Fig. 72.2). The most commonly appreciated abnormality is that which afflicts peripheral sensory nerves. Several types of sensation are involved (pain, proprioception, vibration), and can lead to such uncommon but striking disorders as neuropathic ar-

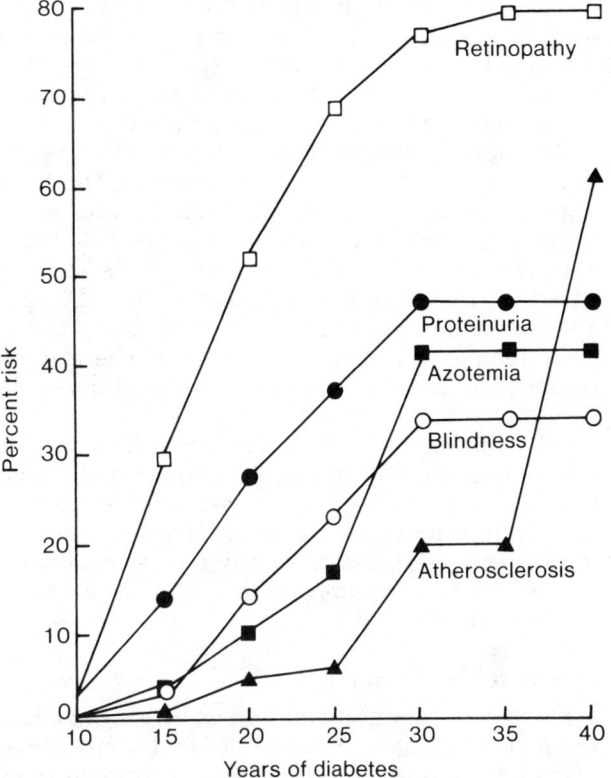

Figure 72.2. Complications of diabetes mellitus as a function of duration of the disease. (From Davidson MB: The continually changing "natural history" of diabetes mellitus. *J Chronic Dis* 34:5, 1981.)

thropathy. Less well appreciated are the autonomic disorders which give rise to disturbances of cardiovascular function (postural hypotension; resting tachycardia), genitourinary function (impotence; bladder dysfunction), and gastrointestinal function (nocturnal diarrhea; fecal incontinence). Motor deficits are much less common but may occur with striking suddenness. Weakness is distal (neuropathic) rather than proximal (myopathic), although a specific type of myopathy also occurs in diabetics (see "Diabetic Myopathy" below).

Peripheral Sensory Neuropathy

Classically, the deficit is distal, with the lower extremities being first affected, followed by the upper extremities. The term "stocking-glove" distribution is appropriate. In more sophisticated terms, the disorder is a symmetric polyneuropathy with a proximal-distal gradient of dysfunction. In severe cases, even the sensory innervation of the trunk is involved; in this instance the most distal fibers are those of the anterior abdomen and low thorax. Rarely, even the distal portion of the cranial nerves is affected (e.g., the distal sensory portion of the trigeminal nerve). The patterns of loss are not specific for diabetes mellitus and can be seen in such diverse states as amyloid neuropathy and toxic (e.g., lead) neuropathies. Whether the process represents a "dying back" of those nerves which are longest or is the cumulative result of randomly scattered lesions along the nerve trunks is not known.

The nerve damage may first produce hyperesthesia and dysesthesia, including tingling and burning sensations. Later, various symptoms are experienced including sensations of numbness or heaviness. Patients often complain that their feet feel "dead" or that they have a sensation of walking on a soft or nonexistent surface. Loss of ability to perceive temperature and firmness gives rise to these complaints. Severe, spontaneous, short lived leg pains and cramps are common.

On neurological testing skin hypesthesia is the commonest finding (pinprick, two-point discrimination, light touch). The hypesthesia and loss of temperature perception lead to unappreciated skin trauma and predispose to infection. The sensory loss in the fingertips can prevent the blind diabetic from learning Braille letters.

Peripheral Motor Neuropathy

Much less common and less well recognized are the motor function abnormalities that occur as part of diabetic neuropathy. The intrinsic muscles of the feet are those most commonly involved. Interosseous atrophy produces inability to separate toes but, more important, allows the foot to assume abnormal positions. When claw or hammer toe develops, new pressure points appear at the tips of the toes and along the dorsal aspects; hyperkeratosis, callus formation, and ulceration follow. The interosseous atrophy that may affect the hands does not lead to total loss of function, but does result in weakness of grip. Diffuse weakness of the legs and upper extremities may also occur.

Neuropathic Foot Ulcers

(See also Chapter 88.)

The combination of sensory loss and motor weakness with anatomical deformity leads to pressure points and to eventual ulceration. Typically, these ulcers occur on the sole of the foot. Remarkably, the ulcers may heal repeatedly only to recur in the same location, but recurrence is not inevitable.

Therapy of Peripheral Neuropathies

The therapy of ulceration is primarily one of local foot care. Since callus formation aggravates the tendency to increase local pressure and worsens ulceration, regular debridement is essential. Some patients can be taught debridement techniques, which may at least delay the intervals between visits for this purpose, but usually periodic professional assistance is essential. Such care is often best provided by podiatrists (see Chapter 102). Fitting of custom-made molded shoes is very helpful and is essential in some cases for prevention of ulceration.

Medical therapy is probably useless, except for analgesics as needed. Codeine or a similar agent is often necessary for relief of pain and it may be required chronically. A number of drugs (phenytoin, amitriptyline, carbamazine, and diphenhydramine) have been recommended for treatment of pain in peripheral neuropathy, but there have been no controlled trials to test their efficacy (see Chapter 84 for additional details). Vitamin therapy is also frequently given, but vitamins are almost certainly useless for this purpose. Prompt and vigorous antibiotic therapy of infection in ulcerated areas is essential.

Mononeuropathies

Mononeuropathy (mononeuritis simplex and multiplex) may occur in any superficial nerve (simplex) or asymmetric simultaneous combination (multiplex). The lower extremities are more commonly involved (femoral, lateral femoral cutaneous, sciatic, peroneal) than the upper (ulnar, radial, etc). Onset is usually sudden with intense, often cramping and lancinating pain (see Tables 84.6 and 84.7). Typically, the pain is worse at night and, when the lower extremities are involved, may be relieved by pacing about.

At onset, diagnosis can only be surmised, although tenderness along a nerve trunk is very suggestive. Herpes zoster may be suspected, especially when hyperesthesia occurs, but when no vesicles appear and muscle weakness and atrophy are eventually evident, the diagnosis becomes obvious. The prognosis is quite good, with complete recovery within a few months being the rule.

Cranial and oculomotor neuropathies. These mononeuropathies are distinguished from other mononeuropathies mainly by their location. Pain and headache may be present. The commonest nerves involved are III (palebral ptosis; pupillary function undisturbed), VI (inward deviation of eye; diplopia), and IV (inward and upward deviations; diplopia). Recovery within 2 months is almost universal. When the facial nerve is involved, distinction from Bell's palsy is not possible (see Chapter 84), although the diabetic variety tends to be less severe and recovery is usually complete.

Abnormal Sweat Production

Almost always associated with other evidence of diabetic autonomic neuropathy, this complication in its typical form produces heat intolerance and increased sweating (hyperhydrosis) of the upper half of the body with decreased or absent sweating (anhydrosis) below the midtrunk. In other cases, anhydrosis is generalized and recognition of the complication may be difficult. In women the condition may be confused with menopausal sweats.

A consequence of impaired sweating includes failure to recognize hypoglycemia (see page 972). This is a serious problem, since one of the warning signals of insulin reaction is lost. Many elderly patients, including those without diabetes mellitus, already have impaired sympathetic responses as a result of aging rather than of diabetes.

Diabetic Myopathy (Amytrophy)

This is a rare but devastating complication of diabetes mellitus which may be confused with diabetic neuropathy. Severe proximal muscle weakness and pain usually affect the pelvic girdle and thigh muscles, although upper truncal musculature can also be involved. The typical patient is an elderly, NIDDM patient with mild disease. Men are more frequently affected than are women. Onset may be fairly rapid, and low grade fever and elevated erythrocyte sedimentation rate may be present. Cerebrospinal fluid protein may be very high. Muscle biopsy shows fiber degeneration. Prognosis for improvement is good, but significant residuals are common.

Cardiovascular Dysfunction

In addition to abnormalities of innervation that result in abnormal cardiovascular reflexes (see below), diabetic cardiac denervation apparently accounts for the phenomenon of painless myocardial infarction, which is said to occur in more than 30% of diabetics who experience an acute event. Diagnosis is difficult unless acute electrocardiographic changes are present. Precipitation of unexplained ketoacidosis or myocardial failure may divert attention to these secondary events.

Resting Tachycardia

Heart rates of 90 to 100 beats/minute are common in patients with autonomic neuropathy; occasionally even higher rates are observed. Parasympathetic damage is the apparent explanation; the sympathetics appear to be less affected. Propranolol is useful if therapy is needed. In severe cases, the tachycardia subsides over the years as denervation becomes more complete and the sympathetics are also lost.

Several noninvasive tests are available to assess the presence of autonomic cardiovascular dysfunction. These include the Valsalva maneuver, beat-to-beat heart rate variation, and the lying-to-standing heart rate response. Such assessments are more subtle indicators of the presence of autonomic dysfunction than is postural hypotension. These tests are rarely of use clinically but do allow objective assessment. The consequences—or at least the associations—of these abnormal cardiovascular reflexes in diabetics are important. Once they have developed, there is a marked decrease of 5-year survival. Sudden death—not attributable to myocardial infarction—has been described in many such patients (5).

Postural Hypotension

The most readily recognized, and a most troublesome, cardiovascular abnormality is postural hypotension (see Chapter 84). The patient may complain merely of dizziness or faintness on standing, or the problem may be more severe, with visual disturbances and syncope. These symptoms may be confused with episodes of hypoglycemia. Remarkably, some patients with fairly marked postural hypotension are asymptomatic.

On initial examination, every diabetic patient should be checked for a postural decrease in blood pressure. In addition, a check for postural hypotension should be made whenever a potentially aggravating condition occurs. The onset or aggravation of postural hypotension is often associated with the beginning of therapy with a variety of drugs often used in diabetics such as antihypertensive drugs, including diuretics, vasodilators/antispasmodics such as nitroglycerin (glyceryl trinitrate), antidepressants (tricyclic), and phenothiazines. Occasional diabetic patients may be unable to tolerate effective doses of these drugs because of this problem.

The mechanism of this disorder is thought to reside in the efferent limb of the baroreceptor arc secondary to damaged sympathetic vasoconstrictor fibers in the splanchnic bed, muscles, and skin. Diminished plasma renin responses to postural change have been noted in such patients, as have abnormalities of plasma norepinephrine, but the role of these defects is not clear.

Various mechanical maneuvers, including the use of antigravity or "space suits," have been recommended but are not useful. Drug therapy with vasopressors such as phenylephrine or combinations of tyramine or amine-containing cheeses and monoamine oxidase inhibitors have had their advocates. For patients with severe postural hypotension, the most useful drug is the mineralocorticoid, fludrocortisone (Florinef). In doses of 0.1 to 1.0 mg/day, the drug is often helpful, but since one of its actions is to expand fluid volume, it can precipitate cardiac failure or produce severe hypertension in the recumbent state. Refractoriness may eventually occur. In mild cases, the simple advice that the patient assume upright positions slowly by sitting on the edge of the bed after recumbency may help to avoid syncopal episodes, while continuing postural hypotension, though easily measured, may not be especially symptomatic (also see Chapter 84).

Digestive System Dysfunction

Most of the disorders of the gastrointestinal tract in diabetes are related to disturbances of motility.

Esophageal motor dysfunction can be demonstrated on testing but is usually not a clinical problem.

Atony of the stomach (gastroparesis diabeticorum) is often asymptomatic but may be troublesome. Diagnosis is apparent—sometimes as an incidental finding—on barium X-ray of the upper gastrointestinal tract. Occasionally a syndrome of vomiting is accompanied by gastric atony, but mere delay and unpredictable emptying of the stomach may produce irregular diabetic control in already difficult to manage patients with IDDM. Metoclopramide (Reglan) is said to be effective in this disorder (see Chapter 36).

Small bowel dysfunction is common and symptomatic, leading to "diabetic diarrhea." Typically the diarrhea is nocturnal. Fecal incontinence may occur and is very distressing. The disorder tends to be episodic, with attacks lasting from a few days to weeks or rarely months. Watery brown diarrhea, usually without steatorrhea, is typical. On barium X-ray studies of the small bowel the findings are those of disturbed motility. Despite the distressing symptoms, the patient appears well; weight loss is uncommon. When steatorrhea occurs, pancreatic exocrine insufficiency and sprue syndrome, more common in diabetics than in the general population, enter the differential. Fully developed sprue is associated with gross evidence of malabsorption. A trial of antibiotic therapy (e.g., tetracycline, 250 mg four times a day for 2 weeks) may improve the diarrhea and the malabsorption if the latter is due to small bowel stasis and bacterial colonization. Symptomatic treatment with antispasmodics (e.g., Lomotil) may be useful, especially when attacks of diarrhea are short lived.

Large bowel complaints, especially of constipation, are common in the elderly. It does not appear that diabetics are especially prone to any additional problems in this regard.

Patients with poorly controlled diabetes may develop fatty changes of the liver. Hepatomegaly and/or elevations of liver enzymes may occur. Effective control of blood sugar results in disappearance of these abnormalities.

Bladder Dysfunction (Neurogenic Bladder)

The symptoms of bladder dysfunction in diabetics are often overlooked [1]. Onset is insidious and occurs over many years. Most patients (80%) will have clinical evidence of neuropathy affecting other systems. The first clinical manifestation of bladder dysfunction is an increase in the interval between voidings until urine is passed only twice or even once daily. A need to strain, slow stream, dribbling, and sensation of incomplete voiding may be present. These symptoms should be routinely solicited from diabetics, especially when there are symptoms or signs of peripheral neuropathy.

Demonstration of residual urine is the hallmark of clinically symptomatic cystopathy, but many diabetic patients, when studied by cystometric techniques, have objective evidence of a neurogenic involvement and a grossly enlarged bladder well before symptoms are evident [1]. At this stage, residual urine is not present and other urinary tract abnormalities (recurrent infections) are not evident. The concept that residual urine invariably leads to bacteriuria and infection is widely held but has been challenged. Bacteriuria is probably better attributed to associated, age-related disorders of bladder outlet (benign prostatic hypertrophy; descensus of the bladder and cystocele).

Various cystometric and other procedures are employed for diagnosis of cystopathy. In recent years gas as a filling medium has been introduced, along with sphincter electromyography, flow measurements (uroflowmetry), and urethral pressure profiles. These procedures are useful in distinguishing diabetic cystopathy from associated nondiabetic disorders and help to determine treatment programs. A long, low pressure curve with lack of sensation until the bladder capacity is reached, together with increased bladder capacity, establishes the diagnosis. These studies require consultation with a urologist.

Therapy is either medical or surgical. When considerable bladder distension is present, a period of decompression, usually with an indwelling catheter, for about 2 weeks, is helpful in re-establishing bladder function. Many relatively early cases can thereafter be managed through forced voiding (as much as is possible) every 3 hours. If residual urine is reduced to 100 ml or less, no further therapy may be needed. Otherwise, parasympathetic drugs such as bethanechol (Urecholine) (10 to 20 mg, three to four times daily, or larger doses twice weekly) may be helpful. Intermittent self-catheterization is also useful. If these maneuvers are not effective, transurethral surgery (vesicle neck resection or limited electroincision) is highly effective in many cases. Urinary incontinence is only rarely a problem with this procedure. Vigorous therapy with antimicrobial drugs is often necessary to prevent recurrent infections and their complications. Long term urological follow-up is mandatory.

Sexual Dysfunction

The frequency of erectile impotence is high in diabetes, perhaps 50 to 60% overall, but it is, like many other complications of diabetes, related to duration of disease. The problem seems to be a type of autonomic neuropathy involving the pelvic parasympathetic nerves.

Impotence is a common problem in nondiabetic men, and the problems leading to such impotence must be included in the differential diagnosis in the diabetic. Psychogenic factors probably account for the large majority of nondiabetic cases. Although no evidence suggests that psychogenic problems are any more common in diabetics, neither are diabetics immune to psychogenic disturbances. The onset of diabetic impotence is usually slow (6 months to several years), often associated with retrograde ejaculation, and impotence eventually becomes complete. Despite this, libido is characteristically retained. While patients with psychogenic impotence often report nocturnal erections and emissions and may retain masturbatory activity, all of these are absent in diabetic impotence.

An important point on clinical examination is that testicular sensitivity to pressure sufficient to cause pain is retained in men with psychogenic impotence, but is often greatly diminished or lost in the diabetic in whom accompanying sensory neuropathy is common.

Endocrinological causes of impotence (see also Chapters 18 and 77) should be considered because they are potentially treatable, but it is rare to find an endocrine basis for impotence in the diabetic. Testosterone secretion, easily verified by plasma testosterone measurement, is invariably normal in diabetics; therefore, as one would expect, testosterone therapy is useless. Prolactin excess has been recently touted as a cause of impotence, but if that is the case, it must be extremely rare.

A variety of drugs, especially ones which are often used in diabetics, may cause impotence. The most common offenders are the nondiuretic antihypertensives (see Chapter 62).

Several studies report that, in contrast to the male, sexual function in diabetic women appears to be unaffected by the disease. Others have asserted that many diabetic women lose ability to achieve orgasm (4).

The differential diagnosis and therapy of impotence are discussed in detail in Chapter 18. In recent years, considerable success has been achieved in diabetics by use of penile implants, including inflatable prosthetic devices.

Neuropathic Arthropathy (Charcot's Joint; Diabetic Charcot's Foot)

This complication of diabetes is frequently unrecognized or misdiagnosed. The disorder is a progressive, degenerative change of the bony structure of the foot, most often involving the tarsal and tarsometatarsal joints (60%), but also the metatarsophalangeal joints (30%) and the ankle (10%). The prevalence has been estimated at 1 in 680 cases, but the disorder is probably more common. The patient presents with a swollen foot, often attributed to or associated with recent trauma. The foot may be painful or may be remarkably free of pain, considering the appearance. Examination shows moderate to gross deformity of the foot with "rocker-bottom" subluxation of the midtarsal region or subluxation

of the metatarsophalangeal joints. Usually the foot is erythematous and warm to the touch. An infected neuropathic ulcer may be present. More often than not, the pulses are intact. Physicians unfamiliar with this presentation are likely to diagnose some other type of inflammatory arthritis or osteomyelitis and their impression may be "verified" by the X-ray findings. In these early stages, the X-rays show severe osteoarthritis, but, as the disease progresses, there is complete destruction of the involved joints with resorption of the metatarsal heads and phalangeal diaphyses. Various other bony changes occur, including fractures, joint effusions, and subluxations. When these changes are at the maximal stage, i.e., when soft tissue involvement is most prominent, the diagnosis of osteomyelitis is frequently entertained, especially when there is an associated, often infected, ulcer. Synovial biopsy showing a thickened synovium containing osseous debris may provide the correct diagnosis and avoid the necessity of embarking on a prolonged and difficult course of antibiotic therapy for suspected osteomyelitis.

Diabetic Charcot's foot may also be confused with the changes associated with osteoarthritis, and gouty, rheumatoid, and psoriatic arthritis. Consultation by an orthopaedic surgeon, rheumatologist, or podiatrist to confirm the diagnosis and to assist with therapy is almost always indicated.

Treatment is based on the cessation of further trauma to the affected area, which is best accomplished by elimination of weight bearing. Hospitalization may be necessary for this purpose. Reduction of edema and signs of inflammation may take several weeks. Immobilization with a cast may be helpful, but should not be undertaken in the acute stage and, if used, should be done with great care to ensure the integrity of the areas covered by the cast. Simpler boot-like devices may also be used. Crutches can be used at this point, followed eventually by a walking cast. Up to 4 months of treatment may be required. Thereafter, molded or contoured shoes are essential to proper long term management. Surgical intervention is inadvisable, although occasionally a stabilization procedure may be required if conservative therapy fails. Amputation is not indicated unless osteomyelitis unequivocally coexists or the entire process fails to respond to prolonged conservative efforts. Despite the discouraging appearance of the foot at its worst stages, sufficient healing and stabilization to produce a useful foot can be anticipated.

Other foot problems in the diabetic. A number of common foot problems (e.g., bunions, calluses, corns, fungal infections, and ingrown toenails) can lead to devastating complications in diabetic patients. Prevention through proper foot care and early recognition and treatment are important considerations in the long term care of every diabetic patient. These problems are discussed in detail in Chapter 102.

Diabetic Nephropathy

Progressive renal failure is another life-threatening complication of diabetes. The relationship between hyperglycemia (or insulin deficiency) and the development of microangiopathy with eventual nodular glomerulosclerosis (Kimmelsteil-Wilson disease) remains to be unequivocally established, but experimental evidence is accumulating in favor of such a relationship. Moreover, from observations in man, it now seems clear that the factor is either hyperglycemia, *per se*, or some other factor in the internal milieu of the diabetic that is responsible for the development of diabetic renal disease, since kidney transplants in diabetic patients often develop typical lesions of diabetes.

The clinical course of diabetic nephropathy and the impact of failing renal function on insulin requirement and the oral hypoglycemic drugs are discussed in Chapter 47.

Infections

Although it has never been unequivocally established that diabetics are more prone to infections than nondiabetics, most clinicians will encounter patients who have experienced repeated bacterial or fungal skin infections (carbuncles, furuncles, external otitis, moniliasis) or gastrointestinal moniliasis at some time before the diagnosis of diabetes was made or in association with uncontrolled hyperglycemia. Most authorities seem to agree that—once established—infections in the diabetic are more difficult than usual to treat and patients are prone to develop complications. Experimentally, hyperglycemia inhibits the phagocytic activity of granulocytes, a factor which may contribute to lowered host resistance. Control of blood sugar, therefore, should be part of any treatment program for an infection.

Urinary tract infections are an especially troublesome problem in diabetics. Although infections are not clearly increased in incidence, a greater prevalence of complications is obvious. Half of all cases of papillary necrosis occur in diabetics. Diabetic patients also seem prone to develop infections with unusual pathogens. However, no statistical case has been made for the desirability of suppression of asymptomatic bacteriuria in diabetics. Development of pyelonephritis is an indication for immediate hospitalization and vigorous antibiotic treatment; risk of renal carbuncle formation is a special hazard for the diabetic.

Diabetic Retinopathy

This complication of diabetes mellitus has become one of the leading causes of blindness in the United States. In IDDM patients retinopathy can be detected by the most sensitive technique, angiography, after as little as 1 to 2 years in 10% of patients. By 10 years, retinopathy is evident in 50% of cases by ophthalmoscopy with a 70% prevalence by angiography. By the time diabetes has been present for 15 to 20 years, about one-third of patients have severe disease and another one-half have obvious but lesser degrees of progressive retinal involvement. Patients with NIDDM also develop retinopathy, apparently with less frequency (3), but when retinopathy does develop in this older group, the process seem to progress even more rapidly than it does in IDDM patients.

Blindness in Diabetic Retinopathy

The visual loss in diabetic retinopathy is potentially even more severe than in blindness due to other causes. Many persons who are legally blind (defined as visual acuity less than 20/200 in both eyes) due to causes other than diabetes have slow onset of visual loss, thus allowing time for adaptation. In addition, they often retain reasonably full visual fields and visual acuity at or close to the legal limit. Such persons can see well enough to ambulate independently and can perform a variety of common activities (self-care, housework). With the aid of special devices they may even be able to read newsprint and can engage in some occupations. In contrast, the visual loss of diabetic retinopathy is often due to sudden hemorrhage or retinal detachment and frequently leaves the patient with only light perception. In addition, the diabetic frequently already has other complications of the disease when blindness develops.

Although total blindness afflicts only a minority of diabetic patients (3), a larger number suffer some degree of loss of visual acuity due to macular edema, the commonest cause of visual loss in diabetics (see below).

Types of Retinal Disease in Diabetics

A crude but convenient classification of diabetic retinal disease is nonproliferative (synonym, "background"), preproliferative, and proliferative retinopathy. The latter, more advanced stage, is the point at which sudden and massive visual loss becomes a problem.

Nonproliferative and preproliferative retinopathy. The earliest lesions—readily visible with an ordinary ophthalmoscope—are the region of the macula: microaneurysms, punctate retinal hemorrhages, hard exudates, soft exudates ("cotton wool"), and so-called intraretinal microvascular anomalies (IRMAs). Both microaneurysms and small intraretinal hemorrhages appear as red dots, and both tend to fade within months. Distinction can best be made by fluorescein angiograms in which only microaneurysms "light up." This procedure often identifies extensive intraretinal disease when only a few abnormalities are evident by ophthalmoscopy.

Hard exudates are glistening yellow or white lipid

deposits located in the outer retinal layers. Soft exudates are areas of ischemia or infarction of the nerve fiber layer; they disappear within a few months. IRMAs are dilated, hypercellular vessels which are thought to represent either dilated capillaries or intraretinal vascular proliferation. These telangiectatic vessels are identifiable using the green filters of an ordinary ophthalmoscope but are best seen in the secondary phase of fluorescein angiograms during which they leak dye into the retina. IRMAs occur adjacent to areas of capillary closure.

While changes of background retinopathy indicate capillary damage and leakage, preproliferative changes (many soft exudates, extensive hemorrhages, IRMAs, and venous bleeding from larger retinal veins) indicate areas of intraretinal vascular occlusion with resulting nonperfusion. Decreased visual acuity at this stage requires an ophthalmologist's examination to determine with stereoscopic techniques whether *macular edema* is present. It is not usually appreciated by general physicians that even without proliferative disease, macular edema may result in visual loss as severe as the 20/200 level. Spontaneous improvement is not common but may occur. Visual acuity can also become poor due to lack of proper perfusion of the perifoveal capillaries. In this instance, visual acuity may be as low as 20/200 in the absence of macular edema. Fluorescein angiography will reveal the cause of poor visual acuity due to the lack of perfusion of the perifoveal capillaries. In the absence of accompanying proliferative disease, patients at this stage can usually ambulate freely and can engage in some occupations. Ability to read a newspaper, except with a vision aid, is unlikely, and the patient will have to relinquish driving a vehicle because driver's license vision requirements will no longer be met.

Eyes with retinal ischemia and moderate to severe preproliferative changes have a 50% chance of developing new vessel proliferation (neovascularization) within 1 year.

Proliferative retinopathy. At this stage of retinal disease, new vessels and accompanying fibrous tissue grow along the posterior suface of the vitreous gel, often causing contraction of the gel and traction on the vessels and the retina. This process creates the conditions for retinal detachment and hemorrhage into the vitreous.

Treatment of Diabetic Retinopathy

Two forms of surgical therapy are now available for the treatment of proliferative retinopathy and its complications. Photocoagulation is of proven value in the prevention of visual loss due to proliferative disease, while vitrectomy restores and appears to stabilize vision after hemorrhage and/or retinal detachment.

Photocoagulation therapy. Since the introduction of the xenon arc photocoagulator in 1959, the approach and rationale of therapy have changed markedly. While the xenon arc polychromatic light source has continued in use, monochromatic devices such as the argon laser have also been extensively used. Initially, therapy was directed at patches of proliferating vessels, but it became apparent that such treatment was not effective in stabilizing proliferative disease. It was noted, however, that in some patients destruction of a large portion of the peripheral retina seemed to arrest the proliferative process. Eventually this approach led to an interinstitutional study called the National Diabetic Retinopathy Study (DRS). One eye of each patient with advanced preproliferative or proliferative retinopathy was treated with either xenon arc or argon laser photocoagulation. The other eye was not treated. Multiple (several hundred) burns were placed in the retinal periphery. Within a few years the efficacy of both light sources was established in treatment of nearly 2000 patients. A reduction of severe visual loss of nearly 60% was apparent in patients with proliferative disease (10).

At this time, the place of laser treatment of macular edema by a study such as the DRS has not been established. Some authorities believe that such therapy is ineffective and may actually decrease central vision, but the issue is not settled. Laser treatment for macular edema and the benefit of earlier use of peripheral retinal laser treatment in reducing visual loss are presently being evaluated in another large collaborative investigation, the Early Treatment Diabetic Retinopathy Study (ETDRS).

Patient experience. Photocoagulation therapy is an office procedure, usually performed in several sessions. Ordinarily only topical (corneal) anesthesia is necessary. Occasionally, some discomfort may be experienced, in which case a local anesthetic is injected into the retroorbital tissues to allow a completed, pain-free procedure.

Vitrectomy for proliferative retinopathy. Hemorrhage into the vitreous is the usual indication for vitrectomy, a procedure which removes old blood and opaque vitreous and can be combined with cataract extraction. Retinal detachment resulting from traction bands that are formed in the vitreous is another indication for vitrectomy. Other repair procedures can be attempted. Recently, as an extension of vitrectomy, the removal of preretinal membranes has been introduced.

The results of vitrectomy are dramatic in restoring sight after vitreous hemorrhage. In addition, stabilization of vision can be expected when the traction process is encroaching on the macula. Remarkably, vitrectomy appears to cause actual regression of proliferative retinopathy. However, it is a formidable procedure and is not currently recommended as a prophylactic intervention. Photocoagulation remains the treatment of choice for proliferative disease with vitrectomy reserved for cases in which photocoagulation has failed to prevent recurrent hemorrhages or vitreous hemorrhage is so severe that it will not clear spontaneously. The benefit of vitrectomy in the earlier stages of proliferative retinopathy is under active investigation in a newly initiated Diabetic Retinopathy Vitrectomy Study (DRVS).

Role of normalization of blood sugar and other measures. Some clinical evidence can be cited to indicate that the development of diabetic retinopathy is related to chronic hyperglycemia. However, *no* convincing evidence is as yet available to show that, once established, diabetic retinopathy can be reversed, stabilized, or improved by normalization of blood glucose. Studies examining this issue are under way. Nonetheless, almost all ophthalmologists urge that every effort be made to normalize blood glucose in the hope of a beneficial effect on the course of the retinopathy.

Every effort should be made to control hypertension in an effort to prevent retinal hemorrhages. Lifting of heavy objects and exposures to high altitudes may also increase the risk of hemorrhages and should be avoided.

Indications for Referral to an Ophthalmologist

All diabetic patients with evidence of background retinopathy or with decreasing visual acuity should be referred for follow-up to an ophthalmologist with expertise in retinal disease. In addition, frequent monitoring of intraocular pressure to detect glaucoma is mandatory in older diabetics (see Chapter 98). Prevention of blindness due to diabetes is now a reality. No longer is ophthalmological referral a mere formality in these cases.

DIABETES DURING PREGNANCY

Fetal Mortality

Statistics vary widely on the effect of diabetes on survival of the fetus. In some studies the more severe the diabetic state, the worse the perinatal survival, but other studies fail to show a close relationship. Agreement is present only in the case of patients with diabetic nephropathy (White Class F) or proliferative retinopathy (Class R). In these individuals perinatal survival appears to be diminished. Overall, and without regard to the severity of the disease, conventional therapy has resulted in 75 to 90% fetal survival. Ketoacidosis occurs in 2 to 10% of diabetic pregnancies and is associated in these cases with fetal losses of 80 to 100%.

Maternal Mortality and Morbidity

Maternal mortality during pregnancy is definitely increased and at 0.5% is about 20 times that in nondiabetics. Most deaths are due to ketoacidosis or to hypoglycemia, the latter usually occurring in the first trimester or immediately postpartum, times at which insulin requirements often decrease. Obviously, optimal management could eliminate most or all of these deaths. Some deaths which may not be preventable include infections following cesarean section or hemorrhage following traumatic delivery of a large infant. Diabetics with overt heart disease (ischemic heart disease, congestive heart failure) have a very high mortality (75%) when allowed to go to term. Such patients should never become pregnant or should have an abortion if pregnancy occurs.

Maternal morbidity also increases during the diabetic pregnancy. Polyhydramnios occurs in 25% of pregnancies (10 times greater incidence than expected). Asymptomatic bacteriuria (20%) and frank pyelonephritis (7%) occur 3 times more often than in the general population. Pyelonephritis is said to occur in 25% of bacteriuric diabetics and is associated with a very high rate of fetal loss.

Implications of Minimal Diabetes for the Pregnancy

Concern over the problems of the overtly diabetic mother and the fetus has resulted in attempts to determine the effects of even minimal diabetes on the pregnant state and in screening for the presence of diabetes by glucose tolerance tests. Identification of such diabetics has led to studies which purport to show increased perinatal mortality up to 3 to 4 times expected for the general population, while other studies have refuted such claims. The most extreme enthusiasts for identification of such individuals sometimes go on to treat with insulin in order to maintain postprandial blood sugar levels which are normal for pregnancy (lower than ordinary normal values; see Table 72.4). Claims have been made that these procedures can be followed in ambulatory patients without undue or unacceptable hypoglycemia. However, unless home blood glucose monitoring and other precautions (page 970) are taken, frequent and sometimes prolonged hospitalizations and multiple episodes of hypoglycemia almost invariably accompany such an approach. Moreover, no evidence has been presented that such therapeutic heroics significantly affect perinatal mortality. At present such therapy for minimal diabetes is experimental and cannot be considered to be established.

Diagnosis of Diabetes during Pregnancy

Diabetes developing *de novo* during pregnancy is termed gestational diabetes (page 957). No diagnostic problem exists when gross hyperglycemia occurs along with glucosuria. However, diagnosis by glucose tolerance testing *during* pregnancy requires special consideration. Since the FPG is normally 10 to 20 mg lower during pregnancy than in the non-pregnant state, special criteria for the diagnosis have been established (see Tables 72.3 and 72.4; note also that the dose of glucose is 100 g). Use of the OGTT for the diagnosis of diabetes is certainly dominant in nonpregnant individuals, but the intravenous glucose tolerance test (IVGTT) has a few strong supporters for pregnant patients. Unfortunately, no studies are available to indicate which test is better able to identify women at risk for diabetic complications of pregnancy.

Indications commonly used for testing include family history of diabetes, previous delivery of a large infant (> 4000 g; 8.8 lb), previous delivery of an infant with a congenital anomaly, previous unexplained stillbirth, polyhydramnios, obesity, and glucosuria. However, the criteria for obesity are vague, and a minor degree of glucosuria is frequent in normal pregnancy and may be seen in 25% of pregnant women, if a sensitive method of testing is used in the postprandial state. Use of these criteria will result in screening 25 to 50% of pregnant women with an OGTT, while only about 3 to 6% of women so tested will be found to be diabetic. Since the figure for the entire population of pregnant women is about 3%, the commonly used screening criteria are obviously not very useful. Others have proposed a preliminary oral glucose load of 50 g combined with a single blood glucose at 1 hour. Only those individuals with a value greater than 130 mg/100 ml are screened by an OGTT. This procedure correctly identifies 80 to 90% of diabetics but has 15 to 20% "false positives."

The rationale for labeling any individual whose OGTT meets the criteria in Table 72.4 as a diabetic is not clear. This approach makes no provision for a state of gestational glucose intolerance. Furthermore, in many studies the prognosis for the pregnant state and the perinatal morbidity of infants born of mothers with an abnormal OGTT but with essentially normal FPG does not differ from normal (see above). If one accepts the claim that perinatal mortality is increased in the infants of women with gestational diabetes discovered by OGTT, the question must then be asked whether therapy beyond that which is normally recommended to prevent excessive weight gain is warranted. The answer to this question receives no consensus. Some obstetricians tend to aggressive management, whereas internists are often reluctant to embark on complicated treatment programs which many consider to be of unproven value.

Management of Overt Diabetes during Pregnancy

Insulin Therapy

Patients with overt diabetes receiving insulin therapy should be monitored to establish optimal control of blood sugar. Although many obstetricians favor hospitalization with frequent daytime blood sugar determinations ("glucose panel") as an aid to establishment of optimal control, the procedure is useless unless patient compliance can be foreseen after the hospitalization.

Several studies have reported that "tight control" is associated with reduction of fetal loss from 25% to 3 or 4%. On the basis of this information, the goal of insulin and diet therapy should be the closest approximation of normalization of blood sugar that is possible while avoiding therapeutic heroics, *i.e.*, multiple and prolonged hospitalizations solely for the purpose of blood sugar control. Normal fasting blood sugar (not exceeding 85 mg/100 ml) and postprandial blood sugars which do not exceed 140 mg/100 ml would be considered "tight control" by most. However, some obstetricians using conventional therapy with insulin strive for blood sugar levels *averaging* 100 mg/100 ml, a goal probably impossible to achieve without prolonged hospitalizations and excessively frequent hypoglycemia. If normalization of blood sugar is attempted, either intensified conventional therapy or an insulin pump should be used in conjunction, of course, with home blood glucose monitoring (see page 970).

Most patients will require at least two doses of intermediate acting insulin or mixtures of intermediate and short acting insulin. A few NIDDM patients may have satisfactory control on a single dose of insulin. It should be kept in mind that insulin requirements often decrease in the first trimester only to rise progressively as pregnancy proceeds and to fall again after delivery. Frequent monitoring of glucosuria and ketonuria is an invaluable guide to ambulatory management, as it is in the nonpregnant patient, but only home glucose monitoring with frequent blood sugar determinations can provide optimal management. Minor ketonuria due to carbohydrate lack is common but can usually be distinguished by rough quantitation of the ketonuria, minimal or absent glucosuria, and, if necessary, measurement of the blood sugar. Determination of plasma bicarbonate and plasma "ketones" should be made if any doubt still exists. The development of ketoacidosis is an indication for immediate hospitalization.

Diet Therapy

Diet therapy is often modified slightly to include increased protein intake. Weight gain of about 25 lb (11.5 kg) is expected and acceptable in both normal and diabetic pregnancies. Severe weight control, previously advocated by some, has been abandoned.

Timing of Delivery

This issue has been argued for decades, since it was recognized that the incidence of stillbirths in diabetics increases beyond the 36th week. However, attempts to deliver infants early (before 40 weeks) has resulted in a high rate of cesarean section and a high rate of neonatal loss due to neonatal respiratory distress syndrome. Attempts have been made to determine fetal lung maturity by amniotic fluid phospholipid measurements (lecithin/sphingomyelin ratios). Other monitoring measurements include the urinary estradiol quantitation. These monitoring issues remain controversial and are largely determined by prevailing obstetrical dogma.

Counseling the Diabetic Woman—Risks of Pregnancy

The issue of the complexity of diabetic management is not likely to deter pregnancy. On the other hand, the possibility of diabetes in the newborn or young child is often of great concern; this issue has already been discussed (see "Inheritance and Genetic Counseling"). Other questions concern maternal and fetal mortality. While the diabetic mother without overt complications suffers little or no increased risk, the fetal issues must be presented with candor. Of special importance beyond that of infant survival is the problem of an increased risk of congenital abnormalities and long term neurological abnormalities in children of diabetic mothers (8). Hyperglycemia during the early weeks of pregnancy appears to account for the increased incidence of congenital malformations in infants born to diabetic mothers. Near normalization of blood sugar prior to conception and continued normalization through the critical first weeks has been reported to reduce this increased incidence to normal. Thus, preconception patient education and intensive therapy appear to be extremely important for young diabetic women who plan to become pregnant.

Whether complications of diabetes are accelerated by pregnancy is not clear. The long term survival of the diabetic with microvascular disease is already significantly compromised and an honest prognosis in this regard may deter pregnancy, not necessarily because of concern over acceleration of the diabetic complications, but out of concern for the future welfare of a child born to a mother whose state of health may be poor and whose survival is threatened.

General References

Davidson MB: *Diabetes mellitus. Diagnosis and treatment.* New York, John Wiley & Sons, 1981, 2 vols, (paperback).

This text contains a wealth of practical information for treatment of the ambulatory patient: numerous references to literature available to patients, diet, sources of aids for the visually impaired, syringe magnifiers, *etc.*

Diabetes Care. A publication of the American Diabetes Association since 1979.

This journal for the practitioner contains reviews and practical articles.

Ellenberg M, Rifkin H: *Diabetes Mellitus, Theory and Practice,* ed 3. Garden City, NY, Medical Examination Publishing Co, 1983.

This is the standard textbook on the subject.

National Diabetes Data Group: Classification and diagnosis of diabetes mellitus and other categories of glucose intolerance. *Diabetes* 28:1039, 1979.

The latest criteria for diagnosis; a milestone in our concepts

of the problem. Many references. Reprints available from: Westwood Building, Room 607, National Institutes of Health, Bethesda, MD 20205.

Podolsky S (ed): *Clinical Diabetes: Modern Management.* New York, Appleton-Century-Crofts, 1980.

A multiauthored text including some outstanding authorities. Many references, diet tables, photographs, *etc.* Especially good portions relevant to management of ambulatory patients.

Schade DS, Santiago JV, Skyler JS, Rizza RA: *Intensive Insulin Therapy.* Garden City, NY, Medical Examination Publishing Co, 1983.

This book presents in great detail the art and practice of intensive therapy with various regimens including insulin pumps.

Specific References

1. Bradley WE: Diagnosis of urinary bladder dysfunction in diabetes mellitus. *Ann Intern Med* 92 (part 2):323, 1980.
2. Cryer PE, Gerich JE: Glucose counterregulation, hypoglycemia, and intensive insulin therapy in diabetes mellitus. *N Eng J Med* 313:232, 1985.
3. Davidson MB: The continually changing "natural history" of diabetes mellitus. *J Chronic Dis* 34:5, 1981.
4. Ellenberg M: Sexual dysfunction in diabetic patients. *Ann Intern Med* 92 (part 2):331, 1980.
5. Ewing DJ, Campbell IW, Clarke BF: Assessment of cardiovascular effects in diabetic autonomic neuropathy and prognostic implications. *Ann Intern Med* 92 (part 2):308, 1980.
6. FILMS: Millner, Fenwick, Inc.: Diabetic Teaching Films. 2125 Greenspring Dr, Timonium, MD. 21093. NEWSLETTERS: *Diabetes in the News.* 233 East Erie Str, Suite 712, Chicago, IL 60611 (no charge; junior high school level or above); *Forecast.* 600 5th Ave., New York, NY 10020 (about $15/year; high school level or above).
7. Goldstein S, Podolsky S: Inheritance of diabetes and genetic counseling. In Podolsky S (ed): *Clinical Diabetes: Modern Management.* New York, Appleton-Century-Crofts. 1980, ch 1, p 1.
8. Haworth JC, McRae KN, Dilling LA: Prognosis of infants of diabetic mothers in relation to neonatal hypoglycemia. *Dev Med Child Neurol* 18:471, 1976.
9. National Diabetes Group: Classification and diagnosis of diabetes mellitus and other categories of glucose tolerance. *Diabetes* 28:1039, 1979.
10. Preliminary report on effects of photocoagulation therapy. *Am J Ophthalmol* 81:383, 1976.
11. Rizza R, Gerich J. Haymond M, *et al*: Control of blood sugar in insulin-dependent diabetes: comparison of an artificial endocrine pancreas, continuous subcutaneous insulin infusion and intensified conventional insulin therapy. *N Engl J Med* 303:1313, 1980.
12. Rushforth NB, Miller M, Bennett PH: Fasting and two-hour post-load glucose levels for the diagnosis of diabetes. *Diabetologia* 16:373, 1979.
13. Schade DS, Santiago JV, Skyler JS, Rizza RA: *Intensive Insulin Therapy.* Garden City, NY, Medical Examination Publishing Co, 1983, p 138.
14. Stamler R, Stamler J (eds): Asymptomatic hyperglycemia and coronary heart disease. A series of papers by the International Collaborative Group, based on studies in fifteen populations. *J Chronic Dis* 32:683, 1979.
15. Weissman PN, Shenkman L, Gregerman RI: Chlorpropamide hyponatremia. Drug-induced inappropriate antidiuretic-hormone activity. *N Engl J Med* 284:65, 1971.
16. West KM: Diet therapy of diabetes: an analysis of failure. *Ann Intern Med* 79:425, 1973.
17. West KM: Diet and diabetes. *Postgrad Med* 60:209, 1976.

CHAPTER SEVENTY-THREE

Thyroid Disorders*

ROBERT I. GREGERMAN, M.D.

INTRODUCTION

Disturbances of thyroid growth and function are among the most common endocrinological disorders encountered in ambulatory practice. Excessive production of the iodine-containing thyroid hormones, thyroxine (T_4) and triiodothyronine (T_3) (Fig. 73.1), results in hyperthyroidism, or thyrotoxicosis; decreased hormone production results in hypothyroidism. Generalized enlargement of the thyroid, regardless of cause, is termed goiter. Focal enlargement of the thyroid is termed a "nodule" and is usually benign. Either goiter or focal enlargement may be associated with abnormal thyroid function. Goiter can produce anatomical changes ranging from simply cosmetic to obstruction of contiguous structures such as the trachea and esophagus.

Thyroid Regulatory Mechanisms

The principal regulatory mechanism of the thyroid is the hypothalamic-pituitary-thyroid negative feedback control system. The hypothalamus secretes thyrotropin-releasing hormone (TRH), which travels *via* the hypophyseal portal system to the pituitary, where it stimulates release of thyroid-stimulating

---

* Substantial portions of this chapter were published in Gregerman RI: The thyroid gland. In Harvey AM, *et al* (eds): *The Principles and Practice of Medicine*, ed 21. New York, Appleton-Century-Crofts, 1984.

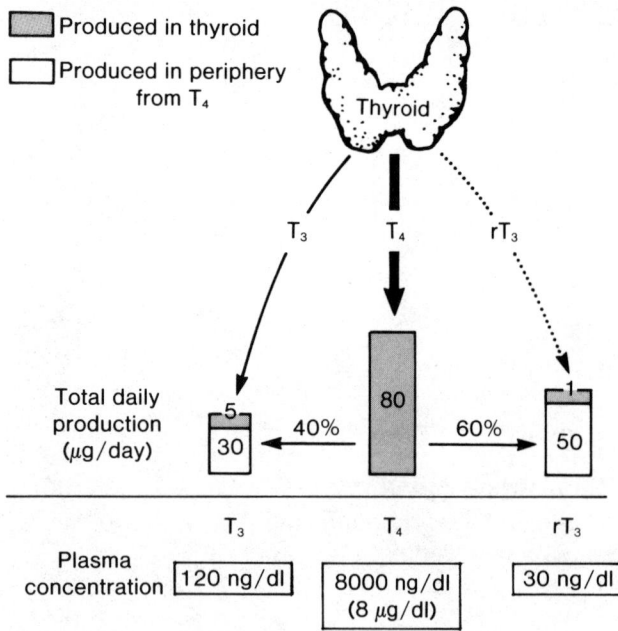

Figure 73.1. Production rates by the thyroid and in the periphery of thyroid hormones and their mean concentrations in the plasma.

hormone (TSH). TSH stimulates many aspects of thyroid activity, including hormone synthesis, thyroid growth, and the release of thyroid hormones. Secretion of TSH by the pituitary is inhibited by the thyroid hormones—thus the term "negative feedback loop."

Iodide from plasma is concentrated by an active process (iodide "pump") which can maintain a thyroid/plasma iodide ratio as high as 500 to 1. Iodide is thereafter converted through a series of enzymatic steps resulting in the formation of T_4 and T_3 within the thyroglobulin sequence. The iodide pump transports a number of anions other than iodide, a phenomenon which has been exploited diagnostically and therapeutically. For example, the pertechnetate anion, TcO_4^-, as the radioactive isotope ^{99m}Tc, has been widely used for thyroid imaging, although ^{123}I is now preferred.

The minimal daily requirement of iodide is only about 100 to 200 μg, an amount which is determined by obligatory loss, mainly through the kidney. The minimal daily requirement is enormously exceeded by dietary intake; for example, iodinated salt provides about 1000 μg in a normal 10-g daily intake. Thus, iodide deficiency, once common in the United States and elsewhere, is essentially unknown except in remote areas of the underdeveloped world.

Any chemical substance that interferes with thyroid hormone function or release may lower blood hormone concentration and induce compensatory hypertrophy of the gland (goiter) *via* stimulation of TSH secretion. Certain substances are known to

prevent iodide accumulation by impairment of the iodide "pump." Other substances interfere with hormone synthesis or inhibit hormone release. Clinically useful agents which have been employed for therapeutic effects in states of excess hormone production (hyperthyroidism) are known to act at one or another of these points. Perchlorate, no longer commonly used therapeutically, inhibits the iodide "pump." The thiocarbamide drugs interfere with hormone synthesis by blockade of incorporation of iodide into the tyrosines ("organification") and of the coupling reactions in iodothyronine formation, but have more effect on coupling than on organification. Lithium ion (currently in wide use for the treatment of affective disorders, Chapter 15), interferes with thyroglobulin proteolysis and hormone release and may result in goiter and, occasionally, hypothyroidism. Iodide itself in pharmacological amounts interferes with hormone formation and release and in some individuals is a goitrogen.

Metabolic Effects of Thyroid Hormone

The thyroid hormones exert their actions through a variety of mechanisms. A classic thyroid hormone effect is on metabolic rate. Measurement of basal metabolic rate (BMR) was the basis for the first laboratory method for clinical assessment of thyroid status. The numerous known actions of thyroid hormone range from specific stimulation of mitochondrial oxidative metabolism to the nuclear regulation of protein synthesis. Thyroid hormones also exert specific regulatory effects on membrane physiology, e.g., potentiation of catecholamine effects. This action of thyroid hormones explains the signs of exaggerated sympathetic activity in hyperthyroidism and the effectiveness of the therapy of this condition by β-adrenergic blockade.

Hormone Transport

The thyroid hormones in the blood are T_4 and a much smaller quantity of T_3. Both hormones are tightly but reversibly bound to several plasma proteins, mainly thyroid hormone-binding globulin (TBG). In the normal person 65 to 70% of the thyroid hormones are bound to TBG, about 15% to the secondary carrier, thyroxine-binding prealbumin (TBPA), and about 15% to albumin. Variations of TBG occur in many clinical states and account for most of the changes in T_4 concentration in plasma that are seen in diseases other than hypo- and hyperthyroidism. Small quantities of T_4 (0.03%) and T_3 (0.3%) are not protein bound but are unbound or "free" and in rapid equilibrium with the protein-bound fraction.

The concentrations of free T_4 and T_3 in plasma are thought to reflect the amount of hormone exerting an effect on tissues. Clinical status in a number of conditions correlates with free T_4 rather than with

Table 73.1.
Factors Affecting Thyroxine-Binding Globulin (TBG)

TBG INCREASED
    Estrogens:
        Oral contraceptives
        Pregnancy
    Hypothyroidism
    Acute hepatitis
    Cirrhosis
    Genetic TBG excess
    Acute intermittent porphyria
    Perphenazine (Trilafon)
TBG DECREASED
    Androgens
    Anabolic steroids
    Cirrhosis
    Glucocorticoids
    Nephrotic syndrome
    Severe chronic nonthyroidal illness
    Cushing's syndrome
    Genetic TBG deficiency

total hormone in plasma. A good example of this correlation is the normal pregnant state in which total T_4 is high, but in which there is no evidence of free thyroid hormone excess. The explanation is that plasma TBG is elevated, a consequence of the hyperestrogenism of pregnancy.

In some pathological states that affect the quantity of TBG in plasma (Table 73.1), and hence the total T_4, the absolute concentration of free T_4 may not adjust to a normal value. During a variety of nonthyroidal illnesses, factors other than the concentration of TBG and TBPA appear to determine the free hormone concentration, presumably by affecting the affinity of the TBG-T_4 interaction.

Metabolism and Interconversion of Thyroid Hormones

Practically all tissues metabolize and degrade the thyroid hormones, but the liver is quantitatively most important as a site at which regulation of hormone degradation occurs. T_4 metabolism is the major source (80%) of circulating T_3 in the normal individual. The normal thyroid secretes mainly T_4 and only a small amount of T_3 (Fig. 73.1). Only in hyperthyroidism, iodine deficiency, and in certain other pathological circumstances is T_3 sometimes the predominantly secreted hormone.

Most of the T_4 secreted (about 85%) is ultimately deiodinated and further degraded. The physiologically most important pathway involves conversion of about 35% of the T_4 to metabolically active T_3, which is itself further deiodinated. About an equal amount of T_4 is converted to reverse T_3 (rT_3) (Fig. 73.1). Although not active in calorigenesis, rT_3 does antagonize a number of the effects of T_3 and thus may have some physiological importance. In a variety of pathological states the formation of T_3 is inhibited, whereas that of rT_3 is reciprocally enhanced. Measurement of rT_3 has some usefulness in the differential diagnosis of the "euthyroid sick syndrome" (see "Differential Diagnosis" under "Hypothyroidism").

LABORATORY TESTS OF THYROID FUNCTION AND OF THYROID DISEASE

Most thyroid "function" tests assess secretory activity of the thyroid gland only indirectly. Measurements of blood hormone concentrations, the most commonly used tests, cannot be equated directly with the rate of hormone production, although they reflect that rate when plasma binding of hormones is normal. However, various illnesses, drugs, and alterations of physiological state affect plasma binding. Accordingly, proper interpretation of plasma hormone concentrations demands concomitant assessment of plasma binding. Thyroid gland function can be assessed somewhat more directly by measurement of thyroidal iodide accumulation ("uptake"; RaIU) using isotopes of iodide (^{131}I, ^{123}I). These tests also must be properly interpreted, since uptake of tracer is only an approximation of the accumulation of stable iodide and of hormone synthesis.

Other laboratory tests are useful in the assessment of thyroid status and in the diagnosis of thyroid disease but are not, strictly speaking, tests of thyroid function. Such tests include measurements of the integrity of the physiological feedback control system (plasma TSH concentration before and after stimulation by administered TRH), thyroid autoantibodies, and the immunoglobulins related to Graves' disease.

Measurements of Plasma Hormones: Plasma T_4 and T_3

The commonly used and important tests of thyroid function are measurements of the levels of T_4 and T_3, as determined by radioimmunoassay or other specific methods. Unlike the case with older techniques, no chemical interference is produced by drugs or iodine-containing substances, but it must be kept in mind that such agents may affect the actual level of thyroid hormones in blood. rT_3 is occasionally also used in differential diagnosis, especially of ill patients. The value of T_4 is certainly the single most important measurement in clinical evaluation of thyroid disease. However, interpretation of a given value (concentration) *must* take into account whether T_4 binding to plasma proteins is normal. Accordingly, T_4 must be measured in conjunction with assessment of hormone binding to plasma proteins or with determination of TBG. In practice this is done by determining the "free T_4" or the "free T_4 index" (see below). Normal values of the common tests are given in Table 73.2.

Table 73.2.
Thyroid Function Tests[a]

	Plasma T_4 (μg/dl)	Plasma T_3 (ng/dl)	T_3 Resin Uptake (T_3U) (%)	T_3 Resin Uptake Ratio (T_3UR)	TSH (μU/ml)	Free T_4 (FT_4) (ng/dl)	Free T_4 Index (FTI)[b]
Normal mean	8	120	30	1		1.5	8.0
Normal range	5–12	80–160	25–35	0.85–1.15	0–6	1.0–2.0	5.8–10.6
Confidence limits	±1	±20	±2	±0.05	±2	±0.3	

[a] See the text for limitations of interpretation of normal ranges. Confidence limits (95%) of a single value are approximate and depend on both the laboratory and the level within the range.
[b] The FTI on any sample is calculated as $T_4 \times T_3$UR, but the normal range for the FTI is determined empirically. The units of the FTI depend on whether the percentage T_3 resin uptake or the T_3 resin uptake ratio is multiplied times T_4.

"Free T_4": Measurement of Non-Protein-Bound Thyroid Hormone in Plasma

The "free T_4" of plasma is estimated by separate measurements of the non-protein-bound T_4 (usually by equilibrium dialysis) and the total T_4; their arithmetic product equals the free T_4. The dialyzable (non-protein-bound) T_4 normally approximates only 0.03% of the total.

The free T_4 hypothesis (see page 988) has been helpful as a physiological concept. Determination of the free T_4 for clinical purposes is often useful, but the measurement has serious limitations. In some states, such as pregnancy or during estrogen therapy, both T_4 and TBG are elevated and thyroid status is accurately reflected by the free T_4. The dialyzable fraction is decreased, but since the T_4 is elevated, the free T_4 is normal. In hyperthyroidism, free T_4 reflects thyroid status better than total T_4; since the altered metabolic state itself lowers TBG; in some cases a normal or borderline elevation of T_4 is associated with an elevated free T_4. In hypothyroidism, TBG is often elevated and the free T_4 is decreased more than is the total T_4.

Problems of interpretation of the free T_4 arise in many seriously ill patients. A variety of nonthyroidal diseases ranging from acute infections to liver disease can result in elevation of the free T_4. In these situations, the patient is usually euthyroid with a normal T_4, the free T_4 is elevated only because the dialyzable fraction is increased. An explanation for this phenomenon is not readily available. Altered concentrations of neither TBG nor TBPA account for the increased free T_4. The appearance of a factor in plasma which interferes with protein binding of T_4 has recently been demonstrated. Thus, an elevated free T_4 is not a specific finding related solely to thyroid status. Moreover, the test is several times more expensive than the "free T_4 index" which is to be preferred as the single most effective screening test of thyroid function (see below).

Estimates of TBG: T_3 Resin Uptake and "Free T_4 Index" (FTI)

The T_3 uptake test (T_3U) is not to be confused with the concentration of T_3 in plasma. The T_3U is not a thyroid function test, but merely provides an indirect estimate of the concentration of plasma TBG. To some extent, T_3U is also influenced by the quantity of T_4 in plasma, i.e., by the degree of saturation of the T_4 (and T_3) binding sites on TBG. The T_3U is beginning to be replaced by direct quantitation of TBG. Technically the T_3U is measured by adding a tracer quantity of T_3 and a nonspecific T_3 binding absorbent(resin) to the sample of plasma to be tested. The tracer distributes itself between nonspecific binding sites on the resin and specific binding sites on TBG. Resin-bound tracer is therefore reciprocally related to the quantity of TBG in the plasma. The test result is expressed either as a percent or as a ratio of the test sample to that of the laboratory's control plasma (T_3U ratio).

The usefulness of the T_3U is in interpreting a given level of T_4. A high (or low) T_4 can be interpreted as reflecting increased or decreased T_4 secretion only if the plasma binding of T_4 is normal, i.e., only if the TBG (T_3U) is normal. Otherwise, to reach a proper conclusion about thyroid function, disturbance of binding must be considered along with the high (or low) T_4. For convenience the T_4 and T_3U have been combined to give a so-called free T_4 index (FTI) by simply multiplying one number times the other. This widely used index "compensates" for the high or low T_4 value which results from abnormality of TBG concentration. In most, but not all, cases, FTI closely parallels free T_4.

In severely ill patients of the type more likely to be hospitalized than to be ambulatory, the FTI may be misleading. In such cases the resin uptake is elevated, not because TBG is low but as the result of the appearance in plasma of a nonspecific inhibitor of hormone binding which affects the distribution of tracer T_3 between sites in plasma and sites on the resin. Both the free T_4 and FTI tests must be interpreted with caution in any patient with severe nonthyroidal illness.

Tests of the Negative Feedback System

Thyroid-Stimulating Hormone

Plasma TSH is invariably elevated in primary hypothyroidism because of reduced feedback inhibition by the decreased concentrations of the thyroid hormones. The measurement of plasma TSH is important both in the diagnosis of primary hypothyroidism and in monitoring the adequacy of thyroid hormone replacement therapy (see below). Elevation of plasma TSH is the most sensitive indicator of hypothyroid status. Elevations of TSH are reliably measured by radioimmunoassay techniques currently available. However, by most assay methods plasma TSH of normal subjects is below the sensitivity of the method; many of the values reported to be within the normal range are nonspecific. Therefore, the plasma TSH, as ordinarily determined, cannot be used to detect secondary hypothyroidism (pituitary TSH deficiency); a "normal" TSH does not exclude this diagnosis.

Suppression Tests: Use of T₄ and T₃

In several thyroid diseases, gland function becomes independent of TSH, i.e., nonsuppressible by amounts of exogenous thyroid hormone that inhibit normal pituitary secretion of TSH. Nonsuppressibility is seen in hyperthyroidism due to any cause, in cases of hyperfunctioning adenoma ("hot nodule") with or without hyperthyroidism, and in 50% of cases of nontoxic nodular goiter. About one-half of patients with Graves' ophthalmopathy without hyperthyroidism have nonsuppressible thyroid function. Return of suppressibility in the course of Graves' disease indicates clinical remission, and the test is therefore a useful guide to therapy as well as to diagnosis. The test has been for the most part superseded by the TRH test (see below). Testing for suppressibility is done with T_3 or T_4 with the use of a 50% decrease of radioiodide uptake as the end point. T_4 is given as a single 3-mg dose or 25 μg of T_3 are given every 8 hours. Radioiodide uptake is measured at 6 to 8 days (see below).

The TRH Test

Parenterally administered TRH produces release of TSH from the pituitary. Response to TRH is abnormal in several clinical circumstances and is diagnostically useful. Confirmation of a diagnosis of primary hypothyroidism is possible when the plasma TSH elevation is borderline, since an exaggerated plasma TSH response will be seen. The *increment* of TSH following TRH does not normally exceed 30 μU/ml, but elevations several times this amount may be seen in cases of borderline hypothyroidism. The most common use of the test is as an alternative to the T_3 suppression test in the diagnosis of hyperthyroidism. Hypersecretion of thyroid hormones producing even minimal elevation of blood hormone levels blunts or abolishes the normal response to TRH. The TRH test is also useful in the differential diagnosis of severely ill patients with low plasma T_4 (see "Hypothyroidism *versus* Euthyroid Sick Syndrome"). The TRH test is of limited use

in the elderly in whom lack of TRH response can be normal.

The test is performed by injecting 500 μg of TRH intravenously. Plasma TSH is measured before injection and at 20 and 30 minutes. A significant response is an increase of more than 2 μU/ml. The general physician can easily perform the TRH test in his office. (The TRH (Thypinone) can be bought through any commercial pharmacy.)

Thyroidal Radioiodide Uptake (RaIU) Tests

The rate of tracer iodide accumulation (^{131}I, ^{123}I) in the thyroid can be measured by using times ranging from a few minutes to the plateau of accumulation (24 hours). These procedures, although still in wide use, have been rendered almost obsolete by the simpler and less expensive measurements of hormone concentrations in plasma. The diagnostic usefulness of the RaIU is also seriously limited by the "saturation" of Western diets with iodide. This has resulted in RaIU values that are too low to discriminate normal function from hypofunction, so that the test is now useless for the diagnosis of hypothyroidism. It is still of use in hyperthyroidism, although, since results are "normal" in up to 50% of cases of hyperthyroidism, a normal RaIU does not exclude the diagnosis. One important use of the test is in patients with hyperthyroidism associated with thyroiditis. If this condition is suspected, an RaIU is important; a low value deters inappropriate therapy. The RaIU is also subject to interference by chemical agents and certain clinical states; both produce false positive and false negative results. The RaIU should no longer be used for the *routine* evaluation of thyroid function.

Immunological Tests

Assay of antibodies to thyroidal antigens (thyroglobulin, microsomes), so-called thyroid autoantibodies, is useful in determining the presence of autoimmune thyroiditis (see below, page 1002, "Hashimoto's Disease"). Measurement of thyroid-stimulating immunoglobulin (TSI) (see "Graves' Disease") is not yet readily available. The long acting thyroid stimulation (LATS) test, still available in some laboratories, is useless. TSI measurements when available, are useful in the pregnant patient, since high levels are associated with an increased likelihood of neonatal hyperthyroidism. A fall in TSI is a good indicator of remission in Graves' disease and will probably be useful for this purpose as the test becomes available.

Other Tests: Imaging and Biopsies

Various *scintiscan or imaging techniques* are available to delineate the anatomy of the thyroid and to distinguish functional from nonfunctional tissue, a consideration in the differential diagnosis of thyroid neoplasms. Currently, ^{99m}Tc pertechnetate (TcO_4^-) is most widely used, but ^{123}I is the imaging agent of choice. (Some tumors will accumulate pertechnetate, thereby obscuring the diagnosis.)

Ultrasound imaging (sonography) is now a routine procedure for distinguishing cystic from solid nodules, an important point in differential diagnosis of these lesions. Moreover, ultrasound can accurately assess the size of nodules, providing an objective basis for evaluation of medical therapy.

Needle biopsy is rapidly assuming the status of a routine procedure in many centers. In proper hands, needle biopsy is a safe, outpatient procedure which gives a diagnosis in most cases. *Fine needle aspiration* with cytological examination is not as reliable as needle aspiration biopsy. Although both procedures may fail to distinguish benign adenomas from well differentiated follicular carcinomas (13), an important limitation of the technique, the procedure undoubtedly helps to avoid many operations and may provide much needed reassurance for the patient. Needle biopsy is performed ordinarily by an endocrinologist or a surgeon who has been trained in the technique. The procedure, performed under local (cutaneous) anesthesia, is ordinarily painless. The only significant complication is local hemorrhage, but this is uncommon and usually of minor degree. Fine needle aspiration is without complications. Neither needle biopsy nor fine needle aspiration should be used unless the pathologist is specifically trained to interpret the biopsy material.

Nonspecificity of Thyroid Function Tests in Nonthyroidal Illness

The clinician should realize that thyroid function tests may be nonspecifically altered in many nonthyroidal diseases, i.e., these tests are *not specific* when severe illness is present (Table 73.3). Moreover, a variety of drugs affect both thyroid function and the function tests (Tables 73.1 and 73.4). Some examples of these considerations are presented below; extensive discussions can be found elsewhere (2, 7, 9, 21, 22).

Table 73.3.
Nonthyroidal Illness: Effects on T_4, Free T_4, and TBG in Plasma[a]

	Effects on T_4	Free T_4	TBG
LIVER DISEASE			
Active hepatitis	↑	↔↑	↑
Cirrhosis	↑↓	↔↑	↑↓
Cholangitis	↑	↔↑	↑
RENAL DISEASE			
Nephrotic syndrome	↔↓	↔	↔↓
Uremia, chronic	↔↓	↔↓	↔↓
INFECTIONS	↓	↑	↔
MALNUTRITION	↔↓	↔↑	↔↓

[a] Most illnesses and even such minor alterations of physiological state as decreased food intake will produce a decrease of plasma T_3.

Table 73.4.
Drug and Hormone Effects on Plasma T_4 and TBG

Gonadal Hormones	Effect on T_4	Free T_4	Effect on TBG
ESTROGENS	↑	↔↓	↑
Oral contraceptives			
Pregnancy			
ANDROGENS	↓	↔	
Testosterone		↑	
Anabolic steroids			
GLUCOCORTICOIDS	↓	↔	↓
Cushing's syndrome			
Pharmacological uses			
PSYCHOTROPIC DRUGS			
Perphenazine (Trilafon)	↑	↔	↑
Amphetamines	↑	↑	↔
ANTICONVULSANTS			
Phenytoin (Dilantin)	↓	↔↓	↔
HEPARIN	↔	↑	↔
ADRENERGIC BLOCKERS			
Propranolol (Inderal)	↔(↓T_3)	↔	↔
ANTIARRHYTHMIC DRUGS			
Amiodarone	↑	↑	↔
GALLBLADDER DYES	↑↔(↓T_3)	↔↑	↔
Iopanoic acid	↑↔(↓T_3)	↔↑	↔
Ipodate	↑↔(↓T_3)	↔↑	↔

Effects of Gonadal and Adrenal Hormones

Estrogens (pregnancy, contraceptives) raise, and androgens lower, T_4 by altering plasma TBG. Glucocorticoids inhibit thyroid activity acutely by interfering with TSH secretion and affect the pituitary's responsiveness to TRH. The plasma T_4 is lowered during chronic glucocorticoid therapy, due mainly to a decrease of TBG. When dexamethasone is given acutely, the plasma T_4 decreases slightly and T_3 falls sharply.

Liver Diseases

Various alterations of thyroid function tests are produced by liver diseases. Early in infectious hepatitis, the T_4 is elevated secondary to an increase of TBG. Chronic liver disease produces many abnormalities in an unpredictable fashion. T_4 may be increased or decreased in parallel with TBG and the T_3U. Free T_4 is often elevated with no obvious relationship to the TBG. T_3 is usually low. A frequent and unexplained abnormality is elevation of TSH, although the response to TRH is not exaggerated as it is in hypothyroidism. RaIU is often elevated in acute alcoholic hepatitis with or without cirrhosis and in some cases of cholangitis. These changes have been attributed both to iodide depletion and to acceleration of T_4 metabolism.

Renal Diseases

The nephrotic syndrome is often associated with depressed T_4, but the decrease is not always explained by a lowering of the TBG. In chronic renal disease, the means of T_4, TBG, and the FTI are not significantly different from normal, but the range is greater and values may exceed the usual normal limits. Some patients with severe chronic renal failure receiving long term dialysis show a progressive decrease of T_4. These patients and those with the nephrotic syndrome may represent examples of the recently recognized "euthyroid sick syndrome" (see "Hypothyroidism"). As one would expect in any chronic illness, the plasma T_3 is depressed.

Infections, Malnutrition, and Drugs

The T_4 may drop early in the course of acute infection and free T_4 may rise. Neither change is accounted for by an alteration of TBG. During starvation, plasma T_3 falls. Free T_4 is often increased without relation to the TBG. Plasma T_3 is often decreased in the elderly, a change which has been attributed to aging, but is in fact due to diminished food intake and nonspecific illness. Closely correlated alterations of T_3U and plasma TBG have been reported in protein-calorie malnutrition. Some pharmacological agents affect the thyroid hormones of plasma (1). Phenytoin (Dilantin) lowers the T_4 and free T_4, often into the hypothyroid range. Although plasma TSH may be somewhat elevated, clinical hypothyroidism is not seen. Heparin acutely elevates the free T_4. The mechanisms of these changes are not known. Propranolol decreases plasma T_3 by inhibition of the normal T_4 deiodination route; rT_3 is increased. A similar decrease of T_3 through reduced hepatic metabolism of T_4 is produced by propylthiouracil, dexamethasone, the antiarrhythmic drug, amiodarone, and the radiopaque contrast media used for visualization of the gallbladder, iopanoic acid and ipodate. In the case of the latter agents, additional mechanisms are operative, since these compounds also elevate T_4 and TSH, an effect attributed to their inhibition of conversion of T_4 and T_3 in the pituitary as well as in the periphery. Amphetamine abuse may increase plasma T_4, presumably by central stimulation of TSH release (2).

Altered Plasma T_4 Due to Inherited Abnormalities of Protein Binding

In addition to those disease states in which T_4 levels are related to altered hormone binding to TBG, other situations that are explicable in terms of altered protein binding include inherited disorders of TBG excess, TBG deficiency, increases of concentration of TBPA, and increases of the number of T_4 binding sites on an albumin variant. The first two conditions are X-linked. The latter two conditions, inherited as autosomal dominants, are rare. Both can produce diagnostic difficulties, however, since neither is detected by the T_3 resin uptake; the free T_4 index is accordingly elevated in both situations, although the free T_4 is normal (2).

Alterations of Plasma T_4 in Nonthyroidal Illness Not Due to Abnormalities of Protein Binding

Elevations of T_4 that are unexplained by changes in thyroxine binding are quite common. These situations are most difficult to distinguish from hyperthyroidism. Included are the elevation of T_4 seen in acute nonthyroidal illness, in psychiatric disease, and as the effect of some drugs. The stress of serious illness may also lower T_4 and simulate hypothyroidism, but such severe illness is not ordinarily encountered in ambulatory patients. An exception may be seen in patients undergoing treatment by dialysis for chronic renal failure. Abnormal thyroid hormone levels in these situations and diseases that are regularly associated with such changes are described briefly below and reviewed in more detail elsewhere (2, 7, 9, 21, 22).

Increase of plasma T_4 during nonspecific illness. Although the phenomenon of decreased T_4 during severe illness is now widely recognized (see above), the frequent occurrence of increased T_4 (and FTI) due to illness is not generally appreciated. The increase of T_4 is modest and the T_4 generally does not exceed about 15 μg. This problem is commonly seen in severely ill elderly patients in whom it raises the issue of hyperthyroidism.

Acute psychiatric illness. Restlessness, hyperactivity, tachycardia, and tremor are often seen as part of severe, acute psychiatric illness. Clinical suspicion of hyperthyroidism leads to thyroid function tests and laboratory results consistent with this diagnosis. Such patients may have elevated T_4, FTI, and T_3. In some series up to one-third of acutely hospitalized psychiatric patients present with an elevated T_4. Although the phenomenon is documented only in hospitalized patients, it might be encountered in any severely disturbed individual. The T_4 returns to normal within 1 to 2 weeks of clinical improvement of the psychiatric disturbance.

Increased plasma T_4 due to resistance to thyroid hormones. A rare but well recognized condition of increased T_4 unaccompanied by binding protein abnormalities is that of peripheral resistance to thyroid hormones. Originally described as a familial syndrome of increased T_4, goiter, deaf mutism, and some degree of hypothyroidism with delayed bone maturation and epiphyseal stippling, the most common situation is actually that of elevated T_4 in a phenotypically normal individual without evidence of hyperthyroidism. The abnormality occurs both sporadically and in familial form and is probably a heterogeneous group of disorders with variable inheritance (23).

Interpretation of Thyroid Function Tests: Statistical Considerations

No single numerical value divides normal from abnormal in any thyroid function test. The upper and lower limits of normal for plasma T_4, free T_4

index, and T_3 are set at ±2 standard deviations from the mean. By definition, therefore, 2.5% of normal persons will have abnormal values at each end of the distribution. To complicate the issue, a small number of hyperthyroid or hypothyroid persons have values that fall within the normal range. In addition to the statistical overlap, one must recall that both biological day-to-day variation and unavoidable analytic error further obscure the dividing line between normal and abnormal. For example, 95% confidence limits of a single T_4 test are ±1 μg/dl at the upper and lower limits of the normal range. For all of these reasons, and because of the occasional instance of laboratory or reporting error, a single determination can neither establish nor exclude a diagnosis with anything more than reasonable statistical certainty. Therefore, all abnormal values should be confirmed before therapy is undertaken.

HYPERTHYROIDISM (THYROTOXICOSIS)

Hyperthyroidism, the clinical state resulting from an excess of thyroid hormone, is the most common functional disorder of the thyroid. Although essentially the same clinical picture results from any of several distinct pathological processes (Table 73.5), selection of proper therapy demands that the correct diagnosis be established. The most common variety of hyperthyroidism is Graves' disease, an autoimmune process also known as diffuse toxic goiter. Only slightly less common is hyperthyroidism due to a hyperfunctioning nodular goiter (toxic nodular goiter). Occasionally hyperthyroidism is due to a solitary hyperfunctioning adenoma. Recently hyperthyroidism has been seen with increasing frequency

Table 73.5.
Causes of Hyperthyroidism[a]

COMMON
  Graves' disease
  Toxic nodular goiter
    Multinodular
    Uninodular
  Hyperthyroidism in association with thyroiditis
  Iodide induced (iodide, iodine-containing drugs and contrast media)
RARE TO VANISHINGLY RARE
  Thyrotoxicosis due to TSH or TSH-like stimulator
    Choriocarcinoma or hydatidiform mole
    Embryonal cell carcinoma of testis
    Pituitary tumor with TSH excess
    Idiopathic TSH excess
  Toxic thyroid carcinoma
  Hyperthyroidism due to exogenous thyroid hormone
    Factitia
    Medicamentosa (iatrogenic)
  Toxic struma ovarii

[a] Listed in approximate decreasing order of frequency.

as a transient phenomenon in the evolution of thyroiditis (8, 15, 20). In addition, the induction of hyperthyroidism by iodide and iodide-containing drugs and contrast media has received considerable attention and should be kept in mind for those patients who have had such exposures (4). The other causes of hyperthyroidism listed in Table 73.5 are so rare that they are not usually encountered in ordinary practice.

Graves' Disease

Graves' disease is a complex disorder comprising toxic goiter, ophthalmopathy, and occasionally dermopathy. At any given time during the course of the disease, one of these manifestations may be an isolated finding. Graves' ophthalmopathy and Graves' dermopathy can occur independently of thyroid hormone excess. Recently, the view has been expressed that ophthalmopathy and dermopathy are closely related but separate and overlapping immunological disorders (19).

Various abnormal immunoglobulins are found in the plasma of patients with Graves' disease. Some of these immunoglobulins have TSH-like activity and are designated thyroid-stimulating immunoglobulins; they are antibodies to the normal receptor sites for TSH. The reasons for development of abnormal immunoglobulins in Graves' disease are not clearly understood. Recent thinking views Graves' disease as a failure of T cell surveillance rather than as a response to thyroid antigens released from thyroid damaged by unknown causes (19).

The plasma of some patients with Graves' ophthalmopathy contains a factor (exophthalmos-producing substance (EPS)), which produces exophthalmos and other abnormalities of orbital tissues in suitable test animals. In Graves' ophthalmopathy, the extraocular muscles show interstitial edema, increased connective tissue, fatty infiltration, and infiltration with lymphocytes. Eventually, gross degenerative changes such as fibrosis may occur (see "Ophthalmopathy of Graves' Disease," below).

Dermopathy, an unique, albeit unusual, finding in Graves' disease, consists of more or less circumscribed areas of mucopolysaccharide deposition, typically over the shins—hence the term "pretibial myxedema." This unfortunate designation unjustifiably suggests a relationship between the very different type of generalized mucopolysaccharide deposition in hypothyroidism and the localized deposition in Graves' disease. No relationship exists between these processes.

Clinical Presentation and Diagnosis of Hyperthyroidism

Historical Features

The presentation of the patient with hyperthyroidism is highly variable (Table 73.6). The severity

Table 73.6.
Signs and Symptoms of Hyperthyroidism

Organ or System	Signs and Symptoms
ADRENERGIC MANIFESTATIONS	Excess sweating, heat intolerance, palpitations, tachycardia, tremor, lid lag, stare, nervousness, and excitability
HYPERMETABOLISM AND CATABO-LISM	Increased appetite, weight loss
ONE SYSTEM PREDOMINANCE	
Eyes[a]	Periorbital edema, exophthalmos (proptosis), chemosis, ophthalmo-plegia, papilledema
Cardiac	Arrhythmia, congestive heart failure
Muscle	Fatigue and weakness, muscle wasting, proximal myopathy, periodic paralysis
Gastrointestinal	Increased frequency of bowel movements, pernicious vomiting
Bone	Acropachy, osteoporosis, hypercalcemia
REPRODUCTIVE	Infertility, abortion, scanty menses, testicular atrophy, gynecomastia
MENTAL	Anxiety, irritability, psychosis, insomnia
SKIN	Onycholysis, "pretibial" myxedema, hyperpigmentation

[a] Graves' disease only.

of the thyrotoxic aspect is determined not only by the degree of hormone excess but also by its rapidity of onset, its duration, and by the age of the patient. The "typical" patient presents with one or more of the following *spontaneous* complaints: "nervousness," weight loss, palpitations (which at first may be intermittent), enlarging neck mass (goiter), change in appearance of eyes (Graves' disease), or symptoms of heart failure. These symptoms usually have been present anywhere from a few weeks to up to a year or longer.

As the disease progresses in severity, skeletal muscle wasting occurs, which tends to involve especially the limb girdle musculature, producing a proximal myopathy. This problem may result in weakness, expressed, for example, as great difficulty in climbing stairs or, on examination, in arising from a squatting position. Exertional dyspnea, without evidence of cardiac failure, is common and may be related to the myopathy.

The "nervousness" is typically irritability, inability to concentrate, restlessness, or overt emotional lability, but it is the tremor that most often leads the patient to express this complaint. Impairment of normal sleep pattern with frequent wakenings is common.

The weight loss classically occurs in the face of increased appetite, although frequently no obvious change in appetite is noticed or there may actually be anorexia, especially in elderly patients. The only prominent gastrointestinal symptom is increased frequency of bowel movements, but true diarrhea is not seen.

The "heat intolerance" of hyperthyroidism is often apparent only on questioning. Commonly the patient will admit to having reduced the number of covers used on the bed at night or to the development of new and unusual habits, such as sleeping in the nude or with feet extended from under the blankets. Sweating is increased but is not usually a spontaneous complaint.

Skin changes are hardly ever noticed by the patient and "silky skin" or hair is only occasionally seen on examination. Hair loss is not infrequent, usually noticed as thinning of the scalp hair by women. Other skin changes include occasional cases in white persons of diffuse hyperpigmentation with darkening noted mostly over extensor surfaces of elbows, knees, and small joints. In black patients, darkening of skin is common.

Physical Findings

The *thyroid* is visibly or palpably enlarged in almost all young patients with hyperthyroidism, but in the elderly the thyroid may not be enlarged. Asymmetric enlargement is common, especially in patients with toxic nodular goiter. Extreme vascularity of the gland may result in palpable or audible blood flow, a bruit, usually heard over the enlarged lobes but occasionally best heard more rostrally over the superior thyroidal arteries. A bruit over the thyroid of a hyperthyroid patient is usually diagnostic of Graves' disease; this finding is not present in patients with toxic nodular goiter.

The *cardiovascular findings* include sinus tachycardia, systolic flow murmurs, and wide pulse pressure, commonly, and atrial fibrillation, occasionally. It is a common belief that most patients with hyperthyroidism have at least a tachycardia; but, in fact only 50% of patients, regardless of age, show this finding. The apex impulse is often prominent and forceful. Cardiac failure may develop in severe cases of long duration, especially in elderly persons.

The *eye findings* can be separated into those that occur as a result of thyroid hormone excess and those that are part of the ophthalmopathy of Graves' disease. Excessive thyroid hormone enhances sympathetic tone. The innervation of the eyelids is partially under sympathetic control. Lid retraction with increased scleral visibility above and below the iris, along with infrequent blinking, leads to the "stare" so commonly seen. Failure of the lid to follow promptly movements of the globe ("lid lag") is another manifestation of the same process. When Graves' ophthalmopathy is present, there is forward protrusion of the globe. This process may be unilateral at first and is often asymmetrical. The protrusion represents true proptosis and contributes an additional component to the stare produced by increased sympathetic tone. Extraocular muscle weakness results in limitation of ability to converge and to perform extreme movements of gaze. Strabismus and diplopia are more severe manifestations. The most serious complications of Graves' ophthalmopathy are infiltrative (page 1000).

The *dermopathy* of Graves' disease occurs most commonly on the legs ("pretibial myxedema") but also can be seen on the dorsum of the foot or on the back, the hands, or even the face. The plaque usually has a sharp, raised margin and may have an orange peel-like appearance. The affected areas are often intensely pruritic.

Clubbing of the fingers and toes is rare (thyroid acropachy) and distinguishable radiographically from that seen in pulmonary disease. A common sign is separation of the distal portion of one or more fingernails from their nailbed (onycholysis).

A *postural tremor*, usually of the hands, is a common physical finding (see Chapter 82).

Diagnosis

Recognition of Graves' disease in a typical case is not difficult, but, because of its frequently insidious onset, an absence of eye findings or of an overtly enlarged thyroid, or because of involvement of one or relatively few organ systems, the diagnosis may be missed for months or years.

The usual thyroid function tests will substantiate the diagnosis in most cases. If the results of the T_4 and free T_4 index are borderline or normal, the plasma T_3 must be measured, since hyperthyroidism may be due to elevation of T_3 alone. "T_3 toxicosis" (see page 1001), however, occurs in less than 5% of cases. Occasionally, all of the tests of thyroid hormone levels are borderline. If the clinical suspicion of thyrotoxicosis is strong, every effort should be made to obtain laboratory confirmation by measurement of RaIU, the TRH test, or the T_3 suppression test (see above). Clinical trials of antithyroid drugs should be avoided.

Differential Diagnosis

In some patients, particularly elderly ones, the clinical picture may not suggest hyperthyroidism and only an astute clinician will promptly consider the correct diagnosis. Such patients may present with only unexplained weight loss or weakness.

Occult neoplasm may first be suspected, and the diagnosis of hyperthyroidism may be missed entirely or considered only after extensive evaluation fails to yield a diagnosis. These are the patients often labeled "apathetic hyperthyroidism." The term implies lethargy—which is, in fact, not often present—but should rather be used to denote that group of individuals who for unclear reasons lack the signs of sympathetic hyperactivity and hence do not exhibit tachycardia, lid retraction, tremor, *etc.*

Congestive heart failure or atrial fibrillation may be the presenting manifestation. So-called thyrocardiac patients have been incorrectly thought to be resistant to ordinary doses of digitalis. This is occasionally true, but a normal response to conventional therapy for cardiac failure or an arrhythmia should not be considered incompatible with a diagnosis of hyperthyroidism.

Some patients with anxiety may present with tachycardia, tremor, irritability, and weakness simulating hyperthyroidism. The "anxiety" of thyrotoxicosis is more likely to appear as irritability and hyperkinesis than as an expressed feeling of anxiety. Primary anxiety disorders are either related to identifiable stresses, coexist with symptoms of depression, or have distinctive characteristics that make them recognizable (see Chapters 12 and 13). In depression, weight loss is invariably accompanied by anorexia, a relatively unusual symptom of hyperthyroidism (see page 995).

The characteristic ophthalmopathy of Graves' disease may offer the first clue to the diagnosis. However, ophthalmopathy may not be accompanied by hyperthyroidism and may be unilateral. The T_3 suppression test or TRH test will substantiate the diagnosis in most but not all cases of euthyroid Graves' ophthalmopathy. Without evidence of either thyroid hyperfunction, disturbance of the negative feedback system, or dermopathy, the diagnosis of Graves' ophthalmopathy cannot be made with absolute assurance. Indeed, other diseases of the orbit or retroorbital space must be considered. Computerized axial tomography of the skull and the orbital contents and high resolution sonography are useful diagnostic tools. These procedures can visualize the enlarged extraocular muscles of Graves' ophthalmopathy, although such enlargement is also seen in pseudotumor. In many cases of Graves' ophthalmopathy, without hyperthyroidism, other aspects of Graves' disease eventually become apparent.

When hyperthyroidism is found in a patient without goiter or exophthalmos, suspicions of factitious hyperthyroidism may be warranted. An RaIU test and scan will establish whether the thyroid is functional, and scintiscan will sometimes give evidence for enlargement that is not palpable. A very low uptake and a normal-sized gland on scintiscan suggest ingestion of thyroid hormone or the presence of thyroiditis with hyperthyroidism (see below, page 1000).

Therapy

Hyperthyroidism due to Graves' disease is frequently a self-limited process that terminates within a year or two in about one-half of patients. This natural history strongly influences selection of therapy. Other therapeutic considerations relate to the age of the patient and the presence or absence of complications.

Since there are currently no means of controlling the underlying cause of the disease, presumably TSI production, therapy is designed to interfere with thyroid hormone synthesis by drugs or by ablation of thyroid tissue by radioiodide or surgery. Opinions differ on approaches, but the views expressed here probably closely approximate a consensus of conservative medical opinion. Each form of therapy has advantages and disadvantages; none provides a simple, definitive solution and none is truly curative. The objective of therapy is to assure minimal morbidity from both the therapy and the disease. The therapy of hyperthyroidism due to causes other than Graves' disease is discussed separately.

Thiocarbamide Antithyroid Drugs

These agents will predictably control excessive production of thyroid hormone in essentially all cases, although in only about one-half of cases will a permanent remission of the hyperthyroidism be seen. Of these latter cases, about one-half will become hypothyroid in the period between 15 to 20 years after successful treatment and onset of remission. Relapses may occur within 6 months to a year or even longer after apparent remission, but such relapses are uncommon except in postpartum patients.

Restoration of the clinically euthyroid state requires at least 4 to 8 weeks, although clinical improvement is usually seen much sooner. Antithyroid drugs are ordinarily the preferred *initial* treatment for children, some young adults without complications or other medical problems, and the pregnant patient. The antithyroid drugs are also routinely used as preliminary therapy in patients who are to be treated by surgery (see below, page 1000). The objective in these cases is to ensure euthyroid status at the time of operation. Patients who are to be treated with radioiodide (see below, page 999) are also frequently treated with an antithyroid drug pre- and/or postablation. Radioiodide is slow in producing its effect and may have to be given in multiple doses; use of an antithyroid drug before or after such therapy is therefore a temporary but useful adjunct.

In the United States, only two thiocarbamide drugs are available, propylthiouracil and methimazole (Tapazole). Propylthiouracil may have an advantage when speed in restoration of euthyroid status is an urgent consideration. Propylthiouracil, unlike methimazole, in addition to its effects in inhibiting thyroid hormone synthesis, also inhibits conversion of T_4 to T_3 in peripheral tissues. Methimazole, on the other hand, is longer acting than propylthiouracil and may be given on a less frequent dosage schedule, thus facilitating compliance. In most adults with hyperthyroidism, 100 to 150 mg of propylthiouracil (available in 50-mg tablets) every 8 hours or 20 to 30 mg of methimazole (available in 5- and 10-mg tablets) every 12 hours will usually suffice as initial therapy, whereas maintenance is often possible with 50 to 100 mg of propylthiouracil twice daily or 5 to 10 mg of methimazole once or twice daily. The T_4 level should be measured after a month of treatment and every 2 to 3 months thereafter. If at these relatively low maintenance doses of antithyroid drug, the plasma T_4 falls below normal, efforts to "titrate" the dose further are frequently tedious and unsuccessful and should be avoided. A euthyroid state can be achieved under these circumstances by the *addition* of oral thyroxine, usually at somewhat less than full replacement dose. Another argument in favor of this approach is that higher doses of methimazole may be associated with higher rates of remission. A simple treatment program is currently gaining favor. After an initial period of treatment with methimazole alone, and at a point when the T_4 has become normal, maintenance is instituted with a *single* daily administration of 60 mg of methimazole plus 0.10 to 0.15 mg of thyroxine.

Although the recommended doses will control the disease in the vast majority of cases, some individuals clearly need higher doses. If the patient is severely ill, larger doses should be given from the beginning. The risk of an adverse drug effect may be increased, but this is not established and should not be a consideration under such circumstances. In order to achieve total blockade of hormone synthesis, as much as 200 mg of propylthiouracil every 4 hours may be necessary. Since methimazole has a longer duration of action, it need not be given so often, but 30 to 40 mg three times daily may be needed in some cases.

Duration of Therapy

Time-honored treatment schedules, strongly favored by the author, use a period of 12 to 24 months of therapy before consideration is given to discontinuation of the drug, although conflicting evidence suggests that lasting remission may not be related to duration of therapy beyond the point at which the patient becomes euthyroid. A few indicators are helpful in predicting success or failure of the outcome of a course of antithyroid drug therapy. Patients who have continued to require large doses of drug are almost certain not to have achieved remission. On the other hand, reduction of thyroid mass during therapy is often predictive of lasting clinical remission. Tests for restoration of the normal negative feedback system at the end of a period of drug therapy (thyroid suppressibility; see above) are of little use in predicting long term remission. For determination of short term status the TRH test is of no use at all, but a test using T_3 or T_4, while not accurately predictive of the long term, may nonetheless be helpful in establishing the clinical status at the time of discontinuation of drug therapy. To perform the test, the antithyroid drug is withheld through the period of the test. The patient is given 75 μg of T_3 (Cytomel) as a single dose daily for 7 days or one 3-mg dose of T_4. RaIU is then determined 1 week after initiation of T_3 administration (or after the single dose of T_4). Low postsuppression 24-hour uptake (< 10%) indicates accurately that the patient is in remission at the time of the test. More significantly, an uptake above the normal range almost invariably indicates continuation of active disease. Intermediate values are not useful. If on clinical grounds, or as a result of testing, continued disease activity seems to be present, discontinuation of therapy is inadvisable and will almost certainly result in clinical relapse and needless morbidity. Measurement of titers of TSI may be useful in predicting relapse, but such measurements are not widely available and are also not accurate predictors.

If the clinical status indicates that remission may have been reached, antithyroid drug therapy is terminated and the patient is observed. Routine determination of plasma T_4 every 3 to 4 weeks for 3 to 6 months allows early recognition of return of thyroid overactivity. If the status is ambiguous, and especially if there is evidence of continued disease activity, antithyroid drug dosage may be reduced to one-half the maintenance level for 3 to 6 months in the expectation that, if recurrence occurs, it will be blunted. Prophylactic use of propranolol (see below) during withdrawal of antithyroid drugs is a useful maneuver that prevents emergence of symptoms of overt hyperthyroidism should relapse occur.

If the hyperthyroid state recurs, treatment with antithyroid drug may be reinitiated for another course (i.e., 1 year) or alternative therapy may be undertaken (^{131}I or surgery). A second course of antithyroid drug has a significant chance of inducing remission. In selected patients, prolonged or even indefinite drug therapy is reasonable, but with most patients such an approach is not desirable.

Minor side effects of drug therapy occur in 1 to 5% of patients. Skin rashes, the most common side effect, are usually seen in the first months of therapy and often disappear even if therapy is continued. Antihistamine drugs are useful in controlling these rashes and the sometimes associated urticaria and pruritus. Leukopenia is not uncommon but is usually not severe and is dose-related. If the absolute number of polymorphonuclear leukocytes falls below 2000, the dose should be reduced or the drug discontinued. If the side effects are not tolerated, a switch to another agent will allow continuation of therapy in about half the cases. *Major complications* of drug therapy occur in less than 0.1% of cases. Agranulocytosis is the most dreaded complication.

Unlike leukopenia, thiocarbamide-induced agranulocytosis due to anti-leukocyte antibodies from thiocarbamides is not dose related and is of such sudden onset that routine blood counts are of no help in prevention. The patient should, however, be instructed to contact the physician promptly if severe sore mouth or sore throat and fever occur. Immediate hospitalization is indicated. Fortunately, most patients with agranulocytosis recover, albeit after a stormy course. Other toxic reactions include drug fever and arthralgias. Elevations of alkaline phosphatase activity are commonly seen in patients receiving propylthiouracil. If other liver enzymes are normal, the drug may be continued, but persistent laboratory evidence of hepatocellular damage is an indication for discontinuation of therapy. White blood count should be monitored after several weeks of therapy and following increases of drug dose. Liver enzymes should be measured every 3 to 6 months.

Adjunctive Drug Therapy

Iodide. Iodide in the treatment of hyperthyroidism should be reserved for patients with severe illness. Occasionally, iodide therapy produces severe dermatitis. Use of iodide may preclude for many weeks the use of radioactive iodide, the uptake of which by the thyroid will be greatly diminished.

Iodide is the best agent available for inhibiting hormone release and is useful in patients who need rapid correction of the hyperthyroid state. Iodide also has a time-honored place in preoperative preparation (see below, page 999) for thyroidectomy, to reduce vascularity of the gland. When given following radioiodide therapy, iodide seems especially effective in accelerating restoration of euthyroid status.

The dose of iodide is one drop of a saturated solution of potassium iodide (50 mg) two times a day; larger doses are often given but are unnecessary. Lugol's solution is an obsolete pharmacological concoction containing iodine and iodide which has no virtue over iodide alone.

Adrenergic antagonists. The symptoms and signs of thyrotoxicosis that are related to sensitization of the sympathetic nervous system are in large measure abolished by β-adrenergic blocking drugs. The current agent of choice is propranolol. Other newer, more selective β-adrenergic antagonists are probably equally effective, although no clear advantage has been demonstrated over propranolol. Some of these agents are partial adrenergic agonists and may prove to be inappropriate for use in hyperthyroidism. The indications for use of propranolol are *severe* tachycardia, tremor, sweating, and agitation. Propranolol is effective for relief of these manifestations of hyperthyroidism, but does not appreciably affect excessive metabolic rate or reverse the catabolic state of severe cases. Propranolol has occasional undesirable side effects and is relatively contraindicated in some individuals (e.g., those with asthma). Concern is often expressed that patients with heart disease may be thrown into congestive heart failure or that heart failure, if present, may worsen. On the other hand, some patients with congestive heart failure may respond well to the drug when excessive heart rate is a major contributing factor. Other uses for propranolol are in the prevention of symptoms during trial withdrawal of an antithyroid drug and while awaiting the effects of ^{131}I therapy. Most patients require propranolol in doses of at least 160 mg daily, but doses up to 720 mg may be necessary. The drug should be discontinued as soon as the patient is rendered euthyroid by other therapy.

Radioactive Iodide Therapy

Radioactive iodide (^{131}I) is uniformly effective therapy; it is simple to administer and inexpensive. It is the preferred form of therapy for most adults with Graves' disease and is much to be preferred over surgery.

The single disadvantage of radioactive iodide is that hypothyroidism is a frequent consequence. For many years, concern was expressed over the possibility of producing carcinoma of the thyroid, leukemia, or genetic damage in the future offspring of women in their childbearing years. All of these concerns have been shown to be groundless. Although low doses of external radiation do produce carcinoma of the thyroid, the higher doses used for treatment of hyperthyroidism do not. Long term follow-up of treated patients over the past 30 years has failed to substantiate any such risk or any increased risk of leukemia. The amounts of radiation to the ovaries from therapeutic doses of radioiodide used for therapy of hyperthyroidism are lower than those delivered by diagnostic X-ray procedures and can be expected to produce no genetic effects. Thus, radioiodide therapy for hyperthyroidism can be considered for any adult patient.

Hypothyroidism follows radioiodide therapy in the immediate few months after therapy in a more or less dose-related fashion. Large doses predictably eliminate hyperthyroidism with certainty but totally ablate the thyroid with great regularity. Small, single doses render the patient euthyroid with 50 to 70% likelihood but unavoidably still produce hypothyroidism within a year in about 10% of cases. Furthermore, of the patients rendered euthyroid, 3 to 4%/year develop hypothyroidism over the ensuing 20 years.

One may question whether the high frequency of post-treatment hypothyroidism constitutes a significant disadvantage of radioiodide therapy. The answer is that, for the majority of those who become hypothyroid, replacement therapy with thyroxine is a trivial inconvenience. For these patients, the advantages of radioiodide therapy far outweigh the one disadvantage. Unfortunately, a few patients, despite warnings to the contrary, discontinue their required lifelong replacement therapy, become lost to follow-up, and suffer all of the consequences of long-standing hypothyroidism and myxedema.

Some physicians advocate the use of deliberately ablative doses of ^{131}I. This approach to therapy certainly greatly simplifies patient management, accelerates restoration of the euthyroid state, and is reasonable in view of the high probability of post-therapy hypothyroidism regardless of dose. Nonetheless, most physicians do not advocate deliberate ablation unless the patient is elderly, has experienced a major complication of hyperthyroidism (e.g., severe heart disease), or has complicating medical problems that demand prompt control. In young patients who are tolerating their disease reasonably well, most physicians prefer to use small doses of ^{131}I, repeated if necessary, until the patient is euthyroid. Such an approach does not, of course, guarantee that hypothyroidism will be avoided.

As discussed below (page 1001), larger (10 to 30 mCi) doses of ^{131}I *are* appropriate initially in the treatment of toxic nodular goiter.

In the past, elaborate schemes have been used to estimate the required dose of ^{131}I. Unfortunately, none of these has proven helpful, since the biological sensitivity to radiation effect, the most important variable, is not measurable. Currently, in a typical "low dose" treatment scheme patients with small glands are given 2 to 3 mCi, while those with moderately enlarged to large glands are given 5 to 10 mCi. Ablative doses approximate 15 mCi. Because of the unpredictable response with nonablative doses, antithyroid drugs are often used initially to render the patient euthyroid. Antithyroid therapy is then interrupted for 48 hours before the ^{131}I is given and reinstituted 24 hours afterward. Alternatively, an antithyroid drug can be initiated 24 to 48 hours following therapy with ^{131}I. Similar approaches combining antithyroid drug and ^{131}I are almost routinely used in patients with severe or complicated hyperthyroidism, e.g., thyrocardiac disease.

Radioactive iodide can be administered only by an appropriately licensed physician—usually an endocrinologist or a nuclear medicine physician. Thereafter, no special precautions need to be taken by the patient.

The undocumented notion has long persisted that radiation thyroiditis may produce excessive release of thyroid hormones 7 to 14 days after therapy, with the possibility of consequent worsening of the clinical state. This complication, if it occurs at all, must be rare. Nonetheless, prudence dictates a conservative approach in precarious patients, e.g., those in congestive heart failure, who are best brought to euthyroid status or who are at least significantly improved by antithyroid drug therapy before ablation with ^{131}I. At 3 months following ^{131}I, when the short term radiation effect becomes maximal, the antithyroid drug can be discontinued or tapered, provided, of course, that the laboratory and clinical evidence indicates return to euthyroid status. Adjunctive therapy with propranolol is useful at this point to ameliorate possible emerging symptoms when the preceding dose of ^{131}I has been inadequate. If the laboratory evidence indicates continuing hyperthyroidism, another dose of ^{131}I will be required.

Therapy with ^{131}I is always successful if enough ^{131}I is given. "Failure" after one or more doses is never an indication for surgery or indeterminate therapy with antithyroid drug. Rather, additional ^{131}I should be given to complete the process.

Surgical Therapy

For many years surgical ablation of the thyroid, e.g., subtotal thyroidectomy, was the main therapy for hyperthyroidism. This procedure still has its advocates, especially for young adults and for children who cannot be successfully treated with antithyroid drugs. In the hands of *experienced surgeons*, subtotal thyroidectomy is certainly effective therapy attended by minimal morbidity. However, complications include the small but real risk of anesthesia/operative mortality, recurrent laryngeal nerve damage with vocal cord paralysis, permanent hypoparathyroidism, and most commonly, hypothyroidism. The latter two complications are, to a certain extent, unavoidable and are not merely the consequence of poor surgical technique. In addition to about a 10% occurrence of immediate postsurgical hypothyroidism, 2 to 3% of patients become hypothyroid each year following surgery, a figure only slightly lower than that following therapy with [131]I. A higher complication rate must be expected when the operation is performed by surgeons with limited experience in thyroid surgery. Surgery also is followed by a significant (5%) rate of recurrent hyperthyroidism, sometimes occurring many years later. In this case, even the most enthusiastic supporters of surgical treatment agree that recurrent hyperthyroidism should never be treated by a second operation, since the frequency of major complications rises to an unacceptable level.

Treatment of Hyperthyroidism during Pregnancy

Hyperthyroidism during pregnancy, almost invariably due to Graves' disease, should be treated with an antithyroid drug. Surgery has been used successfully during pregnancy, but has no advantage and may be associated with increased fetal losses. Radioactive iodide is contraindicated. Therapy with antithyroid drugs during pregnancy is guided by two considerations. First, the antithyroid drugs freely cross the placenta and can, in large doses, produce goiter and hypothyroidism in the infant. Second, thyroid hormones do not cross the placenta from mother to fetus. The dose of antithyroid drugs should be the minimal amount adequate to control the hyperthyroidism. A dose of drug which totally blocks hormone synthesis along with a replacement amount of thyroxine is not appropriate during pregnancy. When ordinary doses of antithyroid drug are used, the fetus is usually born without goiter, but as a precaution the dose is often reduced, if possible, during the last month of pregnancy. Iodide should not be used during pregnancy, since the fetal thyroid is especially susceptible to the goitrogenic effect of iodide. Monitoring the plasma hormone level requires determination of free T_4 or the free T_4 index, since T_4 is normally elevated during pregnancy in association with the increased TBG.

TSIs (see page 991) of Graves' disease cross the placenta and enter the fetal circulation. Occasionally, the newborn infant is hyperthyroid as a result of this passive transfer of antibodies. The physician caring for the newborn should always be alerted to this possibility.

Ophthalmopathy of Graves' Disease

The exact frequency of ophthalmopathy in Graves' disease is not known, but most patients have either no obvious infiltrative eye involvement or show only minimal to moderate proptosis, which generally stabilizes at a tolerable level. Severe exophthalmos occurs in no more than a few percent of cases of Graves' disease. Proptosis becomes more than a cosmetic concern when the eyelids fail to close, setting the stage for corneal ulceration. Paresis of the extraocular muscles producing diplopia can also be troublesome and may require use of an eye patch or corrective surgery. The most disturbing and rarest eye involvement is chemosis or marked inflammation and edema of the conjunctivae and periorbital soft tissues. Ophthalmopathy of this severity is termed malignant or infiltrative exophthalmos. Rarely, optic neuritis leading to blindness occurs. The therapy of severe ophthalmopathy, which may include decompression of the orbit, is accomplished by an ophthalmologist (6, 9).

Graves' ophthalmopathy follows a temporal course which may be totally dissociated from the hyperthyroidism, the treatment of which should be independent of and uninfluenced by the eye disease. Despite claims to the contrary, no form of treatment of hyperthyroidism has any advantage for control of the ophthalmopathy. The notion persists that induction of hypothyroidism may aggravate exophthalmos. Development of clinical hypothyroidism should therefore be avoided, especially when exophthalmos is present.

Hyperthyroidism Associated with Thyroiditis (Lymphocytic Thyroiditis with Spontaneously Resolving Hyperthyroidism; Postpartum Thyroiditis with Hyperthyroidism; Silent Thyroiditis)

Classical subacute thyroiditis (see below, page 1011) has long been known to be associated occasionally with short lived, self-limited hyperthyroidism. The explanation for this phenomenon has been that the destructive inflammatory process causes release of preformed thyroid hormone. The hyperthyroidism invariably disappears within a few months.

In the past few years, another, apparently distinct variant of the thyroiditis-hyperthyroidism syndrome has been recognized. These patients present with a modestly enlarged thyroid gland that is non-tender. No prior history of viral illness can be obtained. The radioiodide uptake is very low, as it is in subacute thyroiditis, while the T_4 and T_3 are high. About one-half of cases have significant elevations of thyroid antibodies, and about one-half of these high titers subside within a few months. A propensity of the condition to occur in the postpartum period has been noted, sometimes in successive pregnancies and sometimes followed by the development of hypothyroidism. On biopsy the changes seen differ from those of the peak phase of classical subacute thyroiditis, but the latter, in its late stages of evolution, may be indistinguishable from that of lymphocytic thyroiditis. Whether lymphocytic thyroiditis with spontaneously resulting hyperthyroidism (silent thyroiditis) is a new disease, as has been suggested by some, or is a newly recognized variant of subacute thyroiditis is a matter of debate (8, 15, 20).

It is important to obtain a radioiodide uptake measurement in all patients with hyperthyroidism who do not clearly have Graves' disease (i.e., who do not have associated eye findings) or toxic nodular goiter. A very low radioiodide uptake will establish the diagnosis of hyperthyroidism associated with thyroiditis and allow the physician to avoid inappropriate therapy (radioiodide or surgery). Treatment with an antithyroid drug *may* be useful; propranolol (see above, page 998) affords symptomatic relief and may be all the treatment that is necessary.

Hyperthyroidism Associated with Nodular Goiter (Toxic Nodular Goiter)

Toxic nodular goiter is usually seen in adults in midlife or in the elderly. While the typical patient with Graves' disease usually relates symptoms extending over a few months to a year, the history in toxic nodular goiter is often much longer. Many years may pass before diagnosis. Because of the patient's age and the duration of illness, severe cardiac or musculoskeletal involvement is common.

Toxic nodular goiter appears to arise in the pathological evolution of some cases of nodular goiter. Most nodular goiters (see below, page 1007) are initially TSH dependent, i.e., suppressible with exogenous thyroid hormone. Eventually, some of these goiters develop autonomous areas, with other regions of relatively decreased activity. Nodular goiters at this stage of evolution do not secrete enough hormone to produce clinical hyperthyroidism but in 20% of cases show nonsuppressible function. A few

of these autonomously functioning goiters evolve to a stage where excessive production of hormone and clinical hyperthyroidism ensue.

If the usual laboratory tests (T_4, free T_4 index) are borderline, special tests such as measurement of T_3, suppression with thyroid hormone (page 991), or TRH stimulation (page 991) should be considered. The suppression test can be undertaken cautiously in the elderly patient without overt heart disease but should not be used if heart disease is obvious. Both tests are more helpful in excluding a diagnosis of hyperthyroidism than in establishing a state of hormone excess, since a significant number of cases of nontoxic nodular goiter are not suppressible. The TRH test is of limited value in the elderly. A normal response to TRH excludes a diagnosis of hyperthyroidism at any age, but failure to respond is a common occurrence in normal elderly persons.

Therapy of toxic nodular goiter is best accomplished with [131]I. Rather large doses, in the range of 10 to 30 mCi, are usually necessary. Hypothyroidism occurs much less frequently following ^{131}I therapy for nodular goiter than for Graves' disease. If the clinical situation demands prompt relief of the hyperthyroidism, an antithyroid drug can be used following the therapeutic dose of ^{131}I, since the response to radioiodide is often slow and multiple doses may be needed. Otherwise ^{131}I given alone is simple therapy, without side effects, and easily monitored by measurements of plasma T_4. Other therapeutic considerations including the use of adjunctive therapy follow those outlined for the therapy of Graves' disease with one exception. In hyperthyroidism due to toxic nodular goiter, antithyroid drugs alone cannot be expected to produce a lasting remission.

Hyperthyroidism Due to Excessive Secretion of T_3; "T_3 Toxicosis"

In most cases of hyperthyroidism, the thyroid secretes excessive quantities of both T_4 and T_3. However, in perhaps 5% of cases, T_3 is the predominant hormone secreted. T_3 toxicosis may occur in hyperthyroidism due to Graves' disease, toxic multinodular goiter, or autonomous adenoma. The patient who appears clinically hyperthyroid but whose T_4 is normal should have plasma T_3 measured. T_3 toxicosis sometimes occurs early in the course of hyperthyroidism due to Graves' disease and can develop during therapy with an antithyroid drug. Continuing clinical findings of hyperthyroidism during such therapy—and despite a normal or low T_4—should raise the possibility that T_3 toxicosis is now present and that more, rather than less, antithyroid drug is needed. The treatment of T_3 toxicosis is the same as is that of other forms of hyperthyroidism.

Thyroid Storm (Thyrotoxic Crisis)

This dreaded complication of hyperthyroidism is now only rarely encountered. When thyroid storm does occur, it is usually in the setting of a severe medical or surgical stress imposed on a patient with uncontrolled or unrecognized hyperthyroidism. Clinical features of full blown thyroid storm include fever, sometimes to the level of extreme hyperpyrexia, marked tachycardia, great irritability, diarrhea, and hypotension. Thyroid storm often progresses rapidly to delirium and coma. Any such severe exacerbation of hyperthyroidism demands hospitalization and urgent consultation with an endocrinologist.

HYPOTHYROIDISM

Hypothyroidism, the metabolic state resulting from deficient thyroid hormones, is relatively common. Most cases can be diagnosed even when symptoms and signs are minimal, provided that the physician considers the diagnosis and seeks appropriate laboratory confirmation. The manifestations of hypothyroidism are varied and to a large measure age dependent. Myxedema is a severe form of hypothyroidism which results in deposition of mucopolysaccharides in the skin and other tissues, producing a characteristic appearance and a constellation of physical findings. The term myxedema is commonly but incorrectly used interchangeably with hypothyroidism. *Primary hypothyroidism* is a term used to indicate that the hormone deficiency results from a disease or other process within the thyroid gland. *Secondary hypothyroidism*, much less common, results from lack of thyrotropin (TSH) secretion, a result of pituitary or, rarely, hypothalamic disease. The thyroid is usually smaller than normal and not palpable. Plasma TSH is low, but low levels cannot be accurately assessed with currently available assays (see "Laboratory Tests of Thyroid Function and of Thyroid Disease"). Almost invariably the hypothyroidism is part of a decrease in pituitary function involving tropic hormones in addition to TSH with consequent hypogonadism and/or adrenal insufficiency. Causes include postpartum necrosis, pituitary tumor, pituitary apoplexy, and granulomatous disease, or may be part of an autoimmune process involving failure of other endocrine glands. Some cases occur without identifiable cause and are termed idiopathic (see also Chapter 74).

Etiology

Currently, the commonest cause of hypothyroidism is iatrogenic, *i.e.*, the result of therapy of hyperthyroidism with radioiodide or by surgery. Spontaneous cases due to thyroid atrophy are also common. A clinical classification is given in Table 73.7.

Idiopathic hypothyroidism in most cases results from autoimmune destruction of the thyroid with subsequent thyroid atrophy. Some cases are the result of long-standing Hashimoto's thyroiditis. Both types occur frequently in association with other autoimmune diseases such as pernicious anemia. In

Table 73.7.
Clinical Classification of Hypothyroidism[a]

HYPOTHYROIDISM WITHOUT GOITER (DECREASE OF THYROID TISSUE MASS)
  Postablative for hyperthyroidism (radioiodide therapy or surgery)
  Idiopathic atrophy
  Developmental defect (congenital)
  Pituitary or hypothalamic disease
HYPOTHYROIDISM WITH GOITER
  Chronic thyroiditis (Hashimoto's disease, *etc*)
  Drug induced (antithyroid drugs, iodide, lithium,[b] sulfonylureas, *etc*)
  Iodide deficiency (remote geographic areas)
  Genetic biosynthetic defects

[a] Hypothyroidism in the United States is now most commonly the consequence of therapy for hyperthyroidism. Hypothyroidism due to idiopathic atrophy of the thyroid is second in frequency. Developmental defects (*e.g.*, lingual thyroid) are rare. Hypothyroidism with goiter is nearly always due to Hashimoto's thyroiditis, rarely to a drug. Genetic biosynthetic defects are rare and usually become manifest in childhood.
[b] Hypothyroidism due to chronic lithium therapy may occur without goiter.

both types, high titers of antibodies to thyroid antigens (thyroglobulin; microsomes) are seen in 90% of cases. As a clinically encountered thyroid abnormality, Hashimoto's thyroiditis is second in frequency only to nontoxic nodular goiter and is by far the most common cause of goitrous hypothyroidism. The clinical distinction between ordinary multinodular goiter and goiters due to Hashimoto's thyroiditis is made by measurement of thyroid autoantibodies.

Drug-Induced Hypothyroidism

A *variety of drugs* can produce hypothyroidism that is invariably associated with goiter formation. Only a few in current use have such an effect. Lithium, currently in wide use for the treatment of manic-depressive illness (see Chapter 15), is one such agent. If goiter occurs, lithium need not be stopped; addition of thyroxine relieves the hypothyroidism and causes regression of the goiter. Overtreatment of hyperthyroidism with an antithyroid drug will, of course, produce hypothyroidism. Iodide in pharmacological amounts is an antithyroid drug and will also occasionally produce goiter and hypothyroidism as in patients given long term iodide therapy for asthma or another chronic lung disease. However, most adults who are susceptible to the antithyroid action of iodide have an underlying thyroid abnormality, such as Hashimoto's thyroiditis (see below, page 1011) or radioiodide-treated Graves' disease.

Clinical Features

Hypothyroidism in the adult is highly variable in presentation. Usually, onset is insidious, often occurring over many years, with the result that the symptoms go unappreciated by patient and physician alike. The nonspecificity of the symptoms also contributes to the delayed diagnosis. No predictable progression of symptoms is apparent, but easy fatigability, lethargy, increased sleep requirement, cold intolerance, muscle aching, and stiffness are perhaps the commonest early symptoms. The skin is dry and scaling. Hair loss is frequent. The eyebrows become sparse, the face is "puffy," i.e., full, with edema of the periorbital areas. The voice often becomes low pitched and rough. Constipation is common and may be severe enough to produce megacolon; sometimes the diagnosis is suggested by the radiologist from the results of a barium enema. Diminished hearing, especially in old persons, is easily overlooked or attributed to "aging." Ordinarily, the affected individual becomes abnormally placid, but agitation or frank psychosis may occur. In the elderly, depression is the commonest psychiatric accompaniment of hypothyroidism. Dementia due to hypothyroidism is rare, but the association of the two processes in the elderly is not uncommon (5). Paresthesias of the hands due to carpal tunnel syndrome are common. Diminished sexual function is the rule. Women often experience menorrhagia. Rarely, galactorrhea may be seen in women of childbearing age. Fertility is diminished, but pregnancy may occur and normal delivery is possible. The newborn is euthyroid, unless the mother's hypothyroidism is drug related or the hypothyroidism is of the rare familial athyrotic variety.

Severe Hypothyroidism with Myxedema

In spontaneous cases of hypothyroidism, only with severe, long-standing disease does extensive deposition of mucopolysaccharide occur, producing the clinical state of myxedema. Rarely, myxedema may develop rapidly after radioiodide or after surgical ablation of the thyroid for hyperthyroidism.

In myxedema, a variety of manifestations can be appreciated on physical examination and, of course, they vary with the severity and duration of the disease. The skin, in addition to being dry and scaling, is typically cool. The scaling may be extensive so that large flakes are shed over the elbows and knees. The subcutaneous tissues may be infiltrated by mucopolysaccharides so that the skin appears to be "thickened" or "doughy." In the elderly, atrophy of the epidermis may occur simultaneously, producing a stiff, translucent, parchment-like appearance. Yellow-orange discoloration of the skin may be evident, especially in the palms. The presence of edema is not obvious, since pitting is not noted except in extreme cases complicated by hypoproteinemia. An exception is the collection around the eyes of "bags of water." This finding is not, however, specific for hypothyroidism. The tongue is sometimes enlarged. The heart rate is usually slow (sinus bradycardia). The heart may appear enlarged, due

either to dilation of the myocardium or to pericardial effusion. Pleural effusions and ascites may also be present, sometimes even in cases that are otherwise not clinically severe. Dilutional hyponatremia, clinically indistinguishable from the syndrome of inappropriate antidiuretic hormone excess, may be present. The deep tendon reflexes characteristically show a delay in their relaxation phase, the so-called "hung-up reflex." This is a highly suggestive finding but may be seen occasionally in other diseases. Mental functioning is slowed, as reflected in the characteristically slow speech. The reading speed may be greatly reduced. Hearing loss may be severe or of a degree apparent only on audiometric testing. Cerebellar dysfunction, if present, is usually evident only on extensive neurological testing, but in rare cases is grossly apparent as ataxia. The unusual aspects of hypothyroidism have been recently reviewed (10).

Myxedema Coma

This severe, often fatal, event is an infrequent complication of long-standing disease and is typically seen in the elderly patient. Myxedema coma is often associated with or precipitated by pneumonia, peritonitis, or some other serious infection. Severe respiratory failure is a major feature and can be due to a variety of factors ranging from upper airway obstruction to impaired chest wall mechanics.

Since elderly patients often become hypothermic on exposure to cold or during sepsis, the diagnosis of myxedema coma is more frequently considered than actually confirmed. Any of these events demands hospitalization.

Laboratory Findings

In primary hypothyroidism, the combination of low plasma T_4, free T_4 index (or free T_4), and high TSH is diagnostic. Difficulties in diagnosis are encountered only in occasional cases. The plasma T_3 is usually low, but since T_3 decreases in a variety of nonthyroidal illnesses ranging from malnutrition to liver disease, its measurement is not useful for diagnosis of hypothyroidism. Furthermore, it is normal in many patients with mild hypothyroidism. In hypothyroidism due to pituitary or hypothalamic disease the TSH is low or "normal." The TRH test is ordinarily not necessary for diagnosis of primary hypothyroidism, but can be helpful when the T_4 and TSH are borderline. In this situation, an exaggerated response to TRH may be seen (TSH increment > 30).

In addition to the definitive diagnostic tests, various other laboratory abnormalities are encountered, although they serve no useful diagnostic purpose. A common laboratory finding is elevation of plasma enzymes which originate in skeletal muscle: creatine kinase (formerly CPK), serum aspartate aminotransferase (formerly SGOT), serum alanine aminotransferase (formerly SGPT), and lactic dehydrogenase (LDH). Fractionation studies show that when these enzymes are elevated in hypothyroidism, they do not originate in cardiac muscle. Other abnormalities include electrocardiographic changes (such as flattened or inverted T waves, minor ST segment depressions, and low amplitude QRS complexes) and abnormalities of blood gas measurements due to hypoventilation. Anemia (see Chapter 49), usually normocytic and normochromic, may be present, as may macrocytic anemia of coexistent vitamin B_{12} deficiency (pernicious anemia). An abnormality of red cell shape (spiculation) also has been described in hypothyroidism.

Differential Diagnosis

The most difficult problem in diagnosis is the simple clinical appreciation of the possibility that the patient may be hypothyroid. Once suspected, the subsequent history, physical examination, and, particularly, laboratory findings will easily establish the diagnosis in all but a few cases. However, some special problems may be encountered. Any elderly patient who is sick, pale, and puffy faced becomes a suspect for the diagnosis, especially if an adequate history cannot be obtained. A patient with atypical chest pain, nonspecific electrocardiographic abnormalities, and elevated creatine kinase or aspartate aminotransferase is not infrequently labeled as having ischemic heart disease and myocardial infarction; the proper diagnosis may be hypothyroidism. A patient with the nephrotic syndrome might be mistaken for one having hypothyroidism. However, although the plasma T_4 may be low (TBG is low in some nephrotic patients), the free T_4 index (or free T_4) is normal. More important, the patient with the nephrotic syndrome will have features characteristic of that disorder, i.e., massive proteinuria and hypoalbuminemia (see Chapter 43).

Diagnosis of Hypothyroidism in Patients Receiving Thyroid Hormone Therapy

Patients are frequently encountered who, having been diagnosed as hypothyroid at some time in the past, are receiving replacement therapy when first seen. Lack of documentation may lead the physician to question the original diagnosis. The physician's alternatives include continuation of therapy despite an uncertain diagnosis, or discontinuation of therapy, a maneuver that will confirm or refute the need for continued treatment. In many instances, continuation of therapy may be simpler, less expensive, and more appropriate than an attempt to resolve the issue, but this can often be easily accomplished, even after many years of treatment, by abrupt discontinuation of hormone therapy. After 5 weeks, determination of plasma T_4 (and FTI) is made. If the value is normal, the patient is considered euthyroid and the original diagnosis is discarded. In contrast,

a low T_4 (and a subsequently determined high TSH) verifies a diagnosis of hypothyroidism.

Occasional euthyroid patients who were inappropriately treated with thyroid hormone for long periods and most hypothyroid patients become symptomatic during the 5-week period of withdrawal. If the physician wishes to avoid the possibility of the development of symptoms as a result of withdrawal, a rapid but expensive way to determine thyroid status while the patient continues to receive full hormone replacement is to administer bovine TSH (10 units intramuscularly) followed 18 hours later by an RaIU test (page 991). A normal or elevated RaIU post-TSH injection indicates normal thyroid function and a previously inappropriate diagnosis of primary hypothyroidism.

Hypothyroidism versus "Euthyroid Sick Syndrome"

The diagnosis of hypothyroidism in severely ill patients presents special problems (6, 21, 22). Patients with the simulating "euthyroid sick syndrome" are usually elderly, and often have sepsis. The T_4 and T_4 indexes are low, TSH is not markedly elevated, and response to TRH is normal or blunted. Plasma rT_3 is often elevated.

Although to date this "euthyroid sick syndrome" has been clearly recognized only in hospitalized, severely ill patients, it probably also occurs in less dramatic form in chronically ill, nonhospitalized individuals. Many patients with chronic renal failure undergoing hemodialysis appear to fall in this group. The mechanisms underlying this phenomenon appear to involve a combination of factors including accelerated T_4 metabolism, impairment of TSH secretion (22), and impairment of T_4 binding to plasma proteins (3).

Treatment

The best preparation for ordinary use is T_4 (levothyroxine; sodium L-thyroxine; Synthroid; Levothyroid). T_3 (liothyronine, Cytomel) is also effective and sometime preferable for treatment of goiter, but has no special advantage for routine therapy of hypothyroidism and has the distinct disadvantage that one cannot monitor the plasma T_4 to determine adequacy of replacement. Combinations of T_4 and T_3 and desiccated thyroid should no longer be used.

Traditionally, initiation of thyroid hormone replacement therapy has been cautious and conservative and has utilized dosage schedules that ensure slow restoration of a normal metabolic state. While the principle is rational, the practice is often faulty. Therapy should be adjusted to the individual case, with several points in mind. If the patient is not elderly and has never had overt cardiac disease, overcautious initiation of therapy will result only in needless prolongation of the hypothyroid state with its attendant morbidity. If the patient has evidence of pre-existing cardiac disease, therapy should be started slowly, but unnecessary delay should be avoided. Only rarely will serious heart disease, such as angina pectoris, prevent at least partial therapy sufficient to eliminate myxedema, if not full correction of hypothyroidism.

The usual hypothyroid patient, without complicating medical problems, may be started on full daily replacement dosage. Even with this therapeutic schedule, the clinical response will be very slow. One can expect several months to pass before restoration of the normal metabolic state.

If the patient is elderly or has known cardiovascular disease, a daily dose of 0.025 to 0.05 mg of T_4 should be started, with 0.05-mg increases at 2-week intervals.

The objective of therapy is to restore the euthyroid state. Enough thyroxine is given daily to maintain the plasma T_4 at the mid to upper range of normal, or, ideally, to the lowest level of T_4 at which the TSH is restored to normal. Most persons need about 0.15 mg/day; only rarely is as much as 0.2 mg necessary and more is hardly ever needed. Elderly patients often require only 0.1 mg daily for maintenance; frequently as little as 0.05 or 0.075 mg may suffice (5).

Recently, concern has been expressed over the bioavailability of hormone in certain generic preparations and even lack of standardization of certain brands of thyroxine, but clinically significant problems are not likely to be encountered with any of these preparations. Determination of plasma T_3 during therapy with T_4 is unnecessary.

Patients with grossly evident hypothyroidism who require surgery are poor risks until their thyroid status is at least partially corrected, a process that requires 3 to 4 weeks with ordinary oral therapy. Elective surgery is best delayed in such patients. In an urgent situation, an intravenous dose of T_4 is probably warranted to prepare the patient for surgery in a few days. The increased susceptibility of severely hypothyroid persons to respiratory depression by conventional doses of many CNS active drugs should be borne in mind. This increased drug sensitivity has been responsible for precipitation of myxedema coma. On the other hand, recent studies indicate that patients with minimal hypothyroidism appear to tolerate ordinary surgical stress quite well.

GOITER

A goiter is an enlarged thyroid gland. The term implies nothing about the functional state of the gland. Goiter is the most common thyroid abnormality. *Diffuse goiter*, also called simple goiter, is a gland that is uniformly and symmetrically enlarged without apparent irregularities. (Some use the term *simple goiter* to denote any nontoxic or non-hyperfunctioning gland, regardless of its anatomy.)

In some areas of the world thyroid enlargement is so common as to be termed *endemic goiter*. Before the widespread introduction of iodized salt these areas were common, but this is no longer the case. Endemic goiter, for practical purposes synonymous with iodine deficiency goiter, is now found only in selected geographically isolated areas of the underdeveloped world. The term *sporadic goiter* refers to thyroid enlargement as now encountered in the United States and other developed areas. Sporadic goiter is seen in a few percent of the population and increases in frequency with age. The cause is unknown.

Causes

Any process that prevents the synthesis of normal quantities of thyroid hormones may produce goiter. If impairment of hormone synthesis is severe enough, goiter formation is associated with reduction of blood hormone levels, eventually to be followed by clinical hypothyroidism. The mechanism of the thyroid enlargement in this situation is increased pituitary TSH secretion *via* activation of the feedback system. The resulting increased thyroid mass is a compensatory mechanism which may allow sufficient hormone synthesis to occur so that the patient remains euthyroid.

Drugs that interfere with thyroid hormone synthesis (thiocarbamides, lithium, iodides, *etc*) can lead to goiter. Withdrawal of a goitrogenic drug results in regression of the goiter, as will administration of enough T_4 or T_3 to suppress endogenous TSH secretion.

Only one well defined, naturally occurring "goitrogen" is known, L-5-vinyl-2-thio-oxazolidone. This substance, with a mechanism of action much like that of the thiocarbamides, is in cabbage, turnips, soybeans, and several other vegetables. Other poorly characterized goiter-producing substances have been detected in the food and water supplies of some areas. No environmental factor has been incriminated, however, as a cause of sporadic goiter, the etiology of which remains obscure.

Recognition

A mass in the base of the neck is the usual mode of presentation of goiter. Occasionally, especially in the elderly, an enlarged thyroid is neither visible nor readily palable but is incidentally found by X-ray of the chest or esophagus when either a retrosternal mass is noted or the trachea or esophagus is found to be deviated. Confirmation of the nature of a neck mass as an enlarged thyroid gland and precise determination of its size are now most economically and accurately performed by ultrasonic examination (sonography). Although radionuclide scanning was previously used for this purpose, it is not as accurate and fails to show nodularity with comparable clarity. Computerized tomography is also quite accurate in delineating the anatomy of goiters and their relationship to contiguous structures but is not indicated on a routine basis.

Except in subacute thyroiditis, pain is not a usual symptom but can develop during cyst formation or hemorrhage, a fairly frequent event usually accompanied by rapid enlargement of a portion of the gland. Obstruction of the trachea or esophagus can be produced, but dysphagia should not be readily attributed to minor degrees of thyroid enlargement. Hoarseness may occur due to involvement of the recurrent laryngeal nerve, but this is rare in benign enlargement, and its occurrence suggests thyroid neoplasm.

Differential Diagnosis

Clinical and laboratory assessment of thyroid function should be made in all cases of goiter. The clinician must recognize that the functional state may change with time, sometimes rather rapidly, and hence the precise diagnosis may not be possible on a single examination. Goiter in association with hyperthyroidism suggests Graves' disease, toxic noduar goiter, or a hyperfunctioning ("hot") nodule. Hypofunction in association with goiter is likely to represent Hashimoto's thyroiditis (see "Hypothyroidism"), but other possibilities, such as drug ingestion, may have to be excluded. Rarities such as an infiltrative process (amyloid disease, metastatic neoplasm) and the inherited defects of hormone synthesis (organification or coupling defects) have to be kept in mind (Table 73.7).

If the clinical and laboratory assessments indicate normal thyroid function, the diagnosis of euthyroid goiter is made. Multinodular enlargement almost always indicates a process of many years' standing. Differentiation of diffuse enlargement from nodular enlargement may require ultrasonic examination since small nodules may be missed on physical examination, while ultrasound may detect nodules as small as 0.5 cm. If the ultrasound image is not helpful, an optimally performed scintiscan may show irregular ("patchy") uptake of tracer, but even the best technique can delineate nodules of only about 0.5 cm in size. A goiter composed of many such small nodules may *appear* to represent a nonnodular thyroid. Antithyroglobulin and antimicrosomal antibodies in serum are readily determined commercially and should be routinely sought in all cases of goiter. Such antibodies are elevated in the blood of 90% of patients with goiters due to Hashimoto's thyroiditis. A proper history will point to possible drug-related goiter. Rapidity of enlargement may help to differentiate benign from malignant lesions, while the presence or absence of pain will help in identifying inflammatory thyroiditis (see below, page 1011).

Treatment

Although thyroid enlargement is idiopathic in sporadic goiter, the process is nevertheless dependent on the presence of TSH. Administration of a physiological quantity of thyroid hormone results in suppression of TSH release. When TSH secretion is chronically suppressed in this manner, the enlarged thyroid eventually regresses or at least ceases to enlarge. This suppression therapy may be accomplished with thyroxine (T_4; sodium L-thyroxine; Synthroid; Levothyroid) or triiodothyronine (T_3; liothyronine; Cytomel). The dose should not be excessive. T_4 at a dose of 0.15 ± 0.05 mg daily is ample. T_3 is given at a dose of 25 to 50 μg daily. Some evidence suggests that T_3 may be effective in a greater proportion of cases.

Suppression therapy must be monitored. The physician must be certain that the gland is suppressible, since 20% of nontoxic nodular goiters are autonomous. Other nonsuppressible goiters may represent inapparent euthyroid Graves' disease. These patients may, if not monitored, develop iatrogenic hyperthyroidism due to the exogenous thyroid hormone. Monitoring of therapy also assures that an adequate amount of hormone is being given. Although regression of goiter is evidence of adequacy of therapy, the physician should be certain that the dose is adequate in those cases that do not show obvious regression.

Although suppression of RaIU was once the standard method of assessing adequacy of dose and suppressibility, the technique is cumbersome, expensive, and less useful now because of the low RaIU so often seen in normal persons. However, the RaIU is still the only currently available method to assess suppression in patients administered T_4. Commercially available TSH determinations are currently too insensitive to measure suppression of TSH to levels below normal.

Suppression therapy with T_3 has the advantage that the plasma T_4 falls to a level below normal if suppression is adequate, thus obviating the need for RaIU testing and assuring patient compliance. When T_4 is used for suppression therapy, a plasma T_4 which is not in excess of normal provides assurance that the dose is not excessive but does not exclude noncompliance. Monitoring of suppression by RaIU should be done no sooner than 3 weeks after beginning suppression therapy with T_4 or 1 week with T_3. If plasma T_4 is monitored during therapy with T_3, at least a month should elapse.

If the treated gland is diffusely enlarged, obvious regression by 6 months is to be expected in about one-half of cases. Nodular glands are less likely to respond, and any response that occurs is slower. Even if complete regression is not accomplished, prevention of further glandular enlargement can be expected. A baseline ultrasound examination—not necessary in every case—and follow-ups at 6-monthly or yearly intervals provide objective assessment of the therapeutic responses but are not always necessary.

Several years may be necessary to discern regression of a long-standing multinodular goiter, and during that time one or more nodules may become more easily palpable as the relatively normal portions of the gland regress. Some confusion may occur if the physician interprets this as a progression of the disease or as the appearance of a malignant area. Ultrasound examinations will help to avoid this error.

Suppression therapy is often properly performed for cosmetic reasons. Suppression therapy is also clearly indicated for individuals with many years of life expectancy during which time mechanical problems may develop. However, little is to be gained by treatment of patients whose glands are known not to have changed in size over many years and who are, therefore, unlikely to develop difficulties. A clear and unequivocal indication is found in the patient who has already had surgery for goiter. Recurrence of goiter is frequent in such persons but can predictably be prevented with suppression therapy.

Once started, suppression therapy is usually continued indefinitely but can be terminated or withdrawn if regression occurs. Some goiters do not recur; in those that do, therapy can be reinstituted. Suppression therapy does not lead to permanent loss of TSH secretion, even after decades of thyroid hormone administration, although rare individuals may manifest a brief period of hypothyroidism when prolonged therapy is withdrawn.

Goiter so large as to produce not merely a deviation but significant tracheal compression, as assessed by plain X-ray views of the trachea, or to interfere with swallowing is now a rarity. In these cases, surgery, although attended by significant morbidity, should be considered, since suppression therapy is unlikely to be effective in significantly reducing the size of such large goiters. Radioiodide therapy can be considered in these cases, especially in the elderly or in individuals with other serious medical problems. Multiple doses are usually required. While the response is slow, useful reduction in the size of the goiter may be achieved.

The frequency of carcinoma in multinodular goiter has been debated for years. Unwarranted concern has resulted in countless unnecessary operations (see page 1010).

THYROID NEOPLASMS

One of the most frequent abnormalities of the thyroid is a localized area of enlargement commonly known as a nodule. In evaluating a thyroid nodule, the possibility of malignancy is the main concern. About 90% are benign adenomas or cysts; the remaining ones are lesions of varying degrees of malignancy.

Benign Thyroid Neoplasms: The Solitary Nodule

Many solitary nodules are true adenomas and are encapsulated. While most benign adenomas are relatively hypofunctioning, follicular adenomas may exhibit normal or greater than normal function, i.e., they take up iodine and elaborate thyroid hormone. The growth of most benign adenomas, hypofunctional though they may be, is dependent on endogenous TSH. Adenomas whose function is independent of TSH are termed autonomous.

Benign thyroid nodules are present in at least 5% of the population, but clinically aggressive thyroid carcinoma is rare. In a group of over 200 patients with thyroid nodules identified in the Framingham study (4% of 5000 patients examined, ages 30 to 60) and followed for 15 years, none developed clinically evident malignancy. In that population, new thyroid nodules continued to appear at a rate of about 1/1000 persons/year, about twice as frequently in women as in men (17).

Clinical Approach

The first point to be established is whether the patient really has only a single nodule. Palpation by an experienced examiner is essential. Frequently, the "solitary" nodule turns out to be one of several nodules in a nontoxic nodular goiter. A single nodule in a clearly enlarged thyroid has a similar connotation, since the enlarged gland is likely to be harboring many small, nondiscrete nodules. Although most patients with a nodule are euthyroid at presentation, T_4 index should be determined for confirmation. If any question about hyperthyroidism exists (see below), plasma T_3 should also be measured.

The next essential question is that of the functional state of the nodule relative to the remaining thyroid tissue, since the hyperfunctioning nodule is almost invariably benign. When scintiscanning is performed, accumulation of isotope in the nodule can approximate that of the surrounding gland ("warm" nodule), be greater ("hot" nodule), or be less ("cold" nodule). A hot nodule can be considered benign (99.8% with ^{123}I). "Warm" nodules are far more likely to be benign than not, but the statistics are not so unequivocal as they are for the hot nodule.

The "hot" nodule. Management of the hot nodule depends on whether an excessive amount of thyroid hormone is being produced. The autonomous hot nodule, if it produces an amount of hormone equal to or greater than that of normal gland output, suppresses TSH; the remaining normal tissue then becomes relatively inactive and may not be visible, or may be only poorly visible, by scintiscan. In cases in which the nodule is hyperactive but has not clearly suppressed the remaining thyroid tissue, demonstration of autonomous function may depend on a scintiscan after a period of suppression (see above, page 1006) with administered thyroid hormone.

If the amount of hormone produced by the adenoma considerably exceeds normal, thyrotoxicosis should be clinically apparent. Usually T_4 and T_3 are produced in excess. However, hyperthyroidism due to T_3 alone (T_3 toxicosis) is fairly frequent with such hyperactive nodules.

The natural history of the hot nodule is variable. Over a 10-year interval about one-third will show little change, one-third will become frankly hyperactive, and the remainder will become "cold," sometimes with obvious hemorrhagic infarction and cystic degeneration. Treatment of the hot nodule that is producing hyperthyroidism can be satisfactorily accomplished with radioactive iodine or surgery. Prophylactic ablative therapy is not indicated. Suppression therapy with thyroid hormone is, of course, not effective and will lead to iatrogenic hyperthyroidism.

The "cold" nodule. Most nodules are "cold", *i.e.*, functionally hypoactive relative to the remainder of the gland. The major concern with most nodules is, of course, malignancy. The diagnostic workup and therapeutic approach to these lesions should be determined by a number of clinical considerations, including the biological potential of the nodule and the age of the patient. In the elderly, even more than in the young, a conservative approach is necessary (5).

Most nodules—variously estimated at 75 to 90%—are benign lesions; most of these are adenomas, but 10 to 15% are cysts. Thus, the overall risk is small. The risk is smaller still when it is realized that the remaining lesions are almost always clinically relatively nonaggressive papillary or follicular carcinomas. These lesions are usually nonlethal (see below) and slow growing, so that a conservative course is always reasonable. Nonetheless, some patients—not to mention physicians—become extremely anxious when faced with the possibility of cancer. If reassurance fails and a conservative approach is insufficient, the patient or physician may wish to proceed with a definitive diagnostic procedure or even excision. However, immediate and indiscriminate excision of all thyroid nodules is irrational and cannot be justified.

Currently, some experts recommend needle biopsy of all nodules as the first diagnostic maneuver, bypassing scintiscanning and sonography. These authorities argue that this approach is more cost effective and helps to avoid unnecessary excisions (18).

Cysts are immediately recognized by preliminary aspiration. Biopsy is by fine needle aspiration for cytological examination, or by aspiration or cutting needle for conventional histological examination. In experienced hands these procedures are safe, direct, and useful, but they have several limitations and go beyond the ability of operator (endocrinologist or surgeon) to obtain a satisfactory specimen. It is probably possible under optimal conditions to make an accurate diagnosis in about 90% of cases examined by biopsy, although both procedures may fail to distinguish benign adenomas from well differentiated follicular carcinomas (13), an important limitation of the technique. However, it must be strongly stressed that the most important consideration in the use of needle aspiration or biopsy is the expertise of the pathologist needed to examine the biopsy material. If a specifically trained pathologist is not available, needle biopsy, especially by fine needle aspiration, should be avoided. Similarly, if the patient is reluctant to undergo the procedure, a conservative approach using suppression therapy should be pursued.

The argument that needle biopsy helps to avoid unnecessary operations is correct if one considers that some physicians have long erroneously held that excision of *all* newly discovered nodules is indicated. However, when physicians have an initial approach that is conservative, universal institution of biopsy for a number of reasons probably adds to the number of unnecessary operative excisions. Reasons include indeterminate pathological diagnoses and discovery of papillary carcinomas that might have been adequately treated by suppression. The issue of whether to biopsy nodules or to treat them conservatively with initial suppression has recently received a detailed decision analysis and statistical treatment. The conclusion of this study is that no "best approach" exists and that continued arguments over this issue will be futile. The decision to operate, suppress, or aspirate is thus a "toss-up," dependent in the individual case upon such subjective factors as psychological disability, relative cost, and attitudes toward operative risk and long term medical therapy (14).

CONSERVATIVE APPROACH TO THERAPY OF COLD NODULES. Initiation of suppression therapy of nodules—with adequate monitoring—is reasonable even without antecedent biopsy scintiscan or sonogram, although most physicians prefer to obtain at least one or the other (14). A sonogram is preferred as the initial procedure. If a cystic lesion is identified, the need for scintiscan is obviated, since a cystic nodule is always "cold." Subsequent scintiscan of solid nodules is useful in identifying the occasionally encountered "hot" lesions. In neither of these two situations is biopsy necessary or helpful.

If a predominantly cystic nodule is identified on sonogram, aspiration and/or suppression therapy can be considered. Some cystic nodules require several aspirations, but most will eventually disappear with this approach. Suppression therapy is rational, since most cysts arise in benign adenomas, but its usefulness is not established. The sonogram provides an objective and accurate measurement of size of cold nodules so that regression or progression of the lesion can be followed during suppression therapy.

Regression of the nodule over a 6-month period indicates clinically benign disease; such patients can be followed indefinitely with continued suppression therapy. Some physicians are satisfied when a nodule at least does not grow larger during suppression therapy. Regression of some nodules will occur, even though some of these are papillary carcinomas. Physicians should not be dismayed by this statement, since suppression therapy is the mainstay of postoperative therapy of such lesions. Considering the probability that 90% of cases treated in this way represent benign disease in the first place and considering the low grade malignancy of almost all of the remaining cases, this approach is reasonable. However, close follow-up is necessary to ensure that appropriate therapy is instituted should the lesion enlarge further during suppression therapy or should lymph nodes become palpable.

Thyroid Carcinomas

General Considerations

About 95% of thyroid carcinomas are of the papillary or follicular variety; of these, 80 to 90% are papillary carcinomas. Anaplastic and medullary carcinomas probably account for no more than 5% of the total. The relative frequency of the various types of thyroid carcinomas is markedly age dependent (see page 1010).

Occult thyroid carcinoma (defined as lesions with the histological appearance of carcinoma, but less than 1.5 cm in diameter) is found in 5 to 10% of US and European populations and in 30% of Japanese samples at autopsy. Death from thyroid carcinoma is as rare in Japan as in the United States. Clearly, occult carcinoma behaves as a benign disease and does not warrant aggressive management.

In the United States, about 10,000 new cases of thyroid carcinoma are seen each year, but only about 1,000 persons die. Most of these deaths result from the aggressive forms of the disease, *i.e.*, anaplastic lesions, the unusually aggressive follicular carcinomas, and a few from the very uncommon aggressive papillary lesions. Only rare deaths are attributable to medullary carcinoma.

Therapeutic Considerations in Thyroid Carcinoma

Papillary carcinoma. Enough information is now available to provide support for a middle-of-the-road approach, one which falls between that which advocated thyroid hormone suppression therapy without surgery and that which has employed radical surgery alone. Long term observations have now also reasonably defined the role of radioiodide ablation therapy (12, 16).

SURGERY FOR PAPILLARY CARCINOMA. Follow-up at 10 years indicates a recurrence rate of about 20% for subtotal resection *versus* 10% for total removal of the gland. Deaths due to carcinoma are 1.5 and 0.5%, respectively. This small difference is reported for one retrospective study to be statistically significant and currently strongly influences the surgical approach. However, the complication rate for total thyroidectomy (hypoparathyroidism, vocal cord paralysis) remains high. As a result, many surgeons have now adopted a modified or "near total" thyroidectomy. In this procedure the affected side is completely removed; most of the contralateral lobe is also removed but the posterior capsule is left, together with the tip of the upper pole. Visibly involved lymph nodes are always removed, but radical neck dissection is not justified even in the presence of obviously involved nodes (12, 16).

The presence of cervical node metastases at operation or the extent of lymphadenectomy does not seem to influence either recurrence or death rate. The death rate in lesions under 2.5 cm without local invasion and without evident distant metastases at the time of surgery is less than 1% in 10 years and is 4 to 8% in the less favorable categories (12, 16).

POSTOPERATIVE THERAPY: TSH SUPPRESSION AND ABLATION WITH RADIOIODIDE. Postoperative therapy with full replacement doses of thyroxine will suppress endogenous TSH and reduce recurrence, and is routine in all cases. In addition, postsurgical ablative therapy with radioactive iodide has a role, although not all cases of localized disease need such therapy. The patient with a minimal papillary lesion needs no such therapy but the patient with a large, locally invasive lesion should receive ablative therapy with ^{131}I. In cases with an intermediate-sized lesion, without invasion of the thyroid capsule and without lymph node metastases, the recurrence rate is greatly reduced by treatment with radioiodide, and deaths from recurrent disease may be completely abolished. The hesitation to use radioiodide routinely stems from the unwarranted fear of radiation-induced leukemia. Doses of ^{131}I smaller than those customarily recommended may be equally effective. In contrast to the constraints on radioiodide therapy of localized disease, known metastatic disease should always be treated vigorously.

Follicular carcinoma. This tumor is somewhat more aggressive than papillary carcinoma, tends to be angioinvasive, and may metastasize to bones and lungs. The tumor may bypass regional lymph nodes, a marked difference from papillary disease. The most important prognostic feature is invasion, either through the tumor capsule or into blood vessels. Unlike papillary carcinoma, primary tumor size at presentation does not appear to influence prognosis (24).

The clinical presentation may be very different from that of papillary disease; the patient may present with metastatic disease involving lungs, bone, brain, or spinal cord. In these cases the primary tumor may be small and initially overlooked. Only rarely do the metastases produce sufficient thyroid hormones to cause thyrotoxicosis.

The surgical approach to follicular carcinoma should be that taken for papillary carcinoma. Suppression therapy with thyroid hormone replacement is routine. Postoperative ablative therapy with radioiodide appears warranted, especially for those patients with overtly invasive disease. However, the case for routine postoperative use of ^{131}I ablation therapy in the treatment of follicular carcinoma is not statistically established (24).

Anaplastic carcinoma. This carcinoma is fortunately distinctly uncommon; its frequency depends on the age of the population. Anaplastic carcinoma is vanishingly rare in children and in adults under the age of 35. By age 50, as many as 10% of cases of thyroid carcinoma are due to anaplastic disease, and by age 80, by which time the overall incidence of thyroid carcinoma has fallen markedly, nearly half of the cases that do occur are of this variety. The disease is locally invasive in a highly aggressive fashion and quickly produces pain, dysphagia, hemoptysis, and hoarseness. Death usually occurs within 6 to 12 months. Surgically resectable disease without evidence of metastases, even if it has extended outside the thyroid capsule, can be associated with long term survival (20 to 30%). It is important to distinguish the small cell type from lymphoma of the thyroid. This rare disease, unlike anaplastic carcinoma, is radiosensitive and amenable to chemotherapy.

Medullary carcinoma. Medullary carcinoma accounts for 1 to 2% of all thyroid cancers. The tumors arise from the parafollicular or C cells and produce thyrocalcitonin. Both sporadic and familial varieties are known. The sporadic case typically presents as a solitary nodule, while the familial variety is often multifocal and part of a multiple endocrine adenomatosis syndrome. Diarrhea occurs in some patients. Thyrocalcitonin in plasma is elevated in the basal state or after stimulation with calcium or pentagastrin infusion. When surgical excision is performed before regional nodes have become involved, 90% of patients survive for 10 years. Once the nodes are involved, only 40% survival can be expected. Medullary carcinoma does not appear to respond to suppression therapy with thyroid hormone.

The Question of Carcinoma in the Multinodular Thyroid

The risk of *clinically significant* carcinoma in a nontoxic nodular goiter is low. Occult carcinoma will be found in a significant proportion of such cases. However, the approach to such occult lesions is no different from that to occult carcinoma in the non-nodular gland. Demonstration of multinodularity by palpation or sonogram or its suggestion by scan leads some physicians, including the author, to a firm recommendation against surgical intervention. Suppression therapy is recommended, but only for prevention of further gland enlargement or to induce regression of symptomatic goiters and not out of concern for malignancy. Others feel that large nonfunctioning nodules within multinodular goiters should be treated with suppression therapy for a period of 6 months. Failure to regress is considered an indication for surgical excision. However, since most large nodules in multinodular goiters do not regress within such a period of time, while a significant number may actually become more prominent as less abnormal tissue regresses, this approach is certain to result in unnecessary surgery. Serial sonographic estimates of nodule size may prove useful in such cases.

Radiation-Associated Thyroid Carcinoma

Low dose irradiation of the thyroid is a stimulus to thyroid carcinogenesis, with a latency period of one to several decades.

In recent years thyroid carcinomas have been reported to occur in increased incidence in patients who received radiation therapy some years earlier for enlarged tonsils, adenoids, or thymus; acne; cervical lymphadenopathy, *etc.* A distinction must be made between treatment with penetrating external radiation and local irradiation with point sources (radium rod and plaque treatment). Thyroid carcinoma has not been related to such limited exposure.

In the reports purporting to show a relationship between external radiation and the development of thyroid carcinoma, as many as one-third of irradiated individuals have been found to develop thyroid carcinoma. Papillary and follicular carcinomas have been seen in about the same ratio as in nonirradiated patients. A relationship between exposure to radiation and development of medullary and anaplastic carcinoma has not been observed. The biological behavior of radiation-induced carcinomas appears to be similar to the behavior of those that appear spontaneously.

Almost as rapidly as this association between clinical radiation therapy to the head and neck and thyroid carcinoma has been noted, reports refuting the association have appeared (see (11) for references). Accordingly, the approach to the patient with a history of irradiation to the head and neck is not currently standardized. If no thyroid abnormality is palpable, re-examination of the patient at 2-year intervals should suffice. Routine scanning procedures for patients with nonpalpable lesions is not indicated. Although many nonpalpable lesions (0.5

to 1.0 cm) can be detected by optimal use of methods now available, and although the frequency of carcinomas in irradiated patients with abnormalities on scan alone is probably smaller to that in patients with palpable disease, the issue at stake here is the natural history of such small lesions. Lesions too small to be palpable are clinically, if not pathologically, benign and should be managed conservatively.

In the postirradiation patient with a palpable nodule, a conservative approach is presently warranted for the following reasons: (a) Even those reports which suggest an association claim no more than an increase of carcinoma from 10% of nodules in nonirradiated persons to 30% of nodules in those radiated. (b) Most nodules that are carcinomas behave in an extremely benign manner. (c) The entire association is in doubt (11). Clearly, prudence demands that these patients should receive the care recommended above for other patients with palpable nodules; but a widespread surgical assault on these cases is not warranted.

THYROIDITIS

Pyogenic (Suppurative) Thyroiditis

Pyogenic or suppurative thyroiditis, also known as acute thyroiditis is very rare, and most physicians will never encounter a case. The thyroid infection usually follows bacteremia, but can occur as an isolated, primary event. The gland shows typical signs of an acute inflammatory process.

Riedel's Thyroiditis

Riedel's thyroiditis is another rare but indolent and painless form of thyroiditis. The intense induration associated with this process makes the clinical differentiation from infiltrating neoplasm difficult.

Hashimoto's Thyroiditis

This entity is common (see "Hypothyroidism"; "Goiter"; and Table 73.7). The process is painless and usually produces only modest enlargement of the thyroid. Nodularity is the rule. Distinction from nontoxic nodular goiter is made by the presence of high titers of thyroid autoantibodies in the serum of 80 to 90% of patients with Hashimoto's thyroiditis.

Subacute Thyroiditis

This entity, also known as granulomatous or de Quervain's thyroiditis, is common. Many mild cases are probably never diagnosed. The term subacute is often deceiving and sometimes inappropriate. Although the onset may be insidious, it is perhaps just as often acute over several days. Many patients give a history of recent antecedent upper respiratory tract infection.

The earliest symptoms may be referred pain, usually to the ear, but pain can appear to originate in the jaw or occiput. This phase may last a few hours or days before tenderness and discomfort in the thyroid area become apparent. Rarely, the patient is concerned only with the referred pain and is unaware of thyroidal tenderness until examination makes it apparent. When the onset is acute, the symptoms and signs are more likely to be severe. Initially, pain and swelling of the thyroid are often unilateral, but the process usually does not remain localized for more than a few days. Systemic symptoms include fever, especially in acute cases, and a sensation of intense fatigue and malaise. The course may be protracted with symptoms persisting for months, although usually they subside within a week or two.

Erythrocyte sedimentation rate is elevated. Early in the disease, the thyroidal radioiodide uptake is depressed, while plasma T_4 may be elevated. Mild cases have no or only borderline abnormalities of the tests. Significant titers of thyroid autoantibodies are not common but can be seen. The radioiodide uptake test is not likely to be useful diagnostically, because in many normal persons the uptake is low (see page 991).

Clinical hyperthyroidism is occasionally seen with subacute thyroiditis (see above). Rarely hypothyroidism occurs and lasts several months. Permanent hypothyroidism is unusual.

Therapy

Therapy for subacute thyroiditis is symptomatic. The patient should be strongly reassured concerning the benign, self-limited character of the disorder. Thyroid tenderness often responds within several days to aspirin in doses sufficient to maintain therapeutic (anti-inflammatory) blood levels. Codeine should be added if neck discomfort is severe. In less than 10% of cases the process may be severe enough to require glucocorticoid therapy (30 to 60 mg of prednisone daily or equivalent). Glucocorticoid produces prompt relief of pain and tenderness but, if the disease is severe enough to require its use, will usually be necessary for weeks to several months. Relapse is common when therapy is discontinued, and retreatment may be necessary.

Lymphocytic Thyroiditis (Silent Thyroiditis)

This newly recognized process occurs in association with hyperthyroidism and is discussed on page 1000.

General References

DeGroot LJ (ed): *Radiation-Associated Thyroid Carcinoma.* New York, Grune & Stratton, 1977.
    An extensive discussion of the development of the subject with additional information on many aspects of thyroid carcinoma. For an update of the radiation-related aspects, see Ref. 11 for additional references.
DeGroot LJ, Larsen PR, Retetoff S, Stanbury JB (eds): *The Thyroid and Its Diseases,* ed 5. New York, John Wiley & Sons, 1984.

Ingbar SH, Braverman LE (eds): *The Thyroid*, ed 5. Philadelphia, JB Lippincott, 1985.
    Comprehensive textbooks on all aspects of the subject.
Felig P, Baxter JD, Broadus AE, Frohman LA (eds): *Endocrinology and Metabolism*. New York, McGraw-Hill, 1981.
Wilson JD, Foster DW (eds): *Textbook of Endocrinology*, ed 7. Philadelphia, WB Saunders, 1985.
    The latest editions of these standard textbooks contain excellent chapters on the thyroid.

Specific References

 1. Anonymous: *Med Lett* 23:30, 1981. Effects of drugs on thyroid function tests.
 2. Borst GC, Eil C, Burman KD: Euthyroid hyperthyroxinemia. *Ann Intern Med* 98:366, 1983.
 3. Chopra IJ, Solomon DH, Chua Teco GN, Eisenberg JB: An inhibitor of the binding of thyroid hormones to serum proteins is present in extrathyroidal tissues. *Science* 215:407, 1982.
 4. Fradkin JE, Wolff J: Iodide-induced thyrotoxicosis. *Medicine* 62:1, 1983.
 5. Gregerman RI: The thyroid gland. In Andres R, Bierman EL, Hazzard WR (ed): *Principles of Geriatric Medicine*. McGraw-Hill, New York, 1984.
 6. Gregerman RI: The thyroid gland. In Harvey AM, Johns RJ, McKusick VA, et al. (eds): *The Principles and Practice of Medicine*, ed. 21. New York, Appleton-Century-Crofts, 1984.
 7. Gregerman RI, Davis PJ: Effects of intrinsic and extrinsic variables on thyroid hormone economy. In Werner SC, Ingbar SH (eds): *Thyroid*. New York, Harper & Row, 1978.
 8. Hamburger JI: Pitfalls in the laboratory diagnosis of atypical hyperthyroidism. *Arch Intern Med* 139:96, 1979.
 9. Ingbar SM, Braverman LE (eds): *The Thyroid*. Philadelphia, JB Lippincott, 1985.
10. Klein I, Levey GS: Unusual manifestations of hypothyroidism. *Arch Intern Med* 144:123, 1984.
11. Maxon HR, Saenger EL, Thomas SR, et al: Clinically important radiation-associated thyroid disease. *JAMA* 244:1802, 1980.
12. Mazzaferri EL, Young RL, Oertel JE, et al: Papillary thyroid carcinoma: the impact of therapy in 576 patients. *Medicine* 56:171, 1977.
13. Miller JM, Hamburger MD, Kini S: Diagnosis of thyroid nodules. Use of fine needle aspiration and needle biopsy. *JAMA* 241:481, 1979.
14. Molitch ME, Beck JR, Dreisman M, et al: The cold thyroid nodule: an analysis of diagnostic and therapeutic options. *Endocr Rev* 5:185, 1984.
15. Nicolai TF, Brosseau J, Kettrick MA, et al: Lymphocytic thyroiditis with spontaneously resulting hyperthyroidism (silent thyroiditis). *Arch Intern Med* 140:478, 1980.
16. Samaan NA, Maheshwari YK, Nader S, et al: Impact of therapy for differentiated carcinoma of the thyroid: an analysis of 706 cases. *J Clin Endocrinol Metab* 56:1131, 1983.
17. Vander JB, Gaston EA, Dawber TR: The significance of nontoxic thyroid nodules. Final report of a 15-year study of the incidence of thyroid malignancy. *Ann Intern Med* 69:537, 1968.
18. Van Herle AJ, Rich P, Britt-Marie EL, et al: The thyroid nodule. *Ann Intern Med* 96:221, 1982.
19. Volpé R: The role of autoimmunity in hypoendocrine and hyperendocrine function. With special emphasis on autoimmune thyroid disease. *Ann Intern Med* 87:86, 1977.
20. Walfish PG, Ginsberg J: Letter. *Ann Intern Med* 88:128, 1978.
21. Wartofsky L, Burman KD: Alterations in thyroid function in patients with systemic illness: "the euthyroid sick syndrome." *Endocr Rev* 3:164, 1982.
22. Wehmann RE, Gregerman RI, Burns WH, et al: Suppression of thyrotropin in the low-thyroxine state of severe nonthyroidal illness. *N Engl J Med* 312:546, 1985.
23. Wortsman J, Premachandra BN, Williams K, et al: Familial resistance to thyroid hormone associated with decreased transport across the plasma membrane. *Ann Intern Med* 98:904, 1983.
24. Young RL, Mazzaferri EL, Rahe AJ, Dorfman SG: Pure follicular carcinoma: impact of therapy in 214 patients. *J Nucl Med* 21:733, 1980.

CHAPTER SEVENTY-FOUR

Selected Endocrine Problems: Disorders of Pituitary, Adrenal, and Parathyroid Glands; Pharmacological Use of Steroids; Hypo- and Hypercalcemia; Osteoporosis; Water Metabolism; Hypoglycemia

ROBERT I. GREGERMAN, M.D.

PITUITARY DISEASES

Disorders of the pituitary gland are manifest by disturbance of function (hyper- or hyposecretion of trophic hormones), by anatomical encroachment on adjacent structures (enlargement of tumors), or by a combination of these processes. Many of the cases of hormone hypersecretion are due to benign tumors—often clinically inapparent microadenomas. Most commonly a small adenoma produces an excess of prolactin with resultant galactorrhea. Most cases of galactorrhea, however, are functional, in some cases idiopathic and in others due to drugs.

When a pituitary tumor is large enough to produce increased pressure within the sella turcica, enlargement and erosion of the bony walls of that structure either produce no symptoms or may cause headache. Tumor enlargement superiorly—the direction of least resistance—leads to encroachment upon the adjacent optic chiasm and may produce visual field defects. Pituitary tumors large enough to be anatomically apparent are frequently associated with failure of hormone secretion (hypopituitarism), a process which results in end organ failure (hypoadrenalism, hypogonadism, and/or hypothyroidism). The pituitary may also be affected by a wide variety of systemic illnesses, including granulomatous, infectious, vascular, and neoplastic processes, but all are extremely uncommon causes of hypopituitarism.

A related problem is that of craniopharyngioma. This developmental abnormality may simulate pituitary tumor. The lesion is usually outside the pituitary and presents as a suprasellar mass lesion readily evident on computerized tomography. Most cases are manifest during childhood.

Clinical Presentations

When a patient presents with evidence of *decreased endocrine function*, routine evaluation must include consideration of whether the process is due to pituitary disease—i.e., "secondary" gland failure—or is "primary"—i.e., in the end organ. For example, in most patients with hypothyroidism thyroid-stimulating hormone (TSH) is elevated due to failure of normal inhibition of the negative feedback loop. However, if TSH is not elevated in the face of hypothyroidism, the possibility of hypopituitarism must then be further evaluated. Similarly, in patients with hypogonadism an easy differential diagnosis can be made, since levels of follicle-stimulating hormone (FSH) and luteinizing hormone (LH) invariably will be elevated if there is primary end organ failure. In patients with adrenal insufficiency, however, the plasma adrenocorticotropic hormone (ACTH) does not always clearly differentiate primary from secondary disease. In cases of *endocrine hyperfunction*, pituitary function may also be evaluated but not necessarily routinely (see "Hyperthyroidism," Chapter 73, page 994; and "Adrenocortical Hyperfunction," page 1019).

Not infrequently, the issue of pituitary disease is raised inadvertently. The patient's complaints lead to radiological examination of the skull because of headaches, suspected sinusitis, injury, or for some other reason. An enlarged or an abnormal sella turcica is noted. The issue then arises concerning further evaluation of what may be an incidental finding. Referral to an endocrinologist is appropriate at this point, but further evaluation by the nonspecialist is also possible.

Evaluation of an Abnormal Sella Turcica

The sella turcica as seen in ordinary X-rays of the skull may appear deceptively normal or may appear abnormal when it is not. Polytomograms are more useful in delineating the anatomy of this structure, but even this procedure is often deceptive. Asymmetry, a double contour, and erosions of the cortical bone forming the sellar outline and of the clinoid processes are all criteria for sellar abnormality. The volume of the sella can be calculated and compared to normal values. Sellar enlargement is probably the most reliable finding on tomography. If the sella is shown to be abnormal, computerized tomography (CT) should be undertaken. For the evaluation of *intrasellar* lesions, CT has not been especially useful until very recently. However, the most advanced CT scanners can show details of intrasellar contents and are probably superior to polytomography for evaluation of the sella itself. CT is essential in evaluation of the possibility of suprasellar extension of tumors. If a suprasellar mass is shown, the patient should be referred for ophthalmological examination of the visual fields, preferably with a red dot, the most sensitive technique for detection of field defects produced by suprasellar masses.

Empty Sella Syndrome

An enlarged sella does not always mean that a pituitary tumor is present. Not infrequently extensive evaluation leads to demonstration of an empty sella turcica. Such patients are often discovered during evaluation of skull X-rays obtained for reasons other than suspected hypopituitarism—usually headache—and, indeed, usually have no clinical endocrine disease. The cause of the empty sella syndrome is not known, but open communication of cerebrospinal fluid through a defect in the diaphragma sellae and/or a ruptured cyst have been postulated. In most cases, a rim of normal pituitary tissue remains and pituitary function, which should be routinely evaluated, is normal; in some there is minimal hypopituitarism and/or a visual field defect for reasons which are not clear but could represent a previous cyst. The diagnosis can be suspected from CT which fails to show enhancement, but definitive diagnosis and differentiation from intrasellar tumor may not be possible without a pneumoencephalogram that demonstrates entry of air into the sella turcica. This procedure is not ordinarily warranted unless the issue is whether surgery or radiation therapy is required for suspected tumor as, for example, when headache is severe and intractable. In such cases, neurological or neurosurgical consultation is indicated.

Chromophobe Adenomas

Chromophobe adenomas, the commonest of the pituitary tumors, account for about 85% of cases;

most occur between ages 30 and 60, not infrequently in association with parathyroid or pancreatic islet cell adenomas and, sometimes, with the Zollinger-Ellison syndrome (see Chapter 36). These associations constitute the syndrome of multiple endocrine adenomatosis (MEA, Type I). When the pituitary is not involved, but pheochromocytoma, medullary thyroid carcinoma, and—occasionally—parathyroid adenomata occur together, the syndrome is termed MEA, Type II.

Chromophobe adenomas are usually noninvasive but may infiltrate local structures and on rare occasions even behave as locally malignant lesions. Long thought to be "functionless," many are now known to be prolactinomas. The term chromophobe adenoma belongs to the era in which pituitary tumors were classified by their histological staining characteristics (chromophobe, eosinophile, and basophile). A more precise classification can now be constructed which is based on the secretory product of the tumor (e.g., somatotrope tumor, growth hormone producing), but the old terms persist.

Pituitary function remains clinically normal until more than 75% of the normal pituitary has been destroyed by the adenoma. Hypogonadism is usually the earliest evidence of a hormone deficiency state (60 to 80% of cases), but hypothyroidism as an initial manifestation is almost as common. Adrenal insufficiency is usually the last problem to develop and is often inapparent except on laboratory testing. In about 10% of cases, diabetes insipidus develops.

Prolactin and Galactorrhea

Bilateral breast discharge may be the first clue to the presence of a prolactin-secreting chromophobe adenoma. In many cases discharge from the breast is minimal and may be apparent only on physical examination when a few drops of milk may be expressable. Breast enlargement may occur in the male, but prolactin excess is an uncommon cause of gynecomastia (Chapter 77). Prolactin secretion appears to inhibit the secretion of gonadotropins and hence may also be associated with evidence of hypogonadism, including impotence and amenorrhea (Chapter 77).

Most cases of galactorrhea are due not to tumor but to a functional disturbance of prolactin secretion, which in turn is either spontaneous or related to the use of certain drugs. In either case, the hallmark of galactorrhea is an increase of the concentration of prolactin in plasma. Radioimmunoassays for prolactin are widely available and present no special problems of interpretation except for the recent demonstration of a high molecular weight form of prolactin in some amenorrheic women. The significance of this material is unknown. The drugs most commonly incriminated in the production of galactorrhea are reserpine, phenothiazines, tricyclic antidepressants, α-methyldopa (Aldomet), and estrogens (oral contraceptives). If no drugs are involved, a functional disorder is still likely, but some cases will be due to chromophobe adenoma. Rarely, galactorrhea occurs secondary to hypothyroidism.

The degree of prolactin elevation is strongly suggestive of the cause of the disorder. Levels of prolactin greater than 200 ng/ml are essentially diagnostic of tumor, even in the absence of changes in the sella. Low levels of prolactin (less than 50 ng/ml) are much more likely to be due to a functional disorder, but in many cases differentiation is not possible by this means. A significant proportion of the normal population harbors a nonsecreting microadenoma which is evident only at autopsy. Other normal persons may have minor abnormalities of the sella on polytomography (2). Hence, demonstration even of such a change does not prove the presence of a functional microadenoma.

Many cases of galactorrhea, with or without microadenoma, can be successfully treated with the drug bromocriptine (Parlodel) which may lower the prolactin, abolish the galactorrhea, and restore normal menses. Treatment with bromocriptine can be undertaken by the nonspecialist provided that tumor is not likely. If prolactin levels are very high or if radiographic evidence of tumor is present, an endocrinologist should be consulted.

The indications for surgical intervention should be anatomical. Small tumors confined to the sella, or even those with some degree of suprasellar extension and associated with limited visual loss, are best treated by trans-sphenoidal surgery (see "Acromegaly"). Microadenomas can often be successfully removed and normal pituitary function restored. With marked suprasellar extension, a transfrontal surgical approach may be needed. This is a much more formidable procedure. In many cases a large tumor cannot be completely removed; postoperative radiation therapy will prevent clinical recurrence in these instances.

Acromegaly

Pituitary tumors that produce an excess of growth hormone result in the clinical state termed acromegaly. If the growth hormone excess occurs before cessation of growth, *gigantism* occurs. When growth hormone excess begins in the adult, the most common clinical feature suggesting the presence of acromegaly is insidious alteration of facial appearance over many years. Old photographs may be useful in helping to identify such changes. The various physical findings include enlargement (lengthening) of the mandible, sometimes with separation of the teeth; coarsening of facial features due both to overgrowth of frontal, malar, and nasal bones and soft tissue overgrowth producing widening of the nose and protrusion of the lips; enlargement of the hands and feet, often noted by increasing glove and shoe size; and dermatological changes which include skin thickening and sebaceous gland enlargement (hydradenitis). Very commonly, patients present with a nerve entrapment (carpal tunnel) syndrome. Osteoarthritis and diabetes mellitus, while frequently seen in this disorder, are too common to provide a clue to the presence of acromegaly. Tumors large enough to produce sellar enlargement may lead to headache; suprasellar extension may result in visual field defects.

The laboratory diagnosis is simple in overt cases but requires dynamic testing in mild cases. Elevation of serum growth hormone (GH) in the fasting, basal state to values consistently greater than 10 ng/ml is strongly suggestive of the diagnosis. However, stress and physical activity may also elevate the GH levels. Elevated values must therefore be confirmed with a test of the ability of glucose to suppress the GH. During a standard glucose tolerance test (Chapter 72), the GH—determined simultaneously with the glucose—should normally fall to a value less than 5 ng/ml. Most acromegalics show no fall of GH, while a few exhibit a "paradoxical" rise during the test. Laboratory evidence of elevated and nonsuppressible GH warrants referral to an endocrinologist, as does the presence of equivocal clinical or laboratory findings.

Treatment of Acromegaly

Treatment should be directed by an endocrinologist. Irradiation of the pituitary, usually by external high voltage techniques, has been standard treatment for years. Such therapy is effective but is usually extremely slow in its effect and may take several years to produce maximal suppression of hormone production. Surgery is indicated when there is a need for rapid reduction of the elevated growth hormone (e.g., for cosmetic reasons in a young woman with early disease; visual field loss; or intractable headache). Trans-sphenoidal operation is now standard for most cases and should, if at all possible, include an attempt at selective removal of a microadenoma. The trans-sphenoidal operation involves minimal morbidity, a very low rate of complications, and essentially no mortality but recurrences are common, leading some authorities to continue to advocate radiation therapy as the first approach for uncomplicated cases.

Cushing's Disease

When evidence is obtained for overproduction of glucocorticoids and testing suggests the presence of adrenal hyperplasia (see "Adrenal Diseases"), X-ray evaluation of the sella turcica is in order. Only rarely will an abnormality be evident, even on CT. Most cases of Cushing's disease with adrenal hyperplasia are, nonetheless, due to a basophilic microadenoma of the pituitary (see page 1020).

PITUITARY FAILURE (HYPOPITUITARISM)

Idiopathic Causes

Patients are occasionally encountered in whom pituitary failure occurs without evidence of pituitary tumor or of another anatomical defect demonstrable by current techniques. Some of these patients are eventually found to have infiltrative processes (sarcoidosis, histiocytosis, lymphoma). Hypopituitarism in these patients is diagnosed by the demonstration of end organ failure occurring in the absence of the expected elevation of trophic hormone. Isolated deficiencies of trophic hormones also occur but are rare. Among these, the most likely to be encountered is hypogonadotropic hypogonadism in the male, sometimes associated with anosmia (Kallmann's syndrome). In these patients, no anatomical basis is apparent.

Sheehan's Syndrome (Postpartum Pituitary Failure)

Massive uterine hemorrhage occurring at delivery occasionally results in pituitary infarction and panhypopituitarism. In this syndrome, failure of postpartum lactation and absence of menses are attended by debility and other evidences of end organ failure. Because of improvements in obstetrical care (prompt treatment of hemorrhage), such cases are now rare.

Pituitary Apoplexy

On rare occasions hemorrhagic infarction of a pituitary tumor may lead to severe headache and/or signs of a rapidly expanding intracranial abnormality. Radiographic examination of the sella turcica is abnormal. Another rare but recently recognized phenomenon is that of pituitary infarction ("apoplexy") occurring during the course of a febrile illness, presumably viral. Intense headache lasts for days and is usually but not always severe enough to require hospitalization. The acute febrile illness subsides with symptomatic therapy and without specific clinical or radiographic findings, only to be followed later by the development of hypopituitarism. Both men and women can be affected.

Hormone Replacement Therapy of Hypopituitarism

Pituitary insufficiency, regardless of the cause, is treated with thyroid hormone (thyroxine, see page 1004) adrenal glucocorticoid (cortisol, see page 1018) and gonadal hormone (testosterone, see page 1086, or an estrogen, see page 1100). At the present time, pituitary trophic hormones are not available for routine clinical use; furthermore, they are not necessary for maintenance of normal health and vigor. Occasionally, young women may be candidates for therapy with gonadotropins in order to produce ovulation and to restore fertility. Such therapy is possible but available at only a few centers. In males, normal libido and sexual performance can be assured with testosterone therapy. Restoration of fertility in the male is also possible with the use of a combination of gonadotropins, but such therapy is not generally available.

Disturbances of Pituitary Function Due to Nonendocrine Disease

Perhaps more common than decreased pituitary function resulting from intrinsic pituitary disease is altered gonadotropin secretion on a functional basis. Many illnesses can affect the functional integrity of the hypothalamic-pituitary-end organ axis. This phenomenon is most obvious as disturbance of menstruation in women (see Chapter 77). Any disease which results in malnutrition can produce decreased gonadotropins and (secondary) amenorrhea. Alcoholism is an outstanding example. Liver disease need not be present in alcoholism in order to produce amenorrhea, but various liver diseases are themselves associated with loss of menses. The common factor seems to be malnutrition.

The classical example of nonendocrine illness that simulates an endocrine disturbance is anorexia nervosa (see Chapter 5). In this psychiatric disturbance, which results in severe malnutrition with resultant weight loss, the most marked disturbance of endocrine function is cessation of menses resulting from a decrease of gonadotropins. Other trophic hormones are not affected. Thyroid function is usually normal. Axillary and pubic hair are retained, giving important clinical evidence for the preservation of adrenal function. Although cortisol secretion is low (urinary steroid excretion is decreased), this results from slow metabolic disposal of cortisol rather than decreased ACTH secretion; plasma cortisol is normal. Growth hormone concentration may be elevated, a consequence of starvation due to any cause. The diagnosis of anorexia nervosa should be based on the association of psychiatric abnormalities and obvious decrease in food intake. The tests described will serve merely to support the diagnosis.

Other diseases may also result in secondary amenorrhea due to failure of gonadotropin secretion. These include such diverse conditions as severe emotional disturbances, marked obesity, poorly controlled diabetes mellitus, and severe chronic infections.

ADRENAL DISEASES

Adrenocortical Insufficiency (Addison's Disease)

In ambulatory patients the clinical presentation of adrenocortical insufficiency is related to a number of chronic complaints which are nonspecific in character. Although a high index of suspicion will certainly result in far more tests than positive diagnoses, detection of this relatively rare problem demands such an approach. The alternative is needless morbidity culminating in acute hospitalization for full blown disease, *i.e.*, vascular collapse with Addisonian "crisis."

Etiology and Association with Other Autoimmune Diseases

Adrenocortical insufficiency is now most commonly due to "autoimmune" disease and is associated with the presence of antibodies to adrenal tissue. Most other cases are secondary to pituitary disease. Tuberculosis, once a common cause, now only rarely produces adrenocortical insufficiency, probably because of decreased frequency of tuberculosis and because of effective therapy. Many cases of autoimmune adrenocortical insufficiency are associated with autoimmune thyroiditis, although the two problems may develop years apart. The simultaneous occurrence of autoimmune thyroid and adrenal disease is termed Schmidt's syndrome. Rarely, autoimmune adrenocortical insufficiency, autoimmune hypothyroidism, and autoimmune gonadal failure occur in the recently recognized syndrome of "polyglandular failure." There is also an association of autoimmune adrenocortical insufficiency with pernicious anemia and Sjögren's syndrome, and probably with systemic lupus erythematosus. Other rare causes of adrenocortical insufficiency include histoplasmosis and sarcoidosis.

Clinical Presentation

Chronic symptoms include anorexia, weight loss, weakness, and decreased physical endurance. Vomiting may occur, and abdominal pain, sometimes resembling that of peptic ulcer disease, can be a presenting feature. Other symptoms include mental sluggishness, irritability, and symptoms of either postural hypotension or of hypoglycemia. In primary adrenal insufficiency, increasing pigmentation (white patients) or further darkening of skin (black patients) may be noted. Loss of axillary and pubic hair—an important finding when present—may occur in females. Such hair loss is commonly overlooked on physical examination and is hardly ever volunteered as part of the history.

Physical examination often shows postural hypotension. Pigmentation is diffuse but in addition is especially evident in creases of the hands, the areolae, over pressure areas (knuckles, elbows), and in new scars. Pigmentation of buccal mucous membranes is a pathognomonic finding in white patients but is a normal finding in blacks. Lymphadenopathy is occasionally seen. When the adrenal insufficiency is secondary to pituitary disease, additional findings may relate to the manifestations of a pituitary tumor (headache visual loss), to hypothyroidism (Chapter 73), and to hypogonadism (Chapter 77).

Laboratory Evaluation

Classically, hyponatremia associated with hyperkalemia and some degree of azotemia provided the clues to the diagnosis. These latter abnormalities are manifestations of severe disease and may be absent in the less severe cases that are likely to be encountered in an ambulatory practice. Various other nonspecific abnormalities occur, occasionally including anemia, lymphocytosis, and eosinophilia.

Laboratory diagnosis of adrenal insufficiency must be made or excluded by determination of plasma cortisol. Determinations of plasma cortisol made without prior adrenal stimulation by injected ACTH have many limitations. In this regard both the normal diurnal rhythm of cortisol and the high degree of variability of plasma cortisol in normal persons must be kept in mind. Plasma cortisol can be initially measured at any time of the day, and a normal value (15 to 25 μg/dl) will exclude the diagnosis. However, afternoon determinations may be "low" simply because of the normal P.M. drop and even the fasting A.M. cortisol is highly variable. Values lower than 5 μg/dl at any time are highly likely to be due to adrenal insufficiency. Intermediate values (5 to 10 μg/dl) may be seen in less severe cases and may overlap those of normals. Thus, measurement of unstimulated plasma cortisol is useful, especially in excluding the diagnosis, but may fail to detect mild cases or may yield indeterminate values.

Plasma ACTH can be determined by radioimmunoassay. An elevated level will be seen in primary adrenal insufficiency because of lack of inhibition of the negative feedback system. However, the high cost and relative lack of reliability make measurement of plasma ACTH only an adjunct to diagnosis which has its major usefulness primarily in establishing a diagnosis of secondary (pituitary) adrenocortical insufficiency.

Evaluation of the significance of low or borderline values of plasma cortisol should always be made by administering exogenous ACTH and then measuring plasma cortisol again—after the adrenal stimulation. The ease with which such testing is performed—and the frequent failure of unstimulated plasma cortisol values to give definitive information—provides a cogent argument for use of ACTH stimulation as the preferred screening procedure for adrenal insufficiency. Many variations of ACTH stimulation tests have been advocated. A simple and reliable procedure is the bolus intravenous injection of 0.25 mg of synthetic ACTH (Cortrosyn) (see below). Plasma cortisol obtained 2 to 3 hours after injection will normally increase 2 to 4 times over baseline and will be above the normal baseline range. Patients with adrenocortical insufficiency do not show a response. If the test is positive (no response), confirmation should be made with an 8-hour intravenous infusion of ACTH (Cortrosyn, 0.25 mg in 500 to 1000 ml of saline or glucose) and at least two plasma cortisols obtained between 6 and 8 hours. Expected increments of cortisol are somewhat greater in the latter test.

Synthetic ACTH (Cortrosyn) is now readily available. This compound is preferred over the older preparations of natural material, since adverse reactions are not seen with the synthetic peptide. If the natural (aqueous) ACTH is used, it is given in a dose of 25 units in the manner described for the synthetic material. Rapid "1-hour" screening tests with either type of ACTH should be avoided, since the increment of cortisol is less than when a longer period is used. The 1-hour test is therefore more difficult to interpret and less reliable. Intramuscular injections of ACTH can be given, but if there is no response, the test must be repeated by intravenous administration. ACTH gel should not be used in testing for adrenocortical insufficiency.

Tests of adrenal function based on urinary excretion of steroid metabolites (17-ketogenic (17-KGS)) or 17-hydroxysteroids (17-OHS)) should be avoided as initial tests for adrenal insufficiency. These tests offer no advantage over plasma cortisol measurements and often yield artifactually low values due to incomplete collection of urine. Following stimulation with ACTH, determinations of urinary steroids can, however, provide useful confirmation of the plasma cortisol response. The adrenal response to ACTH is slow in secondary adrenal insufficiency and requires stimulation for up to 3 days. However, other tests of pituitary function are available and serve better to identify the presence of adrenal insufficiency resulting from pituitary disease (see "Pituitary Diseases").

Although the adrenal mineralocorticoid, aldosterone, may be low in adrenal insufficiency, the hormone is secreted by the zona glomerulosa rather than the more central portion of the adrenal cortex and may be relatively unaffected by processes which destroy much of the adrenal. Therefore, measurements of plasma and urinary aldosterone have no place in routine diagnosis of adrenocortical insufficiency.

Treatment of Addison's Disease

The Addisonian patient should be made to realize the importance of taking hormone therapy regularly and of understanding self-care during situations of stress. Unless both patient and physician cooperate in this effort, the life of the Addisonian patient becomes a series of hospitalizations requiring emergency therapy for crises, most of which should be avoidable.

Steroid replacement therapy. Under normal circumstances patients are given 20 to 30 mg of cortisol (or equivalent) daily. Recommended dosage schemes vary. The simplest and least expensive therapy is 12.5 mg (½ of a 25-mg cortisone tablet) taken twice daily (morning and evening). In another scheme, 10 to 15 mg of cortisol (hydrocortisone) are used on the same schedule. Some authorities prefer to simulate the normal diurnal rhythm of cortisol secretion, although no evidence indicates that this scheme is of any benefit. In this approach, 15 to 20 mg of cortisol are given on arising and 5 to 10 mg in the evening. Equivalent doses of prednisone or another glucocorticoid (see Table 74.2) may be used but have no advantage. Their use may, indeed, dictate a requirement for additional mineralocorticoid therapy, since glucocorticoids such as prednisone, dexamethasone, *etc*, have much less mineralocorticoid activity than does cortisol (or cortisone). Overtreatment with glucocorticoids should be avoided. Frequent increases of dose for treatment of nonspecific complaints are a common practice but are to be deplored, since iatrogenic Cushing's syndrome is a real hazard to the long term well-being of patients with Addison's disease.

The requirement for glucocorticoids (cortisol) is, of course, increased during stress. In the ambulatory patient, minor stress can be handled by a properly instructed and motivated patient. Telephone contact with the physician is also useful—or even essential—on many such occasions, especially in the early months of therapy before the patient's ability to deal with these episodes has been demonstrated. The commonest stress for the ambulatory patient is a nonspecific often viral, febrile illness. Ordinarily, a febrile response to 101°F (38°C) or thereabouts which is unaccompanied by vomiting or diarrhea can be handled by simply increasing the cortisol dose to 50 to 75 mg daily in divided doses. A more severe episode (*e.g.*, bronchitis) may require 100 mg. The occurrence of vomiting or significant diarrhea requires contact with a physician and may demand the use of parenteral glucocorticoids.

The need for hospitalization during stress must be determined by the physician and depends on the circumstances. It is obviously prudent to be cautious, but in this long term, chronic illness frequent and precipitous hospitalizations should be avoided. Many minor events can be handled by judicious increase of steroid dosage. Preoperative management is described elsewhere (Chapter 86).

Although not all patients with fully developed adrenal insufficiency require mineralocorticoid therapy in addition to cortisol replacement, such therapy is usually started when the diagnosis is made. Initial dose is 0.1 mg of fludrocortisone daily (Florinef, 0.1-mg tablets). Aldosterone is not available for therapy of Addison's disease. Only rarely will patients require more than 0.1 mg of fludrocortisone. In the past doses as high as 0.2 mg daily were used, but hypertension and edema were common. Some individuals require as little as 0.05 mg every other day. Adequacy of therapy can be judged by determinations of serum sodium and potassium and clinical parameters, including normalization of blood pressure without postural hypotension. When, during stress, the dose of cortisol is increased beyond 50 to 75 mg daily, fludrocortisone therapy becomes unnecessary, since the mineralocorticoid activity of cortisol is sufficient to maintain salt-balance when taken in greater than baseline physiological amounts.

Patient education. The patient and members of the patient's household should be educated about the symptoms of Addisonian crisis and how to respond in emergencies. In addition, the patient should carry an identification document or wear an inscribed bracelet identifying the Addisonian state and instructing therapy. Appropriate information in addition to name, address, and telephone number should read approximately as follows:

"I am a patient with adrenal insufficiency (Addison's disease). If I am seriously injured, found unconscious, or am vomiting, I should be given an injection of dexamethasone, as emergency treatment for Addisonian crisis. A filled syringe is with my belongings. Notify my physicians [name, telephone number] or other medical authority immediately.

Syringes containing dexamethasone phosphate (4 mg in 1 ml of water) are available for patients and can be conveniently carried.

All patients with Addison's disease should eat a diet which contains a liberal quantity of sodium (100 to 150 mEq/day), regardless of whether mineralocorticoids are used. In event of intercurrent diarrhea or profuse sweating, additional salt should be consumed. Electrolytes should be checked periodically (every 3 to 4 months during the critical first year of therapy). Mineralocorticoid therapy should be cautiously reduced if edema, hypertension, or hypokalemia is noted and salt and/or mineralocorticoid should be increased if postural hypotension, hyponatremia, or hyperkalemia appears. Overtreatment with glucocorticoids should be carefully avoided. Over the long term, it should be borne in mind that, if the Addison's disease is idiopathic (*i.e.*, autoimmune), related diseases and their own manifestations may appear at any time (hypothyroidism, hypoparathyroidism, hypogonadism).

Adrenocortical Hyperfunction

The adrenals produce several steroid products: glucocorticoids (chiefly cortisol), mineralocorticoids (chiefly aldosterone), and so-called adrenal androgens (a group of steroids collectively termed 17-ketosteroids (17-KS)). Clinical disorders are known which affect predominantly the secretion of one or other of these hormones. Table 74.1 lists these disorders of adrenal hyperfunction. Most are rather uncommon or rare, but some essentially functional disorders are frequently encountered. The approach presented here is predominantly oriented to the recognition—or exclusion—and initial evaluation of these diseases in ambulatory patients. Once the practitioner is reasonably certain that a problem

Table 74.1.
Adrenocortical Hyperfunction

GLUCOCORTICOID EXCESS PREDOMINATES
   Adrenal hyperplasia (60–70% of all cases):
     1. Pituitary microadenoma secreting ACTH (most cases
       of adrenal hyperplasia)
     2. Nonendocrine tumor secreting ACTH (rare)
   Adrenal neoplasm (30–40% of all cases):
     1. Adrenal adenoma   } (about equal in frequency)
     2. Adrenal carcinoma
ADRENAL ANDROGEN EXCESS PREDOMINATES
(HIRSUTISM/VIRILISM)
   Some adrenal adenomas
   Some adrenal carcinomas
   Partial adrenogenital syndrome[a]
ALDOSTERONE EXCESS
   Primary aldosteronism:
     1. Adrenal adenoma
     2. Adrenal nodular hyperplasia
   Secondary aldosteronism:
     1. Salt and volume depletion, including diuretic use and
       various disease states causing increased production
       of renin
     2. Juxtaglomerular cell hyperplasia or tumor (rare)

---

[a] Complete enzymatic defects in steroid synthesis are rare and are invariably manifest early in life as adrenal insufficiency and abnormalities of genital development. In ambulatory adults, partial defects of synthesis of cortisol lead to compensatory adrenal hyperplasia with production of excessive quantities of adrenal steroids with weak androgenic activity. Hirsutism, with or without virilism, ensues (see Chapter 77).

exists, detailed evaluation often requires consultation with an endocrinologist and sometimes hospitalization for special procedures. However, many relatively simple tests to define the situation can and should be performed on an ambulatory basis. It must be appreciated that details of diagnostic workups vary widely even among specialists and are in constant evolution as new hormone assays and tests emerge.

Cushing's Syndrome (Glucocorticoid Excess)

Etiology. In this syndrome a supraphysiological amount of glucocorticoid (cortisol) is secreted along with varying amounts of adrenal androgens. Most cases are due to hypersecretion of ACTH from the pituitary with resultant adrenal hyperplasia (Cushing's disease). In recent years it has become apparent that almost all of these cases are due to pituitary microadenomas that produce excessive amounts of ACTH (see "Pituitary Diseases"). A smaller number of these cases are due to adrenal adenoma or carcinoma. Cushing's syndrome may also occasionally be caused by ectopic production of ACTH by malignant tumors. Of these tumors, small cell carcinoma of the lung is most commonly involved. When a tumor causes Cushing's syndrome, the malignancy is usually obvious, although rarely a small neoplasm may be inapparent when the evidence of glucocorticoid excess first appears.

Clinical presentation. The severity of the signs and symptoms depends on the magnitude of the steroid excess, the rapidity with which it develops, and the degree to which androgen production is increased. The signs and symptoms of glucocorticoid excess are familiar to all physicians who have seen the entire picture of this disease emerge as the result of long term treatment of patients with prednisone and similar drugs. Glucocorticoid excess produces increased deposition of subcutaneous fat in the face ("moon facies"), while deposition of fat in the upper body produces "buffalo hump" and truncal obesity. Skin changes include telangiectasia over the face, atrophy and thinning of the skin with easy or spontaneous bruising, ecchymoses, and development of purplish abdominal striae. Hyperpigmentation is sometimes seen. Muscle weakness results from so-called steroid myopathy and is especially prominent in the shoulder and pelvic girdle areas. The extremities become thin as muscle wasting occurs. Eventually bone mineral loss occurs, producing osteoporosis with its resultant back pain. Crush fractures of the vertebrae are common and frequently spontaneous, while hip or wrist fractures may occur following minimal trauma. Hypertension and diabetes mellitus are common. Hypokalemia may occur. Probably less well recognized are the psychiatric disturbances which result from chronic glucocorticoid excess. Lability of mood, depression, mania, and frank psychoses may all be precipitated by glucocorticoid excess.

Androgenic effects occur from both the intrinsic properties of the glucocorticoids and the associated production of adrenal androgens. With glucocorticoid excess alone only mild signs are usually evident, *i.e.*, hirsutism (facial, extremities, truncal) and acne. More profound androgen effects that include virilization suggest adrenal tumor. These signs include frontal baldness in women, oligomenorrhea, increase in muscle mass, and enlargement of the clitoris. Androgenic effects cannot, of course, be appreciated in men.

Differential diagnosis.

OBESITY AND HIRSUTISM. In women obesity is frequently associated with hirsutism, hypertension, and/or diabetes. When weight gain is rapid, striae may appear. These findings often raise the possibility of Cushing's syndrome and provoke laboratory screening for this disorder. Very few such patients will be found to have Cushing's syndrome.

One-half of obese persons have increased cortisol production, which is a phenomenon resulting from the obese state. In these individuals the urinary excretion of steroid metabolites is increased and falls into the range of that seen in Cushing's syndrome. However, in distinction from Cushing's syndrome, such obese individuals have plasma cortisol concentrations which are normal rather than elevated. Furthermore, the suppressibility of the pituitary-adrenal axis in obesity is also normal (see "Laboratory Diagnosis" below). The obesity-related increase of urinary steroid metabolite excretion is one of several reasons why such measurements are to be avoided for screening purposes.

PSYCHIATRIC ILLNESS. Psychiatric symptoms are common in Cushing's syndrome. However, in the past few years it has also been appreciated that depressive illness may be associated with markedly excessive production of glucocorticoids (17). These patients do not appear clinically to have full blown Cushing's syndrome, but at least some clinical features suggest the diagnosis and lead to laboratory investigation. Differentiation from true Cushing's syndrome may be difficult at first, but the differential diagnosis eventually becomes clear, since remission of the psychiatric disturbance results in disappearance of the abnormal laboratory findings.

Laboratory diagnosis.

GENERAL. The tests of adrenal and pituitary function fall into two groups: (a) static measurements of blood or urine steroids or (b) dynamic testing of the pituitary-adrenal axis. Both procedures are useful and may be combined. With regard to the measurements themselves, in blood both plasma cortisol and ACTH can be assayed. In urine, assays are available for cortisol ("free cortisol"), two different groups of cortisol metabolites (17-OHCS and 17-KGS), and the adrenal androgens (17-KS) which also include some cortisol metabolites.

SCREENING FOR SUSPECTED CUSHING'S SYNDROME. Many patients with Cushing's syndrome have mild disease. Steroid production in such individuals is not greatly increased and there is considerable overlap with normal values. Accordingly, determination of plasma cortisol or urinary steroid excretion is not likely to be helpful. Screening can best be performed with an abbreviated suppression test with use of dexamethasone. A single oral dose of 1 mg is given between 11 P.M. and midnight, and the plasma cortisol is measured at 8 to 9 A.M. Normal patients will show suppression of cortisol to less than 5 μg/dl. If the test is abnormal, a more involved but more reliable suppression test is performed in which dexamethasone is given orally at a dose of 0.5 mg every 6 hours for 2 days. Plasma cortisol, urinary 17-OHCS, or both can be monitored by this test. The plasma cortisol at the end of the suppression period should be suppressed to less than 3 μg/dl. Urinary 17-OHCS during the second 24 hours should not exceed 2.5 mg. Suppression is normal in obesity but may be abnormal in patients with psychiatric illness.

OTHER SCREENING PROCEDURES. An alternative screening procedure is measurement of the 24-hour urinary excretion of cortisol (free cortisol). This test is relatively sensitive. Minimal elevations of plasma cortisol tend to result in marked increases of urinary cortisol. The test is not affected by obesity but may be altered in patients with psychiatric illness.

The normal diurnal rhythm of plasma cortisol tends to be obliterated in Cushing's syndrome. In normal individuals, the 4 P.M. cortisol is on an average 50% of that obtained in the early A.M. Although widely advocated for diagnosis, determination of this rhythm by measurement of A.M. and P.M. cortisol is *not a reliable* screening procedure.

Interpreting tests and additional diagnostic maneuvers. Unfortunately, both false positive and false negative screening tests are occasionally seen. If the tests are equivocal and the clinical features strongly suggestive, referral to an endocrinologist is appropriate. In expert hands, a variety of maneuvers can usually establish or exclude the diagnosis and differentiate among the causes of Cushing's syndrome, but familiarity with the specialized test procedures is essential. Often a degree of laboratory precision is required that is not always achieved by ordinary commercial laboratories. Useful tests likely to be employed in such consultations, in addition to those described, include multiple samplings of plasma cortisol throughout the day and night ("integrated blood levels"), determinations of urinary excretion of steroids on multiple occasions, variations of the dexamethasone suppression test with the use of different doses of the steroid, and plasma ACTH measurements by special techniques.

Until strong laboratory evidence is at hand to indicate that steroid production is abnormal, procedures such as X-rays of the skull, tomography of the sella turcica, and CT of the adrenal areas are not justified. These procedures are not useful in screening, although they are important in determining the locus and etiology of steroid excess once this phenomenon has been established.

Treatment of Cushing's syndrome. Surgery remains the treatment of Cushing's syndrome due to an adrenal adenoma. Although surgical removal of the adrenals (bilateral adrenalectomy) has been accepted for years as the most effective therapy for Cushing's disease (adrenocortical hyperplasia), this treatment is being rapidly abandoned. Induction of permanent adrenal insufficiency, the risk of development of an enlarging pituitary adenoma accompanied by hyperpigmentation (Nelson's syndrome), and significant operative mortality and morbidity are drawbacks of adrenalectomy for this condition. However, it has been recently realized that many cases of Cushing's disease can be treated by transsphenoidal surgical removal of a pituitary microadenoma, and this approach has rapidly become the preferred therapy (21). Long term follow-up studies are not yet available, but recent enthusiasm is being rapidly tempered by realization that many cases treated in this manner recur within a relatively short time despite apparently successful removal of a microadenoma. Medical therapy with the adrenolytic agent, mitotane (o,p-DDD), is also effective, either alone or preferably in combination with pituitary irradiation. The selection of the therapeutic approach for the individual patient should be made by an endocrinologist.

Adrenal Androgen Excess

If evidence of Cushing's syndrome coexists with signs of androgen excess, the 24-hour excretion of 17-KS should be measured along with 17-OHCS or 17-KGS. The 17-KS measurement is, however, of no use in *routine* screening for Cushing's syndrome. Elevated values do occur, but do so less frequently than do the other indices of cortisol production. However, an argument can be made for including a single, 24-hour determination of urinary 17-KS in the initial screening workup for Cushing's syndrome, provided there is clinical evidence of androgen excess. When adrenal tumor is present, measurement of urinary 17-KS may be the most abnormal test. Some adrenal tumors (benign adenomas or carcinomas) produce enormous amounts of 17-KS. In suspected cases of adrenal tumor, measurement of 17-KS is specifically indicated. Serum testosterone will also be elevated in women but not in men (see "Adrenal Mass Lesions," below).

HIRSUTISM. Hirsutism without virilism is extremely common (see Chapter 77). The combination of hirsutism plus virilism, which is exceedingly rare, is invariably associated with elevated 17-KS. When such a patient is encountered, referral to an endocrinologist is the most appropriate course. In adults, most cases will prove to be caused by adrenal tumors. Other causes, e.g., entities such as congenital adrenal hyperplasia (female pseudohermaphroditism, isosexual precocity in males, hypertension, and salt loss) all become apparent in childhood. Only a few cases (due to 21-hydroxylase deficiency) have ever been seen in adults.

Other Adrenal Diseases

Mineralocorticoid Excess

The classical condition resulting from mineralocorticoid excess is primary aldosteronism due to a benign adrenocortical adenoma (Conn's syndrome). Clinical features include hypertension and the manifestations of hypokalemia. A significant number of cases are due to bilateral adrenocortical nodular hyperplasia. The evaluation of this condition is described in Chapter 45.

Mineralocorticoid Deficiency

Aldosterone deficiency is part of classical adrenal insufficiency (Addison's disease) but may also occur as a selective, functional deficiency state in the syndrome of hyporeninemic hypoaldosteronism. The identifying feature is hyperkalemia. The syndrome is described in Chapter 47.

Pheochromocytoma

This rare catecholamine (epinephrine, norepinephrine)-producing tumor is usually considered in relationship to the evaluation of hypertension and is described in Chapter 62.

Adrenal Mass Lesions, Incidentally Identified

Adrenal masses were in the past occasionally discovered during intravenous pyelography, but such lesions are now *commonly* recognized during CT of the upper abdomen. When such a lesion is discovered, consideration should be given to the possible presence of Cushing's syndrome, of mineralocorticoid or catecholamine excess producing intermittent or sustained hypertension (pheochromocytoma, aldosteronism), of hirsutism and virilization, and of feminization. Biochemical testing should be initiated as appropriate.

Most of the lesions incidentally encountered during CT are benign, clinically silent adenomas, but a major concern is whether the mass represents a carcinoma. Three considerations are relevant in attempting to make this distinction: biochemical activity, size of the lesion, and the relative incidence rates. Most carcinomas produce biochemically measurable products, e.g., an excess of 17-KS; a few produce 17-KGS but have normal 17-KS; and rarely only testosterone or aldosterone levels are increased. Benign adenomas may also produce excess quantities of steroids. Nevertheless, in general, tumors producing biochemical products should be removed.

If no biochemical abnormality is demonstrable, the size of the lesion gives some indication of whether it is benign or malignant. When discovered, most adenomas are small (< 6 cm diameter), and most carcinomas are large (> 6 cm diameter). However, a conservative approach to all such *biochemically silent* lesions is warranted, because even with tumors over 6 cm, over 60 operations would be necessary to remove one carcinoma, while over 4000 operations would be needed to remove a single carcinoma, if one considers all lesions of diameter greater than 1.5 cm.

Occasionally the adrenal mass is cystic. Large cystic masses can be aspirated by needle puncture; clear fluid indicates a benign lesion, but bloody fluid is indeterminate, and cytology is not helpful. Similarly, needle aspiration biopsy is usually not useful in distinguishing benign from malignant cystic lesions.

In follow-up of biochemically silent adrenal masses, CT scans at 2, 6, and 18 months are indicated. Clear evidence of progressive enlargement is an indication for excision. Lesions that are stable at 18 months can be considered to be benign and should not be removed (7).

PHARMACOLOGICAL USES OF STEROIDS AS ANTI-INFLAMMATORY AND IMMUNOSUPPRESSIVE DRUGS

Most steroid (glucocorticoid) usage is related to treatment of diseases other than adrenal insufficiency. The doses used exceed those of physiological output and are best termed "supraphysiological" or, simply, pharmacological. The anti-inflammatory and immunosuppressive properties of these drugs constitute an invaluable part of the modern therapeutic armamentarium, but such uses, at least when prolonged, are invariably associated with side effects. Short term uses are much safer, if not entirely innocuous. Although the glucocorticoid and mineralocorticoid actions of steroids have been chemically dissociated, no such separation has been possible for desired *versus* undesired effects. All available glucocorticoids share these properties to an equal degree, although potency (effectiveness per milligram) varies widely (Table 74.2). Despite this fact, certain glucocorticoid compounds have tended to become associated with the treatment of particular conditions, e.g., dexamethasone for treatment of cerebral edema. Often no secure pharmacological base supports such practices. On the other hand, legitimate pharmacological differences between available preparations do exist which include different rates of absorption, metabolic disposal, and solubility. Exploitation of such properties is seen in dermatological use. Triamcinolone and fluocinolone acetonides appear to be much more effective than hydrocortisone for cutaneous use, a phenomenon apparently related to properties of absorption (see Chapter 100). Another example is the use of beclomethasone (Vanceril) as an aerosol in the treatment of asthma (see Chapter 55) and allergic rhinitis (see Chapter 23).

Adverse Effects

Untoward effects of glucocorticoids are listed in Table 74.3. These problems are related to dose and—equally important—duration of therapy (9, 12). No contraindication ever exists to a single dose of glucocorticoid, regardless of the size of that dose. Thus, treatment of an allergic reaction with one or a few doses carries no risk. Chronic therapy, however, should be instituted only after consideration of the risk-benefit ratio. Therapy that is not intended as chronic may become so. For example, asthmatic patients may be so impressed by relief afforded by systemic steroids that other modalities are abandoned and the patient becomes totally dependent on glucocorticoids.

Side effects of steroids are closely related to desired effects. Anti-inflammatory effects are obviously desirable when treating a disease such as rheumatoid arthritis. However, many inflammatory

Table 74.2.
Commonly Used Glucocorticoids

Generic Name	Common Trade Name(s)	Equivalent Potency (mg)[a]	Sodium Retention Relative to Cortisol
FOR ORAL USE			
Cortisol (hydrocortisone)	Cortef	20	—
Cortisone[b]	—	25	1
Prednisone	Deltasone Meticorten Delta-Cortef	5	0.1
Prednisolone	Meticortelone Sterane	4	0.1
Methylprednisolone	Medrol	4	0
Triamcinolone	Aristocort, Kenacort	4	0
Dexamethasone[c]	Decadron	0.75	0
Betamethasone[c]	Celestone	0.6	0
FOR PARENTERAL USE			
Cortisol	Solu-Cortef		
Methylprednisolone	Solu-Medrol		
Triamcinolone	Aristocort		
Dexamethasone	Decadron		
Betamethasone	Celestone		
FOR TOPICAL USE			
Triamcinolone	Aristocort, Kenalog		
Fluocinolone	Synalar		
Betamethasone	Valisone		
FOR INHALATION			
Beclomethasone	Vanceril		

[a] Also equivalent to daily physiological replacement when given in divided doses.
[b] Cortisone acetate has long been given parenterally (intramuscular route) as well as orally; however, recent evidence indicates that this compound is unpredictably absorbed from injection sites and cannot be relied upon to produce adequate blood levels.
[c] This compound has a relatively long duration of action and should not be used for alternate-day glucocorticoid therapy.

Most of the compounds listed are available in generic forms. All are marketed as ester derivatives or salts of esters, e.g., cortisol sodium hemisuccinate (Solu-Cortef). For practical purposes, only cortisol and cortisone have significant salt-retaining (mineralocorticoid) action.

responses are beneficial, as for example the inflammatory responses associated with bacterial infection. In this situation, glucocorticoids may inhibit a useful inflammatory response which otherwise would serve to localize the process. Thus, one ordinarily avoids pharmacological doses of glucocorticoids when infection requiring an antibiotic is necessary. Not infrequently, however, patients receiving glucocorticoids develop an infection. Ordinarily, steroid therapy is not discontinued; rather, vigorous antibiotic therapy is instituted and the dose of steroid is kept at as low a level as the clinical situation allows, thus preventing clinical evidence of adrenal insufficiency and the development of nonspecific

Table 74.3.
Untoward Effects of Chronic Glucocorticoid Therapy

ACUTE
   Fluid/electrolyte disturbances
      Sodium retention
      Fluid retention
      Potassium depletion
      Hypokalemic alkalosis
   Gastrointestinal
      Peptic ulcer (hemorrhage, perforation)
      Ulcerative esophagitis
   Endocrine
      Precipitation of diabetes mellitus
   Ophthalmic
      Glaucoma
   Neurological
      Mood swings
      Acute psychosis
      Convulsions
CHRONIC
   Fluid/electrolyte disturbances
      See above, plus hypertension
   Musculoskeletal
      Muscle weakness
      Muscle atrophy
      Steroid myopathy
      Osteoporosis/pathological fractures
      Aseptic necrosis of femoral or humeral heads
      Tendon rupture
   Gastrointestinal
      Pancreatitis
   Dermatological
      Impaired wound healing
      Atrophy of skin (fragility)
      Ecchymoses
      Increased sweating
   Neurological
      Convulsions
      Increased intracranial pressure
      Insomnia
      Euphoria
      Depression
   Endocrine
      Menstrual irregularities
      Carbohydrate intolerance/diabetes mellitus
      Adrenal atrophy/disruption of normal response to stress
        (iatrogenic Addison's disease)
   Ophthalmic
      Cataracts
      Glaucoma
   Hematological
      Thromboembolism
   Other
      Weight gain
      Increased susceptibility to infections

but serious symptoms (see "Steroid Withdrawal Syndrome," page 1025).

Adverse effects of steroids are related not only to duration of therapy but to dose used. Obviously, one should attempt to use a minimally effective dose. Nonetheless, some persons seem especially vulnerable to unwanted side effects. Poorly nourished, debilitated, and elderly patients are all more prone to the muscle-wasting effects of steroids. Postmenopausal women—already prone to develop osteoporosis— are especially vulnerable to the demineralization which accompanies steroid use. Genetically predisposed individuals may develop overt diabetes mellitus when given glucocorticoids. Peptic ulcer disease may be reactivated, and complications such as bleeding or perforation may be precipitated. Tuberculosis, clinically inapparent except for a positive tuberculin test, may become active. The role of isoniazid prophylaxis in this situation is described elsewhere (Chapter 29).

Topical Therapy

Whenever steroids can be used locally, such use is preferred, especially when long term treatment is involved. Although absorption may be complete from a local site, the amount of steroid required is often far less when use is local. One thus avoids—to some extent—systemic effects, side effects, and pituitary-adrenal suppression. In addition to dermatological use of topical steroids, treatments of some ophthalmological conditions, allergic rhinitis, asthma, and localized joint disease are examples of this principle.

Intermittent Therapy

Usually, severe disease requires initiation of steroid therapy given as multiple daily doses. When the disease intensity has waned (e.g., 1 to 2 weeks), conversion to alternate-day therapy can be made. Intermittent therapy of this type should always be considered whenever long term use is contemplated. Such therapy is to be preferred because pituitary-adrenal suppression is not likely and the adverse effects of glucocorticoids are minimized (9, 12). When initiating intermittent therapy the daily divided dose is given as a single morning dose. After this dose has been shown to be tolerated for several days, the single daily dose may be doubled and given as a single dose every other day. Thereafter, the dose given every other day can be reduced slowly, as clinically indicated. The "off" day, particularly when alternate-day therapy is first started, may result in the patient becoming symptomatic. To handle this situation small doses of glucocorticoid may be given on this day. Nonsteroidal anti-inflammatory agents may also be helpful in ameliorating symptoms at this time and in easing the transition.

Use of Adrenocorticotropic Hormone

The clinical indications for use of ACTH rather than a glucocorticoid are practically nonexistent. ACTH was available for clinical use even before cortisone. It is clear that in sufficient amounts (100 units) long acting preparations (gel or zinc suspensions) given once daily are capable of stimulating adrenal secretion of up to 300 mg of cortisol daily. However, disadvantages are multiple: the route is parenteral; magnitude of response is unpredictable; mineralocorticoid effects (salt and fluid retention, potassium wasting) are considerable; response in patients previously treated with glucocorticoids is slow and unpredictable. The only advantage is that adrenal responsiveness is maintained during therapy. Combined ACTH-glucocorticoid therapy has been advocated for this reason, as has the occasional injection of ACTH to prevent adrenal atrophy. The advantage of such an approach over that of intermittent glucocorticoid therapy is not clear. Moreover, when ACTH is used alone in high doses for a prolonged period, pituitary suppression occurs even though adrenal suppression does not. Another disadvantage of ACTH therapy is failure to produce more than the equivalent of 300 mg of cortisol (60 mg of prednisone) despite maximal stimulation of the adrenals. Such a dose, while considerable, may be insufficient to produce the desired anti-inflammatory effect. The only current, fairly widespread use of ACTH is in the treatment of multiple sclerosis. It is not clear that such use is supported by anything more than anecdote.

Withdrawal from Chronic Glucocorticoid Therapy

Treatment with glucocorticoids (cortisone, hydrocortisone, prednisone, *etc*) produces suppression of the hypothalamus-pituitary-adrenal axis; the output of ACTH falls and there is subsequent adrenal atrophy and an inability to respond to stress with increased cortisol output. The time required for initial suppression is highly variable, but all patients receiving daily pharmacological doses of glucocorticoids for more than 1 week should be presumed to have a suppressed response to stress (18). If stressed by surgery, trauma, or severe infection these patients should be treated with replacement glucocorticoids as if they had Addison's disease. On the other hand, glucocorticoids may be discontinued abruptly after 2 to 4 weeks of pharmacological steroid therapy provided that the patient is not under stress, since baseline—as opposed to stress-related—adrenal function will almost always be adequate. Patients who have been treated with alternate-day steroid therapy are not at risk, since pituitary-adrenal function seems well preserved in these individuals (9, 12).

When it becomes desirable to terminate glucocorticoid therapy, the question arises of how to accomplish this goal while avoiding adrenal insufficiency. In the presence of active underlying disease, for which the glucocorticoids may have been given in the first place, a dilemma quickly becomes apparent. The nonspecific symptoms of adrenal insufficiency may be similar or identical to those of the disease that was under treatment. In addition, the occurrence of the "steroid withdrawal syndrome" (see below) may further compound the issue.

Withdrawal Schedule

No single scheme can solve this difficult clinical problem although many have been proposed (3). However, a few general points can be made. First, even after prolonged therapy, in the absence of active underlying systemic disease, symptoms of adrenal insufficiency should not be expected until the daily dose of glucocorticoid drops below physiological replacement (30 mg of cortisol, 7.5 mg of prednisone, or equivalent; see Table 74.2). At this point most patients will tolerate a single 20- to 30-mg daily dose of cortisol (or 5 to 7.5 mg of prednisone). Continuation for 2 months at this level should ensure some degree of recovery of pituitary-adrenal function. Further withdrawal begins to re-establish the normal pituitary-adrenal relationship. Additional reductions of 5 mg of cortisol can be made every 2 to 3 weeks over the next 2 months or, alternatively, an every-other-day program can be tried over the same period; the glucocorticoid can then usually be stopped without producing symptoms. Assessment of the functional status of the patient's adrenals at this point is described elsewhere (see "Assessment of Recovery from Pituitary-Adrenal Suppression" below).

Steroid Withdrawal Syndrome

Abrupt withdrawal of pharmacological doses of glucocorticoids, even after months of therapy, does not always produce chemical evidence of adrenal insufficiency. Nonetheless, the patient may experience many of the symptoms of adrenal insufficiency, e.g., lethargy, malaise, anorexia, nausea, vomiting, myalgias, fever, and—in severe cases—desquamation of skin in a manner resembling exfoliative dermatitis. Such patients may be found to have normal or elevated levels of cortisol. This phenomenon is not simply adrenal insufficiency, but rather is a pharmacological withdrawal syndrome. Symptoms subside promptly with reinstitution of glucocorticoid therapy (1).

Recovery from Pituitary-Adrenal Suppression

After long term glucocorticoid therapy (pharmacological doses for a year or more), recovery of normal pituitary-adrenal responsiveness does not occur readily (10). At least several months must elapse, even if the patient receives no exogenous steroid therapy during that time. In the first month after withdrawal, both pituitary and adrenal function remain depressed (low plasma ACTH and low plasma cortisol). Over the following 4 months, pituitary function recovers (plasma ACTH is elevated), but adrenal function remains subnormal (plasma cortisol is lower than normal). Eventually, adrenal function recovers (plasma cortisol levels normalize) while elevated plasma ACTH returns to normal. The entire process may require up to 9 months. During this interval the patient may fare well, provided there is no stress, but replacement therapy with glucocorticoids may become necessary at any time. Accordingly, no patient should be considered to have normal pituitary-adrenal function unless at least 1 year has elapsed after complete withdrawal of chronic glucocorticoid therapy. Occasional patients seem never to recover normal responsiveness. Ideally, therefore, all patients with a history of chronic steroid therapy should be tested for normal responsiveness 1 year after withdrawal.

Assessment of a glucocorticoid-treated patient's adrenal function under baseline conditions is not difficult. Both plasma cortisol measurements and urinary excretion of steroid metabolites give a reasonable estimate of such baseline function. However, predicting the response to stress is more difficult. Since hypothalamic-pituitary function usually recovers first, followed by adrenal function, a normal response to exogenous ACTH usually indicates recovery of the entire axis (see page 1018 for details of testing with ACTH). A more complete assessment of the integrity of the axis can be made by induction of hypoglycemia with insulin (insulin tolerance testing). Hypoglycemia triggers ACTH release and the adrenal's cortisol secretory response. A normal insulin tolerance test assures that if the patient is subjected to stressful circumstances, replacement therapy with steroids will not be necessary. If neither an ACTH nor an insulin tolerance test has been done, clinical assessment, including perhaps plasma cortisol determinations or empirical treatment with glucocorticoids, becomes necessary. In the suppressed individual, testing with metyrapone (Metopirone), an adrenal 11-hydroxylase inhibitor sometimes used for evaluation of the integrity of the hypothalamic-pituitary-adrenal axis, may be misleadingly normal.

HYPOCALCEMIC STATES

Hypocalcemia is a relatively uncommon problem in ambulatory patients. The classic cause of hypocalcemia is idiopathic hypoparathyroidism, but most cases encountered are a consequence of inadvertent surgical ablation of the parathyroids during thyroidectomy or of a metabolic disturbance such as renal failure. The causes of hypocalcemia are listed in Table 74.4.

Clinical Manifestations of Hypocalcemia

The symptoms of hypocalcemia are primarily neuromuscular and are not usually evident until the serum calcium falls below about 8 mg/dl and often considerably lower. Mild symptoms are totally nonspecific and include psychological manifestations (irritability; mood changes; depression), paresthesias, and muscle cramps. More severe symptoms are delirium, psychosis, tetany (including laryngeal stridor), and seizures. Neuromuscular irritability can

Table 74.4.
Causes of Hypocalcemia[a]

HYPOCALCEMIA WITH HIGH SERUM PHOSPHATE
  Postablative hypoparathyroidism (post-thyroidectomy)
  Idiopathic hypoparathyroidism
  Pseudohypoparathyroidism
  Renal failure
HYPOCALCEMIA WITH LOW OR NORMAL SERUM PHOSPHATE
  Malabsorption (vitamin D deficiency)
  Magnesium deficiency (alcoholism)
  Renal rickets (renal tubular acidosis; phosphate diabetes; cystinosis; Fanconi's syndrome; vitamin D-resistant rickets)
  Medullary carcinoma of thyroid

[a] The serum alkaline phosphatase activity is elevated whenever severe metabolic bone disease is present. Parathyroid hormone levels are depressed in idiopathic hypoparathyroidism and may be depressed in magnesium deficiency. Parathyroid hormone levels are regularly elevated in renal failure and in pseudohypoparathyroidism. Urine calcium is depressed in most hypocalcemic states, except when the rare renal tubular calcium-wasting syndromes are responsible for the hypocalcemia.

often be demonstrated by the twitching which is induced by tapping over the facial nerve just anterior to the ear. A positive response is contraction of the facial muscles around the lip (Chvostek's sign). Another clinical maneuver is compression of the upper arm by a blood pressure cuff with the pressure elevated above the systolic pressure. A positive response is spasm of the hand induced within 3 minutes (Trousseau's sign). Signs of chronic hypocalcemia include patchy hair loss, scaling of skin, atrophy and brittleness of fingernails, and cataract formation. Candidiasis is common. Calcification of the basal ganglia may be seen on X-ray examination of the skull. Either osteosclerosis or osteopenia may occur depending on the etiology of the hypocalcemia.

Laboratory Findings

Hypocalcemia can be said to be present when the serum calcium falls below 8.5 mg/dl. However, since almost half of serum calcium is protein bound, reduction of serum protein by 1 g/dl lowers the serum calcium by about 0.8 mg/dl. The level of serum calcium must, therefore, always be evaluated in the context of the serum protein concentration; the serum magnesium concentration should also be evaluated at the same time (see below, "Other Causes of Hypocalcemia"). Plasma parathyroid hormone (PTH) levels are low or nondetectable in idiopathic or postablative hypoparathyroidism and in some cases of hypocalcemia due to magnesium deficiency, but they are elevated in pseudohypoparathyroidism, renal failure, malabsorption, and vitamin D deficiency. The interpretation and indications for determination of PTH levels are discussed below.

Idiopathic Hypoparathyroidism

This condition is rare. Although most patients are diagnosed in childhood, some do not exhibit the disease until adult life. Occasionally familial, the idiopathic disease is autoimmune, frequently associated with high titers of antibodies to parathyroid tissue, and may be seen in association with other autoimmune endocrine diseases (adrenal insufficiency, Hashimoto's thyroiditis) and pernicious anemia.

Post-thyroidectomy Hypoparathyroidism

Probably the most common cause of hypoparathyroidism, this condition is a complication of surgical thyroidectomy. The hypocalcemic state may become evident immediately after surgery, but often takes many years to develop, presumably due to slowly progressive interference with the blood supply to the parathyroids. Routine screening of serum calcium in patients who have had thyroidectomy will reveal many asymptomatic patients. Most of these individuals will seem to need no therapy, but in view of the subtle neuromuscular changes which can result from hypocalcemia, careful consideration should always be given to this issue. Hypoparathyroidism does not occur following radioiodide therapy of thyroid disease, even if hypothyroidism has been produced.

Pseudohypoparathyroidism

This is a rare disorder of genetic origin (X-linked dominant trait). In addition to hypocalcemia and its manifestations, there are associated skeletal developmental defects which result in short stature, shortening of metacarpals and metatarsals, and round face. Clinical manifestations attributable to hypocalcemia may not appear until adult life. The biochemical basis of the hypocalcemia is end organ resistance to the action of PTH. The combination of hypocalcemia, elevated level of parathyroid hormone, and typical skeletal abnormalities is virtually diagnostic. In the absence of skeletal abnormalities, diagnosis depends on demonstration of resistance to administered PTH, a specialized procedure requiring referral to an endocrinologist.

Treatment of Hypoparathyroidism and Pseudohypoparathyroidism

The treatment of all forms of hypoparathyroidism is similar. A few patients with idiopathic or post-ablative PTH deficiency can be managed with calcium supplements alone. The dose is 1 to 2 g of calcium daily. Since calcium gluconate and lactate contain only about 10% calcium, one must administer 10 to 20 g of these salts; the carbonate contains 40% calcium. Numerous tablets must be taken; patient compliance is a common problem. Every effort should be made to work out an acceptable, palatable, and economic program with a consistently available preparation for what is invariably lifelong therapy.

The second mainstay of therapy is vitamin D. The most commonly used preparation in the past has been ergocalciferol (vitamin D_2; Calciferol). The dose is usually 50,000 or 100,000 units daily, although higher doses may be necessary. The compound is available in 50,000-unit (1.25-mg) capsules. The sole advantage of ergocalciferol is cost; it is by far the least expensive form of vitamin D therapy. The disadvantage of ergocalciferol is somewhat unpredictable toxicity with resultant hypercalcemia and all of its manifestations (see page 1029). Because vitamin D is fat soluble, toxicity may last for many weeks or even months after discontinuation of therapy. Glucocorticoids are effective therapy for hypercalcemia due to vitamin D toxicity.

A preferable vitamin D preparation is its synthetic analog, dihydrotachysterol (DHT; Hytakerol). The dose varies from 0.2 to 2 mg daily. The compound is available as tablets and as an oil. The advantage of therapy with DHT is more rapid onset of action than D_2 and more rapid reversibility of toxicity upon withdrawal of the drug. The only disadvantage of DHT is its relatively high cost. Yet another effective compound is 1,25-dihydroxyvitamin D_3 (calcitriol; Rocaltrol), the natural, active form of vitamin D. This compound is more rapid than DHT in onset and has a shorter duration of effect but has the disadvantage of even greater cost. The dose is 0.25 to 1.0 μg daily. Both 0.25- and 0.5-μg tablets are available.

The approach to chronic therapy of hypoparathyroidism is institution of a relatively fixed calcium intake at a total level of about 2 g, which is about 1 g over regular dietary intake. Thus, a patient whose normal daily calcium intake approximates 1 g needs an additional 1 g of calcium in the form of supplementary calcium salts (see above). Instruction of the patient by a dietician is essential. Vitamin D, in whatever form is selected, is given simultaneously, with adjustments of dose at weekly or biweekly intervals depending on the serum calcium level. The goal of therapy is a serum calcium concentration of 8.5 to 9.5 mg/dl. Hypercalcemia is to be avoided. Once a stable level of serum calcium is reached (1 to 2 months), the patient can be monitored at monthly intervals and eventually every 3 to 4 months. The possibility of toxicity due to hypercalcemia is always to be kept in mind. Even mild hypercalcemia predisposes to nephrocalcinosis and nephrolithiasis in these patients.

Hypocalcemia Due to Other Causes

When hypocalcemia is related to malabsorption, efforts to correct that situation should be undertaken, but simultaneous treatment with vitamin D and calcium may be indicated.

One relatively common cause of hypocalcemia is alcoholism with resultant magnesium deficiency. Overt malnutrition need not be present. The mechanisms by which alcohol abuse produces magnesium depletion include decreased dietary intake and alcohol-facilitated renal excretion of magnesium. Magnesium depletion results in both impaired secretion of PTH and impaired PTH action. Intramuscular magnesium therapy normalizes the serum calcium within hours.

Other diseases associated with hypocalcemia include osteomalacia (vitamin D and/or calcium deficiency) and variants of Fanconi's syndrome (a spectrum of renal tubular abnormalities). The hypocalcemia associated with renal failure is described in Chapter 47.

HYPERCALCEMIC STATES

In recent years routine, automated blood analyses have come to include determinations of serum calcium. This development has led to the detection of many cases of hypercalcemia, most of them mild and asymptomatic. The demonstration of hypercalcemia always requires investigation.

Etiologies

In an ambulatory setting the most common cause of minimal, asymptomatic hypercalcemia may be that associated with use of thiazide diuretics, although the precise incidence is really not known. The problem is fully reversible upon withdrawal of the drug. Once established as the cause of the hypercalcemia, thiazide therapy may be continued if otherwise clinically indicated and the hypercalcemia is minimal. In the rare case where the serum calcium exceeds 12 mg/dl, one may switch to an alternative, nonthiazide diuretic.

Another common cause of benign hypercalcemia in ambulatory patients is hyperparathyroidism. Small, indolent, probably harmless parathyroid adenomas produce hypercalcemia in 1 of 1000 patients screened (11). The approach to such patients is described below (see page 1029).

Some ambulatory patients who are found to have hypercalcemia will have weight loss, anorexia, *etc*. A calcium elevation in this setting is ominous. Since minimal elevations of calcium (less than 12.0 mg/dl) are ordinarily asymptomatic, the patient's symptoms of anorexia, weight loss, *etc*, are more likely attributable to the underlying disease, rather than to the incidental and associated but minimal hypercalcemia. The calcium elevation, however, is a finding which suggests a malignant process, e.g., carcinoma of the lung or breast, *etc*. These patients are usually promptly hospitalized for diagnostic procedures and therapy of the underlying disease.

In the event that malignancy is not apparent, the differential diagnosis includes primary hyperparathyroidism (see below). At this point, determination of PTH concentration is useful in elucidating the cause of the hypercalcemic state. However, one should not rely on only a PTH assay to determine the cause of the hypercalcemia. A normal PTH on repeated determinations excludes a diagnosis of hyperparathyroidism (see below), but an elevated PTH does not necessarily indicate its presence. PTH assays do not always reliably differentiate between hypercalcemia due to hyperparathyroidism and that due to PTH-producing tumor. Elevations of PTH are often due to ectopic PTH production by tumors. Although tumor-produced PTH is not identical to normal PTH, the antibodies used to quantitate PTH often fail to distinguish between these substances. Recent improvements in PTH assays with more specific antibodies have improved diagnostic accuracy, but absolute specificity is not yet possible (19). Results will vary with the laboratory and depend on the assay used. Information concerning specificity may not be available from a particular commercial laboratory.

Various other circumstances produce hypercalcemia. These are listed in Table 74.5.

Therapy of Hypercalcemia

The treatment of hypercalcemia due to hyperparathyroidism is discussed elsewhere (see "Primary Hyperparathyroidism").

Table 74.5.
Causes of Hypercalcemia

Condition	Comment
COMMON CAUSES	
Thiazide drugs	Mild elevation (not > 12.5 mg/dl); requires 2 or more weeks to subside
Hyperparathyroidism	Frequently asymptomatic; commonly discovered on routine blood test
Malignancy	Commonest cause in hospitalized patients; may lead to initial encounter in ambulatory patients
Spurious	Inappropriate technique while drawing blood (venous stasis produces hemoconcentration)
RARE CAUSES	
Multiple myeloma	Severe disease is evident
Milk alkali syndrome	Requires use (abuse) of both alkali ($NaHCO_3$) and large quantities of milk or calcium salts
Hypervitaminosis D	Usually 50,000 units or more daily
Thyrotoxicosis	Severe disease is evident
Paget's disease of bone	Immobilization necessary
Immobilization	Body cast in adolescent males; patients with Paget's disease of bone; quadriplegia
Sarcoidosis	Hyperglobulinemia usually present
Chronic renal failure	Very uncommon; may exacerbate after transplantation or during hemodialysis
Adrenal insufficiency	Hemoconcentration present
Idiopathic elevation	Mild elevation in postmenopausal women; may revert to normal with physiological estrogen therapy

Therapy to control hypercalcemia is not commonly initiated in ambulatory patients. Most often the hypercalcemia or its underlying cause will have required initial therapy in a hospital. However, when the acute symptoms of hypercalcemia have been controlled during hospitalization, long term palliative therapy may be needed for the ambulatory patient.

In malignancy, glucocorticoids (20 to 60 mg of prednisone daily) may control hypercalcemia, as may indomethacin (100 to 200 mg daily) in a small proportion of cases. Mithramycin is an effective agent for control of hypercalcemia of any cause, but this drug is ordinarily used only for the treatment of hypercalcemia due to tumor. Usually such therapy is given in a hospital, but ambulatory treatment is also feasible. The drug is given intravenously. At a dose of 25 μg/kg (15 μg/kg if hepatic disease is present or bone marrow function is impaired by disease or other drugs) side effects are not usually seen. Several days are often needed for a response to become apparent, but the effect often lasts for many days or even weeks. Calcitonin (Calcimar) is an effective calcium-lowering agent for many hypercalcemic states and can be self-administered. This hormone must be given subcutaneously on a daily or several times weekly schedule. The principal use of calcitonin is in the treatment of Paget's disease of bone. The major side effects are nausea and vomiting in a small percentage of cases. Glucocorticoids are often effective in lowering hypercalcemia due to sarcoidosis, vitamin D intoxication, and the milk-alkali syndrome. Mild hypercalcemia in elderly postmenopausal women may sometimes respond to physiological amounts of estrogen (16). Treatment of hypercalcemia with phosphates administered orally is sometimes possible, especially in mild hyperparathyroidism (see below). Often partial control of hypercalcemia is sufficient to relieve symptoms; complete normalization of calcium level is often neither desirable nor necessary.

Primary Hyperparathyroidism

The term primary hyperparathyroidism refers to autonomous hyperfunction of one or more parathyroid glands. Hypercalcemia is the hallmark of this disorder. Secondary hyperparathyroidism, on the other hand, is a physiological or pathophysiological homeostatic response to situations that lower blood calcium.

The most common cause of primary hyperparathyroidism is a solitary benign adenoma (85% of patients). In a small proportion of patients more than one adenoma is present, and in the remainder the cause is idiopathic hyperplasia. Carcinoma of the parathyroid is rare (less than 1% of patients). Hyperparathyroidism may be familial and may occur as part of the syndrome of multiple endocrine adenomatosis (MEA; page 1015).

Diagnosis

Most patients are now detected by routine automated analysis of blood electrolytes. The symptoms or sequelae of hypercalcemia may also alert the physician to the diagnosis (Table 74.6). Once the diagnosis is suspected, it is most important to establish beyond any doubt the presence of hypercalcemia. Multiple determinations of serum calcium should be made in a laboratory where a high degree of precision is assured. Because of spontaneous fluctuations of the serum calcium and because of analytical error, values that are only minimally elevated (10.5 to 12.0 mg/dl) must be repeated many times. The resulting *mean* level should be used for diagnostic purposes, not the last—sometimes normal—value obtained.

Once hypercalcemia is established as being present (greater than 10.5 mg/dl on multiple determinations), the next (or simultaneous) step is to determine the likelihood of the presence of other causes of hypercalcemia (see Table 74.5). Finally, assay of PTH in blood should be performed (see below).

Other routine laboratory studies may include low serum phosphorus and, in severe cases with bone involvement, elevation of serum alkaline phosphatase activity. Other more elaborate indirect tests of PTH hyperfunction—none of which is useful for screening purposes—include the calculation of the tubular resorption of phosphate (TRP) and determination of urinary excretion of cyclic adenosine monophosphate (cyclic AMP). These tests, if they are to be used at all, are best performed by specialists. Other abnormalities in laboratory tests occur but are not useful for screening or in differential diagnosis, since they occur nonspecifically. Patients with hypercalcemia, regardless of cause, usually

Table 74.6.
Symptoms and Signs of Hypercalcemia

SHORT TERM (READILY REVERSIBLE)
  General: weakness, anorexia, weight loss, fatigue
  Gastrointestinal: nausea, vomiting, constipation
  Genitourinary: polyuria, azotemia
  Musculoskeletal: bone aches
  Neurological: lethargy, sleepiness, difficulty concentrating, confusion, psychosis
  Cardiovascular: bradycardia, electrocardiographic abnormalities (short Q-T, arrhythmias, digitalis toxicity)
  Ophthalmological: difficulty focusing
  Dermatological: pruritis
LONG TERM (IRREVERSIBLE OR SLOWLY REVERSIBLE)
  Gastrointestinal: peptic ulcer, pancreatitis
  Genitourinary: renal calculi (colic, hematuria); nephrocalcinosis; polyuria
  Skeletal: bone loss (osteopenia); subperiosteal resorption, bone cysts, pseudogout
  Neuromuscular: muscle atrophy
  Ophthalmological: band keratopathy; conjunctival calcifications (usually require slitlamp examination)

show hypercalciuria, but hypercalciuria may also occur without hypercalcemia. Increased excretion of hydroxyproline occurs, as it does in other bone diseases.

In severe cases of long duration, X-ray studies of various bones will reveal a variety of changes suggestive but not diagnostic of hyperparathyroidism. Demineralization (osteopenia) and subperiosteal resorption are most obvious in the clavicles and the hands, while the lamina dura of the teeth may be resorbed. Cystic changes occur in skull and long bones. None of these changes is likely to be seen in mild cases. X-ray studies are not useful for screening purposes.

Parathyroid hormone assays. These radioimmunoassays, now widely available from commercial laboratories, are quite useful but have several limitations. Specificity of the assay varies among laboratories, due to the use of different antibodies. Some laboratories offer several different PTH assays, each of which has its own advantages and limitations. The most commonly used procedure, the so-called "C-terminal" assay, measures a peptide fragment derived from PTH. This assay, as performed on peripheral venous blood (plasma or serum), is the most sensitive test for detecting hyperparathyroidism, but it is also elevated by impaired renal function, due in part to decreased peptide fragment excretion, and is frequently elevated in normal elderly persons, especially women over about age 65. The elevations seen in primary hyperparathyroidism are often only modest (e.g., 50% greater than the upper limits of normal). Accordingly, at least two or three assays should ordinarily be obtained. The assay also measures PTH-like materials produced by tumors.

Several other assays are also available; these measure "intact" hormone or N-terminal fragment(s). Interestingly, although these assays are more specific and less likely to be elevated in cases of ectopic (tumor) production of PTH, they are also less sensitive in detecting primary hyperparathyroidism, being normal in nearly half of cases. In chronic renal failure, where secondary hyperparathyroidism is invariably present, the "intact hormone" assays are not artifactually raised by retention of PTH fragments, as are the C-terminal assays, and more or less reflect the degree of secondary hyperparathyroidism.

Steroid suppression test. Although most cases of hyperparathyroidism and of other hypercalcemic states can be diagnosed by the means described, the etiology of occasional cases of hypercalcemia remains in doubt. In these, a short course of prednisone therapy (30 to 40 mg daily for 10 to 14 days) may help diagnostically. The hypercalcemia of hyperparathyroidism does not respond to such therapy. While only about one-half of cases of hypercalcemia due to malignancy respond, hypercalcemia due to diseases that are not always apparent—such as sar-

coidosis, vitamin D intoxication, and milk-alkali syndrome—responds consistently. Daily determinations of blood calcium should always be obtained during such a test.

Further evaluation. Having established the presence of hypercalcemia and elevation of PTH, and having excluded by appropriate means malignancy, impaired renal function, and other conditions in Table 74.5, the diagnosis of hyperparathyroidism is reasonably well established. However, the urinary excretion of calcium should be determined at this point. Recently, benign familial hypercalcemia due to parathyroid hyperplasia has been described. These patients—for reasons which are not understood—do not have hypercalciuria or other complications of minimal hypercalcemia and do not need surgical intervention. In most cases of hyperparathyroidism referral to an endocrinologist should be made if the diagnosis is in doubt or if surgery is contemplated.

Therapy

In diagnosed patients the main question is whether surgical intervention is warranted. The rate of development of complications (urolithiasis, emotional disorders, bone disease, decreased renal function, peptic ulcer, pancreatitis) in patients with asymptomatic hypercalcemia is quite low. However, the decision for or against surgery will obviously be based not only on the presence of such problems, but on such factors as patient age, associated medical illness, *etc* (6, 11). In occasional patients, medical management of the hyperparathyroidism may be indicated (see below).

Surgical Therapy

If a decision is made to treat the patient surgically, referral to a surgeon experienced in parathyroid/thyroid exploration is warranted. In such experienced hands, an adenoma, if present, will be located and easily removed in 90 to 95% of cases. Parathyroid hyperplasia, which accounts for 10% of cases of hyperparathyroidism, is usually easily identified. In such cases, the surgeon should be prepared to perform a near total parathyroidectomy. Second neck explorations are technically difficult and may result in unnecessary morbidity (damage to the recurrent laryngeal nerve). Accordingly, any hyperplastic parathyroid tissue that is left behind should be identified with clips. As an alternative, many surgeons are now removing all parathyroid tissue from the neck and transplanting a portion of one hyperplastic gland to an accessible location, usually a sternocleidomastoid muscle or into the forearm.

Failure to identify an adenoma and absence of hyperplasia may require partial thyroidectomy—the adenoma may be embedded in the thyroid—or exploration of the anterosuperior mediastinum. This procedure may be performed at the time of initial surgery or at some time later. Such "details" obviously involve the surgeon's preference and experience, but should be considered and discussed before surgery. If the neck has already been explored unsuccessfully, a selective venous catheterization study with sampling of PTH levels is a useful procedure for preoperative localization of the tumor. Only a few major medical centers can perform this procedure. Such localization studies are not indicated before initial surgery.

Medical Therapy

The medical therapy of hyperparathyroidism with phosphate is ordinarily limited to those patients in whom surgery is not desirable but who require therapy. Although intravenous phosphate therapy carries the risk of soft tissue calcium deposition, no such problem attends the use of phosphate given orally. Sodium-potassium phosphate salts given orally (K-Phos; Neutra-Phos) may produce diarrhea. Dosage should be titrated upward as tolerated. A sodium-free preparation is also available (Neutra-Phos-K) for use in patients whose sodium intake should be restricted. Asymptomatic patients with mild hypercalcemia should probably not be treated with phosphate.

OSTEOPOROSIS (14)

Epidemiology and Manifestations

Primary osteoporosis is an age-related disorder characterized by a generalized decrease in bone mass (both the osteoid matrix and the inorganic macrocrystalline component) and increased risk of developing fractures in the absence of other known causes of bone loss. It is an important public health problem, affecting nearly 15 to 20 million persons in the United States. Approximately 1.3 million fractures related to osteoporosis occur annually in individuals beyond the age of 45. An estimated 32% of women and 17% of men who live to age 90 will experience a hip fracture. Among people so afflicted there is a 12 to 20% mortality within the first 3 to 4 months postfracture, and the physical, psychological, and socioeconomic toll on those who survive is formidable. In the United States alone, the annual cost of osteoporosis is about $3.8 billion.

The proportions of the two major forms of bone, cortical (compact) bone and trabecular (medullary) bone, vary at different anatomical sites. Vertebral bodies contain mostly trabecular bone, while the proximal femur and radius contain mostly cortical bone. The responses ot the two forms of bone to mechanical forces, hormones, and local regulatory factors and their susceptibility to fracture differ. Peak bone mass is achieved at about age 35 for cortical bone and several years earlier for trabecular bone. Multiple factors, including heredity, sex, race, nutritional status, level of physical activity, and general health influence peak bone mass. Bone mass is about 30% greater in men than in women, and 10% greater in blacks than in whites. Throughout life, the normal process of bone remodeling exists as a dynamic equilibrium between bone formation and bone resorption.

After reaching its peak, bone mass decreases steadily throughout adult life due to an imbalance in remodeling. The two major etiologies of primary osteoporosis are estrogen deficiency (see Chapter 77 for details) and aging. Known risk factors for osteoporosis include a sedentary life style, prolonged bed rest, chronic cigarette smoking, nulliparity, diabetes mellitus, Caucasian race, and chronic glucocorticoid therapy. In women, bone mass decreases rapidly during the first 3 to 7 years after natural or surgical menopause or any other cause of estrogen deficiency. As a result, osteoporosis and fractures are more common in women than in men, and in whites than in blacks. During the first 15 to 20 years after the menopause, vertebral fractures predominate, whereas in elderly women and in men, fractures of the hip and distal radius are more common. Optimal, cost-effective use of radiological techniques (photon absorptiometry and CT scanning) for diagnosing early or established osteoporosis or following progression of the process remains to be defined. It is clear, however, that osteoporosis is quite advanced when it is detectable on plain X-rays.

Prevention of Osteoporosis

Patient management should emphasize the prevention of osteoporosis. The treatment of symptoms due to vertebral compression fractures is palliative (see Chapter 65, Low Back Pain).

Estrogen therapy begun at or within 5 to 6 years of the menopause is highly effective in preventing osteoporosis in women. Such treatment decreases bone resorption and postmenopausal bone loss and has been shown in case-controlled studies to reduce the incidence of hip and wrist fractures and vertebral fractures as well. Use of added progestin decreases the risk of endometrial cancer. However, since the risks and acceptability of long term therapy with estrogen and progestin in postmenopausal women have not been defined, an unequivocal recommendation for such therapy should probably be reserved for women at high risk for developing osteoporosis, such as those with premature menopause. (Chapter 77 contains a detailed discussion of estrogen replacement in the menopause.)

Most adults consume diets deficient in calcium and dairy products. In the absence of contraindications (e.g., history of hypercalcemia, kidney stones, or kidney failure), it is recommended that after the age of 40 calcium be taken in amounts sufficient to meet the daily nutritional calcium requirements of 1200 mg for premenopausal women and estrogen-treated postmenopausal women, or 1500 mg for non-estrogen-treated postmenopausal women and for men, especially Causasian men with risk factors for osteoporosis. Such calcium therapy has been shown to retard age-related bone loss greatly and, in preliminary studies, to decrease the rate of hip fractures in patients with established osteoporosis. When postmenopausal women take calcium supplements in addition to estrogen replacement, these two modalities have an additive favorable impact on reducing the rate of vertebral fractures by nearly one-half (15). The major sources of calcium in the United States diet are milk and dairy products. Each 8-ounce glass (240 ml) of milk contains 275 to 300 mg of calcium. Skim or low fat milk is preferred to minimize fat intake. For those unable to take 1000 to 1500 mg of calcium by diet, supplementation with calcium tablets is recommended, with special attention to their elemental calcium content. Nonprescription oral calcium supplements, such as calcium carbonate, phosphate, lactate, or gluconate, can supplement a calcium-poor diet. The carbonate preparation has the highest percentage of calcium, containing 40% elemental calcium by weight; and calcium gluconate has the lowest percentage, only 9%. Patient compliance is greatest with the carbonate preparations, because fewer tablets are needed to achieve recommended calcium intake. However, the carbonate preparation can cause bloating, flatulence, and constipation, and some patients prefer calcium lactate or gluconate. Moreover, absorption of calcium from the carbonate form depends on the presence of gastric hydrochloric acid. Achlorhydria becomes common in older patients, so calcium carbonate may prove to be unsatisfactory for precisely those patients having the greatest need for calcium supplementation. Because the cost of calcium products varies greatly, patients should be told to take a recommended amount of *elemental* calcium and encouraged to shop for the least expensive preparation. Tables 74.7 and 74.8 list practical information about a number of calcium-containing foods and calcium supplements.

Other measures which may be important in preventing osteoporosis are modest weight-bearing exercise, such as walking; avoidance of prolonged bed rest following acute illness; smoking cessation; avoidance of prolonged glucocorticoid treatment; and treatment of any co-existing conditions which are known to cause or accelerate osteoporosis.

DISORDERS OF WATER METABOLISM

The combination of excess thirst, increased intake of water, and increased output of urine is a common clinical presentation of a number of conditions (Table 74.9). In most of these, the symptoms are related to some event which results in excessive loss of fluid *via* the kidney. For example, hyperglycemia results in a large solute load (glucose) being presented to

Table 74.7.
Calcium Content of Some Foods[a]

Food	Serving Size	Calcium Content (mg)
Sardines, canned in oil	8 medium	354
Spinach, frozen chopped, cooked	½ cup	113
Turnip greens, cooked	½ cup	246
Cheddar cheese (American)	1 ounce	211
Creamed cottage cheese	1 cup	211
Muenster cheese	1 ounce	203
Milk, whole	1 quart	1152
Milk, skim	1 quart	1212
Yogurt (lowfat, fruit flavored)	1 cup	345
Chocolate fudge	3 ½ ounces	100

[a] From Calcium for postmenopausal osteoporosis. *Med Lett* 24:105, 1982.

Table 74.8.
Commercially Available Calcium Supplements[a]

Drug	Tablet Size	Equivalent of 1 G of Calcium/ Day
Calcium carbonate (40% calcium)		
Generic—Lilly	600 mg	4 tablets
—Rugby	600 mg	4 tablets
Alka-2—Miles	500 mg	5 tablets
Amitone—Norcliff Thayer	350 mg	7 tablets
Equilet—Mission	500 mg	5 tablets
Dicarbosil—Norcliff Thayer	500 mg	5 tablets
Mallamint—Mallard	420 mg	6 tablets
OsCal-500—Marion	1250 mg	2 tablets
TUMS—Norcliff Thayer	500 μg	5 tablets
Calcium gluconate (9% calcium) generic	600 mg	18.5 tablets
	1000 mg	11 tablets
	930 mg	12 tablets
Calcium lactate (13% calcium) generic	600 mg	12 tablets
Dibasic calcium phosphate (31% calcium) generic	500 mg	7 tablets
Chelated calcium (20% calcium)		
generic—Arco	750 mg	7 tablets
—Nature's Bounty	750 mg	7 tablets

[a] Adapted from Calcium for postmenopausal osteoporosis. *Med Lett* 24:105, 1982.

the renal tubules; an obligatory loss of water (osmotic diuresis) ensues. Hypercalcemia produces abnormalities of renal tubular function which result in impaired ability to concentrate urine. Lithium, widely used for treatment of bipolar affective disorders (manic-depressive illness), impairs the action of antidiuretic hormone and thereby produces water loss. Table 74.9 lists some of the conditions producing polyuria and their mechanisms.

Table 74.9.
Causes of Polyuria[a]

Disorder	Mechanism
Glucosuria (diabetes mellitus)	Osmotic diuresis
Excessive intake of water	Psychogenic
Various drugs	Often due to anticholinergic effects producing dryness of mouth; possible central effects
Decreased antidiuretic hormone (ADH) effect	Deficiency of ADH secretion (idiopathic diabetes insipidus or due to pituitary-hypothalamic disease); nephrogenic diabetes insipidus
Renal disease, plus renal effects of potassium depletion, hypercalcemia, and lithium therapy	In all of these disorders, impairment of renal concentrating ability is present
Hyperthyroidism	Impairment of urinary concentrating ability; decreased salivary flow

[a] Disorders associated with increased urine volume.

Disorders of water metabolism are uncommon in ambulatory patients, but the commonest is probably that of psychogenic water drinking. In this disorder, the patient's psychiatric state alters normal behavior in such a way as to produce compulsive water drinking. Many of these patients have poorly defined psychiatric disorders. Occasional individuals begin excessive water intake on receiving "health advice" from a lay source, i.e., the notion that drinking large quantities of water is healthful. Regardless of the cause, one such behavior is started, a compulsive behavior pattern tends to persist and is reinforced by a pathophysiological mechanism. Whatever the cause, large urine output, if it persists for a long time, produces a reversible impairment of urine-concentrating ability due to washout of renal medullary solutes. Thus, the behavior pattern, though basically of psychogenic origin, may become self-perpetuating. Attempts to have the patient restrict water intake when urinary concentrating ability is impaired under these conditions lead to continued water loss, and the resulting hyperosmolality leads to intense thirst. "Weaning" from excessive water intake may be very difficult.

A rare disorder of water metabolism in ambulatory patients is diabetes insipidus, a deficiency of antidiuretic hormone (ADH, arginine vasopressin, AVP). This condition is either idiopathic—in which case it is unassociated with other evidence of pituitary-hypothalamic disease—or, more commonly, is secondary to pituitary disease (tumor) or other disease in the hypothalamic-pituitary stalk-pituitary area (craniopharyngioma; aneurysm). Other rare causes include a variety of infiltrative diseases (sarcoidosis, tuberculosis), head trauma—especially with basal skull fracture or neurosurgical procedures, and central nervous system infections. The most common illness mimicking diabetes insipidus is the drug-related disorder which results from use of lithium for bipolar affective illness. Another very rare condition resembling lack of ADH results from an inherited renal tubular resistance to antidiuretic hormone, nephrogenic diabetes insipidus.

Approach to the Patient with Polydipsia and Polyuria

The history should be corroborated by family or friends if possible. Important historical points are rapidity of onset of symptoms, a preference for use of iced water, and nocturnal drinking habits. Sudden onset and preference for iced water are classical for diabetes insipidus. Numerous spontaneous awakenings at night in order to drink and urinate also strongly suggest this diagnosis, while absence of such nocturnal events is in favor of functional disease. A careful psychiatric history is important. The use of drugs should be noted (8).

Initial laboratory workup should be simple. Urine glucose should be measured. An A.M. serum sodium and/or osmolality determination along with serum potassium, calcium, urea nitrogen, and creatinine should be made. The patient should collect all urine over one or two 24-hour periods. The sample should be examined to determine the volume, osmolality, and total creatinine excretion, the latter serving as a marker for completeness of the collection. Measurement of urine specific gravity is obsolete and should not be used.

These preliminaries will define the problem and provide an insight into the diagnosis. Unless considerable glucosuria is present, the patient's problem is not due to uncontrolled diabetes mellitus, even if blood glucose is incidentally elevated. The presence of a normal serum sodium and/or osmolality indicates only that the process is not severe enough to have overwhelmed the ability to excrete water or the homeostatic (thirst) mechanism. Elevated serum osmolality strongly suggests diabetes insipidus; the opposite finding indicates psychogenic water drinking. The presence of normal serum calcium and potassium concentrations excludes several metabolic problems, while abnormalities of calcium, of potassium, or of renal function will make it clear that the problem is not primarily one of water metabolism (see Table 74.9).

At this point most patients will have normal findings in serum but a large volume of urine with low osmolality. Normal urine volume ranges up to 2500 ml; urine osmolality is decidedly low when the value is well below that of serum, i.e., less than 300 mOsm/kg (the urine is maximally dilute at 50 to 70 mOsm/kg). In both diabetes insipidus and psychogenic water drinking urine volume will usually exceed 4 liters daily. Values less than 5 to 6 liters daily do not distinguish between these possibilities but do indicate less than complete diabetes insipidus, in which urine volumes approach 10 to 12 liters daily, as they may in cases of severe psychogenic water drinking. If the serum sodium/osmolality is low and the urine volume is large with low osmolality, a diagnosis of psychogenic water drinking is likely.

Diabetes Insipidus *versus* Psychogenic Water Drinking

Having established the presence of a large urine volume of low osmolality together with normal serum electrolytes, additional testing is necessary to establish a diagnosis. Referral to an endocrinologist or nephrologist is appropriate at this juncture, although under optimal conditions further efforts to establish the diagnosis on the ambulatory patient may be undertaken before referral (see below). Hospitalization for testing under "metabolic" conditions is nearly always to be preferred in these cases; however, most *ordinary* hospital conditions are not appropriate for the gathering of definitive information on water handling.

The first additional test is that of water deprivation. Best performed during the day when monitoring is possible, the patient remains recumbent and refrains from fluid intake; all urine is collected in hourly batches for 6 hours. Volumes and osmolalities are determined on each sample. Body weight is determined hourly. When the urine volume and osmolality seem to have stabilized after several hours, antidiuretic hormone (ADH, Pitressin) is given (5 units, aqueous, subcutaneously). Urine osmolality and volume are then determined every 30 minutes for an additional 90 to 120 minutes. If at any point drop in body weight exceeds 3%, the ADH should be injected and the test terminated over the next 90 minutes.

In the normal individual, urine volume will fall and osmolality will rise over several hours. Urine osmolality will exceed 500 mOsm/kg. Administration of ADH produces an additional increase in urine osmolality, but the increase will be small if the level is already high. In the patient with partial diabetes insipidus, the plateau is at 300 mOsm/kg with an increase to at least 500 mOsm/kg after ADH; some patients will not respond maximally (osmolality 1000 mOsm/kg). Patients with nephrogenic diabetes insipidus will not respond to ADH. A prompt fall of urine volume and an increase of urine osmolality may not occur in some patients with psychogenic water drinking. These patients are often overhydrated and may not reach plateau levels for as long as 12 hours. If the diagnosis is still doubtful at this point, referral for consultation should be made. Further tests can be performed to provoke ADH release by infusion of hypertonic saline. Administra-

tion of intravenous ADH and other special maneuvers may be necessary. X-rays of the sella turcica and CT scans of the area of the sella, although usually negative, are important in cases of diabetes insipidus to rule out space-occupying lesions. Anterior pituitary function must be assessed when diabetes insipidus is diagnosed.

Treatment

The treatment of psychogenic water drinking involves psychiatric counseling. These patients are difficult to manage, especially if they become severely hyponatremic. "Weaning" such patients from water may also be a slow process not only because of the profound nature of their psychiatric disturbance, but because of their acquired inability to concentrate urine, a process which is only slowly reversible.

The treatment of diabetes insipidus involves use of ADH in some form. Until the last few years Pitressin Tannate in oil was the preferred agent. This material is given intramuscularly. Great care must be taken to suspend the insoluble hormone before injection. The usual dose is 5 units every 24 to 72 hours, depending on the duration of effect in a particular individual. Antidiuretic hormone may also be administered as a nasal spray. Two forms are available; lysine vasopressin, with an effect which lasts only 4 to 6 hours, has been largely replaced by the synthetic analog, desmopressin (DDAVP). This material acts for 12 hours or longer. DDAVP is a great advance in the therapy of diabetes insipidus. Nasal absorption may be impaired by rhinitis or respiratory tract infections, during which treatment with Pitressin Tannate may be necessary. Patients with partial diabetes insipidus can sometimes be managed with chlorpropamide (Diabinese; 250 to 500 mg daily), a drug which potentiates endogenous ADH. However, hypoglycemia is a significant hazard. Clofibrate (Atromid-S) is another drug which has been used to treat diabetes insipidus. Nephrogenic diabetes insipidus, both idiopathic and secondary to lithium, is partially responsive to thiazide diuretics (13).

Syndrome of Inappropriate Secretion of Antidiuretic Hormone (SIADH)

The clinical manifestations of this disorder are due to hyponatremia and the diagnosis is based on that finding. The causes are multiple. Classically, the disturbance was related to ectopic production of ADH by a neoplasm. The tumor most likely to produce this syndrome is a small cell (oat cell) carcinoma of the lung, but many other tumors have also been shown to produce the same syndrome. The presence of a tumor is usually obvious, but occasionally it may be clinically occult. In addition, a variety of acute and chronic diseases of the central nervous system can produce an identical syndrome. Drugs, acting centrally, may also produce ADH hypersecretion (morphine, barbiturates (13)). The best described drug-related SIADH which is likely to be encountered in an ambulatory patient is that due to chlorpropamide (Diabinese) during the therapy of diabetes mellitus (Chapter 72). In this case, the disturbance is due to potentiation of ADH action, although increased ADH release may also be involved (13).

Treatment

The treatment of SIADH is usually that which is related to the underlying disease or involves withdrawal of drug therapy (e.g., chlorpropamide, Diabinese; see Chapter 72). Water restriction is effective but is difficult to maintain in an ambulatory setting. Lithium has been occasionally useful. Demeclocycline, a tetracycline analog, is an ADH antagonist and is effective in some cases. An ADH peptide analog which blocks ADH action has been recently developed and offers promise for therapy, but the agent is not yet available for clinical use.

HYPOGLYCEMIA

Since the symptoms of hypoglycemia are rather nonspecific, hypoglycemia is properly more often suspected than present. Chemical hypoglycemia, defined as a plasma sugar of less than 50 mg/dl, may not be symptomatic, although levels less than 30 mg/dl are nearly always associated with symptoms (see Chapter 72 for discussion of plasma *versus* blood glucose values).

Hypoglycemia produces symptoms by two mechanisms: (a) by triggering the release of epinephrine, one of several homeostatic responses which tend to normalize a low blood sugar, and (b) by deprivation of the nervous system of its essential energy source.

The causes of hypoglycemia are numerous, but by far the most common is a benign functional disturbance of insulin secretion which is temporally associated with absorption of food from the gastrointestinal tract. Most other hypoglycemic events are seen in diabetics being treated with insulin. A few other conditions producing hypoglycemia are associated with insulin overproduction, the rarest of which is an insulinoma. In most situations hypoglycemia is due not to insulin excess but to disturbances of glucose production, as in ethanol ingestion, or rarely to glucose overutilization, as in the presence of certain extrapancreatic tumors. The causes of hypoglycemia are listed in Table 74.10.

Clinical Diagnosis

Presentation of the Problem

In some patients the history will suggest to the physician that the patient is experiencing periodic hypoglycemia. Other patients will themselves suggest to their physician that hypoglycemia accounts

Table 74.10.
Causes of Hypoglycemia

POSTPRANDIAL STATE
Reactive (idiopathic)
Early diabetes mellitus
Ethanol ingestion
Postgastrectomy state
FASTING STATE
Insulin excess:
1. Insulin injection
2. Sulfonylurea ingestion[a]
3. Miscellaneous drugs[b]
4. Insulinoma
Alcohol ingestion
Hormonal deficiencies:
1. Adrenal insufficiency
2. Pituitary insufficiency
Prolonged fasting in normal women
Liver disease
Extrapancreatic tumors
Renal failure (chronic end stage)

[a] Many drugs, including such diverse compounds as anti-inflammatory agents, antibiotics, and lipid-lowering agents, potentiate the effects of sulfonylureas and may cause hypoglycemia.
[b] Haloperidol, propoxyphene, salicylates, *etc.*

for the symptoms. Much has been written in the lay literature about hypoglycemia, and many books attribute the entire range of human miseries to this disorder. Needless to say, the case has been overstated. The physician encountering such a patient may find mere reassurance ineffective, so convincing is some of the lay literature in this area and so obsessed are some patients. However, the physician inevitably embarks on a search, either to confirm or to refute the suspected diagnosis. Unfortunately, failure to document the presence of hypoglycemia may not serve to dispose of the issue, while generation of dubious or equivocal laboratory results may merely serve to prolong the preoccupation, initiate useless diets, or even delay diagnosis of serious but unrelated disease.

"Nonhypoglycemia"

The frequency with which self-diagnosis of hypoglycemia occurs depends on the population, but in one study from Los Angeles, the problem was very common. The condition has been termed "nonhypoglycemia" and extends the concept of "nondisease," as it originates from misattributes of the physician, such as misinterpretation of laboratory values, to misattributes of the patient (20). Identification of such individuals is important, as is their re-education (4). The ready acceptance by patients of hypoglycemia as a diagnosis is perhaps related to its social acceptability, the comfort received from attributing vague symptoms (e.g., fatigue, mental "fogginess") to a "real" disease, the satisfaction of an escape into dietary rituals, and possibly relief from the anxiety that life-threatening or at least serious disease may be lurking.

The recognition of "nonhypoglycemia" requires a careful history which fails to demonstrate the legitimate symptoms of hypoglycemia as well as a clear demonstration that glucose metabolism is normal (see below). Exclusion of other organic disease is routine (Table 74.10). Distinction from the idiopathic postprandial syndrome must be made (see below). Finally, psychiatric disease must be considered, based on positive findings rather than merely on an exclusion of apparent organic illness.

If the evaluation fails to establish the presence of *bona fide* hypoglycemia, the physician is left with the issue of the therapy of "nonhypoglycemia." This difficult problem includes at least three steps which have been termed (a) disattribution, (b) explanation and ventilation, and (c) reattribution (20). Disattribution involves confrontation of the patient with the results of the test procedure. For some patients the mechanics or ritual of the procedure itself are impressive and therefore helpful. If the patient clings to the diagnosis of hypoglycemia despite strong evidence to the contrary, the physician should attempt to explore the reason for the patient's need to do so. During this process, an effort should be made to have the patient fully explain his notions about hypoglycemia and ventilate about what might happen if those notions are challenged. Finally, the physician must either provide an alternate explanation for the symptoms—reattribution—along with a treatment plan or be prepared to assist the patient in accepting an uncertain and ambiguous situation. Unless grossly apparent emotional problems become evident during this process, psychiatric referral should be made after considerable deliberation and only after an effort has been made by the internist to resolve the problem. (Chapters 10 and 11 describe in detail interviewing and psychotherapeutic techniques for working with patients such as these.)

Defining Hypoglycemic Symptoms

Because laboratory confirmation may be extremely difficult in some cases, an extraordinarily careful history is essential. The degree to which the history is convincing will determine the vigor with which a rather nebulous diagnosis is to be pursued. Two issues guide the process. First, what exactly are the symptoms? Second, do the symptoms occur postprandially or in the fasting state?

Adrenergic versus neuroglycopenic symptoms. Two groups of symptoms and signs are associated with hypoglycemia. Many of the symptoms of hypoglycemia relate to stimulation by low blood glucose of the release of epinephrine. These comprise the first group and are termed *adrenergic* or sympathetic. Usually these symptoms are of rapid onset and more than one is ordinarily present. Ordinarily they last only 15 to 30 minutes and include sweating, tremor ("shakiness") a sensation of hunger, and anxiety. Irritability and palpitations are often mentioned

but are rarely spontaneous or prominent complaints.

The second group of symptoms is related to glucose deprivation of the central and, to a lesser extent, peripheral nervous systems. These symptoms may be termed *neuroglycopenic* and when severe mimic those of central nervous system hypoxia. Minimal symptoms are headache, mental dullness, and sudden fatigue. Confusion and visual disturbances (blurring, dimming of vision) are associated with moderate to severe hypoglycemia, while unconsciousness and seizures are indications of very severe hypoglycemia.

While adrenergic symptoms are mainly postprandial, neuroglycopenic symptoms, especially those of severe variety, are seen in association with fasting hypoglycemia. Minor neuroglycopenic symptoms may also be seen in the postabsorptive state, but symptoms severe enough to cause loss of consciousness are rare and should not be readily attributed to this cause. When severe symptoms do occur in the postprandial state, great difficulty in establishing a diagnosis may be encountered. The duration of this type of hypoglycemia is so short that, by the time the patient is seen by a physician and a blood sugar determination is obtained, the glucose has often returned to normal.

Postprandial versus fasting hypoglycemia. An accurate history is essential in order to identify the hypoglycemia as either postprandial or fasting. The subsequent evaluation and the diagnostic possibilities segregate clearly once this distinction is made. If a distinction can be made based on the history, the alternate type of hypoglycemia should no longer be considered since the two types do not coexist.

Postprandial (reactive) hypoglycemia. In this situation the patient has no problem on arising and before breakfast. Similarly, no difficulty is experienced if the patient sleeps late. The symptoms usually develop 2 to 5 hours after a meal.

Inquiry concerning the patient's dietary habits may be revealing. Some patients restrict carbohydrate intake intermittently. When this is done and a large carbohydrate meal follows, hypoglycemia may be precipitated. A history of previous gastrointestinal surgery (gastrectomy) is also important. The amount of alcohol consumed should be noted, since ethanol ingestion may precipitate hypoglycemia, even in the nonfasting patient (see below). Often the patient may recall milder symptomatic episodes experienced over a long period, since the intensity of postprandial hypoglycemia tends to wax and wane over the years. A family history of diabetes should be sought. Postprandial hypoglycemia can be an early manifestation of diabetes mellitus of the non-insulin-dependent type (see Chapter 72). Although symptoms and signs of anxiety or depression may be present, they have no diagnostic usefulness.

General physical examination can be expected to be negative. Even when early diabetes mellitus is found by glucose tolerance testing to be the cause of the hypoglycemia, complications of diabetes that can be found on physical examination (retinopathy, neuropathy) will not be present.

Postprandial Hypoglycemia

Laboratory Evaluation

Although ordinary meals do not consist of carbohydrate alone, the only practical and standardized test for detection of postabsorptive hypoglycemia is the glucose tolerance test. For this purpose, the test as described for diagnosis of diabetes mellitus (Chapter 72) is modified to include more frequent sampling (30-minute intervals) and a longer period (5 hours). The patient is observed during the entire test. Correlation of blood sugar values with clinical symptoms is essential. If the patient develops hypoglycemia associated with typical adrenergic symptoms and signs which reproduce those ordinarily experienced, a diagnosis of postabsorptive hypoglycemia can be considered established. A more precise diagnosis depends on the type of curve observed (see below). If symptoms without signs occur in the absence of hypoglycemia, the diagnosis is psychiatric. If hypoglycemia is seen but no symptoms occur, the hypoglycemic response may simply not have been severe enough to have triggered symptoms. The diagnosis then remains presumptive. A repeat test may succeed in reproducing the clinical situation.

Criteria for diagnosis of hypoglycemia. Plasma glucose values are greater than 50 mg/dl during glucose tolerance testing in 75% of *normal, asymptomatic* persons. However, some *normal* individuals show values which fall to 50 mg/dl or somewhat lower and may exhibit hypoglycemic symptoms during the test, even though they never have such symptoms spontaneously. Thus, even a finding of hypoglycemia during testing should not be used to explain atypical symptoms. In addition, occasional normal individuals may reach levels below 35 mg/dl without any symptoms at all. Recently, the plasma epinephrine response during glucose tolerance testing has been proposed as a measure of "hypoglycemic" response, which exceeds the usually accepted glucose cut-off of 50 mg/dl. In individuals who develop typical adrenergic symptoms and signs, an increase of plasma epinephrine can be documented even though the glucose concentration never reaches a diagnostic level for hypoglycemia (5). This phenomenon appears to provide an objective criterion for what has been termed "idiopathic postprandial syndrome" (see below).

Determinations of plasma insulin, growth hormone, glucagon, and norepinephrine in connection with the glucose tolerance test are of no particular use in interpreting the results. Variability is very great and in no sense diagnostic.

Types of hypoglycemic response during glucose tolerance testing.

EARLY DIABETES MELLITUS. The fasting glucose concentration is normal. In the first 2 hours, values diagnostic of diabetes mellitus are reached, although the highest values are usually between 200 and 250 mg/dl (Chapter 72). Thereafter, between 3 and 4 hours, the glucose concentration falls to its lowest value and below 50 mg/dl.

POSTGASTRECTOMY STATE. Plasma glucose concentration rises rapidly and may reach a peak over 300 mg/dl by 1 hour, following which a rapid decline occurs. The lowest value is seen at 2 to 3 hours.

IDIOPATHIC. In this response the blood glucose values in the first 2 hours are normal, but at about 3 hours a fall to hypoglycemic levels occurs. Values usually return to baseline by 5 hours.

Management of Hypoglycemia

Early diabetes mellitus. If the patient is obese, weight reduction may normalize the glucose tolerance and abolish the hypoglycemic episodes. If the patient is not obese, dietary manipulation can be attempted, but no standardized approach is available. The diet most likely to succeed is one which simulates that now recommended for diabetes generally, *i.e.,* a diet which contains a high proportion of complex carbohydrates rather than simple sugars (Chapter 72). Also important is the distribution of food intake into small meals—often as many as six. Alcohol may be an aggravating factor in producing hypoglycemia and should be restricted, at least on a trial basis. Caffeine (coffee, tea) need not be restricted. Sulfonylurea drugs are not useful.

Postgastrectomy state. As many as 75% of asymptomatic patients who have had a gastrectomy will show reactive hypoglycemia during a glucose tolerance test. The therapy of symptomatic patients is similar to that described above: frequent small meals and restriction of simple sugars. The anticholinergic drug propantheline (Pro-Banthine), 7.5 mg taken 30 minutes before meals, may be helpful. This drug inhibits gut motility and delays gastric emptying. At this dose, side effects (blurred vision; dry mouth) are minimal. Propranolol (Inderal) often blocks symptoms but does little to affect hypoglycemia and therefore may be hazardous.

Idiopathic hypoglycemia. The course of this disorder is obscure. Some patients may present with anxiety and/or depression in association with onset of hypoglycemic symptoms. Although diet manipulation and/or propantheline therapy as described above may ameliorate the hypoglycemia, additional treatment may be needed for the psychological aspects. Recent introduction of high protein, low carbohydrate diets for weight reduction has also led to difficulties in some persons. Carbohydrate restriction followed by carbohydrate ingestion leads to the hypoglycemia in these individuals. Ethanol (doses of 3 ounces of gin or equivalent) may potentiate reactive hypoglycemia in normal subjects.

Idiopathic Postprandial Syndrome

In this situation patients complain of typical adrenergic symptoms and show objective signs, but during glucose tolerance testing (see below) never achieve diagnostic levels of hypoglycemia. This condition has been termed "idiopathic postprandial syndrome." Recently, plasma epinephrine has been shown to increase abnormally in such persons. In these individuals, or in some diabetics (see page 972) the release of epinephrine appears to be triggered at levels of blood glucose (50 to 70 mg/dl) not ordinarily considered to be in the "hypoglycemic" range. Determination of plasma epinephrine during the performance of the glucose tolerance test has been proposed as an objective criterion for this disorder (5). Whether release of epinephrine is caused by change of blood glucose concentration or some other mechanism is not clear. It should be stressed that affected individuals have *typical* adrenergic symptoms and signs; their complaints are not to be confused with the vague symptoms of "nonhypoglycemia" (see above).

Fasting Hypoglycemia

The classical entity associated with fasting hypoglycemia is the insulinoma, but such insulin-secreting tumors are very rare, and other causes of fasting hypoglycemia should be eliminated before embarking on the difficult task of establishing the presence of an insulinoma.

Fasting hypoglycemia in a well nourished or obese individual suggests insulinoma, drug (sulfonylurea) ingestion, or insulin self-administration. Debilitation suggests hepatic disease (most often related to chronic alcohol abuse) or, rarely, extrapancreatic tumor. The history, physical examination, and routine laboratory studies will readily identify patients with chronic congestive heart failure or chronic renal disease, two other conditions occasionally associated with fasting hypoglycemia. Other aspects of these problems as well as endocrine deficiencies and alcohol abuse as causes of hypoglycemia are discussed below.

Laboratory Evaluation

When symptoms of hypoglycemia occur in the fasting state (usually overnight but in any case longer than 4 hours following a meal) a number of diagnostic possibilities more serious than those associated with postprandial hypoglycemia must be considered. However, the first step in evaluation of the problem is to establish the existence of hypoglycemia. Assuming that the symptoms are not so profound as to have caused coma, in which case hospitalization is mandatory, an overnight fast followed by determination of plasma glucose is the simplest screening procedure. This procedure may have to be repeated several times. If hypoglycemia cannot be documented in this way, the period of fasting may have to be extended to 24, 48 or even 72 hours. Hospitalization and close monitoring are necessary under these circumstances.

A sex difference in response to fasting is well established. Normal males may fast for up to 72 hours and will not show fasting plasma glucose (FPG) below 50 mg/dl. In contrast, women often exhibit a progressive fall in the concentration of plasma glucose during prolonged fasting. At 72 hours the majority of premenopausal women have a concentration of glucose less than 50 mg/dl and some as low as 25 mg/dl. Thus, prolonged fasting to establish the diagnosis of fasting hypoglycemia is not always useful, since so many normal women will become hypoglycemic.

Insulinoma

This tumor occurs with equal frequency in men and women and at any age. Symptoms of headache on arising, confusion before breakfast, or nocturnal or early A.M. seizures may be present for years before the diagnosis is suspected. Hyperinsulinism may produce abnormal hunger, weight gain, and obesity. Neuropsychiatric symptoms may lead to neurological or psychiatric evaluations or to hospitalizations. In some of these cases, permanent neurological deficits have been seen and are presumably related to long duration of symptomatic hypoglycemia before diagnosis.

Diagnosis. In addition to the demonstration of hypoglycemia, the determination of plasma insulin is important. During fasting in normal persons both glucose and insulin levels decline and the ratio of immunoreactive insulin (IRI) and glucose (G) is maintained at less than 0.3 (milliunits of IRI/milligrams of G/dl). In most patients with insulinoma an abnormally high ratio of IRI/G is apparent after even overnight fasting. These determinations should be made repeatedly, since fasting hypoglycemia and an abnormal ratio of IRI/G often occur only intermittently even in patients with subsequently proven insulinomas. In addition, a single abnormal ratio determination never establishes the diagnosis. The physician should be very cautious in accepting the accuracy of IRI values obtained from commercial laboratories. Proinsulin levels are elevated in patients with insulinoma and can be a useful adjunct. A variety of other useful procedures should, if necessary, be conducted by an endocrinologist. If fasting fails to provoke hypoglycemia (see above), the patient should exercise as vigorously as tolerable. Up to 2 hours of exercise should be completed with sampling for glucose every 15 to 20 minutes before concluding that hypoglycemia does not develop. A bicycle exerciser, jogging, or vigorous calisthenics may be used. Exercise raises glucose levels in normal persons but lowers plasma concentration further in patients with insulinoma. Provocative tests of insulin secretion (tolbutamide, leucine, glucagon) can be utilized with appropriate caution. Suppression of endogenous insulin C-peptide is another useful procedure in difficult cases, but requires induction of hypoglycemia by infusion of insulin under controlled conditions, a procedure which must be performed by an endocrinologist in a hospital. Computerized axial tomography and sonography can localize tumors of 2- to 3-cm size. Selective angiography can sometimes identify even smaller tumors. These procedures must not be used as alternatives to the tests described above but should be performed after demonstration of abnormal secretion of insulin. The definitive treatment of an insulinoma is surgical.

Insulin and Sulfonylurea Self-administration

Occasional nondiabetic patients, usually family members of diabetics or persons with medically related occupations (nurses, technicians), engage in surreptitious insulin administration. Physican examination may reveal needle marks. Other clues can be provided by the presence of antibodies to insulin, which are present only in persons given insulin of animal origin, or by the measurement of insulin C-peptide. In persons who are secreting insulin, C-peptide is also produced concomitantly, but C-peptide is not present in commercial insulin and will be very low or absent when hypoglycemia is induced by exogenous insulin.

Oral hypoglycemic drugs (sulfonylureas; see Chapter 72), like insulin, may occasionally be abused and cause fasting hypoglycemia. The drug can be detected by analysis of the blood, although only specialized laboratories perform these measurements.

Alcohol Abuse

This problem probably produces hypoglycemia more commonly than any other single cause. As stated above, ingestion of ethanol can produce postprandial hypoglycemia in normal, well nourished persons who engage in "social" drinking. However, fasting hypoglycemia related to ethanol ingestion occurs in chronic alcohol abusers and especially in those who are malnourished. The situation most likely to provoke hypoglycemia is cessation of food intake and continued ingestion of ethanol over the ensuing 10 to 20 hours. Under these circumstances, ethanol intoxication, i.e., drunkenness, may mistakenly be thought to be responsible for the symptoms.

Liver Disease and Chronic Congestive Heart Failure

Although hypoglycemia can be seen in the course of severe, acute hepatitis or as a result of chronic passive congestion in long-standing congestive heart failure, liver disease does not usually produce hypoglycemia. Patients with severe cirrhosis may occasionally have fasting hypoglycemia, but the development of hypoglycemia in such a patient should suggest the presence of a hepatoma. In patients with well differentiated hepatoma, hypoglycemia may be an early symptom.

Endocrine Disease

Glucocorticoids and growth hormone are important regulators of glucose metabolism. Thus, either pituitary insufficiency or adrenal insufficiency (primary or secondary to hypopituitarism) can result in hypoglycemia as a presenting manifestation. The diagnosis of these disorders is described elsewhere in this chapter.

General References

DeGroot LJ (ed): *Endocrinology*. New York, Grune & Stratton, 1979, vols 1–3.
    A comprehensive, multivolume textbook containing a great deal of information. Poorly indexed.
Felig P, Baxter, JD, Broadus, AE, Frohman, LA (eds): *Endocrinology & Metabolism*. New York, McGraw-Hill, 1981.
    A textbook of manageable proportions.
Hershman JM (ed): *Management of Endocrine Disorders*. Philadelphia, Lea & Febiger, 1980.
    A short textbook.
Wilson JD, Foster DW (eds): *Williams' Textbook of Endocrinology*, ed 7. Philadelphia, WB Saunders, 1985.
    The latest edition of this standard textbook contains detailed coverage of most aspects of the topics considered in this chapter.

Specific References

1. Amatruda TT Jr, Hurst MM, D'esopo ND: Certain endocrine and metabolic facets of the steroid withdrawal syndrome. *J Clin Endocrinol Metab* 25:1207, 1965.
2. Burrow GN, Wortzman G, Rewcastle NB, et al: Microadenomas of the pituitary and abnormal sellar tomograms in an unselected autopsy series. *N Engl J Med* 304:156, 1981.
3. Byyny RL: Withdrawal from glucocorticoid therapy. *N Engl J Med* 295:30, 1976.
4. Cahill GF, Soeldner JS: A noneditorial on nonhypoglycemia. *N Engl J Med* 291:905, 1974.
5. Chalew SA, McLaughlin JV, Mersey JH, et al: The use of the plasma epinephrine response in the diagnosis of idiopathic postprandial syndrome. *JAMA* 251:612, 1984.
6. Coe FL, Favus MJ: Does mild, asymptomatic hyperparathyroidism require surgery? *N Engl J Med* 302:224, 1980 (editorial); and rebuttal (letters), Incidence of primary hyperparathyroidism. *N Engl J Med* 302:1312, 1980.
7. Copeland PM: The incidentally discovered adrenal mass. *Ann Intern Med* 98:940, 1983.
8. Davis FB, Davis PJ: Water metabolism in diabetes mellitus. *Am J Med* 70:210, 1981.
9. Fauci AS, Dale DC, Balow JE: Glucocorticoid therapy: mechanisms of action and clinical considerations. *Ann Intern Med* 84:304, 1976.
10. Graber AL, Ney RL, Nicholson WE, et al: Natural history of pituitary-adrenal recovery following long-term suppression with corticosteroids. *J Clin Endocrinol Metab* 25:11, 1965.
11. Heath H III, Hodgson SF, Kennedy MA: Primary hyperparathyroidism. Incidence, morbidity, and potential economic impact in a community. *N Engl J Med* 302:189, 1980.
12. Melby JC: Systemic corticosteroid therapy: pharmacology and

endocrinologic considerations. *Ann Intern Med* 81:505, 1974.

13. Miller M, Moses AM: Drug-induced states of impaired water excretion. *Kidney Int* 10:96, 1976.

14. Osteoporosis (NIH Consensus Conference). *JAMA* 252:799, 1984.

15. Riggs BL, Seeman E, Hodgson SF, *et al*: Effect of the fluoride/calcium regimen on vertebral fracture occurrence in postmenopausal osteoporosis. *N Engl J Med* 306:446, 1982.

16. Roof BS, Gordan GS: Hyperparathyroid disease in the aged. In Greenblatt RB (ed) *Geriatric Endocrinology*, vol 5, *Aging*, p 33. New York, Raven Press, 1978.

17. Sachar EJ (ed): *Hormones, Behavior, and Psychopathology.* New York, Raven Press, 1976.

18. Spielgel RJ, Vigersky RA, Oliff AI, *et al*: Adrenal suppression after short-term corticosteroid therapy. *Lancet* 1:630, 1979.

19. Stewart AF, Horst R, Deftos LJ, *et al*: Biochemical evaluation of patients with cancer-associated hypercalcemia. *N Engl J Med* 303:1377, 1980.

20. Yager J, Young RT: Nonhypoglycemia is an epidemic condition. *N Engl J Med* 291:907, 1974.

21. Zervas NT, Martin JB: Management of hormone-secreting pituitary adenomas. *N Engl J Med* 302:210, 1980.

CHAPTER SEVENTY-FIVE

Clinical Implications of Abnormal Lipoprotein Metabolism

MARC R. BLACKMAN, M.D., DAVID E. KERN, M.D., AND
ANDREW P. GOLDBERG, M.D.

Interest in plasma lipids, lipoproteins, and apoproteins stems from their strong relationship to the development of atherosclerosis of the coronary and peripheral vasculature (2, 4). At a time when it is possible to reduce the frequency of premature death and disability from atherosclerotic disease, the physician should be knowledgeable about and capable of diagnosing and treating the major abnormalities of lipoprotein metabolism.

LIPOPROTEIN NOMENCLATURE AND COMPOSITION (Table 75.1)

Lipids by definition are insoluble in the aqueous plasma medium. They circulate in plasma as component parts of macromolecules that consist of a nonpolar hydrophobic lipid core of cholesterol esters and triglycerides and a polar hydrophilic monolayer surface coat of protein, phospholipid, and unesterified cholesterol (Fig. 75.1). These macromolecules, which are made miscible in plasma by their surface coat, are called lipoproteins.

Lipoproteins have traditionally been classified as a family of molecules containing the same basic constituents, but in different proportions (Table 75.1). The major classes of lipoproteins can be separated from each other by differences in density (ultracentrifugation), net surface charge (electrophoresis), size, and composition. Ultracentrifugation, which provides the most useful means of classification, separates lipoproteins into five principal classes. From the least dense and largest to the most dense and smallest, these are the chylomicrons, very low density lipoproteins (VLDL), intermediate density lipoproteins (IDL), low density lipoproteins (LDL), and high density lipoproteins (HDL) (16).

Each lipoprotein contains characteristic proportions of lipids and type-specific apoproteins (apos) such that, with increasing lipoprotein density, the relative amount of lipid decreases and that of (apo)protein increases (Table 75.1). Thus, triglycer-

Table 75.1.
Classification of Plasma Lipoproteins by Physical and Chemical Characteristics

Lipoprotein Fraction (Ultracentrifugation)	Density (g/ml)	Migration (Electrophoresis)	Composition as Percent Total Mass			
			Cholesterol	Triglyceride	Apoprotein	Phospholipid
Chylomicron	0.95	Origin	2–7	80–90	2 (A, B-48, C, E)	3
Very low density (VLDL)	< 1.006	Pre-β	10–22	50–70	6 (B-100, C, E)	14
β-very low density (β-VLDL or VLDL₂)	< 1.006	β	30–40	45	12 (B-100, B-48, C, E)	15
Intermediate density or remnant (IDL)	1.006–1.019	Slow pre-β	30–40	40	18 (B, E)	22
Low density (LDL)	1.019–1.063	β	45–50	5–10	21 (B-100)	22
High density (HDL)	1.063–1.21	α	15–25	3–5	50 (A, C, E)	28

ide is the major lipid component in chylomicrons and VLDL, while cholesterol is the major component of LDL. Intermediate density or remnant lipoproteins are catabolic products of chylomicrons and VLDL and contain similar amounts of both lipids and apo (see below, "Normal Physiology of Lipoprotein Transport"). The HDL are the densest lipoproteins; they contain the most apos and ordinarily consist of 15 to 25% cholesterol and a small amount of triglyceride in the core. HDL are further subdivided into HDL₂ and HDL₃. The former is more buoyant as reflected by its higher lipid to protein ratio and richer apo A-I and apo C and E content, relative to the more dense HDL₃ which has a lower lipid to protein ratio and a higher apo A-II than A-I composition. The strong inverse relationship of coronary risk to plasma concentrations of HDL₂ and apo A-I relates to the heightened capacity of the latter molecules to transport cholesterol from cells (19).

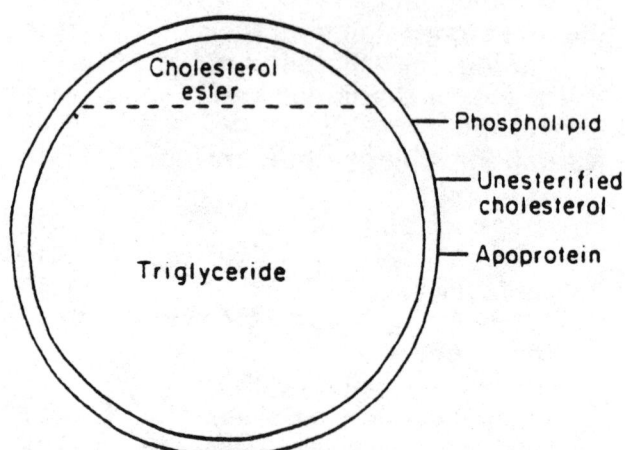

Figure 75.1. Structure of the lipoprotein macromolecule with the nonpolar lipids, cholesterol ester and triglyceride, in the lipoprotein core surrounded by a monolayer composed of specific (apo) proteins and the polar lipids, unesterified cholesterol and phospholipid.

PLASMA LIPOPROTEINS AS RISK FACTORS FOR ATHEROSCLEROSIS

The risk factor concept, which developed as an outgrowth of the Framingham study and other large epidemiological studies, is based upon the strong association between certain characteristics in people and the increased likelihood of developing cardiovascular disease (14). Among the most formidable risk factors for atherosclerotic vascular disease, the most clearly established ones at this time are plasma total cholesterol levels (and plasma LDL and HDL content), hypertension, and cigarette smoking. Each has been clearly implicated and makes a sizable independent contribution to the overall risk of developing coronary artery disease (CAD).

Evidence from several large prospective and retrospective epidemiological studies among diverse populations has demonstrated that variations in plasma levels of certain lipids and lipoproteins are associated with an increased likelihood of developing or having CAD. *Hypercholesterolemia*, for example, is strongly associated with the subsequent development of CAD. The relationship is uniformly

consistent, dose related, and independent of sex. The predictive value of the plasma level of total cholesterol is somewhat limited, however, by the fact that it reflects the opposing influences of *LDL and HDL cholesterol*. Levels of LDL correlate positively, while those of HDL are inversely related to CAD risk. The negative correlation between HDL levels and CAD depends mainly on its subfraction, HDL₂, which may provide, along with its major protein component, apo A-I, a better index of risk than the total plasma level of HDL (19). Over the range of plasma levels of total cholesterol or of HDL cholesterol levels found in an average American population, the risk of CAD varies roughly 5-fold. Plasma levels of total cholesterol have less predictive value beyond the age of 50 or 60, but HDL cholesterol levels and the ratio of LDL to HDL cholesterol remain useful predictors in this age group. The relationships between plasma levels of total cholesterol, LDL cholesterol, and HDL cholesterol and CAD are *independent* ones, in that the associations remain significant even after statistical adjustment for the contributions of other risk factors (such as cigarette smoking, hypertension, obesity, impaired glucose tolerance, and other lipoprotein levels).

Elevated fasting levels of plasma *triglyceride* and its major lipoprotein transporter, *VLDL*, also correlate with an increased risk of atherosclerotic disease. However, in most large epidemiological studies, the association does not appear to be an independent one. In certain subgroups of patients, however, such as those with familial combined hyperlipoproteinemia or familial dysbetalipoproteinemia, the hypertriglyceridemia may reflect altered lipoprotein and apoprotein composition and metabolism (25) and seems causally related to the development of premature atherosclerosis (4). In addition, hypertriglyceridemia may be prognostically important in patients with diabetes mellitus (27) or end-stage renal disease (8).

Not only do these lipoprotein and apoprotein abnormalities seem to increase one's predisposition to CAD, there is a parallel increased risk for cerebrovascular disease (11, 14) and peripheral vascular disease as well (11).

Plasma levels of other lipoproteins and apos also correlate with atherosclerotic disease. Elevated plasma concentrations of *LDL apo B* appear to discriminate between patients with and without atherosclerosis of the coronary and peripheral vasculature, even in the presence of normal plasma levels of total cholesterol and LDL cholesterol (4, 5, 25). The determination of plasma LDL apo B concentrations may prove useful in assessing risk in hypertriglyceridemic patients (4, 25). In familial dysbetalipoproteinemia, a genetic disorder characterized by elevated plasma levels of *IDL* and an abnormally migrating *β-VLDL* (20), there is an increased risk of both peripheral and coronary atherosclerotic disease. In contrast, fasting *chylomicronemia* is associated with recurrent episodes of abdominal pain and pancreatitis, but not with the early development of atherosclerosis.

In several epidemiological studies, plasma levels of total cholesterol below 180 to 195 mg/dl have been associated with an increased risk of cancer, especially cancer of the colon. The evidence does not, however, suggest a significant causal link, since (a) in most, but not all, studies the association was strongest in the first year of follow-up, then attenuated and disappeared in subsequent years, suggesting that preclinical cancer might have lowered levels of plasma cholesterol rather than *vice versa*; (b) studies comparing populations have shown a positive rather than a negative association between dietary fat intake and risk for major cancers, such as breast and colon cancer; and (c) the relationship was generally weak, present in a minority of studies, and demonstrated no consistent relation between cholesterol level and cancer risk (15).

RATIONALE FOR DIAGNOSIS AND TREATMENT

The need for a preventive approach to the control of atherosclerotic disease becomes clear when one considers the following facts: At present atherosclerotic disease constitutes the leading cause of death and disability in western industrialized societies. In the United States, approximately 725,000 individuals die annually from atherosclerotic disease, 550,000 of them from CAD. Many of the deaths occur suddenly and unexpectedly in otherwise apparently healthy people. Despite medical advances in the treatment of symptomatic disease, more than 40% of patients who sustain a myocardial infarction still die, with more than half of the deaths occurring outside the hospital before medical care is available. Complications and disability from atherosclerotic disease, once established, are seldom fully reversible. The economic costs are formidable, with more than $60 billion being spent annually in direct health care costs and lost wages and productivity.

The prevention, diagnosis, and treatment of plasma lipoprotein abnormalities constitute a major component of an overall effort to prevent atherosclerotic disease. The measurement of plasma concentrations of lipids and lipoproteins can identify asymptomatic individuals at high risk. A large and increasing body of data derived from pathological, genetic, metabolic, epidemiological, animal, and clinical studies has demonstrated that certain abnormalities in plasma lipoproteins (such as elevated levels of total cholesterol and LDL cholesterol) actually promote or cause atherosclerosis. It is equally well established that both exogenous factors (such as diet, drugs, exercise, and cigarette smoking) and endogenous metabolic factors (which are genetically determined and may be affected by various diseases) determine plasma levels of lipids and lipoproteins.

The "lipid hypothesis," based upon the data described above, postulates that favorable alteration of plasma lipoprotein levels by diet, drugs, or other therapy reduces the risk of atherosclerosis in humans. While there had been much suggestive data based upon animal studies, clinical trials of diet and drug therapy, and observations of falling CAD mortality in the United States concurrent with widespread changes in dietary habits (as well as with the reduction of other risk factors), evidence supporting the lipid hypothesis was inconclusive until the recent completion of the Lipid Research Clinics Coronary Primary Prevention Trial (18). This trial was a prospective, randomized, double-blinded, multiinstitutional trial of therapy with cholestyramine and diet *versus* placebo and diet in 3806 healthy hypercholesterolemic men aged 35 to 59 followed for an average of 7.4 years. During the study period, 155 of 1906 (8.1%) men in the cholestyramine group experienced definite CAD death and/or definite nonfatal myocardial infarction (the primary end points) as opposed to 187 of 1900 (9.8%) men in the placebo group. The resulting 19% reduction in the frequency of the primary end points in the treated group was accompanied by decreases in the development of new angina (by 20%), a positive exercise stress test (by 25%), and incidence of coronary bypass surgery (by 21%). There was a 2% reduction in overall CAD risk for each 1% reduction in plasma level of total cholesterol; thus in men compliant with the prescribed dose (24 g/day), a 25% decrease in total cholesterol level resulted in a 50% decrease in overall CAD risk. Another recently completed double-blinded, 5-year prospective, randomized study examined the effect of cholestyramine plus diet *versus* placebo plus diet on the angiographic progression of CAD in 116 hypercholesterolemic patients with prior angiographic evidence of CAD (1). The cholestyramine group evidenced a suggestive decrease in "definite" CAD progression and a significant decrease in "definite and probable" CAD progression. Favorable alterations in the ratios of plasma levels of total (or LDL) cholesterol to HDL cholesterol correlated significantly with a decrease in CAD progression, however defined.

NORMAL PHYSIOLOGY OF LIPOPROTEIN TRANSPORT (Fig. 75.2)

Plasma lipoproteins arise from both exogenous dietary sources and from endogenous hepatic sources (Fig. 75.2). They function as efficient vehicles for the transport of their nonpolar core components, triglyceride and cholesterol ester, to tissues.

After the ingestion of fat, *dietary triglycerides* are hydrolyzed in the gut and absorbed by *intestinal enterocytes*. Triglyceride, as apo B-48 containing *chylomicrons*, is formed in these cells, secreted into lymphatic vessels, and enters the plasma *via* the thoracic duct. Chylomicrons function as a system of high energy caloric transport, allowing calories ingested in excess of the immediate needs of the body to be transferred to sites of storage for use between meals. Absorbed *dietary cholesterol* is also esterified and transported in chylomicrons.

Other *triglyceride-rich lipoproteins* are synthesized from *endogenous sources* by the liver and intestine. Insulin and glucagon-regulated processes that occur in these organs include: uptake of fatty acids and glucose from the blood stream, synthesis of fatty acids from glucose and acetate, and esterifi-

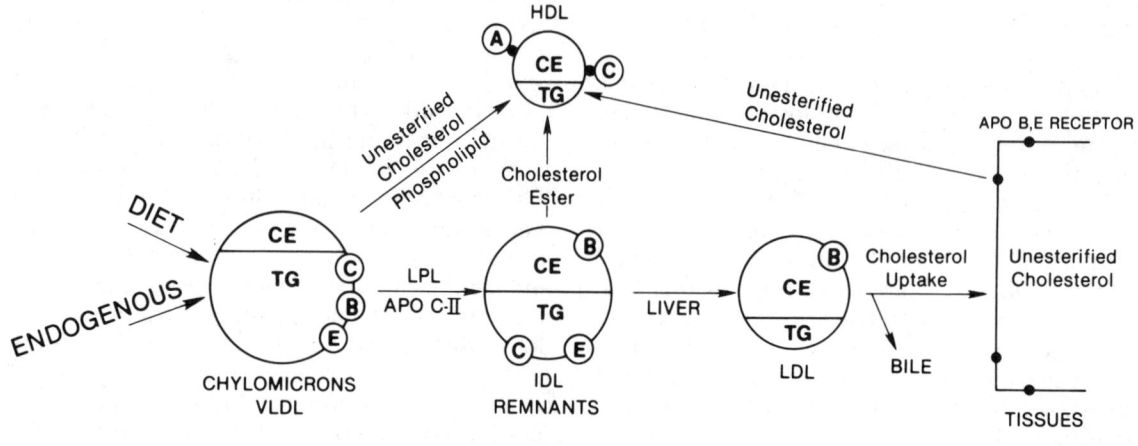

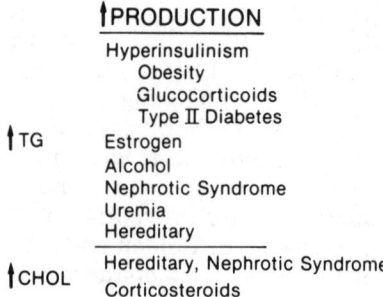

↑PRODUCTION	↓REMOVAL

↑TG   Hyperinsulinism
      Obesity
      Glucocorticoids
      Type II Diabetes
   Estrogen
   Alcohol
   Nephrotic Syndrome
   Uremia
   Hereditary
	Untreated Diabetes (Type I)
	Hypothyroid
	Renal Failure
	Dysgammaglobulinemia
	Dysbetalipoproteinemia
	Familial LPL Deficiency
	Apo C-II Deficiency

↑CHOL Hereditary, Nephrotic Syndrome Corticosteroids	Hereditary (FH), Dysbetalipoproteinemia Hypothyroid, Nephrotic Syndrome

Figure 75.2. The normal physiology of lipoprotein transport is illustrated schematically in the *upper portion* of the figure (see pages 1044 to 1046 for details), while a pathophysiological classification of the major disor-

ders of lipoprotein metabolism is depicted in the *lower portion* of the figure (see pages 1048 to 1054 and Table 75.5 for details).

cation of fatty acids with glycerol to form triglycerides. Cholesterol synthesis from acetate also occurs in the liver and is regulated by the enzyme hydroxymethylglutaryl (HMG) CoA reductase. Triglycerides synthesized in the liver combine with cholesterol ester and are enveloped in a lipoprotein monolayer composed of phospholipid, unesterified cholesterol, and apo B-100 prior to secretion into the hepatic venous outflow system as *endogenous triglyceride-rich VLDL.*

Chylomicrons and VLDL are transported to adipose tissue and muscle for storage and utilization. The uptake and storage of triglyceride are regulated by *lipoprotein lipase* (LPL). LPL is secreted by cells in virtually all parenchymal tissues and migrates to the endothelial cells of local capillary beds where it is activated by the apo C-II peptide normally found on chylomicrons, VLDL and HDL. It hydrolyzes triglyceride and surface components (apo C and phospholipids) from chylomicrons and VLDL to transform them into *remnant lipoproteins* (Fig. 75.2). The fatty acids released during this reaction migrate to muscle cells for combustion or to adipose cells for resynthesis and storage as triglyceride (21). The *remnant lipoproteins* are smaller, denser, and relatively enriched in cholesterol, apo B, and apo E compared to the chylomicrons and VLDL from which they derive. They are taken up by apo B-E receptors in the liver where their apo E composition serves as a signal for binding. The chylomicron remnants are further degraded, while the VLDL remnants are processed into IDL and cholesterol-rich LDL (Fig. 75.2). Apo C-II and apo C-III (which stimulate and inhibit, respectively, the hepatic uptake of apo E-containing lipoproteins), and the phospholipids and free cholesterol released during the LPL reaction are transferred to HDL for utilization. The surface material generated by LPL-mediated removal of core triglyceride from VLDL and chylomicrons is the substrate (apo A-I is the cofactor) for the enzyme *lecithin-cholesterol acyl transferase* (LCAT), which converts nascent HDL to mature spherical HDL and plays a major role in reverse cholesterol transport (see below).

Hepatic triglyceride lipase, like LPL, is released into plasma by heparin administration, hence the term *postheparin lipolytic activity* (PHLA). Hepatic lipase and LPL differ in composition, yet both are involved in the regulation of the plasma concentration of HDL_2 and in the catabolism of triglyceride-rich lipoproteins. Hepatic lipase promotes the hepatic removal of phospholipids and cholesterol from HDL_2 to form either HDL_3 (which re-enters the circulation) or irreversible catabolic products of HDL. Like LPL, it also hydrolyzes additional triglyceride from remnant lipoproteins and, by preserving apo B, converts remnants to LDL.

The *LDL* are the principal carriers of *cholesterol* in plasma. Cholesterol is a major structural component of all cell membranes and is a precursor for steroid hormone synthesis by the adrenal glands and gonads. The *LDL cholesterol-rich particles* are derived mainly from VLDL and their catabolic remnants *via* the action of LPL, hepatic lipase, and the hepatic conversion of remnants to LDL containing only apo B-100 and cholesterol ester (fig. 75.2). The principal removal of LDL occurs in the periphery by cells having a specific cell surface receptor (2) that recognizes all forms of apo B and is currently referred to as the *apo B-E (LDL) receptor* (Fig. 75.2). After specific cell receptor binding, LDL are internalized by receptor-mediated endocytosis and carried to lysosomes, where apo B is irreversibly degraded to amino acids and LDL cholesterol ester is hydrolyzed to free cholesterol. The free cholesterol is transported to an intracellular cholesterol pool where it regulates, by a cellular feedback pathway, the resynthesis of cholesterol, cholesterol ester, and apo B-E (LDL) receptors (13).

The cholesterol content of the cell is also regulated by a *removal system involving HDL* as a vehicle for cholesterol transport. This process is mediated by a distinct extrahepatic cell surface receptor that promotes the efflux of cholesterol from the cell, followed by a reaction involving HDL_3 and LCAT, whereby cholesterol is transported from peripheral to hepatic cells by HDL_2 for catabolism and excretion into bile directly or after conversion to bile acid (13, 22). This *reverse cholesterol transport system* provides an efficient mechanism for the removal of cholesterol arising from cell membrane turnover and cell death.

Continued LDL catabolism in excess of that performed by hepatic and other parenchymal cells occurs in macrophages *via* a *scavenger pathway*. The latter is the predominant mechanism for LDL catabolism in persons with homozygous familial hypercholesterolemia (2).

An apparent antiatherogenic alteration in both the lipoprotein and apoprotein composition of HDL, the formation of HDL_c, occurs during high cholesterol feeding and represents one pathway by which the body can enhance its capacity to clear excess cholesterol from cells (13). Thus, the dynamic equilibrium between plasma and extracellular LDL and HDL, and their interaction with the apoproteins, enzymes, and receptors involved in lipoprotein transport are necessary for the homeostatic maintenance of the intracellular and extracellular cholesterol pools and the control of the atherogenic process.

Apoproteins occupy specific domains on the three-dimensional structures of the individual lipoproteins (Table 75.2). Alterations in lipid-protein interactions occur during the normal metabolism of lipoproteins, resulting in changes in the association of apoproteins with lipoproteins. Abnormalities in lipoprotein transport occur when the domains of apo-

Table 75.2.
Apoproteins: Nomenclature and Metabolic Role

Apoprotein	Lipoprotein Association	Concentration in Plasma (mg/dl)	Metabolic Role
A-I	HDL, chylomicron	110–120	LCAT activator
A-II	HDL, chylomicron	25–50	Unknown
A-IV	Chylomicron, HDL d > 1.21	8	Unknown
B-100 } B-74 } Hepatic B-26 }	VLDL, LDL	90	Transports lipids from the liver as VLDL, β-VLDL, LDL to peripheral cells where they are recognized by cellular LDL apo B-E receptors
B-48} Intestinal	Chylomicron	5	Transports lipids from cells in the intestine
C-I	Chylomicron, VLDL, HDL	4	
C-II	Chylomicron, VLDL, HDL	4	Activates lipoprotein lipase
C-III	Chylomicron, VLDL, HDL	12	Inhibits activation of lipoprotein lipase by apo C-II, inhibits recognition of apo E by cell receptors
D	HDL, d > 1.21	8	Transfers cholesterol esters between lipoproteins as part of a transfer complex composed of apo A-I-D-LCAT
E	Chylomicron, VLDL, β-VLDL, IDL, HDL	5	Recognized by the apo B-E receptor on cells and in the liver; role in LDL, β-VLDL, HDL catabolism
Transfer proteins	HDL, d > 1.21	2	Several proteins which transfer cholesterol esters, phospholipids, and triglycerides between lipoproteins in plasma

proteins are altered by substitutions or deletions in amino acids. For example, the abnormal recognition of β-VLDL by the apo B-E receptor on cells occurs due to an abnormality in apo E in dysbetalipoproteinemia (see below, "Pathophysiology of Lipoprotein Disorders"), while abnormalities in the apo B-E receptors are responsible for the defect in familial hypercholesterolemia (2, 20).

HYPERLIPOPROTEINEMIA

Definition

Hyperlipoproteinemia is defined as the excessive accumulation in the blood of one or more of the lipoprotein classes of lipid-transporting macromolecules. The diagnosis of *hyperlipoproteinemia* is based upon plasma levels of lipids or lipoproteins above the 95th percentile of those found in a reference population. The distributions of plasma levels of total cholesterol, LDL cholesterol, total triglyceride, VLDL triglycerides, and HDL cholesterol among North American participants in the Lipid Research Clinics Prevalence Study have been published (17, 26). While the participants in that study did not

represent a random sample of the entire North American population, they did encompass a broad range of sociodemographic groups and thus provide the best available reference values for lipoproteins. Because lipoprotein values vary with age, sex, and race, these must be considered when assigning a range of normal or a percentile to an individual's lipid levels (Table 75.3).

Based upon the results of recent treatment trials (18), the arbitrary use of a 95th percentile cut-off point in the diagnosis of hyperlipoproteinemia has some utility in suggesting the need for drug therapy in hypercholesterolemic patients. However, it should not be considered the dividing point between "diseased" and "healthy" individuals, since CAD risk seems to increase continuously over a broad range of lipid values. Furthermore, lipid distributions vary between and within populations. For example, levels of total cholesterol (and the prevalence of CAD) are much higher in North American and Northern European populations than they are in the Japanese population. Many people diagnosed as normolipidemic in the United States would probably be classified as hyperlipidemic in Japan.

Decreased as well as increased plasma levels of

Table 75.3.
Fasting Plasma Concentrations (mg/dl) of Lipoprotein Lipids in North Americans[a]

Caucasians[b]

Age	Men TC[c] 5th%	Mean	95th%	LDL-C 5th%	Mean	95th%	TG 5th%	Mean	95th%	HDL-C 5th%	Mean	95th%
15–19	118	153	191	62	94	130	38	78	143	30	46	63
20–24	118	162	212	66	103	147	44	89	165	30	45	63
25–29	130	179	234	70	117	165	45	104	204	31	45	63
30–34	142	193	258	78	126	185	46	122	253	28	46	63
35–39	147	201	267	81	133	189	52	141	316	29	43	62
40–44	150	205	260	87	136	186	56	152	318	27	44	67
45–49	163	213	275	98	144	202	56	143	279	30	45	64
50–54	156	213	274	89	142	197	63	153	313	28	44	63
55–59	161	215	280	88	146	203	60	134	261	28	48	71
60–64	163	217	287	83	146	210	56	131	240	30	52	74
65–69	166	221	288	98	150	210	54	139	256	30	51	78
70+	144	210	265	88	143	186	63	133	239	31	51	75

Age	Women TC[c] 5th%	Mean	95th%	LDL-C 5th%	Mean	95th%	TG 5th%	Mean	95th%	HDL-C 5th%	Mean	95th%
15–19	118	159	207	59	96	137	36	73	126	35	52	74
20–24	121	170	237	57	104	159	37	87	168	33	53	79
25–29	130	179	231	71	110	164	42	87	159	37	56	83
30–34	133	179	228	70	111	156	40	86	163	36	56	77
35–39	139	190	249	75	120	172	40	98	205	34	55	82
40–44	146	198	259	74	125	174	45	98	191	34	58	88
45–49	148	206	268	79	129	186	44	113	223	34	59	87
50–54	163	217	281	88	138	201	53	116	223	37	62	92
55–59	167	229	294	89	146	210	59	133	279	37	62	91
60–64	172	232	300	100	152	224	57	132	256	38	64	92
65–69	167	234	291	92	154	221	56	137	260	35	63	98
70+	173	225	280	96	149	206	60	128	289	33	61	92

Blacks

Men

Age	TC[c,d] 5th%	Mean	95th%	TG[d] 5th%	Mean	95th%		HDL-C[e] Age	Mean ± SD
10–19	120	160	205	31	59	102		15–19	53 ± 11
20–29	—[e]	179	—	—[d]	81	—		20–24	—
30–39	138	192	253	42	107	224		25–29	58 ± 15
40–49	148	207	—	52	126	294		30–34	54 ± 13
50–59	—	207	—	—	142	—		35–39	53 ± 16
60+	—	221	—	—	109	—		40–44	58 ± 20

Women

Age	TC[c,d] 5th%	Mean	95th%	TG[d] 5th%	Mean	95th%		HDL-C Age	Mean ± SD
10–19	124	165	211	36	65	110		15–19	54 ± 11
20–29	124	177	235	38	77	137		20–24	—
30–39	132	185	243	38	80	150		25–29	57 ± 10
40–49	146	202	268	43	99	188		30–34	60 ± 13
50–59	—	217	—	—	104	—		35–39	59 ± 15
60+	—	234	—	—	120	—		40–44	62 ± 19

[a] 5th%, 5th percentile; 95th%, 95th percentile; TC, total cholesterol; LDL-C, low density lipoprotein cholesterol; HDL-C, high density lipoprotein cholesterol; TG, total triglycerides.
[b] Adapted from reference 24, visit 2.
[c] Levels determined routinely by clinical laboratories are often higher (up to 30 mg/dl or more) than those determined by a standardized laboratory (e.g., Centers for Disease Control). Check how your laboratory is standardized.
[d] Adapted from reference 16, visit 1.
[e] Adapted from references 16 and 26.

certain lipoproteins can also pose a threat of atherosclerosis. Specifically, plasma levels of HDL cholesterol and apo A-I are inversely correlated with the risk for CAD, with the 5th rather than 95th percentile being the arbitrary cut-off point to distinguish those at greatest risk.

Classification

Primary versus Secondary

For clinical purposes hyperlipoproteinemic states should be classified as primary (hereditary or sporadic genetic disorders of metabolism), secondary, or both. Secondary hyperlipoproteinemia is associated with an identifiable disease or condition and is reversible with control or eradication of that disease or condition. The major causes of secondary hyperlipoproteinemia are listed in Table 75.4, and their usual hyperlipidemic patterns are displayed in Table 75.5.

Phenotypic versus Genotypic and Pathophysiological

In the 1960s, it was popular to classify the various hyperlipidemic states *phenotypically*, based upon

Table 75.4.
Causes of Secondary Lipoprotein Disorders

Exogenous	Alcohol, oral contraceptives, estrogens, androgens, corticosteroids, diuretics (thiazides, chlorthalidone), β-adrenergic blocking agents, obesity, nutritional (diet high in cholesterol/saturated fat)
Endocrine-metabolic	Diabetes mellitus, hypothyroidism, Cushing's disease, Addison's disease, acromegaly, hypopituitarism
Hepatic	Obstructive or parenchymal disease, hepatoma
Renal	Nephrotic syndrome, chronic renal failure, hemodialysis
Acute stress situations	Acute myocardial infarction, sepsis, burns
Pregnancy	
Pancreatitis	
Dysgammaglobulinemias	Multiple myeloma, macroglobulinemia
Systemic lupus erythematosus	
Gout	
Viral infections	
Other	Glycogen storage disease, lipodystrophies, progeria, acute intermittent porphyria, anorexia nervosa, Klinefelter's syndrome

specific concentrations of lipids and lipoproteins and electrophoretic patterns (Table 75.6). While the *phenotypic* classification describes in abbreviated fashion the plasma lipoproteins that are present in elevated or low concentrations, it does not reflect the genetic mechanisms or pathophysiology of the lipoprotein disorders (10). It is desirable to classify patients *pathophysiologically* (Table 75.5) and *genotypically* (Table 75.6) in order to diagnose and treat lipoprotein disorders accurately. Since apoproteins, enzymes, and cellular receptors are the major regulators of lipoprotein metabolism, it is appropriate to categorize lipoprotein disorders wherever possible in terms of pathophysiological defects in the structure, function, and metabolism of these molecules, rather than by using a rigidly fixed phenotypic classification. Often, the pathophysiological and genotypic classification can be surmised from a patient's phenotypic pattern, medical history, family history, and physical examination. Sometimes family members must be studied and/or more sophisticated laboratory analyses performed, necessitating referral to a specialist in endocrinology and metabolism.

PATHOPHYSIOLOGY OF LIPOPROTEIN DISORDERS

The abnormal accumulation of lipoproteins in plasma results from their excessive production, defective removal, or both. Lipoprotein disorders may be primary (usually genetic), may be secondary to certain diseases (especially diabetes mellitus, chronic renal disease, hypothyroidism, dysglobulinemia) or drugs (corticosteroids, estrogens, thiazide diuretics), or may represent an interaction between primary and secondary factors. A pathophysiological approach to understanding the regulation of plasma lipoprotein metabolism is outlined in Figure 75.2 and Table 75.5. Abnormalities can occur in (*a*) triglyceride-rich lipoprotein synthesis, (*b*) lipoprotein lipase-mediated triglyceride catabolism, (*c*) remnant lipoprotein catabolism, (*d*) cholesterol-rich lipoprotein catabolism, and (*e*) cholesterol-rich lipoprotein (LDL cholesterol) synthesis and absorption.

Increased Triglyceride Synthesis

The majority of triglyceride input is from the diet in normal individuals. However, abnormalities in the regulation of the endogenous production of triglyceride-rich VLDL are fairly common and are the most frequent causes of hypertriglyceridemia. They are associated with an increase in plasma levels of VLDL (type IV) or VLDL plus chylomicrons (type V). The underlying metabolic cause for endogenous hypertriglyceridemia is usually related to insulin, specifically hyperinsulinemia and insulin resistance, due most often to obesity, the ingestion of excessive calories or alcohol, or the use of estrogens or corticosteroids.

Table 75.5.
Pathophysiological Approach to the Management of Hyperliproproteinemia

Pathophysiological Classification[a]	Predominant Lipoprotein (Usual Phenotype)	Cholesterol	Triglyceride	Underlying Cause	Diet Therapy[c]	Drug Therapy[d]
↑ Triglyceride synthesis	VLDL (IV) or VLDL + chylomicrons (V) when severe	↔, ↓ or ↑	↑ to ↑↑↑	*Primary genetic* Familial hypertriglyceridemia (1/100)[b] Familial combined hyperlipidemia (1/100)[b] *Secondary-acquired* Caloric excess Alcohol ↑ Insulin—obesity, type II diabetes mellitus Nephrotic syndrome Corticosteroids, estrogens	Loss of excess weight ↓ Alcohol ↓ Saturated fat, cholesterol ↓ Simple sugars	1. Fibric acid derivatives or nicotinic acid
↓ Triglyceride removal	VLDL (IV) or VLDL + chylomicrons (V) when severe	↔ or ↑	↑ to ↑↑↑	*Primary genetic* LPL deficiency (rare) Apo C-II deficiency (rare) *Secondary* ↓ Insulin—type I diabetes mellitus ↓ Thyroxine Renal failure (dialysis) Dysglobulinemia (rare)	↓ Total fat Medium chain triglycerides Loss of excess weight if ↑ VLDL ↓ Saturated fat, cholesterol if ↑ VLDL	1. Replacement of insulin or thyroid hormone deficiency 2. Fibric acid derivatives or nicotinic acid
↓ Remnant removal	Remnants (III) + VLDL and chylomicrons when severe	May be normal or ↑ to ↑↑	↑ to ↑↑↑	*Primary genetic* Dysbetalipoproteinemia (1/5000)[b] *Secondary* Hypothyroidism, obstructive liver disease End-stage renal disease	↓ Saturated fat, cholesterol Loss of excess weight ↓ Simple sugars	1. Fibric acid derivatives 2. Nicotinic acid 3. Estrogen (see the text)
↓ LDL removal	LDL (IIa)	↑ to ↑↑↑	↔ to ↑	*Primary genetic* Familial hypercholesterolemia (monogenic homozygous—1/1,000,000 or heterozygous—1/500)[b] *Secondary* Hypothyroidism	↓ Saturated fat, cholesterol ↑ P/S ratio ↓ Calories (weight loss) ↑ Fiber, soy protein	1. Bile acid sequestering resin 2. Combination therapy (see the text)
↑ Cholesterol synthesis	LDL (IIa) or LDL + VLDL (IIb)	↑ to ↑↑↑	↔ to ↑↑	*Primary genetic* Familial hypercholesterolemia Familial combined hyperlipidemia (1/100)[b] *Secondary* Obesity Nephrotic syndrome Corticosteroids	Loss of excess weight ↓ Saturated fat, cholesterol ↑ P/S ratio ↑ Fiber, soy protein	1. Bile acid sequestering resin 2. Combination therapy (see the text)
↑ Cholesterol absorption	LDL (IIa)	↑	↔	Dietary excess	↓ Saturated fat, cholesterol ↑ P/S ratio Loss of excess weight ↑ Fiber, soy protein	1. Bile acid sequestering resin 2. Nicotinic acid 3. Other (see the text)

[a] Combinations of these mechanisms and patterns are common: *e.g.,* ↑ triglyceride synthesis plus ↑ cholesterol synthesis produces ↑ VLDL + ↑ LDL.
[b] Frequencies refer to the prevalence (gene frequency) of the disorder in the general population.
[c] Dietary measures are listed in order of importance (see the text).
[d] Drugs are listed in order of recommended use (see the text).

The primary forms of endogenous hypertriglyceridemia, familial hypertriglyceridemia and primary familial combined hyperlipidemia, also appear to be related to an increase in the synthesis of triglyceride-rich lipoproteins (Table 75.5). Familial hypertriglyceridemia results in an increase in the endogenous synthesis of large triglyceride-rich VLDL. Many such patients are obese and exhibit

Table 75.6.
Classification of Lipoprotein Disorders by Phenotypes and Genotypes and Corresponding Clinical Manifestations

Phenotype	Lipoprotein in Excess	Plasma Lipid Levels[a]		Plasma Appearance[a]	Genotype	Age of Onset (Primary Form)	Xanthomas[b]	Other Clinical Manifestations
		Cholesterol	Triglyceride					
I	Chylomicrons	Normal or ↑	↑↑↑ lipemia	Clear plasma, creamy supernatant	Familial lipoprotein lipase deficiency, Apo C-II deficiency	Infancy or childhood	Eruptive, tuberoeruptive	Recurrent abdominal pain, other gastrointestinal symptoms, lipemia retinalis, hepatosplenomegaly
IIA	LDL	↑↑↑	normal	Clear	Familial hypercholesterolemia; Familial combined hyperlipidemia; Polygenic and sporadic hypercholesterolemia	Childhood for homozygous FHC,[c] late childhood to middle age for heterozygous FHC, adulthood for others	Tendinous, xanthelasma, tuberous; planar (homozygous)	Premature CAD,[c] arcus corneae, aortic stenosis (homozygous FHC), arthritic symptoms
IIB	LDL + VLDL	↑↑	↑	Clear	Familial combined hyperlipidemia; Familial hypercholesterolemia			
III	β-VLDL, IDL	↑↑	↑↑	Slightly turbid	Familial dysbetalipoproteinemia	Adulthood (occasionally late adolescence)	Planar (especially palmar), tuberous	Premature CAD and peripheral vascular disease, male > female, obesity, abnormal glucose tolerance, hyperuricemia, aggravated by hypothyroidism, good response to therapy
IV	VLDL	Normal or ↑[d]	↑↑	Turbid	Familial hypertriglyceridemia; Familial combined hyperlipidemia; Sporadic hypertriglyceridemia	Early to late adulthood	Usually none; rarely eruptive, or tuberoeruptive	CAD and peripheral vascular disease, obesity, abnormal glucose tolerance, hyperuricemia, arthritic symptoms, gallbladder disease
V	Chylomicrons + VLDL	Normal or ↑	↑↑↑	Turbid plasma, creamy supernatant	Homozygous familial hypertriglyceridemia	Childhood to middle age, usually adulthood	Eruptive, tuberoeruptive	Recurrent abdominal pain, other gastrointestinal symptoms, lipemia retinalis, hepatosplenomegaly, peripheral paresthesias, abnormal glucose tolerance, hyperuricemia

[a] Plasma obtained after 12 hours of fasting, left undisturbed in refrigerator overnight.
[b] Seen only in a minority of patients, but the frequency increases as plasma lipid levels rise.
[c] FHC, familial hypercholesterolemia; CAD, coronary artery disease.
[d] Cholesterol normal if triglycerides < 400 mg/dl.

mild glucose intolerance, hyperinsulinemia, and clinical evidence of diabetes mellitus, conditions which contribute to the excessive hepatic production of VLDL triglyceride. An especially insulin-sensitive lipoprotein receptor for VLDL triglyceride synthesis seems operative.

In contrast, patients with familial combined hyperlipidemia (multiple lipoprotein type hyperlipidemia) exhibit an increase in the production of apo B, which can appear in VLDL, LDL, or both. Various lipoprotein types are found in patients with familial combined hyperlipidemia, and the presenting sign can be an increase in either VLDL triglyceride or LDL cholesterol, or both. The clinical expressions of this disorder vary among individual patients depending on diet, the degree of obesity, the level of physical activity, and the concomitant use of other drugs. In both of the above lipoprotein disorders, LDL and remnant lipoprotein catabolism, as well as LDL receptor function, appear to be normal.

Familial hypertriglyceridemia and familial combined hyperlipidemia are inherited as separate autosomal dominant disorders, each occurring in approximately 1% of the general population. Familial hypertriglyceridemia is not associated with xanthomas unless hyperchylomicronemia supervenes. Basal concentrations (after a 12-hour fast) of total triglycerides and VLDL triglycerides are characteristically elevated, but plasma levels of total and LDL cholesterol are normal or low unless levels of VLDL cholesterol are also increased. Familial hypertriglyceridemia is not associated with an increased incidence of premature CAD; however, patients with familial combined hyperlipidemia are at high risk, primarily due to their increased plasma levels of apo B and abnormalities in the composition of HDL, reduced levels of apo A-I and HDL_2 (4). Familial combined hyperlipidemia may be present in as many as 10% of the survivors of myocardial infarction under the age of 60 and thus represents a common and important risk for atherosclerosis.

The diagnosis of these disorders of lipoprotein metabolism and their exact definition can only be established by family studies. As noted above, phenotypic expressions of combined hyperlipidemia are varied (IIA, IIB, or IV), while those for familial hypertriglyceridemia are consistently an increase in VLDL triglyceride and low or normal levels of LDL cholesterol. A strongly positive family history of atherosclerosis favors the diagnosis of familial combined hyperlipidemia in those hypertriglyceridemic patients in whom secondary causes for hyperlipidemia have been excluded. Differentiating between these two disorders of lipoprotein metabolism is important in the evaluation of a patient with hyperlipidemia, particularly with regard to deciding whether therapeutic intervention is warranted for the prevention of CAD and its complications.

Occasionally, patients present with marked hypertriglyceridemia and hyperchylomicronemia (triglyceride levels greater than 1000 mg/dl), pancreatitis, eruptive xanthomas, and lipemia retinalis. Coexistence of familial hypertriglyceridemia or familial combined hyperlipidemia with either obsesity, uremia, untreated diabetes mellitus, chronic alcoholism or the use of corticosteroids, thiazide diuretics, or estrogens can result in this syndrome. The chylomicronemia syndrome requires immediate treatment with elimination of dietary fat, nasogastric suction, and treatment of the secondary causes. Prevention is the primary means to avoid recurrences, and frequently patients with primary hypertriglyceridemia receive lipid-lowering agents prophylactically (13).

Decreased Lipoprotein Lipase-Mediated Triglyceride Catabolism

LPL is the rate-limiting enzyme for the uptake and storage of triglyceride by adipose tissue or muscle tissue and for the processing of triglyceride-rich lipoproteins to chylomicrons and VLDL remnants. A defect in the LPL reaction may occur due to a reduction in the activity of the enzyme or an abnormality in the interaction between the enzyme and its triglyceride-rich substrate, most often because of a derangement in the lipoprotein and apo structure of the VLDL-triglyceride moiety. However, other abnormalities in the interaction between LPL and triglyceride-rich lipoproteins may occur and cause hypertriglyceridemia despite a normal postheparin plasma lipoprotein lipase activity. For example, in patients with the autosomal recessive trait of apo C-II deficiency, LDL activity is normal, but marked hypertriglyceridemia is present (13). In contrast, in the more frequently encountered (yet also rare) autosomal recessive syndrome of familial LPL deficiency, marked hypertriglyceridemia and chylomicronemia are both evident and LPL activity is absent. The type I phenotypic pattern is more likely to occur in patients with the familial form of LPL deficiency, rather than in those with apo C-II deficiency, yet both conditions manifest themselves in childhood with episodes of eruptive xanthomas and with the acute abdominal pain of pancreatitis. Most adult patients who have an acquired impairment in LPL function usually have moderately severe diabetes mellitus, hypothyroidism, end-stage renal disease, or dysgammaglobulinemia, or are receiving corticosteroids or thiazide diuretics. The severity of the lipoprotein abnormality seems to be directly related to the decrease in LPL activity in postheparin plasma and adipose tissue.

In all of these disorders of defective triglyceride-rich lipoprotein clearance, hypertriglyceridemia can be controlled by restriction of dietary fat and substitution of carbohydrates or medium chain triglycerides as energy sources. Effective treatment of diabetes mellitus with diet, insulin, or an oral sulfonyl-urea normalizes LPL activity and plasma triglyceride levels within 3 months. Similar changes are seen after appropriate therapy of hypothyroidism with thyroxine or uremia with renal transplantation.

LPL also plays a role in the formation of HDL_2 (see "Normal Physiology of Lipoprotein Transport" above). This mechanism appears to mediate the increase in HDL_2 seen in endurance-trained athletes (6) and in patients with primary hypercholesterolemia treated with colestipol. Hence, diseases associated with abnormalities in LPL frequently have concomitant reductions in HDL cholesterol.

Defective Remnant Lipoprotein Catabolism and Dysbetalipoproteinemia

Excessive accumulation of lipoprotein remnants in plasma is usually caused by a defect in their removal due to an autosomal recessive derangement in the structure of apo E (20). Apo E3, identified by isoelectric focusing to be the predominant form of apo E in the normal population, is absent in patients with the classic form of dysbetalipoproteinemia (type III hyperlipoproteinemia). The mutation causing this syndrome results in the occurrence of an abnormal form of apo E, referred to as apo E2/E2 homozygosity. Of the 1% of individuals homozygous for this condition, only 1 to 2% will exhibit hyperlipoproteinemia clinically.

Of the multiple alleles for the apo E isoforms, only those producing certain amino acid sustitutions are associated with abnormal apo E binding to hepatic membranes and result in the phenotypic expression of dysbetalipoproteinemia (20). Consequently, most affected individuals do not have hyperlipoproteinemia; rather, they have low plasma levels of LDL cholesterol, presumably due to defective conversion of remnants to LDL. Although some patients exhibit hypertriglyceridemia, recent information suggests that an additional underlying lipid disorder is usually necessary for the clinical and hyperlipidemic expression of dysbetalipoproteinemia. The activity of adipose tissue LPL is normal in this disorder, while abnormalities in postheparin hepatic triglyceride lipase have been reported, probably due to abnormalities in apo E.

Dysbetalipoproteinemia (remnant removal disease or broad β disease) has served as a prototype for the study of remnant lipoprotein metabolism. It appears that several defects in lipoprotein metabolism are required before excessive accumulation of IDL and of cholesterol-enriched β-VLDL, can occur. The diagnosis is suggested by the initial findings of β (rather than pre-β)-VLDL and similarly elevated plasma concentrations of cholesterol and triglyceride. It is made more likely by the finding of an abnormally cholesterol-rich VLDL fraction (ratio of VLDL cholesterol to VLDL triglyceride of > 0.42). The presence of tuberous and planar xanthomas (Fig. 75.3) is virtually pathognomonic for the disorder. Definitive diagnosis, however, requires separation of VLDL by preparative ultracentrifugation followed by isoelectric focusing and apo analysis of VLDL to demonstrate the absence of apo E3. A strong association between this lipoprotein disorder and atherosclerosis of the coronary arteries and peripheral vessels has been reported and appears to diminish during treatment.

The accumulation of remnants in plasma is also found in certain patients with hypothyroidism, end-stage renal disease, and liver disease. The latter disorders are associated with an increase in the activity of the enzyme hepatic lipase, suggesting that a relationship may exist between this enzyme and the catabolism of remnant lipoproteins by the liver.

Increased Cholesterol Synthesis

The accumulation of cholesterol-rich LDL can occur as a result of an increased input of cholesterol into the plasma from dietary or endogenous sources. The latter occurs because of an increase in HMG CoA reductase activity and enhanced synthesis of cholesterol from acetate, or as a consequence of a primary genetic increase in the synthesis of apo B and cholesterol within the liver. The resulting apo B-enriched lipoprotein, usually of the VLDL class, is then metabolized in the liver to an apo B-enriched LDL. The presence of apo B-enriched VLDL is highly suggestive of a genetic disorder of overproduction of apo B, as compared with the overproduction of VLDL triglyceride in familial hypertriglyceridemia.

The overproduction of apo B-containing LDL and VLDL leads to an increased propensity for the development of atherosclerosis (4). Moreover, the coexistence of obesity promotes the overproduction of apo B-enriched VLDL and cholesterol in these individuals. Finally, the augmented intake of dietary cholesterol usually contributes to the hypercholesterolemia characteristic of these patients.

Primary (sporadic) forms of hypercholesterolemia, with a genetic defect in the steps controlling the rate of hepatic synthesis of cholesterol from acetate, lead to an overproduction of cholesterol and resultant hypercholesterolemia. Usually dietary therapy involving an increase in polyunsaturated fat and a reduction in sucrose and simple carbohydrates is helpful in the treatment of these disorders; rarely are drugs required. Hypercholesterolemia in obese hyperinsulinemic patients with type II diabetes mellitus is decreased by hypocaloric diets and the return of body weight toward normal. In patients noncompliant with dietary measures, therapy with cholestyramine or nicotinic acid is usually effective in lowering plasma levels of cholesterol.

Defective Removal of Low Density Lipoproteins

Isolated primary elevations of plasma LDL or combined elevations of LDL and VLDL can be seen in

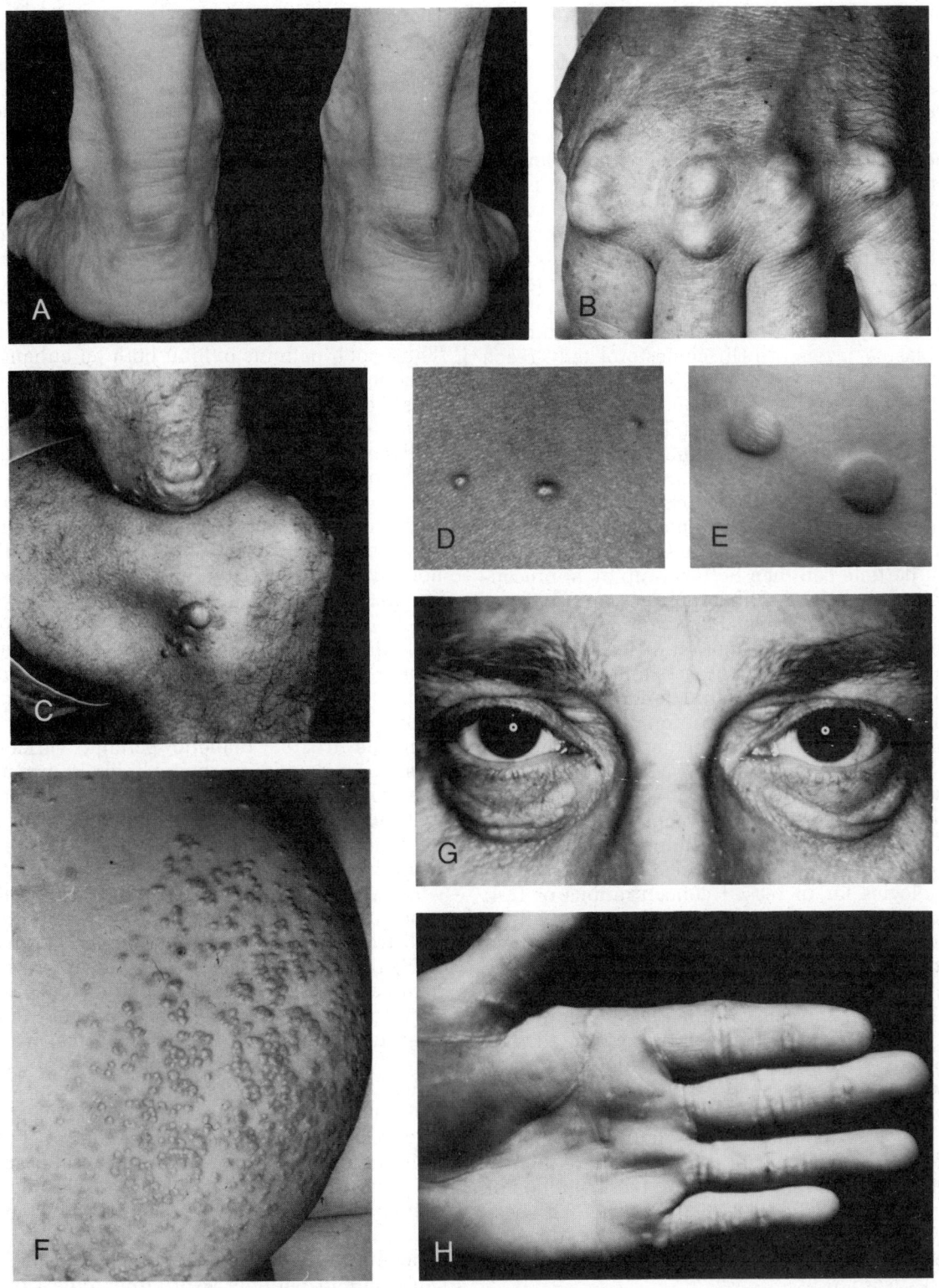

Figure 75.3. Dermatological manifestations of lipid disorders. *A.* Tendinous xanthomas. *B.* Tuberous xanthomas. *C.* Tuberous xanthomas. *D.* Eruptive xanthomas. *E.* Planar xanthomas. *F.* Eruptive xanthomas. *G.* Planar xanthoma on eyelids (xanthelasma). *H.* Planar xanthomas confined to palm creases (xanthoma striata palmaris).

affected members of families with familial hyper-cholesterolemia (2). While the cells of some homozygous patients may be totally lacking in identifiable LDL (apo B-E) receptors, in other patients, these receptors are present but functionally defective. The resultant excess accumulation of LDL in the plasma varies with the severity of the defect in receptor number and/or function as well as with the level of cholesterol synthesized by the liver. Individuals heterozygous for familial hypercholesterolemia exhibit greater than a 50% reduction in LDL receptor number or a 50% defect in receptor-mediated catabolism; commonly their plasma levels of LDL cholesterol are elevated above 400 mg/dl regardless of their level of cholesterol synthesis. In patients who are homozygous, plasma levels of LDL cholesterol may reach 1000 mg/dl (13).

Cultures of skin fibroblasts and certain other tissues confirm that the cellular LDL receptors are defective or absent in individuals with the above disorder. Additionally, the retarded plasma clearance of LDL in these patients causes LDL to accumulate in plasma and to be identified by its interaction with other tissues and cells. The altered LDL protein particle can then be taken up by nonreceptor-mediated pathways (macrophages or scavenger cells) in the arterial wall. The accumulation of cholesterol results in the formation of foam cells that accelerate the atherogenic process and promote the deposition of cholesterol in skin, tendons, and arteries (xanthomatosis). The deposition of lipid deposits in tendons is virtually pathognomonic for the disorder. Documentation of abnormal receptor binding, however, is necessary for the precise diagnosis of individuals with familial hypercholesterolemia.

While primary causes (including familial combined hyperlipoproteinemia) predominate, secondary etiologies for increased concentrations of LDL cholesterol occur in patients with hypothyroidism, nephrotic syndrome, multiple myeloma, obstructive liver disease, and porphyria and in patients who have ingested excessive amounts of dietary cholesterol. Whatever the cause of the LDL accumulation in the plasma, the primary forms are associated with marked susceptibility to CAD and a high frequency of complications associated with early mortality, such as myocardial infarction, stroke, and severe peripheral vascular disease. The hallmark of these disorders is the tendon xanthomas which frequently affect the Achilles tendon or the extensor tendon of the forearm and hand (Fig. 75.3). Patients with secondary hypercholesterolemia appear not to develop atherosclerosis at as high a rate as people with the primary disorders.

COMMON SECONDARY DISORDERS OF LIPOPROTEIN METABOLISM

Several disease states are commonly associated with increased plasma levels of VLDL, elevated levels of both VLDL and LDL, or decreased levels of HDL cholesterol.

Diabetes Mellitus

Abnormalities in fat transport are frequently noted in patients with diabetes mellitus and are related to abnormalities in insulin action or insulin availability that lead to increased production and/or decreased removal of plasma lipoproteins. For example, in patients with type II diabetes mellitus, which is characterized most often by obesity, hyperinsulinemia, and insulin resistance, endogenous triglyceride production is increased and LPL-mediated triglyceride clearance is usually saturated. Thus, such patients exhibit both an enhanced production and reduced plasma clearance of triglycerides. These patients also have abnormalities in HDL cholesterol, since the ability to catabolize VLDL triglyceride-enriched lipoproteins affects the synthesis of HDL$_2$. In contrast, the hypertriglyceridemia that occurs in patients with insulin-dependent (type I) diabetes mellitus is due to markedly reduced levels of LPL activity, since insulin is required for normal synthesis of the enzyme (13). The diabetic lipemia syndrome is characterized by low or absent levels of LPL in the plasma and tissues of these patients. Although the underlying enzyme deficiency can be reversed after insulin repletion, normalization of the lipoprotein abnormalities can take as long as 3 months.

In the treated diabetic patient, variability in plasma levels of lipoprotein lipids is primarily related to dietary factors, body weight, physical activity, and the degree of glycemic control. If glucose tolerance deteriorates because of inadequate insulin administration or increased insulin resistance, severe hypertriglyceridemia may ensue and alter the concentrations of other classes of lipoproteins. In well treated type I diabetic patients, plasma levels of HDL cholesterol are increased; in contrast, patients with type II diabetes usually have low plasma levels of HDL cholesterol. Regardless of the specific treatment or type of diabetes mellitus, women ordinarily exhibit higher plasma levels of VLDL triglyceride and LDL cholesterol, and lower levels of HDL cholesterol, than do diabetic men (27). This may explain the increased prevalence of atherosclerosis in diabetic women and the disappearance of the usual preponderance of atherosclerotic disease in men compared with premenopausal women (14).

Hypercholesterolemia, with increased plasma concentrations of LDL cholesterol and apo B, also can occur in patients with either type I or type II diabetes mellitus, and is usually induced by diet. However, in patients with type II diabetes and hyperinsulinemia, the synthesis of LDL from VLDL is increased, while glycosylation of the LDL molecule impairs receptor-mediated LDL catabolism to some extent. Intensive therapy with diet, exercise, and insulin usually normalizes lipoprotein levels unless a genetic lipoprotein disorder coexists.

Hyperlipidemia in the patient with diabetes mellitus increases the risk for the major complications of atherosclerosis, CAD, cerebrovascular disease, and peripheral vascular disease. The severity of peripheral vascular disease has been associated with the lipoprotein abnormalities in diabetic women. Whether treatment of the lipid abnormalities in diabetic patients will decrease their risk for CAD and other arteriosclerotic complications remains to be tested.

Chronic Uremia and Treatment with Dialysis

Many patients with chronic uremia have increased plasma levels of VLDL triglycerides and decreased levels of HDL cholesterol (8). These abnormalities persist during maintenance hemodialysis or peritoneal dialysis. The accelerated atherosclerosis observed in white *versus* black men undergoing chronic hemodialysis appears to be related to the abnormal composition of HDL_2 cholesterol in the plasmas of white men. These lipoprotein abnormalities result from defects in LPL-mediated triglyceride removal and in the formation of HDL cholesterol. A sedentary life style, obesity, high fat diets, or treatment with corticosteroids, β-blockers, or androgens worsens the lipoprotein profiles in these patients, whereas effective reversal of these secondary causes improves the lipid profile (8).

Hypothyroidism

Adequate levels of thyroid hormone appear to be necessary for the proper function of the lipoprotein cascade. Decreases in LDL receptor function, abnormalities in LPL and hepatic lipase-mediated metabolism of triglycerides and HDL, and reduced LCAT activity have been demonstrated in some patients with hypothyroidism. Consequently, increased plasma levels of VLDL, IDL, and LDL and reduced levels of HDL cholesterol have all been reported in patients with this disease. Treatment with thyroid hormone improves LDL receptor function, increases the activity and function of LPL and LCAT, and normalizes lipoprotein profiles.

Other Common Secondary Causes of Hyperlipidemia

Patients with the *nephrotic syndrome* frequently lose apo C-II in the urine, thus decreasing LPL-mediated triglyceride clearance. The hypoalbuminemia which accompanies the nephrotic syndrome increases hepatic VLDL synthesis, thereby elevating plasma levels of VLDL triglyceride and LDL cholesterol. Treatment of the primary disease causing the nephrotic syndrome usually corrects the lipoprotein abnormalities, but drug and diet (low fat) therapy may be required.

Hypercortisolemia of endogenous or exogenous origin increases hepatic synthesis of VLDL, LDL or both. Kidney transplant recipients treated with high doses of corticosteroids frequently exhibit elevated plasma levels of both VLDL and LDL as well as reduced levels of HDL cholesterol. The atherosclerosis that develops in such patients is probably related to these lipid abnormalities, which should be treated accordingly.

Obesity, androgen administration and alcohol ingestion tend to increase hepatic lipoprotein synthesis, but have different effects on levels of HDL cholesterol and LDL cholesterol. In obese individuals, plasma levels of VLDL triglyceride and LDL cholesterol are increased, while those of HDL are decreased. Mild alcohol ingestion (up to 2 ounces/day) increases levels of VLDL triglyceride and HDL cholesterol but lowers levels of LDL cholesterol. Exogenous androgens raise levels of LDL cholesterol by increasing hepatic processing of VLDL to LDL and lower HDL cholesterol levels by enhancing the catabolism of HDL by hepatic lipase. *Diseases affecting the liver*, such as hepatitis or cholelithiasis, alter lipoprotein metabolism. Diseases causing an obstruction in the hepatobiliary system tend to elevate plasma LDL, IDL, and remnant lipoproteins and cause abnormal lipoproteins (Lp X) to accumulate in plasma. Inflammatory processes usually lower levels of HDL and LDL cholesterol and raise VLDL depending on the nutritional state of the patient. *Drugs* used to treat hypertension, particularly thiazide diuretics and β-adrenergic blockers, raise levels of VLDL and LDL and lower levels of HDL cholesterol. Weight loss or the discontinuation of alcohol or these drugs usually normalizes lipoprotein profiles.

Hyperlipidemia occurs in patients with *systemic lupus erythematosus* or *dysgammaglobulinemia*. This may be related to interactions among amyloid protein, certain immunoglobulin fractions, and various steps in the lipoprotein cascade.

Table 75.4 lists common secondary causes for disordered lipoprotein metabolism. The pathophysiological mechanisms of some of these are shown in Table 75.5. Finally, Table 75.7 lists the effect of several exogenous and endogenous factors on plasma levels of HDL cholesterol.

CLINICAL MANIFESTATIONS OF LIPOPROTEIN DISORDERS

Adverse clinical sequelae of the lipoprotein disorders most frequently manifest themselves as disorders of the vascular, dermatological, and gastrointestinal systems. The clinical manifestations associated with each of the major disorders of lipoprotein metabolism are outlined in Table 75.6.

Vascular

As discussed previously, elevated levels of total cholesterol, LDL cholesterol, and apo B-enriched

Table 75.7.
Factors That Affect HDL Cholesterol Levels

Increase	Decrease
Exercise	Androgens (male sex, drugs)
Estrogens (female sex)	In males, puberty
Alcohol	In females, menopause
Familial (hyperalphalipoproteinemia)	Obesity
Leanness	Hypertriglyceridemia
Antihyperlipidemic drugs:	Type II diabetes mellitus
Nicotinic acid, colestipol, Clofibrate, gemfibrozil	Familial hypoalphalipoproteinemia
Insulin	(Tangier's disease)
IV Heparin	Cigarettes
	Sedentary life style
	Probucol
	Uremia
	Vegetarian diet
	Progestogens

lipoproteins, and decreased levels of HDL cholesterol, HDL_2, and apo A-I, contribute to the development of atherosclerotic disease. The earlier the onset of symptomatic disease of the coronary, cerebral, or peripheral vasculature, the more likely it is that a lipoprotein abnormality and/or another major risk factor (cigarette smoking, hypertension, diabetes) is present (14). In the most severe form of hypercholesterolemia, homozygous familial hypercholesterolemia, plasma levels of total cholesterol vary from 600 to 1200 mg/dl, CAD generally develops in childhood, and very few patients survive past age 30. In heterozygotes, plasma levels of total cholesterol vary from about 270 to 550 mg/dl, and the time of onset of CAD varies between early adulthood and late middle age, with about 50% of men and women becoming symptomatic by age 50 and 60, respectively. Patients with monogenic familial combined hyperlipoproteinemia exhibit elevated levels of VLDL, LDL, or both, as well as abnormalities in HDL, apo A, and apo B; most patients manifest symptoms of CAD by age 60. Individuals with familial dysbetalipoproteinemia develop premature peripheral vascular disease and CAD at about equal rates, with the mean age of onset in both men and women of about 40. Such patients seem to be especially amenable to therapy. Individuals with monogenic familial hypertriglyceridemia or with fasting chylomicronemia do not appear to be at increased risk for CAD unless other risk factors for atherosclerosis are also present.

Dermatological

Xanthomas may occur in all of the hyperlipidemias; however, they are present in a minority of hyperlipidemic individuals. They occur with increasing frequency as the plasma lipid levels rise. They are present predominantly in the primary forms of hyperlipoproteinemia: familial hypercholesterolemia, familial dysbetalipoproteinemia, and familial LPL deficiency. Xanthomas are cutaneous and/or subcutaneous papules, plaques, or nodules characterized histopathologically by localized collections of lipid-laden histiocytes (foam cells). The presence or absence of xanthomas should always be noted. If present, their appearance (see below) can provide useful information about the nature of the underlying lipid disorder (Table 75.7). Unless tendons (especially the Achilles tendon) are palpated, tendon thickening characteristic of tendon xanthomas may be missed. Xanthomas are divided morphologically into several types:

1. *Tendinous* (Fig. 75.3A)—firm subcutaneous masses, which arise in tendons and occasionally in ligaments, fascia, or periosteum. They characteristically move in concert with the associated tendon, and can appear as diffuse thickenings of the tendon. They most often occur on the Achilles tendons and the extensor tendons of the hands, knees, and elbows. The overlying skin is normal in color.

2. *Tuberous* (Fig. 75.3, *B* and *C*)—soft cutaneous and subcutaneous nodules which may harden with age and increasing fibrosis. Occasionally, they occur as superficial extensions of tendon xanthomas. They can also form from the confluence of eruptive xanthomas, an intermediate stage being called *tuberoeruptive* xanthomas. They occur most often on extensor surfaces and areas subjected to trauma, such as the elbows, knees, dorsa of the hands, heels, and buttocks. The overlying epidermis can be normal in color or have a yellow or orange hue.

3. *Eruptive* (Fig. 75.3, *D* and *F*)—small (1 to 4 mm) cutaneous papules, which tend to appear in crops, often coincident with an abrupt rise in plasma triglyceride levels. Compared to the other types of xanthomas, they contain more inflammatory cells, free fatty acids, and triglycerides and fewer foam cells and cholesterol esters. They most often occur over pressure areas, such as the buttocks, parts of the trunk, elbows, and knees. They often have a yellow center and red halo.

4. *Planar* (Fig. 75.3, *E G*, and *H*)—flat, slightly elevated cutaneous lesions, which occur most often

in skin folds and scars but which can be more widely distributed. When present on the eyelids, they are called *xanthelasma*. When located on the palms, they are called palmar xanthomas, and when confined to the palmar creases, *xanthoma striata palmaris*. They tend to be yellow or yellow-brown.

Hypercholesterolemia is associated with tendinous, planar, and tuberous xanthomas. Severe hypertriglyceridemia and chylomicronemia are associated with eruptive and occasionally tuberoeruptive or tuberous xanthomas. Palmar xanthomas are characteristic of familial dysbetalipoproteinemia and florid obstructive liver disease. Planar xanthomas on the body or palms in the presence of a type II lipid profile suggest homozygous monogenic familial hyperchholesterolemia. The presence of tendinous or tuberous xanthomas or premature xanthelasma with a type II lipid profile suggests either heterozygous or homozygous monogenic familial hypercholesterolemia, as opposed to the polygenic or nongenetic forms. Tendon xanthomas are found in one-third to one-half of heterozygotes, while tuberous xanthomas are seen most often in patients with familial dysbetalipoproteinemia. The usual relationships between lipoprotein disorders and xanthoma type are outlined in Table 75.6.

Occasionally, xanthomas appear in the absence of a hyperlipidemic state. For example, xanthelasma occur commonly in normolipidemic older individuals and in nonwhites, whereas planar xanthomas can occur in patients with lymphoma, leukemia, or myeloma. Recently, studies in normolipidemic individuals with xanthelasma have revealed abnormalities in apo B and E suggestive of familial dysbetalipoproteinemia and/or elevated levels of LDL apo B, suggesting that these individuals may be at an increased risk of developing atherosclerosis.

Differences exist in the responses to treatment of the various hyperlipidemia-associated xanthomas. Thus, tendon xanthomas are the most resistant to treatment and, in practice, seldom disappear. In contrast, eruptive and planar xanthomas can disappear within a few weeks after return of plasma lipid levels toward normal.

Gastrointestinal

As many as 35 to 55% of patients with fasting chylomicronemia experience episodes of recurrent abdominal pain. Symptoms are ordinarily associated with marked elevations of plasma triglyceride levels (greater than 1000 to 2000 mg/dl). Abdominal pain may be so severe that it prompts unnecessary surgery, particularly if the lipid disorder is not suspected. The pain is often associated with pancreatitis, although the responsible pathogenetic mechanism is not well understood. It should be noted that routine serum amylase determinations are frequently subject to technical artifact when hyperlipidemia is present, due to the presence of an amylase-inhibiting factor that may or may not be triglyceride.

In such cases, a more reliable estimate of the serum amylase value can be obtained by determining amylase levels on serial dilutions, until the value obtained no longer changes with further dilution. Another cause of abdominal pain may be rapid hepatic or splenic enlargement with capsular distension due to triglyceride deposition in reticuloendothelial cells. Often the cause is unclear. Gastrointestinal symptoms other than abdominal pain, such as nausea, vomiting, borborygmi, and diarrhea, also occur.

Other Clinical Associations

Other clinical concomitants of hyperlipidemia include the following: premature arcus corneae (grayish-white corneal ring due to lipid droplets) in hypercholesterolemia (elevated LDL); aortic stenosis in homozygous monogenic familial hypercholesterolemia; Achilles tendonitis in heterozygous monogenic familial hypercholesterolemia; obesity, glucose intolerance, hyperinsulinemia, hyperuricemia, and perhaps cholelithiasis in association with hypertriglyceridemia and elevated VLDL; recurrent polyarthralgias, arthritis, tenosynovitis, and sicca-like syndromes in hypertriglyceridemia (elevated VLDL) or hypercholesterolemia (elevated LDL); lipemia retinalis (cream-colored retinal vessels) in chylomicronemia (evident when plasma triglycerides rise above 3,000 mg/dl; obvious when they exceed 10,000 mg/dl).

DIAGNOSIS

Indications for Evaluation

The level of plasma total cholesterol should be determined on every patient under the age of 55, regardless of family or personal medical history. Measurement of the HDL cholesterol level is also desirable; but, because of the unreliability of many clinical laboratories and the added expense, it is not yet practical to use this test for the purpose of routine screening. When risk analysis is desired in a patient over the age of 55, however, the level of HDL cholesterol must be determined along with that of total cholesterol, since the utility of using the ratio of total (or LDL) cholesterol to HDL cholesterol for risk analysis continues while total cholesterol level alone loses its predictive value (Table 75.3). Although determination of the fasting plasma triglyceride level is somewhat inconvenient to the patient, it is inexpensive, provides further prognostic information, and may identify a patient who would benefit from hypolipidemic therapy. Not only is this case-finding activity valuable in detecting individuals who might benefit from hypolipidemic therapy, but it also forms part of an overall risk assessment (including determination of cigarette smoking, alcohol, and exercise history, blood pressure determination, weight, *etc*) that provides important prognostic information and permits the physician to individualize strategies for management.

A more complete evaluation including measurement of plasma levels of total cholesterol, HDL cholesterol, and fasting triglyceride and calculation of the level of LDL cholesterol (see below), is desirable when (a) abnormalities are detected on screening; (b) there is a high suspicion of lipoprotein abnormalities (premature CAD, strong family history, xanthomata, etc); or (c) conditions coexist that could cause secondary abnormalities in lipoprotein metabolism. Although the frequencies with which certain drugs (e.g., thiazide diuretics, antihypertensives, oral contraceptives) adversely affect lipoprotein metabolism is unknown, and direct causal interrelationships between such drug-associated lipid abnormalities and premature atherosclerosis are unproved, it seems prudent also to consider the more complete evaluation before therapy is initiated with these drugs. The utility of the more complete evaluation, given a screening total cholesterol level of 280 mg/dl, is depicted in Table 75.8.

Laboratory Evaluation

Baseline plasma (or serum) lipid levels should be repeated at least once to account for laboratory variability and physiological instability. In the absence of marked hypertriglyceridemia, determinations of plasma total cholesterol and HDL cholesterol may be performed in the nonfasting state. However, plasma triglyceride determinations require a 12- to 15-hour overnight fast because of physiological postprandial hypertriglyceridemia. Since levels of total (and LDL) cholesterol fall during the first few days after myocardial infarction (9), it is recommended that cholesterol determinations be made either within 24 hours of a severe acute myocardial infarction (when they are still valid) or postponed until 3

to 4 weeks after recovery. Fasting triglyceride (and VLDL) levels tend to rise slowly after a myocardial infarction, peaking at about 3 to 4 weeks and returning to baseline by 8 to 12 weeks. Triglyceride levels should, therefore, be obtained either within 24 hours of the acute event or delayed for 8 to 12 weeks.

The *determination of HDL cholesterol* is the measurement most subject to laboratory error. The precision of its measurement was inadequate in the majority of clinical laboratories recently surveyed by the Centers for Disease Control, Atlanta. It is, therefore, important for each physician periodically to assess his laboratory's performance against one that is rigidly standardized. Repetition of the baseline measurement provides a further safeguard. Such measures to enhance validity are important, since there is a relatively narrow range of HDL cholesterol values within which even small differences are prognostically important. For example, a reduction in the level of HDL cholesterol of 5 mg/dl from 40 to 35 mg/dl increases the risk for CAD by about 25%. When triglyceride levels exceed 400 mg/dl, the standardized techniques for the precipitation of VLDL and LDL are ineffective and HDL cholesterol levels are unreliable. The plasma can be ultrafiltered to remove the interfering VLDL. If this is required, the physician should consult the laboratory. Despite these problems, the level of HDL cholesterol represents a potent index of CAD risk, an aid to diagnosis (Table 75.8), and an important measure to follow during therapy. It also allows one to calculate LDL cholesterol (LDL-C) levels (provided triglyceride level is below 400 mg/dl) by the formula: LDL-C = TC-(TG/5 + HDL-C), where TC is plasma level of total cholesterol, TG is fasting plasma triglyceride level, and HDL-C is the level of HDL cholesterol.

Table 75.8.
HDL Cholesterol in the Diagnosis of Hyperlipoproteinemia[a]

A. 50-year-old man			
TG	150	150	150
Chol	280	280	280
HDL-C	70	20	100
LDL-C	180	230	150
Diagnosis	Normal	Hypercholesterolemia (type IIA)	Hyperalphalipoproteinemia
B. 50-year-old man			
TG	350	350	350
Chol	280	280	280
VLDL-C	70	50	125
HDL-C	45	20	35
LDL-C	165	210	120
Diagnosis	Hypertriglyceridemia (type IV)	Combined (multiple phenotype) Hyperlipidemia (types IIB, III, IV)	Dysbetalipoproteinemia (type III)

[a] TG, triglyceride; C, cholesterol; VLDL, very low density lipoproteins; LDL, low density lipoproteins; HDL, high density lipoproteins.

Observation of a fasting plasma sample, which has been left undisturbed overnight in a refrigerator at 4°C, is indicated in the presence of a significantly elevated fasting plasma triglyceride level. Elevated levels of total (or LDL) cholesterol do not affect the appearance of plasma, whereas hypertriglyceridemia associated with increased levels of VLDL imparts uniform turbidity to plasma, and hypertriglyceridemia associated with chylomicronemia is characterized by a creamy supernatant fraction which floats on the top of plasma.

A marked abnormality in serum lipid levels, especially marked hypertriglyceridemia (triglyceride > 2000 mg/dl), can affect the validity of other laboratory tests. Marked hypertriglyceridemia has an inhibitory effect on the serum amylase assay, interferes with the measurement of liver enzymes (aspartate aminotransferase, alanine aminotransferase) and calcium by autoanalyzer, and causes artifactual reductions in the serum concentration of molecules restricted to the aqueous phase, such as sodium. Ultracentrifugation of plasma, with the removal of chylomicrons, permits these measurements to be performed accurately; but sometimes serial dilutions of the plasma are necessary, particularly for the measurement of amylase (the level of which increases upon dilution).

Clinical Evaluation

Clinical data contribute substantially to the diagnosis of specific lipoprotein disorders. History, physical examination, and indicated laboratory evaluation are required to rule out secondary causes of hyperlipidemia (Table 75.4). A positive family history, the presence of premature atherosclerotic disease, and the presence of specific dermatological manifestations may permit the diagnosis of a primary form of hyperlipoproteinemia (see Table 75.6).

Referral

When laboratory and clinical evaluations do not result in a clear-cut diagnosis of a lipoprotein disorder, referral to a specialist in endocrinology and metabolism is indicated. Such specialists can perform (or readily obtain) and interpret more sophisticated tests, such as ultracentrifugal quantification of lipoprotein levels, apoprotein measurement, receptor analysis, and determination of LPL activity. They may also assist in the evaluation of family members, so that the presence of a genetic disorder can be accurately diagnosed.

TREATMENT

General Considerations

The first step in the management of a lipoprotein disorder is accurate diagnosis. Secondary causes should be identified (Table 75.4) and treated. If the secondary cause is not reversible or a primary disorder exists, treatment may be required that is specifically directed at the abnormal lipoprotein pattern.

Such treatment should be part of the comprehensive management of other coexisting CAD risk factors (such as cigarette smoking, hypertension, diabetes mellitus, obesity, and inactivity). It will likely require behavioral change on the part of the patient and lifelong management, emphasizing the need for a positive patient-physician relationship, appropriate patient education, and skill on the part of the physician in using maneuvers to improve patient compliance (see Chapters 3 and 4). The long term follow-up and monitoring of various parameters in such patients are necessary to enhance compliance, assess the effectiveness of therapy, and detect drug toxicity or the effect of concomitant therapy on plasma lipids (e.g., diuretics and other antihypertensive agents).

Because of the need for long term use of drugs with known and potential toxicities, pharmacological therapy should generally be reserved for patients with plasma lipoprotein levels above the 90th or 95th percentile for the appropriate sex, age, and race (Table 75.3). On the other hand, the physician should have a low threshold for recommending nonpharmacological maneuvers that are safe, favorably alter plasma lipoprotein levels, and may have other health advantages. This is so since plasma total cholesterol, LDL cholesterol, and HDL cholesterol affect CAD risk over a wide range of values. For example, the incidence of CAD increases proportionally as the mean plasma total cholesterol level of populations rises above 200 mg/dl. Levels between 180 and 200 mg/dl are associated with low incidences of both CAD and other diseases.

Management of hypertriglyceridemia must be individualized. When familial combined hyperlipidemia or familial dysbetalipoproteinemia is diagnosed, specific treatment is required. Patients with fasting triglyceride levels above 500 mg/dl sometimes accumulate chylomicrons and develop pancreatitis. The risk becomes substantial when triglyceride levels exceed 1000 mg/dl. The plasma triglyceride level should therefore be lowered in these patients. Individuals with familial hypertriglyceridemia or fasting triglyceride levels in the 250 to 500 mg/dl range in the absence of other CAD risk factors do not seem to be at increased risk of CAD or pancreatitis. Treatment is recommended only when risk factors coexist, such as (a) a family history of premature CAD; (b) abnormal levels of total (or LDL) cholesterol, HDL cholesterol, or apoproteins; (c) concomitant CAD, diabetes, end-stage renal disease, smoking, or obesity; and (d) young age. Isolated fasting triglyceride levels below 250 mg/dl do not require treatment.

Table 75.9.
Single Diet Treatment of Hyperlipoproteinemia[a]

American Heart Association Dietary Phase	Fat (% of Calories)	Carbohydrate (% of Calories)	Protein (% of Calories)	Cholesterol (mg/day)	Polyunsaturated: Saturated Fat (P/S) Ratio
I	30–35	45–50	20	230–300	1.0
II	30	50	20	150–200	1.0
III	20–25	55–60	20	100–110	>1

[a] Note: Caloric allowance is adjusted to ensure loss of excess weight or maintenance of ideal body weight (see Chapter 76).

Nonpharmacological Therapy

Diet (Tables 75.9 and 75.10)

It is now well established that plasma lipid levels can be altered by dietary manipulations. Under strictly controlled conditions (such as in a metabolic unit), elevated (> 95th percentile) plasma levels of total (or LDL) cholesterol may be reduced by as much as 30% or more and levels of triglyceride or VLDL (in the presence of marked elevations) by as much as 80% or more. Fasting chylomicronemia can also be eliminated. Under ambulatory conditions, where diets tend to be less restrictive and noncompliance more common, reductions in lipid levels are less dramatic. For example, among prospective studies of cholesterol-lowering diets, the decrease in plasma cholesterol averaged 15% (range 8.5 to 22%).

Single diet approach (Table 75.9). It is now appreciated that one diet can be used to treat all of the common forms of hyperlipoproteinemia. As recommended by the American Heart Association (AHA), the diet consists of caloric restriction to attain ideal body weight (see Chapter 76), reduction of cholesterol intake to less than 300 mg/day, a decrease in total fat to less than 30 to 35% of total calories, and restriction of saturated fat to no more than 10% of calories, so that a P/S (polyunsaturated/saturated fat) ratio of 1:1 is achieved. There is a concomitant increase in the proportion of complex carbohydrate and fiber in the diet. Sodium intake is also reduced. Using the principle of "graduated regimen implementation" (see Chapter 4), the diet can be introduced in three phases, with each phase introducing further restrictions in dietary total fat, saturated fat, and cholesterol (Table 75.9). Phase I represents the AHA "prudent diet" which is recommended for the entire American population. When severe chylomicronemia is present, more severe restriction of dietary fat is required (see below).

The AHA publishes useful booklets on this diet for the patient, physician, and nutritionist (see "General References"). Most patients with hyperlipoproteinemia will benefit from referral to a suitably trained dietitian.

The single diet actually incorporates several nutritional strategies, each of which tends to have a selective effect on plasma lipoprotein levels. It is helpful to consider each strategy separately.

Cholesterol reduction (Table 75.9). Diets designed

Table 75.10.
Nutritional Strategies Utilized in Single Diet Approach

REDUCTION OF PLASMA CHOLESTEROL (LDL) LEVEL

1. Reduction in saturated fat to < 10% of total calories
2. Cholesterol restriction (100–300 mg/day)
3. Increase in polyunsaturated fats (see the text)
4. Loss of excess weight
5. Fiber

The above objectives may be achieved by monitoring the following foods:

Foods to limit (partial list): meat, especially nonlean and organ meat, shellfish (high in cholesterol, low in fat); fat; egg yolk; cream; whole milk; butter; ice cream; most cheeses; artichoke; avocado; coconut; cocoa butter; palm oil.

Foods allowed (partial list): fish, deskinned chicken; egg white and egg substitutes; soy protein; skim milk; sherbert; low fat cottage cheese; ricotta, mozzarella, and Parmesan cheeses in small amounts; yogurt made from skim milk; vegetable oil (especially safflower, corn and cottonseed oil); vegetable margarines; vegetables other than those listed above.

REDUCTION OF PLASMA TRIGLYCERIDE (VLDL) LEVEL

1. Loss of excess weight (total calories restricted)
2. Alcohol restriction, if needed
3. Low cholesterol, low saturated fat, increased polyunsaturated fat diet, if needed
4. Sucrose restriction

ELIMINATION OF FASTING CHYLOMICRONEMIA

1. Fat restriction (5–20% of total calories)
2. Medium chain triglycerides allowed (see the text)
3. Vegetable fat (5 g) to supply essential fatty acids
4. Loss of excess weight and elimination of alcohol are indicated when plasma VLDL triglyceride elevations accompany the chylomicronemia (see the text)

Note: Shellfish (high in cholesterol but low in fat) are allowed.

INCREASE OF PLASMA HDL CHOLESTEROL LEVEL

1. Loss of excess weight
2. Diet to correct coexistent hypertriglyceridemia

to lower plasma cholesterol levels are characterized by a restriction of *dietary cholesterol* to 100 to 300 mg/day and a reduction of *saturated fat intake*, with or without a marked increase in dietary *polyunsat-*

urated fat. Restrictions in dietary cholesterol and saturated fats independently contribute to the reduction in plasma cholesterol levels. An increase in dietary polyunsaturated fat will result in further, though less marked, reduction in plasma cholesterol level. The influence of *dietary fiber* on plasma cholesterol levels is complex, dependent on the type of fiber, and somewhat controversial. Guar, pectin, and unprocessed high fiber food, such as legumes and oats, lower plasma total cholesterol levels, whereas other fibers, such as wheat bran, do not. Effects on levels of HDL cholesterol and triglyceride are minimal. In the amounts consumed in a palatable diet, fiber plays a minor role compared to control of dietary fats and cholesterol. Lecithin, a phospholipid derived from soybeans, is a widely publicized popular remedy for hypercholesterolemia commonly sold in health food stores. Since it is not absorbed as such from the gastrointestinal tract, any hypocholesterolemic effect probably derives from its high content of linoleic acid, a *polyunsaturated fatty acid.* Use of a liquid polyunsaturated vegetable oil would be a less expensive and more effective substitute.

The typical North American diet has a quite unfavorable *P/S ratio* of 0.4. On the other hand, there is no historical precedent that attests to the safety of diets very rich in polyunsaturated fats (e.g., P/S ratio ≥ 1.5). It does appear that the latter diets can promote formation of lithogenic bile and actually increase the incidence of symptomatic biliary tract disease. Although the data from at least one study suggested that such diets are associated with an increased risk of malignant disease, this finding was not supported when data from several trials were pooled (7). Another disadvantage to substantially increasing dietary intake of polyunsaturated fat is that the resultant high caloric intake might promote obesity. For these reasons, a P/S ratio of about 1.0 is recommended in most hypocholesterolemic diets.

Maximal effect of hypocholesterolemic diet usually occurs within 6 weeks. Dietary therapy alone is often sufficient in the approximately 85% of hypercholesterolemic patients with polygenic or nonhereditary forms of hypercholesterolemia. While diet usually reduces cholesterol levels in patients with monogenic hypercholesterolemia, concomitant drug therapy is almost always required.

Triglyceride reduction. Diets designed to reduce plasma triglyceride and VLDL levels emphasize the *loss of excess weight* by total caloric restriction. Plasma triglyceride levels usually fall, often to normal, after a few days of caloric restriction. The reduction is maintained as long as weight loss continues at a rate of 1 to 2 pounds (0.5 to 1 kg)/week. If normal weight is attained and maintained, further therapy may not be necessary. If hypertriglyceridemia persists or occurs in individuals of normal weight, a *cholesterol-lowering diet,* as outlined above, may be effective. *Alcohol* intake should be

restricted since it can cause a striking rise in triglyceride levels in some patients with hypertriglyceridemia. Although extreme increases in the carbohydrate content of a diet can cause transient and, rarely, sustained hypertriglyceridemia, there is no firm evidence to suggest that total carbohydrate restriction is helpful in the treatment of hypertriglyceridemia. There are conflicting data regarding the effect on plasma triglyceride level of excessive intake of *sucrose* (common sugar) and simple sugars. In most studies, especially in patients who are already hypertriglyceridemic, they do raise plasma triglyceride levels and lower those of HDL cholesterol, but the effect is small. The rationale for dietary restriction of sugar is based more upon the need to avoid excessive caloric intake (and to prevent caries), than on its having a direct effect on plasma lipids. Like alcohol, sucrose provides "empty" calories in that it contains none of the valuable nutrients, such as protein, fiber, minerals or vitamins. For this reason the substitution of complex (e.g., starches) for simple carbohydrates in the diet is recommended. A triglyceride-lowering diet should favorably affect plasma HDL cholesterol levels in most individuals, since obesity and triglyceride levels are inversely correlated with the levels of HDL cholesterol, and since plasma HDL levels usually rise during weight reduction. Plasma levels of total (and LDL) cholesterol often fall with loss of excess weight; when they rise, familial combined hyperlipoproteinemia may be present.

Chylomicron reduction. Treatment of fasting chylomicronemia (type I) involves the *restriction of dietary fat intake* to 5 to 20% of total calories (0.5 g of fat/kg of body weight is a reasonable starting point). The fat deficit should be corrected predominantly by substitution of complex carbohydrates. Since medium chain triglycerides are transported directly from the intestine to the liver in the portal circulation without incorporation into chylomicrons, they (available as MCT oil) may be added to the diet to provide calories. The recommended dose of MCT oil (available at most pharmacies) is 1 tablespoonful three to four times daily, mixed with foods. Five grams of vegetable fat rich in polyunsaturates should be included to prevent essential fatty acid deficiency.

Dietary fat is severely restricted until fasting chylomicronemia is eliminated and clinical symptoms are prevented or reduced in frequency; dietary fat is then chronically restricted to whatever degree is necessary to prevent fasting chylomicronemia. The efficacy of fat restriction in preventing recurrent abdominal pain is supported by clinical observations in individual patients.

When fasting chylomicronemia is accompanied by elevation of VLDL triglyceride levels, therapy is initiated with restriction of dietary fat intake and correction of coexistent secondary causes for the disorder. Once chylomicronemia has been eliminated, a triglyceride-requiring diet with a modest reduction in total fat intake (to approximately 30% of total calories) is all that is usually required to prevent recurrence. Total abstinence from alcohol is usually necessary.

Diets to raise levels of HDL. A dietary approach to the patient with an HDL cholesterol level below the 5th percentile involves treatment of concomitant hyperlipoproteinemia and *loss of excess weight.* While moderate alcohol consumption (2 to 3 ounces/ day) is positively correlated with HDL cholesterol level and negatively correlated with CAD, it is not recommended for three reasons: (*a*) excessive use (greater than two or three drinks/day) increases the overall risk of morbidity and mortality; (*b*) its use may interfere with attempts to control obesity and hypertriglyceridemia; and (*c*) evidence is not conclusive that modest intake results in an overall health advantage.

Exercise

Evidence has accumulated over the past decade that regular isotonic exercise favorably affects plasma lipid levels. Most of the exercise programs that have been evaluated, including jogging, rapid walking, swimming, bicycling, cross-country skiing, and mountain climbing, have involved 30 minutes or more of continued effort at 70 to 85% of maximal heart rate at least three times weekly. In most studies, levels of HDL cholesterol have been shown to rise (approxmately 20%) and triglyceride levels to fall (approximately 25%) with exercise (6). While levels of LDL cholesterol usually do not fall in normal subjects, significant reductions may occur in individuals with hypercholesterolemia.

That individuals who exercise regularly are at a reduced risk for CAD has been demonstrated in both cross-sectional and longitudinal epidemiological studies. Exercise also improves glucose metabolism, assists in weight reduction, and may reduce blood pressure (23).

Thus, exercise counseling (see Chapter 58) is a part of the management of patients with abnormalities in lipoprotein metabolism.

Smoking Cessation

Plasma levels of HDL cholesterol have been found to be lower and levels of VLDL triglyceride higher in people who smoke cigarettes than in nonsmokers or ex-smokers. Moreover, an inverse relationship exists between the number of cigarettes smoked daily and the level of HDL cholesterol. Smoking cessation has been associated with a modest rise in plasma HDL level. It is not known what proportion of the increased risk of CAD associated with smoking is mediated through alteration in the plasma lipids or *via* other mechanisms. There is, however, substantial evidence that smoking cessation reduces CAD risk. There is also evidence that physician counseling of patients increases cessation rates. Therefore, all patients who smoke cigarettes should be counseled, regardless of their lipoprotein profile (see Chapter 20).

Drugs

In general, drug therapy is recommended only after an initial 6-week to 3-month trial of nonpharmacological therapy (diet and exercise) has proved unsuccessful. Moreover, diet therapy should be continued during drug treatment since the effects of each are often additive. Information on drugs with which the general physician should be familiar is displayed in Table 75.11. The particular drug used depends upon the type of hyperlipoproteinemia present (Table 75.5).

Hypercholesterolemia

The *bile acid-binding resins, cholestyramine and colestipol,* are the drugs of choice for patients with primary hypercholesterolemia. They enhance LDL catabolism and excretion and prevent intestinal absorption by diverting cholesterol and bile acids into the feces. They also increase HDL, particularly HDL$_2$. In doses of 20 to 24 g/day, a 20 to 30% reduction in LDL cholesterol may be achieved, but the expense is high ($50.00/month). While these resins may be the safest of all the hypolipidemic drugs, compliance is a problem because taste and gastrointestinal side effects prevent many patients from taking a full dose. Gradual increase of dose, continuation of therapy, and concomitant symptomatic management of constipation may diminish side effects.

Combination therapy of a bile acid-sequestering resin with nicotinic acid (3) or the experimental drug mevinolin (12) has been reported to reduce plasma levels of LDL cholesterol by about 50% in patients heterozygous for familial hypercholesterolemia. Probucol may also be used in combination with a resin, but it seems less effective than the above regimens. Patients with homozygous familial hypercholesterolemia may respond less well to treatment with drugs and diet than do patients with heterozygous monogenic, polygenic, or nonhereditary hypercholesterolemia.

Nicotinic acid (3 to 6 g/day) significantly lowers plasma levels of LDL and VLDL while raising the level of HDL cholesterol. Its use is limited, however, by unpleasant side effects and the frequent presence of coexisting contraindications. By starting at a very low dose of 100 to 200 mg daily and gradually increasing the dose of the drug and adding aspirin, increased tolerance often develops to the common side effects of cutaneous flushing, rashes, hives, and pruritis. Nicotinic acid is inexpensive, with monthly costs averaging $5.00 at a dose of 2 to 4 g daily.

Probucol is better tolerated than the bile acid-

Table 75.11.
Commonly Used Lipid-Lowering Drugs

BILE ACID SEQUESTERING RESINS (Cholestyramine, Colestipol)

Mechanism: Anion exchange resins that bind bile acids, resulting in increased hepatic synthesis of cholesterol and bile acids, increased apo B catabolism, increased fecal excretion of cholesterol, increased LDL receptor activity, and usually a net reduction of plasma cholesterol levels.

Efficacy: Decreases total and LDL cholesterol up to 25–40% (onset 4–7 days, maximal effect within 2 weeks). In the LRC trial, mean reductions in experimental group of total and LDL cholesterol were 13.4 and 20.3%. Apo B level falls, while HDL level rises slightly. VLDL is unchanged or increased.

Pharmacokinetics: Not absorbed, but may bind other drugs (*e.g.*, thiazides, digitalis preparations, anticoagulants, phenobarbital, thyroxine, phenylbutazone, iron).

Side Effects: (a) Common—unpleasant sandy/gritty preparations, gastrointestinal (constipation, nausea, abdominal discomfort, flatulence, *etc.*, often resolve with continued therapy and/or treatment of constipation), lowered serum folate levels; (b) uncommon—gastrointestinal (steatorrhea), hyperchloremic acidosis (small patients on high doses), fat-soluble vitamin deficiency; (c) possible—(?) increased risk of cholelithiasis.

Administration: (a) Cholestyramine—12–32 g/day, given twice daily to four times daily before or during meals; supplied as Questran 9-g packets each containing 4 g of active drug; (b) colestipol—15–30 g/day, given twice daily to four times daily before or during meals; supplied as Colestid in 5-g packets or 500-g bottles.
Preparations should be taken in water or juice to prevent esophageal irritation or blockage. Other medicines should be taken 1 hour before or 4 hours after dosage. Monitor serum folate levels and consider supplemental multivitamins with folic acid.

Clinical Use: Drugs of first choice in the treatment of hypercholesterolemia, because of their relative safety and efficacy.

FIBRIC ACID ANALOGS (Clofibrate, Gemfibrozil, *etc*)

Mechanism: Increases clearance of VLDL by enhancing lipolysis, may increase lipoprotein lipase activity, reduces hepatic cholesterol synthesis, and increases cholesterol excretion in the bile.

Efficacy: Clofibrate—decreases triglycerides/VLDL within 2–5 days (mean reduction 22% in Coronary Drug Project, up to 80% reduction in some patients), may decrease or increase LDL cholesterol (mean decrease in total cholesterol of 6% in Coronary Drug Project), reduces IDL in type III. Gemfibrozil and the newer analogs tend to raise HDL more consistently and are less likely to raise LDL than clofibrate. In familial combined hyperlipoproteinemia, however, use of any fibric acid analog is likely to raise LDL cholesterol.

Pharmacokinetics: Clofibrate—completely absorbed, rapidly hydrolyzed to an active metabolite; peak concentration within 4 hours; metabolized in liver and excreted in urine; elimination divided into two kinetic phases, with half-lives of 1.7 and 15 hours. Gemfibrozil—peak concentration within 2 hours; half-life 1.5 hours; 70% excreted unchanged, primarily in urine. Both may enhance the action of oral anticoagulants, phenytoin, and hypoglycemic agents, and of furosemide by displacing them from albumin-binding sites.

Side Effects: (a) Usually—well tolerated; (b) occasional—2- to 3-fold increase in the incidence of cholelithiasis (may be less with gemfibrozil and newer analogs); other gastrointestinal (nausea, diarrhea, weight gain); reduced libido, impotence; unusual flu-like syndrome; (c) uncommon—rash, alopecia, breast tenderness, reversible abnormality in liver function, hepatomegaly, myositis, increased plasma glucose, *etc*; (d) unknown—(?)thromboembolism, (?)intermittent claudication, (?)dysrhythmia, (?)neoplasia.

Administration: Clofibrate (Atromid-S, 500 mg)—2 g/day in two or three divided doses. Gemfibrozil (Lopid, 300 mg)—600 mg twice daily (½ hour before meals). Some recommend periodic monitoring of aspartate aminotransferase (formerly SGO-T), alanine aminotransferase (formerly SGP-T), and creatine kinase (formerly CPK).

Clinical Use: Drugs of choice in the treatment of elevated VLDL triglyceride; of particular utility in type III. Use with caution in the presence of hepatic or renal insufficiency. Gemfibrozil has a more favorable effect on HDL and may be less lithogenic than clofibrate, but there is less long term experience with this drug.

NICOTINIC ACID (such as Nicobid (time-released), 125, 250, or 500 mg, or Nicolar, 500 mg)

Mechanism: Diverse effects on lipid metabolism: decreases LDL and apo B synthesis by decreasing hepatic synthesis of VLDL, increases synthesis of HDL, inhibits lipolysis in adipose tissue, increases lipase activity.

Efficacy: Decreases VLDL triglycerides within 1–4 days (mean 26% in Coronary Drug Project, range up to 80% depending on pretreatment levels); decreases LDL cholesterol, onset 5–7 days, maximal effect 3–5 weeks (mean decrease 10% in Coronary Drug Project, range up to 30%). Favorable impact on total and LDL cholesterol, triglyceride, VLDL, HDL, apos A-I and B.

Pharmacokinetics: Well absorbed by mouth; in the high doses used it is partially metabolized in liver and partially excreted unchanged in urine; plasma half-life is about 45 minutes.

Side Effects: (a) Common—cutaneous flushing and pruritis, which diminish after several weeks of therapy; gastrointestinal (nausea, diarrhea, abdominal pain, abnormal liver function); (b) less common—dermatological disorders (*e.g.*, increased pigmentation); activation of peptic ulcer; dysrhythmia; gout; urinary frequency and dysuria; glucose intolerance, etc.

Administration: Gradual increase over 1–3 weeks from 300 mg/day to 2–9 g/day; given in three times daily dosage; give with meals to diminish side effects. Flushing may be ameliorated by concomitant use of aspirin 324 mg twice daily. Administer with caution in presence of coronary artery disease.

Clinical Use: Second-line (because of side effects) but effective drug in the treatment of elevated LDL cholesterol or VLDL triglyceride. Contraindications include peptic ulcer disease, dysrhythmia, liver disease, diabetes mellitus, hyperuricemia, and gout.

sequestering resins and nicotinic acid. Its hypocholesterolemic effect is accompanied, however, by a reduction in plasma levels of HDL cholesterol and decreased apo A-I synthetic rates. The decrease in the ratio of LDL cholesterol to HDL cholesterol is often smaller than desired due to the concomitant decrease in HDL levels during therapy. Moreover, because this drug is lipid soluble and stored in body fat, it has an unusually long biological half-life; hence, its long term safety has not been established.

Estrogen therapy frequently lowers levels of LDL cholesterol and raises HDL cholesterol levels in post-menopausal women, but the doses required for these effects exceed those used for physiological "replacement therapy." Hence, there is a potential for significant side effects that warrant careful monitoring. *Neomycin* is effective in lowering cholesterol levels in hypercholesterolemic patients by enhancing the fecal excretion of neutral sterols. However, patients frequently develop diarrhea. Since neomycin is an aminoglycoside, renal function must be monitored during therapy. Treatment with *dextrothyroxine* should not be given because of its potential for inducing cardiac dysrhythmias.

The newer, experimental agents, *compactin and mevinolin*, look especially promising for lowering levels of total (or LDL) cholesterol. They are powerful competitive inhibitors of the enzyme, HMG CoA reductase, the rate-limiting enzyme in the synthesis of cholesterol. They also increase LDL removal from the circulation, apparently due to increased LDL clearance by LDL receptors. Since hepatic cholesterol synthesis often rises during resin therapy in patients with familial hypercholesterolemia, a disorder characterized by deficient LDL cellular receptors, these drugs offer considerable hope for the reduction of CAD risk in these patients.

Hypertriglyceridemia

Drugs which decrease hepatic production of VLDL and apo B, enhance VLDL clearance by stimulating LPL activity, or both are generally effective in treating hypertriglyceridemia. The fibric acid derivatives (clofibrate, gemfibrozil, bezafibrate, fenofibrate) and nicotinic acid do both.

Although *nicotinic acid* may be most efficacious, its use is limited by its side effects and the presence of coexisting contraindications. The *fibric acid derivatives* are, therefore, the drugs most commonly used. Gemfibrozil may be preferable to clofibrate, since it more consistently raises plasma levels of HDL, is less likely to raise the plasma LDL level, and may be less lithogenic. It is a new agent, however, and long term experience with it is limited. While the fibric acid drugs are generally well tolerated, an acute myositis which occasionally progresses to renal failure may occur, particularly in patients with impaired renal clearance or hypoalbuminemia. These drugs either should not be used or their dose

reduced by 70 to 90% in azotemic patients. Frequent monitoring of muscle enzymes (creatine kinase, aldolase) is required to avoid toxicity. When the level of LDL cholesterol rises in a patient on a fibric acid drug, the diagnosis of familial combined hyperlipoproteinemia should be considered.

In compliant patients who remain hypertriglyceridemic with diet and a single drug, combined therapy with a fibric acid drug and nicotinic acid may be useful. Rarely, after consultation with a specialist in lipid disorders, the progestational agent, norethidrone acetate, or the androgenic anabolic steroid, oxandrolone, may be required to treat persistent hypertriglyceridemia plus chylomicronemia in women or men, respectively.

Dysbetablipoproteinemia

The decreased remnant catabolism characteristic of this clinically uncommon disorder can be corrected or improved by drug therapy. Clofibrate or gemfibrozil appears to normalize lipid levels and to enhance remnant clearance in patients with dysbetalipoproteinemia. They are the drugs of choice in this disorder. Furthermore, a reduction in peripheral vascular disease has been demonstrated during clofibrate therapy. Ethinyl estradiol has a similar and even more dramatic effect, but in doses that greatly exceed those used for postmenopausal replacement therapy. Hence, its use requires careful monitoring for possible adverse estrogenic effects that would lead to discontinuation of the drug. Nicotinic acid is the drug of second choice.

Surgery and Other Therapies

More experimental forms of therapy (such as ileal bypass, portacaval shunt, plasma exchange and extracorporeal hemoperfusion) exist for the severely hypercholesterolemic patient who is resistant or only partially responsive to diet, exercise, and lipid-lowering drugs. These therapies should be implemented only in consultation with a specialist in lipid disorders.

Obtaining Consultation

The Lipid Metabolism Branch, National Heart, Lung and Blood Institute, National Institutes of Health, Bethesda, MD 20205, can provide the names of research centers in each geographic area where sophisticated evaluation of lipoprotein abnormalities, consultation services, and experimental forms of therapy are offered.

Additional information for the management of patients with hyperlipoproteinemia and other risk factors for CAD is available from both regional and the national offices of the American Heart Association. This agency can provide information about diet, drugs, and exercise in the treatment of hyperlipidemia, hypertension, cigarette smoking, and obesity.

General References

Ad Hoc Committee to Design a Dietary Treatment of Hyperlipoproteinemia: Gotto AM, Bierman EL, Connor W, *et al*: Recommendations for treatment of hyperlipidemia in adults: a joint statement of the Nutrition Committee and the Council on Arteriosclerosis. *Circulation* 65:1067, 1984.
> Excellent detailed yet practical treatise on the management of patients with lipoprotein disorders.

AMA Council on Scientific Affairs: Dietary and pharmacologic therapy for the lipid risk factors. *JAMA* 250:1873, 1983.
> Concise review of the lipoprotein risk factors and recommendations for management.

American Heart Association Booklets
> *Eating for a Healthy Heart, Dietary Treatment for Hyperlipidemia.*
>> Booklet for patients on the American Heart Association (AHA) single diet approach to improving plasma lipoprotein levels.
> *Counseling the Patient with Hyperlipidemia.*
>> Short booklet for the physician or nutritionist on implementing the AHA diet.
> *Heart to Heart, Nutrition Counseling for the Reduction of Cardiovascular Disease Risk Factors.*
>> Detailed book for the physician or nutritionist on counseling patients regarding the AHA diet.
> (All are available from your local chapter of the American Heart Association.)

Brunzell JD: Physiologic approach to hyperlipidemia. In Schwartz TB (ed): *The Year Book of Endocrinology*, Chicago, Year Book Medical Publishers, 1984, p 11
> Well written, readily understandable, insightful physiological approach to lipoprotein metabolism and its relationship to atherosclerosis.

Kaplan NM, Stamler J: *Prevention of Coronary Heart Disease, Practical Management of the Risk Factors*. Philadelphia, WB Saunders, 1983.
> Excellent book which reviews numerous risk factors (including lipoprotein abnormalities, cigarette smoking, hypertension, physical inactivity, psychosocial factors, *etc*) and their management in a thorough, yet concise and practical manner.

Lipid Research Clinics Program: *Manual of Laboratory Operations* Vol 1: *Lipid and Lipoprotein Analysis*. Washington, DC, US Government Printing Office, DHEW publ no. (NIH) 75-625, 1974.
> The methods book for lipoprotein analysis. A good reference to assist you in checking your local laboratory's methodology and standardization.

NIH Consensus Conference: Treatment of hypertriglyceridemia. *JAMA* 251:1196, 1984.
> Excellent discussion of when and how to treat the patient with hypertriglyceridemia.

NIH Consensus Conference: Lowering blood cholesterol to prevent heart disease. *JAMA* 253:2080, 1985.
> Recommendations on screening, treatment, and public health policy.

Specific References

1. Brensike JF, Levy RI, Kelsey SF, *et al*: Effects of therapy with cholestyramine on progression of coronary arteriosclerosis: results of the NHLBI type II coronary intervention study. *Circulation* 69:313, 1984.
2. Brown MS, Goldstein JL: How LDL receptors influence cholesterol and atherosclerosis. *Sci Am* 251:58,1984.
3. Brown WV, Goldberg IJ, Ginsberg HN: Treatment of common lipoprotein disorders. *Prog Cardiovasc Dis* 27:1, 1984.
4. Brunzell JD, Sniderman AD, Albers JJ, Kwiterovich PO, Jr: Apoproteins B and A-1 and coronary artery disease in humans. *Arteriosclerosis* 4:79, 1984.
5. Campeau L, Enjalbert J, Lesperance J, *et al*: The relationship of risk factors to the development of atherosclerosis in saphenous-vein bypass grafts and the progression of disease in the native circulation: a study 10 years after aortocoronary bypass surgery. *N Engl J Med* 311:1329, 1984.
6. Dufaux B, Assmann G, Hollman W: Plasma lipoproteins and physical activity: a review. *Int J Sports Med* 3:123, 1982.
7. Ederer F, Leren P, Turpeinin O, Frantz ID Jr: Cancer among men on cholesterol-lowering diets. *Lancet* 2:203, 1971.
8. Goldberg AP: Lipid abnormalities in hemodialysis: prevalence, implications and treatment. *Perspect Lipid Disord* 2:17, 1984.
9. Gore JM, Goldberg RJ, Matsumoto AS,, *et al*: Validity of serum total cholesterol level obtained within 24 hours of acute myocardial infarction. *Am J Cardiol* 54:722, 1984.
10. Havel RJ: Classification of the hyperlipidemias. *Annu Rev Med* 28:195, 1977.
11. Heiss G, Johnson NJ, Reiland S, *et al*: The epidemiology of plasma HDL cholesterol levels. The Lipid Research Clinics Prevalence Study. Summary. *Circulation* 62 (suppl IV) IV:116, 1980.
12. Illingsworth DR: Mevinolin plus colestipol in therapy for severe heterozygous familial hypercholesterolemia. *Ann Intern Med* 101:598, 1984.
13. Havel RJ (guest ed): Symposium on lipid disorders. Med Clin North Am 66:319, 1982.
14. Kannel WB, Schatzkin A: Risk factor analysis. *Prog Cardiovasc Dis* 26:309, 1983.
15. Levy RI: Consideration of cholesterol and nonvascular mortality. *Am Heart J* 104:324, 1982.
16. Lindgren FT, Jensen LC, Hatch FT: The isolation and quantitative analysis of serum lipoproteins. In *Blood Lipids and Lipoproteins: Quantitation, Composition, and Metabolism*. New York, John Wiley & Sons, 1972, p 181.
17. Lipid Research Clinics Populations Studies Data Book, vol I: *The Prevalence Study*. US Department of Health and Human Services, Public Health Service, National Institutes of Health, NIH publ no. 80-1527, 1980.
18. Lipid Research Clinics Coronary Primary Prevention Trial Results: I. Reduction in incidence of coronary heart disease. II. The relationship of reduction in incidence of coronary heart disease to cholesterol lowering. *JAMA* 251:351, 365, 1984.
19. Maciejko JJ, Holmes DR, Kottke BA, *et al*: Apolipoprotein A-I as a marker of angiographically assessed coronary artery disease. *N Engl J Med* 309:385, 1983.
20. Mahley RW, Angelin B: Type III hyperlipoproteinemia: recent insights into the genetic defect of familial dysbetalipoproteinemia. *Adv Intern Med* 29:385, 1984.
21. Nilsson-Ehle P: Regulation of lipoprotein lipase: triacylglycerol transport in plasma. In Carlson LA, Pernow B (eds): *Metabolic Risk Factors in Ischemic Cardiovascular Disease*. New York, Raven Press, 1982, p 49.
22. Oram JF, Brenton EA, Bierman EL: Regulation of high density lipoprotein activity in cultured human skin fibroblasts and human arterial smooth muscle cells. *J Clin Invest* 72:1611, 1983.
23. Paffenberger RS, Hyde RT, Wing AL, Steinmetz CH: A natural history of athleticism and cardiovascular health. *JAMA* 252:491, 1984.
24. Rifkind BM, Segal P: Lipid Research Clinics Program reference values for hyperlipidemia and hypolipidemia. *JAMA* 250:1869, 1983.
25. Sniderman AD, Wolfson C, Teng B, *et al*: Association of hyperbetalipoproteinemia with endogenous hypertriglyceridemia and atherosclerosis. *Ann Intern Med* 97:833, 1982.
26. Tyroler HA, Hess G, Schonfeld G, *et al*: Apoprotein A-I, A-II and C-II in black and white residents of Evans County. *Circulation* 62:249, 1980.
27. Walden CE, Knopp RH, Wahl PW, *et al*: Sex differences in the effect of diabetes mellitus and lipoprotein triglyceride and cholesterol concentrations. *N Engl J Med* 331:953, 1984.

CHAPTER SEVENTY-SIX

Obesity

MARC R. BLACKMAN, M.D.

Obesity, defined as an excess of total body fat, is one of the most prevalent chronic medical disorders in the world. Moreover, its incidence and prevalence appear to be increasing, particularly in the highly industrialized nations (see below). Numerous complex, as yet ill understood, interactions among predisposing genetic and environmental factors influence the initiation, development, and persistence of excess adiposity. Although controversy exists about the exact health risks associated with mild obesity (3, 18, 28, 29), in more obese patients, morbidity and mortality vary directly with the amount and topographical distribution of excess body fat, as well as with certain associated medical and behavioral abnormalities. Newer classification schemes need to be devised so that rational therapeutic interventions can be more specifically targeted toward those obesity syndromes associated with increased risk for morbidity and mortality. In so doing, perhaps both short and long term treatment results will improve substantially. In any event, there remains an urgent need to promote a variety of effective societal and individual approaches for prevention of excess adiposity.

DEFINITION

Obesity *versus* Overweight

Obesity must be distinguished from overweight, which refers to an increase in body weight due to increased bone, muscle, or fat. Although the two terms are often used synonymously, errors do occur in equating obesity with overweight, as for example in the muscular athlete with normal or decreased body fat. Since body composition and, in particular, body fat normally vary with age, sex, diet, physical activity, and population group, it is important to compare measurements of body fat in individual patients with those derived from appropriate control groups.

Methods for Quantifying Adiposity

Numerous methods exist for assessing and quantifying adiposity, but the simplest, most common, and most reliable clinical approaches to date involve either determination of relative weight or measurement of skin-fold thickness. In the former approach, a patient's weight is expressed as a percentage or ratio of an "ideal," "desirable," or "acceptable" weight, such as that issued in the Metropolitan Life Insurance Company's Build and Blood Pressure Study of 1959 (30) and updated recently in the Metropolitan's Height and Weight Tables of 1983 (26). Of the various indices of weight and height tested, the body mass index [weight/(height)^2] has the highest correlation with other measures of body fat (see Fig. 76.1). Although measurements of skin-fold thickness (using standardized calipers) are useful in assessing body fat in population studies, the technique is often less reliable in individual patients than are direct measurements of weight and height.

CLASSIFICATION

The heterogeneous nature and the many approaches to evaluation and management of the obesity syndromes have made classification schemes necessary but nonuniform. Thus, various classification systems might serve different purposes, as for example (a) to identify subpopulations of obese individuals at risk for increased morbidity and mortality, in whom therapeutic interventions might be beneficial and (b) to distinguish among primarily genetic, environmental, and combined genetic plus

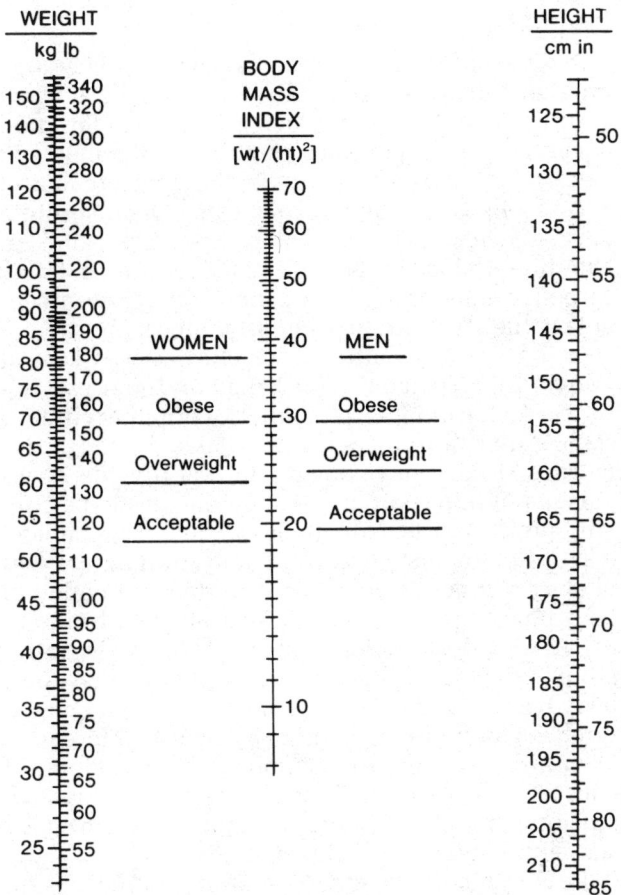

Figure 76.1. Nomogram for body mass index. (From Bray GA (ed): *Obesity in America*, DHEW publ no. (NIH) 79-359. Washington, DC, US Government Printing Office, 1979.)

environmental etiologies. With regard to the former, recent research suggests that patients with predominantly upper body obesity (*i.e.* increased fat in the back of the neck, shoulder areas and abdomen) exhibit an increased frequency of metabolic concomitants of obesity and an enhanced risk for developing diabetes mellitus, hyperlipidemia, and cardiovascular disease (11, 20, 23, 25). In contrast, patients with predominantly lower body obesity (*i.e.,* increased fat in the hips, thighs, and buttocks) are metabolically stable and are not at significantly enhanced risk for such diseases. Further research is necessary to discern whether therapeutic interventions should be targeted mostly toward patients with upper body obesity, and whether doing so will improve short and long term treatment results. With regard to the latter, categorization can be conveniently based upon anatomical/developmental and etiological criteria.

Anatomical/Developmental

Until recently, it was thought that the number of fat cells in healthy individuals increased steadily through the first few years of life, again increased slightly during the peripubertal years, and remained fixed thereafter. Subsequent gains or losses of body fat in adulthood were considered to result solely from corresponding increases or decreases in fat cell size. Recognition that patients with *youth onset* (< 15 to 20 years old) obesity more often had generalized obesity with both hyperplasia and hypertrophy of their adipocytes, whereas patients with *adult onset* (> 15 to 20 years old) obesity more often had a centripetal distribution of excess fat and adipocyte hypertrophy without an increase in the number of fat cells (5, 17) tended to confirm this hypothesis.

With the increasing awareness of the considerable overlap between these two groups, the concept of hyperplastic *versus* hypertrophic obesity has undergone further revision. Thus, it is currently appreciated that, in any given individual, fat cell number can increase at any stage of life if a critical (presumably genetically determined) fat cell size has been surpassed. One future therapeutic goal might be to identify and treat patients prior to their irreversible conversion from adipocyte hypertrophy to hyperplasia.

Other, much less common types of obesity fall within the anatomical classification. The *lipodystrophies* are localized accumulations of excess fat, most commonly single or multiple lipomas. The latter are inherited as an autosomal dominant trait. *Dercum's disease* (adiposis dolorosa) and *Weber-Christian disease* are two rare illnesses of unknown etiology characterized by focal (occasionally painful) distributions of single or multiple nodules of histologically normal fat.

Etiological

Various organic and environmental factors, none mutually exclusive, are included within the etiological classification of obesity.

Organic Factors

As already noted, even in patients with an apparently genetic predisposition to obesity, environmental influences seem to be important determinants of body weight (see below).

In both experimental animals and in man, certain *primary endocrine disorders* are important causes of obesity. These include hyperinsulinism, hypercortisolism, and deficiencies of growth hormone, thyroid hormone, or sex steroids.

Hyperinsulinemia can result from appropriate or surreptitious use of exogenous insulin, or from insulin hypersecretion by benign or malignant pancreatic neoplasms.

Hypercortisolism most often is iatrogenic, resulting from excess administration of exogenous glucocorticoids. Much less commonly, true Cushing's disease or syndrome is responsible.

Since *growth hormone* exerts an influence on conversion of fat stores into energy for body growth and protein deposition, its absence, either due to pituitary dysfunction or removal, leads to increased adiposity which is reversible by administration of the hormone.

Although *thyroid hormones* directly modulate the overall basal metabolic rate (BMR), hypothyroidism *per se* is most often associated with modest or no weight gain. Morbid obesity (defined below) due solely to hypothyroidism has not been documented, whereas moderate weight loss because of anorexia disproportionate to the decrease in BMR is occasionally seen.

The *polycystic ovary (Stein-Leventhal) syndromes*, a fairly common group of disorders in young women, is characterized by mild obesity, hirsutism, oligomenorrhea, and infertility in association with mild hypothalamic-pituitary-ovarian (and possibly adrenal) dysfunction. The obesity and the menstrual abnormalities are often ameliorated after ovarian wedge resection.

Hypothalamic obesity is a rare disorder associated most often with the presence of a craniopharyngioma or, less often, with other neoplastic or inflammatory diseases near the hypothalamic ventromedial nuclei, sites in the brain that appear to be involved in the control of normal feeding and satiety.

Of uncertain etiology, but increasingly recognized, are the primary eating disorders of bulimia (binge eating) and anorexia nervosa (self-induced starvation). Although the true incidence and prevalence of these conditions are unknown, bulimia is thought to occur in fewer than 5% of obese persons and in as many as 50% of patients with anorexia nervosa. It is generally refractory to most forms of medical and psychiatric management. In one study, Dilantin therapy was found to be helpful in controlling symptoms in about one-third of bulimics (34).

In addition to insulin and glucocorticoids, other *pharmacological agents* induce increases in food intake and body fat. The most commonly used are phenothiazines, oral contraceptives, and the antihistamine, cyproheptadine (Periactin). Weight gain associated with the latter drug probably results from its antiserotoninergic properties.

Most chronic cigarette smokers weigh less than age- and sex-matched nonsmokers, but gain weight after they stop smoking. The weight gain frequently leads to resumption of smoking with its attendant risks for developing cardiovascular disease, emphysema, or cancer. Although the mechanisms responsible for weight loss during active cigarette smoking remain unknown, it has recently been shown that there is a strong positive correlation between the activity of the enzyme, adipose tissue lipoprotein lipase, in the fasting state and the amount of weight regain during the first 2 to 3 weeks after smoking cessation (9).

Environmental Factors

In view of the obvious imbalance between energy input and expenditure in obese individuals, it is not surprising to find numerous clinical studies that document the importance of nutritional habits and patterns of physical activity in the development of excess adiposity. The adverse effects of an absolute or relative excess in total caloric intake, of a maldistribution of foodstuffs (especially too much fat or carbohydrate), and of the general increase in sedentary life styles are particularly important.

In contemporary affluent societies, obesity is most frequently associated with behavioral and psychological determinants that affect both the circumstances and substance of food intake. Although numerous studies have sought to identify the obese persona, it appears that no such diagnostic personality profile exists. Nonetheless, a major psychological distinction between youth and adult onset types of obesity may reside in the distorted perception of body image that is frequently associated with obesity in childhood and adolescence. Thus, in the latter group, affected individuals often believe that their body habitus and weight are normal, a phenomenon rarely encountered in adult onset obesity. Moreover, in contrast to certain commonly held notions, it appears that obese individuals are often depressed, are unhappy about being fat, and are relieved by successful and sustained weight loss.

Socioeconomic factors exert strong influences on the development and persistence of obesity in individuals as well as in population groups. In the United States obesity is more common in (a) children and adults from the lower socioeconomic groups, (b) black *versus* white women, (c) white *versus* black men, and (d) first generation Americans *versus* their descendants. Interestingly, when body weights of women of similar ages were compared, those women born later in this century were less heavy than women born in the early 1900s; the opposite trend appeared true for men. The reason for this is unclear, but may be related to the steadily increasing fashion consciousness and emphasis on exercise among American women, and to the generally more sedentary work habits and life styles of men.

Morbid Obesity

Morbid obesity defines a subset of patients who are 50 to 100%, or 100 lb (45.5 kg), above their "ideal," "desirable," or "acceptable" body weights. A predominantly genetic origin, with onset of disease in youth, a generally relentless progression through life, and a long term cure rate of less than 5% are characteristic. In contrast, the onset and progression of the usual forms of mild to moderate adult onset obesity are influenced more by psychosocial factors. Whereas patients with youth onset morbid obesity often suffer from distorted perceptions of body image, this has not been true of patients with adult onset disease. The latter group, however, has been characterized as generally lacking in internal cues that control food intake, thus being more susceptible to external, environmental eating cues. This observation, confirmed in numerous psychological studies, has exerted a major influence upon the philosophy and design of behavior modification programs.

PREVALENCE

Before the true prevalence of obesity in any population group can be ascertained, several general methodological concerns must be addressed. (a) A practical, standardized definition of obesity or overweight must be available and utilized. (b) The study population should be representative of the larger population group of which it is a part. (c) The presence and significance of coexistent morbid diseases or other conditions that may affect body weight must be known. (d) The effects of sex, age, socioeconomic, religious, ethnic, and other related factors must be considered (e) The effects of confounding variables, such as cigarette smoking, should be analyzed. (f) Both cross-sectional and long term longitudinal data should be collected. (g) Methods used for quantifying body fat in epidemiological studies, such as relative weight (e.g., body mass index) should be further refined to more closely approximate the most accurate known measures of adipose tissue mass. (h) The prevalence and significance of topographical variations in the distribution of body fat (i.e., upper versus lower body obesity) need to be assessed. Although many excellent, large scale demographic surveys have been reported, to date no single study has satisfied all of the above criteria.

Comparative data on weight and height derived from three major cross-sectional surveys of the US population have been published by the National Center for Health Statistics, and are in Table 76.1. Examination of the table reveals that for both men and women, weights and heights were greater in the periods from 1971 to 1974 and from 1976 to 1980 than they were from 1960 to 1962. These findings have been replicated in numerous studies, particularly in the Build Study of 1979 (8), a survey of 4.2 million generally healthy, middle class persons insured by 25 US and Canadian insurance companies. Data from this latter study have been widely publicized by the Metropolitan Life Insurance Company as the 1983 Metropolitan Height and Weight Tables (26), and have led to upward revisions of the widely used "desirable" weights previously derived from the Build Study of 1959 (30). Since weights in these latter tables were not derived from a representative sample of the North American population, they should not be considered "desirable" and are therefore not labeled as such.

There is now widespread recognition that with advancing age, there are physiological alterations

Table 76.1.
Mean Weights and Heights by Age and Sex in Three Populations[a,b]

Age Group	Men			Women		
	HES	NHANES I	NHANES II	HES	NHANES I	NHANES II
Weight (kg)						
18–24 years	71.7	74.8	73.9	57.6	59.9	60.8
25–34 years	72.6	79.8	78.5	60.8	63.5	64.4
35–44 years	77.1	80.7	80.7	64.4	67.1	67.1
45–54 years	77.1	79.4	80.7	65.8	67.6	68.0
55–64 years	74.4	77.6	78.9	68.0	67.6	68.0
65–74 years	71.7	74.4	74.8	65.3	66.2	66.7
18–74 years	75.3	78.0	78.0	63.5	64.9	65.3
Height (m)						
18–24 years	1.74	1.77	1.77	1.62	1.63	1.63
25–34 years	1.76	1.77	1.77	1.61	1.63	1.63
35–44 years	1.74	1.76	1.76	1.60	1.62	1.61
45–54 years	1.73	1.75	1.75	1.58	1.60	1.60
55–64 years	1.71	1.73	1.74	1.56	1.58	1.58
65–74 years	1.70	1.71	1.71	1.60	1.62	1.62
18–74 years	1.73	1.75	1.76			

[a] From Simopoulos AP, Van Itallie TBV: Body weight, health, and longevity. *Ann Intern Med* 100:285, 1984.
[b] The three populations are from the National Health Examination Survey (HES), 1960 to 1962 and the National Health and Nutrition Examination Surveys (NHANES) I, 1971 to 1974, and II, 1976 to 1980. Two pounds were deducted from HES data to allow for weight of clothing; total weight of all clothing for NHANES I and II ranged from 0.1 to 0.3 kg and was not deducted from weights in table. Height was measured without shoes. Data are preliminary. Age-adjusted mean values and estimates of variation (standard error) about the mean estimates are not currently available.

Table 76.2.

Comparison of the Weight for Height Tables from Actuarial Data (*Build Study* 1979): Non-Age-Corrected Metropolitan Life Insurance Company and Age-Specific Gerontology Research Center Recommendations[a]

HEIGHT (Feet Inches)	Metropolitan 1983 Weights[b]		Gerontology Research Center[b]				
	Men	Women	Age-Specific Weight Range for Men and Women				
	25–59 yr		25 Yr	35 Yr	45 Yr	55 Yr	65 Yr
4 10		100–131	84–111	92–119	99–127	107–135	115–142
4 11		101–134	87–115	95–123	103–131	111–139	119–147
5 0		103–137	90–119	98–127	106–135	114–143	123–152
5 1	123–145	105–140	93–123	101–131	110–140	118–148	127–157
5 2	125–148	108–144	96–127	105–136	113–144	122–153	131–163
5 3	127–151	111–148	99–131	108–140	117–149	126–158	135–168
5 4	129–155	114–152	102–135	112–145	121–154	130–163	140–173
5 5	131–159	117–156	106–140	115–149	125–159	134–168	144–179
5 6	133–163	120–160	109–144	119–154	129–164	138–174	148–184
5 7	135–167	123–164	112–148	122–159	133–169	143–179	153–190
5 8	137–171	126–167	116–153	126–163	137–174	147–184	158–196
5 9	139–175	129–170	119–157	130–168	141–179	151–190	162–201
5 10	141–179	132–173	122–162	134–173	145–184	156–195	167–207
5 11	144–183	135–176	126–167	137–178	149–190	160–201	172–213
6 0	147–187		129–171	141–183	153–195	165–207	177–219
6 1	150–192		133–176	145–188	157–200	169–213	182–225
6 2	153–197		137–181	149–194	162–206	174–219	187–232
6 3	157–202		141–186	153–199	166–212	179–225	192–238
6 4			144–191	157–205	171–218	184–231	197–244

[a] From Andres R: Mortality and obesity. The rationale for age-specific height-weight tables. In Andres R, Hazzard WR, Bierman E (eds): *Principles of Geriatric Medicine.* New York, McGraw-Hill, 1985.
[b] Values in this table are for height without shoes and weight without clothes.

both in body weight (which increases gradually until the fifth to sixth decade, then tends to plateau) and body composition (with progressive loss of lean body mass and absolute or relative increase in total body fat). Table 76.2, originally reported by Andres (3), illustrates comparative weight for height data derived from the 1983 Metropolitan Height and Weight Tables (uncorrected for age) and from the Baltimore Longitudinal Study of Aging, conducted at the Gerontology Research Center of the National Institute on Aging. Perusal of these data reveals that, for most of the heights reported, the Metropolitan optimal weights for men and women are similar to those for the age-adjusted weights of individuals in their thirties and forties. Therefore, the Metropolitan tables overestimate the "norms" for younger adults but underestimate the corresponding "norms" for elderly people. In the age-adjusted data from the Gerontology Research Center, there is an increased weight allowance of about 10 pounds/decade.

In the US Public Health Service Ten State Nutrition Survey of 1968 to 1970 (16), the prevalence of obesity in adolescents was determined by measurement of triceps skin-fold thickness. With use of the criterion of skin-fold thickness greater than the 85th percentile of adult values (18.6 mm in men and 25.1 mm in women), obesity in adolescents was found to vary with age from 11 to 39% for white males and from 9 to 19% for white females. White male adolescents were more obese than their black counterparts. In this study there were no consistent rela-

Table 76.3.

Prevalence of Overweight and Obesity in Groups of Men from Seven Countries[a]

Country	Percent of Sample	
	Overweight[b]	Obese[c]
Japan	2	2
Greece	11	11
Finland	15	14
Yugoslavia	19	29
Italy	33	28
Netherlands	13	32
United States	32	63

[a] Data adapted from Keys (19), from Bray GA: The obese patient. In Smith LH (ed): *Major Problems in Internal Medicine,* Philadelphia, WB Saunders, 1976, vol 9.
[b] Overweight = men 10% or more over standard weight.
[c] Obesity = men with sum of triceps and subscapular skinfold > 28 mm.

tionships between obesity and socioeconomic status. However, Stunkard et al (32) have emphasized the importance of social factors in the prevalence of obesity or overweight in childhood. In one study overweight children from lower socioeconomic groups were identified by age 6, whereas overweight children from upper socioeconomic groups could not be identified until age 8, and there were fewer at later ages in childhood.

The Seven Country Study of Keys et al (19) (Table 76.3) provided comparative data on obesity and overweight, utilizing criteria of skin-fold thickness and relative weight; by either criterion men from the United States were among the most corpulent examined.

PATHOGENESIS

Energy Intake

In the United States the typical diet is composed of approximately 40 to 45% carbohydrate, 40% fat, and 15 to 20% protein. Energy intake that exceeds energy expenditure is the cardinal pathogenetic mechanism promoting an increase in body fat. Although there is evidence to support the idea that, in healthy people, body weight is fairly closely regulated over long periods of time, body composition changes considerably with age, as noted previously. The numerous factors controlling normal food intake and distribution, storage, and expenditure of energy represent a complex, highly integrated series of events, as yet only partially understood.

Until recently, it was thought that normal control of hunger and satiety in man resided in certain nuclei of the lateral and medial hypothalamus, respectively, and that other neural, nutritional, endocrine-metabolic, gastrointestinal, and psychological factors exerted their influences by impinging upon these sites. Current evidence favors a more diffuse localization of feeding and satiety "centers" involving not only the perihypothalamic area but portions of the limbic system and cerebral cortex as well.

The application of contemporary techniques of cell, tissue, and organ culture has allowed for novel approaches to examine directly the basic cellular processes occurring in various tissues and cells (e.g., adipocytes, hepatocytes, etc) known to be affected by metabolic derangements in obesity, in both humans and experimental animals. Data derived from such studies will undoubtedly provide important new information pertinent to understanding the pathophysiological derangements in cellular uptake, storage, and expenditure of energy in human obesity.

Energy Expenditure

Even after adjustments for differences in age, sex, and body weight, energy expenditure varies considerably among normal adults. Under resting conditions, there are adaptations to the amount and type of food ingested that allow for increased or decreased utilization of nutrients and that maintain a stable weight in most people. For example, after increased food intake above that required for maintenance of normal weight, healthy individuals exhibit an initial increase in weight followed by a new plateau of weight despite continued overeating, a phenomenon referred to as luxuskonsumption, or dietary-induced thermogenesis (DIT). Current evidence favors the hypothesis that DIT is an important factor in regulating body weight and, that the "missing energy" is

burnt off in "brown fat," metabolically more active than the usual "white fat" (13).

In our sedentary society physical exercise plays a relatively minor role in energy expenditure. Short term vigorous exercise such as weight lifting, competitive contact sports, etc often leads to increases in dietary intake, utilization of muscle glycogen stores, and muscle mass. In contrast, frequent, sustained, moderate aerobic exercise, such as jogging, swimming, etc, mobilizes fat stores.

Despite the apparent long term control of general energy balance and body weight in normal persons, there is no conclusive evidence of an endogenous set-point (e.g., glucostatic, lipostatic, or thermostatic) that modulates adipose tissue mass. However, Schwartz and Brunzell have reported that the activity of adipose tissue lipoprotein lipase (LPL), the rate-limiting enzyme in the uptake and storage of lipoprotein triglyceride in adipose tissue, is increased in obese Caucasians and that enzyme activity increases, rather than decreases, after weight loss (27). Moreover, there appear to be demographic/genetic differences in the occurrence of this phenomenon. These authors have proposed that adipose tissue LPL may exert a counterregulatory role in preventing deviation from a set-point for fat cell size or mass, thus predisposing to return to the original obese state (27). As noted above (see page 1068), the correlation between baseline adipose tissue LPL activity and the amount of weight gained after cessation of cigarette smoking further supports this hypothesis.

Recently, certain indices of cellular sodium potassium ATPase activity have been reported to be increased (6), decreased (10), or unchanged (4) in red blood cells or liver from obese subjects, as compared with controls. Further investigation is necessary to clarify whether alterations in the activity of this critical cellular enzyme contribute to the pathophysiological mechanisms by which cellular thermogenesis, and therefore the efficiency of energy expenditure, might be perturbed in human obesity.

The observation that most obesity in adult men is upper body in distribution, while that in most adult women is lower body in distribution, suggested that sex hormones might influence body fat topography and function. Recently, increased androgenic activity has been reported in the blood of women with upper versus lower body obesity and has been shown to correlate with abnormalities in fat cell size and biochemical function (11). Moreover, abdominal adipocytes from patients with upper body obesity are metabolically active, whereas abdominal adipocytes from patients with lower body obesity, and thigh adipocytes from patients with upper or lower body obesity, are metabolically relatively stable.

NATURAL HISTORY

Much information has been adduced to show that obese infants and children become obese adults more often than do their lean counterparts. In addition, youth onset obesity tends to be more severe and persistent, and more resistant to treatment, than are the usually milder forms of later onset. This may be due to the fact that weight loss and decrease in adiposity *per se* result predominantly from a decrease in adipocyte size and not number, so that adipose hyperplasia (regardless of age of onset) (see page 1067) is ordinarily irreversible. In contrast, there is greater therapeutic promise for the more common normocellular adult onset obese population.

Metabolic Concomitants

Although the exact roles of all organic and environmental factors in the pathogenesis of obesity remain to be elucidated, certain metabolic concomitants of excess adiposity have been characterized. Numerous studies document the close association between obesity and *diabetes mellitus* and suggest that obesity *per se* is diabetogenic. Obesity leads to increased pancreatic insulin production and hyperinsulinemia, both basally and after stimulation by ingestion of glucose, amino acids, *etc.* Evidence exists that the hyperinsulinemia and concurrent glucose intolerance are due to insulin resistance at the tissue level (e.g., liver, adipose tissue, and skeletal muscle) (21), caused in some individuals by a decrease in the number of cell surface receptors for insulin, and in others by aberrant, insulin-dependent intracellular glucose metabolism. Finally, it has been proposed that chronic hyperinsulinemia leads to a further decrease in the number of cell surface insulin receptors (i.e., "down-regulation"), the latter serving as an adipocyte response to prevent episodes of hypoglycemia.

There is a significant association between obesity and the presence of *hyperlipidemia*, especially hypertriglyceridemia. This latter relationship probably results, at least in some patients, from the hyperinsulinemia-induced increase in hepatic triglyceride synthesis and formation of triglyceride-rich very low density lipoproteins (VLDL), although this hypothesis requires further confirmation. Increased endogenous cholesterol synthesis is also more frequent in obese patients, leads to increased circulating concentrations of total cholesterol and low density lipoprotein (LDL) cholesterol and decreased concentrations of high density lipoprotein (HDL) cholesterol, and may be responsible for the increased risk of cholesterol gallstones.

Many patients with adult onset upper body obesity appear cushingoid. Simple obesity is associated with an *increased cortisol production rate* leading to increased hepatic steroid metabolism and increased urinary excretion of certain steroid conjugates. Such patients typically have increased urinary 17-hydroxycorticoids; however, plasma cortisol, urinary free cortisol, and overnight dexamethasone suppression tests are usually normal.

Salt and water retention is a common problem in obese patients, and is in part mediated by increases in aldosterone secretion induced by dietary carbohydrate and, to a lesser extent, protein intake.

Onset of normal menarche does not occur until a critical body weight is reached (usually 40 to 45 kg), a finding that explains the *earlier menarche* in women with youth onset obesity. *Menstrual abnormalities*, such as dysfunctional uterine bleeding, amenorrhea, and infertility, are also more common in obese women, and are often associated with aberrant cyclical reproductive hormone function (subnormal levels of follicle-stimulating hormone (FSH) in the follicular phase, and of progesterone in the luteal phase).

Other important endocrine or metabolic sequelae of obesity, the mechanisms for which are unclear, are *decreased growth hormone responses* to provocative stimuli (including the recently isolated hypothalamic growth hormone-releasing hormone) and *hyperuricemia*. The former, by decreasing the availability of a lipolytic hormone, permits excess fat accumulation, while the latter is responsible for the increased prevalence of gout in obese individuals.

Risks

A large body of research and anecdotal data has suggested that obesity and overweight exist as graded phenomena, and that there is strong positive correlation between the degree of excess adiposity and increased morbidity and mortality, the latter particularly from cardiovascular and cerebrovascular diseases. It now appears that this hypothesis must be somewhat modified.

Critical analysis of data derived from retrospective life insurance studies (28) suggested that there was no significant increase in mortality until body weight rose to values greater than 30% above ideal body weight. Data from a large number of prospective studies also suggest that severe to extreme, but not mild to moderate, obesity is associated with decreased longevity. More recent reanalyses of data from various large scale epidemiological studies have led several investigators to conclude that the "mortality for weight" curves are often "J-" or "U"-shaped, in that the highest mortality rates occur at both extremes of relative weight (e.g., body mass index), whereas the lowest mortality rates occur at intermediate weights (29). Andres has demonstrated that the body mass index associated with lowest mortality itself increases with advancing age, both in men and women, and has thus emphasized the need for age-specific weight-height tables (3). It is also evident, as noted above (page 1067), that the risks of obesity vary not only with the amount, but also with the topographical distribution, of excess body fat. Finally, data recently published as part of a 26-year follow-up of subjects in the Framingham study (18) reveal that obesity *per se* is an independent risk factor for premature dying; it exerts its deleterious effects, in addition, by influencing known risk factors, such as hypertension, hyperlipidemia, and diabetes mellitus. It seems likely that public health and other officials, as well as individual physicians, will become more cautious in their advice regarding evaluation and management of patients with mild to moderate obesity, particularly if it is lower body in distribution.

Medical Consequences

The major physiological and medical concomitants of moderate to extreme obesity are depicted in Table 76.4. Although a direct pathophysiological link between obesity and these conditions has not been unequivocally established, in each instance, the morbidity associated with the condition is pro-

Table 76.4.
Possible Medical Consequences of Obesity

ENDOCRINE-METABOLIC:
  Hyperglycemia, hyperinsulinemia, insulin resistance
  Hypertriglyceridemia, hypercholesterolemia ($\uparrow$VLDL $\uparrow$LDL $\downarrow$HDL)
  $\uparrow$ Cortisol production but normal plasma cortisol, diurnal rhythm, urine free cortisol and overnight dexamethasone suppression
  Early menarche, menstrual abnormalities, hirsutism
  $\downarrow$ Growth hormone, basally and after provocative stimuli
  Hyperuricemia, gout
CARDIOVASCULAR:
  Hypertension
  Coronary artery disease
  Congestive heart failure
  Varicose veins
  Cerebrovascular disease
PULMONARY:
  Hypoventilation (*e.g.*, Pickwickian) syndromes
  Sleep apnea syndrome
  Chronic respiratory infections
GALLBLADDER:
  Cholelithiasis (cholesterol gallstones)
MUSCULOSKELETAL:
  Osteoarthritis
  Chronic orthopaedic problems
  $\downarrow$ Ambulation
RENAL:
  Nephrotic syndrome (normal or nonspecific biopsy)
ONCOLOGICAL:
  Endometrial and (?) breast carcinoma
DERMATOLOGICAL:
  Acanthosis nigricans
  Chronic skin infections
PSYCHOSOCIAL:
  Depression, loss of self-esteem
  $\downarrow$ Employability
PREGNANCY:
  Worsen underlying hypertension, diabetes mellitus
  $\uparrow$ Maternal mortality
SURGERY (especially under general anesthesia)
  Increased perioperative morbidity and mortality

portional to the degree of excess adiposity and is partially or totally reversed after successful weight loss. In addition, obesity, particularly when severe, frequently exacerbates or complicates the course of a variety of other conditions—for example, by delaying surgical procedures, enhancing peri-operative risks, prolonging convalescence from many illnesses, worsening pregnancy-associated problems, and exacerbating unstable behavioral patterns.

EVALUATION AND MANAGEMENT

Evaluation

The initial evaluation of the obese patient should include a medical and psychosocial history, physical examination, and appropriate laboratory and other studies. The history will usually indicate whether the patient has youth onset or adult onset obesity, and will often provide important information regarding usual or unusual dietary practices, as well as patterns of physical activity. It is particularly important to identify any medical or psychological factors that may motivate the patient to lose weight or that militate for or against certain treatment plans. The physical examination should include an assessment of whether the patient has primarily upper or lower body obesity by measuring the ratio of the minimum circumference at the waist to the maximum circumference at the hips with the patient in the standing position. A waist to hip ratio (WHR) greater than 0.85 indicates definite upper body obesity, while a WHR less than 0.76 indicates lower body obesity.

Although secondary obesity is rare, its importance lies in its reversibility after identification and specific therapy of the underlying medical or pharmacological disorder. Special emphasis should therefore be placed on screening an obese patient for any contributing endocrine-metabolic process and on obtaining a history of medication use.

Evidence of glucose intolerance should be sought by obtaining fasting blood glucose levels with the patient on a regular (or, preferably, high carbohydrate) diet, and comparing the results with those from age- and sex-matched controls. The oral glucose tolerance test is not ordinarily necessary to make the diagnosis of adult onset diabetes mellitus. Hypercortisolemia should be suspected in any plethoric, hypertensive patient with upper body obesity, hypokalemia, and glucose intolerance. A normal overnight dexamethasone suppression test (*i.e.*, 1.0 mg of oral dexamethasone at 11 P.M., followed by an 8 A.M. plasma cortisol < 5 μg/dl) ordinarily eliminates the diagnosis of endogenous hypercortisolemia with a reasonable degree of certainty. Clinically significant hypothyroidism can usually be ruled out when the free thyroxine index (*i.e.*, serum $T_4 \times$ resin T_3 uptake) is normal. On occasion, hyperthyroid patients "outeat" their increased BMR and complain to the physician of weight gain. The finding of menstrual irregularities, mild hirsutism (but not virilization), and obesity in a young woman prompts suspicion of the polycystic ovarian syndrome, a diagnosis made more likely by the additional findings of a mildly elevated serum testosterone level (60 to 100 ng/dl), flat basal body temperature curve (i.e., no ovulation), and palpable abnormalities on pelvic examination. Diseases of the hypothalamic-pituitary region should be considered in obese patients with otherwise unexplained neuroendocrine abnormalities. Certain rare syndromes, such as the Prader-Willi syndrome (obesity, short stature, hypogonadism, and mental retardation), are usually recognized in childhood by their characteristic clinical presentations.

In addition to the above, fasting blood samples should be sent for determinations of triglyceride, total cholesterol, HDL cholesterol, and uric acid levels. Most patients with hyperlipidemia have acquired (i.e., secondary), not genetic (i.e., primary) hyperlipidemias, and will respond to appropriate diet regimens (see Chapter 75). Finally, in patients with clinically apparent or suspect hypoventilation syndromes or sleep-disordered breathing, pulmonary function should be tested.

A useful algorithm for the outpatient evaluation of the obese patient has been published by Bray and Teague (7). Initial experience with this algorithm, as applied to 234 obese women and 27 obese men, led to detection of the following significant abnormalities: hypertension (16%), hypertriglyceridemia (25%), glucose intolerance (25%), hypercholesterolemia ($\uparrow$ total cholesterol, 11%), and hyperuricemia (7%). In 2 of 57 patients studied, T_4 values were abnormal; one was high and one low.

Management of Mild to Moderate Obesity

Based upon the initial assessment of the patient, the physician should ascertain the type, topographical distribution, and degree of obesity, including the medical or psychological urgency for weight loss, the patient's motivation and readiness for weight loss, and the most suitable treatment plan. Since the usual form of simple adult onset, mild to moderate lower body obesity appears not to carry an increased risk of morbidity or mortality (see pages 1072 to 1073), it should probably not be treated at all. On the other hand, until the possible risks of mild to moderate upper body obesity are more clearly defined, it would seem prudent to treat it with a combination of moderate diet, regular exercise, and patient-motivated nutritional education and behavioral relearning. There is no justification for the use of anorexigenic drugs in the treatment of the problem. If the patient asks for them, the physician should explain that they are modestly effective, are of little or no help in maintaining long term weight loss, and that many of them are potentially danger-

ous (see below, page 1078). Moreover, the patient should be cautioned against the purchase of patent medicines. It is now clear that several lay organizations for weight reduction (e.g., Weight Watchers and Take Off Pounds Sensibly (TOPS)) are as capable as health professionals in effecting weight loss in this category of obese patient.

For most adults, a balanced diet containing 1500 to 1800 calorie/day is necessary for maintenance of optimal body weight under conditions of basal activity. Thus, modest caloric restriction to 900 to 1200 calories/day for women and 1200 to 1500 calories/day for men is appropriate, with small increases proportionate to increases in levels of physical activity. It is often useful to advise patients who are motivated to diet to purchase one of the readily available, inexpensive calorie counters and to use the information to limit their daily diet to a specific number of calories. In general, daily modest exercise programs should be tailored to the individual patient's ability and enjoyment. Regular physical conditioning will facilitate weight loss, as well as decrease or abolish obesity-associated hyperinsulinemia, insulin resistance, glucose intolerance, hypertriglyceridemia, hyperuricemia, and systolic and diastolic hypertension and will improve cardiovascular, respiratory, and musculoskeletal problems. A goal of a loss of 1 or 2 pounds (0.5 to 1 kg) a week is appropriate whenever a patient embarks on a weight reduction program.

Improved nutritional understanding often results from effective and practical dietary counseling. Diet sheets and booklets that set forth easy to understand and follow recommendations, particularly when attuned to the sociocultural and economic characteristics of the patient, are especially valuable. Improved patterns of eating behavior should be encouraged. Specific suggestions should include smaller, more frequent, or regular meals, eaten more slowly, in defined surroundings. Use of food diaries is especially helpful (Fig. 76.2), particularly in identifying abnormal behavioral patterns leading to excess food intake. For the patient who makes a significant effort, reinforcement of the improved eating behavior by his physician is important in maintenance of weight reduction. Usually, formal consultation with a professional behavioral therapist is not required.

Management of Morbid Obesity

Morbid obesity (see page 1068), particularly of the upper body variety, is associated with a measurably increased morbidity and mortality, as well as with a generally poor response to conventional methods of moderate caloric restriction. Although there are hazards associated with each of the more intensive forms of treatment, in many severely obese patients the risks and disadvantages of being overweight greatly exceed those of treatment. In some individ-

FRANCIS SCOTT KEY MEDICAL CENTER
WEIGHT CONTROL PROGRAM

Name: _____Date: _____

Day: Mon.   Tues.   Wed.   Thurs.   Fri.   Sat.   Sun.   (circle one)

Exercise or activity: A. Type_____   Minutes_____   B. Type_____   Minutes_____

Time	Minutes	Food Type	Amount	Meal/ Snacks	Hunger Yes No	Body Position	Activity while Eating	Location of Eating	Eating (with Whom)	Feeling

Time: starting time for a meal or snack; Meal/snack: indicate type of eating by the appropriate letter—M (meal) or S (snack).
Hunger: check yes or no.

Figure 76.2. Food diary for identification of abnormal behavioral patterns leading to excess food intake.

uals, behavioral modification (see below), alone or in combination with other therapies, may offer an effective and safe management option.

Diet

Significant weight loss (up to 5 to 6 kg/week) can be achieved by prolonged (4 to 8 weeks) *starvation* of motivated, hospitalized morbidly obese patients. Within 1 to 2 years following such treatment, however, fewer than 25 to 30% of these patients have maintained their initial weight loss, and in the long term, fewer than 5% attain and maintain their "ideal" body weight. A major hazard of such treatment is the extensive loss of lean body mass, and thus negative nitrogen balance, that occurs predictably within the first 1 or 2 weeks of starvation, and continues at a somewhat lower rate thereafter. Other complications of this technique include orthostatic hypotension, ketoacidosis, electrolyte and vitamin deficiencies, weakness, decreased libido and impotence, menstrual irregularities, hyperuricemia and acute gout, renal uric acid calculi, emotional disturbances, and, rarely, sudden death. Despite these potential disadvantages, the need for hospitalization and the high incidence of recidivism, total fasting appears to be a generally safe and efficacious technique for inducing significant short term (e.g., presurgical) weight loss when supervised by physicians experienced in the technique.

Supplemented fasting is a technique that exploits in an ambulatory setting several of the advantages of total fasting, particularly those of significant short term weight loss and high patient adherence. In general, patients consume 1 to 1.5 g of protein/kg of desirable body weight, enough to prevent loss of lean body mass, in a hypocaloric (e.g., 300 to 500 calories/day) diet supplemented by adequate hydration, potassium salts, and other vitamins and minerals. In one study of nearly 1200 patients who were followed clinically and biochemically at frequent intervals, approximately 75 to 80% of the patients lost more than 40 lb (18 kg) (14). Moreover, hypertension and glucose intolerance, as well as the need for appropriate medications, disappeared or diminished in the majority of affected patients; other benefits, such as improved exercise tolerance, ambulation, pulmonary function, psychosocial and employment status also became evident. The disadvantages of the technique are similar to, but of lesser magnitude than, those described above for total fasting; there have been, in addition, several sudden cardiac deaths in patients without known pre-existing heart disease. A major problem with supplemented fasting is that the initial success rate drops to about 25% on subsequent attempts at fasting after major weight regain.

A variant of the supplemented fast, the "*liquid protein*" diet, has been widely used in this country in recent years, and consists of a very poor quality protein, collagen hydrolysate, supplemented with tryptophan. Because of the ready commercial availability of this diet, many obese patients have consumed it without appropriate vitamin or mineral supplementation or medical supervision. In one report (33), more than 60 sudden cardiac deaths were documented during or shortly after discontinuation of this diet. Although electrocardiograms often showed prolonged QT intervals, decreased QRS voltages, and refractory ventricular dysrhythmias, electrolyte abnormalities such as hypokalemia and hypocalcemia were not invariably present. Some autopsy studies have revealed a nonspecific cardiac muscle atrophy similar to that seen in protein-calorie malnutrition states in man and experimental animals. More recently, transient, potentially life-threatening cardiac dysrhythmias were detected by 24-hour Holter monitoring, but not by standard 12-lead electrocardiograms, in three of six morbidly obese, hospitalized patients followed for 40 days on a commercially available liquid protein diet (24). In none of the six patients was there an antecedent history of cardiac disease, and in all of the patients Holter monitoring was normal before and after the study diet. Except for mild hypokalemia in one of the affected patients, none of many routine chemical or metabolic parameters distinguished between patients with and without cardiac abnormalities. In a subsequent related study, six additional morbidly obese but otherwise healthy patients were hospitalized and fed for 40 days with a markedly hypocaloric (470 Kcal/day) experimental diet containing 60% high quality protein, 25% carbohydrate, and 15% fat, and supplemented with the Recommended Daily Allowances or more of all essential minerals, trace elements, vitamins, and essential fatty acids (1). No dysrhythmias were detected on 24-hour Holter monitoring, nitrogen balance remained positive, and the previously noted electrolyte abnormalities were reversed or decreased. It thus appeared that appropriate supplementation of even a markedly hypocaloric diet was safer than the nutritionally inadequate liquid protein diet. The Food and Drug Administration requires that warning labels be placed on all protein-supplemented diets and has suggested restricting such diets to certain individuals, all of whom should be aware of the potential hazards and should be followed by physicians experienced in using such diets. However, in view of the above observations, it appears prudent to discontinue use of liquid protein diets until the mechanisms of their cardiac toxicity are elucidated.

There are numerous, palatable balanced and unbalanced low calorie diets in common use. Many patients find it easier to follow regimens that limit caloric intake by eliminating entire food groups, such as carbohydrates, or by providing nutritionally adequate food homogenates. Perhaps the benefits of these approaches derive both from a perception that they are more "medicinal" and from diminution in external feeding cues.

Diets that are very low in calories (fewer than 800 calories/day) and carbohydrates are usually ketogenic. They are particularly popular because of the commonly held ideas that (a) nutritional ketosis exerts an anorexic effect, (b) greater weight loss ensues than after a balanced diet containing an equal number of calories, and (c) such diets spare body protein better than do balanced diets. There are no unequivocal data to support the first two notions. Although low carbohydrate, low caloric diets do generally cause a more profound early (1- to 2-week) diuresis of salt and water than do balanced diets, the rate of fat loss is no greater. Moreover, hypocaloric, low carbohydrate diets, like fasting and supplemented fasting, are associated with weakness, dehydration, postural hypotension, and occasional hyperuricemia and acute gout.

In conclusion, the safest diets are balanced and contain more than 800 calories daily. Table 76.5 illustrates several popular fad diets that are nutritionally unbalanced and/or hypocaloric. Use of the numerous other related fad diets that are hypocaloric and unbalanced, particularly when medically unsupervised, should be avoided.

How effective are dietary attempts at long term weight loss? Although quantitation of successful weight loss has been defined differently by various investigators, numerous studies confirm that at most only 10 to 20% of obese patients who initially lose significant amounts of weight on diets maintain or increase that weight loss several years later. Although all factors that promote such success or failure remain unknown, it has been shown that ability to continue in a diet program (nearly 25% of patients drop out within the first few weeks) and emotional stability are important. The appearance of pathological depression during or after dietary weight loss is well recognized, and is more common in juvenile onset obese patients, in whom the baseline distortion of body image is often accompanied, paradoxically, by a perception of larger body size with progressive weight loss. It is to be hoped that improved classification schemes will better identify subpopulations of obese patients more amenable to specifically defined therapeutic programs.

Behavior Modification

The basis for behavior modification therapy in the management of obesity rests upon the finding that many obese patients, particularly those of adult onset, respond predominantly to external, rather than internal, feeding cues. Both classical aversive conditioning and operant conditioning have been used successfully. The latter approach, which offers rewards or contracts, or modification of the environment, to change eating behavior, has been associated with greater patient satisfaction and, correspondingly, lower dropout rates. Weight loss resulting from behavior modification, unlike that produced by dietary, pharmacological, or surgical therapy, has not been associated with serious adverse side effects. Although these techniques offer great therapeutic promise, particularly when used in conjunction with diet and exercise programs, not all obese indi-

Table 76.5.
Characteristics of Several Widely Used Fad Diets

Diet	Composition	Deficiencies	Side Effects and Potential Hazards	Other Comments
HIGH PROTEIN/KETOGENIC DIETS Dr. Atkin's Revolutionary Diet The Drinking Man's Diet The Scarsdale Diet Dr. Stillman's Quick-Weight-Loss Diet	High protein Moderate to high fat Low carbohydrate Caloric intake varies from 1000–2000 calories	Likely deficiencies: Dietary fiber Calcium Riboflavin Folic acid Vitamins A, C Thiamine Iron	Potential exists for: Ketosis, anorexia, fatigue, dehydration, postural hypotension, hypokalemia/sodium loss, hyperlipidemia, hyperuricemia, constipation, halitosis	Long term maintenance unrealistic. NOT RECOMMENDED especially during pregnancy, in kidney disease, diabetes mellitus, lipid disorders. Can precipitate an acute attack of gout. Effectiveness due to high satiety values of foods consumed in diet. Large initial weight loss felt to be due to loss of body water. No greater actual fat loss than with balanced diet of equal calories.
PROTEIN-SPARING MODIFIED FAST (PSMF) Liquid Protein Diet The Last Chance Diet Cambridge Diet	Variation to total fast. Maximize fat loss but minimize lean body mass lost by adding 1.0 to 1.5 g of variable quality protein/kg of ideal body weight ~400 calories (300–700 calories) e.g., 330 calories/day 31 g of protein 44 g of CHO 2 g of fat and vitamin and mineral supplements	If poor biological quality protein, tryptophan deficiency. Likely deficiencies in poorly supplemented regimens: Potassium Phosphorus Calcium Magnesium Vitamin A Riboflavin	Ketosis Dehydration Hypokalemia Postural hypotension Cold intolerance Constipation Rarely—sudden death, felt to be secondary to cardiac arrhythmias	Unrealistic for long term maintenance. Not recommended for ambulatory management since needs careful medical monitoring. Tolerated more by morbidly obese than by mildly to moderately overweight individuals. Some programs do include instructions on nutrition, exercise, mental conditioning, life style modifications.
Pritiken Diet	80% complex CHO 10% fat 10% protein 650–1000 calories/day	Likely to be deficient in calcium, B_{12}, iron (slightly). Does not meet FDA's requirement for protein (especially high quality protein)	Dry skin, flatulence, gastric distress secondary to high fiber content	Long term compliance unlikely because of extreme change from average American diet. Exercise is encouraged.
Fasting	Fluid/electrolytes/vitamin and mineral supplementation	Extensive	Extensive	Inappropriate for ambulatory management. Needs to be done on metabolic ward only

viduals will respond, even in the short term, to this form of therapy, a fact which underscores the need for improved categorization and prognostication of obesity subtypes.

The short and long term efficacy of group therapy for obesity has also been examined and appears to be similar to that of individual therapy, a finding that should prompt more effective use of trained therapists. Data published by two of the most popular lay, self-help groups that advertise success at weight reduction, Weight Watchers and TOPS, confirm prior anecdotal impressions by experienced therapists that these groups achieve short term results as good as, and long term results as poor as, those in medically supervised programs.

Pharmacological Therapy

There is no known pharmacological agent for the treatment of obesity that is reliably effective, devoid of short and long term adverse side effects, inexpensive, and readily available. The anorexigenic derivatives of phenethylamine (Table 76.6), which include the amphetamines and fenfluramine, are the most commonly prescribed drugs. All possess certain pharmacological properties like those of epinephrine and norepinephrine; however, their various chemical modifications have led, to differing extents, to decreased cardiovascular and central nervous system toxicity and to preservation of anorexigenic properties. For the amphetamines, appetite suppression is probably mediated primarily by catecholaminergic pathways, whereas for fenfluramine, these

Table 76.6.
Anorectic Agents Currently Employed for the Treatment of Obesity in the United States[a]

Generic Name	Proprietary Name	DEA Schedule[b]
d,l-Amphetamine	Benzedrine and others	II
Methamphetamine	Desoxyn and others	II
Phenmetrazine	Preludin	II
Phendimetrazine	Plegine	III
Benzphetamine	Didrex	III
Chlorphentermine	Pre-State	III
Clortermine	Voranil	III
Mazindol	Sanorex	III
Fenfluramine	Pondimin	IV
Diethylpropion	Tenuate, Tepanil	IV
Phentermine	Fastin, Ionamin (resin)	IV

[a] From Bray GA (ed): *Obesity in America*. DHEW publ no. (NIH) 79-359. Washington, DC, US Government Printing Office, 1979.
[b] Drug Enforcement Administration: The schedules of the Controlled Substances Act are numbered in order of decreasing potential for abuse; drugs in Schedule II (amphetamine, methamphetamine, and phenmetrazine) are the most restricted.

Table 76.7.
Drugs of Unproved Efficacy or Safety in the Treatment of Obesity[a]

Human chorionic gonadotropin
Cholecystokinin
Glucagon
Indomethacin
Biguanides
Neomycin, cholestyramine
Diuretics, laxatives
Bulk fillers (methylcellulose)
L-Dopa
Hydroxycitrate
Amylase inhibitors
Thyroid hormones

[a] Adapted from Bray GA (ed): *Obesity in America*. DHEW publ no. (NIH) 79-359. Washington, DC, US Government Printing Office, 1979.

effects probably result from activation of serotonergic pathways. In a detailed analysis of the safety and efficacy of this group of drugs, the Food and Drug Administration has examined clinical data from nearly 10,000 patients reported in a large number of double-blind and two-drug comparison studies. At the end of 20 weeks, patients on drug and placebo had equal dropout rates, while patients taking drugs averaged about ½ pound (0.25 kg)/week greater weight loss. Moreover, there were no significant differences in weight loss when any drugs in this class were used. Intermittent therapy (2 to 4 weeks on, 1 to 2 weeks off) was often as effective as uninterrupted treatment, except with fenfluramine, which sometimes led to depression after the drug was stopped.

It should be noted that the above data from the Food and Drug Administration represent the analysis of pooled results of group performance, averaged over many weeks, using fixed dosages of drugs. It is evident, however, that individual patients exhibit considerable variations in short and long term responsivity to these drugs, and that patients often derive improved benefit, and avoid tolerance to the drug, after even small increases in their dosages. Thus, there seems to be a role for the judicious use of these anorexigenic agents in carefully selected patients followed in medically supervised, comprehensive, therapeutic programs that include diet, exercise, etc.

Although the most frequent side effects of the anorexigenic drugs are insomnia and dry mouth, and, for fenfluramine, depression and diarrhea, the major obstacle to their more widespread use is their potential for inducing physical and/or psychological dependence.

Table 76.7 lists other drugs, purported to promote weight loss, which are of unproved efficacy or safety in humans and should not be used in the management of obesity.

Surgical Therapy

Because of the increased morbidity and mortality associated with extreme degrees of obesity, and the generally unsatisfactory results produced by more conservative therapies, several surgical techniques have been devised to effect substantial weight loss in massively obese patients. Although some controversy exists regarding optimal selection criteria, surgery should in general be reserved for psychologically stable, motivated patients with (a) massive obesity (usually 100 pounds (45 kg) or more above ideal body weight) and repeated failures on strict diet and other therapies; (b) severe medical consequences of obesity (e.g., hypertension, diabetes mellitus, hyperlipidemia, orthopaedic problems) refractory to conventional therapy alone; and (c) unremitting, severe obesity-related despair and loss of self-esteem.

Until recently, the most frequently used procedure was *jejunoileostomy*, performed by anastomosing the distal jejunum to the terminal ileum either as an end-to-side or end-to-end procedure; in the latter approach, the defunctionalized bowel was drained with an ileocolonic anastomosis. The major benefits from successful surgery have been (a) permanent (if no reanastomosis) weight loss varying from 10 to 15 to 100 kg within 1 to 3 years postoperatively; this weight loss resulted primarily from a marked decrease in food intake (despite normal appetite), and only secondarily from an iatrogenic chronic malabsorption syndrome; (b) substantial improvement in blood pressure, hyperinsulinemia, and glucose intolerance, hyperlipidemia, *etc*; and (c) dramatic improvement in sense of well-being and self-esteem.

Unfortunately, the list of adverse effects associated with the intra- or postoperative course of jejunoileostomy patients has grown progressively more formidable. Even in large medical centers with experienced personnel, the overall mortality rate following surgery has varied from 3 to 5%. Serious perioperative complications have included pulmonary embolus, renal failure, wound infection, gastrointestinal bleeding, and pancreatitis. Among the adverse long term effects have been chronic diarrhea and flatulence, malabsorption with electrolyte and vitamin imbalance, cholelithiasis, urinary tract stones (calcium oxalate), hyperuricemia, polyarthralgias, intestinal bacterial overgrowth (pseudo-obstructive megacolon and bypass enteropathy), and progressive hepatic dysfunction leading to hepatic failure. In one large series (15) 58% of patients experienced potentially life-threatening complications or major reoperations; 17% of patients required surgical reversal of reanastomosis, usually because of severe hepatic cirrhosis and failure.

Gastric bypass surgery and its variants (e.g., gas-troplasty), currently more popular than jejunoileostomy (2, 22), induce significant weight loss by promoting decreased oral food intake while preserving normal gastrointestinal absorptive and digestive function. In the gastric bypass procedure, the proximal 10% of the stomach is fashioned into a 25- to 50-ml pouch by anastomosis to the jejunum through a 0.9- to 1.2-cm channel, thus producing rapid gastric filling, slow emptying, and prolonged satiety. One year postoperatively, weight loss in one review of approximately 1500 reported patients averaged 30 to 35% of baseline weight, with one-third of patients losing 50 kg or more. Although carbohydrate and bile acids are absorbed normally after gastric bypass, glucose intolerance and hyperlipidemia (especially hypertriglyceridemia) are, nonetheless, substantially improved; in addition, liver function does not worsen and malabsorption, electrolyte and vitamin imbalance, and kidney stones do not occur. By taking frequent small feedings of high caloric foods, it is possible for patients to "outeat" the bypass. Within the first postoperative month, vomiting occurs two to three times weekly in nearly 65 to 70% of patients. However, this complication becomes progressively less frequent, so that by 2 years postoperatively, it occurs in fewer than 10% of patients. Other complications of the procedure include channel ulcers or obstruction, bile reflux, and the dumping syndrome. In centers with experienced personnel, the overall mortality rate has been reduced from 3 to 1%, but remains as high as 8 to 10% in patients over 50 years old. Reoperation necessitated either by surgical complications or unsatisfactory weight loss appears to be uncommon, and "takedown" of the gastric bypass has been described in fewer than 1% of patients. The major variant of the gastric bypass, the gastroplasty (2), involves creation of a 0.9- to 1.2-cm stoma separating a 25- to 30-ml gastric pouch from the distal stomach. Thus, the distal 80 to 90% of the stomach is no longer excluded from the flow of nutrients, and gastrointestinal continuity is maintained.

Although more research is needed to determine the long term efficacy and safety of gastric bypass surgery and its variants, it appears that these procedures may be of benefit in the treatment of selected morbidly obese patients. In contrast, the striking complication rates associated with jejunoileal bypass procedures militate strongly against use of this technique in all but the most extreme instances.

PREVENTION OF OBESITY

As is evident from the preceding discussion, psychological and sociocultural factors play prominent roles in the development and maintenance of nearly all types of obesity. Since the long term results of therapy for both mild to moderate and morbid obesity are so unsatisfactory, much more attention should be paid to prevention of excess body fatness.

The finding that behavior modification techniques can benefit not only individual obese patients, but also groups of such people, even in commercially run weight-reducing programs, is provocative and suggests that this approach to weight reduction may have much wider application. The ability to modulate community awareness of, and responsivity to, the need for maintenance of, optimal weight has been proved in several large scale community studies, including that of the Stanford Heart Disease Prevention Program, which succeeded in a highly coordinated effort to decrease various of the risk factors of cardiovascular disease in three demographically matched communities (12).

Stunkard has suggested a variety of new, imaginative approaches to obesity prevention that could be initiated, singly or in combination (31). For example, organized industry, given the proper (financial) incentive, could (a) increase the number and availability of quality, commercially run weight reduction programs and provide data regarding their short and long term efficacies; (b) develop new, more nutritious low calorie food products; (c) offer a wide variety of reasonably priced health foods throughout the general restaurant and food service (e.g., vending machines) industries; (d) increase, perhaps with aid from the sporting goods industry; the number of health and sports clubs; and (e) promote widespread improvement in general health habits by decreasing life insurance premiums for individuals who maintain normal body weight, blood pressure, etc. Analogous untapped potential for fostering good general health patterns, including the maintenance of optimal body weight, resides in other influential segments of our society, such as the media, education establishment, government, work site, and various volunteer agencies.

General References

Bray, GA: The obese patient. In Smith LH (ed): *Major Problems in Internal Medicine*, Philadelphia, WB Saunders, 1976, vol 9.
> Major text, comprehensive and lucidly written.

Bray, GA (ed): *Obesity in America*, DHEW publ no. (NIH) 79–359. Washington, DC, US Government Printing Office, 1979.
> Valuable resource, summary of NIH symposium.

Buchwald H (ed): Morbid obesity. *Surg Clin North Am* 59: no. 6, 1979.
> Good account of a multidisciplinary approach to the extremely obese patient.

Greenwood, MRC (ed): Obesity. In *Contemporary Issues in Clinical Nutrition*, New York, Churchill Livingstone, 1983, vol. 4.
> Excellent reviews of new directions in obesity-related research and treatment.

Stunkard, AJ (ed): *Obesity*. Philadelphia, WB Saunders, 1980.
> An important, comprehensive clinical text.

Specific References

1. Amatruda JM, Biddle TL, Patton ML, Lockwood DH: Vigorous supplementation of a hypocaloric diet prevents cardiac arrhythmias and mineral depletion. *Am J Med* 74:1016, 1983.
2. Andersen T, Backer OG, Stokholm KH, Quaade F: Random-ized trial of diet and gastroplasty compared with diet alone in morbid obesity. *N Engl J Med* 310:352, 1984.
3. Andres R: Mortality and obesity. The rationale for age-specific height-weight tables. In Andres R, Hazzard WR, Bierman, E (ed): *Principles of Geriatric Medicine*. New York, McGraw-Hill, 1985.
4. Beutler E, Kuhl W, Sacks, P: Sodium-potassium-ATPase activity is influenced by ethnic origin and not by obesity. *N Engl J Med* 309:756, 1983.
5. Bjorntorp, P: Effects of age, sex and clinical conditions on adipose tissue cellularity in man. *Metabolism* 23:1091, 1974.
6. Bray GA, Kral JG, Bjorntorp P: Hepatic sodium-potassium-dependent ATPase in obesity. *N Engl J Med* 304:1580, 1981.
7. Bray GA, Teague RJ: An algorithm for the medical evaluation of obese patients. In Stunkard AJ (ed): *Obesity*. Philadelphia, WB Saunders, 1980.
8. *Build Study 1979*: Chicago, Society of Actuaries and Association of Life Insurance Medical Directors of America, 1980.
9. Carney RM, Goldberg AP: Weight gain after cessation of cigarette smoking: a possible role for adipose-tissue lipoprotein lipase. *N Engl J Med* 310:614, 1984.
10. DeLuise M, Blackburn GL, Flier JS: Reduced activity of the red-cell sodium-potassium pump in human obesity. *N Engl J Med* 303:1017, 1980.
11. Evans DJ, Hoffmann RG, Kalkhoff RK, Kissebah, AH: Relationship of androgenic activity to body fat topography, fat cell morphology and metabolic aberrations in premenopausal women. *J Clin Endocrinol Metab* 57:304, 1983.
12. Farquhar JW, Maccoby N, Wood PD, *et al*: Community education for cardiovascular health. *Lancet* 1:1192, 1977.
13. Garrow JS: Luxuskonsumption, brown fat and human obesity. *Br Med J* 286:1684, 1983.
14. Genuth SM, Castro JH, Vertes V: Weight reduction in obesity by outpatient semistarvation. *JAMA* 230:987, 1974.
15. Haverson JD, Wise L, Wazna MF, Ballinger WF: Jejunoileal bypass for morbid obesity. A critical appraisal. *Am J Med* 64:461, 1978.
16. Health Services and Mental Health Administration: *Ten State Nutrition Survey 1968–1970*. DHEW publ no. (HSM) 72-8130. Washington DC, US Government Printing Office, 1972.
17. Hirsch J, Batchelor, B: Adipose tissue cellularity in human obesity. *Clin Endocrinol Metab* 5:299, 1976.
18. Hubert HB, Feinleib M, McNamara PM, Castelli WP: Obesity as an independent risk factor for cardiovascular disease: a 26 year follow-up of participants in the Framingham heart study. *Circulation* 67:968, 1983.
19. Keys A (ed): *Coronary Heart Disease in Seven Countries*. American Heart Association Monograph No. 29, 1970.
20. Kissebah AH, Vydelingum N, Murray R, *et al*. Relation of body fat distribution to metabolic complications of obesity. *J Clin Endocrinol Metab* 54:254, 1982.
21. Kolterman OG, Insel J, Saekow M, Olefsky J: Mechanisms of insulin resistance in human obesity: evidence for receptor and postreceptor defects. *J Clin Invest* 65:1272, 1980.
22. Kral JG: Surgical therapy. In Greenwood MRC (ed): *Obesity*. Contemporary Issues in Clinical Nutrition. New York, Churchill, Livingstone, 1983, vol 4.
23. Krotkiewski M, Bjorntorp P, Sjostrom L, Smith U: Impact of obesity on metabolism in men and women—importance of regional adipose tissue distribution. *J Clin Invest* 72:1150, 1983.
24. Lantigua RA, Amatruda JM, Biddle TL, *et al*: Cardiac arrhythmias associated with a liquid protein diet for the treatment of obesity. *N Engl J Med* 303:735, 1980.
25. Larson B, Svardsudd K, Welin L, *et al*: Abdominal adipose tissue distribution, obesity, and risk of cardiovascular disease and death: 13 year follow-up of participants in the study of men born in 1913. *Br Med J* 288:1401, 1984.
26. Metropolitan Height and Weight Tables, 1983: *Stat Bull Metrop Life Found* 64 (Jan–June):2, 1983.
27. Schwartz RS, Brunzell JD: Increase of adipose tissue lipoprotein lipase activity with weight loss. *J Clin Invest* 67:1425, 1981.

28. Seltzer CC: Some re-evaluations of the build and blood pressure study, 1959, as related to ponderal index, somatotype and mortality. *N Engl J Med* 274:254, 1966.

29. Simopoulos AP, Van Itallie TBV: Body weight, health, and longevity. *Ann Intern Med* 100:285, 1984.

30. Society of Actuaries: *Build and Blood Pressure Study.* The Society, Chicago, 1959, vol 1.

31. Stunkard AJ: Obesity and the social environment: current status, future prospects. *Ann NY Acad Sci* 300:298, 1977.

32. Stunkard AJ, d'Aquili E, Fox S, Filion RDL: Influence of social class on obesity and thinness in children. *JAMA* 221:579, 1972.

33. Van Itallie, TB: Liquid protein mayhem. *JAMA* 240:144, 1978.

34. Wermuth BM, Davis KL, Hollister LE, Stunkard AJ: Phenytoin treatment of the binge-eating syndrome. *Am J Psychiatry* 134:1249, 1977.

CHAPTER SEVENTY-SEVEN

Common Problems in Reproductive Endocrinology: Hypogonadism, Gynecomastia, Impotence, Hirsutism, Galactorrhea, Frigidity, Menopause, Menstrual Abnormalities

S. MITCHELL HARMAN, M.D., PH.D., J. COURTLAND ROBINSON, M.D., M.P.H., AND MARC R. BLACKMAN, M.D.

Few general physicians feel comfortable or competent with sexual and reproductive medicine. This is in part because neither medical school nor postgraduate training has given sufficient emphasis to this subject to engender the confidence that comes with familiarity. Thus, most physicians view complaints involving the reproductive system as esoteric or rare, and hence the province of the specialist (*i.e.*, endocrinologist, urologist, or gynecologist). Also, the subject of sex, although more openly dealt with than in former years, still may produce feelings of embarrassment in both patient and physician.

In fact, sexual and reproductive dysfunction is not rare in the general population. Nearly 50% of men will experience one or more periods of impotence between the ages of 20 and 50 (8); as many as 10% of married couples will have difficulty with conception; and approximately 1 in 400 male births will have Klinefelter's (XXY) syndrome (7).

Furthermore, the new freedom with which sex and reproduction are discussed socially and treated in the popular media, and the advent of scientific investigation of human sexuality have altered the expectations of the patient population. "Normal" sexual function is now an objective of many men and women and dysfunction is legitimately viewed as a health problem. Such problems are now more likely to be brought openly to a physician than in former times, when reticence and modesty were the social norm. Thus it is important that the generalist be familiar with the major disorders of reproductive function and have adequate knowledge of the points of history, techniques of physical diagnosis, and modes of laboratory investigation to allow him to distinguish patients who require reassurance or can be treated simply in the office from those who need referral to a specialist for more complex testing and therapy.

SEXUAL AND REPRODUCTIVE PHYSIOLOGY

Levels of Sexual Differentiation

The sexual differentiation of individuals can be viewed as a continuum proceeding in time from conception to adulthood and in biological "depth" from genetic to social and psychological as follows: (a) *genetic sex* is determined at conception when the egg, bearing an X chromosome, is fertilized by a sperm bearing either a Y (XY = male) or X (XX = female) chromosome. The genetic sex determines (b) *gonadal sex*—the development of an ovary or testis from the undifferentiated primitive gonad. (c) *Primary sex*—the embryonic testis secretes testosterone, which in turn causes the development of a penis and scrotum. In the absence of a testis the embryo develops a uterus and fallopian tubes, and, without androgen, female external genitalia form, so that the primary sex is female. The primary sex characteristics identify the individual's sex at birth. (d) *Secondary sex* changes occur at puberty and are the result of greatly increased secretion by the gonads of sex steroid hormones. In males growth of body and pubic hair, beard growth, increase in muscle mass, deepening of voice, and onset of male libido with ejaculations and increased frequency of erections are characteristic effects of testosterone. In the female, rounding of body contours with breast growth and subcutaneous deposition of fat in the hips and buttocks, and also the onset of menses, are effects of cyclic estrogen secretion, while growth of pubic and axillary hair and probably libido are manifestations of adrenal androgen secretion. Both sexes experience a spurt of body growth at puberty, which is then followed by closure of epiphyses and cessation of growth of long bones. It is the hormone-dependent secondary sex characteristics which provide clues to adult sexual identity and which form the underpinning of (e) *tertiary sex* which is the way in which an individual identifies him or herself. There are few mammalian species whose level of sexual dimorphism is as extreme as that of humans. This is reflected by the fact that our identification as man or woman is crucial to balanced psychological and social function and is a critical component of our self-image. The physician must bear in mind that any change which seems to alter a patient's masculinity or femininity is perceived as profoundly threatening and has power to harm well beyond its biological manifestations.

Male Reproductive Physiology

Activity of the male reproductive system is regulated by the hypothalamus which produces, at irregular intervals of 40 to 120 minutes, surges of secretion of a decapeptide, luteinizing hormone-releasing hormone (LHRH), into capillaries of the median eminence, which drain into the pituitary portal veins. LHRH induces pituitary gonadotropic cells to episodic secretion of two glycoprotein hormones, luteinizing hormone (LH) and follicle-stimulating hormone (FSH). FSH induces spermatogenesis in the seminiferous tubules while LH acts on the Leydig (interstitial) cells of the testis to stimulate testosterone secretion. Testosterone, the major circulating androgenic steroid, is partially bound in plasma to a protein, sex hormone-binding globulin (SHBG), which decreases its clearance rate and also serves as a testosterone reservoir. In most target cells testosterone is reduced to 5α-dihydrotestosterone which binds to specific cytoplasmic hormone receptor proteins and is translocated to the cell nucleus. Once in the nucleus the testosterone-receptor complex activates particular genes which in turn leads to specific protein synthesis and to altered cellular

activity. In addition to its masculinizing activity, testosterone also acts in concert with FSH on the seminiferous tubules to induce growth, lumen formation, and spermatogenesis. Testosterone is needed for growth of and secretion by the prostate and seminal vesicles. More general body effects include positive nitrogen and calcium balance (with bone and muscle formation) and increased function of apocrine and sebaceous glands of the skin, which often results in comedones and acne. Another important effect of testosterone is to "feed back" to the hypothalamus and pituitary to inhibit secretion of gonadotropins. Thus, the reproductive hormones form a "closed loop" autoregulated system.

Female Reproductive Physiology

The hypothalamic pituitary relationship is similar to that of males, except that the complex modulation of hormone secretion in women normally results in a cyclic rather than tonic reproductive pattern. In women LH stimulates the interstitial-thecal tissue to make androgen and, to some extent, the estrogens estradiol and estrone. In concert with FSH these steroids produce growth of ovarian follicles by proliferation of granulosa cells. Granulosa cells convert thecal androgens to estradiol and a dominant follicle emerges as the major source of estradiol secretion, while adjacent follicles undergo atresia. Rising estrogen secretion in this follicular phase of the cycle induces proliferation of the uterine endometrium, and by a "positive feedback" effect, a sudden surge of LH secretion around day 14 of the cycle. This LH surge results in ovulation. LH then induces the follicle to become a functioning corpus luteum producing both estradiol and progesterone during the latter half, or luteal phase, of the cycle. Progesterone acts to produce a secretory endometrium, rich in glycogen and, in concert with estrogen, causes a negative feedback effect which gradually reduces the secretion of LH and FSH. With loss of gonadotropic support, the corpus luteum involutes, steroid secretion diminishes, the endometrium, left without estrogen and progesterone stimulation, sloughs off as the menstrual flow, and the stage is set for the next cycle. Ovarian estradiol is the major estrogen during the reproductive period and is primarily responsible for inducing and maintaining female secondary sex characteristics. Some estrogen, mainly estrone, is formed peripherally in fat, liver, kidney, and other tissues by conversion of adrenal and ovarian androgenic precursors. The secretion of these androgens also increases at puberty.

Male and Female Hormones and Libido

The reader is referred to Chapter 18 (Sexual Disorders) for a description of the stages of the sexual response which characterize sexual physiology in men and women. It is not clear in humans precisely to what extent sex hormones influence these events. There is no doubt that men completely deprived of testosterone (*i.e.*, chemical or physical castration) experience a gradual loss (over 1 to 2 years) of interest in sex, reporting an absence of sensations of arousal in response to sexual cues (*e.g.*, female nudity) and also loss of erections and ejaculation. Many also report heightened emotional sensitivity, weepiness, and loss of aggressive interest, ability to concentrate or drive toward career goals, *etc.* Experimental evidence suggests a direct effect of testosterone on the central nervous system (6). In women, there is no such obvious relationship between libido and sex hormones, but some data exist to suggest that women are more likely to initiate sexual contact during phases of the menstrual cycle when androgen activity is highest (1), and women with androgen-secreting tumors often report heightened sex drive with increased sexual content of dreams and fantasies. It has also become apparent in recent years that the pituitary hormone, prolactin, which in women is responsible for lactation, is probably an "antisexual" hormone which reduces libido and potency in both sexes (4). In women, estrogens are necessary to maintain the vagina and the external genitalia in their mature reproductive states. In the absence of adequate estrogen, genital atrophy may result in pain on intercourse, with resultant loss of interest in sexual activity (see below).

SEXUAL AND REPRODUCTIVE DYSFUNCTION IN THE MALE

Hypogonadism

Etiologies

Failure of the testicle to secrete adequate testosterone to develop or to maintain male secondary sex characteristics and libido results in the syndrome of male hypogonadism. In order to investigate and diagnose these patients it is helpful to classify the failure as shown in Table 77.1.

Central. An example of *central, genetic, primary* hypogonadism is Kallmann's syndrome, which is characterized by hyposmia, and is due to a defect in hypothalamic LHRH secretion. *Acquired* hypothalamic failure may occur with diencephalic tumors. Pituitary hypogonadism is also *central* and usually *acquired.* Etiology may be infectious (*e.g.*, tuberculosis or mycosis), traumatic, vascular (as in infarction with pituitary apoplexy), or most commonly neoplastic (either chromophobe adenoma, or craniopharyngioma). *Central* hypogonadism may also be associated with functioning pituitary tumors, such as those which secrete prolactin (prolactinoma) or growth hormone (acromegaly). Occasionally pituitary hypogonadism is congenital and idiopathic.

Gonadal. Acquired causes of *gonadal* hypogonadism include trauma and infection (usually viral or granulomatous). Autoimmune damage to the testis may occur either alone or as part of a complex of multiple endocrine failure (Hashimoto's thyroiditis, idiopathic Addison's disease, adult onset diabetes mellitus, hypoparathyroidism, or pernicious anemia). Occasionally a varicocele will produce partial hypogonadism. Whether these entities result in *secondary* or *primary* failure depends on the time of life at which the damage occurs.

The most common cause of *genetic gonadal* hypogonadism is Klinefelter's syndrome which is due to chromosomal nondisjunction producing XXY genetic sex. These patients have very small, firm testes and gynecomastia. They usually enter puberty, but fail to progress fully and present as phenotypic males with impotence, small phallus, and, often, gender confusion. *Genetic gonadal* hypogonadism may also occur if one or more critical enzymes in the steroid synthetic pathway leading to sex hormones is miss-

Table 77.1.
Classification of Male Hypogonadism

Classification	Criteria
ACCORDING TO LOCATION OF LESION	
Central (hypothalamic or pituitary)	Gonadotropins ↓ or →
	Testosterone ↓
Gonadal (testis)	Gonadotropins ↑
	Testosterone ↓
Peripheral (failure of end organ response)	Gonadotropins ↑
	Testosterone ↑ or →
ACCORDING TO ETIOLOGY	
Genetic	History, (especially family history)
	Buccal smear, karyotype
Acquired	History, physical examination, radiology
	Evidence of infection, trauma, neoplasia, etc.
ACCORDING TO TIME OF ONSET	
Primary (failure of pubertal development)	History, physical examination
Secondary (loss of previously developed libido and secondary sex characteristics)	

ing. Usually such defects are common to the adrenal gland and testis and produce female primary sex in XY individuals.

Peripheral. Peripheral hypogonadism is always genetic and causes a continuum from complete androgen insensitivity or "testicular feminization" in which the phenotype is female (with normal estrogenization at puberty but lacking a uterus, and hence menses) through varying degrees of partial sensitivity in which midline fusion of labioscrotal structures is highly variable (Reifenstein's syndrome) producing gender confusion, and ending with minor defects such as hypospadias and cryptorchidism.

Approach to the Patient

The approach to the patient should be directed first at determining whether hypogonadism truly exists, then at its etiological classification, and finally at providing appropriate therapy and/or referral for the specific condition diagnosed.

Patient presentations. Patients are frequently brought to the attention of physicians by parents concerned with failure of pubertal onset or progression (see also Chapter 5). *Primary* hypogonadism may stem from almost any of the etiologies cited above and must be differentiated from so-called "constitutional delayed puberty" which is an idiopathic self-limited, familial condition. A strong family history of "late blooming" and beginning enlargement of the testicles are reassuring in this regard. A set of standards for pubertal development of adolescent boys is available (23) (see Chapter 5, Table 5.5). In general, any boy reaching 17 years of age without signs of pubertal onset, or who begins but does not proceed through puberty, or who has other associated signs or symptoms (e.g., severe headaches) of disease (e.g., a pituitary tumor) which produces hypogonadism deserves further investigation. Another presentation is genital intersexuality. A finding of hypospadias, cryptorchidism, or ambiguous genitalia in a patient with complaints suggesting hypogonadism should lead to further diagnostic procedures. The gradual loss of male secondary sex characteristics and libido is a third presentation of male hypogonadism. This may be so insidious as to be taken for "normal" by the patient, especially one progressing from middle toward old age, so that it is only noticed in association with the investigation of some related condition, such as hypothyroidism, adrenal failure, severe headaches, renal tuberculosis, *etc.* Finally, and probably most common, is the complaint of impotence which may be the earliest manifestation of hypogonadism, but is also seen in various other physical and psychological conditions. Impotence is discussed more completely below and also in Chapter 18.

History. A proper history should include a chronicle of pubertal progression, with time of onset of pubic hair, beard growth, voice change, growth spurts, erections, and ejaculations recorded as accurately as recollection allows. Of critical interest are loss or diminishment of libido and erections or ejaculations, slowing of beard growth, thinning of body and pubic hair, changes in the breast (*i.e.,* swelling or tenderness), and loss of aggressive impulse or drive. The presence of headaches, double vision, or reduced peripheral vision may give clues to a pituitary tumor. Symptoms of hypothyroidism, adrenal failure, acromegaly, diabetes, anemia, pulmonary disease, and autoimmune disease should be sought. A history of urological problems, cryptorchidism, hypospadias, or episodes of orchitis is important. Finally, a family history of delayed puberty or of other endocrine abnormalities may be revealing.

Physical examination. The physician should first note the body habitus and facies. Does the patient look mature or babyish, masculine or feminine? A lower body segment (greater femoral trochanter to floor) longer than the upper segment and arm span greater than height comprises "eunuchoid" proportions and suggests pubertal or prepubertal hypogonadism. Good muscle mass and axillary hair militate against long-standing hypogonadism. Male pattern baldness is an androgen-dependent process. The presence of comedones, especially in the tragus of the ear (a very common location), is a good sign of androgen activity. Complexion should be noted, since increased pigmentation suggests primary adrenal failure, and dry flaky skin, hypothyroidism. Vital signs should be taken and the presence of hypertension or of postural hypotension should be noted as possible indicators of adrenal enzyme defects or of Addison's disease. Special attention should be paid to the eyes for limitation of extraocular movements, papilledema, or restriction of visual fields, all suggestive of an intracranial tumor. Examination of the male breast should include careful palpation for the subareolar thickening and nodularity which may be the only evidence of gynecomastia (see page 1087), and squeezing of the nipple to elicit galactorrhea, which, though rare in males, is pathognomonic of a prolactinoma. Careful attention should be paid to the genitals, with observation of pubic hair pattern (which should extend up the linea alba to the umbilicus), penis size and location of urethral meatus, scrotal rugation and pigmentation, and size and turgor of the testicles. The normal adult testis should be no less than 15 ml in volume (approximately 4.0×3.0 cm) and have the resistance to palpation cf a firm ripe plum. An "overripe" softer feeling strongly suggests testicular atrophy. Careful palpation of the left side of the scrotum while the patient performs a Valsalva maneuver may reveal the presence of a varicocele; significant varicoceles are always on the left and approximately 5% of them are associated with lower testosterone production from both testes (venous drainage from the left testis crosses over to the right). Rectal examination should assess prostate size, since the prostate shrinks with testosterone deficiency. Careful neurological examination should include testing of the sense of smell to detect Kallman's syndrome.

Differential Diagnosis

The two basic hormone tests which give the most information about suspected male hypogonadism are the serum *testosterone* and *gonadotropin* measurements. These are readily available from most commercial laboratories and are generally accurate within 20%. Normal adult males will have morning serum testosterone levels not less than 300 (and usually 450 to 700) ng/dl in most laboratories. Borderline values between 250 and 350 ng/dl are suspicious. It is important that testosterone levels be determined in the morning since the diurnal variation in testosterone can produce an afternoon and evening decrement in testosterone concentration of as much as 200 ng/dl. Abnormal or suspicious determinations should be repeated at least once for confirmation since there is considerable variability both in radioimmunoassay determination and from time to time within individuals. Serum LH usually is from 2 to 30 mIU/ml and FSH from 2 to 16 mIU/ml, but different assays will have different ranges of normal. Low or *normal* LH and FSH in the presence of subnormal testosterone defines central hypogonadism. Elevated gonadotropins indicate gonadal failure. Peripheral hypogonadism is characterized by elevated gonadotropin levels and normal or elevated testosterone levels. Table 77.1 shows the male hormonal patterns typical of central, gonadal, and peripheral hypogonadism.

Further investigation of patients with proven hypogonadism should probably be undertaken by a specialist in endocrinology. Table 77.2 lists various investigative procedures and types of patients for whom they are pertinent.

Referral to a urologist for testicular biopsy may be helpful in diagnosing traumatic or infectious damage. Biopsy shows shrinkage and hyalinization of tubules in Klinefelter's syndrome. This procedure can often be done on an ambulatory basis under local anesthesia. However, it may cause hemorrhage and considerable pain and about a week is required for full recovery. Therefore, it usually should be undertaken only after at least a telephone consultation with an endocrinologist.

Therapy

There are three basic aims of therapy in patients with central hypogonadism. The first is to suppress or remove any intracranial mass whose size or extent threatens vision or brain function. This may be accomplished by neurosurgery or radiation therapy depending on the type and size of the lesion. The second aim, to suppress abnormal hormone secretion, is applicable to prolactinomas too small to threaten vision or brain function. Treatment with bromocriptine (Parlodel) a synthetic dopamine agonist, 2.5 mg, three times daily, with meals and continued indefinitely, has proven effective in lowering serum prolactin, increasing gonadotropins and testosterone, and restoring libido (4). Unfortunately, bromocriptine has a high incidence of gastroenteric side effects, with dyspepsia, nausea, vomiting, cramping, and diarrhea in up to 10 to 12% of patients. In addition, in high doses, it has been associated with symptoms of depression and bizarre dreams or nightmares. The drug should be started at a dose of one 2.5-mg tablet/day (with food or antacid) and the dosage increased by one tablet/day each week up to a maximum of three/day to obtain the desired effect. The third aim, which is to replace deficient androgen, may be necessary in either central or gonadal hypogonadism. This is best accomplished by intramuscular injection of 200 to 300 mg of testosterone enanthate in oil (such as Delatestryl) every 2 to 4 weeks. The dose may be started at 200 mg every 4 weeks, after which the dose and interval can be adjusted depending on duration of the symptomatic (libido, sexual potency) therapeutic effect. Oral androgen preparations are generally less effective. Interestingly, the mere replacement of testosterone by injection has not restored sexual competence so long as prolactin levels remained elevated. In *central* hypogonadism, three times weekly injec-

Table 77.2.
Additional Investigations Useful in the Evaluation of Hypogonadism

Type of Failure	Radiological Procedures	Hormone Measurements	Other Tests
Central	Skull film (sella)	Prolactin	Visual fields (formal)
	Polytomography	Thyroxine	Clomiphene test
	CT scan with contrast	TSH	LHRH test
	Pneumoencephalogram (rarely)	Cortisol (A.M.)	
	Cerebral angiogram (rarely)		
Gonadal	Bone age (if primary)	Thyroxine	Buccal smear
		Cortisol (A.M.)	Karyotyping
			Gonad biopsy

tions of 2000 to 4000 IU of human chorionic gonadotropin (hCG) (such as Pregnyl or Follutein) will normalize testosterone levels, generally within a month of initiation of therapy, and may also stimulate spermatogenesis. hCG is used because of its LH-like activity. Human LH is otherwise not available. Because of the requirement for more frequent injections as compared to testosterone, hCG should replace testosterone only in those patients with central hypogonadism who want to have children. Follow-up of treated patients should include questions about sexual function, assessment of habitus, beard growth, and depth of voice. Libido and potency usually return within a few weeks of initiating treatment, while secondary sex characteristics improve gradually over 6 months to a year. Determination should be made as to whether gynecomastia or prostate enlargement with symptoms of urethral obstruction are occurring as a side effect of therapy.

Gynecomastia

Importance

Significant enlargement of the male breast is a phenomenon which requires a physician's attention so that those cases with a serious hormonal and/or neoplastic etiology can be distinguished from the common benign idiopathic form.

Etiologies

Gynecomastia is common as sex steroids rise in early adolescence (up to 65% of boys age 14), but it regresses spontaneously (to less than 15%) by age 17. The incidence increases again in the twenties, remains stable around 25%, and increases again to about 60% in the fifties. This idiopathic gynecomastia is nearly always less than 5 cm in diameter and causes no symptoms (26). Neoplastic hormone secretion is a rarer but important cause of breast enlargement. Noticeable gynecomastia of > 5 cm in diameter may be the first clue to the presence of an adrenal or testicular neoplasm or to a prolactinoma. In the case of adrenal tumors there is usually, but not always, an associated Cushing's syndrome. Various malignant tumors may secrete chorionic gonadotropin, which can overstimulate testicular steroid production and thus lead, indirectly, to gynecomastia. Hypo- and hyperthyroidism have been associated with breast enlargement. The taking of exogenous estrogen either purposely (by individuals with gender confusion or with prostate carcinoma) or incidentally because of estrogenic activity of various medications (e.g., diazepam, cimetidine, spironolactone, digitalis glycosides) should always be considered. Another iatrogenic cause is peripheral conversion to estrogens of excess androgens from testosterone or hCG therapy. Gynecomastia is also common in liver failure. Finally, true gynecomastia must be differentiated from the "gynecoid" breast seen in obesity and/or old age, which contains increased fatty tissue, but not glandular breast tissue, and also from carcinoma of the male breast.

Approach to the Patient

History. The duration and age of onset of breast swelling is important. The presence of tenderness or discharge and the quality of the discharge (clear, turbid, bloody) should be noted. Any symptoms of hypogonadism (see above) should be elicited, as should symptoms of hypothyroidism (see Chapter 73) or Cushing's disease (see Chapter 74). Careful medication history and sexual history may reveal an exogenous etiology.

Physical examination. In general the examination should be the same as for hypogonadism (see above) with the addition that signs of Cushing's disease and thyroid disease should be emphasized (see Chapter 73). Deep palpation of the upper abdomen may reveal an adrenal tumor or downward displacement of the kidney by such a tumor. Careful bimanual palpation of the testicles may detect a secretory tumor (androblastoma). A useful formal system for staging breast development has been described by Marshall and Tanner (22). Briefly, at stage I there is minimal proliferation of glandular tissue just beneath the areola. At stage II a flat pad of glandular tissue spreads beyond the bounds of the areola (i.e., > 5 cm). At stage III this pad rounds up, lifting the breast area forward from the chest wall in a cone shape with the nipple at the tip. At stage IV the areola spreads laterally as subareolar gland proliferation gives the breast a "double-contoured" appearance. Finally further maturation with increase in fatty tissue results in the mature single contour of stage V (see Fig. 5.2, page 65). Examination of the breast must also be directed at differentiating between presence of breast tissue (firm, slightly lobulated, and symmetrically distributed from the nipple outward with a limited boundary); fat (softer, diffusely distributed, and with no clear separation from surrounding subcutaneous adipose); and tumor (hard, nodular, frequently tender, often fixed to skin or underlying muscle, asymmetric with regard to the nipple). Milky nipple discharge on firm squeezing suggests prolactinoma; clear or bloody discharge suggests breast cancer. Unilateral breast enlargement should increase the suspicion of neoplasia, but asymmetry is not uncommon (10 to 15%) in patients with idiopathic gynecomastia. The decision whether further investigation is required depends on the age of the patient, the rapidity of enlargement of the breast, and the degree of such enlargement. Men between 18 and 45 years of age with recent onset of rapidly enlarging mammary glands, or glandular breast tissue diameter greater than 5 cm, or with symptoms or signs suggesting hypogonadism, hypothyroidism, or Cushing's disease should receive further attention.

Diagnostic Procedures

Determinations of serum estradiol, testosterone, and gonadotropin (LH and FSH) are indicated as are serum prolactin and specific determination of serum hCG. If the serum estradiol is greater than 50 pg/ml and if the testosterone/estradiol ratio is reduced to less than 100:1, the diagnosis of estrogen-secreting testicular tumor is strongly indicated (3). Elevation of 24-hour urinary 17-ketosteroids indicates an adrenal etiology in which case adrenal hyperfunction should be investigated with the diagnosis of adrenal neoplasm in mind (see Chapter 74). A low or low normal testosterone level with elevated FSH and LH suggests the diagnosis of Klinefelter's syndrome (XXY trisomy). Elevated serum hCG should prompt a search for occult malignancy with particular attention to gonads, lungs, and gastrointestinal tract. Elevated prolactin levels could be associated with taking certain medications (especially major tranquilizers, see Chapter 13) or with adenoma of the pituitary (see Chapter 74 and Table 77.2). The possibility of hypothyroidism should be evaluated by T_4, T_3, and TSH determinations. Finally, patients with firm, nodular, unilateral enlargement should be referred for surgical biopsy of the breast.

Therapy

Drug-induced gynecomastia remits gradually (several months) if the drug can be discontinued. Treatment of primary endocrine disease (e.g., prolactinoma, adrenal tumor, hCG-secreting carcinoma, etc) should usually be undertaken by an appropriate specialist once the diagnosis is clear. When "idiopathic" gynecomastia is a cosmetic problem, plastic surgical excision of breast tissue is usually the therapeutic method of choice. It is important to bear in mind that breast development which has progressed beyond Tanner stage II (see Fig. 5.2, page 65) will never fully regress even if the proximate cause is corrected, and therefore will require surgical intervention if complete cosmetic correction is desired.

Impotence

In this section, impotence and loss of libido will be considered only as they relate to physical disorders. For more general treatment of sexual dysfunction the reader is referred to Chapter 18. Briefly, impotence is the inability to achieve or maintain erection satisfactorily to effect penetration and ejaculation. Transient or occasional impotence is common and not evidence of a medical problem, but a pattern of repeated (> 25% of opportunities) episodes over more than a month should be investigated. Impotence may or may not be accompanied by loss of sexual desire, depending on the etiology.

Etiologies

A disorder of any of the systems which maintain the sexual response and apparatus may lead to impotence: (a) psychological (see Chapter 18); (b) vascular—diminished blood supply to the pelvic area (e.g., aortic atherosclerosis or peripheral vascular disease) may result in impotence with intact libido; (c) neuropathic—damage to the peripheral pelvic autonomic nerves (e.g., peripheral neuropathy due to diabetes mellitus or heavy metal poisoning) or damage to the central nervous system (e.g., spinal injury due to tumor, trauma, or multiple sclerosis, or brain damage from a variety of causes) may inhibit or obliterate the sexual response; (d) toxic—various drugs, especially alcohol and opiates, can acutely and chronically diminish sexual ability (other medications affecting the autonomic and central nervous system, especially tranquilizers and all sympatholytic antihypertensives, may be associated with impotence); (e) debilitative—various severe and chronic medical illnesses (e.g., malignancy, renal failure) are commonly accompanied by loss of sex drive and/or impotence; and (f) endocrine—hypogonadism (see page 1084) and prolactinoma (see page 1084) have been discussed as causes of impotence. Other endocrine diseases frequently producing reduced sexual function are hyper- and hypothyroidism, Cushing's syndrome, and acromegaly. In one series of patients referred to a major diagnostic center for persistent symptoms without apparent psychiatric etiology, 35% were found to have endocrine disorders (30).

Approach to the Patient

History. The duration of symptoms, the frequency with which intercourse is attempted, and the percent of attempts ending in erectile failure should be recorded in order to determine whether the impotence is absolute or relative and if it is progressing. Impotence unaccompanied by loss of libido suggests a neurological or vascular problem, whereas loss of interest in sexual activity is consistent with either hypogonadism or a psychological etiology. Normal men frequently awaken in the morning with an erection. This is a local response to a full bladder and detumesces with urination. Preservation of morning erections is evidence against vascular or neuropathic disease; however, in the cited series (30) 14% of patients with an endocrine etiology still had morning erections. A history of medication use and substance abuse should be diligently sought. The physician should also ask about symptoms of hypo- or hyperthyroidism, Cushing's disease, and diabetes, peripheral neuropathy (paresthesia, hyperesthesia, burning or shooting pains) or central nervous system disease, and vascular disease (claudication, angina, cold extremities, skin ulcers).

Physical examination. The physical examination should pay particular attention to the manifestations of hypogonadism described above (page 1085), to signs of thyroid or adrenal disease (Chapters 73 and 74) and also signs of peripheral vascular disease (peripheral pulses, skin temperature, skin atrophy or hair loss) (Chapter 87) and central or peripheral neuropathy (Chapter 84).

Diagnostic Procedures

Hormone determinations should be used to investigate for hypogonadism (page 1086) or prolactinoma (page 1084). If historical or physical findings lead to a suspicion of thyroid or adrenal disease, appropriate tests should be undertaken (Chapters 73 and 74). A fasting blood sugar should always be obtained. If peripheral neuropathy seems a likely etiology, this can often be confirmed by referral to a urologist for bladder manometrics and to a neurologist for nerve conduction velocity measurements (see also Chapter 84). Diagnosis of vascular causes may require Doppler estimation of penile blood flow and/or selective angiography. Measurement of nocturnal penile tumescence in a sleep laboratory may also be useful.

Therapy

Therapeutic efforts should be directed at the specific entity underlying the impotence, whenever one can be found. Psychological impotence may respond to various therapeutic modalities depending on its severity and associated problems (see Chapter 18). Vascular causes may require revascularization by surgery or implantation of a penile prosthesis. Neuropathic impotence is occasionally reversible with removal of the inciting lesion (e.g., spinal cord tumor) but, if irreversible, may also be treated with an implantable penile prosthesis, though results will vary depending on whether the spinal ejaculatory center or afferent pathways are damaged. Drug-induced impotence will usually be reversed by discontinuation of the offending agent. Therapy of hypogonadism has been discussed (see page 1086). If sexual function does not improve within 6 weeks after specific therapy for an organic cause has been instituted, consideration should be given to the possibility that the experience and expectation of sexual failure are inhibiting the response even though the primary etiology is no longer present. Such "secondary" psychological impotence may respond to psychological or behavioral therapy (see Chapter 18).

Aging

A series of investigations conducted from 1966 to 1976 found that men's testosterone levels declined with age and protein binding of testosterone to sex hormone-binding globulin increased with age, resulting in a profound decrease in mean free (bioavailable) testosterone. These changes were accompanied by an increase in circulating estrone and estradiol and in gonadotropins (11). More recent work, in which older men were carefully selected to match the younger men in terms of health, obesity, alcohol intake, social class, *etc* revealed only

an increase in gonadotropins and minimal increase in SHBG but no change in total or free sex steroids with age (12). Thus, there does not appear to be "male menopause" in healthy middle class American men. Despite the stability of serum testosterone and other sex steroids, these same men, and men in many other studies, have reported a steady decrease both in sexual appetite and ability with decreases in frequency of intercourse from an average of 2.6 events/week to less than 2/month by age 70 to 75 (24). This decrease cannot be blamed on hypogonadism, but probably reflects changes in other (i.e., nervous and vascular) systems occurring with age. There are no satisfactory scientific data to support a beneficial effect of administration of androgens in aging men whose testosterone levels are normal. Until and unless such data become available, this practice should be discouraged. Older men with abnormally low testosterone levels should be investigated in the same way as are patients with suspected male hypogonadism (see page 1085) and treated appropriately.

SEXUAL AND REPRODUCTIVE DYSFUNCTION IN WOMEN

Common Problems

Hirsutism and Virilization

Growth of coarse dark hair (terminal hairs) in various body areas (except the scalp and eyebrows) depends on the action of androgens. The pattern of appearance of hair reflects the relative sensitivity of different skin zones to androgen effect. While pubic and axillary hair appear in both sexes, further hair growth diverges due to different androgen levels. Although male patterns vary, maximum expression of androgen effect includes terminal hair development over the face, limbs, chest, superior pubic triangle, linea alba, and back. In those carrying genes for "male pattern baldness," high levels of androgens are also associated with loss of scalp hair, first at the temporal hairline and later at the crown.

Most women (80%) develop some dark hair growth over the legs and forearms without much facial hair, while about one-third have some hair on the chest or extending along the linea alba. Abnormally high levels of plasma androgens can result in the male distribution of hair growth, the state of "hirsutism." Very high levels of androgen production also lead, over time, to virilization with increased muscle mass and decreased subcutaneous fat in hips and breasts ("male habitus"), clitoral enlargement (> 2.0 cm), deepening of voice, male pattern baldness, development of acne, and malodorous perspiration.

Excess body hair without signs of virilization is termed "simple" hirsutism. Hirsutism with virilization is rare and almost always is due to adrenal or ovarian tumor, congenital adrenal hyperplasia, or male pseudohermaphroditism. Therefore, virilized patients should be referred directly to an endocrinologist.

Hirsutism without virilization. Although simple hirsutism may be an early manifestation of Cushing's syndrome or an adrenal or ovarian neoplasm, most cases will fall into a group termed "idiopathic" or "constitutional." The prevalence of simple hirsutism has been estimated to be as high as 10% of adult North American women (25). This typically develops during the late teens, although slow progression may not produce troublesome amounts of hair for 10 years after onset of menses. In half to two-thirds of these patients somewhat excessive ovarian production of androgens (testosterone and/or androstenedione) is demonstrable, and is usually associated with oligomenorrhea and decreased fertility. Ovarian structure may show hyperthecosis or polycystic ovarian disease. The combination of hirsutism, obesity, acne, amenorrhea, and polycystic ovaries is known as the Stein-Leventhal syndrome. These individuals produce excessive quantities of estrogen precursors (testosterone and Δ^4-androstenedione) and normal quantities of estrogen.

In perhaps half of all cases of simple hirsutism, elevated serum testosterone is not demonstrable, but recently, about one-half of these cases have been shown to have increased plasma "free" (*i.e.,* nonprotein-bound) testosterone due to reduced sex hormone-binding globulin. Increased hair follicle conversion of testosterone to the more potent dihydrotestosterone has been demonstrated in some of the remaining cases and other causes of increased sensitivity of hair follicles to androgens have been postulated.

Racial and ethnic factors are also important determinants of hair growth. Women of Asian ancestry and Caucasian women of northern European origins usually have relatively little facial or extremity hair. In contrast, Caucasian women of Mediterranean origins frequently develop mustache, beard, or sideburn hair. The immediate family history is also important (*e.g.,* hirsutism in an individual of Mediterranean origins with a strong family history is most unlikely to require laboratory studies). The timing of onset is also important. Sudden develpoment of hirsutism, many years after onset of menses, is likely to be due to tumor.

Transitory hirsutism may occur during pregnancy and occasionally during menopause. A number of pharmacological agents can produce hirsutism, including glucocorticoids, phenytoin (Dilantin), minoxidil, diazoxide, and phenothiazines. Drug-induced hirsutism is characterized by the fact that increased hair growth is not limited to the androgen-sensitive areas of the skin. Rare cases include chronic local skin trauma and porphyria cutanea tarda.

Differential diagnosis. A careful ethnic and family history is essential. The temporal evolution of the process should be noted, including the menstrual history. On physical examination one should carefully note the distribution and density of terminal hairs in the sideburn and mustache areas, the periareolar and midsternal regions, and over the back and buttocks. Particular attention should be paid to the pattern of pubic hair. In the female the pubic hair forms an inverted triangle in the inferior pubic region only. The male escutcheon is a rhomboid space with terminal hairs filling the superior pubic triangle and extending up the linea alba to the umbilicus. A male type escutcheon in a female is a good presumptive sign of hyperandrogenism. Physical signs of virilization (see above) should be sought. Cases with virilism need referral to an endocrinologist, while those with severe ovarian dysfunction may require the attention of a gynecologist for therapy of abnormal menstruation or impaired fertility. Finally, signs of Cushing's syndrome (in which hirsutism may occasionally be more prominent than the classic changes) should also be sought.

The decision to proceed with laboratory testing depends on the severity of the hirsutism. Laboratory studies can be performed sequentially, if financial considerations are dominant, or simultaneously. Plasma testosterone, which is of ovarian and rarely adrenal origin, is measured first. Normal serum testosterone suggests idiopathic hirsutism and excludes major ovarian disorders. Not excluded are mild cases of ovarian hyperthecosis with abnormal androstenedione production or decreased sex hormone binding globulin (increased "free" or bioavailable androgen). The uncovering of such borderline cases is usually not worthwhile since management would be unaffected. Also, excess production of weak androgens (*e.g.,* androstenedione, dehydroepinandrosterone) by the adrenal remains a consideration and can be confirmed by appropriate plasma assays. Large increases in serum dehydroepiandrosterone-sulfate (DHEA-S) or 24-hour urinary excretion of 17-ketosteroids (17-KS) suggests adrenal disease (neoplasia, rare enzyme deficiencies) and should be evaluated by an endocrinologist.

If the testosterone is elevated to between 85 and 200 ng/dl, a diagnosis of ovarian hyperthecosis or polycystic ovaries (Stein-Leventhal) is most likely. These patients should have determinations of serum FSH and LH. Normal values suggest ovarian hyperthecosis, while increased LH and low-normal or reduced FSH are highly suggestive of polycystic ovary disease.

Levels of testosterone greater than 200 ng/dl suggest a diagnosis of ovarian neoplasm and further diagnostic workup should be directed by specialists. This may include sonography, computerized axial tomography, and/or ovarian vein catheterization.

Therapy. The therapy of simple hirsutism is usually local and essentially cosmetic, even when there is a hormonal abnormality, because medical reduction of androgen excess does not rapidly affect the presence of existing hair and is often incomplete.

Local measures include bleaching, wax stripping, shaving, plucking (tweezing), the use of hair removal creams (depilatories), and electrolysis. Contrary to popular belief, such measures do not accelerate the growth rate of hair. Plucking may cause local infection. Wax applications or hair removal creams are effective but may be irritating and must be used with care. All of these procedures must be repeated at intervals. Electrolysis and thermolysis are effective procedures for permanent removal of hair, but are expensive and uncomfortable. Effectiveness and safety (avoidance of burns, scarring, and infection) are dependent on the technique of the operator. Referral of the patient requires that the physician be familiar with the electrologist's skill. Under the best of circumstances, electrolysis is generally successful in destroying about 50% of the follicles treated at one time. Thus, several repetitions are invariably required.

Patients on medical therapy should be cautioned not to expect rapid results, since dedifferentiation of androgenized follicles may require 6 to 18 months, even when androgen excess is totally eliminated. The major benefit to be expected is prevention of progression of the hirsutism, with variable degrees of reversal coming later as therapy is continued. Medical therapy is directed toward the suppression of androgen production. Although such therapy appears more rational when androgen excess is demonstrable, idiopathic cases may occasionally respond. Adrenal suppression, although introduced on the erroneous assumption that androgens of adrenal origin were responsible for most cases of hirsutism, is, nonetheless, effective in about one-third of cases. This seems to be due to reduction of ovarian androgen production which is either directly dependent on ACTH or indirectly dependent on ovarian conversion of circulating adrenal steroids. Adrenal suppression is directly effective in cases of congenital adrenal hyperplasia. This form of therapy is simple and usually free from side effects. Dexamethasone is given as a single dose of 0.5 mg orally at bedtime which reduces the morning peak of ACTH secretion. Signs of glucocorticoid excess are unlikely to occur, nor is chronic adrenal suppression with adrenal insufficiency a problem. Normal adrenal responsiveness is restored within a few days of discontinuation. Insomnia and appetite stimulation may occur.

The alternative form of medical therapy, suppression of ovarian androgen production with a cyclically administered estrogen-progestin combination (oral contraceptive), is effective in about one-half of cases. Estrogens also increase concentration of plasma sex hormone binding globulin, reducing the circulating free androgens. Since progestins have some intrinsic androgen-like activity on hair follicles, a combination which minimizes the content of progestational agent may be the most appropriate. Agents containing 2 mg or less of norethindrone or 0.5 mg or less of norgestrel are acceptable. When used, oral contraception should be given on the usual schedule recommended for fertility control for the particular preparation (see Chapter 93).

Disadvantages of oral contraceptives include their cardiovascular and other undesirable effects. The multiple disadvantages of administering these agents must be weighed when they are to be prescribed for an essentially benign problem. Suppression of ovarian androgen production by oral contraceptives precludes pregnancy. Thus therapy must be interrupted when fertility is desired and the drug withheld until pregnancy is terminated. Hirsutism may recur during this time. Rarely, combined adrenal-ovarian suppression may be used if neither alone is effective.

Several other agents have been used successfully for the medical therapy of hirsutism. Medroxyprogesterone acetate (Provera), 100 mg intramuscularly every 2 weeks, or 30 to 40 mg orally reduces testosterone production and interferes with testosterone action at the tissue level. A variety of side effects may be encountered and this mode of therapy is not recommended by the authors. Spironolactone (Aldactone) at a generally well tolerated dose of 25 mg twice daily, also appears to suppress ovarian androgen production and may additionally antagonize androgen action at the hair follicle (28). Cyproterone acetate is a competitive inhibitor of androgen action at the level of the hair follicle and has been used successfully outside of the United States in the treatment of hirsutism. Although none of the latter three agents is currently approved in the United States for the treatment of hirsutism, the authors believe that a trial of spironolactone therapy may be justified in more severe cases of hirsutism, unresponsive to ovarian and adrenal suppression. Contraindications to spironolactone include concomitant taking of potassium supplements or renal insufficiency, either of which may predispose to hyperkalemia.

Dysmenorrhea

Dysmenorrhea, painful menstruation, is a very common problem. It is considered *primary* when it appears within a year or two of the menarche, a problem therefore beginning in the teenage years. When the painful menstruation appears for the first time or suddenly intensifies in a mature women, it is referred to as *secondary dysmenorrhea* and is nearly always a result of a specific pathological process, such as fibroids, endometriosis, pelvic inflammatory disease, or an intrauterine contraceptive device. Therefore, in secondary dysmenorrhea, the physician should seek an initiating cause, as the problem will not resolve without control of the inciting disorder. Patients with secondary dysmenorrhea should generally be referred to a gynecologist. Typical primary dysmenorrhea consists of the development within 1 or 2 days of the onset of menstruation of either crampy or sustained lower abdominal and pelvic pain which may radiate into the legs and which may be associated with nausea, vomiting, irritability, or abdominal distension. In a few patients, symptoms may be so severe that performance of their usual daily activities is not possible. Usually the discomfort is most severe during the initial several hours and then begins to fade and is usually gone within 2 or 3 days. The episodes tend to become less severe with increasing age and often disappear spontaneously within 5 or 10 years after the menarche or after pregnancy. The pathogenesis of primary dysmenorrhea is not completely understood, but it requires ovulation and it is felt to result from excessive myometrial contractions, possibly due to an excess formation of uterine prostaglandins.

Mild forms of dysmenorrhea require only mild analgesic therapy, such as aspirin or acetaminophen, and reassurance from the physician that the symptoms reflect only uterine spasm associated with shedding of the endometrium. There are a number of preparations available without prescription which are marketed for menstrual cramps. Most are combination tablets and none are proven to be more effective than aspirin or acetaminophen alone. Examples of these combination tablets are: Femcaps (aspirin, phenacetin, citrate, ephedrine, and atropine) and Midol (aspirin, caffeine, and cinnamedrine). These preparations work best when taken promptly at or slightly before the onset of menses and continued regularly (every 4 to 6 hours), rather than when necessary for pain.

When symptoms are more severe or incapacitating, therapy with nonsteroidal anti-inflammatory agents with antiprostaglandin activity greater than that of aspirin should be tried and will be effective in approximately one-half of the patients. Ibuprofen (Motrin, 400 mg, four times/day, for 5 to 6 days) and mefenamic acid (Ponstel, 250 mg, four times/day, for 5 to 6 days) have been approved by the FDA for use in dysmenorrhea. Other nonsteroidal anti-inflammatory agents such as indomethacin (Indocin, 25 mg, four times/day for six doses) and naproxen (Naprosyn, 500 mg, two times/day for five doses) have been shown to be effective in the treatment of dysmenorrhea but have not been studied as extensively and have not yet been approved as analgesics by the FDA. These drugs are most effective if given just before menstrual flow begins and continued for 2 to 3 days thereafter. However, because of the uncertainty of the effects of these agents in early pregnancy, it is suggested that their use be delayed until the beginning of menstrual flow in those patients who are sexually active and who are not using effective means of birth control. The patient should use one agent as a trial for three cycles and then

this should be discontinued if there has been an inadequate response in controlling the symptoms. It is currently unknown whether one nonsteroidal anti-inflammatory agent might be effective when another has failed.

Oral contraceptive agents suppress ovulation and thereby dramatically control dysmenorrhea; these agents may occasionally be necessary for management of this problem when it is severe. The use of oral contraceptive agents is fully discussed in Chapter 93.

The unusual patient who does not respond to these therapies should be seen by a gynecologist for evaluation for an undetected problem causing secondary amenorrhea or to provide more experienced guidance in the drug therapy of primary amenorrhea.

Premenstrual Tension Syndrome

The premenstrual tension syndrome is an ill defined complex of signs and symptoms that occurs to some degree in approximately 30% of women of reproductive age. Symptoms include irritability and increased aggressiveness, cravings for sweet or salty foods, nervousness, depression, tearfulness, mood swings, difficulty in concentrating, headaches, fullness and tenderness of the breasts, fatigue, and abdominal bloating. A significant minority of affected women find such symptoms severely disruptive to their lives. Any or all of the symptoms may be present, and the characteristic complaints vary from patient to patient, but the hallmark of the syndrome is that these problems appear during the latter half (luteal phase) of the menstrual cycle, disappear with the onset of menstruation, and are absent during the first part (follicular phase) of the cycle.

Investigations of the etiology of this entity have not been very rewarding. No typical pattern of hormone or electrolyte changes has been found that sets symptomatic women apart from asymptomatic women. Nonetheless, it is clear that when ovarian function is suppressed (as by inhibition of pituitary function with an LHRH agonist compound), symptoms are abolished. It seems likely that the symptoms stem from an "abnormal" physical response to an essentially normal pattern of steroid hormone fluctuations during the menstrual cycle.

There is, at this time, no effective or accepted treatment for the premenstrual tension syndrome. Although progesterone supplementation, pyridoxine, minor tranquilizers, and thiazide diuretics have all been tried, their effectiveness has not been substantiated in clinical trials, nor is there a definite rationale for the use of any of these agents. Until such time as the pathophysiology of the syndrome has been better elucidated, it will remain a puzzling and frustrating clinical problem. The practitioner is advised to treat the most prominent symptoms empirically, while reassuring the patient that she is not mentally ill, but rather the victim of a common, hormonally mediated malady with no serious physical consequences.

Abnormal Vaginal Bleeding before Menopause

During the 35 to 45 years of menstruation nearly all women will have occasional variations in bleeding pattern. In women approaching the menopause, irregularity of the menstrual cycle is typical, as described below. In younger women, most changes in bleeding pattern will be of the type called dysfunctional uterine bleeding (DUB), which is defined as abnormal bleeding for which no anatomical source can be found. Most DUB is related to anovulation, generally as a manifestation of alterations in pituitary-gonadal physiology described as hypothalamic oligomenorrhea" (see below). DUB may also be seen in the hirsutism-anovulation syndrome (e.g., Stein-Leventhal syndrome). A variety of physical and emotional stresses can precipitate DUB. In a few patients, abnormal vaginal bleeding will be related to unsuspected pregnancy or to anatomical problems.

Women frequently describe abnormal bleeding first to their general physician, and will often be concerned about cancer. Therefore, it is important for the general physician to have a systematic approach to this problem. With careful history taking and a limited evaluation, a working diagnosis and plan can usually be developed in the office.

Table 77.3 lists the various causes of abnormal vaginal bleeding in the premenopausal woman.

History. The patient should be asked how the abnormal bleeding differs from that which occurs during her normal cycle in terms of volume, timing, and quality, and when the normal pattern changed. *Menorrhagia* is present when menstruation occurs at the usual time or is extended by only a few days and blood loss is greater than usual (e.g., the patient has to change pads more frequently, pads contain more blood than usual). This characteristic is consistent with DUB, leiomyomata uteri, endometrial polyps, or an underlying medical problem (e.g., hypothyroidism). *Metrorrhagia* is present when the patient has vaginal bleeding (usually spotting) between otherwise normally spaced periods. This characteristic may be found with leiomyomata, polyps, or local vulvar vaginal problems, but carcinoma of the endometrium or cervix and breakthrough bleeding related to oral contraceptives may also present this way. *Menometrorrhagia* indicates the presence of both menorrhagia and metrorrhagia. *Polymenorrhea* is present when menstruation occurs at intervals of less than 21 days. *Oligomenorrhea* is present when menstruation occurs at intervals of greater than 35 days. The latter two patterns are more commonly associated with alterations in hormone balance (i.e., DUB), often precipitated by physical or emotional stress.

The history can also provide *evidence of ovulation.* This may be very helpful since most DUB is usually associated with failure to ovulate. Features associated with ovulation include (a) mittelschmerz (mild or moderate pain in one iliac fossa at midcycle, indicating rupture of an ovarian follicle), (b) increased midcycle mucus (due to the secretory effect of progesterone), (c) premenstrual molimina (abnormal fullness, headaches, and irritability immediately preceding the onset of bleeding), (d) dysmenorrhea, and (e) a biphasic basal body temperature pattern (at time of ovulation, the temperature usually rises 1°F or ½°C and remains elevated until the onset of bleeding).

Sexually active women should be asked what type of contraception they are using and questioned regarding symptoms suggesting pregnancy. Breakthrough bleeding (metrorrhagia) is not uncommon in women using oral contraceptives, especially during the first year of use. Pregnancy-related bleeding is a problem in the first trimester, when it may be difficult to distinguish clinically whether the patient is pregnant. Almost always, the patient will have missed her period, and she may have morning sickness, frequent urination, and other early symptoms of pregnancy. Bleeding in the pregnant patient may be due to one of several conditions. *Threatened abortion* is characterized by bleeding before the loss of the fetus; this occurs in 10% of pregnancies and ultimately about half of these women will have healthy babies. *Spontaneous abortion* is characterized by intense cramping and bleeding with passage of clots. The abortion may be complete (the uterus is empty and no further management may be needed) or incomplete (partial loss of uterine contents and need for prompt attention by a gynecologist). *Ectopic pregnancy*, a life-threatening medical emergency, must be seriously considered. It is characterized by a missed period followed by abnormal bleeding which may range from spotting to heavy

---

Table 77.3.
Causes of Abnormal Vaginal Bleeding in the Premenopausal Woman

1. Dysfunctional uterine bleeding (hypothalamic idiopathic anovulation)
2. Perineal causes: bladder pathology, hemorrhoids
3. Vulvar causes: infection, laceration, tumor
4. Vaginal causes: infection, laceration, tumor, foreign body
5. Cervical causes: infection, erosion, polyp, carcinoma
6. Uterine causes: infection, polyp, leiomyomata, carcinoma, intrauterine device (IUD)
7. Ovarian causes: infection, polycystic ovary (Stein-Levinthal syndrome)
8. Pregnancy: threatened abortion, complete abortion, ectopic pregnancy
9. Oral contraceptive pills
10. Systemic medical conditions: bleeding diathesis (especially thrombocytopenia), thyroid disease, others

bleeding. There may also be associated unilateral pelvic pain.

The history should include inquiry about an *abnormal vaginal discharge* or other symptoms of pelvic infection or irritation (Chapter 94). A chronic pelvic infection may cause any of the abnormal bleeding patterns described above.

In patients with menorrhagia, polymenorrhea or oligomenorrhea, the history should include a brief inquiry about several medical conditions. Severe *thrombocytopenia* may cause menorrhagia, but coagulation abnormalities, including anticoagulant therapy, rarely cause abnormal vaginal bleeding. The patient with abnormal vaginal bleeding due to thrombocytopenia will usually have other manifestations of this problem (Chapter 50). *Hypothyroidism* may cause menorrhagia while hyperthyroidism tends to be associated with oligomenorrhea. The patient's history should therefore include a check for symptoms of thyroid disease (Chapter 73).

When *dysfunctional uterine bleeding* is suspected (absence of features of ovulation and lack of evidence for other causes), the patient should be asked about recent changes in her general health and in her daily activities. Among the factors which may precipitate DUB are diet change, weight gain or loss, emotional stress, jogging and other strenuous activities, sleep loss, mental strain, chronic medical conditions, and alcohol or illicit drug use.

Physical examination. All patients complaining of abnormal vaginal bleeding should have a pelvic examination to look for obvious anatomical causes of the bleeding. It is important not to defer the examination because of the bleeding. Hemorrhoids, vulvar conditions, vaginitis and cervicitis, cervical polyp or cervical erosion, and leiomyomata uteri are the principal anatomical problems which may be identified. Vulvovaginal and cervical sources of bleeding should be suspected especially in patients who describe metrorrhagia or postcoital bleeding.

The patient should also be checked for ecchymoses and petechiae, especially in the lower extremities, and for physical signs of thyroid disease.

Laboratory tests. A hemoglobin concentration or a hematocrit value should always be obtained, and, in an actively bleeding patient, orthostatic blood pressure and heart rate should be checked. In addition, every woman with a change in her bleeding pattern should have a Pap smear evaluated (Chapter 95). Sexually active women should always have a pregnancy test.

If the history or physical examination suggests the possibility of a bleeding diathesis, a platelet count, bleeding time, prothrombin time, and partial thromboplastin time should be obtained (Chapter 50). Thyroid function tests should be obtained if thyroid disease is suspected on clinical grounds.

Working diagnosis and managment.

ANATOMICAL CAUSES. The general evaluation described above is sufficient to identify most of the anatomical causes for abnormal bleeding in the premenopausal woman. A history of typical ovulatory symptoms increases the likelihood that the bleeding is due to an anatomical problem or a chronic medical condition. Because uterine problems (e.g., fibroid tumors, and, much less commonly, endometrial cancer) are more frequent in women over 35, these patients should be evaluated by a gynecologist if they develop *any* unexplained change in their bleeding pattern, especially if a change persists for more than two cycles. When definite pelvic disease or pregnancy is detected or suspected, the patient should be referred promptly to a gynecologist, except in the case of vaginitis or cervicitis, which may be treated by the general physician (Chapter 94). The evaluation which a gynecologist will perform for possible gynecologic cancer is described in Chapter 95.

When a primary medical condition seems to explain the patient's problem, this condition should be managed appropriately (thrombocytopenia: see Chapter 50; thyroid disorders: see Chapter 73).

DYSFUNCTIONAL UTERINE BLEEDING. For the large number of women in whom the working diagnosis is dysfunctional uterine bleeding, the general physician may elect to manage the problem himself or refer the patient to a gynecologist. The most common cause of DUB is anovulation. In this case no corpus luteum is formed so that a progesterone-primed endometrium is not produced. If levels of estrogen are fairly high, the endometrium will continue to proliferate, become hyperplastic, then break down irregularly and bleed.

When dysfunctional bleeding has been a problem for a brief period (two to four cycles), appropriate management consists of explaining the problem to the patient and having her modify obvious precipitating factors whenever this is possible. If her menorrhagia is particularly heavy and is interfering with her usual activities, the problem can be controlled promptly by prescribing a 21-day package of a combination oral contraceptive such as Ovral-21. She should be given the following written instructions: take the first three tablets immediately, then take one tablet twice daily for the next 9 days. Within 24 hours, the current bleeding will be suppressed, and she will then have withdrawal bleeding at the end of the 9-day course. If the primary stress causing her DUB is not modified, the DUB will persist, and referral to a gynecologist is appropriate.

Patients with persistent DUB, especially those in whom there is a problem of infertility, should be referred to a gynecologist or a reproductive endocrinologist. Two objective findings which help to confirm the absence of ovulation are the lack of a biphasic basal body temperature pattern described above and a failure of serum progesterone to rise during the patient's menstrual cycle. The two pieces of data should be obtained if possible before referral. DUB will occur in some women in whom these data indicate ovulation. The usual explanation is that there has not been adequate progesterone produced to promote proper shedding of the endometrium. An endometrial biopsy will often be performed by the consulting gynecologist. This biopsy can confirm either the absence of ovulation (the endometrium will be proliferative, indicating only an estrogen effect) or the presence of ovulation (the endometrium will be secretory, reflecting a progesterone effect, or it may show a mixture of proliferative and secretory changes). Depending upon these findings and additional investigations, the gynecologist will develop a management plan for the patient.

Oligomenorrhea

Gonadal dysfunction in women nearly always presents as alteration of the menstrual pattern, either irregular and infrequent menses (oligomenorrhea) or cessation of menses (amenorrhea). Oligomenorrhea (the syndrome of few or no periods) may be classified (see Table 77.4) as primary or secondary; as juvenile, feminized, or masculinized; as central, gonadal, peripheral, or exogeneous, and finally as congenital or acquired.

Primary. Primary *central amenorrhea with maturational failure* suggests idiopathic or genetic gonadotropin deficiency of pituitary or hypothalamic origin. A patient with *primary gonadal failure* is likely to have Turner's syndrome (XO sex chromosomes and no ovaries). *Primary amenorrhea with normal maturation* may be due to *peripheral* causes as simple as imperforate hymen with obstruction of menses, or as serious as congenital uterine agenesis. A

special case of this latter kind is testicular feminization (see page 1085).

Secondary. Feminized patients with *central secondary amenorrhea* may have brain tumors or anorexia nervosa, but most commonly, have hypothalamic amenorrhea, another type of central failure. Pituitary amenorrhea is usually *acquired* and is frequently accompanied by deficiencies in other hormone axes (adrenal, thyroid). Etiologies are the same as in the male (see above).

Gonadal secondary amenorrhea can be due to infection (e.g., tuberculosis), neoplasm (Krukenberg tumor—metastasis of gastrointestinal neoplasm to ovary), trauma, surgery, or an autoimmune disorder. This latter category is often associated with a syndrome of polyglandular failures (see page 1084) and is the most common cause of "idiopathic premature menopause."

Exogenous. Exogenous amenorrhea may be caused by hyper- or hypothyroidism, liver failure, or renal failure. Hypothalamic (secondary, central, acquired) amenorrhea is also often exogenous in that there is a proximate cause such as weight loss, vigorous exercise, pathological obesity, or severe stress, as in grief or mental illness. Another form of exogenous interrruption may come from consumption of substances of abuse (opiates, alcohol) or prescribed medications (major tranquilizers, estrogens).

Galactorrhea

Galactorrhea (also see page 1097) is the production of milk (confirmed by demonstrating fat after staining the fluid with Sudan stain) by a non-nursing individual who is not recently postpartum. *Secondary central* amenorrhea is frequently (15%) accom-

Table 77.4.
Classification of Female Hypogonadism (*i.e.*, Oligomenorrhea)

Classification	Criteria
ACCORDING TO TIME OF ONSET	
Primary (no onset of menses)	History
Secondary (cessation of established menses)	
ACCORDING TO SOMATOTYPE	
Maturation failure (juvenile)	Physical examination
Feminized (normal secondary sex)	
Masculinized (hirsute, deep voice, increased muscle mass, clitoromegaly)	
ACCORDING TO LOCATION OF LESION	
Central (hypothalamic or pituitary):	Gonadotropins ↓ or →
a. Without galactorrhea	
b. With galactorrhea	
Gonadal (ovarian failure)	Gonadotropins ↑
Exogeneous (disruption of menses by drugs, stress, or illness of other than reproductive organs)	History, physical examination, various laboratory and radiological tests
ACCORDING TO ETIOLOGY	
Genetic (chromosomal or familial)	History, buccal smear, karyotype
Acquired (infectious, neoplastic, traumatic, surgical, hemorrhage or infarction, autoimmune)	History, physical examination, radiology, other special procedures

panied by galactorrhea. Galactorrheic amenorrhea is often (42%) due to the presence of a prolactin-secreting pituitary adenoma which may or may not be readily detectable (macro versus microadenoma) (18). Other causes of galactorrheic amenorrhea include medication (INH (isoniazid), phenothiazines), recent pregnancy, hypothyroidism, and idiopathic hypothalamic dysfunction. It is not uncommon for a woman who has nursed to have mild persistent galactorrhea (without amenorrhea) for up to 5 years after weaning. In these cases prolactin levels are normal (< 30 ng/ml).

Approach to Women with Reproductive Endocrine Dysfunction

The diagnostic approach to female reproductive disturbances is aimed at classifying the kind of disorder (see above), identifying or eliminating specific disease entities which require medical or surgical treatment, and, having done this, determining to what extent the remaining symptoms represent a problem to the patient and treating these problems appropriately.

History

The physician should determine whether the problem is primary or secondary. A chronicle of pubertal events should be recorded including earliest budding of breast tissue (thelarche), pubic hair darkening and lengthening (pubarche), onset of menstrual flow (menarche), and time of growth spurt and its cessation. A menstrual history includes the average interval between menses, their regularity and when irregularity developed, date of last period and previous period before that, the duration of flow and its magnitude, the presence of ovulatory pain (mittelschmerz), premenstrual tension, and dysmenorrhea. The latter three findings suggest ovulatory cycles. A pregnancy and nursing history (mature and premature deliveries, abortions, success with and duration of lactation, and living children's ages) and history of gynecological surgery (including dilation and curettage) are pertinent. A history of breast changes (swelling, tenderness, discharge) should be determined. The physician should ask whether the patient is troubled by growth of excessive hair, and if so, the duration of symptoms, the location and severity of the problem, and the treatment used, if any. Also of interest are symptoms of masculinization: increased libido with greater sexual appetite or increased sexual dreaming and fantasies, voice deepening, and frontal hair loss. Symptoms of estrogen deficiency (hot flashes, vaginal discharge with dyspareunia, and breast atrophy) are important. A careful history of medication and drug use, including oral contraceptive agents, may be helpful. A further general history should include weight gain or loss, dietary habits (especially rigorous dieting), strenuous exercise (e.g., running, ballet,

gymnastics), symptoms of diabetes, adrenal or thyroid disease, and history of tuberculosis or hepatic, renal, or neurological problems. A family history should include ethnic origin and familial occurrence of reproductive and other endocrine dysfunctions (e.g., hirsutism, oligomenorrhea, hypothyroidism).

Physical Examination

On inspection the physician should note body habitus (obese or wasted, mature or child-like, masculine or feminine). The presence or absence of pubic and axillary hair, distribution of coarse dark hair on chest (periareolar, midsternal), abdomen, buttocks, and extremities, and the density of such hair must be noted. The equality of the patient's voice should be evaluated. Examination of breasts and pubic hair should include an estimate of their stage of maturity based on available standards (22) (see also Chapter 5, Fig. 5.2 and Table 5.5). Nipples should be squeezed to look for galactorrhea. On pelvic examination it is important to look for clitoromegaly (> 2.0 cm in length), state of the vaginal mucosa (dry versus moist, thick and rugated versus thin and atrophic), discharge, presence or absence and size and consistency of cervix and uterus, and also to attempt to estimate whether ovaries are enlarged (cystic) or not. In primary amenorrhea without maturation, signs of Turner's syndrome (wide set eyes, shield chest, wide set nipples, "webbing" of neck, short fourth metacarpal, and signs of aortic coarctation) should be sought. The remainder of the general physical examination (eyes, abdomen, etc) should be as described in the evaluation of male hypogonadism (see page 1085) looking especially for signs of an intracranial mass lesion and thyroid or adrenal disease.

Diagnostic Procedures

All women with secondary amenorrhea should be considered pregnant until proven otherwise (even if sexual activity is not admitted, as, in adolescence, it may not be). Specific hCG assay is the most sensitive test for pregnancy (see Chapter 93). Further testing should be delayed until pregnancy is ruled out.

Serum estrogen determinations by radioimmunoassay have now improved to the point that one can generally distinguish low normal from definitely low (values less than 40 pg/ml are suspect and less than 25 pg/ml are low), but, estrogen status may also be assessed by vaginal cytology and by the provocation of withdrawal bleeding. Cells for vaginal cytology should be obtained at the time of pelvic examination so that a maturational index can be estimated (see Chapter 94). A progesterone withdrawal test (7 days of 10 mg of medroxyprogesterone acetate (Provera) orally or a single 100-mg dose of progesterone in oil intramuscularly) will result in withdrawal bleeding within a few days (2 to 5 if oral and 7 to 10 if intramuscular) after the drug is administered if estrogen levels are adequate. If there is no bleeding, a 21-day course of estrogen (0.02 or 0.05 mg of ethinyl estradiol (Estinyl)/day) with 5 to 10 mg of medroxyprogesterone acetate (Provera) for the last 7 days should be administered. Absence of vaginal bleeding at this point indicates an absent or severely damaged endometrium, sometimes secondary to previous overvigorous dilation and curettage (Asherman's syndrome).

Serum or urinary gonadotropins are used to classify hypogonadism as gondal (elevated) or central (low or normal). The investigation of central hypogonadism should include a serum prolactin level, especially if galactorrhea is present. Prolactin values between 30 and 100 ng/ml are elevated but may be consistent with prolactinoma or hypothalamic (idiopathic) galactorrhea. Values greater than 100 ng/ml nearly always mean that a prolactinoma is present (18). Further testing should be undertaken by appropriate specialists and is similar to that outlined for patients with male hypogonadism (Table 77.2). If hirsutism is present, the serum testosterone and urinary 17-ketosteroids should be measured (see page 1090).

Therapy in Women with the Oligomenorrhea Syndrome

Absence of Menses

The mere fact of amenorrhea is disturbing to some women, but not to others. Women with idiopathic oligomenorrhea who desire regular periods can be treated with low dose estradiol plus progestin regimens in cyclic fashion as outlined below. Where fertility is an issue, appropriate referral should be made.

Galactorrhea (See Also page 1095)

Women with hyperprolactinemia can be treated by trans-sphenoid removal of an adenoma (if present) or by suppression with bromocriptine (Parlodel) 2.5 mg, two or three times a day, which treatment frequently also restores libido (see "Frigidity and Female Endocrine Dysfunction," below), suppresses lactation and restores menses and fertility. Surgery is successful in restoring menses and reducing or eliminating galactorrhea in about 80% of cases. Risks of surgery include meningitis and CSF leakage into the sphenoid sinus, or permanent damage to the pituitary gland (hypogonadism about 5%, other axes, less than 2%), as well as the usual anesthetic and hemorrhagic risks of any surgical procedure. Risks of bromocriptine therapy have been described above (page 1086). When tolerated, this agent is 85 to 90% effective.

Intracranial Tumor

If vision or brain function is threatened, surgery or radiotherapy is indicated. Recent studies have shown that bromocriptine shrinks prolactin-secreting adenomas in size by reducing the volume (but not the number) of cells, so that it may be helpful, even in patients with suprasellar extension of tumor and visual symptoms, as emergency therapy prior to surgery. If only a microadenoma is present, it may be legitimate simply to follow visual fields and serial CT scans at intervals of 6 months to 1 year and to treat hormone deficiency appropriately.

Estrogen Deficiency State

Estrogen deficiency is not a frequent occurrence in young women with central secondary amenorrhea, but may occur in some women, especially those with hyperprolactinemia (19). It may be defined by a failure to develop withdrawal bleeding after progestin administration, by plasma estrogen levels less than 25 pg/ml, and/or by failure to ovulate and menstruate after being given clomiphene citrate (Clomid) 50 to 100 mg/day for 5 days. Estrogen deficiency is invariable in gonadal hypogonadism. Symptoms, complications, and therapy are discussed in the section on menopause (see below).

Frigidity and Female Endocrine Dysfunction

Definition

As in the male, female hyposexuality can be divided into reduced sexual interest or appetite (inhibition of desire), failure of arousal (inhibition of excitement), and anorgasmia (for a more complete discussion, see Chapter 18). Discussion below will be limited to physical and especially endocrine etiologies.

Etiologies

Organic etiologies of female hyposexuality include diabetes mellitus with peripheral neuropathy, hyperprolactinemia, hypogonadism with estrogen deficiency, and organic disease of the vagina, uterus, fallopian tubes, or ovaries with resultant dyspareunia. Various endocrine (e.g., hyper- or hypothyroidism) and other systemic debilitating diseases can also cause loss of interest in sexual activity.

History

Questions should be the same as those asked of the patient with female hypogonadism (see above). Additional questions should be asked about dyspareunia. If there is pain or discomfort on intercourse, it is important to know if it occurs with attempts at penetration (local vaginal or vulvar problems) or only after deep penetration (pelvic disease—e.g., leiomyoma, endometriosis, salpingitis). The physician should determine whether there was a previous history of satisfactory sexual activity, and if so, the time and circumstances of onset of its deterioration. Careful questioning should reveal to what extent the problem is one of loss of interest, excitation (lubrication and heightened pelvic blood flow), or orgasm. A history of symptoms of diabetes or peripheral neuropathy and of thyroid, adrenal, or other serious systemic disorders should be obtained. Medication use (tranquilizers, oral contraceptives) and substance abuse (opiates, alcohol) are also pertinent.

Physical Examination

The physical examination should be conducted in the same way as for patients with female hypogonadism (see page 1096). Careful attention should be given to the genitalia, uterus, and adnexa for evidence of infection, atrophy, or neoplasia. Endometriosis is sometimes detected on rectovaginal examination by palpation of nodules in the space between the rectum and vagina (pouch of Douglas). Testing of peripheral sensation should be thorough.

Diagnostic Procedures

If evidence of hypogonadism exists, appropriate tests should be made (see page 1096). Measurement of serum prolactin level may be helpful even in patients without apparent galactorrhea or amenorrhea (see page 1097). Patients with pelvic disease should be referred to a gynecologist for further evaluation and therapy.

Therapy

Therapeutic efforts should be directed at the specific organic etiology whenever possible. Estrogen deficiency should be corrected (see below) and hyperprolactinemia should be treated surgically or medically (see above). When no organic cause is evident after careful examination, consideration of various modes of psychological diagnosis and treatment is appropriate (see Section 2, Psychiatric and Behavioral Problems).

Problems of Menopause

Definition

Menopause is the irreversible cessation of the female reproductive cycle and menses that follows from a permanent loss of ovarian response to gonadotropins. This change generally occurs spontaneously between the ages of 45 and 55 in American women, with an average age of 50. Destruction or cessation of function of the ovary prior to age 40 is referred to as premature menopause. Hysterectomy terminates menstrual bleeding, but not ovarian function, and hence, does not constitute a true menopause. In any year between 1981 and 2000, there will be approximately 30 million women of postmenopausal age (roughly one-third of the female population in the United States). Thus, an understanding of the medical problems of the menopausal period is important for all general physicians.

Physiology

Although it has long been known that the menopausal ovary is nearly depleted of primary follicles, the hormonal events of the perimenopausal period have only recently been elucidated. The work of Sherman and Korenman (29) and others has shown that after age 35 to 40 there is a tendency for serum estradiol to decrease, probably reflecting a reduction in the responsive cohort of follicles at onset of a cycle. This results in less feedback inhibition which in turn raises FSH levels and leads to a shortened follicular phase of the cycle (earlier ovulation), so that women in their late thirties may go from a regular 28- or 29-day menstrual interval to one of 25 to 27 days. In the early forties the luteal phase may also become inadequate with lower progesterone levels and early dissolution of the corpus luteum, resulting in further shortening of the cycle. Estradiol levels continue to decline. Next, anovulatory cycles and "missed" cycles, with long quiescent periods in which gonadotropins are high and estradiol very low, begin to occur. For a year or two menses are irregular and occur with reduced frequency, but occasional ovulatory cycles are seen. Finally cyclic bleeding ceases. FSH and LH levels become greatly elevated in serum and urine. Usually the FSH increase is greater. The ovary may still contain a few follicles, but these do not respond to gonadotropin. Estradiol levels become extremely low and adrenal estrone becomes the major estrogen.

Psychological Symptoms

Epidemiological and clinical studies have shown that there is not an increase in mental illness attributable to menopause and that, in particular, women who develop depression during the menopausal years do not have a distinct syndrome but rather are characterized by a previous history of depressive illness or symptoms and/or the presence of situational factors (e.g., late life divorce, the empty nest, etc) commonly associated with depressive episodes (33). There are, however, many cultural misconceptions about this period (e.g., expectations of loss of sexual interest and ability and expectations of an increased incidence of mental illness), and often these misconceptions propagate feelings of inadequacy, somatic symptoms such as fatigue, and other complaints. The organic changes of the menopause may reinforce these symptoms, and many women have had their symptoms worsened even further by the comment from a physician that the phemomenon is "an expected part of aging."

In spite of the lack of evidence that psychological symptoms accompanying menopause are due to estrogen deficiency, many women have been given estrogens for their psychological complaints. Reported benefits are probably due to a placebo effect. The physician should try to educate each patient about the menopause and should evaluate her for any underlying psychological disturbances. Women who develop significant psychological problems during the menopause should be managed appropriately, as described in the chapters in Section 2 of this book.

Estrogen Deficiency State

Ovarian estrogen production is minimal after the menopause. Ovarian interstitial and hilus cells still retain some secretory capacity, but produce mainly small amounts of testosterone and androstenedione. Most estrogen is therefore formed from peripheral conversion of androgen, 75% of which comes from the adrenal. There is evidence that this rate of conversion is greater in obese women, who therefore tend to have higher estrogen levels postmenopausally. Estrogen deficiency results in various symptomatic manifestations in approximately 70% of postmenopausal women.

Hot flashes. Nearly 50% of menopausal women complain of a sudden sensation of flushing and extreme warmth, followed by profuse sweating and sometimes shaking or tremor. These episodes occur at irregular intervals from a few to many times a day and may awaken the patient at night. In about 15% they are severe enough to limit normal daily activities. It is important to remember that this, and other menopausal symptoms, may have their onset prior to actual cessation of the menses, since estrogen levels fall progressively in the premenopausal period. Recent investigations have shown that these episodes, objectively identifiable by altered skin and core temperature and skin resistance, are closely related temporally to episodic gonadotropin secretion by the pituitary gland. They precede LH and FSH secretory rises by just a few minutes (32). LH and FSH secretory episodes are generally increased in amplitude, but not frequency during the menopause, probably reflecting derepression of neurosecretory activity of the hypothalamus by loss of estrogen feedback. It is theorized that this exaggerated excitation of neurosecretory nuclei may spread to the adjacent thermoregulatory centers in the hypothalamus, setting off the "hot flash" (which is thus a sort of "hypothalamic seizure").

Genital and breast atrophy. The female reproductive organs undergo striking changes at the time of the menopause. Pubic hair becomes sparse and lank, and may turn gray. The labia majora lose their fullness as subcutaneous adipose is withdrawn from them and the mons veneris, thus exposing the labia minora. The skin and mucous membranes of the genitalia become thin and dry. The vaginal pH becomes more alkaline as glandular secretion of glycogen is lost. This change and the mucosal atrophy may result in a chronic vaginitis with itching, discharge, and local tenderness (see Chapter 94). Many women report decreased lubrication at intercourse and complain of dyspareunia. The cervix, uterus, and fallopian tubes also shrink. Estrogen deprivation also is implicated in the relaxation of pelvic ligaments and muscles which may result in uterine or bladder prolapse and contributes to the disturbing

symptom of stress incontinence. At the same time glandular breast tissue atrophies, the breasts lose adipose and become shrunken and pendulous. There is a decrease in the erectile response of the nipple.

Osteoporosis

Loss of calcium from bone begins as early as age 35. The rate of mineral loss is highly variable, but is greater in women (about 1%/year) than men. Accelerated rate of demineralization occurs with premature menopause (or with any other cause of severe estrogen deficiency) and has been well documented in a number of studies (15). Although the exact mechanism by which estrogen deficiency leads to increased calcium loss from bone remains incompletely understood, the consequences are clear. Accompanying this process is an age-related decrease in the efficiency of calcium absorption by the gastrointestinal tract. As a result, postmenopausal women exhibit higher daily dietary calcium requirements (1500 mg/day) than do their premenopausal counterparts (1200 mg/day). Because of their common consumption of calcium-deficient diets (400 to 600 mg/day), many women are in a state of markedly negative calcium balance.

During the first 15 to 20 years after the menopause, calcium loss is primarily from trabecular bone (e.g., vertebrae), whereas later, calcium loss occurs nearly equally from trabecular and cortical bone (e.g., hip and long bones). Eventually, fractures occur. Crush fractures of the vertebral bodies predominate, causing back pain, loss of height, and stooped posture (dowager's hump). Fractures of the hip and forearm (e.g., distal radius or Colles') fractures are common. The incidence of fractures is greater in white than in black women, probably reflecting greater peak bone mass at maturity in blacks. Clinically significant fractures are 5 to 8 times more common in women than in men. Other known risk factors for osteoporosis include a sedentary life style, prolonged bed rest, chronic cigarette smoking, nulliparity, diabetes mellitus, and chronic glucocorticoid therapy.

It has been estimated that if a white woman lives to be 90 years of age she has a 32% chance of hip fracture. About 1 million bone fractures occur annually in women over 45 years of age; 150,000 are hip fractures. The death rate within 3 months of hip fracture is a staggering 12 to 20%, usually from complications of surgery and/or prolonged hospitalization. Repeated fractures are all too likely in survivors. With approximately 30 million women at risk in the United States in any year until 2000 A.D., postmenopausal osteoporosis is a public health problem of major magnitude.

Optimal, cost-effective use of sophisticated radiological techniques (photon absorptiometry and computed tomographic scanning) for diagnosing early or established osteoporosis remains controversial, and recommendations for general use of these techniques await the results of further investigation.

Endometrial Hyperplasia and Carcinoma

With loss of regular progesterone-induced maturation and subsequent shedding of the endometrium, the incidence of endometrial hyperplasia, due to the unopposed tonic effects of residual (adrenal) estrogen, begins to rise. This lesion is rarely seen in cyclic premenopausal women, but occurs frequently in young women with a pattern of irregular anovulatory bleeding since these women also lack progesterone. Hyperplasia also appears to be more common in obese postmenopausal women, probably because of increased aromatization of androgens to estrone in fatty tissue. Endometrial hyperplasia, especially the atypical adenomatous pattern, characteristic of unopposed estrogens, appears to be a precursor of endometrial carcinoma. It is therefore not surprising that the latter lesion is also more common in young anovulatory and postmenopausal obese women (17).

The incidence of endometrial carcinoma begins to rise at age 45, reaches a peak at about 0.08% (80/100,000) at age 70, and falls off thereafter. It is usually detected because of postmenopausal vaginal bleeding, is invasive (into myometrium and vessels) in only about 10% of cases, and has a relatively good prognosis if treated promptly by hysterectomy. It results in very few deaths, being relatively rare and frequently curable.

Estrogen Replacement Therapy

Benefits. It is clear that use of estrogen is highly effective, compared with placebo, in suppressing the symptoms of the "hot flash" (20). Even low doses (0.02 mg/day of ethinyl estradiol (Estinyl) or 0.625 mg/day of Premarin), which have no measurable effect on circulating serum gonadotropins, have been found effective. Such therapy is often given for 6 months to a year and then tapered; hot flashes recur in about 50% of cases, however. In this instance, a more prolonged course of low dose estrogens, cyclic or progestin-opposed estrogen therapy (see below) may be useful. Genital atrophy, vaginitis, and dyspareunia are all relieved by estrogen therapy, which may be systemic or local (by means of estrogen-containing cream). This latter form of therapy, is not necessarily advantageous in preventing systemic effects of estrogen, since estrogens are taken up through the vaginal mucosa in unpredictable but significant amounts (27). Finally, estrogen replacement has been shown to be effective in reducing calcium loss and decreased bone density (14) and also the actual number of fractures (2) in estrogen-deficient women. Thus, there is no longer any doubt that estrogens are highly efficacious in reducing the major problems associated with menopausal estrogen deficiency.

Risks. The risk of estrogen therapy of greatest current concern to the practicing physician and patient population is endometrial carcinoma (see above). A number of recent studies have demonstrated that postmenopausal estrogen therapy, as commonly practiced in the United States, *i.e.,* 0.625 to 1.25 mg of oral conjugated estrogens (Premarin) given daily without interruption, is associated, after 2 or more years of therapy, with a 6- to 8-fold increase in the incidence of endometrial carcinoma (21). However, Hulka *et al* (16) demonstrated that monthly interruption (see below) of therapy and/or use of nonconjugated estrogen reduces the relative risk of invasive carcinoma to about 1.3 (not statistically significant). Furthermore, it is apparent from other studies that the use of an oral progestin for 7 to 10 days of the cycle to mature the endometrium does not produce any excess endometrial hyperplasia or endometrial carcinoma (10, 31). It is also of interest that women treated for up to 10 years with cycles of combined estrogen-progestin for birth control have not shown an increased rate of development of endometrial carcinoma, despite the high doses of estrogen employed. Thus it appears that cyclic, progestin-opposed estrogen therapy is free of this risk. One objection to this mode of therapy is that many women will find continuation or resumption of monthly vaginal bleeding unacceptable. Another is that such bleeding will be confusing to the physician trained to assume that postmenopausal bleeding indicates disease. It can be pointed out, however, first, that continued menstruation may be a small price to pay for even partial protection from osteoporosis and its distressingly frequent complications, not to mention prevention of genital atrophy, *etc*, and, second, there is no reason why regular monthly bleeding should be any more confusing to the physician in a 70-year-old women than in a 35-year-old. In either case, it is intermenstrual spotting or unexpectedly heavy flow that should alert the physician to the necessity for investigation. Furthermore, even if this mode of therapy should result in some slight increase in the risk of endometrial carcinoma, comparison of incidences of morbidity and mortality show that endometrial carcinoma is a relatively rare and infrequently fatal disease, while osteoporotic fractures are very common and often crippling or fatal.

Although data have been presented on both sides of the issue, the best current information supports the conclusion that estrogens, whether used for oral contraception or for postmenopausal replacement therapy (13), are not associated with an increased incidence of breast cancer. In fact, a single study (9) suggests that the use of cyclic progestin in combination with estrogen by postmenopausal women may actually reduce the incidence of breast cancer. The high doses of estrogen in oral contraceptives have been shown to have a number of pharmacological side effects, which are fully discussed in Chapter

93. Because orally administered estrogens reach the liver first in high concentration, there is no dose of oral estrogen which will provide precise physiological replacement and also will avoid the potential for harmful side effects. Even though only one of the known complications (gallbladder disease) has actually been found with estrogen replacement therapy, these effects, which include increased risk of thromboembolic disease, hypertension, and atherosclerosis are a legitimate consideration. Development of a convenient method of administering systemic (rather than portal) estrogen in physiological doses cyclically for 3 weeks at a time would probably minimize these risks, but as yet such a method is not available. The physician must therefore weigh the risks and benefits in his own mind. We believe the current evidence favors the use of estrogen replacement therapy continuously after the menomenopause, especially in women with premature loss of ovaries (under age 40) and in white women, especially those at high risk for osteoporosis (see above). This therapy is contraindicated in known cases of breast cancer and probably in women with a high risk of breast cancer (see Chapter 89), and in women who have suffered from stroke, phlebitis, or pulmonary emboli. The use of progestin is not necessary in those women who have had a hysterectomy. A regimen of 24 days of 1 mg of micronized estradiol (Estrace), 0.02 mg of ethinyl estradiol (Estinyl), or 0.625 mg of conguated estrogens (Premarin and others) with the addition of a suitable progestin (e.g., 5 to 10 mg of medroxyprogesterone acetate, Provera) for the last 12 days is recommended. This is followed by 5 to 6 days without therapy before resumption of the cycle. Current cost for such a regimen is approximately $12.00 per month. Treatment should be begun after the third missed period in symptomatic women, or in asymptomatic women with negative pregnancy tests. The use of androgens adds little or nothing to this form of therapy and is not justified. Until further evidence confirms the absence of risk of endometrial carcinoma, an endometrial biopsy should probably be done on such patients at the initiation of therapy and every 2 years thereafter or if "intermenstrual" bleeding occurs (see Chapter 95).

Alternatives to Estrogen Therapy

There is no good alternative to estrogen for genital atrophy. As noted above, local estrogen cream produces unpredictable systemic estrogen absorption and thus has only illusory advantages over systemic therapy. Traditional modes of therapy for prevention of osteoporosis have included regimens of increased weight-bearing exercise, supplementation of diet with approximately 1500 mg of calcium (see Chapter 74, Tables 74.7 and 74.8 for practical details) and use of vitamin D (1000 units/day). However, in older patients vitamin D increases resorption of calcium from bone, despite its stimulatory effect on calcium uptake from gut, with a net loss of bone mass. Therefore, supplemental vitamin D is not recommended in postmenopausal patients at present. On the other hand, weight-bearing exercise (e.g., walking, but not swimming) and calcium supplementation have shown considerable benefit in reducing bone loss, and, in preliminary studies, calcium supplementation has been associated with a decreased rate of hip fractures and vertebral fractures. Thus, these two modalities are strongly recommended in conjunction with estrogen or alone, when estrogen therapy is unacceptable or contraindicated (5).

Postmenopausal Bleeding

Postmenopausal bleeding is defined as any vaginal bleeding which occurs in a woman who had had no menstrual periods for 1 year.

Postmenopausal bleeding must always be investigated because approximately 10% of women with such bleeding will be found to have a malignant process of some kind. The remainder have various problems such as endometrial hyperplasia, polyps, infections, traumatic lacerations, *etc.* It is important that patients be educated that any bleeding after 1 year of menopause is abnormal and needs to be reported to the physician.

History

The management of postmenopausal bleeding begins with a careful review of the history with respect to duration, frequency, and the characteristics of the bleeding in terms of color, amount, and flow. The presence or absence of hormone therapy is important. Even if cyclic hormones are being used, heavy bleeding or bleeding at unexpected times in the cycle should still be investigated.

Physical Examination

A careful physical examination should be undertaken. The abdomen must be evaluated for suprapubic masses and lower abdominal tenderness. The external genitalia must be inspected for neoplasia and/or atrophic changes. The vaginal mucosa should be inspected for atrophy or lacerations. The cervix must be visualized and a Pap smear obtained if needed. The size, shape, and position of the uterus must be noted and the adnexae evaluated for enlargement or tenderness. A rectal examination may reveal the presence of hemorrhoids and/or fissures. Samples of stool and of urine should be obtained for analysis for occult blood. These latter procedures may suggest the rectum or bladder rather than the uterus or genitals as the source of bleeding.

Diagnostic Procedures

Patients with obvious lesions of the vulva, vagina, or cervix should have a direct biopsy taken for histological evaluation. Where there is no obvious lesion of the cervix, culposcopy (rather than biopsy) is indicated. Patients with significant adnexal disease should be further investigated by intravenous pyelogram, barium enema, flat plate of the abdomen, and sonography. Bleeding from nonmalignant causes such as atrophic vaginitis, or traumatic lacerations secondary to intercourse, should not postpone the next and most important step, namely referral of the patient to a gynecologist for dilatation and curettage (if the uterus is present).

Cervical biopsies are indicated only if the Pap smear is borderline or abnormal. The physician and patient should know that general anesthesia for a dilatation and curettage may be recommended by the gynecologist for patients who are obese, who have a low tolerance for pain, or who are new to the consultant. In those patients who have been seeing the physician for annual examinations and who have negative Pap and pelvic examinations over a number of years, a D and C under local anesthesia is usually a very satisfactory procedure and requires minimal hospital time.

General References

Eskin BA (ed): *The Menopause, Comprehensive Management.* New York, Masson, 1980.
> Excellent summary of pertinent clinical issues and menopausal physiology.

Gregerman RI, Bierman EL: Aging and hormones. In Williams RH (ed): *Textbook of Endocrinology,* ed 6. Philadelphia, WB Saunders, 1981.
> Thorough discussion of endocrine relationships involved in osteoporosis and of effects of aging on reproductive endocrinology.

Paulsen CA: The testis. In Williams RH (ed): *Textbook of Endocrinology,* ed 6. Philadelphia, WB Saunders, 1981.
> Definitive chapter on pathophysiology of the male reproductive system.

Ross GT, Vande Wiele RL: The ovaries. In Williams RH (ed): *Textbook of Endocrinology,* ed 6. Philadelphia, WB Saunders, 1981.
> Detailed step-by-step instruction on diagnosis and management of disturbances of female reproductive endocrinology.

Specific References

1. Adams DB, Gold AR, Burt AD: Rise in female-initiated sexual acfivity at ovulation and its suppression by oral contraceptives. N Engl J Med 299:1145, 1978.
2. Aitken JM, Hart DM, Lindsay R: Estrogen replacement therapy for the prevention of osteoporosis after oophorectomy. Br Med J 3:515, 1973.
3. Bercovici JP, Nahoul K, Tater D, et al: Hormonal profile of Leydig cell tumors with gynecomastia. J Clin Endocrinol Metab 59:625, 1984.
4. Carter JN, Tyson JE, Tolis G, et al: Prolactin secreting tumors and hypogonadism in 22 men. N Engl J Med 299:847, 1978.
5. Council on Scientific Affairs, American Medical Association: Estrogen replacement in the menopause. JAMA 249:359, 1983.
6. Davidson JM: Hormones and sexual behavior in the male. Hosp Pract 10:126, 1975.
7. Federman D: *Abnormal Sexual Development.* Philadelphia, WB Saunders, 1968, p 27.
8. Frank E, Anderson C, Rubinstein D: Frequency of sexual dysfunction in normal couples. N Engl J Med 299:111, 1978.
9. Gambrell RD, Maier RC, Sanders BI: Decreased incidence of breast cancer in postmenopausal estrogen-progesterone users. Obstet Gynecol 62:435, 1983.
10. Gambrell RD, Massey FM, Castaneda TA, et al: Reduced incidence of endometrial cancer among postmenopausal women treated with progestogens. J Am Geriatr Soc 27:389, 1979.
11. Harman SM: Clinicl aspects of aging of the male reproductive system. In Schneider E (ed): *The Aging Reproductive System,* New York, Raven Press, 1978, p 29.
12. Harman SM, Tsitouras PD: Reproductive hormones in aging men: I. Measurement of sex steroids basal luteinizing hormone and Leydig cell response to human chorionic gonadotropin. J Clin Endocrinol Metab 51:35, 1980.
13. Hoover R, Gray IA, Cole P, MacMahon B: Menopausal estrogens and breast cancer. N Engl J Med 295:401, 1976.
14. Horsman A, Gallagher JC, Simpson M, Nordin BEC: Prospective trial of estrogen and calcium in postmenopausal women. Br Med J 2:789, 1977.
15. Horsman A, Jones M, Francis R, Nordin C: The effect of estrogen dose on postmenopausal bone loss. N Engl J Med 309:1406, 1983.
16. Hulka B, Kaufman DG, Fowler WC, et al: Predominance of early endometrial cancers after long-term estrogen use. JAMA 244:2419, 1980.
17. Judd HL, Lucas WE, Yen SSC: Serum 17β-estradiol and estrone levels in postmenopausal women with and without endometrial cancer. J Clin Endocrinol Metab 43:272, 1976.
18. Kleinberg DL, Noel GL, Frantz AG: Galactorrhea: a study of 235 cases, including 48 with pulmonary tumors. N Engl J Med 296:589, 1977.
19. Klibanski A, Neey RM, Beitins IZ, et al: Decreased bone density in hyperprolactinemic women. N Engl J Med 303:1511, 1980.
20. Lauritzen C, VanKeep PA: Proven beneficial effects of estrogen substitution in the postmenopause: a review. Front Horm Res 5:1, 1978.
21. Mack TM, Pike MC, Henderson BE: Estrogen and endometrial cancer in a retirement community. N Engl J Med 294:1262, 1976.
22. Marshal WA, Tanner JM: Variations in pattern of pubertal changes in girls. Arch Dis Child 44:291, 1969.
23. Marshall WA, Tanner JM: Variations in pattern of pubertal changes in boys. Arch Dis Child 45:13, 1970.
24. Martin CE: Sexual activity in the aging male. In Money J, Musaph N (eds): *Handbook of Sexology,* New York, Elsevier-North Holland, 1977, p. 813.
25. Muller SA: Hirsutism. Am J Med 46:803, 1969.
26. Nutall FQ: Gynecomastia as a physical finding in normal men. J Clin Endocrinol Metab 48:338, 1979.
27. Schiff I, Tulchinsky D, Ryan KJ: Vaginal absorption of estrone and 17β-estradiol. Fertil Steril 28:1063, 1977.
28. Shapiro G, Evron S: A novel use of spironolactone: treatment of hirsutism. J Clin Endocrinol Metab 51:479, 1980.
29. Sherman BM, Korenman SG: Hormonal characteristics of the human menstrual cycle throughout reproductive life. J Clin Invest 55:699, 1975.
30. Spark RF, White RA, Connolly PB: Impotence is not always psychogenic. Newer insights into hypothalamic-pituitary-gonadal dysfunction. JAMA 243:750, 1980.
31. Sturdee DW, Wade-Evans T, Paterson MEL, et al: Relations between bleeding pattern, endometrial histology, and estrogen treatment in menopausal women. Br Med J 1:1575, 1978.
32. Tataryn IV, Meldrum DR, Lu KH, et al.: LH, FSH, and skin temperature during the menopausal hot flash. J Clin Endocrinol Metab 49:152, 1979.
33. Weissman MM: The myth of involutional melancholia. JAMA 242:742, 1979.

SECTION 11

Neurological Problems

CHAPTER SEVENTY-EIGHT

Evaluation of the Patient with Neurological Symptoms*

MARGIT L. BLEEKER, M.D., PH.D., and BARRY GORDON, M.D., PH.D.

This chapter describes approaches to history taking, physical examination, and laboratory evaluation that are most useful in ambulatory patients with neurological symptoms. One or more of these approaches is appropriate in patients with each of the neurological problems discussed in subsequent chapters (headache, seizures, dizziness, vertigo, syncope, tremor, Parkinson's disease, cerebrovascular disease, peripheral neuropathy).

NEUROLOGICAL HISTORY AND PHYSICAL EXAMINATION

General Principles

Four types of information should be obtained (or inferred) whenever there is a new neurological symptom: the temporal evolution of the symptom,

---

* Alfred C. Server, M.D., Ph.D. contributed to this chapter in the first edition of this book.

any associated symptoms, the specific abnormality of neurological functions, and the anatomical localization of the problem. Figures 78.1 and 78.2 summarize those facts that are most often needed for anatomical localization. Additional details regarding the anatomical relationships of peripheral nerves are shown in Chapter 84, Figures 84.1 and 84.2

It is important to remember that most individual neurological symptoms or signs are not specific for one functional or anatomical disturbance or for one etiology (e.g., loss of a reflex is not necessarily due to motor nerve damage, a hemiparesis is not necessarily due to cerebrovascular disease, and a resting tremor is not necessarily due to Parkinson's disease). The constellation of findings from the history and physical examination, however, is often quite specific. Therefore, a good history and physical examination are adequate for making a working diagnosis for most neurological problems encountered in office practice. For example:

A physically active patient with a history of recurrent low back pain for many years gives a 3-day history of increased back pain, numbness on the back of the right leg extending to the foot, and some clumsiness of the leg. Symptoms began about 1 day after he dug up his garden. Physical findings are consistent with lower motor neuron impairment at the level of S1. Working diagnosis: herniated disc at the L5-S1 level.

Depending on the circumstances, either a brief (but adequate) examination of each general neurological function may be required or only selected areas of the nervous system may need evaluation.

Brief Neurological History

Higher Functions and Consciousness

Handedness. Are you right-handed or left-handed?

Language. Have you had any problems with your thinking or with your speech? (Minor difficulty in finding words is very common in normal people, as are brief lapses of memory.)

Memory. How is your memory? What kind of things do you forget? (To the family: Have any problems with concentration, memory, or general abilities been noted?)

Acute cerebral dysfunction. Have you ever fainted,

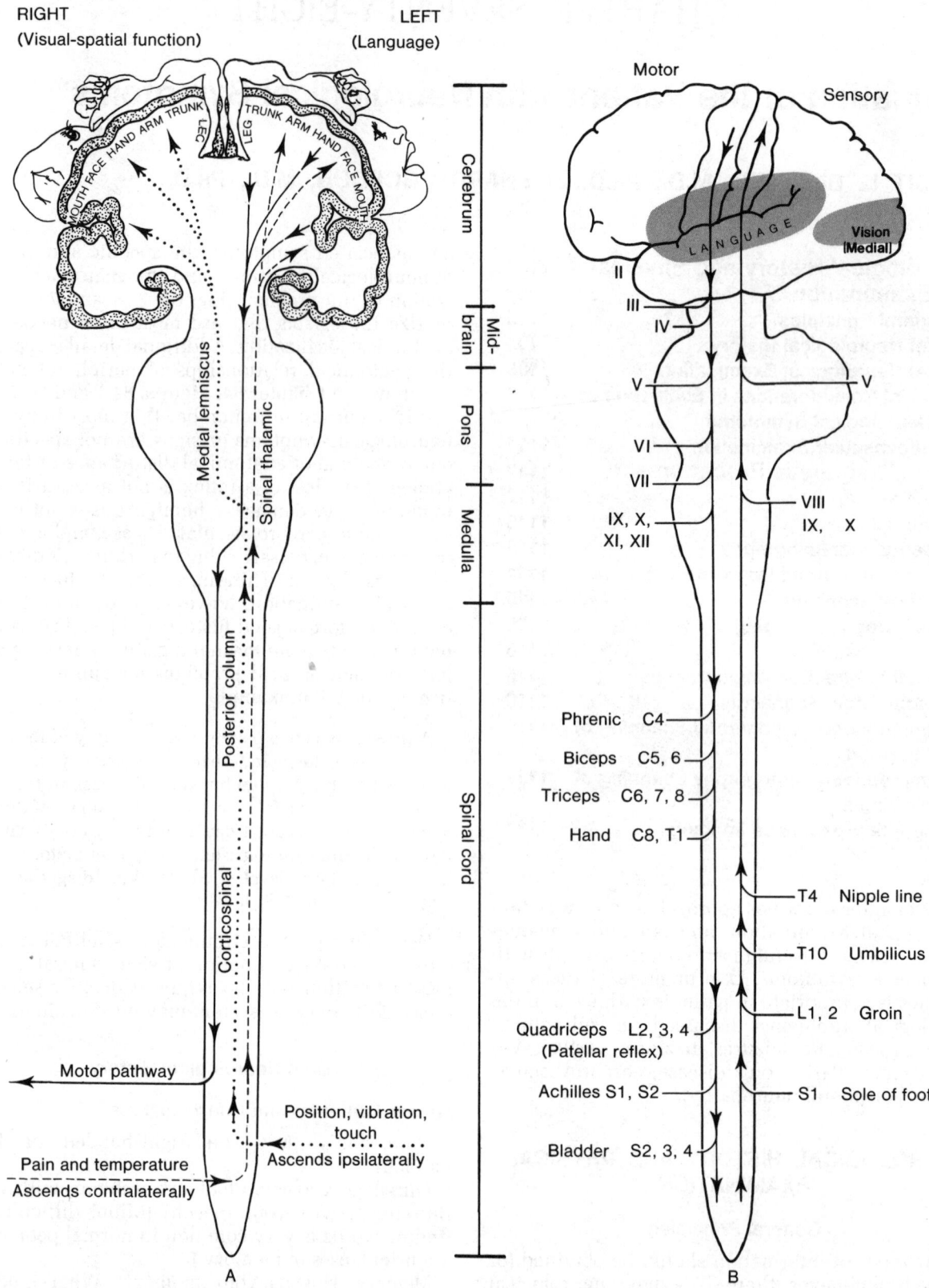

Figure 78.1. Schematic of neurological localization. Anterior (A) and lateral (B) schematics of central nervous system localization. Upper motor neuron signs and nonradicular sensory signs can only define the *side* of the lesion (A); in general, they do not reveal the *level* of the lesion. The presence or absence of other neurological signs or symptoms can help to specify the *level* of a localized neurological problem (B).

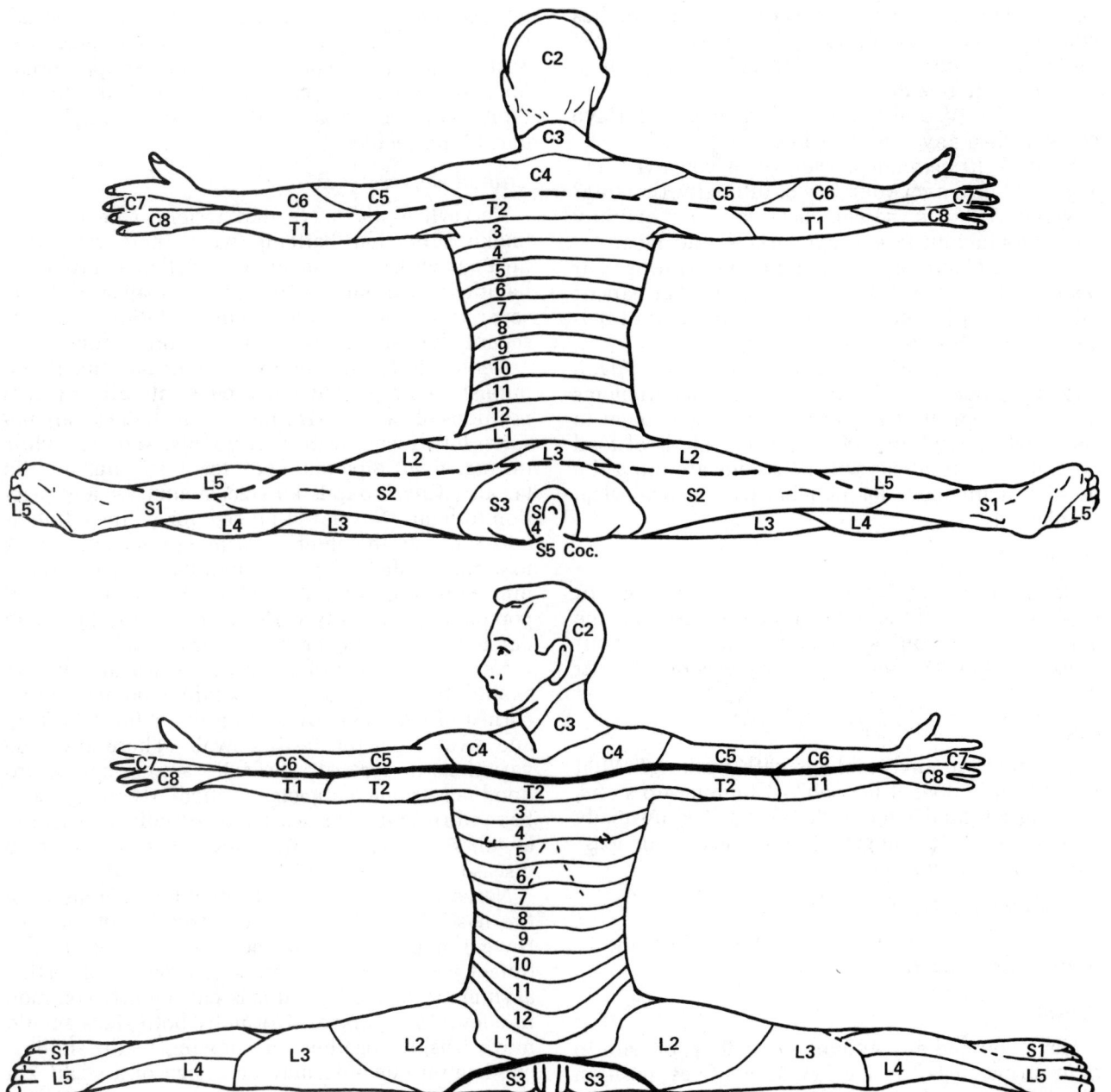

Figure 78.2. Cutaneous innervation areas of dermatomes. The numbers correspond to the spinal cord level of the dermatome. *C*, cervical; *T*, thoracic; *L*, lumbar; *S*, sacral. (From Haymaker W, Woodhall B: *Peripheral Nerve Injuries*, ed 2. Philadephia, WB Saunders, 1962.)

lost consciousness, felt dizzy, or had a seizure (fit, convulsion)?

Mood. How are your spirits? Do you feel depressed? Are you worrying a great deal? How do you feel about the future? About yourself (confident, hopeless, helpless, guilty)?

Hallucinations/delusions. Have you seen or heard things that are unusual or that you think are not there? Does your imagination seem to play tricks on you? What do you feel is wrong? Is there anything or anybody affecting you?

Cranial Nerves

Nerve I (olfactory). Not tested in brief history and physical unless patient specifically mentions it.

Nerve II (optic nerve and vision). How is your

vision? Do things seem blurred or are there patches where it is hard for you to see? Have you ever lost the vision in one eye or had trouble seeing out of one side or in one direction?

Nerves III, IV, and VI (extraocular motions). Have you ever had any double vision?

Nerve V (trigeminal nerve). Have you ever had any numbness over your face or difficulty chewing?

Nerve VII (facial nerve). Have you ever had any weakness in your face or paralysis of your face?

Nerve VIII (auditory-vestibular nerve). How is your hearing? Have you had any ringing in your ears or difficulty hearing out of one side? Any loss of balance, spinning sensations, or dizziness?

Nerves IX, X, and XII (glossopharyngeal, vagal, and hypoglossal nerves). Have you had any problems chewing or swallowing your food? Does it seem to get caught anywhere? Where? What kinds of food do you have problems with? (Liquids are often the most difficult foods for patients with neurological problems.)

Motor

Have you noted any weakness in your arms or legs? Is it there all the time, or does it seem to come and go? Have you noted any twitching in your muscles? Where? How often? Any wasting of your muscles?

Gait

Do you have any problems with walking? What kind? Where does it happen?—Climbing up stairs, walking certain distances, *etc?* Do you feel unsteady on your feet? Do you get any cramps in your legs? Under what circumstances?

Fine Motor and Cerebellar Function

Have you noticed any shaking or any difficulty in writing, drawing, buttoning, *etc?*

Sensation

Have you had any numbness, tingling, or pain in your arms, legs, or feet? Where? Does position change or any other factor seem to bring it on?

Bladder/Bowel

Have you had any problems in starting to urinate or in urinating? Any difficulty with constipation or diarrhea? Any uncontrolled urination or stool evacuation? If so, was it associated with the urge to urinate/defecate, or was it spontaneous?

Brief Neurological Examination

Higher Functions and Consciousness

The questions suggested in the history plus observations made throughout the history and physical examination are usually sufficient for determining level of consciousness, language functioning, visual-spatial functioning, mood, and level of intelligence. Systematic mental status examinations appropriate for patients with psychiatric problems and for patients with dementia are described in Chapters 10 and 17, respectively.

Cranial Nerves

Nerve II (optic nerve and vision). Check vision (make sure that patients wear their glasses, if needed) with the use of the Snellen chart or by having the patient read from a newspaper, each eye separately. Check fields by confrontation (each eye separately) using finger wiggle. Examine fundi.

Nerves III, IV, and VI (extraocular movement and pupils). Make patient move eyes into all principal positions of gaze (horizontal, vertical, diagonal), observe for dysconjugate movements, and ask, while testing, about diplopia. Look for nystagmus and lid lag also. Check pupils for size, symmetry, and reaction to light. (Normal pupil size for young adults is 3 to 5 mm. In the elderly, normal pupils are often 2 to 3 mm. A slight degree of pupillary asymmetry, 1 mm or less, is present in about 5% of the normal population; it usually varies from hour to hour and day to day, and it decreases in bright light.)

Nerve V (trigeminal nerve). Corneal reflexes should be tested at corresponding points on the cornea of each eye, by having the subject look up and away from the testing swab. (There are wide variations in corneal sensitivity among normal individuals; some subjects, particularly those who have worn contact lenses, have virtually no response at all. Asymmetry is the most important clue to disease.)

Nerve VII (facial nerve). Inspect for asymmetry of the nasolabial folds when the face is not moving. Have the patient show teeth, close eyes, frown. (Intact persons may have a slight degree of resting asymmetry of the face; this is particularly common in edentulous persons. Normally both sides should move briskly together on showing teeth, smiling, *etc.* Lag on one side may be a sign of a slight 7th nerve palsy, central or peripheral.)

Nerves IX and X (glossopharyngeal and vagus nerves). Inspect the uvula for position and for motion with "Ahh." Test the gag reflex on both sides of the pharnyx, looking for asymmetry of response. (Some people have asymmetry of the resting uvula. Also, bilaterally hyperactive to bilaterally absent gag responses are within the normal range.)

Nerve XI (accessory nerve). Observe shoulder shrug; it should be symmetric.

Nerve XII (hypoglossal nerve). Inspect the tongue at rest in the mouth; have the patient protrude it and move it to both sides. (The tongue normally has small twitches which are not pathological fasciculations; it should protrude in the midline.)

Motor Examination

Adventitious movements. Observe for tremor and other spontaneous movements. (See additional details in Chapter 82, Common Disorders of Movement.)

Bulk. Examine for asymmetries of muscle mass. (Denervation will cause loss of muscle bulk, reaching a maximum by 4 months; disuse over months to years will also cause a decrease in muscle bulk, e.g., in the legs of patients who are permanently bedridden.)

Muscle tone (resistance to passive motion). Test tone by passively flexing and extending the upper and lower extremities. Normal tone is a slight firmness of muscles and slight resistance to passive motion. In *hypotonia*, the muscles are flaccid, without resistance to passive motion. This may mean lower motor neuron or cerebellar disease.

There are several subtypes of *hypertonia*:

Rigidity is increased resistance to passive motion throughout the whole range of motion around a joint.

In *spasticity*, the initial passive motion is easy, but then there is a tightening of the muscle ("spastic catch") possibly followed by a sudden release ("clasp-knife effect"). Spasticity usually affects only one set of muscles around a joint (in the upper extremities, the biceps, forearm pronators, and finger flexors; in the lower extremities, the quadriceps, hamstrings, and plantar flexors).

In *gegenhalten or paratonia*, resistance is present in all directions, but varies with the examiner's force and speed. It often seems to be voluntary ("fighting back"). Gegenhalten is seen normally in infants, but appears pathologically in adults with dementias or frontal lobe disease.

Voluntary strength. Voluntary strength should be sampled in several major muscle groups. Test elbow extension and flexion, hand and finger extension, grip strength (with two fingers), hip flexion (with patient sitting), knee flexion, knee extension, and foot dorsiflexion. Also observe the patient's gait (see below).

If desired, the following rating scale can be used:

0 = No movement
1 = Flicker
2 = Able to move with gravity eliminated (e.g., lateral motion of arm when recumbent)
3 = Able to move against gravity
4 = Able to move against resistance
5 = Normal strength.

(In conversion reactions and malingering, strength on formal testing is usually jerky or "giving." With sudden passive motions in the opposite direction, the examiner may be able to demonstrate that the muscles can produce normal force. The examiner may note that the subject can do some voluntary activities, e.g., combing hair, reaching for objects, getting up or sitting down, *etc*, with muscles which the patients states are "too weak" to use for such motions on formal testing.)

Reflexes

The most important reflexes to test are the biceps (C5-6), triceps (C6-8), patellar (L2-4), Achilles tendon (S1-2), and plantar flexion ("Babinski"). (Activity of the reflexes varies widely among patients and can vary in the same individual depending upon his emotional status and upon his ability to relax his muscles. As in the rest of the examination, asymmetries between two sides generally carry more weight than symmetric reflex changes; comparison must be made with the muscles relaxed to a similar degree and with the two extremities in identical positions. A *decrease* in the reflex or reflexes is generally due to disruption of the sensory or motor nerves (or both) of the reflex loop itself. Sometimes decreased reflexes are seen immediately after a cerebrovascular accident, in which case interpretation does not depend on the reflexes alone. *Increased* reflexes mean upper motor neuron (UMN) disease located anywhere from just above the anterior horn cell to the cerebral cortex. A *Babinski* response is dorsiflexion of the big toe, which may be associated with dorsiflexion and spreading of the other toes and dorsiflexion of the foot. The classic Babinski response is slow and deliberate. Nonspecific withdrawal may resemble the Babinski reflex, but it is usually rapid and the patient usually complains of subjective distress; a reliable Babinski sign can and should occur in the absence of any patient discomfort from the stimulus. A Babinski sign may be found in the absence of other UMN signs, as an indicator of UMN disease.)

Sensation

The patient should be tested for symmetry and for differences in proximal and distal perception, in all four extremities. Sensitivity to pinprick (lateral spinothalamic tract) should be tested, as should both proprioception and vibratory sense (posterior column). (There are normal differences in pinprick perception over different areas of the body—for example, it is decreased over the beard area—but patients generally ignore these differences. Patients who do not can give very confusing responses and must be told to ignore small subjective differences. Repeat testing is often important to determine the reliability of a patient's response. Vibration sense should be tested with a 128 cycles/second (cps) tuning fork. Loss of vibration sense is often the earliest detectable abnormality in peripheral neuropathy. Mild distal loss of pin and vibration sense is very common in otherwise normal elderly patients.)

Fine Motor and Cerebellar

The patient should be told to touch his thumb sequentially to each of the fingers of each hand separately and the speed, effort, and rhythm should be observed. Finger-to-nose-to-finger should be tested (subject has to touch examiner's moving finger, then touch his own nose, then touch the examiner's finger again, *etc*) for speed, rhythm, intention tremor, and inaccuracy (dysmetria). The subject should be asked to tap each foot separately, and differences in speed, ease, and rhythm should be observed. (In these tests, normal subjects show equal ability with either side or are slightly better on the side of their preferred hand. Slowness and subjective effort on repetitive movements, without a loss of rhythm, are characteristic of UMN lesions. Relatively preserved speed with erratic movements and loss of rhythm may be seen in cerebellar disease. Finger-nose-finger testing may be affected by tremor of various types as described in Chapter 82).

Station and Gait

Any tendency to list or any need for support while sitting, standing, or walking should be observed. The patient should be asked to walk normally and to walk on his heels and toes (tests strength and balance). A Romberg test should be performed (feet together in young patients, slightly apart in older patients).

In *cerebellar disease*, there is a wide base (legs widely separated), unsteadiness, and lateral reeling (lateral reeling can be evaluated by having the patient walk around a chair in both directions; he will tend to walk into the chair when it is on the affected side and to veer away from the chair when it is on the unaffected side). Because of his fundamental abnormality of motor coordination, the patient with cerebellar disease affecting the lower extremities cannot participate in a Romberg test, which requires standing with the two feet together; this is not an "abnormal Romberg test."

In *sensory ataxia* (loss of proprioception), there is uncertainty, slapping or stamping of the feet, and a "positive" Romberg test (the patient loses his balance with eyes closed but can avoid falling when his eyes are open because of visually mediated vestibular or cerebellar compensation).

In a *spastic gait* (in UMN disease), the leg does not flex but circumducts, and there is foot dragging (the toe of the sole of the patient's shoe becomes disproportionately worn); there is also loss of arm swinging on the spastic side.

In a *parkinsonian gait*, there is unilateral or bilateral loss of arm swinging; the patient is bent forward; and there is rigidity, shuffling, and festination (the upper part of the body advances ahead of the lower extremities; gait becomes faster as if to catch up).

In *lower motor neuron (LMN) paralysis* of the pretibial and peroneal muscles, there is drop-foot; hip flexion is preserved, and the patient lifts the foot very high, advances it by swinging it forward, then slaps it down.

In *frontal lobe disease*, gait may be wide based, shuffling, and slow, and turning is very slow, but there is no weakness or loss of sensation.

Special Considerations in Evaluation of Neurological Symptoms

The neurological symptoms seen in ambulatory patients are often less florid than are those of patients hospitalized for neurological disease, and many of these symptoms are related to prior acute neurological events. There are two important considerations in the evaluation of ambulatory patients with neurological symptoms: the variability in patient performance over time and the difference between the manifestations of UMN and LMN lesions.

Variability over Time

In dealing with abnormalities of the peripheral nerves, spinal cord, and brainstem, the physician can expect symptoms and signs to remain about the same after the basic problem has stabilized; subsequently, alterations of the findings usually reflect a change in the patient's disease. On the other hand, the performance of patients with ostensibly stabilized cerebral disease may vary greatly from minute to minute, hour to hour, or day to day. The variability affects the psychomotor domain, e.g., performance of everyday tasks, memory, speech and language, and mood. For example:

1. The patient may be able to dress, fix breakfast, and bring in the mail one morning; be incapable of these tasks the next morning; and perform them correctly on the third morning.
2. The patient may remember his wife's name in the morning but not in the evening of the same day.
3. The aphasic patient may be able to say something one minute and be unable to say it several minutes later.
4. The stroke survivor's affect may vary from depressed to euphoric from hour to hour and day to day.

As a result of this type of variability, members of the patient's family may become confused and, often, quite angry. They may frequently contact the physician to inquire whether a change in behavior means that the disease is getting worse, or they may conclude that the patient is capable of doing certain tasks but "just not trying" sometimes. When the pattern is clearly one of waxing and waning, the family should be reassured that, just as intact individuals have their "good days" and "bad days," brain-damaged subjects do also, but in exaggerated and different ways. The evaluation and management of behavior changes of patients with cerebral damage are discussed in more detail in Chapters 17 (dementia) and 83 (stroke).

Difference between UMN and LMN Symptoms

The manifestations and the course of UMN and LMN damage differ fundamentally. UMN lesions affect the pathways bringing a command from the cortex to the anterior horn cell. UMN function depends upon integrity of the cortex and the corticospinal and corticobulbar tracts. LMN lesions affect the final common pathway for muscle movements. LMN function depends upon the integrity of the anterior horn cell in the spinal cord and its nerve fiber for carrying impulses to the muscle cell. A number of points are helpful in recognizing or distinguishing these common problems when they are less overt, which is often the situation in patients seen in office practice.

UMN lesion syndrome. If a UMN lesion is total, movements will be absent. However, there may be preservation of involuntary movements, such as those associated with yawning, laughing, crying, or anger.

When there is weakness (paresis) rather than paralysis due to UMN damage, the following patterns of weakness are seen.

In the face, the lower muscles are usually involved. There is variable but often some involvement of the orbicularis oculi (producing a widened palpebral fissure and weakness of eye closure), but the forehead is completely spared. This is in contrast to LMN (peripheral) 7th nerve damage where usually both the upper and lower facial muscles are involved (although sometimes mild peripheral 7th nerve weakness—e.g., early Bell's palsy, an LMN lesion—can mimic this pattern). One additional differential point is that the LMN lesion will produce the same amount of weakness with both a voluntary and an involuntary movement (e.g., laughing). A UMN 7th nerve paresis (from a stroke, for example) may not be apparent when the patient is laughing or crying involuntarily but may only be present when the patient is asked to smile voluntarily.

In the arm and leg, distal muscles are affected by UMN lesions much more than proximal muscles. In addition, some specific motor functions are affected more than others: in the arm, shoulder abduction and external rotation; in the forearm, extension and supination; in the wrist and finger, extension; in the hip, flexion; in the knee, flexion; and in the foot and toe, dorsiflexion.

Whether or not the muscles are weak in a UMN lesion, voluntary movements are typically slowed and require greater effort than usual, and the affected limb's ability to make fine movements is lost. A patient with a very mild hemiparesis may be able to squeeze the examiner's hand with normal strength, but his movements are slower and clumsier than usual; he may be unable easily to use his fingers individually; also, when asked to extend both arms with his eyes closed, there may be downward and inward drift of the weak arm (pronator sign). In the lower extremity, a patient with such a mild defect may be able to dorsiflex his foot voluntarily. However, he may not be able to do this very rapidly (as revealed on attempted foot tapping), and the movement may not be automatically coordinated with walking, resulting in a "drop foot."

Typically (but not invariably), UMN lesions are accompanied by spasticity and hyperreflexia.

LMN lesion syndrome. Weakness resulting from a permanent LMN lesion is fixed and unchanging. Only those muscles served by the involved spinal cord segment or peripheral nerve are weak. There are none of the widespread effects characteristic of an UMN lesion. Atrophy is usually apparent within several weeks after a LMN lesion, in contrast to UMN lesions where atrophy is slight and late (many months). Pathological fasciculations may be present in affected muscle groups, distinguishable from benign occasional muscle twitching by the fact that they are frequent and occur only in the denervated muscles. Muscles are usually flaccid and hyporeflexic or areflexic. If a peripheral nerve has been involved, there may be associated hypesthesia or anesthesia.

Mixed UMN and LMN lesions. In some situations, UMN and LMN lesions may occur together. For instance, *spinal cord injury* will typically give signs of a LMN lesion at the level of the injury, due to localized destruction of the anterior horn cells and their nerve roots; below the level of the injury, there may be a partial or complete UMN syndrome with spasticity, hyperreflexia, and preserved involuntary reflexes. Likewise, *amyotrophic lateral sclerosis,* an idiopathic degenerative disease, affects both pyramidal tract cells and anterior horn cells. Along with LMN type weakness, fasciculations, and wasting (more pronounced in the upper extremities), these patients often have lower extremity hyperreflexia and Babinski signs.

Neurovascular Examination

This section describes a systematic approach to the neurovascular examination. This examination is especially important in patients in whom cerebrovascular disease or an increased risk of cerebrovascular disease is the problem (see Chapter 83). The examination includes an assessment of the heart and peripheral vasculature with emphasis on the vessels of the head and neck.

Heart and Peripheral Vessels

The radial arteries should be simultaneously palpated at both wrists to determine any asymmetry in pulse amplitude or timing (pulse delay). The brachial arterial blood pressure should be measured in both arms with the patient supine, sitting, and standing. Unequal blood pressures in the two arms (≥ 20 mm Hg difference in systolic and diastolic pressure) are suggestive of a stenotic lesion of the subclavian artery on the side with the lower pressure. Orthostatic hypotension, defined as a fall in systolic pressure of greater than 15 mm Hg on moving from a supine to an upright position, may be important in explaining symptoms in some patients.

A detailed cardiac examination can provide evidence of cardiomegaly, valvular disease, or an arrhythmia, each of which may predispose a patient to having a stroke. Finally, a complete assessment of the peripheral vasculature, for evidence of widespread atherosclerosis, should include palpation and auscultation of the femoral arteries and palpation of the arterial pulses in the feet.

Vessels of Head and Neck

The evaluation of the vessels of the head and neck should follow the time-honored format of inspection, palpation, and auscultation.

Inspection. Prominence of the superficial *temporal artery* with erythema, and, occasionally, ulceration of the overlying skin, in a patient with persistent malaise is suggestive of giant cell arteritis, an inflammatory process which can lead to retinal and/or cerebral infarction (see Chapter 79).

Dilation of the *episcleral arteries* of an eye can result from occlusion of the ipsilateral internal carotid artery (in this instance, the hemisphere on the side of the occlusion is being supplied in a retrograde fashion by the external carotid artery through enlarged ophthalmic arteries). The *funduscopic examination* allows direct visualization of the retinal vessels, and changes resulting from atherosclerosis, hypertension, or diabetes can be detected. Moreover, the absence of an expected change can be informative, as in the case of the hypertensive patient with normal retinal vessels on the side of a severely stenosed carotid artery (in this instance, occlusive disease of the ipsilateral carotid artery protects the retina from the effects of chronic hypertension). A detailed funduscopic examination may also demonstrate emboli, seen as white or refractile elements in the retinal arterioles (see Figure 83.1). These emboli may be composed of cholesterol, platelets and fibrin, or calcium and are suggestive of atherosclerotic carotid occlusive disease or cardiac valve disease.

Palpation. The value of palpation of the cervical vessels has been the subject of debate. Reports of embolic stroke following firm palpation of a diseased carotid artery have left many clinicians with a sense of trepidation regarding manipulation of this vessel. The current consensus, however, is that gentle palpation of the carotid artery can be performed with limited risk and will occasionally provide useful information about the status of the vessel. Perhaps more valuable and certainly less dangerous is palpation of the superficial temporal and facial arteries, which are branches of the external carotid artery. A

weak or absent pulse in these arteries on one side of the head is suggestive of ipsilateral occlusive disease of the external or common carotid artery. In contrast, an increase in pulsation in these vessels may result from stenosis or occlusion of the ipsilateral internal carotid artery causing collateral flow through the external system. Finally, the finding of a tender superficial temporal artery with decreased pulsation may support other data consistent with the diagnosis of giant cell arteritis.

Auscultation. Following auscultation of the heart to rule out the possibility of a transmitted cardiac murmur, the examiner should proceed to the following sites: the clavicular regions over the subclavian arteries; the lateral and anterior aspects of the neck along the paths of the vertebral arteries (as they course through the cervical vertebrae) and of the carotid arteries up to their bifurcation at the angle of the jaw; the occipital, temporal, and parietal regions of the cranium; and the orbits. The finding of a cephalic bruit in an adult raises the possibility of an arteriovenous malformation, while a cervical bruit is suggestive, but not diagnostic, of atherosclerotic occlusive disease. In addition to its location, a bruit can be characterized on the basis of its duration, loudness, and pitch. These parameters can provide information on the degree of stenosis of the involved vessel (Fig. 78.3). Moreover, by following these parameters in subsequent examinations, a progression to greater stenosis over time can be detected.

USE OF DIAGNOSTIC PROCEDURES

The general physician or a consulting neurologist may refer a patient for any of several diagnostic procedures in evaluating a neurological problem. For the majority of these procedures currently available for ambulatory application, the following information is provided here: definition, principal indications, limitations, and a description of what the patient experiences during the procedure. For nerve conduction tests and electromyography, this information is provided in Chapter 84.

Skull X-rays

Definition of Procedure

The term "routine skull X-rays" refers to a set of films which include three standard views: lateral, anteroposterior (AP), and inclined AP. Many other views are possible and may be indicated in specific conditions (e.g., basal skull views for a patient with atypical trigeminal neuralgia).

Principal Indications

1. Known or suspected significant head trauma.
2. Minimal or possible head trauma, for medicolegal reasons.

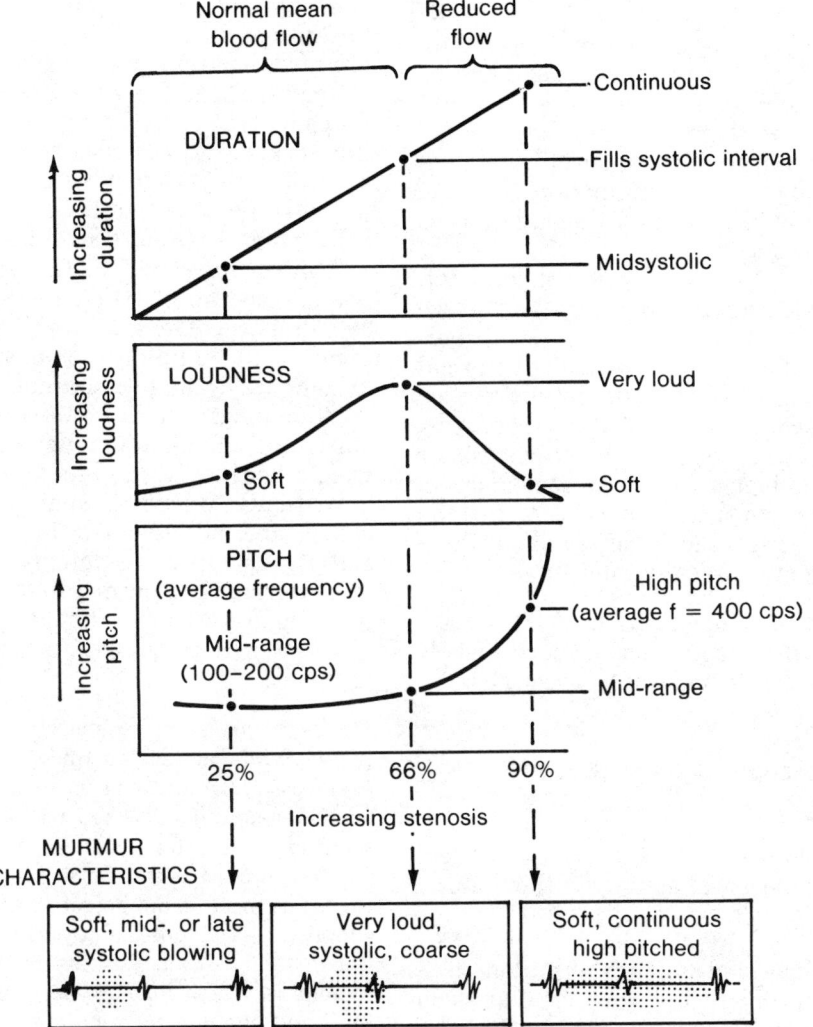

Figure 78.3. Effect of increasing stenosis on the duration, loudness, and pitch of a murmur. (From Toole JF, Patel AN: *Cerebrovascular Disorders*, ed 2. New York, McGraw-Hill, 1974.)

3. Suspected pituitary tumor.

4. Suspected problems involving the bones—e.g., metastatic tumor (osteoblastic or osteolytic), myeloma, or Paget's disease.

Limitations

The skull X-ray has very little value anymore as a general screening test for intracranial disease. Relatively few neurological conditions are associated with bony changes; even when such changes are present, they can generally be evaluated better by procedures with greater sensitivity, specificity, and often nearly equivalent cost and risk, such as computerized tomography (see below).

Patient experience. The patient should be informed that he will be asked to keep his head in several uncomfortable positions for short periods of time; accurate positioning might be impossible for patients who have neck problems or who are old.

Spine Films

Definition of Procedure

Standard spine films are usually AP and lateral views; oblique and flexion/extension views usually must be ordered specifically.

Principal Indications

1. Suspected cervical spondylitic radiculopathy—in this case, oblique films are necessary to examine the intervertebral foramina through which the roots pass.

2. Suspected cervical or lumbar stenosis or spondylolisthesis.

3. Suspected vertebral fracture.

4. Suspected metastatic tumor.

5. To rule out other problems, such as tumor, fracture, and infection, in patients with suspected spondylosis or disc disease.

Limitations

Interpretation of "positive" findings: asymptomatic cervical spondylosis and interspace narrowing due to disc degeneration are so common after age 40 (see Chapter 64) that their presence has limited usefulness in the absence of more specific findings from the history and physical examination. Negative films provide good evidence against spondylosis as the cause of radicular symptoms.

X-rays are indirect studies; they do not show soft tissue or the actual status of the cord and nerve roots; these must be inferred. In patients with herniated intervertebral discs, films are usually normal or show only nonspecific intervertebral narrowing. However, patients with congenitally small bony canals (cervical or lumbar stenosis) are at high risk for these soft tissue problems occurring secondary to degenerative changes in the disc and ligaments; the radiologist should be specifically asked about these possibilities if they are clinically relevant.

Patient experience. The patient must cooperate for several views. Patients with neck problems or who are elderly may be unable to position themselves for adequate cervical spine films.

Electroencephalography (EEG)

Definition of Procedure

This is a record of the minute (1 to 50 μV) electrical rhythms and other electrical activity of the brain.

Principal Indications

1. Known or suspected seizure disorders (see Chapter 80). (Recording during sleep or after sleep deprivation significantly increases the chances of a useful diagnostic examination; for complex partial seizures, nasopharyngeal leads record from the medial temporal regions where most of these seizures originate and, therefore, can slightly increase the yield of the study.)
2. Confirmation of focal brain lesions in the absence of other evidence (e.g., to help localize a stroke).
3. Confirmation of diffuse brain disease, such as dementia, delirium, cerebral vasculitis, drug effect or withdrawal. (Because the general criteria for normal are broad, serial EEGs on the same subject are most helpful in these situations to confirm/disprove pathology.)
4. Sleep disorders (see Chapter 85)—routine and special EEG recording techniques are often indicated.

Limitations

General. An EEG records only relatively gross waves of electrical activity. Only one-third of the cerebral cortex is accessible to standard surface EEG recording, and disturbances have to extend over a wide area of cortex before they can be recorded. Furthermore, many different etiological processes produce the same kind of electrical disturbances.

Negative EEG. Since the EEG is not very sensitive, a single negative EEG is not convincing evidence for the absence of most diseases. For example, up to 20% of patients even with known epilepsy have normal interictal records. Serial or repeated negative EEGs may be far more significant.

"Mildly abnormal" EEG. Depending upon the reader and the classification scheme, many (5 to 30% or more) of normal adult EEGs can be classified as minimally or mildly but nonspecifically abnormal in some way. The relevance of these interpretations must be judged in the context of the patients' problems, but should often not be given very much weight because of the broad range of normal. This is particularly true in infancy, childhood, adolescence, and old age. For instance, temporal slow activity (usually on the left, occasionally on the right or bilaterally) is a normal finding after the age of 40 in as many as 30 to 40% of subjects; it may be confused with the slowing produced by a focal brain lesion.

Patient experience. Subjects are asked to lie down or recline while surface electrodes are attached with electrode paste (which tenaciously clings to hair, so that women should not get their hair done before coming for the study). The total procedure takes an average of about 40 to 60 minutes, with 20 to 30 minutes of actual recording time. For most of the actual recording, the patient will simply be asked to lie calmly with his eyes closed. Additional studies which most laboratories routinely perform include recording during hyperventilation (for 3 to 5 minutes) and photic simulation with a repetitive flash. (For many tracings, subjects will be encouraged to fall asleep if they can. Some laboratories induce sleep with oral chloral hydrate.)

The EEG is extremely sensitive to patient movement, sweating, or muscle tension; any of these may make a tracing uninterpretable.

For sleep-deprived EEGs. The patient is generally asked to stay up all night the night before, and the EEG is done in the laboratory first thing in the morning.

Nasopharyngeal leads are generally applied through the nostrils after local anesthesia of the nasopharynx by spray; they may be annoying and they may interfere with nasal breathing, but they should not hurt.

Periorbital Carotid Doppler Examination

Definition of Procedure

The carotid Doppler examination is an ultrasonic study of blood flow in the supraorbital artery, with and without superficial temporal artery compression. The supraorbital artery is a branch of the internal carotid, and it also has anastomotic connections with the superficial temporal artery. With a patent internal carotid, flow through the supraorbital artery should be unaffected by compression of the temporal artery (the direction of flow may transiently reverse as the internal carotid supply compensates). However, with significant compromise of the internal carotid circulation, supraorbital artery flow becomes totally dependent upon the superficial temporal artery supply and will be abolished by compressing it. It is this that the Doppler study assesses. This study is, therefore, dependent both upon a hemodynamically significant alteration of flow in the internal carotid (usually meaning a greater than 90% stenosis) and upon the "normal" pattern of vascular supply to the supraorbital artery.

Principal Indications

Suspected significant internal carotid artery stenosis (carotid bifurcation): a Doppler study has approximately 90% sensitivity and specificity as an indicator of significant (greater than 90%) carotid bifurcation stenosis.

Limitations

This procedure is not useful for suspected vertebrobasilar disease. It often is normal if there is less than 90% occlusion. It does not reveal plaque ulceration or intracranial vascular disease in the carotid siphon or middle cerebral artery. A negative Doppler study does not completely rule out significant stenotic disease; 10% of even highly stenotic lesions will be missed by the Doppler because of collateral flow to the supraorbital artery. It is never a substitute for thorough investigation of suspected cerebrovascular disease.

Patient experience. Subjects sit or recline with their eyes closed while an ultrasound-conducting gel is applied to the supraorbital region. An ultrasonic probe is then held over the artery for a few minutes while the temporal artery is being compressed and released. There is no appreciable discomfort or risk.

Periorbital Doppler examination, and other tests which measure pressure and flow changes in the oribital circulation, are used to evaluate vascular collateralization distal to high grade stenosis or occlusion of the carotid system. The following noninvasive imaging modalities allow direct investigation of the cervical carotid arteries.

B-Mode Scanning

Definition of Procedure

The B-scanner registers echoes that are related to variations in acoustical impedance of tissues. High resolution B-scan units provide instantaneous images of the vessel wall in real time, *i.e.*, the vessel can be seen pulsating. No information is given about blood velocity. If the bifurcation and adjacent segments of the internal, external, and common carotid areas are within reach of the transducer head, a stenosis of 50% of the luminal diameter or greater will be detected in more than 80% of cases.

Principal Indications

This noninvasive screening technique may be used in the evaluation of asymptomatic carotid bruits, TIAs, and/or in patients with relative contraindications to arteriography. With use of this procedure, stroke-prone patients may be better selected for hospital admission and arteriography.

Limitations

No more than 3 cm of the internal carotid artery can be imaged above the bifurcation. The distal common carotid is imaged for a variable distance, depending on its tortuosity. Calcified atheromatous plaque may accentuate the ultrasonic beam and make it impossible to evaluate the contour of the lumen.

Patient experience. A comprehensive B-scan examination of the carotid arteries takes approximately 15 minutes. The small transducer head is held over the carotid bifurcation at the angle of the mandible. There is no appreciable discomfort or risk.

Direct Doppler Imaging

Definition of Procedure

The Doppler imaging device registers echoes that are related to flow velocity. Spectrum analysis of the Doppler signal increases the sensitivity of detection of an increased blood velocity and turbulence in the vicinity of mild stenosis or placques. Another Doppler system involves scanning of the neck with a positron-sensitive probe, providing a series of transverse scans from which longitudinal images of the carotid arteries can be reconstructed and color coded in accordance with areas of relative differences in blood velocity. Because high velocity regions occur immediately proximal and distal to a zone of stenosis, hemodynamically significant lesions are detectable in more than 80% of cases with this technique.

Principal Indications

See B-mode scanner. Direct Doppler examination at the bifurcation can provide data to help identify lesions causing proximal (arch) and distal hemodynamic changes as well as local disturbances in flow characteristics. It is most useful when the residual lumen is approximately 3.5 mm or less in diameter.

Limitations

Doppler system provides no images of deranged morphology in diseased carotids; it outlines the vessel wall by constructing profiles of a moving blood column.

Patient experience. See "B-Mode Scanning."

Duplex Scanning

This technique combines real-time B-mode ultrasound with Doppler scanning, providing both structural and hemodynamic information. It cannot distinguish *complete* occlusion from a very high grade stenosis in the carotid.

These tests, combined, have about 80% sensitivity for detecting significant carotid stenosis, *i.e.*, greater than 70% narrowing.

Digital Subtraction Angiography

Definition of Procedure

Digital angiography was developed when it was demonstrated that good hard copy images could be made through electronic imaging in which amplifiers and other detectors were substituted for film-screen combinations. In comparison with conventional arteriography, the contrast sensitivity with digital imaging is higher and the total dose of radiation to the patient is significantly reduced, but the spatial resolution is also reduced. The increased contrast sensitivity in digital imaging provides an improved radiographic contrast resolution of anatomical structures. Also contrast-medium levels 10 to 20 times lower than those achieved with direct arterial injection are used.

In digital subtraction an image made before the injection of an iodinated contrast medium is stored in the computer, and a postcontrast injection image is subsequently subtracted from it.

Principal Indications

Digital subtraction angiography can be substituted for catheter angiography in the study of carotid artery disease. Because of its safety and good patient tolerance, digital subtraction angiography can be used for the evaluation of ambulatory patients with transient ischemic attacks and with asymptomatic carotid bruits. Stenosis of any degree, as well as ulceration, can be detected.

Limitations

One of the greatest problems with digital subtraction angiography lies in artifacts produced by swallowing. Although this technique is adequate for many examinations, it will probably not substitute entirely for catheter angiography in situations where a higher degree of spatial resolution is required. Even direct arteriography fails to reveal 40% of cases of known carotid embolic disease originating from sites in the neck.

Patient experience. Digital angiography, unlike catheter studies, can be done on an ambulatory basis. The major discomfort results from venipuncture and the placement of an intravenous catheter into an antecubital vein. Contrast material is given by single bolus. The patient must lie on a table for approximately 30 minutes.

Isotope Brain Scanning

Definition of Procedure

Normally, the blood-brain barrier is impervious to the carrier of the radioactive isotope used in brain scanning. Breakdown of the blood-brain barrier caused by infarct, tumor, or other disease permits migration of the isotope carrier into the brain and, if enough breakdown has occurred, the brain scan is positive in that region.

Principal Indications

Isotope brain scanning is not the procedure of choice for any suspected diagnosis except early brain abscess. For most other suspected intracranial disease, computerized tomography is preferable (and no more costly).

Limitations

The isotope scan has comparatively low sensitivity and spatial resolution (limited to lesions >2 cm). It has limited discriminating power, *i.e.*, infarct, abscess, and tumor can give a similar appearance. Timing of the scan is important. For example, in a brain infarction, the isotope scan is usually not positive for the first 10 days to 2 weeks; it then becomes positive but reverts back to "normal" a few weeks later. It is not useful for intracerebral hematomas; it is unreliable for subdural hematoma (except when large); it gives poor visualization of the cerebellum; it gives no effective visualization of the brainstem; and it is not useful for hydrocephalus, atrophy, old infarction, or other quiescent structural damage. Finally, scalp and skull lesions (bruises, contusions, Paget's disease) can produce prominent artifacts.

Patient experience. Patients may be given sodium perchlorate orally shortly before the injection of isotope to block carrier uptake in the choroid plexus. Then the patient is required to lie still for the (variable) period of time it takes to accomplish each scan by overhead scintillation counters (usually a fairly massive piece of machinery which is moved over the patient's head). There are no appreciable risks.

Computerized Tomography (CT) Scanning of the Head

Definition of Procedure

Computerized tomography uses narrow X-ray beams to exploit the differences in X-ray absorption between different kinds of intracranial tissues. Without contrast, the CT scanner can differentiate between the density of bone, calcified tissue, blood, grey matter, white matter, cerebrospinal fluid (CSF), and air. Its resolving power is proportional to how marked these density differences are; modern CT scanners can reveal hematomas only several millimeters wide, and infarcts of perhaps 1 to 1.5 cm wide. Although CT scan results are typically presented as horizontal slices through the brain, present technology allows slices to be reconstructed in the vertical or in any other plane to give a better perspective on abnormal findings.

Intravenous injection of dye (usually Renografin) is used to enhance the X-ray contrast of vascular lesions and will diffuse into an area of blood-brain barrier breakdown to increase the X-ray absorption density there.

CT scanning is highly sensitive and often diagnostic; as such, it has a place in both screening and in specific investigation. When done without contrast injection, it is essentially free of risk. When done with contrast, the risk is that of the contrast material itself—frequently, a warm flush in the face, nausea, and sometimes vomiting. In approximately 1 case in 100,000 there is the possibility of death from the contrast injection. Many conditions can be screened for without the use of radiographic contrast; this should be strongly considered in patients where the most common abnormalities do not require contrast for visualization (e.g., dementia syndrome evaluation) and in the elderly where the risks are somewhat greater.

Principal Indications

Evaluation of intracranial problems where structural alteration is known or suspected—e.g., tumor, ischemic cerebrovascular disease, hemorrhagic cerebrovascular disease, atrophic degenerative disease (Alzheimer's, Huntington's), hydrocephalus, or subdural hematoma.

Limitations

CT scanning is neither 100% sensitive nor infallible. For instance, a CT scan after a transient ischemic attack may be normal; this finding does not detract from the significance of the event and the need for further study. Furthermore, a negative CT scan does not exclude actual structural damage. The lesion site may not have been included in the slices done as part of a routine examination, or the damage may not have caused enough change in local absorption density to contrast with its surroundings. (This is not uncommon in cerebral infarction a week or so after the initial insult, when the original edema has cleared, and new vessel formation (and phagocytosis) have not yet begun to affect brain density). A CT scan can also be negative because the damage is in an area of the brain that is poorly seen, such as the brainstem or spinal cord, or outside of the brain tissue itself.

Patient experience. The patient is asked to lie down with his head inside what looks like a washing machine. In some scanners, a bag of water is pumped up around the head, but there is no direct contact. Straps will usually be applied over the forehead to prevent motion. (Patient motion will seriously impair the quality of the scanning and may make the scan uninterpretable). Contrast mate-

rial may be given intravenously, by single bolus, or by intravenous drip. The procedure takes 5 to 20 minutes, depending upon the scanner.

Computerized Tomography Scanning of the Spine

Definition of Procedure

See "Computerized Tomography Scanning of the Head."

Principal Indications

CT is the most important diagnostic modality for studying the spine; it shows both the osseus and soft tissues of the spine better than conventional radiographic techniques, including myelography, without morbidity and without excess cost or exposure to radiation. Indications for primary CT of the spine include suspected disc herniation, spinal dysraphism, and facet joint pathology. Since 90% of herniated lumbar intervertebral discs occur at L4-L5 or L5-S1, a CT scan of these two levels can be performed quickly. In cases of spinal fractures it may demonstrate lesions missed by conventional tomography besides showing traumatic injuries of the spinal soft tissues. Spinal stenosis, narrowing of the spinal canal, or narrowing of the neural foramen and lateral recess may be most accurately diagnosed with CT. Other spinal lesions, including arteriovenous malformation, syringomyelia, spinal neoplasms, inflammatory processes, bone mineral analysis, and metabolic disease are accurately evaluated with CT.

Limitations

If the spinal region to be studied spans three or more vertebrae, myelography is more practical than is CT. Diagnostic accuracy of CT presupposes use of a localizer image for accurately selecting the plane and angle of the slice besides a relatively thin slice thickness and optimal resolution. CT diagnosis of a herniated disc is inaccurate in patients with a previous laminectomy. If clinical criteria do not permit the selection of appropriate levels for scanning, CT may be a less satisfactory technique than myelography for examining the cervical spine. The major impediment to greater use of CT in imaging of the spine is probably the unavailability of adequate scanning facilities.

Patient experience. See "Computerized Tomography Scanning of the Head."

Magnetic Resonance Imaging (MRI)

Definition of Procedure

The basis of magnetic resonance imaging is the property of all nuclei with an odd number of protons, neutrons, or both to act as magnets. Hydrogen, because it is the most sensitive of the stable nuclei to a magnetic resonant effect, and because it is also the most abundant nucleus in the body, is ideally suited for MRI. Through the use of magnetic fields whose strength varies with their position, it is possible to define both the location and concentration of resonant nuclei, such as those of hydrogen, and to create thereby images that reflect the distribution of these nuclei in the tissues. Two concepts are particularly important to an understanding of MRI: (a) Because the radio waves emitted by nuclei in the magnetic fields commonly used in MRI are between 10 and 100 m in length, the images in this technique cannot be made through an optical process. (b) The intensity of the signal is not simply a reflection of the hydrogen density; rather, the observed intensity is actually the hydrogen density strongly modulated by local physical and chemical factors.

Principal Indications

MRI is a novel noninvasive imaging technique which gives better contrast and sensitivity than does X-ray CT. Many cranial abnormalities can be demonstrated with MRI, including intra- and extracranial tumors (especially posterior fossa), early cerebral infarctions, aneurysms, hydrocephalus, sinusitis, white matter disease (multiple sclerosis), and spinal cord abnormalities.

In several aspects of brain imaging, MRI has already shown itself to be superior to CT. First, MRI provides better imaging of the posterior fossa than does CT because the surrounding bone causes no streak artifacts. Second, the soft tissue contrast with MRI is better than that with CT. As a result, gray matter and white matter are much better delineated in magnetic resonance images, and the extent of certain diseases is better appreciated with MRI. For example, MRI can reveal many more of the lesions of multiple sclerosis than can CT. Third, coronal and sagittal plane views can be made directly with MRI, rather than requiring the reformatting of serial transverse plane views, as required in CT. Fourth, major blood vessels can be identified with MRI without the need for contrast media because the flowing blood, as a result of its velocity, appears dark. The common carotid, internal carotid, external carotid, vertebral, and basilar arteries are easily seen. Aneurysms of the internal carotid artery have been detected and a thrombus in the lumen of the artery can be identified.

MRI will probably replace CT evaluation of the nervous system in many instances simply because of its ability to detect lesions not visible on the latter. For instance, in the evaluation of dementia, enlarged ventricles secondary to loss of parenchyma can be differentiated from enlarged ventricles secondary to increased pressure (normal pressure hydrocephalus) by the appreciation of increased transependymal fluid.

Limitations

MRI has high sensitivity for disease detection in the central nervous system, but it does not detect a signal from calcium deposits. Further, MRI does not have the sensitivity to describe glucose metabolic rate, neurotransmitter concentration, or amino acid transport with the spatial resolution of positron emission tomography, another novel technique.

MRI is presently available only at large medical centers. In 1985, third party payers did not cover the cost of the procedure.

The known hazards of MRI are due to the force and torque exerted by the field on ferromagnetic objects brought into the vicinity of the magnet and on patients' prostheses, such as surgical clips, pacemakers, and joint replacements. Cardiac pacemaker function can be disrupted and false signals produced, and ferromagnetic metal clips, such as those on cerebral aneurysms, may be dislodged.

Patient experience. The patient lies down on a table identical to the CT scanner, only the head holder consists of a plastic coil which passes very close to the nose of the patient. The entire table is then moved into a larger tunnel. The patient may experience claustrophobia and feel very warm. A knocking sound is heard during data collection, at which time the patient must remain absolutely still. Presently at the National Institutes of Health, 3 to 5% of patients refuse testing once they have seen the machine.

General References

Ackerman RH: Noninvasive carotid evaluation. *Stroke* 11:675, 1980.
> Brief review of Doppler studies.

Baker AB, Baker LH (eds): *Clinical Neurology* (3 volumes). Hagerstown, MD, Harper & Row, 1976 (with yearly updates).
> Although not the most comprehensive survey of neurological diagnosis and practice, many of its chapters are well recognized for their succinctness and clarity, and yearly updates of this loose-leaf book keep the information up to date. Some specific chapters of interest:

Dejong RN: Case taking and the neurologic examination.

O'Leary JL, Landau WM: Electroencephalography and electromyography.
> Short introduction to EEG and EMG.

Heinz ER: The *Clinical Neurosciences*, vol 4 (*Neuroradiology*). Rosenberg RN, Grossman RG, Heinz ER, Willis WD (eds). New York, Churchill Livingstone, 1984.
> Comprehensive description of neuroradiological procedures including all of the newer techniques covered in this chapter. Good background reading for a more thorough understanding of the technological advances made in this field.

Weisburg LA: Computer tomography in the diagnosis of intracranial disease. *Ann Intern Med* 91:87, 1979.
> Good general review.

CHAPTER SEVENTY-NINE

Headaches and Facial Pain

BARRY GORDON, M.D., PH.D., L. RANDOL BARKER, M.D., AND
MARGIT L. BLEECKER, M.D., PH.D.

EPIDEMIOLOGY

While epidemiological surveys of headache are not always comparable or consistent with one another, all agree on the magnitude of the problem: 80 to 90% of the normal adult population reports recurrent headache, and in 30 to 50% of this population headaches are described as severe or disabling at times. Women clearly suffer disproportionately from headaches, both in terms of numbers affected and in severity of headaches; the reported prevalence in women varies from slightly higher to as much as 3 times higher than in men (8, 16, 20). The majority of headache sufferers depend chiefly on self-care with over-the-counter remedies rather than on visits to their doctors to deal with their headache problems.

Findings from the 1977 to 1978 National Ambulatory Medical Care Survey (NAMCS) provide a profile of that subset of headache sufferers who do go to a physician for headache. In this survey of office practice, headache was the seventh most frequent symptomatic reason for visits to all physicians; it accounted for approximately 2% of all visits to internists, general practitioners, and family practitioners. Table 79.1 adapted from the NAMCS, indicates the differences in visit rate for headache with respect to age group and sex of patients. Table 79.2 shows the distribution of headache duration reported by these patients; almost one-half of visits were for headache of less than 1 week's duration.

One aspect of the epidemiology of headache which deserves emphasis is the lower prevalence of recurrent headache in persons 65 and older. Fifty-seven percent of men and 43% of women in this age group report themselves as headache free, and only 18 to 30% report disabling or severe headaches (NAMCS). On the other hand, as indicated in Table 79.1, the frequency of visits to physicians by those persons who do have headache increases with age.

Of all patients with headache, 80% or more will have what has been described as tension (muscle contraction) headache. Two to 7% will have migraine headaches, usually common migraine. In practice, physicians see a disporportionate number of patients with migraine, since these individuals are much more likely to seek medical attention than are those with tension headache (16). In addition, the physician is likely to see a number of patients with nonmigrainous vascular headaches due to systemic infections with fever (2). Likewise, the relatively uncommon organic syndromes associated with significant headache (such as cluster headache, exertional headache, temporal arteritis, and sinusitis) are likely to be overrepresented in a physician's office.

Life-threatening causes of headache are rare. In a study of a community hospital emergency department, 1% of patients complaining of acute headache had a subarachnoid hemorrhage or meningitis (2).

Table 79.1.
Average Annual Rate of Office Visits for Headache, According to Sex and Age of Patient: United States 1977–1978[a]

Sex and Age (yr)	Average Annual Visit Rate/1000 Persons
BOTH SEXES	
All ages	43.2
Under 15	17.6
15–24	31.4
25–44	53.8
45–64	60.2
65 and over	63.9
FEMALE	
All ages	55.4
Under 15	15.8
15–24	40.8
25–44	67.0
45–64	82.0
65 and over	81.8
MALE	
All ages	30.3
Under 65	19.4
15–24	21.7
25–44	39.7
45–64	36.3
65 and over	38.4

[a] Adapted from Cypress BK: Headache as the reason for office visits, National Ambulatory Medical Care Survey: United States, 1977–1978. *Advance Data, Vital and Health Statistics of the National Center for Health Statistics.* Number 67, January 7, 1981.

In specialized headache clinics, which provide consultation for preselected patients, serious conditions (usually tumors, increased intracranial pressure, arteriovenous malformations, and the like) are found in about 5% of referrals. However, not surprisingly, such conditions (especially brain tumor) are often the major concerns of patients who come to a physician for evaluation of acute or chronic headaches.

GENERAL APPROACH TO THE PATIENT WITH HEADACHE

History

The history provides by far the most useful information for evaluating headache, particularly a careful account by the patient of the current or most recent episode. The following questions are especially helpful in the differential diagnosis of headache (the interpretation of the patient's answers to these questions is discussed in detail in the sections on specific headache syndromes):

1. *Associated factors.* Is there any warning of the attack (prodromal feeling, focal numbness or weakness, or visual symptoms including the fortification hallucinations of classic migraine)? Is the patient aware of any factors that can bring on these headaches (alcoholic ingestion, vasodilator use, psychosocial stresses, perimenstrual period, foods, drug use, position, sexual intercourse, exertion, tobacco)? What drugs is the patient taking for other conditions? To what does the patient attribute the headache? Does the patient fear a dreaded cause such as a tumor?

2. *Temporal features.* How does the headache begin—suddenly, or by building up slowly over a period of several hours or even days? When does the headache occur? Does it waken the patient from sleep or is it present on awakening? What is the frequency of headaches (have the patient recount the past month's and the past year's pattern)? How long do the headaches last (maximum, minimum, average)? Have there been intervals of weeks or months without the headache?

3. *Character and location of pain.* What kind of pain is the patient experiencing with the current headaches (band like, squeezing, pressure, pounding, or throbbing)? Where is the pain located (one side of the head, all over the head, in the eyes, radiating up the back of the neck, *etc*)? Does the pain radiate anywhere or seem to spread during the course of attack? How severe can the headaches be (on a scale of 1 to 10)? How does the patient rate this headache pain to the pain of other headaches or other situations (e.g., is it the "worst ever" or the "worst pain in my life")?

4. *Aggravating and alleviating factors.* Does anything make the headache pain worse (bending, sneezing, straining, coughing)? What factors seem to help the headache (lying down, pressing on the temples, avoidance of work, simple analgesics, narcotics, or other medications)? How is the patient currently treating the headache?

5. *Environmental exposures.* Does the headache occur predictably after exposure to an environment that may have elevated carbon monoxide levels (e.g., a closed room heated by a space heater)? Did the headache start after the patient began work (or activities at home) that entails exposure to fumes or dust containing lead? These and other environmental exposures that may cause headache are listed in Table 7.3, page 102.

Table 79.2.
Percentage of Office Visits with Headache as a New Problem with Respect to Sex of Patient and Time Since Onset of Complaint: United States, 1977–1978[a]

Time Since Onset of Complaint	Female (%)	Male (%)
Less than 1 week	43.9	49.3
1–3 weeks	16.3	22.7
1–3 months	16.1	13.6
More than 3 months	20.5	13.7

[a] Adapted from Cypress BK: Headache as the reason for office visits, National Ambulatory Medical Care Survey: United States, 1977–1978. *Advance Data, Vital and Health Statistics of the National Center for Health Statistics.* Number 67, January 7, 1981.

6. *Associated neurological symptoms.* Does the patient have associated symptoms during the headaches such as spots before the eyes (very common in both tension and migraine headaches); inability to tolerate light, sound, touch or movement; nausea and/or vomiting; focal numbness or weakness?

7. *Prior evaluation.* Has the patient been evaluated for the headaches and what has he been told as a result of this evaluation? It is important to request previous records for all patients who give a history of severe, disabling headache, irrespective of the reported duration of the present headache problem or the nature of the previous evaluation; sometimes even just requesting the records reminds the patient of a 10- or 20-year history of severe headache and of multiple visits; sometimes the previous records confirm this despite a patient's poor recall. In either case, this information can be particularly valuable in evaluating a patient who describes recent onset of severe headaches.

8. *Functional impact.* How are the headaches currently affecting the patient (work and social relationships)?

9. *Family and household history.* Is there any history of headaches in the parents, siblings, children, or other people living in the patient's household? What type?

Physical and Laboratory Examination

As stated, information obtained in the history will usually suggest the probable basis for a patient's headache. Appropriate physical examination and laboratory examination are described under each type of headache below. The extent of the physical examination indicated may vary from no examination (e.g., in a patient with headache following vasodilator therapy), to an examination focused upon structures which may be the source of the headache (e.g., sinuses), to an extensive neurological and laboratory examination (e.g., the patient with new onset or marked change in prior headache pattern).

Principles of Initial Treatment

Most patients with headache can be treated presumptively for tension or migraine headache, as described below. A fuller investigation should be carried out in patients who show either of the following situations after initial treatment: (a) Those patients who fail to respond to treatment of the presumed condition. Even in this situation, the extent of the evaluation should be tempered by the circumstances and the patient's expectations. For example, a middle-aged patient who fails a conservative treatment regimen for recent onset of what appear to be migraine headaches should have an earlier and more extensive evaluation than a middle-aged patient with 20 years of apparent tension headaches, and a repeatedly normal examination,

who has not responded to the full spectrum of therapeutic options. (b) Those patients who show significant changes in complaints or physical findings which point to one of the less common causes of headache discussed below.

Treatment Expectations

A recent study compared physicians' expectations in the management of headaches with the expectations of their patients (11). The majority of the physicians in this study expected that their patients would demand pain relief and not care very much about getting an explanation of their problems or medications. In contrast, only 31% of the patients themselves stated that pain relief was most important; 46% rated an explanation of their problem as their most important concern.

When treating the usual tension or migraine headache, the physician should neither expect always to achieve total relief of headache pain, nor should the patient be misled into thinking that this is always possible. The patient must be educated to understand realistically the limitations of drug therapy and the potential for drug side effects, which, in some cases, can be more distressing than the headaches. Selection of a treatment regimen is complicated by the high placebo response rate (20 to 40%) and by the variable natural history of headaches. Because of this variability, a detailed baseline history of the patient's headache problems is important for subsequent assessment of the patient's response to treatment.

SPECIFIC HEADACHE SYNDROMES

Tension (Muscle Contraction) Headache

In the absence of any rigorous criterion or physiological markers, the term "tension headache" has been applied to what is probably a heterogeneous group of headache syndromes.

Pathogenesis

The symptoms of this type of headache are presumed to be caused by contraction of scalp and neck muscles. The muscle contraction is thought to be a somatic consequence of coexisting psychosocial stress in the patient's life, although the stress cannot always be identified. Neither increased muscle tension nor precipitating stress is specific for tension headaches; both are also common in migraine, which is the prototype of vascular headache (see below). Table 79.3 summarizes the data obtained by Friedman *et al* in 1954 (3) on the frequency of several characteristics in a large number of patients and shows considerable overlap between tension and migraine headaches. Depressed mood is associated with chronic tension headache but the causal relationship between headache and depression is con-

Table 79.3.
Characteristics of Migrainous and Tension Headaches[a]

	Migraine (%)	Tension (%)
Age at onset		
<20 years	55	30
>20 years	45	70
Premonitory symptoms	60	10
Frequency		
Daily	3	50
<Weekly	60	15
Duration		
Constant, daily	0	20
1–3 days	35	10
Throbbing pain	80	30
Location		
Unilateral	80	10
Bilateral	20	90
Vomiting with attacks	50	10
Family history of headache	65	40

[a] Adapted from Raskin NH, Appenzeller O: *Headache*. Philadelphia, WB Saunders, 1980; as modified from Friedman AP, *et al*: *Neurology* 4:773, 1954.

troversial, with some believing it to be the cause while others consider it to be secondary to headaches.

Presentation

Tension headache is usually described as a squeezing, "band-like" tightness or pressure sensation which is felt bilaterally and which may be generalized, occipital, frontal, or bitemporal. However, some patients with otherwise typical tension headaches complain in addition of throbbing pain (suggestive of vascular headache), or sharp shooting pain (suggestive of neuralgia); these may be the only manifestations of tension headache in occasional patients. Patients frequently complain of spots before their eyes when the pain is intense, but these are not the true fortification hallucinations of migraine (see below). The duration of the headache varies from minutes to hours to days. Some patients complain of continuous headaches which have been unremitting for years; this kind of headache is almost always due to tension. Moreover, a history of increased psychosocial stress will often be associated with headache episodes. Finally, the patients may report some relief of pain with massage of their scalp (as may patients with migraine headache).

Physical examination is unremarkable except for neck or scalp muscle tenderness, in some patients, and occasionally an exaggerated physiological tremor (see Chapter 82) due to anxiety.

Treatment

Nonpharmacological. It is usually helpful to explain to the patient the presumed pathogenesis of tension headache, *i.e.*, scalp and neck muscle con-

traction or "tension." This information helps the patient to understand both the benign nature of his headache and its possible relationship to psychosocial stress. As explained elsewhere (Chapter 11), concerned listening to a patient's story often helps to reduce somatic symptoms due to stress. The physician can also help by encouraging any effort made by the patient to reduce the stressful situations. For patients seeking nonpharmacological relief of symptoms, massage of the scalp and neck muscles by another person or use of relaxation techniques (see Chapter 13) can be recommended; in addition, any other procedure which the patient may have found helpful should be encouraged by the physician (as long as he believes it to be harmless).

Pharmacological. Symptomatic treatment with drugs is an important adjunct to the general measures just described; for selected patients, prophylactic drug treatment can also be tried. Most patients will have used headache remedies containing aspirin or acetaminophen before consulting their physician about treatment. For mild to moderate headaches, however, an additional trial of these mild analgesics should be recommended if they have not been taken at the usual effective dose (600 mg every 4 to 6 hours).

A number of drugs are widely prescribed for patients with moderately severe intermittent headaches unresponsive to aspirin or acetaminophen. These drugs include codeine sulfate; propoxyphene (Davron); and two products which contain combinations of analgesics, sedatives, and caffeine: Fiorinal (butalbital, caffeine, aspirin); and Percodan (oxycodone, aspirin). Each of these drugs can lead to habituation and dependency (see Chapter 22). Therefore, it is unwise to initiate treatment with these drugs unless it is clear that the patient can use them appropriately for limited periods.

Prophylaxis can also be tried for the occasional patient whose tension headaches are very severe or very frequent. The best results (60% improved *versus* 22% on placebo) have been obtained with the tricyclic antidepressant amitriptyline (Elavil), given in daily doses of 50 to 100 mg at bedtime (7). (A detailed discussion of the use of the tricyclics is found in Chapter 15). Somewhat less benefit was obtained with prophylactic benzodiazepine anxiolytic drugs (diazepam and chlordiazepoxide) in the same study.

Migraine

Migraine headache is divided into two subgroups—*classic migraine*, which denotes a syndrome of headache with associated characteristic premonitory sensory, motor, or visual disturbances; and *common migraine*, which denotes a syndrome in which there is no neurological disturbance preceding the headache.

Pathogenesis

The symptoms of a migraine headache are attributed to sequential changes affecting intracranial and extracranial arteries.

The initial change is *vasoconstriction*, which, when it produces brain ischemia, is responsible for the fortification hallucinations (see below), transient hemiparesis or hemiparesthesias, confusion, and vertigo that can be seen in classic migraine. While vasoconstriction presumably also occurs in common migraine, it seems to be below the threshold necessary to produce obvious symptoms and instead is perhaps responsible for the prodomal unease and warning that these patients may experience. Vasoconstriction is thought to last from ½ hour to several hours in a typical migraine attack.

The initial vasoconstriction is followed by *vasodilation* of the affected vessels, resulting in typical "vascular headache" pain—pain which throbs in unison with the pulse. Some patients even report noticing dilated, throbbing, aching vessels over one side of the scalp during an episode. Patients often report some relief during the attack by pressure on the temples, which presumably decreases blood flow to the dilated temporal arteries.

Usually the vasoconstrictive symptoms are resolving or have resolved by the time the headache (vasodilation symptoms) starts. In some patients, however, these symptom groups overlap, perhaps because some vessels remain vasoconstricted while others are becoming vasodilated.

Epidemiology and Natural History

The lack of a simple, specific test for migraine headache and variations in the definition of migraine headache make it difficult to determine the prevalence and natural course of this condition. Nevertheless, some characteristics are clear.

From 20 to 50% of migraine headache sufferers have a positive family history for migraine, usually in one parent. This seems to be particularly true with patients who have classic migraine.

The onset of migraine is usually between the ages of 15 through 25 and the headaches are more common in women. Recurrence is a hallmark of migraine headache. The majority of migraine sufferers have several attacks each year, while some have one or more episodes per week and some have only rare episodes or even only a single typical episode in their lives. Migraine episodes usually become less frequent and less severe with age.

The perimenstrual period (particularly before the onset of bleeding, when levels of estradiol are falling), oral contraceptives (particularly off-days, presumably due to falling estrogen levels), and menopause are associated with migraine headaches. The following substances may initiate headaches in susceptible subjects: vasodilators (nitrates and antihypertensives); alcohol; chocolate; cheeses, wines, and other foods containing tryamine; and monosodium glutamate. Withdrawal of caffeine or of ergotamine can also cause headaches (presumably by rebound vasodilation). The patient should be asked about these associations and any others which he may have noted.

Diagnosis and Differential Diagnosis

The following are reasonably well established criteria for the working diagnosis of a migraine headache:

1. *Prodromal warning* of some kind, ranging from vague malaise to focal neurological symptoms. So-called fortification hallucinations are almost specific for classic migraine; these are slowly enlarging scotomata which are surrounded by luminous angles and which slowly change shape and appear to move across the visual fields (see Fig. 79.1) (rarely occipital lobe tumors or arteriovenous malformations may produce the same effects).

2. *Unilateral head pain* during any one attack. The pain usually increases gradually, reaching a peak in several hours and lasting for several hours to a day in typical cases. Attacks lasting 2 to 3 days are not uncommon, and some migraine attacks last for 1 to 2 weeks. The pain is usually described as "pounding" or "throbbing." Although headaches are typically unilateral during a single attack, most patients will have attacks on both sides of the head. However, in 20% of patients, headaches will always be on the same side.

Even these criteria are not broad enough to encompass all of the manifestations of migraine headache. Other frequent symptoms include photopho-

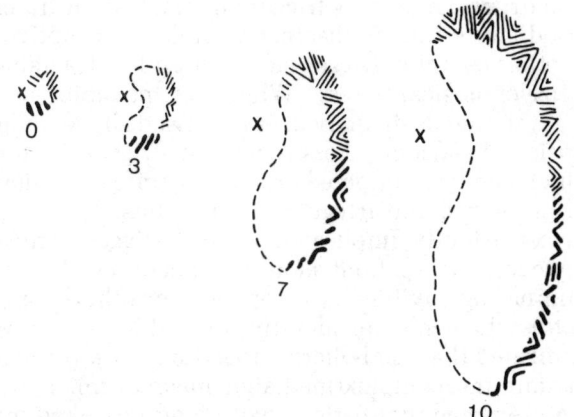

Figure 79.1. Lashley's maps of the progression of his own fortification spectra at varying time intervals after the onset of a migrainous attack. The *X* in each instance indicates the visual fixation point. The numbers represent minutes. (From Raskin NH, Appenzeller O: *Headache.* Philadelphia, WB Saunders, 1980; as appeared in Lashley KS: *Arch Neurol Psychiatry,* 46:331, 1941.)

bia, sonophobia, nausea, vomiting, and generalized malaise. The headache itself is usually described as throbbing but may also be described as aching or stabbing. Furthermore, scalp muscle contraction may occur, so it is not unusual for a patient with migraine to develop bilateral headache and scalp tenderness, features typical of tension headache. In this instance, the headache is referred to as "mixed headache" or "migraine/tension variant headache."

In the *differential diagnosis* of migraine, the most important considerations are transient ischemic attacks (TIAs) or other cerebrovascular events, particularly in middle-aged and older patients (see Chapter 83 for details). Migrainous ischemia usually occurs in patients with a prior history of similar attacks, often in young adulthood; the family history in these cases tends to be particularly strong. Symptoms of migrainous vasoconstriction typically last ½ hour to several hours; TIAs usually last minutes to several hours. Headaches should be a prominent component of the migrainous ischemic event; while headache may occur in up to 25% of patients with transient ischemic events, it is usually relatively mild and transitory. Some patients with suspected migrainous ischemic events, particularly those with "migraine equivalents" (ischemic symptoms without headache) should be evaluated for TIA before their symptoms are attributed to migraine.

Treatment

The vast majority of migraine sufferers can be helped by treatment, principally pharmacological treatment.

Nonpharmacological. The most useful nonpharmacological treatment is elimination of avoidance of known trigger factors, when this is possible. Common drugs which may trigger an attack are nitrates, vasodilators, indomethacin, and oral contraceptives. Another common trigger factor, often less tractable, is psychological stress. Whenever possible such stress should be decreased, as discussed above under tension headache. Less common trigger factors which can be eliminated are excess coffee use, dental problems, and irregular sleep habits. There are no consistently implicated dietary trigger factors; however, each patient should be encouraged to try eliminating any dietary component or other trigger factor which he can identify. Recent studies have confirmed that food-allergic reactions arise through an immune complex-mediated mechanism. It has been reported that patients with food-provoked migraine refractory to drug therapy may be protected by sodium cromoglycate (Cromolyn), known to prevent the hypersensitivity mechanism of mast cell degranulation (10).

During an established attack, a patient usually feels better reclining in a dark cool room. This is the only practice other than drug treatment which appears to be helpful.

Pharmacological: mild attacks. Patients with mild migraine attacks often obtain relief from aspirin or acetaminophen, used as described above under tension headache.

Moderate and severe attacks. At the start of an attack in a patient with moderate to severe migraine, ergotamine tartrate is the agent of choice. Because of its relative specificity, ergotamine may be administered at the onset of symptoms as a therapeutic trial to confirm a clinical suspicion of migraine headache. The action of ergotamine has traditionally been attributed to its vasoconstrictor property, but the reason for its effectiveness in aborting migraine symptoms is not understood clearly.

Ergotamine is available in preparations which permit administration by multiple routes (see Table 79.4). The ideal route is one which is convenient, leads to prompt absorption of the drug, and is not affected by vomiting. Both suppositories and sublingual preparations meet these criteria well. Ingested tablets may be vomited and are therefore less reliable. Recommended schedules for ergotamine administration are summarized in Table 79.5. The objective of these schedules is to attain a total dose which is effective, but which is below the dose that produces nausea and vomiting. Traditionally this has been accomplished by taking additional doses at 30 and 60 minutes if the first dose is ineffective.

Because of the variability of response to ergotamine, each patient should be told how to determine the dose which produces nausea for him (the nauseating dose). This is done by following the traditional schedule on a headache-free day; the cumulative dose attained just prior to the nauseating dose is the appropriate total therapeutic dose (the subnauseating dose) for that patient to take (all at once) at the onset of future attacks.

A number of points are important in instructing a patient about the use of ergotamine. Above all, the patient should understand that ergotamine is not a "pain killer," but that it is used to interrupt the vascular events causing migraine pain. He should understand that for maximum benefit he *must* take ergotamine at the onset of prodromal symptoms or headache (waiting for the headache to become well established is a common problem in patients who report no benefit from ergotamine). In order to assure immediate access to his medicine, the patient should be advised to carry some with him at all times. The patient should be informed that taking more than the recommended maximum daily dose (see Table 79.5) carries the risk of peripheral vasoconstriction in addition to nausea and vomiting. Because ergotamine preparations have a short shelf life, the patient should be instructed to obtain a new supply if he fails to obtain benefit from his medicine or if he has not used it for many months. Finally, patients should be warned not to use ergotamine more than twice in the same week.

Table 79.4.
Ergot-Containing Drugs[a]

Brand and Generic Names	Route[b]	Ergot Alkaloid	Caffeine	Belladonna	Other
Bellergal	p.o.	Ergotamine 0.3 mg		0.1 mg	Phenobarbital 20 mg
Bellergal-S	p.o.	Ergotamine 0.6 mg		0.2 mg	Phenobarbital 40 mg
Cafergot	p.o.	Ergotamine 1 mg	100 mg		
Cafergot	p.r.	Ergotamine 2 mg	100 mg		
Cafergot-PB	p.o.	Ergotamine 1 mg	100 mg	0.125 mg	Phenobarbital 30 mg
Cafergot-PB	p.r.	Ergotamine 2 mg	100 mg	0.25 mg	Phenobarbital 60 mg
D.H.E. 45	i.m./i.v.	Dihydroergotamine mesylate 1 mg/ml			
Ergomar	s.l.	Ergotamine 2 mg			
Ergonovine	p.o.	Ergonovine 0.2 mg			
Ergostat	s.l.	Ergotamine 2 mg			
Ergotamine	s.c./i.m.	0.25 mg/0.5 ml or 0.5 mg/1 ml			
Ergotamine	Inhal.	0.36 mg/puff			
Ergotamine	p.o.	1 mg			
Ergotrate	p.o.	Ergonovine 0.2 mg			
Gynergen	p.o.	Ergotamine 1 mg			
Medihaler Ergotamine Aerosol	Inhal.	Ergotamine 0.36 mg/puff			
Migral	p.o.	Ergotamine 1 mg	50 mg		Cyclizine 25 mg
Wigraine	p.o.	Ergotamine 1 mg	100 mg	0.1 mg	Phenacetin 130 mg
Wigraine	p.r.	Ergotamine 1 mg	100 mg	0.1 mg	Phenacetin 130 mg

[a] Adapted from Raskin NH, Appenzeller O: *Headache.* Philadelphia, WB Saunders, 1980.
[b] p.o., *per os*; p.r., per rectum; i.m., intramuscular, i.v., intravenous; s.l., sublingual; s.c., subcutaneous; Inhal., inhalation.

Table 79.5.
Recommended Schedules of Ergotamine for Treating a Migraine Attack

Route	Strength per Dose	Initial Dose[a]
Sublingual (s.l.)	2 mg (tablet)	2 or 3 mg (1 or 1½ tablets)
Rectal (p.r.)	1 mg (suppository) 2 mg	1 or 2 mg
Oral (p.o.)	1 mg (tablet) 2 mg	1 or 2 mg
Aerosol (inhal.)	0.36 mg/puff (fine powder in cannister)	1 or 2 puffs

[a] Repeated at 30 and 60 minutes if necessary. This constitutes the maximal total dose for 1 day.

Occasionally the patient has *side effects* from ergotamine even when taken at the subnauseating dose. These include abdominal cramps, vertigo, diarrhea, and distal paresthesia; less commonly, syncope, tremor, angina pectoris, and claudication may occur. Most patients, however, tolerate the drug well.

Serious adverse effects, including mental changes, edema, peripheral vascular occlusion, and distal gangrene, can occur if the daily dose of ergotamine exceeds 6 mg or the weekly dose exceeds 10 mg on a chronic basis.

The relative contraindications to ergotamine use are established angina and symptomatic peripheral arterial disease. Traditionally, hypertension has been named as a contraindication, but the risk has probably been overemphasized (see Raskin and Appenzeller, "General References"). Whenver there is concern about the effect of ergotamine on the blood pressure of an individual patient, the blood pressure response to ergotamine should be measured in the physician's office, following the protocol for determining the subnauseating dose of ergotamine outlined above.

For an *established, severe migraine headache,* simple analgesics usually do not help. For this reason, reliable patients should be given small supplies of either codeine (60 mg) or meperidine hydrochloride (Demerol) (50 to 100 mg), to be taken as needed if ergotamine and other measures have failed to abort an attack. This measure may save a patient many unnecessary trips to the physician's office.

Prophylactic Therapy

Prophylactic therapy for migraine should be considered when the patient has two or more attacks/week or when he has less frequent attacks which cannot be controlled with ergotamine and which disrupt employment or social life.

The decision regarding prophylaxis must be the patient's after the distinction between symptomatic and prophylactic therapy has been explained clearly. Even a patient who has not had adequate relief from routine measures may forego prophylactic treatment because of continuous drug therapy. Furthermore, for each of the drugs used prophylactically for migraine, a relatively long trial period (up to several months) may be necessary to assess its effectiveness; and trials with a number of drugs may be necessary. These facts should also be explained to the patient. Finally, the patient should understand that during the trial of prophylaxis he can continue the usual measures for treating his migraine attacks.

Those drugs which have been effective in migraine prophylaxis together with dose ranges and common side effects are listed in Table 79.6. Calcium channel blockers are the drugs most recently added to the list.

The following general conclusions can be drawn about migraine prophylaxis (13):

1. Fifty percent or more of patients report some improvement in their migraine syndrome during the first year, compared with a reported improvement in 25% of "control patients" (patients who choose not to take prophylaxis); during the second year of prophylaxis, the response rate may be lower.

2. Most of the improvement consists of a decrease in frequency or severity of headaches—freedom from headaches occurs in only a minority of patients.

3. Each of the drugs which has been tried (Table 79.6) gives similar results; failure of one drug does not predict response to another, so that a sequential trial of different drugs is reasonable.

4. Those drugs which are known best to the physician should be tried first for at least 2 to 3 months (for the generalist, these are propranolol, amitriptyline, and calcium channel blockers).

Each patient who chooses prophylactic therapy should be asked to keep a log in which to record the frequency and severity of headaches and the nature of any associated factors. As stated, improvement may occur either as a decrease in frequency of attacks or a decrease in the severity of the attacks, or both; the patient's log will determine whether any improvement has occurred.

The Patient with Intractable Migraine Headaches

A small number of migraine sufferers do not obtain relief from intractable and disabling headaches, even after prolonged and thorough attempts at therapy. For a complete assessment and an adequate trial of therapy, these patients should be referred to a neurologist. During particularly incapacitating episodes, hospital admission should be considered to provide adequate rest and treatment with potent analgesics.

Cluster Headache

Cluster headache is probably a variant of migraine (7). It has previously been designated by a number of names, e.g., Horton's headache, histamine headache (a misnomer), and migrainous cranial neuralgia. Episodes of pain occur in clusters extending over days to weeks, thus giving the syndrome its name. Most episodes last from 4 to 6 weeks and are followed by long pain-free intervals. The intervals between episodes range from 3 months to 5 years, and occasionally longer; most patients, however, have one or two episodes/year. Eventually the problem ceases altogether.

Cluster headache is much less frequent than mi-

Table 79.6.
Interval Therapy of Migrainous Attacks—Prescribing Information[a]

Drug	Tablet Size(s)	Daily Dose Range	Commonest Side Effects
Ergonovine	0.2 mg	0.4–2.0 mg	Nausea, abdominal pain, leg "tiredness"
Amitriptyline	10, 25, 50 mg	10–175 mg	Sedation, dry mouth
Propranolol	10, 20, 40, 80 mg	40–320 mg	Lethargy, insominia, constipation, lightheadedness
Papaverine	150, 300 mg	300–900 mg	Nausea
Cyprohepatdine	4 mg	12–32 mg	Sedation, weight gain
Ergotamine-phenobarbital-belladonna	tabs	1–4 tablets	Nausea, sedation
Phenelzine	15 mg	15–75 mg	Insomnia, light-headedness, constipation
Methylsergide	2 mg	2–8 mg	Nausea, abdominal pain, muscle cramps, insomnia, weight gain, edema, peripheral vasoconstriction, retroperitoneal fibrosis
Propranolol LA	80, 120, 160 mg	80–240 mg	Bradycardia, light-headedness, insomnia, nausea, short term memory loss
Verapamil[b]	80, 120 mg	240–640 mg	Hypotension, dizziness, constipation, skin rash
Nifedipine[b]	10 mg	20–60 mg	Hypotension, dizziness, flushing, nausea

[a] From Raskin NH, Appenzeller O: *Headache*. Philadelphia, WB Saunders, 1980.
[b] Not approved by the Food and Drug Administration for use in headache therapy.

graine in the population. It occurs predominantly in middle-aged men. Onset usually occurs between the age of 20 and 50. There is no evidence for a familial basis for cluster headache.

Manifestations

In a typical attack, there is sudden stabbing or burning pain in the eye, orbit, and cheek on one side. The pain is usually excruciating. Unlike patients with migraine, patients with cluster headaches are usually agitated and they often pace the floor during the attack. Characteristically, the patient also describes ipsilateral lacrimation, rhinorrhea, and conjunctival injection. Ipsilateral ptosis and miosis may also occur; this is thought to be due to compression of the sympathetic plexus by the dilated carotid artery, which produces a partial Horner's syndrome. Usually the same side is involved during a cluster of attacks.

Attacks last from 30 minutes to 2 hours (mean 45 minutes); occasional mild attacks may last only 10 minutes. The attacks range in frequency from six/day to one/week during a cluster; and they tend to occur at the same time each day, most commonly in the evening just after the patient has gone to bed. In some patients, alcohol may be a particularly potent trigger factor; nitrates and vasodilator drugs may also induce attacks. Therefore, there should be a full inquiry about the use of drugs in evaluating these patients.

These characteristics describe the typical syndrome of cluster headache. Some individuals have less well defined episodes, whereas other patients may have almost daily attacks of pain for a number of years, a syndrome known as "chronic paroxysmal hemicrania" (9).

Except during an attack, when the unilateral findings described above are present, the physical examination in patients with cluster headache is unremarkable.

Differential diagnosis. Cluster headache must be carefully distinguished from tic douloureux (see below); acute glaucoma (by the presence of miosis, normal tonometry, no lasting visual impairment); sinusitis (by lack of history of upper respiratory infection, lack of purulent rhinorrhea or sinus tenderness, and by negative X-rays); from peripheral dental abscess (by the absence of tenderness on tooth percussion); and from atypical facial neuralgia (see below).

Treatment

Because attacks may be short, lasting only 30 minutes, drug treatment may be ineffective in ameliorating an *acute episode*. The preferred method of aborting short attacks is 100% oxygen, administered for approximately 15 minutes at a 7 liters/minute flow rate (6). Oxygen is a potent cerebral vasoconstrictor and that may explain its effect in patients

with this condition; it will abort or diminish pain in about 75% of patients. Ergotamine, administered by inhaler or sublingually, may also be effective abortive therapy for cluster headaches. When administered by inhaler the dose is one puff every 5 minutes until a maximum of six puffs a day or 18 puffs a week is reached. A sublingual preparation of ergotamine containing 2 mg may be given at the beginning of the attack and repeated twice, at 30-minute intervals. No more than 6 mg should be taken in a 24-hour period, nor more than 10 mg/week.

The drug of choice in *preventing* episodic cluster headache is prednisone, 60 mg a day in divided doses, and tapered over 1 month (1). Prednisone shortens the duration of the cluster episode and decreases the severity and frequency of the attacks. A maximum effect occurs within 2 or 3 days after initiation of therapy. While side effects arising from a short course of prednisone are unusual, they do occur, and include weight gain, salt retention, and emotional lability. Prednisone therapy should not be utilized in pregnant women or in patients with brittle diabetes, congestive heart failure, uncontrolled hypertension, or severe osteoporosis. (See additional information on prescribing and tapering of corticosteroids, Chapter 74.) There are anecdotal reports of effective prophylaxis for cluster headache by treatment with propranolol, amitriptyline, and cyproheptadine, in doses similar to those used in migraine (see Table 79.6).

In addition, for the rare patient who suffers from almost daily cluster headache (chronic paroxysmal hemicrania) lithium carbonate, 300 mg three times a day, has been used successfully. Most patients with chronic cluster headache seem to be controlled at serum levels below 0.8 mEq/liter. Contraindications to lithium use include renal disease, congestive heart failure, dehydration, pregnancy, and concomitant diuretic administration. Major side effects relating to neurotoxicity include tremor, lethargy, and confusion. There must be a frequent check for polyuria, a symptom suggesting the onset of nephrogenic diabetes insipidus. Dermatological reactions include acne-like lesions and thinning of the hair. Lithium carbonate therapy is generally effective within 5 to 7 days. If lithium fails to control daily cluster headache, ergotamine tartrate may be added. Methysergide (see Table 79.6), either alone or with ergotamine, may be used if control still has not been achieved.

The patient in whom neither treatment nor prophylaxis with the above regimens helps should be referred to a neurologist or to an internist with wide experience in headache management.

Sinus Headache

The pain of *acute sinusitis* may be described by the patient as headache. The diagnosis is based upon the other manifestations of acute sinusitis and on the reproduction or exacerbation of the patient's "headache" by applying pressure to affected sinuses (see Chapter 28 for a full account).

Chronic sinusitis is often cited by patients as the reason for their headaches; it is actually a relatively uncommon cause for chronic intercurrent headache. Chronic sinusitis can present diagnostic difficulties, particularly when it involves the sphenoid sinus (causing a dull boring pain behind the eyes). The physician's suspicions should be aroused if there is a history of preceding acute sinusitis, especially if there is not a long history of headache. The diagnosis and management of chronic sinusitis are discussed in Chapter 28.

Acute Exertional Headache (Orgasmic, Cough, Sneeze)

The features of acute exertional headache are (a) that is of sudden (or almost instantaneous) onset and (b) that it is directly related to exertion of some kind (orgasm, coughing, sneezing, straining, bending, running, lifting, *etc*). It may last from minutes to ½ hour, rarely longer (14). In 90% of patients the headache is presumably due to intracranial-spinal pressure dissociations, and the course is benign. In 10% of patients significant organic disease has been found (Arnold-Chiari malformation, hydrocephalus, tumor, and subarachnoid hemorrhage).

Exertional headache must be differentiated chiefly from the headache of *subarachnoid hemorrhage*. The headache of major subarachnoid hemorrhage is usually far more persistent and is often associated with fever, stiff neck, progressive clouding of consciousness, and focal neurological signs. Exertional headaches may be quite severe, but they are brief and they recur with the trigger activity. Because it may be impossible to distinguish the first episode of exertional headache from a minor subarachnoid hemorrhage, and because of the 10% risk of another organic basis for the headache, computerized tomography (CT), with and without contrast because of the possibility of tumor or arteriovenous malformation (see "Patient Experience," Chapter 78), should be considered when patients initially report the problem.

If CT findings are normal, the benign nature of the condition should be explained to the patient. The patient will usually find ways to avoid some of the activities which produce headache. If desired, propranolol, 40 to 80 mg twice/day, or indomethacin, 25 mg three times daily, can be tried for prophylaxis.

Temporomandibular Joint Syndrome

On history and examination, some patients complaining of headache will have the stigmata of this common syndrome—pain brought on by motion of the jaw and tenderness of the temporomandibular joint. The epidemiology, course, and management of this syndrome are described in Chapter 101.

Headache Due to Drugs

Headache is listed as an occasional side effect of many drugs. Among those commonly used drugs for which headache is more than an occasional side effect are indomethacin (Indocin), nalidixic acid (NegGram), trimethoprim-sulfamethoxazole (Bactrim, Septra), oral contraceptives, and vasodilators. Therefore, as noted earlier, it is important to ask the patient routinely about new drugs when evaluating a headache of recent onset.

A throbbing vascular type headache frequently occurs shortly after initiation of treatment (or a dose increase) with a *vasodilator* drug. The most common offenders are the short and long acting nitrates, calcium channel blockers, and the vasodilators used to treat hypertension (hydralazine and minoxidil). The management of this problem depends upon the importance of the drug and the severity of the headache. Some patients, if informed in advance of the possibility of headache, will choose to take the drug anyway; this is particularly true of sublingual nitrates administered for angina. For the long acting nitrates, dose reduction may effectively reduce headache for some patients, while alternate antianginal treatment will be needed for others (see Chapter 57). The headache associated with antihypertensive vasodilators can usually be prevented by treating the patient with a β-blocker before the vasodilator is added (see Chapter 62).

Headache in Acute Febrile Illnesses

Acute febrile illnesses may cause vascular type throbbing headaches that remit when the illness resolves. A febrile patient in whom the headache is the major symptom and in whom nuchal rigidity or other manifestation of meningeal irritation is present requires a cerebrospinal fluid examination to exclude meningitis.

Giant Cell Arteritis and Polymyalgia Rheumatica (4, 5)

Giant cell arteritis (GCA) is a vasculitis which affects large arteries throughout the body. Clinical manifestations, however, are usually due to involvement of branches of the external carotid artery and the most common syndrome is headache. GCA has also been called temporal arteritis (TA) because temporal headaches and a positive temporal artery biopsy are the findings which are most typical of the disease. The etiology of GCA is unknown.

Polymyalgia rheumatica (PR), a debilitating condition which presents with stiffness and aching of the neck and shoulder muscles, occurs in about 50%

of patients with GCA. PR may also occur in patients who do not have GCA.

Epidemiology

GCA is almost exclusively a disease of persons over the age of 50; the average age of onset is 65. It is very uncommon in black individuals. It is somewhat more common in women than in men. In the single reported community study of GCA, it was found that the yearly incidence in persons over 50 was approximately 17/100,000 and the prevalence, 130/100,000 (5).

Manifestations

Giant cell arteritis. The headache of GCA does not have specific features which distinguish it clearly from other headaches. It is temporal in over one-half of patients; however, it may be frontal, occipital, parietal, or holocephalic. The patient usually reports that it involves the surface and is not intracranial. It may be made worse by hair brushing, resting the head on a pillow, and, at times, by exposure to cold. It is usually not described as throbbing. It is often described as being worse at night, and building up gradually over a number of hours. Because these symptoms are not specific, the most important factors in suggesting the diagnosis of GCA are a number of associated findings, listed in Table 79.7. It is important to inquire specifically about pain (claudica-

Table 79.7.
Clinical Features of Giant Cell Arteritis[a]

Common Features (% of Patients with Feature at Initial Evaluation)		Less Common but Characteristic Features
Headache	(85)	Raynaud's phenomenon of limbs or tongue
Temporal artery tenderness	(70)	
Jaw claudication	(65)	Tender scalp nodules
Lingual, limb or swallowing claudication	(20)	Thick, tender occipital arteries
Brachiocephalic bruits	(50)	Necrotic lesions of scalp, tongue
Thickened or nodular temporal artery	(45)	Carotid artery tenderness
Pulseless temporal artery	(40)	
Visual symptoms	(40)	Swelling of the hands
Fixed blindness, partial or complete	(15)	Taste, smell disturbances
Polymyalgia rheumatica	(40)	Distended, beaded retinal veins
Weight loss > 6 kg	(35)	
Erythrocyte sedimentation rate		Diminished or absent radial artery pulses
>50 mm/hour	(95)	Mononeuropathy—median, peroneal, cervical root
>100 mm/hour	(60)	
Fever (>37.7°C)	(20)	
Abnormal liver function	(50)	
Anemia (hematocrit <35%)	(50)	

[a] Adapted from Raskin NH, Appenzeller O: *Headache*. Philadelphia, WB Saunders, 1980.

tion) associated with chewing, swallowing, and arm or tongue motion, as these symptoms are highly suggestive of GCA. The combination of one or more of the findings listed in Table 79.7 with a new headache in an older individual is sufficient to suspect GCA.

Polymyalgia rheumatica (PR). This condition is insidious in onset. The chief complaints are aching and stiffness of the shoulder girdle and, less commonly, of the thigh muscles. These symptoms may make it particularly hard for the patient to get up in the morning. Associated low grade fever, weight loss, and anorexia are common. On physical examination, there may be some tenderness of the shoulder and neck muscles, but there is no significant loss of muscle strength.

Diagnosis

Whenever GCA or PR is suspected, the erythrocyte sedimentation rate (ESR) measured by the Westergren method is the most useful screening test. The vast majority of patients will have a markedly elevated ESR (often 100 or greater). Since the upper limit of normal for persons over 60 may be as high as 40, an ESR of 40 to 60 is less informative than is a very high rate. *Definitive diagnosis of GCA* is made with a temporal artery biopsy. Because the typical histological changes (inflammatory cells, edema, and giant cells) are patchy in distribution, examination of serial sections of the resected segment of artery is essential; in occasional patients with GCA, even extensive sampling of one temporal artery does not yield a positive biopsy and the other artery must also be examined by biopsy.

Patient experience. A temporal artery biopsy can be done in an ambulatory surgery facility (by a general surgeon, vascular surgeon, plastic surgeon, or neurosurgeon). The scalp hair is shaved, the skin is anesthetized with Xylocaine, and the segment of artery (4 to 6 cm) is excised. The entire procedure requires about ½ hour. There are no serious sequelae.

The *diagnosis of polymyalgia rheumatica* is based on the combination of the typical symptoms, a high ESR, and exclusion of other explanations for the patient's symptoms. If a patient with typical PR has manifestations suggesting GCA (see Table 79.7), a temporal artery biopsy is indicated, since the recommended treatment for the two conditions is different.

Course and Treatment

Both GCA and PR are self-limited conditions, lasting up to 2 years. Treatment with corticosteroids produces dramatic symptomatic relief in patients with both conditions. More important, treatment appears to prevent almost entirely the most serious complication of GCA, blindness due to ischemic optic neuropathy. In untreated persons with GCA, unilateral or bilateral blindness occurs in 20 to 30% of patients.

If the diagnosis of GCA is strongly suspected, treatment should be initiated immediately and the temporal artery biopsy should be obtained within 3 to 4 days. The initial treatment is high dose prednisone (60 to 80 mg daily in four divided doses) for 4 to 6 weeks. During this time, symptoms usually remit entirely and there is a significant decrease in the ESR. After this initial period, the prednisone should be tapered weekly by about 10% until a dose of 10 to 15 mg daily has been reached. This dose should be continued for about 2 years, being discontinued by gradual tapering at the end of the second year (see Chapter 74 for details regarding long term steroid therapy).

If the patient has isolated PR, the treatment is 10 to 15 mg of prednisone daily, from the outset. Treatment is also continued for approximately 2 years, with gradual discontinuation at the end of that time. The symptoms of PR, and the ESR, respond to this regimen within a few days to a week.

Although the symptoms of both GCA and PR may respond to aspirin and other nonsteroidal anti-inflammatory agents, these agents have not been shown to prevent the progressive vasculitis in GCA that may lead to blindness. The evidence for the efficacy of prednisone therapy in preventing blindness is based not upon controlled trials but upon the dramatic difference in the occurrence of blindness in untreated patients before prednisone was used (20 to 30% of patients) and in prednisone-treated patients (little or no occurrence of blindness).

The diagnosis and treatment of typical cases of GCA and PR can be accomplished readily by the generalist in the ambulatory setting. Whenever there is some question about the diagnosis or an unsatisfactory response to treatment, the opinion of a rheumatologist should be obtained.

Benign Intracranial Hypertension (Pseudotumor Cerebri) (12, 15)

Benign intracranial hypertension, is thought to result from idiopathic swelling of the brain tissue and/or an increase in brain vascular volume. The net result of either of these processes is a generalized increase in intracranial pressure. Headache in this condition is presumably due to stretching of the dura and perhaps the large vessels. Papilledema is a direct result of the increased pressure. The paucity of focal neurological symptoms and signs is due to the generalized nature of the pressure increase. Those focal signs that do appear (for example, 6th nerve palsies producing horizontal diplopia) are probably related to stretching of the involved structure.

This condition may occur *de novo* or may appear in association with a number of purported contributing factors (obesity, menstrual irregularity, steroid therapy or steroid withdrawal, oral contraceptives, nalidixic acid, vitamin A intoxication, venous sinus thrombosis).

Manifestations

The prototypical patient is an obese young woman who develops progressively more severe headaches, nausea, vomiting, dizziness, and blurred vision. In approximately one-half of patients, onset is abrupt, while the rest develop symptoms progressively over several weeks or months. The headache always precedes visual symptoms. It is usually generalized, constant or throbbing, and episodic; it is often more severe in the morning and is aggravated by coughing, straining, or position change. The diagnosis is suggested strongly by these historical characteristics coupled with a physical examination which shows papilledema (plus retinal hemorrhages in about one-fourth of patients) without focal neurological signs. Visual fields may be constricted and the blind spot enlarged. Rarely the papilledema involves the macular area, resulting in blindness (15).

The diagnosis of pseudotumor is always one of exclusion, as its name implies. The most important considerations in the *differential diagnosis* are intracranial mass lesion, hydrocephalus, and hypertensive encephalopathy. To exclude an intracranial mass or hydrocephalus, a contrast CT scan (see "Patient Experience," Chapter 78) should be obtained in pseudotumor. The scan may show small ventricles and no evidence of a mass lesion. Following a negative scan, a lumbar puncture should be performed; in pseudotumor, the cerebrospinal fluid (CSF) pressure is high (200 to 400 mm H_2O or more) and the content of CSF protein is normal or low. The diagnosis of hypertensive encephalopathy should be made if the patient has the typical clinical features of pseudotumor, severe diastolic hypertension (equal to or greater than 120 mm Hg), and a negative CT scan. In a very obese woman, with a history of amenorrhea for many months, it is also important to consider pregnancy-induced hypertension (toxemia), which is ruled out by a negative pregnancy test (see Chapter 93).

For less clear-cut cases, such as a typical clinical presentation in an older male patient, referral to a neurologist is indicated.

Treatment and Course

Most patients recover completely from pseudotumor within several weeks, or months. Because the disease itself is self-limited, it is difficult to assess the role of treatment in recovery.

Treatment of the syndrome is aimed at reducing CSF pressure, to avoid progressive visual loss. In the very obese, weight reduction is recommended. Steroids (Decadron 6 to 12 mg daily) or diuretics (Diamox 2 to 4 g/day) have been used with some success in patients with persistent elevated pressure. Steroid withdrawal must occur gradually over at least 1 month.

Absence of response to drug therapy has resulted in the use of repeated lumbar punctures for decompression. The value of removing 10 to 50 ml of CSF when 500 ml are produced daily is dubious. Most patients rebel against this treatment, and the pressure usually returns to its initial high level within 24 or 48 hours. In patients with a serious threat to vision, caused by pressure, a CSF shunting procedure, such as a lumboperitoneal shunt, is required. Management of these patients is difficult and requires the attention of neurologists and neurosurgeons experienced in handling this disorder.

Post-traumatic (Postconcussive) Headache

Manifestations

Head trauma, which may or may not have been severe enough to cause loss of consciousness, may be followed by a number of symptoms which have been collectively entitled the postconcussive syndrome: headache, vertigo (often positional, see Chapter 81) light-headedness or giddiness, poor concentration and memory, lack of energy, irritability, and anxiety. There is convincing evidence that these varied symptoms may be organic consequences of the injury, even though their exact causal mechanism is not understood. Raskin and Appenzeller (see "General References") provide an excellent review of the syndrome with the focus on headache.

Headache is the most frequent and often the most troubling manifestation of this syndrome. It typically begins within 24 hours of the trauma, as a dull, constant, generalized aching or cephalic discomfort which may wax and wane through the day or become concentrated at different points on the head (bifrontal or unilateral). During exacerbations, the pain typically becomes more vascular, with a throbbing quality. Headache may be worsened by sneezing, coughing, stooping, straining, or rapid head motions and changes in body position; it may be accompanied by nausea and vomiting.

Typically, these headaches worsen over days to weeks, then resolve over weeks or months; in some patients (roughly 15%) headache and other postconcussive symptoms continue for more than a year. It is now appreciated that minor head trauma in individuals with no prior headache history may lead to chronic recurrent headaches typical of classic or common migraine. Propranolol or amitriptyline used alone or in combination (see Table 79.6) has resulted in a dramatic reduction in frequency and severity of the headaches in some patients (19).

Differential Diagnosis

Subdural hematoma and other expanding mass lesions. Although postconcussive syndrome is a far

more likely explanation of post-traumatic headache and ill defined intellectual impairments than subdural hematoma, the seriousness of this possibility and the ease of ruling it out with CT scan make it an important consideration.

Post-traumatic dysautonomic cephalgia. Predominantly vascular (throbbing) headache pain associated with sweating of one side of the face, pupillary dilation, and sometimes, carotid bifurcation tenderness, may represent a lesion of the carotid sympathetic plexus produced by whiplash-like injury (17). This condition may respond well to propranolol (see Table 79.6).

Pre-existing *migraine* or chronic *tension headaches* will have to be excluded by history; furthermore, post-traumatic headaches may make a preexisting headache condition temporarily worse.

Cervical spine injury. See Chapter 64.

Objective Tests

In addition to the neurological history and examination, a number of currently available objective tests may be helpful for confirming the diagnosis of postconcussive syndrome: electroencephalography; vestibular function tests; electronystagmography; and auditory and visual evoked potentials. These tests, when positive, may be helpful medically and medicolegally. Because the abnormalities in these patients may be below the threshold of detectability, negative test results do not exclude an organic explanation of the patient's symptoms.

Treatment

For some patients with postconcussive headache, treatment similar to that used for migraine, with ergotamine and other agents (see page 1124), may occasionally be successful. In most patients, the course of the illness is self-limited even though fairly lengthy.

Characteristics of Headache Due to a Mass Lesion

For both the headache sufferer and the physician, concern about the possibility of a brain tumor often dominates the situation. A number of clinical clues suggest that one is not dealing with a benign process; the most important clue to the presence of an intracranial lesion in a headache sufferer is the simultaneous onset of headache and focal neurological signs/symptoms or a change in mental status. In a person over the age of 50, the onset of persistent headache for the first time, especially in the absence of psychosocial stress, is also very worrisome.

A number of other features, none of them specific, may be clues to the presence of an intracranial mass lesion:

1. Although the headache associated with a mass lesion can initially be intermittent, mild, and responsive to mild analgesics, typically it becomes

more continuous and intense and, at the same time, less responsive to analgesics.

2. The headache may wake the patient from sleep or be present on waking every day. The value of these characteristics is somewhat diminished by the comparatively larger number of patients with chronic tension headache, migraine, and cluster headache who are also awakened by or wake up with headache. True sinus headache may also be worse in the morning due to lack of postural drainage during the night.

3. Coughing, sneezing, and straining may aggravate a persistent headache due to a mass lesion, presumably by transiently increasing intracranial pressure and accentuating the stretching of pain-sensitive structures. Again, however, migraine headaches can show the same features.

4. Anorexia, nausea, and vomiting may accompany the headache, but these symptoms are not distinguishable from those caused by severe migraine headache. Projectile vomiting is rarely seen in adults with intracranial masses.

Except when there are focal neurological signs or symptoms, the decision to evaluate a patient for a mass lesion will usually be made after an initial period of observation and a trial of analgesics. A CT scan with contrast (see "Patient Experience," Chapter 78) is the diagnostic procedure of choice when the decision is made to evaluate for a mass lesion. Because of its safety, high sensitivity, and moderate specificity, this procedure is the only screening test usually needed in the search for a mass lesion. When the CT scan is positive for intracranial disease, the patient should be referred to a neurologist or a neurosurgeon for definitive care.

FACIAL PAIN SYNDROMES

Idiopathic Trigeminal Neuralgia (Tic Douloureux)

Manifestations

Trigeminal neuralgia is a problem seen almost exclusively in patients over the age of 40, most of them elderly. It has several distinguishing features: the pain is severe, paroxysmal, and lancinating; it lasts only a few seconds to a minute. The patient's face usually contorts with the pain, and the patient may find it impossible to control his emotional response. Between attacks the patient is usually pain free, although some patients may have a dull ache in the area. The interval between paroxysms is usually at least 2 or 3 minutes. The frequency of paroxysms is highly variable; some individuals have hundreds each day.

The pain is usually felt in those structures innervated by the second and third divisions of the trigeminal nerve (lips, gums, cheek, chin). There is a slightly greater tendency for tic to affect the right side of the face than the left. The pain is typically unilateral in a single attack, and in 95% of patients it remains unilateral. It is exceedingly uncommon for attacks to involve both sides of the face simultaneously.

The patient frequently can identify trigger points on the face or in the mouth, which, when touched (even by contact with a gust of cold air) or moved, precipitate pain.

A few patients with idiopathic trigeminal neuralgia will have some areas of slightly decreased sensation which may be difficult to distinguish from normal; however, there is generally no objective decrease in sensation (in men, no more decrease than would normally be observed over the beard area).

Differential Diagnosis

A syndrome identical to or similar to idiopathic trigeminal neuralgia can be produced by a number of known conditions (secondary trigeminal neuralgia), e.g., multiple sclerosis, acoustic neurinoma, aneurysms, trigeminal neuromas, meningiomas, and others. These conditions should be considered, particularly if the patient is under 40 years, and has any of the following: pain predominantly in the upper division of the trigeminal nerve (forehead and eye); bilateral pain; or evidence of bilateral sensory loss or associated motor signs (e.g., weak jaw, facial weakness, swallowing difficulty).

In a patient with a typical clinical presentation, medical therapy (see below) can be initiated without further workup. If medical therapy is ineffective, or if there are any atypical features, referral to a neurologist is appropriate. He will usually request X-ray views helpful in evaluating the divisions of the trigeminal nerve which are clinically most involved (for the first division, the superior orbital fissure; for third division, the foramen ovale). A contrast CT scan (see "Patient Experience," Chapter 78) may also be obtained to check for a neuroma or a meningioma involving the trigeminal or other nerves.

Treatment

Advances in drug therapy have made the treatment of idiopathic trigeminal neuralgia relatively easy. The patient should initially be given carbamazepine (Tegretol, 200-mg tablets) ½ tablet (100 mg) twice daily, with meals, increasing every 2 to 3 days to a three times daily schedule and a total dose of 300 to 600 mg. An occasional patient may need doses as high as 1200 mg/day; in these cases, blood levels should be monitored to confirm the adequacy of the drug trial. Sixty to 70% of patients can expect excellent to satisfactory relief with carbamazepine. Benign side effects of the drug include nausea, vomiting, ataxia, vertigo, and transient leukopenia. The most serious side effects seem to be either allergic or idiosyncratic, including persistent leukopenia and aplastic anemia. Patients must be informed of these possible risks, the incidence of which is unknown but which appears to be quite low. Because of these risks, patients should have serial hemograms performed, weekly for the first 3 months, and monthly thereafter. Because trigeminal neuralgia may remit spontaneously after 6 months to a year, cautious withdrawal from drug therapy should be attempted at periodic intervals (3 months).

If the patient fails to improve with carbamazepine or fails to tolerate the drug, he should be referred to a neurosurgeon for percutaneous radiofrequency treatment of the trigeminal ganglion on the affected side. This procedure has essentially no morbidity or mortality. It can be repeated if pain relief is not achieved or if pain recurs.

Atypical Facial Pain

"Atypical facial pain" is a collective term for a variety of painful facial symptoms which do not meet the diagnostic criteria for any recognized entity (18). If untreated, most patients with this problem continue to complain of it for many years. The management of these patients involves excluding all reasonable possibilities; a one-time referral to a dentist and to an otolaryngologist should be part of this evaluation.

Most of these patients whose workup is negative have psychosocial problems and may improve with psychotherapy, provided either by the general physician or a psychiatrist. For additional details, see the discussion of the patient with chronic pain in Chapter 12.

General References

Caviness VA, O'Brien P: Current concepts—headache. *N Engl J Med* 302:446, 1980.

A succinct review of several types of headache and recent therapeutic modalities.

Delassio DJ (ed): *Wolff's Headache and Other Head Pain*, ed 4. New York, Oxford University Press, 1980.

The most recent edition of the classic reference work on headache.

Diamond S, Delessio DJ: *The Practicing Physician's Approach to Headache*, ed 2. Baltimore, Williams & Wilkins, 1978.

A good general reference by two authorities in the field.

Diamond S, Medina JL: Review article: Current thoughts on migraine. *Headache* 20:208, 1980.

A practical and up to date review.

Packard RC (ed): *Neurologic Clinics. Symposium on Headache.* Philadelphia, WB Saunders, 1983, vol 1.

A comprehensive update on new developments in the field of headache, with practical information and techniques for headache diagnosis and management.

Raskin NH, Appenzeller O: *Headache.* Philadelphia, WB Saunders, 1980.

Extensively referenced book on selected headache syndromes (migraine, tension headache, cluster headache, post-traumatic headache, giant cell arteritis).

Specific References

1. Clinical Conferences at The Johns Hopkins Hospital: Cluster headache. *Johns Hopkins Med J* 150:246, 1982.
2. Dhopesh V, Anwar R, Herring C: A retrospective assessment of emergency department patients with complaint of headache. *Headache* 19:37, 1979.
3. Friedman AP, von Storch TJC, Merritt HH: Migraine and tension headaches: a clinical study of 2,000 cases. *Neurology* 4:773, 1954.
4. Hamilton CR, Jr, Shelley WM, Tumulty PA: Giant cell arteritis: Including temporal arteritis and polymyalgia rheumatica. *Medicine* 50:1, 1971.
5. Huston KA, Hunder GG, Lie JT, et al: Temporal arteritis: a 25–year epidemiologic, clinical and pathologic study. *Ann Intern Med* 88:162, 1978.
6. Kudrow L: Response of cluster headache attacks to oxygen inhalation. *Headache* 21:1, 1981.
7. Lance JW, Curran DA, Anthony J: Investigations into the mechanism and treatment of chronic headache. *Med J Aust* 2:909, 1965.
8. Markush RE, Karp HR, Heyman A, O'Fallon WM: Epidemiologic study of migraine symptoms in young women. *Neurology* 25:430, 1975.
9. Price RW, Posner JB: Chronic paroxysmal hemicrania; a disabling headache syndrome responding to indomethacin. *Ann Neurol* 3:183, 1978.
10. Monro J, Carini C, Brostoff J: Migraine is a food-allergic disease. *Lancet* 2:719, 1984.
11. Packard RC: What does the headache patient want? *Headache* 19:370, 1979.
12. Johnston I, Patterson A: Benign intracranial hypertension. *Brain* 97:289, 1975.
13. Raskin NH, Schwartz RK: Interval therapy of migraine: long-term results. *Headache* 20:336, 1980.
14. Rooke ED: Benign exertional headache. *Med Clin North Am* 52:801, 1968.
15. Rush JA: Pseudotumor cerebri, clinical profile visual outcome in 63 patients. *Mayo Clin Proc* 55:541, 1980.
16. Schnarch DM, Hunter JE: Migraine incidence in clinical versus nonclinical populations. *Psychosomatics* 21:314, 1980.
17. Vijayan N, Dreyfus PM: Post-traumatic dysautonomic cephalalgia. *Arch Neurol* 32:649, 1975.
18. Weedington WW, Blazer D: Atypical facial pain and trigeminal neuralgia: a comparison study. *Psychosomatics* 20:348, 1979.
19. Weiss H, Stern BJ, Goldberg J: Chronic migraine after minor head trauma. *Ann Neurol* 16:113, 1984.
20. Ziegler DK, Hassasein RW, Cough JR: Characteristics of life headache histories in a nonclinic population. *Neurology* 27:265, 1977.

CHAPTER EIGHTY

Seizure Disorders

ROBERT S. FISHER, M.D., Ph.D

Approximately 0.5 to 1% of the United States population, as many as 2 million Americans, are believed to have epilepsy. Many additional patients who do not carry the diagnosis of epilepsy present to their personal physicians or to emergency rooms for evaluation and management of seizures. Convulsive disorders are estimated to account for about 5% of visits to all physicians in private practice and for 20% of visits to neurologists (15). Because seizures are so common and the potential consequences of the disease which they cause are so serious, all physicians should be familiar with the basic principles of their diagnosis and management.

DEFINITION AND MECHANISM OF SEIZURES

The precise definition of a "seizure" is not easy, in part because no single behavior or laboratory result is pathognomonic. One approach is to define a seizure as an episode, with a clear start and finish, which affects motor control, sensation, speech, or consciousness and which is associated with certain characteristic electrical abnormalities of the brain. Most patients are relatively normal during the period between seizures (the interictal period), and their electroencephalograms (EEGs) may be normal as well.

The term "epilepsy" describes the condition of recurrent seizures due to primary (and persisting) nervous system disease. Therefore, single or even multiple seizures which occur as a result of temporally limited circumstances (such as high fever) should not be labeled as "epilepsy."

Although many predisposing factors are known, the basic mechanisms of seizures are still uncertain. Until a clear understanding of these mechanisms emerges, all classification schemes must be empirical. A widely accepted, clinically relevant scheme is shown in Table 80.1.

About 75% of all people with epilepsy can easily be classified according to this scheme. About 22% of classifiable patients over the age of 15 have generalized epilepsy and 78% have partial epilepsy.

Table 80.1.
Classification of the Epilepsies[a]

PRIMARY GENERALIZED EPILEPSY
    Tonic-clonic (grand mal)
    Absence (petit mal)
    Myoclonic
    Akinetic, others
PARTIAL (FOCAL) EPILEPSY
    With elementary symptomatology
        Focal motor
        Focal sensory
        Vegetative
        Psychic
        Mixed
    With complex symptomatology
        Partial complex (psychomotor)
SECONDARY GENERALIZED
UNCLASSIFIABLE

[a] Adapted from Dreifuss FE: Proposal for revised clinical and electro-encephalographic classification of epileptic seizures. *Epilepsia* 22:489, 1981.

Complex partial seizures, labeled in the past "temporal lobe epilepsy," "psychomotor epilepsy," or "limbic epilepsy," are the most common form of seizures in adults. Specific causes of these different categories of seizures are considered below.

CLINICAL PRESENTATIONS OF THE EPILEPSIES

The clinical manifestations of a seizure depend upon several factors: the degree of maturity of the nervous system, the location of the initial abnormal electrical discharges, and the manner in which these discharges spread. A seizure focus in the motor cortex will produce jerking of those parts of the body normally governed by the region of the focus; a seizure in a "sensory region" of the brain will generate abnormal sensation; a seizure in the so-called areas of "higher function" leads to complex cognitive and behavioral manifestations (see Fig. 80.1). Certain types of seizures present with sudden changes in consciousness rather than with focal motor or sensory signs or symptoms.

Generalized Tonic-Clonic (Grand Mal)

In patients with grand mal (now called "primary generalized tonic-clonic") epilepsy, seizure discharges present nearly synchronously in widespread regions of the cortex. The term "grand mal" should not be applied to seizures having focal onset and secondary generalization. These latter events should be called "generalized seizures" or "major motor seizures" instead of "grand mal," because the latter connotes initial generalization of seizure activity.

Grand mal seizures typically begin with an arrest of activity and sudden loss of consciousness, followed by trembling, tonic stiffening of the upper and lower extremities, then clonic rhythmical jerking of the limbs, followed by waxing and waning to a state of flaccidity. The usual duration of the sequence is 2 to 5 minutes. After a seizure, the patient may remain stuporous for minutes to hours. During the seizure loss of consciousness is invariable; consequently, production of speech, purposeful eye movements, or subsequent recall for events during the seizure are features which rule out the diagnosis of grand mal epilepsy. Although a general sensation of unease may warn of an impending grand mal attack, a definite sensory, motor, or psychological aura should raise strong suspicion of a partial (focal) seizure that has become secondarily generalized. Common associated findings during both grand mal or secondary major motor seizures include incontinence, sweating, tachycardia, elevated blood pressure, and minor cardiac arrhythmias.

Grand mal seizures may first develop at any age, though onset is rare after about age 35. Frequency may range from one seizure in an entire lifetime to several seizures a day.

Generalized Absence (Petit Mal)

Petit mal (now designated "absence, typical") is another example of primary generalized epilepsy. It comprises about 10% of seizures, but it is primarily a disease of children, with onset usually between 4 and 12 years of age. The clinical presentation of petit mal seizures is quite distinct from grand mal. Petit mal is an entity in its own right and not a "little grand mal." Similarly, the use of the term "petit mal" to describe any brief lapse of consciousness or attention is a misnomer and an invitation to inappropriate therapy. Petit mal seizures present with absence attacks (i.e., lapses of consciousness) lasting about 3 to 30 seconds. There is no tonic-clonic phase, nor loss of posture. Slight rhythmic twitching of the mouth or periorbital musculature may be observed. If petit mal seizures are atypical, with prolonged duration or notable automatisms, the distinction

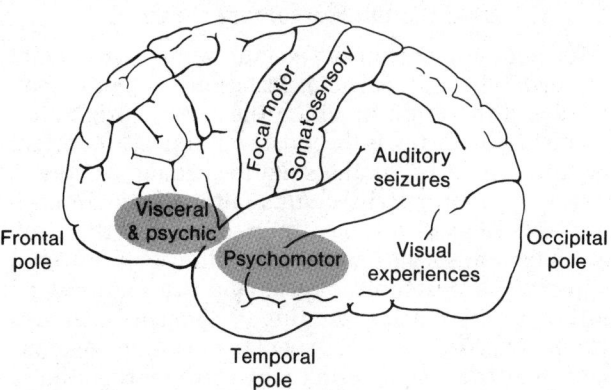

Figure 80.1. Relation of local seizure phenomena to brain topography.

from temporal lobe ("partial complex") seizures can be quite difficult. After a petit mal seizure, recovery of awareness occurs within seconds, but amnesia for events during the seizure is lasting. Petit mal seizures can occur over 100 times/day. Children who suffer such frequent seizures may be labeled daydreamers or slow learners, until a correct diagnosis is made.

The EEG during a petit mal seizure shows a characteristic 3/second spike-wave pattern. Interictal EEGs in children with petit mal epilepsy are often normal. Sometimes hyperventilation or stimulation with regularly flashing lights may bring out abnormalities. Both clinical and EEG findings should be used to secure a diagnosis of petit mal epilepsy: neither alone is diagnostic.

About three of four children outgrow petit mal by age 20, but up to 50% (especially among those with atypical absence) may later develop grand mal seizures.

Myoclonic Seizures

Myoclonus consists of involuntary nonrhythmic jerking of limbs, trunk, or head, which is usually not fully synchronous (i.e., all parts do not move at the same time). When a series of frequent myoclonic jerks occurs in a limited period of time—exact criteria are arbitrary—the term "myoclonic seizure" is applied. Myoclonus is encountered by general physicians as a consequence of diffuse cortical injury from such causes as anoxia, hypoglycemia, severe renal or hepatic failure, or drug toxicity. In these conditions myoclonic seizures are often self-limited and resolve as the underlying illness stabilizes. Primary neurological disease, e.g., viral encephalitis, Jakob-Creutzfeldt disease, Huntington's chorea, or Wilson's disease, also may present in part with myoclonus.

Cases of familial myoclonus with associated neurological symptoms may be parceled into several different syndromes. These patients are generally managed in consultation with a neurologist.

Partial (Focal) Elementary Seizures

Focal motor or sensory seizures may present at any age. The clinical manifestations depend upon the site of the brain in which the seizure originates.

The motor cortex is the most common site of origin for focal seizures; as the seizure discharges spread across the motor strip, clonus (alternating contraction and relaxation) may "march" across the limb and face. Sensory seizures most often begin from a focus in the postcentral gyrus and are manifest by numbness in the face or fingers. Sensory seizures can also involve areas of special sensation. A focus in or near the visual cortex may cause perception of spots and lights, similar to the experience of patients suffering from classic migraine. Buzzing or ringing may be generated from a focus in the superior temporal lobe. Gustatory and olfactory sensations are components of partial complex (temporal lobe) seizures. Seizures dominated by vestibular symptoms are rare.

Retention of awareness is characteristic of focal seizures, so that patients may walk, talk, and think normally during a seizure—accomplishments that would be impossible during a generalized seizure. However, a large focus in the dominant hemisphere may generate seizures which blunt awareness.

After a focal motor seizure, there may be weakness of the body parts that have been involved. This so-called "Todd's paralysis" usually resolves within a few hours or, in unusual cases, after a few days. Distinction between cerebrovascular ischemic events with associated seizures and seizures with Todd's paralysis may be impossible without clues from the past history. Presence of a Todd's paralysis has localizing value and is good evidence that a seizure was focal.

Electroencephalography will not necessarily reveal a seizure focus, especially if it is small, particularly during the interictal stage.

Partial (Psychomotor) Complex Seizures

"Partial complex epilepsy" may be considered synonymous with "temporal lobe epilepsy," "psychomotor epilepsy," and "limbic epilepsy." This category of seizures is important for several reasons: the condition is common in the adult population; psychomotor seizures are often misdiagnosed; and correct diagnosis leads to a search for potentially correctable lesions and to effective therapy. Complex partial epilepsy is classified as a focal epilepsy because of clinical evidence linking these seizures with foci in or near the temporal lobe.

The presentation of partial complex epilepsy is more varied than that of the other forms of epilepsy and may include autonomic, psychic, visceral, sensory, or motor symptoms. Warning of an impending seizure may be signaled by an "aura." The classic aura of olfactory or gustatory hallucination is actually less common than is an aura of nondescript unpleasant visceral sensations or a sense of unease. There is, in general, no clear boundary between the aura and the seizure itself, particularly when seizures feature distorted visual or auditory sensations, or vertigo or general disequilibrium. Arrest of motor activity, rigid posturing of the head and eyes, and slow repetitive limb movements may occur and are easily distinguished in most cases from the tonic-clonic sequence of major motor attacks. Autonomic instability, including fluctuating heart rate or blood pressure, flushing, sweating, salivating, alterations in pupillary reactions, or incontinence of urine or feces, has been described in patients with temporal lobe seizures. The term "psychomotor epilepsy" derived from the frequent mental changes that characterize this form of epilepsy. Patients often say that they feel strange, in a "dream," or experience inappropriate emotions such as intense dread or strange serenity. During the seizure, consciousness is impaired to a variable extent; if they can talk, patients may portray what appears to be a primarily psychiatric illness. The distinction between partial complex epilepsy and psychosis may be obscured further in patients whose interictal personality is abnormal. Such individuals can easily be misdiagnosed as schizophrenic.

In a condition whose presentation may range from apparent appendicitis to apparent schizophrenia the physician must make special efforts to elicit a detailed history of a "spell" and, when possible, to observe one personally. Complex partial seizures should have a definite start and finish; they should be associated with some impairment in ability to register and process information during the seizure; and they should be relatively stereotyped from episode to episode. Observations of automatic behavior, such as repetitive mouth smacking, raising and lowering the arm, buttoning and unbuttoning a shirt, or pacing in circles, may secure the diagnosis of a partial complex seizure disorder, for such "automatisms" are common in psychomotor epilepsy and uncommon in other forms of seizures.

The standard EEG is abnormal in only about half of patients with partial complex seizures. The yield may be increased to 80 to 90% by recording EEGs during sleep and by using special electrodes positioned in the nasopharynx close to the undersurface of the temporal lobe.

Although partial complex seizures may begin at any age, the majority begin before age 20. Adult onset of temporal lobe epilepsy carries the same significance as does a new onset of any focal seizure; a significant structural lesion must be ruled out. Patients with onset of temporal lobe seizures, who come to surgery or to postmortem, may show either no histological abnormality of the brain or may have tumors, infarcts, granulomas, or infections, or more often a generalized gliosis of the mesial temporal lobe ("mesial temporal sclerosis"). It is not known whether gliosis causes temporal lobe seizures or follows from them.

Prognosis for spontaneous remission of complex partial seizures is not as favorable as it is for grand mal seizures.

Secondarily Generalized Seizures

Secondarily generalized seizures begin clinically as focal seizures (including those beginning as partial complex seizures) and then generalize to seizures indistinguishable from grand mal attacks. The focal onset can be as fleeting as a few tremors in an arm, numbness of the hand or one side of the face, or marked conjugate deviation of the eyes or head. Sensory or visceral auras are also evidence of focal

onset, as is preservation of consciousness during the early part of a seizure.

Complex electrophysiological mechanisms govern whether seizure discharges remain in a local focus, spread along certain prescribed anatomical pathways, or generalize to much of the brain. A focal seizure may generalize when conditions of overall brain excitability are "right." Conversely, anticonsulsive therapy may convert a secondarily generalized seizure into a focal seizure. It is not known how often grand mal attacks are actually secondarily generalized seizures with occult primary origins.

The treatments for secondarily generalized seizures are the same as those for grand mal seizures (see pages 1144–1148), except for the need to treat, if possible, any structural lesions responsible for the focal origins.

Unclassifiable Seizures

With an adequate history, most seizures should be classifiable by the scheme given above. Unfortunately, the history is sometimes lacking, as when observers report "falling down and shaking," but cannot describe the full sequence of events. In these instances it is best to list the seizure as "unclassifiable" or to use nondescript terms such as "tonic-clonic" or an "absence attack" (if there was a brief lapse of consciousness), until the specific seizure type becomes evident.

EPIDEMIOLOGY AND PROGNOSIS OF SEIZURES

The reported yearly incidence of new onset epilepsy is approximately 20 to 50/100,000 population, and the prevalence is between 2 and 10 (0.2 to 1%)/ 1,000 population (30). Treiman (27) reviewed three series published since 1975, comprising 4,751 adult cases, to determine the relative frequency of the different types of epilepsy. Overall 67% were partial in onset, 20% generalized, and 13% unclassified. Partial complex (previously designated "psychomotor") seizures were the most prevalent, at 41% of the entire seizure group; partial simple (focal motor or sensory) seizures were next, at 15%; primary generalized tonic-clonic (grand mal) and secondarily generalized each comprised about 11%; myoclonic seizures accounted for about 4%. At the younger end of the age spectrum, partial seizures are less frequent and generalized absence seizures more frequent than is represented by these averaged percentages.

The natural history of epilepsy is difficult to determine because all modern studies include heterogeneous mixes of treated and untreated patients. After a first unprovoked seizure the cumulative risk of recurrence is 16% at 1 year, 21% at 2 years, and 27% at 3 years (9). The role of treatment in reducing this risk is presently uncertain. If a person suffers a second, unprovoked seizure, then the risk for further seizures is high.

Once two spontaneous seizures have occurred, epilepsy is considered to exist, and the epidemiological focus switches to the possibility for remission. Before the development of anticonvulsant medication, the spontaneous remission rate for all types of seizures was about 10 to 32%. A study from the Mayo Clinic in Minnesota (3) showed that the remission rate, defined as 5 consecutive years seizure free (on or off therapy), was 70% at a time 20 years after diagnosis of epilepsy. Studies on prognosis have not yet clarified the role of treatment in the long term outcome. It is useful to know that the probability of 5 years without seizures is 42% at 1 year and 51% at 2 years after diagnosis of epilepsy. The probability of being in remission at 20 years was 80 to 85% for patients with primary generalized epilepsies, but only 65% for those with partial complex epilepsies. Slightly less than half of the Mayo Clinic patient group remained on medication at 20 years. A British study (7) has showed the following to be poor prognostic factors in becoming seizure free for at least 2 years while on therapy: continuing seizures for the initial 2 years of treatment, presence of partial seizures, a high frequency of tonic-clonic seizures before treatment, a neuropsychiatric deficit, and positive family history for epilepsy.

It is generally possible to reassure a person with epilepsy that the long term prognosis for remission is likely to be good; however, except for the primary generalized epilepsies in children, the remission can be expected to require many years.

Serious injury or death rarely occurs as a direct consequence of epilepsy, although anecdotal instances of sudden unexplained deaths in people with epilepsy have been reported.

ETIOLOGY OF SEIZURES

General Comments

Classification of seizures, as given above, depends upon clinical and EEG observation of the patient. A seizure represents a symptom: once the presence of a seizure has been established and the seizure classified, an etiology must be sought. How likely this search is to be successful is difficult to ascertain from the medical literature, because of serious biases in selecting populations for study.

Epilepsy secondary to identified causes is sometimes called "symptomatic" as opposed to "essential," "cryptogenic," or "idiopathic" epilepsy. It is agreed that most cases of primary generalized epilepsy are cryptogenic, so that a child presenting with typical petit mal or grand mal seizures, in the context of a normal examination, normal screening laboratory tests (see below), and a positive family history for similar seizures, would not warrant an extensive search for underlying causes. The yield is

higher from investigation of partial or atypical generalized seizures (25); without a computerized tomographic (CT) scan a lesion can be demonstrated about 50% of the time; with a CT scan, about 65 to 70% of the time (16).

Table 80.2 lists specific etiologies which should be considered for different types of seizures at various ages; the diagnoses are listed from top to bottom roughly in the order of their frequency (except that "idiopathic" is placed at the end of each list because it is a diagnosis of exclusion). It is worth emphasizing that all of the partial epilepsies can become secondarily generalized, and that the focal onset may be obscured. Therefore, the clinician should give some though to "focal etiologies" even in apparently generalized seizures.

Special issues are raised by *seizures that are manifest for the first time in the elderly*. First, most seizure disorders have onset in the first three decades of life, and onset of the primary generalized forms of epilepsy almost never occurs after this age. Second, cerebrovascular disease accounts for 30 to 60% of all new seizures in the elderly population (23). Tumors, the major cause of focal seizures in the middle-aged, cause 2 to 30% (23) of seizures in the elderly; however, brain tumors in this age group are very likely to be malignant. Infection, trauma, metabolic disease, hypertensive encephalopathy, and degenerative conditions are all documented causes of seizures in the geriatric population, but a cause is not found to explain seizures in half or more of this group. When an elderly patient presents with seizures, a special effort should be made to rule out treatable conditions—carotid artery occlusions, cardiac arrhythmias, infection, and toxic-metabolic derangements.

Some classes of seizures are so commonly encountered by the primary physician that detailed consideration of them is warranted.

Post-traumatic Seizures

According to the National Head and Spinal Cord Injury Survey of the National Institutes of Health (1) 422,000 patients were hospitalized in 1974 for head injuries, 200/100,000 US population. Four to 5 times that number of head injuries are sustained by people who are not hospitalized but who still have a significant risk of brain damage (4). The incidence of post-traumatic epilepsy depends upon several factors: the population under study, the severity of the injury, the duration of follow-up, and the criteria used to label a seizure as a manifestation of epilepsy. In patients with a mild injury (brief unconsciousness or amnesia) risk of later epilepsy is not increased significantly above baseline, whereas severe injuries (intracranial hematomas, focal neurological signs, unconsciousness for more than 24 hours) result in epilepsy in 7% of patients after 1 year and in 11.5% after 5 years (2). Moderately severe injuries (skull

Table 80.2
Etiological Factors for Seizures with Onset at Various Ages[a]

Adolescent (12–21 yr)	Adult (21–65 yr)	Elderly (65+ yr)
Common Causes		
Genetic (g)	Alcohol withdrawal (g)	Cerebrovascular (m)
Mesial temporal sclerosis (f)	Toxins or drugs (g)[c]	Thrombotic
Infection (m)	Drug withdrawal (g)	Embolic
Meningitis	Tumor (f)	Hemorrhagic
Viral encephalitis	Trauma (f)	Cardiac arrhythmia
Abscess	Scar	Trauma (f)
TORCHS[b]	Subdural hematoma	Scar
Parasites	Mesial temporal sclerosis (f)	Subdural hematoma
Hysteria/factitious (m)	Genetic (g)	Tumor (f)
Toxins or drugs (g)[c]	Hysteria/factitious (m)	Infection (m)
Drug withdrawal (g)	Infection (m)	Meningitis
	Meningitis	Viral encephalitis
	Viral encephalitis	Abscess
	Abscess	Syphilis
	Syphilis	Parasites
	Parasites	
Occasional Causes		
Metabolic (g)	Metabolic (g)	Alcohol withdrawal (g)
Hypoglycemia	Hypoglycemia	Toxins or drugs (g)[c]
Hyponatremia	Hyponatremia	Drug withdrawal (g)
Hypocalcemia	Hypocalcemia	Hypoxia (g)
Porphyria	Hypomagnesemia	Metabolic (g)
Trauma (f)	Hypoxia (g)	Hypoglycemia
Scar	Cerebrovascular (m)	Hyponatremia
Subdural hematoma	Thrombotic	Hypocalcemia
Tumor (f)	Embolic	
Arteriovenous malformation (f)	Hemorrhagic	
Subarachnoid hemorrhage (m)	Cardiac arrhythmia	
Eclampsia (m)	Renal failure (g)	
Renal failure (g)	Eclampsia (m)	
Rare Causes		
Collagen disease (m)	Collagen disease (m)	Hypertensive encephalopathy (m)
Hepatic failure (g)	Hypertensive encephalopathy (m)	Hyperosmolar (m)
Multiple sclerosis (f)	Hyperosmolar (m)	Renal failure (g)
	Multiple sclerosis (f)	Hepatic failure (g)
	Degenerative (m)	Degenerative (g)
		Factitious (m)
Idiopathic	Idiopathic	Idiopathic

[a] f, usually focal; g, usually generalized; m, often mixed.
[b] TORCHS, toxoplasmosis, rubella, cytomegalovirus, herpes, syphilis.
[c] See list of occupational exposures which may cause seizures, Table 7.3.

fractures or unconsciousness for 30 minutes to 24 hours) impose an intermediate risk. Injuries over the vertex are more epileptogenic.

The value of prophylactic therapy (20) in preventing post-traumatic seizures has not been firmly established. Until more data become available, a reasonable approach for clinicians includes the following elements: patients with minor scalp lacerations or brief loss of consciousness should not be considered to have a significantly increased risk of epilepsy. A single seizure occurring during the first 2 weeks after head injury, or while the patient is still suffering from the acute effects of injury, should not

be an indication for long term therapy. A second seizure in this setting might be grounds for treatment. Patients with brain injuries should be given a 2- to 4-year course of prophylactic phenytoin (unless there are particular contraindications to chronic medication), especially if consciousness has been lost for more than 24 hours, if the dura has been penetrated (by trauma or by surgery), or if the vertex has been involved. If a patient has a "spontaneous" seizure more than 2 weeks after a head injury, he should be evaluated and treated as would any other patient with a new onset of seizure disorder—the seizure should not be attributed to a recent or remote episode of head trauma until other treatable causes of seizures have been ruled out.

Alcohol-Related Seizures

Alcohol withdrawal is a very common cause of seizures: almost all of them occur within the first 48 hours of abstinence and most of them are generalized. In some series up to 25% of seizures have been focal, presumably because of a concomitant old cortical scar from trauma, infection, or vascular disease. If a known alcoholic has had a prior withdrawal seizure, presents a typical picture of a generalized seizure without focal features, has a normal examination and no complications, then investigations may be limited. More often, the history is imprecise and findings are equivocal, or the patient has a fever or an elevated leukocyte count. In these instances lumbar puncture, EEG, and continued observation are indicated. A CT scan is likely to be of use when focal seizures, focal neurological deficits, or signs of acute head trauma are present.

Treatment of alcohol withdrawal seizures is controversial, because the majority of patients (approximately 95%) in a state of withdrawal do not have seizures, or have them only once or twice. Many of the standard medications, such as chlordiazepoxide (Librium), which are used to treat the abstinence syndrome, have anticonvulsant properties as well. Nevertheless, the value of these medications (or of phenytoin) in the prevention of seizures is uncertain (13). Alcoholics with no prior seizure history should not be given prophylactic phenytoin during withdrawal. If a patient who is entering alcohol withdrawal gives a history of prior seizures, then a 5-day course of phenytoin (300 mg/day) may prevent the occasional seizure with its attendant risks of aspiration pneumonias and falls. Long term therapy with anticonvulsants is not recommended.

Alcohol abusers are sometimes abusers of other drugs. Withdrawal from barbiturates or tranquilizers at the same time as withdrawal from alcohol may cause fulminant seizures.

For the alcoholic, ability to abstain is the principal determinant of seizure frequency. There is a strong relationship in this population between drinking and seizure frequency. On the other hand, nonalcoholic people with epilepsy can usually tolerate occasional alcohol and should be permitted to drink alcohol unless they clearly have seizures more often when they drink.

Seizures and Brain Tumors

Brain tumor is a relatively uncommon cause of epilepsy, but epilepsy is a common symptom of brain tumors. About one-third of intracranial and one-half of intrahemispheric tumors are associated with seizures. Slow growing tumors appear to be more epileptogenic: seizures occur in 90% of patients with

oligodendrogliomas, 69% of patients with astrocytomas, 34% of patients with glioblastomas, 37% of patients with meningiomas, and 41% of patients with metastases to the brain (18).

The prevalence of brain tumors among people with epilepsy varies from 2 to 12% (22) depending upon the population studied and on the type of seizures. Young and middle-aged adults with new onset of focal seizures have the greatest chance of harboring a tumor, with rates quoted at 35% (27). The following features suggest that seizures may be associated with a brain tumor: onset after 20 years of age, presence of focal neurological signs, increased intracranial pressure, focal unilateral slow waves on the EEG, asymmetry of fast activity on the EEG, and inducibility by hyperventilation (29). If a tumor is suspected, a CT scan, with and without contrast, is the test of choice.

Seizures and Cerebrovascular Disease

Cerebrovascular disease is the most common, and epilepsy the second most common, of the serious neurological illnesses. The two conditions are found together fairly often. It is generally assumed in such patients that ischemia leaves a damaged area of brain, which then somehow "matures" into an epileptic focus. One series (14) reported an overall incidence of seizures of about 8% in patients with stroke, 4% in those with bland infarction, and 10% in those with hemorrhage. The seizures are more likely to be focal (60%) than generalized (40%). In 40% of the patients, seizures occur at the onset of the deficit or within the first 2 weeks; only a few of these patients later develop recurrent epilepsy. However, most patients who have seizures after the second week do develop epilepsy. Consequently, early seizures after stroke do not mandate the use of anticonvulsants, but late seizures should be treated as epilepsy.

As discussed above (page 1138), seizures in the elderly should raise the suspicion of cerebrovascular disease and may be the first clue to the presence of transient ischemia or of impending stroke. In young patients, cerebral vascular disease is uncommon, but a seizure may lead to a diagnosis of an arteriovenous malformation, an aneurysm, collagen vascular disease, or a rare case of cortical thrombophlebitis.

Seizures and Infections

A seizure may be one of the first manifestations of bacterial meningitis, particularly in the very young and in the very old patient in whom the classic signs of meningitis may be lacking. Less fulminant forms of meningitis, such as cryptococcal or tuberculous meningitis, have been known to produce seizures which recur over weeks or months. Viral encephalitides—for example, herpes simplex encephalitis—may also produce seizures. Meningoencephalitis can scar the cortex, so that an epileptic focus is established which remains symptomatic years after the infection is eradicated.

For reasons which are poorly understood, systemic infections may trigger seizures in susceptible patients, even if the infection does not directly involve the central nervous system. However, when a patient presents with a seizure and signs of infection, especially if the seizure is focal or if focal signs are detected on neurological examination, the possibility of brain abscess must be explored.

EVALUATION OF A PATIENT WITH SEIZURES

When a physician evaluates a patient for a possible seizure disorder, three questions must be answered: First, was the event a seizure? Second, if so, what type of seizure was it? Third, are there clues in the history, physical examination, or laboratory tests which point to an etiology of the seizure?

Because the answers to these questions are derived from the standard history and physical examination, initial data should be gathered by the primary physician. In certain instances referral to a neurologist for a consulting opinion may be warranted. Threshold for referral will depend upon the practitioner's own desires and experiences, but many obtain neurological consultation before performing lumbar puncture or a CT scan, or initiating long term therapy in all but the most straightforward cases. This is particularly true if there is uncertainty about the nature of the "seizure," its etiology, and the need for special diagnostic tests, or if the examination or EEG has focal features (see page 1142).

Differential Diagnosis of Seizure-Like Behavior

Determination of the nature of a seizure-like episode may be difficult (Table 80.3). Unless the physician has observed an attack, the patient and surrogate observers must specify whether or not it represented an episode "punched out in time" with specific signs of neurological dysfunction. The features which are most helpful in confirming that a

Table 80.3.
Differential Diagnosis of Seizure-Like Behavior

Condition	See Chapter
Syncope	81
Cerebrovascular disease	83
Migraine	79
Narcolepsy	85
Fluctuating delirium	17
Paroxysmal vertigo	81
Breath-holding spells	
Episodic movement disorders	82
Functional episodes	12
Hysteria	12

seizure has occurred include tonic-clonic sequences, with or without tongue biting and incontinence; rhythmic jerking of a limb or of the face; and speech and motor arrest followed by automatisms. The differential diagnosis is dependent upon the character of the attack. Loss of consciousness raises the possibility of syncope (see Chapter 81); if a careful observer can specify sudden loss of consciousness and tone with no abnormal motor activity, syncope is a much more likely diagnosis than is seizure. Transient numbness, weakness, speech or vision problems, or dizziness may occur as part of a cerebrovascular syndrome (see Chapter 83), including transient ischemic attacks, stroke, bleeding from an arteriovenous malformation or from an aneurysm, or a classic migraine. Context may help to distinguish seizure from cerebrovascular disease, but particularly in the elderly, where the two conditions are linked, a firm diagnosis may have to be deferred.

Narcolepsy (see Chapter 85) is relatively uncommon disorder in which people suddenly lapse into REM (rapid eye movement) sleep with associated inhibition of muscle tone ("cataplexy"). These patients can be aroused from their sleep, will often report that they dreamed during the attack, and will deny postictal confusion. A waxing and waning organic mental syndrome (see Chapter 17) with occasional motor manifestations, such as might be produced by renal failure or by a drug intoxication, may superficially resemble a seizure, but the episode will usually lack both the stereotypical aspects of a seizure and its clear start and finish.

Vertigo, from disease of the inner ear, can present paroxysmally and may be confused with epilepsy (see Chapter 81). Certain adults have tics, which, unlike a true seizure, may be brought in part under voluntary control and often occur at predictable times.

In an office practice, the most common problem in seizure diagnosis is making a distinction between a functional spell and a true seizure. Anxiety attacks can produce recurrent, fulminant, and moderately stereotyped symptomatology, all of which may be seen in patients with partial complex seizures. Since seizures may have emotional concomitants (for example, an aura of extreme fear) and may be triggered by stressful situations, it is evident how difficult the differential diagnosis may be. If a diagnosis of functional problems can be supported on other grounds, if the attacks are strongly linked to preceding anxiety, and if automatisms are lacking, then a functional spell becomes more likely.

Hysterical seizures represent extreme, but common, examples of functional seizure-like behavior. Unlike a malingerer, the patient with hysterical pseudoseizure has no clear awareness of "faking" a spell. Observation of a generalized attack may reveal features unlikely to be part of physiological seizures—for example, retention of protective reflexes such as blink reflex, or breathing effort when the airway is briefly occluded, or speech, or directed eye movements. The motor activity may lack the organized tonic-clonic stages seen with grand mal epilepsy, unless the patient is sophisticated and has observed seizures before (unfortunately, this is often the case). Hysterical psychomotor spells may be the most difficult to diagnose. As a general rule, purposeful, goal-directed behavior, such as driving, shopping, talking in full sentences, or committing acts of specific violence, should not be considered to be part of the seizure unless there is strong supporting evidence. As with simple functional spells, positive features suggestive of hysteria—presence of secondary gain, "la belle indifference," inappropriate reactions to stress—may contribute to a correct diagnosis. Consultation among primary physician, neurologist, and psychiatrist may be required for proper diagnosis and management (see also Chapter 12).

Classifying the Seizure

In actual practice, classifying a seizure (see page 1135) goes hand in hand with establishing that a seizure has, in fact, occurred. Emphasis should be placed on a careful description of the start of the episode, because a fleeting focal onset or an aura may be the only indication that a seizure was a secondarily generalized rather than a grand mal seizure.

Establishing an Etiology

The history usually supplies the main clues to the etiology of a seizure. Careful note should be taken of any birth trauma or perinatal illness, febrile convulsions, past head trauma, prior stroke or intracranial hemorrhage, previous encephalitis or meningitis, cancers, and any prior seizures. A family history of seizures is pertinent, because there is increased risk particularly with primary generalized epilepsies, for seizures in relatives of people with epilepsy. Use of alcohol and/or barbiturates and of seizurogenic drugs, such as amphetamine, phenothiazines, tricyclic antidepressants, anticholinergics, or aminophylline, must be ascertained. Many patients know of factors that precipitate their attack. Most commonly, visual flashing at a rate of about 10/second is a precipitant, but a small percentage of individuals with epilepsy have idiosyncratic precipitants, such as touch of certain regions of skin, loud sounds, or even such complex activities as reading, calculating, laughing, eating, or listening to music. These so-called "reflex seizures" may be aborted in some instances by avoiding the offending stimuli.

Physical examination will reveal whether a seizure patient is neurologically normal. Subtle asymmetries on the neurological examination may lead to diagnosis of a structural lesion which is generating the seizures. Furthermore, the general physical examination may give clues to an underlying cause (Table 80.4). A physician should be wary of findings occurring in the immediate wake of a seizure and should take the opportunity to recheck them in a few hours or a few days.

Laboratory Diagnosis of a Patient with Seizures

Laboratory tests are not very helpful in determining whether a seizure has taken place, but they may be useful in establishing an etiology and in patient management.

Routine Laboratory Tests

The data base should include a hematocrit value, a white blood cell and differential count, a measurement of blood urea nitrogen or of serum creatinine, serum glucose, and serum electrolytes. Other tests (for example, measurements of blood gases and of liver function) should be ordered only if there is some suspicion that they may be abnormal. A number of striking abnormalities (metabolic acidosis, marked leukocytosis) may develop transiently immediately after an attack. A baseline electrocardiogram is useful, although immediately after a seizure it may show ST-T wave changes or arrhythmias which are quite transient and which are results of, rather than causes of, seizure activity.

Electroencephalography

The EEG is the most useful of the laboratory studies in the diagnosis of seizure disorders. An EEG may show generalized or focal epileptiform activity or, even in the absence of such activity, may demonstrate asymmetries of basic rhythms, focal slow waves, or diffuse slowing, all of which may give direction to further investigation. In general, the EEG should not be relied upon to make a diagnosis of a seizure but to confirm a clinical impression derived from the history. When history and EEG are at variance, primacy should go to the history. Patients should not be treated for epilepsy because of an abnormal EEG alone, since interictal epileptiform discharges may be seen in 0.4% of the healthy population, in 2.2% of patients with nonepileptic neurological disease, and in 3.5% of asymptomatic relatives of people with epilepsy (10). On the other hand, a clinician should not be dissuaded from a clear impression of a seizure disorder just because the EEG is negative. Interictal EEGs are usually normal in children with petit mal epilepsy, and they may be normal in from 10 to 50% of individuals with grand mal or partial elementary or partial complex seizures, depending upon the conditions of recording, the duration of recording, and the vagaries of any sampling process (5, 18). Where EEG confirmation of seizure activity is needed (for example, when the history is equivocal) repeated studies, 24-hour monitoring of tracings with concomitant

Table 80.4.
General Physical Signs Suggesting Causes of Epilepsy[a]

System	Signs	Disease
Skin and membrane	Petechiae	Subacute bacterial endocarditis (SBE), blood dyscrasias, leukemia, thrombocytopenic purpura, fat emboli
	Cyanosis	Cyanotic congenital heart disease, pulmonary disease
	Icterus	Liver disease, sickle cell disease, thrombotic thrombocytopenic purpura (Moschowitz)
	Malar skin rash	Systemic lupus erythematosus
	Facial port wine stain	Sturge-Weber-Dimitri disease
	Café au lait spots	Neurofibromatosis
	Depigmented spots	Tuberous sclerosis
Head	Head circumference ↑ or ↓	Hydrocephalus, macrocephaly, microcephaly
	Bruit	Arteriovenous malformation
Fundi	Papilledema	↑ intracranial pressure—brain tumor, hemorrhage
	Hemorrhage	Subarachnoid hemorrhage, hypertension, systemic bleeding tendency
	Exudate	SBE, diabetes mellitus, hypertension
	Retinal lesions	Intrauterine infections, tuberous sclerosis
Neck	Meningeal signs—stiff neck	Meningitis, subarachnoid hemorrhage, fractured odontoid, herniated cerebellar tonsils
	↓ Carotid pulses or bruit	Cerebrovascular disease
Circulation	Hypertension	Renal disease, cardiovascular disease, coarctation of aorta, collagen disease
	Arrhythmia	Cardiac disease—congenital, rheumatic, arteriosclerotic heart disease
Abdomen	Organomegaly	Liver disease, neoplasm, hematological disease
	Mass	Neoplasm
Bones and joints	Clubbing	Lung carcinoma, cyanotic congenital heart disease

[a] From Solomon GE, Plum F: *Clinical Management of Seizures.* Philadelphia, WB Saunders 1976.

observation of behavior, recordings after sleep deprivation, stimulatory techniques, such as hyperventilation or flash, or use of nasopharyngeal or sphenopalatine leads may be indicated.

Epileptiform EEG discharges can usually be observed in the presence of anticonvulsant drugs, although some generalized discharges may be blunted. Medications should not be altered for the first EEG. If tracings are repeatedly negative and a suspicion of epilepsy remains, then admission to a hospital, rapid tapering of medicines in concert with EEGs, and direct observation off medicines may clarify the picture. Among patients with epilepsy, the pattern of generalized EEG slowing without seizure discharges is a fairly common finding, usually resulting from medication intoxication or a postictal state.

Since EEGs can remain abnormal for a few weeks after a major seizure, any findings should be confirmed with repeat studies. An EEG is without risk, unless there are consequences from an injudicious interpretation (see "Patient Experience," Chapter 78).

Lumbar Puncture

Certain conditions which lead to seizures may require examination of cerebrospinal fluid to secure a diagnosis; chronic meningitis is an example. Data are not available from the medical literature on the yield of lumbar puncture in investigation of patients with various types of seizures; consequently, it is not possible to be dogmatic about whether this test is a requirement for all patients with seizures. The context of the seizure often resolves the issue. A normal child with classic petit mal epilepsy probably does not need a lumbar puncture. A patient with a strongly suspected mass lesion should not have a routine spinal tap until other studies have given information on the risk of cerebral herniation. Most other patients, with focal or generalized seizures of uncertain etiology, should undergo spinal fluid analysis.

After prolonged generalized seizures the cerebrospinal fluid may show a pleocytosis of up to 100 cells, presumably from a transient breakdown of the blood-brain barrier (21). Clearly, however, infection must be the diagnosis of first concern in this setting.

Computerized Tomographic Scans

Computerized tomographic scans (see "Patient Experience," Chapter 78) of patients with primary generalized seizures are abnormal (excluding nonspecific atrophy) in about 10% of instances (19). Scans of individuals with focal motor or secondarily generalized seizures show a focal abnormality about 65% of the time (16). Patients with partial complex seizures show abnormalities about 36% of the time. If the neurological examination reveals focal signs the CT scan is especially likely to be positive.

The following recommendations seem reasonable: All patients with focal or secondarily generalized seizures or with an abnormal neurological examination should have a CT scan with (unless there is a contraindication) contrast injection. In patients with a negative examination and in children the decision to perform a scan should be individualized. Lastly, CT scanning may be indicated when a stable pattern of seizures deteriorates.

Other Diagnostic Tests

"Traditional" neuroradiological studies—skull X-rays, radionuclide brain scan, pneumoencephalography, and arteriography—have to a great extent been supplanted by CT scanning in the initial evaluation of a seizure disorder, but each still has its own special indications which will be pointed out when appropriate by the consulting neurologist.

TREATMENT OF EPILEPSY

Except in unusual instances, epilepsy cannot be "cured." In about three of four patients it can, however, be controlled so that patients experience no seizures or only a very rare seizure. Most attention in the medical literature has been focused on details of pharmacological management for seizures, but the importance of a comprehensive approach cannot be overemphasized: an individual who is seizure free, but so toxic from medicines that employment is impossible, is at best a dubious success. Employment problems and other social aspects of managing epilepsy are considered below. General measures of therapy should not be neglected. Removal of precipitating factors for seizures, reduction of stress, provision for adequate amounts of rest, and attention to proper diet can all be important in control of epilepsy.

General Principles of Drug Therapy

It has been said that half of those patients who have generalized seizures monthly or more frequently are probably undertreated. In contrast, other patients are maintained on unnecessary or improper regimens of anticonvulsants. To achieve the ideal goal of seizure control without toxicity, clinicians should follow the general principles listed in Table 80.5.

In deciding whether to treat a first seizure, the physician should recall that a single seizure does not necessarily mandate a diagnosis of epilepsy nor a need for chronic therapy. As noted previously, early seizures after head trauma or stroke, or seizures in association with some clear precipitant should in general be treated conservatively. The more difficult decision involves the patient with a single "idiopathic" convulsion, because the risk of having a second seizure is small but real (see above). Some patients are so frightened of the possibility of having another seizure with potential repercussions for employment, social relations, and license to drive, that they are willing to accept the inconvenience and morbidity of chronic medication. Other patients would prefer not to be medicated until they have another seizure. Clearly, the decision to treat after a first seizure must be individualized. After a second attack, most physicians would initiate therapy.

To treat the patient appropriately, the physician must know the type of seizure under consideration. The drugs of choice differ for the different categories of epilepsy (Table 80.6). In several instances, more than one drug may be considered the "drug of choice" in terms of efficacy, in which case the selection can be made on the basis of personal familiarity with the drug or on the relative risk of side effects. For a review of compared controlled trials of anticonvulsants, the reader is referred to Gram and associates (11).

Table 80.5.
Principles of Drug Therapy

Decide whether to treat.
Select the proper drug for the particular form of epilepsy.
Start drugs slowly and build up levels gradually, to avoid toxicity.
Start with one drug, and use it to effect or toxicity before adding another.
Choose the simplest regimen possible.
Suspect compliance problems in treatment failures.
Monitor blood levels in problem cases.
Withdraw medications gradually.
Decide how long to treat.

Table 80.6.
Drugs of Choice

Seizure Category	Drugs of Choice	Alternates
Grand mal	Phenytoin Phenobarbital Valproic acid	Carbamazepine Primidone
Petit mal	Ethosuximide	Valproic acid
Myoclonic	Clonazepam	Valproic acid
Partial simple	Phenytoin Carbamazepine	Phenobarbital Valproic acid
Partial complex	Carbamazepine Primadone	Phenytoin Phenobarbital Valproic acid
Mixed forms	Valproic acid Carbamazepine Clonazepam	Phenytoin Phenobarbital

Drugs should be initiated at one-quarter or one-half of the anticipated maintenance dosage (except for phenytoin and phenobarbital—see below), and the dosage should be built up over several weeks, in order to avoid significant early toxicity which might discourage the patient from continuing with treatment. Since some of the medications remain in the blood for some time, it may take several days before the effects of a dosage adjustment are manifest.

There is a long and deplorable tradition of treating epilepsy with several drugs simultaneously, stemming from times when most patients were started automatically on phenytoin, 100 mg, and phenobarbital, 32 mg, each three times a day. There is no evidence that two drugs in subtherapeutic doses are better tolerated or more effective than one drug in full dose. Shorvon and colleagues (24) have argued that about 90% of new onset seizures can be controlled with one drug (in their study, phenytoin or carbamazepine), and that, when one drug is unsuccessful, addition of a second helps in only 36% of cases.

Compliance is a major factor in success of drug therapy for epilepsy (also see Chapter 4, Patient Compliance with Medical Advice). Every effort should be made to simplify the dosage regimen. Phenobarbital and certain formulations of phenytoin can be given in a once daily dose. Therefore, medicines such as carbamazepine, primidone, and valproic acid, which must be given in divided doses, should be employed only when there is an identifiable advantage over phenytoin or phenobarbital. At each visit a patient (or the responsible person) should be asked to report on the exact medication regimen; all too often the answer indicates a need for better spoken and written communication with the patient. Physicians should have some familiarity with cost of medicines because patients may be hesitant to purchase an expensive medicine, unless the need is clearly explained. In general, poor compliance is the most common cause of treatment failure; when in doubt, the serum levels of drugs should be measured.

The optimum dose of an anticonvulsant medication may vary several-fold among different patients. Determination of serum levels of medicines (Table 80.7) is now a reliable way to measure how much medication is circulating, but such measurements should not be ordered indiscriminately. If a patient has a good response and little toxicity from a drug regimen, measurement of a serum level is wasteful and might even encourage the physician to alter a successful regimen. If control is not optimal, drug levels can document inadequate compliance or absorption, or highlight the occasional case where drug toxicity is manifest by increased seizures. The levels can also provide guidance for patients with symptoms which might or might not be due to drug intoxication. Practitioners should be aware that with some anticonvulsants, particularly phenytoin, drug dose and drug level are not linearly related: a saturation point is reached above which minor increments in daily dose (for example, increasing from 400 to 500 mg a day of phenytoin) may lead to major increases in serum level and in side effects. A level is most informative if measured in the "steady state" (see Table 80.7), which requires a stable dosage for about four or five half-lives of the medicine before measurement.

The determination of how long to maintain treatment with anticonvulsants is a difficult issue, because seizures remit over time, and thus freedom from seizures may or may not be due to the medicine. About one-half to two-thirds of patients will be entirely seizure free for 2 years with therapy. If an adult patient is seizure free for about 5 years on medication and stops treatment by gradual tapering, there is a 30 to 50% chance of relapse in the next 5 years (12). About 90% of the relapses are registered within the first 2 years after discontinuing medication. As with the decision to initiate therapy, the decision to terminate anticonvulsant therapy must be individualized. A patient who was very difficult to control initially, who has an underlying structural lesion, or a persistently abnormal EEG may benefit from lifelong therapy. In contrast, a patient with idiopathic epilepsy who has been well and seizure free for 2 to 5 years and who is willing to accept an increased risk of having a seizure may be a candidate for drug withdrawal. If more than one drug has been prescribed, the medications should be tapered one at a time, each over a period of several months, and reinstated rapidly if seizures recur.

Surprisingly few studies exist to establish firmly the value of one anticonvulsant over another. Table 80.6 represents a general, but not unanimous, consensus of opinion on drugs of choice and alternates for the main forms of epilepsy. Dosages, half-lives, serum levels, and main potential side effects of the drugs are given in Table 80.7.

Phenytoin (Diphenylhydantoin, DPH, PHT, Dilantin)

Since its introduction in 1938, phenytoin has been one of the two major drugs used to treat seizures. It is most useful in grand mal epilepsy, partial simple epilepsy, and secondarily generalized epilepsy. Although it is often used for partial complex seizures, it is not as effective as carbamazepine for psychomotor spells. Phenytoin may make petit mal worse.

Phenytoin is absorbed from the gastrointestinal tract in 4 to 8 hours. Without a loading dose, a full week is required to reach therapeutic levels, but a load of 3 times the daily maintenance, given in the first day, will achieve immediate therapeutic levels. The mean half-life is 22 hours, with a range from 7 to 42 hours. Phenytoin is 90% protein bound, so that low serum albumin can lead to an increased concen-

Table 80.7.
Major Antiseizure Medications

Medication (Brand Name)	Available Strengths (mg)	Typical Adult Dose and Range	Half-life (hr)	Levels (mg/liter[e])	Major Side Effects
Phenytoin (Dilantin)	100 capsules	300 mg 1 time daily[b] (200–500 mg)	22	10–20	Ataxia Cosmetic changes Rash Rare blood changes Osteomalacia
Phenobarbital (Luminal)	15, 30, 60, 100 tablets	100 mg 1 time daily	72	15–40	Sedation Hyperactivity Confusion Mood change
Primidone (Mysoline)	50, 250 scored tablets	250 mg 4 times daily (500–1500 mg)	3–12[c] 72[d]	6–12[c] 15–40[d]	Sedation Hyperactivity Mood change
Carbamazepine (Tegretol)	200 tablets (100 chewable)	200 mg 4 times daily (400–2000 mg)	10–25	4–12	Gastrointestinal (GI) distress Ataxia Blurred vision Blood changes Hepatotoxicity
Ethosuximide (Zarontin)	250 capsules	250 mg 4 times daily (500–1500 mg)	30	50–100	GI distress Sedation Headache Dizziness
Valproic acid (Depakene)	250 capsules	250 mg 4 times daily (500–4000 mg)	8–12	50–100	GI distress Drowsiness Ataxia Alopecia Tremor Blood changes Rare liver toxicity Rare pancreatitis
Clonazepam (Clonopin)	0.5, 1, 2 tablets	2 mg 3 times daily (2–20 mg)	20–40	0.05–0.7	Drowsiness Ataxia Behavior change Dizziness

[a] These doses are usually attained gradually over days to weeks. The ranges are relatively rough guidelines; because absorption varies, serum levels are better guides to dosage.
[b] Only for Dilantin capsules.
[c] For primidone.
[d] For phenobarbital.
[e] Lab may report same figures as micrograms per milliliter.

tration of the free agent and to increased toxicity. The drug is metabolized in the liver and is not excreted by the kidney. Dosage should only be lowered in renal failure to compensate for a severe decrease in serum protein, and then about a 25% reduction usually suffices. In renal failure drug-binding proteins may be deficient, resulting in a low measured total serum level with an adequate free drug serum level. Phenytoin is partially removed by hemodialysis.

The usual starting dose of phenytoin is 300 mg/day. This medication can be given once a day if it is given as Dilantin capsules, for this preparation is manufactured in slow release form. Other preparations are fast release capsules. They are slightly less expensive but must be given in divided doses (i.e., 100 mg three times a day). The therapeutic level for phenytoin is generally between 10 and 20 mg/liter; the toxic range is usually over 20 mg/liter, but patients show fairly wide individual susceptibility to side effects. The lethal dose may range from 2 to 20 g.

Several drugs elevate phenytoin plasma levels: disulfiram and isoniazid, commonly; coumadin, chloramphenicol, methylphenidate, phenothiazines, benzodiazepines, and propoxyphene, less often. Other drugs may lead to increased phenytoin metabolism, resulting in decreased phenytoin levels: alcohol, folic acid, pyridoxine, theophylline, and occasionally carbamazepine, cimetidine, oral contraceptives, and sulfonamides. These potential drug interactions may be managed best by patient and physician awareness and by observation of serum drug levels during times of medication changes.

There are many potential *undesirable effects* of phenytoin. Dose-related acute effects include nystagmus (seen at therapeutic levels), ataxia (usually above 30 mg/liter), lethargy and paradoxical tendency to increased seizures at higher toxic levels (usually above 40 mg/liter), and allergic reactions. Chronic side effects of phenytoin generally manifest after a few months to several years of daily ingestion. Chronically progressive cosmetic changes can be vexing in young women. Gum hypertrophy occurs in about 30%; it may be forestalled by good oral hygiene, but once established may regress only partially; hirsutism is seen in 5% overall, but in 30% of young women. Even more disconcerting are facial changes due to thickening of subcutaneous tissue about the nose and eyes, the so-called "leonine faces." Skin rash occurs in 2 to 10% of users, with a peak incidence about 2 weeks into the course. Stevens-Johnson syndrome occurs rarely. Lymphadenopathy develops in 2 to 5%, sometimes in association with fever, arthralgia, eosinophilia, and hepatosplenomegaly, presenting a picture of "pseudolymphoma" and, very rarely, true lymphoma. Hepatitis and a variety of blood dyscrasias have been reported. Megaloblastic anemia may occur, which responds to folate. Many patients develop measurable antinuclear antibodies in the serum; a minority of this group progresses to irreversible clinical systemic lupus erythematosus. Peripheral neuropathy with loss of muscle stretch reflexes can be documented in about 20% of chronic users. Occasional pulmonary infiltrates and fibrosis have given rise to the term "Dilantin lung." Phenytoin can induce liver enzymes, thereby secondarily affecting metabolism of numerous hormones and drugs. Induced inactivation of vitamin D leads to radiological or biochemical evidence of bone disease in one of every three chronically treated patients. Teratogenic effects of phenytoin are strongly suspected (see below, page 1151).

Phenobarbital

Phenobarbital competes with phenytoin as the drug of choice for generalized tonic-clonic seizures. It is particularly useful in the pediatric age group, where it may be better tolerated than phenytoin because it does not cause cosmetic side effects; it may, however, cause significant behavioral side effects (hyperactivity in up to 40% of children).

Phenobarbital is a long lasting drug. The gastrointestinal absorption is slow so that levels reach a peak in 10 to 12 hours after an oral dose, compared to 20 minutes after an intravenous dose. The drug is detoxified by the liver and excreted by the kidney, but the dosage need be only slightly reduced in renal failure. The serum half-life is about 72 hours, ranging from 37 to 96 hours. Therapeutic levels are 15 to 40 mg/liter. Phenobarbital is a potent inducer of liver enzymes and leads to rapid tolerance, as well

as to alteration of kinetics of numerous other medications. The dose of phenobarbital is 1 to 3 mg/kg/day, or about 100 mg/day for the average adult. Little justification can be made for giving it in divided doses.

The main acute side effect of phenobarbital in adults is sedation. After a few weeks, partial tolerance to the sedation usually develops. In elderly patients phenobarbital can cause confusion and respiratory depression. Subtle or overt personality changes due to phenobarbital probably occur more often than is generally recognized, especially in the elderly. Ataxia and nystagmus are common in all patients at high doses. Occasionally, there is idiosyncratic allergy, with accompanying dermatitis or gastrointestinal symptoms. Phenobarbital must not be administered to potential drug abusers or to unreliable patients who might precipitously discontinue their medicine.

Primidone (Mysoline)

Primidone is a barbiturate which is used for treatment of partial complex seizures (usually as a second choice after carbamazepine (see below). It has also been used in place of phenobarbital for treatment of grand mal or focal seizures, when the latter drug has failed, but it should not be a drug of first choice for these conditions. Primidone is excreted in part unchanged and is in part metabolized to phenobarbital and to phenylethylmalonic acid (PEMA). Primidone and PEMA are cleared in hours, whereas the phenobarbital persists for days. Serum levels of primidone and PEMA can be ascertained, but it often suffices just to confirm that a therapeutic steady state level of phenobarbital is present. In order to benefit from the short lived primidone and PEMA, each of which has some anticonvulsant action, primidone must be given in three or four divided doses. A therapeutic dose is usually around 250 mg orally three or four times a day, but the initial doses should be much lower to avoid inducing extreme sedation. It is reasonable to start with 125 to 250 mg daily, with increments each week, until therapeutic effect, therapeutic levels, unacceptable sedation, or the maximum dose of 2 g/day is reached. The dosage should be reduced by about half in patients with significant renal failure.

Side effects of primidone parallel those of phenobarbital, except that primidone tends to be more sedating.

Carbamazepine (Tegretol)

Carbamazepine is one of the newest of the major anticonvulsants used in the United States, but over a decade of use for seizures and for treatment of chronic neuropathic pains has proven it to be a safe and effective medicine. Carbamazepine is the drug of choice in partial complex epilepsy. It has efficacy probably equal to that of phenytoin in the treatment of focal and of generalized seizures. The adult dose is 400 to 2000 mg/day. Tablets come in 200-mg (or 100-mg chewable) sizes, and it is advisable to initiate therapy with no more than 200 to 400 mg/day, building up to the full dose over a week or two. The half-life is about 10 to 25 hours, and dosage should be divided into three or four times a day regimens. If compliance is a problem, sometimes a twice daily dosage will suffice. Therapeutic serum levels are about 4 to 12 mg/liter.

The side effects of carbamazepine include fatigue (although it is not very sedating), nystagmus, diplopia, dizziness, ataxia, dysarthria, rash, (including rarely the Stevens-Johnson syndrome), inappropriate secretion of antidiuretic hormone, occasionally abnormal liver function tests, and an infrequent lupus-like syndrome. Gastrointestinal distress is the most common side effect, particularly if the medication is initiated too rapidly. Reversible leukopenia or thrombocytopenia is seen in 5 to 10% of patients, so that blood counts should be monitored weekly at the start of therapy and then every few months. This drug has had a reputation for causing aplastic anemia, based largely on six cases of this complication that were reported in the 1960s (even though a causal relation to carbamazepine was not established). The actual incidence of aplastic anemia is not known, but it is thought to be very rare (8).

Ethosuximide (Zarontin)

Ethosuximide is the drug of choice for treatment of petit mal epilepsy or absence spells in children. It has little efficacy in other types of seizures.

Valproic Acid (Sodium Valproate, Depakene, Depakote)

Valproic acid is a recent addition to the list of major drugs used to treat seizures. Its effectiveness is quite broad, but it is thought to be particularly valuable for absence attacks in children. Some groups favor its use as a first line agent for tonic-clonic or myoclonic seizures (5), though it is not approved formally for use in these conditions.

Valproic acid is a fatty acid, structurally dissimilar from all other common anticonvulsants. It comes in 250-mg capsules (also as coated tablets purported by the manufacturer to cause less gastrointestinal upset) and as an elixir. Peak serum levels are reached in 1 to 4 hours after ingestion, and the half-life is about 8 to 12 hours. The drug is metabolized in the liver and excreted in the urine in modified form. Serum levels may be measured, but at present have limited utility. The approximate therapeutic range is 50 to 100 mg/liter. The manufacturer suggests initiation of therapy with a dose of about 10 to 15 mg/kg/day, to be increased at weekly intervals by

about 5 to 10 mg/kg/day to a maximum dose of 60 mg/kg/day. A common final regimen is 250 to 500 mg orally, two to four times/day.

In studies on several thousand patients abroad, before the release of the drug in the United States in 1978, valproic acid proved to be quite safe. About one in five patients had significant side effects—commonly gastrointestinal upset, drowsiness, rash, reversible hair loss, weight loss or gain, ataxia, tremor, or hyperactivity. A limited number of studies suggest that valproic acid inhibits platelet aggregation and may prolong the bleeding time, but this effect is poorly documented. Less commonly, valproate may produce frank thrombocytopenia. After release in this country, there have been several dozen reported cases of liver toxicity in association with administration of valproic acid. Several patients have developed serious episodes of pancreatitis. Because of these recently discovered toxicities, and because of high cost, valproic acid has not yet replaced ethosuximide as the drug of choice for petit mal epilepsy.

Clonazepam (Clonopin)

Clonazepam is a benzodiazepine drug, closely related to diazepam, and is used principally for treatment of myoclonus. It is not approved for treatment of motor or psychomotor seizures but has been used effectively for these conditions in Europe. Clonazepam is an oral medicine, with a serum half-life of 20 to 40 hours, Serum levels vary from 5 to 70 ng/ml and correlate only very roughly with clinical effect. Because of the sedative effect of the medicine, therapy is usually initiated very gradually, beginning with 0.01 to 0.15 mg/kg, increased each third day to clinical effect or to maintenance at 0.1 to 0.2 mg/kg/day. In adults the daily maximum dose is 20 mg. Clonazepam commonly produces drowsiness, ataxia, and behavioral changes and can also cause dizziness and decreased muscle tone.

Other Anticonvulsants

No attempt has been made to catalog all of the agents used as anticonvulsants; only the major drugs of choice for the common types of seizures have been discussed. Ineffectiveness of the standard agents, when applied in accordance with the general therapeutic principles given previously, is certainly an indication for specialty referral and for possible trials of the more unusual therapies. Practitioners frequently use diazepam or chlordiazepoxide to treat seizures, and although these drugs do have some efficacy, this practice cannot be condoned except in special cases, such as ethanol withdrawal or status epilepticus. Benzodiazepines (other than clonazepam) have drawbacks for chronic therapy; anticonvulsant effects tend to diminish as sedative effects accumulate (26).

REFERRAL TO A NEUROLOGIST

The use of a neurologist for help with therapy of epilepsy depends upon the experience of the primary physician. There are a number of common management problems for which referral may be helpful (Table 80.8): patients who need adjustment of a complex polypharmaceutical regimen; patients who do not respond to, or experience significant side effects from, the "drug of choice" for a seizure type; patients with seizures during pregnancy (see page 1150); patients in whom discontinuation of medication is being considered; and, lastly, patients having a change in the frequency of type of seizures.

HOSPITALIZATION

Few general statements can be made about the need for hospital admission of seizure patients, because availability of monitoring systems, emergency room "holding rooms," and availability of inpatient beds vary from locale to locale. Nonetheless, a set of reasonable guidelines is shown in Table 80.8. Individuals brought to offices or emergency rooms after a first seizure are usually admitted in order to facilitate the diagnostic workup and to observe the patient in case a serious underlying cause, for example meningitis or subdural hematoma, is present. This

Table 80.8.
When to Refer or to Hospitalize the Patient with Seizures

DIAGNOSTIC ISSUES
   Question about whether a seizure took place
   Abnormal physical examination
   Questionable focal findings
   Focal seizures
   Focality on the EEG
   Need for special diagnostics (lumbar puncture, CT scan)
   Uncertainty about etiology
THERAPEUTIC ISSUES
   Adjustment of an existing drug regimen which is complex
   Patient does not respond to a drug of choice
   Patient has significant medication side effects
   Patient wishes to become pregnant
   Patient wishes to taper off medication
   Significant change in the pattern of seizures
WHEN TO HOSPITALIZE
   Most new onset seizures
   New focal signs on examination
   Obtunded or prolonged "postical" patients
   Febrile patients
   Crescendo pattern of seizures
   All cases of status epilepticus
   Barbiturate withdrawal seizures
   Possibility of rapidly expanding mass lesion
   Seizures after recent head trauma
   Need for special inpatient studies
   Consideration for neurosurgery
   Monitoring of compliance

principle has exceptions. A young patient with a normal examination, positive family history for epilepsy, and a reliable family may be evaluated in an ambulatory setting. Any patient with new focal signs on examination should be admitted, as should obtunded patients, febrile patients, or those whose postictal lethargy persists for over ½ hour. A patient with a crescendo pattern of seizures, with several in one day, especially if tonic-clonic, should be admitted to a hospital immediately. Status epilepticus, where continuous or back-to-back seizures occur without intervening return of consciousness, is a true medical emergency and requires immediate hospitalization. Barbiturate withdrawal seizures may become fulminant; therefore, patients having seizures in this setting should be admitted. If the possibility exists of a rapidly expanding mass lesion, such as tumor, abscess, or possible hematoma after head trauma, then admission should not be delayed. Legitimate reasons for elective admissions include a need for special inpatient studies (arteriography, continuous monitoring), for evaluation for possible neurosurgical procedures for intractable epilepsy, and, lastly, for trials of supervised drug management to rule out noncompliance as a factor in treatment failure.

Admission is usually not needed for those patients who are known to have chronically recurrent seizures, whose pattern of seizures is stable, whose etiology is established or is thought to be idiopathic on the basis of a prior thorough workup, who have fully recovered from recent seizures, who have normal examinations (or static documented old deficits), and who are reliable enough to return for follow-up.

SOCIAL ISSUES

Once a serious underlying etiology has been ruled out, the physician tends to view epilepsy as a benign disease. From the viewpoint of the patient, this is often far from the case. Seizures are distressing for every patient. Fear of having a seizure can cause people with epilepsy to withdraw from society, and those who are willing to compete may be faced with nearly insurmountable discrimination. Physicians must be sensitive to these issues.

The Commission for the Control of Epilepsy and Its Consequences (1977) found that the unemployment rate among those with epilepsy is twice the national average, and the underemployment rate is even higher. Suspension of a driver's license may make it nearly impossible to get to work. Children may be denied participation in sports or moved unnecessarily to "special sections" in school. People with epilepsy marry less often than matched cohorts; a significant fraction of the public believes that individuals with epilepsy are likely to be physically unattractive. Because of the social stigma associated with epilepsy, the physician caring for these individuals must take special efforts to focus on the patient's overall social setting, rather than simply on seizure control. The patient and family should be counseled regularly to address those concerns that limit full participation in society.

Patients should be told that epilepsy is a medical illness, for too many carry notions, passed down from centuries of medical unenlightenment, that it is a punishment for some past abuse. Whereas a single seizure should not be labeled as "epilepsy," definite epilepsy should not be mislabeled as something else, to avoid facing the correct diagnosis. The patient should know that individual seizures do not cause measurable brain damage and that the condition does not lead to mental deterioration. Several great historical figures, including Julius Caesar, Emperor Charles V, Dostoevski, Flaubert, and possibly the prophet Mohammed, achieved high stations while suffering from frequent seizures. The prognosis of epilepsy is good.

Restrictions of Activity

Patients often ask for guidelines about what they can and cannot do. Maximal activity consistent with avoidance of personal injury should be the goal. The specifics must be formulated by a physician familiar with the individual patient and his pattern of seizures. Patients with nocturnal seizures need not be restricted during the day. Contact sports are safe for people with infrequent seizures. Common sense dictates limits on activities during which a seizure could be fatal, for example, flying, rock climbing, or scuba diving. Some potentially hazardous activities, such as swimming, are acceptable if provisions can be made for proper supervision. Seizures are not contraindications to strenuous activities, including sex. Alcohol consumption (in moderation) can be enjoyed by most with impunity (see above, page 1140).

Driving a Motor Vehicle

Overall, motor vehicle accident rates for people with epilepsy are about twice the rates in control subjects. The actual rate of traffic accidents caused by people with epilepsy is low, estimated at 1/10,000 accidents (28). By comparison, it is estimated that 6/10,000 of these accidents are due to deaths from natural causes and that 5,000/10,000 are due to alcohol use. Approximately 12 to 20% of accidents in persons with epilepsy occur with the patient's first seizure. Despite these statistics, seizures at the wheel do occur and can represent both personal and public dangers. The key element of increased risk is blunting or loss of consciousness. Seizures without this element—for example, partial simple motor seizures—do not affect the risk of driving and affected patients are usually exempted from regulations.

Some states require that physicians directly report occurrence of seizures to the Department of Motor Vehicles; others require only documentation in the medical record that the patient has been informed of the risks for traffic accidents and has been instructed to contact the Motor Vehicle Department for a hearing. Patients and physicians should be honest in their communications; both are potentially liable for consequences of inaccurate or incomplete information. In general, the physician should address the medical facts of a case and leave the final determination of licensing to the state authorities. Often, if an applicant has regular lapses of consciousness, the license will be suspended until a period of from 3 months to 2 years without seizures has elapsed (depending upon the state), but the recent national trend has been to consider shorter periods of suspension.

Employment

It is now illegal to discriminate against handicapped individuals, including people with epilepsy, in the job marketplace. If an individual with seizures is unemployed or dissatisfied with work, the primary physician should be quick to refer to a local rehabilitation agency for possible retraining, patient and employer education, or advice on legal action. The Epilepsy Foundation of America (1828 L Street NW, Washington, DC 20036) is a central nonprofit organization that can serve as a source for information and action on social aspects of epilepsy; at least one chapter exists in each state. Their training and placement service (TAPS) has been effective in training people with epilepsy for work and in finding them employment, either in the general work pool or in sheltered workshops. The same local organizations may further aid patients and physicians with regular group counseling for those who cannot live independently, or in providing for regular home visits by visiting nurses and other medical personnel.

Some patients with difficult to control seizures should be advised to apply for medical disability under Social Security (see criteria in Table 9.4).

Pregnancy

Special problems are raised by a woman with epilepsy who is, or wishes to become, pregnant. About 0.4% of all pregnancies occur in mothers with seizures. In women with epilepsy childbearing carries an above average risk for toxemia, vaginal hemorrhage, and complicated labor. The rate of premature births and perinatal deaths is elevated. Seizures become more difficult to control during pregnancy in about 50% of cases, easier to control in about 10%, and unchanged in the rest. Rarely, pregnancy can induce a new onset of recurring idiopathic seizures. Antiepileptic medications—phenytoin, carbamazepine, valproic acid, and to a lesser extent all of the other agents—are believed to be teratogenic. Studies suggest that the incidence of congenital abnormalities, particularly cleft lip, cleft palate, and cardiac defects, is 2 to 6 times more common in offspring of drug-treated mothers with epilepsy. Valproate has specifically been associated with neural tube closure defects.

Unfortunately, no study has yet been able to specify the relative contribution of medication and of epilepsy itself to this increased incidence. Authorities agree that major motor seizures can produce anoxic, ischemic, or traumatic damage to a fetus and that this risk must be balanced against the teratogenic potential of medication. The best solution to the above dilemma is careful advance planning. Physicians should not only ask their patients to plan pregnancies, but to alert them to the plan months in advance. Prior to pregnancy special efforts can be made to taper medications or to switch to phenobarbital or carbamazepine, which may be less teratogenic than phenytoin or valproate. Brief psychomotor or absence seizures pose no known risk to a fetus, and a decision may be made that the patient should tolerate them during pregnancy. If pregnancy is unexpected, an ongoing successful regimen of anticonvulsants should probably be continued, to avoid the possibility of fulminant withdrawal seizures during a critical obstetrical stage. Ultimately, all of these relative risks must be discussed among primary and specialist physicians, patient and husband, so that a mutually satisfactory plan can be derived. The problems of childbearing are increased for mothers with epilepsy, but not greatly, and only the severely disabled epileptic woman should be flatly discouraged from having children.

Mothers taking anticonvulsants who wish to breast-feed may do so, because the amount of antiepileptic medications excreted in breast milk is too low to affect the infant.

Potential parents wonder about the likelihood that their child will have epilepsy if they or a previous child have epilepsy. Although there are methodological problems in performing studies to answer this question, it can generally be said that there is about a 1 in 40 risk of transmitting primary tonic-clonic epilepsy (the risk is primarily from the mother, not the father), and that a positive family history increases the risk 2- to 4-fold (17). When seizures result from head trauma, tumor, drug withdrawal, or other identified causes, then the hereditary risk is not above baseline.

Family Counseling

Families must be told how to behave during a seizure; too often, frantic efforts to "treat" the seizure result in extreme anxiety and broken teeth. Seizures should be allowed to run their course; unless convulsions become nearly continuous (status epilepticus) they are not dangerous, and no first aid can shorten them. The mouth should not be forced open so that matchbooks, pencils, or other objects can be pushed in. The family should be informed that it is impossible to swallow the tongue. It is advisable to move the individual undergoing a seizure away from sharp corners and heights and to turn him on his side to decrease the risk of aspiration. Forcible restraint during a tonic-clonic phase is of no value, and during the automatisms of partial complex seizures restraints may increase agitation. There is little need to fear behavior during automatisms, because directed violence is extremely rare.

Concerned family members may be very helpful in promoting improved seizure control. They should be encouraged to discuss compliance, the cost of a medicine regimen, and how the seizures and/or drug toxicities affect school, work, and social relations. Patients may wish to keep a log of their seizures, medication times, side effects, and possible precipitating stresses. Perfect control of epilepsy with no toxicity is an ideal attained in only a minority of cases; in the remainder, patient, family, and physician can decide in concert how to balance the inconvenience of seizures against the unpleasant effects of medication and thereby achieve the best possible results.

General References

Drugs for epilepsy. *Med Lett* 21:25, 1979.
    Tabular summary of antiseizure medicines.
Epilepsy Foundation of America: *Basic Statistics on the Epilepsies.* Philadelphia, FA Davis, 1975.
    Epidemiological sourcebook.
Laidlaw J, Richens A: *A Textbook of Epilepsy*, New York, Churchill Livingstone, 1982.
    A detailed general textbook about all aspects of clinical epileptology.
Niedermeyer E: *Compendium of the Epilepsies.* Springfield, IL, Charles C Thomas, 1974.
    A succinct overview of diagnosis and treatment of epilepsy.
Penry JK, Newmark ME: The use of antiepileptic drugs. *Ann Intern Med* 90:207, 1979.
    A review of antiseizure medication, written for practicing physicians.
So EL, Penry JK: Epilepsy in adults. *Ann Neurol* 9:3, 1981.
    An excellent, well referenced review.
Solomon GE, Plum F: *Clinical Management of Seizures: A Guide for the Physician.* Philadelphia, WB Saunders, 1976.
    Pithy summary of seizure therapeutics.
Temkin O: *The Falling Sickness: A History of Epilepsy from the Greeks to the Beginnings of Modern Neurology.* Baltimore, The Johns Hopkins Press, 1971.
    The definitive history of epilepsy from ancient to modern times.

Specific References

1. Anderson DW, McLawsin RL: The national head and spinal cord injury survey. *J Neurosurg* 53:51, 1980.
2. Annegers JF, Grabow JD, Grover RV, et al: Seizures after head trauma: a population study. *Neurology* 30:683, 1980.
3. Annegers JF, Hauser WA, Elveback LR: Remission of seizures and relapse in patients with epilepsy. *Epilepsia* 20:729, 1979.
4. Caveness WF: Epilepsy, a product of trauma in our time.

Epilepsia 17:207, 1976.

5. Delgado-Escueta AV: Epileptogenic paroxysms: modern approaches and clinical correlations. *Neurology* 29:1014, 1979.

6. Dreifuss FE: Proposal for revised clinical and electroencephalographic classification of epileptic seizures. *Epilepsia* 22:489, 1981.

7. Elwes RDC, Johnson AL, Shorvon SD, Reynolds EH: The prognosis for seizure control in newly diagnosed epilepsy. *N Engl J Med* 311:944, 1984.

8. Hart RG, Easton JD, Carbamazepine and hematological monitoring. *Ann Neurol* 11:309, 1982.

9. Hauser WA, Anderson VE, Loewenson RB, McRoberts SM: Seizure recurrence after a first unprovoked seizure. *N Engl J Med* 307:522, 1982.

10. Gastaut H, Tassinari CA: Epilepsies. In Remand A (ed): *Handbook of EEG and Clinical Neurophysiology*. Amsterdam, Elsevier, 1975, vol 13, part A.

11. Gram L, Bentsen KD, Parnas J, Flachs H: Controlled trials in epilepsy: a review. *Epilepsia* 23:491, 1982.

12. Juul-Jensen P: Frequency of recurrence after discontinuance of anticonvulsant therapy in patients with epileptic seizures: a new follow-up study after 5 years. *Epilepsia* 9:11, 1968.

13. Kaim SC, Klett CJ, Rothfeld B: Treatment of the acute alcohol withdrawal state: a comparison of four drugs. *Am J Psychiatry* 125:1640, 1969.

14. Louis S, McDowell F: Epileptic seizures in nonembolic cerebral infarction. *Arch Neurol* 17:414, 1967.

15. Masland RL: Commission for the control of epilepsy. *Neurology* 28:861, 1978.

16. McGahan JP, Dublin AB, Hill RP: The evaluation of seizure disorders by computerized tomography. *J Neurosurg* 50:328, 1979.

17. Metrakos JD, Metrakos K: Genetics of convulsive disorders. II. Genetic and electroencephalographic studies in centrencephalic epilepsy. *Neurology* 11:474, 1961.

18. Niedermeyer E: *Compendium of the Epilepsies*. Springfield, Il, Charles C Thomas, 1974.

19. Ramirez-Lassepas M, Cipolle RJ, Morillo LR, Gumnit RJ: Value of computed tomographic scan in the evaluation of adult patients after their first seizure. *Ann Neurol* 15:536, 1984.

20. Rapport RL II, Penry JK: Pharmacologic prophylaxis of posttraumatic epilepsy; a review. *Epilepsia* 13:295, 1972.

21. Schmidley JW, Simon RP: Postictal pleocytosis. *Ann Neurol* 9:81, 1981.

22. Schmidt RP, Wilder BJ: *Epilepsy*. Philadelphia, FA Davis, 1968.

23. Schold C, Yarnell PR, Earnest MP: Origin of seizures in elderly patients. *JAMA* 238:1177, 1977.

24. Shorvon SD, Chadwick D, Galbraith AW, Reynolds EH: One drug for epilepsy. *Br Med J* 1:474, 1978.

25. Sumi SM, Teasdall RD: Focal seizures: a review of 150 cases. *Neurology* 13:582, 1963.

26. Theodore WH, Porter RJ: Removal of sedative-hypnotic antiepileptic drugs from the regimens of patients with intractable epilepsy. *Ann Neurol* 13:320, 1983.

27. Treiman DM: Seizure types and causes of epilepsy. *Semin Neurol* 1:65, 1981.

28. van der Lugt PJ: Traffic accidents caused by epilepsy. *Epilepsia* 16:747, 1975.

29. Vignaendra V, Ng KK, Lim CL, Loh TG: Clinical and electroencephalographic data indicative of brain tumors in a seizure population. *Postgrad Med J* 54:1, 1978.

30. Zielinsky JJ: Epidemiology. In Laidlaw J, Richens A (eds): *A Textbook of Epilepsy*. New York, Churchill Livingstone, 1982, p 16.

CHAPTER EIGHTY-ONE

Dizziness, Vertigo, Motion Sickness, Near Syncope, Syncope, and Disequilibrium

L. RANDOL BARKER, M.D., HAMILTON MOSES, III, M.D., AND
WARREN ROTHMAN, M.D.

Dizziness, vertigo, and syncope are common conditions. Nearly everyone has experienced them in certain circumstances; but about 10% of adults report that dizziness is chronic or recurrent (19). The symptoms may be severe and be indicative of no serious condition (as in vasovagal syncope), or they may be mild and yet indicate a serious problem, such as a cardiac arrhythmia or a transient ischemic attack. Proper diagnosis is usually possible when careful attention is paid to the history and the patient is examined with special attention to cardiovascular and neurological abnormalities. A limited number of diagnostic studies can aid the evaluation of selected patients, but these can only be interpreted properly in the light of information gained from the patient.

DELINEATING THE MECHANISM FOR A PATIENT'S DIZZINESS

Patients who complain of dizziness usually mean that they are uncertain of their position or their motion in relation to the environment—they are spatially disoriented. A large number of terms may be used to describe this sensation (see Table 81.1). However, sometimes the "dizzy" patient is not even referring to spatial disorientation but to fatigue, dysphoric mood, and other subjective states. Drachman and Hart (5) have pointed out that dizziness due to spatial disorientation may be related to one of the following *three mechanisms*: (a) the illusion that the patient or the environment is moving or rotating (vertigo), (b) a sensation of impending faint or loss of consciousness (near syncope, syncope), and (c) disequilibrium or loss of balance without vertigo or near syncope (cerebellar ataxia, multiple sensory deficits, and miscellaneous other causes). These authors also point out that there are patients with ill defined "light-headedness" other than vertigo, presyncope, or disequilibrium and that the basis for their complaint may be impossible to establish. They emphasize that as many as 25% of patients with chronic dizziness have it on the basis of hyperventilation, which may produce a typical presyncopal pattern or may present as ill defined dizziness.

In taking a history from the patient with dizziness, the first objective should be to determine the probable mechanism for the complaint. Initially it is important to determine the true character of the patient's symptoms. The patient should be asked to use words more specific than "dizziness" (Table 81.1), and he should be asked to *describe a discrete recent episode*. Vertigo is defined as a hallucination of movement and may be described either as a sensation as if the external world were turning around the patient (objective vertigo) or as if the patient himself were turning in place (subjective vertigo). This sensation is similar to that experienced after being on a merry-go-round or after spinning in place for several minutes. This should be differentiated from light-headedness and loss of consciousness. Questions about associated auditory symptoms, or neurological symptoms, may further help

Table 81.1.
Terms That Patients May Use to Describe Spatial Disorientation

Dizziness	Blurred vision	Staggering
Vertigo	Whoozy	Weaving
Unsteadiness	Poor equilibrium	Moving
Imbalance	Drunk feeling	Blackout
Spinning	Haziness	Passing out
Floating	Weird feeling	Tilting
Fainting	Fuzzy-headed	Listing
Light-headed	Bouncing	Rocking
Swaying	Falling	Rolling
Twisting	Swimming	

to classify the patient's problem more specifically (peripheral *versus* central vertigo, metabolic *versus* vascular presyncope, *etc*). If the patient's brief account does not point to the probable mechanism, the following questions may help:

1. (Positive response favors vertigo). Is there actually the sensation of movement or rotation of your head or your body?

2. (Positive response favors presyncope). Is is like the sensation you might get if you stand up too quickly after resting? A sensation as if you might black out?

3. (Positive response favors disequilibrium). Is it a sensation of unsteadiness on your feet? A sensation that you are not sure where your hand or body is and that you cannot quite catch your balance and might fall?

For a patient whose history does not establish the probable mechanism, asking *if he can reproduce his symptoms* may be more efficient than exhaustive questioning.

The patient who says that he is dizzy "right now" while sitting before the physician should

1. Be checked for hypotension, first while seated, then recumbent and standing;

2. Be observed for hyperventilation (slow, hyperpneic breathing, not overt tachypnea); if hyperventilation seems likely, he should be instructed to control his breathing and then to hyperventilate (see further description Chapter 13);

3. Be examined for nystagmus (see below).

A patient who produces "dizziness" by turning his head should then be asked to elaborate on his symptoms; vertigo (positional) and presyncope (due to compromise of cerebral blood flow) are the two problems most likely to be described.

If the patient reports typical dizziness on rising from his chair, orthostatic hypotension is likely; this can be confirmed by measuring the blood pressure before and after he stands up. If the patient demonstrates gait ataxia (see Chapter 78) or reports dizziness as he turns while walking, the problem may be disequilibrium rather than vertigo.

As part of this preliminary inquiry, it is important to ask the patient whether his dizziness has interfered with his usual activities. This information will be important in the management of the patient, regardless of the mechanism of dizziness.

VERTIGO

It has been estimated that somewhat less than a quarter of the patients who visit physicians for dizziness have vertigo (5). Most vertigo is due to conditions affecting labyrinthine structures or the vestibular nerve (peripheral vertigo); although these conditions are distressing and at times disabling, they are usually self-limited.* In some patients, however, vertigo is a manifestation of progressive disease of the central nervous system (central vertigo) or is a secondary manifestation of a systemic condition. The major causes of vertigo in these three categories are listed in Table 81.2.

Vestibular Reflexes

In evaluating the patient with vertigo, it is helpful to have an understanding of the principal reflexes involved in vestibular function. The vestibular system functions through the vestibulospinal and vestibulo-ocular reflexes. The *vestibulospinal reflex* uses information from the sensory structures contained in the bony labyrinth (semicircular canals, utricle, and saccule) to determine the orientation of the head with respect to the ground and to promote appropriate postural adjustments to keep the body upright. The *vestibulo-ocular reflex* uses information from these sensory structures to detect rotational movements of the head and to generate appropriate compensatory eye movements which are exactly equal and opposite to head movements. This reflex permits maintenance of ocular fixation during head movements. All reflex arcs between the vestibular sensory structures and the central nervous system utilize the vestibular branch of the 8th cranial nerve and the four vestibular nuclei of the brainstem.

In these reflex systems there is a tonic discharge from each vestibular sensory organ that elicits a perfectly balanced motor response in the central nervous system. When the head is moved in any direction, the labyrinthine output from one side increases while the output from the other side decreases; this temporary imbalance of sensory input elicits the compensatory motor commands for vestibulospinal and vestibulo-ocular reflexes. If the input from the labyrinths or its central processing becomes disordered, abnormal subjective states (*i.e.*, vertigo) and motor responses (*i.e.*, nystagmus and loss of balance) occur.

---

* See Figure 96.1 (anatomy of the ear and 8th cranial nerve).

Table 81.2.
Major Causes of Vertigo[a]

PERIPHERAL CAUSES OF VERTIGO
  "Benign" positional vertigo
  Post-traumatic vertigo
  Peripheral vestibulopathy (labyrinthitis, vestibular neuroni-
    tis, acute and recurrent peripheral vestibulopathy)
  Vestibulotoxic drug-induced vertigo (aminoglycosides)
  Ménière's syndrome (endolymphatic hydrops)
  Inflammatory labyrinthitis (syphilis, vasculitis)
  Other focal peripheral disease (acute and chronic otitis
    media, cholesteatoma, tumor, fistula, genetic anomalies,
    rarely focal ischemia and others)
CENTRAL CAUSES OF VERTIGO
  Brainstem ischemia and infarction
  Cerebellopontine angle tumor (acoustic neurinoma, menin-
    gioma, metastatic tumor, etc)
  Demyelinating disease (multiple sclerosis, postinfectious
    demyelination, remote effect of carcinoma)
  Cranial neuropathy with focal involvement of 8th nerve
  Intrinsic brainstem lesions (tumor, arteriovenous malfor-
    mation, trauma, etc)
Other posterior fossa lesions (primarily other intrinsic or extra-
    axial masses of the posterior fossa, such as meatoma,
    metastatic tumor, and cerebellar infarction)
  Seizure disorder (temporal lobe epilepsy)
  Migraine
  Heredofamilial disorders (spinocerebellar degenerations:
    Friedreich's ataxia, olivopontocerebellar atrophy, etc)
SYSTEMIC CAUSES OF VERTIGO AND DIZZINESS
  Drugs (anticonvulsants, hypnotics, antihypertensives, al-
    cohol, analgesics, tranquilizers)
  Infectious disease (viral and bacterial meningitis, and sys-
    temic infection)
  Endocrine disease (diabetes and hypothyroidism particu-
    larly)
  Vasculitis (systemic lupus erythematosus, giant cell arteri-
    tis, and drug-induced vasculitis)
  Other systemic conditions (polycythemia, anemia, dyspro-
    teinemia, Paget's disease of the bone, sarcoidosis, gran-
    ulomatous disease, and systemic toxins)

[a] Adapted from Troost BT: Dizziness and vertigo in vertebrobasilar
disease. *Curr Concepts Cerebrovasc Dis* 14:21, 1979.

Approach to the Patient

Initial Office Evaluation

A systematic approach to the history and physical examination should be utilized for all patients with vertigo. Even when a working diagnosis of a self-limited peripheral vertigo is made, follow-up is needed for confirmation, since there is significant overlap in the symptoms and signs produced by peripheral and central vertigo. The following information should be obtained in the initial office evaluation of the patient (the presentation and course of the major causes of vertigo are described on subsequent pages):

History.
  1. Was the onset gradual or sudden?

  2. Are symptoms severe, moderate, or mild?
  3. Are symptoms constant or episodic?
  4. How long do symptoms last?
  5. How frequently do symptoms occur?
  6. Is there anything that brings on the attack (i.e., change in position, stress, etc)?
  7. Is there anything that makes symptoms worse or better?
  8. Does the patient tend to fall, and to which side?
  9. Is there associated nausea or vomiting?
  10. Is this a first episode or a recurrent episode of illness?
Associated Auditory Symptoms.
  1. Is there a hearing impairment (unilateral or bilateral)?
  2. Is tinnitus present (pulsatile or constant)?
  3. Is there a history of prior ear infections or draining ears?
  4. Is there a sensation of aural pressure?
  5. Is there a history of prior head or neck trauma, recent barotrauma, or recent viral illness?
  6. Has the patient been exposed to any ototoxic drugs?
Associated Neurological Symptoms.
  1. Are there changes in vision (diplopia, blurring of vision, flashing lights, etc)?
  2. Is there numbness of face or extremities?
  3. Is there weakness in arms or legs (unilateral or bilateral)?
  4. Is there clumbsiness in the arms or legs?
  5. Is there confusion or loss of consciousness?
  6. Is there slurring of speech?
  7. Is there difficulty with swallowing?
Examination.
  1. Inspection of external auditory canal and tympanic membrane (see Chapter 96).
  2. Simple office assessment for hearing impairment (see Chapter 96).
  3. Observation for spontaneous nystagmus (see below).
  4. Tests for positional vertigo and positional nystagmus (see below).
  5. Selective neurological and neurovascular examination (cranial nerves, particularly 5 and 7; cerebellar tests, gait testing, Romberg test; motor testing—see Chapter 78 for recommended brief neurological and neurovascular examination).

Laboratory tests. Because luetic labyrinthitis and hypothyroidism can cause peripheral vertigo, a serological test for syphilis (FTA-ABS, since nonreponemal tests may be negative in tertiary syphilis; see Chapter 30) and a T4 level should be obtained on patients with peripheral vertigo. In addition, a hematocrit and a fasting blood sugar should be ordered to check for anemia and diabetes. There are no other routinely indicated laboratory tests in the initial office evaluation of vertigo. Several tests of vestibular function may be utilized by a consulting otolaryngologist (see below, page 1161). With the exception of hypothyroidism, most of the systemic causes of vertigo listed in Table 81.2 will present with other symptoms in addition to the vertigo. Rarely, vertigo and decreased hearing may be the only symptoms described by a hypothyroid patient.

Evaluation of Nystagmus

Nystagmus is rhythmic movement of the eyes. When it is *pendular* (to-and-fro movements about equal in amplitude and speed), it is usually due to disturbance of central vision. *Jerk nystagmus* (having a slow and a quick component) is typically, but not exclusively, a sign of vestibular disease; every patient complaining of vertigo should be checked for this type of nystagmus. It is important to know how to recognize and test for jerk nystagmus since it is the only objective indicator of vestibular dysfunction.

Spontaneous Nystagmus

In patients with peripheral or central vestibular dysfunction, nystagmus may be present with the eyes in midposition or in any direction of gaze. The nystagmus may be detected even when the patient is not experiencing vertigo. During an episode of acute vertigo, there should usually be accompanying nystagmus if the vertigo is due to organic disease. Absence of nystagmus suggests that one of the other mechanisms for dizziness described above is present. Spontaneous nystagmus should be sought in five positions of gaze: straight ahead, right, left, up, and down. The patient should be instructed to turn his eyes only about 30° from midline, since extreme lateral gaze may produce end-position nystagmus in normal individuals. Visual fixation tends to suppress the spontaneous nystagmus of peripheral vestibular disease. Therefore, if spontaneous nystagmus is not observed, the patient should close his eyes (to eliminate visual fixation) and be observed for nystagmus through the eyelids, again in each of the five positions of gaze. Preferably, he can be examined with eyes open through Frenzel lenses (special 10-diopter lenses that distort the patient's view, making fixation impossible). If spontaneous nystagmus is present with the eyes open, the patient should be asked to fixate on a nearby object: *suppression of nystagmus with fixation favors peripheral vestibular disease*, while persistence or enhancement of the nystagmus is typical of central disease.

Features which distinguish peripheral from central spontaneous nystagmus are summarized in Table 81.3.

Positional Nystagmus

Positional nystagmus (and vertigo) is that which is produced by a sudden change in head or body position. The patient with positional vertigo usually

Table 81.3.
Features of Spontaneous Nystagmus

Feature	Peripheral	Central
Direction	Usually horizontal-rotatory	Any direction
	Never purely vertical	May be purely vertical
Direction of fast component	Away from side with disease	Toward side with disease (or direction changing)
Effect of visual fixation	Suppressed	Not suppressed (may be enhanced)
Usual anatomical location of problem	Labyrinth or vestibular nerve	Brainstem or cerebellum

gives a history of symptoms brought on by such changes as lying back in bed, turning the head while lying, arising from bed, or bending over, but it usually does not occur when the body is erect or when the head is not in motion. The purposes of provocative testing are (a) to replicate the patient's symptoms, (b) to demonstrate nystagmus as objective evidence for vestibular impairment, and (c) to determine whether the nystagmus is fatigable.

The test utilized to detect positional vertigo was described by Bárány in 1921 (1) and is illustrated in Figure 81.1. The patient sits close enough to one end of the examining table so that his head would be over the edge if he were lying down. He is asked to keep his eyes open during the maneuver and to report any sensations (vertigo, nausea, *etc*) that he experiences. Frenzel lenses are used, if available, to prevent suppression of the nystagmus. The patient is asked to turn his head to one side. Then, while the examiner supports the head and shoulders, the patient is quickly brought to a reclining position with his head still rotated to one side and hanging over the end of the table. This position should be maintained for 20 seconds. In addition to listening to the patient's symptoms, the examiner should observe his eyes for nystagmus. If nystagmus appears, the examiner should note its time of onset (relative to the start of the maneuver), the direction of eye motion (horizontal, vertical, rotatory, or mixed), the nature of associated symptoms, the adaptability of nystagmus (does it disappear despite maintaining the same head position?), and its fatigability on repeated testing. The maneuver should then be repeated with the head turned in the opposite direction. In particular, if nystagmus was present in one position, the physician should pay careful attention to any change in its direction or amplitude when tested in the opposite direction.

Features which distinguish peripheral from central positional nystagmus are summarized in Table 81.4.

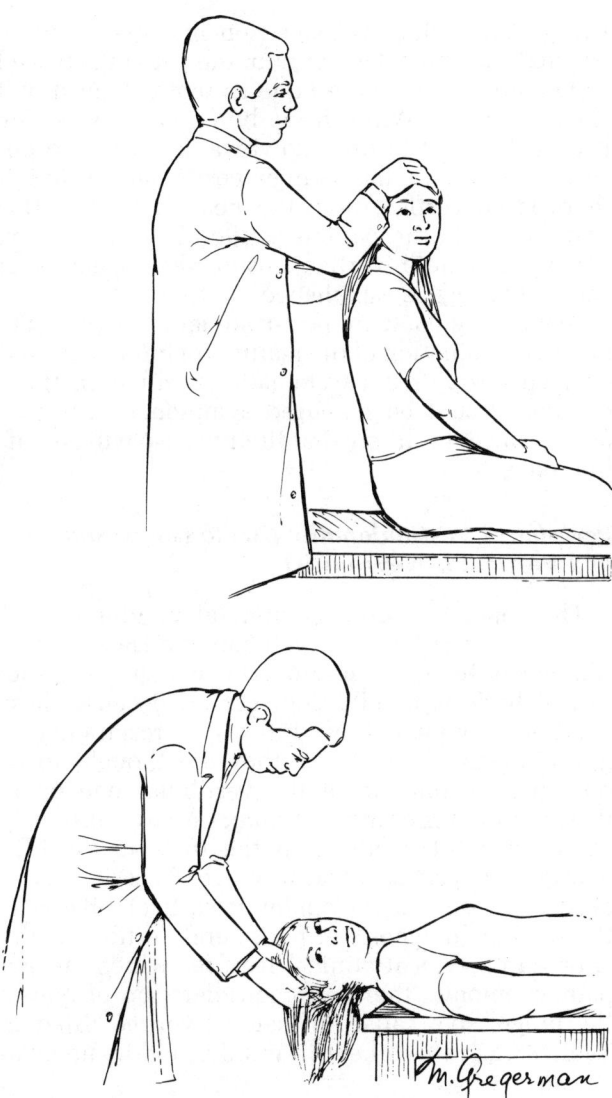

Figure 81.1. Bárány maneuver for testing a patient for positional vertigo and nystagmus.

Peripheral Causes of Vertigo

Idiopathic Benign Positional Vertigo (BPV)

This is probably the most common type of vertigo seen in adult patients. It occurs at all ages but is most common after the fourth decade and in persons with recent head trauma. The pathological basis for idiopathic BPV is not known. The differentiation of BPV from post-traumatic cervical vertigo, endolymphatic hydrops (Ménière's disease) and vertebral-basilar insufficiency is often the principal challenge for the physician.

Symptoms are first noted when the head is turned (a) as the patient is assuming a recumbent position, (b) when the patient is already recumbent, or (c) when the patient is rolling over in bed. The episodes of vertigo are brief (usually lasting less than 1 minute), and they are always brought on with a change in head position. If the vertigo is related to trauma (see below), it may begin immediately after the trauma or days to weeks later. Typically, patients with BPV do not complain of tinnitus or of hearing impairment. They may, however, have nausea during episodes of vertigo.

On examination, spontaneous nystagmus (see above) is *not* present. A positive positional test of the peripheral type (see Table 81.4) with the absence of other otological or neurological findings supports the working diagnosis of idiopathic BPV.

BPV is usually self-limited; however, symptoms may persist for weeks or months, and episodes may recur in later years. Because positional vertigo is observed in other conditions besides BPV, it is important to re-evaluate the patient serially, following the systematic approach utilized initially and looking for ancillary evidence for one of the other causes of vertigo listed in Table 81.2. Any patient whose course is atypical should be seen in consultation by an otolaryngologist or a neurologist.

BPV is usually treated with *positional exercises*. The patient should be instructed to do these exercises on a bed. He is instructed to assume the head position that will initiate symptoms and to maintain this position until the vertigo disappears; then to sit upright for a few seconds; then to repeat the exercise multiple times (usually 5 times) until the exercise produces no symptoms. This should be done three or four times a day. Most patients report excellent relief of symptoms after utilizing these exercises for about 2 weeks (3). Younger patients tend to improve more rapidly than older ones.

Individuals with BPV who work at heights (repairmen, roofers, *etc*) may have to curtail these activities until the symptoms have abated. Sympto-

Table 81.4.
Features of Positional Nystagmus Elicited by the Bárány Maneuver

Feature	Peripheral	Central
Time to onset after quick position change (latency)	3–20 seconds	Immediate
Duration	Less than 1 minute (often only a few seconds)	Persists longer than 1 minute
Fatigability	Marked (may not be present on immediate repetition)	None
Subjective vertigo	Often marked	Often minimal or absent
Nystagmus direction	Fixed irrespective of head position	Changing with change in head position
Usual anatomical location of problem	Labyrinth or vestibular nerve	Brainstem or cerebellum

matic treatment may be helpful, although this has never been confirmed in a controlled trial (see below, page 1160).

Post-traumatic Vertigo (8)

Vertigo is very common after both blunt head trauma and whiplash (flexion-extension) injury to the neck. The basis for the vertigo may be disruption of the utricular otolithic membrane (so-called "cupulolithiasis"), hemorrhage into the endolymph or into the eighth nerve, or fracture of the temporal bone, causing damage to the nerve.* Clinically, it may be impossible to determine which of these mechanisms is responsible for a patient's symptoms. However, there are two typical patterns which are thought to suggest the dominant problem.

The first pattern is *immediate* post-traumatic vertigo, with associated spontaneous nystagmus (beating away from the side of injury), nausea and vomiting, positional nystagmus, and either conductive or sensorineural hearing loss. This pattern suggests temporal bone fracture and is typical of moderately severe trauma to the temporal bone or occiput. A history of brief unconsciousness, the presence of Battle's sign (postauricular hematoma), and bleeding in the external auditory canal are other findings which suggest this diagnosis. Computerized tomographic scanning of the temporal bone is needed to detect the fracture. Because there is the possibility of finding surgically correctable damage, these patients should always be evaluated immediately by an otolaryngologist. Based upon this evaluation, an exploratory tympanotomy may be recommended. These patients must be carefully examined also for facial nerve paralysis. In general, immediate palsy requires immediate decompression, whereas delayed palsy may be followed conservatively, as in Bell's palsy (see Chapter 84).

In the majority of patients with immediate post-traumatic vertigo, the vestibular symptoms improve rapidly over the first few days and they are gone entirely within 6 to 12 weeks. Symptomatic treatment (see below) may be helpful.

The second common pattern is that of *delayed onset* (latent period of days to weeks) of post-traumatic vertigo, which presents in the same way as idiopathic BPV (see above). This pattern is more typical of minor head or whiplash injury and is thought to be due to cupulolithiasis. BPV, without spontaneous vertigo or nystagmus and without hearing deficit, is the typical finding on physical examination. The course and management are similar to those of idiopathic BPV.

Some patients with injuries of the cervical spine may experience *cervical vertigo*. This may be distinguished from benign positional vertigo by a modification of the Bárány maneuver. To test for cervical

vertigo the patient is placed on his side with the affected ear down. Once again, the patient is placed sufficiently high on the table so that the head will clear the table. While he is lying on his side, the head is allowed to drop downwards. If vertigo ensues, the patient has benign positional vertigo. If there is no vertigo, then the head is held in this position while the patient is allowed to lie flat on his back. Should vertigo ensue, the diagnosis of cervical vertigo is established.

Some patients with post-traumatic vertigo may have a combination of the features of immediate and delayed vertigo. After systematic examination, these patients should be managed symptomatically (see below) since it is likely that their vertigo will be self-limited.

Peripheral Vestibulopathy (Acute Labyrinthitis and Vestibular Neuronitis)

The collective term "peripheral vestibulopathy" has been suggested by Drachman and Hart (5) for a number of benign conditions for which the pathological basis is chiefly conjectural. Because these conditions often follow viral upper respiratory or gastrointestinal infections, they are thought to be due to inflammation of the vestibular end organ (labyrinthitis) or of the vestibular nerve (neuronitis). They are most common in the third to the fifth decade but may occur at any age. Occasionally, a cluster of cases occurs (epidemic vertigo). Like BPV, the working diagnosis of peripheral vestibulopathy is based on typical clinical features which are not pathognomonic; therefore, consideration of one of the progressive causes of central vertigo listed in Table 81.2 must be kept in mind in follow-up evaluation.

Typically, there is a sudden onset of moderate to severe spontaneous vertigo. Often there is accompanying nausea and vomiting, and symptoms are made worse by any change in position. The initial symptoms usually persist for several days, during which they may be incapacitating. A patient may describe tinnitus, but there is usually no complaint of hearing loss. There may be a tendency for the patient to fall when he tries to walk.

On systematic examination spontaneous nystagmus with peripheral features (see above) is present. This is an important feature differentiating peripheral vestibulopathy from BPV in which spontaneous nystagmus is not present. Since involvement is often unilateral, there may be a typical nystagmus pattern in which (a) the fast component is away from the side of the lesion when the subject is asked to look away from the lesion, and (b) the nystagmus may lessen or cease when the subject looks toward the side of the lesion. Caloric testing after recovery from the acute episode (see below) shows an absence or decreased response on the affected side, but this test is not needed routinely. Positional testing (if performed) may produce a positive response with peripheral characteristics (see Table 81.4). There is usually no hearing loss, and the neurological and neurovascular examinations are unremarkable.

The vertigo of peripheral vestibulopathy usually resolves within 6 weeks, although nystagmus may be demonstrated for several months, especially if electronystagmography (ENG) is performed (see below). In occasional patients, the vertigo may also persist for more than 6 weeks. Such patients should be systematically re-examined for evidence of a central cause of vertigo, in particular acoustic neurinoma and brainstem or inferior cerebellar infarction (see below).

There is no specific treatment. Patients should be told that the worst symptoms will last only a few days, that all symptoms usually resolve within 1 month to 6 weeks, and that they should adjust their usual activities according to how they feel (during the first few days, many patients will require strict bed rest for symptomatic relief). Antivertigo drugs may be helpful (see page 1160). Diazepam (Valium) 5 mg three times daily, may also be useful in patients with peripheral vestibulopathy. An occasional patient may require hospital admission for intravenous hydration if nausea and vomiting are severe.

Vertigo Due to Vestibulotoxic Drugs (9)

Ototoxicity is an occasional complication of aminoglycoside antibiotics, salicylates, and potent diuretics (ethacrynic acid and furosemide). Most of these drugs are cochleotoxic and produce sensorineural hearing loss and tinnitus (see Chapter 96). Two aminoglycosides, streptomycin and gentamicin, are vestibulotoxic. The basis for aminoglycoside ototoxicity seems to be that these drugs are concentrated in the inner ear. Pathologically, there is destruction of the sensory hair cells of either the cochlea or the labyrinth. Ototoxicity due to an aminoglycoside can usually be prevented by avoiding serum concentrations above the therapeutic range and by limiting the duration of therapy.

In office practice, vestibular toxicity due to an aminoglycoside may appear shortly after the patient has been treated with an aminoglycoside drug while in hospital. Because these drugs produce bilateral, symmetrical damage, the patient will usually not describe frank vertigo, but will have unsteadiness and intolerance to motion and may describe difficulty walking in the dark. The pathological changes produced by aminoglycosides are permanent, and the symptoms usually persist indefinitely. Fortunately, most patients with vestibular toxicity are able to adjust to their problem, and hearing aids may help those with cochlear toxicity.

Mild vertigo or disequilibrium may occur as a side effect of a number of drugs (Table 81.2) that do not produce permanent pathological damage; these side effects remit promptly after stopping the drug.

Ménière's Syndrome (Endolymphatic Hydrops)

This condition is described in Chapter 96. Ménière's syndrome should always be considered in the differential diagnosis of a patient with the acute onset of severe vertigo with peripheral characteristics. The features which distinguish it from other causes of vertigo are the spontaneous onset of attacks, the limited duration of symptoms during each discrete attack (minutes to hours, not 1 or more days as seen with peripheral vestibulopathy), the associated tinnitus and sensorineural hearing loss (may vary in severity from day to day) found in most patients, and normal brainstem and cerebellar function. At times, Ménière's syndrome may present initially with only vertigo (isolated hydrops of the labyrinth) or only hearing loss (isolated hydrops of the cochlea). Serial observation is therefore important. In clinically suspected cases of isolated hydrops, a trial of diuretic treatment may be helpful.

Inflammatory Labyrinthitis

Labyrinthitis may occur, although rarely, as a manifestation of *secondary* or *tertiary syphilis*. It is always important to consider this etiology, as it may mimic other forms of peripheral vertigo and it requires antibiotic treatment. Typically, the patient has a combination of (a) sensorineural hearing loss, which may be unilateral or bilateral and fluctuating or sudden, (b) impaired ability to understand speech (loud enough but not clear), and (c) peripheral type vertigo which is not positional. As noted earlier, this problem should be sought by sending a serological test for syphilis routinely (always including an FTA-ABS) in every patient with new peripheral type vertigo. If the test is positive, the patient should have a cerebrospinal fluid FTA-ABS determination and be treated according to the stage of the disease (see Chapter 30).

Systemic lupus erythematosus, polyarteritis nodosa, and other causes of vasculitis may present with vertigo or loss of hearing. Nearly always other manifestations of the disease will also be apparent simultaneously or will be evident from the history.

Central Causes of Vertigo

Table 81.2 lists the principal central causes of vertigo. Most are uncommon. The important clues to the presence of one of these conditions are the finding of associated neurological signs and symptoms, the presence of nystagmus with central characteristics (see Tables 81.3 and 81.4), or deviation of the patient's presentation and course from that expected for the common peripheral causes of vertigo.

Whenever a central cause for vertigo is suspected, the patient should be referred for evaluation to a neurologist or an otolaryngologist. When the onset of symptoms is acute or there is evidence of rapidly progressive neurological symptoms, the patient should be hospitalized.

The principal manifestations of the two types of central vertigo that a generalist is most likely to see (tumor and vascular disease) are described here.

Cerebellopontine (CP) Angle Tumor

Acoustic neurinoma, the commonest CP angle tumor, is described in Chapter 96. The usual manifestations of these tumors are due to compression of the auditory component of the 8th nerve (sensorineural hearing loss) and, much later, to compression of adjacent structures (the 5th and 7th cranial nerves in particular). Frank vertigo and nystagmus are present in a minority of patients. A vague complaint of unsteadiness, however, is present in almost half of the patients when they are first seen. Most patients complain of unilateral hearing loss and tinnitus. They generally have a great deal of difficulty in understanding speech in the affected ear. The electronystagmogram (see description below) usually shows a markedly decreased or absent response in the affected ear. The symptoms of CP angle tumor typically are insidious in onset (usually confined to sensorineural hearing loss for a prolonged interval), constant, and progressive. This time course distinguishes them from the periodic or severe symptoms typical of most peripheral vertigo and of the central vertigo of transient ischemia. Occasionally onset of vertigo may be acute, but even then hearing loss will have been apparent earlier.

As pointed out elsewhere (Chapter 96), consultation with an otolaryngologist is the most appropriate plan for a patient who may have a CP angle tumor. The consultant should determine which of a large variety of otoneurological tests is appropriate in pursuing this diagnosis (7).

Vertebrobasilar Arterial Disease

Cerebrovascular ischemia may cause vertigo. When this symptom is due to atherosclerosis, there are almost always symptoms or signs of other brainstem involvement, in particular clumsiness or weakness, loss of vision, diplopia, perioral numbness, ataxia, drop attack (sudden loss of motor tone in the lower extremities, without loss of consciousness), or dysarthria.

When these symptoms are *transient*, they may be due (a) to a transient ischemic attack (TIA) (see Chapter 83), (b) to mechanical compromise of the vertebrobasilar circulation (see Fig. 81.2) brought on by rotation of the neck (detected either in the history or by having the patient replicate hs symptoms in the office), or (c) to diversion of blood from the brainstem to an arm during use of that arm—the

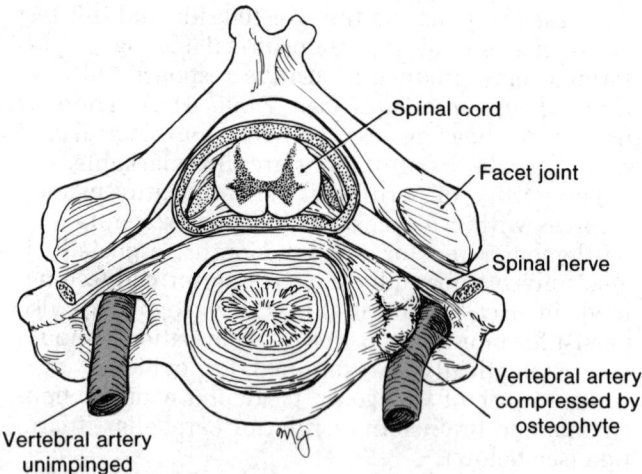

Figure 81.2. Anatomical relationship of the vertebral artery in a transverse foramen. The artery lies alongside the uncinate portion of the vertebra, the most common site of degenerative changes due to cervical spondylosis with osteophyte formation. (From Sheehan S, Bauer RB, Meyer JS: Vertebral artery compression in cervical spondylosis. *Neurology* 10:968, 1960.)

subclavian steal syndrome (suspected on the basis of history and of the finding of a subclavian artery bruit or a decreased blood pressure in the symptom-provoking arm). When the symptoms are abrupt in onset and *persistent*, they may be due to infarction of the brainstem or cerebellum. Insidious onset of persistent symptoms would be more suggestive of tumor. Acute cerebellar infarction in the distal territory of the posterior inferior cerebellar artery (PICA), a relatively uncommon problem, may initially mimic acute vestibulopathy, presenting as sudden marked vertigo, nausea, and vomiting. Usually infarction due to PICA occlusion will involve the brainstem, so that other neurological signs will be present (ipsilateral loss of pain and temperature sense of the face and contralateral loss of these sensations in the rest of the body, cerebellar ataxia, or ipsilateral Horner's syndrome).

Sudden vertigo and unilateral hearing loss may occur due to *selective occlusion of the internal auditory artery*; in such patients, a condition affecting small arteries (syphilitic arteritis or other vasculitides, or microembolism) is a more likely cause than atherosclerosis.

Symptomatic Treatment of Vertigo

When the working diagnosis is peripheral vertigo of any type, treatment with one of the "antivertigo" antihistamines may provide symptomatic relief. There have been no systematic studies to evaluate the efficacy of these drugs. It is hypothesized that these agents work both by suppressing the vestibular end organ receptors and by inhibiting activation of

Table 81.5.
Drugs for Symptomatic Treatment of Vertigo

Type of Action	Generic (Trade Name)	Available Preparation	Dose and Schedule
Labyrinthine suppressants (antihistamines)	Meclizine (Antivert, Bonine)	12.5 and 25-mg tablets	12.5–25 mg 3 or 4 times daily
	Dimenhydrinate (Dramamine)	50-mg tablets	50 mg 3 or 4 times daily
Antiemetics	Prochlorperazine (Compazine)	5- and 10-mg tablets	5–10 mg every 4 hours as needed
		10- and 25-mg suppositories	10 mg 4 times daily or 25 mg twice daily
	Trimethobenzamide (Tigan)	250-mg capsule	3 to 4 times daily
		200-mg suppository	3 to 4 times daily
Sedative	Diazepam (Valium)	5, 10 mg	3 times daily

vagal responses. Commonly recommended drugs in this group are listed in Table 81.5, with appropriate doses and schedules. Because peripheral vertigo from common causes is usually self-limited, the patient should be instructed to take an antivertigo agent only for a few weeks and then to try discontinuing the drug. The major side effects of these drugs are dry mouth and sedation.

When nausea and vomiting are pronounced, in either peripheral or central vertigo, an *antiemetic* can be tried. It is hypothesized that these agents work by suppressing central vestibular pathways which activate vagal responses. Commonly recommended antiemetic drugs are listed in Table 81.5. The major side effect occurring with short term use is sedation; with the phenothiazine antiemetic, prochlorperazine, acute dystonias may occur in occasional patients (see Chapter 16 for a full discussion of phenothiazine side effects).

Patients with persistent and disabling vertigo should be referred to an otolaryngologist for definitive evaluation and management. For permanent relief of symptoms, some persons will require surgery, which may consist of sectioning of the vestibular nerve, repair of an inner ear fistula, labyrinthectomy, or lymphatic shunt. Several of these procedures produce unilateral deafness.

Tests Utilized in Evaluation of Vertigo

When a patient with vertigo that is difficult to diagnose is referred to a neurologist or an otolaryngologist, one or more of the studies listed in Table 81.6 will usually be conducted. A combination of results from several tests may support a specific diagnosis.

Audiometry (16)

A number of audiological tests are usually performed in evaluating vertigo (i.e., puretone audiometry, speech audiometry, tone decay testing, acoustic reflex testing, and others). Typically, there is no audiometric abnormality in the most common

Table 81.6.
Tests Used in the Evaluation of Vertigo

Audiometry (puretone, speech, tone decay, brainstem evoked potentials, *etc*)
Caloric tests
Electronystagmography
Skull X-rays
Mastoid X-rays
Polytomogram of temporal bone and internal auditory canal
CT scan
Air contrast myelogram, with CT scan

forms of peripheral vertigo (BPV and peripheral vestibulopathy), while there are typical patterns of hearing loss in Ménière's syndrome (low frequency hearing loss), acoustic neurinoma (high frequency hearing loss), with poor discrimination), and a variety of middle ear disorders (conductive hearing loss).

Patient experience. These tests are performed in a small soundproof testing room. There is no significant discomfort for the patient. Complete testing may take up to 1 hour.

Caloric Stimulation (13)

This is the only test that evaluates individually the vestibular end organs on each side of the head. The test is based upon the fact that the intact labyrinth responds to caloric stimulation with a typical pattern, *i.e.*, warm water induces horizontal nystagmus with the rapid phase toward the stimulated ear, and cool water produces nystagmus in the opposite direction. Vertigo may be induced with both hot and cold stimulation. Under certain circumstances, electronystagmography is utilized (see below) in addition to direct observation during caloric stimulation. Ideally, the water temperatures are set at 30°C and 44°C; these are equidistant from normal body temperature, constitute equal stimuli, and produce less distress than more extreme temperatures. Absence of the normal caloric response or deviation from the normal response may be helpful in diagnosis. Vestibular neuronitis and acoustic neurinoma are examples of conditions in which the normal response to caloric stimulation is absent or decreased on the involved side.

Patient experience. The patient lies on his side with the head positioned comfortably at an angle of about 30°. Flowing water is introduced into the external auditory canal for 30 seconds. For optimal testing, there should be about a 30-minute wait between irrigations. During caloric stimulation, the patient will experience vertigo. An absent caloric response signifies vestibular disease.

Electronystagmography (ENG) (17)

ENG records changes in the electrical potential between the cornea and the retina; when the eye moves, characteristic changes in electrical potential can be picked up (and recorded with a penwriter) in the skin adjacent to the eye. ENG has two advantages over direct inspection in detecting nystagmus. First, it is more sensitive than simple inspection and can confirm the presence of nystagmus when simple inspection is equivocal (often because the patient fixates and suppresses nystagmus under these conditions). Second, it can provide serial tracings which permit comparison of a patient's nystagmus pattern over time. The disadvantages of ENG are that it requires considerable cooperation from the patient and skill from the operator both for correct conduction of the test and for proper interpretation. The principal value of ENG is in picking up subtle spontaneous nystagmus and in differentiating peripheral from central nystagmus, usually by caloric stimulation.

Patient experience. The patient is recumbent. Small electrodes are taped to the skin on either side of the eye. Nystagmus is measured under a number of conditions, including caloric stimulation (see above), optokinetic testing (the patient is asked to follow the stripes on a rotating drum), and others. The entire procedure may take up to 1 hour. The major discomfort is that associated with caloric stimulation (vertigo).

MOTION SICKNESS

Motion sickness is experienced by most normal persons when they are exposed to conditions analogous to those of severe storm conditions at sea. About one-third of people experience symptoms when exposed to the equivalent of moderate sea conditions such as may occur with automobile travel and air travel, as well as with boating. Normal vestibular function is necessary for an individual to experience motion sickness. Visual stimuli are contributory but not necessary for the experience of motion sickness (for example, looking out of the window of a vehicle on a curving or undulating road).

Manifestations

The symptoms of motion sickness vary from person to person, but an individual usually experiences the same symptoms each time. Malaise and nausea are always present, and vomiting is common. Other symptoms may include drowsiness, salivation, swallowing, hyperventilation, headache, flushing, and diaphoresis. There is a major psychological component in motion sickness; for example, some persons develop their typical symptoms in anticipation of an air flight or a boat ride. Vertigo is usually not present.

Most people adapt fairly rapidly to motion. After the first few days of a sea voyage, for example, they are able to tolerate the motion that made them ill at the beginning of the voyage.

Treatment (20)

In tests simulating sea conditions, a number of drugs have been shown to be quite effective in preventing motion sickness. These drugs are much less effective if taken after the onset of symptoms. Because all drugs which prevent motion sickness are sedating, individuals should not operate cars, boats, planes, or potentially dangerous machines while taking these drugs.

Antihistamines

Either meclizine (Antivert, Bonine), 25 to 50 mg, or dimenhydrinate (Dramamine), 50 to 100 mg, can be used. For persons who routinely get moderate or marked motion symptoms, taking one of these drugs about 1 hour before embarking in a car, plane, or boat may be very helpful. The protective effect from meclizine lasts from 12 to 24 hours, while that from dimenhydrinate lasts only 4 hours. The principal side effect is drowziness; because this is more prominent with dimenhydrinate, meclizine is the better choice for persons who wish to remain alert during travel; others may prefer the greater sedating property of dimenhydrinate.

Scopolamine

The anticholinergic drug scopolamine prevents severe motion sickness in a high percentage of persons known to suffer from this problem. Scopolamine is available in tablet form and in the form of a plastic disc for continuous administration through the skin. A 0.4-mg tablet can be taken 1 hour before travel or boating. Alternatively, the button-sized disc (Transderm-SCOP) can be applied behind the ear. The disc works optimally when applied a number of hours before travel or boating. It is designed to deliver 0.5 mg of scopolamine over a period of 3 days. Dry mouth, sedation, and impaired visual accommodation may occur, probably more frequently with the oral preparation. Known closed angle glaucoma and benign prostate hypertrophy are relative contraindications to the use of this and all anticholinergic drugs.

SYNCOPE AND NEAR SYNCOPE

Definitions and Normal Physiology

Many patients have as their principal symptom loss of consciousness. They may be unconscious for a few seconds or minutes (*syncope*) or may be unconscious for many minutes, hours, or longer (*stupor or coma*). The patient may or may not have symptoms just before he becomes unconscious. If symptoms are recalled they are particularly important to note, for their timing and character will often indicate the cause. Similarly, symptoms during the period of recovery from unconsciousness are also important and may indicate whether a primary neurological event has occurred or whether the explanation lies in the cardiovascular system or elsewhere.

Some patients report transient dizziness or lightheadedness without frank loss of consciousness. This may be referred to as *near syncope* or impending syncope. Near syncope is far more common than syncope. The physiological changes leading to both syncope and near syncope are identical; they are simply shorter in duration or less severe in the person who becomes dizzy without actually losing consciousness. Further, since near syncope may occur before frank syncope, these symptoms should be seriously considered so that a proper diagnosis can be made.

Unconsciousness implies that either both cerebral hemispheres have become impaired or that certain critical structures in the brainstem have failed. In general, unilateral diseases of the cerebral hemispheres do not lead to unconsciousness unless the brain becomes more generally affected.

Causes

Syncope and near syncope are caused by four general classes of abnormalities: hypotension, cardiac disease, metabolic derangement, and primary intracranial conditions (see Table 81.7).

Based on reports of large numbers of patients with syncope, hypotension is the cause in about two-thirds of patients, heart disease in about 10%, intracranial disease in about 10%, and metabolic disorders in about 5%. The remaining patients have syncope in which no cause can be discerned. The single most common cause of syncope is the common faint or vasovagal episode. Orthostatic hypotension due to many causes is also very common. The commonest cardiac causes are ventricular arrhythmias, cardiac pain from angina or myocardial infarction, and, less often, aortic stenosis or ventricular outflow obstruction. Epilepsy and cerebrovascular disease account for most syncope due to primary neurological abnormalities. Hyperventilation is a very common cause of dizziness (through hypocapnea) but rarely leads to frank syncope. It is the only common metabolic cause of transient unconsciousness. Hypoglycemia rarely leads to syncope, although it frequently causes dizziness that is associated with other characteristic symptoms (palpitations, diaphoresis, hunger, *etc*; see Chapter 72).

The management and prognosis of the patient with a history of syncope or near syncope depend on correct identification of the underlying cause. The following discussion focuses chiefly upon the diagnostic evaluation of the patient. Appropriate management for the common causes of these problems is discussed elsewhere in the book, as indicated by cross-referencing.

General Approach to the Patient

Most patients who come to a physician after an episode of syncope or near syncope do so after their symptoms have resolved. The physician should obtain the history both from the patient and from anyone who observed the episode. The inquiry should focus upon the events immediately preceding and following the attack; upon associated problems that may have been present for days to weeks before the episode; and upon evidence of significant trauma, neurological deficit, or aspiration complicating the current episode of syncope. The objectives of these initial steps are (*a*) to reach a working diagnosis or to decide what further evaluation is needed to do so and (*b*) to decide upon the appropriate initial management for the patient. Appropriate management may range from reassurance (for example, the patient with vasovagal syncope) to volume expansion (for example, the patient with a diarrheal illness) to hospital admission for observation, prompt diagnostic testing, and necessary treatment (for example, the patient with a history suggesting recurrent life-threatening arrhythmias or the patient with a fracture or an aspiration pneumonia complicating syncope).

History

Current Episode

The patient should always be questioned about what position he was in immediately before the attack. Syncope from most causes does not occur unless the patient is in the upright position. If the attack occurred when the patient first stood up, orthostatic hypotension due to venous pooling, loss of intravascular volume, or autonomic failure should be considered. If exercise preceded the attack, a number of cardiopulmonary abnormalities are likely, including aortic stenosis, idiopathic hypertrophic subaortic stenosis, arrhythmia, or pul-

Table 81.7.
Causes of Syncope/Near Syncope[a]

HYPOTENSION	**CARDIAC DISEASE**
Simple faint (vasovagal syncope)	*Arrhythmia (heart block, brady- and tachyarrhythmias)*
Vasodilating drugs	*Outflow obstruction*
1. Angiotensin converting enzyme inhibitors	1. Aortic stenosis
2. Calcium channel blockers	2. Idiopathic hypertrophic subaortic stenosis
3. Nitroglycerine preparations	3. Aortic dissection
4. Vasodilator antihypertensives	4. Myxoma
Drugs affecting autonomic function	*Acute myocardial infarction*
1. Sympatholytic antihypertensives	*Mitral valve prolapse*
2. Neuroleptics	*Cyanotic congenital heart disease*
3. Tricyclics and monoamine oxidase (MAO) inhibitors	*Cardiac tamponade*
4. Levodopa	**METABOLIC CONDITIONS**
5. Cholinergic agents	*Hypoglycemia*
Autonomic neuropathy	1. Exogenous insulin
Peripheral neuropathy	2. Reactive
Postsympathectomy	3. Starvation (islet cell tumor)
Tabes dorsalis and diabetic pseudotabes	4. Dumping syndrome
Parkinsonism (Shy-Drager syndrome)	*Hypocapnia (hyperventilation)*
Idiopathic	*Hypoxia*
Decreased blood volume	1. Anemia
1. Hemorrhage	2. Airway obstruction
2. Salt and water deficit (diarrhea, vomiting, perspiration, diuretics, hyperglycemia)	3. Carbon monoxide
3. Fasting	*Hyperviscosity*
4. Adrenal insufficiency	*Electrolyte derangements (hyponatremia, hypokalemia, hypocalcemia, hyperglycemia)*
5. Hypoalbuminemia	*Drug overdose*
Venous pooling	1. Sedatives and ethanol (venous pooling)
1. Prolonged immobility while standing	2. All drugs causing autonomic impairment (see above)
2. Severe varicose veins	**INTRACRANIAL CONDITIONS**
3. Late pregnancy	*Seizure disorder*
4. After exercise	*Subarachnoid hemorrhage*
Mobilization after bed rest	*Cerebral embolism or thrombosis*
Orthostasis of aging	*Migraine*
Valsalva maneuver	*Acutely increased intracranial pressure*
1. Tussive	1. Tumor
2. Micturition	2. Trauma
3. Defecation (with straining)	3. Ventricular obstruction
4. Intermittent positive pressure breathing	4. Hypertensive encephalopathy
Compromise of cerebral blood flow due to cervical osteoarthritis or subclavian steal	*Brainstem compression*
Carotid sinus hypersensitivity	1. Cervical or odontoid fractures
Pulmonary embolism	2. Metastasis
Severe pain of visceral origin	3. Cysts or anomalies of the posterior fossa
	4. Platybasia

[a] Modified from Lee JE, Killip T, Plum F: Episodic unconsciousness. In Baron JA (ed): *Diagnostic Approaches to Presenting Syndromes.* Baltimore, Williams & Wilkins, 1971.

monary hypertension. If syncope was associated with micturition, cough, or passing stool, this suggests diminished venous return due to a Valsalva maneuver. If there was psychological stress (*e.g.*, an argument, fear associated with a medical or other procedure, *etc*), vasovagal syncope is highly likely. In each case, the patient will usually recall feeling dizzy, that events were moving very slowly and that he was distant from them, that his limbs became heavy, and his vision dimmed or objects lost their color and seemed tinted just before loss of consciousness. Nausea, usually without vomiting, is quite characteristic of vasovagal syncope, syncope associ-

ated with bradyarrhythmias, and syncope associated with loss of intravascular volume.

Syncope which occurs when the patient is *seated or recumbent* should suggest hypoglycemia, carotid sinus hypersensitivity, cardiac arrhythmia, hyperventilation, a seizure, or hysteria. Syncope or dizziness occurring with position change while recumbent should always be distinguished from benign positional vertigo, which occurs most frequently in the recumbent position (see above).

Other manifestations just before syncope may suggest the diagnosis. Hunger may indicate hypoglycemia. Headache or characteristic visual disturbances may precede migrainous syncope. Hemiparasis, paraparesis, diplopia, dysarthria, or other neurological abnormalities may precede syncope/near syncope due to transient occlusion of the basilar artery or to vasospasm associated with migraine.

The physician should always take advantage of *observations made by others* who witnessed the period of unconsciousness. Particular attention should be paid to the duration of the spell, whether a convulsion occurred, if incontinence was noted, the sequence of events, and how the patient seemed during the period of recovery. In general, recovery of consciousness is swift. Slow recovery of clear consciousness (recovery after more than 5 minutes should raise suspicion of a seizure, hypoglycemia, or an occluded intracranial vessel.

Associated Recent History

Information about the patient during the hours, days, or weeks preceding syncope/near syncope is often very helpful in the differential diagnosis.

A large proportion of patients will give a history of episodic near syncope. The patient will usually use the word "dizziness" or one of the other terms listed in Table 81.1. The circumstances surrounding these episodes may support a working diagnosis for a current episode of frank syncope. For example, the patient may have started, or increased the dose of, a drug known to cause orthostatic hypotension (see Table 81.7); or there may be a history of a problem leading to volume deficit, e.g., diarrhea, heat exposure, diuretic use; increased polyuria (in a diabetic), or melena. A patient convalescing from recent illness may relate his symptoms to beginning to be up and around after bed rest. An insulin-using diabetic or a patient with reactive or starvation hypoglycemia may describe episodic hypoglycemic symptoms, successfully aborted with carbohydrate intake, during the week(s) prior to frank syncope. In the absence of any relevant changes in the patient's circumstances, a history of recent near syncopal episodes is suggestive of arrhythmia, transient cerebral ischemia, or chronic idiopathic orthostatic hypotension.

A second group of patients will describe prior episodes of frank syncope, without prodromal near syncope. Most often, these will be patients with a history, often long-standing, of syncope due to vasovagal attack brought on by psychological or physical stress. A history of recurrent syncope without near syncopal episodes and without the features of vasovagal attacks is most suggestive of arrhythmia, transient cerebrovascular occlusion, or a seizure disorder.

Physical Examination

General Examination

The physical examination after an attack should include a systematic search for abnormalities in the blood pressure, heart and great vessels, abdomen, and central and peripheral nervous system. In particular, the blood pressure should be measured after the patient has been recumbent for several minutes, again after he is seated, and finally while he is standing. The character, volume, and timing of the carotid pulses should be appraised, and any bruits should be noted. The pulse should be palpated for 1 to 2 minutes to look for irregularities. The heart should be carefully examined for murmurs, systolic clicks, or gallop rhythms. Abdominal examination may reveal a large bladder or signs of a visceral catastrophe. If unexplained orthostatic hypotension has been found, a rectal examination should be performed to check the stool for occult or gross blood.

Neurological Examination

A brief examination of the major components of the nervous system (see Chapter 78) may reveal evidence of either pre-existing neurological disease or of an acute insult related to the current episode of syncope/near syncope. Orientation, speech, memory for the event itself as well as for general information, and judgment should be noted. The fundi may reveal microemboli (see Fig 83.1) or subhyaloid hemorrhages (a sign of subarachnoid hemorrhage). Nystagmus, ophthalmoplegia, or abnormalities of the pupils, facial movement and sensation, the corneal reflexes, speech, or movement of the palate or tongue indicate involvement of the midbrain, pons, or medulla. Weakness, sensory abnormalities, and pathological reflexes found in a general neurological examination may indicate a lesion elsewhere in the central nervous system. Any neurological abnormalities should raise the suspicion of cerebrovascular disease, a mass causing an epileptic focus, subarachnoid hemorrhage, or central nervous system infection. If trauma has occurred in the recent past or if a fall was sustained during the syncopal episode, subdural or epidural hemorrhage should be considered.

Significance of Seizures and Neurological Deficits

Seizure activity may occur after syncope due to any of the common causes, including the simple faint, hyperventilation, orthostatic hypotension, or venous pooling. This is not surprising since unconsciousness signifies a major disruption in normal brain function. A single tonic convulsion is the commonest type of postsyncopal seizure; less often a focal seizure or a generalized convulsion may occur. In all three of these instances, the patient's evaluation should include routine tests for a seizure focus (see Chapter 80).

Minor neurological signs, such as slight focal weakness, reflex asymmetries, or pathological reflexes, may also occur following syncope from any cause. These findings may be present particularly if the patient is examined immediately after recovering consciousness, and they rarely persist for more than a few minutes. If such signs persist longer, are more profound, or occur in a constellation which suggests a particular anatomical lesion, they warrant further pursuit. However, one should not be surprised if a source is not found even after a thorough search is completed, since neurological abnormalities are not uncommon after general ischemic or metabolic insults to the brain.

Laboratory Tests

No laboratory test is indicated routinely in the evaluation of syncope/near syncope, although an electrocardiogram will often be indicated if the cause of the patient's problem is not obvious. Noble (15) estimates that the carefully taken history with a screening physical examination, plus an electrocardiogram, will lead to the correct diagnosis in most patients. The indications for other laboratory tests are cited in the discussion of specific problems which follows.

Features of Common Causes of Syncope/Near Syncope

Hypotension

Because of autoregulation, cerebral blood flow is protected over a wide range of systemic blood pressure. In normal persons, a critical decrease in CNS blood flow (clinically producing near syncope or syncope) does not occur until the mean blood pressure is below 50 mm Hg. Under a number of circumstances (e.g., sympatholytic drug treatment, cerebrovascular disease, aging), however, the minimum tolerated blood pressure may not be this low. Therefore, symptomatic failure of the systemic circulation may occur over a relatively wide range of blood pressures.

Simple Faint

The simple faint (vasovagal episode) has long been known to afflict young people; it is particularly apt to occur in the setting of anxiety, tension, fatigue, or during venipuncture or other painful procedures. The simple faint is not just a disease of the young but can occur in older patients in identical settings. Early theories suggested that bradycardia due to vagal overactivity was the initial event; but it is now known that venous pooling due to peripheral arterial constriction with venous dilation occurs in the first phase, with a vagal phase (bradycardia) occurring only after the faint itself. Vasovagal attacks nearly always occur while the patient is upright, but may occur while he is seated; and consciousness is nearly always regained promptly when the patient becomes recumbent. Typically there is a prodromal warning period, at times lasting 3 to 5 minutes, during which the patient feels dizzy, light-headed, and flushed

and has palpitations, often with a tightness in his throat or mild nausea. If the subject assumes a recumbent position during this stage, he may avoid loss of consciousness. An observer will note cold hands, pale skin, and tachycardia just before the patient loses consciousness. After the faint, when the patient is usually recumbent, a flush replaces the pallor and a bradycardia replaces the tachycardia. If the patient is unable to lie flat, recovery may be prolonged; and an occasional death has been noted, as in a faint occurring in a telephone booth or if the person is held upright during the spell. Bradycardia may persist for up to ½ hour after a simple faint. During this time the patient should remain in a recumbent position. The examination is otherwise normal unless there has been trauma or aspiration.

Autonomic Impairment

Syncope/near syncope due to autonomic impairment is always associated with orthostatic hypotension. To document this problem, blood pressure must be taken while the patient is supine, seated, and standing. In some patients, exercise while standing (walking for a few minutes, for example) may be required for a significant orthostatic drop (20 mm Hg systolic) to occur.

The most common cause of this problem nowadays is *antihypertensive drug use*; most syncope due to these drugs is preventable if these drugs are prescribed cautiously and the standing blood pressure, after exercise, is monitored routinely. Other drugs may also produce orthostatic symptoms (see Table 81.7). The initial management of drug-induced orthostasis is described in Chapter 62 (Hypertension); definitive management requires discontinuation or reduced dose of the offending drug.

Orthostatic hypotension can also be due to *autonomic neuropathy*. In patients suspected of having this problem, the integrity of the autonomic nervous system can be tested by noting the size and reaction of the pupils, the distribution of sweating, and the response to a Valsalva maneuver (6, 10, 11). The Valsalva maneuver is performed by having the patient expire against a closed glottis for 20 to 30 seconds, then release air from the chest (see Table 81.8). This maneuver creates a sudden reduction in cardiac output, stimulating vagal (afferent) and sympathetic (efferent) responses. Absence of the reflex tachycardia (phase II) and/or absence of the blood pressure overshoot and reflex bradycardia (phase IV) indicate autonomic impairment.

Sympathetic failure commonly occurs late in diabetic peripheral neuropathy (Chapter 72), but may be the presenting feature of amyloidosis or the neuropathy associated with various neoplasms. The Shy-Drager syndrome, which occurs in late life, is due to failure of certain central autonomic neurons and causes orthostatic hypotension, parkinsonism,

Table 81.8.
Four Phases of a Normal Valsalva Maneuver

ONSET	*Phase I: A sharp rise* in systolic pressure caused by an abrupt increase in intrathoracic pressure and emptying of the pulmonary bed during forced expiration against a closed glottis.
(20–39 seconds)	*Phase II: A gradual fall* in systolic pressure and a concomitant narrowing of peripheral pulse pressures caused by decrease in pulmonic and systemic venous return. *Heart rate increases* during this phase.
RELEASE	*Phase III: A sudden further drop* in blood pressure occurs. Pulse pressure may be very narrow for the few beats during refilling of pulmonary venous reservoir.
	Phase IV (overshoot): Cardiac output increases with the increase in ventricular filling. Within 30 seconds of release of intrathoracic pressure, blood pressure *rises above its original level* because of reflex vasoconstriction initiated by small pulse pressure during phase III. The pressoreceptor stimulation in phase IV results also in *transient bradycardia slowing.*

and other autonomic symptoms in varying combinations. Sympathectomy, particularly when done bilaterally or in the lumbar segments, may be followed immediately by orthostatic hypotension and syncope, though usually venous tone recovers several weeks after the operation. Tabes dorsalis and more commonly diabetic pseudotabes may present with lighting pains and autonomic failure. The management of orthostasis due to autonomic neuropathy is symptomatic; it is summarized in Chapter 84.

Decreased Intravascular Volume

Decreased intravascular volume due to hemorrhage or to salt and water loss (*e.g.*, of gastroenteritis, heat exposure, diuretics, *etc*) is recognized by the combination of orthostatic hypotension and an associated basis for the volume deficit. Hot weather and exercise predispose to volume depletion and thereby to syncope, particularly after vigorous exercise. Prolonged fasting, as in anorexia nervosa or with fad diets, also may produce syncope through volume depletion. Adrenal insufficiency due to pituitary or primary adrenal disease may produce syncope, due to the combination of chronic volume deficit and the loss of vascular tone; the syncope is often precipitated by an intercurrent illness which would not produce syncope in a healthy person. Hypoalbuminemia due to liver disease, enteropathies, or chronic disease can also lead to syncope/presyncope due to intravascular volume deficit. Volume expansion, either by increased salt and water ingestion or by intravenous fluids, is the initial treatment; the choice of ambulatory or hospital management and the planning of definitive treatment de-

pends upon the severity and the primary cause for the volume deficit.

Venous Pooling

Venous pooling prevents return of blood to the heart, lowering cardiac output, at times sufficiently to produce near syncope or syncope. Symptoms may occur after prolonged standing in one position, particularly after exercise, as in recruits standing at attention. Severe dependent varicose veins or the compression of pelvic veins by a fetus or a large abdominal mass may produce symptoms due to a similar mechanism. Syncope 15 to 30 minutes after exercise has been attributed to dilation of the splanchnic circulation before blood flow to the skeletal muscles has completely returned to normal. Management of patients with these conditions is chiefly by avoidance of the precipitating circumstances after an initial episode. Supportive elastic stockings may be helpful for patients with marked pooling due to varicose veins (see Chapter 88).

Orthostatic Syncope/Near Syncope after Bed Rest

This problem is due to the combined effects of venous pooling, relative hypovolemia, and probably to some degree of lowered sensitivity of the baroreceptor system. It is a very common occurrence and should be anticipated in any person who has been at bed rest for more than a few days, in the hospital or at home; moreover, it may persist for 1 or 2 weeks, occasionally longer, after mobilization begins. Orthostatic symptoms may be minimized or prevented by having the patient gradually stand only after several minutes of sitting on the bed with his legs dependent. Practical exercises which may help convalescing patients in overcoming postural weakness and hypotension are illustrated in Figure 81.3.

Orthostasis of Aging

Transient orthostatic symptoms are relatively common among older persons. An orthostatic fall of 30 mm Hg in systolic pressure is found in approximately 10% of healthy older persons (4). Recently, it has been shown that a significant fall in systolic blood pressure is common in elderly patients, in the sitting position, shortly after eating (14). This response may make elderly subjects especially susceptible to presyncope or syncope when getting up after a meal. The physiological basis for orthostatic blood pressure fall in the elderly is not established, although studies of small numbers of elderly persons have shown an impaired Valsalva response (11), indicating autonomic dysfunction. This often asymptomatic condition is important insofar as it increases the risk associated with drugs and conditions which may cause orthostatic hypotension. Clearly, older persons should have their standing blood pressure checked whenever they complain of even mild orthostatic symptoms and should be mon-

LEG EXERCISES

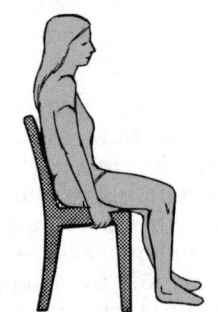
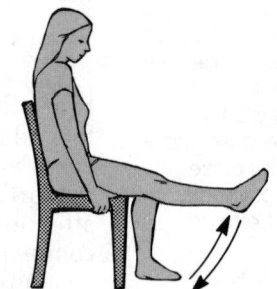
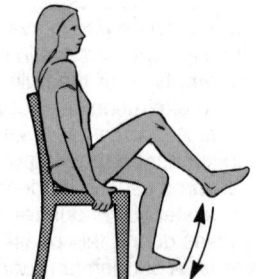

Starting position: Sitting in chair, exercise one leg at a time

Raise leg up and down. Repeat 10 times

Keeping knee bent, raise leg up and down

ARM EXERCISES: To increase effectiveness, hold a soup can in each hand for weight

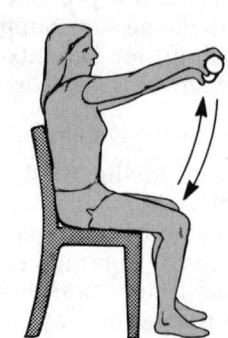
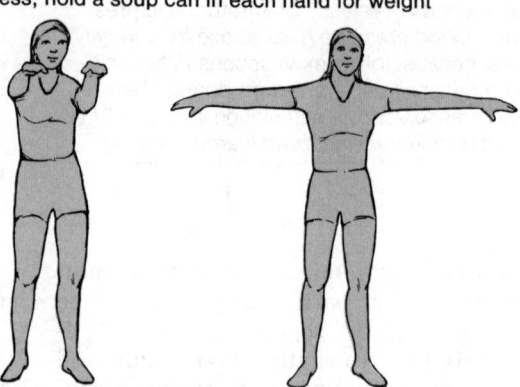

Start with arms straight out in front. Raise arms up and down, only to chin level. Repeat 10 times

Start with arms straight out in front. Swing arms out to sides and return to front. Repeat 10 times

RISING EXERCISE

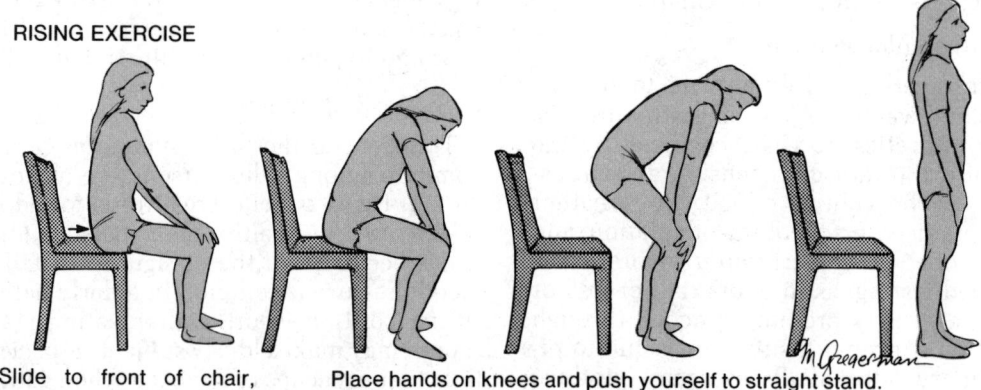

Slide to front of chair, keeping legs apart

Place hands on knees and push yourself to straight stand. Sit down, using hands on knees to help

Repeat 3–5 times using hands less and legs more each time. Repeat exercise without using hands to help

Figure 81.3. Exercise for weakness and orthostatic hypotension after prolonged bed rest. Patient must be out of bed 2 hours a day, morning, afternoon, and evening (for meals). Exercises are done three times a day. (Courtesy of Ms. Karen Ryder, Registered Occupational Therapist.)

itored similarly whenever a drug in one of the groups listed in Table 81.7 is prescribed. Those who are troubled by orthostatic symptoms should be advised to follow the steps recommended above for patients convalescing from bed rest.

Micturition Syncope (13a)

Micturition syncope, defined as syncope occurring at the beginning of, during, at the termination of, or immediately after urination, occurs typically in two types of subjects: (a) Young men who are otherwise healthy. Both the Valsalva mechanism and direct vagal stimulation have been hypothesized as the basis for this form of syncope. Alcohol, because it causes venous pooling, may be a predisposing factor in some patients. (b) Older men and women, many of whom have baseline orthostasis related to drugs or to aging. Persons with micturition syncope should be evaluated for orthostasis, and when this is found any factors contributing to it should be modified. In addition, all patients with recurrent micturition syncope should be advised to sit while urinating and to remain seated for a minute after urination.

Other Forms of Syncope Related to Systemic Circulation

Tussive syncope may follow a prolonged bout of coughing in otherwise normal individuals; in these persons, the syncope is thought to be due to the Valsalva mechanism (see above). Tussive syncope may also occur after only a slight cough in persons with obstructive airways disease; abnormalities of pulmonary and pleural vagal receptors in such individuals may aggravate their tendency to faint. Syncope during *positive pressure breathing* occurs by similar mechanisms.

Hypersensitivity of the carotid sinus is a controversial entity and probably an uncommon cause of syncope. Stimulation of the baroreceptors in the carotid sinus may provoke sympathetic relaxation and lead to hypotension with a normal heart rate; it may increase vagal activity leading to bradycardia without hypotension; or it may provoke abnormalities in the brainstem which lead to syncope without a change in circulatory dynamics. These mechanisms have been invoked in patients with longstanding and severe hypertension or with coronary or carotid arteriosclerosis. Older men wearing tight collars, women with cumbersome necklaces, or patients having large masses in the neck are predisposed to the problem. In some patients thought to have carotid sinus hypersensitivity, compression of the common or internal carotid arteries (or the external carotid, an important collateral in the case of a carotid occlusion) may lead to the symptoms of cerebral ischemia if the contralateral artery is not fully patent. Some authorities recommend provoking syncope by unilateral or bilateral carotid mas-

sage. This may be a dangerous maneuver, and it should be performed only in an emergency department or in the hospital, with intravenous fluid running, ECG monitoring, and atropine at hand.

Syncope with *pulmonary embolism* is estimated to occur in 15 to 20% of cases (18). It may lead to prolonged unconsciousness, at times lasting for 10 to 15 minutes and often accompanied by a small seizure, and it may be followed by minor neurological abnormalities, even when paradoxical embolization has not occurred.

Severe pain arising from any site may be followed immediately by a faint, occurring probably by a vasovagal mechanism.

Cardiac Abnormalities

Rhythm Disturbances

Heart block may reflect ischemic, infiltrative, or neoplastic lesions of the heart and may lead to syncope when the heart rate falls below 40/minute or if ineffective ventricular contraction occurs. Likewise, brady- or tachyarrhythmias without block may lead to cerebral symptoms or to syncope. Cardiac arrhythmias should be strongly considered in older patients and in patients who have syncope while seated or recumbent. A number of drugs may cause arrhythmias (e.g., quinidine, digitalis, tricyclic antidepressants, neuroleptics). Though premonitory warnings may be recalled (particularly grayouts, sweating, mild nausea, and fear), patients' reports regarding palpitations are notoriously unreliable and should not be used to substantiate or refute the diagnosis of a cardiac arrhythmia. Most patients with cerebral symptoms due to cardiac arrhythmias have normal resting ECGs, or at most minor PR or QT prolongations (12). Therefore, 24-hour cardiac monitoring is usually essential in confirming this diagnosis. Particular attention should be paid to sustained tachycardia, bradycardia, paroxysmal blocks, and spells of asystole. Details regarding the diagnosis and management of patients with these problems are found in Chapter 59.

Outflow Obstruction

An obstruction to ventricular outflow due to rheumatic or calcific *aortic stenosis* may lead to syncope in older individuals. It nearly always follows exertion and is usually associated with chest pain. Unconsciousness may be prolonged and may be followed by neurological abnormalities. Similarly, idiopathic *hypertrophic subaortic stenosis* in patients of any age may lead to syncope by outlet obstruction after exercise or due to an arrhythmia at any time. The diagnostic approach to patients thought to have outflow obstruction from these causes is described in Chapter 60. *A left atrial myxoma* (very rare) may cause syncope by obstruction of blood flow when a patient leans over or exerts himself. *Cyanotic congenital heart disease* also leads to syncope after exercise or, rarely, during an airplane flight. Hypoxia and increased blood viscosity are contributing factors.

Myocardial Infarction

Acute myocardial infarction may present with syncope, which may result from arrhythmia, low cardiac output, or severe pain. Embolization from a mural thrombus should be considered when syncope occurs during recovery from myocardial infarction.

Metabolic Abnormalities

Since some metabolic derangements (e.g., hypoglycemia or hypoxia) may lead to lasting damage, the physician should be very alert to the possibility of these problems in patients with syncope who have features or abnormalities characteristic of these derangements in their history or examination.

Hypoglycemia

Hypoglycemic syncope may occur in the adult when the blood glucose level is below 40 mg/100 ml. Hunger, palpitations, sweating, and anxiety nearly always occur 5 to 15 minutes before the patient loses consciousness. As the brain can survive for only about 10 minutes with a blood glucose of 20 mg/100 ml, the prophylactic administration of glucose is warranted in anyone who remains unconscious long enough for the physician to prepare the solution. Convulsions and incontinence commonly accompany hypoglycemic coma. The evaluation and management of hypoglycemia due to *exogenous insulin* are described in Chapter 72. *Reactive hypoglycemia and starvation* hypoglycemia (which may be due to insulinoma) usually produce near syncope but not unconsciousness. These problems are described in Chapter 74. Mild hypoglycemic symptoms may also occur postprandially in patients who have had ulcer surgery, as part of the *dumping syndrome* (see Chapter 36).

Hypocapnia

Hypocapnia due to *hyperventilation* leads to syncope/near syncope by decreasing cerebral blood flow through vasoconstriction of small arterioles throughout the brain. A pCO_2 of 25 mm Hg is sufficient to lower cerebral blood flow to levels at which symptoms occur; such a value may be produced in some persons by a few very deep breaths. Athletes preparing to race, musicians playing wind instruments, or anyone who is fearful or anxious may develop transient symptoms in this way. Tetany or carpopedal spasm may or may not precede the cerebral symptoms. Recovery is prompt if ventilation is slowed. The diagnosis and management of hyperventilation related to anxiety, the commonest cause of this problem, are described in Chapter 13.

Hypoxemia

Hypoxemia due to any primary cause may cause syncope/near syncope. *Severe anemia* (see Chapter 49) may sufficiently deprive the brain of oxygen to lead to syncope after exercise; it may also predispose to syncope from any other cause. Asphyxiation due to *obstruction of the upper airway* should be considered in small children, patients with bad teeth, or patients with masses about the neck. The "cafe coronary" due to laryngeal aspiration of food is usually betrayed by sudden collapse at the table. Patients with esophageal diverticula, however, may choke hours after a meal. Poisoning with *carbon monoxide* is suggested by a history of intentional or unintentional exposure to products of combustion (e.g., poorly ventilated space heaters, gas-burning engines in closed spaces). Manifestations may include prodromal headache and confusion plus bright pink color and prolonged unconsciousness.

Seizures are very common in patients with acute hypoxemia, and neurological sequelae are the rule after unconsciousness lasting more than 1 or 2 minutes. The management of hypoxemic syncope depends entirely on prompt and accurate diagnosis in order to prevent recurrence or worsening of the primary cause of hypoxemia.

Drug Overdose

Overdose of some drugs may cause syncope/near syncope due to orthostatic hypotension. These drugs include sedatives, which may produce venous pooling (particularly chloral hydrate, paraldehyde, and ethanol, and less often benzodiazepines and barbiturates) and all of the drugs listed as potential causes of autonomic impairment in Table 81.7. Stupor or coma due to the sedating effects of drug overdose is more common than are transient cerebral symptoms (syncope/near syncope) due to acute orthostatic hypotension.

Intracranial Abnormalities

Seizure

A seizure may occur with or without warning in any position and may be the primary event leading to an episode of syncope. The diagnosis and management of seizure disorders are described in detail in Chapter 80.

Subarachnoid hemorrhage. A brief period of unconsciousness at the beginning of subarachnoid hemorrhage is the rule. This diagnosis is strongly suggested when the constellation of headache, confusion, and neck stiffness follows shortly after a syncopal episode. Any patient who is confused and who develops headache during initial evaluation demands more scrutiny, even if meningismus has not yet developed. Such patients should be admitted for observation and evaluation.

Embolism or Thrombosis

Cerebral embolism or thrombosis may cause brief (TIA) or prolonged (cardiovascular accident) unconsciousness if the basilar artery is affected. Rarely, a carotid occlusion may cause unconsciousness initially, even if the remaining vessels are patent. A carotid occlusion likewise may cause syncope or coma if the contralateral carotid is already occluded; in this instance, the period of unconsciousness is usually prolonged and seizures may occur; neurological symptoms and signs nearly always are present simultaneously (near syncope) or after the patient awakens (syncope). The ambulatory diagnosis and management of cerebrovascular disease are described in detail in Chapter 83.

Migraine

Migraine (see Chapter 79) may produce syncope/ near syncope, albeit rarely, due to spasm of the basilar artery or of the posterior cerebral arteries. Syncope that occurs with migraine is more often due to hyperventilation or to a vasovagal mechanism than to a central abnormality.

Increased Intracranial Pressure

Increased intracranial pressure, whether due to a brain tumor, trauma, or an obstruction to the ventricular system, may result in syncope when a Valsalva maneuver is performed such as during straining at stool or bending over. The hallmarks are preexisting symptoms, papilledema, or neurological signs.

Brainstem Compression

Rarely, brainstem compression due to a displaced fracture of C1 or of the odontoid process or to metastatic tumors or cystic anomalies of the posterior fossa may lead to syncope with movement of the neck causes transient compression of critical structures of the brainstem. Associated neurological abnormalities are the rule. The diagnosis and management of patients thought to have this problem require prompt hospital admission.

Overall Prognosis

The overall prognosis of syncope and near syncope depends ultimately on the underlying disorder and upon any trauma or other morbidity which may have occurred as a consequence of losing consciousness. The simple faint, hyperventilation, venous pooling, or syncope with a Valsalva maneuver may occur repeatedly when the patient finds himself in the same circumstance and can be prevented if he avoids it. Drug-provoked syncope/near syncope can be eliminated by discontinuating or decreasing the dose of the offending drug; and syncope due to intravascular volume deficit is usually amenable to therapy. While limiting exercise may prevent syncope due to cardiac outflow obstruction, surgical therapy is usually needed (particularly for aortic stenosis), and the prognosis depends on the outcome of the surgery. Cerebral symptoms due to cardiac arrhythmias can usually be eradicated by pacemaker or antiarrhythmic treatment. Similarly, most symptoms due to common metabolic or intracranial abnormalities are amenable to treatment.

Selected Conditions That May Mimic Syncope

Hysterical Faint

Sudden, dramatic fainting was very common in the 19th century, especially in women. Today fainting preceded by hyperventilation is more common. Usually the fainting occurs in a manner to avoid injury, an important distinguishing feature from true syncope. The patient crumples to the ground with a limp body and shallow respirations. Recovery is usually immediate. Quite often, the faint may be embellished with movements that resemble seizures (referred to as pseudoseizures), but more often voluntary movements are the rule. Hyperventilation or coaxing may reproduce the spell. Chapter 12 provides additional detail regarding the evaluation and management of such patients, whose physical symptoms are often due to emotional factors.

Drop Attack

Older patients, especially men, may report sudden and unprovoked falls to the ground. Consciousness is not lost, and the patients can usually remember the entire episode. This maintenance of consciousness distinguishes drop attacks from syncope. Ischemia of the lower brainstem is thought to cause drop attacks, and occasionally patients will report other symptoms coincidentally that suggest vertebrobasilar ischemia. Management is identical to that of TIAs occurring in the posterior circulation (see Chapter 83).

Cataplexy

Cataplexy is a special kind of drop attack, not due to ischemia, that occurs as part of the syndrome of narcolepsy (see Chapter 85). The patient falls suddenly to the ground because of a loss of extensor muscle tone but without loss of consciousness. These spells are usually provoked by a sudden startle, a joke, laughing, or sneezing. They may be effectively managed by tricyclic agents. *Sleep paralysis* (paralysis of the limbs for a minute or two upon awakening) and peculiar visual hallucinations on awakening or before falling asleep may also accompany narcolepsy. (See Chapter 85 for additional details.)

DISEQUILIBRIUM OF MISCELLANEOUS ORIGINS

Some patients with relatively persistent "dizziness" do not have manifestations which make it possible to classify their problem as vertigo or near syncope. Most of these persons have disequilibrium, or a sense of imbalance, which may be due to one of the following problems: cerebellar ataxia (see Chapter 78 for physical findings); multiple sensory deficits (2) (e.g., partial hearing, visual, and proprioceptive impairment); lower extremity weakness (e.g., from an old stroke or from disuse after a fracture or after a period of bed rest); pain in a weight-bearing joint; recently initiated drugs, especially sedatives; or the onset of a progressive central nervous system disease such as parkinsonism (see Chapter 82), normal pressure hydrocephalus (see Chapter 17), or CP angle tumor (see Chapter 96). These problems often occur in older persons, in debilitated persons (particularly chronic alcoholics), or in patients with long-standing diabetes. In these persons, cerebrovascular disease or autonomic neuropathy may cause periodic vertigo and near syncope to be superimposed on their day-to-day problem with imbalance.

The evaluation of persons describing imbalance consists chiefly of obtaining a history of the duration, progression, and day-to-day characteristics of the problem, focusing upon the limitations imposed upon the usual activities and upon any falls or near accidents which may have occurred. In the physical examination, it is important to determine which of the many problems listed above may be contributing to the patient's symptoms.

Depending upon the individual patient, management by the generalist may include (a) referring the patient for correction of deafness or cataract (see Chapters 96 and 97); (b) obtaining a consultant's opinion whenever unexplained progressive symptoms are found (for example, cerebellar ataxia in a relatively healthy person); (c) obtaining the help of a physical therapist if weakness or the need for selecting a cane or a walker is apparent; (d) discontinuing any drugs which may be contributing to the patient's symptoms and avoiding drugs which may worsen symptoms (see Tables 81.2 and 81.7).

CHRONIC DIZZINESS: GENERAL MEASURES IN MANAGEMENT

Patients with chronic dizziness or disequilibrium will have a far better prognosis if their physicians assure that their home environments are safe and that others in their households are aware of risks which should be avoided and of devices which may be helpful. A number of general measures important for these patients are the following: the use of night-lights, tacking down loose carpeting and floorboards, use of canes or walkers, installation of special railings in the bathroom, and proper selection of footwear. These measures can be accomplished most effectively if the physician or a visiting nurse evaluates the patient in his (the patient's) home.

General References

Baloh RW, Honrubia V: *Clinical Neurophysiology of the Vestibular System.* Philadelphia, FA Davis, 1982.
> Excellent review of vertigo.

Kapoor WN, Karpf M, Wiland S, et al: A prospective evaluation and follow-up of patients with syncope. *N Engl J Med* 309:197, 1983.
> A concise discussion of diagnostic studies and prognosis.

Lee JE, Killip T, Plum F: Episodic unconsciousness. In Baron JA (ed): *Diagnostic Approaches to Presenting Syndromes.* Baltimore, Williams & Wilkins, 1971.
> A detailed discussion of normal physiology and specific causes of syncope.

Wolfson RJ: Symposium on vertigo. *Otolargynol Clin North Am* 6: No. 1, 1973.
> Excellent coverage of all aspects of vertigo.

Specific References

1. Bárány R: Diagnosis of disease of the otolith apparatus. *J Laryngol Otol* 36:229, 1921.
2. Brandt T, Daroff RB: The multisensory physiological and pathological vertigo syndromes. *Ann Neurol* 7:195, 1980.
3. Brandt T, Daroff RB: Physical therapy for benign paroxysmal positional vertigo. *Arch Otolaryngol* 106:484, 1980.
4. Caird Fl, Andrews GR, Kennedy RD: Effect of posture on blood pressure in the elderly. *Br Heart J* 35:527, 1973.
5. Drachman DA, Hart CW: An approach to the dizzy patient. *Neurology* 22:323, 1972.
6. Ewing DJ, Campbell IW, Clarke BF: Assessment of cardiovascular effects in diabetic autonomic neuropathy and prognostic implications. *Ann Intern Med* 92:308, 1980.
7. Glassock ME III, Hayes JW: Pitfalls in the diagnosis of acoustic and other cerebellopontine angle tumors. *Laryngoscope* 83:1038, 1973.
8. Hart CW: Evaluation of post-traumatic vertigo. *Otolaryngol Clin North Am* 6:157, 1973.
9. Hybels RL: Drug toxicity of the inner ear. *Med Clin North Am* 63:309, 1979.
10. Ibrahim MM: Localization of lesion in patients with idiopathic orthostatic hypotension. *Br Heart J* 37:868, 1975.
11. Johnson RJ, Smith AC, Spalding JMK, Wollner L: Effect of posture on blood-pressure in elderly patients. *Lancet* 1:731, 1965.
12. Jonas S. Klein I, Dimant J: Importance of Holter monitoring in patients with periodic cerebral symptoms. *Ann Neurol* 1: 470, 1977.
13. Jongkees LBW: The caloric test and its value in evaluation of the patient with vertigo. *Otolaryngol Clin North Am* 6:73, 1973.
13a. Kapoor WH, Peterson JR, Karpp M: Micturition Syncope. *JAMA* 253:796, 1985.
14. Lipsitz LA, Nyquist RP, Wei JY, Rowe JW: Postprandial reduction in blood pressure in the elderly. *N Engl J Md* 309:81, 1983.
15. Noble RJ: The patient with syncope. *JAMA* 237:1372, 1977.
16. Page JM: Audiologic tests in the differential diagnosis of vertigo. *Otolaryngol Clin North Am* 6:53, 1973.
17. Rubin W: Electronystagmography and its value in the diagnosis of vertigo. *Otolaryngol Clin North Am* 6:95, 1973.
18. Thames MD, Alpert JS, Dalen JE: Syncope in patients with pulmonary embolism. *JAMA* 238:2509, 1977.
19. Weiss NS: Relation of high blood pressure to headache, epistaxis, and selected other symptoms. *N Engl J Med* 287:631, 1972.
20. Wood CD, Graybiel A: The antimotion sickness drugs. *Otolaryngol Clin North Am* 6:301, 1973.

CHAPTER EIGHTY-TWO

Common Disorders of Movement: Tremor and Parkinson's Disease

MAHLON R. DELONG, M.D., BARRY GORDON, M.D., PH.D., AND
L. RANDOL BARKER, M.D.

TREMOR

Definition and Classification

Tremor, a common symptom, is defined as the involuntary rhythmic or semirhythmic oscillations of a body part, resulting from contractions of antagonistic muscle groups.

Clinically, there are three major types of tremor—resting, postural, and intention (see Table 82.1—which can be identified readily by history and examination. Each type of tremor points to a group of specific underlying conditions (Table 82.2), the diagnosis of which may lead to therapy that will control the tremor.

Evaluation of the Patient with Tremor

History

The history is useful both in assessing the significance of the tremor to the patient and in classifying the type of tremor. The following questions may be particularly useful:

1. How long ago did the tremor begin? How did it begin (slowly and insidiously, or suddenly)? Where did the tremor begin? To which muscle groups did it spread, and over what time period? (Parkinsonian tremor often begins unilaterally)

2. What parts of the body are affected by the tremor and under what circumstances (rest, motion, active reaching)?

3. Has the tremor interfered with such activities as eating, dressing, or handwriting? Has it caused the patient to modify significantly his usual activities, especially socially valued activities, such as playing cards, engaging in sports, or going to social gatherings?

4. What medication(s) is the patient taking currently, and what is the temporal relationship to the onset of the tremor?

Almost all tremors are made worse by anxiety and disappear during sleep, so these are not important historical points in differentiating the type of tremor.

Examination

The classification of tremors is based upon findings in the physical examination, specifically upon the character of the tremor in the resting state, in posture in which gravity is opposed, and during voluntary motion.

Examination for resting tremor. The patient should sit with his hands resting on his lap and his head unsupported. Often it is best to have the subject distracted by conversation. Under these conditions, relatively slow (3 to 5/second) flexion-extension tremor of the metacarpophalangeal joints ("pill-rolling" tremor), pronation-supination of the forearm, or flexion-extension of the wrists or feet may be seen. If the patient becomes too relaxed, the tremor may lessen or disappear; typically, it disappears during sleep. Resting tremor is typical of Parkinson's disease (see below, page 1177) and of other conditions affecting the basal ganglia.

Examination for postural tremor. The patient should hold his hands outstretched, with eyes closed. The physician should note whether there is any temor in the hands, arms, or head. A relatively rapid (6 to 12/second) medium to high amplitude tremor is abnormal. Some degree of hand or finger tremor is normal (physiological tremor). Postural tremor is typical of exaggerated physiological and essential tremor. A side-to-side tremor of the head (titubation) may also be noted; usually this is an expression of essential tremor.

Examination for intention tremor. The patient

Table 82.1.
Principal Features of Common Tremors

Feature	Three Major Types of Tremor		
	Resting	Postural	Intention
Situation(s) in which the tremor is present	Resting posture, in awake patient; extinguished or decreased with purposeful movement; absent during sleep	Posture involving effort against gravity (e.g., outstretched arms, holding an object); not present in resting limb	Purposeful movement of extremity from one point to another
Frequency of tremor	Usually 3–6/second	6–12/second	3–5/second
Clinical conditions	Parkinsonian syndrome	Exaggerated physiological tremor Essential tremor	Cerebellar dysfunction

Table 82.2.
Conditions Associated with the Three Major Types of Tremor[a]

RESTING TREMOR
  Parkinson's disease
  Secondary parkinsonism: postencephalitic, toxic (phenothiazines, reserpine, carbon monoxide, manganese, carbon disulfide), tumor, trauma, vascular, metabolic (hypoparathyroidism, chronic hepatocerebral degeneration)
  Heterogeneous disorders with parkinsonian features: striatonigral degeneration, olivopontocerebellar atrophy, progressive supranuclear palsy, Wilson's disease, Huntington's disease, normal pressure hydrocephalus
POSTURAL TREMOR
  Exaggerated physiological tremor
    Stress-induced; anxiety, fright, fatigue
    Endocrine: thyrotoxicosis, hypoglycemia, pheochromocytoma
    Drugs: any sympathomimetics, caffeine, theophylline, levodopa, lithium, tricyclic antidepressants, phenothiazines, butyrophenones, thyroid hormone, hypoglycemic agents, withdrawal from alcohol and sedative-hypnotic drugs
  Essential tremor
    Familial (may be autosomal dominant)
    Sporadic
    Senile
    With other movement disorders: parkinsonism, torsion dystonia, spasmodic torticollis
INTENTION TREMOR (CEREBELLAR DYSFUNCTION)
  Cerebellar degeneration, atrophy, infarction
  Multiple sclerosis
  Wilson's disease
  Drugs—toxins: phenytoin, barbiturates, lithium, alcohol, mercury, 5-fluorouracil
  Miscellaneous cerebellar and cerebellofugal lesions

[a] Adapted from Jankovic J, Fahn S: Physiologic and pathologic tremors: diagnosis, mechanism and management. *Ann Intern Med* 93:460, 1980.

should reach for the examiner's finger with his hands (finger-nose-finger testing) or feet (toe-to-finger testing). Normal subjects frequently have a very fine lateral tremor of the distal limb during purposeful motion. Exaggeration of this tremor, with worsening as greater precision is demanded and often with continuation for a fraction of a second after the action is completed, is characteristic of an intention tremor. The combination of intention tremor and dysmetria (inaccuracy in actually touching a point at the termination of a voluntary movement) is typical of cerebellar disorders.

Common Conditions Presenting as Tremor

Parkinson's Disease

The typical resting tremor of Parkinson's disease is discussed on page 1177.

Physiological and Exaggerated Physiological Tremor

Most individuals have a barely perceptible postural tremor that may be best appreciated by placing a piece of paper over their outstretched hands. Exaggeration of this physiological tremor is usually due to a transient condition, such as occurs with stress, after ingestion of caffeine or another stimulant, in withdrawal from alcohol or other sedating drugs (where an underlying essential tremor may also be unmasked), as a side effect of a prescribed drug, or as part of a variety of generalized metabolic or systemic illnesses (see Table 82.2). With severe disease, this kind of tremor becomes generalized, and there is widespread hyperexcitability. Other manifestations of this central excitatory state include myoclonic jerks, delirium, hallucinations, and seizures. A florid example of this state is delirium tremens; less extreme forms are very common.

Treatment

The major step in management is identification and removal of the offending cause; resolution of the tremor confirms the diagnosis of exaggerated physiological tremor. Discontinuation of tremor-producing drugs usually leads to prompt resolution of the problem. With severe metabolic disturbances, it may take 1 to 2 weeks for the tremulousness to subside, even after the underlying abnormalities have been corrected. If the underlying condition cannot be eliminated, propranolol (see dosage information below) usually abolishes the tremor; in fact, if it does not do so, the tremor is probably misclassified. For persons subject to situational anxiety, manifested as exaggerated physiological tremor and/or heightened perception of cardiac activity, prophylactic treatment with propranolol before an anxiety-producing situation (for example a public address) may be helpful (see Chapter 13).

Essential Tremor (Senile Tremor, Familial Tremor)

In its prototypical form, this is a marked bilateral and symmetrical postural tremor in the hands. It may also involve the head (typically with side-to-side rotatory tremor). This tremor resembles an exaggerated physiological tremor. A major difference is that essential tremor is a relatively constant problem while exaggerated physiological tremor is usually related to a transient condition. Frequently, intention tremor (see below) is present as well.

Essential tremor is quite common; in various forms, it has been reported in up to 8% of a normal population. The family history is positive in 25 to 50% of cases, and many families show autosomal dominant transmission. Onset is insidious, starting anywhere from childhood (familial) to old age (senile). There is a wide spectrum of severity. In some patients, the tremor is totally disabling, making self-care and self-feeding almost impossible. When the tremor has had its onset in late middle life, its progression is typically quite slow, and years pass before deterioration becomes apparent. With aging, the frequency of the tremor may diminish while the amplitude increases. When the condition begins earlier, an accurate prognosis is difficult; however, when there is a family history of essential tremor, the experience of others in the family is helpful in anticipating a patient's course.

Many patients report that alcohol markedly reduces the amplitude of their tremor within 15 to 30 minutes (10). Some patients use alcohol as a method of treatment without consulting a physician; this may lead to alcohol addiction and should be considered in the evaluation of alcoholic patients.

As with most tremors, anxiety and situational stress markedly enhance the symptom. Essential tremor can occur in association with tics, dystonic motions of the head or feet, choreiform movements, and even resting tremors (4).

Some older patients with essential tremor, especially those who may have had a prior stroke or other incapacitating illness, are mistakenly thought to have Parkinson's disease. However, the patient with essential tremor can usually be distinguished readily from a patient with Parkinson's disease by checking for other distinctive features of extrapyramidal disease (see below).

Treatment

When essential tremor is mild, reassurance and treatment of transient situation-specific anxiety with agents such as diazepam (Valium), 2.5 to 5 mg once or twice daily, may be sufficient. Used judiciously, small amounts of alcohol (e.g., one glass of wine) can be quite helpful in many of the situations where tremor would be particularly bothersome (10).

If the condition is significantly symptomatic, propranolol is usually quite effective in reducing the amplitude of the tremor to the point where it no longer interferes with writing, eating, drinking, and other daily activities (20). It is best to begin with a small initial dose (10 mg, two or three times daily), increasing to a maximum of 300 to 400 mg daily while monitoring benefits and side effects. Contraindications to propranolol are: (a) congestive heart failure, especially if poorly controlled; (b) second or third degree atrioventricular block; (c) asthma; and (d) insulin-dependent diabetes mellitus. For patients intolerant of propranolol, the more selective β-blocker, metaprolol (Lopressor), may be a suitable substitute. Precautions and additional information about the use of these two β-blocking agents are found in Chapter 62.

Another recently recognized and often highly effective treatment for essential tremor is primidone, a drug used primarily in the treatment of epilepsy (see Chapter 80 for details). Since some patients who respond to primidone may be highly sensitive to its side effects, the initial dose should be very low (e.g., one-half of a 250-mg tablet at bedtime). The dose should then be increased slowly each week to a total of 125 to 250 mg two or three times daily. Acute side effects include dizziness, ataxia, dysarthria, lethargy, and confusion. These usually decrease with time. Long term side effects are infrequent with primidone.

When essential tremor is extremely severe or disabling and is not responsive to symptomatic therapy, referral to a neurologist is indicated. For selected patients, stereotactic surgery may be recommended.

Tremor Due to Cerebellar Dysfunction

The finding of intention tremor points to cerebellar or cerebellar-related disease. Conditions which superficially may mimic this aspect of cerebellar disease are marked physiological tremor or essential tremor (which may impair purposeful movements) and proprioceptive sensory neuropathy. Careful assessment of all of the patient's signs and symptoms usually enables the physician to distinguish these conditions from cerebellar dysfunction (see Table 82.3, which compares cerebellar and posterior column incoordination). Some patients with cerebellar-related disease have a low frequency (3 to 5/second) postural tremor as well as a typical intention tremor.

Unilateral intention tremor in a hand and/or leg

points to ipsilateral disease of the cerebellar hemisphere; infarction is the most frequent cause. When tremor is bilateral, it may reflect more generalized cerebellar degeneration (carcinomatous, drug induced) or reversible drug effect (particularly phenytoin (Dilantin)). Disease of the anterior midline cerebellum more typically presents as gait ataxia (common etiologies in adults are alcoholic cerebellar degeneration and carcinomatous cerebellar degeneration); and disorders of the inferior midline cerebellum present typically as posture imbalance (in adults, an infarct involving the posterior inferior cerebellar artery is the most common cause).

With the exception of drug-induced cerebellar dysfunction (see Table 82.2), which should be managed by discontinuation or dose reduction of the drug, a patient with newly diagnosed cerebellar disease should be referred promptly to a neurologist for help in obtaining an accurate diagnosis and prognosis. Most of the diseases producing cerebellar dysfunction are not amenable to treatment, and there is little that can be done but to treat the coordination problems symptomatically.

PARKINSON'S DISEASE AND RELATED DISORDERS

Definitions

A *parkinsonian syndrome* may result from several processes which affect the basal ganglia (see Table 82.2).

Parkinson's disease is a specific clinical and neuropathological entity which is manifested clinically by akinesia (poverty of movement), bradykinesia (slowness of movement), rigidity, and resting tremor together with abnormalities of gait and posture. It is a sporadic disease of unknown etiology. Neuropathologically, there is degeneration of the dopamine-containing cells of the substantia nigra. In most patients, the disease begins after the age of 40, with the peak incidence in the sixth and seventh decades. The approximate prevalence of Parkinson's disease in persons over 50 is 1%. The problem is equally common in men and women.

Postencephalitic Parkinson's disease was seen in a large number of victims of the global epidemic of encephalitis following World War I. Although not a cause of new cases at present, presumably some new cases are due to sporadic encephalitides which have occurred since the epidemic.

Drug-induced parkinsonism is very common in persons taking neuroleptic antipsychotic drugs. This problem is usually transient and reversible. It is described in Chapter 16.

Differential Diagnosis

Parkinson's Disease

The diagnosis of Parkinson's disease is based entirely on the clinical evaluation of the patient. When slowly progressive tremor, rigidity, and bradykinesia are present in a person over 50, the diagnosis is simple to make. Prompt improvement when antiparkinsonian drugs are initiated helps to confirm the diagnosis. Failure to respond to treatment together with atypical signs (oculomotor, autonomic, or pyramidal signs) should alert one to other causes of the parkinsonian syndrome (see below).

Drug-Induced Parkinsonism (See Chapter 16)

The diagnosis of neuroleptic-induced parkinsonism is not difficult. This problem usually commences within 1 to 4 weeks of initiating or increasing the dose of a neuroleptic antipsychotic drug. A similar problem was seen in the past in psychotic patients treated with high doses of reserpine, a practice which has been virtually discontinued.

Other Conditions

A variety of disease processes that affect the basal ganglia can produce a parkinsonian syndrome. In

Table 82.3.
Characteristics of Cerebellar and Sensory Posterior Column Incoordination

Observation or Examination	Cerebellar	Sensory and/or Posterior Column
Influence of vision	Elimination of visual aid (night, eyes closed) does not affect symptoms or signs	Symptoms and signs markedly increased by eliminating visual aid
Sensation	No necessary sensory problems (although may be superimposed, as in alcoholic cerebellar degeneration and sensory neuropathy)	Impaired position and vibration sense is *sine qua non* for diagnosis
Finger-nose-finger and/or toe-finger testing of coordination	Could be marked intention tremor and dysmetria (inaccuracy); affected limbs depend upon site of lesion(s)	Marked intention tremor and dysmetria (inaccuracy), usually most marked in legs
Gait	Wide based, asynchronous limb movements (depending upon nature of the lesion)	Wide based, high stepping, foot-slapping (steppage) gait (often due to foot drop from motor neuropathy)
Romberg testing	Patient equally unsteady with eyes open or closed (uninterpretable Romberg)	Patient can find a stable position with eyes open, but becomes markedly unsteady with eyes closed (positive Romberg)

any patient with presumed Parkinson's disease in whom the disorder is atypical (e.g., very early or very late age of onset, striking predominance of one of the principal manifestations of parkinsonism, rapid onset, marked asymmetry, prominent neurological findings in addition to extrapyramidal manifestations, or a poor response to antiparkinsonian medication), another condition should be considered. Because accurate diagnosis is essential to both prognosis and management, these atypical patients should be referred to a neurologist for evaluation. For most of the conditions causing or resembling parkinsonism other clinical clues may be noted on initial evaluation.

Wilson's Disease (Hepatolenticular Degeneration)

This is an autosomal recessive condition characterized by copper accumulation throughout the body, which is expressed clinically in the liver, the eyes, and the central nervous system; and blood ceruloplasmin levels are low. Parkinsonian features in a patient under the age of 40, particularly under the age of 30, should prompt an investigation for this condition. Chronic liver disease may be present at the onset of neurological symptoms. Kayser-Fleischer rings (green or golden deposits of copper in Descemet's membrane of the cornea), blood ceruloplasmin level less than 20 mg/100 ml, and urine copper in excess of 100 μg/day are the usual criteria for this diagnosis.

Degenerative Diseases

HUNTINGTON'S CHOREA. This autosomal dominant condition is due to degeneration of the caudate nucleus, the putamen, and the cerebral cortex. It usually begins in midlife with symptoms of dementia and with abnormal movements (tics, chorea, athetosis), but it may begin with or include prominent rigidity and bradykinesia.

ALZHEIMER'S DISEASE (see Chapter 17). This disorder can present at times with a parkinsonian-like syndrome associated with dementia evolving over years. However, usually tremor is not present; the rigidity is actually "gegenhalten" (*i.e.*, resistance to passive motion is present in all directions but varies with the force and speed applied by the examiner); and intellectual deterioration is extremely marked. It is important to note that this diagnosis does not exclude coexisting Parkinson's disease, since, as noted below, Alzheimer's and Parkinson's diseases may occur in the same patient.

Other degenerative conditions involving the basal ganglia, such as progressive supranuclear palsy, the Shy-Drager syndrome, pallidal atrophy, and some atypical spinal-cerebellar syndromes may present as a parkinsonian syndrome. These conditions often have other clinical features, a positive family history, or unresponsiveness to L-dopa, which should alert the clinician to the possibility of an alternate diagnosis.

HYDROCEPHALUS AND NORMAL PRESSURE HYDROCEPHALUS. Frontal lobe-like apathetic and immobile behavior, apraxic gait, and rigidity have sometimes led to the mistaken diagnosis of Parkinson's disease in patients with these conditions.

Subdural Hematomas and Multiple Cerebral Infarctions

Sometimes the demented, immobile, and spastic/rigid state resulting from these conditions can mimic Parkinson's disease. Pyramidal tract signs are important clues to the presence of one of these conditions.

Metabolic Disorders

Subacute metabolic encephalopathies (hepatic, pulmonary, or renal) can produce symptoms which superficially resemble Parkinson's syndrome. The metabolic abnormality underlying the patient's neurological manifestations should easily be recognized in these patients. Some patients with severe hepatic failure, especially patients with portocaval shunts, may have degeneration of the basal ganglia, producing a parkinsonian picture (hepatocerebral degeneration).

Manifestations of Parkinson's Disease

The onset of symptoms is insidious; the patient usually cannot specify a beginning of his disease and is often not initially fully aware of its extent. Most of the time, the earliest presentation of symptoms is asymmetric or even clearly unilateral. The patient may notice, for example, tremor and rigidity of only one limb; the physician, on closer examination, may discover mild signs on the contralateral side to confirm the diagnosis. As the disease progresses, these asymmetries may or may not be maintained. Many patients, even with advanced disease, recognize that one side is worse than the other.

Resting Tremor

Tremor is the initial complaint in 70% of patients with Parkinson's disease. It is a relatively slow tremor with a 3 to 5/second rate, usually most prominent in the hands as a "pill-rolling" (metacarpophalangeal flexion and extension) or in the arms, as forearm pronation and supination. Sometimes it involves the lips and tongue, but it is relatively uncommon for it to involve the whole head. The latter feature, plus the fact that it is present at rest and usually decreases or disappears when the limb is used, distinguishes the parkinsonian tremor from essential tremor (see above, page 1175). The tremor is accentuated when the patient becomes excited or uses the opposite limb. Frequently a postural tremor (see above, page 1173) may be present as well.

Rigidity

Rigidity is the abnormal resistance to passive movement, which is typically present throughout the whole range of motion, in both extensor and flexor muscle groups. Therefore, the limb gives the examiner a feeling of a plastic or lead pipe resistance. "Cog-wheel rigidity" is the ratcheting sensation often superimposed on this type of rigidity; it is not an expression of the resting tremor (a common misconception), but instead seems to be a separate kind of subclinical tremor. "Cog-wheeling" is not specific for Parkinson's disease.

Akinesia and Bradykinesia

Patients with Parkinson's disease have difficulty initiating movements and their movements are slow. In contrast to the almost unconscious way that normal persons utilize their limbs, the Parkinson's patient must consciously force the limb to move; and what movements do occur are usually quite slow. Speech gradually becomes soft and slow and is delivered in a monotone. Even automatic movements such as blinking and facial expression are suppressed. When akinesia is extreme, the patient may sit helplessly immobile for hours, expressionless and unblinking.

Since rigidity and akinesia can occur independently of each other, akinesia is not solely due to rigidity. This becomes apparent when treatment markedly decreases a patient's rigidity but has no effect on his akinesia.

Postural Abnormalities

Patients with Parkinson's disease sit and stand with a stooped, flexed posture of the head, trunk, arms, and legs. Abnormalities of small muscle tone may produce an ulnar flexion deformity of the fingers, distinguished from that of rheumatoid arthritis by the lack of demonstrable joint and synovial disease.

Gait Abnormalities

Parkinsonian patients may have a great deal of difficulty initiating gait. They may be unable to rise from a chair or, once standing, be unable to initiate stepping motions (apraxia of gait). For a variety of reasons, they have poor control of balance with a tendency to fall forward and backward; typically, they will be aware of beginning to fall but will be unable to make corrective movements to prevent the fall. When the patient with Parkinson's disease does begin to walk, his steps are short and shuffling. The tendency to fall forward and the partial attempt to prevent falling, may lead to a festinating ("hurrying") propulsive gait. Even after walking is initiated, the patient may suddenly freeze while going through doorways or while attempting to make a turn. This transient freezing may throw the patient completely off balance.

Other Associated Symptoms or Signs

Seborrhea and *excessive perspiration* are both common; the former may be due to hypothalamic release of excess sebotrophic hormone and the latter to disordered central temperature regulation.

Constipation is quite prominent in many patients, representing both inactivity and the side effects of anticholinergic drugs. Constipation can progress to obstipation, large bowel obstruction, megacolon, and volvulus of the sigmoid.

Dysphagia is a common complaint in Parkinson's disease. Some patients become completely incapable of swallowing. This problem may be due to incoordination of the inferior pharyngeal constrictors and perhaps of the other muscles involved in swallowing.

Sialorrhea (increased salivation) is probably explained by decreased swallowing, rather than by overproduction of saliva.

Urinary hesitancy/retention may be due to the disease itself, but it may also be due to other urinary problems which afflict older patients (such as prostatic hypertrophy) and which are aggravated by immobility and by anticholinergic drugs.

Orthostatic hypotension is common and may be caused by the disease itself, by inactivity, or by levodopa therapy (see below). The degenerative process in Parkinson's disease may affect not only the substantia nigra but also other regions of the brainstem and spinal cord, including the intermediolateral sympathetic column of the spinal cord. In this respect, Parkinson's disease might be included on a continuum of orthostatic conditions along with the Shy-Drager syndrome and idiopathic orthostatic hypotension. The Shy-Drager syndrome (17) begins with evidence of autonomic dysfunction (*i.e.*, episodes of hypo- and/or hypertension or impotence). It progresses after several years to show many of the features of Parkinson's disease, particularly rigidity, which may respond to levodopa. The intermediolateral cell column and the basal ganglia show pathological changes. In patients with isolated idiopathic orthostatic hypotension, often only the intermediolateral cell column is found to be diseased (2).

Sensory symptoms. Many patients with Parkinson's disease complain of a tightness or a pulling sensation in their affected extremities without objective sensory deficit. The basis for these symptoms is not clear, but treatment of the disease often alleviates them.

Two *abnormal reflexes* are usually found in parkinsonian patients: (*a*) the palmomental reflex (contraction of the ipsilateral mentalis muscle, producing wrinkling of the chin, elicited by stroking the palm near the base of the thumb), and (*b*) an exaggerated glabellar reflex (contraction of the orbicularis oculi muscles after repeatedly tapping the frontal bone superior to the bony septum of the nose; in a normal person, this reflex fatigues after repeated tapping). Neither of these reflexes is specific for Parkinson's syndrome.

Depression (14). A large proportion of parkinsonian patients develop a depressive illness having either predominantly endogenous or reactive features (see Chapter 15). Some studies have found a close correlation between the severity of depression and the severity of physical impairment; others have found these two manifestations to be independent of each other.

Dementia (16). Up to 30% of patients with Parkinson's disease will develop an irreversible dementia syndrome. The dementia in many patients seems to be due to typical Alzheimer's disease, which for some reason occurs with a higher than expected frequency with Parkinson's disease (11). A parkinsonian patient who develops dementia should be evaluated like any other demented patient, in order to rule out potentially treatable conditions (see Chapter 17). The relationship of cognitive deterioration to antiparkinsonian drugs should always be considered, as the problem may be reversible (see below, page 1183). Delirium, as discussed below, is seen occasionally in patients with Parkinson's disease—but as a drug side effect, not as a manifestation of the disease itself.

Course of Parkinson's Disease

The course of Parkinson's disease varies substantially among individual patients. This variation is due to a combination of the temporal progression of the disease itself; the variable impact of treatment on individual symptoms (see below); the patient's mental adaptation to his illness (as distinct from those mental changes which may be part of the disease); the amount of social and rehabilitative support the patient receives; the complications of bradykinesia, especially falls and prolonged bed rest; and drug side effects.

Table 82.4 divides the "typical" course of Parkinson's disease into five stages, indicating for each stage the principal manifestations of the disease and the impact on the patient's overall function. These stages of parkinsonism occur eventually in most patients, usually over a time span of 5 to 15 years. As discussed in the following section, drug treatment and supportive therapy can significantly modify the course of Parkinson's disease; however, neuronal degeneration progresses despite treatment, and the patient's symptoms ultimately fail to respond to treatment.

A rough indication of the prognosis of "untreated" patients with Parkinson's disease comes from a study of patients followed before the L-dopa era (3). In this study, the average survival after diagnosis was 9 years; the prognosis was best when tremor was the major manifestation at the time of diagnosis. Twenty-five percent of patients were severely disabled or dead 5 years after the diagnosis; 66% after 10 years; 80% after 15 years. There was a small, very atypical group, still ambulatory 20 years after the diagnosis of Parkinson's disease. Deaths are generally due to bronchopneumonia, urinary tract infection, thromboembolism, or severe malnutrition.

Pharmacological Management

Overview

The current pharmacotherapy of Parkinson's disease is based upon what is known of neurotransmission in the basal ganglia. Two major neurotransmitters found in these regions are dopamine and ace-

Table 82.4.
Five Stages of "Typical" Parkinson's Disease[a]

Stage	Principal Manifestations	Overall Functional Status
1	Unilateral involvement, blank facies, affected arm in semiflexed position with tremor and diminished swing, patient leans to affected side; gait slightly affected or normal	Patient can continue most activities as usual except those requiring quick motor responses (playing tennis, for example). Social embarrassment may be a problem.
2	(Usually within 1 to 2 years of stage 1.) Bilateral involvement with early postural changes (stooped); slow shuffling gait with decreased excursion of legs; executes turn slowly and deliberately	Patient usually must retire, if still working. High risk of becoming withdrawn (reactive depression) and abandoning valued social and recreational activities (although physical impairment may not prohibit them).
3	Pronounced gait disturbance with postural instability and tendency to fall	Patient begins to need assistance with some tasks because of slowness in accomplishing them (*e.g.,* dressing, packing a suitcase).
4	Significant disability; ambulation limited and only with assistance because of marked difficulty in standing and tendency to fall	Patient needs almost constant supervision and requires assistance in completing most activities of daily living.
5	Complete invalidism; confined to bed or chair; unable to stand or walk even with assistance; head becomes flexed on trunk; speech barely audible; face expressionless and blinking infrequent	Patient requires total care; death from aspiration or other form of infection related to immobolization.

[a] Adapted from Duvoisin R: Parkinsonism. In *Clinical Symposia.* Summit, NJ, CIBA Pharmaceutical Co, 1976, vol 28, no. 1.

tylcholine. It is hypothesized that the smooth control of voluntary movements depends upon a delicate balance between dopaminergic and cholinergic activity. Imbalance in these transmitter systems is the apparent basis for some movement disorders. Parkinson's disease, in which dopamine depletion follows damage to the source of dopamine (the substantia nigra), is attributed to a deficiency of dopamine and a relative excess of cholinergic activity.

The antiparkinsonian drugs currently used are either *anticholinergic* or *dopaminergic*; the fact that drugs in these two groups ameliorate the symptoms of Parkinson's disease supports the pathophysiological concept of neurotransmitter imbalance.

To obtain the best results with drug therapy for Parkinson's disease, the *approach to each patient must be individualized.* Systematic monitoring for the benefits and side effects of treatment and careful (often frequent) adjustment of the medical regimen are the mainstays of this approach. Combination treatment with dopaminergic and anticholinergic agents is needed for optimal results in most patients with moderately advanced symptoms. Even the most skillfully tailored regimen rarely controls *all* symptoms of Parkinson's disease, and it is important to explain this to the patient and his family from the outset.

There is evidence that L-dopa, the most effective of the available drugs for Parkinson's disease, becomes much less effective after 3 or 4 years of use in most patients (8), although some investigators have disagreed with this view (13). The progressive loss of effectiveness seems to be further complicated by increasing sensitivity to the side effects of this drug. Therefore, it seems prudent to limit the initial use of L-dopa, reserving this drug for a time when the patient's disease begins to interfere appreciably with his life. Since many patients (or their families) will have heard about L-dopa and will expect it to be prescribed from the onset of treatment, it is essential for the physician to explain to the patient

and the patient's family the sequence of drug therapy which will be tried.

Table 82.5 summarizes a *stepwise approach to medical management* that most authorities would recommend; and Table 82.6 summarizes practical information about currently available drugs. For persons who are minimally affected at the time of diagnosis, it may be reasonable to delay medical treatment and to encourage the patient to decide when symptoms are interfering with valued activities; however, only a small proportion of patients are likely to be in this category at the time of diagnosis, as most will wait until their symptoms are troublesome before consulting their physician. Once the symptoms of Parkinson's disease begin to interfere with valued activities, drug treatment should be initiated. At this point, individual consideration is essential in deciding whether to use L-dopa from the outset. For most persons, a trial of anticholinergics alone or in combination with amantadine (Symmetrel) should be the first step in treatment. Anticholinergics are particularly effective for tremor but have little or no effect on akinesia. In situations where prompt control of symptoms is essential, *e.g.*, for public figures, technical workers who depend on fine manual skills, or persons threatened with job loss due to their impairment, initial therapy with L-dopa (as carbidopa/levodopa, Sinemet, see below) is appropriate.

It is impossible to predict with certainty the degree and duration of amelioration of symptoms which an individual patient can expect. Overall, however, most patients should have significant improvement in tremor, rigidity, and bradykinesia (in this order) and in activities affected by these symptoms. Anticholinergic therapy is effective in this respect in about one-half of patients, while L-dopa produces good results in approximately 80%. Apart from reactive depression, mental deterioration usually does not respond to antiparkinsonian drugs. Depression which persists despite physical improvement, how-

Table 82.5.
Recommended Steps in Drug Therapy for Parkinson's Disease

Step	Patient Status	Treatment
1	Very mild symptoms which do not interfere with usual activities	None (explain rationale to patient and his family)
2	Neurological symptoms are troublesome but do not threaten income, psychological well-being, or social activities	Anticholinergic agent (substitute or add amantadine if patient is unable to tolerate anticholinergic or if patient's symptoms are transiently worse)
3	Disease advanced at the time of diagnosis; control inadequate with step 2 strategy; or symptoms threaten employment or valued social activities	Add Sinemet to step 2 regimen (and attempt to decrease dose of anticholinergic) or begin Sinemet alone
4	Initial response to Sinemet inadequate or diminished after good response (usually after 2 or more years)	Consider adding bromocriptine; consultation with a neurologist advised

Table 82.6.
Drugs Used for Parkinson's Disease

Drug	Available Preparation (mg)	Schedule	Starting Dose (mg)	Usual Daily Dosage Range (mg)
ANTICHOLINERGIC AGENTS				
Trihexyphenidyl (Artane)	Scored tablets—2, 5 Elixir—2/5 ml	3 or 4 times daily (after meals and bedtime)	2	1–10
	Timed-release capsule—5	Once daily (after breakfast)	(Substitute for tablets, same total amount, after appropriate dose found)	
Benztropine mesylate (Cogentin)	Tablets—0.5, 1, 2	Once daily (bedtime)	1	1–2 (0.5–6)
Procyclidine (Kemadrin)	Scored tablets—2, 5	3 times daily (after meals)	2	1–10
Biperiden (Akineton)	Scored tablets—2	3 or 4 times daily	1	1–10
Cycrimine (Pagitane)	Tablets—1.25, 2.5	3 times daily	1.25	1.25–10
Diphenhydramine hydrochloride (Benadryl)	Capsules—25, 50 Elixir—12.5/5 ml	3 or 4 times daily	50	50–200
DOPAMINERGIC AGENTS				
Levodopa (Larodopa, Dopar)	Tablets, capsules—100, 250, 500	4 times daily (with meals)	100	1500–6000
Carbidopa/levodopa (Sinemet)	Scored tablets—10/100, 25/250, 25/100	3 or 4 times daily (with meals; more often in selected patients)	10/100	40–200 carbidopa/400–2000 levodopa
Bromocriptine (Parlodel)	Tablets—2.5	3 times daily	2.5	10–50
Amantadine (Symmetrel)	Capsule—100	Twice daily	100	200–400

ever, may respond to tricyclic antidepressants (1) (see Chapter 15).

Anticholinergic Drugs

Practical information about commonly prescribed drugs in this category is contained in Table 82.6. All of these agents cross the blood-brain barrier and are thought to work by blunting the cholinergic activity of the basal ganglia. The first five drugs listed in the table belong to the antimuscarinic class of anticholinergic agents. None of these five drugs is known to be superior to the others in the management of Parkinson's disease. They differ principally in the schedules recommended. Two of them, Cogentin tablets and Artane sustained-action capsules, offer the advantage of once daily administration. A patient who shows little response to one anticholinergic *may* rarely respond to another. Therefore, a 2- to 4-week trial of several of these agents is reasonable in a patient with mild disease. In general, these drugs may be tested at the starting dose and increased every few days until the maximum recommended dose is reached or until the patient shows a response or unacceptable side effects. The maximum recommended doses are shown in the table. Some patients do not develop therapeutic anticholinergic levels and improvement in extrapyramidal symptoms until they are taking a relatively high

dose; patients with neuroleptic-induced parkinsonism (see Chapter 16), in particular, should be given a trial of high dose anticholinergic treatment (19).

The antihistamine-anticholinergic diphenhydramine (Benadryl) has the least antiparkinsonian effect; it may be useful, however, because of its sedating property, in patients who are agitated and in patients who cannot tolerate the more pronounced side effects of the antimuscarinic drugs.

When L-dopa or amantadine is added to anticholinergic therapy, it is advisable to try to reduce the total daily dose of anticholinergic; usually this step will not alter the effect on parkinsonian symptoms, but it will decrease the risk of mental confusion, a side effect which may attend all of the antiparkinsonian drugs.

The common *side effects* of anticholinergic drugs include dry mouth (which may be an advantage if the patient has marked sialorrhea), blurred vision, urinary retention, constipation, confusion, and agitation. The risk of these problems is increased if the patient is taking other drugs with anticholinergic properties, such as antihistamines, tricyclic antidepressants, or antispasmodics. As noted earlier, the patient should be questioned routinely about side effects with each increase in dose of anticholinergic drugs. Because other options are available, these drugs should be discontinued or the dose reduced whenever side effects add to the patient's distress. Angle closure glaucoma is an absolute contraindication to antimuscarinic agents.

Compared to other antiparkinson drugs (see below), the anticholinergics are relatively inexpensive (less than $10/100 tablets or capsules).

L-Dopa and Carbidopa/L-Dopa (Sinemet)

Levodopa (L-dopa) penetrates the blood-brain barrier and is decarboxylated to dopamine, the neurotransmitter which is deficient in Parkinson's disease. When L-dopa alone is given, most of the drug is converted by enzymes outside the central nervous system into metabolites which are responsible for many of the "peripheral" side effects of the drug. Carbidopa is a peripheral decarboxylase inhibitor which is combined with L-dopa (usually in a 1:10 ratio) in Sinemet. Seventy to 100 mg of carbidopa/day will effectively saturate the extracerebral decarboxylating enzymes, thereby decreasing the severity of the peripheral side effects of L-dopa and permitting more of the administered dose of L-dopa to reach the brain. Because of these advantages, Sinemet is recommended when a patient requires L-dopa treatment. The principal disadvantage of Sinemet is the greater cost of this drug to the patient (in the range of $25/100 tablets, as compared to approximately $10/100 tablets of L-dopa).

Initiation and Adjustment of Treatment

Sinemet is available in scored tablets containing carbidopa/L-dopa (in milligrams) in the following ratios: 10/100, 25/250, and 25/100. The usual starting dose is 10/100, three times daily. The dosage of Sinemet should be increased until side effects appear or until the patient shows a satisfactory response. The daily dose should be increased no more frequently than every 3 days, since it may take several days for full clinical improvement to be seen or for side effects to be fully evident. Elderly patients or patients felt to be potentially more sensitive to the side effects of the drug should have their dose increased less often. Dosage can be increased to a total of six 10/100 tablets daily; at that point Sinemet 25/250 can be substituted, and increments of ½ to 1 tablet/day can be added, if needed, every 3 days until a satisfactory response or the usual maximum dose (8 tablets) is reached. The increased dose should be given at the time of day when the patient reports that his symptoms are worst.

For patients being *converted from L-dopa to Sinemet*, the L-dopa must be discontinued at least 8 hours before initiation of Sinemet, as the decarboxylase inhibitor will significantly potentiate the effects of any L-dopa remaining from the last dose. Usually the transfer is best accomplished by having the patient take an evening dose of L-dopa and then beginning therapy with the combination tablet on the following morning. The starting dose of Sinemet (in 1:10 ratio) should contain approximately 25% of the previous L-dopa dose. After this transfer, the usual plan for increasing Sinemet should be followed.

Various problems and side effects are associated with the use of L-dopa; most patients will experience some of them.

Peripheral Side Effects

Nausea, vomiting, anorexia, and cardiac arrhythmia are side effects of L-dopa therapy that are mediated principally by peripheral mechanisms. They occur early in L-dopa treatment. They can be largely prevented or greatly reduced by using Sinemet because peripheral metabolism is impeded. Since approximately 100 mg/day of carbidopa are needed to block peripheral decarboxylation of L-dopa, the 25/100 preparation of Sinemet may be useful in a patient who responds to a relatively small dose of L-dopa. The peripheral side effects can be minimized also by having the patient take the drug with meals or with a snack, and by temporarily reducing the total dose of Sinemet if side effects become a problem. Eventually, patients become tolerant to most of the peripheral side effects.

Orthostatic hypotension is an important side effect which appears to be partly due to peripheral actions and partly due to central actions of L-dopa; it may be reduced but not eliminated by the use of Sinemet. It is critical to measure the patient's standing blood pressure before initiating L-dopa, as orthostatic hypotension may also occur as part of the parkinsonian syndrome in some patients. Whether disease or drug-induced, orthostatic hypotension can be managed by having the patient gradually change position from lying to standing; by avoiding other drugs which may exacerbate hypotension; by recommending increased salt intake and use of elastic stockings; and, if necessary, by prescribing fluorocortisone, 0.1 mg to 1 mg daily (see Chapter 84, Table 84.8).

Central Side Effects

In general, the centrally mediated side effects occur after the patient has taken L-dopa at relatively high doses for several years. They occur with both L-dopa alone and with Sinemet.

Dyskinesias (involuntary movements of the limbs, hands, trunk, and lingual-buccal-facial musculature) occur in 40 to 90% of treated patients. Their occurrence and severity seem related to the total duration of therapy and/or disease, and they become progressively worse with time. The longer they have been present, the smaller is the dose of L-dopa needed to produce them; this observation suggests that they are due to a denervation hypersensitivity of dopamine receptor sites. Dyskinesias improve with a reduction of the total daily L-dopa dose, but this also diminishes the antiparkinsonian effect.

When dyskinesias first appear, it is important to

determine whether they show a stereotyped relationship to each dose of drug (15). Some patients may report the following sequence after taking the drug; (a) initial improvement in parkinsonian symptoms, (b) dyskinesias, and (c) resolution of the dyskinesia but continued antiparkinsonian effect. In this instance, the total daily dose of L-dopa should be taken on a more frequent schedule, avoiding the peak doses which apparently provoke the patient's dyskinesia. A less common sequence is (a) dyskinesia immediately after taking a dose, (b) resolution of dyskinesia as antiparkinsonian effect occurs, and (c) return of dyskinesia as the drug level falls. In this situation, a higher total daily dose may preserve the clinical effect and eliminate the dyskinesia.

Mental Disturbances

L-Dopa should be used cautiously in schizophrenic patients, as it may cause psychotic deterioration in these persons. On the other hand, patients who develop marked drug-induced parkinsonian symptoms may be treated judiciously with L-dopa if other treatments are not effective. At times, a patient with no psychiatric history may develop a florid schizophreniform psychosis, usually after an increase in the dose of L-dopa. Confusion, bizarre dreams, hallucinations, delirium, and paranoid ideation may also occur as dose-related side effects in patients on long term therapy. These problems may be produced either by L-dopa alone or by the combined effect of L-dopa and any of the other antiparkinsonian agents, usually after a small increment in the dose of any of these drugs. Management consists of prompt reduction, but not discontinuation, of L-dopa, followed by either careful redistribution of the previous dose in more frequent, smaller doses or by prescription of a smaller daily dose. Disruptive behavior can be treated with diphenhydramine (Benadryl) or thioridazine (Mellaril) for 1 or 2 days while awaiting resolution of the side effect.

Fluctuations in Response to L-Dopa

At least two distinct patterns of transient worsening of symptoms may occur during L-dopa therapy.

1. "Wearing off" refers to a loss of effect hours after taking a dose. If a patient reports a pattern of recurring symptoms before each scheduled dose of L-dopa, the problem can be eliminated usually by administering the dose more frequently or by adding a dopamine agonist (bromocriptine).

2. The "on-off effect" refers to distressing episodes of sudden freezing or bradykinesia, lasting minutes to hours and not occurring in a predictable temporal relationship to a prior dose of L-dopa. This side effect is usually first seen after several years of therapy. At times, fluctuating dose levels may play a role, and the problem may be eliminated by more frequent doses, again keeping the daily dose unchanged (7); in addition, amantadine or bromocriptine (see below) may ameliorate the problem in some patients. Transient freezing may, however, be unresponsive to treatment and may in some patients represent progression of the parkinsonian state.

Interaction with Other Drugs

Coadministration of a number of drugs may diminish the antiparkinsonian effect of L-dopa (see Table 82.7), either by decreasing absorption, by antagonizing its effects in the central nervous system, or by other mechanisms. Apart from the neuroleptic drugs, the other drugs listed can be given with L-dopa and the dose can be adjusted as necessary. Monoamine oxidase inhibitors should not be given with L-dopa, as this can precipitate a hypertensive crisis. Potential drug interactions that may exacerbate the side effects of L-dopa have been mentioned above.

Progressive Loss of Responsiveness

After several years of disease and/or L-dopa treatment, the symptoms of Parkinson's disease become less responsive to medication, and side effects often increase at a dose that was previously tolerated. This seems to represent not only progression of the disease but also a change in the patient's responses to medicine (12). For optimal medical management at this stage, consultation with a neurologist is advisable. Some patients who reach a plateau or show deterioration in their response to L-dopa may regain responsiveness to the drug after a gradual reduction in their daily dose or after a 5- or 10-day "drug holiday" (5). This latter maneuver must be undertaken in the hospital under the supervision of a physician acquainted with the technique, for the patient temporarily becomes immobilized by severe parkinsonism and requires excellent supportive care and judicious reinstitution of L-dopa therapy.

Amantadine (Symmetrel) (18)

This drug was developed as an antiviral (A-2 influenza) agent and was found to have antiparkinson-

Table 82.7.
Drugs That May Diminish the Antiparkinsonian Effect of L-Dopa

Drug	Probable Mechanism
Anticholinergics	Decreased levodopa absorption
Antidepressants, tricyclic	Decreased levodopa absorption
Benzodiazepines	Not established
Clonidine	Not established
Methionine	Not established
Papaverine	Not established
Neuroleptics	Inhibition of dopamine uptake
Phenytoin	Not established
Pyridoxine[a]	Enhancement of decarboxylation of levodopa at periphery

[a] Not a problem if the patient is taking Sinemet.

ian properties. It is thought to promote dopamine release from intact dopaminergic terminals remaining in the nigrostriatum. Amantadine is *useful chiefly as an adjunct* to either anticholinergic or L-dopa treatment. Its effects are often self-limited; patients improve within a few days, but show a loss of responsiveness after about 2 months. Therefore, it may be useful periodically for a few weeks in a patient who appears to be transiently worsening on his usual regimen. Amantadine is also useful for short term management of neuroleptic-induced parkinsonism in patients who cannot tolerate anticholinergics (6) (see additional details in Chapter 16).

Amantadine is available in 100-mg capsules. It should be given as 100 mg daily for the first 1 or 2 weeks, then increased to 100 mg twice daily. Higher doses may cause unpleasant side effects, including depression, confusion, nausea, headaches, amblyopia, edema, orthostatic hypotention, and urinary retention. As noted earlier, amantidine must be used carefully with anticholinergics, as both groups of drugs may produce mental confusion. Like Sinemet, this is a relatively expensive drug.

Bromocriptine (Parlodel) (9)

This drug is an ergot derivative which was developed for use in the amenorrhea-galactorrhea syndrome; it also acts as a dopamine agonist. In Parkinson's disease, it is useful chiefly as an adjunct in patients whose symptoms are not adequately controlled with L-dopa. Fifty percent of patients show initial improvements in a variety of symptoms (tremor, bradykinesia, rigidity, freezing), although only about one-third of patients show sustained improvement with high doses (25 to 50 mg/day). There is a very high incidence of side effects (approximately 70% of patients), which are similar to the peripheral and central side effects of L-dopa described above. This greatly limits the usefulness of the drug. Recent studies with lower doses (10 to 25 mg/day) indicate a lesser frequency of side effects.

Bromocriptine is available in 2.5-mg tablets. Therapy should be initiated with a test dose of ½ tablet because occasionally orthostatic hypotension with this drug can be quite severe. If the test dose is tolerated, treatment is initiated at 2.5 mg, three times daily, increasing every 4 to 5 days up to a dose of 25 to 50 mg. Lower doses (10 to 25 mg) may be adequate for milder cases. The dose of L-dopa can usually be decreased concomitantly with increases in bromocriptine.

Other Aspects of Management

General Management

The patient's physician, aware of the prognosis of Parkinson's disease, can provide much helpful advice to prevent the patient from withdrawing from valued activities and to ensure that he avoids unsafe activities. Duvoisin has written a book explaining the disease in a way useful for the patient and his family (see "General References").

Physical activities should be encouraged, particularly activities which require walking. However, activities that can be dangerous if balance is imperfect or motor response is delayed should be avoided (e.g., skiing, bicycling, driving in heavy traffic, using electric tools, *etc*).

Weak or *slow speech and poverty of facial expression* can produce the impression of lack of interest during a conversation. Therefore, the patient should be advised tactfully to make a conscious effort to let others know that he is interested, despite his lack of facial expression. Having the patient practice speech by reading aloud and by recording and listening to his voice may help to overcome his reticence to speak.

Fear of falling is experienced by virtually all parkinsonian patients. Walking with hands clasped behind the back or using a walker (but not a cane) may improve stability. The patient's living environment should be free of obstacles which may cause him to stumble and he should avoid walking in places where he is apt to encounter obstacles (rocky terrain, for example).

When the patient becomes progressively disabled, the *assistance of others* is necessary to avoid as much as possible the complications of bradykinesia and of sedentary living. Such assistance includes periodic change in the patient's position to avoid skin breakdown, passive range of motion of the limbs and digits to avoid flexion contractures, and as much mobility and social or intellectual stimulation as possible.

General Surgery

Special considerations in the parkinsonian patient who must undergo surgery are discussed in Chapter 86.

Stereotactic Surgery

Twenty percent of patients with Parkinson's disease do not respond significantly to L-dopa from the outset. In others, L-dopa and other therapy ameliorate only some of their symptoms. In some of these patients, stereotactic surgery can be considered. This approach seems especially useful in the relatively uncommon patient in whom uncontrollable parkinsonian tremor alone is disabling; surgery does not seem to be useful for akinesia. Consultation with a neurologist or a neurosurgeon should be obtained in patients who may meet the criteria for consideration of surgery.

General References

Tremor

Jankovic J, Fahn S: Physiologic and pathologic tremors: diagnosis, mechanism, and management. *Ann Intern Med* 93:460, 1980.

Useful review article.

Parkinson's Disease

Boshes B: Sinemet and the treatment of parkinsonism. *Ann Intern Med* 94:364, 1981.
> Critical and practical review of Sinemet.

Duvoisin R: Parkinsonism. In *Clinical Symposia.* Summit, NJ, CIBA Pharmaceutical Co, 1976, vol 28, no. 1.
> Well illustrated account of clinical and physiological aspects of parkinsonism.

Duvoisin RC (ed): *Parkinson's Disease: A Guide for Patient and Family,* ed 2. New York, Raven Press, 1984.
> Two hundred-page book with abundant detail for patients and families.

Lieberman AN, Gopinathan G, Neophytides A, Goldstein M (eds): *Parkinson's Disease Handbook: A Guide for Patients and Their Families.* New York, American Parkinson's Disease Association, 1985.
> Helpful 37-page booklet available free from the American Parkinson Disease Association, Inc., 116 John Street, New York, NY 10038; (toll-free number 1-800-223-APDA).

Pallis CA: Parkinsonism: natural history and clinical features. *Br Med J* 3:683, 1971.
> Extensively referenced review of clinical features of parkinsonism; includes useful information about conditions which mimic parkinsonism.

Specific References

1. Andersen J, Aabro E, Gulmann N, *et al*: Anti-depressive treatment in Parkinson's disease: a controlled trial of the effect of nortriptyline in patients with Parkinson's disease treated with L-dopa. *Acta Neurol Scand* 62:210, 1980.
2. Bannister R, Oppenheimer R: Degenerative diseases of the nervous system associated with autonomic failure. *Brain* 95:457, 1972.
3. Barbeau A: Six years of high-level levodopa therapy in severely akinetic parkinsonian patients. *Arch Neurol* 33:33, 1976.
4. Critchley E: Clinical manifestations of essential tremor. *J Neurol Neurosurg Psychiatry* 35:365, 1972.
5. Direnfeld LK, Feldman RG, Alexander MP, Kelly-Hayes M: Is L-dopa drug holiday useful? *Neurology* 30:785, 1980.
6. DiMascio A, Bernardo DL, Greenblatt DJ, Marder JE: A controlled trial of amantadine in drug-induced extrapyramidal disorders. *Arch Gen Psychiatry* 33:599, 1976.
7. Fahn S: "On-off" phenomenon with levodopa therapy in parkinsonism. *Neurology* 24:431, 1974.
8. Fahn S, Calne DB: Considerations in the management of parkinsonism. *Neurology* 28:5, 1978.
9. Fahn S, Cote LJ, Snider SR, et al: The role of bromocriptine in the treatment of parkinsonism. *Neurology* 29:1077, 1979.
10. Growdon JH, Shahani BT, Young RR: The effect of alcohol on essential tremor. *Neurology* 25:259, 1975.
11. Hakim AM, Mathieson G: Dementia in Parkinson disease: a neuropathologic study. *Neurology* 29:1209, 1979.
12. Lesser RP, Fahn S, Snider SR, et al: Analysis of the clinical problems in parkinsonism and the complications of long-term levodopa therapy. *Neurology* 29:1253, 1979.
13. Markham CH, Diamond SG: Evidence to support early levodopa therapy in Parkinson's disease. *Neurology* 31:125, 1981.
14. Mindham RHS: Psychiatric aspects of Parkinson's disease. *Br J Hosp Med,* March: 411, 1974.
15. Muenter MD, Sharpless NS, Tyce GM, Darley FL: Patterns of dystonia ("I-D-I" and "D-I-D") in response to L-dopa therapy for Parkinson's disease. *Mayo Clin Proc* 52:163, 1977.
16. Pollock M, Hornabrook RW: The prevalence, natural history and dementia of Parkinson's disease. *Brain* 89:429, 1966.
17. Shy GM, Drager CA: A neurological syndrome associated with orthostatic hypotension: a clinical-pathologic study. *Arch Neurol* 2:511, 1960.
18. Timberlake WH, Vance MA: Four-year treatment of patients with parkinsonism using amantadine alone or with levodopa. *Ann Neurol* 3:119, 1978.
19. Tune LE, McHugh PR, Coyle JT: Management of extrapyramidal side effects induced by neuroleptics. *Johns Hopkins Med J* 148:149, 1981.
20. Winkler GF, Young RR: Efficacy of chronic propranolol therapy in action tremors of the familial, senile or essential varieties. *N Engl J Med* 290:984, 1974.

CHAPTER EIGHTY-THREE

Cerebrovascular Disease

THOMAS J. PREZIOSI, M.D., AND L. RANDOL BARKER, M.D.*

OVERVIEW

Cerebrovascular disease is a major cause of disability and the third leading cause of death in the United States. The impact on society is far-reaching with an estimated annual cost of greater than 7.3 billion dollars. According to a survey published in 1980 (33), the *annual incidence* of first stroke is 150 per 100,000 population; about 80% of strokes are due to thrombotic or embolic cerebral infarction, 12% to cerebral hemorrhage, and 8% to subarachnoid hemorrhage. As shown in Table 83.1, approximately 75% of strokes occur in individuals who are 65 or older. The *annual death rate* from stroke is 75/100,000 population with a disproportionately greater number of early deaths among patients with hemorrhage as compared to patients with infarction. Data on *the prevalence of stroke* suggest that in a population of 100,000 there are approximately 500 stroke survivors at any particular time.

The incidence of stroke declined by more than 50% in one population (Rochester, Minnesota) dur-

ing the 5-year period 1975 to 1979 compared to the 5-year period 1945 to 1949 (21). The decline was found for all age groups. Subsequent studies have shown that stroke incidence has decreased on a nationwide and indeed worldwide level (24, 50). Factors that may have contributed to the decline include more aggressive treatment of hypertension, more effective and early delivery of health care, and better management and recognition of the cardiogenic sources of cerebral embolization.

Cerebrovascular disease presents *two major challenges in ambulatory practice*: First, the prevention of stroke in the large number of individuals with risk factors that make them stroke prone; and second, the optimal care of the many stroke survivors in each community.

RISK FACTORS

A major goal of patient evaluation in ambulatory practice is the identification of the individual with an increased risk of stroke. Patients who have previously suffered a stroke constitute an important subgroup of this high risk population. A community-based study of the natural history of stroke in Rochester, Minnesota, has shown that the first year recurrence rate among survivors of a first stroke was 10% and that the 5-year recurrence rate was 20% (37). In addition to a previous history of stroke, other factors predispose a patient to stroke. Epidemiological data indicate that the incidence of stroke and the associated death rate increase markedly with age. Three other factors, all amenable to therapy, have also been found to correlate strongly with stroke occurrence: transient episodes of focal cerebral dysfunction of vascular origin called transient ischemic attacks (TIA), hypertension, and certain types of cardiac disorders.

TIA

Approximately one-third of patients with a TIA subsequently develop a stroke and the TIA provides a significant warning of impending infarction. The etiology, natural history, and treatment of TIA are discussed in detail later in this chapter (page 1194).

Hypertension

Data accumulated during the Framingham study indicate that the risk of both nonhemorrhagic and

---

* Alfred Server, M.D., Ph.D. contributed to this chapter in the first edition.

Table 83.1.
Percentage Distribution of Stroke Occurrence by Age Group[a]

	Percentage of Total Persons in Each Age Group[b]							
	All ages	Under 35	35–44	45–54	55–64	65–74	75–84	84+
US population	100.0	58.3	10.4	11.4	9.5	6.6	3.3	1.0
Stroke patients	100.0	1.2	2.0	6.8	15.6	28.3	33.4	12.7

[a] From National Survey of Stroke, US Department of Health, Education and Welfare, Public Health Service National Institutes of Health, NIH publ no. 80-2069; January 1980.
[b] Note that while the age group 65 years and older constitutes only 10.9% of the population, approximately three-fourths (74.4%) of all strokes occur in this age group.

hemorrhagic stroke are strongly related to *hypertension*. Atherothrombotic brain infarction occurred in hypertensive subjects (blood pressure greater than 160/95) 4 times more often than in normotensive subjects (31). Moreoever, the available evidence suggests that stroke risk is significantly reduced by the treatment of hypertension in all patients including those with a history of cerebrovascular disease (6, 11, 48, 49) (see below page 1194). The evaluation and long term management of hypertension is discussed in detail in Chapter 62.

Cardiac Impairment

Cardiac impairment clearly predisposes to stroke. It has long been known that the heart is often the source of emboli that lodge in cerebral vessels and lead to infarction. However, this type of stroke is thought to be relatively uncommon, constituting only 3 to 8% of all cerebral infarctions. Data from the Framingham study have identified cardiac impairment as a significant risk factor in the occurrence of the more frequently encountered nonembolic atherothrombotic brain infarction (ABI) (52). Subjects with electrocardiographic evidence of left ventricular hypertrophy (LVH) were 9 times more likely to develop ABI than individuals without this abnormality. Patients with coronary artery disease (CAD) had 5 times the risk of ABI and those with radiographic evidence of cardiomegaly had 3 times the risk. When the contribution of concomitant hypertension was eliminated, LVH and CAD were each associated with a 3-fold increase in the risk of ABI; the contribution of cardiomegaly on X-ray was not found to be significant when other variables were controlled. On the basis of these findings it was concluded that cardiac impairment, especially if associated with hypertension, significantly heightens the risk of stroke occurrence. It is not clear that cardiac abnormalities, once established, can be modified so that the risk of subsequent stroke is reduced.

Other Factors

A number of other factors have been associated with an increased incidence of stroke: family history of vascular disease, elevated serum glucose concentration, elevated serum lipid levels, cigarette smoking, elevated blood hemoglobin and hematocrit levels, and the presence of a cervical bruit. To date, it is not known whether modification of any of these risk factors reduces the likelihood of stroke and each requires some qualification. Data on *family history* are incomplete, although the available evidence suggests that the parents of stroke patients have a higher mortality from vascular disease. With regard to *diabetes mellitus*, prospective data from the Framingham study indicated an increased risk of cerebral infarction in subjects with even a modest abnormality of glucose tolerance (29). This study also demonstrated that *elevated serum lipid levels* were associated with increased stroke risk, but only in subjects under the age of 50. The contribution of *cigarette smoking* to the risk of stroke occurrence remains controversial. However, in the Framingham study male cigarette smokers had a 3-fold greater risk of cerebral infarction than nonsmokers. The data on female smokers was too limited to draw a valid conclusion. *Elevated blood hemoglobin and hematocrit levels* have also been implicated as possible risk factors, but a cause and effect relationship has not been established (30, 47). *Oral contraceptive use* is associated with a 5- to 10-fold increase in risk of vascular diseases, including stroke (see details in Chapter 93). Finally, it is generally accepted that the presence of an *asymptomatic cervical bruit* correlates with an increased incidence of subsequent stroke, but there is controversy regarding the appropriate management of patients with this finding (see below, page 1198).

CLASSIFICATION OF CEREBROVASCULAR EVENTS

Type of Event

Symptoms and signs of vascular origin are characterized by their relatively rapid onset. The following classification has been developed based upon their duration.

A *transient ischemic attack* is defined as a transient episode of focal cerebral dysfunction, rapid in onset (from no to maximal symptoms in less than 5 minutes) that usually lasts from 2 to 15 minutes but always resolves completely within 24 hours.

A *reversible ischemic neurological deficit* (RIND) is defined as an episode of focal cerebral dysfunction that lasts longer than 24 hours but resolves completely within 3 weeks.

A *completed stroke* is defined as an episode of focal cerebral dysfunction that has stabilized and may have improved but has not resolved completely after 3 weeks. The term "stroke in evolution" is used to describe a vascular syndrome that is acute in onset and worsens during the period of observation.

Vascular Territory

Cerebrovascular events are also classified on the basis of the vascular territory involved. Symptoms and signs referable to the two major vascular territories are listed in Table 83.2. There is some overlap in the symptom complexes, making the distinction between carotid and vertebrobasilar disease difficult at times. However, frequently the history alone provides the physician with the evidence necessary to diagnose a cerebrovascular episode and to identify the arterial territory involved.

Another group of ischemic events, presenting as *lacunar syndromes*, is due to occlusion of penetrating nonanastamosing branches of the major cerebral arteries. The pathology of the involved vessels has been characterized; occlusion is due either to miniature atherosclerotic plaques at the origin of vessels 400 to 1000 μ in diameter or, more commonly, to a degenerative process called lipohyalinosis affecting vessels 200 μ or less. These changes correlate strongly with the presence of hypertension. At least 20 clinical lacunar syndromes have been described (18); lacunar infarctions may also be silent, identified only by computed tomographic (CT) scan. The common syndromes are the following:

Pure motor hemiparesis (internal capsule or pons): hemiplegia or hemiparesis involving the face, arm, and leg without sensory deficit, dysphasia, or hemianopsia.

Pure sensory stroke (thalamus): numbness of the face, arm, and leg on one side without weakness or hemianopsia.

Homolateral ataxia and crural paresis (pons): cerebellar ataxia, weakness, and pyramidal signs involving the limbs on the same side, the lower extremity more than the arm.

The *dysarthria-clumsy hand syndrome* (pons): dysarthria, facial weakness, clumsiness of the hand with little or no weakness, a slight imbalance, and a Babinski sign on the affected side.

Multi-infarct dementia: a dementia syndrome characterized by stepwise progression (see description of dementia, Chapter 17).

COMPLETED STROKE

Any occlusive arterial disease may lead to a completed stroke. The vast majority of strokes are due to atherosclerosis, lipohyalinosis, or emboli from the heart. A number of conditions may produce a syndrome resembling a completed stroke, RIND, or TIA. These are summarized in the discussion of the differential diagnosis of TIA (see below, page 1194).

Both the diagnostic evaluation and initial care of the patient with a new stroke should be accomplished in the hospital. This includes patients with lacunar syndromes, which vary as to their etiology and their appropriate treatment (18). Following hospital discharge, ambulatory or home care for the stroke survivor requires the collaboration of the patient, the family, the physician, and other professionals, as explained below.

Natural History

The major studies on the natural history of stroke differ with regard to two important variables: the type of stroke patient studied and the treatment available to the study population. The few studies that attempted to restrict the variables under consideration were performed before the advent of cerebral CT scanning and were therefore marred by a significant degree of diagnostic inaccuracy. Despite these criticisms, the extensive body of literature on the "natural history" of stroke provides useful information.

Early Prognosis

There is general agreement that *age* influences greatly the early prognosis for the patient who sustains a stroke, regardless of the type. The older the patient, the less likely he is to survive (see Table 83.3). Studies that classify strokes on the basis of *etiology* indicate that the early prognosis is much better for thrombotic or embolic disease than for hemorrhage. During the interval 1955 to 1969, 82% of stroke patients from the Mayo Clinic with a clinical diagnosis of cerebral thrombosis and 67% of those with cerebral embolism were alive 30 days after the acute episode (37). These values compare favorably with the 1-month survival of 48% observed for subarachnoid hemorrhage and 16% observed for intracerebral hemorrhage.

Morbidity in Stroke Survivors

A number of studies have evaluated stroke survivors on the basis of the degree of neurological, functional, and psychosocial impairment.

Table 83.4 shows the spectrum and frequency of

Table 83.2.
Clinical Features of Ischemia Involving the Major Vascular Territories

CAROTID ARTERIAL DISEASE
  Paresis (mono- or hemi-)
  Sensory loss or paresthesias (mono- or hemi-)
  Speech or language disturbances
  Loss of vision in one eye or part of one eye (amaurosis fugax)
  Homonymous hemianopsia
  Cognitive impairment
VERTEBROBASILAR ARTERIAL DISEASE
  Vertigo, diplopia, dysphagia, or dysarthria when two occur together or when one occurs with any of the following:
  Paresis (any combination of the extremities)
  Sensory loss or paresthesias (any combination of the extremities)
  Ataxia
  Homonymous hemianopsia (unilateral or bilateral)

Table 83.3.
Percentage Distribution of Stroke Survivors by Age Group[a]

Age Group	Percentage Surviving									
		Days				Years				
	Onset	30	60	90	180	1	2	3	4	5
Under 65	100.0	73.7	71.1	69.4	65.9	63.2	57.6	57.6	52.0	49.2
65–74	100.0	75.6	69.5	65.2	63.1	59.4	52.9	46.1	42.7	34.5
75–84	100.0	68.1	62.1	57.6	52.4	45.7	37.2	30.0	23.1	21.9
85+	100.0	52.4	45.8	37.2	33.0	27.8	20.7	15.1	9.2	7.4

[a] From: National Survey of Stroke, US Department of Health, Education and Welfare, Public Health Service National Institutes of Health, NIH publ no. 80-2069, January 1980.

neurological impairments found in stroke survivors in the Framingham study (23). Study subjects were living at home or in institutions at the time of functional evaluation. The interval between the stroke and the functional assessment ranged from 6 months to 33 years (mean, 7 years). It is notable that half of these individuals (63 of 123) had no motor deficit. These community-based data are probably representative of the situation in other communities.

In an extensive study of *overall function*, Katz et al (32) found that, of the patients who survive a stroke, approximately 50% are independent 2 years later and are able to ambulate and perform activities of daily living with minimal or no assistance. Spontaneous improvement is most rapid in the first few months after the stroke and is rarely noted after 2 years. Only a small percentage of stroke survivors remain bedridden and completely dependent. These findings are supported by results from the Mayo Clinic where only 4% of the survivors of a stroke required total care at 6 months; 36% had some degree of neurological deficit, yet were able to work; and 29% were functioning normally (37). On the basis of the authors' assessment, 54% of their patients may have benefited from rehabilitative care, including the 10% who were aphasic.

The Framingham study provided information on the equally important *social and psychological sequelae* of stroke (23). A significant decrease in the levels of vocational function and socialization outside the home was noted among stroke survivors as compared to age and sex-matched controls (see Table 83.5), and the decrease exceeded that anticipated based on the levels of neurological deficit. In a more recent study in Monroe County, New York, the social and psychological difficulties facing the stroke survivor were evaluated prospectively (17). Within the first 6 months after hospital discharge, 37% of the patients demonstrated moderate or severe depression, 32% anger and/or anxiety, 56% social isolation, 43% reduction in community involvement, 46% economic strain causing life style alteration, and 52% disruption of normal family functions. Additional longitudinal studies have (a) confirmed the high incidence of moderate or severe depression in the first year following stroke; (b) shown that the risk of depression is particularly high in patients with damage in the left frontal hemisphere; and (c) shown that this depression responds well to tricyclic antidepressants, especially nortriptyline (41, 42). Recognition and treatment of the psychosocial prob-

Table 83.4.
Prevalence of Neurological Deficits in the 123 Survivors of Completed Stroke, Framingham Study (1972 to 1974)[a]

Type of Peripheral Motor Deficit	Survivors	No. Surviving with:			
		Sensory deficit	Hemi-anopsia	Dys-arthria	Dys-phasia
No motor deficit	63	3	5	2	10
Left hemiparesis	28	13	6	3	2
Right hemiparesis	27	10	5	13	9
Bilateral motor deficit	4	4	3	2	1
No data	1	1	1	1	1
Total survivors	123	31	20	21	23

[a] From Gresham GE, Fitzpatrick TE, Wolf PA, et al: Residual disability in survivors of stroke—the Framingham study. *N Engl J Med* 293:954, 1975.

Table 83.5.
Prevalence of Four Types of Functional Disability in 119 Survivors of Completed Stroke and in 119 Controls, Framingham Study (1972 to 1974)[a]

Type of Disability	Survivors		Matched Controls[b]		P Value
	No.	%	No.	%	
All persons examined for functional disability	119	100	119	100	—
Dependent in activities of daily living	37	31	9	8	<0.0001
Dependent in mobility	24	20	6	5	<0.0001
Decrease in level of vocational function[c]	85	71	49	41	<0.0001
Decrease in socialization outside home	74	62	37	31	<0.0001

[a] Gresham GE, Fitzpatrick TE, Wolf PA, et al: Residual disability in survivors of stroke-the Framingham Study. *N Engl J Med* 293:954, 1975.
[b] Matched for age and sex.
[c] Either stopped working or incomplete resumption of homemaking activities.

lems of the stroke patient and his family are discussed below.

Mortality in Stroke Survivors

The death rate among stroke survivors is significantly greater than that expected for the general population matched for age and sex. The 5-year cumulative mortality is approximately 50 to 60%, with the greatest number of deaths occurring in the first year. With time, however, the mortality rate approaches that of the general population and in at least one study the accelerated rate of death following a stroke subsided completely after 24 to 30 months (32). There is evidence to suggest that the etiology of a stroke (occlusive versus hemorrhagic) is a less reliable predictor of late prognosis than early prognosis. Eisenberg et al (15) reported that while cerebral hemorrhage was more lethal acutely than cerebral thrombosis, those cerebral hemorrhage victims who lived 1 month had a 5-year survival equal to or better than cerebral thrombosis victims. The leading cause of death in stroke survivors is cardiovascular disease, with cardiac-related deaths exceeding deaths attributed to cerebrovascular disease by a factor of 2 to 1. Thorough evaluation and management of cardiac disease are, therefore, of great importance in the care of stroke survivors.

Management

Management of the patient who has survived a stroke involves the evaluation and treatment of any physical and psychosocial sequelae and the selection of appropriate therapy to lessen the risk of stroke recurrence. Once the patient has been discharged from the hospital, his personal physician plays a critical role in coordinating his care. Reduction in a patient's disability and dependency frequently requires the concerted efforts of the patient's family; physical, occupational, and speech therapists; and occasionally a psychiatrist. Stroke patients with significant deficits persisting for 3 months or longer may qualify for Disability Insurance under Social Security (see Table 9.3).

Role of the Family

At the time of discharge from the hospital, appropriate education is especially important for the stroke survivor and his family. It is during this period that the patient is confronted with the full extent of his functional loss and that the actions of well meaning but uninformed family members can increase the patient's feeling of inadequacy. The physician must dispel myths regarding stroke and supplant them with accurate and useful information. The American Heart Association (AHA) has produced a series of invaluable booklets that discuss stroke and its sequelae in lay terms and provide guidelines for the home management of the stroke

patient. The titles of these publications are listed in Table 83.6. Table 83.7 shows, as an example, the table of contents of *Up and Around*, a booklet designed to assist in restoration of mobility. The AHA booklet entitled *Strokes—A Guide for the Family* provides the following general suggestions for the family of a stroke patient with residual disability:

Divide duties so that the full burden of care does not fall on one person.

Help the patient take responsibility for doing his exercises regularly.

Allow the patient to take on responsibilities for self-care and other activities gradually and by easy steps. It calls for fine judgment to encourage independence and still not to frustrate a patient with overdifficult tasks; to stimulate progress and still not to encourage unrealistic expectations.

Praise any successful efforts that he makes, don't be discouraged by failures. Recovery from a severe stroke is a slow process.

Have him participate in as many family activities and as much family planning as he can. Feeling useful is a tremendous morale builder.

Help him keep in contact with the world he has known.

Don't relegate him to the side lines and leave him with only television and radio to occupy himself. Encourage him to develop a hobby. Spend time with him . . .

Table 83.6.
Booklets Published by the American Heart Association[a]

Strokes: A Guide for the Family—a brief overview of the mechanisms causing strokes and general suggestions for care of the patient at home

Strike Back at Stroke—a well illustrated booklet prepared for the physician, the patient, and the patient's family demonstrating the following aspects of home care of the stroke patient: postion of the patient in bed, passive exercises that must be done for the patient, active exercises that the patient can do, methods for getting out of bed, standing, use of a sling, and walking with the assistance of a cane or other devices

Up and Around—an extensively illustrated booklet written for the physician, the patient, and the patient's family, on ways in which the patient can regain activities of daily living (see "Table of Contents" in Table 83.7)

Do It Yourself Again—well illustrated booklet on self-help devices for eating, grooming, dressing, using the bathroom, reading, writing, telephoning, preparing food, cleaning, sewing, walking, and selecting and using a wheelchair

Stroke: Why Do They Behave That Way?—a detailed booklet providing recommendations for the care of the patient who has completed most of his spontaneous recovery of higher functions and has major residual deficits (see "Summary of Recommendations" in Table 83.8)

Aphasia and the Family—explains many of the problems in aphasia and suggests practical ways in which the family can help the aphasic patient

[a] Available without charge from local AHA chapters.

Table 83.7.
Table of Contents of US Public Health Service Publication Entitled *Up and Around—A Booklet to Aid the Stroke Patient in Activities of Daily Living* **(Available from American Heart Association)**

Encourage visitors if his condition warrants it. Make him feel wanted and a part of the social picture.

Check with the doctor regularly. Get in touch with him if things are not going as you think they should.

Role of Rehabilitation

Success in stroke rehabilitation is often dependent upon the extent of permanent central nervous system damage and the patient's ability to utilize alternative methods of function to compensate for fixed deficits. As noted above, spontaneous improvement in the stroke survivor may continue to occur for the first 6 to 12 months after the stroke, yet the mechanisms underlying such gains remain obscure. Lehmann and his colleagues (34) have studied the important question of whether or not an intensive program of rehabilitation will result in functional gains after the period of spontaneous improvement. They found that even among significantly impaired patients admitted to a rehabilitation program 12 months after a stroke, marked improvement was attainable in dressing skills, bladder and bowel function, and walking. These findings formed the basis for their conclusion that a program of rehabilitation does improve the outcome of the stroke survivor. Furthermore, they estimated that the savings derived in returning a patient to his family or to independent living more than equaled the costs of rehabilitation.

It is clear that not all patients in a rehabilitation program show significant functional improvement. A number of patient characteristics correlate with poor rehabilitation results, including bowel and bladder incontinence, low self-care status on admission, right hemispheric involvement, intellectual and perceptual deficits, heart failure, signs of generalized arteriosclerosis, and lower educational levels (7, 35). However, since none of these factors correlates strongly with poor outcome, the best approach is to offer rehabilitation services whenever possible to each stroke survivor with significant functional impairments.

It is generally agreed that, except for patients with evidence of subarachnoid bleeding, for whom bed rest and mild sedation are indicated, a program of functional rehabilitation should begin as soon as possible after a stroke occurs. *There are several reasons for the early initiation of a program of rehabilitation.* First, it is generally accepted that patients who are provided with rehabilitation services early are likely to experience greater long term functional improvement. Second, early transfer from bed to chair coupled with physical therapy reduces the complications that can develop in the immobile bedridden patient and that can subsequently limit the extent of functional recovery. Stretching of tight muscles, passive range of motion, and active or resistive exercises minimize the degree of muscle atrophy and prevent the development of contractures. In addition, even limited mobility of the patient will reduce the risk of circulatory complications such as thrombophlebitis, postural hypotension, and pressure sores. Third, early rehabilitation is of particular benefit to the patient who demonstrates an impaired ability to communicate due either to dysphasia or to dysarthria. Approximately one-third of stroke patients exhibit some form of communication disorder and many of these remain severely impaired beyond the period of spontaneous recovery (45). Such patients may feel desperately isolated because of their sudden loss of ability to communicate. Therapists who specialize in speech and hearing are skilled in the evaluation and management of these problems and play an integral role in daily interactions with the patient and in recommending appropriate strategies to the patient's family and physician.

Everyone involved in the rehabilitation process must appreciate the significance of the functional losses sustained by the patient and to do so, the losses must be viewed from the patient's perspective. This requires an *awareness of the patient's usual activities before the stroke*; this essential information should be obtained in conjunction with a social worker who can evaluate the patient's role at home prior to the stroke and can project how the stroke will alter that role when the patient returns to his home.

Ideally, the *rehabilitation initiated in the hospital is continued in the patient's home or in ambulatory care facilities*. Many communities have physical, occupational, and speech therapists available for both home and ambulatory follow-up. The patient, his family, and the patient's personal physician should be acquainted with the goals and plans for rehabilitation before discharge to home or to a rehabilitation facility. The comprehensive text of Licht (see "General References") provides details about the many individualized approaches available for rehabilitation.

Management of Psychological and Behavioral Sequelae

The high incidence of psychological and behavioral problems among stroke survivors has been noted above. These problems often hinder rehabilitation efforts. Fear of a second stroke and depression due to loss of functional ability are readily understandable in the context of the patient's predicament. Appropriate counseling (as outlined above) of the patient and his family, coupled with participation in an active rehabilitation program, are the best ways to minimize these adverse psychological reactions to a stroke.

A number of stroke survivors experience *disturbances of mood that do not correlate with the level of functional disability*; and there is evidence that for many patients the mood disorder is a specific complication of cerebral damage rather than simply a reaction to functional loss (19, 41, 42). These findings expand earlier observations that showed that the type of mood disorder is dependent upon the side of the brain affected by the stroke. Gainotti (20) re-

ported that behavior denoting a catastrophic reaction (see Chapter 17; page 210) and anxious depressive orientation of mood (anxiety reactions, bursts of tears, provocative utterances, depressed renouncements, or sharp refusals to go on with the examinations) are more frequent among patients with left (dominant) hemisphere damage. Symptoms denoting an opposite emotional reaction (denial of illness, minimization, indifference reactions, and tendency to joke) and expressions of hate toward the paralyzed limbs are more frequent among patients suffering from a lesion of the right (minor) hemisphere. Most authorities agree, however, that both psychological and physiological factors contribute to the development of mood disorders following strokes. Tricyclic antidepressants have been shown to benefit patients with poststroke depression (41, 42). Practical information about these drugs is found in Chapter 15, Affective Disorders.

The AHA booklet *Stroke: Why Do They Behave That Way?* is particularly helpful for the family and for health care professionals caring for the patient who has survived a major stroke involving the cerebral cortex. Table 83.8 contains summaries of the recommendations for dealing with permanent behavioral problems in these patients.

Management of Late Complications

There are a number of late complications that may occur during the months to years following a stroke.

Shoulder Problems

The *painful shoulder* is one of the most disturbing complications encountered in the stroke patient with a residual hemiparesis. Shoulder pain is frequently caused by increased traction on the shoulder capsule secondary to abnormal positioning of the paralyzed arm. The normal alignment of the joint can be restored through the use of a sling and proper positioning of the arm at night. Physical therapy, following initial symptomatic treatment with analgesics and the application of heat, can limit the extent of permanent structural damage (see Chapter 63, Shoulder Pain, for additional detail).

The *shoulder-hand syndrome*, also called reflex sympathetic dystrophy, occurs in approximately 5% of stroke patients. It is characterized by the occurrence of a painful shoulder associated with stiffness and swelling of the hand and fingers. Onset is acute or subacute (developing over a 3- to 6-month period), and may involve the hand and shoulder simultaneously or one followed by the other. While a number of conditions can result in shoulder discomfort, the dystrophic changes in the hand are characteristic of the shoulder-hand syndrome. There is swelling below the wrist but no pitting edema, and the skin of the hand is warm and pink. With time, the intrinsic muscles of the hand atrophy and extension deform-

Table 83.8.
Recommendations for Dealing with Behavioral Problems Associated with Permanent Loss of Higher Functions in Stroke Patients[a]

LEFT HEMISPHERE DAMAGE

Right hemiplegics will often have difficulties with speech and language. They also tend to be somewhat cautious, anxious, and disorganized when attempting a new task. Keep in mind the following suggestions:

1. Do not underestimate the patient's ability to learn and communicate even if he cannot use speech.
2. If he cannot use speech, try other forms of communication. Pantomime and demonstration are often useful.
3. Do not overestimate his understanding of speech and overload him with "static."
4. Do not shout. Keep messages simple and brief.
5. Do not use special voices.
6. Divide tasks into simple steps.
7. Give much feedback and many indications of progress.

RIGHT HEMISPHERE DAMAGE

If the patient is having difficulty with self-care activities, you can expect spatial-perceptual deficits. He will tend to talk better than he can actually perform. He may be impulsive or careless. Remember, when working with the patient who has significant spatial-perceptual deficits:

1. Do not overestimate his abilities. Spatial-perceptual difficulties are easy to miss.
2. Use verbal cues if he has difficulty with demonstration.
2. Break tasks into small steps and give much feedback.
4. Watch to see what he can do safely rather than taking his word for it.
5. Minimize clutter around him.
6. Avoid rapid movement around the patient.
7. Highlight visual reference points.

ONE-SIDED NEGLECT

One-sided neglect is a problem that involves more than a simple visual field cut or hearing loss. It can occur in both right and left hemiplegics but seems to be more common and more persistent among left hemiplegics. When dealing with a neglect problem, you should:

1. Keep the unimpaired side toward the action unless specifically working with neglected side.
2. Avoid trapping the patient in an unnecessarily confined environment.
3. Avoid nagging but give frequent cues to aid orientation.
4. Provide reminders of the neglected side.
5. Arrange the environment to maximize performance.

MEMORY PROBLEMS

Some memory problems can be expected in most stroke patients. When working with memory deficits, you can often increase the patient's ability to perform if you:

1. Establish a fixed routine whenever possible.
2. Keep messages short to fit his retention span.
3. Present new information one step at a time.
4. Allow the patient to finish one step before proceeding to the next.
5. Give frequent indications of effective progress; he may forget his past "successes."
6. Train in settings that resemble, as much as possible, the setting in which the behavior is to be practiced.
7. Use memory aids such as appointment books, written notes, and schedule cards whenever possible.
8. Use familiar objects and old associations when teaching new tasks.

[a] Adapted from *Stroke: Whey Do They Behave That Way?* American Heart Association.

ities in the metacarpophalangeal joints develop. At this stage radiographic examination of the hand often shows spotty demineralization of the carpal bones. The severe pain associated with this condition greatly hinders rehabilitation efforts. Therefore, early recognition and treatment are important. Ross and Chipman (43) offer the following plan for the management of this condition. Begin treatment with analgesics and with heat to the shoulder; then carefully initiate and gradually increase abduction and external rotation exercises of the arm (described in Chapter 63). If there is no significant improvement after 1 month, the patient should be referred to a neurosurgeon for stellate ganglion block, followed by a course of oral corticosteroids if symptoms persist.

Complications of Inactivity

The partially paralyzed stroke survivor often leads a sedentary existence. This life style is conducive to the development of vascular complications such as *thrombophlebitis* and *pressure sores*. Appropriate use of elastic stockings and frequent repositioning of the immobile patient by an informed family member will minimize these problems.

Neurological Complications

Prolonged pressure on a paralyzed limb may lead to a *peripheral nerve lesion*, which may be difficult to recognize when superimposed on brain damage resulting from the stroke. An awareness of this potential complication can expedite its recognition and electrodiagnostic studies can confirm the lower motor neuron damage (see Chapter 84). Once a diagnosis is made, prompt initiation of physical therapy will limit the degree of functional loss resulting from this usually reversible lesion.

Approximately 2.5 to 5% of stroke survivors develop *focal or generalized recurrent seizures* (epilepsy) as a late complication. Patients with damage to their sensorimotor cortex are the most likely to develop epilepsy, with the first seizure usually occurring 6 to 12 months after the stroke (36, 40). Transient neurological dysfunction following a seizure in a stroke survivor is often attributed to a second stroke. The rapid resolution of symptons and electroencephalogram (EEG) evidence of an epileptogenic focus point to seizure activity rather than ischemia as the cause. Recurrent seizures in the stroke survivor confirm the diagnosis of epilepsy.

Seizure control can usually be achieved through the use of anticonvulsant medication (see Chapter 80).

Finally, *stroke-related deficits may transiently worsen* when the patient develops a major intercurrent illness such as pneumonia or myocardial infarction. In this instance, neurological status returns to baseline after resolution of the intercurrent illness (See discussion of upper motor neuron symptoms in Chapter 78).

General Surgery

The approach to general surgery in the stroke patient is discussed in Chapter 86.

Prevention of Stroke Recurrence

The selection of appropriate therapy to lessen the risk of stroke recurrence is based on the pathophysiology of the initial stroke and upon the presence of any risk factors (see above) that can be modified. In this section only the most frequently advocated forms of preventive treatment are discussed.

Antihypertensive Therapy

In a prospective randomized clinical trial, Carter (11) assessed the efficacy of antihypertensive therapy in the treatment of hypertensive patients who had sustained a nonembolic ischemic stroke. He reported that 44% of the untreated patients, as compared to 20% of the treated patients, suffered another major stroke. At the end of a 2- to 5-year follow-up period 46% of the untreated patients and 26% of the treated patients had died. While the number of recurrent strokes was too small to allow a valid comparison, the difference in mortality was statistically significant in favor of the treated group at the 0.05 level. Moreover, no treated patient sustained a major neurological complication as a result of a documented hypotensive episode.

Two subsequent studies of the effect of antihypertensive treatment on stroke recurrence included patients with hemorrhagic as well as ischemic strokes. Beevers *et al* (6) noted that the stroke recurrence rate varied inversely with success in controlling blood pressure. In patients with good, fair, and poor control of hypertension, the recurrence rates were 16, 32, and 55%, respectively. In contrast, the Hypertension-Stroke Cooperative Study Group (27) failed to demonstrate a significant reduction in stroke recurrence in treated as compared to control patients, although the incidence of congestive heart failure was reduced among the treated patients. In comparing their results to those reported by Beevers *et al*, the Study Group noted that their patients were less hypertensive. They suggested that "... when stroke survivors with blood pressures considerably higher than those that prevailed in our study are given antihypertensive therapy, a beneficial effect on stroke recurrence can be obtained."

In summary, despite the differences in the studies cited above, critical assessment of the data yields the conclusions that antihypertensive medication can be safely administered to hypertensive stroke survivors and that it is indicated for these patients to reduce cerebrovascular and cardiovascular sequelae. (See Chapter 62) for details on the treatment of hypertension.)

Anticoagulant and Antiplatelet Agents

Anticoagulant and antiplatelet agents have been extensively evaluated for their efficacy in the prevention of stroke recurrence. There is evidence from noncontrolled studies that patients with ischemic infarcts due to emboli from the heart will benefit from long term anticoagulation with Coumadin (13). However, for the large majority of stroke survivors, those with completed strokes due to atherothrombotic cerebrovascular disease, anticoagulation does not result in a significant reduction in the incidence of stroke recurrence or death and is frequently associated with hemorrhagic complications (22).

Data on the antiplatelet agents are somewhat more encouraging (see Chapter 51). Several studies have reported that aspirin, 1000 to 1200 mg/day, prevented strokes as well as death from cerebral vascular disease in patients who had had TIAs or partial completed strokes (10) or completed strokes (8). In one of these studies the benefit was limited to men (10); in the other, it was observed in both men and women (8). At present, many investigators recommend the use of aspirin (and dipyridamole—although its efficacy has not been established) for both men and women with documented thromboembolic cerebral vascular disease (38, 44).

Carotid Artery Surgery

Based upon careful analysis of a number of studies, Kistler *et al* (see "General References") concluded that carotid artery surgery may benefit a carefully selected group of patients with a completed stroke. According to these authors, carotid endarterectomy can be recommended to patients with a small infarct in the carotid system who have surgically correctable arterial lesions appropriate to the deficit (e.g., a large ulcerated plaque or stenosis of greater than 60%) and who are otherwise in good health and neurologically stable. Angiography and surgery should only be performed by a team of specialists with a record of documented success in the evaluation and treatment of occlusive cerebrovascular disease.

TRANSIENT ISCHEMIC ATTACK (TIA)

As noted earlier, TIAs are defined as transient episodes of focal cerebral dysfunction, rapid in onset (no to maximal symptoms in less than 5 minutes), with symptoms referable to the carotid or vertebrobasilar arterial territory (see Table 83.2), which resolve completely within 24 hours.

Early studies on the pathophysiology of TIAs suggested that they are primarily caused by vasospasm or hypotension. However, according to Barnett (3) "subsequent observations have led to the firm conviction that these ischemic events result from a variety of conditions, including hemodynamic factors, cardiac emboli, extracranial mechanical interference with arteries, altered coagulability, thrombocytosis, nonarteriosclerotic vasculopathies, lacunar infarction, and artery to artery emboli." Artery to artery emboli resulting from atherosclerotic disease of intra- and extracranial cerebral vessels are currently considered the most common cause of TIAs (3).

Differential Diagnosis

Before the diagnosis of TIA is made, other conditions that can produce transient neurological dysfunction must be considered. *Epileptic seizures* (see Chapter 80) can result in transient neurological symptoms, but the history of either a grand mal seizure with loss of consciousness, clonic movement of a subsequently weakened limb, or a rapid march of sensory symptoms will aid in reaching the correct diagnosis. *Migraine attacks* (see Chapter 79) are occasionally associated with sensory or motor symptoms that resemble TIAs. With migraine, however, the patients are usually younger, headache is almost invariably present, and the spread of symptoms often occurs with a characteristic march over minutes to hours. *Disorder of a vestibular end organ* (see Chapter 81) can lead to dizziness or vertigo suggestive of the brainstem ischemia of a vertebrobasilar TIA. However, as noted earlier, brainstem ischemia usually results in additional symptoms such as diplopia, dysphagia, dysarthria, weakness, sensory changes, ataxia, or loss of vision. A *mass lesion* such as a tumor or subdural hematoma will occasionally present with recurrent transient neurological symptoms. A careful examination of the patient may reveal mild persisting neurological signs that progress over time, and the lesion can often be detected by CT scan (see "Patient Experience," Chapter 78). *Hypoglycemia* can lead to transient neurological symptoms, which may be focal if the hypoglycemia is superimposed on existing occlusive cerebrovascular disease. Finally, transient neurological abnormalities may be present for a short interval *following syncope due to any cause* (see Chapter 81).

Natural History

The natural history of TIAs has long been debated. In his review of 27 articles on this subject Brust (9) concluded that "differences in definition, patient selection, therapy, duration of follow-ups, patient age, socioeconomic status, associated disease and other factors, leave considerable uncertainty about the natural history of TIA." Despite this variability in the published reports, the available data indicate that TIAs represent a significant warning of impending stroke, with between 25 and 40% of patients experiencing a cerebral infarction within 5 years of their first TIA (39). The 15-year experience (1955 to 1969) of the Mayo Clinic perhaps provides the best information on natural history. During this period the average annual incidence of first TIA in Rochester, Minnesota, was 31/100,000 population with the rate increasing with age (51). While long term survival after the first TIA was not significantly different from that anticipated for the general population matched for age and sex, the risk of stroke occurrence was markedly increased. Specifically, 36% of patients with TIAs experienced a stroke over an average follow-up of 7.5 years; this was an incidence 9 times greater than the incidence in subjects without a history of TIAs. A large percentage of the strokes occurred in the first few months after the onset of TIAs indicating that this was a particularly high risk period. The risk was similar for TIAs in the carotid and vertebrobasilar territories.

Evaluation and Management

The patient who experiences an episode of transient focal neurological dysfunction should be hospitalized for observation and evaluation. A detailed personal and medical history is essential to identify risk factors for cerebrovascular disease and to classify the presenting symptoms (see above). During the general physical and neurologic examination the physician should seek evidence of hypotension, hypertension, cardiac disease, peripheral vascular disease, and persisting neurologic disability. Auscultation of the head and neck should be performed to detect the presence of a bruit (see details, Fig. 78.3). The patient should also have a careful funduscopic evaluation to assess the status of the retinal vessels and to detect emboli (see example, Fig. 83.1) that suggest atherothrombotic carotid occlusive disease or cardiac valve disease. (See detailed description of the neurovascular exam in Chapter 78.) If there is clinical evidence of heart disease, an echocardiogram should be obtained. Holter monitoring is frequently used to detect significant cardiac arrhythmias that may contribute to the patient's symptoms.

Selected patients with TIAs should have a noninvasive carotid evaluation (ophthalmodynamometry or Doppler studies—see "Patient Experience," Chapter 78) to detect evidence of a stenotic and hemodynamically significant arterial lesion (1). Laboratory evaluation should routinely include a complete blood count, prothrombin time, erythrocyte sedimentation rate, serum glucose and lipid profile, se-

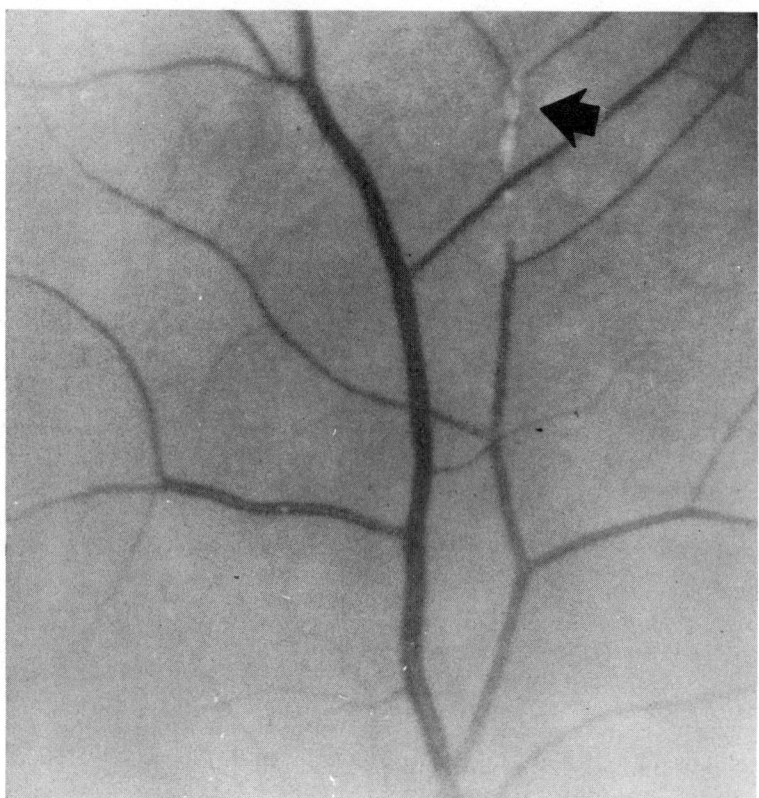

Figure 83.1. Atheromatous debris embolus lodged in retinal arteriole (*arrow*) in patient with recurrent hemisphere TIA and amaurosis fugax. These emboli persist for hours to weeks, and even permanently, while the platelet-fibrin emboli are fleeting and gone within a few minutes. (From Meyer JS, Shaw T: *Diagnosis and Management of Stroke and TIAs.* Baltimore, Williams & Wilkins, 1982.)

rological test for syphilis, serum creatinine, and urinalysis. In selected patients, valuable information may be provided by additional studies such as EEG, cerebral CT scan, vestibular and auditory function tests.

The data generated in the initial workup are often sufficient to allow an accurate diagnosis of the disorder underlying the transient neurological symptoms. Although the most common type of TIA results from artery to artery emboli, optimal treatment for this condition remains controversial. Despite the extensive data generated on this subject, the proponents of the use of anticoagulants, antiplatelet agents, and surgery continue to disagree. The following guidelines are based on recommendations by Sandok *et al* (44) and McDowell *et al* (38).

Patients with a diagnosis of artery to artery embolic TIA who demonstrate evidence of an active process (*i.e.*, multiple recurrent events) should be hospitalized and started on intravenous heparin therapy, if there are no contraindications, while their evaluation proceeds.

Those patients with typical symptoms referable to the distribution of the carotid artery, who would accept surgery and who have a reasonable surgical risk (see Chapter 86), should have *angiography* to determine whether there is a localized, extracranial, surgically accessible lesion of the artery. Angiography should also be considered for patients with less typical symptoms who have markedly positive carotid noninvasive studies. For ambulatory patients, *digital venous subtraction angiography* can be considered (see description, Chapter 78). Its advantages over arterial angiography are that there is less risk and the patient does not have to be hospitalized. It requires more contrast material, does not visualize the intracranial vessels, and is only sensitive enough to detect high grade stenosis. *Digital arterial subtraction angiography* is currently the optimal technique, offering higher resolution with lesser amounts of contrast material and a lower complication rate than conventional arteriography.

Patient experience. The patient can expect the following experience when admitted for four-vessel conventional carotid angiography: He is allowed nothing by mouth for 12 hours before the study and will usually receive premedication consisting of either an analgesic or an anxiolytic drug before going to the radiology suite. After local anesthesia, a catheter-containing needle is inserted percutaneously into a femoral artery. Substantial time is devoted to the positioning of catheters, under fluoroscopic guidance. Dye is injected into both vertebral and both carotid arteries—also into the aortic arch when an arch study is included. For about 30 seconds after each dye injection the patient feels intense warmth in a location adjacent to the injection (the neck, the face, or the substernal area). Nausea may also occur. Throughout the procedure, the patient is supine and his head is immobilized in a soft mold. Total time in the radiology suite is about 1½ hours. The reported incidence of neurological complications from angiography in TIA or stroke patients varies from 1 to 12%; a small proportion of these complications may leave permanent deficits (14, 16).

Carotid endarterectomy, with or without long term antiplatelet therapy, can be recommended to those patients whose angiograms show a significant arterial lesion that is at the carotid bifurcation and that could account for the patient's clinical symptoms. If stenotic disease is more severe in the intracranial carotid artery or the middle cerebral artery, then surgery of the carotid in the neck should not be recommended. If there is additional less severe disease in other extracranial or intracranial vessels, then, following surgery, long term antiplatelet therapy is recommended.

Surgical revascularization has been successfully performed with acceptably low morbidity (less than 5%) in patients in whom the carotid artery is totally occluded or the severe stenotic lesion is inaccessible (e.g., in the intracranial portion of the internal carotid or the middle cerebral artery) (5). This procedure is known as the external carotid internal carotid bypass and consists of anastomosing branches of the external carotid artery (usually the superficial temporal) to branches of the middle cerebral artery (usually the angular branches) through a craniectomy. The efficacy of this procedure in preventing strokes in the long term is currently being evaluated in a randomized trial (4). Preliminary results indicate no benefit from this procedure in the long term prevention of stroke except perhaps in a very small subgroup of patients which has yet to be identified.

In severe cases of basilar vertebral insufficiency with recurrent strokes in the basilar vertebral territory and arteriographic evidence of bilateral vertebral compromise or high grade basilar stenosis, other bypass procedures have been undertaken. These procedures require the skill of a highly competent neurovascular surgeon and are used as last resorts. Bypasses have been successfully completed under the above conditions between the occipital artery and the posterior inferior cerebellar artery, the occipital and the anterior inferior cerebellar artery, and the superficial temporal artery and the

superior cerebellar artery. Their efficacy has not yet been established, although they have been successfully completed with relatively low morbidity in small numbers of patients (12).

Patients with a history of recurrent TIAs who are not candidates for surgery must be managed medically. Those initially treated with heparin should be switched to coumadin, with close follow-up, for a period of 1½ to 3 months. Thereafter, they should be treated indefinitely with aspirin, 650 mg twice daily. In contrast to antiplatelet therapy, Coumadin has not been proven in controlled trials to be efficacious in long term stroke prevention. It is, however, frequently used where antiplatelet therapy has failed.

Patients with a single TIA who do not require anticoagulants or those for whom these medications are contraindicated should be treated with aspirin or other antiplatelet agents (see Chapter 51).

These guidelines for the management of patients with TIAs due to artery to artery emboli are not comprehensive and the reader is referred to the excellent review by Sandok et al (44). Treatment must be individualized to meet the unique needs of each patient. Decisions regarding management, especially in an area as controversial as this, often require input from a neurologist who specializes in the field of cerebrovascular disease.

ASYMPTOMATIC CERVICAL BRUIT

The asymptomatic patient with a cervical bruit is encountered commonly in ambulatory practice. For example, 4.4% of subjects over the age of 45 had asymptomatic cervical bruits in a population-based study in Evans County, Georgia, and the majority of the bruits were heard anteriorly in the neck over the location of the carotid artery (25). Although atherosclerosis probably accounts for most of these bruits, a number of other mechanisms are possible (see Table 83.9).

Natural History

Prospective studies of asymptomatic patients with an anterior cervical bruit have demonstrated an increased risk of cerebrovascular disease. There is disagreement, however, as to (a) whether the initial neurological deficit in the patient who becomes symptomatic is more likely to be transient or permanent and (b) whether the side of the bruit is of any predictive value in determining the location of the initial neurological event. At one extreme is the view that the initial deficit is often permanent and is most likely to occur in the vascular territory distal to the carotid artery with the bruit. At the other extreme is the belief that the initial event is almost invariably transient and can occur with equal fre-

Table 83.9.
Possible Causes of Cervical Bruit

Physiological murmur
Venous hum
Transmitted cardiac murmur
Atherosclerosis of carotid, vertebral, subclavian, or innominate artery
Loops, kinks, inflammation, fibromuscular dysplasia of carotid artery
Arteriovenous fistula
Angiomatous malformation
Intracranial neoplasm
Paget's disease of the skull

quency in the distribution of the affected or contralateral carotid artery. It is clear from a review of the available data that further studies are required to resolve these critical issues, which bear directly on the need for aggressive management of these asymptomatic patients.

Evaluation and Management

The physical examination of the neurovascular system is described in detail in Chapter 78. At times, the auscultatory characteristics of a cervical bruit can help to estimate its importance (see Fig. 78.3).

The evaluation and treatment of the asymptomatic patient with an anterior cervical bruit is controversial. Many authorities believe that there is no role for cerebral angiography and surgical intervention in the management of these patients (25), while others feel that for certain "high risk" patients these invasive procedures may be indicated (26). According to the latter view, a patient whose bruit is in the location of the carotid bifurcation (near the angle of the jaw) should have a careful funduscopic examination to look for emboli (see Fig. 83.1) as well as a noninvasive carotid evaluation (ophthalmodynamometry and Doppler studies (see "Patient Experience," Chapter 78); and angiography should be considered for those patients with markedly positive noninvasive studies, those with retinal emboli seen on funduscopic examination, or those scheduled for major vascular surgery in the thorax or abdomen that might result in transient intra- or postoperative hypotension. Considerable difference of opinion exists about the benefits of carotid endarterectomy in patients with high grade stenosis, shown by arteriography, who are asymptomatic. No controlled studies have been completed that support a decrease in the occurrence of stroke when endarterectomy has been done either as a prelude to major vascular surgery, coronary artery bypass surgery or in the uncomplicated asymptomatic patient. Despite this, carotid endarterectomy is often performed in instances where high grade carotid stenosis does exist in the asymptomatic patient. Such an approach should be considered only where an experienced team of neurologists and neurovascular surgeons is available.

There is general agreement that patients who do not undergo surgery must be followed closely for any change in the character of their bruit suggestive of progressive disease and for the occurrence of symptoms referable to an underlying arterial lesion. These patients should also be followed by interval noninvasive studies of carotid flow. When and if these studies become positive, serious consideration should be given to further evaluation of the extent of the disease with cerebral arteriography. It is reasonable to prescribe aspirin for these patients, although to date no study has assessed its role in this situation. Because serial angiographic studies have suggested that the rate of atheromatous change at the carotid bifurcation is directly related to hypertension (28), antihypertensive treatment is important in patients with asymptomatic bruits and high blood pressure; in these patients, it is particularly important to avoid the orthostatic hypotension which may accompany use of any antihypertensive drug.

General References

Benton AL (ed): *Behavioral Changes in Cerebrovascular Disease.* New York, Harper & Row, 1970.
    A detailed account of psychological problems complicating stroke.
Kistler JP, Ropper AH, Heros RC: Therapy of ischemic cerebral vascular disease due to atherothrombosis. *N Engl J Med* 311:27, 1984.
    Thorough review of the subject, extensively referenced.
Licht S (ed): *Stroke and Its Rehabilitation.* Baltimore, Williams & Wilkins, 1975.
    A detailed, well illustrated, and extensively referenced resource on all aspects of the rehabilitation of stroke patients.
Sessler GJ: *Stroke—How to Prevent It/How to Survive It.* Englewood Cliffs, NJ, Prentice-Hall, 1982.
    A comprehensive discussion of stroke and its prevention for the physician and potential patient.

Specific References

1. Ackerman RH: Noninvasive carotid evaluation. *Stroke* 11:675, 1980.
2. Ausman J, Diaz F, DeLos RA, et al: Extracranial intracranial anastomoses in the posterior circulation. In Berguer R, Bauer, RD (eds): *Vertebrobasilar Occlusive Disease: Medical and Surgical Management,* New York, Raven Press, 1984, p 313.
3. Barnett HJM: The pathophysiology of transient cerebral ischemic attacks. Therapy with platelet antiaggregants. *Med Clin North Am* 63:649, 1979.
4. Barnett HJM, Peerless SJ: Collaborative EC/IC bypass study: the rationale and a progress report. In Massey J, Reinmuth OM (eds): *Cerebrovascular Diseases.* New York, Raven Press, 1981, p 271.
5. Barnett HJM, Plum F, Walton JM: Carotid endarterectomy—an expression of concern. *Stroke* 15:941, 1984.
6. Beevers DG, Fairman MJ, Hamilton M, Harpur JE: Antihypertensive treatment and the course of established cerebrovascular disease. *Lancet* 1:1407, 1973.
7. Bourestom NC: Predictors of long term recovery in cerebro-

vascular disease. *Arch Phys Med Rehabil* 48:415, 1967.

8. Bousser MG, Eschwege E, Haguenau M, *et al*: "AICLA" controlled trial of aspirin and dipyridamole in the secondary prevention of athero-thrombotic cerebral ischemia. *Stroke* 14:5, 1983.

9. Brust JCM: Transient ischemic attacks: Natural history and anticoagulation. *Neurology* 27:701, 1977.

10. Canadian Cooperative Study Group: A randomized trial of aspirin and sulfinpyrazone in threatened stroke. *N Engl J Med* 299:53, 1978.

11. Carter AB: Hypertensive therapy in stroke survivors. *Lancet* 1:485, 1970.

12. Chambers BR, Norris JW: The case against surgery for asymptomatic carotid stenosis stroke. *Stroke* 15:964, 1984.

13. Easton JD, Sherman DG: Management of cerebral embolism of cardiac origin. *Stroke* 11:433, 1980.

14. Eisenberg RL, Bank WO, Hedgcock MW: Neurologic complications of angiography for cerebrovascular disease. *Neurology* 30:895, 1980.

15. Eisenberg H, Morrison JT, Sullivan P, Foote FM: Cerebrovascular accidents: incidence and survival rates in a defined population. Middlesex County, Connecticut. *JAMA* 189:883, 1964.

16. Faught E, Tarder SD, Hanna GR: Cerebral complications of angiography for transient ischemia and stroke: prediction of risk. *Neurology* 29:4, 1979.

17. Feibel JH, Berk S, Joynt RJ: The unmet needs of stroke survivors. *Neurology* 29:592, 1979.

18. Fisher CM: Lacunar strokes and infarcts: a review. *Neurology* 32:871, 1982.

19. Folstein MF, Maiberger R, McHugh PR: Mood disorders as a specific complication of stroke. *J Neurol Neurosurg Psychiatry* 40:1018, 1977.

20. Gainotti G: Emotional behavior and hemispheric side of the lesion. *Cortex* 8:41, 1972.

21. Garraway NW, Whisnant JP, Drury ID: The continuing decline in the incidence of stroke. *Mayo Clin Proc* 58:520, 1983.

22. Genton E, Barnett HJM, Fields *et al*: XIV: Cerebral ischemia: the role of thrombosis and of antithrombotic therapy. *Stroke* 8:147, 1977.

23. Gresham GE, Fitzpatrick TE, Wolf PA, *et al*: Residual disability in survivors of stroke—the Framingham study. *N Engl J Med* 293:954, 1975.

24. Hachinski V: Decreased incidence and mortality of stroke. *Stroke* 15:376, 1984.

25. Heyman A, Wilkinson WE, Heyden S, *et al*: Risk of stroke in asymptomatic persons with cervical arterial bruits: a population study in Evans County, Georgia. *N Engl J Med* 302:838, 1980.

26. Hurst JW, Hopkins LC, Smith RB: Noises in the neck. *N Engl J Med* 302:862, 1980.

27. Hypertensive-Stroke Cooperative Study Group: Effects of antihypertensive treatment on stroke recurrence. *JAMA* 229:409, 1974.

28. Javid H, Ostermiller WE, Hengesh JW, *et al*: Natural history of carotid bifurcation atheroma. *Surgery* 67:80, 1970.

29. Kannel WB: Current status of the epidemiology of brain infarction associated with occlusive arterial disease. *Stroke* 2:295, 1971.

30. Kannel WB, Gordon T, Wolf PA, McNamara PM: Hemoglobin and the risk of cerebral infarction: the Framingham study. *Stroke* 3:409, 1972.

31. Kannel WB, Wolf PA, Verter J, McNamara PM: Epidemiologic assessment of the role of blood pressure in stroke. *JAMA* 214:301, 1970.

32. Katz S, Ford AB, Chinn AB, Newill, VA: Prognosis after strokes: II. Long term course of 159 patients. *Medicine* 45:236, 1966.

33. Kurtzke JF: Epidemiology of cerebrovascular disease. In Siekert RG (ed): *Cerebrovascular Survey Report*. Rochester, Minn. Whiting Press, 1980.

34. Lehmann JF, DeLateur BJ, Fowler RS, *et al*: Stroke: does rehabilitation affect outcome? *Arch Phys Med Rehabil* 56:375, 1975.

35. Lehmann JF, Delateur BJ, Fowler RS, *et al*: Stroke rehabilitation: outcome and prediction. *Arch Phys Med Rehabil* 56:383, 1975.

36. Louis S, McDowell F: Epileptic seizures in nonembolic cerebral infarction. *Arch Neurol* 27:414, 1967.

37. Matsumoto N, Whisnant JP, Kurland LT, Okazaki H: Natural history of stroke in Rochester, Minnesota, 1955 through 1969: an extension of a previous study, 1945 through 1954. *Stroke* 4:20, 1973.

38. McDowell FH, Millikan CH, Goldstein M: Treatment of impending stroke. *Stroke* 11:1, 1980.

39. Millikan C: The transient ischemic attack. *Adv Neurol* 25:135, 1979.

40. Richardson EP, Jr, Dodge PR: Epilepsy in cerebral vascular disease: a study of the incidence and nature of seizures in 104 consecutive autopsy-proven cases of cerebral infarction and hemorrhage. *Epilepsy* 3:49, 1954.

41. Robinson RG, Starr LB, Kubos KL, Price TR: A two-year longitudinal study of post-stroke mood disorders: findings during the initial evaluation. *Stroke* 14:736, 1983.

42. Robinson RG, Starr LB, Lipsey JR, *et al*: A two-year longitudinal study of post-stroke mood disorders: dynamic changes in associated variables over the first six months of follow-up. *Stroke* 15:510, 1984.

43. Ross GS, Chipman M: The neuralgias. In Baker AB, Baker LH (eds): *Clinical Neurology*. Hagerstown, Harper & Row, 1974, vol. 3.

44. Sandok BA, Furlan AJ, Whisnant JP *et al*: Guidelines for the management of transient ischemic attacks. *Mayo Clin Proc* 53:665, 1978.

45. Sarno MT: Disorders of communication in stroke. In Licht S (ed): *Stroke and Its Rehabilitation*. Baltimore, Williams & Wilkins, 1975.

46. Sorenson PS, Pedersen H, Maquardsen J, *et al*: Acetylsalicylic acid in the prevention of stroke in patients with reversible cerebral ischemic attacks. A Danish cooperative study. *Stroke* 14:15, 1983.

47. Tohgi H, Yamanouchi H, Murakami M, *et al*: Importance of the hematocrit as a risk factor in cerebral infarction. *Stroke* 9:369, 1978.

48. Veterans Administration Cooperative Study Group on Antihypertensive Agents: Effects of treatment on morbidity in hypertension. Results in patients with diastolic blood pressures averaging 115 through 129 mm Hg. *JAMA* 202:1028, 1967.

49. Veterans Administration Cooperative Study Group on Antihypertensive Agents: Effects of treatment on morbidity in hypertension. II. Results in patients with diastolic blood pressure averaging 90 through 114 mm Hg. *JAMA* 213:1143, 1970.

50. Whisnant JP: The decline of stroke. *Stroke* 15:160, 1984.

51. Whisnant JP, Matsumoto N, Elveback LR: Transient cerebral ischemic attacks in a community. *Mayo Clin Proc* 48:194, 1973.

52. Wolf PA, Kannel WB, McNamara PM, Gordon T: The role of impaired cardiac function in atherothrombotic brain infarction: the Framingham study. *Am J Public Health* 63:52, 1973.

CHAPTER EIGHTY-FOUR

Peripheral Neuropathy

LORRAINE F. JOSIFEK, M.D., AND MARGIT L. BLEECKER, M.D., PH.D.

DEFINITIONS AND PATHOPHYSIOLOGY

A peripheral nerve is a bundle of fibers called axons; the large and medium-sized axons are normally covered with a layer of myelin. Most peripheral nerves are mixed nerves carrying both incoming sensory information (afferent fibers) and outgoing motor and autonomic impulses (efferent fibers). Large diameter afferent fibers convey information about position and vibration; large diameter efferent fibers innervate the muscles themselves. Small diameter, often unmyelinated, fibers convey pain and temperature sensation, as well as autonomic information.

Peripheral neuropathies result from disease processes which involve nerve axons or their myelin encasements. Axonal neuropathies are the result of processes which primarily affect the cell body and axon, whereas demyelinating neuropathies result from processes which primarily affect the myelin sheath. Often, especially in chronic disorders such as diabetes, irrespective of the initial type of pathological process, the interdependence between axon and myelin produces secondary changes which, on biopsy, reveal a mixed pathological picture. The etiological diagnosis of peripheral neuropathies, therefore, usually depends upon their clinical features and on other supportive laboratory findings.

The three major patterns of peripheral nerve disease may be distinguished by clinical presentation: mononeuropathy, multifocal neuropathies (mononeuropathy multiplex), and polyneuropathy. *Mononeuropathies* are lesions of individual nerve roots or peripheral nerves; they usually are due to local causes such as trauma or entrapment (compression of a nerve by adjacent structures). *Multifocal neuropathy* (also called mononeuropathy multiplex) refers to involvement of two or more discrete nerves, usually asymmetrically and not contiguously, either at the same time or sequentially. This less common pattern is usually caused by systemic diseases such as polyarteritis nodosa or diabetes which may affect several nerves focally. *Polyneuropathy* is the result of a generalized disease process affecting the peripheral nerves in a symmetrical distal distribution. In both axonal and demyelinating diseases the longer and larger axons (nerves) are involved earlier and more severely than the shorter ones. In demyelinating neuropathies, this is because the longer axons have more potential sites for demyelination; in the axonal neuropathies, the longer axons require more metabolic support and are therefore more susceptible to curtailment of this support. Therefore, symptoms of both types of neuropathies tend to appear first in the feet and then in the hands. Most polyneuropathies indiscriminately affect both the sensory and the motor nerve fibers (mixed polyneuropathies or sensorimotor neuropathies). However, clinically (and occasionally pathologically), in some patients there will be a predilection for either the sensory nerves (sensory polyneuropathies) or motor nerves (motor polyneuropathies).

APPROACH TO THE PATIENT

History and Physical Examination

Symptoms of peripheral neuropathy include loss of sensation (sometimes accompanied by pain), weakness, muscle cramps and symptoms of autonomic dysfunction (impotence, urinary retention or overflow incontinence, constipation or diarrhea, and orthostatic hypotension). In patients with polyneuropathy, paresthesias (pins and needles) located in the feet are the most common presenting complaint. Many other sensory misperceptions occur and are difficult for the patient to describe. Frequently the patient is bothered by non-noxious sensory stimuli (e.g., light touch perceived as burning), and they may be somewhat relieved by pacing the floor, by firm massage, or by cold (e.g., leaving the legs outside the covers at night). Complaints of heaviness or coldness of the extremities are also common.

The major *signs* of peripheral neuropathy are sensory loss, weakness, muscle atrophy, diminished or absent tendon reflexes and trophic changes in the skin. The most common sensory modalities diminished in polyneuropathy are pain and vibration, in a symmetrical stocking-glove distribution. Temperature is usually also affected but is harder to document in the clinical setting. In polyneuropathies the weakness is most often distal, affecting the intrinsic muscles of the feet, causing inability to spread the toes and difficult walking on uneven surfaces. In long-standing neuropathies the muscle imbalance causes high arched feet and hammer toes. Eventually the shin may appear prominent because of atrophy of the tibialis anterior muscle and there may be striking wasting of the small muscles of the hand. The skin of the lower extremities may appear shiny, scaling, and atrophic. Marked loss of proprioception in the feet may be manifest as unsteadiness, ataxia, or a positive Romberg test (see Chapter 78 for additional details about neurological signs).

Distinctive Features

While a limited number of conditions produce mononeuropathy and multifocal neuropathy (Table 84.1), there are many etiologies of polyneuropathy (Table 84.2). Diagnosis often depends on obtaining a thorough history (for example, of alcoholism or of occupational exposure to toxins) or on finding a relevant systemic condition (for example, diabetes). Therefore, the physician must be alert to distinctive features in the history or on physical examination that suggest a specific diagnosis. Table 84.3 summarizes the distinctive clinical features of a number of polyneuropathies.

Table 84.1.
Common Causes of Neuropathy

MONONEUROPATHY
    Trauma—direct (occupational, recreational) (*e.g.,* ulnar or peroneal nerve), compression and entrapment (carpal tunnel, root compression, *etc*)
    Infection—herpes zoster
    Toxins (*e.g.,* penicillin injection into a sciatic nerve)
    Vascular—vasculitis, diabetes mellitus
    Neoplasm—lymphoma, neurofibroma
MULTIFOCAL NEUROPATHY
    Diabetes mellitus
    Vasculitis
POLYNEUROPATHY
    Multiple etiologies (see Table 84.2)

Time Course

Mononeuropathies are often acute in onset; that is, the patient remembers the time of onset. The most common of the acute polyneuropathies is the Guillain-Barré syndrome but other processes—metabolic, infectious, or toxic—may cause severe neurological dysfunction rapidly, sometimes within-hours. Most toxic neuropathies (lead poisoning, for example) develop somewhat more slowly—within weeks—as do neuropathies associated with malnutrition (e.g., thiamine deficiency). The most common of the chronic neuropathies (gradual progression over months to years) are associated with diabetes mellitus (see Chapter 72) and with alcoholism (see below); and, in an unselected population, these are the most common of the polyneuropathies in general.

Patients with hereditary neuropathies sometimes may be unaware that they suffer from a long-standing progressive disorder. A history of a lack of athletic ability in school or difficulties with maneuvers in the military or of problems fitting shoes may be a useful clue in that regard. High arched feet and hammer toes reflect long-standing disease and may point to the diagnosis of one of these hereditary processes.

Patterns of Involvement

Mononeuropathy usually produces both motor and sensory involvement in the distribution of the affected nerve root or peripheral nerve (see below, Tables 84.6–84.7).

Most polyneuropathies produce both sensory and motor disturbances. Polyneuropathy with predominantly sensory involvement suggests diabetes, carcinoma, amyloidosis, dysproteinemia, and alcoholism. Occasionally, sensory losses are dissociated; that is, the patient has diminished appreciation of pain and temperature but preserved appreciation of

Table 84.2.
Distinctive Features, by Etiology, of the Polyneuropathies

Etiology	Dominant Pathology	Involvement	Typical Distribution	Typical Time Course
METABOLIC/DEFICIENCY				
Diabetes mellitus:				
Polyneuropathy	Axonal	Sensory	Distal symmetric	Chronic
Mononeuropathy and mononeuropathy multiplex	Ischemic	Sensorimotor	Cranial III, VI, VII, lumbar plexus	Acute or sub-acute
Autonomic	Neuronopathy	Autonomic	Bladder, gastrointestinal, peripheral vessels	Chronic
Alcoholism and vitamin deficiency	Axonal	Sensorimotor, autonomic	Distal, symmetric	Chronic/subacute
Uremia	Axonal and segmental demyelination	Sensorimotor	Distal, symmetric	Chronic/subacute
Hypothyroidism	Axonal and demyelination	Sensory > motor	Distal, symmetric, carpal tunnel	Subacute/chronic
Porphyria	Axonal	Motor > sensory	Proximal	Acute
Toxin[a]:				
Lead	(?)Axonal	Motor	Asymmetrical, radial wrist-drop	Subacute
Pyridoxine	Neuronopathy	Sensory	Distal	Subacute
Most other toxins and drugs	Axonal	Sensorimotor	Distal	Subacute
INFECTION				
Diphtheria	Demyelination	Motor	Bulbar and Distal	Acute 30–50 days following pharyngitis
Leprosy	Demyelination	Sensory	Distal, temperature areas	Chronic
Herpes zoster	Neuronitis	Sensory	Cranial nerves and roots	Acute
INFLAMMATORY				
Guillain-Barré syndrome	Demyelination	Motor	Ascending proximal, bulbar	Acute
Recurrent inflammatory polyneuropathy	Demyelination	Motor	Proximal	Relapsing
COLLAGEN VASCULAR				
Systemic lupus erythematosus, polyarteritis nodosa	Ischemic	Sensorimotor	Mononeuropathy multiplex	Acute/subacute
TUMOR				
Carcinomatous, sensory	Neuronopathy	Sensory, painful	Distal	Subacute
Carcinomatous, sensorimotor	Axonal	Sensorimotor	Distal	Subacute
Paraproteinemia (e.g., myeloma, primary amyloidosis)	Axonal	Sensorimotor	Distal, carpal tunnel	Chronic
HEREDITARY				
Charcot-Marie-Tooth syndrome	Axonal or demyelinating	Motor	Distal	Very chronic
Amyloidosis	Compressive, axonal, ischemic	Sensorimotor, autonomic	Distal or entrapment, carpal tunnel	Chronic

[a] See list of toxins and drugs causing neuropathy, Table 84.5.

Table 84.3.
Differential Diagnosis of Polyneuropathies[a, b]

COURSE
  Acute (days):
    Guillain-Barré syndrome
    Porphyric neuropathy
    Diphtheritic neuropathy
    Some toxins (*e.g.*, triorthocresyl phosphate)
  Subacute (weeks):
    Many toxins
    Nutritional neuropathies
    Carcinomatous neuropathies
    Uremic neuropathy
  Relapsing:
    Relapsing inflammatory neuropathy
    Refsum's disease
  Chronic (many months or years):
    Diabetic motor-sensory neuropathy
    Alcoholic neuropathy
    Chronic inflammatory neuropathies
  Very chronic (childhood onset):
    Heritable motor-sensory neuropathies (*e.g.*, Charcot-Marie-Tooth disease)
SELECTIVE FUNCTIONAL INVOLVEMENT[c]
  Predominately motor:
    Guillain-Barré syndrome
    Relapsing and chronic inflammatory neuropathy
    Acute intermittent porphyria
    Lead neuropathy
    Heritable motor-sensory neuropathies (Charcot-Marie-Tooth)
    Diphtheritic neuropathy
  Predominately sensory:

Global loss:
  Diabetes
  Carcinomatous sensory neuropathy (ganglioradiculitis)
  Paraproteinemic and cryoglobulinemic neuropathy
  Tabes dorsalis
Dissociated loss of pain and thermal sensibility:
  Diabetes (small fiber type)
  Amyloidosis
  Hereditary sensory neuropathies
  Lepromatous leprosy
Dissociated loss of joint position and vibration sensibility:
  Subacute combined degeneration
  Friedreich's ataxia
Autonomic neuropathy:
  Diabetes
  Amyloid
  Acute, chronic, and relapsing pandysautonomia
  Dysautonomia (Riley-Day)
DISTRIBUTION[d]
  Proximal weakness:
    Guillain-Barré
    Porphyria
    Carcinomatous neuropathy with proximal weakness ("carcinomatous neuromyopathy")
    Spinal muscular atrophies
  Proximal sensory loss:
    Porphyria
    Tangier disease (analphalipoproteinemia)
  Temperature-related distribution:
    Lepromatous leprosy

---

[a] Adapted from Griffen JW: Peripheral neuropathies. In Harvey AM *et al* (eds): *Principles and Practice of Medicine*, ed 21. New York, Appleton-Century-Crofts, 1984.

[b] The most common etiologies are set in *italic*.
[c] Most polyneuropathies produce sensory and motor disturbances.
[d] Most polyneuropathies produce distal involvement.

---

light touch and joint position; this pattern is typical of small fiber neuropathies. When pain sensation is lost but position sense is preserved, vitamin B_{12} deficiency (usually pernicious anemia) or, much more rarely, Friedreich's ataxia should be considered. In polyneuropathy, predominantly motor involvement suggests the Guillain-Barré syndrome, hereditary neuropathies, lead intoxication, and acute intermittent porphyria. Predominantly autonomic involvement suggests diabetes, amyloidosis, alcoholism, dysautonomia, and dysproteinemia.

INVESTIGATIONS

Laboratory

It is important to identify the cause of a peripheral neuropathy because often neurological dysfunction will persist unless the underlying disease can be treated. The common causes of polyneuropathy (shown in *italics* in Table 84.3) are usually obvious to the physician; but sometimes, even these require direct questioning (concerning alcoholism, for example) or specific laboratory tests (for example, measurement of serum glucose or of thyroid func-

tion) before they are appreciated. If the cause of the neuropathy is not obvious, routine screening tests should include erythrocyte sedimentation rate, fasting blood glucose, serum urea nitrogen or serum creatinine, thyroxine (T_4), a complete blood count (CBC), a chest X-ray, and, in patients over the age of 40, a serum protein electrophoresis. There are many relatively unusual conditions that may be associated with neuropathy, but an extensive screening program to rule out all of these processes would be expensive and almost always unrewarding unless there is some clue in the history or physical examination to warrant a particular test (for example, measurement of blood lead in a patient with a history of occupational exposure). If, after evaluating a patient with neuropathy, no cause of the process has been identified, consultation with a neurologist should be considered.

Nerve Conduction Studies

The measurement of nerve conduction velocity is helpful in establishing the diagnosis, severity, and location of the neuropathy. A baseline measurement makes it possible to differentiate progression of the peripheral neuropathy from other clinical conditions at future points in time. Although there are laboratories that will perform nerve conduction studies upon demand, it is prudent to let a neurologist decide about the usefulness and the interpretation of the procedure.

Nerve conduction velocity measurements involve stimulating a nerve at one point and recording the response, either at the muscle, or at some distance along the nerve. The former applies to motor nerve and the latter to sensory nerve conduction rates. The results of nerve conduction studies usually include latency of response, conduction velocity, and amplitude of response. The latency of response refers to the time elapsed between the start of the stimulus and the muscle response (muscle fiber depolarization) or nerve response (sensory nerve action potential). By subtracting the latencies determined by stimulating the same nerve at two different sites, the nerve conduction velocity for the segment between the two points is obtained. The conduction velocity is calculated by dividing the distance between two points of stimulation by the difference between the latencies (time) obtained by stimulating at the two points. In this way, the conduction velocity is determined between two points along the nerve and is always expressed in meters per second. In sensory conduction studies, the latency can also be measured by stimulating the trunk of a mixed nerve and recording the nerve potential to the second point along the same nerve trunk. Since large diameter sensory fibers have lower thresholds and conduct faster than motor fibers by about 5 to 10%, the mixed nerve potentials allow determination of the faster sensory nerve potentials.

Conduction disturbances of the peripheral nerve may be localized, as in an entrapment syndrome, or may involve nerves more diffusely as in polyneuropathies. In general, early axonal degenerations are associated with normal conduction and the presence of denervation on electromyography (EMG, see below), whereas demyelination is characterized by slowing of nerve conduction and normal EMG studies.

The procedure has several limitations. First, nerve conduction velocities (NCVs) only test directly that portion of the nerve between the two sites; they generally do not detect damage more distal than (e.g., muscle) or more proximal to (e.g., nerve root) the segment tested. F waves may detect proximal segment pathology but are not performed routinely. The standard test is therefore not directly applicable to such common clinical situations as spondylosis or lumbar or cervical disc disease (see Chapters 64 and 65). Second, NCVs measure the speed of conduction in the largest and fastest conducting fibers of peripheral nerves. Therefore, nerve conduction studies are only sensitive to diseases which involve such fibers.

It is important for the clinician to be able to specify as precisely as possible the clinical problem and question to be addressed; stating only "numbness in the upper extremities" or "test nerves in lower extremities" without any specific guidance is likely to be both unpleasant for the patient and unproductive for the physician.

Patient experience. With the patient comfortably positioned paste is applied over the sites to be tested and electrodes are taped over the appropriate muscles and nerves. The shocks may be mildly unpleasant. Usually the nerves on both sides of the body are compared. Testing takes approximately 20 to 60 minutes.

Electromyography

Electromyography (Table 84.4) is not often helpful in the diagnosis of peripheral neuropathy; the sensitivity and specificity of the procedure are relatively low. It is useful primarily in situations in which the distinction between neuropathy and myopathy is difficult (polyneuropathy *versus* polymyositis, for example) and in confirming the diagnosis of an entrapment syndrome (see below). Since EMG is unpleasant, the physician should consider carefully whether the information to be gained from it

Table 84.4.
Electromyography

Disorder	Insertional Activity	Complete Rest (Spontaneous Activity)	Action Potentials	Interference Pattern
Denervation[a]	Increased	Fibrillations, positive waves, fasciculations	High amplitude, long duration, polyphasic	Reduced or incomplete with fast firing rate
Myopathic				
Myopathy	Normal	Normal or rare fibrillations	Small amplitude, short duration polyphasic	Full, small amplitude
Myositis	Increased	Fibrillations, positive waves	Small amplitude, short duration polyphasic	Full, small amplitude

[a] Neuropathy, radiculopathy, disc disease.

is likely to benefit the patient. Consultation with a neurologist is advised in helping to make this decision.

EMG involves the insertion of needles into a muscle to record electrical activity directly. During complete rest, no electrical activity should be observed. *Spontaneous fibrillation* potentials are the action potentials of single fibers that are twitching spontaneously in the absence of innervation. Fibrillation potentials are usually, but not invariably, a good indication of primary denervation (they also occur in polymositis and more rarely in other myopathic processes.) *Fasciculations* are the spontaneous firings of whole motor units (all of the muscle fibers innervated by a single nerve fiber). Fasciculations may be seen in normal individuals, although they are more frequent and likely to be more polyphasic in states of denervation. Therefore, the presence of fasciculations is only moderately useful in diagnosing denervation.

Muscle action potentials are examined individually by asking the patient to move only slightly. Large amplitude, long duration polyphasic potentials suggest a denervating process. Small amplitude, short duration polyphasic potentials are associated with myopathic processes.

The *interference pattern* is the pattern produced when the subject is asked to contract the muscle fully. A "full" interference pattern is normal. Anything less may indicate less than maximal effort (hysteria, malingering), poor conduction of nerve impulses to the muscle (denervation), or poor ability of the muscle to respond (myopathy).

The highest yield of useful information with EMG is from moderately affected muscles. The physician should expect a low yield from muscles that are clinically normal or only minimally involved and should anticipate uninterpretable results from muscles that are severely involved, as end-stage muscle disease of almost any cause ultimately presents the same EMG picture.

The physician should remember that the EMG electrodes damage and inflame the muscles into which they have been inserted (note—serum creatine phosphokinase activity is not altered by this procedure). Thus, if there is a possibility that a muscle biopsy will be required, the muscle that may be examined by biopsy should not be tested by EMG.

Patient experience. There is usually discomfort with the initial insertion of the needles and also during movement of the muscles when the needles are in place. As the needles are very thin and only penetrate skin and muscle, the risks of infection or hemorrhage are almost nil. The procedure takes 30 to 90 minutes.

Nerve Biopsy

Nerve biopsy should be reserved for those patients in whom a specific histological diagnosis is a possibility (for example, amyloidosis or vasculitis). In general the procedure has limited usefulness, since the pathology is usually nonspecific; also the nerve tested by biopsy is usually a sensory nerve (the sural) and may not reflect a disease process which has affected the motor nerves. The biopsy may lead to painful sequelae in the distribution of the tested nerve (usually the sural distribution on the dorsolateral foot). If the nerve biopsy is done, the specimen must be specially processed for maximum information at centers which are familiar with nerve pathology. Consultation with a neurologist will be helpful in deciding whether a nerve biopsy is indicated.

COMMON PROBLEMS

Guillain-Barré Syndrome

Most cases of the Guillain-Barré syndrome (2) follow a mild viral illness (by 10 to 12 days); the syndrome also may be associated with pregnancy, the postoperative period, and with recent influenza immunization. There is rapid progression of symmetric motor weakness (usually moving from the lower extremities to the upper extremities) accompanied by loss of deep tendon reflexes. Although acute pain or paresthesias in the back and posterior legs may be prominent early symptoms, objective evidence of sensory loss is minimal. Cranial nerve weakness may be present, with bilateral facial nerve palsy, in 40% of patients. NCVs may be abnormal, and the cerebrospinal fluid may show increased protein with normal cell counts (cytoalbumin dissociation). Because of rapid progression of the disease, patients suspected of having this disorder should be admitted to the hospital for close monitoring for potential respiratory distress and autonomic disturbances (hypotension, hypertension, cardiac arrhythmias, hyperpyrexia) which are often part of the course. Recent evidence suggests that plasmapheresis early in the course shortens the period of disability. Recovery is complete in about half the patients (although it may take 6 to 18 months); most of the remainder have only mild residual deficits; but 10% have severe permanent disability. The patients may remain at a plateau of function and then suddenly recover. Splints to avoid contractures and passive range of motion should be employed until the recovery period is complete. The differential diagnosis includes diphtheria, botulism, and porphyria.

Diabetic Neuropathy

The prevalence of diabetic neuropathy (5, 13) is not known precisely, but it is clearly one of the more common neuropathies. The problem is discussed in detail in Chapter 72, Diabetes Mellitus.

Alcoholic Neuropathy

Neuropathies associated with alcoholism (3) and with associated vitamin deficiencies usually occur in the fourth to seventh decades with a slow onset over a period of months. The presenting symptoms are varied, but they often reflect a distal, motor and sensory, symmetric polyneuropathy with pain and paresthesias in the feet and legs. Autonomic features, including impotence, bladder dysfunction, and orthostatic hypotension, may also be seen. Malnutrition and vitamin deficiencies (particularly thiamine deficiency) probably make a major contribution to the neuropathy, although there is evidence that alcohol has a direct toxic effect on peripheral nerves.

Treatment is aimed toward improved nutrition and vitamin replacement as well as toward effective treatment for the alcoholism (see Chapter 21). The paresthesia of a mild neuropathy can be expected to improve with good nutrition and abstinence from alcohol. However, with moderate to severe sensorimotor and autonomic neuropathy, significant residual symptoms and findings will persist.

Carcinomatous Neuropathy

Carcinomatous neuropathy (9, 14) (excluding nerve damage from direct invasion of nerves by tumor) occurs most commonly in association with cancer of the lung, sometimes years before the tumor has been diagnosed.

Distal Sensorimotor Neuropathy

This is primarily an axonal process in which the sensory loss predominates in the lower extremities. It develops over weeks or months, and often becomes stationary, or, if the underlying cancer responds to treatment, it may improve.

Carcinomatous Sensory Polyneuropathy

This has the uncommon but distinctive patterns of progressive sensory polyneuropathy beginning in adulthood. The neuropathy usually begins distally and asymmetrically. Over many weeks this process spreads more proximally with the development of profound sensory loss, sometimes accompanied by pain and pseudoathetosis (seemingly purposeless movements that, in reality, are due to loss of position sense). Proprioceptive loss may become generalized so that the patient may be unable to stand or walk unassisted. The face is seldom involved (9). NCV may show normal motor potentials but unobtainable sensory potentials. The neuropathy is usually irreversible, even if an underlying malignancy is successfully treated. A common chemotherapeutic agent in the treatment of ovarian cancer, cis-platinum, produces a similar clinical picture.

Paraproteinemic Neuropathies

Peripheral neuropathy is commonly associated with paraproteinemic and dysglobulinemic disorders. Often there are features of distal burning dysesthesias and autonomic dysfunction. Although the course is usually one of steady progression, improvement in the neuropathy may occur following the successful treatment of the underlying disease.

Toxic Neuropathy

Toxic neuropathies are becoming increasingly more frequent. They are important to recognize since they are potentially reversible if the toxin can be identified. The diagnosis may be made easily if there is a history of drug exposure (e.g., isoniazid, hydralazine, vincristine) or of industrial exposure (see Table 84.5). Since these neuropathies have no distinguishing features on routine history or on physical examination, a detailed history of exposure to drugs and of the patients occupation and recreational habits is important. Axonal involvement in the spinal cord may occur with the toxic neuropathy but be masked by the presence of the latter. In these cases, a residual spastic paraparesis becomes apparent when the peripheral neuropathy has resolved. Toxic neuropathies are classically associated with chronic low dose exposure (months to years), though they may appear within days to weeks with high level exposure. A delayed neuropathy associated with organophosphates develops 10 to 14 days following exposure while Vacor, a rodenticide, produces an acute toxic neuropathy within 2 to 3 days.

A recently recognized toxicity with megadose pyridoxine consumption produces a gradually progressive sensory ataxia and profound distal limb impairment of position and vibratory sense (12). General acceptance of vitamin B_6 therapy as safe and that "more might be better" by the public makes direct questioning about vitamin habits necessary. Since the original description, some patients have been reported who have injested lower daily doses in the range of 0.5 to 1.0 g/day.

Table 84.5.
Toxins Associated with Peripheral Neuropathies

INDUSTRIAL
  Pesticides—organophosphates, dichlorophenyoxyacetate (2, 4-D), Vacor rodenticide
  Metal work—lead, arsenic, mercury, thallium, methyl bromide
  Plastics, synthetic fabrics—n-hexane, methyl n-butyl ketone, acrylamide, carbon disulfide, perchlorethylene, trichlorethylene, dimethylaminoproprionitrile
  Gases—carbon monoxide, ethylene oxide
EUPHORIANTS
  Glue sniffing—n-hexane, solvents
  Nitrous oxide inhalation—whipped cream dispensers, dental offices
PHARMACOTHERAPEUTIC AGENTS
  Antimicrobial—isoniazid, nitrofurantoin, metronidazole (Flagyl)
  Cardiovascular—hydralazine, procainamide, amiodarone
  Other—phenytoin, disulfiram (Antabuse), pyridoxine

Compression and Entrapment Neuropathies

When a peripheral neurological abnormality occurs in one upper or lower extremity, the abnormality is usually due to nerve entrapment or compression, although polyneuropathy and mononeuropathy may present initially as a focal deficit in one extremity. With careful evaluation, it is usually possible to determine whether the patient's problem is due to nerve or root damage or to damage to a peripheral nerve or one of its branches. Tables 84.6 and 84.7 and Figures 84.1 and 84.2 summarize the information needed to make this distinction, i.e., distribution of sensory, motor, and reflex deficits; common causative lesions; and critical anatomical relationships.

Several commonly encountered entrapment neuropathies are discussed here. Root compression symptoms due to cervical and lumbar spine disease are discussed in Chapters 64 (Neck Pain), 65 (Low Back Pain), and 68 (Degenerative Joint Disease).

Median Nerve (Carpal Tunnel Syndrome)

Etiology

Carpal tunnel syndrome (CTS) is a very common pressure neuropathy in which median nerve injury results from compression by neighboring anatomical structures. The carpal canal or tunnel is formed by the concave arch of the carpal bones and is roofed by the transverse carpal ligament. These structures form a rigid compartment through which nine tendons and the median nerve must pass. Conditions which cause a decrease in the size of the carpal canal (e.g., Colles' fracture, rheumatoid arthritis, congenital carpal canal stenosis), enlargement of the median nerve (e.g., endoneural edema in diabetes, amyloid, neuroma), or increase in the volume of other structures within the canal (e.g., tenosynovitis, ganglion, lipoma, urate deposits in gout, hematoma, fluid retention in pregnancy) may all have one common result, namely, compression of the median nerve. Many cases previously classified as idiopathic

Table 84.6.
Comparative Data on Root and Nerve Lesions in the Upper Extremity[a, b]

Root	Sensory Loss	Motor Loss	Tendon Reflex	Causative Lesion
C5	Lateral upper arm	Deltoid, some biceps infra- and supraspinatus	Slight ↓ biceps	Cervical spondylosis
C6	Dorsolateral forearm and thumb	Biceps, brachioradialis, some deltoid	Biceps, brachioradialis	Cervical spondylosis, disc disease
C7	Mid-dorsal forearm and middle finger	Triceps, wrist and finger extensors	Triceps	Disc disease, cervical spondylosis
C8	Medial forearm, ring and small fingers	Thenar eminence	Finger jerk	Thoracic outlet syndrome, neoplastic disease at apex of lung or in cervical nodes
T1	Medial arm, axilla	Interossei of hand	None	

[a] See dermatomal patterns, Table 78.1.
[b] Pain distribution is usually from the neck along area of muscles supplied to the distal areas of sensory loss

Common Entrapments of the Upper Extremity			
Peripheral Nerve	Sensory Loss	Motor Loss	Comment
Median	Lateral 3½ digits	Thenar	+ Tinel at wrist
At wrist (carpal tunnel)			
At forearm anterior interosseous	None	Flexor digitorum longus, Flexor digitorum profundus, Pronator quadratus	Tenderness in volar forearm at entrapment site
Pronator teres	Lateral 3½ digits	Pronator teres plus distal muscles listed above	
Ulnar		Variable	
At wrist (Canal of Guyan)	Variable, Medial 1½ digits	(Flexor digitorum profundus remains strong)	Local tenderness (Bicycling)
At elbow (cubital tunnel)	Medial 1½ digits	Intrinsics of hand	Paresthesias with palpation at elbow
Radial		Extensor carpi ulnaris	Tenderness over forearm 1–2 inches distal to epicondyle
At forearm (posterior interosseous)	None	Extensor digitorum profundus	
At arm	Dorsal lateral hand	Supinator of wrist, finger extensors and triceps	

Table 84.7.
Comparative Data on Root and Nerve Lesions in the Lower Extremity[a]

	Sensory Loss	Motor Loss	Tendon Reflex	Predominant Causative Lesion
L2	Upper and medial thigh	Iliopsoas (Hip flexion)	None	Neoplastic disease
L3	Anterior thigh	Quadriceps (knee extension) Adductor	Adductor	Neoplastic disease Rare disc lesions
L4	Lateral thigh to medial knee	Quadriceps (knee extension) Anterior tibial (dorsiflexion of foot)	Knee	Neoplastic disease Disc lesions
L5	Lateral leg to dorsum of foot	Great toe extensor Anterior tibial (dorsiflexion of foot)	Medial hamstring	Disc lesions Local metastatic
S1	Posterior leg to plantar aspects of foot	Gastrocnemius (plantar flexion of foot) Biceps femoris (flexion of knee)	Ankle	Other neoplastic diseases

Common Neuropathies of the Lower Extremity			
Peripheral Nerve	Sensory Loss	Motor Loss	Comment
Tibial			
Tarsal tunnel	Plantar aspect of foot (burning pain) Tips of toes	Usually none detected	+ Tinel at medial malleolus Medial arch support may help Good response to surgery
Peroneal			
Compression at knee	Dorsum of foot and lateral leg May spare deep branch at first web space	Anterior tibial (Dorsiflexion of foot)	Cock-up foot splint helps ambulation
At dorsal ankle	First web space "Tightness" of dorsum of foot	Extensor digitorum brevis (toe spreading)	Direct trauma to dorsum of ankle or violent plantar flexion at foot
Femoral			
At inguinal ligament	Anterior-medial thigh	Quadriceps (knee extension) Iliopsoas (hip flexion)	Loss at knee reflex To be distinguished from more usual diabetic plexopathy
Lateral femoral cutaneous (meralgia paresthetica)	Upper-lateral thigh usually 10–12 inches below iliac crest	None	Usually conservative management Weight loss

[a] See dermatomal patterns, Table 78.1.

are explained by occupational factors. CTS in the workplace is associated with occupations in which the wrist position deviates from the normal straight alignment and with occupations involving the use of greater hand force in all wrist positions (e.g., meat processing, fruit packing, upholstering, and waiting on tables). Median nerve compression can also be caused by tasks that require a sustained or repeated stress over the base of the palm, such as that caused by the use of screwdrivers, scrapers, paint brushes, and buffers. Vibration exposure (low frequency 10 to 40 Hz), is another well recognized risk factor for carpal tunnel syndrome (air-powered tools). Repetitive wrist and hand movements leading to CTS may also occur in activities such as knitting, crocheting, hooking rugs, playing a musical instrument, painting, woodworking, gardening, and lifting weights.

Manifestations and Evaluation

Unless associated with direct trauma, the onset of symptoms of CTS is usually nocturnal and insidious. Symptoms in the hand may initially be described as episodic tingling and numbness with gradual progression to more severe symptoms referred to as burning, aching, pricking, or as a painful numbness in the fingers and deep in the palm. With the pain

and tingling there is a subjective feeling of uselessness in the fingers, which are sometimes described as feeling swollen, even though, on inspection, little swelling is apparent. Many patients will have accompanying pain in the forearm, sometimes reaching the shoulder and described as a dull aching pain felt deeply in the limb.

Color changes in the fingers have been described, particularly with exposure to cold, but they are not related to the attacks. Also, excessive sweating and mild degrees of edema are related to the vasomotor imbalance known to occur in CTS.

As CTS progresses, the nocturnal pain and tingling may begin to wake the patient after a few hours' sleep. Relief may be obtained by hanging the arm out of bed or shaking or rubbing the hand, but as symptoms increase, patients often get out of bed and walk about until the symptoms have eased. At this stage episodic tingling may develop during the day, but the associated pain in the arm occurs less often during the day than at night. In addition to sensory symptoms, there may be clumsiness and difficulty in performing certain tasks, such as unscrewing bottle tops, turning a key, or crocheting.

Objective changes in sensation and strength may appear in the hand, but some patients may suffer

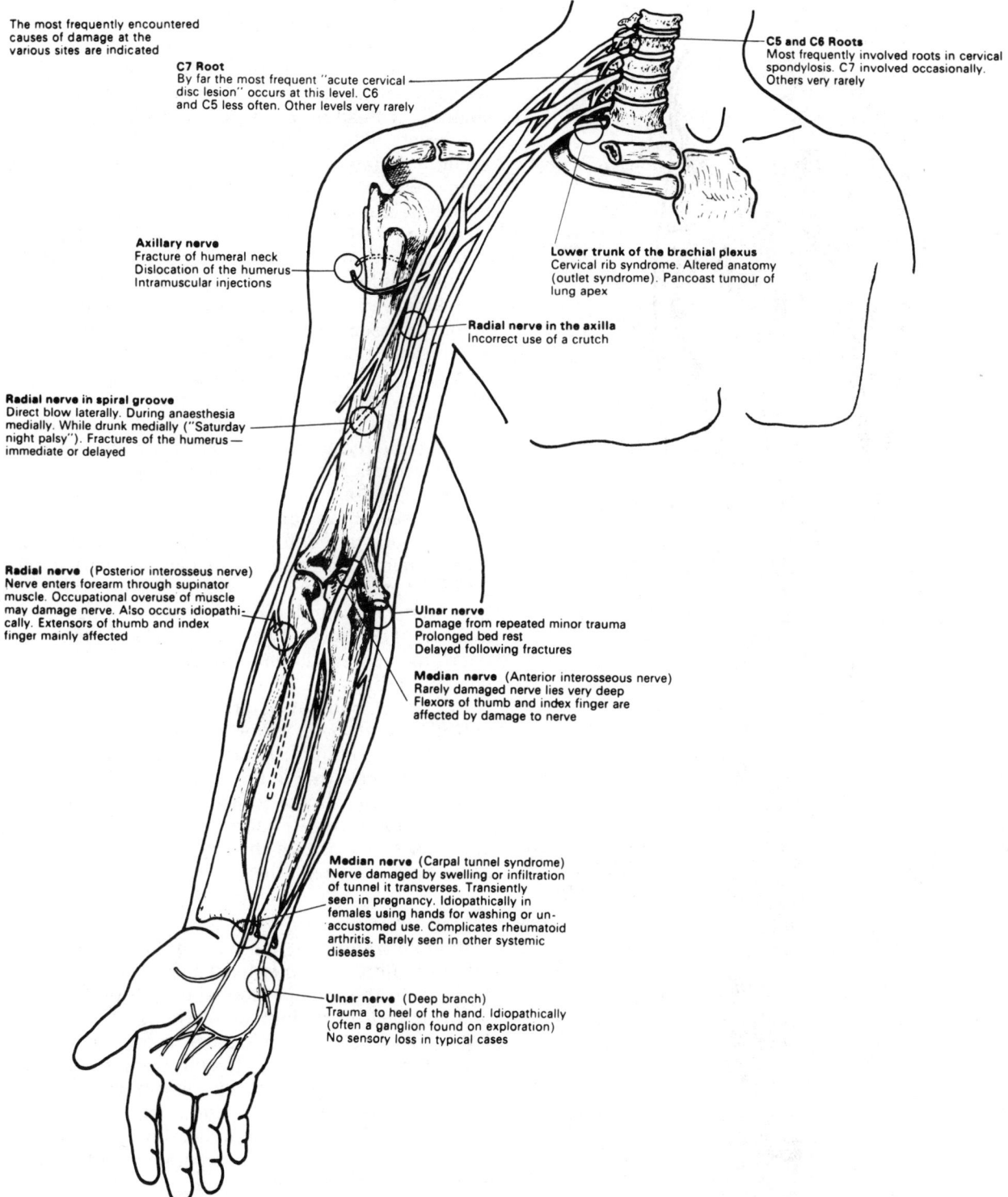

The most frequently encountered causes of damage at the various sites are indicated

C7 Root
By far the most frequent "acute cervical disc lesion" occurs at this level. C6 and C5 less often. Other levels very rarely

C5 and C6 Roots
Most frequently involved roots in cervical spondylosis. C7 involved occasionally. Others very rarely

Axillary nerve
Fracture of humeral neck
Dislocation of the humerus
Intramuscular injections

Lower trunk of the brachial plexus
Cervical rib syndrome. Altered anatomy (outlet syndrome). Pancoast tumour of lung apex

Radial nerve in the axilla
Incorrect use of a crutch

Radial nerve in spiral groove
Direct blow laterally. During anaesthesia medially. While drunk medially ("Saturday night palsy"). Fractures of the humerus — immediate or delayed

Radial nerve (Posterior interosseus nerve)
Nerve enters forearm through supinator muscle. Occupational overuse of muscle may damage nerve. Also occurs idiopathically. Extensors of thumb and index finger mainly affected

Ulnar nerve
Damage from repeated minor trauma
Prolonged bed rest
Delayed following fractures

Median nerve (Anterior interosseous nerve)
Rarely damaged nerve lies very deep
Flexors of thumb and index finger are affected by damage to nerve

Median nerve (Carpal tunnel syndrome)
Nerve damaged by swelling or infiltration of tunnel it transverses. Transiently seen in pregnancy. Idiopathically in females using hands for washing or un-accustomed use. Complicates rheumatoid arthritis. Rarely seen in other systemic diseases

Ulnar nerve (Deep branch)
Trauma to heel of the hand. Idiopathically (often a ganglion found on exploration) No sensory loss in typical cases

Figure 84.1. Anatomical relationships of nerves to the upper extremity. (From Patten J: *Neurological Differential Diagnosis.* New York, Springer-Verlag, 1977.)

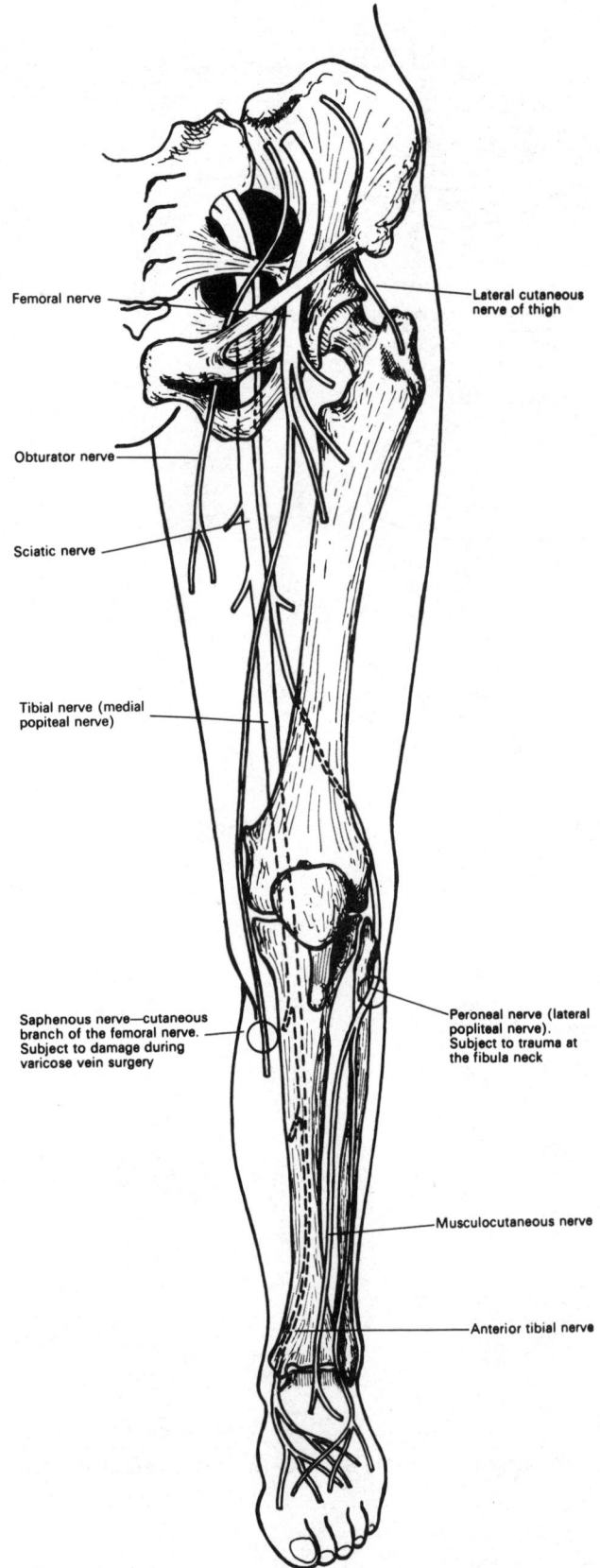

Femoral nerve

Lateral cutaneous nerve of thigh

Obturator nerve

Sciatic nerve

Tibial nerve (medial popliteal nerve)

Saphenous nerve—cutaneous branch of the femoral nerve. Subject to damage during varicose vein surgery

Peroneal nerve (lateral popliteal nerve). Subject to trauma at the fibula neck

Musculocutaneous nerve

Anterior tibial nerve

Figure 84.2. Anatomical relationships of nerves to the lower extremity. (From Patten J: *Neurological Differential Diagnosis.* New York, Springer-Verlag, 1977.)

severe attacks of pain for many years without developing abnormal neurological signs. Sensory signs within the median nerve distribution (see Table 84.6) are best sought for in the fingertips, where impairment is, as a rule, more pronounced. Occasionally, instead of decreased sensation, there is an overreaction to cutaneous stimuli in the median innervated lateral three and a half fingers. Isolated thenar wasting or sensory impairment in the distribution of one of the lateral three digital nerves may be the presenting feature of median nerve lesions at the wrist. Mild weakness of the abductor pollicis brevis or of the opponens pollicis muscle (see "General Reference," Medical Research Council) is frequently present with no visually apparent atrophy. Manual pressure over the flexor aspect of the wrist or prolonged hyperextension or hyperflexion of this joint may reproduce sensory symptoms (Phalen's sign). Tinel's sign, consisting of shock-like pain and tingling elicited by percussion of the median nerve at the wrist, is a less common finding.

Although abnormalities of the nerve conduction studies (see above) are more likely to be found in the presence of a defect on clinical examination in CTS, a significant number of patients with typical CTS symptoms have no abnormalities other than those detected on electrodiagnostic testing. Abnormalities of conduction in motor fibers of the median nerve in the carpal canal are frequent and are important findings in CTS, but abnormalities of sensory fibers occur with even greater frequency. Nearly 90% of patients have abnormalities on sensory nerve conduction studies from the index finger, and in some instances, this is the only objective evidence to support the clinical diagnosis. Needle-electrode examination of the thenar eminence is uncomfortable and less sensitive in CTS than are the routine nerve conduction studies.

Treatment

Immobilization of the wrist with a close-fitting anterior splint (extends from the upper part of the forearm to the metacarpophalangeal joints), which is worn by the patient at night or when resting, holds the wrist immobilized in a neutral position. This often will alleviate all symptoms, but if symptoms persist after a few weeks, additional therapy is indicated. Local corticosteroid injections or a trial of oral anti-inflammatory medication is frequently used but generally yields temporary relief at best.

Indications for *carpal tunnel release* include the failure of nonoperative treatment or clinical evidence of thenar atrophy. A relative indication is the persistence of sensory loss, especially if it is long standing. The surgical treatment for CTS is one of the most successful operations that can be performed on the hand. The operation demands care and skill by an orthopaedic, plastic, or neurological surgeon who is performing hand surgery regularly. Complications of the operation or poor results are almost uniformly related to poor surgical technique (*i.e.*, reflex sympathetic dystrophy, severance of median nerve branches, hypertrophic scar, adherent flexor tendons). The usual postoperative recovery time is 6 to 8 weeks. An additional month may be needed for occupational rehabilitation.

Ulnar Nerve

Etiology, Manifestations, Evaluation

Ulnar nerve compression occurs most often at the elbow. The *cubital tunnel* refers to the area of entrapment of the ulner nerve at the elbow as it runs beneath the aponeurosis of the flexor carpi ulnaris muscle just distal to the medial epicondyle. Minor pressure directly over the cubital tunnel during anesthesia, intoxication, stupor, coma, or by trauma may subsequently cause symptoms.

Cumulative trauma to the ulnar nerve at the elbow may occur with activities requiring repeated flexion and extension of the elbow. Hypermobility of the ulnar nerve in these cases results with hypesthesia in the fifth digit often associated with elbow flexion.

Patients may awaken at night with elbow pain, shooting pain in the hand or fifth digit, and paresthesias and hypesthesias in the ulnar nerve distribution. These symptoms usually improve with elbow extension. The amount of pain and paresthesia varies, and for some the sensory loss is not bothersome. Patients usually see a physician when they experience motor dysfunction, such as weakness of grasp and pinch or loss of dexterity.

Ulnar sensory loss (see Table 84.6) is easiest to establish over the distal two phalanges of the little finger with two-point discrimination. Transition between the ulnar territory over the hypothenar eminence and the medial cutaneous nerve (branch from the brachial plexus) of the forearm is often detected at the skin crease at the wrist. Motor disability is manifested as decreased pinch strength which is related to the degree of intrinsic atrophy of the involved muscles, and as impaired coordination and dexterity. Grasp may be decreased if the interossei and flexor digitorum profundus to the fourth and fifth digits are weak. One of the earliest signs of ulnar nerve entrapment is weakness of the third palmar interosseus manifested by an abducted posture of the fifth digit.

Ulnar neuropathy distal to the elbow occurs at the wrist or in the hand and must be considered if there is no weakness in the flexor digitorum profundus (see "General References," Medical Research Council). This is most often caused by a ganglion, rheumatoid arthritis, or by trauma (such as long distance bicycling). Often lesions in the wrist or hand produce no paresthesias or sensory loss. Depending upon the level of entrapment at the wrist either all the ulnar innervated muscles may be weak or there may be selective preservation of hypothenar function (*i.e.*, abductor digiti quinti).

Focal slowing of the ulnar motor or sensory nerve conduction across the elbow is found with nerve conduction studies (see above) in one-third to one-half of patients, depending upon the severity. False positive findings may be obtained and, therefore, close correlation with the clinical findings is mandatory. Increased distal latencies are found with entrapment at the wrist but must be correlated with EMG to determine the actual site of the lesion.

Treatment

Nonsurgical treatment is indicated for the patient with intermittent symptoms, acute or chronic mild neuropathy, or mild neuropathy associated with an occupational cause. For a mild ulnar neuropathy, splinting the elbow at night in an extended position may be helpful. An easy way to splint the elbow is to strap a pillow around it. Splinting should be continued for 2 to 3 months, especially if the symptoms are intermittent or show improvement. For ulnar compression at the wrist, whether due to a single traumatic event or to chronic trauma, conservative treatment with a splint is generally adequate. Surgical intervention is not necessary as long as symptoms do not progress and especially as long as there is no motor involvement or objective sensory loss. Surgical approaches to lesions of the ulnar nerve at the elbow depend on the etiology and the surgeon. These include simple release of the cubital tunnel, medial epicondylectomy, and anterior transplantation of the nerve. Detailed description with associated complications may be found in the "General References" (see Dawson *et al* on entrapment neuropathies). Complications from any of the surgical approaches include persistent or recurrent symptoms due to inadequate surgery or to recurrent scarring of the nerve.

Radial Nerve

Etiology, Manifestations, Evaluation

Radial nerve lesions are the least common of the major upper extremity nontraumatic compression neuropathies. Radial nerve entrapment or compression usually involves the radial nerve either at or proximal to the elbow (see Fig. 84.1).

Besides traumatic conditions such as humeral fractures, radial nerve injuries can occur after the arm has been held in a hyperabducted position during surgery or sleep, is seen in patients who have lain unconscious for a long time in abnormal positions ("Saturday night palsy"), and may occur with axillary pressure due to incorrect use of a crutch (central palsy).

Depending on the location of a high radial compression, the triceps function may or may not be affected. Elbow flexion and supination may be slightly weaker. The most obvious finding in a radial palsy is wrist drop and digital extensor paralysis (see "General References," Medical Research Council).

The radial nerve is predominantly a motor nerve. High radial nerve lesions may produce sensory loss over the dorsum of the hand. Pain, tenderness, and a positive Tinel's sign in the area of nerve damage may be present with radial nerve compression injuries. Nerve conduction studies (see above) can be helpful in localizing and quantifying radial nerve compression. For example, Saturday night palsy causes focal slowing of conduction at the site of pressure injury, but normal motor and sensory conduction below this lesion.

Treatment

The treatment of traumatic radial nerve compression is generally conservative. Cockup splint for the wrist joint should be accompanied by a spring-loaded extensor brace for the fingers if the weakness is long lasting. Individually constructed splints made by the occupational therapist are superior to those obtained from a surgical supply house. Treatment of compression of the posterior interosseus nerve (branch of radial nerve in the forearm) is surgical in most instances.

Peroneal Nerve

Etiology, Manifestations, Evaluation

The most common mechanism of damage to the peroneal nerve is compression at the head of the fibula (see Fig. 84.2) which may result from improperly applied plaster casts, tight stockings, bandages, and garters. Falling asleep with the side of the leg resting against a sharp or protruding object may occur in drug- or alcohol-induced stupor and even in the weakened bedridden patient. Occupations that require sitting, squatting, or kneeling may provoke peroneal compression. Entrapment may also occur in the fibular tunnel formed by the peroneus longus muscle.

Peroneal palsy produces foot drop due to weakness in the dorsiflexors of the foot, which may be accompanied by weakness of eversion (see Table 84.7). Symptoms usually consist of painless loss of motor power with partial sensory loss when acute compressive lesions exist. Entrapment, however, does produce radiating pain with slowly progressive motor and sensory disturbances.

Nerve conduction studies can detect focal slowing across the fibular head as compared to the leg segment.

Treatment

Because the gait is quite unstable in the presence of foot drop, a rigid plastic splint worn in the shoe or a spring-loaded brace attached to the shoe is required. Compressive lesions of the peroneal nerve can be watched for several months before any consideration of a surgical approach is made. Entrapment presenting with pain and progressive motor and sensory loss is an indication for relatively early surgical exploration.

Tibial Nerve (Tarsal Tunnel Syndrome) (7)

Etiology, Manifestations, Evaluation

The tarsal tunnel is located at the inferoposterior margin of the medial malleolus (see Fig. 84.2) and is formed by bones of the ankle and the flexor retinaculum (fibrous sheath from medial malleolus posteroinferior to the medial side of the calcaneus). In addition to the posterior tibial nerve the tunnel contains the posterior tibial artery and three long flexor tendons.

Enlarged tortuous veins within the tarsal tunnel, fracture or dislocation at the ankle, and nonspecific tenosynovitis may affect the other contents of the tarsal tunnel and lead to compression of the nerve trunk. Prolonged standing and walking often aggravate the pain, indicating that stasis or engorgement within the tunnel is likely to play some role. Also, sensory symptoms are made worse by the venous stasis and engorgement that occur at night during sleep. Except for a high prevalence in jockeys, no clear occupational factors have been identified.

The primary symptom of tarsal tunnel syndrome (TTS) is pain and dysesthesia in the sole of the foot. The burning pain (description by patient may vary, i.e., walking on knives or pins, sole feels very thick) worsens with rest after a day of activity, and nocturnal pain is characteristic. Any or all of the three divisions (medial plantar, lateral plantar, and calcaneal) of the tibial nerve may be affected, resulting in sensory disturbance over the entire plantar surface or only one portion of it.

Specific points of the examination which help to confirm the diagnosis are the presence of a Tinel's sign, i.e., shooting pain to the plantar surface, produced by gentle percussion over the tarsal tunnel, below and behind the medial malleolus. Sensory loss, if present, is found over the plantar surface of the foot. It is easier to test sensory function over the tips of the toes (the sural and peroneal territories on the dorsum of the foot do not include the tips of the toes). Weakness in the intrinsic muscles of the foot may lead to a change in configuration of the foot and to instability of the phalanges, which impairs the pushing-off phase of walking. In contrast to carpal tunnel syndrome, tarsal tunnel syndrome is usually unilateral.

Nerve conduction studies for distal motor latency (see above) are done by stimulation proximal to the tarsal tunnel, and recordings are taken over the abductor pollicis brevis or abductor digiti quinti. Prolongation of motor latency or absence of motor potential may be recorded; however, sensory conduction studies appear to be much more sensitive than the motor studies in confirming the diagnosis.

Treatment

It may be possible to splint the foot or employ orthotic devices such as arch supports or heel wedges to reduce the stretch on the tibial nerve.

Temporary response has also been obtained with corticosteroid injections. The definitive treatment of tarsal tunnel syndrome is surgical release of the flexor retinaculum which can result in dramatic relief of symptoms if localized compression neuropathy is present.

Lateral Femoral Cutaneous Nerve (Meralgia Paresthetica)

This nerve may be compressed or stretched at the anterior superior iliac spine at the lateral end of the inguinal canal (see Fig. 84.2), causing burning pain, paresthesia, and decreased sensation over the lateral thigh. The sensory involvement is more lateral than that in femoral neuropathy (see Table 84.7), and there is *no motor involvement* or loss of patellar reflex. Point tenderness can usually be elicited at the passage of the nerve at the ipsilateral anterior iliac crest. Common causes include pelvic tilt, acute abdominal enlargement (ascites, pregnancy), external mechanical trauma (girdle, utility belt), and diabetes. The nerve compression may be relieved by weight loss or correction of the aggravating condition. Pain may respond to medical management (see below). If the pain is severe, local injection of an anesthetic may provide relief for long periods; sectioning of the ligament over the canal is only rarely needed. Paresthesias and pain usually disappear gradually, but an asymptomatic sensory loss in the lateral thigh may persist.

Bell's Palsy

Paralysis of the facial muscles due to inflammation and swelling of the 7th (the facial) cranial nerve (Bell's palsy) is seen occasionally in a general medical practice. One large series reported an incidence of 23 cases/100,000 population/year (8). There is no predilection for a particular sex, age group, or race. The cause of the condition is unknown. Although involvement of the facial nerve results in the predominant signs and symptoms, the process is actually a polyneuropathy that subclinically affects other cranial nerves as well. Usually patients will note the sudden onset, within hours, of a unilateral paralysis of a facial nerve: the eyebrow sags; the eye cannot be closed; the nasolabial fold disappears; and the mouth appears drawn to the unaffected side. Less commonly, there is loss of taste on the anterior two-thirds of the tongue, and there is hyperacusis (an accentuation of loud sounds) in the affected ear. There may be pain behind the ear. Most patients recover spontaneously within weeks to a few months; approximately 15% recover incompletely, but severe residual weakness is rare (8). There is, in those who do not recover completely, a considerable risk of synkinesis, a contraction of all of the facial muscles on the affected side when the patient attempts to move just one or a few of them.

Corticosteroids appear to reduce the incidence of incomplete recovery (1, 15) of patients with Bell's palsy. Thus, it is reasonable to administer prednisone for 9 days after diagnosis—60 mg for 3 days, and then tapered by 10 mg a day—starting within 3 days of onset. If pain behind the ear recurs during the tapering, the prednisone should be increased and a neurologist should be consulted. Some advocate early surgical decompression of the facial nerve in patients who demonstrate by EMG complete or nearly complete denervation (6), but most neurologists believe that the data do not support this radical approach.

THERAPEUTIC PRINCIPLES

General

Treatment of peripheral neuropathies first requires identifying and treating any underlying cause if possible. Efforts should be made also to prevent further damage; for example, patients with an underlying generalized polyneuropathy are more prone to pressure palsies, and it is important to educate them about habits that could be injurious (such as leaning on elbows or crossing legs). The daily administration of multivitamins is prudent to prevent any contributing nutritional deficiencies. Avoidance of potential toxins, such as alcohol, is also important since it may have a synergistic effect.

For entrapment and compression neuropathies, eliminating pressure on the affected nerve is the primary mode of treatment, as discussed above. For deficits which are partial or recent in onset, recovery of function usually occurs within about 6 weeks after eliminating nerve entrapment or compression.

Symptomatic Treatment

Polyneuropathy is often irreversible and progressive. Symptomatic therapy and rehabilitative measures are, therefore, fundamental in helping these patients.

Motor

In most polyneuropathies, weakness usually affects dorsiflexion of the feet early (causing foot drop); ambulation can be greatly improved by a rigid plastic splint worn in the shoe or by a spring-loaded brace attached to the shoe obtained from a physical therapist. Fine motor weakness in the hands can be aided by special tools and other devices provided by occupational therapists.

Sensory

Anesthetic limbs are vulnerable to repeated, unrecognized trauma. The patient should always check the temperature of bath water, pot handles, *etc* with parts of his body that have normal sensation. Small hard objects (keys, faucet handles) can be built up with soft materials. Occupational therapists can make useful suggestions in this regard. Meticulous care should be given to feet and toenails (see Chapter

102). Moisturizing cream for dry, insensitive skin will reduce serious abrasions.

Pain associated with sensory neuropathies is usually chronic and difficult to treat. Simple analgesics (aspirin), whirlpool, and massage may help to relieve relatively mild pain. Narcotics should be avoided, because of the potential for addiction. Phenytoin (Dilantin), 300 to 500 mg/day to yield a serum level of 15 to 20 μg/ml, may provide relief of refractory pain and thus is worth a therapeutic trial. Details regarding the use of phenytoin are found in Chapter 80. If phenytoin has been maintained in the therapeutic range for 2 weeks and still proves unsuccessful, it should be discontinued and a trial of carbamazepine (Tegretol), 200 to 1000 mg/day in divided doses (two or three times a day), should be tried. This drug is started at 100 mg twice a day and is increased slowly (200 mg every 4 days in divided doses). Intolerance to carbamazepine (ataxia, drowsiness, and nausea) is especially likely in the older patient. Hematological values and liver function tests must be checked periodically (see details in Chapter 80). Tricyclic antidepressants (such as amitriptyline, 25 to 75 mg at bedtime) may also be tried.

Autonomic

Autonomic dysfunctions should also be approached symptomatically. The *hypotonic bladder* may be treated by drugs that increase bladder tone (urecholine, 10 to 25 mg every 8 hours), by biofeedback, or with surgery to decrease resistance to bladder emptying. Details regarding the evaluation and management of the hypotonic bladder are found in Chapter 6. *Sexual impotence* cannot be helped directly, although penile prostheses have been helpful for selected patients (see Chapter 18). The knowledge that sexual dysfunction has a neurological basis may relieve the anxiety that accompanies the prob-

lem. A check for medications that may be contributing to impotence is important (see Chapter 18). *Orthostatic hypotension* may be treated with salt supplementation and a volume-expanding mineralocorticoid (fludrocortisone, 0.1 to 0.2 mg daily) in patients without congestive heart failure and hypertension. Most patients tolerate support stockings (e.g., Jobst) poorly; but learning to arise slowly, maintaining active ambulation, and sleeping with the head of the bed on blocks (to stimulate renin release) may help. Table 84.8 summarizes the practical ways to manage patients with this vexing problem.

OTHER PROBLEMS

Restless Legs Syndrome

This is a common syndrome and an important cause of insomnia (see Chapter 85) which is often unrecognized or attributed to "hysteria" or "malingering." Patients complain of cold, unpleasant, sometimes painful crawling sensations in their legs at rest or in the early stages of sleep. The sensations are usually bilateral, symmetrical, and most frequently in the lower leg; they are described as "deep inside" the muscles or bones. Movement of the limbs provides some relief; affected patients usually find it impossible to keep their limbs still.

In one survey 5% of a group of otherwise healthy subjects had recognizable symptoms of the restless legs syndrome (4). The syndrome has been related in some patients to a mild neuropathy; it can be seen in diabetes, after gastrectomy, and in uremia. Sometimes the condition seems hereditary, in that it is present in several family members. There seems to be a relationship between iron deficiency anemia and restless legs in some patients. In a series of 77 patients with the syndrome, one-fourth had definitely decreased serum iron levels, whereas in a series of patients with iron deficiency anemia one-fourth had restless legs (4). Correction of the iron deficiency improved symptoms in these patients. In some patients diazepam (Valium) and clonazepam (Clonopin) may relieve the restless legs syndrome.

Muscle Cramps

Cramps are localized involuntary painful contractions of skeletal muscles and produce a visible and palpable hard and bulging muscle. They must be distinguished from the sensation of cramp such as that described with intermittent claudication.

Ordinary muscle cramps are common and may be stopped by stretching the affected muscles. Cramps are associated with fatiguing exercises, salt depletion, dehydration, pregnancy, hypothyroidism, alcoholism, uremia, hypomagnesemia, myopathy, or denervation. Patients with frequent daytime cramps and no contributing factors should be referred to a neurologist for evaluation of the rare muscle enzy-

Table 84.8.
Management of Patients with Orthostatic Hypotension Due to Autonomic Neuropathy

Avoid sudden changes in position
Avoid excessive intake of alcohol
Avoid diuresis
Correct hypovolemia
Discontinue or reduce the dosage of drugs known to cause orthostatic hypotension:
    Antihypertensive drugs
    Nitroglycerine
    Diuretics
    Neuroleptics
    Tricyclic antidepressants
    CNS depressants (opiates, alcohol)
    Levodopa
Prescribe mineralocorticoid
Supplement diet with salt
Tilt up the head of the bed (may stimulate renin release)
Use elastic support stockings

matic defects (*e.g.*, phosphorylase, phosphofructo-kinase, or carnitine palmatyltransferase deficiency). If no associated condition exists, these patients may be given a therapeutic trial of phenytoin, carbamazepine, or amitriptyline (see above for dosages).

Nocturnal cramps occur in 15% of healthy young adults and are more common in the elderly. Two drugs have proved effective in a double-blind trial against placebo: quinine sulfate, 200 mg at bedtime, and chloroquine phosphate, 250 mg a day (10, 11). Relief occurred in 1 to 3 weeks and often lasted several months after treatment ended. Even though cramps are more often associated with muscular dysfunction, nocturnal cramps (frequently in one leg) are a common presentation for entrapment of the tibial nerve (see above).

General References

Asbury A, Johnson P: *Pathology of Peripheral Nerves.* Philadelphia, WB Saunders, 1978.
>A standard reference.

Dawson D, Hallett M, Millender L: *Extrapment Neuropathies.* Boston, Little, Brown, and Co, 1983.
>Thorough and readable review of clinical experience.

Dyck P, Thomas PK, Lambert EH, Bunge R (eds): *Peripheral Neuropathy.* ed 2. Philadelphia, WB Saunders, 1984.
>An excellent comprehensive review.

Medical Research Council: *Aids to the Examination of the Peripheral Nervous System.* London, Her Majesty's Stationary Office, 1976.
>A complete pictorial demonstration for individual muscle testing.

Schaumburg HH, Spencer PS, Thomas PK: *Disorders of Peripheral Nerves.* Philadelphia, FA Davis, 1983.
>A short work organized by disease processes that involve peripheral nerves.

Specific References

1. Adour KK, Wingerd J, Bell DN, *et al*: Prednisone treatment for idiopathic facial paralysis (Bell's palsy). *N Engl J Med* 287:1268, 1972.
2. Asbury AK, Arnason BG, Karp HR, McFarlin DE: Criteria for diagnosis of Guillian-Barré Syndrome. *Ann Neurol* 3:565, 1978.
3. Behse F, Buchthal F: Alcoholic neuropathy: Clinical, electrophysiological and biopsy findings. *Ann Neurol* 2:95, 1977.
4. Ekbom KA: Restless legs. In Vinken PJ, Bruyn GW (eds): *Handbook of Clinical Neurology.* New York, American Elsevier, 1970, vol 6, p 311.
5. Ellenberg M: Diabetic neuropathy: clinical aspects. *Metabolism* 25:1627, 1976.
6. Fisch U: Surgery for Bell's palsy. *Arch Otolaryngol* 107:1, 1981.
7. Goodgold J, Kopell HP, Spielholz NI: The tarsal tunnel syndrome. *N Engl J Med* 273:742, 1965.
8. Hauser WA, Karnes WE, Annis J, Kurland LT: Incidence and prognosis of Bell's palsy in the population of Rochester, Minnesota. *Mayo Clin Proc* 46:258, 1971.
9. Horwich MS, Cho L, Porro RS, Posner JB: Subacute sensory neuropathy: a remote effect of cancer. *Ann Neurol* 2:7, 1977.
10. Moss HK, Herrman LG: Night cramps in human extremities. A clinical study of the physiologic action of quinine and prostigmine upon the spontaneous contractions of resting muscles. *Am Heart J* 35:403, 1948.
11. Parrow A, Samuelsson SM: Use of choloroquine phosphate. A new treatment for spontaneous leg cramps. *Acta Med Scand* 181:237, 1967.
12. Schaumberg H, Kaplan J, Windebank A, *et al*.: Sensory neuropathy from pyridoxine abuse—a new megavitamin syndrome. *N Engl J Med* 309:445, 1983.
13. Spritz N: Nerve disease in diabetes mellitus. *Med Clin North Am* 62:787, 1978.
14. Wilkinson M, Croft PB, Urich H: The remote effects of cancer on the nervous system. *Proc R Soc Med* 60:683, 1967.
15. Wolf SM, Wagner JH, Davidson S, Forsythe A: Treatment of Bell's palsy with prednisone: a prospective, randomized study. *Neurology* 28:158, 1978.

CHAPTER EIGHTY-FIVE

Sleep Disorders

RICHARD P. ALLEN, Ph.D., AND PHILIP L. SMITH, M.D.

EPIDEMIOLOGY AND CLASSIFICATION

Recent population studies indicate that approximately one in three adults in America has trouble sleeping within a given year (11). Of these, about one in six actually reports the problem to his physician. Moreover, 4% of adults use prescription sleep medication at some time each year, and 1% of these report using prescription sleep medication on consecutive nights for 2 months or more (2, 15).

The sleep-related problems described by patients should be regarded as symptoms rather than diagnoses *per se*. In recent years, a classification of sleep disorders has been developed which enables physicians to formulate and to manage their patients' sleep problems appropriately (1). The four major categories in this classification are: (*a*) disorders of initiating and maintaining sleep—DIMS (the insomnias), (*b*) disorders of excessive somnolence—DOES (the hypersomnias), (*c*) disorders of the sleep-wake cycle, and (*d*) parasomnias (sleepwalking, sleep terrors, enuresis, *etc*). A number of discrete entities have been identified within each of these categories.

PHYSIOLOGICAL PATTERNS OF NORMAL SLEEP

The fundamental sleep-wake cycle is maintained by at least two physiologically and neurologically distinct control mechanisms.

1. *Homeostatic mechanism*: establishes a balance between wake and sleep time over a period of 1 or 2 days (sleep-wake cycles). This balance varies greatly with species, but for adult humans is set at about 30 to 40% sleep (7 to 9 hours/day). Establishing this balance within a time frame of a few days appears more important than making up for loss of sleep.

2. *Circadian oscillator*: establishes a sleep tendency variation over the normal 24-hour day. This oscillator also modulates core temperature and the activity levels of a large number of neurological hormonal functions (e.g., serotonin and cortisol levels). Without time cues, this oscillation cycles for man every 25 hours and needs to be reset daily by 1 hour. Intense light and perhaps activity help to reset this clock.

These mechanisms each produce a drive for sleep (sleepiness or lack of it) which are usually in stable harmony (e.g., circadian oscillators and homeostatic mechanisms both increasing at the end of the day).

The normal sleep cycle is characterized by two physiologically different states: rapid eye movement (REM) sleep and nonrapid eye movement (NREM) sleep. Initially, sleep consists of the four successively "deeper" stages of NREM sleep. During each of these four stages, there is generally much less fluctuation in heart rate, blood pressure, and respiratory rate than that which occurs during REM sleep. The presleep wake stage and each sleep stage have additional distinctive clinical and electroencephalographic (EEG) characteristics.

Presleep wake (sleep latency period). As the patient begins to fall asleep, eye blinks, limb movements, and moderate tone in skeletal muscles are accompanied by either low voltage, mixed frequency EEG or the characteristic alpha pattern (basic posterior rhythm).

Stage 1. This represents light sleep with slow rolling eye movements (pursuit eye movements). The alpha pattern disappears with lower frequency and usually higher voltage than the wake EEG. Sudden limb jerks may occur episodically, particularly during early stage 1 sleep.

Stage 2. Eye movements become infrequent or absent and muscle tone is usually reduced. The EEG shows characteristic occasional sleep spindle bursts, vertex sharp waves, K complexes, and some slow waveforms.

Stages 3 and 4. Slow wave sleep muscle tone is variable. The EEG high voltage, slow wave activity predominates. Arousal is difficult from these deeper sleep stages.

At 1 to 2 hours after sleep onset, the first period of REM sleep occurs with a characteristic marked decrease in muscle tone and bursts of rapid (saccadic) eye movements. During REM sleep there is a paralysis of major skeletal muscles punctuated by occasional episodes of muscle twitches; hypercapneic and hypoxic respiratory drive are decreased; core body temperature fluctuates with ambient temperature; heart rate and blood pressure are extremely variable; and penile erections occur. Dreaming is also most closely related to REM sleep but may occur, usually less vividly, at other times.

On a typical night, a subject passes through three to five cycles of NREM and REM sleep. Typical sleep patterns for young healthy adults and for healthy elderly adults are shown in Figure 85.1. The major differences between the two age groups are (a) the greater frequency and longer intervals of REM sleep in young adults and (b) the decreased amount of EEG slow wave sleep (stages 3 and 4) plus more frequent awakenings and decreased total sleep time in elderly subjects. During the day, young adults require 10 to 15 minutes to fall asleep for a nap, older adults fall asleep more easily. As discussed later in this chapter, deviations from the normal sleep cycles are helpful at times in establishing the correct diagnosis for a sleep disorder.

GENERAL APPROACH TO DIAGNOSIS AND MANAGEMENT OF SLEEP DISORDERS

Although patients with significant sleep disorders or relatives of such patients will usually report the problem to the physician, it is important for physicians to inquire at least briefly about sleep in taking the medical history of any patient. Four questions will detect the presence of most significant sleep disorders:

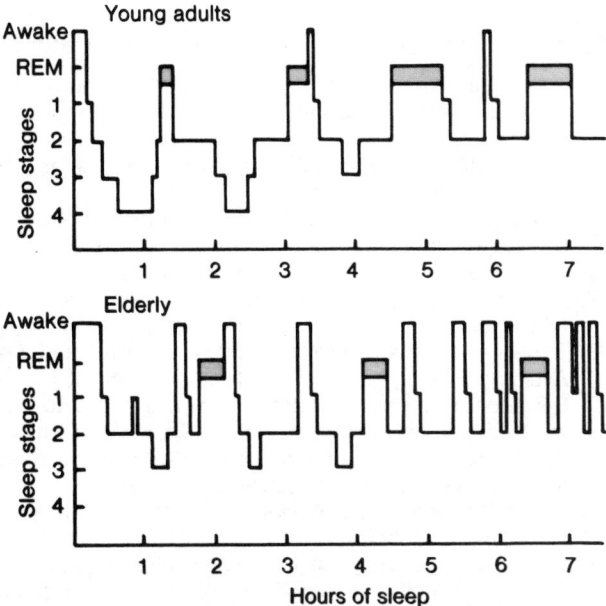

Figure 85.1. Normal sleep cycles in healthy young and elderly subjects. *Darkened area* indicates REM sleep. (Adapted from Kales A, Kales JD: Sleep disorders: recent findings in the diagnosis and treatment of disturbed sleep. *N Engl J Med* 290:487, 1974.)

1. *Do you have trouble sleeping—either falling asleep, staying asleep, or getting enough sleep?* (Positive response suggests a DIMS.)

2. *Do you or others notice that you are disturbed by excessive sleepiness when engaged in your usual daytime activities?* (Positive response in a patient reporting no difficulty initiating or maintaining sleep suggests a DOES.)

3. *Do you or your bed partner notice that you have any problem with unusual movement at night?* (Positive response suggests sleep disorder, especially if there is daytime sleepiness, insomnia, or parasomnia.)

4. *Do you snore or note any abnormalities in breathing?* (Positive response raises the possibility of sleep-associated respiratory impairment and further questions should be asked, especially about excessive daytime sleepiness.)

It is very important at the outset to distinguish genuine sleepiness from other problems perceived by the patient as "sleepiness." Sleepiness by definition involves the need to fall asleep, and the patient usually reports some relief of the symptom after sleeping. Muscle weakness, loss of interest in usual activities, exertional dyspnea, postural dizziness, and other symptoms may be referred to as sleepiness, tiredness, or fatigue. By having the patient describe concrete circumstances in which the symptom occurs, these problems can usually be distinguished from true sleepiness.

Table 85.1.
Strategies Which May Be Useful for Patients with Sleep Disorders

1. Sleep in the same room consistently, preferably not a room utilized for most wake time activities.
2. Develop a regular bedtime, with lights out or dimmed and a regular waking time, and avoid sleeping longer than usual except occasionally.
3. Adjust total sleep time to fit your needs—may be as little as 4 hours or as much as 10 hours.
4. Avoid routine daytime naps.
5. Plan regular daily exercise, preferably in the evenings and preferably exercising leg and arm muscles; no exercise for 30 minutes before bed.
6. Sleep in a cool room, avoiding temperature extremes.
7. Avoid heavy meals within 2 hours of bedtime; however, a light snack such as milk, cheese, and crackers at bedtime may be soporific.
8. Take no more than one alcoholic drink (equivalent of 2 ounces, 90 proof) after dinner.
9. Avoid stimulants, particularly within 8 hours of bedtime (*e.g.*, no coffee, cola drinks, tea, cocoa, chocolates, *etc*).
10. For poor sleep onset, do not stay awake in bed for more than 30 minutes. Instead, get out of bed, read, or engage in another quiet but productive activity. Try sleep again in an hour; if still unable to sleep, repeat this cycle.
11. For troublesome recurrent thoughts disturbing sleep onset, write them down with a possible plan of action. Try to start thinking about simpler, less troubling matters.
12. Accept an occasional night with sleeplessness; it is a normal healthy bodily adjustment to various conditions and provides extra time for hobbies, work, *etc*.
13. Use sleep medications, including bedtime alcohol, only rarely and never for more than 4 days out of a week or for more than 2 consecutive weeks without consulting your doctor.
14. Unless you are unable to stay awake, do not alter your daily activities because you feel tired. You may think you are less alert than others do.

A number of strategies are helpful in assuring effective sleep for most people. These are summarized in Table 85.1. Counseling about the value of such strategies is often helpful for patients with a history of insomnia and poor sleep habits. In general, patients with excessive waketime sleepiness should be cautioned against driving a car, operating heavy machinery, and working in high places or other activities, where decreased attention or sleepiness could be dangerous.

SLEEP CENTER REFERRAL

For a number of the problems discussed in this chapter, referral for expert evaluation and management is recommended. Referral can be made to individual physicians who are expert in managing sleep disorders or, ideally, to a regional sleep disorders center. Table 85.2 lists the accredited sleep disorders centers active in 1984. Access to the centers has become increasingly available; nevertheless, discussion about particular patients by telephone may be as useful prior to referral.

Patient experience. When a patient is evaluated at a sleep center, he undergoes a careful historical review of his sleep problem and a general physical examination; frequently, he may have one or more all-night sleep studies in order to evaluate his sleep objectively. The sleep study is performed using noninvasive simultaneous measurements of a number of physiological activities during sleep: eye movements, brain activity by EEG, submental and anterior tibialis muscle activity, respiratory air flow and effort, cardiac rhythm, and continuous blood oxyhe-

moglobin saturation. Sometimes additional parameters are recorded such as rectal temperature, esophageal pH, and penile circumference.

DISORDERS OF INITIATING AND MAINTAINING SLEEP (DIMS)

Patients with DIMS have difficulty initiating sleep, intermittent disruption of sleep, or early waking with difficulty returning to sleep. These problems are usually secondary to underlying psychological or medical conditions. Some persons who report difficulty initiating sleep in fact have normal objective sleep; they appear to suffer from a heightened perception of wakefulness, requiring unusually long periods of deeper objective sleep before they perceive themselves as being asleep.

Transient Psychophysiological Insomnia

This is the most common sleep disorder in our society, even though the majority of affected persons do not seek medical help. By definition, transient psychophysiological insomnia lasts less than 3 weeks and, characteristically, has an abrupt onset related to an identifiable precipitating stressor (usually a domestic or occupational problem). The third edition of the American Psychiatric Association's *Diagnostic and Statistical Manual of Mental Disorders* classification for an episode of marked insomnia related to a stressor is adjustment disorder (see Chapter 12). These patients usually recover spontaneously, either because stress subsides or the patient adapts to it. Prophylactic treatment may be useful

Table 85.2.
Sleep Disorders Centers, 1984[a]

State	Location
FULL ACCREDITED CENTERS	
Alabama:	Baptist Medical Center Montclair, Birmingham, (205) 592-5650
Arizona:	Good Samaritan Medical Center, Phoenix, (602) 239-5815
California:	Holy Cross Hospital, Mission Hills, (213) 365-8051, Ext. 1497
	Scripps Clinic and Research Foundation, La Jolla, (619) 455-8087
	Stanford University Medical Center, Stanford, (415) 497-7458
	UCLA School of Medicine, Los Angeles, (213) 206-8005
	University of California Irvine Medical Center, Orange, (714) 634-5777
Colorado:	Presbyterian Medical Center, Denver (303) 839-6447
Connecticut:	The Griffin Hospital, Derby, (203) 735-7421
Florida:	Mt. Sinai Medical Center, Miami Beach, (305) 674-2613
Hawaii:	Straub Clinic and Hospital, Honolulu, (808) 523-2311
Illinois:	Rush-Presbyterian-St. Luke's, Chicago, (312) 942-5440
	University of Chicago, Chicago, (312) 962-1780
Kansas:	Wesley Medical Center, Wichita, (316) 688-2660
Kentucky:	Humana Hospital Audobon, Louisville, (502) 636-7459
Maryland:	Francis Scott Key Medical Center, Baltimore, (301) 955-0571
Michigan:	Henry Ford Hospital, Detroit, (313) 876-2233
Minnesota:	Hennepin County Medical Center, Minneapolis, (612) 347-6288
	Mayo Clinic, Rochester, (507) 284-8403
	Deaconess Hospital, St. Louis, (314) 645-8510
	St. Louis University Medical Center, St. Louis, (314) 771-6400
New Hampshire:	Dartmouth Medical School, Hanover, (603) 646-7521
New York:	Montefiore Hospital, Bronx, (212) 920-4841
	SUNY at Stony Brook, Stony Brook, (516) 246-2561
Ohio:	Ohio State University, Columbus, (614) 421-8296
Oklahoma:	Presbyterian Hospital, Oklahoma City, (405) 271-6312
Pennsylvania:	Crozer-Chester Medical Center, Upland-Chester, (215) 847-1184
	The Medical College of PA, Philadelphia, (215) 842-4250
	Western Psychiatric Institute, Pittsburgh, (412) 624-2246
Tennessee:	Baptist Memorial Hospital, Memphis, (901) 522-5704
Texas:	Baylor College of Medicine, Houston, (713) 799-4886
	Metropolitan Medical Center, San Antonio, (512) 223-4057
	Presbyterian Hospital, Dallas, (214) 696-8563

[a] For further information, including location of new centers accredited after 1984, contact: Assocition of Sleep Disorders Center, c/o Stanford Sleep Center, Stanford University Medical Center, Stanford, CA 94305.

when patients appear vulnerable to recurrence. Therapy includes short term counseling (see Chapter 11), sleep hygiene advice (Table 85.1), and judicious use of hypnotic-sedative medications (see below). When frequent recurrent episodes of transient insomnia occur, a sleep cycle disturbance is likely. Personality or depressive disorders may also be present (see Chapters 14 and 15).

Another common cause of transient insomnia is periodic or permanent reduction or discontinuation of addictive substances, such as tobacco, alcohol, or antianxiety drugs. In mild cases, only transient insomnia occurs, but in more severe cases insomnia may become persistent and difficult to treat. These problems are discussed in Chapters 20, 21, and 22.

Persistent Insomnia

By definition, these patients have insomnia lasting more than 3 weeks. This problem may be seen in a number of situations.

Psychological Problems

These constitute the most common reasons for persistent insomnia. The sleep-related symptoms usually decrease as the primary psychological problem improves. Psychophysiological insomnia can become persistent but similar to transient DIMS noted above has an abrupt onset, a precipitating event, and usually a good response to supportive therapy and adaptation to the stressor. A sedative-hypnotic should be used cautiously since dependence is likely to develop. When counseling and sleep hygiene fail, the use of a sleep restriction procedure may help. Referral to a sleep center is recommended.

Affective disorders (see Chapter 15) often present initially with insomnia. Patients with unipolar depressions have less difficulty with sleep onset than with repeated awakenings and difficulty returning to sleep after awakening; patients with bipolar depressions commonly have episodic hypersomnia with complaints of awakening tired. In manic states, there is a profound inability to fall asleep, but even brief periods of sleep seem to restore wakefulness completely. Depression secondary to other medical or psychiatric conditions (reactive or neurotic depression) may also present with daytime sleepiness associated with premature arousals and sleep onset problems. These patients, however, show distinctive REM sleep characteristics on a nocturnal sleep study. A formal sleep study may occasionally be helpful in establishing the diagnosis of depression (6). Management of persistent insomnia includes appropriate treatment of the affective disorder as well as improvement in sleep habits (Table 85.1) and possible sleep cycle adjustment.

Patients with *personality problems* (see Chapter 14), particularly those with obsessive thoughts, and patients with *phobias* (see Chapter 13) frequently have insomnia associated with excessive ruminating thoughts at sleep onset. These patients usually require psychotherapy. Hypnotics should be avoided because of their abuse potential in these patients. On the other hand, judicious use of 25 to 50 mg of amitriptyline (Elavil) may be effective (see below, page 1230).

Occasionally, patients will describe *anxiety only at sleep onset* and not in relation to other life events. The patients fear they will not sleep and, thus, become too conscious of trying to sleep, noting every few minutes that they remain awake. Such patients may be very sleepy and even fall asleep in their chair watching television; however, when they attempt to sleep in bed, they suddenly become wide awake as if conditioned not to sleep in bed. Many have poor sleep hygiene (see Table 85.1), while others may have minor depressive symptoms. Generally, these patients are helped by sleep cycle adjustment and/or relaxation training (see Chapter 13). If minor depression is suspected, low dose (25 to 75 mg) amitriptyline (Elavil) 2 hours before bed can be tried (see below). Benzodiazepines, barbiturates, and related medications should be used cautiously because of the possibility of serious dependence with prolonged use of these drugs.

In many cases, the insomnia may have been precipitated by a transitory condition that leads to a persistent disruption of the sleep cycle. These patients demonstrate decreased waketime activity. Appropriate sleep cycle adjustment is available through sleep disorders centers. Since the diagnosis and management of chronic insomnia are difficult, consultation with a sleep specialist is recommended.

Chronic Sedative-Hypnotic Use

Protracted use of sedative-hypnotic medication paradoxically may cause poor sleep onset with repeated premature awakenings (9). This condition develops in patients with both transient and persistent insomnia who continue to use medication. The diagnosis is based on a history of prolonged sedative-hypnotic use with concomitant worsening insomnia. Treatment is usually difficult since drug withdrawal is mandatory in spite of the attendant transient worsening of symptoms. When withdrawal from medication is attempted, the patient must be told his sleep disorder will temporarily worsen and that overall improvement may not occur for several weeks, and in some cases months, after the drug has been stopped. The patient should be reassured that if his problem continues thereafter (i.e., it is not due solely to sedative abuse), the appropriate diagnosis and treatment can be accomplished after withdrawal. It is generally advised that the medication be stabilized for a fixed dosage and then gradually reduced, by one therapeutic dose per week. During withdrawal, frequent support and reassurance can be provided by brief contacts with the physician, either at weekly office visits or by telephone calls. More focused psychotherapy (Chapter 11) may be necessary in more difficult cases.

Sleep Apnea and Sleep-Induced Respiratory Impairment

This disturbance of respiration during sleep usually presents with hypersomnia and is discussed under DOES (page 1222). However, some patients with persistent insomnia, especially those with short sleep onset but frequent awakenings, may have this condition. As noted below, this condition will be exacerbated if treated with hypnotics, sometimes with serious complications (7).

Medical Conditions (16)

Patients with most symptomatic medical conditions may describe persistent insomnia associated with their underlying condition, but only occasionally is insomnia a major presenting symptom. The sleep disturbance, while probably related to the pathophysiology of the disease in some conditions, is due to nonspecific psychological or physical distress in most situations. For example, patients with recurrent paroxysmal nocturnal dyspnea associated with either underlying congestive heart failure or obstructive pulmonary disease will note characteristic difficulties with recurrent arousals secondary to manifest shortness of breath. Similarly, patients who experience worsening daytime asthma will often note repeated awakenings at night and the need for bronchodilators before sleep can again be initiated. Thus, insomnia in this clinical setting generally improves or worsens with the course of the associated medical condition. Sedative-hypnotic drugs (see below) should be reserved for patients whose insomnia is due to stress associated with their illness.

Periodic Leg Movements (Sleep-Related Myoclonus)

Periodic leg movements (also known as sleep-related myoclonus) are characterized by rhythmic, stereotyped leg kicks or arm jerks occurring every 20 to 40 seconds for much of the sleeping time. Unlike other movement disorders, periodic leg movements begin after sleep onset, may appear in clusters for 15 to 30 minutes, or in severe cases persist throughout sleep. The movements typically involve flexion at the ankle and knee (occasionally also at the hip) with extension of the big toe. Arm movements are less common. The etiology, prevalence, and course of this condition are not well known. Prevalence is age related, occurring rarely before age 40 but commonly (about 30%) after age 65. Once established, these movements persist with only rare spontaneous remission. This diagnosis should be suspected if the patient reports repeated nocturnal awakenings and very active sleep, or if a bed partner reports that the patient moves excessively in sleep, kicking his legs frequently.

Differential diagnosis includes normal twitches associated with REM sleep, sleep onset leg kicks, which cease after sleep is well established, and epileptic seizure activity during sleep. Diagnosis of periodic leg movement requires a nocturnal sleep study (10).

Treatment should be planned in consultation with a sleep disorders specialist and usually involves exercise and moderate doses of short acting benzodiazepines that suppress the associated arousal from sleep but do not reduce the frequency of leg movements. Clonazepam (Clonopin), oxazepam (Serax), or baclofen (Lioresal) before bed may also be effective, and tolerance is not a major problem.

"Restless legs" (see also Chapter 84) is a wake time disorder; almost all patients also have periodic leg movements during sleep (although most patients with periodic leg movements do not have daytime restless legs). The patient with restless legs reports deep, unpleasant leg muscle sensations that are resolved by moving the legs. Inactivity and tiredness exacerbate the problem. This condition has a strong familial incidence and generally becomes progressively worse with age. Treatment of the sleep-associated periodic leg movements is important in order to decrease wake time tiredness, but morning or wake time drowsiness may occur due to the medication used to treat the excessive movements.

Sleep Disorders which Mimic DIMS

Disorders of excessive somnolence or DOES (see details below) may present commonly with disturbed nocturnal sleep and are occasionally misdiagnosed as DIMS. This problem is exacerbated by the patient's tendency to minimize wake time sleepiness and to emphasize disturbances of nighttime sleep. When there is a history of napping, particularly with an irresistible need to nap, DOES must be considered as the primary diagnosis.

Sleep-wake schedule disturbance (see details below) can also be confused with DIMS. Again, it is crucial that wake time functioning be carefully assessed. In patients who report marked drowsiness and impaired functioning in a particular part of the day associated with a progressive delay in sleep onset, a sleep-wake schedule disturbance should be considered.

Natural short sleepers who are more commonly adult males may also present with DIMS symptoms. Again, the significant information relates to wake time functioning. The amount of sleep needed by any person varies considerably; there are recorded examples of patients who sleep very little and appear to function without difficulty (8). A short sleeper awakens refreshed with little difficulty functioning during the day. Generally, sleep onset time is minimal and there are few awakenings during the night. Furthermore, the short total sleep time remains constant over weekends and holidays and will have been stable since late adolescence. The patient usually seeks consultation either because others have convinced him that his sleep is abnormal and might cause medical problems or because he has trouble using his wake time when others are asleep. Since his sleep restores wakefulness, he can be reassured that he has no sleep problem and can be advised to use his extra wake time constructively.

DISORDERS OF EXCESSIVE SOMNOLENCE (DOES)

Diagnostic Evaluation

Symptoms of hypersomnia, unlike symptoms of insomnia, are often difficult to elicit with certainty from the patient (5). Once reported, either by the patient or a reliable observer, the symptoms deserve attention for they may indicate the presence of life-threatening sleep apnea. To assess symptom severity, behavior must be observed and recorded systematically. This is done by having either an observer or the patient himself complete for 1 or 2 days an hourly check of alertness using a scale such as that used in the Hopkins Alertness Report (see Fig. 85.2). Excessive wake time sleepiness is present when the patient reports no decrease in the amount of sleep he gets but has periods of very low alertness, significant sleepiness, and even takes naps during wake time. The patient's prior sleep history serves as the baseline for his "normal" amount of sleep, as there are no established sleep time norms that can be applied to patients, generally. In severe cases, there may be a history of accidents that can be attributed to the excessive sleepiness. Wake time activities that are associated with sleepiness in normal individuals result in pathological sleepiness in patients with these disorders. These activities include watching television, riding in or driving a car, reading, sitting in a conference, waiting to be seen at a physician's office, and relaxing soon after a large meal.

Definitive assessment of excessive somnolence re-

HOPKINS ALERTNESS REPORT	Patient Name: John Doe																						Date: 1/10/81
	Time																							
Behavior	(A.M.)											(Noon)	(P.M.)											Mid-night
	1	2	3	4	5	6	7	8	9	10	11	12	1	2	3	4	5	6	7	8	9	10	11	12
6. *Wide Awake: Alert* — Active, moving a lot, talking, listening, interacting, actively working—continually									√	√	√	√	√		√	√	√							
5. *Awake: Quiet* — Sitting, resting or leaning. Not participating in conversation or activities—only listening or watching. Working some—but not all the time (less than 50%)								√										√	√		√			
4. *Awake: Inattentive* — Not listening or following conversation or activity. Not working (more than 15% of time) Staring, lack of facial expression. Decreased body movements							√							√										
3. *Possibly dozing* 10% of time. Head dropping, eyes closing momentarily (less than 1 min) during 10–20% of time																						√		
2. *Definitely dozing* 20% of time. Head drops, eyes close for brief *naps* (less than 5 min) during at least 20% of time																					√			
1. *Asleep-Napping:* 20–50% time. Total nap time at least 12 min (20% of hr) or one nap of more than 5 min																								
0. *Asleep* for at least 50% of time	√	√	√	√	√	√																		√

Figure 85.2. Example of an alertness report which can be completed by a patient being evaluated for a sleep disorder. The example shows a normal sleep-wake pattern. (From the Johns Hopkins Sleep Disorder Center located at the Francis Scott Key Medical Center, Baltimore.)

quires observation such as that provided in a sleep disorders center (see above). If access to a center is not easily available, telephone consultation with the nearest center is often the most practical plan.

Transient Hypersomnia

Excessive daytime somnolence lasting less than 3 weeks is usually due to a psychological response to stress. Onset is abrupt, symptoms consist of persistent fatigue and loss of energy, and behavior is characterized by long periods of time in bed, as a result of an identifiable precipitating event. In contrast to other patients with DOES, these patients spend excessive time in bed and generally do not express significant drive or effort to leave the bed. The condition should improve simultaneously with improvement in the psychological problem; however, if the patient's sleep problem persists, an alternate diagnosis should be considered. In particular, drug abusers may present with DOES symptoms in an effort to obtain stimulant medication; therefore, physicians must use judgment in treating patients complaining of hypersomnolence who are not well known to them.

Persistent Hypersomnia

By definition, persistent hypersomnia is present when symptoms last longer than 3 weeks.

Sleep Apnea and Sleep-Induced Respiratory Impairments (5)

Definitions

These are by far the most serious disorders associated with sleep. They are characterized by breathing abnormalities that vary from reduction to complete cessation of airflow (hypopnea and apnea, respectively). The sleep apneas can be distinguished as *central apnea* (cessation of respiratory effort and, thus, no airflow) and *obstructive apnea* (occlusion of upper airway with continued respiratory effort). Isolated central apneas are usually associated with coexisting symptoms of insomnia, while obstructive apneas present typically with symptoms of excessive wake time somnolence. Importantly, all types of sleep-related apnea can be associated with hypoxemia and sleep fragmentation that lead to the systemic cardiovascular alterations and cognitive dysfunction noted in these individuals.

Epidemiology

The prevalence of sleep apnea is not well established; although it is suspected that as many as 1 to 2 million obese American men may have some degree of obstructive apnea. Recently, more young children are being diagnosed with obstructive sleep apnea. The typical patient with obstructive sleep

Table 85.3.
Disorders Associated with Sleep Apnea

OBSTRUCTIVE SLEEP APNEA
  Narrowing of upper airway
    Nasal abnormalities (deviation, polyps)
    Oral abnormalities (tonsillar hypertrophy, acromegaly)
    Bony abnormalities (micrognathia)
  Muscular abnormality
    Shy-Drager
    Myotonic dystrophy
  Hypothyroidism
CENTRAL SLEEP APNEA
  Central nervous system disorders (stroke)
  Brainstem-spinal defect (polio, infarction, neoplasia, surgery)
  Cardiovascular disorders (decreased cardiac output)

apnea is a middle-aged, mild to moderately obese man (male to female ratio of 20 to 30:1); however, this disorder is often associated with specific abnormalities of the upper airway or metabolic dysfunction (Table 85.3). By contrast, central sleep apnea occurs most commonly in either infants or normal individuals over 65. Frequently, central apnea may occur as a result of major central nervous system disease or brainstem spinal defects (Table 85.3).

Presentation

Characteristically, patients with obstructive apnea present with significant snoring or daytime hypersomnolence. The snoring is characteristically loud, intermittent, and often punctuated by respiratory efforts unaccompanied by obvious airflow. The snoring is associated with arousals and twitching at the termination of the apneas which cause demonstrable sleep fragmentation with subsequent daytime hypersomnolence. This sleepiness may range from subtle decreases in alertness toward the end of the day to onset of sleep in the middle of a conversation. Since most patients are unaware of their breathing pattern and often underestimate the severity of daytime somnolence, unless extreme, it is imperative that a bed partner or other observer be present for the initial evaluation. Other clinical manifestations include choking or gasping episodes at night, systemic and pulmonary hypertension, and, in severe cases, cor pulmonale. By contrast, patients with central apnea will usually be observed to cease breathing with no associated respiratory efforts. In adults, there may be associated snoring, gasping for air, and arousal from sleep since often the central apnea occurs in combination with obstructive events; thus, it is often not possible clinically to distinguish the two forms of apnea.

The physical examination is usually not diagnostic in patients with obstructive apnea, although patients with narrowing of the upper airway are at significantly higher risk. In particular, children and adults who demonstrate a compatible history and marked tonsillar hypertrophy or retrognathia should be suspected of having this disorder. In elderly individuals with central apnea, the physical examination is normal, while patients with neurological or cardiovascular pathology will usually demonstrate obvious localizing signs (e.g., stroke) or cardiomegaly (cardiomyopathy).

Course

The course of obstructive sleep apnea appears to be chronic, although not necessarily progressive if body weight remains stable. Some patients clearly develop progressive cardiopulmonary decompensation manifested by worsening hypercarbia and hypoxemia which can be associated with cor pulmonale and life-threatening arrhythmias. Nevertheless, these complications are the exception and tend to occur in the more severely obese individuals after many years of disease. By contrast, the course of central apnea is determined by the underlying pathological process. Thus, if reversible central nervous system or cardiovascular disease exists, central apnea may resolve entirely. In normal elderly individuals with central apnea, the course and prognosis are unknown.

Diagnosis

A working diagnosis of sleep apnea can be made by direct observation of the patient during sleep, either at home or in a general hospital. However, even with ideal observation, clinically significant apnea may not be appreciated (7a). Definitive diagnosis requires a sleep study (see above) that monitors the various parameters previously outlined. Other laboratory studies such as arterial blood gases and routine pulmonary function provide information about mechanical or gas exchange abnormalities useful in therapy but not diagnosis. Flow volume curves may demonstrate fluttering during expiration associated with evidence of variable extrathoracic obstruction in patients with obstructive apnea. Although this test is quite specific it is not very sensitive; therefore, it is not recommended to screen patients. Finally, computerized tomography of the upper airway consistently demonstrates narrowing of the upper airway in patients with obstructive sleep apnea. Nevertheless, it is unclear at the present time how this information can be best utilized in the management of these patients. Therefore, patients with suspected sleep apnea should either be managed empirically (see below) or referred for definitive evaluation in a sleep laboratory.

Management

The treatment of obstructive sleep apnea continues to evolve and, thus, consultation with a certified sleep center or pulmonologist experienced in this disorder will be useful. Table 85.4 summarizes a

Table 85.4.
Approaches to Management of Obstructive Sleep Apnea

GENERAL
    Avoid CNS depressants
    Weight loss
UPPER AIRWAY MEASURES
    Tracheostomy
    Palatopharyngoplasty
    Constant positive airway pressure (CPAP)
MEDICATIONS
    Medroxyprogesterone
    Protriptyline
OXYGEN

number of the approaches that have been tried. Ambulatory medical therapy dominates the management of these patients. Initial management should emphasize correcting associated medical conditions such as hypothyroidism (12) or anatomical factors such as severe tonsillar hypertrophy, control of weight, and the avoidance of CNS depressants. Although the mechanism for improvement in obstructive apnea is not entirely known, it is clear that as little as 10% weight loss may markedly improve the severity of the apneas (14). Since most patients are 30 to 40% above ideal body weight, the minimal amount of weight reduction expected does not represent an unrealistic goal. Patients should adopt a life style change that allows slow (about 1 lb/week) and progressive weight loss that can be maintained over a long period of time rather than attempting rapid weight loss (see practical approaches in Chapter 76, Obesity). Patients and their families usually note that symptoms such as snoring and wake time sleepiness begin to improve after approximately a 5% loss of body weight. In those individuals who can return to within 10% of ideal body weight, there can be total resolution of apneas and associated symptoms.

Selection of *surgical measures* to alter upper airway anatomy requires consultation with an otolaryngologist. While tracheostomy was once employed regularly in the treatment of this syndrome, it is infrequently performed now because of the newer forms of medical therapy and the associated psychosocial adjustments and physical discomfort. Palatopharyngoplasty and constant positive airway pressure (CPAP) should be considered new procedures and should be performed only at institutions that are systemically evaluating these forms of therapy.

Medications such as medroxyprogesterone and protriptyline have been used to treat obstructive sleep apnea, but it is still unclear which patients will respond to pharmacological therapy (13). In general, protriptyline has been shown more consistently to reduce the snoring and severity of sleep apnea, while improving daytime hypersomnolence

in people with mild to moderately severe obstructed apnea. The initial dosage is 5 to 10 mg given at bedtime or early in the morning if sleep onset is delayed as a result of the medication. In general, 30% of patients experience side effects that include dry mouth, difficulty initiating micturition in older men, and constipation. Since protriptyline is a mild appetite suppressant, it may facilitate weight reduction.

Presently, it is unclear which patients respond best to oxygen therapy; however, individuals with significant cor pulmonale appear to benefit the most. Patients usually will have evidence of resting, awake, and nocturnal hypoxemia; therefore, continuous 24-hour oxygen therapy will occasionally be required.

As a general rule, all forms of therapy discussed will reduce but not eliminate episodes of obstructive sleep apnea, except when the airway is bypassed (e.g., tracheostomy and CPAP). After therapy is initiated, bed partners should be instructed to observe changes in frequency of apneas as well as improvements in snoring, but they should be told not to expect complete elimination of these breathing irregularities. Furthermore, any changes in breathing pattern with alterations in diet or medications for other conditions should be noted.

Presently, there are no therapies for central apnea that consistently produce a reduction in frequency of events. Administration of oxygen will, however, almost always reverse any associated hypoxemia and bradyarrhythmias. Various respiratory stimulants have produced conflicting results, and there are too few studies evaluating diaphragmatic pacing.

Narcolepsy and Idiopathic Hypersomnolence (17)

These are perhaps the best recognized primary disorders of excessive somnolence, even though they remain difficult to diagnose. Both narcolepsy and idiopathic hypersomnolence are characterized by irresistible need for wake time naps. The naps vary in duration from 30 seconds to 15 minutes and yet the subject awakens refreshed only to become somnolent with 2 to 3 hours. Most patients will report frequent near accidents and socially embarrassing situations related to their uncontrollable hypersomnolence. Narcolepsy also involves REM disturbances not seen in idiopathic hypersomnolence.

Narcolepsy

The prevalence of narcolepsy is approximately 4/10,000. It is equally common in men and women. Symptoms usually develop in the second decade of life and are relatively stable once the wake time sleepiness has developed fully. There is a probable genetic linkage with HLA-DW2 for at least Japanese and Caucasians. The pathogenesis also probably involves abnormal control of REM sleep.

In narcolepsy, excessive wake time sleepiness is

Table 85.5.
Drugs for Narcolepsy

Drug	Available Strengths (mg)	Minimum Effective Dose (mg)	Maximum Effective Dose (mg)	Time for Dose Effect
FOR HYPERSOMNOLENCE				
Dextroamphetamine (Dexedrine, generics)	5, 10, 15	5, every day	20, 3 times daily	3 days
Magnesium pemoline (Cylert)	18.75, 37.5	37.5, every day	112.5 every day	1 week
Methylphenidate (Ritalin, generics)	10, 20	10, twice daily	30, 3 and 4 times daily	3 days
FOR CATAPLEXY				
Protriptyline (Vivactil)[a, b]	5, 10	5, twice daily	10, 4 times daily	1 week
Imipramine (Tofranil, generics)[b]	25	25, twice daily	25, 4 times daily	1 week
Desipramine (Norpromin, Pertofrane)[b]	25, 50	25, twice daily	50, twice daily	1 week

[a] May also help reduce wake time sleepiness.
[b] For details on the use of tricyclics, see Chapter 15.

usually accompanied by one or more of the following symptoms: (a) *cataplexy*—a transitory sudden loss of postural muscle tone, sometimes causing collapse without loss of consciousness and often precipitated by an emotional response such as laughing, crying, or anger; (b) *sleep paralysis*—awakening with a transitory inability to move or speak, sometimes associated with dream-like hallucinations (this symptom is different from the sleep palsies experienced occasionally by most people—transient sensorimotor palsies of the ulnar, radial, and peroneal nerves which are subject to prolonged compression during deep sleep); (c) *hypnagogic hallucinations*—dream like, usually visual, hallucinations occurring at the transition from wakefulness to sleep; and (d) *disturbed nocturnal sleep*—frequent brief awakening during a night's sleep. In some narcoleptic patients, these associated symptoms may occur before the development of wake time sleep attacks; in others they may never occur. Conditions which may be found in association with narcolepsy include sleep apnea (see above), sleep-related myoclonus (see above), and automatic behaviors, all of which occur more commonly in patients with narcolepsy than in the general population.

A working diagnosis of narcolepsy can be made on the basis of the history given by the patient and other observers. The definite diagnosis must be based upon characteristic findings in the napping tests performed in a sleep laboratory after other sleep disorders have been excluded by a nocturnal sleep study.

The treatment of narcolepsy utilizes both pharmacological and environmental measures to correct the two major symptoms, sleepiness and cataplexy. Before initiating treatment, the patient's usual pattern of daytime hypersomnolence should be documented to provide a baseline for assessing the response to therapy. Any of three stimulant drugs—magnesium pemoline (Cylert), methylphenidate (Ritalin), dextroamphetamine (Dexedrine)—and one

tricyclic—protriptyline (Vivactil)—will provide relief from the wake time sleepiness. Tolerance is a major problem for all stimulants, and weekend drug "holidays" are advised. A minimally effective dose should be initiated with gradual increases in dosage every 1 to 2 weeks until symptom relief or side effects occur (see Table 85.5). Environmental management focuses on diet and planned wake time naps. Patients should avoid large meals and significant alcohol intake since both will exacerbate an underlying tendency for sleepiness. The cataplexy associated with narcolepsy is most effectively controlled by the tricyclics, imipramine (Tofranil) and protriptyline (Vivactil) (see Table 85.5). A regimen that was particularly effective in one large group of patients with sleep attacks plus cataplexy was treatment with imipramine, 25 mg, and methylphenidate, 5 to 10 mg three times daily (17). However, desipramine (Norpramin) and protriptyline (Vivactil) may be more effective than imipramine for reducing cataplexy with less sedation (see Chapter 15 for additional details about tricyclic antidepressants).

Idiopathic Hypersomnolence (IPH)

Approximately 10% of patients presenting with excessive daytime hypersomnolence will be diagnosed as having idiopathic hypersomnolence. As opposed to narcolepsy, idiopathic hypersomnolence is not associated with inappropriate REM sleep during the daytime. These patients report a more pervasive sleepiness with less benefit from naps and less dreaming during naps than do narcoleptics; they also do *not* report the other symptoms of narcolepsy—sleep paralysis, hypnogogic images, and cataplexy. Treatment includes use of stimulants, although the response is less consistent than in patients with narcolepsy.

In light of the difficult diagnosis, the variable response to treatment, and the significant risk of a false historic reporting by individuals seeking stimulant medications, patients with suspected narcolepsy or idiopathic hypersomnolence should be discussed with a specialist in sleep disorders (see Table 85.2).

Medical and Environmental Causes (16)

Causes for hypersomnia not due to a specific sleep disorder are varied and usually result in persistent wake time sleepiness. The more common medical conditions which should be considered are hypothyroidism (or apathetic hyperthyroidism in the elderly), hypoglycemia, anemia, uremia, hypercapnia, hypercalcemia, liver failure, and a number of neurological abnormalities (epilepsy, neurosyphilis, multiple sclerosis, chronic brain syndrome, brain tumors involving the brainstem and third ventricle, and progressive hydrocephalus from any cause). Progressive hydrocephalus may present initially as excessive somnolence without localizing findings; and sleepiness after head trauma may not develop until 6 to 18 months after the trauma.

Iatrogenic hypersomnia may accompany the use of a number of drugs with sedating side effects including centrally acting antihypertensives (reserpine, methyldopa, clonidine, β-blockers), antihistamines, anxiolytic agents, tricyclic antidepresssants, neuroleptics, sedative-hypnotic drugs, and barbiturates used in epilepsy.

Physical confinement and reduced environmental stimulation may lead to excessive somnolene. For example, in the elderly, there is a natural tendency toward wake time sleepiness, which in combination with some restrictions on activities, promotes excessive somnolence.

In each of these conditions, improvement in hypersomnolence depends largely upon improving the primary conditions. Thus, proper diagnosis, appropriate therapy, and discontinuation or adjustment of sedating medications will generally reduce but seldom completely reverse the sleepiness unless the primary condition is resolved (e.g., hypothyroidism).

Psychological Conditions

Psychosocial stress, affective disorders, and *schizophrenia* may present with persistent wake time sleepiness. Patients will usually note precipitating stressful events or will demonstrate evidence of significant clinical depression. Moreover, the wake time status often involves a feeling of general fatigue and loss of energy, without need for sleep to restore wakefulness. These patients require management with a combination of psychotherapy and appropriate medications (see Chapters 12, 15, and 16).

Voluntary insufficient sleep occurs in our industrialized society, apparently related to social demands. For example, when college students are examined within the laboratory environment, they often demonstrate significant daytime hypersomnolence. With increased sleep time to approximately 9 or 10 hours, this sleepiness resolves. Thus, it is important to review the social and occupational circumstances under which the excessive daytime somnolence is occurring.

Other Sleep Disorders That Mimic DOES

Sleep-wake schedule disturbances (see below) may be incorrectly diagnosed as hypersomnia since these patients sleep late in the day and report an inability to stay awake for a large part of society's normal workday. In severe cases, the patient may have occasional reversal of the sleep-wake cycle with very long periods of sleep, short periods of wakefulness, and a complaint of never feeling very much awake. Sleep-related myoclonus (see above) often presents with wake time sleepiness and in extreme cases may be confused with narcolepsy. Minor symptoms generally associated with DIMS (insomnia) or DOES are present in wake time, e.g., morning malaise, minor irritations, diplopia, irritability, and multiple somatic complaints. Unlike DIMS, there is no problem initiating and maintaining sleep.

Natural long sleepers (usually adult females) also complain of excessive somnolence, sometimes because they have insufficient sleep owing to requirements of daily living, but more often because they feel they need too much sleep. The total sleep time required by a small subgroup of individuals (less than 2% of the adult population) is greater than 9 hours. When not under pressure, these individuals may sleep as much as 12 to 14 hours/day. This trend develops by early adolescence and remains stable throughout life. Therefore, when sleep time increases significantly later in life, it should not be attributed to this condition. Adequate protracted sleep, in one consolidated sleep period each day, serves as both the diagnostic test and treatment for natural long sleepers. In difficult cases, sleep center referral should be considered to evaluate the patient for one of the causes of DOES.

DISORDERS OF THE SLEEP-WAKE SCHEDULE

Transient Problems

The homeostatic and circadian oscillation control of sleep and waking are usually well linked in a stable 24-hour pattern corresponding to social demands. Certain conditions may disrupt these relations leading to disorder of the sleep-wake cycle usually characterized by sleepiness at inappropriate times. Transient disturbances of the circadian cycle are well known to occur with transmeridian jet travel and with shiftwork. Recent understanding of these problems has led to improved techniques for reducing these types of sleep impairments.

For *jet travel,* short acting sedative-hypnotics, such as triazolam (see Table 85.6), have been shown

Table 85.6.
Sedative-Hypnotic Benzodiazepine Drugs (in Order by Increasing Duration of Action)

Drug	Rate of Absorption or Appearance[d]	Half-life[e] (hr)	Available Strengths (mg)	Minimum Effective Dose (mg)	Maximum Recommended Dose (mg)
SHORT ACTING					
Midazolam (Versed)[a]	Fast	1.5–3.5	7.5, 15	7.5	15
Triazolam (Halcion)[b]	Intermediate	1.5–5.0	0.25, 0.5	0.125	0.5
Brotizolam[a]			0.25, 0.5	0.25	0.5
INTERMEDIATE ACTING					
(half-lives usually 10–20 hours)					
Oxazepam (Serax)[c]	Slow	4–15	10, 15, 30	10	30
Lorazepam (Ativan)	Intermediate	10–20	0.5, 1, 2	0.5	4
Estazolam[a]	Intermediate	10–20	1, 2	1.0	2.0
Temazepam (Restoril)[c]	Slow	8–22	15, 30	15	30
Clonazepam (Clonopin)			0.5, 1, 2	0.5	1.5
LONG ACTING					
Diazepam (Valium)	Rapid	40–120	2, 5, 10	2	15
Chlordiazepoxide (Librium)		36–200	5, 10, 25	5	25
Flurazepam (Dalmane)	Rapid	36–200	15, 30	15	30

[a] These medications were not available in the US market at the time this table was prepared.
[b] This medication commonly used at 0.125 mg starting dose for patients over 45, and 0.25 mg for younger patients.
[c] These medications have have a somewhat delayed onset of action and should be taken about 1 hour before bedtime.
[d] Rate for most rapid significantly active compound in blood; correlates with onset of sedating action.
[e] Half-life for longest significantly active compound in blood.

to permit sleep at the new time schedule and to facilitate wakefulness during the next day. Medication should be used for only 3 to 5 days. This treatment is useful for travel from east to west or west to east.

Shift workers demonstrate poor sleep during the daytime with subsequent sleepiness during the evening or night shift. The sleep-wake difficulties can be minimized by adjusting the sleep schedules with a forward rotation. In other words, an evening shift should be followed by night followed by day and not in the reverse order, which is the more typical manner. In addition, adjustments to a new shift require 4 to 5 days; therefore, new changes in work shifts should be maintained for a minimum of 2 weeks before another change is initiated. In one study, this has clearly resulted in increased worker productivity with a concomitant decrease in accidents (4). Shift workers on night shift will generally do better sleeping in the afternoon than in the day.

Persistent Problems

Persistent disruption of the normal sleep-wake cycle has only in recent years been recognized as a biologically based sleep disorder. This disorder may begin in childhood but usually develops in young adult life following some change in living schedule. The prevalence is unknown since the disorder has only been recognized recently.

Mechanism and Manifestations

The circadian biological rhythms of all species exert a major influence upon sleep. In an environment free of all time cues (e.g., prolonged living in a cave with constant light), the circadian rhythm for man runs slightly longer than 24 hours (about 24.5 to 25.5 hours). Under normal circumstances, the internal clock in each individual is reset evey 24 hours in response to external cues. For reasons that are not clear, some people fail to entrain their internal cycle to the socially prescribed 24-hour clock. They either lose a stable cycle (progressive sleep cycle delay) or the cycle becomes fixed, unfortunately, out of phase with social demands. In the former case, the patient's sleep period changes rapidly, with occasional periods of prolonged sleepiness. In the latter case, the patient attempts sleep when he is physiologically most active and, therefore, finds sleep difficult to establish. Conversely, during the daytime, he must struggle to stay awake when he is physiologically ready for sleep. Under these circumstances, it is understandable why there are complaints about both insomnia and daytime sleepiness.

In contrast to most other sleep disorders, patients with sleep cycle disturbances report normal, good quality sleep when they are allowed to sleep for a few days on their own schedule, such as on nonworking days. Most report a nearly fixed delay in sleep onset (several hours after the expected bedtime), plus an ability to sleep late and to feel refreshed on the late awakening. Some report an advance in their cycle so that they are sleepy too early in the evening and unable to sleep in the early morning. Less commonly, the patients report the following cycle in their sleep disturbance: a period of insomnia with wake time sleepiness, followed by a period of premature sleepiness with premature awakenings. There is a brief period of normal sleep which ends in a repetition of the entire cycle beginning with insomnia with wake time sleepiness. Compared to the fixed sleep cycle delay, this progressive sleep cycle delay is an extremely unusual conditon diagnosed by the characteristic history.

Diagnosis

A sleep-wake log (see Fig. 85.2) and a temperature record assist in the diagnosis. For 2 consecutive days, the patient is instructed to keep an oral temperature record for every 2 hours when not asleep. The temperature should not be taken within 10 minutes of consuming hot or cold beverages or food nor within 30 minutes after physical exercise. Body temperature fluctuates 1 to $2°F$ (about 0.5 to $1°C$) during the day, reaching a peak during the time of greatest alertness and dropping off just before sleep onset. A temperature record showing no relative decrease before the planned bedtime supports the diagnosis.

Differential Diagnosis

This disorder is commonly misdiagnosed as insomnia or as a problem of excessive somnolence. Both of these are excluded, if during extended sleep the patient sleeps well with good restoration of wakefulness. In some psychological disturbances, particularly manic type bipolar affective disorders and neurotic depression (see Chapter 15), sleep onset is delayed for a few hours. However, in these patients, the total sleep time is usually markedly reduced.

Schizophrenia may present with a sleep cycle disruption which resembles this disorder, but usually the underlying psychosis is diagnosed early. Some patients seen after chronic sedative-hypnotic (or stimulant) use may indeed have a primary disturbance in the sleep-wake cycle, a diagnosis which becomes apparent once the sleep-wake medication has been discontinued.

Treatment

Patients with the working diagnosis of fixed sleep-wake cycle delay can be placed on "chronotherapy." The first night the patient sleeps at the time suited for his internal clock. Each consecutive day, the bedtime and wake time are advanced to 2 hours later, until after 8 to 10 days the desired bedtime is reached. Good sleep habits (Table 85.1) are then recommended to maintain the desired bedtime. Use of sedative-hypnotics or stimulants in this group of patients will not reset the sleep cycle and will seriously complicate the treatment. Unfortunately, chronotherapy is not effective in patients with the progressive sleep cycle delays or sleep cycle advance; these conditions are often difficult to manage. The best plan is referral to a sleep center (see Table 85.2) for diagnosis and individualized environmental management without medication.

DYSFUNCTIONS ASSOCIATED WITH SLEEP (PARASOMNIAS)

There are a number of miscellaneous problems associated with sleep, including three major disorders associated with incomplete arousal, usually from deep sleep. These incomplete arousals are increased by stress and tend to co-occur in the same person, who is often seen as a "deep" sleeper. There is a familial tendency for these disorders, and they occur most often in childhood.

Sleepwalking

Sleepwalking occurs in the first third of the sleep period with partial or total amnesia for the event on awakening. It is most common between ages 6 and 12, when it resolves. Occasionally, sleepwalking occurs in adults, although there is an antecedent history in childhood with complete remission until a recurrence in the late twenties or thirties when it may persist for several years. During sleepwalking, arousal from sleep can be difficult and the walking is complicated by associated clumsiness and accidents. Measures should, therefore, be taken to reduce the risks of accidents (e.g., ensure closed lower windows, restricted access to stairways, and cleared floor areas). Parents can be reassured that sleepwalking is otherwise of little concern, even though patients may report that it is worse during stress. In adults, however, there is usually an associated psychological problem requiring evaluation and appropriate psychotherapy. The possibility of sleep-induced seizures—particularly temporal lobe seizures in the REM stage of sleep—should be excluded (see Chapter 80). Sleepwalking in the elderly (over 65) is rare unless precipitated by sedative-hypnotic use.

Sleep Terrors (3)

Sleep terrors occur in childhood as loud and uncontrollable screaming usually during the first third of the sleep period, but occasionally repeating later in sleep. Throughout an episode, the child is generally uncontrollable until shortly before he returns to sleep. Fortunately, there is complete amnesia for the event, although the behavior is very disturbing to the family. Adults also experience sleep terrors characterized by sudden awakenings in the first third of the night accompanied by a profound sense of dread but not by the loud scream. Marked autonomic activity (tachycardia, diaphoresis) occurs in both children and adults. Sleep terrors occur in 1 to 4% of children beginning between ages 1 and 12 and ceasing by early adolescence. Adult onset is less common but does occur in the twenties or thirties but almost never after 40. Treatment of children includes reassurance of the family that the condition is benign. When the problem is very disrupting, a low dose anxiolytic agent, such as 2 to 5 mg of diazepam (Valium), at bedtime usually provides complete remission. Treatment for adults includes psychotherapy and a short course of treatment with a benzodiazepine agent. Bedtime doses of tricyclic antidepressants and neuroleptics should be avoided since exacerbation of the sleep terrors may result. The differential diagnosis includes sleep apnea, sleep-related epilepsy, and dream anxiety attacks. When sleep terrors persist in adults, sleep center referral (see above) should be considered to ensure correct diagnosis. For children, a referral should be considered if the condition is extreme and persistent.

Sleep-Related Enuresis (3)

Persistent sleep-related enuresis is relatively common in childhood, occurring at age 5 in 15% of boys and 10% of girls. By puberty, the problem usually remits. Unless the sleep-related enuresis is associated with other problems, persists beyond puberty, or recurs after remission of several months, it can be considered benign. For adult onset or for recurring enuresis, the most important possibilities in the differential diagnosis are epilepsy, psychological disturbance, neurogenic bladder, dementia, and sleep apnea. Behavioral treatment for childhood enuresis is preferred to medication because it is more effective and safer.

SLEEP MEDICATIONS

Sedative-Hypnotic Drugs

As noted in previous sections, sedative-hypnotic drugs may be useful in dealing with a number of sleep disorders. The benefits from these medications reported by patients may be very significant, even though the overall effects on sleep are a 10- to 30-minute reduction in sleep onset time and a 20- to 40-minute increase in total sleep time (15). The most important contraindication for sedative-hypnotic drug use is any symptom or sign of unexplained respiratory problems at night, including a history of heavy snoring or significant wake time sleepiness, as these may indicate sleep apnea (see above, page 1222).

Selection and Use

The sedative-hypnotics of first choice are the *benzodiazepines*. Table 85.6 summarizes available tablet sizes and recommended doses for sleep medications in this group. There is very little reason to select barbiturates or other sedative-hypnotics due to their significantly lower toxic to therapeutic ratio.

Since tolerance may develop to all sedative-hypnotics, the daily use of any of these drugs should be limited to 4 weeks. It is best to start at the minimum effective dose (see Table 85.6) and to permit an increase in dose, if necessary, every 3 to 4 days until the effective dose is found or the usual maximum dose is reached. Most patients can titrate their own dose for symptom relief, but the dosage should not be increased once tolerance to an effective dose occurs. Even in the most unusual case, increasing doses more than twice is likely to create a new problem of drug dependence and does little to solve the patient's sleep problem.

In adjusting dosage, particular attention should be given to wake time function. Several of the popular benzodiazepines (flurazepam, diazepam, chlordiazepoxide) along with their active metabolites have long half-lives which may produce continuing daytime sedation even after one dose. When taken daily, the cumulative effects of these medications may lead to drowsiness during waking hours. Under these circumstances, the dosage should be decreased. For the longer acting benzodiazepines, such as flurazepam (Dalmane), diazepam (Valium), and chlordiazepoxide (Librium), weekend drug-free intervals are recommended; alternatively, the shorter acting benzodiazepines, triazolam (Halcion), oxazepam (Serax), lorazepam (Ativan), and temazepam (Restoril) may be considered. Very short acting benzodiazipines, such as triazolam (Halcion), cause little or no wake time sedation. They have, however, been reported to produce a *rebound insomnia* (insomnia after stopping the medication which is worse than that before treatment). Studies reporting this finding have methodological problems, and often studies have failed to confirm the existence of a rebound form of insomnia. If this problem occurs, it appears to be rare and lasts only 2 days after stopping the medication.

The barbiturate sedative-hypnotics have three distinct disadvantages in comparison with the benzodiazepines: the frequent occurrence of hangover after only one dose, the development of physiological dependence with the accompanying risk of a severe withdrawal reaction, and the low toxic to therapeutic ratio. A number of other sedative-hypnotics (chloral hydrate, glutethimide, meprobamate, methaqualone, and methyprylon) have been shown to be effective, but are associated with especially high potential for lethal respiratory depression with overdose. Therefore, there is little reason to select one of these agents or a barbiturate instead of a benzodiazepine. Of the entire group, chloral hydrate (500 to 1000 mg) is perhaps the safest if an alternative to the benzodiazepines is needed.

Information to Patients

When prescribing a sedative-hypnotic medication, it is recommended that sleeping medications be taken 10 to 60 minutes before bedtime, depending on the rate of absorption of the medication (see Table 85.6). The patient should be warned of the following: (*a*) the risk of tolerance and dependence with later withdrawal problems (especially with barbiturates and the short acting benzodiazepines) and the risk of developing the "sleeping pill habit" and never adequately resolving the sleep problem; (b) potential problems of interaction with other drugs, particularly alcohol (alcohol abstinence, particularly after dinner, is essential and the patient should generally not take more than one sedating medication in the same day); (c) hangover effects and the possibility of becoming sleepy while driving, especially after the first few days on the longer acting benzodiazepines or barbiturates; and (d) the uncertain knowledge about effects on pregnancy.

Sedative-Hypnotic Withdrawal

For patients taking too much sleeping medication, the withdrawal must be gradual, particularly if the patient has been on a regimen for several months. These patients may report worsening insomnia due to chronic use of the medication (see above, page 1220) or develop physiological dependence and risk serious withdrawal symptoms. Nevertheless, withdrawal should be attempted and the patient informed that he will become temporarily worse before improving. The dosage of medication should be reduced by one therapeutic dose per week. If more than one medication is involved, one medication at a time should be reduced. Contact with the physician is essential in order to avoid relapses during this trying experience. Difficult but motivated patients may need expert assistance from a psychotherapist with broad experience in managing withdrawal from drugs (see Chapter 22).

Over-the-Counter Sleep Medications and Antihistamines (Table 85.7)

Over-the-counter (OTC) sleep medications and antihistamines are effective for many patients with transient insomnia and may be as effective as low doses of the commonly prescribed sedative-hypnotics. The OTC medications contain small amounts of antihistamines.

The prescription sedative-antihistamines include diphenhydramine (Benadryl), 25 to 50 mg, and hydroxyzine (Vistaril and Atarax), 25 and 50 mg. These drugs are more potent sedatives than the OTC sleeping medications. They may be particularly useful in patients with chronic obstructive pulmonary disease, for whom benzodiazepines are hazardous because they can suppress respiration.

Tricyclic Antidepressants

The most sedating of the tricyclic antidepressants, such as amitriptyline (Elavil) and imipramine (Tofranil), are useful in low doses for the management of persistent insomnia associated with those psychological conditions in which there is a depressive or obsessive-compulsive component. These medications are particularly effective either when sleep onset is disturbed by anxiety or ruminating thoughts or when sleep is interrupted in the later part of the sleep period by dreams characterized by anxiety.

Table 85.7.
Constituents of Commonly Used Over-the-Counter Sleep Remedies

Product Name	Constituent	
Miles Nervine[a]		
Sleep-Eze	Pyrilamine maleate[b]	25 mg
Sominex[c]		
Nytol		
Unisom Night-time Sleep Aid	Doxylamine succinate[d]	25 mg

[a] This product no longer contains bromine.
[b] Antihistamine of the ethylenediamine class.
[c] This product no longer contains scopolamine.
[d] Antihistamine of the ethanolamine class.

Under these conditions, the tricyclics are preferable to sedative-hypnotics both because of better efficacy and the lesser probability of dependence. Usual dose is 25 to 75 mg about 1 to 2 hours before bed. At this dose, the side effects are usually minimal. Additional information about tricyclics is found in Chapter 15.

General References

Chase MH, Weitzman ED (eds): *Sleep Disorders: Basic and Clinical Research*, vol 8. *Advances in Sleep Research* (Weitzman ED, senior Ed). New York, Spectrum, 1983.
> Very good technical but readable articles on the scientific basis for sleep disorders. Excellent section on hypnotics.

Coats TJ, Thoresen CE (eds): *How to Sleep Better: A Drug-Free Program for Overcoming Insomnia*. Englewood Cliffs, NJ, Prentice-Hall, 1977.
> Useful self-help book emphasizing self-regulation techniques.

Guilleminault C (ed): *Sleeping and Waking Disorders: Indications and Techniques*. Menlo Park, CA, Addison-Wesley, 1982.
> Basic text on methodology and treatment.

Hauri P (ed): *The Sleep Disorders, Current Concepts*. Kalamazoo, MI, Upjohn, 1982.
> A useful general introductory work to sleep, sleep disorders, and their treatment. (The Upjohn Company provides copies of this small booklet.)

Lamberg L (ed): *American Medical Association Guide to Better Sleep*. New York, Random House, 1984.
> Nontechnical introduction to sleep disorders written for the general public, but so well done it is useful as a secondary reference.

Phillipson DA, Bowes G: Sleep disorders. In Fishman AP (ed): *Update: Pulmonary Diseases and Disorders*. New York, McGraw-Hill, 1982, p 256.
> Excellent review of pathophysiology and diagnosis of obstructive sleep apnea.

Specific References

1. Association of Sleep Disorders Centers: Diagnostic classification of sleep and arousal disorders. *Sleep* 2:1, 1979.
2. Bixler EO, Kales A, Soldatos CR, et al: Prevalence of sleep disorders in the Los Angeles metropolitan area. *Am J Psychiatry* 136:1257, 1979.
3. Broughton R: Sleep disorders: disorders of arousal? *Science* 159:1070, 1978.
4. Czeisler CA, Moore-Ede C, Coleman RM: Rotating shift work schedules that disrupt sleep are improved by applying circadian principles. *Science* 217:460, 1982.
5. Dement WC, Carskadon MA, Richardson G: Excessive daytime sleepiness in the sleep apnea syndrome. In Guilleminault C, Dement WC (eds): *Sleep Apnea Syndromes*. New York, Alan R Liss, 1978, p 23.

6. Gilin JC, Duncan W, Pettigew DK, *et al*: Successful separation of depressed, normal and insomniac subjects by EEG sleep data. *Arch Gen Psychiatry* 36:85, 1979.

7. Guilleminault C, Eldridge FL, Dement WC: Insomnia with sleep apnea: a new syndrome. *Science* 181:856, 1973.

7a. Haponik E, Smith PL, Bleeker FR: Diagnosis of obstructive sleep apnea: is polysommography necessary? *Chest* 84:354, 1983.

8. Jones H, Oswald I: Two cases of healthy insomnia. *Electroencephalogr Clin Neurophysiol* 24:378, 1968.

9. Kales A, Bixler EO, Tan TL, *et al*: Chronic hypnotic drug use: ineffectiveness, drug withdrawal insomnia and hypnotic drug dependence. *JAMA* 227:513, 1974.

10. Lugaresi E, Coccagna G, Gambi C, *et al*: Symond's nocturnal myoclonus. *Electroencephalogr Clin Neurophysiol* 23:289, 1967.

11. National Center for Health Statistics: *Selected Symptoms of Psychological Distress*. US Public Health Service Publication 1000, series II, no. 37. Washington, DC, US Department of Health, Education and Welfare, August, 1970.

12. Rajagopal KR, Abbrecht PH, Derderian SS, *et al*: Obstructive sleep apnea in hypothyroidism. *Ann Intern Med* 101:491, 1984.

13. Smith PL, Haponik EF, Allen RP, Bleecker ER: The effects of protriptyline in sleep-disordered breathing. *Am Rev Respir Dis* 127:8, 1983.

14. Smith PL, Haponik EF, Gold AR, Bleecker ER: The effect of weight loss on sleep disordered breathing. *Am Rev Respir Dis* 129:A59, 1984.

15. Solomon F, White CC, Parron DL, Mendelson WB: Special report: sleeping pills, insomnia and medical practice, from the Institute of Medicine of the National Academy of Sciences. *N Engl J Med* 300:803, 1979.

16. Williams RL: Sleep disorders in various medical and surgical conditions. In Williams RL, Karacan I (eds): *Sleep Disorders* New York, John Wiley & Sons, 1978.

17. Zarcone V: Narcolepsy. *N Engl J Med* 288:1156, 1973.

SECTION 12

Selected General Surgical Problems

CHAPTER EIGHTY-SIX

Preoperative Planning for Ambulatory Patients

RICHARD J. GROSS, M.D., L. RANDOL BARKER, M.D., AND
EVERETT K. SPEES, M.D., PH.D.

PREOPERATIVE PLANNING: OVERVIEW

The general physician often invests substantial time and effort in preoperative planning for a patient with a problem amenable to surgery. He schedules tests to confirm the initial diagnosis, discusses the findings with the patient and the patient's family, proposes consultation with a surgeon, and consults on the care of the patient's medical problems in the perioperative period. Most preoperative planning should be done in the ambulatory setting. Increasingly large proportions of operations are performed in ambulatory surgery units, which require outpatient preoperative "clearance" based on an office visit (14, 25).

In general, the surgeon expects the referring physician to have made an independent assessment of the need for surgery *and of the patient's general fitness for surgery.* Although the surgeon obtains the actual consent for the surgical procedure, the patient's expectations and assumptions are often based upon the counseling provided by his personal physician. The referral itself is usually understood by the patient and his family as an endorsement of the importance of a surgical opinion and of the competence of the consulting surgeon. For these reasons, the general physician should know the place of surgery in the management of a broad array of conditions (or should discuss the possibility of surgery with a surgeon whenever he is uncertain) and should be aware of the competence of the surgeon whom he selects. Two recently published books which summarize the probability of success and failure in a large variety of surgical procedures are especially useful (8, 9).

In counseling the patient and his family, the general physician, as well as the surgeon, should explain clearly the objective and the expected outcome of the operation. This is especially important for surgical procedures which are undertaken for asymptomatic conditions (such as elective cholecystectomy) and for procedures which may be disfiguring (such as mastectomy or amputation). Preoperative counseling should be documented in the patient's record, and this documentation should always include any special issues raised by the patient and how they were resolved (such as obtaining additional consultations or providing supportive counseling). A description of the surgical procedure written for the lay person can be a useful adjunct to the verbal explanation provided by the patient's physician(s). In this regard, a useful book is *The Surgery Book* (see "General References"), which provides well illustrated information about more than 100 common operations.

Approximately 50% of adults who undergo surgery are ostensibly in good general health; the other 50% have various medical problems (the percentages vary depending upon the age of the population). In perhaps 5 to 10% of patients, new medical problems will be identified during preoperative evaluation, a small proportion of which will have implications for the planning of surgery. For every patient, the general physician should complete an appropriate preoperative evaluation (see below) and should assure that existing medical conditions that may affect the outcome of surgery are optimally controlled. These steps should be taken before admission for surgery, and specific recommendations should be communicated to the surgeon regarding the care of the patient's medical problem(s) during the perioperative period. This chapter provides guidelines for these steps in the management of patients with a number of common medical problems.

GENERAL PREOPERATIVE EVALUATION

There is no consensus on the makeup of a general preoperative evaluation. For adult patients undergoing general or spinal anesthesia, most physicians currently perform a history and physical examination and order a number of routine laboratory tests (e.g., chest X-ray and electrocardiogram in patients over 40; and complete blood count, tests of hemostasis, electrolytes, glucose, measurement of blood urea nitrogen or creatinine, and urinalysis in all adults). This complete workup has been criticized for having a low yield and for being unnecessarily costly (25).

The large number of factors that influence the preoperative evaluation make a consensus unlikely. The patient's age, the nature of the planned surgery (major or minor), the type of anesthesia to be used (general, spinal, regional, or local), and the interval since the patient's last comprehensive evaluation are all relevant in the preoperative evaluation of every patient. In addition, one or more of the following considerations is often pertinent: estimating operative risk, establishing a baseline for expected postoperative changes or possible complications, avoiding harm to other patients or medical personnel (e.g., hepatitis, tuberculosis), documenting selected information for medicolegal reasons, determining drug dosage, and detecting rare but potentially catastrophic circumstances (e.g., thrombocytopenia in a patient scheduled for a craniotomy) (14). A practical approach for the individual patient is to select one of the two general types of preoperative evaluation as summarized in Table 86.1, *i.e., a limited or a comprehensive workup.* Guidelines for choosing between these alternatives are summarized in Table 86.2. Selected screening tests should be added to either workup in order to avoid potential catastrophes associated with certain high risk situations (see Table 86.3).

CURRENT MEDICATIONS AND KNOWN ALLERGIES

All drugs that a patient is taking and any known drug allergies should be specified at the time of referral for surgery. Planning should be initiated at that time, for the following reasons: to avoid possible

Table 86.1.
Two Types of General Preoperative Evaluation

Component of Workup	Limited Workup[a]	Comprehensive Workup[a]
History	Heart, lungs, hemostasis, medications, allergies, and new symptoms (especially upper respiratory infection)	Brief review of all systems, medications, allergies, past operations
Physical examination	Vital signs, oral cavity, chest, heart, and abdomen	Vital signs, eyes, oral cavity, neck, chest, breast, heart, peripheral pulses, abdomen, nervous system
Laboratory[a]	Hematocrit value, urinalysis, pregnancy test[b]	Chest X-ray, ECG (>age 40), complete blood count, serum electrolytes, blood urea nitrogen or serum creatinine, serum glucose, urinalysis, pregnancy test[b]

[a] Basic evaluation for screening and baseline data. Other tests may be added to evaluate known disease in a patient or to follow-up findings in the preoperative history and physical examination.
[b] Women in childbearing age group.

Table 86.2.
Guidelines for Selecting the General Preoperative Evaluation

Limited Workup	Comprehensive Workup
Age < 40	Age > 40 (especially > 60)
Local, regional, or spinal anesthesia	General anesthesia
Minor procedure	Major procedure (especially thoracic, abdominal, neurosurgical)
Well patient	Patient with moderate-severe major organ disease
	No, old, or inadequate data base

Table 86.3.
Additional Preoperative Screening Tests for Common High Risk Situations

High Risk Situation	Screening Tests
Patient undergoing neurosurgical, cardiac, vascular, or major abdominal procedure	Tests of hemostasis: platelet count, prothrombin time, partial thromboplastin time
Patient with increased risk of chronic pulmonary disease (e.g., smoker with ≥10 pack years) who is undergoing general anesthesia	Pulmonary function tests (see Table 86.12)
Patient with increased risk of active liver disease (e.g., alcoholism, drug addiction, homosexuality, dialysis patient) who is undergoing general or spinal anesthesia	Liver function tests: serum aminotransferases, alkaline phosphatase, bilirubin hepatitis-associated antigen
Patient with increased risk of tuberculosis (e.g., known exposure, underprivileged population)	Chest X-ray, purified protein derivative skin test
Patient with increased risk of coronary artery disease (i.e., smoker, hypertensive, strong family history, diabetic, hyperlipidemia)	ECG

interactions with anesthetic agents and possible complications during surgery; to manage the patient when an essential drug cannot be administered orally during the perioperative period; and to avoid exposure to drugs to which the patient is allergic. The patient should be asked specifically about nonprescription drug use, which, although very common, is often not mentioned spontaneously (particularly aspirin-containing compounds, which may potentiate postoperative bleeding; and sedatives which may interact with anesthetic drugs); about prior allergic reactions to drugs (especially penicillin and other antibiotics which may be indicated postoperatively at a time when a patient is unable to provide information); about use of corticosteroids within the past year (particularly patients with obstructive airways disease or seasonal allergy); and about current use of recreational substances which may affect the patient's course during or after surgery (alcohol, tobacco, illicit drugs).

For patients taking one or more drugs regularly, preoperative office management should include a careful review of all medications including over-the-counter preparations (especially aspirin). Other specific perioperative recommendations regarding medication should be communicated to the surgeon. Modification of chronic medications for surgery is best done before the patient is hospitalized rather than the night before surgery at the hospital, in order to allow time to detect unanticipated effects (Table 86.4). Most medications have a duration of action between 6 and 12 hours, and omission of one or more doses may precipitate symptoms. For patients who are expected to be awake and to be able to take oral medications within this time span, it is appropriate to recommend giving a dose, with a small amount of water (1 ounce or less) in the morning before the induction of anesthesia and resuming the medication orally 6 to 12 hours later. When oral medications cannot be continued throughout the perioperative period, alternate medications or routes of administration should be recommended.

THE PATIENT WITH CARDIOVASCULAR DISEASE (15)

Overview

Most forms of general anesthesia may cause cardiovascular stresses (decreased myocardial contractility, arrhythmias, hypotension); and spinal or epidural anesthesia may cause hypotension. These factors and the stresses associated with surgery itself probably account for the greatly increased risk of surgery for patients with underlying cardiovascular disease. Knowledge of the risks of surgery and of the appropriate preoperative management for patients with established cardiovascular disease is needed frequently by the general physician.

Ischemic Heart Disease

Size of the Risk (15, 28)

Ischemic heart disease poses two major risks perioperatively in the patient undergoing general anesthesia: myocardial infarction and death. These risks depend upon the patient's preoperative status. Overall, the risks for patients with arteriosclerotic heart disease are 2 or 3 times those of patients of the same age without cardiac disease.

The increased risk posed by ischemic heart disease is dependent on preoperative cardiac status (see Table 86.5). *Stable angina pectoris* represents only a small increase in risk. The risk attending *severe* or *unstable angina* cannot be estimated accurately because of varying definitions and the small number of patients reported in the medical literature; but there is a significantly increased risk. A *myocardial infarction within 6 months* before surgery represents a very high risk, particularly in the 3 months follow-

Table 86.4.
Management of Drugs in the Surgical Patient[a]

Drug Class	Anticipated Problems	Recommendations to Surgeon for Perioperative Period
CARDIOVASCULAR		
Antihypertensives[b]	Interaction with anesthetics, hypotension	Inform anesthesiologist of use
	Inability to give orally	Plan postoperative regimen with alternative agents if needed
Antiarrhythmics[b]	Inability to give orally	ECG monitor in operating room and postoperatively, use alternative parenteral agents
β-Blockers[b]	Myocardial depression, bradycardia	Continue intravenously (propranolol, 1–2 mg every 6 hours), taper to lower dose, or discontinue depending on circumstances
Digitalis[b]	Toxicity	Obtain serum levels preoperatively
	Inability to give orally	Give 75% of daily oral dose of digoxin intravenously each day
Long acting oral nitrates[b]	Inability to give orally	Substitute transdermal nitroglycerine
GASTROINTESTINAL		
Antacids[b]	Inability to give orally	Intravenous cimetidine, nasogastric suction (if patient has active peptic ulcer disease)
ANTIBIOTICS		
Tetracycline	Risk of renal failure if given with methoxyflurane	Use alternative antibiotic or anesthetic
CORTICOSTEROIDS[b]	Adrenal insufficiency	Plan coverage (with intravenous corticosteroids) adequate for the stress of surgery
	Poor wound healing	Discuss with surgeon
NEUROLOGICAL		
Levodopa/Carbidopa[b]	Interaction with anesthetics (hypertension or hypotension), inability to give orally	Inform anesthesiologist of use; resume orally as soon as possible after surgery
Barbiturates	Increased CNS depression by anesthesia, inability to give orally	Inform anesthesiologist of use; give daily dose intramuscularly
Dilantin	Inability to give orally	Give daily dose slowly intravenously (or substitute phenobarbital before admitting patient for surgery)
BRONCHODILATORS		
Theophylline[b]	Inability to give orally	Switch to intravenous aminophylline
β₂-Sympathomimetics[b]	Inability to give orally	Switch to aerosolized or subcutaneous β₂-agent
PSYCHIATRIC		
Antidepressants[b]	Hypotension or hypertension, arrhythmias	Inform anesthesiologist of use; withhold monoamine oxidase inhibitors 1–2 weeks preoperatively; withhold other agents 24 hours preoperatively.
Neuroleptics (i.e., phenothiazines and haloperidol)[b]	Arrhythmias, enhancement of neuromuscular blocking agents, hypotension	Inform anesthesiologist of use; withhold 24 hours preoperatively in some cases.
Benzodiazepines	Increased CNS depression by anesthesia	Inform anesthesiologist of use
Lithium[b]	Myocardial depression, hypernatremia	Inform anesthesiologist of use; determine blood levels; withhold 24 hours preoperatively; avoid diuretics and nonsteroidal anti-inflammatory agents
ANALGESICS		
Narcotics	Decreased cough reflex, increased CNS depression by anesthesia, hypotension	Inform anesthesiologist of use
Aspirin compounds[b]	Increased bleeding	Discontinue 1–2 weeks before surgery

Table 86.4—cont.

Drug Class	Anticipated Problems	Recommendations to Surgeon for Perioperative Period
ANTICOAGULANTS		
Warfarin[b]	Increased bleeding	Discontinue 48 hours before surgery, vitamin K_1 if needed, check prothrombin time before operation
DIURETICS	Electrolyte abnormalities, hypotension, inability to give orally	Obtain electrolytes and check blood pressure (lying, standing) within 24 hours preoperatively, use intravenous furosemide if needed
GOUT		
Benemid, allopurinol	Inability to give orally	Observe, treat acute gout with intravenous colchicine
DIABETES		
Oral hypoglycemics[b]	Inability to give orally	Switch to insulin preoperatively in selected patients
Insulin[b]	Risk of hyper- or hypoglycemia	Give one-third to one-half of usual dose preoperatively
THYROID THERAPY		
Thyroid hormone[b]	Inability to give orally	Usually can be discontinued for up to 7–10 days
Antithyroid drugs[b]	Inability to give orally	Use parenteral iodides or propranolol if necessary
TOPICAL DRUGS FOR GLAUCOMA		
Timolol	Systemic β-blockage	Notify anesthesiologist preoperatively
Phospholine iodide	Prolonged muscle relaxant activity	Discontinue 7–10 days preoperatively
RECREATIONAL DRUGS		
Alcohol	Affect drug metabolism, drug interactions, withdrawal syndrome, impaired respiratory function	If possible, have patient discontinue use 1 or more weeks before admission for surgery; inform anesthesiologist and surgeon of recent use
Illicit drugs		
Tobacco[b]		

[a] If the patient will be able to take medication orally within 12 hours postoperatively, most maintenance drugs can be given at that time. If a shorter interval is crucial, a maintenance drug can be given with less than 1 ounce of water, before anesthesia, and the drug can be resumed orally after surgery.
[b] See additional details in subsequent section of this chapter.

Table 86.5.
Approximate Cardiovascular Risk in Relation to Preoperative Cardiac Status

Patient Preoperative Status	Approximate Risk of Postoperative Myocardial Infarction (%)	Approximate Mortality Risk (%)
No "cardiac" disease	0.2–2[a]	3[a]
"Cardiac disease" present	6	5
Angina (stable)	3	3–10
Postmyocardial infarction		
<6 months	25	18–20
<3 months	30–35	25–40
3–6 months	15–20	10–20
>6 months	5	No data

[a] Risk varies with age of population studied.

ing infarction. Preliminary evidence (24) suggests that aggressive perioperative management may significantly lower cardiovascular risk (e.g., reduce recurrent myocardial infarction risk from 30 to 4%); but this remains to be confirmed. Even 6 months after an infarction, the risk of a perioperative myo-cardial infarction is considerably larger than the risk in a control population.

In addition to a recent myocardial infarction, a number of factors contribute to the risk of perioperative cardiac complications or mortality. The most important of these factors are decompensated congestive heart failure, arrhythmias, and significant chronic obstructive lung disease. These and other factors have been incorporated into a *cardiac risk index* (Tables 86.6 and 86.7) (12). Until this cardiac risk index is validated in other studies, it should not be used as an absolute classification; however, it provides helpful guidelines for assessing the significance of multiple risk factors.

Preoperative Planning

Office evaluation. Patients with established ischemic heart disease should have a comprehensive preoperative evaluation (see Table 86.1). Noninvasive tests of cardiac function including echocardiography, nuclear scanning, and stress tests should be reserved for situations where the presence or severity of cardiovascular disease is questioned.

Table 86.6.
Cardiac Risk Factors in Surgical Patients[a]

Risk Factors	Points for Cardiac Risk Index (see Table 86.7)
HISTORY	
Myocardial infarction in past 6 months	10
Age >70	5
PHYSICAL	
S_3 gallop or jugular venous distention	11
Significant aortic stenosis	3
ECG	
Rhythm other than sinus or premature atrial contractions on last preoperative ECG	7
>5 premature ventricular contractions/minute any time preoperatively	7
OTHER ORGAN SYSTEMS	
$pO_2 < 60$, $pCO_2 > 50$	
$K < 3.0$, $HCO_3 < 20$ mEq/dl	
BUN > 50	
CR > 3.0 mg/dl	
Signs of chronic liver disease or elevated aminotransferase	3 (each factor)
Bedridden from noncardiac causes	
OPERATION	
Intraperitoneal or intrathoracic	3
Emergency	4
TOTAL POSSIBLE	53

[a] Adapted from Goldman L, Caldera DL, Nussbaum SR, *et al*: Multifactorial index of cardiac risk in noncardiac surgical procedures. *N Engl J Med* 297:845, 1977.

Based upon the preoperative evaluation, the risk of general anesthesia and surgery should be estimated for each patient. For patients with recent myocardial infarction (within less than 6 months), with unstable angina, or with less severe coronary artery disease and multiple other risk factors (see Table 86.6), only urgent lifesaving surgery should be undertaken until the risk is lowered. Surgery may be done 3 months after infarction when the risk of waiting the additional 3 months is thought to be significant (e.g., recurrent cholecystitis). Patients with stable angina or uncomplicated recovery from myocardial infarction more than 6 months previously have an increased risk that does not decline further with time; thus, necessary operations need not be postponed.

Coronary artery bypass surgery should be considered before elective noncardiac surgery, in consultation with a cardiologist, only in patients who have other indications for bypass surgery (see Chapter 57).

Table 86.7.
Cardiac Risk Index (Based on a Prospective Study of Patients at the Massachusetts General Hospital)[a]

Class	Point Total[b]	No or Moderate Complication (N = 943)[c] (%)	Life-Threatening Complication (N = 39)[d] (%)	Cardiac Deaths (N = 19)[e] (%)
I	0–5	99	0.7	0.2
II	6–12	93	5	2
III	13–25	86	11	2
IV	≥26	22	22	56

[a] Adapted from Goldman L, Caldera DL, Nussbaum SR, *et al*: Multifactorial index of cardiac risk in noncardiac surgical procedures. *N Engl J Med* 297:845, 1977.
[b] See Table 86.6.
[c] New or worsened heart failure without pulmonary edema, supraventricular tachyarrhythmia, or intraoperative or postoerative ischemia (as indicated by chest pain or ECG changes) without documented myocardial infarction.
[d] Documented intraoperative or postoperative myocardial infarction, pulmonary edema, or ventricular tachycardia without progression to cardiac death.
[e] Deaths due to arrhythmia or to low output heart failure.

Recommendations to the surgeon. A baseline ECG should be obtained before surgery for all patients with known coronary artery disease and for all patients over age 40. Routine postoperative ECGs should be obtained only in high risk patients (i.e., all patients with known coronary artery disease and any adults who develop hypotension during surgery), since the yield of useful information from them is low.

For patients taking a long acting oral nitrate for angina, the drug should be administered on the morning of surgery with a sip of water. While the patient is unable to take medications orally, nitroglycerine paste or a transdermal patch should be substituted; because there is no simple way to determine the paste dose equivalent to an oral nitrate, an intermediate dose equivalent to 1 to 2 inches of nitroglycerine paste every 4 to 6 hours should be recommended.

For patients taking a β-blocking agent for angina, intravenous small doses of propranolol (i.e., 1 to 2 mg every 6 hours) should be substituted, given by a physician, while the patient is unable to take medications by mouth. This should protect the patient from the risk of acute cardiac ischemia, which occasionally follows abrupt cessation of a β-blocking agent. Patients able to resume oral intake within 12 to 24 hours usually can be observed without intravenous propranolol.

Calcium blocking agents should usually be given orally up to the morning of surgery. Another type of antianginal medication must be used postoperatively until the patient can resume oral intake.

Intensive intraoperative monitoring using Swan-Ganz and radial artery catheters should be considered for patients who are very sensitive to volume

Table 86.8.
Risk of Perioperative Cardiac Complications in Patients with Mild to Moderate Hypertension[a]

Preoperative Characteristics	Mean Point Total[b] (± SEM)	Patients with No Cardiac Complication (%)	Patients with Minor Complications Only (%)	Patients with Major Nonfatal Complications (%)	Patients with Cardiac Death (%)
Normal blood pressure No history of hypertension	4.3 ± 0.3	89	9	2	0.2
Hypertension controlled Taking antihypertensive drug(s)	6.9 ± 0.6	76	15	8	1
Hypertensive Taking antihypertensive drug(s)	4.4 ± 0.5	93	8		1
Hypertensive Not taking antihypertensive drug(s)	5.5 ± 0.6	88	9	1	1

[a] Adapted from Goldman L, Caldera DL: Risks of general anesthesia and elective operation in the hypertensive patient. *Anesthesiology* 50:285, 1979.
[b] See Tables 86.6 and 86.7 for risk factor index.

changes, such as those in congestive heart failure (see below) and for operations where loss and replacement of large volumes of fluid are expected (e.g., aneurysm repair).

Hypertension

Size of the Risk (11, 15)

Controversy still exists about whether mild to moderate hypertension (diastolic ≤ 110 mg Hg) increases anesthetic and surgical risks. The only prospective study showed no correlation between uncontrolled diastolic pressures in this range and the risk of perioperative cardiac, renal, or cerebrovascular events (11). Patients in this study often had other cardiac risk factors which did correlate with the incidence of perioperative cardiac morbidity (see Tables 86.6 and 86.8).

Too few patients have been studied to define adequately the risk for persons operated on when their diastolic pressure exceeds 110 mm Hg, but there is probably an increased risk (23). Likewise, control of hypertension may be more important in selected patients with severe cardiac, renal, or cerebrovascular disease.

Preoperative Planning

Office evaluation. The basic preoperative evaluation in the hypertensive patient should determine whether there is end organ damage (renal: serum creatinine concentration and urinalysis; cerebrovascular: history, neurological and neurovascular examination; and cardiovascular: history, cardiac examination, chest X-ray, and ECG). Blood pressure and pulse measurements should be made with the patient lying, sitting, and standing (after brief exercise, to identify the maximum orthostatic fall in patients taking antihypertensive drugs); the preoperative status of blood pressure control may then be classified as untreated, hypertensive despite therapy, or controlled.

Patients who are controlled, or patients who are partially controlled and have diastolic pressures ≤ 110 mm Hg should be continued on their prescribed antihypertensive medication. Two exceptions to this rule are guanethidine and monoamine oxidase inhibitors. A patient taking either of these should be switched to a different drug as both of these drugs may cause markedly labile blood pressure during anesthesia.

Untreated patients with diastolic pressures ≤ 110 mm Hg may undergo surgery, with institution of antihypertensive therapy after convalescence from surgery.

Individual judgments must be made about patients with diastolic pressures ≥ 110 mm Hg, depending on the severity and duration of hypertension, the presence of end organ damage, and the extent of planned surgery. Patients with severe hypertension (i.e., diastolic ≥ 120 mm Hg) should have their blood pressure at least partly controlled before admission for nonurgent surgery (23), although there are no studies proving that such control modifies risks. Attempts to control blood pressure too rapidly (for example, rapid increases in diuretic treatment over several days) may result in volume depletion, hypokalemia, or hypotension at the time of surgery. Therefore, these patients should have their blood pressure stabilized during 1 to 2 weeks before admission for surgery.

Recommendations to the surgeon. For all hypertensive patients it is important to advise the surgeon to avoid significant intravascular volume expansion or contraction, as these conditions may either cause a significant rise in blood pressure (volume expansion) or fall in blood pressure (volume contraction, especially in the patient who is taking antihypertensive drugs).

Current antihypertensive medications should be continued through the morning of surgery and resumed postoperatively when the patient is stable and can take oral medications (diuretics are usually withheld the morning of surgery). Because of bed rest and inactivity during convalescence, some patients will require less antihypertensive medication postoperatively and during the first few weeks following major surgery.

In some patients, chronic hypertension will require treatment postoperatively, before oral medication can be resumed. For such patients, the surgeon should know that there are now several regimens that will reliably control the blood pressure when carefully administered and adjusted (15). These regimens are: (a) propranolol (1 to 2 mg intravenously every 4 to 6 hours) plus hydralazine (5 to 50 mg intravenously every 4 to 6 hours); (b) nifedipine (contents of a 10-mg capsule sublingually every 4 to 6 hours); (c) methyldopa intravenously; and (d) transcutaneous clonidine (one or more patches, lasting up to 7 days), especially for patients who were taking clonidine before surgery and are at risk of rebound hypertension and tachycardia due to clonidine withdrawal. Intravenous furosemide and short acting antihypertensives, such as nitroprusside, also aid in postoperative management of hypertension.

Further details about antihypertensive drugs are found in Chapter 62.

Valvular Heart Disease

Size of the Risk

The risk of surgery in the patient with valvular heart disease varies with the valve affected (aortic *versus* mitral), the nature (stenosis *versus* insufficiency), and the severity of the lesion (13, 15). The severity of valvular lesions as judged clinically by New York Heart Association (NYHA) classification (see Table 61.3, Chapter 61) provides a reasonable indication of surgical risk, with the exception of aortic stenosis.

Valvular heart disease poses two major surgical risks: cardiac death and congestive heart failure. The presence of aortic stenosis of any degree of hemodynamic significance poses a high risk of surgical mortality. Mild to moderate mitral lesions or aortic insufficiency represent only slightly increased risks of cardiac death; however, hemodynamically severe valvular disease (i.e., NYHA class 3 or 4) due to these lesions creates major risks. In addition to increasing the risk of perioperative mortality, significant valvular disease poses an increased risk of decompensated heart failure.

No specific information exists regarding the risks associated with prolapsed mitral valve or with hypertrophic cardiomyopathy. It is reasonable to assume that the risk in patients with prolapsed mitral valve depends upon the degree of mitral regurgitation. Patients with hypertrophic cardiomyopathy may be very sensitive to volume contraction and are probably best managed with a Swan-Ganz catheter in place during major procedures associated with rapid volume changes.

Patients with artificial heart valves, patients with any evidence of valvular heart disease (including mitral prolapse and hypertrophic cardiomyopathy), and patients with congenital structural defects (e.g., patent ductus arteriosis, ventricular septal defect) have a small but definite risk of acquiring bacterial endocarditis when they undergo procedures in the oral cavity and upper respiratory, gastrointestinal, or genitourinary tracts.

Preoperative Planning

Office evaluation. The basic cardiac evaluation should delineate the nature and severity of the valvular disease and should identify any associated cardiac conditions. The uses of echocardiography and cardiac catheterization to evaluate valvular heart disease are described in Chapter 60. Patients with severe valvular disease should have corrective cardiac surgery followed by a period of convalescence before they undergo elective major noncardiac operations.

Recommendations to the surgeon. Patients undergoing procedures attended by a risk of endocarditis should receive antimicrobial prophylaxis as summarized in Table 86.9.

The preoperative management of congestive heart failure, arrhythmia, or anticoagulant therapy (in patients with artificial valves) is described in subsequent sections of this chapter.

Congestive Heart Failure

Size of the Risk

Information on the risk of developing congestive heart failure (CHF) perioperatively is limited because of the few studies available. However, the best prospective studies (13, 15) closely correspond to general clinical experience. The most significant risk factors for postoperative CHF are decompensated failure preoperatively and, to a lesser extent, prior CHF that is clinically stable preoperatively (Table 86.10). However, only 40% of patients who develop perioperative CHF have had prior failure. The best predictors for the other 60% of patients are age greater than 60, major surgery (especially abdominal aortic aneurysm repair or major abdominal surgery), and nonspecific electrocardiographic abnormalities.

Patients with postoperative pulmonary edema have a high total mortality (20 to 57%), most of which is cardiac. Patients who develop less severe postoperative CHF do not have an increased risk of postoperative cardiac death, although the overall mortality from all causes is increased. Most postop-

Table 86.9.
Prevention of Bacterial Endocarditis in Patients with Valvular Heart Disease, Prosthetic Heart Valves, and Other Abnormalities of the Cardiovascular System[a,b]

	Dosage for Adults
DENTAL AND UPPER RESPIRATORY PROCEDURES[c]	
Oral[d]	
Penicillin V	2 g 1 hour before procedure and 1 g 6 hours later
Penicillin allergy:	
Erythromycin	1 g 1 hour before procedure and 500 mg 6 hours later
Parenteral[d]	
Ampicillin	1 g IM or IV 30 minutes to 1 hour before procedure and repeat once 8 hours later
or aqueous penicillin G	2 million units IM or IV 30 minutes to 1 hour before procedure and repeat once 8 hours later
plus gentamicin	1.5 mg/kg IM or IV 30 minutes to 1 hour before procedure and repeat once 8 hours later
Penicillin allergy:	
Vancomycin	1 g IV infused *over 1 hour* beginning 1 hour before procedure and repeat once 8–12 hours later[f]
GASTROINTESTINAL AND GENITOURINARY PROCEDURES[c,g]	
Parenteral	
Ampicillin	2 g IM or IV 30 minutes to 1 hour before procedure and repeat once 8 hours later
plus gentamicin	1.5 mg/kg IM or IV 30 minutes to 1 hour before procedure and repeat once 8 hours later
Penicillin allergy:	
Vancomycin	1 g IV infused *over 1 hour* beginning 1 hour before procedure and repeat once 8–12 hours later
plus gentamicin	1.5 mg/kg IM or IV 30 minutes to 1 hour before procedure and repeat once 8–12 hours later[f]
Oral[d]	
Amoxicillin	3 g 1 hour before procedure and 1.5 g 6 hours later[f]

[a] Modified from *Med Lett* 26:4, 1984; see also Prevention of bacterial endocarditis. *Circulation* 70:1123A, 1984.
[b] For patients with valvular heart disease, prosthetic heart valves, most forms of congenital heart disease (but not uncomplicated secundum atrial septal defect), idiopathic hypertrophic subaortic stenosis, and mitral valve prolapse.
[c] Data are limited on the risk of endocarditis with a particular procedure. For a review of the risk of bacteremia with various procedures, see Everett ED, Hirschmann JV: *Medicine* 56:61, 1977.
[d] An oral regimen is safer. Parenteral regimens are more likely to be effective; they are recommended especially for patients with prosthetic valves, those who have had endocarditis previously, or those taking continuous oral penicillin for rheumatic fever prophylaxis. Oral regimen should be used only for minor procedures in low risk patients.
[e] Parenteral regimens are more likely to be effective.
[f] Although the second dose is given "8–12 hours" later for vancomycin-gentamicin regimens in most recommendations, the usual interval for vancomycin dosage is 12 hours based on its half-life.
[g] In patients with renal insufficiency, the second dose may need to be modified in terms of timing or dose for gentamicin and vancomycin.

erative CHF occurs during or within several hours of surgery.

Preoperative Planning

Office evaluation. Patients with compensated CHF should have a comprehensive preoperative evaluation (see Table 86.1). This evaluation should include a meticulous assessment of volume status (lying and standing blood pressures, inspection of neck veins, determination of whether edema is present) and examination for cardiac gallops and for rales. Laboratory data should include a digoxin level if that drug is being administered. Noninvasive methods for assessing left ventricular function (see Chapter 61) may be useful when the degree of cardiac dysfunction is uncertain.

Although there are no definitive studies in this regard, it is prudent to *digitalize* patients with a confirmed history of moderate or severe CHF, ideally during the week before admission. Most controversy about preoperative digitalization has concerned the patient who has a past history of no or minimal CHF, but a "risk" of developing CHF because of an enlarged heart or because the surgery will involve major volume shifts. Although data are lacking, it is likely that digitalis does not help the latter type of patient and that the risk of digitalis toxicity is not warranted (7).

Patients with decompensated CHF should have all but lifesaving surgery postponed until the failure is controlled, either in the office or in the hospital.

Recommendations to the surgeon. Patients with controlled CHF should be maintained on their usual oral regimen until midnight before surgery and

Table 86.10.
Risks of Developing Congestive Failure (CHF) in Perioperative Period[a, b]

Patient Characteristics	Size of Risk	
	All CHF (%)	Pulmonary edema (%)
No prior CHF	4	2
Past CHF:		
All—now compensated	16	6
Past pulmonary edema (regardless of current status)	32	23
Decompensated CHF preoperatively	21	16
Preoperative physical findings:		
S₃ gallop	47	35
Jugular venous distention	35	30
New York Heart Association class preoperatively (see Table 61.3)		
1	5	3
2	7	7
3	18	6
4	31	25

[a] Adapted from Goldman L, Caldera DL, Southwick FS, *et al*: Cardiac risk factors and complications in non-cardiac surgery. *Medicine* 57:357, 1978.
[b] Based upon 1001 consecutive patients undergoing general surgery, orthopaedic surgery, or urological surgery (transurethral resection of the prostate omitted because of existing evidence of its safety even in elderly patients).

maintained with intravenous diuretics and digoxin (75% of the oral dose) during the immediate postoperative period.

Arrhythmias

The arrhythmias which are encountered most frequently in ambulatory patients are described in detail in Chapter 59.

Size of the Risk (10, 15)

Patients with arrhythmias before surgery have significantly increased risks of cardiac morbidity and death. These risks have not been quantified for subgroups of patients with specific arrhythmias, except as indicated in the cardiac risk index shown in Tables 86.6 and 86.7. Patients with complete heart block, Mobitz type II second degree block, and sick sinus syndrome have a significant risk of complications during anesthesia if a pacemaker is not inserted. On the other hand, there is little or no increased risk associated with bi- or trifascicular block on ECG in patients who are asymptomatic.

Arrhythmias do occur in approximately 20% or more of adult patients during general anesthesia; however, most of these patients do not have preoperative arrhythmias. Most intraoperative arrhythmias are supraventricular, transient, related to specific anesthesic or surgical manipulation, and do not

require specific therapies. The number of arrhythmias that are detected clinically, without the use of continuous monitoring, is lower: supraventricular arrhythmias are detected clinically in 4% of patients and other arrhythmias in 11% (13, 15).

Preoperative Planning

Office evaluation. Patients with arrhythmias should have the comprehensive preoperative evaluation (Table 86.1) expanded in several ways. The probable etiology of the arrhythmia should be delineated (see Chapter 59). If the arrhythmia is intermittent or control is not certain, 24-hour Holter monitoring should be done. Drug levels of antiarrhythmic drugs that are being administered should be obtained. In general, this entire evaluation should be accomplished before admission for surgery.

Patients with *supraventricular arrhythmias* should have their ventricular rates controlled or should be converted to more stable rhythms. Except for atrial fibrillation, this usually means conversion either to normal sinus rhythm or to atrial fibrillation, since other supraventricular arrhythmias are either hemodynamically unstable or give an unpredictable ventricular response even with appropriate drug therapy. Patients with atrial fibrillation should have their rates slowed but should be able to accelerate their heart rate under stress as indicated by their ability to raise their pulse rate more than 10 points by mild exercise.

Established indications for *preoperative digitalization* in patients with arrhythmias are control of rate in atrial fibrillation and prophylaxis of supraventricular arrhythmias in selected patients (e.g., patients with past histories of supraventricular arrhythmias, especially atrial fibrillation or flutter, who remain at high risk for recurrence; and patients with significant mitral stenosis).

Patients with *premature ventricular contractions* (PVCs) or other ventricular arrhythmias should be treated according to the criteria outlined in Chapter 59.

Recommendations to the surgeon. Antiarrhythmic drugs should be continued orally through the morning before surgery, after which the following intravenous treatment should be substituted until the patient is able to take oral medications again: intravenous digoxin (75% of the oral dose) for patients on digoxin, and intravenous lidocaine or procainamide for patients taking quinidine or disopyramide for ventricular arrhythmias.

There is general agreement that patients undergoing general anesthesia should have a *prophylactic or therapeutic pacemaker* inserted for the following conditions:

1. Symptomatic or significant dysfunction of the sinoatrial node;

2. Idioventricular rhythm;

3. Current or past history of third degree or Mobitz type II second degree atrioventricular (AV) block;

4. Some instances of Mobitz type I second degree AV block;

5. A few instances of trifascicular block (right bundle branch block plus left anterior hemiblock plus first degree AV block; alternating left and right bundle branch block; or left bundle branch block and first degree AV block) especially in the presence of severe valvular disease, ischemic disease, or congestive failure;

6. A history of Stokes-Adams attacks.

Patients with findings suggesting bradyarrhythmias (especially a history of syncope or near syncope, and an underlying ECG abnormality) probably should have a temporary pacemaker recommended if a full workup to evaluate the etiology of the symptoms cannot be performed preoperatively or is not revealing. Isolated conditions for which a pacemaker is more controversial, but probably not indicated, include bifascicular block, bundle branch block, first degree AV block, and sinus bradycardia that is asymptomatic.

THE PATIENT WITH PULMONARY DISEASE (33, 34)

Overview

Patients with significant pulmonary disease have an increased mortality and morbidity during surgery. The increased risks are due chiefly to the following physiological changes produced by the effects of anesthesia, sedatives, and analgesics: (a) abnormalities of pulmonary gas exchange, causing hypoxemia; (b) depression of the cough reflex and decrease in clearance of respiratory secretions; (c) respiratory depression; and (d) loss of sighing and normal lung inflation—each of which increases the risk of atelectasis and pneumonia. In addition, normal breathing and voluntary coughing are decreased after surgery because of pain and discomfort, especially after upper abdominal and thoracic surgery. Optimal preoperative treatment of pulmonary disease can reduce perioperative morbidity and possibly mortality.

Chronic Obstructive Pulmonary Disease (COPD)

Size of the Risk (31, 34)

The precise risk of perioperative death from pulmonary causes for patients with COPD is not known because of the lack of information regarding patients with mild lung disease. In patients with moderate to severe COPD, pulmonary deaths occur in about 4% (versus 0 to 2% of unselected patients) and pulmonary complications in 36% (versus 9% of unselected patients) (34).

The presence of a smoking history, dyspnea, cough, or abnormal spirometry increases the risk of minor postoperative pulmonary complications (i.e., atelectasis or infection without significant respiratory compromise). The risk of respiratory failure requiring vigorous postoperative respiratory therapy is increased in patients with an FEV_1 (forced expiratory volume in 1 second) less than 1.5 liters. A FEV_1 less than 1.0 liter or a pCO_2 greater than 45 mm Hg defines a high risk group with a marked increase in perioperative pulmonary mortality and in the incidence of postoperative respiratory failure requiring prolonged mechanical ventilation.

A number of *nonpulmonary factors* are helpful in predicting postoperatve pulmonary complications in patients with COPD (see Table 86.11). The greatest risks are in patients who are older than 60, who undergo upper abdominal and thoracic operations or operations under general anesthesia lasting more than 3 hours, or who have repeat operations within 1 year. A much lower risk is posed by operations on the extremities, back, breast, and central nervous system. Lower abdominal surgery represents an intermediate risk. Combining these factors with the pulmonary factors listed above increases the physician's ability to predict operative morbidity.

The *type of anesthesia* may affect the risk of pulmonary complications. Local anesthesia creates very little risk; if the patient is heavily sedated, however, there may be temporary deterioration in respiratory control and there may be a suppression of the cough reflex. Spinal anesthesia has been reported to be associated with a relatively low mortality rate in patients with COPD (31) in some studies. Because of the simultaneous use of sedatives and because the patient must ventilate in the supine position, spinal anesthesia creates a significant risk of intraoperative and postoperative respiratory complications; this is especially true of obese patients with chronic pulmonary disease. Because of these problems, general anesthesia, which permits control of ventilation and clearance of secretions, is often preferable to spinal

Table 86.11.
Nonpulmonary Factors Which Increase Pulmonary Risks during General Surgery

MOST IMPORTANT
Age over 60
Upper abdominal or thoracic operation
Repeat operations within 1 year
OTHER
General anesthesia lasting more than 3 hours
Obesity
Abnormal ECG
Poor patient effort/cooperation
Narcotic analgesics
Minor upper respiratory illness

anesthesia in patients with moderate or severe COPD.

Preoperative Planning

Office evaluation. Patients with known COPD should have a comprehensive preoperative evaluation (see Table 86.1) and if they are taking aminophylline, measurement and adjustment of the serum aminophylline concentration. Any history of smoking, chronic or intermittent sputum production, recent upper respiratory infection, dyspnea on effort, or concomitant cardiovascular disease is particularly pertinent. Ideally smokers should stop smoking 2 weeks before admission for surgery to be performed under general or spinal anesthesia, and patients with upper respiratory infections should have surgery postponed at least 2 weeks, regardless of how minor the episode.

Table 86.12 summarizes for patients undergoing general or spinal anesthesia the principal indications for preadmission spirometry alone (forced vital capacity (FVC) and FEV_1)) or for spirometry plus lung volumes and arterial blood gases. Unfortunately, major operations are often performed without pulmonary function testing, despite the fact that even experienced clinicians sometimes misjudge the severity of obstructive lung disease. Spirometry will clarify the presence and severity of lung disease in questionable cases.

Pulmonary consultation should be obtained for patients whose FEV_1 is less than 1.0 liter and for patients with less severe pulmonary disease who are being evaluated for thoracic or upper abdominal surgery.

Recommendations to the surgeon. After admission to the hospital, the patient should be instructed preoperatively about coughing and deep breathing exercises; as well as the use of devices such as an incentive spirometer that will be used postopera-

Table 86.12.
Indications for Evaluation of Patients with Pulmonary Disease

SPIROMETRY ONLY (FEV_1 and FVC)
  Smokers (>10 pack years)
  Any pulmonary symptoms (*e.g.*, dyspnea, wheezing, cough, or sputum production)
  Upper abdominal surgery
  Age > 60
  Repeat surgery within 1 year
  Multiple other risk factors (obesity, recent upper respiratory infections, narcotics abuse, abnormal ECG)
SPIROMETRY, LUNG VOLUMES, AND ARTERIAL BLOOD GASES
  Thoracic surgery
  Upper abdominal surgery and pulmonary disease
  Patients with restrictive lung disease
  Patients with chronic obstructive pulmonary disease with FEV_1 < 1.0 liter

tively. Patients already taking bronchodilators should continue their regimen through the morning of surgery; patients who have a history of intermittent airways obstruction should also be started on a theophylline compound before surgery. In order to prevent bronchospasm, especially in the immediate postoperative period, inhaled specific β_2-sympathomimetics and intravenous aminophylline should be administered, and the serum aminophylline level should be kept in the therapeutic range (10 to 20 mg/liter), during the time that the patient cannot take oral medications. Patients who have received corticosteroids for more than 2 weeks during the year before surgery should be appropriately covered for stress with parenteral steroids (see below). Patients with chronic purulent sputum production should receive a 5- to 7-day course of broad spectrum antibiotics (tetracycline, ampicillin, or trimethoprim-sulfamethoxazole) to decrease the quantity and purulence of secretions. Finally, arterial blood gases should be checked in all patients with moderate to severe COPD just before and just after surgery. There is some dispute about the efficacy of most of these individual measures. However, controlled trials combining bronchodilators, antibiotics, lung expansion, and mobilization of secretions have been shown consistently to decrease the number of perioperative complications (29, 31, 34).

Lung Resection and COPD (16, 34)

Overall mortality rates for lung resection are about 5% for lobectomy and about 15% for total pneumonectomy. The mortality and morbidity rates for lung surgery vary widely depending upon patient factors (particularly age and pulmonary function), type of operation (pneumonectomy, lobectomy, segmental resection), and experience and skill of the surgical team.

Assessment of pulmonary function in the patient with COPD who has an indication for lung resection (usually a tumor) can be performed in the ambulatory setting. Use of the following criteria to select candidates for lung resection has reduced mortality for patients with COPD.

For *pneumonectomy*, the major critiera for operability are $FEV_1 \geq 2$ liters and FVC $\geq 50\%$ of predicted. Patients with an FEV_1 less than 2 liters should have quantitative perfusion lung scanning to determine the FEV_1 that can be expected following pneumonectomy (e.g., if 30% of perfusion and ventilation goes to the affected lung, the patient's pulmonary function will be decreased by approximately 30% postoperatively). Those with a predicted postoperative remaining FEV_1 greater than 0.8 to 1 liter by quantitative lung scanning can undergo pneumonectomy, although their mortality risk is probably increased.

Patients not meeting the criteria for pneumonectomy may tolerate *lobectomy or segmental resection*.

Most patients with a preoperative $FEV_1 \geq 1.5$ liters can tolerate a lobectomy. The patient may undergo resection if removal of the segment or lobe will leave him with an FEV_1 greater than 0.8 to 1 liter.

Other measures in the preoperative planning for the patient with COPD undergoing pulmonary resection are similar to those described for such patients in the preceding section.

Asthma

Size of the Risk

Asthma effects approximately 3% of Americans, which makes it one of the most common pulmonary diseases (see Chapter 55). It is difficult to give a firm estimate of the operative risks posed by asthma because in most reports data on asthma are pooled with results for other types of obstructive airways disease. The most dangerous period for the asthmatic is not usually the period during general anesthesia, since the anesthetic may be an effective bronchodilator, but the immediate postoperative period. The major risks are severe bronchospasm and inspissation of thick secretions.

Preoperative Planning

Office evaluation. The asthmatic patient should have a comprehensive evaluation (see Table 86.1) in the office before admission for surgery. This allows adequate time for changes in chronic management prior to admission. The patient should stop smoking 2 weeks before surgery.

Recommendations to the surgeon. Spirometry (FEV_1 and FVC) should be performed in all asthmatic patients the day before the operation. Arterial blood gases should be measured in patients who are not in their stable baseline state or who have significant abnormalities in FEV_1. β_2-Sympathomimetics can be continued, as inhaled aerosols, until the induction of anesthesia and can be resumed in the recovery room. The concentration of aminophylline in the serum should be measured in all patients preoperatively because of the large number who have subtherapeutic or toxic levels on standard doses; planning for the immediate preoperative period should include continuation of oral bronchodilators through the morning of surgery and scheduling of surgery early in the day to avoid the need for preoperative intravenous aminophylline. In very severe asthmatics, a constant infusion of aminophylline should be recommended for the preoperative period and for the period when the patient is unable to take medicine by mouth; other patients are adequately managed by resuming aminophylline, intravenously, in the recovery room. Patients taking maintenance corticosteroids or who have been taking systemic corticosteroids for more than 2 weeks during the previous year should receive doses of parenteral steroids sufficient to cover the stress of surgery (see below) (22).

THE PATIENT WITH RENAL DISEASE (4, 5)

Size of the Risk

The size of the operative risk for patients with chronic renal disease depends upon the severity of their disease (see Chapter 47). Overall, the surgical mortality following major surgery in patients with severe renal disease (*i.e.*, creatinine clearance less than 10 to 15 ml/min including patients on dialysis, is about 2 to 4% when these patients are managed carefully. In patients not requiring dialysis, postoperative acute renal failure is the gravest complication, as it carries a high mortality (4, 5).

The major complications associated with surgery in the patient with moderate to severe renal disease are electrolyte disturbances (especially acidosis and hyperkalemia), volume contraction, volume overload, toxicity due to agents that are nephrotoxic or that are excreted by the kidneys, and bleeding. Volume contraction, with the risk of ischemic cerebral, cardiac, or renal damage, is a particular risk in patients with the nephrotic syndrome; these patients usually have a slightly contracted intravascular volume at baseline and are at risk of hypovolemia if an effort is made to decrease their edema with potent diuretics preoperatively. Toxic renal damage may follow the use of two agents which are frequently used in the perioperative period: radiocontrast agents and aminoglycoside antibiotics.

Preoperative Planning

Office evaluation. Before admission for surgery, patients with chronic renal failure should have the comprehensive evaluation outlined in Table 86.1, and current volume status should be documented. Radiocontrast studies should be avoided, if at all possible, in the preoperative workup of patients with serum creatinine concentrations greater than 4.5 mg/100 ml, since the subsequent risk of acute renal failure is about 30% (4, 35).

Recommendations to the surgeon. The most important consideration in perioperative management of patients who do not require dialysis is avoidance of fluid imbalance. When the surgery carries a risk of significant volume shifts, Swan-Ganz catheterization should be considered to assure close monitoring of the intravascular volume. Administration of drugs such as antihypertensives should follow the guidelines stated elsewhere in this chapter. Adjustments in the doses of drugs should be appropriate for the patient's degree of renal insufficiency (2). The concentration of electrolytes and creatinine in the serum should be monitored carefully before and after surgery, to detect, particularly, hyperkalemia and deterioration of renal function. Patients with renal failure frequently have a metabolic acidosis

Table 86.13.
Management of Diabetes on Day of Surgery

Surgical Procedure	Treatment Required to Control Glucose Preoperatively		
	Diet Only	Oral Hypoglycemic Agent	Insulin
Minor	Observe	Withhold until after procedure	Withhold until after procedure or use "major" protocol
Major	Observe	Change to long acting insulin (achieve control with insulin before operation)	*Preferred regimen:* One-half to two-thirds of total long acting insulin dose preoperatively; regular insulin only if needed *OR* One-third of total long acting insulin dose preoperatively; one-third postoperatively; regular insulin only if needed *OR* Continuous low dose infusion of regular insulin *OR* Regular insulin in each liter of dextrose 5% in water (D_5W)

compensated by hyperventilation; postoperatively continued appropriate hyperventilation will be necessary to avoid a potential precipitous fall in arterial pH. Preoperative prophylactic dialysis is not generally recommended in the patient not already on chronic dialysis. Furthermore, patients with a chronic anemia secondary to renal failure usually are well compensated and do not require preoperative transfusion unless they are symptomatic from the anemia or a large blood loss is expected during surgery.

In general, the nephrologist caring for patients on chronic dialysis should coordinate the medical management of these patients throughout the surgical episode. Although these patients have a very high postoperative complication rate (due to hyperkalemia, bleeding, arteriovenous fistula thrombosis, pneumonia, wound infection, and arrhythmias), their risk of dying due to surgery remains in the 2 to 4% range if they are carefully managed (3).

THE PATIENT WITH ENDOCRINE DISEASE

Diabetes

Size of the Risk (36)

Total surgical mortality for all diabetic patients is about 2 to 4%; less than 0.3% die as a result of poor control of their diabetes. About 14% of diabetics have postoperative complications which may be related to diabetes, particularly wound infection.

Preoperative Planning

Office evaluation. Each diabetic patient should have the comprehensive preoperative evaluation outlined in Table 86.1. Patients controlled with diet alone or with oral agents may be hospitalized the day before surgery if their diabetes is mild or if the

planned procedure is minor. Otherwise they should be admitted earlier so that adequate time is allowed for switching to insulin. In general, insulin-dependent diabetics should be admitted 1 to 2 days before surgery in order to assure satisfactory preoperative control of their diabetes.

Recommendations to the surgeon. Measurements of fasting blood sugars should be obtained on all diabetics on the day before and on the day of surgery, and their state of hydration should be evaluated to assure that they are not significantly volume contracted. Elective surgery should not be undertaken until diabetes is at least reasonably controlled (i.e., fasting blood sugar of 250 mg/100 ml or less for 2 or more days).

The appropriate perioperative treatment of diabetes depends upon the type of surgical procedure planned and upon the preadmission regimen, as summarized in Table 86.13).

Diabetics who are controlled by diet can be monitored with daily fasting blood sugars throughout the operative episode and treated with insulin if unacceptable rises in glucose occur.

Management of *patients taking oral agents* varies because they represent a heterogeneous group. Patients with mild elevations of glucose who are undergoing minor procedures that will allow them to eat the same day can take their hypoglycemic drug on the day *before* surgery and resume it when they begin eating on the day of surgery. The exception is the patient taking chlorpropamide (Diabinese), which should be withheld on the day before surgery because of its long half-life. If the patient is to undergo a major procedure, oral agents should be discontinued because they have long half-lives, control is less predictable, and the drugs cannot be given parenterally. Therefore, such a patient should be switched to management by diet only or to insulin.

For the patient who is *taking insulin before surgery*, one of several strategies is recommended for the preoperative period (see Table 86.13). Because of its simplicity and the small risk of hypoglycemia, the first regimen (giving one-half to two-thirds of the usual total daily dose of long acting insulin preoperatively) is the preferred regimen. Postoperative management is easiest with a single morning dose of long acting insulin, with the dose adjusted according to the metabolic status and calorie intake; supplemental regular insulin may be given as needed. Blood sugars by a bedside technique (Dextrometer, Accu check) is recommended; measurement of a fasting glucose and of electrolytes by the clinical laboratory should be obtained daily in the immediate postoperative period.

Adrenal Insufficiency and Chronic Steroid Therapy (36)

Size of the Risk

Too few patients have been adequately studied to estimate the increased surgical risks or the risk of precipitating an Addisonian crisis in patients who are currently taking or who have recently taken corticosteroids. It is generally agreed that patients who are currently taking *a pharmacological dose* of corticosteroids (*i.e.*, more than the equivalent of 20 to 30 mg of hydrocortisone daily) or who have taken corticosteroids at a pharmacological dose for 2 or more weeks in the past year require additional steroid coverage for surgery. Patients who are receiving *replacement doses* for adrenal insufficiency also require additional coverage, as these patients cannot produce the extra steroids needed during the stress of surgery (see Chapter 74 for additional details).

Preoperative Planning

Office evaluation. These patients should have a comprehensive evaluation before admission (see Table 86.1). For patients with adrenal insufficiency, the evaluation should include particular attention to factors that may reflect the adequacy of corticosteroid replacement (*i.e.*, lying and standing blood pressure, concentration of serum urea nitrogen and/or serum creatinine, glucose, and electrolytes). Some authorities suggest adrenocorticotropic hormone (ACTH) stimulation or insulin-hypoglycemia testing to determine the need for steroid coverage in patients who are no longer receiving steroids but who have received large doses of steroids in the past; however, these tests cannot be recommended for routine use since adequate evidence that a normal response precludes the need for steroid coverage during surgery is lacking.

Recommendations to the surgeon. The patient may receive his usual steroid dose by mouth the day before surgery. On the day of surgery, the patient should be given hydrocortisone, 100 mg intrave-

nously, at 6:00 A.M.; a second 100 mg is infused continuously during surgery; then a 100-mg dose is given intravenously every 6 hours for the first 24 hours following surgery followed by 50 mg every 6 hours for the second 24 hours after surgery, and 25 mg every 6 hours for the third 24-hour period. The patient may then return to his preoperative medical regimen.

There are two exceptions to these guidelines. First, the regimen is based on the assumption that there is no prolonged stress after surgery; if this occurs, higher doses of steroids must be continued for a longer time postoperatively. Second, for minor procedures, the patient may return to his usual dose within 24 to 48 hours postoperatively.

Hypothyroidism (36)

Size of the Risk

The major potential complications of surgery in hypothyroid patients are increased sensitivity to and prolonged half-life of anesthetic agents, hypoventilation and respiratory arrest in the immediate postoperative period, hyponatremia due to decreased free water clearance, and myxedema coma.

Preoperative Planning

Office evaluation. Hypothyroid patients should be evaluated carefully before admission for surgery. The patient should have the comprehensive evaluation outlined in Table 86.1 and the thyroxine (T_4) level should be checked (unless a value from the past 2 months is available). The serum thyroid-stimulating hormone (TSH) concentration should be obtained in newly hypothyroid patients and in patients in whom there is a question about the adequacy of their replacement dose of thyroid hormone (see Chapter 73 for details).

Recommendations to the surgeon. Specific recommendations for preoperative management depend upon the status of the patient's hypothyroidism. Patients with previously known and adequately treated hypothyroidism can undergo surgery. The half-life of administered thyroxine is about 7 days. Therefore, oral thyroxine can usually be discontinued before surgery and resumed when the patient is able to take oral medication. The stress of major surgery or of severe infection may accelerate the turnover of thyroxine, necessitating daily treatment with intravenous thyroxine (one-half the oral dose) in patients in either of these situations.

If the hypothyroidism has been effectively treated for a long period (as indicated by only minor symptoms or only a slightly decreased level of T_4), the patient can usually tolerate surgery and thyroid replacement can be adjusted postoperatively. For hypothyroid patients who have not been treated or who remain significantly hypothyroid because of inadequate replacement therapy, surgery should be postponed because of the risks listed above. Such patients should receive adequate thyroid replacement for a minimum of 1 to 2 months before elective surgery (4 to 6 months for patients with profound myxedema). Surgery required before this period (especially minor surgery under local anesthesia) may be performed, if the patient can be started on a total replacement dose immediately and if there is prompt improvement in signs and symptoms of hypothyroidism (see Chapter 73 for additional details).

When a patient with previously undiagnosed hypothyroidism requires immediate major surgery, an endocrinologist should be consulted regarding perioperative treatment and monitoring.

Hyperthyroidism (36)

Size of the Risk

The major risk of operation in patients with uncontrolled hyperthyroidism is thyroid storm. In one series, there were only 25 episodes of thyroid storm after 1383 operations on thyrotoxic patients (20). However, surgery accounts for up to one-third of the cases of thyroid storm reported.

Preoperative Planning

Office evaluation. The patient with known hyperthyroidism should be reassessed clinically and with thyroid function tests before admission for surgery. In previously undiagnosed patients, the usual approach should be used in diagnosis (see Chapter 73).

Recommendations to the surgeon. The treatment of the hyperthyroid patient during surgery depends on his current thyroid status. Patients previously diagnosed and adequately treated should take their current treatment until midnight the night before surgery and should resume treatment when they can take substances by mouth again. Patients with new, known, or recurrent hyperthyroidism who are not euthyroid should be brought to a euthyroid state with thyroid blocking agents and/or iodides (see Chapter 73). Ideally, surgery should be postponed for several months in these patients until a consistent euthyroid state is attained.

An endocrinologist should be consulted regarding the treatment and monitoring of any patient with uncontrolled hyperthyroidism who requires urgent surgery.

THE OBESE PATIENT

Size of the Risk

Massive obesity significantly increases the mortality risk associated with surgery. In one study, for example, women undergoing surgery for adenocarcinoma of the uterus had a 20% operative mortality if they weighed more than 300 lb (136 kg), compared to a 1.5% mortality for obese women weighing between 200 and 240 lb (91 and 110 kg) (30). Less severe obesity probably does not increase mortality risks.

Moderate or massive obesity also increases the risk of a number of perioperative problems, including difficult intubation, difficulty in ventilating the patient during anesthesia, the need for a large amount of anesthesia during induction, potential delay in anesthesia washout because of slow release of anesthetic agents from adipose tissue, postoperative atelectasis and pneumonia, thromboembolism, difficult postoperative mobilization when the patient is unable to help himself, nosocomial wound infection (particularly when there is increased moisture due to pannus adjacent to the surgical incision), wound dehiscence, and late incisional hernia.

Preoperative Planning

Office evaluation. For massively obese persons, a program of gradual weight reduction (see Chapter 76) should be planned before any elective operation; this may require up to 6 months. When prompt surgery is needed, these patients should have a comprehensive evaluation (see Table 86.1). In particular these patients should be checked for uncontrolled diabetes and significant hypoventilation (by history and arterial blood gases), two common complications of obesity which increase the risk of surgery. Either of these two problems should be managed preoperatively as discussed above.

Recommendations to the surgeon. Massively obese patients should be given preoperative instruction in deep breathing and in the use of the incentive spirometer or of other devices designed to prevent pulmonary complications postoperatively. Other recommendations for perioperative management depend upon the obesity-associated conditions, such as diabetes, which the patient may have.

THE PATIENT WITH GASTROINTESTINAL DISEASE

Peptic Ulcer Disease

Size of the Risk

Data are lacking on the risk and the management of surgery in patients with active peptic ulcer disease.

Preoperative Planning

Office evaluation. Patients with active ulcer disease should have elective non-ulcer surgery postponed until the ulcer heals. The average time required for the healing of uncomplicated ulcers is 4 to 6 weeks for duodenal ulcer and 6 weeks for gastric ulcer (see Chapter 36). There is no consistent relationship between disappearance of ulcer symptoms, ulcer healing, and recurrence. Therefore, it is best to wait several weeks after all symptoms have disappeared and 2 to 3 months from the beginning of an episode before admission for elective non-ulcer surgery. If surgery cannot be deferred this long or if ulcer recurrence is suspected, endoscopy should be performed preoperatively. Before admission, these patients should also have the comprehensive medical evaluation summarized in Table 86.1 and multiple stool samples should be checked to exclude active bleeding.

There are no empirical data to confirm these guidelines, nor to indicate whether surgery can be done safely as soon as an ulcer has healed (as shown by endoscopy). If abdominal surgery must be performed in a patient with active ulcer disease, consideration should be given to surgical treatment for the ulcer as well (see detailed discussion of indications for and types of surgery, Chapter 36).

Recommendations to the surgeon. Patients with remote or inactive ulcer disease require no special therapy preoperatively or postoperatively.

Patients with recently active ulcer disease should continue their current therapy until midnight the day before surgery. Because cimetidine can be given intravenously (300 mg every 6 hours), it should be utilized throughout the period when the patient cannot take medicines by mouth; nasogastric suctioning should also be recommended during this period.

Hepatitis

Size of the Risk

General anesthesia and surgery during acute hepatitis are associated with a high mortality and morbidity (17). The major problem accounting for these risks is postoperative hepatic encephalopathy and its complications. The catabolic effects of surgery, hypotension during anesthesia, and hepatic toxicity from anesthetic agents are the principal factors which may precipitate hepatic encephalopathy.

Preoperative Planning

Office evaluation. Patients with a history of acute hepatitis should have a comprehensive evaluation (see Table 86.1) and liver function tests (serum aminotransferases, bilirubin, alkaline phosphatase, al-

bumin, globulin, and prothrombin time) obtained before admission for surgery. Tests for hepatitis B antigen should also be performed (see Chapter 42). Liver biopsy is only necessary if the diagnosis or activity of the disease is uncertain.

Ideally, surgery should be postponed for a minimum of 6 to 12 months after all laboratory evidence of active liver disease has returned to normal. This cautious approach is advised because there is a risk of exacerbating hepatic injury if surgery is performed earlier. Only urgent, lifesaving surgery should be performed during the acute phase of hepatitis whatever its etiology.

Recommendations to the surgeon. Anticipation of postoperative complications (particularly bleeding and encephalopathy) is important in the patient with active hepatitis who must undergo surgery. For the patient with an abnormal prothrombin time (less than 50% of normal), fresh frozen plasma should be given throughout the immediate perioperative period. When immunological tests or epidemiological information indicates infectious hepatitis (see Chapter 42), the surgical team should be notified in order to minimize the risk of spreading infection.

Cirrhosis

Size of the Risk

Most of the quantitative data regarding the risks of surgery in the cirrhotic patient have been collected in trials of portal-systemic shunts; therefore, these data may not accurately reflect the risks of surgery unrelated to the liver. The most widely used measure of the mortality risk from shunt procedures is Child's index, which incorporates measurements of serum bilirubin, albumin, ascites, encephalopathy, and nutrition (see Table 86.14). The perioperative complications encountered in these patients are those associated with chronic cirrhosis: encephalopathy, jaundice, gastrointestinal hemorrhage, infection, and hepatorenal syndrome.

Regional and spinal anesthesia do not entirely eliminate the risks of complications in cirrhotic patients. For example, increased morbidity and mortality due to liver disease have been associated even

Table 86.14.
Child's Classification of Operative Risk in the Cirrhotic Patient[a]

	Group		
	"A" Minimal	"B" Moderate	"C" Advanced
Bilirubin (mg/100 ml)	<2.0	2.0–3.0	>3.0
Serum albumin (g/100 ml)	>3.5	3.0–3.5	<3.0
Ascites	None	Controlled	Poorly controlled
Encephalopathy	None	Minimal	Coma
Nutrition	Excellent	Good	Poor ("wasted")
Operative mortality	0%	9%	53%

[a] From Siefkin AD, Bolt RJ: Preoperative evaluation of the patient with gastrointestinal or liver disease. *Med Clin North Am* 63:1309, 1979.

with hernia repair under local anesthesia in some patients (1). The stress of the procedure itself and complications such as hypotension and wound infection may worsen hepatic function, even in the absence of toxic general anesthetics.

Preoperative Planning

Office evaluation. In addition to a comprehensive preoperative evaluation (see Table 86.1), patients with cirrhosis should have liver function tests (serum aminotransferases, bilirubin, alkaline phosphatase, albumin, and prothrombin time). Liver biopsy is indicated in selected patients to establish the presence of cirrhosis, to provide an additional indicator of the severity of liver damage, or to exclude active hepatitis. Liver scan is only occasionally needed to exclude other causes of hepatomegaly. In the history and physical examination, a careful search should be made for complications of cirrhosis, especially encephalopathy, bleeding, varices, and ascites.

The expected benefits of surgery must be weighed carefully against the risks in patients with cirrhosis. In general, risks are higher and only essential surgery should be performed. There are stable patients with mild cirrhosis, however, who have no ongoing injury (e.g., due to removal of a toxin or to discontinuation of alcohol) and in whom standards may be liberalized.

Recommendations to the surgeon. A number of precautions should be emphasized in the cirrhotic patient who does require surgery. Local (or, as a second choice, spinal) anesthesia may be safer than general anesthesia, although data are lacking. Therapy to prevent complications of liver disease, such as postoperative bleeding (fresh frozen plasma for the patient with an abnormal prothrombin time or partial thromboplastin time) and encephalopathy (see Chapter 42), should be established and maintained throughout the operative period, and the patient should be repeatedly checked for evidence of these two problems. The occasional patient who is taking chronic, corticosteroid therapy for liver disease should have his steroids increased during the perioperative period as described above.

THE PATIENT WITH AN IATROGENIC IMPAIRMENT OF HEMOSTASIS

All anticoagulants increase the risk of intraoperative and postoperative bleeding and should be discontinued before any type of surgery. Patients receiving anticoagulants should have a comprehensive preoperative evaluation (see Table 86.1) before admission for surgery, and an appropriate plan for perioperative management of anticoagulation should be communicated to the surgeon.

Coumadin

A reasonable protocol for discontinuing anticoagulation with coumarin derivatives is to stop treatment 48 hours preoperatively for most patients, including those with artificial heart valves (15, 32). If there is less time or if the prothrombin time does not return rapidly enough to normal or near normal (less than 1½ times normal), vitamin K₁ (Aquamephyton), 10 mg, can be given orally, subcutaneously, or intravenously over 10 to 15 minutes; the prothrombin time will usually return to normal within 24 to 36 hours. Where there is a particularly high risk of clotting, such as in patients with artificial heart valves who have developed emboli in the past, anticoagulation can be stopped 24 to 36 hours before surgery, followed by intravenous vitamin K₁; when the prothrombin time becomes subtherapeutic (usually within 12 hours), full anticoagulation should be resumed with heparin and continued until 6 hours before surgery. In all of these situations, the prothrombin time (and if heparin is given, the clotting time and the partial thromboplastin time) should be normal before surgery.

Warfarin (Coumadin) ordinarily can be resumed 24 hours after surgery, at the preoperative dose if all surgical bleeding is controlled. Patients who have undergone intracranial, spinal, or opthalmological operations probably should not be anticoagulated for 48 to 72 hours after surgery. For patients with a high risk of thromboembolism (artificial mitral valves, active venous thromboembolic disease), heparin can be reinstituted 12 to 24 hours postoperatively, if the surgeon is confident that hemostasis is assured, and continued until full anticoagulation with warfarin has been re-established. After the administration of vitamin K₁, the patient may be relatively refractory to the administration of warfarin for a week or more.

Aspirin

Aspirin prolongs the bleeding time and may increase blood loss during and after operation in some patients. Generally, if aspirin is not being used as a critical therapy, it should be discontinued 1 week preoperatively since aspirin continues to affect platelets for this period of time. Discontinuation of aspirin is particularly important prior to procedures where hemostasis is critical, such as neurosurgical operations.

THE PATIENT WITH CHRONIC BACTERIAL INFECTION

Two types of chronic bacterial infection pose risks to the patient and to others in the operating room and therefore require appropriate management before surgery—staphylococcal skin infections and pulmonary tuberculosis.

Skin Infections

Chronic bacterial skin infections (usually due to staphylococci) pose a high risk for wound sepsis and may be the source of infections in other patients (19). Therefore, they should be suppressed or eradicated prior to admission of the patient for an elective operation. Chapter 25 describes the antibiotic treatment of the various types of staphylococcal skin infection.

Tuberculosis

Active pulmonary tuberculosis poses a problem for the surgical patient because of the general debilitation it causes. It also creates the risk of infection for others in the operating room. Therefore, adult patients with a history of unexplained chronic cough or with a prior history of tuberculosis should be evaluated for active tuberculosis before admission for surgery. Patients with active pulmonary tuberculosis should be stable and have negative sputum cultures before admission for elective surgery. The ambulatory treatment of tuberculosis is described in Chapter 29.

THE PATIENT WITH NEUROPSYCHIATRIC DISEASE (37)

Neuropsychiatric problems present ill defined risks during surgery and the postsurgical period. The major concerns are worsening of mental status due to both metabolic changes and psychological stresses. The patient with psychiatric disease may decompensate postoperatively, making care difficult and jeopardizing wound healing.

Cerebrovascular Accident

Size of the Risk

Patients with recent strokes have a significant risk of worsening focal deficits during carotid artery surgery, but this cannot necessarily be extrapolated to other types of surgery. Patients with recent strokes (less than 6 weeks' duration) also have a risk of deterioration in their general mental status, regardless of the status of their focal deficits, if they undergo major surgery; but firm data are lacking on the size of this risk.

Preoperative Planning

Patients with recent strokes should have a comprehensive preoperative evaluation (see Table 86.1), emphasizing documentation of the preoperative neurological impairment. The data regarding the course of the patient's stroke should be reviewed and additional testing (see Chapter 83) should be performed if necessary to exclude a treatable etiology.

No specific perioperative therapy for the patient with a stable completed stroke is needed. In general, it is prudent to delay elective, noncarotid surgery at least 6 weeks after a completed stroke, although no firm data are available to support this practice.

Asymptomatic Cervical Bruit

Size of the Risk

Cervical bruits are present in about 4% of persons over the age of 45 (18). These bruits may be due to a number of processes (see Table 83.9, Chapter 83) including common or internal carotid stenosis. In the patient with an asymptomatic cervical bruit, there is slight or no increased risk of cerebrovascular accident during surgery (6, 26).

Preoperative Planning

Apart from a careful history and physical examination to exclude evidence of a prior stroke or a transient ischemic attack (TIA) related to the cervical bruit, there is no special approach needed for these patients. Hypotension and excessive neck manipulation should be avoided in these patients during surgery. The patient with a history of symptoms possibly related to the bruit should be evaluated as described in Chapter 83.

Parkinson's Disease

Size of the Risk

The perioperative risks in patients with Parkinson's disease derive from the rigidity, which may impair voluntary postoperative ventilation, mobilization, and swallowing. The rigidity of patients taking antiparkinsonism medication may recur after the patient has missed several doses. Despite this potential problem, most patients with Parkinson's disease do tolerate anesthesia and temporary omission of medications (21).

Preoperative Planning

The patient should have a comprehensive preoperative evaluation (see Table 86.1), and the antiparkinsonian regimen should be tailored to provide the best possible relief of his symptoms (see Chapter 82). For patients taking an anticholinergic agent, the drug may be continued until midnight before surgery and resumed when the patient is able to take oral medications. L-Dopa or Sinemet (L-dopa/carbidopa), should be continued up until induction of anesthesia, and the drug should be resumed as soon as possible after surgery. Postoperative physical therapy to maintain range of motion may help the patient until he is able to take oral medication.

Dementia and Organic Brain Syndrome

Size of the Risk

Patients with dementia have an increased risk of mortality and morbidity during surgery. The increase in mortality is due to lack of cooperation (e.g., with postoperative respiratory care). Much of the morbidity is related to worsening mental status due to anesthesia and surgical stress. Because surgery is always a difficult process for a demented patient and because the degree of increased risk is ill defined, the potential benefits of surgery should be carefully reviewed before the final decision to operate is made.

Preoperative Planning

The patient should have a comprehensive evaluation (see Table 86.1) before admission for surgery. A careful search for metabolic abnormalities that may worsen cerebral function should be made before admission, just before surgery, and throughout the postoperative period. Emphasis should be placed on detecting and correcting hypovolemia, electrolyte abnormalities, and hypoxia. Before major surgery, it is advisable to document the patient's mental status formally (see Mini-Mental Status Exam, Table 17.1) so that altered mental status following surgery can be compared with baseline status.

For patients undergoing major procedures, constant observation is recommended for the first 24 to 48 hours after surgery.

Other Psychiatric Problems (37)

Size of the Risk

The major problems associated with general surgery in psychiatric patients are lack of cooperation with postoperative care, postoperative psychosis, and interactions between psychotropic medications and anesthetic agents. The degree of cooperation that can be expected postoperatively can generally but not always be predicted on the basis of the patient's past behavior and his preoperative mental status.

Preoperative Planning

Office evaluation. A careful history of past psychiatric illness should be obtained. The patient's mental status should be documented preoperatively (see Chapter 10) so that it can be compared to postoperative changes. A psychiatric consultation should be obtained in all patients with psychosis or with other severe psychiatric problems. Additional issues that must be dealt with by the patient's personal physician and surgeon are the ability of the patient to give informed consent (see Chapter 10) and the effect of the patient's psychiatric state on the surgical evaluation (such as evaluating symp-

toms in a patient with hysteria or evaluating the need for cosmetic surgery).

Careful explanation of the operation is especially crucial to management of patients with psychiatric disorders or with anticipated stress reactions to surgery. The procedure should be explained in language the patient can understand. After the explanation, the patient should be asked to express any concerns which he has about the planned surgery, and his comprehension of the planned surgery should be assessed. The need to ventilate about anxiety associated with disfiguring surgery (e.g., mastectomy, amputation, *etc*) and with the fear of "not waking up" is particularly common in both anxiety-prone patients and in persons who are usually free of anxiety.

Patients with severe psychosis should be in a stable, manageable state before admission for elective surgery; this should be accomplished through close collaboration between the primary physician, the surgeon, and a psychiatrist.

Patients with mild to moderate anxiety or depression can be managed by supportive counseling, use of support by family members, selective use of antidepressants or minor tranquilizers, and careful explanation of the procedure to the patient. These interventions should be initiated before hospital admission, not at the last minute before surgery.

Recommendations to the surgeon. The principal recommendation for the perioperative period is that the patient's use of psychotropic drugs should be communicated to the anesthesiologist.

Neuroleptics and tricyclic antidepressants can interact with anesthetics to cause increased sedation, hypo- or hypertension, and arrhythmias. Small to moderate doses of phenothiazines, haloperidol, and tricyclic antidepressants should be continued until about 12 hours before surgery. In the occasional patient taking very high doses of these agents, it is recommended that the drug be stopped about 24 hours before surgery, except in patients who have severely decompensated in the past when their medication has been changed.

The dose of benzodiazepines does not need to be changed unless it is very high.

Lithium carbonate can prolong the action of muscle relaxants, and cause myocardial depression and hypernatremia. Lithium should be discontinued 24 hours preoperatively; however, the anesthesiologist should be aware that it has been administered recently. A blood lithium level and electrolyte measurements should be obtained before surgery as a guideline. Additional information about lithium is found in Chapter 15.

Monoamine oxidase (MAO) inhibitor antidepressants can lead to an enhancement of the effect of sympathomimetic agents, to enhanced sympathetic responses to anesthesia, and to a decrease in the rate of elimination of certain anesthetic agents. Because of these problems, MAO inhibitors should be discontinued at least 1 to 2 weeks before surgery, and the anesthesiologist must be informed of their recent administration.

SURGERY IN THE ELDERLY PATIENT (14a)

Size of the Risk

The mortality risk associated with anesthesia and surgery is increased in the elderly. However, the risk in elderly patients has fallen substantially over the past 10 to 20 years and is lower than many physicians think. The overall mortality risk for major surgery in patients under 65 is about 1%; the risk is about 5% between ages 65 and 80. Patients over age 80 have a 10% risk, although recently mortality as low as 6% has been reported (7a).

A number of factors besides age itself increase surgical risk in older patients. These other factors are important because some can be modified (unlike age), and they account for wide variations in surgical risks among patients of the same age. The most important factors are general overall health, nutrition, type of surgery (body cavity versus non-body cavity; elective versus emergency), type of anesthesia, and coexisting conditions (cardiac, infectious, renal, pulmonary) (Table 86.15) (14a).

The most frequent causes of death in elderly surgical patients are uncorrectable surgical lesions, such as infarcted bowel or ruptured aneurysm. The next most important cause is cardiac disease, followed by infections (especially pneumonia), renal disease, and pulmonary disease. In the preoperative evaluation, attention should be focused on these problems, since they account for most perioperative deaths.

Certain common procedures can be performed at low risk in the elderly, often without general anesthesia. These low risk operations include cataract surgery, simple hernia repair, and transurethral prostate resection. The risks of some major surgical procedures in the elderly have fallen greatly over the past few years; examples include elective abdominal aortic aneurysm repair and repair of hip fractures.

Preoperative Planning

Office evaluation. The elderly patient undergoing major surgery should have a comprehensive preoperative evaluation (see Table 86.1) because of the wide variety of coexisting, often unrecognized, medical conditions found in older individuals. The workup should be reviewed specifically for risk factors listed above (Table 18.15). Any major preoperative risks must be weighed against the benefits of the operation, with attention to the fact that quality of life may be as important as longevity in this age

Table 86.15.
Known Factors Increasing Operative Risk in the Elderly (in Addition to Age)[a]

A. Patient
  1. ? Sex
  2. General health (ASA status; healthy *versus* chronic disease)
  3. General condition
    Nutrition (malnutrition)
    Activity (debility, inanition)
    Psychological status (attitude toward surgery, will to live, social situation)
B. Specific Organ Disease
  1. Cardiac (coronary artery disease, congestive heart failure)
  2. Infection or sepsis (especially pneumonia)
  3. Renal disease
  4. Less important or common: chronic obstructive pulmonary disease, liver disease, dementia
C. Type of Surgery
  1. Body cavity *versus* non-body cavity
  2. Elective *versus* emergency
  3. Type of anesthesia

[a] From Kammerer WS, Gross RJ (eds): *Medical Consultation*. Baltimore, Williams & Wilkins, 1983, p 464.

group. An accurate estimation of average future longevity for the patient's age group is important; this is often *underestimated.*

Preoperative cardiac evaluation is discussed above. Clues to occult infection (including simple upper respiratory infections) should be carefully sought, since classic signs may not be present in the elderly. Spirometry should be performed routinely in patients over age 65 if there is any suggestion of pulmonary disease, because of the increased incidence of pulmonary complications in older patients. It should be remembered that serum creatinine may be falsely low in elderly patients due to reduced muscle mass; therefore, a creatinine clearance should be obtained if the state of the patient's renal function is not certain, because of the importance in determining drug dosages. Finally, a brief formal mental status examination (see Table 17.1) should be routinely obtained to serve as a baseline, since postoperative changes in mental status occur frequently in the elderly. If there is hearing impairment preoperatively, the patient should be checked for cerumen impaction.

Recommendations to the surgeon. Elderly patients often have limitations of understanding because of memory deficits, hearing problems, and education. Since these are often known to the primary physician, communication to the surgeon of these limitations will improve the effectiveness of his explanation of the procedure. Explanation of what to expect during hospitalization and surgery is even more important in the elderly, to avoid fear and confusion and because of outdated conceptions of the nature of surgery among the elderly.

Simple measures may help to reduce the high incidence of postoperative confusion in older patients. Such measures include allowing family members to stay beyond visiting hours, returning the patient to the same room postoperatively, allowing the presence of familiar objects, leaving a night light on, and avoiding unnecessary instrumentation. Tranquilizers, sedatives, hypnotics, and pain medications should be used in reduced doses and *for appropriate indications, not routinely*. Haloperidol in small doses (0.5 to 1 mg) is effective in agitated patients; benzodiazepines should be avoided in older patients.

Mobilization postoperatively of the elderly patient should be planned preoperatively. In general, ambulation should be as early as possible, but not so early that the patient has inadequate pain relief, is too weak, has orthostatic hypotension, or becomes symptomatic from underlying cardiac disease.

Finally, postoperative care of the elderly patient, in whom problems with pre-existing medical conditions unrelated to surgery are as common as surgical complications, is a joint responsibility of both the primary physician and the surgeon. Careful attention needs to be paid to routine care, such as fluid-electrolyte orders, since major complications may result from minor errors in management that would not affect younger patients. Meticulous follow-up is necessary to allow early detection of complications, since the elderly tolerate delay in diagnosis of postoperative problems poorly, especially infections.

SURGERY IN THE PREGNANT PATIENT

Size of the Risk

Up to 2% of women require nonobstetric surgery during pregnancy. Risks posed to the mother and fetus include complications from the surgical problem, effects of anesthesia and medication (including teratogenicity), and precipitation of premature labor. Because of these problems, women of childbearing age who are not known to be pregnant should be screened for pregnancy before surgery. History, pelvic examination, and sensitive serum human chorionic gonadotropin pregnancy tests will usually suffice, but very early pregnancy may still be missed. If it is uncertain whether a woman is pregnant, nonurgent surgery should be postponed for 2 to 3 weeks until the situation is clarified; more urgent surgery requires judgment on an individual basis.

Few data exist to prove or quantitate the risk to mother and fetus of surgery during pregnancy. For acute surgical problems, such as appendicitis, the illness clearly is a greater risk to both the mother and the fetus than is the surgery itself. Thus, correct diagnosis and prompt, appropriate surgical treatment are the most important factors in the urgent situation. For less acute problems, prudence would dictate consideration of potential adverse effects of surgery on the pregnancy, including increased maternal mortality, fetal mortality, teratogenicity, and premature labor.

Physiological alterations in pregnancy which may complicate anesthetic-surgical management are listed in Table 86.16. Two common changes of pregnancy should be taken into account when evaluating the patient preoperatively: The "normal" creatinine is lower in pregnancy, and an S_3 gallop or edema is commonly present in the pregnant patient without cardiac disease.

Fetal risks include teratogenicity of drugs and anesthetics, risk of diagnostic X-rays, premature labor, and fetal death. No definitive evidence exists that any one inhalational anesthetic is safer than another for the fetus.

Preoperative Planning

Preoperative planning for the pregnant surgical patient involves a number of complex issues (see review by Barron, "General References"), which can only be summarized here. Considerations should include:

1. *Urgency of the surgery.* Can it be postponed until after delivery or is it urgent, e.g., acute appendicitis, where delay will increase fetal-maternal mortality? In general, emergency surgery should not be delayed because of pregnancy, and totally elective surgery should be postponed until the postpartum period. In intermediate situations, the duration and risk to the mother of waiting must be balanced against the risk of immediate surgery.

2. *Testing.* Tests should be carefully planned to allow a precise diagnosis with minimal risk, especially risk from X-ray exposure. Whenever possible, other tests should be substituted for radiological procedures (e.g., a T_3 radioimmunoassay instead of I^{131} uptake in suspected hyperthyroidism or gallbladder sonogram instead of oral cholecystogram in suspected cholelithiasis). Routine X-rays, such as chest films or flat abdominal films, should be avoided. When these X-rays are unavoidable, use of lead screening, collimated equipment with minimal exposure, and few films can minimize fetal exposure. Avoidance of X-ray exposure should be remembered in the postoperative as well as the preoperative period. The parents should be aware of exposure and risks, for both ethical and legal reasons.

3. *Medications.* Drugs required during the perioperative period should be anticipated. The potential effects on the fetus should be ascertained from obstetrical colleagues or available reference sources, and the least toxic alternative should be used. Routine drugs prescribed postoperatively should be avoided unless they are believed to be absolutely necessary.

Table 86.16.
Physiological Alterations in Pregnancy and Their Relevance to the Surgical Patient[a]

System	Change	Clinical Implications
Cardiovascular	Uterine compression of vena cava and aorta in supine position	Decreased cardiac output and uterine perfusion; avoid supine recumbency; tilt hip 15° in perioperative period
	Decrease in blood pressure in early-mid gestation	Altered criteria for diagnosis of hypotension
	Presence of dyspnea, third heart sound and edema	No known increased risk, and such findings are not an indication for diuretic therapy or delay of surgery
Respiratory	Decreased arterial pO_2 when patient is in the supine position	Avoid supine recumbency
	Decreased pulmonary functional residual capacity and increased O_2 consumption	Increased risk of hypoxia perioperatively; avoid hypoventilation and increase inspired O_2 content prior to procedures inducing apnea (intubation or tracheal suctioning)
Arterial	Arterial pCO_2 and serum HCO_3 decrease to 30 mm Hg and 20 mmol/liter, respectively	Maternal and fetal acidosis may occur in patient ventilated to "normal," nonpregnant values of arterial pCO_2; normal values for pregnancy should be used to guide diagnosis and therapy of acid-base disturbances
Hematological	Decreased venous flow in legs and increased levels of clotting factors	Increased risk of thromboembolism; avoid supine position and consider use of support stockings, pneumatic compression device, or prophylactic heparin
	Proximity of fetal and maternal circulations	Risk of isoimmunization; $Rh_0(D)$ immune globulin should be considered when uterine trauma is likely
Gastrointestinal	Decreased gastric motility and reduced competency of gastroesophageal sphincter	Increased risk of aspiration; preoperative antacids should be considered
Renal	Dilatation of urinary collecting system	Increased risk of urinary infection, and hence catheterization should be avoided when possible
	30 to 50% increase in glomerular filtration rate and renal plasma flow with a concomitant decrease in serum creatinine and urea nitrogen to 0.5 mg/dl and 9 mg/dl, respectively	Serum creatinine above 0.8 mg/dl may reflect impaired renal function; the clearance of many drugs is increased, and dosage schedules may require alteration

[a] From Barron WM: The pregnant surgical patient: medical evaluation and management. *Ann Intern Med* 101:683, 1984.

4. *Anesthesia.* A decision on the type of anesthesia is usually best left to the anesthesiologist and obstetrician in the absence of any data unequivocally supporting one type of agent. Local or regional anesthesia would presumably be safer than general or spinal anesthesia, but no data exist to support this impression.

5. *Monitoring of fetal status* by the obstetrician should be planned throughout the perioperative period.

PROBLEMS FOLLOWING DISCHARGE

Miscellaneous Problems

During the weeks and months after surgery, patients will often have questions about incisional pain, about various symptoms in the system which was operated on, and about restrictions of activity. These questions are best answered by the surgeon. In addition, patients who have major surgery will often complain of postoperative fatigue, a problem which can usually be handled by the patient's regular physician or by the surgeon.

Postoperative Fatigue

Patients with postoperative fatigue may describe any of a number of symptoms: the need for increased sleep, weakness of the arms and legs when resuming usual activity, symptoms of orthostatic hypotension, and loss of interest in resuming usual activities (27). The physiological changes responsible for these symptoms have not been well defined.

Although the symptoms of postoperative fatigue often last for 1 or more months, it is important to evaluate each symptom carefully in order to identify drugs or underlying medical problems which may be contributing to the problem. Sleepiness may be related to sedatives, tranquilizers, or analgesics prescribed at the time of discharge and may improve with discontinuation of these drugs. The patient with orthostatic symptoms may have had a drug prescribed that can produce this problem (diuretics, antihypertensives, long acting nitrates, antidepressants); because bed rest alone may cause orthostasis, it is important to resume these drugs cautiously in a patient who has had recent major surgery and to try discontinuing the drug or reducing the dose whenever the patient complains of orthostatic symptoms. Loss of interest may also be secondary to drugs prescribed after surgery (see list of drugs producing dysphoria, Table 12.1, Chapter 12). Alternatively, this symptom may represent a minor mood disturbance in a patient who has had similar problems at previous times of stress (see Chapter 12); or it may represent a reactive depression, similar to a grief reaction (see Chapter 19), which is related to disfiguring surgery.

When evaluation of postoperative fatigue does not disclose contributing factors that can be treated, the patient should be reassured that the problem will gradually resolve; he should also be given a rough timetable for a return to regular activities that is realistic both in terms of the surgical procedure and of the fact that postoperative fatigue may take a number of months to resolve entirely. Simple exercises for patients convalescing from bed rest are illustrated in Chapter 81, page 1168. For selected patients, these or similar exercises can be recommended during the period of recovery from postoperative fatigue.

General References

Barron WM: The pregnant surgical patient. Medical evaluation and management. *Ann Intern Med* 101:683, 1984.
> A comprehensive and up-to-date review of the subject.

Corman LC, Bolt RJ (eds): Symposium on medical evaluation of the preoperative patient. *Med Clin North Am* 63:1129 (entire issue) 1979.
> Reviews many common medical conditions in the preoperative patient.

Gross RJ, Kammerer WS: Medical consultation on surgical services: an annotated bibliography. *Ann Intern Med* 95:523, 1981.

Kammerer WS, Gross RJ (eds): *Medical Consultation: The Role of the Internist on Surgical, Obstetric, and Psychiatric Services*, Baltimore, Williams & Wilkins, 1983.
> A comprehensive multicontributor book, extensively referenced.

Smith NT, Miller RD, Carbascio AN (eds): *Drug Interactions in Anesthesia*. Philadelphia, Lea & Febiger, 1981.
> Detailed account of interactions of commonly prescribed drugs with anesthetic agents.

Spees EK, Youngstein K: *The Surgery Book*. New York, Simon & Schuster, Poisidon Press, 1986, in press.
> Written for laypersons. Systematic coverage for more than 100 common operations of the following: the nature of the problem, symptoms, diagnosis, treatment alternatives, indications for surgery, contraindications for surgery, type of surgery, type of facility, preoperative care, description of the operation, postoperative care, complications, going home, long term outlook.

Vandam LD (ed): *To Make the Patient Ready for Anesthesia: Medical Care of the Surgical Patient*. Reading, MA, Addison-Wesley, 1980.
> Brief, practical recommendations for preoperative management of most common medical problems.

Specific References

1. Baron HC: Umbilical hernia secondary to cirrhosis of the liver. *N Engl J Med* 263:824, 1960.
2. Bennett WM, Muther RS, Parker RA, *et al*: Drug Therapy in renal failure; dosing guidelines for adults. Part 1 and Part 2. *Ann Intern Med* 93:62, 286, 1980.
3. Brenowitz JB, Williams CD, Edwards WS: Major surgery in patients with chronic renal failure. *Am J Surg* 134:765, 1977.
4. Briefel G, Turer P: Renal disease. In Kammerer WS, Gross RJ (eds): *Medical Consultation*. Baltimore, Williams & Wilkins, 1983, p 138.
5. Burke GR, Gulyassy PF: Surgery in the patient with renal disease and related electrolyte disorders. *Med Clin North Am* 63:1191, 1979.
6. Corman LC: The preoperative patient with an asymptomatic cervical bruit. *Med Clin North Am* 63:1335, 1979.
7. Deutsch S, Daten JE: Indication for prophylactic digitalization. *Anesthesiology* 30:648, 1969.
7a. Djokovic JL, Hedley-White J: Prediction of outcome of surgery and anesthesia in patients over 80. *JAMA* 242:2301, 1979.
8. Eisman B (ed): *Prognosis of Surgical Disease*. Philadelphia, WB Saunders, 1980.
9. Eisman B, Watkins RS (eds): *Surgical Decision Making*. Philadelphia, WB Saunders, 1978.
10. Goldman L: Supraventricular tachyarrhythmias in hospitalized adults after surgery. *Chest* 73:450, 1978.
11. Goldman L, Caldera DL: Risks of general anesthesia and elective operation in the hypertensive patient. *Anesthesiology* 50:285, 1979.
12. Goldman L, Caldera DL, Nussbaum SR, *et al*: Multifactorial index of cardiac risk in noncardiac surgical procedures. *N Engl J Med* 297:845, 1977.
13. Goldman L, Caldera DL, Southwick FS, *et al*: Cardiac risk factors and complications in non-cardiac surgery. *Medicine* 57:357, 1978.
14. Gross RJ: Evaluation of medical risks in surgical patient. In Kammerer WS, Gross RJ (eds): *Medical Consultation*. Baltimore, Williams & Wilkins, 1983 p 13.
14a. Gross RJ, Kammerer WS: Special topics. In Kammerer WS, Gross RJ (eds): *Medical Consultation*. Baltimore, Williams & Wilkins, 1983, p 458.
15. Gross RJ, Kern D: Cardiovascular disease. In Kammerer WS, Gross RJ (eds): *Medical Consultation*. Baltimore, Williams & Wilkins, 1983, p 86.
16. Harman E, Lillington G: Pulmonary risk factors in surgery. *Med Clin North Am* 63:1289, 1979.
17. Harville DD, Summerskill WHJ: Surgery in acute hepatitis *JAMA* 184:257, 1963.
18. Heyman A, Wilkinson WE, Heyden S, *et al*: Risk of stroke in asymptomatic persons with cervical arterial bruits: a population study in Evans County, Georgia. *N Engl J Med* 302:838, 1980.
19. Hiral D: Nasal *Staphylococcus aureus* and postoperative infection. *Am Surg* 46:310, 1980.
20. McArthur JW, Rawson RW, Means JH, Cope O: Thyrotoxic crisis: an analysis of the thirty-six cases seen at the Massachusetts General Hospital during the past twenty-five years. *JAMA* 134:868, 1947.
21. Ngai SH: Medical intelligence: parkinsonism, levodopa, and anesthesia. *Anesthesiology* 37:344, 1972.
22. Oh SH, Patterson R: Surgery in corticosteroid-dependent asthmatics. *J Allergy Clin Immunol* 53:345, 1974.
23. Prys-Roberts C: Hypertension and anesthesia—fifty years on. *Anesthesiology* 50:281, 1979.
24. Rao Tadikonda LK, Jacobs K, El-Etr A: Reinfarction following anesthesia in patients with myocardial infarction. *Anesthesiology* 59:499, 1983.
25. Robbins JA, Mushlin AI: Preoperative evaluation of the healthy patient. *Med Clin North Am* 63:1145, 1979.
26. Ropper AH, Wechsler LR, Wilson LS: Carotid bruit and the risk of stroke in elective surgery. *N Engl J Med* 307:1388, 1982.
27. Rose EA, King TC: Understanding postoperative fatigue. *Surg Gynecol Obstet* 147:97, 1978.
28. Rose SD, Courman LC, Mason DT: Cardiac risk factors in patients undergoing noncardiac surgery. *Med Clin North Am*

63:1271, 1979.

29. Stein M, Cassara EL: Preoperative pulmonary evaluation and therapy for surgery patients. *JAMA* 211:787, 1970.

30. Strauss RJ, Wise L: Operative risks of obesity. *Surg Gynecol Obstet* 146:286, 1978.

31. Tarhan S, Moffitt ED, Sessler AD, *et al*: Risk of anesthesia and surgery in patients with chronic bronchitis and chronic obstructive pulmonary disease. *Surgery* 74:720, 1973.

32. Tinker JH, Tanhan S: Discontinuing anticoagulant therapy in surgical patients with cardiac valve prostheses. *JAMA* 239:738, 1978.

33. Tisi GM: Preoperative evaluation of pulmonary function; validity, indications, and benefits. *Am Rev Respir Dir* 119:293,

1979.

34. Trautlein JJ: Preoperative pulmonary evaluation. In Kammerer WS, Gross RJ (eds): *Medical Consultation*. Baltimore, Williams & Wilkins, 1983, p 45.

35. Van Zee BE, Hoy WE, Talley T, Jaenike JR: Renal injury associated with intravenous pyelography in nondiabetic and diabetic patients. *Ann Intern Med* 89:51, 1978.

36. White VA, Kumager LF: Preoperative endocrine and metabolic considerations. *Med Clin North Am* 63:1321, 1979.

37. Woodcock J: Psychiatry. In Kammerer WS, Gross RJ (eds): *Medical Consultation*. Baltimore, Williams & Wilkins, 1983, p 403.

CHAPTER EIGHTY-SEVEN

Peripheral Vascular Disease and Arterial Aneurysms

CALVIN B. ERNST, M.D.

Most people, if they live long enough, develop arterial disease. Each specific disease entity is only an isolated clinical manifestation of a generalized atherosclerotic process, and evaluation and management of specific problems of arterial disease must be viewed in this context. Quality and quantity of life may be improved by recognition, thorough evaluation, and appropriate therapy of peripheral arterial diseases. The purpose of this chapter is to provide guidelines for recognition and management of the more commonly encountered arterial problems: acute and chronic occlusive disease and abdominal and peripheral aneurysms.

ACUTE ARTERIAL OCCLUSION OF LOWER EXTREMITIES

Acute ischemia of the legs demands immediate recognition and management since late recognition and treatment may eventuate in loss of limb or loss of life. If collateral circulation is not well developed, muscle necrosis and other irreversible changes may occur as early as 4 to 6 hours following acute arterial occlusion.

The two major causes of acute arterial occlusion

are emboli and thromboses. Since surgical management of these two entities may be quite different, it is important to distinguish between them. Embolism demands immediate operation because pre-existing collaterals are scanty, and relief of ischemia is easily accomplished by a simple operation involving extraction of the clot using local anesthesia. Thrombosis usually can be managed under less emergent conditions than embolus because pre-existing collateral channels stimulated by chronic underlying occlusive arterial disease provide marginal but adequate blood flow. Furthermore, management of ischemia secondary to thrombosis requires complex reconstructive surgical procedures which are best performed under elective conditions after adequate evaluation, which includes arteriographic study. Attempted thrombectomy of a badly diseased artery is doomed to failure and may preclude subsequent reconstructive procedures. However, faced with a nonviable extremity, immediate operation for thrombosis is mandatory.

Over 90% of the time, acute embolic occlusion may be distinguished from acute thrombotic occlusion on clinical grounds alone (see below). In instances in which doubt exists about the etiology, arteriography is key in distinguishing embolus from thrombosis (see below, "Laboratory and X-ray Studies").

Etiology

The majority of arterial emboli originate in the heart. In a series of 338 patients, Fogarty and Buch (9) ascribed 94% of emboli to cardiac disease. Whereas several years ago a preponderance of patients had rheumatic heart disease, in recent years peripheral embolization associated with the sequelae of arteriosclerotic cardiac disease has predominated (2). Arrhythmias secondary to coronary insufficiency, recent myocardial infarction with mural thrombosis, or old myocardial infarction with ventricular aneurysm are sources of emboli. Less common sources include proximal arterial lesions such as aortic aneurysms or large thrombo-ulcerative mural aortic plaques. Such lesions cause arterioarterial emboli. Left atrial myxomas, debris from prosthetic heart valves, paradoxical emboli (venous clots passing through a congenital cardiac defect into the arterial circulation), and foreign body emboli, although quite rare, all have been implicated in sudden arterial occlusion.

Although most acute arterial occlusions follow emboli, *in situ* thrombosis of an arteriosclerotic lesion accounts for approximately 25% of acute occlusive events. Such thrombotic complications are most likely to occur in segments of severe stenosis such as the aortic bifurcation, iliac bifurcation, common femoral bifurcation, and the superficial femoral artery just above the knee. Concomitant problems such as hypovolemia from volume depletion or hem-

orrhage, congestive heart failure, polycythemia, or trauma all have profound influences on management.

Clinical Manifestations

Emboli lodge at arterial bifurcations: abdominal aortic (saddle embolus), 14%; iliac, 18%, common femoral, 46%; popliteal, 11% (Fig. 87.1). The brachial artery in the antecubital fossa is the most common site of embolism in the upper body. Approximately 20% of upper body emboli go to the cerebral circulation. Ten percent travel to the abdominal viscera. Multiple emboli result from a "shower discharge" of clots from the heart. Recurrent embolic episodes, during the same hospitalization, may affect 15% of patients. Therefore, although the legs are affected most often, there may be symptoms and signs of ischemia elsewhere.

Clinical manifestations vary depending on the adequacy of pre-existing collateral circulation and on the site of occlusion in the lower extremities. If pre-existing collateral vessels, stimulated by underlying occlusive arterial disease, are present, acute ischemic symptoms may be mild; however, total arterial occlusion of a previously normal arterial tree causes severe symptoms. Cardinal features include the six "P's" of arterial occlusion: pulselessness, pallor, poikilothermia, pain, paralysis, and paresthesias. The latter three P's reflect neurophysiological sequelae of ischemia, while the former three result from mechanical occlusion of an artery. Three-quarters of patients complain of pain, but 20% note numbness as the first manifestation of sudden arterial occlusion. Initially, pain may be mild; but as the ischemic process progresses, pain worsens only to subside late in the course of the disease as anesthesia and paralysis develop.

Additional findings other than the six "P's" include poor capillary filling and collapsed or severely sunken veins on the dorsum of the foot. Although pedal edema rarely, if ever, accompanies embolic occlusion, it may be noted among individuals with thrombotic occlusion who have had nocturnal ischemic rest pain and who attempt to gain relief by sleeping sitting or by dangling their leg over the edge of the bed.

Cardiac examination may reveal atrial fibrillation, a diastolic rumble or the opening snap of mitral stenosis, or a gallop associated with congestive failure. Recent history of chest pain or electrocardiographic evidence of myocradial infarction implicates a cardiac origin of acute leg ischemia.

Laboratory and X-ray Studies

Laboratory studies usually are not helpful in making the diagnosis of acute arterial ischemia of the lower extremities. Arterial blood gases and pH should be obtained to serve as baseline studies for subsequent comparative measurement as well as to

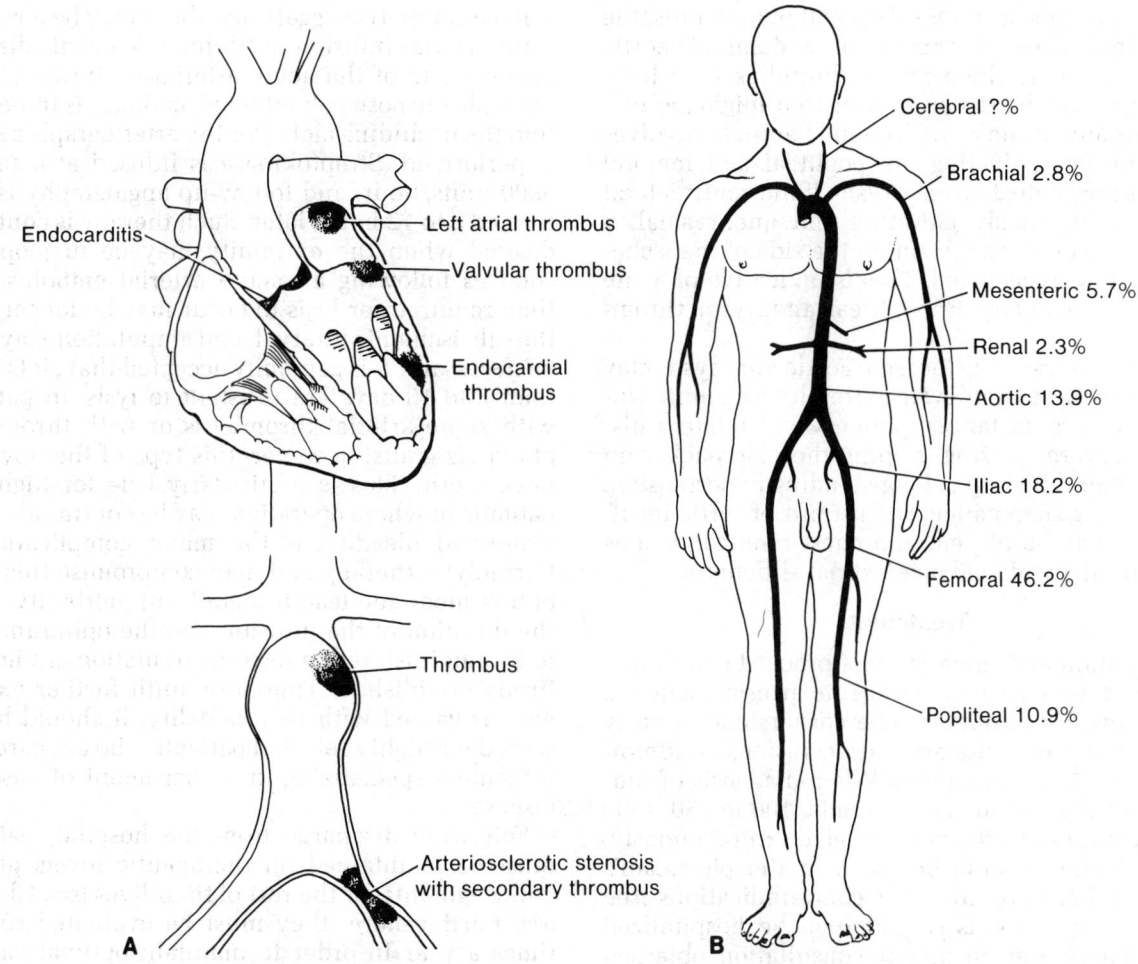

Figure 87.1. *A.* source of arterial emboli in 338 patients. Over 90% originate in the heart. *B.* distribution of arterial emboli in the same group. Over 90% impact in the distal aorta or lower extremities. (Adapted from Rutherford RB (ed): *Vascular Surgery*, ed 2. Philadelphia, WB Saunders, 1984.)

identify metabolic acidosis from muscle ischemia which might require correction prior to operation. Hyperkalemia may be manifest, particularly if advanced muscle ischemia has occurred. A roentgenogram of the chest may document cardiac enlargement or congestive heart failure. All of these studies should be obtained after the patient is hospitalized.

Arteriography is not routinely performed except, occasionally, in instances of modest ischemia when it is needed to distinguish between thrombosis and embolus (see below). Evidence of generalized and severe arteriosclerosis, tapered occlusions of arteries, and of well developed collateral vessels indicates acute thrombotic occlusion. Normal appearing arteries with scanty collateral circulation and an occlusion with an inverted meniscus configuration indicate embolic occlusion.

Other studies, such as Doppler ultrasonic velocity detection of peripheral blood flow, plethysmography studies, and other noninvasive evaluation procedures serve only to confirm the clinical impression already evident and therefore are not required.

Differential Diagnosis

The most important differential, because surgical management depends upon it, is to distinguish embolus from thrombosis. History is often quite helpful in separating these two entities. History of intermittent claudication or rest pain would implicate arterial thrombosis as the acute ischemic event. Complete lack of history of intermittent claudication usually indicates embolus. However, approximately 25% of patients who suffer acute superficial femoral arterial occlusion secondary to thrombosis have never had symptoms of intermittent claudication prior to the sudden occlusive event. On physical examination classic findings of chronic ischemia such as loss of hair on the toes and dorsum of the foot and the shin, along with nail, skin, and muscle atrophy may be noted. Such findings also suggest arterial thrombosis rather than embolus. A pulsatile abdominal mass diagnostic of abdominal aortic aneurysm from which mural thrombus may have discharged to the distal arterial tree might be evident. Finally, if the acute ischemic episode involves only one leg, palpating the popliteal and femoral arteries may detect an aneurysm. If the contralateral vessel is vigorously pulsating and aneurysmal, a thrombosis of an aneurysm on the side of the ischemia may have occurred. This is indicative of acute ischemia secondary to popliteal aneurysm thrombosis.

An acute dissecting thoracic aortic aneurysm may present as unilateral lower extremity ischemia. Under these circumstances, patients will relate a history of severe, searing, ripping thoracic back pain and provide a history of long-standing hypertension. Also, among such patients a murmur of aortic insufficiency may be present and chest roentgenograms may reveal a widened mediastinal silhouette.

Treatment

Evaluation and therapy must proceed simultaneously in the management of acute arterial ischemia of the lower extremities. The cornerstone of early management of acute arterial occlusions is administration of heparin sodium. When diagnosis of sudden arterial ischemia is first made, 100 to 150 units of heparin sodium/kg must be given intravenously. This injection should be given in the physician's office, if there are no major contraindications (see Chapter 51). Patients should then be hospitalized immediately and an urgent consultation obtained with a vascular surgeon.

Introduction of the balloon-tipped embolectomy catheter by Fogarty and his co-workers in 1963 revolutionized management of acute embolic occlusion (10). Adoption of the balloon-tipped catheter converted a previously complex undertaking to a simple operative procedure which invariably can be performed under local anesthesia. Consequently, since introduction of this device, improved survival and limb salvage rates have been reported from many centers. Practically any patient, no matter how ill, may be operated upon using this device.

The surgeon must be knowledgeable of vascular reconstructive techniques so that, should acute arterial thrombosis be encountered rather than acute arterial embolus, definitive treatment may be employed which will usually require arterial reconstruction. In a critically ill patient in whom sufficient time has not been available for proper preoperative preparation, because the acutely ischemic limb mandates immediate management, aortofemoral bypass reconstruction may carry prohibitive operative risks. Under such circumstances, extra-anatomical arterial reconstructive procedures such as axillofemoral, axillobifemoral, or femoral-femoral bypass may be warranted.

Recent reports suggest that there may be a role for intra-arterial infusion of *fibrinolytic agents* directly into the site of the acute arterial occlusion (16). A multiple purpose polyethylene catheter is imbedded into the occluding clot after the arteriographic study is performed. Streptokinase is infused at a rate of 5000 units/hour, and follow-up angiography is performed 8 to 12 hours later. Such therapy is contraindicated when the extremity may be in jeopardy, such as following an acute arterial embolus. The time required for lysis to occur may be longer than the safe ischemic interval, and amputation may then be necessary. It is generally accepted that clots older than 7 to 10 days are resistant to lysis. In patients with acute arterial thrombosis or with thrombosis of bypass grafts, however, this type of therapy may have merit. This is particularly true for high risk patients in whom operation may be contraindicated. Untoward bleeding is the major complication of fibrinolytic therapy and may compromise this form of treatment and lead to significant morbidity. Also, the duration of the infusion and the optimum dose to be administered to restore circulation are not yet firmly established. Therefore, until further experience is gained with this modality, it should be reserved for highly selected patients who are cared for in centers specializing in management of vascular disease.

Following discharge from the hospital, patients must be maintained on therapeutic levels of oral anticoagulants for the rest of their lives (see Chapter 51). Furthermore, they must be evaluated several times a year in order to maintain optimal cardiac function and for continued evaluation of their peripheral circulation.

Results

In spite of improved diagnosis, preoperative care, operative management, and postoperative support, mortality from acute lower extremity ischemia continues to be discouraging. Prior to 1963 mortality following arterial embolectomy ranged between 34 and 63%. Mortality since 1963 has remained high and ranges between 10 and 40% (13, 21). Death associated with acute arterial occlusion of the lower extremities has been unrelated to surgical intervention. Virtually all deaths are related to complications of cardiovascular disease (11). Such findings reinforce the contention that recognition and correction of causes of embolism or thrombosis represent an important aspect in the management of such patients.

If the patient does not succumb to complications secondary to diffuse arteriosclerosis, limb salvage exceeds 95% in most series. Likelihood of successful limb salvage is directly related to time between arterial occlusion and restoration of blood flow. Therefore, it is improbable that a 100% limb salvage rate will ever be achieved.

CHRONIC ARTERIAL OCCLUSIVE DISEASE OF LOWER EXTREMITIES

In contrast to the management schema for acute arterial occlusion, which requires emergent or urgent treatment, chronic arterial occlusive disease, manifest by symptoms covering the spectrum from mild intermittent claudication to rest pain and gangrene, almost never requires emergent treatment. By virtue of development of collateral channels which bypass slowly developing atherosclerotic lesions, chronic arterial occlusive disease may be approached in an unhurried and organized fashion, often by nonoperative management. Thorough knowlege of the natural history of chronic arterial occlusive disease is key to proper management of patients suffering such problems. In an era of vascular surgery when practically any arterial circuit may be successfully reconstructed, and sophisticated diagnostic procedures offer objective data confirming clinical impressions and results of treatment, perspectives are occasionally distorted and operative management is enthusiastically overadopted.

Etiology and Pathophysiology

Atherosclerosis is the cause of chronic arterial occlusive disease affecting the legs in the vast majority of affected individuals. The symptoms and signs of the disease are unusual before the fifth decade. The disease process is influenced significantly and adversely by the presence of diabetes mellitus, hypertension, hyperlipoproteinemia, use of tobacco, factors affecting blood viscosity such as polycythemia, and by reduction in cardiac output. Furthermore, symptoms of arterial insufficiency of the legs are only regional manifestations of a generalized disease process.

Although atherosclerosis is a generalized disease, it has a remarkably segmental distribution. Arteriosclerosis is prone to develop at major arterial bifurcations, in areas of arterial fixation, and at points of marked arterial angulation such as the distal superficial femoral artery as it enters Hunter's canal, the bifurcation of the common femoral artery, the aorta distal to the renal arteries and, most commonly, at its bifurcation, and the common iliac bifurcations.

With gradual development of such lesions, the formation of collateral vessels compensates for segmental obstructive processes, and in many instances collaterals are sufficient to provide adequate blood flow even during moderate exercise. On the other hand, sudden occlusion of a previously unobstructed vessel may not be compensated by immediate collateral blood flow so that tissue necrosis and gangrene ensue. When collateral channels are adequate, no or only minimal symptoms may be present. However, as progressive main arterial involvement occurs, collateral channels may be progressively lost, and symptoms of severe and significant exercise ischemia (intermittent claudication) occur which may progress to gradual development of rest pain and tissue necrosis. The spectrum, then, of symptomatic arterial occlusive disease to the legs extends from mild exercise ischemia to severe rest pain and frank gangrene of the toes and forefoot or to ulceration of the ankle (see Chapter 88).

Diabetes mellitus (see Chapter 72) has a unique influence on the pathogenesis of atherosclerosis. Diabetic patients manifest atherosclerosis of a more severe degree and at an earlier age than nondiabetic individuals. Furthermore, distribution of the atherosclerotic process in the lower extremity of a diabetic compared to a nondiabetic is different in that distal vessels such as popliteal, peroneal, and tibial arteries are more commonly involved than are aortoiliac segments. Microangiopathy also affects peripheral nerves as well as nutrient vessels to skin and muscle which may result in insensitivity and progressive ischemia and in lack of natural protective mechanisms in the diabetic foot. Breakdown of skin and entry of bacteria with subsequent infection may cause extensive damage, since normal sensation is lost and significant symptoms may be obscured. Diabetic neuropathy (Chapter 72) also involves the sympathetic nervous system, and many of these patients have undergone autosympathectomy at the time they are initially seen by a clinician.

Buerger's disease, thromboangiitis obliterans, is a severe chronic panarteritis leading to fibrosis and obliteration of small vessels at the tibial and pedal levels. It is an infrequent cause of lower extremity arterial insufficiency in the United States. This entity affects young men in their twenties and thirties and is almost always associated with severe tobacco addiction. Successful management hinges on cessation of use of all forms of tobacco.

Natural History

The studies of Boyd (1) Imparato and co-workers (14), and Juergens and co-workers (15), are remarkably similar in documenting the natural history of occlusive arterial disease, in particular, intermittent claudication. These investigators concluded that intermittent claudication is a relatively benign condition; approximately one-third of patients with claudication improve; one-third remain stable and tolerate their symptoms; and one-third deteriorate and require operation. Relentless deterioration of the lower extremity associated with intermittent claudication is unlikely in most nondiabetic patients, particularly if use of all tobacco products is discontinued. The chance of amputation occurring among individuals initially seen with intermittent claudication is approximately 1%/year. Patients with ischemic rest pain or gangrene, however, are at very high risk for amputation if surgical management is not employed.

The overall 5-year survival rate among individuals with intermittent claudication approximates 70%. The 10-year survival rate is approximately 40%. Of note is that of those individuals dying, three-quarters succumb to complications of coronary artery disease.

Clinical Manifestations

Symptoms among individuals suffering occlusive arterial disease to the legs range from mild pain in the calves on exercise to severe rest pain and gangrene. Such individuals should be carefully questioned for symptoms involving other arterial circuits such as transient cerebral ischemic attacks. The distance a patient walks before developing claudication should be documented. Men should be questioned specifically about impotence. Patients with rest pain will often note that they can alleviate their pain by dangling their legs over the side of a bed or a chair.

On *physical examination*, in the mildest form of the disease, only a diminution in intensity of peripheral pulses may be noted. Complete vascular examination should be performed noting locations of bruits, blood pressure measurements in both upper extremities, and the recording of all peripheral pulses. Among individuals with mild intermittent claudication, the skin of the feet may appear normal; there may be hair growth on toes; nails may appear normal; and there may even be faintly palpable dorsalis pedis and posterior tibial pulses. With progressive arterial involvement, however, trophic changes may involve the lower extremities with loss of hair on toes and anterior tibial areas. Poor skin nutrition is reflected by thin parchment-like skin. Lack of pulses below the inguinal ligaments, blanching and pallor with elevation of the extremity, and dependent rubor all indicate advanced ischemia. Gangerous areas may be evident involving digits. The typical locations of ischemic ulcers are over the calcaneus, the lateral malleolus, and the dorsum of the foot (see Chapter 88).

Laboratory and X-ray Studies

The distribution and severity of peripheral arterial disease can be determined objectively by noninvasive Doppler flow studies. These studies are performed by the consulting vascular surgeon. A sphygmomanometer cuff is placed immediately above the malleoli and the cuff is inflated to above systolic pressure. As it is slowly deflated, with the Doppler velocity detector placed over the dorsalis pedis or the posterior tibial artery, pulsatile sounds will occur at systolic opening pressure. The highest pressure recorded is utilized to compare with brachial arterial systolic pressure and the ankle/arm pressure index is determined. Normal individuals have a mean index of over 1; for individuals suffering intermittent claudication the mean index is 0.59; for those with rest pain, 0.26; and patients suffering impending gangrene have a mean ankle/arm blood pressure index of 0.05 (25).

A Doppler study of lower extremity blood flow, although important, is not needed in evaluating all patients with lower extremity arterial occlusive disease. However, noninvasive testing is very helpful in distinguishing vascular insufficiency from other causes of leg pain (e.g., neurogenic claudication secondary to cauda equina compression from spinal stenosis). In the latter, Doppler ankle/arm indices are normal and, of particular note, remain normal after exercise. Noninvasive studies can also provide data which objectively document whether or not nonoperative therapy is effective in management or if deterioration of circulation is progressive. In addition, comparison of preoperative and postoperative noninvasive data are useful in documenting effectiveness of operative therapy.

The most important laboratory study, if it is determined the patient is a candidate for operation, is arteriography (see below). Although risks are very small in experienced hands, arteriography is utilized only when operation is indicated and agreed to by the patient.

Treatment and Results

Treatment for arterial insufficiency of the legs may be either operative or nonoperative. Knowing the natural history of the occlusive process aids significantly in determining whether or not the patient's symptoms warrant operative intervention in light of associated risk factors and life expectancy. Except for very poor surgical candidates, individuals with ischemic rest pain, pregangrenous changes, or gangrene, always require operative intervention.

There are patients, however, who are not, and probably never will become, candidates for operation. This group includes individuals whose symptoms are not severe enough to warrant operation and those whose symptoms, although they may be severe, are of such recent onset that sufficient time has not elapsed to determine whether or not development of collateral circulation will cause symptoms to lessen or significantly abate. Indications for operation are shown in Table 87.1. Patients should be managed by nonoperative therapy unless one of these indications is present.

General Measures

Much can be recommended to control or improve symptoms; and an itemized list of recommendations, written in layman's language, is often very helpful in managing such individuals. Such recommendations should first be reviewed with the patient, after which the patient should be given the list for ready reference (Table 87.2). Many of these recommenda-

Table 87.1.
Indications for Operation

Claudication that is intolerable
Rest pain in good risk patient
Impending gangrene in good risk patient

Table 87.2.
Advice Which Should Be Given to Patients with Arterial Insufficiency

QUIT SMOKING—Use NO tobacco in ANY form.

If overweight—lose weight.

Exercise (walk) to the point of discomfort or at least 2 miles a day.

Keep feet very clean. Bathe at least daily in LUKEWARM water.

Gently apply lanolin or mild hand cream to feet after bathing.

Use a night light to avoid hitting toes or shins.

Wear clean, preferably cotton, socks daily (cotton does not retain moisture).

Avoid injury to feet. Wear proper fitting shoes to prevent calluses, corns, blisters.

Place lamb's wool (available from pharmacies) between overriding toes.

Avoid extremes of temperature. Do not put feet in hot water or use heating pads on lower extremities. In cold weather, wear socks to bed to warm feet. Do not get feet cold or wet.

If feet hurt at night, raise head of bed 6–10 inches (15–25 cm) on blocks.

For any sudden change in symptoms such as prolonged pain, numbness or tingling, or inability to move foot or leg, consult your physician *immediately.*

tions pertain to protection of the feet. It should be emphasized that avoidance of trauma to the feet from ill fitting shoes and avoidance of extremes of temperature are very important in the management program. If the patient finds that his feet are cold, particularly at night, he should be told not to use heating pads or hot water bottles since these may cause tissue breakdown and ulceration. A warm pair of socks or a muffler is advised. Patients should bathe their feet at least once a day in lukewarm water (tested by the hand) and thereafter apply lanolin or hand cream to the skin to keep it soft and pliable, thereby avoiding cracking and fissuring, particularly between the toes, which might lead to skin breakdown.

Other measures that significantly affect outcome include improving cardiac output, if congestive heart failure is present (see Chapter 61) and controlling diabetes mellitus. Very important, the patient should be advised to *exercise* to tolerance every day to stimulate collateral channel development. Exercise tolerance can be improved in up to two-thirds of individuals in this way. Also, it is most important to urge strongly the cessation of use of all tobacco products. It must be emphasized to patients that

smoking accelerates atherogenesis, causes further hypoxia because of carbon monoxide poisoning, and causes vasospasm secondary to nicotine which may last up to 1 hour after each cigarette. Patients must be admonished that nicotine in any form is absorbed through the buccal mucosa, be it pipe, or cigarette smoke, or tobacco juice.

Management of coexistent hypertension is sometimes challenging because among such patients, if blood pressure is too well controlled, symptoms may increase. Therefore, when managing hypertension in such individuals, one often must settle for less than ideal blood pressure control.

Pharmacological Management

There is little objective evidence to suggest that *vasodilating drugs* offer significant benefits to patients with symptomatic peripheral arterial insufficiency. Since all systemic vessels may be dilated by these drugs, blood flow to the involved extremity may actually decrease and vasodilators may have the paradoxical effect of causing further ischemia. Furthermore, ischemia probably produces more effective and complete local vasodilation than can be achieved by drugs. Therefore, vasodilator therapy should not be used in the treatment of patients with occlusive vascular disease.

Similarly, except for heparin anticoagulation in hospital among patients who suffer acute deterioration of their peripheral circulation, long term anticoagulation with oral agents has not been shown to have any beneficial effect on retardation of atherosclerosis or on improving symptoms. Oral anticoagulants in elderly, forgetful, and unreliable individuals may pose significant hazards from complications of anticoagulation therapy (see Chapter 51). Platelet-inhibiting agents have not been shown to be effective in management of lower extremity arterial occlusive disease (see Chapter 51).

Although drug therapy has been disappointing in the past there has been recent enthusiasm for using drugs that improve blood flow through the microcirculation by a direct effect on the membrane of the red cell. It has been shown that erythrocytes from patients with obstructive arterial disease have a decrease in membrane flexibility and consequently may not deform adequately to squeeze through capillaries with a diameter of 4 to 5 μm. A new drug, pentoxifylline (Trental) that returns erythrocyte deformability to almost normal has been recently approved for use in the United States. It is a xanthine derivative whose precise mechanism of action is as yet undefined but probably is related to its inhibition of phosphodiesterase in red cells, thereby increasing intraerythrocyte cyclic AMP (red cells depleted of cyclic AMP are more rigid). A recent randomized double-blind parallel group evaluation of the efficacy of pentoxifylline in the treatment of intermittent claudication documented that statistically significant improvement in claudication distance was found in individuals taking pentoxifylline (20). Further clinical experience must be reported to determine the efficacy of this drug but it appears for the first time agents may be available to improve perfusion of the microcirculation.

Pentoxifylline is available in 400-mg tablets, usually prescribed in a dosage of one tablet three times a day with meals. A positive effect, if it occurs, will be seen in 1 to 2 months. The major side effects of the drug are nausea, dyspepsia, and dizziness and often may be relieved by reducing the dose to one tablet twice a day.

Operative Intervention

It is only upon failure of nonoperative therapy or among individuals with clear indications for operation that arteriographic studies are obtained. It must be understood that arteriography serves as a guide for the vascular surgeon when reconstructing the vascular tree. There are no characteristic arteriographic findings which distinguish between patients with intermittent claudication, those with ischemic rest pain, and those suffering from gangrene and ulceration. As a generalization, however, patients who have intermittent claudication usually have hemodynamically significant proximal arterial occlusive lesions affecting the iliofemoral system or the femoral-popliteal-tibial system. Characteristically, such individuals have reasonably good outflow with two or more crural vessels patent. Individuals with advanced ischemic changes will be found to have diffuse multisegment involvement and none or only one patent vessel in the lower leg or foot. However, overlap between various groups is wide and no single arteriographic finding consistently characterizes any one symptom complex.

Occasionally arteriography documents distribution of arterial involvement which is either too extensive or too peripheral to permit reconstruction. Under these circumstances, nonoperative therapy usually is recommended; but if ischemic rest pain and tissue necrosis are present, both patient and family are informed that when an operation is required, amputation is all that may be offered.

Indications for operation among patients with intermittent claudication relate mainly to rehabilitation to retain or gain employment. Trivial claudication and even mild ischemic rest pain, controlled by non-narcotic analgesics, are not indications for operation, particularly in high risk individuals. A trial of conservative management is particularly important if other risk factors, such as recent myocardial infarction, are present (see Chapter 86, Preoperative Planning for Ambulatory Patients).

When it is determined that the condition of the patient warrants operative intervention and when arteriography documents repairable vessels, a number of options for arterial reconstruction are open to the vascular surgeon. Procedures employed include bypass reconstruction by use of a prosthetic graft and endarterectomy. In the past decade definite preference for bypass reconstructive procedures over endarterectomy has become apparent, and endarterectomy is rarely used at the present time. Reconstructive procedures include aortofemoral bypass, femoral-popliteal bypass and femoral-tibial bypass. Recently, there has been enthusiasm for extra-anatomical reconstruction, bypassing the diseased aortoiliac arterial tree, particularly among individuals deemed to be at great risk from a major intra-abdominal procedure. Such extra-anatomical reconstructive procedures include axillounifemoral bypass, axillobifemoral bypass, and femoral-femoral bypass.

It is not appropriate to compare results between various surgical modalities and various patient populations because of variability among patient groups. As a generalization, however, operative mortality for aortofemoral bypass reconstruction is approximately 5%. The patency rate for aortofemoral bypass reconstruction using grafts as well as endarterectomy is approximately 80 to 90% at 5 years. Operative mortality rates for extra-anatomical reconstruction are slightly less than aortofemoral reconstruction, but graft patency rates are significantly worse.

Operative mortality for autogenous vein femoral-popliteal bypass procedures ranges from 0.5 to 1% depending on the general condition of the patient. Five-year patency rates for such procedures vary between 60 and 70%, but it should be emphasized that patency varies directly with the extent of the disease in the vessel being reconstructed.

In general, in contrast to arterial reconstruction for aneurysmal disease, arterial reconstruction for occlusive disease is at best palliative and does not significantly increase the patient's life expectancy because most individuals have significant coincident coronary artery disease. However, the quality of life is vastly improved, particularly among those individuals who would have undergone amputation if successful arterial reconstruction had not been feasible.

Patients with aortofemoral arterial occlusive disease, but without coronary artery disease or diabetes, have survival rates that equal those of the normal age- and sex-adjusted population. Observed differences in life expectancy between "normal" populations and those undergoing arterial reconstructive procedures are usually due to the high prevalence of associated coronary artery disease and diabetes mellitus. It appears that the presence of coronary artery disease reduces life expectancy approximately 10 years, and the presence of diabetes mellitus reduces life expectancy by an additional 15 years (18).

Percutaneous Angioplasty

Since the mid-1970s *percutaneous transluminal arterial dilation*, as an alternative to surgical reconstruction, has been available for highly selected patients with arterial occlusive disease. Its advantages include low morbidity, low mortality, lower cost than arterial reconstruction, shorter hospital stay, repeatability, low complication rate, and patient acceptability. It must be understood that patients who are not candidates for arterial reconstruction, but may be candidates for percutaneous transluminal dilation, may also require operation for complications of transluminal dilation. Therefore, a cooperative team approach between the angiographer and vascular surgeon is mandatory to provide optimal results and minimize complications.

There is limited experience with transluminal angioplasty used as an adjunct to surgical reconstruction. Although the role of adjunctive angioplasty has not yet been defined, it will probably find greatest use among patients with multisegment tandem stenotic lesions. Most authors agree that the best results with percutaneous transluminal dilation are obtained in the iliac arterial segment where success rates at 1 year range from 76 to 93% and at 2 years range from 66 to 92%. The reported success rates for femoropopliteal disease range between 51 and 80% at 1 year and 46 to 75% at 2 years. There is general agreement that results are less satisfactory if the runoff, documented by arteriography, is poor. Recent evidence suggests that in the properly selected patient, the probability of early success of percutaneous transluminal dilation is high if the vessel is stenosed, the involved vessel is the iliac, and the runoff is good (17). Results are less satisfactory when multiple iliac dilations or multiple femoropopliteal dilations are required. Some surgeons are reluctant to dilate occluded vessels for fear of perforating the artery or reluctant to dilate long stenoses for fear of early occlusion.

For isolated unilateral or bilateral iliac stenoses less than 5 cm long, angioplasty provides excellent results. Longer stenoses and occlusions have less favorable results but in very poor risk patients may be an alternative to reconstruction. In the femoropopliteal arterial system, ideal lesions for dilation should be localized and not diffuse. Occlusions less than 5 cm long and stenoses less than 10 cm long appear to be the outer limits for successful percutaneous arterial dilation.

The role of percutaneous transluminal dilation has not yet been firmly established but it appears that in properly selected patients, it serves not only as a valuable therapeutic tool but is an adjunct to arterial reconstruction. It is appealing to believe that percutaneous transluminal arterial dilation can be substituted for arterial reconstruction. However, indiscriminate use of such a therapeutic modality without the same rigid indications required for reconstructive surgery is certainly to be condemned.

Amputation

Occasionally the only form of therapy that can be offered is *amputation*. Debilitated patients with frank gangrene or continuous ischemic rest pain are not candidates for arterial reconstruction or arterial dilation and amputation is the only feasible alternative. The object of amputation is to relieve the patient of disabling pain, remove nonviable and potentially infected tissue, and to select a level which will provide the greatest chance of healing with maximum rehabilitation. Requirements which must be kept in mind when selecting amputation level are (a) the amputation must remove all necrotic and painful ischemic tissue, (b) the amputation stump must be able to be fitted with a functional and easily applied prosthesis, and (c) the blood supply to the skin at the level of the amputation must be adequate to permit primary skin healing.

If the gangrenous process is dry and does not involve the great toe, either autoamputation may be allowed to occur or formal surgical amputation may be performed. If pulses are palpable in the foot and the ischemic process affects the tips of the digits, primary healing will usually occur following toe amputation. In addition, neurotrophic (nonischemic) ulcers on the plantar aspects of the foot in diabetic patients will frequently heal if the head of the metatarsal is removed to relieve the pressure necrosis which occurs as a result of the diabetic neuropathy.

Mortality for amputation is directly related to the preoperative condition of the patient and to other complicating diseases. Mortality rates for amputations performed for occlusive arterial disease have been reported to be as high as 30% with the higher mortality rates recorded in the more proximal amputations.

Following successful amputation, one of the most important aspects of therapy is rehabilitation. To this end, the more distal the amputation, the easier the rehabilitation. In addition, close cooperation between the surgeon and a rehabilitation center is essential to provide the greatest chance of functional ambulation with a minimum of delay. Although it is difficult to predict precisely which amputees will be able to use a prosthesis successfully, in general, patients who have had above-the-knee amputation, who are elderly, who are obese, or are diabetic adjust less well to attempts to restore ambulatory function.

ABDOMINAL AORTIC ANEURYSMS

Abdominal aortic aneurysm is the most commonly encountered aneurysm of the arterial tree. It is encountered 2 to 3 times more often than popliteal arterial aneurysm, the second most common aneurysm. Abdominal aortic aneurysms have been found in almost 2% of consecutive postmortem studies (3).

Men are affected by aneurysmal disease 10 times more often than women. Occurrence of abdominal aortic aneurysms increases with age.

Although it is not possible to implicate precisely a single etiology of abdominal aortic aneurysm, most are arteriosclerotic in origin. The infrarenal abdominal aorta is more susceptible to aneurysmal degeneration than are other arterial segments, although the reasons for this are unknown. Only about 5% of abdominal aortic aneurysms encroach upon visceral vessels, most commonly the renal arteries.

The *natural history* of untreated abdominal aortic aneurysms was unknown until the report of Estes (8) in 1950 which documented, for the first time, the grave consequences of this disease. Five-year survival of patients with untreated aneurysms approximates only 20%. Forty to 50% of patients with untreated abdominal aortic aneurysms die of rupture; and 30% die of other causes, usually from complications of diffuse arteriosclerosis, most notably myocardial infarction. In recent years, multiple groups have presented corroborating data emphasizing the improved life expectancy following surgical treatment of this condition (4, 5, 12, 23) (see below).

Clinical Manifestations

History

The presentation of an abdominal aortic aneurysm depends upon whether complications have occurred. Over 50% of abdominal aortic aneurysms are asymptomatic when first discovered. Asymptomatic aneurysms may be noted during routine examination by a physician for another problem or may be found by the patient. Occasionally, patients complain of a "second heart" in the abdomen after they palpate a pulsatile epigastric mass.

The patient may complain of abdominal, flank, or back pain as the aneurysm expands and becomes symptomatic. Such symptoms are a harbinger of disaster because rupture may follow at an unpredictable time after onset of symptoms.

Rupture. Most aneurysms rupture into the retroperitoneal space, affording lifesaving tamponade after blood pressure falls sufficiently. Under these circumstances, the patient presents with a history of syncope, flank, or back pain, and in a hypovolemic-hypotensive state. Most patients suffering intraperitoneal rupture of abdominal aortic aneurysms are dead by the time medical therapy is available. However, a few do present for treatment; such individuals are profoundly hypotensive and require immediate operative intervention, in spite of seemingly lethal coincidental problems. Aneurysms may rupture also into an adjacent vein, causing a large

arteriovenous fistula (such as an aortocaval or aortorenal fistula); or they may rupture into the gastrointestinal tract, usually duodenum, causing an aortoenteric fistula.

Other complications. If aneurysms are large enough, they may compress adjacent structures, such as ureter, duodenum, vena cava, or vertebral column, with production of appropriate symptoms (for example, symptoms of gastric outlet obstruction in patients with duodenal compression).

Dislodgement of laminated clots from the wall of the aneurysm may cause peripheral embolization to femoral, popliteal, or distal vessels. When emboli occur, patients may complain of symptoms of sudden leg ischemia as the first indication of an abdominal aortic aneurysm (see below). If embolic bits of debris are small and distal vessels are patent, patients may complain of small areas of tissue necrosis such as digital gangrene of the tip of a toe, or small punctate pretibial ischemic lesions.

Finally, aneurysms which suddenly thrombose may present with abrupt ischemia of a lower extremity that can be confused with the presentation resulting from cardiac or from arterial emboli.

Although the incidence of the various complications (other than rupture) is not known, they do underscore the pessimistic natural history of untreated abdominal aortic aneurysms. After seeking specific historical information regarding the aneurysm itself, it is important to question the patient regarding other symptoms of arteriosclerosis so that an estimate of the extent of involvement is obtained; this information will frequently influence recommendations for or against surgical therapy (see Chapter 86). Symptoms of transient cerebral ischemia or previous stroke, angina pectoris or previous myocardial infarction, or symptoms of cardiac decompensation such as significant severe shortness of breath, ankle edema, orthopnea, and paroxysmal nocturnal dyspnea all are especially important in determining the risks in this group of patients.

Physical Examination

Physical examination is the single most valuable source of information in the diagnosis of infrarenal abdominal aortic aneurysms and has been reported to be accurate in almost 90% of cases (8). Depending on the clinical presentation, either complicated or uncomplicated, physical examination will vary. As noted, most patients present with asymptomatic abdominal aortic aneurysms which are discovered on routine physical examination during evaluation for other problems. Under these circumstances, an epigastric pulsatile mass usually is felt. However, in extremely obese individuals or in those with very small aneurysms, a mass may not be palpable. Among these individuals asymptomatic aneurysms may be discovered when X-rays are obtained for other intra-abdominal conditions such as peptic ulcer or renal or colonic disease.

It is important to palpate the epigastrium since the bifurcation of the abdominal aorta is at the level of the umbilicus. Only rarely when palpating inferior to the umbilicus will one identify an abdominal aortic aneurysm unless both common iliac arteries are also greatly aneurysmal. The laterally pulsatile nature of an abdominal aortic aneurysm is key to differentiating it from a mass which might feel pulsatile because it overlies the aorta. Lesions confused with abdominal aortic aneurysm include pancreatic neoplasms, pancreatic pseudocyst, horseshoe kidneys, neoplasms of the stomach or transverse colon, and retroperitoneal soft tissue tumors. Not uncommonly, a normal but prominently pulsatile abdominal aorta in a healthy individual is confused with an abdominal aortic aneurysm. Furthermore, in elderly patients an undilated but tortuous aorta may simulate an abdominal aortic aneurysm. In this circumstance, the pulsatile mass is felt to the left of the midline but not to the right. One should palpate the abdomen by approaching the midline both from the right and from the left to identify the laterally pulsatile characteristic of an aneurysm.

Risk of rupture correlates best with the size of the aneurysm (see below). Estimation of the size by physical examination alone, however, is so variable that it is completely unreliable.

One-quarter to one-third of patients have significant associated occlusive arterial disease as well as the abdominal aortic aneurysm; therefore, a systematic evaluation of all peripheral pulses should be performed. Systemic blood pressure in *both* arms should be measured because many patients with aortic aneurysms have hypertension. By listening with a stethoscope (the bell is most efficient) over the carotid bifurcations the physician may determine if concomitant carotid arterial occlusive disease is present. When examining the lower extremities, particular attention should be directed to the character of the femoral, popliteal, and pedal pulses. In a small percentage of patients (probably less than 10%) there may be coexistent peripheral aneurysms involving the popliteal or femoral arteries.

Laboratory and X-ray Studies

It is particularly important that the suspicion, on physical examination, of an abdominal aortic aneurysm be confirmed by roentgenography. Confirmation is readily accomplished by use of standard X-ray techniques since approximately 70 to 80% of abdominal aortic aneurysms are calcified. Anteroposterior and cross table lateral films of the abdomen document abdominal aortic aneurysms in such individuals (Fig. 87.2). If anteroposterior, cross table lateral, or oblique abdominal X-rays do not substantiate an aneurysm, ultrasonic B-mode scanning may

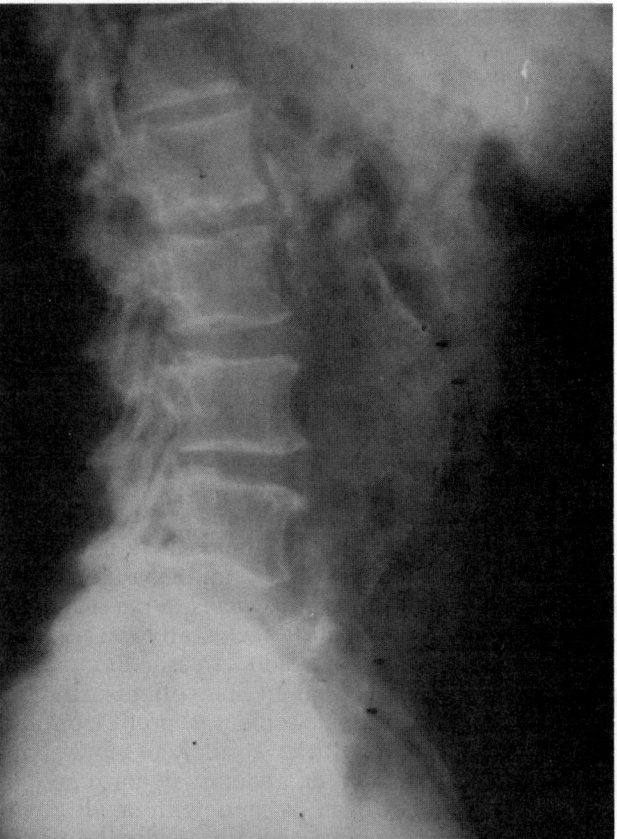

Figure 87.2. Cross table lateral abdominal X-ray documenting calcified abdominal aortic aneurysm.

prove helpful. The accuracy of ultrasonic diagnosis of abdominal aortic aneurysms approaches 98% (19, 24). Since the size of the aneurysm may affect therapy, particularly in asymptomatic and in very poor risk individuals, reliance on accurate ultrasonography or on X-ray assumes great importance. Although there are certain pitfalls in ultrasonography (e.g., the size of the aneurysm is often underestimated), it is an excellent technique, not only for detection of abdominal aortic aneurysms but for following patients who are not candidates for operation; repeated studies every 3 to 6 months are helpful in monitoring the size of the aneurysm.

Computed tomography has provided a new and useful means of assessing abdominal aortic aneurysms, which are seen on computed tomograms as areas of increased diameter. An advantage of CT scanning is that it delineates both the lumen and the outer wall of the aneurysm with the intervening mural thrombus. Computed tomography also may document chronic aortic rupture with a contained hematoma as well as a very thin walled aneurysm that may have a propensity for rupture.

It is useful, also, to have an objective measurement of peripheral pulses in the lower extremities to gauge the results of therapy or to follow the progression of coexistent occlusive arterial disease. This measurement is best made by the vascular surgeon by use of a Doppler blood velocity detection device.

Treatment and Results

Once the presence of an abdominal aortic aneurysm has been verified by either plain abdominal X-rays or ultrasound, a decision regarding therapy must be made. The risk of catastrophic rupture among patients with aneurysms greater than 6 cm in transverse diameter is so great that almost all such individuals must be considered candidates for operation. Aneurysms less than 6 cm in transverse diameter (small aneurysms) are less prone to rupture than aneurysms greater than 6 cm (large aneurysms). However, small aneurysms grow and, if thin walled, also may rupture. If patients have significant life-limiting concurrent disease and small asymptomatic abdominal aortic aneurysms, a close follow-up program can be instituted. Operative candidates should, of course, be referred to a vascular surgeon; the general physician might, in patients that he thinks are not operative candidates, profit from telephone consultation with a vascular surgeon.

The natural history of abdominal aortic aneurysms dictates that even patients with small aneurysms should be treated surgically unless the risk is prohibitive. Szilagyi and co-workers' classic study (23) comparing nonoperative *versus* operative therapy is summarized in Figure 87.3. Even with the worst operative mortality (13%), survival following surgical management of small aneurysms is better than nonsurgical management. As operative mortality declines, the disparity becomes greater. When dealing with large aneurysms, even assuming an operative mortality rate of 13%, surgical therapy is clearly superior to nonsurgical therapy. Over the last two decades, operative mortality has declined to between 2 and 5% for elective aneurysmectomy (4, 7). Should operation be delayed until the aneurysm ruptures, operative mortality increases to a formidable 60 to 80%, particularly if the patient arrives at the hospital in hypovolemic shock. Even when such patients can be resuscitated adequately prior to operation, operative mortality remains approximately 50%.

Age in itself is not a determinant of indication for operation. Elective aneurysmectomy can be performed in a very elderly individual with an operative mortality rate comparable to a similar operation in younger individuals, provided the patient is a satisfactory operative candidate. Furthermore, as a group patients with major complications of their aneurysm (see above) do better with surgical therapy than they do without surgical therapy (22).

Therefore, it is generally advised that aneurysmectomy be performed in all individuals with a

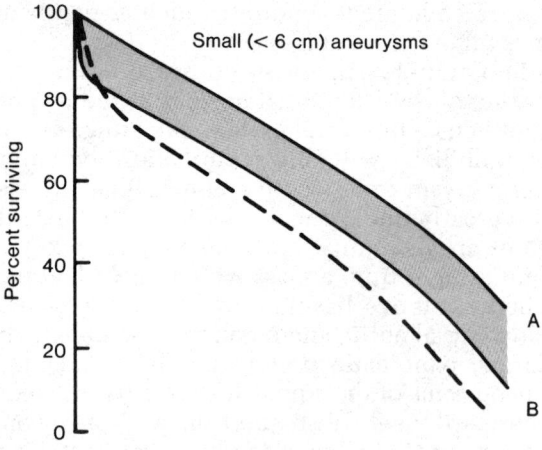

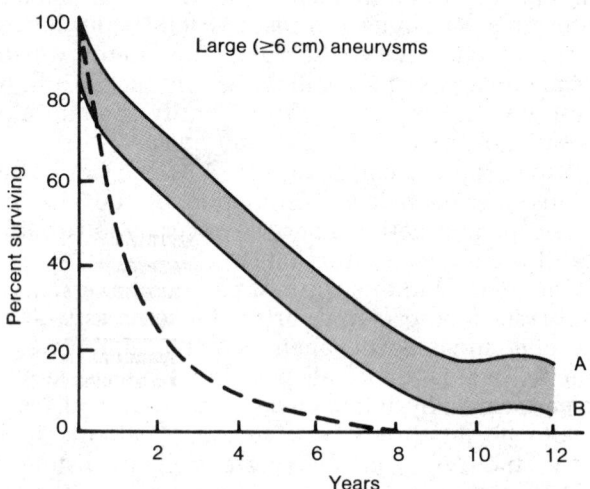

Figure 87.3. Survival curves for surgical and nonsurgical patients with large and small aortic aneurysms. The *dashed lines* represent mortality rates in the nonsurgical groups; the bands, in the surgical groups (the top of the bands (*A*) assumed no operative mortality; the bottom (*B*), a 13% operative mortality). (Modified by Rutherford from data provided by Szilagyi). Even with 13% operative mortality, surgical treatment is better than nonsurgical treatment (Adapted from Rutherford RB (ed): *Vascular Surgery*, ed 2. Philadelphia, WB Saunders, 1984.)

reasonable life expectancy who, in the judgment of the physician and surgeon, would tolerate the operative procedure with an operative mortality of less than 5%. Clearly, operation is mandatory for any individuals who have complications of their aneurysms (see above).

Controversy exists regarding routine use of preoperative aortography among patients with abdominal aortic aneurysms. Although some surgeons routinely recommend aortography, the majority employ aortographic studies selectively. One thing is clear—aortography should neither be used to confirm the diagnosis of an abdominal aortic aneurysm nor to make the diagnosis. Because of laminated clots within the aneurysmal sac, abdominal aortography may actually be misleading, giving an impression of an aneurysm which is actually smaller than it is or even giving the impression that an aneurysm is not present.

Under certain circumstances, abdominal aortographic studies are helpful and even mandatory. Indications for aortography include the possibility of the involvement of other blood vessels, either by the aneurysm itself encroaching upon the renal arteries or by concomitant occlusive arterial disease involving inferior mesenteric, superior mesenteric, or celiac vessels. It is important to determine the extent of reconstruction necessary so that these occlusive lesions do not go untreated and thereby jeopardize the overall result following aneurysmectomy. Drug-resistant hypertension, possibly on a renovascular basis, is another indication for aortography to document renal arterial involvement which might be correctable during abdominal aortic aneurysmectomy. Also, if aneurysmal disease is associated with extensive involvement of the iliac vessels, aortography is indicated. If there is suspicion of congenital arterial anomalies or other congenital defects such as horseshoe kidneys, abdominal aortography is helpful to delineate variances in blood supply associated with such abnormalities and to facilitate operative correction.

It is essential to inform the patient and family of various risks of operative *versus* nonoperative therapy. Equally important is explaining what complications may occur in the postoperative period. Although this is primarily the responsibility of the operating surgeon, it is appropriate for the primary physician to discuss with the patient what is likely to occur. The patient should know that a Dacron or Teflon prosthesis will be used to replace the abdominal aorta and that such arterial grafts are durable and, in general, never need to be replaced. Complications, fortunately, are very rare and in aggregate probably occur less than 2 to 3% of the time. Such complications include paraplegia from spinal cord ischemia, renal failure, loss of one or both legs, graft infection, ischemic colitis, and aortoenteric fistula development. In addition, approximately one-quarter of male patients may develop impotence following abdominal aortic reconstruction. It should be stressed to the patient and family that postoperative complications of abdominal aortic aneurysmectomy are magnified by the urgency of the operative procedure.

If, for any reason, operation is not recommended or accepted, patients should be evaluated at 3- to 6-month intervals for progression of disease or for improvement of coincidental problems, either of which might mandate operation. Since abdominal aortic aneurysms do not dissect, symptoms mimicking dissecting thoracic aneurysms, such as pain shooting into the legs, do not occur. Most commonly, a patient with a rupturing or symptomatic aneurysm will complain of steady, dull abdominal, flank, or back pain. If such pain occurs or if a change in existing symptoms is noted in a patient being followed with an abdominal aortic aneurysm, he and his family should be instructed to seek surgical attention promptly.

PERIPHERAL ARTERIAL ANEURYSMS

Peripheral arterial aneurysms may involve the carotid, subclavian, brachial, iliac, femoral, and popliteal arteries. Over 90% of peripheral aneurysms involve either popliteal or femoral arteries. Popliteal arterial aneurysms predominate. More commonly, tortuous vessels presenting as serpiginous pulsations under the skin, are mistaken for peripheral aneurysms. The most noted example of this is a tortuous subclavian or common carotid artery in an elderly, hypertensive individual which may be confused with a carotid or subclavian artery aneurysm.

Most peripheral arterial aneurysms are arteriosclerotic in origin although mycotic, traumatic, and syphilitic aneurysms are seen occasionally. Peripheral arteriosclerotic aneurysms are localized manifestations of a generalized disease process. This is underscored by noting that, among patients who have femoral arterial aneurysms, 95% have another aneurysm elsewhere; and, more important, 92% have abdominal aortic aneurysms (6). Almost 60% of femoral arterial aneurysms are bilateral. Similarly, among individuals with popliteal arterial aneurysms, almost 80% have another aneurysm elsewhere; two-thirds have abdominal aortic aneurysms; and about half have another popliteal arterial aneurysm (6). Therefore, upon identifying a peripheral arterial aneurysm, the physician should routinely look for a potentially lethal abdominal aortic aneurysm.

Femoral and, particularly, popliteal arterial aneurysms are associated with a very high incidence of distal thromboembolism and of eventual limb loss. Untreated peripheral aneurysms may eventuate in limb loss approximately 75% of the time from either distal embolization or acute thrombosis. On the other hand, rupture with exsanguinating hemorrhage from femoral or popliteal arterial aneurysm is not a major risk.

Clinical Manifestations

Most patients presenting with peripheral arterial aneurysms are elderly, and many may be asymptomatic. Femoral arterial aneurysms usually are quite evident, particularly when they measure 4 or 5 cm in diameter. Similarly, popliteal arterial aneurysms, if they are large, are easily identified. However, popliteal arterial aneurysms may be overlooked because many clinicians do not routinely palpate the popliteal fossa during a physical examination.

Clinical manifestations depend upon whether or not complications are associated with peripheral aneurysms. Patients may present with sudden acute ischemia of an extremity because of thrombosis of the popliteal or femoral arterial aneurysm and manifest any of the six "Ps" of acute arterial ischemia: pallor, pulselessness, poikilothermia, pain, paresthesia, or paralysis. Among individuals in whom complications of peripheral aneurysms develop, successful limb salvage is significantly less likely than among patients in whom surgical therapy is offered before the development of such complications.

Similar to abdominal aortic aneurysms, lateral expansileness of a prominent femoral or popliteal pulse makes the diagnosis of a femoral or popliteal aneurysm. A bruit may be associated with the aneurysm but it is of no clinical significance. Diagnosis of femoral arterial aneurysm is easily made on clinical examination alone. The diagnosis of popliteal aneurysm may be more difficult. When palpating the popliteal fossa, it is helpful to have the patient relax his leg in a passively flexed position to allow the examiner's fingers access to the fossa. If an unusually prominent popliteal fossa is palpated and the examiner suspects aneurysm, the patient may be placed in the prone position and the lower leg supported by the examiner's arm to facilitate popliteal arterial palpation. If diagnosis of politeal arterial aneurysm is in doubt, X-rays of the popliteal region may be obtained since approximately 25 to 30% of popliteal arterial aneurysms are calcified and may be identified on standard X-ray films. B-mode ultrasonography may be a helpful adjunct but is required only rarely. Occasionally, the only manifestations of a popliteal arterial aneurysm are small punctate necrotic areas of skin over the anterior tibial region or small gangreous areas of the tips of toes. This "blue toe syndrome" is a result of microemboli from the aneurysm that have showered to the periphery.

Once the diagnosis of a peripheral arterial aneurysm is made, the patient should be referred to a vascular surgeon. Although arteriography is not required, but is highly recommended in management of abdominal aortic aneurysms (see above), arteriography is mandatory in management of peripheral aneurysms and in particular, of popliteal arterial aneurysms. The arteriogram is used not so much to make the diagnosis but to document patency of arteries distal to the aneurysm, information which is critical to the vascular surgeon in planning arterial reconstruction.

Treatment and Results

Treatment of peripheral aneurysms is indicated in all instances in which it is the physician's esti-mate that the patient has a reasonable life expectancy. Since the natural history of peripheral aneurysms is one of eventual limb loss, it is important to offer surgical therapy to maintain or improve quality of life by avoiding amputation. If however, patients have concurrent significant disease or are bedridden for other reasons, operation is not justified. Surgical correction includes replacement of femoral arterial aneurysms with Dacron grafts or with segments of reversed autogenous saphenous vein. Similarly, popliteal arterial aneurysms are managed by bypassing the diseased segment, preferably with autogenous saphenous vein but, if vein is not available, with any suitable prosthetic material.

Operative mortality for management of peripheral aneurysms approximates 1 to 3%. Limb salvage is obtained in over 90% of cases and is related to the degree of arterial involvement peripheral to the aneurysm. In almost all series reporting repair of popliteal arterial aneurysms, amputations in the postoperative period have been associated with severe occlusive arterial disease manifest by gangrene and rest pain preoperatively.

General References

Boyd AM: The natural course of arteriosclerosis of the lower extremities. *Angiology* 11:10, 1960.
> This study of 1440 patients with intermittent claudication, carefully evaluated and followed over an interval of 15 years, for the first time documented the natural history of intermittent claudication. This study provides the control data base against which results of surgical and nonsurgical therapy are judged.

Crawford ES, Saleh SA, Babb JW III, et al: Infrarenal abdominal aortic aneurysm; factors influencing survival after operation performed over a 25-year period. *Ann Surg* 193:699, 1981.
> Experience of an outstanding vascular surgeon evaluating 920 consecutive patients operated upon for abdominal aortic aneurysm. This paper will become the "gold standard" by which others will measure results.

Dent TL, Lindenauer SM, Ernst CB, Fry WJ: Multiple arteriosclerotic arterial aneurysms. *Arch Surg* 105:338, 1972.
> Evaluation of 57 patients with peripheral aneurysms among 1488 having aneurysmal disease. Importance of coincidental multiple aneurysms when encountering patients with aneurysmal disease stresses need for thorough vascular evaluation.

Rutherford RB (ed): *Vascular Surgery*, ed 2. Philadelphia, WB Saunders, 1984.
> The first comprehensive text of vascular surgery. Specific disease entities are extensively discussed including nonoperative as well as operative aspects. Basic pathophysiological concepts are lucidly presented. This work should be in the library of all interested in vascular diseases.

Specific References

1. Boyd AM: The natural course of arteriosclerosis of the lower extremities. *Angiology* 11:10, 1960.
2. Campbell HC, Hubbard SG, Ernst CB: Continuous heparin anticoagulation in patients with arteriosclerosis and arterial emboli. *Surg Gynecol Obstet* 150:54, 1980.
3. Carlsson J, Sternby NH: Aortic aneurysms. *Acta Chir Scand* 127:466, 1964.
4. Crawford ES, Saleh SA, Babb JW III, et al: Infrarenal abdom-

inal aortic aneurysm; factors influencing survival after operation performed over a 25-year period. *Ann Surg* 193:699, 1981.

5. DeBakey ME, Crawford ES, Cooley DA, Morris GC Jr: Aneurysm of the abdominal aorta; analysis of results of graft replacement therapy 1 to 11 years after operation. *Ann Surg* 160:622, 1964.

6. Dent TL, Lindenauer SM, Ernst CB, Fry WJ: Multiple arteriosclerotic arterial aneurysms. *Arch Surg* 105:338, 1972.

7. DeWeese JA, Blaisdell FW, Foster JH: Optimal resources for vascular surgery. *Arch Surg* 105:948, 1972.

8. Estes JE: Abdominal aortic aneurysm. A study of 102 cases. *Circulation* 2:258, 1950.

9. Fogarty TJ, Buch WS: The management of embolic and thrombotic arterial occlusion. In Rutherford RB (ed): *Vascular Surgery*, Philadelphia, WB Saunders, 1977, p 423.

10. Fogarty TJ, Cranley JJ, Krause RT, *et al*: A method for extraction of arterial emboli and thrombi. *Surg Gynecol Obstet* 116:241, 1963.

11. Fogarty TJ, Daily PO, Shumway NE, Krippaehne W: Experience with balloon catheter technique for arterial embolectomy. *Am J Surg* 122:231, 1971.

12. Foster JH, Bolasny BL, Gobbel, WG Jr, Scott HW Jr: Comparative study of elective resection and expectant treatment of abdominal aortic aneurysm. *Surg Gynecol Obstet* 129:1, 1969.

13. Hardin CA, Hendren TH: Arterial embolism. *Vasc Dis* 2:11, 1965.

14. Imparato AM, Kim G-E, Davidson T, Crowley JG: Intermittent claudication; its natural course. *Surgery* 78:795, 1975.

15. Juergens JC, Barker NW, Hines EA: Arteriosclerosis obliterans. Review of 520 cases with special reference to pathogenic and prognostic factors. *Circulation* 21:188, 1960.

16. Katzen BT, Edwards KC, Albert AS, VanBreda A: Low-dose direct fibrinolysis in peripheral vascular disease. *J Vasc Surg* 1:718, 1984.

17. Lally ME, Johnston KW, Andrews D: Percutaneous transluminal dilatation of peripheral arteries: an analysis of factors predicting early sucess. *J Vasc Surg* 1:704, 1984.

18. Malone JM, Moore WS, Goldstone J: Life expectancy following aortofemoral arterial grafting. *Surgery* 81:551, 1977.

19. Nusbaum JW, Freimans, AK, Thomford NR: Echography in the diagnosis of abdominal aortic aneurysm. *Arch Surg* 102:385, 1971.

20. Porter SM, Baur EM. Pharmacologic treatment of intermittent claudication. *Surgery* 92:966, 1982.

21. Satiani B, Gross WS, Evans WE: Improved limb salvage after arterial embolectomy. *Ann Surg* 188:153, 1978.

22. Szilagyi DE, Elliott JP, Smith RF: Clinical fate of the patient with asymptomatic abdominal aortic aneurysm and unfit for surgical treatment. *Arch Surg* 104:600, 1972.

23. Szilagyi DE, Smith RF, DeRusso FJ, *et al*: Contribution of abdominal aortic aneurysmectomy to prolongation of life. *Ann Surg* 164:678, 1966.

24. Winsberg G, Cole-Beuglet C, Mulder DS: Continuous ultrasound "B" scanning of abdominal aortic aneurysms. *AJR* 121:626, 1974.

25. Yao JST: Hemodynamic studies in peripheral arterial disease. *Br J Surg* 57:561, 1970.

CHAPTER EIGHTY-EIGHT

Lower Extremity Ulcers and Varicose Veins

ANDREW MUNSTER, M.D., AND CALVIN B. ERNST, M.D.

LEG ULCERS

Ulceration of a lower extremity is a common and important problem in ambulatory medical practice. Accurate diagnosis is based mainly on history and physical examination and is essential for appropriate treatment. Often the management of various types of leg ulcers is completely different so that inappropriate therapy can lead to the loss of a toe or even of a limb. Generally it is necessary for the physician (a) to give detailed instructions to the patient and (b) to have a great deal of patience.

History

In addition to a complete general medical history, specific attention should be paid to the following; duration of ulceration; symptoms of peripheral arteriosclerotic vascular disease, such as intermittent calf claudication, intermittent thigh or gluteal claudication, impotence, rest pain, and feelings of coldness and tingling in the legs; a history of previous ulceration or of injury to the lower extremities; a history of discomfort associated with footwear; a history of chronic swelling; and if swelling has occurred, whether it has been alleviated by lying down.

Rest pain is usually a symptom of advanced arteriosclerotic vascular disease, and it is characteristically alleviated if the patient dangles his feet over the edge of the bed, or sits in a chair when awakened at night by ischemic pain. In contrast, the common nocturnal leg cramps that occur in many individuals with no evidence of peripheral vascular disease are usually accompanied by palpable hardening of the calf muscles, and by involuntary muscle contraction of the extensor muscles of the toes. The cramps usually are relieved if the patient gets out of bed and walks around. Examination of the extremities in these patients (see below) is usually normal.

Physical Examination

A thorough physical examination of the patient should be undertaken in conjunction with the examination of the lower extremities, particularly searching for abdominal aneurysm and other intrabdominal masses, as well as for signs of hypertension, cardiac disease, lymphatic masses in the groin, and for the other stigmata of vascular disease.

Examination of the Lower Extremities

The patient should be undressed and both lower extremities should be bared. Initial examination is performed while the patient is supine. Both legs are examined and compared. Particular points to be noted are: (a) the presence of either pitting or nonpitting edema. Pitting edema is a sign of chronic venous obstruction or of an acute inflammatory process. Nonpitting edema is a sign of lymphatic obstruction. If edema is present, it is important to note whether it is unilateral, and if it is bilateral, whether it is asymmetrical or symmetrical; (b) the presence of hemosiderin deposited in the skin of the ankles (a sign of venous insufficiency); (c) the general appearance and quality of the skin, including hair growth (hair loss may signify arterial insufficiency); (d) evidence of fungal infection (scaling, apparently pruritic lesions); and (e) the status of the nails.

Following inspection of the feet and legs, a vascular examination of the lower extremities should be conducted. Femoral, popliteal, dorsalis pedis, and posterior tibial pulses should be palpated and the capillary refill time following pressure on the toes should be observed (normally less than 10 seconds). Auscultation from the midabdomen down to the popliteal regions should be performed to detect bruits that are produced by narrowed atherosclerotic arteries. The temperature of the legs should be felt with the dorsum of the hand, both descending from the thigh to the foot and symmetrically from side to side, comparing one side to the other. Evidence of varicose veins is best sought with the patient standing.

Inspection of Ulcer or Ulcers

Ulcerated areas on the legs are often very tender; and palpation, although necessary, should be done gently, with the gloved hand.

Site. An accurate description of the site of the ulcer, preferably with reference to some immovable anatomic landmark—e.g., the medial or the lateral malleolus—should be made, and the findings should be recorded.

Size. The size of the ulcer must be documented, and the vertical and horizontal diameter in centimeters should be noted in the patient's record for future reference.

Shape. It should be noted whether the ulcer is regular or irregular in outline, whether the edges are undermined, whether the base is clean or covered with exudate, and what type of tissue is at the base of the ulcer (clean fascia, granulation tissue, dirty exudate, debris, *etc*).

Mobility. With the gloved hand, an attempt should be made to move the ulcer over the underlying tissue. It is important to know whether the ulcer is attached to the deep fascia of the leg and particularly to the bone, or whether it moves freely with its surrounding skin over the underlying structures.

Examination of edge of ulcer. It should be noted whether the edges are raised, heaped, everted, or flat and whether there is any evidence of epithelial ingrowth from the edge of the ulcer toward the center—i.e., healing.

Tenderness. If the ulcer is tender, it should be determined whether it is *very* tender such as in an acute inflammatory process or only mildly tender as in a neuropathy with loss of superficial sensation.

Changes in adjoining skin. It should be noted whether there are fluctuant areas of purulence near the ulcer, particularly on the sole of the foot, whether there are any callosities surrounding the ulcer, and whether there is a heavy deposition of pigment near the ulcer.

When this examination is complete, the patient should stand, preferably on a stool, and face the examiner. Edema should now be looked for together with the appearance of varicose veins along the course of the short and long saphenous veins on the front and back of the legs (see Fig. 88.1). In particular, the appearance of perforator varicosities (see below, page 1280) should be noted, usually above the medial malleolus, and the relationship of these perforators to ulcerated areas should be sought.

Types and Characteristics of Leg Ulcers

The principal characteristics of common ulcers are shown in Table 88.1.

Venous—Associated with Varicose Veins

Ulcers associated with varicose veins (see pages 1278–1282) characteristically occur in the presence of advanced varicose veins, usually affecting the long saphenous system (Fig. 88.1). Such varicosities should be apparent when the patient has stood for a few minutes. Ulcerations associated with varicose veins occur where the deep perforators meet the long saphenous or the accessory long saphenous system just above, or 3 or 4 cm higher, than the medial malleolus. Edema and hemosiderin deposition are usually absent or minimal and there are no signs of peripheral arterial insufficiency. The ulcers are characteristically fairly shallow, regular, and tender; they are usually initiated by minor trauma. They move with the skin and fascia over the underlying tissues. The edges are not undermined. There may be evidence of varicose veins on the nonulcerated side of the extremity. The patient will complain that the ulcer hurts and that he has a feeling of heaviness in his legs. Claudication and chronic edema are usually absent.

Venous—Associated with Chronic Venous Insufficiency ("Stasis")

Chronic venous insufficiency is the commonest cause of leg ulcers. The disorder probably follows deep venous thrombophlebitis with destruction of valves in the deep venous system and reversal of normal superficial-to-deep flow of blood in the perforating veins. The muscular action of the calf be-

Table 88.1.
Characteristics of Common Leg Ulcers

Type of Ulcer	Usual Location	Edema	Pigmentation	Evidence of Arterial Insufficiency
Varicose	Medial leg	0 to +	0 to +	0
Stasis	Medial leg	++ to ++++	+++	0 to +
Arterial	Lateral leg, foot	0 to +	0	++++
Dystrophic	Sole, tip of toe	++	0	0
Traumatic	Midleg, toe	0	0	0 to ++++
Diabetic	Toes, dorsum of foot	++	0	+ to +++
Factitious	Anywhere	+	0	0

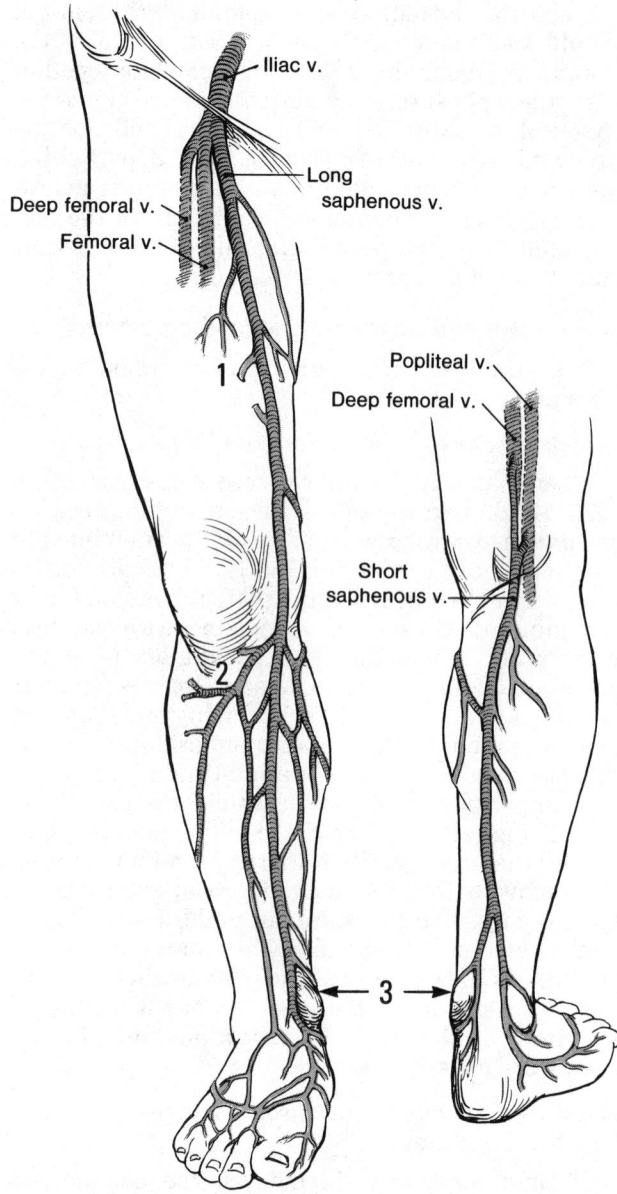

Figure 88.1. Venous circulation of the lower extremity. *1*, Hunter's canal perforator; *2*, anterior communicating vein of the leg; and *3*, ankle perforators.

comes ineffective and blood flows to the superficial veins instead of in the usual centripetal direction through the deep venous system. Valves in the superficial (saphenous) system become incompetent, thereby raising the hydostatic venous pressure at the ankle. As a result, small venous capillaries rupture and an extravasation of red cells takes place; hemoglobin from these red cells is processed locally by macrophages and is deposited in the tissues, causing pigment deposition (hemosiderosis). The pigment acts as an irritant to the tissues, causing further collagen deposition which results in strangulation of the nutrient arteriolar circulation to the

skin. Both venous stasis and arterial capillary nutrient insufficiency therefore relate eventually to ulceration.

The patient usually gives a history of long-standing swelling of the affected leg. Often, there is a history of minor trauma at the site of the ulcer. The physical examination reveals edema, hemosiderin deposition, and ulceration, usually in line with the long saphenous vein, the short saphenous vein, or over a medial ankle perforator (Fig. 88.1). Arterial circulation in the leg may be entirely normal. Varicosities may or may not be present. The ulcer is usually fairly superficial and involves the skin, with irregular margins and with exudate covering the floor of the ulcer. The ulcer is usually moveable with the skin and is tender. In grossly neglected cases, the ulceration may be massive and may involve most of the circumference of the leg. Occasionally, cellulitis may be evident, with erythema, tenderness, and fever secondary to superimposed bacterial infection (see Chapter 25).

Ulceration Associated with Arterial Insufficiency

Arterial insufficiency (see also Chapter 87) is the second most common cause of leg ulcers and, with the ulcer of venous insufficiency, accounts for the great majority of leg ulcers. Ulcers associated with peripheral arterial occlusive disease usually begin with trauma and therefore appear at sites which are most subject to trauma—i.e., on toes, over the lateral or medial malleolus, at the base of the fifth metatarsal, at the head of the first metatarsal, on the heel or the ball of the foot, and in the distal pretibial region. However, occasionally, ulceration occurs in the untraumatized leg, in which case it is more likely to involve the lateral rather than the medial malleolar region, the common site of venous ulceration. Ulcers secondary to occlusive arterial disease are characteristically quite painful, and may be surrounded by cellulitis. Edema is usually absent. The foot may appear atrophic with shiny, fragile transparent hairless skin; the nails are often hypertrophied and deformed. Other hallmarks of arterial, insufficiency—e.g., pulselessness and coolness— may be present. Because some patients are relieved of rest pain when they dangle the ulcerated leg, dependent edema may be present.

Dystrophic Ulcers

A neuropathic or dystrophic ulcer is usually associated with somatic or sympathetic neurological dysfunction. The precise pathogenesis of these ulcers is not known. Perhaps sympathetic dysfunction causes a reduction of arterial blood flow to local areas of skin resulting in ulceration, or hypesthesia or anesthesia renders the patient more susceptible to trauma. Dystrophic ulcers are most commonly associated with peripheral neuropathies (see Chapter 84) and the neuropathies of congenital or acquired disease of the spinal cord, such as Friedreich's ataxia, syringomyelia, or multiple sclerosis. Peripheral neuropathies due to vitamin deficiency or to injuries may also result in ulcers. Ulceration almost always occurs in areas of pressure. The patient may complain of pain in the ulcer, but the ulcer is usually insensitive to light touch. There may be deformity in the foot associated with the neuropathy (talipes calcaneovalgus or equinus) or there may be a back deformity or a surgical scar as might occur in a patient with a meningomyelocele. Usually, neurological examination of the lower extremity will be abnormal, revealing decreased proprioception, decreased cutaneous sensation, and perhaps impaired movement. The ulcer may be undermined and there may be subcutaneous tracking of infected material into adjacent tissues which, on pressure, will exude loculated pus from the undermined border of the ulcer. If the neuropathy is severe, the patient may be ambulating without pain, yet show quite advanced ulceration of the sole of the foot.

Post-traumatic Ulcers

Post-traumatic ulcers are common and usually are associated with impairment in nerve or vascular supply of the leg. Minor injury to the toe of a patient with arteriosclerotic occlusive vascular disease, or a leg injury in an individual with chronic venous insufficiency, may lead to ulceration. However, such ulcers may develop in the legs of otherwise healthy individuals, particularly after major injuries, such as fractures, which involve areas where vascular supply is normally marginal. The most susceptible site is the junction of the middle and lower third of the subcutaneous surface of the tibia. In this situation, most traumatic ulcers, even in healthy youngsters, heal with some difficulty, and in older patients and in those with even minimal arterial insufficiency, injury at this site resolves with great difficulty. Post-traumatic ulcers may be accompanied by problems of chronic infection and present with tenderness and local cellulitis.

Diabetic Ulcers

Diabetic ulcers have features of dystrophic, traumatic, and arterial ulcers since all three factors contribute to their development. The characteristic location of such an ulcer is in an area of pressure, such as a corn or a callosity (see Chapter 102). The ulcer is fairly insensitive, often heavily infected, with undermined edges, and tracks under the plantar fascia or proximally on the dorsum of the foot. Although usually patients are aware that they are diabetic, some are not, and a thorough evaluation upon suspicion of diabetes is mandatory since control of the ulcer will depend to a large extent on control of the diabetes. Radiological examination is important, for the bone underlying the ulcer may be the site of chronic osteomyelitis that will necessitate surgical intervention (see example, Fig. 31.1B, page 384).

Factitious Ulcers

Factitious ulcers commonly occur in the legs of addicts who inject drugs into slightly varicose leg veins. Perhaps the most common drug in this regard is pentazocine (Talwin) which, when either extravasated or injected in the suspension form, made by emptying the capsule into some water, is a strongly thrombogenic agent causing widespread skin necrosis. The distribution of these ulcers is usually bizarre. They may be multiple and bilateral; and, if the history can be obtained, the diagnosis is easily made. Factitious ulcers may also occur in patients with poor hygiene or who have disorders associated with itching, such as scabies, which has led to excoriation.

Neoplastic Ulcers

Neoplastic ulcers of the leg are rare; but when they do occur, they are usually either basal cell or squamous cell carcinomas and have the usual characteristics of these tumors (see Chapter 100). They have elevated or rolled edges, are anesthetic, and are usually attached to deeper tissue. Marjolin's ulcer, a rare form of squamous epithelioma occurring in healed burn scars, also may be seen on the legs.

Miscellaneous

Ulceration of the legs may occur in sickle cell disease, in polyarteritis nodosa and other collagen diseases, and in other systemic conditions (e.g., ulcerative colitis). In these instances, the diagnosis depends on making the diagnosis of the systemic disorder.

A toxic cause of skin ulceration is the brown recluse spider bite, common in the southeastern United States. The poison of the brown recluse spider contains a necrotizing enzyme which causes a rounded sloughing ulcer of approximately 3 to 4 cm with an indurated edge. The patient may not be aware that he has been bitten by a spider. These ulcers are refractory to healing by use of conservative measures, and should be surgically excised and closed.

In the tropics, ulceration of the foot and leg may occur from local mycoses such as maduromycosis; these conditions should be kept in mind when an individual is returning from a prolonged sojourn in a tropical climate.

Laboratory Aids in Diagnosis

Bacteriology

Leg ulcers are often infected and almost invariably contaminated, usually with enteric organisms. Infections are particularly hazardous in the diabetic and in the patient with chronic arterial insufficiency. Cultures of the ulcer bed are useful, and cultures of obviously purulent ulcers are mandatory since antibiotic therapy is an important part of management (see Chapter 25). If fungal infection is suspected (unusual degree of scaling and of excoriation), unless the physician is experienced in the scraping of lesions and in the microscopic identification of fungi, dermatological consultation is indicated.

Biopsy

Biopsy, by a surgeon or a dermatologist, is indicated if neoplastic or obscure fungal disease is suspected. Biopsy may be performed in the office under local anesthesia, and should include a wedge-shaped section of the edge and floor of the ulcer.

Laboratory Tests for Systemic Disease

These tests are performed as dictated by the clinical diagnosis, when the ulcer is suspected to be part of a systemic disorder—e.g., diabetes, polyarteritis nodosa, sickle cell disease, etc.

Noninvasive Vascular Testing

When ulceration is noted in a patient with occlusive arterial disease, he should be referred to a vascular laboratory for testing. This is more fully discussed in Chapter 87.

Natural History and Management

Venous Ulcers Associated with Varicose Veins

These lesions will invariably heal with elevation and appropriate elastic compression to counteract the increased hydrostatic pressure in the varicose venous system. If the patient is at home, he should be at bed rest for a period of 2 weeks with only bathroom privileges. A Telfa gauze pad is placed over the ulcer and the leg is carefully wrapped in Ace bandages. Alternatively the leg may be wrapped in gauze impregnated with a zinc-gelatin dressing (Unna boot). If an Unna boot is used (the impregnated gauze is commercially available), it should be removed within 48 hours to ascertain that the compression is adequate, since either too tight or too loose compression will result in treatment failure. The bandage may then be reapplied and changed weekly, and healing will usually result. If the ulcer is grossly infected, a Unna boot should not be used. Following adequate bacteriological cultures, it is best to treat an infected ulcer with a suitable topical antibacterial preparation such as Bacitracin-Neomycin cream, a Telfa pad on the ulcer, and Ace bandage compression. The dressing should be reapplied twice a day. It is important *never to apply a Unna bandage to a leg when peripheral arteriosclerotic vascular disease is suspected or cannot be excluded.*

The patient should be followed at twice weekly intervals in the physician's office. After healing of the ulcer, the patient should be referred for surgical opinion about whether stripping and ligation of the long saphenous vein and ligation of the incompetent perforators are indicated to prevent recurrence. If the ulcerations do not heal in 2 to 3 weeks, hospitalization and surgical consultation are indicated.

Ulceration of Chronic Venous Insufficiency ("Stasis" Ulcer)

There is probably no other form of ulcer which taxes the patient or the physician as much as stasis ulcer. The mainstays of therapy are elimination of infection, cleansing of the ulcer bed to facilitate healthy tissue growth, and reduction of edema by elevation and compression. The patient should be at bed rest, and the ulcer should be treated with dressings and with topical antibacterial agents, if appropriate (see Chapter 25).

The patient should be instructed to apply and change the dressing twice a day. One of the following approaches can be used: (a) A sterile gauze pad, moistened in normal saline (not soaking wet, as this can cause maceration) is secured over the ulcer (with an elastic bandage, not with an adhesive tape as this can damage the skin adjacent to an ulcer) and left to dry; necrotic tissue and other debris will be removed when the dry dressing is removed, gently, at the end of each dressing interval. This procedure is appropriate early in ulcer management when there is substantial exudate and debris to remove. (b) When the ulcer is clean, or if it is quite shallow to begin with, a debriding procedure that is less likely to disrupt the growth of granulation tissue is to apply a gauze pad soaked in normal saline for 10 to 20 minutes, then to remove it and cover the ulcer with Telfa gauze (does not adhere) until the next dressing change. (c) In patients with particularly dirty or wet ulcers, the use of a hydrophilic agent (e.g., Debrisan beads) or a proteolytic enzyme (Travase or Elase) for a few days may be helpful. These agents should be used according to the manufacturer's instructions.

Resolution of edema usually can be accelerated with the use of diuretics even when no element of cardiac or renal failure exists; but, to avoid the danger of volume depletion, elastic stockings should be tried first. If the edema can be controlled, the ulcers usually can be healed, although several weeks to months may be required. Following healing, the patient must be advised to keep the leg elevated, if possible, when sitting down and to wear some form of elastic compression permanently: preferably, a made to measure, elastic support garment such as a Jobst stocking.

If, with the above measures, the ulcer still fails to heal, then skin grafting may be required along with venous ligation and stripping. This will require surgical consultation and hospitalization.

Arterial Ulcers

Arterial ulcers are almost impossible to heal unless a surgical procedure can improve blood flow to the area. Therefore, if there is any suspicion of arterial insufficiency, the patient should be referred for surgical evaluation. If the patient's lesion is unsuitable for surgical correction, or if the patient has already had an operation but ulceration persists, the ulcer can sometimes be healed with painstaking debridements every 2 or 3 days. This treatment, however, requires expertise; in case of doubt, surgical referral should be made. A pair of sharp scissors is used to remove the dry eschar that covers the ulcer and to remove the necrotic edges of the ulcer carefully without causing bleeding, and wet to dry dressings are then applied, using a topical antibiotic solution such as Polymixin-Bacitracin 5% aqueous suspension to set the bandages. The patient is instructed to apply the bandage wet with antibiotic solution, in the morning, and to remove it in the evening after it has been allowed to dry. This has the effect of debriding the ulcer, and allowing the delicate epithelial edges the best chance for ingrowth.

If there is a great deal of debris in the ulcer bed, twice daily application of a debriding agent such as Debrisan (hydrophilic beads), Travase (proteolytic enzymes), or Elase (fibrinolytic enzymes), applied for a few days under Telfa gauze or simple sterile gauze, will usually help to clear the thick debris from the ulcer. In conjunction with these measures, meticulously compulsive foot protection, soft footwear, elevation of the extremity, and avoidance of weight bearing are mandatory.

Dystrophic Ulcers

Dystrophic ulcers are a real threat to the limb because infection will often advance unnoticed by the patient until there is considerable spread of pus around and under the ulcer. Treatment consists of bed rest, appropriate antibiotic therapy as indicated following culture (see Chapter 25), debridement of necrotic skin edges (which can be done without anesthesia in the office), and wet to dry dressings as described above. Dystrophic ulcers probably take the longest of all to heal, perhaps several months. If, despite office measures and adequate bed rest at home, no progress seems to be made, the patient should be hospitalized in a setting where debridement can be performed once or twice a day by a skilled individual.

Traumatic Ulcers

Traumatic ulcers will usually heal by avoidance of weight bearing, elevation, appropriate topical antibiotic therapy, and protection of the ulcer by dressings. If no progress is made within 2 to 3 weeks, the patient should be seen by a surgeon for possible operative debridement and surgical closure of the wound.

Diabetic Ulcers

An ulcer in the diabetic foot imposes such serious risk of limb loss that the majority of these patients should be hospitalized.

In the hospital, diabetes can be more meticulously regulated; any pockets of suppuration can be drained, and treatment of osteomyelitis in the metatarsals, and proper debridement can be carried out.

Factitious Ulcers

Factitious ulcers will usually heal if the cause can be found and controlled.

Neoplastic and Other Ulcers

Neoplastic and other unusual ulcers, such as the previously mentioned brown recluse spider bite, are a surgical problem; and these patients should be referred promptly for consultation.

Prevention and General Foot Care in Susceptible Patients (See Chapter 102)

Foot and leg ulcers from any cause often recur after healing, since, with the exception of varicose veins and factitious ulcers, the underlying disease is difficult to reverse. It is therefore mandatory to be familiar with the principles of foot care, and patients must understand and carry out instructions aimed at minimizing exposure to trauma. Patients with peripheral arterial disease or diabetes should wear very comfortable footwear, even if it is not fashionable. The front of the shoe should be broad so that the toes can spread. Areas of pressure caused by foot deformities should be corrected by orthopaedic shoes with appropriate fittings—e.g., insoles or metatarsal bars; these problems should be referred to an orthopaedic surgeon or to a podiatrist. Patients should be instructed to keep their feet very clean— i.e., at least once-daily showers or footbaths in tepid water; nails should be very carefully trimmed, preferably with clippers; under no circumstances should sharp scissors be used to trim the sides of nails, as they may cause injury to the delicate nail fold and become a portal of entry for infection and consequent laceration. Patients can protect their toes during walking by the insertion of small, fluffy pieces of cotton wool between them. Lanolin or other emollient creams are useful in preventing cracking of hardened areas of skin, and in keeping the skin soft and supple. Patients should avoid extremes of temperature, and reduce exposure to trauma (e.g., a night light in the bedroom to avoid "stubbing" a toe). With attention to these small details, recurring trouble can often be prevented.

VARICOSE VEINS

Causes

Varicose (dilated) veins of the lower extremities are common, affecting females more often than males, and usually become symptomatic between the ages of 20 and 40. They are due to an incompetence of the valves of the long or short saphenous veins (see Fig. 88.1), permitting retrograde or downward flow of blood, or simply stagnation of the normal centripetal flow. In the perforator system, which is a system of veins communicating between the deep and the superficial veins, destruction of valves interferes with the unidirectional movement of blood from superficial to deep.

The disorder is aggravated, indeed may be caused, by conditions elevating intra-abdominal pressure, such as pregnancy, large intra-abdominal tumors, conditions causing chronic straining—e.g., prostatic obstruction, carcinoma of the sigmoid colon, and occasionally, by mechanical interference with venous return in the venous system itself such as thrombosis of the pelvic veins.

Symptoms

The symptoms of uncomplicated varicose veins usually consist of heaviness and aching in the area of the veins or in the calves. The patient may complain of mild edema at the end of a long day's work. Occasionally, patients will complain of varicose veins for cosmetic reasons and desire treatment. Patients with uncomplicated varicose veins do not complain of intermittent claudication or severe pain; in the presence of these symptoms, other causes must be carefully sought. Occasionally, thrombophlebitis will supervene in a varicose vein and can cause severe pain; the culpable vein is then palpable as an inflamed cord. Following bed rest, elevation, application of local heat, and appropriate anti-inflammatory therapy (e.g., aspirin), thrombophlebitis in the varicose veins will result in cure of that particular varix.

Physical Examination

It is useful to have some idea of the anatomy of the venous system of the leg (Fig. 88.1). This will enable the clinician to judge the patient's symptoms on the basis of an anatomical abnormality detected by physical examination. There are several types of varicose veins which conform to the underlying anatomic arrangement of these veins.

Subcutaneous Varicose Veins ("Sunburst" Varices)

These are not, in the true sense of the word, varicose veins, but rather dilations of subcutaneous venous plexuses which have a spider-like arrangement and an unsightly purple color. These veins are quite frequently the object of cosmetic complaints by patients. Otherwise, they are essentially asymptomatic.

Varicosities of Long Saphenous System

These are the most common type of varicose veins. The long saphenous vein begins anterior to the medial malleolus at the ankle, courses superficially to the medial side of the knee and then curves upwards to enter the deep system just below the inguinal ligament medial to the femoral artery. The vein has several tributaries in the calf and in the thigh which are superficial, and it is also joined by several perforating veins from the deep venous system; the valves at these junctions can become incompetent and lead to focal varicosities (Fig. 88.1). There are three or four consistent perforators—three above the medial malleolus at a distance separated by approximately 3 cm, and a fourth just above the knee joint. If varicosities appear in this situation, then the perforator system is almost certainly incompetent. Otherwise, varicosity of the long saphenous vein is clearly visible with the patient standing.

Varicosities of Short Saphenous System

The short saphenous vein arises behind the lateral malleolus and courses upward behind the calf to join the popliteal vein in the popliteal space (Fig. 88.1). Varicosities of this system are best seen with the patient standing with his back to the examiner.

Perforator Varicosities

As mentioned above, perforator incompetence is usually noticed in the long saphenous vein where the ankle perforators and the above-the-knee perforator join the vein; however, perforators join other superficial veins which in turn, join the long and short saphenous system. Examination may reveal that there is no incompetence of the short or long saphenous veins, only of the perforators.

Clinical Testing to Determine Level of Incompetence

One or two easy clinical tests can be performed in the office which will aid in the determination of the severity of the problem and in the selection of appropriate treatment.

Trendelenburg's Test

The patient lies on his back and raises his leg to empty the veins. A venous tourniquet is applied just below the saphenous opening about 3 inches (7.7 cm) below the inguinal ligament and the patient then stands up. Constriction is released; if the saphenofemoral valve is incompetent, the veins will fill immediately from above; if not, the veins fill slowly from below. If the veins fill rapidly from above *before* the release of the tourniquet, this indicates an incompetent valve at the entry of the long saphenous vein into the femoral vein and signifies major long saphenous incompetence. This test is now repeated at successively lower levels in the leg; and thereby, the location of incompetence may be mapped.

Perthes' Test

This is a test for deep venous thrombosis in association with varicose veins. A tourniquet is lightly applied below the inguinal ligament as in Trendelenburg's test and the patient is instructed to walk in place. If varicose veins are accompanied by a thrombosed deep femoral system, the varicose veins will become very prominent after this exercise.

Treatment

Subcutaneous Varicosities Asymptomatic Except for Cosmetic Appearance

If the offending venous plexus is deemed large enough to accommodate a 25 gauge needle, a sclerosing solution may be injected. The technique is described below. Other treatments such as freezing with carbon dioxide snow, cautery under local anesthesia, and even laser therapy have been advocated, but their use requires a great deal of skill, and unnecessary skin scarring may result which is, in the end, more unsightly than the original vein. Probably the safest treatment of this kind of vein is the use of masking cosmetic creams, together with reassurance.

Localized Small Varicosities Not Accompanied by Major Long Saphenous or Short Saphenous Incompetence

These veins are suitable for treatment by a sclerosing injection and compression therapy. The procedure can easily be performed in the office by anyone skilled with a needle; however, the patient should be warned that several sittings may be required for complete elimination of the veins.

Technique. The patient stands with a tight tourniquet around the thigh, just enough to make the vein prominent. The area of the vein is lightly prepped with a suitable antiseptic and 0.5 ml of sclerosing solution is injected by use of a 2-ml syringe, following initial aspiration to make sure the needle is in the vein. Immediately after the end of the injection, the needle is withdrawn; and the vein is gently compressed with a 2- × 2-inch gauze for 3 minutes, after which the tourniquet is released and compression continued for 2 minutes more. The patient now wears an Ace bandage on the area for approximately 4 hours. The sclerosant produces an inflammatory reaction in the intima which obliterates the vein by phlebitis. Failure to use a tourniquet may release an unnecessarily large amount of sclerosant into the major veins of the leg and cause undesirable thrombosis at distant sites. The patient should be warned that extravasation of the sclerosant is a possibility and may cause a small skin slough. There are several commercially available sclerosant solutions, morrhuate sodium and sodium tetradecyl sulfate (Soltradecal) which are suitable for injection.

Major Long or Short Saphenous Varicosities, or Perforator Varicosities in Symptomatic Patients

Symptomatic patients should be referred for surgical consultation. Attempts to inject and compress veins associated with clear-cut varicosities of the major superficial systems are doomed to failure without surgical intervention.

If an operation has been performed on either the long or short saphenous system or both, there are often residual varicosities of a minor degree requiring additional injection therapy which may be performed in the office. The recurrence rate of major varicosities after operation is only approximately 10%.

Varicose veins should *not be treated* in individuals who have an underlying cause associated with increased intra-abdominal pressure, until the primary cause has been removed. The wearing of elastic stockings may, however, give comfort during this time. Such stockings may be advisable for support in any individual with varicose veins in whom other treatment is either undesirable or contraindicated.

Patient experience. Outpatient surgery is often adequate for varicose vein operations on one leg, but hospitalization is recommended when both legs are to be operated. For minor varicose veins local anesthesia may suffice. For more extensive varicose veins, or those involving both legs, general or spinal anesthesia is necessary. The patient is instructed to shower or to bathe the legs and groin several times with surgical soap before operation to reduce the bacteria colonizing the skin. Usually the upper end of the vein is tied off in the groin to stop backflow of blood in the upper vein due to a defective valve. Next the lower end of the vein is identified and an incision is made in the skin. The vein is opened and a hard plastic or metal wire is inserted into the vein and passed all the way up to the groin. Next all enlarged branches of the varicose vein and all defective valve areas that have been marked before operation are opened and the smaller veins at these sites are tied off and removed, and the incisions are closed with sutures. Then, a ball is screwed onto the wire at the distal incision which allows the vein to be uprooted, the leg is elevated and wrapped with elastic dressings and the vein stripper is slowly pulled upward, removing the varicose vein through the proximal incision. After varicose vein removal the legs are kept elevated for 6 to 8 hours. Walking is permitted with elastic wrapping of the legs. Elastic wraps or elastic stockings are continued for at least 6 weeks after operation and the patient is instructed to elevate the legs periodically during the day. The patient is advised to avoid prolonged sitting or standing, but walking is encouraged. The patient can return to light work after a few days' convalescence but should not return to heavy lifting or hard manual labor for a month or so. Bleeding under the skin is the most frequent complication, but it is usually not serious. Infection occurs rarely and is treated with antibiotics and local application of heat. Damage to nerves can occur if the saphenous or sural nerves, located just under the skin, are injured during the process of making incisions or stripping the veins. This can cause pain or numbness over part of the lower leg, which usually resolves within a few weeks. About 10% of varicose veins will return after surgical treatment. These are usually the result of failure to tie off all of the communicating branches to varicose veins.

General References

Bailey JL: Leg ulcers. *Nurs Time* 72:1752, 1976.

> Primarily directed to nurses, it carries some practical suggestions on equipment and on dressing techniques for dealing with leg ulcers in the office.

Beninson J: Medical management of the peripheral vascular ulcer. *Angiology* 30:48, 1979.

> A simple, sensible description of management by a physician who has over 30 years' experience running a major leg ulcer clinic. Some very practical suggestions on basic advice to the patient with leg ulcers.

Litchfield R, Wolfson P, Haspel L, Dunlap S: Differential diagnosis of leg ulcers. *J Am Osteopath Assoc* 78:204, 1978.

> An excellent series of photographs showing various types of ulceration and a good description of the clinical features of the more common ulcers.

Robson MC, Edstrom LE: Conservative management of the ulcerated diabetic foot. *Plast Reconstr Surg* 59:551, 1977.

> An article on a currently controversial subject, the management of diabetic ulcer. It points out the disastrous complications of mismanagement, and the excellent results that can be obtained from meticulous conservative therapy.

Young JR: Differential diagnosis of ulcers on legs of vascular cause. *J Dermatol Surg Oncol* 4:687, 1978.

> A useful discussion of vascular ulceration.

CHAPTER EIGHTY-NINE

Diseases of the Breast

ROBERT M. QUINLAN, M.D., AND CALVIN B. ERNST, M.D.

A mass is the most common symptom of breast disease that causes women to seek help from their physician. Although the majority of these masses are benign, 90% of breast cancers are discovered by the patient. No mass, therefore, is too trivial to be investigated.

One in every 13 women develops breast cancer; it is the leading cause of cancer death in women, claiming almost 40,000 lives in this country each year. Approximately one-third of the 120,000 new cases each year present at an advanced stage, often because of delays by either patients or physicians. The primary physician must have a rational approach to the diagnosis and treatment of breast masses and to other, nonspecific, complaints referred to the breast. A surgeon usually enters into the diagnostic and treatment plan since the most definitive diagnostic test for a breast mass is biopsy and histological review. A reassuring patient-doctor relationship is critical in dealing with this emotionally charged area, and although this relationship should be shared by all of the physicians involved in this case, the role of the primary physician is critical.

NORMAL ANATOMY AND PHYSIOLOGY OF THE BREAST

The breast is a modified sweat gland, situated in a fascial envelope on the anterior chest wall. There is an extension of breast tissue reaching toward the axilla. There are 12 to 20 acini arranged like a bunch of grapes with draining ducts emptying into openings on the nipple. These ducts are lined by two layers of epithelium, one of which serves as a basement membrane and source of epithelial cell reproduction. It is this "reverse layer" which can proliferate in certain pathological conditions (20). Surrounding each duct is a specialized periductal fibrous layer, which is under hormonal influence.

Only ducts are present at birth. At puberty, under stimulation of estrogen and progesterone, these ducts branch into surrounding stroma and acini bud from them. With each menstrual cycle, a fall in hormonal activity at the menses results in the desquamation of duct lining, which proliferates again at the cessation of menses. Increases in periductal vascularity and lymphocytic infiltration accompany this proliferation. During pregnancy, with prolonged hormonal stimulation, the ducts and acini proliferate maximally, often never returning to normal in the postpartum period. In many parts of the breast the glandular hypertrophy will remain until it involutes at menopause. At that time there is a loss of parenchyma and an increase in fat, especially in the periductal region. The lobular anatomy slowly disappears. It is thought that variations in hormonal balance can result in various benign pathological conditions occurring during the active menstrual childbearing years and at menopause. It is important to realize that anatomic changes associated with normal hormonal fluctuations during a menstrual cycle do not all occur to the same degree in all areas of the breast. This accounts for the asymmetric palpatory findings in the normal breast, which is often very "lumpy."

SCREENING PROCEDURES

The Health Insurance Plan (HIP) Study, a major randomized controlled trial initiated in 1963, documented a 23% decrease in mortality from breast cancer, over a 14-year period, in women over the age of 50 who were involved in a screening program (physical examination and mammography) (13,14). The recently reported Swedish randomized controlled trial of screening mammography and two large case control studies from the Netherlands (one on mammography and one on mammography plus physical examination) reported in 1984 corroborated the HIP findings; additional randomized controlled trials in progress are addressing the role of breast self-examination, and optimal age and frequency of screening for breast cancer (see "General References," entitled Screening for Breast Cancer).

In the trials reported to date, there has been no definite survival benefit from screening in women under 50 years of age, although the most recent HIP report, based on 14 years of follow-up, showed a possible trend favoring younger screenees as deaths from breast cancers accumulated (14). It is important to remember these facts when considering how to advise women about screening and to consider as well the possible drawbacks of screening procedures: increased anxiety, unnecessary biopsies, false reassurance, and radiologically induced cancer. However, it is important to stress to the patient the possible reduction in morbidity if lesions are detected earlier so that treatment is less deforming (6).

Self-examination

There has been no definitive evidence that breast self-examination (BSE) decreases the mortality from breast cancer (8). However, since the procedure imposes no risk, it is worthwhile encouraging women to perform it. There is, however, a major problem of patient compliance with BSE which limits its effectiveness. It is well known that twice as many women will practice BSE if it is taught by a physician or his designee.

The premenopausal woman should be instructed to examine her breasts approximately 7 to 10 days after her menses. The menopausal or postmenopausal woman should examine her breast on a convenient day once a month, such as the first calender day. BSE should be done both in the sitting or standing and in the supine positions. Instructions (19) should be kept simple: for example, "palpate the breast in a clockwise fashion." The physician should perform the initial instructional self-examination with the patient so that she can answer questions which might arise concerning the normal "lumpy" character of the breast. The appropriate technique for BSE is well illustrated in brochures available without charge from local chapters of The American Cancer Society and from the National Cancer Insti-

tute (write to Office of Cancer Communications, NCI, Bethesda, MD 20205). Ideally, the patient should be given one of these brochures when she is taught self-examination.

Mammography

The controversy surrounding screening with mammography (X-rays of the breast) stems from concern about radiologically induced breast cancer. It has been estimated that the risk from radiation is equivalent to six cases of breast cancer for each million women irradiated with 1 rad each (18). With increased technological improvements, the standard two mammographic views can now be obtained with good quality images using less than 1 rad for both exposures. The physician should be aware of how his radiology consultants accomplish mammography. The American Cancer Society and National Cancer Institute have suggested the following guidelines for mammography screening for breast cancer:

1. Women over age 40 should have physical examinations yearly and mammograms every 1 to 2 years.

2. Women ages 35 to 39 should have baseline mammography, annual physical examinations, and follow-up mammography only if a suspicious lesion is detected during the annual examination.

Widespread use of mammography in asymptomatic women has resulted in the identification of radiographic abnormalities which are "suspicious for carcinoma." Such findings include asymmetry in breast densities, skin retraction and/or skin thickening, and a mass with irregular borders or a sharply outlined mass with one indistinct order. Even in the absence of a palpable mass, these findings usually mandate biopsy. If all patients with suspicious mammograms, but negative physical examinations, are examined by biopsy, cancer is diagnosed 8 to 10% of the time (RM Quinlan, unpublished data).

3. Women less than 30 should not have routine mammography screening.

In summary, screening for breast cancer should include BSE monthly, mammography (according to the guidelines listed above), and annual breast examination by a qualified medical professional. More frequent examinations by a physician might be suggested for patients at increased risk of developing breast cancer (11) (see below, page 1287)

CLINICAL CHARACTERISTICS OF COMMON DISEASES OF THE BREAST

Benign Tumors

Fibroadenoma

Fibroadenoma is the most common unilateral discrete mass in the 15- to 35-year-old age group. The peak incidence is from 21 to 25 years of age. In 10 to 15% of cases, there will be multiple tumors. Rapid growth during pregnancy, just prior to menopause, and in animals given estrogen, all support a concept that fibroadenomas are under hormonal control.

The patient with a fibroadenoma usually complains only of the mass and denies pain, nipple discharge, or other breast changes. On physical examination, the lesion is usually firm, but not rock hard; it is smooth and well circumscribed, nontender, and easily movable. It often rolls about in the breast, mimicking a very large marble. In some adolescents, giant fibroadenomas can be confused with virginal hypertrophy; despite the adenoma's size, however, it is usually more discrete than is diffuse hypertrophy.

A fibroadenoma has both fibrous and epithelial components. The tumor probably arises from terminal ducts and lobules, and the rare finding of lobular carcinoma rather than intraductal carcinoma within or in the vicinity of fibroadenoma (5) is consistent with such an origin.

Although no definite evidence exists, there is suspicion that *cystosarcoma phylloides*, a noncarcinomatous neoplasm of the breast, arises from fibroadenomas (17). The overgrowth of stroma in cystosarcoma is the main difference between it and a fibroadenoma. The best estimates suggest a malignancy rate of between 20 and 30% in cystosarcomas; only 2 to 3% of these tumors will metastasize. Nevertheless, there is a high rate of local recurrence even with the benign type of cystosarcoma. The rate of local recurrence increases with increasing tumor pleomorphism regardless of the extent of surgical excision. Currently, wide local excision would be favored for benign cystosarcoma and modified radical mastectomy for the malignant tumor. In tumors of questionable histology, the more extensive procedure would be appropriate. The criteria of malignancy in this disease are often difficult for the pathologist to define.

The natural history of fibroadenoma is of a tumor growing old with the patient, perhaps calcifying in the postmenopausal woman, and rapidly growing in the pregnant patient. Because of the rare possibility of simultaneous lobular carcinoma or of progression to cystosarcoma phylloides and the inability to exclude definitively carcinoma in a breast mass, the physician should recommend excisional biopsy (see page 1289).

Intraductal Papillomas

Intraductal papillomas often present with serosanguinous, spontaneous, recurrent, or persistent nipple discharge from a single duct. These small tumors are not palpable, but their location can usually be determined by applying pressure on various quadrants of the areolocutaneous margin and noting which quadrant produces the discharge. An intraductal papillary cancer is a possibility that must be excluded. Surgical exploration and excision are performed by removing a small pie-shaped segment in the area producing the discharge.

Fibrocystic Disease

Cystic and proliferative changes in the breasts are common: autopsy studies have revealed them in 4 to 90% of women, depending on the criteria that are applied. The incidence of fibrocystic disease, like that of breast cancer, increases between the ages of 30 and 50. It is reasonable to assume that approximately 50% of women will be affected during their reproductive years. After menopause fibrocystic disease usually disappears, as the disproportionately increased fibroepithelial tissue is replaced by fat.

The disease is usually bilateral, and frequently multiple lesions are found in each breast; however, unilateral discrete lesions are seen occasionally. Diffuse lesions (5 cm or more) are more easily distinguished from cancer than are discrete lesions (less than 5 cm).

The patient with fibrocystic disease usually complains about dull, aching pain in the area of most pronounced nodularity; and this pain is often more prominent just before menses. It is possible that much of the pain related to fibrocystic disease is due to cancer phobia, and it does often lessen with improvement in the doctor-patient relationship (12). Some patients will not have pain and will complain only of a mass or of nipple discharge. Many patients are only first aware of a fibronodular mass in their breast after being examined for another reason. At other times, when patients are asked about the "lumps" in their breasts, they reassure the doctor that they have been present for many years.

The cause of fibrocystic disease is unknown, but is suspected to be linked to changes in the activity of female sex hormones. The great majority of lesions appear benign when examined histologically, but approximately 30% of the time (4a) epithelial hyperplasia or cellular atypia is seen which causes the pathologist and the clinician to worry about the potential for malignant transformation. If such epithelial changes are seen, there is a 2 to 5 times greater risk of breast cancer developing eventually (women with fibrocystic disease without such changes are not at increased risk) (4a). This information and the inability to exclude cancer in a discrete unilateral fibrocystic lesion are the reasons why biopsies are performed so commonly in women with this condition. A general surgeon interested in breast disease will biopsy 10 to 20 benign lesions for every malignant one. Often clinical examination is consistent with fibrocystic disease (bilateral, upper outer quadrant, diffuse, tender, easily movable masses), but the patient has a persistent *localized* symptom of pain or unilateral discharge. In these patients, if there is a family history of breast cancer or a suspicious area on a mammogram, a biopsy is often recommended. In addition to excluding carcinoma, the physician will be able better to evaluate the epithelial component of the fibrocystic change and thereby plan more appropriate follow-up with clinical examination and mammography.

Sometimes fibrocystic disease is associated with *duct ectasia*, usually heralded by spontaneous discharge of thick, gray-green fluid from multiple dilated ducts. At other times duct ectasia and discharge may be present in the absence of palpable fibrocystic lesions. In the first instance, a biopsy should be done to rule out carcinoma; in the second, the administration of estrogen may stop the discharge. If it does, mammography should be performed and then a biopsy should be considered.

Cancer

Unfortunately, one-third of patients with breast cancer present with advanced disease. Their case histories are often replete with multiple risk factors; and physical findings are unmistakable (for example, nipple retraction; marked skin changes; mass fixation to the chest wall; hard, matted axillary nodes). Other patients (85% of the remainder) will present with a painless, hard, irregular mass, less than 5 cm in size, frequently (37%) located in the upper outer quadrant. Again it is the latter group who can be confused with patients with the discrete type of fibrocystic disease (see above). The patient with a carcinoma will often have subtle skin dimpling or nipple retraction even with a mass less than 5 cm.

A lesion which mimics the rock hard texture of a carcinoma, although generally more mobile, is *traumatic fat necrosis*. This lesion can be even more worrisome on mammography where the small microcalcifications of fat necrosis are similar to those found in carcinoma.

Because surgical intervention is so common, the natural history of breast cancer is not known. A report from the Middlesex Hospital in England demonstrated a median survival of 2.7 years from the first symptom in 250 untreated patients seen between 1805 and 1933. Five percent of patients died from causes other than breast cancer, and the last death did not occur for almost 20 years (Fig. 89.1) (2). These patients were not staged according to extent of disease. Prognosis with current treatment modalities is dependent upon the stage of the disease at the time of diagnosis.

The American Joint Committee on Cancer Staging has devised a clinical staging for breast cancer based on tumor size, nodal status, and the presence or absence of metastases (Table 89.1). In addition, histologic evaluation of removed axillary lymph nodes provides the most precise data on survival and is independent of tumor size.

Despite this elaborate clinical and histological staging there are qualitative differences in biological

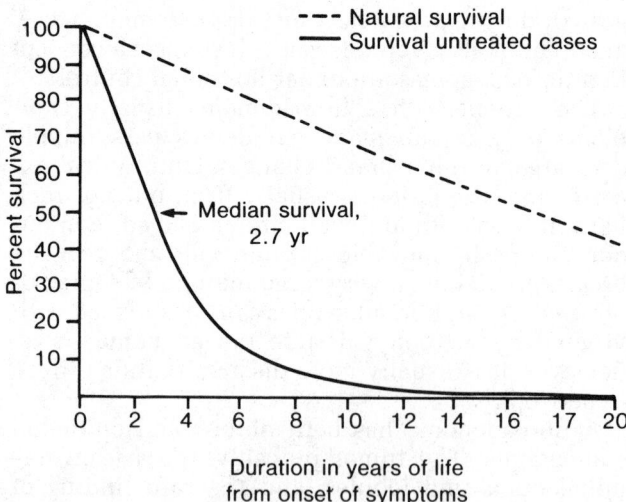

Figure 89.1.   Survival of untreated breast cancer. Middlesex Hospital, 1805–1933 (250 cases). (Adapted from Bloom HJG, Richardson WW, Harries EJ: Natural history of untreated breast cancer (1805–1933). Comparison of untreated and treated cases according to histologic grade of malignancy. *Br Med J* 2:213, 1962.)

Table 89.1.
Survival of Patients with Breast Cancer Relative to Clinical and Histological Stage[a]

Clinical Staging (American Joint Committee)	Crude 5-Year Survival (%)	Range of Survival (%)
STAGE I	85	82–94
Tumor < 2 cm in diameter		
Nodes, if present, not felt to contain metastases		
Without distant metastases		
STAGE II	66	47–74
Tumor < 5 cm in diameter		
Nodes, if palpable, not fixed		
Without distant metastases		
STAGE III	41	7–80
Tumor > 5 cm or,		
Tumor any size with invasion of skin or attached to chest wall		
Nodes in supraclavicular area		
Without distant metastases		
STAGE IV	10	
With distant metastases		

Histological Staging (NSABP[b])	Crude Survival (%) 5-Year	Crude Survival (%) 10-Year	5-Year Disease-Free Survival (%)
All patients	63.5	45.9	60.3
Negative axillary lymph nodes	78.1	64.9	82.3
Positive axillary lymph nodes	46.5	24.9	34.9
1–3 positive axillary lymph nodes	62.2	37.5	50.0
>4 positive axillary lymph nodes	32.0	13.4	21.1

[a] From Henderson IC, Canellos GP: Cancer of the breast; the past decade. *N Engl J Med* 302:17, 1980.
[b] National Surgical Adjuvant Breast Project.

potential of breast cancers in similar stages. Bloom (1) in a study of 1250 patients, matched for stage, noted a decrease in 5-year survival with patient delay of up to 6 months prior to consulting a physician; yet with delays greater than 6 months, there were smaller adverse effects on survival. Patients delaying more than a year had results as good as those seeking prompt therapy. This would imply more and less aggressive types of tumors. Currently, these distinctions are not made in reporting end results of treated patients.

Premature Hyperplasia

A concentric swelling can occur unilaterally beneath the nipple before puberty in girls. This commonly occurs during ages 7 to 9. The lump can be 1 to 2 cm in diameter and is usually nontender. Within a year, a contralateral lump will appear and often both lumps remain static until puberty. A biopsy is *contraindicated* and would be equivalent to total mastectomy.

Gynecomastia

The main differential in male breast masses lies between gynecomastia (see Chapter 77) and male breast cancer. The latter is extremely rare, accounting for approximately 1% of all breast cancers. Although gynecomastia has many causes, its physical characteristics are usually unvaried. Gynecomastia presents as a breast mass beneath the areola, is usually slightly tender, and is easily movable. It is never associated with ulceration or nipple retraction. If gynecomastia is ruled out, a breast mass in a male should be examined by biopsy.

EVALUATION OF A BREAST MASS

History: Risk Factors (Table 89.2) and Symptoms

A *family history* of breast cancer increases a woman's risk of developing breast cancer when compared to the general population. The relative risk is 1.5 for women with an affected aunt or grandmother, 2 to 3 for women with an affected mother or sister, and 11.0 for women with proliferative fibrocystic disease (see above) and a positive family history (4a, 12a).

A detailed past medical history of *previous breast problems* should be obtained. It should include de-

Table 89.2.
Risk Factors for Carcinoma of the Breast

Factors	Relative Risk
Positive family history	1–5 (see the text)
Early menarche and late menopause (cyclic ovarian activity greater than 30 years)	Slight
Nulliparity	3
Previous breast cancer	5
Benign disease of the breast	2½–3 (see the text)
Radiation	Dependent on dose

tails of previous symptoms, masses, mammograms, biopsies, other operations, and any known pathological findings. A previous breast cancer will increase a woman's risk 5-fold of developing cancer in the contralateral breast. Likewise, certain proliferative ductal changes of fibrocystic disease found on previous biopsy place the patient in a higher risk category for breast cancer (see page 1285).

The *menstrual and reproductive history* is also important. Early menarche and late menopause (i.e., prolonged duration of cyclic ovarian activity—greater than 30 years) have been associated with a slightly increased risk of developing breast cancer. Surgical menopause (bilateral oophorectomy) before age 40 reduces the risk of breast cancer by 75%. The risk of breast cancer is increased 3-fold in nulliparous women, while a full term pregnancy before age 25 offers some protective benefit.

The patient should be asked about the presence of other *symptoms* (pain, discharge) related to a breast mass, the duration of those symptoms if present, and if the discovery of the mass or onset of the other symptoms was associated with changes in the menses, injury to the breast, pregnancy, or to changes in medication.

Nipple discharge is the second most frequent symptom of breast cancer. Nonlactational nipple discharge can be unilateral or bilateral, spontaneous or evoked only by pressure and massage, and persistent or recurrent. If the discharge is associated with a mass on physical examination, then the mass should be the primary concern.

Nipple discharge in women over 50 years old must be viewed with more suspicion than in younger women, regardless of its presentation.

Discharge evoked only by trauma, massage, or pressure has no clinical importance. Spontaneous, recurrent, or persistent discharge from one or two ducts not associated with a mass requires surgical exploration of the duct to differentiate benign papilloma (see page 1285) from intraductal papillary carcinoma. Both are possible without a presenting mass lesion. The character of the discharge cannot help in distinguishing benign from malignant conditions.

Physical Examination

The patient should be seated undressed to the waist on an examining table, in a warm, well lit room. Inspection and palpation of the nodal drainage areas (supraclavicular, infraclavicular, and axillary) should be performed. Inspection and palpation of nipples, areolae, and breasts are done next. While the patient is sitting, her arm on the side being examined can be raised by the physician to allow palpation high into the axilla. The examination should then be repeated with the patient in the supine position with her arm raised over her head so that the breast flattens on the chest wall.

If the clinician cannot appreciate a mass noted by the patient, it is critical to allow the patient sufficient time to find the lesion herself rather than to dismiss the complaint. If both the patient and the physician cannot locate the mass, the patient should be reassured that benign fibrous masses often disappear spontaneously.

Initial Management

The three most common masses producing lesions in the breast are fibroadenoma, fibrocystic disease, and carcinoma. Each of these common lesions has a peak incidence at different ages; yet there is a high degree of overlap. It is because of this overlap and the clinician's inability to distinguish with certainty the lesions clinically that a biopsy is usually the only definitive test to rule out carcinoma.

Ages 15 to 30

An easily movable, nontender, smooth, marble-like mass in a woman less than 30 years of age is most likely to be a fibroadenoma. The mass should be electively excised. In a teenager, excision can be delayed several months until a school vacation if the mass is not growing rapidly and if there are no other risk factors.

A mammogram should not be obtained in the evaluation of a discrete mass in this age group. In all likelihood, the mass will be excised regardless of mammographic findings. If carcinoma, rather than fibroadenoma, is found on histological examination, mammography to search for multicentric or contralateral nonpalpable lesions can be easily obtained. Even in the absence of a palpable mass, but with symptoms referred to the breast (pain, tenderness, nipple discharge), mammography is rarely indicated in patients less than 30 years of age. Perhaps a young obese patient with very large pendulous breasts that are difficult to examine, a persistent symptom (3 months' duration) but no mass, and a strong family history of breast cancer (mother or sister) deserves a mammogram. Generally, however, the tissue is much too dense in these years to make mammography worthwhile.

Ages 30 to 50

If a discrete mass is noted during the reproductive years and is clinically suspicious for fibrocystic disease, a watch-and-wait policy through one or two menstrual periods might be justified. Significant risk factors for developing breast cancer would make such a policy unreasonable (see Table 89.2). Mammography would be appropriate if the patient had previous benign breast biopsies unless a mammogram had been obtained within the previous year. If a previous biopsy had revealed high risk epithelial changes, the patient should be referred to a surgeon for possible repeat biopsy. If the previous biopsy was benign without epithelial changes or if a mammo-

gram at that time revealed no worrisome changes, it would be reasonable to follow the lesion through one or two menstrual cycles.

Any patient with a persistent (1 to 3 months' duration) discrete mass, compatible with fibrocystic disease, which has never been examined by biopsy, should be referred for surgical consultation. A mammogram need not be obtained before this consultation. If the patient presents with complaints related to the breast, not associated with a mass, and any one of the following conditions exists, a mammogram is appropriate before consultation: (a) risk factors for breast cancer; (b) large, pendulous, breasts that are difficult to examine; or (c) absence of a baseline mammogram in a patient over 35 years old. Mammography, however, should not be obtained within a year of a previous study, regardless of presentation, without surgical consultation.

Ages 50 and Over

A patient with a mass very suspicious for breast cancer should be referred to a surgeon as soon as possible. Mammography is not necessary since a suspicious discrete mass will be tested by biopsy after which mammography can be obtained to search for multicentric or contralateral disease. However, many surgeons do obtain prebiopsy mammography to screen for nonpalpable suspicious abnormalities which could be examined at the time of biopsy of the palpable mass.

All Ages

In summary, the preferred treatment of discrete breast masses in the absence of a recent (less than 2-year interval) previous benign breast biopsy is excision of the mass under *local* anesthesia. If the mass is too large (greater than 2 cm in diameter) to be easily excised *in toto*, incisional biopsy is appropriate. A Tru-cut needle biopsy is obtained of the mass that is highly suspicious for malignancy. This type of biopsy results in less tumor spill and does not interfere as much as does open biopsy with planning for the incision for the definitive mastectomy. A needle biopsy is *only* definitive if carcinoma is found. If malignancy is not found on the frozen section of the needle biopsy, formal excisional or incisional biopsy should be performed. Tumor tissue must be submitted at some time for estrogen and progesterone receptor analysis (patients with cancers that have such receptors have a more favorable prognosis and, if they develop recurrent disease, have a better response to hormonal manipulation) and if this is not done at the time of needle biopsy, some of the excised surgical specimen must be saved.

Simultaneous biopsy, frozen section, and mastectomy should be discouraged. Not only is frozen section analysis of breast tumors sometimes difficult, but many patients require time to deal with the realization that they have breast cancer. Problems with self-esteem, body image, and dependence are especially common at this time. By helping the patient take an active role in carefully weighing all the options of treatment, once a diagnosis of carcinoma is established on permanent section, her acceptance of recommended therapy is facilitated.

Needle Aspiration

The primary physician should not attempt needle aspiration of discrete breast masses. Even with extensive clinical experience, it is often difficult to distinguish solid and cystic breast masses. Ultrasound is being used increasingly (15) to help in this differential diagnosis. If the surgeon decides the mass is cystic, based on clinical or sonographic examination, he will attempt needle aspiration. This is accomplished in the surgeon's office by sterile technique, under local anesthesia. If fluid is obtained and the mass disappears, the patient will be requested to return in 2 to 3 weeks.

Before aspiration is attempted, the patient must understand that if the mass is solid, if it does not completely disappear following aspiration, if aspirated fluid is bloody, or if the mass recurs within 2 weeks, formal biopsy will be required.

Surgical Biopsy

It is important not only for the referring physician to inform the patient of the plan for surgical consultation, but also for the physician to state clearly the likelihood of the need for a minor surgical procedure. The patient will often ask questions about the biopsy before any firm decision has been made; yet she will be somewhat reassured to hear some initial information from her personal physician.

Preparation. Most biopsies can be carried out on an outpatient, ambulatory surgery schedule. Either local (preferred) or general anesthesia can be used. The patient should not eat or drink after 12 midnight on the night before operation.

Operation. Local anesthetic is infiltrated into the skin around the tumor, causing mild to moderate transient burning. Accompanying sedation can be given intravenously. A 1- to 3-inch (2.5 to 7.5 cm) incision is used to allow an adequate biopsy to be made and to be cosmetically satisfactory. The biopsy may remove the entire mass or only a segment of it. This should be explained to the patient, along with reassurance that there is no ultimate difference to her health. In addition to the possible residual mass, there is often a ridge of tissue secondary to sutures and scar remaining after the operation. Removal of a large mass might necessitate a small drain, which is withdrawn in the office 1 or 2 days following the biopsy.

Follow-up. Ecchymoses or hematoma (5% of patients) and wound infection (1 to 2% of patients) are the two main complications of breast biopsy. A large hematoma may require evacuation, but this usually can be done in the office. Exercise and strenuous activities should be avoided for 7 to 10 days following a breast biopsy to guard against late bleeding.

The long term sequelae of breast biopsy are minimal; the only one worth noting is a residual mass secondary to chronic scar formation, which may cause some difficulty with follow-up examinations and mammograms. Detailed descriptions of this biopsy site must be noted in the chart by all physicians on follow-up, and details of the previous biopsy should be conveyed to the radiologist responsible for reading future mammograms.

FOLLOW-UP MANAGEMENT OF A BREAST MASS

Fibroadenoma

After excision of a fibroadenoma, the patient should have routine yearly follow-up, but should be seen more often if there are high risk factors for developing breast cancer. The patient should be reassured there is no increased risk of malignancy because of the fibroadenoma.

Fibrocystic Disease

Pathologists should be requested to determine the presence or absence of proliferative epithelial changes in any fibrocystic tissue. If there are no epithelial changes of concern, then the patient should be reassured that no special follow-up is necessary. If there are proliferative changes (see above, page 1285), the physician, should stress the importance of breast self-examination *monthly*, a physician examination *twice* yearly, and periodic mammography according to specified guidelines.

As mentioned above (page 1285), the pain associated with fibrocystic disease is often ameliorated once a cancer has been excluded. If pain continues, the patient should be advised to wear a brassiere both day and night. Many patients will try this on their own. A number of pharmacological and dietary strategies have been said to be effective in the management of patients with fibrocystic disease, usually without adequate supporting evidence (10). However, Danazol, a weakly androgenic steroid, has been shown to decrease pain and nodularity in up to 70% of patients with fibrocystic disease when used in doses of 100 to 400 mg a day for 4 to 6 months (4). Side effects are relatively minor—weight gain, acne, and amenorrhea being the most common.

Cancer

If the biopsy is consistent with carcinoma, definitive staging and treatment should be instituted within 1 to 2 weeks. Once clinical staging (Table 89.1) is complete, bilateral mammography is necessary to identify multicentric or contralateral non-palpable lesions. In addition, certain other studies are useful (Figs. 89.2 and 89.3). It has been well documented that bone scans or liver scans in the absence of symptoms or of abnormal liver function tests are not useful in stage I or II breast cancer. Although a bone scan is routinely recommended in stage III patients, liver scan is not.

The treatment of operable breast cancer has changed as the result of several recent controlled clinical studies. The following statements can be made:

1. Radical mastectomy, the standard procedure for many years, is now performed very rarely, if at all, since modified radical mastectomy (pectoral muscle remains) affords comparable survival.

2. The National Surgical Adjuvant Breast Project (NSABP) (Fig. 89.4) has provided convincing evidence (4b) that limited surgery followed by breast irradiation (9) (see below) is as effective as modified radical mastectomy for many women with stage I or II disease (Table 89.1). Precisely what therapy should be recommended depends on a number of variables, including the size and resectability of the tumor (see below) as well as the personal preference of each patient. Also, which subset of patients will benefit the most from which therapeutic approach is still to be defined. Women with breast cancer should be made aware, however, that therapeutic options now often exist.

3. Knowledge of the extent of nodal involvement is the best prognosticator of tumor recurrence (Table 89.1) and aids the oncologist in planning possible adjuvant therapy. All premenopausal women with stage I or II disease should undergo axillary dissec-

tion as should postmenopausal women, if they are candidates for experimental protocols that are assessing the value of adjuvant therapy (see below, "Follow-up of Patients with Breast Cancer").

4. Surgery is not primary treatment for inflammatory carcinoma of the breast.

Modified Radical Mastectomy and Axillary Dissection

The operation requires general anesthesia, and hospitalization varies from 1 to 2 weeks. Most patients are ambulating and eating normally within 24 hours of the operation. Rarely, early postoperative bleeding will necessitate reoperation (less than 1%). Skin necrosis at the wound edge and prolonged serous drainage are more common complications but still occur in less than 5% of patients. Limited skin necrosis requires minimal wound debridement by the surgeon and wet to dry dressings at home by the patient. Secondary healing occurs in 3 to 6 weeks. Serous fluid may accumulate under the skin flaps even after drains are removed, and may require aspiration under sterile conditions. Aspirations may be done in the surgical office and the patient suffers no long term sequelae.

In the early postoperative period the patient may be inconvenienced with arm and shoulder discomfort, but is able to use the arm normally within 2 to 3 weeks.

Since recurrent breast cancer, when it develops, usually occurs within the first few years, close follow-up with physical examination is recommended every 3 to 6 months for the first several years. Chest X-ray and contralateral mammogram are obtained yearly. Bone scan should be added for stage III pa-

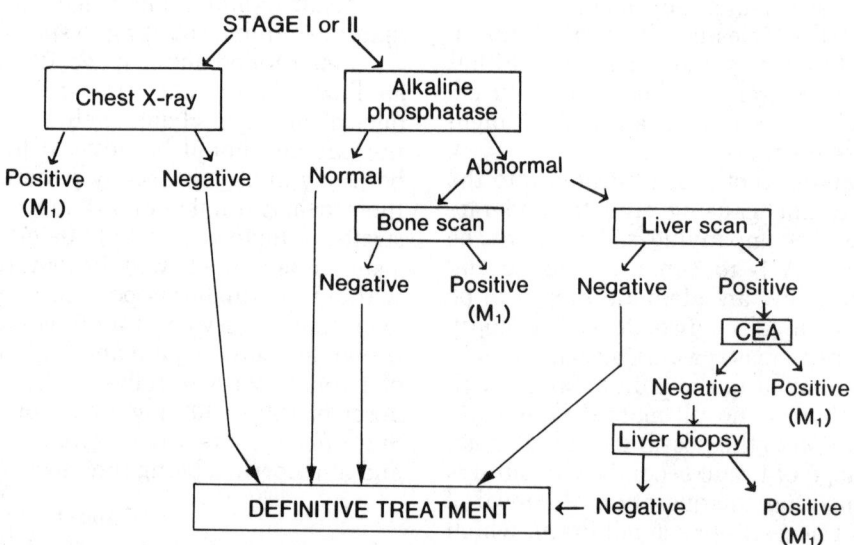

Figure 89.2. Clinical assessment of patients with stages I and II breast cancer. Negative = no evidence of metastases; positive = evidence of metastases; M₁ = distant metastases; CEA = carcinoembryonic anti-

gen. (Adapted from Baker RB: Preoperative assessment of the patient with breast cancer. *Surg Clin North Am* 58:689, 1978.)

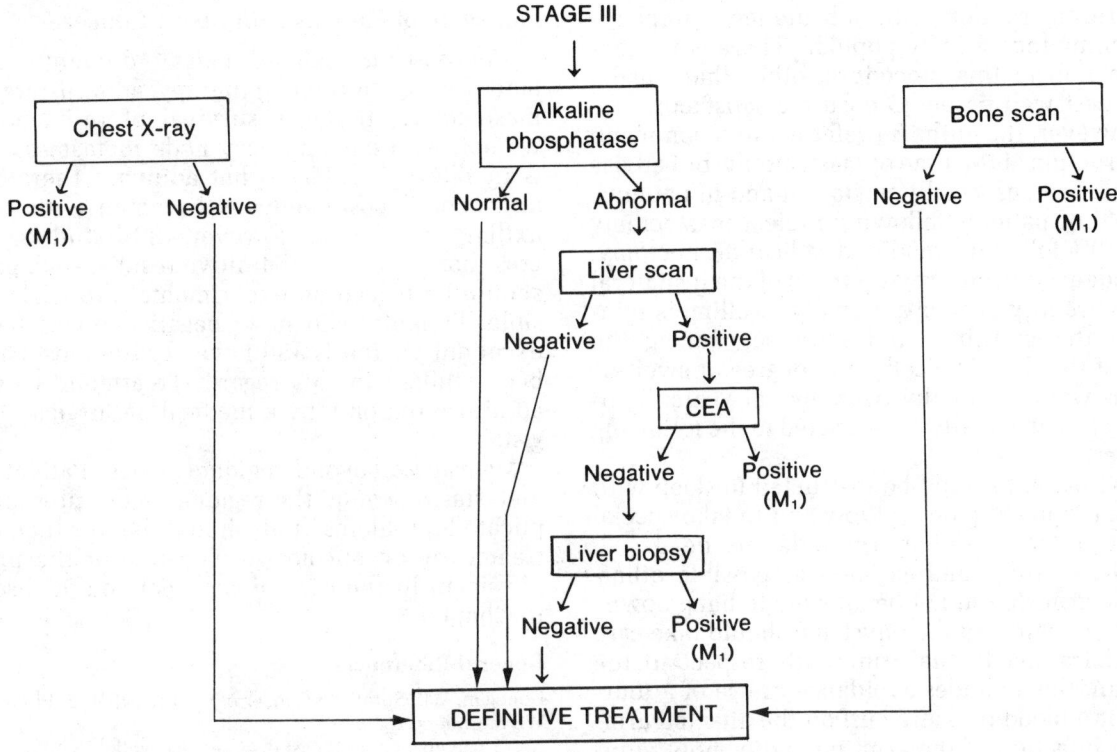

Figure 89.3. Clinical assessment of patients with stage III breast cancer. See Figure 89.2 for definitions. (Adapted from Baker RB: Preoperative assessment of the patient with breast cancer. *Surg Clin North Am* 58:689, 1978.)

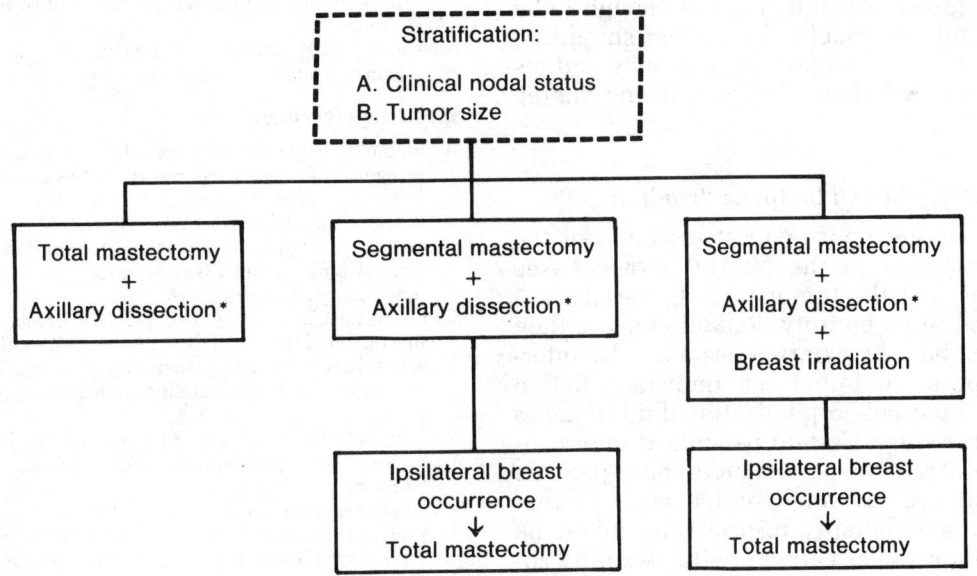

Figure 89.4. National Surgical Project for Breast Cancers schema. [*All patients with histologically positive nodes receive chemotherapy.] (Adapted from Fisher B, Redmond C, Fisher ER: Clinical trials and the surgical treatment of breast cancer. *Surg Clin North Am* 58:723, 1978.)

tients or if symptoms occur. Liver and brain scans are obtained only for appropriate symptoms or signs.

Within 3 to 6 weeks of operation, most patients can be fitted with a breast form if skin healing is complete. These forms can be obtained in retail stores. Most hospitals have a representative from the American Cancer Society's Reach for Recovery program who is of considerable assistance in this regard.

Breast reconstruction with subcutaneous implants is becoming increasingly popular. There is no contraindication to this procedure, other than inadequate chest wall tissue, to ensure a satisfactory result. However, the authors prefer not to recommend reconstruction at the time of mastectomy, but advise waiting a year, especially in stage II and III patients.

In 30% of patients following radical mastectomy and in 10% following modified radical mastectomy, lymphedema (pitting or nonpitting) of the ipsilateral upper extremity develops. Usually swelling is minimal in the mornings and increases during the course of the day. Typically, the degree of swelling becomes worse gradually over several years. Management (7) can usually be restricted to the following measures:

1. The patient should be instructed to sleep with her arm propped up on a pillow and to take special care not to sleep with her arm under her head.

2. When sitting, and as often as possible otherwise, the arm should not be allowed to hang down.

3. The patient and the physician should take care to avoid trauma to the arm. With respect to the physician, this includes avoidance of use of a tourniquet or a blood pressure cuff on the affected arm.

4. An infection of the arm, no matter how minimal, should be seen as soon as possible by the physician and treated aggressively (see Chapter 25). (Cellulitis is the major complication of lymphedema.)

5. If the degree of swelling is great enough to be unsightly or uncomfortable, the patient should be fitted with a Jobst sleeve (available in Jobst outlets in most cities), which should be worn during waking hours.

Limited Surgery followed by Breast Irradiation (3)

Segmental mastectomy or local resection of the tumor as described in the NSABP protocol (see above) means that the tumor mass (generally < 5 cm) is excised in its entirety. Radiotherapy is then usually given, both by external beam and by interstitial implant, to the tumor bed. Implant radiation requires 2 to 3 days of hospitalization if it is done as a separate procedure. Certain patients are not candidates for local resection and radiotherapy: patients whose breasts are too small or too large so that surgery and radiotherapy, respectively, might be technically impossible; patients with centrally located lesions; patients with lesions equal to or greater than 5 cm in diameter; and patients whose tumors are fixed to the chest wall or to the skin.

Limited surgery followed by breast irradiation is not complicated by postoperative lymphedema nor does the radiation impair wound healing. The radiated breast will atrophy gradually over a number of months.

Follow-up of Patients with Breast Cancer

Metastases to regional nodes. Adjuvant cytotoxic (and possibly hormonal) therapy, administered after mastectomy, prolongs survival of premenopausal women who have axillary node metastases. There is increasing evidence that adjuvant therapy may also benefit postmenopausal women with positive axillary nodes (16). However, until studies in progress have achieved definitive results, such patients should be placed on experimental protocols if possible. Patients who have negative nodes have an excellent prognosis and have, for the most part, not been studied in this regard. Treatment should be administered only by a medical or surgical oncologist.

Metastases beyond regional nodes. Patients with metastases beyond the regional nodes present complicated problems and should be evaluated and treated by an oncologist. The role of the primary physician in the care of such patients is discussed in Chapter 8.

General References

Donegan, WL, Spratt JS: *Cancer of the Breast*, ed 2. Philadelphia, WB Saunders, 1979.
    Covers benign breast disease very well.
Henderson JC, Canellos GP: Cancer of the breast: the past decade. *N Engl J Med* 302:17, 78, 1980.
    An excellent critical review.
Screening for Breast Cancer, *Lancet* 1:851, 1985.
    Well-referenced editorial summarizing all completed studies and studies in progress related to screening for breast cancer.
Townsend CM: Breast lumps. *Ciba Clin Symp* 32:3–32, 1980.
    Concise review of the subject.

Specific References

1. Bloom HJG: The influence of delay on the natural history and prognosis of breast cancer; a study of cases followed for five to twenty years. *Br J Cancer* 19:228, 1965.
2. Bloom HJG, Richardson WW, Harries EJ: Natural history of untreated breast cancer (1805–1933). Comparison of untreated and treated cases according to histologic grade of malignancy. *Br Med J* 2:213, 1962.
3. Bluming AZ: Treatment of primary breast cancer without mastectomy: review of the literature. *Am J Med* 72:820, 1982.
4. Brookshaw JD: Danazol treatment of benign breast disease: a survey of U.S.A. multicenter studies. *Postgrad Med J* 55:52, 1979.
4a. Dupont WD, Page DL: Risk factors for breast cancer in women with proliferative breast disease. *N Engl J Med* 312:146, 1985.
4b. Fisher B, Redmond C, Fisher ER, *et al*: Ten-year results of a randomized clinical trial comparing radical mastectomy and total mastectomy with or without radiation. *N Engl J Med* 312:674, 1985.
5. Fondo EY, Rosen PP, Fracchia AA, Urban JA: The problem of carcinoma developing in a fibroadenoma; recent experience at Memorial Hospital. *Cancer* 43:563, 1979.
6. Foster RS, Lang SP, Costanza MC, *et al*: Breast self-examination practices and breast-cancer stage. *N Engl J Med* 229:265, 1978.
7. Grabois M: Rehabilitation of the postmastectomy patient with lymphedema. *CA* 26:75, 1976.
8. Greenwald P, Nasca PC, Lawrence CE, *et al*: Estimated effect

of breast self-examination and routine physician examinations on breast cancer mortality. *N Engl J Med* 299:271, 1978

9. Harris JR, Levene MB, Hellman, S: Primary radiation therapy for breast cancer. *Annu Rev Med* 32:387, 1981.

10. London RS,, Sundaram GS, Goldstein PJ: Medical management of mammary dysplasia. *Obstet Gynecol* 59:519, 1982.

11. Mahoney LJ, Bird BL, Cooke GM: Annual clinical examination; the best available screening test for breast cancer. *N Engl J Med* 301:315, 1979.

12. Peacock EE, Jr: Management of benign disease of the breast. *Am Surg* 44:626, 1978.

12a. Sattin, RW, Rubin, GL, Webster LA, *et al*: Family history and the risk of breast cancer *JAMA* 253:1908, 1985.

13. Shapiro S: Evidence on screening for breast cancer from a randomized trial. *Cancer* 39:(6 Suppl) 2772, 1977.

14. Shapiro S, Venet W, Strax P, *et al*: Ten- to fourteen-year effect on screening on breast cancer mortality. *JNCI* 69:349, 1982.

15. Teixidor HS: The use of ultrasonography in the management of masses of the breast. *Surg Gynecol Obstet* 150:486, 1980.

16. Tormey DC *et al*: A randomized trial of five- and three-day chemotherapy and chemoimmunotherapy in women with operable node positive breast cancer. *J Clin Oncol* 1:138, 1983.

17. Treves N: A study of cystosarcoma phylloides. *Ann NY Acad Sci* 114:922, 1964.

18. Upton AC, Beebe GW, Brown JM, *et al*: Report of the N.C.I. Ad Hoc Working Group on the risks associated with mammography in mass screening for the detection of breast cancer. DHEW publ no. (NIH) 77-1400, March 1977.

19. Venet L: Self-examination and clinical examination of the breast. *Cancer* 46:930, 1980.

20. Wilson RE: The breast. In Sabiston DC (ed): *Davis-Christopher Textbook of Surgery*, ed 11. Philadephia, WB Saunders, 1977.

CHAPTER NINETY

Diseases of the Biliary Tract

ROBERT M. QUINLAN, M.D., ESTEBAN MEZEY, M.D., AND CALVIN B. ERNST, M.D.

Diseases of the biliary tract are encountered commonly in ambulatory practice. Many patients will be discovered to have asymptomatic gallstones during the course of evaluation of another condition; others will be found to have symptomatic chronic cholecystitis. Less commonly, patients will present with an acute illness due to acute cholecystitis or to common bile duct obstruction. This chapter describes the cause, diagnosis, and treatment of these various conditions.

CHOLELITHIASIS

Epidemiology

It is estimated from autopsy studies that there are 10 to 15 million people with gallstones in the United States, but only about 2 to 3 million (20%) are recognized to have cholelithiasis—either incidentally or because they are symptomatic—during their lives. About 300,000 individuals, 2 to 3% of the total population with gallstones, undergo a cholecystectomy each year.

Ninety percent of gallstones found in patients in

this country are cholesterol gallstones; 10% are pigment (bilirubinate) stones. The prevalence of gallstones is greater in women than in men and increases with age. In the United States 10% of men and 20% of women between the ages of 55 and 65 are affected (3). The prevalence of cholesterol gallstones is particularly high in the Southwest Indians of the United States; for example, 70% of Pima women over age 25 have cholelithiasis (13).

Gallstone Formation

Bile is produced in the liver and excreted into the duodenum. Bile contains bile acids (primarily cholic, deoxycholic, and chenodeoxycholic acid), phospholipids (primarily lecithin), and cholesterol. The solubility of cholesterol depends on its incorporation with bile and phospholipids into a micelle. In the intestinal tract, bile salts are necessary for the absorption of dietary fats; they solubilize fatty acids and monoglycerides into micellar solutions. The fatty acids are absorbed in the jejunum, while the bile salts are absorbed in the ileum and enter an enterohepatic circulation.

There are three major types of gallstones that form in human bile: cholesterol stones (> 70% cholesterol), mixed stones (50 to 70% cholesterol), and pigment stones (12% cholesterol). These stones probably develop in three stages: first, the formation of a supersaturated bile; second, the crystallization or initiation of stone formation; and third, the growth of the stone to a certain detectable size before crystals in the bile are expelled into the intestine. It is likely, but not clearly established, that one of these stages is more important in the formation of certain types of stones than in others. The formation of pigment or bilirubinate stones may depend more on crystallization and growth and cholesterol stones more on supersaturation.

Cholesterol Stones

An alteration of the critical relationship between bile salts, phospholipids, and cholesterol can produce bile which is supersaturated with cholesterol and therefore predisposed to the development of cholesterol stones (12). At a low rate of bile flow, the ratio of cholesterol to bile salts and phospholipids increases, favoring supersaturation. Bile flow can decrease because of (a) excess loss of bile salts from the body (after ileal resection or bypass); (b) inability to synthesize normal amounts of bile acids in the liver (i.e., the rare disease of cerebrotendinous xanthomatosis—characterized by xanthomatous deposits in the tendons, lung, and brain); or (c) from a faulty regulatory system which does not increase bile acid production in the liver appropriately when there is a decrease in the enterohepatic circulation of bile salts. If the enterohepatic feedback system is faulty, a diseased gallbladder which does not empty

appropriately may trap bile salts and prevent them from participating in the enterohepatic circulation.

Once supersaturated bile is present in the gallbladder, desquamated mucosal cells, bacteria, parasites, foreign bodies, or other random crystals may provide a nidus for crystallization of gallstones. Growth of these stones may then occur, especially in a dyskinetic gallbladder, one in which contraction is impaired—such as in diabetes, celiac disease, or pregnancy. However, if there is normal enterohepatic regulation of bile flow, even with a sluggish gallbladder, bile salt excretion will increase with an eventual increase in the total bile acid pool and, consequently, less lithogenic bile.

Pigment Stones

Formation of pigment stones is probably initiated by supersaturation of unconjugated bilirubin in the gallbladder and common bile duct. Unconjugated bilirubin, like cholesterol, is relatively insoluble in water. An increased concentration of unconjugated bilirubin in bile results either from formation of unconjugated bilirubin from conjugated bilirubin in the biliary tree through the action of a glucuronidase (perhaps of bacterial origin, in patients with infected bile, see below) or from increased production of unconjugated bilirubin by the liver (e.g., in patients with hemolytic anemia). Unlike the formation of cholesterol stones, a diseased gallbladder is probably not a factor in the formation of pigment stones.

Risk Factors

Since most patients with cholelithiasis are asymptomatic, it is difficult to evaluate risk factors precisely. Known risk factors for the development of cholesterol and pigment stones are listed in Table 90.1 (1).

Cholesterol Stones

The demography of cholesterol stones probably reflects, in part, a genetic predisposition and, in part, nongenetic ethnic characteristics. For example, it is known that obese people, and nonobese people who eat a high calorie diet, secrete relatively more cholesterol into their bile than does the average person. Therefore, populations in whom obesity is common (e.g., the Indians of the American Southwest) or who consume high calorie diets (occidental societies in general) are more susceptible to cholelithiasis.

The reasons for the increasing incidence of gallstones in middle-aged and elderly people are unknown but may be related to the time that elapses, first, between formation of supersaturated bile and formation of stones, and second, between formation of stones and recognition of them.

The influence of estrogens on the secretion of cholesterol in bile is reflected in the increased prevalence of gallstones in women (between puberty and

Table 90.1.
Risk Factors for Gallstones[a]

CHOLESTEROL STONES
  Demography: Northern Europe, North and South America more than the Orient; American Indians; probably familial predisposition
  Obesity
  High caloric diet
  Drugs used in the treatment of hyperlipidemia: clofibrate, cholestyramine, and colestipol
  Gastrointestinal disorders involving major malabsorption of bile acids; ileal disease, resection or bypass; cystic fibrosis, with pancreatic insufficiency
  Female sex hormones: women more at risk than men, use of oral contraceptives and other estrogenic medications
  Age, especially among men
  Probable but not well established: pregnancy, diabetes mellitus, and polyunsaturated fats
PIGMENT STONES
  Demography: oriental more than occidental; rural more than urban
  Chronic hemolysis
  Alcoholic cirrhosis
  Biliary infection
  Age

[a] After Bennion LJ, Grundy SM Risk factors for the development of cholelithiasis in man. *N Engl J Med* 299:1161, 1978.

menopause) compared to men (see above) and in women who take estrogenic preparations compared to women who do not (see Chapter 93).

Finally, there are a number of ways by which the concentration of bile acids in bile is reduced, favoring the formation of gallstones: drugs utilized to treat hyperlipidemia, such as clofibrate, cholestyramine, and colestipol (see Chapter 75), decrease bile acid secretion; and certain disorders of the gastrointestinal tract (ileal resection, Crohn's disease of the ileum) reduce bile acid resorption.

Pigment Stones

The demography of pigment stones is entirely different from that of cholesterol stones. The propensity of orientals to develop pigment stones is not entirely understood, but it may be attributable to the higher prevalence of bacterial infection of the bile (usually *Escherichia coli* infections), and of *Ascaris* infestation, in the Orient compared to the Occident. In the United States, patients with pigment gallstones do not usually have infected or infested bile. The recognized risk factors in this country—hemolysis and alcoholic cirrhosis—are unexplained. Like cholesterol stones, pigment stones are more common with advancing age; and for the same reasons that may pertain to cholesterol stones (see above). Unlike cholesterol stones, endogenous and exogenous estrogens or obesity have no influence on the development of pigment stones.

Natural History

Many attempts have been made to study the natural history of gallstones among the 2 to 3 million people in this country known to harbor them. Thirty percent of these people are asymptomatic, having had gallstones discovered incidentally on abdominal film (10 to 15% are radiopaque) or during celiotomy or treatment of another condition. The other 70% are symptomatic: *i.e.*, gallstones are discovered during evaluation of the typical or atypical abdominal pain of cholecystitis (see below).

Approximately 18% of individuals with "silent" gallstones will develop symptoms in 15 to 20 years, and 3% will develop complications of biliary tract disease: acute cholecystitis, pancreatitis, or jaundice (4). The risk of developing complications is unrelated to the severity of symptoms but does increase with the length of time symptoms have been present. Most complications occur only among symptomatic patients. However, 20% of the time acute cholecystitis is the first indication of cholelithiasis. If complications occur, they usually occur within 5 years of the discovery of gallstones. Causes of death related to cholelithiasis among patients not having cholecystectomy are acute cholecystitis, cholangitis with liver abscess, necrotizing pancreatitis, gallbladder carcinoma, and gallstone ileus with mechanical small bowel obstruction. In Lund's study of the natural history of cholelithiasis, 2.7% of the deaths among patients not operated upon were attributed to gallbladder disease (7).

The Asymptomatic Patient

It cannot be predicted, on the basis of the size, number of stones, sex, or age of the patient, which asymptomatic patients are likely to become symptomatic (16). Whether or not asymptomatic patients should undergo elective cholecystectomy, therefore, depends largely on the bias of the general physician and of the consulting surgeon. About 18% of patients become symptomatic (see above), sometimes at a point in their lives when operation is more dangerous because of age, intercurrent illness, or the presence of acute cholecystitis. The risk of complications of cholelithiasis, other than acute cholecystitis, is negligible in the asymptomatic patient. Carcinoma of the gallbladder is more common among people with gallstones but the risk—0.3 to 1% over a lifetime—is approximately the same as is the operative mortality from cholecystectomy. If the gallbladder is calcified, risk of cancer is markedly increased, however, and cholecystectomy should be performed.

Over the past several years bile acids have been available—first chenodeoxycholic acid and then ursodeoxycholic acid—which reduce the hepatic synthesis and the concentration of cholesterol in bile and ultimately dissolve gallstones (5).

Chenodeoxycholic acid (Chenix) is marketed as a 250-mg tablet; the recommended dose is 15 mg/kg in two divided doses (morning and night). It is recommended that treatment be begun in a dosage of 250 mg twice a day for 2 weeks increasing by 250 mg a day thereafter until the desired dosage is achieved. Ursodeoxycholic acid is not yet released for noninvestigative use; but since chenodeoxycholic acid, but not ursodeoxycholic acid, causes diarrhea in approximately 10% of patients and hepatotoxicity in 3% of patients, if ursodeoxycholic acid becomes available, it probably will be the drug of choice. The cost of therapy with either drug is about $750/year.

In a large multicenter study, chenodeoxycholic acid therapy for 2 years resulted in complete or partial dissolution of stones in 11 and 30% of patients, respectively. Dissolution occurred more frequently in women, thin patients, and in patients with small or with floating gallstones (11). At the end of 2 years, treatment should be discontinued, even if stones have not totally dissolved, since the safety of a longer course of treatment is not established. Oral cholecystography or sonography should be done every 6 to 9 months to monitor the progress of therapy. It is recommended also that liver function tests be done monthly for the first 3 months of treatment and every 3 months thereafter and that if aminotransferase activity is greater than 3 times the upper limit of normal, the treatment be stopped permanently. Intermediate increases in aminotransferase activity dictate also that the treatment be stopped but if liver function returns to normal, another trial of therapy is probably safe. In those patients whose stones *have* completely dissolved, there is a 25% recurrence rate within 2 years and a 50% recurrence rate within 5 years.

Ultimately the administration of bile acids may become the treatment of choice for asymptomatic or mildly symptomatic patients who, because of their age or physical condition, are poor operative risks. Patients with cholecystitis (see below) do not respond to treatment with bile acids because the diseased gallbladder does not concentrate the bile acids sufficiently.

CHOLECYSTITIS

The hallmark of cholecystitis is abdominal pain, often epigastric at onset, but localizing within a few hours to the right upper quadrant. The pain is characteristically, but not always, severe and unremitting with only slight variations in intensity. Use of the term "biliary colic," therefore, is not precise because colic is defined as pain that waxes and wanes. Some patients describe the pain as heavy and aching; some, as knife-like. Occasionally it radiates into the right side of the back or, less often, into other parts of the abdomen. The pain usually begins abruptly, within 1 to 3 hours of eating a meal. Patients may also complain of being awakened in the middle of the night. Pain is often accompanied by slight nausea. A typical attack subsides spontaneously within 2 to 3 hours. The frequency of such attacks is extremely variable, from every few days to once or twice a year.

A patient who presents this history is very likely to have gallstones. However, the degree of inflammation of the gallbladder often cannot be determined from the history: there may be gallstones without any inflammation at all; there may be acute inflammation; or there may be chronic inflammation with fibrosis. The severity of the symptoms and the presence or absence of signs of inflammation and/or of biliary obstruction determine the physician's response (see below).

Acute Cholecystitis

Pathophysiology

Acute cholecystitis is caused over 90% of the time by a gallstone which obstructs the cystic duct. Acalculous cholecystitis occurs primarily in patients who have sustained major trauma, including major operations, or in patients with emphysematous cholecystitis due to infection with gas-forming bacteria. Inflammation of the gallbladder in early acute cholecystitis is probably due to irritation by concentrated static bile. In some cases, as the process progresses, infection may play a role; bile cultures are positive in only 20 to 30% of patients during the first few days of an attack but, by 7 to 10 days, almost 80% of biliary cultures are positive. In certain patients, e.g., diabetics, mural ischemia might also play a role.

The difference between the presentation of acute and chronic cholecystitis (see below) is probably due to the length of time the cystic duct has been totally obstructed and to the intensity of the inflammation.

Signs and Symptoms

The pain of classical acute cholecystitis is severe and persistent. It is usually accompanied by nausea and fever (99 to 102°F; 37 to 39°C) and less often, by vomiting. Unless treated, the symptoms are likely to persist for up to a week.

The severity and persistence of the pain will usually cause the patient to call or see his physician (see Chapter 35 for a general discussion of abdominal pain). On examination, the patient is restless. There is considerable right upper quadrant abdominal tenderness, associated with involuntary guarding of the abdominal wall. This guarding, indicative of early peritoneal inflammation, is particularly important to recognize. It is not a feature of less acute disease (see below). *Murphy's sign*, the sudden involuntary arrest of inspiration (because of pain), when the examiner palpates the right upper quadrant during inspiration, is caused by the abutment of the inflamed gallbladder against the examiner's fingers as it moves downward with expansion of the chest cavity. This sign is more often elicited after several days of inflammation. In one-third of the patients, the gallbladder is palpable during an attack of acute cholecystitis, if the physician probes the right upper quadrant very gently. Occasionally patients are mildly jaundiced (see below).

Laboratory Tests

Leukocytosis (12,000 to 15,000 white blood cells/mm^3) due to a neutrophilic granulocytosis is common. Serum amylase activity may be increased, in the absence of other evidence of acute pancreatitis. Often, serum aminotransferases (aspartate aminotransferase and alanine aminotransferase) are increased as well. Twenty percent of patients have mild hyperbilirubinemia (< 4 mg/100 ml).

A TcHIDA or PIPIDA radioisotopic study is the test of choice in the diagnosis of acute cholecystitis (TcHIDA and PIPIDA are ^{99m}Tc-labeled derivatives of iminodiacetic acid, a compound concentrated in bile). The study requires injection of isotope intravenously and evaluation of uptake of the isotope by the gallbladder. If the cystic duct is obstructed, because of acute inflammation, or because of a common duct stone, uptake does not occur. The test is performed in the nuclear medicine department of a hospital and takes 1 to 4 hours to complete. A positive study shows isotope in the biliary tree and in the duodenum but not in the gallbladder. A negative study shows isotope in the gallbladder as well. If isotope is not excreted, the test is uninterpretable; but, if it *is* excreted, the sensitivity of the test is extremely high (essentially 100%). Specificity also is high (95%), but false positive results may occur in patients with chronic cholecystitis or with acute biliary obstruction due to pancreatitis.

Differential Diagnosis

The differential diagnosis must include those disorders which might cause severe right upper quadrant abdominal pain and, usually, leukocytosis and slightly abnormal hepatic function: acute pancreatitis, appendicitis, hepatitis, hepatic abscess, a perforated or penetrated peptic ulcer, acute pyelonephritis, myocardial infarction, and right lower lobe pneumonia or pleuritis. Because of the severity of the illness, these distinctions should be made in the hospital.

Treatment

The patient suspected of having acute cholecystitis should be hospitalized for observation, hydration, and further diagnostic procedures (see below, page 1298 and Chapter 35 for a discussion of these procedures as they pertain to ambulatory patients). If the pain is intolerable, the physician can administer meperidine parenterally. Since this drug may increase biliary pressure by causing spasm of the sphincter of Oddi, it is reasonable to administer 0.6 mg of atropine along with the narcotic to prevent that effect. The patient should be told that he will be fed intravenously, rather than by mouth, and that a nasogastric tube will be passed. Antibiotics may be administered, depending on the severity of the inflammatory response. If the temperature, white blood count, and pulse rate increase further and if abdominal tenderness and guarding increase as well, emergency operation will be required to prevent acute gangrenous cholecystitis and perforation. This progression of signs and symptoms occurs in 30 to 40% of patients. On the other hand, if the patient improves and the diagnosis is confirmed, elective cholecystectomy may be performed within a few days. A randomized prospective study which compared early and delayed cholecystectomy for acute cholecystitis concluded that the duration of hospitalization and the duration of disability were significantly reduced by early operation (6). Because of an increased likelihood of rapid progression of the disease to gangrene and perforation in elderly or diabetic patients (9, 10), cholecystectomy should be performed in these patients as soon as they can be prepared for it (assuming that they are considered able to tolerate an operation). Similarly, the presence of emphysematous cholecystitis due to gas-forming bacterial infection dictates emergency operation (air bubbles in the right upper quadrant on a plain film of the abdomen indicate the diagnosis).

A discussion of surgery of the biliary tract and of the results and complications of operations is provided below (pages 1300 and 1301).

Chronic Cholecystitis

Pathophysiology

Symptomatic chronic cholecystitis is associated with gallstones over 95% of the time; the remaining cases are due to other diseases of the gallbladder, such as cholesterolosis (the appearance of macrophages laden with cholesterol crystals in the wall of the gallbladder—often without stones). Recurring attacks of relatively mild acute cholecystitis cause eventual fibrosis so that the gallbladder empties poorly. The symptoms of chronic disease, like those of acute cholecystitis, are due to obstruction by a gallstone of the cystic duct. In chronic recurrent cholecystitis obstruction of the cystic duct is relatively short (probably no more than a few hours) compared to the length of time of obstruction in acute cholecystitis, and therefore, inflammation is less intense. Chronicity of symptoms may also be related to gallbladder dyskinesia secondary to mural fibrosis.

Signs and Symptoms

Many patients who complain of biliary pain for the first time probably already have chronic gallbladder inflammation. The character and location of the pain are identical to those of acute cholecystitis. Pain is variably associated with nausea and, occasionally, vomiting. Unlike classical acute cholecystitis, fever is unusual with chronic disease. Typically, pain follows eating, beginning 1 to 6 hours after a meal (see above)—and lasts for 2 to 3 hours. Nonspecific symptoms—vague postprandial pain, bloating, belching, flatulence, so-called fatty food intolerance—thought by many to suggest gallbladder disease, are extremely common in the general population and therefore are not helpful diagnostically.

The patient with chronic cholecystitis usually seeks the physician less urgently than does the patient with acute cholecystitis. On examination during the attack, although there is tenderness to deep palpation in the right upper quadrant of the abdomen, there is no muscle guarding as there is in patients with acute inflammation. *Murphy's sign* (see above) is absent, the gallbladder is rarely palpable, and jaundice usually is not present. Between attacks, there is no abdominal tenderness.

Laboratory Tests

The white blood count, serum amylase, serum aminotransferases, and serum bilirubin are usually normal.

Unlike patients with acute cholecystitis, patients with symptoms due to chronic cholecystitis can be evaluated further in an ambulatory setting.

Oral cholecystogram. The oral cholecystogram (OCG) is the mainstay in the diagnosis of gallbladder disease. The patient is given 3 g of iopanoic acid (Telepaque) in the evening after dinner and is instructed not to eat overnight; films of the abdomen are taken the following morning. If the gallbladder fails to visualize, the patient is given another 3 g of Telepaque and X-rays are repeated the following day. The patient should be warned that he may experience mild diarrhea for up to a day after the ingestion of the Telepaque.

Approximately 75% of gallbladders are visible on the first dose and another 15% will become visible on the second dose. Although, as stated above, 10 to 15% of gallstones are radiopaque and can be seen on plain film, confirmation of their location in the gallbladder should be obtained by OCG. The OCG is reliable only if the Telepaque is ingested at the proper time, retained in the gastrointestinal tract, absorbed from the small bowel, transported to the liver, esterified to glucuronide, and excreted by the liver into the bile. Therefore, gastrointestinal or hepatic disease may cause a false positive study. However, the specificity of the test is high (4% false positive) if either radiolucent stones are present in an opacified gallbladder or if the gallbladder fails to concentrate contrast material after the second Telepaque dose. The sensitivity of the test is lower (10% false negative) and therefore OCG should be followed by sonography if the gallbladder is visualized and no stones are seen.

Ultrasound. The detection rate for gallstones 3 mm or greater in diameter is between 89 to 96% by ultrasound with 93 to 97% specificity (3 to 7% false positive) (2). In a fasting patient, failure to identify the gallbladder by ultrasonography also suggests gallbladder disease. The advantages of ultrasound are that it exposes the patient to no radiation; it is much quicker (5 to 10 minutes); and it has no side effects. It also is not influenced by associated gastrointestinal or hepatic disease. Because of familiarity with the technique, however, and its lower cost, most surgeons still prefer OCG as the initial diagnostic test except in patients who are pregnant or who have concomitant gastrointestinal or hepatic disease. It is reasonable to perform ultrasonography in patients whose gallbladders fail to opacify by OCG and in patients with typical symptoms of gallbladder disease who have a normal OCG.

CT scan. Computerized tomography accurately identifies gallstones 80% of the time. Currently, it has no advantages over OCG and ultrasonography in the diagnosis of gallbladder disease. CT scans might be useful occasionally, however, if both the oral choelcystogram and ultrasound are equivocal.

Upper gastrointestinal series (UGI). Many patients are evaluated with a UGI series in addition to an oral cholecystogram, especially if symptoms are atypical of biliary tract disease. Max and Polk (8) reported 250 patients who underwent cholecystectomy, 145 of whom had a UGI and 105 of whom did not. Of the 145 patients selectively chosen for UGI only 39 had positive findings. In only seven of these patients was an associated gastroduodenal operation done at the time of cholecystectomy. Of these seven only three patients had any new information added by UGI. Based on these data, Max and Polk suggested guidelines for selectively choosing patients who might benefit from a UGI (Table 90.2).

Duodenal drainage. Patients with symptoms suggestive of biliary tract disease who have a normal OCG, a normal abdominal sonogram, and a normal abdominal CT scan may have biliary sludge or stones too small to be detected. In such patients, duodenal drainage, ordinarily done by a consulting gastroenterologist, may prove useful by identifying cholesterol crystals or bilirubin granules in the bile indicative of supersaturation. The test is performed by having the patient swallow a plastic tube with a double lumen weighted at the end by a mercury-filled bag. There are holes in the tube above the bag. When the bag has passed into the second portion of the duodenum (documented by fluoroscopy), mag-

Table 90.2.
Suggested Indications for Upper Gastrointestinal Series in Patients with Documented Biliary Tract Disease [a]

Older patients (>50 years)
Men
Previous gastroduodenal operations
Previously documented upper gastrointestinal disease
History of pancreatitis
History or presence of jaundice
Long atypical history

[a] After Max MH, Polk HC: Routine preoperative upper gastrointestinal series (UGIS) in patients with biliary tract disease; a plea for more selectivity. *Surgery* 82:334, 1977.

nesium sulfate is injected into one lumen of the tube to stimulate contraction of the gallbladder. Duodenal contents are then aspirated and the sediment is separated by centrifugation, and examined under a microscope. In the absence of hepatic disease (which may produce abnormal bile even though the gallbladder is normal), a positive duodenal drainage is highly suggestive of gallbladder disease.

TcHIDA or PIPIDA scan. Radioisotopic imaging of the gallbladder (see page 1297) is useful in the diagnosis of symptomatic chronic cholecystitis if the patient is experiencing pain at the time of the study (*i.e.*, if there is acute inflammation of the gallbladder or obstruction of the cystic duct).

Treatment

The treatment of choice of symptomatic chronic cholecystitis is elective cholecystectomy (see below). Patients who cannot tolerate an operation are candidates for therapy with bile acids to dissolve the gallstones (see above, "The Asymptomatic Patient"). Risks of not treating, surgically or medically, patients with chronic cholecystitis include gangrene and perforation of the gallbladder, choledocholithiasis (see below), pancreatitis, and, rarely, gallstone ileus (the obstruction of the small bowel by a large gallstone passed through an acute fistula which has formed between the gallbladder and the duodenum).

CHOLEDOCHOLITHIASIS

Epidemiology

Common duct stones occur in approximately 15% of patients with chronic cholecystitis, either before or after cholecystectomy. The incidence increases with age and length of time symptoms of gallbladder disease have been present. There are three categories of common duct stones: (*a*) concomitant gallbladder stones and common duct stones; (*b*) retained stones found in the common duct soon after cholecystectomy and/or common duct exploration; and (*c*) common duct stones identified long after chole-

cystectomy and/or common duct exploration. The incidence of common duct stones decreases exponentially in the first year after cholecystectomy only to rise again, reaching a peak at 3 years. In one study 26% of symptomatic common duct stones occurred 10 or more years after cholecystectomy (14). Also, patients with congenital agenesis of the gallbladder have a 20% incidence of common duct stones. These observations support the concept that common duct stones originate either in the gallbladder or in the intrahepatic or common bile duct.

Signs and Symptoms

Approximately 6% of patients with common duct stones are asymptomatic. More typically patients develop severe colicky right upper quadrant pain, often associated with jaundice, mild fever, and nausea and vomiting. The pain usually begins abruptly and lasts up to an hour. If nothing is done, attacks recur at variable periods of time. Eventually cholangitis will develop, manifest by persistent malaise and anorexia and intermittent fever, chills, and jaundice—associated with persistently high serum alkaline phosphatase activity. Suppurative ascending cholangitis characterized by right upper quadrant pain, high fever, shaking chills, and jaundice (Charcot's triad) is life threatening and constitutes a surgical emergency.

On physical examination, if the patient is asymptomatic, no abnormal signs are elicited. If the patient is symptomatic, right upper quadrant abdominal tenderness and muscle guarding are usually present—similar to the findings in patients with acute cholecystitis. The patient is usually mildly to moderately jaundiced.

Laboratory Tests

Because of the acute onset of symptoms and the severity of pain in patients with choledocholithiasis, laboratory studies in the ambulatory setting are usually not appropriate. If such studies are done, leukocytosis and increases in serum alkaline phosphatase activity, serum bilirubin, serum aminotransferase activity, and serum amylase activity are likely to be observed.

Treatment

If common duct stones are discovered during cholecystectomy, they are removed. If the patient presents to the physician with severe right upper quadrant pain, tenderness, guarding, and/or jaundice, he should be hospitalized for further diagnostic studies and for treatment. If sonography or CT scan shows a dilated biliary tree, cholangiography should be performed. The patient should be aware that percutaneous transhepatic cholangiography is the likely procedure unless the serum bilirubin concentration is under 3 mg/100 ml, in which case intravenous cholangiography is possible. The patient experience during transhepatic cholangiography is essentially the same as it is during liver biopsy (see Chapter 42), except that the former procedure is done in the radiology department. Common duct stones must be removed, either by operation (see below), or, if possible, by endoscopic retrograde cholangiopancreatography (ERCP). (ERCP is performed only in the hospital, usually in the radiology department since fluoroscopy and X-rays of the cannulated duct are required. The patient experience during the procedure is essentially the same as it is during other kinds of upper endoscopy (see Chapter 35), except that ERCP usually lasts for 30 to 60 minutes and may be complicated 5 to 10% of the time by postendoscopic infection, especially if the common duct is manipulated, and by pancreatitis.)

BILIARY TRACT OPERATIONS

The general physician should be aware of the mechanics of biliary surgical procedures so that he can inform and reassure the patient who is to be referred to a surgeon.

Cholecystectomy

Elective cholecystectomy has a mortality rate of 0.5% or less. Urgent or emergency operation for acute cholecystitis associated with common duct stones in an elderly patient with cardiac and/or pulmonary disease has a mortality rate of 10%. The morbidity of cholecystectomy primarily relates to superficial wound infection (< 5 to 7%). Wound infection is more common if the operation lasts longer than 2 hours, if the patient is obese or diabetic, and if the patient has acute, rather than chronic cholecystitis. Other possible but rare (< 1%) immediate complications of cholecystectomy are postoperative bleeding, postoperative bile leak, injury to biliary ducts (common hepatic or common bile duct), and overlooked common duct stones. A drain may be left in place for 24 to 48 hours after operation.

Cholecystostomy

This operation may be required in the patient who is critically ill from acute cholecystitis and who has associated severe cardiac, pulmonary, or renal disease which contraindicates the use of general anesthesia. Another less often cited indication for cholecystostomy is inability to detect normal biliary anatomy because of a severe inflammatory process near the main bile ducts. Rather than risk possible injury to structures in the porta hepatis, a cholecystostomy may be performed.

A cholecystostomy can be done through a small incision in the right upper quadrant under local anesthesia. A large drainage tube is inserted into the gallbladder through a stab wound in the fundus. The tube is brought through the abdominal wall and allowed to drain freely. An attempt should be made to empty the gallbladder of stones before placing the tube. If a stone is impacted at the cystic duct, future cholecystectomy will be necessary or a mucous fistula will persist after the tube is removed. If, however, *all* stones are removed, only 30 to 50% of patients will develop recurrent symptoms of cholelithiasis within 2 years after the tube is removed. The operative mortality is very high from cholecystostomy, not because of the operation, but because of the patient's critical condition.

Choledochotomy

Common duct exploration or choledochotomy, whether combined with a gallbladder operation or as an isolated operation, has a higher morbidity and mortality rate than does simple cholecystectomy. The operation takes longer than cholecystectomy and patients are generally older, two factors very important in determining morbidity and mortality. Generally the patient will be hospitalized 3 to 5 days longer for common duct exploration than for cholecystectomy alone (see below).

COURSE AFTER OPERATION
Normal Course

The patient is usually discharged 5 to 10 days following an uncomplicated biliary tract operation. Skin sutures will have been removed and the patient will be allowed to bathe. Usually patients are requested to avoid driving and sexual relations for 2 to 3 weeks from the day of discharge. Patients are also advised to avoid heavy (approximately 15 pounds (7 kg) or more) lifting for 6 weeks. The incidence of incisional hernia (see Chapter 91) is very low following a right subcostal oblique incision, slightly higher with a vertical midline incision, and highest with vertical paramedian incisions. The patient returns to the surgeon's office for evaluation at 3 to 6 weeks after operation. The drain site and wound should be healed unless there has been wound infection. The patient should have been able to resume an unrestricted regular diet within a few days of operation without difficulty. Stools should be at preoperative frequency and of normal color.

The patient should be expected to complain about pulling sensations in the area of the incision since the right rectus muscle has been divided and resutured. If the subcostal incision has made close to the costal margin, the patient will often complain also about discomfort on bending or sitting. The area just below a right subcostal incision is apt to be numb for several months because of interruption of a cutaneous sensory nerve to this area. Sensitivity does

Table 90.3.
Frequency of Postcholecystectomy Syndrome (PCS) and Distribution of its Etiology[a]

	Bodvall and Oevergaard (1967)	Stefanini et al (1974)	Hess (1977)	Brandstatter et al (1976)
Number of patients with cholecystectomy	1930	800	919	—
PCS total	764(40%)	249(31%)	241(26%)	—
Mild PCS	660(35%)	317(27%)	—	—
Severe PCS	104(5%)	32(4%)	—	—
Etiology:				
Organic total	—	—	58%	66%
Organic biliary	9%	14%	4.5%	43%
Organic extrabiliary	—	—	53.5%	23%
Nonorganic total	—	—	42%	34%

[a] After Tondelli P, Gyr K, Stalder GA, Allgöwer M: The biliary tract. Part I. Cholecystectomy. *Clin Gastroenterol* 8:487, 1979.

return, however, in the majority of cases. It is not surprising to find patients gaining weight after cholecystectomy, especially if they had lost weight preoperatively.

Postcholecystectomy Syndrome

About 90% of patients operated upon for symptomatic biliary tract disease become asymptomatic or have relatively trivial symptoms (occasional dyspepsia, for example). The other 10% may continue to be symptomatic either because they were treated for the wrong disease or because they have developed a postoperative complication. In the former category are patients who had gallstones but whose symptoms actually emanated from another disease (e.g., recurrent pancreatitis, peptic ulcer disease, angina, reflux esophagitis, or hiatus hernia).

Postoperative problems associated with the operation itself include retained common duct stones, an excessively long cystic duct remnant, and common duct injury with eventual bile duct stricture and recurrent pancreatitis.

Tondelli et al (15) have collated data from a number of series on the incidence and cause of the postcholecystectomy syndrome (PCS) (Table 90.3). Mild PCS refers to symptoms of dyspepsia, constipation, diarrhea, and intolerance to certain foods. Severe PCS refers to severe upper abdominal pain, cholangitis, or biliary fistula. Organic biliary etiologies include retained common duct stones, papillary stenosis, bile duct stricture, cystic duct remnant, chronic pancreatitis, or bile duct tumor. Organic extrabiliary etiologies include esophagitis, ulcer disease, pancreatitis, liver disease, heart disease, colon or urinary tract disease, and adhesions. Nonorganic disease includes irritable bowel syndrome and psychiatric or metabolic disease.

Specific References

1. Bennion LJ, Grundy SM: Risk factors for the development of cholelithiasis in man. *N Engl J Med* 299:1161, 1978.
2. Ferruci T: Body ultrasonography. *N Engl J Med* 300:538, 590, 1979.
3. Friedman GD, Kannel WB, Dawber TR: The epidemiology of gallbladder disease; observations in the Framingham study. *J Chronic Dis* 19:273, 1966.
4. Gracie WA, Ransohoff DF: The natural history of silent gallstones. The innocent gallstone is not a myth. *N Engl J Med* 307:798, 1982.
5. Hofman AF: The medical treatment of cholesterol gallstones. A major advance in preventive gastroenterology. *Am J Med* 69:4, 1980.
6. Järvinen HJ, Hastbacka J: Early cholecystectomy for acute cholecystitis; a prospective randomized study. *Ann Surg* 191:501, 1980.
7. Lund J: Surgical indications in cholelithiasis; prophylactic cholecystectomy elucidated on the basis of long-term followup on 526 nonoperated cases. *Ann Surg* 151:153, 1960.
8. Max MH, Polk HC: Routine preoperative upper gastrointestinal series (UGIS) in patients with biliary tract disease; a plea for more selectivity. *Surgery* 82:334, 1977.
9. Morrow DJ, Thompson J, Wilson SE: Acute cholecystitis in the elderly, a surgical emergency. *Arch Surg* 113:1149, 1978.
10. Mundth ED: Cholecystitis and diabetes mellitus. *N Engl J Med* 267:642, 1962.
11. Schoenfield LS, Lachin JL: The Steering Committee, The National Gallstone Study Group: Chenodiol (chenodeoxycholic acid) for dissolution of gallstones: the National Cooperative Gallstone Study: a controlled trial of efficacy and safety. *Ann Intern Med* 95:257, 1981.
12. Small DM, Rapo S: Source of abnormal bile in patients with cholesterol gallstones. *N Engl J Med* 283:53, 1970.
13. Thistle JL, Schoenfield LJ: Lithogenic bile among young Indian women; lithogenic potential decreased with chenodeoxycholic acid. *N Engl J Med* 284:177, 1971.
14. Thurston OG, McDougall RM: The effect of hepatic bile on retained common duct stones. *Surg Gynecol Obstet* 143:625, 1976.
15. Tondelli P, Gyr K, Stalder GA, Allgöwer M: The biliary tract. Part I. Cholecystectomy. *Clin Gastroenterol* 8:487, 1979.
16. Way LW, Sleisenger MH: Cholelithiasis and chronic cholecystitis. In Sleisenger MH, Fordtran JS (eds): *Gastrointestinal Disease. Pathophysiology, Diagnosis, Management*, ed 2. Philadelphia, WB Saunders, 1978.

CHAPTER NINETY-ONE

Abdominal Hernias

W. ROBERT ROUT, M.D., AND CALVIN B. ERNST, M.D.

DEFINITIONS

A hernia is a protrusion of any part of the body from the compartment that ordinarily contains it. Most commonly, the term is applied to a protrusion frm the abdominal cavity. The site at which the protrusion occurs defines the hernia further: epigastric, umbilical, incisional, inguinal, femoral, *etc.* If the protrusion can be pushed back into the abdominal cavity, the hernia is said to be *reducible:* if it cannot, it is said to be *irreducible* or *incarcerated.* If the blood supply to the herniated part is occluded, the hernia is said to be *strangulated* (all strangulated hernias are incarcerated).

This chapter describes the more common types of hernias and discusses the role of the general physician in their diagnosis and treatment.

HERNIAS OF THE GROIN

Inguinal Hernias

Inguinal hernias (Fig. 91.1, *A* and *B*) are classified either as direct or indirect; the great majority (over two-thirds) are indirect. Direct hernias are portions of the bowel and/or omentum which protrude directly through Hesselbach's triangle (the triangle formed by the inguinal ligament inferiorly, the lateral border of the rectus muscle medially, and the inferior epigastric vessels laterally) to emerge at the external inguinal ring (Fig. 91.2). Indirect hernias enter the inguinal canal through its internal ring, lateral to the inferior epigastric vessels (the lateral boundary of Hesselbach's triangle), traverse the canal, and emerge also at the external inguinal ring (Fig. 91.2).

Epidemiology and Etiology

Inguinal hernia is a common problem in ambulatory practice: it accounts for approximately 75% of all abdominal hernias. Approximately 85% of inguinal hernias are in men. At some time in their lives, about 5 to 10% of men in the United States will develop an inguinal hernia. Even in women, inguinal hernia accounts for more than half of the abdominal hernias. Although femoral hernias (see below) are much more common in women than in men, the most common groin hernia in women is an indirect inguinal hernia. Less than 10% of inguinal hernias in adults are bilateral when the patient is first seen. The chance of later developing a contralateral hernia is the same whichever side is affected first.

All *indirect inguinal hernias* are due to a congenital defect in which the processus vaginalis remains patent. Under such circumstances, a tract lined with peritoneum extends from the abdominal cavity into the scrotum. With time this may enlarge, and abdominal contents may herniate into it. Occasionally, however, only intra-abdominal fluid may gravitate into the scrotum, causing scrotal swelling while the patient is erect but draining back into the abdominal cavity when the patient is supine. Such a lesion is termed a *communicating hydrocele* and is more commonly seen in children than adults. The severity of the combination of a congenital abnormality and a predisposing acquired condition which increases intra-abdominal pressure (such as obesity, chronic obstructive airway disease, ascites, chronic constipation with straining at stool, prostatism with straining at urination, and hard physical labor) determine when an inguinal hernia develops.

Direct inguinal hernias are acquired lesions and are not only influenced by changes in intra-abdominal pressure but also by progressive attenuation of the inguinal structures as part of the normal aging process. Occasionally, inherited defects in collagen synthesis (e.g., Marfan's syndrome) provide an obvious explanation for accelerated weakening of these structures.

Direct hernias are for the most part problems of the middle-aged and elderly. Indirect hernias, since they are associated with a congenital defect, are more likely to develop in younger people, but these too increase in incidence with advancing age and are about 4 to 5 times more common after the age of 50 than before.

History

Most patients complain of a dull ache in the groin and of a bulge, either localized to the groin or ex-

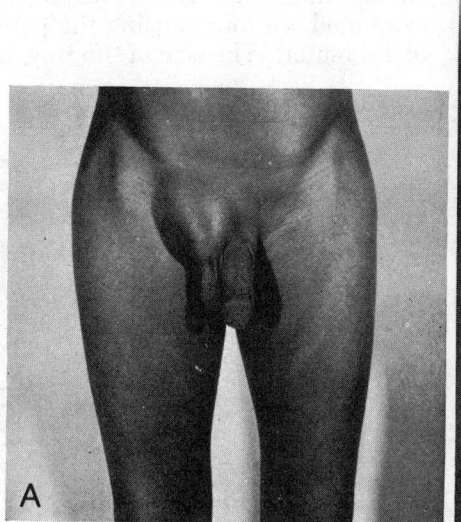

Figure 91.1. *A.* Right inguinal hernia in young adult male. *B.* Left scrotal hernia. (From Zimmerman LM, Anson BJ: *Anatomy and Surgery of Hernia*, ed 2. Baltimore, Williams & Wilkins, 1967, p 152.)

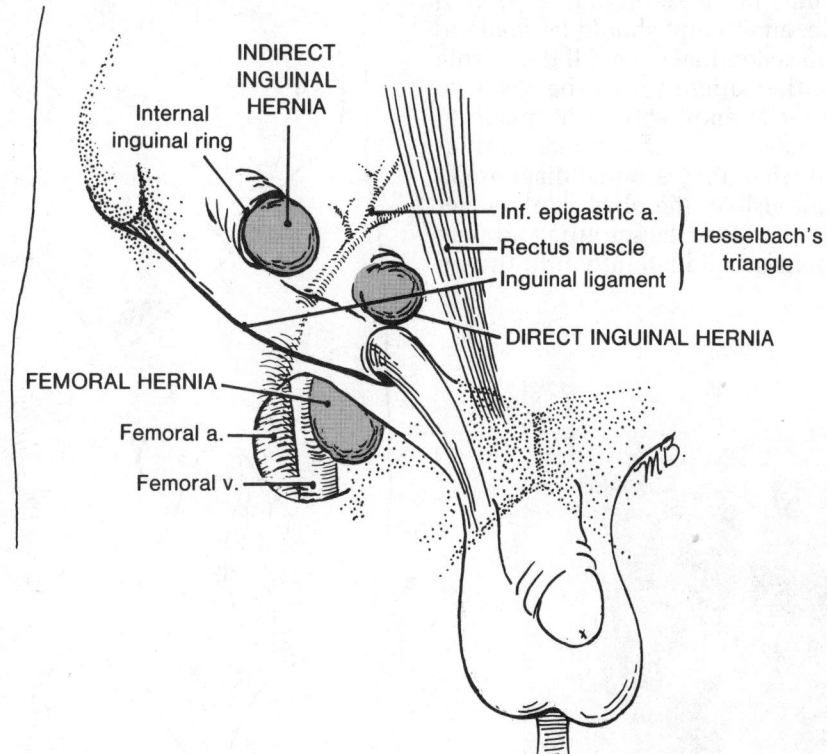

Figure 91.2. Artist's rendition of groin region illustrating femoral hernia and indirect and direct inguinal hernias. (Modified from Dunphy JE, Botsford TW: *Physical Examination of the Surgical Patient*, ed 3. Philadelphia, WB Saunders, 1964, p 118.)

tending into the scrotum (in women, the labia are the anatomical counterpart of the scrotum). Sometimes pain precedes discovery of the mass by some months (perhaps because a piece of omentum has become pinched in the canal before the bowel has followed it). Occasionally a patient will recall a short burning pain during straining, which represents the initial herniation. Often the patient, or the physician, notices the herniated mass, but no pain has been experienced. If the hernia becomes large enough, it may cause a dragging sensation when the patient walks. Small reducible indirect hernias may be noticed intermittently, at times of increased intra-abdominal pressure.

If a hernia incarcerates, it may become more painful, although many patients with chronically incarcerated hernias are pain free. Indirect hernias have an approximately 10% chance of incarcerating; direct hernias incarcerate less often. Strangulated hernias are always symptomatic: the hernia becomes extremely painful and tender; and nausea, vomiting, and fever (with granulocytosis) are common.

Physical Examination

The patient should first be examined while he is standing. An indirect hernia sometimes can be distinguished from a direct hernia by inspection: an indirect hernia, once it has entered the inguinal canal, presents as an elliptical swelling descending toward or even into the scrotum (Fig. 91.3). A direct hernia presents as an isolated oval swelling near the pubis; it rarely is found in the scrotum (Fig. 91.4). If the hernia is visible, an attempt should be made to push it back into the abdominal cavity. If the hernia cannot be reduced, the patient should be asked to lie down and another attempt should be made to reduce it. Approximately 10% of inguinal hernias will be incarcerated when they are first diagnosed.

If the hernia is not visible, the physician's finger should be placed at the base of the scrotum and then gently advanced cephalad and laterally into the inguinal canal (Fig. 91.5). The external ring can be examined without causing the patient a great deal of discomfort. The size of the ring, in itself, does not

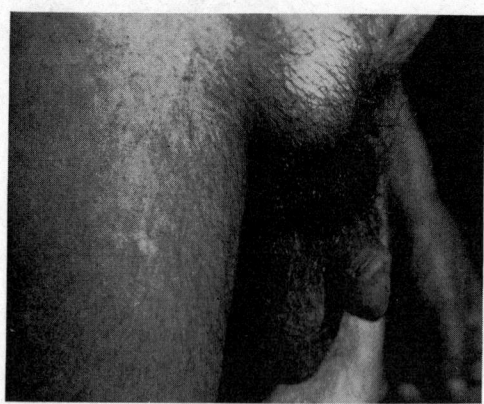

Figure 91.4. Direct inguinal hernia. Note medially situated globular swelling. (From Zimmerman LM, Anson BJ: *Anatomy and Surgery of Hernia*, ed 2. Baltimore, Williams & Wilkins, 1967, p 154.)

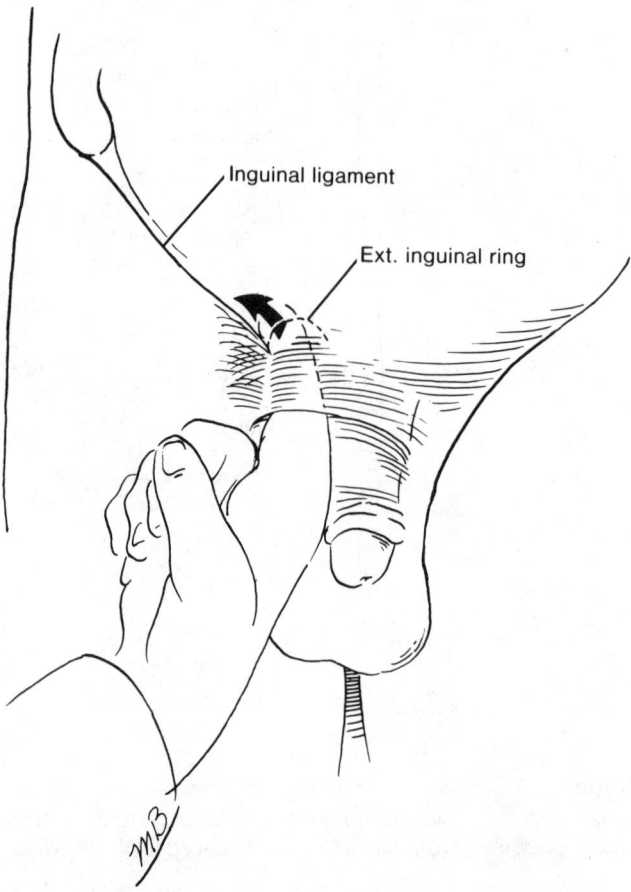

Inguinal ligament

Ext. inguinal ring

Figure 91.5. Examination of the inguinal canal. The examining finger gently invaginates the scrotum into the inguinal canal. (Modified from Dunphy JE, Botsford TW: *Physical Examination of the Surgical Patient*, ed 3. Philadelphia, WB Saunders, 1964, p 116.)

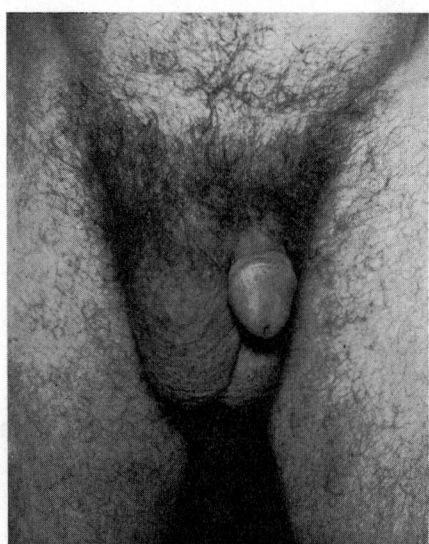

Figure 91.3. Indirect inguinal hernia. Swelling is oblique, cylindrical, and extends into scrotum. Zimmerman LM, Anson BJ: *Anatomy and Surgery of Hernia*, ed 2. Baltimore, Williams & Wilkins, 1967, p 155.)

predict the presence of a hernia or the propensity to develop one because the external ring is an opening in the external abdominal oblique aponeurosis which does not contribute to the integrity of the inguinal floor. Further palpation will identify the crest of the pubic bone, the fibers of the external inguinal ring, the spermatic cord, and weakness in the posterior inguinal canal. When the examining finger has been directed through the external ring, having the patient increase intra-abdominal pressure by coughing or straining will cause a hernia to protrude and to be felt as an impulse or bulge at the tip of the examining finger.

Occasionally, contents of the hernia sac may be determined by physical examination: omentum may feel nodular and pliant; intestine, smooth and tense. Occasionally intestinal gas can be palpated as it moves through the bowel; also, a gas-filled loop of bowel may be tympanitic and on auscultation, bowel sounds may be heard within it.

Differential Diagnosis

An incarcerated scrotal hernia must be distinguished from other scrotal lesions (Fig. 91.6). One of the most common of these is a *hydrocele*, a tense, slightly fluctuant mass that can be distinguished from a hernia and from solid masses by transillumination (the mass is made tense between examining fingers and, with the room darkened, a flashlight is pressed into the side of it; light passes through the hydrocele, but not through other masses).

Another common scrotal mass is a *varicocele*, an enlarged venous plexus that on palpation feels soft and worm-like and that extends from the testicle up toward the spermatic cord. It does not transilluminate and, when the patient lies down, it collapses. If a varicocele is of recent onset in the adult, occurs on the left, and does not disappear in the supine position, one must suspect obstruction of the left spermatic vein (which enters the left renal vein) by retroperitoneal neoplasm or renal tumor.

A *spermatocele* is a localized but vaguely circumscribed mass that also does not transilluminate and that persists when the patient lies down.

Apart from distinguishing a hernia from another kind of scrotal mass, an important component of the physical examination is the examination of the testicle and its surrounding structures. In that way epididymal cysts, epididymitis, orchitis, testicular torsion, and testicular tumors can be detected. *Epididymal cysts* may be in any portion of the epididymis and may be smooth or lobulated; some of them transilluminate; they are innocuous and require no treatment. *Epididymitis* presents as a tender, swollen epididymis. The inflammation, if untreated, may spread to the testicle (orchitis); see Chapter 27 for a discussion of this problem. Frequently, elevation and immobilization of the scrotum will relieve the pain associated with an inflammatory process. In contrast, the pain produced by *torsion of the testicle*

is unremitting. Sudden onset of testicular pain in an otherwise healthy person is characteristic of this problem. On examination, the testicle is enlarged and exquisitely tender. The patient should be referred immediately to a general surgeon or to a urologist. *Testicular tumors* can involve the entire testicle or simply protrude as a small nodule from the testicular surface. These masses are more indurated than the common benign scrotal masses and usually lack the slight tenderness of the normal testicle. Patients with suspected tumors should be referred as soon as possible to a urologist.

Management and Course

Almost all inguinal hernias should be repaired. Severe coexistent illness is the only real contraindication to herniorrhaphy (see Chapter 86 for a discussion of anesthesia/surgery risks in patients with coexistent medical conditions). Nonoperative therapy should be discouraged; the wearing of a truss is potentially dangerous and does not guarantee that a hernia will remain reduced. Also, the pressure of the truss on the margin of a large defect will eventually lead to atrophy of the fascial and aponeurotic (broad tendinous) layers, causing the hernia to enlarge. Subsequent repair will be more difficult and, therefore, will carry a greater risk of recurrence.

Elective herniorrhaphy precludes acute incarceration (and strangulation) and the necessity to perform an emergency operation. If the hernia is chronically incarcerated and there are no symptoms of strangulation (strangulation is primarily a risk in acutely incarcerated, relatively small hernias), repair may still be scheduled electively. If the hernia has incarcerated acutely, the patient must be hospitalized and attempts made to reduce the hernia before operation. If the hernia is strangulated, an operation must be performed immediately.

If there are bilateral hernias, depending on their size, the type of repair required, the age of the patient, and coexistent problems, they may be repaired as staged procedures or at one operation. If the patient is elderly, and the hernias are large and require complex repair, herniorrhaphies should be staged, 4 to 6 weeks apart. Bilateral repairs of indirect inguinal hernias in children or young adults are routinely done at one operation.

One concern of the patient with a hernia is the type of anesthesia that will be administered. Currently, general, spinal, or local anesthesia is used, depending on the preference of the surgeon. Local anesthesia is becoming more popular; the patient is rarely uncomfortable during the procedure and usually can leave the hospital within 48 hours (see below). Also, postoperative complications (atelectasis, for example) are less likely.

No matter which anesthesia is employed, certain *complications of herniorrhaphy* are possible (in about 7% of patients): urinary retention, wound

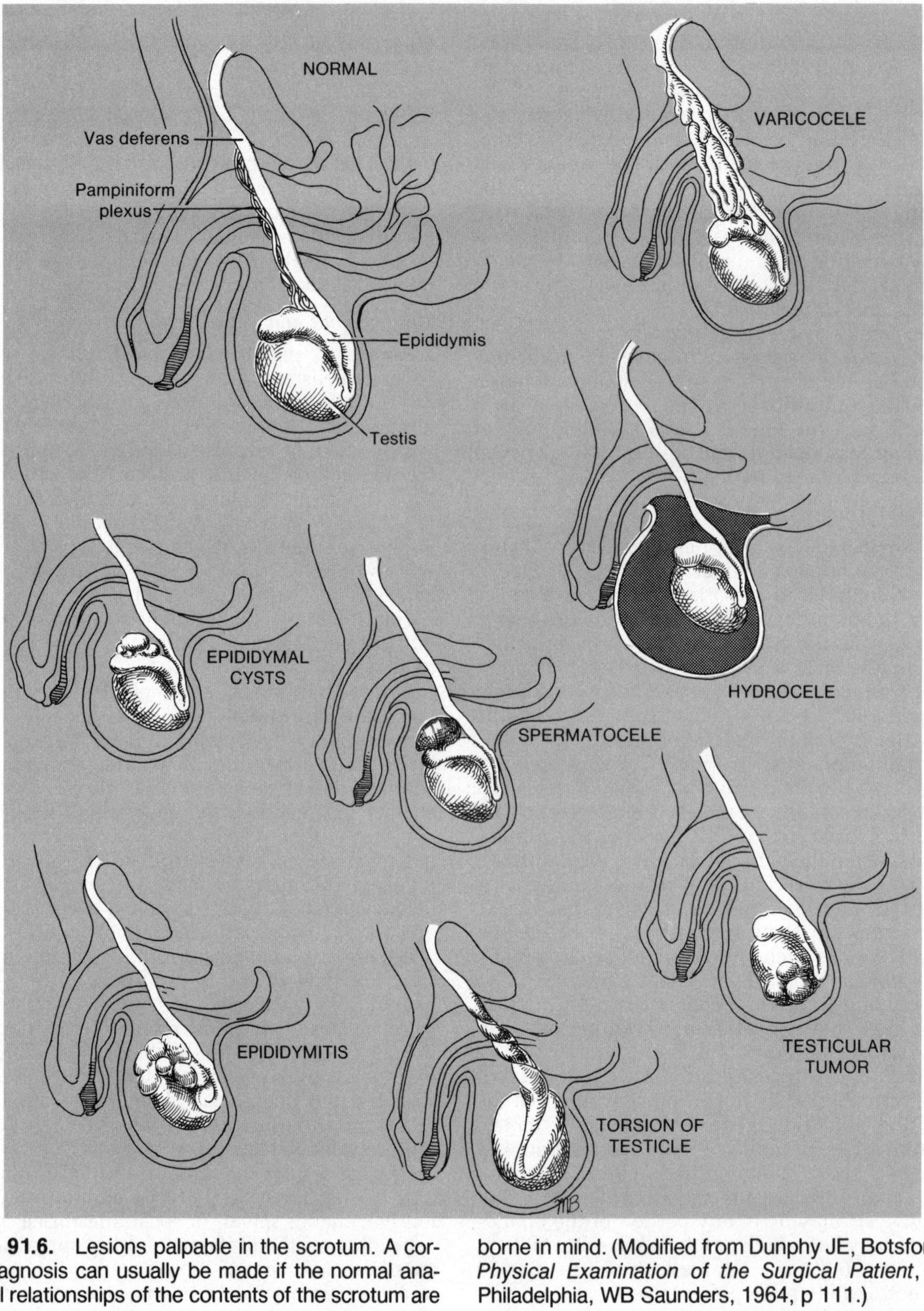

Figure 91.6. Lesions palpable in the scrotum. A correct diagnosis can usually be made if the normal anatomical relationships of the contents of the scrotum are borne in mind. (Modified from Dunphy JE, Botsford TW: *Physical Examination of the Surgical Patient*, ed 3. Philadelphia, WB Saunders, 1964, p 111.)

infection, hydrocele formation, femoral neuritis, and, rarely, unilateral testicular atrophy. The general physician and the surgeon should discuss these complications with the patient before the operation and assure him that, if they do occur, they are usually treatable or transient problems.

When the patient is discharged from the hospital, he is ambulatory and usually requires no more than codeine for relief of pain. The time of discharge is determined by the patient's response to pain and by his ability to ambulate. For the first 2 to 4 weeks, he is told to avoid lifting or straining and to use a stool softener and a mild laxative (see Chapter 38). The patient can return to light work (and light activity such as long walks) within another 2 weeks, but an occupation that requires heavy lifting or considerable exertion requires a total convalescence of about 6 weeks. Driving a car during this time should be discouraged, not because it is a form of strenuous activity, but because the patient, fearing pain or injury, may not react to crisis situations such as stepping on the brake vigorously enough or soon enough to avoid a collision. Sexual activity should be avoided for about 4 weeks. Resumption of normal recreational and work activities requires common sense. Most patients are fully rehabilitated and working 2 months following herniorrhaphy. Since recurrence may be related to premature untoward exertion, patients must be cautioned to avoid strenuous activity for 2 to 3 months. However, most episodes of recurrence result from wound infection or from operations performed with poor technique.

Approximately 1 to 7% of indirect and 4 to 10% of direct inguinal hernias recur. Over 50% of the recurrences will occur within 5 years of the initial repair. Unfortunately, the recurrence rate after repair of a recurrent hernia is very high, ranging from 5 to 35%. Apart from advising patients with a recurrent hernia that has been repaired to avoid straining and heavy lifting and to lose weight if they are obese, there is no special advice that these patients can be given.

Femoral Hernias

Epidemiology and Etiology

A femoral hernia is a protrusion of omentum and/or bowel through the femoral canal (Fig. 91.2). It is the second most common type of abdominal hernia, accounting for 10% of all abdominal hernias. It is much more common in women than in men; 33% of abdominal hernias in women, but only 3% of abdominal hernias in men, are femoral hernias. The incidence increases with increasing age, presumably again because of the degradation of collagen and tissue attenuation that accompanies aging (see above, "Inguinal Hernia"). It is likely, however, that a contributing cause of a femoral hernia is a congenitally large femoral ring. Preperitoneal fat, forced through the large ring, enlarges it further. Increased pressure produced by straining or by pregnancy undoubtedly contributes to femoral herniation.

History

The primary symptom of a femoral hernia is a bulge in the groin. A dull pain may be experienced, but less commonly than in patients with an inguinal hernia. About 20% of femoral hernias incarcerate (twice the rate of indirect inguinal hernias). The symptoms of incarceration and of strangulation are the same as they are in patients with inguinal hernias.

Physical Examination

A mass is often palpable, medial to the femoral vessels and inferior to the inguinal ligament. The mass is usually reducible, and occasionally it is tender. Despite careful examination, the hernia frequently is difficult to detect, especially in obese women, even if it is incarcerated or strangulated. Therefore, women who present with signs and symptoms of unexplained intestinal obstruction should be examined carefully for evidence of a femoral hernia which has strangulated.

Differential Diagnosis

A femoral hernia must be distinguished from an enlarged lymph node, a lipoma, a saphenous varix, and a direct inguinal hernia. The first three of these possibilities are not reducible. A lymph node or lipoma may not transmit an impulse to the examiner's finger when the patient coughs. A saphenous varix may simulate a hernia impulse, however, since increased venous pressure induced by the Valsalva maneuver is transmitted to the varix. A lymph node or a lipoma is more movable than a hernia; and a varix can be collapsed by compression of the saphenous vein. The distinction between a femoral and other groin hernias sometimes can be made only at operation.

Management and Course

Femoral hernias should be repaired unless the patient is unable to tolerate an operation. The operative and postoperative considerations of inguinal hernia (see above) apply to femoral hernias as well. From 1 to 7% of femoral hernias recur; and, like inguinal hernias, 5 to 35% of repaired recurrent hernias also recur.

INCISIONAL HERNIAS

An incisional hernia is the protrusion of omentum and/or bowel through a surgical incision. Unlike the other types of abdominal hernia, a congenital weakness of the abdominal wall does not contribute to the development of the hernia. Any abdominal incision may be the site of a hernia. The major risk factors leading to the development of an incisional hernia are poor surgical technique, wound infection, and obesity. With the increasing use of chronic ambulatory peritoneal dialysis to treat patients in chronic renal failure (see Chapter 47), it has become apparent that incisional hernias (as well as inguinal hernias) are particularly common in this group of patients.

The hernia usually presents as a bulge through

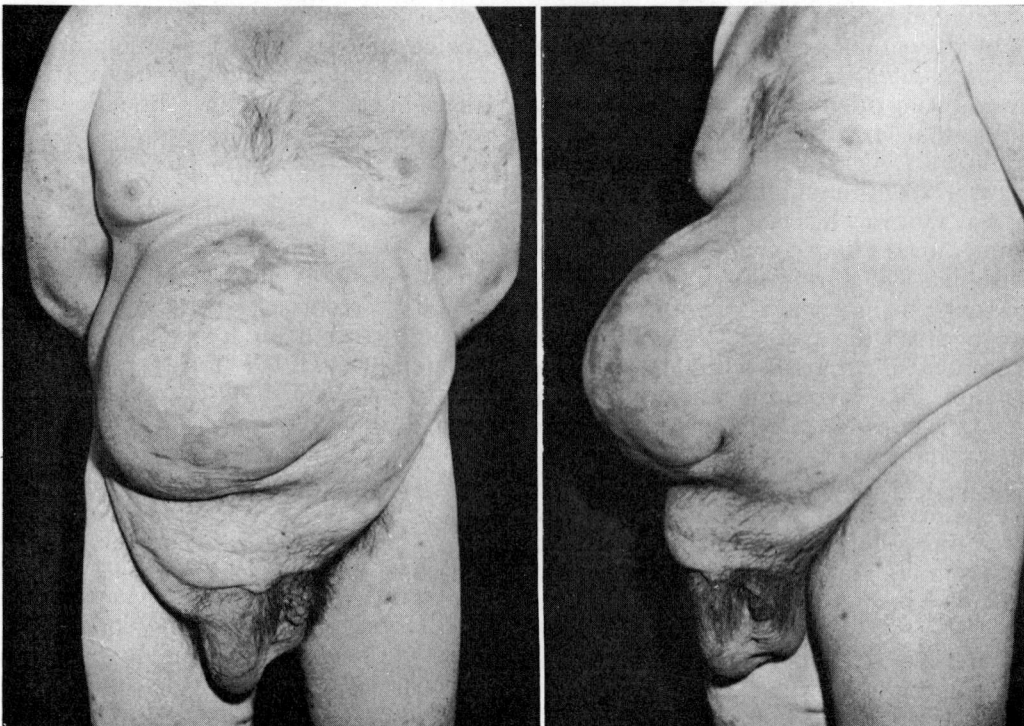

Figure 91.7.   Large postoperative hernia after chole-cystectomy. (From Zimmerman LM, Anson BJ: *Anat-omy and Surgery of Hernia*, ed 2. Baltimore, Williams & Wilkins, 1967, p 287.)

the incision that may enlarge if neglected (Fig. 91.7) and may even lead to intestinal obstruction. It should be repaired soon after the diagnosis is made to avoid the development of a larger defect, which will complicate repair and will be more likely to recur. If possible, an obese patient should lose weight before the operation (see Chapter 76).

UMBILICAL HERNIAS

An umbilical hernia is a protrusion of omentum and/or bowel through the umbilical ring. These hernias are probably due to congenital defects. Among adults, they appear most often in middle-aged multiparous women, in patients with cirrhosis of the liver and ascites, and in old, malnourished, chronically ill people.

Most umbilical hernias are obvious as an enlargement of the umbilical ring with protrusion of in-traabdominal contents through it. However, a few patients present with only the complaint of vague intermittent pain and tenderness in the region of the umbilicus. On examination, a small defect is usually found that contains a small piece of omentum, pre-peritoneal fat, or a knuckle of bowel. If the patient is placed in the supine position and is asked to raise his head and cough, the hernia can be palpated.

The most common complication of umbilical hernia is incarceration with or without strangulation. For that reason, unless the patient simply cannot tolerate an operation, all umbilical hernias should be repaired. Morbidity and mortality from such an operation are much lower if it can be done electively rather than in response to acute incarceration or strangulation.

EPIGASTRIC HERNIAS

An epigastric hernia is a protrusion of fat or omentum through the linea alba between the umbilicus and the xiphoid cartilage. A congenital defect in the linea alba is probably the major disposing factor. Epigastric hernias most commonly appear between the ages of 20 and 50 and are 3 times more common in men than in women.

Most patients complain of a small painless sub-cutaneous mass, most often just to the left of the midline. Usually the hernia consists of preperitoneal fat or of fat of the falciform ligament. Larger defects also contain omentum and, sometimes, small bowel.

Complications are more common in patients with small hernias, because these are more likely to in-carcerate. When this happens, there is usually local pain and tenderness and, less often, deep epigastric pain, abdominal distention, and nausea and vomiting.

Treatment must be individualized. Small asymptomatic hernias require no treatment; an asymptomatic hernia greater than 1.5 cm in diameter should be repaired. Incarceration of a small hernia is an indication for operation. The recurrence rate following epigastric herniorrhaphy is approximately 10%

and usually can be attributed to failure to appreciate multiple defects in the linea alba at the time of the initial operation.

General References

Halverson K: Hernia. In Goldsmith HS (ed-in-chief): *Practice of Surgery*. Vol 3: Bryne JJ (ed): *General Surgery*. Philadelphia, Harper & Row, 1984, chap 9, p 1.

    A succinct, well illustrated summary.

Nyhus LM (ed): *Hernias* 64: April, 1984.

    Seventeen articles on different aspects of hernias

Nyhus LM, Condon RE (eds): *Hernia*. Philadelphia, JB Lippincott, 1978.

    A definitive text.

CHAPTER NINETY-TWO

Benign Conditions of the Anus and Rectum

W. ROBERT ROUT, M.D., CALVIN B. ERNST, M.D., AND JOHN R. BURTON, M.D.

Anorectal disorders are often encountered in ambulatory practice. This chapter describes four particularly common problems—pruritis ani, anal fissure, hemorrhoidal disease, and perirectal abscess. Also included, because of their importance to the general physician are somewhat less common problems, such as proctalgia fugax and rectal prolapse. Cutaneous disorders that affect the perianal area, such as psoriasis, are discussed in Chapter 100 (Common Problems of the Skin). The common venereal diseases as they affect the anus and the rectum are discussed in Chapters 27 and 94 (Genitourinary In-

fections and Benign Vulvovaginal Conditions) and in Chapter 30 (Syphilis). In addition to the more common venereal diseases that affect the anus and rectum, proctitis characterized by rectal pain, tenesmus and often an anal discharge may also be caused by unusual organisms. In gay men, symptoms suggesting proctitis should raise suspicion of the *gay bowel syndrome*, a form of proctitis that results from the sexual transmission of a variety of pathogens (bacteria, helminths, protozoa, and viruses) (4). Because of the difficulty in establishing a specific diagnosis, patients suspected of having this syndrome should be referred to a gastroenterologist or an infectious disease specialist. Other conditions that may affect the rectum are discussed in Chapters 26 (Acute Gastroenteritis and Associated Conditions) and 38 (Constipation and Diarrhea).

PRURITUS ANI

Definition

Pruritus ani, a distressing perianal itch, is a very common complaint, paticularly in men. The intensity of the symptom is variable but is usually greatest at night. Often the itching abates spontaneously only to recur after widely variable asymptomatic periods.

Etiology

Although the cause of pruritis ani is often unknown (50 to 75% of the time), the symptoms may be a manifestation of many anorectal disorders (Table 92.1). Whatever the cause, the itching is frequently associated with fecal contamination of moist macerated skin, often complicated by excoriation and secondary infection.

Diagnosis

Whenever a patient complains of perianal itching, specific historical information should be obtained and several observations should be made to aid in establishing a diagnosis.

History

A limited dietary history is important since occasionally an excess intake of milk, coffee, tea, alcohol, cola, and spices may be associated with pruritus ani. It is important to review the drugs the patient is taking since medications, such as laxatives or col-

Table 92.1.
Common Problems Associated With Pruritus Ani

DERMATOLOGICAL DISORDERS
  Psoriasis
  Atopic dermatitis
  Contact dermatitis
  Lichen planus
  Condylomata
  Venereal warts
  Herpes simplex
  Tumors
DIARRHEA
FISSURES
FISTULAS
INFECTION
  Fungi and yeast (especially in diabetic patients) (see
    Chapter 100, Common Problems of the Skin)
  Erythrasma
  Scabies (see Chapter 100, Common Problems of the
    Skin)
  Pinworm infestation—more common in children—*Entero-
    bius vermicularis*
  Vaginal infections (see Chapter 94, Benign Vulvovaginal
    Disorders)
OBESITY
POOR ANAL HYGIENE
RECTAL PROLAPSE
PROLAPSED HEMORRHOIDS (most often hemorrhoids are
    not associated with pruritus and other causes should be
    sought)

chicine, which casuse gastrointestinal irritation may be associated with perianal itching.

General Examination

The patient should be examined for the presence of a dermatological problem such as psoriasis, scabies, or fungal infection (Table 92.1) that may be associated with pruritus ani. In addition, in women, a pelvic examination should be performed because of the occasional association of vaginal infection with pruritus ani (see Chapter 94).

With the patient in the lateral decubitus or the knee-chest position and with the buttocks separated, the perianal area should be inspected. During the inspection the patient should be asked to strain, a maneuver that may demonstrate prolapse or fecal or flatal incontinence.

If skin lesions are identified, appropriate evaluation (such as a KOH preparation) to establish a diagnosis (such as *Tinea* or *Candida*) should be done in order to initiate definitive therapy (see Chapter 100). If no lesions are visualized, or if only excoriated skin or hemorrhoids are seen,the evaluation should include a series of three to five cellophane tape preparations in an attempt to demonstrate the ova of pinworms (see below).

Rectal Examination

Digital rectal examination should always be accomplished using a well lubricated gloved finger.

Evaluation must be gentle in order to avoid spasm of the anal sphincter which will preclude adequate examination. At initiation of the examination, the patient should be asked to bear down, which will minimize discomfort. Excessive pain or tenderness of one area should alert the physician to the presence of an anal fissure (see below). All structures of the anal canal within the limits of the reach of the finger should be assessed (the anus, the distal rectum, the prostate gland, the cervix).

Anoscopy

After rectal examination, and without laxative or enema preparation, an anoscopy (with the use of an instrument that permits a side or oblique view) should be performed. A well lubricated anoscope should be inserted gently, while the patient bears down to minimize discomfort. The instrument should be inserted slowly as deeply as possible. Then, after removal of the obturator, the rectum should be inspected using adequate light. Visualization is possible only through the side or oblique aspect of the instrument as it is withdrawn gradually. It is important to avoid rotation of the anoscope, which will be uncomfortable and which may actually tear the anal mucosa. For adequate inspection of all quadrants of the anal canal, the instrument must be reinserted and withdrawn three or four times.

Cellophane Tape Examination for Pinworms

This is easily accomplished by the patient at home or by the physician in the office. Swabs are commercially available (Pinworm Diagnostic Tapes, Parke-Davis), but they are also easily made by folding clear cellophane tape, sticky side out, over a tongue blade. At night pinworms migrate from the anal canal to the perianal area, where they deposit eggs. Therefore, the swab should be obtained upon arising, before a bowel movement, and before the perianal area is cleansed. The swab is placed at the anal verge and then the tape is mounted onto a glass microscopic slide. A specimen obtained in this way will keep for several days. The slides should be examined under the low power (× 10) objective of the microscope searching for the typical ova of pinworm (Fig. 92.1).

Treatment

General Measures

Most patients with pruritus ani can be diagnosed and treated adequately by the general physician. Even when the evaluation is inconclusive, except for the identification of excoriation, symptoms can be controlled by relatively simple measures:

Tepid sitz baths for 15 to 20 minutes provide excellent temporary relief (for example, at bedtime). If used several times daily at the outset of symptoms,

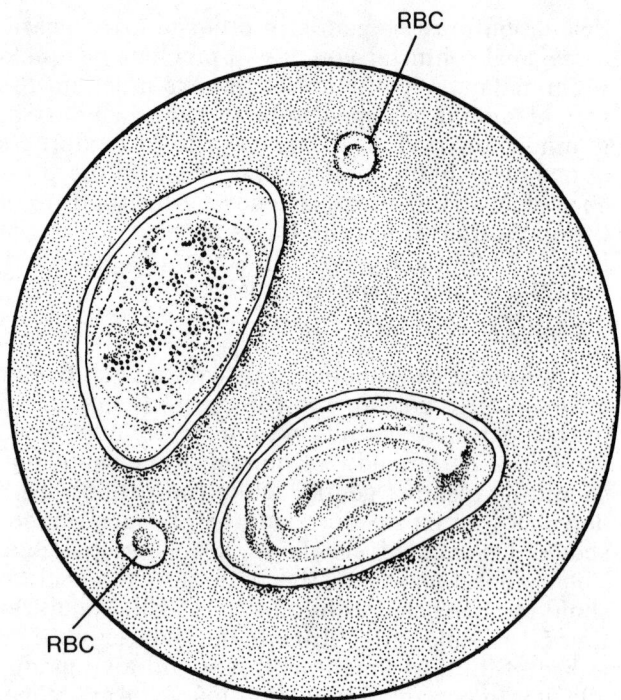

RBC

RBC

Figure 92.1. Appearance of the eggs of *Enterobius vermicularis* (pinworm). The egg is approximately 20 to 50 μm and typically has one relatively flattened side.

sitz baths may be sufficient to control pruritus ani. However, often the patient will find frequent sitz baths impractical.

Anal cleanliness is mandatory; it should be thorough but gentle. After a bowel movement the anus should be cleaned with soft, white, nonperfumed toilet tissue (colored or perfumed tissue is potentially allergenic or irritative and should be avoided). If paper is too irritating, cotton swabs moistened with warm water or with glycerin may be used (cotton fiber is less irritating than paper fiber). Glycerin-witch hazel wipes (Tucks, available without prescription) are helpful to cleanse the anal area. The patient should discontinue the use of these preparations if he notices intense burning and use plain glycerin (available without prescription) instead.

The anal area should be cleaned once or twice a day with plain soap, such as Ivory or Purpose, or plain shaving cream and should be kept dry between times by the application of plain talc (such as Johnson's Baby Powder); cornstarch is not a good substitute as it may promote the growth of microorganisms, which could compound the problem. At night, zinc oxide paste (available without prescription) may be substituted for talc. This should be applied thickly to the anal area where it will absorb moisture and provide comfort. In the morning it may be removed with soap and water, mineral oil, glycerin, or Tucks, or it may be reapplied in the morning and after each bowel movement.

The patient should use *cotton underwear* to provide better ventilation and should avoid polyester clothing. Prolonged sitting, especially on synthetic materials (such as vinyl seats), which prevent proper ventilation, should be avoided.

Specific Measures

If a rectal problem is identified during the initial evaluation of a patient with pruritus ani (Table 92.1), it must be treated (see below or the chapters on dermatology (Chapter 100) and on benign vulvovaginal disorders (Chapter 94) or the section on gastrointestinal problems (Section 4)).

When the pruritis is severe, commonly at night, the patient may gain relief by the temporary application of a minimal amount of *hydrocortisone cream*, 0.5% (available without prescription) or 1% (requires a prescription). Chronic use of fluorinated steroids should be avoided because of their tendency to cause atrophy and telangiectasias. Topical steroids will help the patient to *avoid scratching* the anal area, reducing trauma and subsequent injury.

The diet, when found to contain foods thought to be associated with pruritus ani (see above), may be modified, at least on a trial basis. If a food is incriminated, the patient may find that symptoms will not resolve for 1 or 2 weeks after the diet is appropriately modified. Moreover, the patient will note recurrence of symptoms, usually within 24 to 48 hours, after the reinstitution of an offending food.

Diarrhea and/or constipation should be controlled (see Chapter 38); stool softeners such as psyllium (Effersyllium or Metamucil), which are not irritating and which absorb mucus, a possible irritant to the sensitive perianal tissue, are preferred.

Occasionally these relatively simple measures do not provide adequate relief and it may be necessary to acidify the stool. There is evidence that in some patients with pruritus ani the stool pH is alkaline (pH 9 to 10) instead of slightly acid (pH 6 to 7) as it is normally. The stool pH may be measured in the office by using litmus paper or a urine dipstick after mixing some water with the stool specimen. If the pH is high, therapeutic acidification of the stool is indicated. Acidifiction may be accomplished with *Lactobacillus acidophilus* (such as Acidophilus, Bacid, or DoFus, all available without prescription), 1 to 2 capsules three times/day or with malt soup extract (Maltsupex) available without prescription in powder, liquid, or tablet form.

Occasionally antipruritic sedatives such as diphenhydramine (Benadryl), 25 to 15 mg, or trimeprazine (Temaril), 2 to 5 mg, taken before bed may be helpful in controlling nocturnal symptoms.

Referral

Should a patient with idiopathic pruritus ani not be responsive to these therapies, he should be referred to a gastroenterologist.

Enterobius Vermicularis (Pinworms)

Because the infestation is passed *via* the fecal-oral route and because the ova may remain alive on bed clothing for up to 3 weeks, dissemination of the disorder within families readily occurs. Once the problem is identified, all members of the household should be evaluated with the cellophane tape test.

The drug of choice to eradicate this infestation is pyrantel pamoate (Antiminth). It is available as an oral suspension (50 mg/ml) and is given as a single oral dose (11 mg/kg, not to exceed a total dose of 1 g). An alternative drug, mebendazole (Vermox), 100 mg, is given as a single oral dose; it should not be used in infants or in pregnant women. These agents approach 100% effectiveness in killing the worms, and symptoms usually subside within 48 hours. The patient is no longer infective once the deposited eggs are removed from the perinal area and clothing by cleaning. Both drugs are well tolerated but may be occasionally associated with mild, transient gastrointestinal distress. Pyrantel pamoate may occasionally be associated with transient elevation of liver enzymes, and its use should be avoided in patients with known liver disease.

Patients who have been identified to have pinworm infection should launder their clothing and bed linens with detergent and hot water on the same day that they have received oral treatment. All infected members of the household should be treated simultaneously. Reinfection is common and re-evaluation is appropriate whenever symptoms recur. Retreatment is necessary with recurring infestation.

ANAL FISSURE

Definition

An anal fissure is a painful elliptical tear, usually located in the posterior portion of the anal canal where the mucosa is relatively fixed. The problem is very common and is observed with equal frequency in men and women. Fissures can extend to the pectinate line (Fig. 92.2) from their origin at the anal verge. A primary fissure represents a tear in the mucosa which occurs because of trauma associated with the passage of a hard stool or with another similar insult.

Secondary fissures are much less common. They result from inflammatory bowel disease, infections, such as syphilis, gonorrhea, or tuberculosis, or an anatomical anal abnormality, such as scarring that may occur after a hemorrhoidectomy.

Presentation

An acute anal fissure presents with the sudden onset of sharp rectal *pain*, especially during defecation and often is followed by a more dull *discomfort* which may persist for several hours. A fissure may be associated with *spotty bleeding,*usually noticed as red staining of the toilet tissue or as blood on the surface of the stool. Occasionally, *pruritus ani,* (see above) is the major symptom associated with a fissure, in which case a mucus discharge is almost always present.

If the buttocks are gently retracted, thereby everting the anal mucosa, many anal fissures can be readily visualized, usually at the posterior margin of the anal verge. During this examination it is important to avoid inducing pain, which will result in spasm of the anal sphincter, increasing discomfort and masking the findings. Occasionally anoscopy (using a side view instrument) will be required to identify the fissure.

If an anal fissure is identified, and if it is necessary to perform a rectal examination despite the presence of such a fissure (e.g., if a rectal cancer is suspected), a cotton pledget saturated with Xylocaine gel may be placed over the fissure before the examination. During digital rectal examination the examining finger should be pressed away from the fissure. If anoscopy is required, abundant Xylocaine gel should be used.

A chronic fissure, less common than an acute fissure, may be recognized by its indurated edges and especially by a collection of redundant tissue at the outer lip (the sentinel pile). If anal intercourse has been practiced, a venereal disease should be considered (see Chapters 30 (Syphilis), 27 (Genitourinary Infections), and 94 (Benign Vulvovaginal Disorders)).

Either acute or chronic fissures may be associated with development of a perianal abscess, readily recognized as an area of intense inflammation and fluctuation (see below).

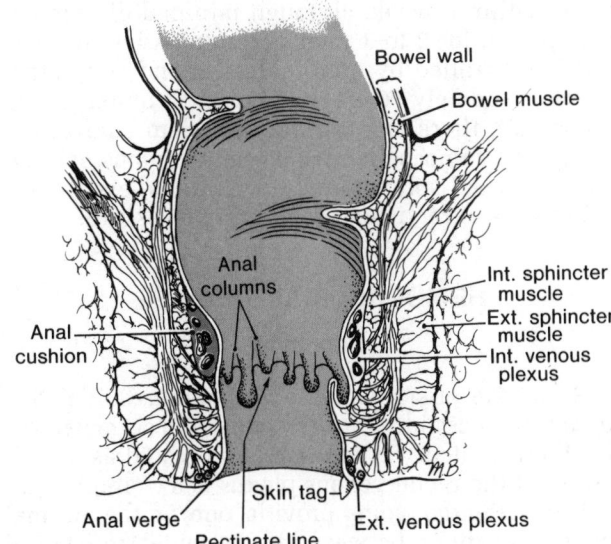

Figure 92.2. Important structures of the anal area.

Treatment

Many patients with an acute anal fissure can be made comfortable within a day or two and cured within 3 weeks by use of conservative therapy. Bulk laxatives such as Effersyllium or Metamucil should be taken as necessary to provide a soft stool. Irritant cathartics, such as Dulcolax, magnesia, and cascara, should be avoided as they exacerbate the problem. Once the fissure has healed, it is important for the patient to continue ingesting a high fiber diet and to continue using a stool softener as necessary.

Anal discomfort may be relieved by the use of showers or sitz baths for 15 to 20 minutes two to three times/day, followed by the application of ½% hydrocortisone cream (available without prescription) or 1% hydrocortisone cream (requires a prescription) or by the use of topical anesthetics such as Nupercainal cream, ointment, or suppositories or Perifoam aerosol (both available without prescription). Anesthetic agents may occasionally be associated with a contact allergy and should be immediately discontinued should the patient notice intensification of symptoms or a rash after their use. Topical corticosteriods and anesthetics should be used only on a temporary basis (i.e., 2 to 3 weeks).

If after 3 or 4 weeks of therapy the fissure has not improved or if initially the fissure appears to be chronic (see above), the patient should be referred to a surgeon, because in these instances conservative therapy is not likely to be successful.

If the problem is found to be primary, the surgeon may perform an internal sphincterotomy often without having to remove the actual fissure. This procedure is usually done in an ambulatory surgery center, is well tolerated, and is quite successful. An uncommon but important postoperative complication is anorectal abscess (see below).

After this procedure, patients generally return to work within a week, although minimal discomfort may persist for 2 to 3 weeks. Postoperative discomfort is controlled by oral analgesics and sitz baths. In approximately 70% of patients who undergo this procedure, there is a transient problem controlling flatus and some patients have mild mucus soiling. After internal sphincterotomy, there is less than a 3% chance of recurrence of a primary fissure.

HEMORRHOIDAL DISEASE

Definition

A precise characterization of hemorrhoidal disease is not possible since the pathogenesis has never been elucidated. To define a hemorrhoid as a varicosity of the rectal venous plexus is too simplistic.

Hemorrhoidal veins provide one of the normal communications between the systemic and portal venous systems. These veins have the tendency to dilate and develop into a tortuous plexus. Anal cushions are part of the normal anatomy of the anal canal (Fig. 92.2). These cushions, which consist of hemorrhoidal venous and arterial plexuses, smooth muscle, and connective tissue, lie under the mucosa. The cushions apparently permit the passage of variable sized stools without disruption of the rectal mucosa. Hemorrhoidal disease is thought to be the result of displacement of these vascular anal cushions. The three cushoins that are most likely to be involved are found in the right anterior, right posterior, and left lateral portions of the anal canal (Fig. 92.3). Venous drainage from these cushions is into the portal venous system.

Many physicians classify hemorrhoids as being external or internal; most of the time the diagnosis of external hemorrhoids is incorrect. Often the term is being used to describe redundant skin tags at the anal verge (Fig. 92.2). A small plexus of veins at the anal verge communicates with the systemic venous system. Dilation of these veins is uncommon and is usually associated with an internal hemorrhoid; however, isolated thrombosis may occur, and, while causing only minor discomfort, it may result in the development of a skin tag (Fig. 92.2).

A classification of hemorrhoidal disease is outlined in Table 92.2.

Pathogenesis

Internal hemorrhoidal disease (or piles) occurs when an anovascular cushion prolapses through the anal canal and becomes entrapped and congested by the internal anal sphincter. Prolapse is believed to be initiated by a shearing force produced by the passage of a large firm stool, from urgent defecation that may occur with explosive diarrhea, or with some form of partial obstruction of the anal canal. Increased portal or systemic venous pressure may predispose to development of hemorrhoids. This increase in pressure might occur from congestive heart failure, pregnancy, portal hypertension, or pelvic inflammatory or neoplastic disease. Straining at micturition because of urethral or bladder outlet obstruction or straining that occurs with lifting or defecation has been implicated in causing hemorrhoids. Carcinoma of the rectum may be associated with hemorrhoidal development because of straining with bowel movements and local obstruction of venous outflow.

Epidemiology

Asymptomatic hemorrhoids are present in half of the population over age 50, but are uncommon in individuals under the age of 25 to 30 except in women who have been pregnant. A more precise definition of hemorrhoids—one in which *symptoms* are associated with these normal vascular plexuses—reduces the prevalence to approximately 5% of the population over age 50.

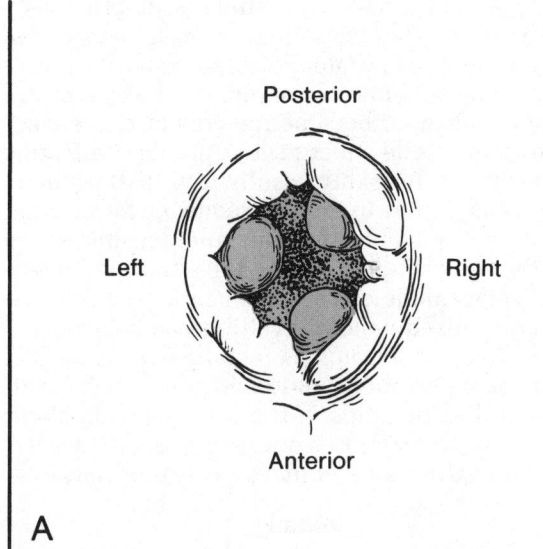

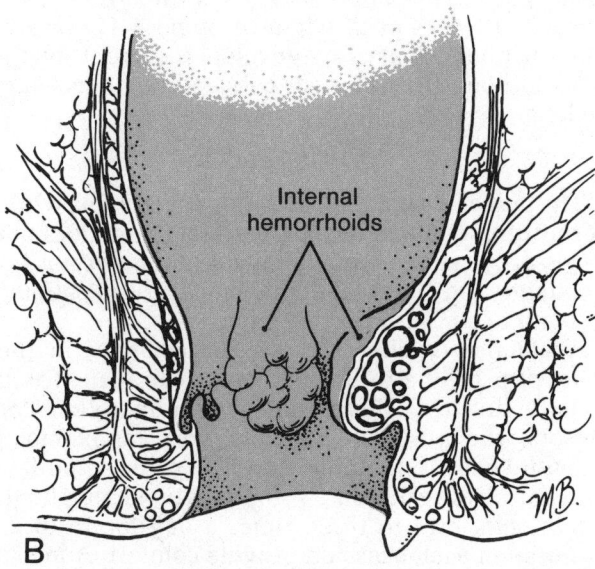

Figure 92.3. *A.* Common sites of hemorrhoids. *B.* Protrusion of anal cushions.

Presentation

Asymptomatic "hemorrhoids" noticed incidentally during an examination should not be considered a problem and should not be treated. Symptomatic hemorrhoids result in pain, bleeding, and prolapse. Symptoms that follow persistent prolapse, such as fecal soilage, mucus production, or pruritus ani, symptoms of localized infection, or rarely portal venous infection (pylephlebitis) may also occur.

External Hemorrhoids

External hemorrhoids are covered by pain-sensitive skin. The most common manifestation, there-fore, is pain, which results from thrombosis in the external venous plexus. Pain is perianal in location and can be exacerbated by defecation. The patient may be aware of a tender perianal lump.

Internal Hemorrhoids

Internal hemorrhoids are covered by pain-insensitive mucosa, produce symptoms primarily from bleeding or prolapse, and are only painful in the event of thrombosis or strangulation (ischemia caused by constriction of a prolapsed hemorrhoid) with or without associated ulceration and infection.

Bleeding

Characteristically the bleeding from hemorrhoids is intermittent, bright red, and spots toilet tissue or the surface of the stool. Occasionally it may be sustained and described as a dripping of blood. Rarely, massive hemorrhage may occur, particularly among patients with portal hypertension. Bleeding may also be occult; but because of their common occurrence, hemorrhoids should never be considered the cause of occult bleeding until other causes of gastrointestinal blood loss have been ruled out by appropriate evaluation. Gastrointestinal bleeding is fully discussed in Chapter 37.

Prolapse

Prolapse of internal hemorrhoids produces the sensation of fullness in the anal canal, especially after defecation. Usually prolapsed hemorrhoids will reduce spontaneously. Occasionally prolapse is more severe and manual reduction may be necessary. When reduction is not possible, prolapse may be associated with fecal soilage, mucus accumula-

Table 92.2.
Classification of Hemorrhoids

EXTERNAL SKIN TAGS: Small discrete skin tags arising from the anal verge
EXTERNAL HEMORRHOIDS: Hemorrhoids arising from the inferior hemorrhoidal plexus exterior to the anal verge, covered by pain-sensitive skin
INTERNAL HEMORRHOIDS: Hemorrhoids arising from the vascular cushions, normal structures, lying above the anal verge, covered by pain-insensitive mucosa. Internal hemorrhoids may be classified further:
First degree: Hemorrhoids bulging into the lumen of the anal canal that produce bleeding
Second degree: Hemorrhoids that prolapse during defecation but that reduce spontaneously
Third degree: Prolapsed hemorrhoids that require manual reduction
Fourth degree: Hemorrhoids that are irreducibly prolapsed
THROMBOSED HEMORRHOIDS: An internal hemorrhoid may prolapse and strangulate, which leads to thrombosis, an excruciatingly painful condition. If swelling progresses, gangrene of the hemorrhoids with ulceration, local infection, or pylephlebitis (septic phlebitis of the portal venous system) may result

tion, and the development of pruritus ani (see above).

Pain

Pain from internal hemorrhoids suggests thrombosis or strangulation, and referral to a surgeon is necessary. Thrombosis and strangulation occur when prolapse of a hemorrhoid through the anal canal is followed by increasing congestion created by spasm of the entrapping anal sphincter. If the hemorrhoid strangulates, it may ulcerate and cause infection, which is usually localized or which rarely may spread through the portal venous plexus, resulting in pylephlebitis.

Examination

Hemorrhoids are readily visualized by observing the anal canal in good light after the patient gently retracts his buttocks and strains as if having a bowel movement. This maneuver produces slight eversion of the anal canal and enables the examiner to see the internal hemorrhoidal plexus.

An external hemorrhoid will be seen as a mass just outside the anal verge and will usually be tender.

If the patient is in severe pain from thrombosis, strangulation, or ulceration, no further evaluation is necessary and urgent referral to a surgeon is appropriate (see below). If the patient is not in severe pain, a more thorough evaluation of the anal canal should be accomplished by anoscopy (using a side view instrument). It is important that this procedure be done carefully as described above. Anoscopy is the definitive diagnostic procedure for establishing the diagnosis of internal hemorrhoids.

Sigmoidoscopy should be performed in patients with recent onset of symptomatic hemorrhoidal disease because of the possibility that sigmoid or rectal carcinoma has caused the development of hemorrhoids. The need for additional evaluation of the colon by barium enema, air contrast barium enema, or colonoscopy must be determined on an individual basis; it is mandatory if there has been significant or repeated bleeding (see Chapter 37).

Differential Diagnosis

Several problems may be confused with hemorrhoidal disease:

Hypertrophied anal papilla (sentinel pile) occurs along the pectinate line (Fig. 92.2) in association with an anal fissure (see above), Crohn's disease, or without obvious cause. These papillae usually are asymptomatic and require no therapy unless they have become particularly large, eroded, or infected, or unless they bleed. Sentinel piles are easily differentiated from hemorrhoids by their location and by the absence of a vascular swelling.

Anal skin tags are very common. They appear as small projections of redundant skin external to the anal verge. They may be remnants of previously active external hemorrhoidal disease, associated with internal hemorrhoidal disease, or with Crohn's disease. They are of no consequence unless they are very large, bleed, or become infected or excoriated.

Prolapse of rectal mucosa is a problem affecting the elderly and probably results from pathogenetic mechanisms similar to those responsible for internal hemorrhoids, except that the anal cushions are small. Prolapse is identified by the abnormal downward displacement of rectal mucosa without evidence of localized venous swelling (see below).

Protruding tumors such as rectal polyps, anal carcinoma, or, in women, endometriosis can be confused with hemorrhoids. If there is suspicion about the diagnosis, referral to a surgeon or a gastroenterologist for evaluation and biopsy is appropriate.

Course

Without treatment, symptoms due to hemorrhoids usually resolve spontaneoulsy within several days to several weeks even when thrombosis is present. Most patients, however, develop recurrent symptoms, although the intervals between symptoms may be long.

Treatment

The aim of treatment is to relieve symptoms while permitting spontaneous healing; treatment does not necessarily reduce venous bulges, although not infrequently they regress spontaneously. Most patients respond to conservative therapy:

Avoidance of direct pressure is essential in the relief of pain due to hemorrhoids. The patient will usually find a position that gives him relief. For persons who must sit (doing desk work, for example) a donut-shaped inflatable ring is usually helpful in preventing pressure on a symptomatic hemorrhoid.

Sitz baths two to three times a day for 15 to 20 minutes on each occasion provide comfort. A moist, warm wash cloth, firmly applied between the cheeks of the buttocks, may also provide good temporary relief of symptoms.

Stool softeners are mandatory, if stools are hard, to reduce straining with defecation and to prevent evacuation of hard stools that may prolapse the mucosa. Bran-containing breakfast cereal and/or whole wheat bread help to maintain soft stools. An alternative is daily ingestion of a bulk laxative-stool softener such as Effersyllium, Metamucil, Colace, or Peri-Colace (see also Chapter 38). Instructing the patient to increase fluid consumption, especially water, facilitates effectiveness of stool softeners. Use of stool softeners should continue, even after the resolution of the acute problem, as it may help to prevent recurrence.

Topical preparations may provide relief of pain or pruritis. *Hydrocortisone-containing rectal preparations*, such as Anusol-HC cream, Protofoam-HC aerosol, or Wyanoids-HC ointment (all require prescription), used three to four times a day, may provide symptomatic relief. Cream, foam, or ointment is preferred to suppositories, which tend to be expelled or drawn up in the rectum and, therefore, have less local effect. One-half percent (available without prescription) or 1% (requires a prescription) hydrocortisone cream (generic) is also useful.

Analgesic rectal preparations are also useful when pain is prominent, but they may occasionally result in contact allergy. Preparations such as Nupercainal (available without prescription) or Xylocaine 2.5% ointment (requires a prescription) used three to four times a day may provide relief of rectal discomfort, particularly over the first several days when the discomfort tends to be most intense.

There is no acceptable evidence that Preparation H, which contains the antiseptic phenylmercuric nitrate, 3% shark liver oil, and "live yeast cell derivative," can shrink hemorrhoids, reduce inflammation, or heal injured tissue (5).

Bed rest for several days may help to reduce prolapse and will avoid the exacerbation of discomfort associated with "upright" daily activities.

Systemic analgesics, such as meperidine (Demerol), 50 to 100 mg every 4 to 6 hours, may occasionally be necessary for pain associated with hemorrhoids. Severe pain is usually associated with thrombosis, which may be more effectively treated by a surgeon by thrombectomy (instant relief of pain) as compared to conservative therapy (4 to 5 days before pain is relieved). Systemic analgesics such as codeine or meperidine may be associated with constipation; therefore, they should be used in conjunction with laxatives.

Referral for Surgical Management

Patients should be referred to a surgeon for evaluation whenever there is doubt about the diagnosis (see above), if the patient does not respond within 1 or 2 weeks to conservative therapy, if pain is severe as may occur with thrombosis, or if there is evidence of strangulation, ulceration, or perianal infection. When uncomplicated hemorrhoids are recurrently symptomatic, the patient should be referred to a surgeon for definitive treatment.

The surgeon will evaluate the patient, confirm the diagnosis, and then consider several therapeutic options that are not normally provided by general physicians (6):

Injection of Sclerosing Agents

The submucosal injection of a symptomatic hemorrhoid with several milliliters of a sclerosing solution causes fibrosis and retraction of the hemorrhoid. This procedure is ideal therapy for small internal hemorrhoids; it is simple, requires no anesthesia, and can easily be performed in the office (requires only a few minutes). There may be a period of several days during which the patient experiences a sensation of anal fullness. This symptom is usually well tolerated or is easily controlled by use of sitz baths three to four times/day and by mild analgesics, such as acetaminophen or aspirin. After this procedure the patient usually requires no recovery period and can return to work immediately.

It is important that the physician peforming this procedure be experienced with its use. If the solution is improperly injected, severe pain, necrosis, and rectal stenosis may occur. Sclerotherapy is rarely associated with the development of infection, an oleoma, or an oil embolus. Injection of sclerosing agents generally provides temporary relief, but it does not prevent the development of subsequent hemorrhoids. The procedure may be repeated several times. However, it produces an area of fibrosis and if repetitively used, may result in rectal stenosis.

Rubberband Ligation

Rubberband ligation of hemorrhoids is a relatively simple office procedure used primarily for the treatment of mild hemorrhoids that have not responded to conservative therapy (2, 3). The patient requires no special preparation, and usually the only discomfort results from anoscopy required during the procedure. No anesthesia is necessary although some surgeons administer a local analgesic before "banding." With use of an anoscope and a special instrument one or two rubberbands are applied near the base of one or two and occasionally three hemorrhoids which are at least 0.5 cm above the pectinate line. Constriction by the rubberband results in ischemic necrosis of the hemorrhoid, which eventually sloughs and is passed in the stool. Sloughing usually occurs between the 5th and 10th day after banding and is associated with passage of a small amount of blood. Occasionally, bleeding may be massive and urgent reassessment by the surgeon is necessary to control the bleeding by electrocautery or by ligation.

Usually, following rubberband ligation of hemorrhoids, the patient is not disabled and has only minimal discomfort characterized by a sensation of rectal fullness, a symptom which is usually well controlled by the use of sitz baths and/or mild oral analgesics, such as acetaminophen or aspirin. If the rubberband is improperly placed below the pectinate line, the patient may experience considerable pain, in which case reassessment by the surgeon is appropriate.

Following rubberband ligation the patient should suppress having a bowel movement for 12 hours. A bulk-forming stool softener such as Effersyllium or Metamucil should be prescribed to prevent straining. This will be necessary for several weeks and should be continued as long term therapy to prevent straining, which may predispose to the subsequent developent of new hemorrhoids.

Complete healing after this procedure occurs within 4 to 6 weeks, after which the patient may be treated with further rubberband ligations if there are other symptomatic hemorrhoids. Banding provides good temporary relief of hemorrhoidal disease approximately 70 to 90% of the time. Mild symptoms may recur in as many as 60 to 70% of patients. Should there be recurrence, the hemorrhoidal symptoms may be treated conservatively (see above) and if this is unsuccessful, referral to a surgeon may be necessary.

Manual Dilation of the Anus

This procedure is predicated on the belief that hemorrhoids result from partial anal canal obstruction necessitating increased pressure for evacuation of the bowel. The pressure is transmitted to the anal vascular cushion, resulting in the development of hemorrhoids. Dilation is used occasionally in the United States, is popular in England, and is considered by some (1) to be an acceptable, cost-effective, short term treatment alternative to hemorrhoidectomy. The patient requires general anesthesia with good muscle relaxation. The dilation is performed in an ambulatory surgery center or in a hospital. In the latter instance hospitalization is usually limited to 1 or 2 days. The surgeon manually dilates the anus up to the size of six to eight fingers. This disrupts the muscular fibers and relieves the partial obstruction. The procedure is well tolerated with only minimal discomfort of rectal fullness for several days following the procedure. Frequently there is a 2- to 4-day period of incontinence of flatus and occasionally of stool. After dilation the patient is required to perform anal dilation, using a special device, daily for at least 2 weeks and then occasionally for as long as 6 months.

Despite reports of 75 to 85% initial satisfactory results with anal dilation, the procedure has not been widely accepted. Complications occur because the dilation is not well controlled and may be excessive, causing long term anal sphincter incontinence. Up to 25% of patients develop persisting incontinence of flatus following dilation. Chronic postoperative incontinence tends to be highest in the elderly, especially in females with atrophy of the perineum. Rectal mucosal prolapse can occur. Recurrence of hemorrhoids, despite claims to the contrary, is quite common. If the anal sphincter is excessively disrupted, anal stenosis may occur secondary to scarring.

Partial Internal Sphincterotomy

This procedure is based on the same logic as manual anal dilation: that relief of partial anal sphincter obstruction, which leads to increased straining during defecation thus causing the development of hemorrhoids, will cure the hemorrhoids.

This procedure may be performed under local or general anesthesia and usually is done in an ambulatory surgery center. The surgeon divides portions of the internal anal sphincter. Following this procedure the patient is usually able to return to his usual activities within a few days and the associated local discomfort is usually short lived and easily controlled by sitz baths and oral analgesics. The major complication of this relatively simple procedure is incontinence, which may occur in up to 25% of patients, but is usually minimal or transient.

Reccurence of hemorrhoids following this procedure is high and the procedure is inferior to rubberband ligation in the relief of symptoms in patients with first and second degree hemorrhoids (see Table 92.2)

Cryotherapy

This procedure is practiced in the United States by only a few surgeons. A freezing probe destroys the hemorrhoid, which in time sloughs off. Usually the procedure is done in a surgeon's office without anesthesia. After the procedure there is often an uncomfortable, profuse, foul-smelling anal discharge that persists until the necrotic hemorrhoid sloughs off, which usually occurs on about the 14th day. At this time bleeding may occur and is usually minor. However, in an occasional patient bleeding can be marked and will require re-evaluation with subsequent cauterization or ligation. After this procedure the patient is unable to return to his usual activities for a period of 2 to 3 weeks, primarily because of the anal discharge. Healing generally is complete by 6 weeks. Postoperatively, the patient is required only to take sitz baths and oral analgesics in addition to stool softeners.

Hemorrhoidectomy

Hemorrhoidectomy is usually performed for treatment of large hemorrhoids. This procedure requires general or spinal anesthesia and the patient is usually hospitalized for 2 to 3 days, although good risk patients with less severe hemorrhoids may be able to have the surgery performed in an ambulatory center. The patient is prepared for the procedure by taking stool softeners for approximately a week before the procedure and is given a laxative the evening before the operation. The purpose of the operation is to remove hemorrhoidal tissue and to appose the skin and mucus membrane. Usually postoperative discomfort is not severe and is easily controlled by sitz baths, oral analgesics, and stool softeners. An uncommon but important postoperative complication is anorectal abscess (see below).

Following hemorrhoidectomy there is a recovery period of 3 to 4 weeks before the patient is able to return to his usual activities.

When hemorrhoidectomy is performed by an experienced surgeon, the complications of infection, fistula formation, fissure development, significant bleeding, or acute thrombosis of an external hemorrhoid occur only rarely (less than 1%). Minor bleeding is more common but is usually present during the first 2 weeks. Acute urinary retention following hemorrhoidectomy occurs in about 10% of individuals and may require the short term use of an indwelling catheter. Late complications of incontinence or of anal stenosis are quite rare. Skin tags are usually excised with the hemorrhoids, although small ones may develop after hemorrhoidectomy and are usually of no consequence (see above).

Following hemorrhoidectomy the surgeon will usually evaluate the patient weekly for two to three visits until healing is complete and before the patient returns to work. The patient is seen 6 months following hemorrhoidectomy to be examined for the presence of additional hemorrhoids, stenosis, stricture, or skin tags.

Hemorrhoidectomy offers the best chance of long term control with less than a 5% late recurrence rate. Its use is limited because of the associated short term morbidity and the observation that many hemorrhoids can be eliminated by less traumatic procedures.

Special Considerations

Because of an increased rate of complications associated with operative procedures in individuals with severe congestive *heart failure or debilitating disease*, the treatment of hemorrhoids in these patients should be as conservative as possible. Patients who have *portal hypertension* present a special risk because of the frequent association of a coagulopathy and because operative hemorrhoidectomy in a few instances can diminish shunting between the portal and systemic systems and result in a rise in portal pressure that on occasion may be associated with esophageal or gastric variceal bleeding.

Hemorrhoids are very common in *pregnancy* and are best managed conservatively. They frequently resolve spontaneously after delivery. Occasionally, development of strangulated hemorrhoids requires surgical evaluation during the pregnancy. Patients with *inflammatory bowel disease* and hemorrhoidal disease should be managed in consultation with a gastroenterologist and a surgeon.

ANORECTAL ABSCESSES AND ANORECTAL FISTULAS

Definition

An anorectal abscess is an abscess involving the perineum and perianal structures. Abscesses are classified by their anatomical location (Fig. 92.4). *Low intramuscular or perianal abscesses* are located

in the subcutaneous tissue immediately surrounding the anus, which is the site of 50 to 75% of all anorectal abscesses. An *ischiorectal abscess* is located in the ischiorectal fossa, a fat-filled space present between the levator ani (external anal sphincter) and the ischial tuberosity, and accounts for 20 to 40% of anorectal abscesses. *Intersphincteric, high intermuscular, pelvirectal, and submucosal abscesses* are far less common and account for about 10% of all abscesses. Anorectal abscesses are common, and the general physician should be familiar with presentation of such an abscess so that patients suspected of having this problem are promptly referred to a surgeon. Most anorectal abscesses are associated with anal fistulas. Occasionally, anorectal abscesses occur in association with other anal and perianal disorders (Table 92.3).

An *anorectal fistula* (fistula-in-ano) is a tract lined by granulation tissue having an internal opening in the anal canal and an external opening in the perianal skin. The internal opening is usually located in one of the anal crypts. If only one opening is identifiable, it is termed an *anorectal sinus*.

Etiology

Anorectal abscesses are more common in men. Most often they represent a primary bacterial infection of anal glands and ducts. Anal glands, thought to be diverticula of the anal canal mucosa, are located along the pectinate line. Many of these glands pass through the internal sphincter into the intersphincteric space. It is presumed that muscle tone in the internal sphincter prevents discharge from the glands causing stasis, dilation, and eventual infection. Bacterial cultures from the abscesses frequently isolate *Staphylococcus aureus, Escherichia coli, Bacteriods* species, *Proteus* species, *Streptococcus* species, or a mixed flora. Since anal glands in the adult are concentrated more in the anterior and posterior walls of the anus, abscesses and fistulas tend to occur in these areas. The majority of abscesses are located in the posterior rectal wall.

Most anorectal fistulas result from abscess formation in the anal glands and drainage through the perianal skin. Therefore, bacterial flora of fistulas are similar to those of anorectal abscesses. Some fistulas are not pyogenic in origin and are associated with inflammatory bowel disease or tuberculosis. Fistulas that do not originate in anal glands may result from diverticular disease, neoplastic disease, or trauma.

Diagnosis

History

Most commonly, a patient with an anorectal abscess will describe an abrupt onset of perianal pain described as full or throbbing and often intensified by sitting, walking, coughing, or defecating. Sys-

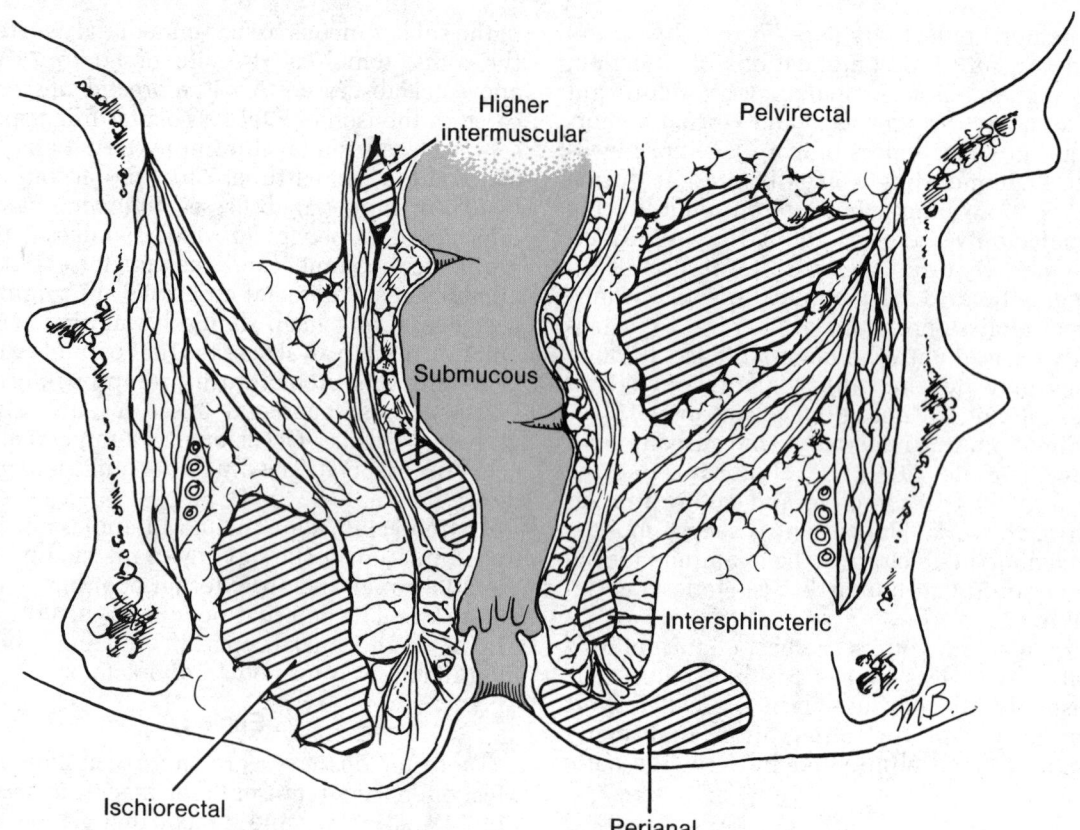

Figure 92.4. Anatomical classification of common anorectal abscesses.

Table 92.3.
Conditions Which May Be Complicated by Anorectal Abscess and Fistula-in-Ano

INFLAMMATORY BOWEL DISEASE
CHRONIC SPECIFIC INFECTIONS (uncommon)
   Actinomycosis
   Tuberculosis
   Lymphogranuloma venereum
   Schistosomiasis (rare)
   Amebiasis (rare)
INFECTION ANATOMICALLY ADJACENT TO THE RECTAL
   AREA AND PRESENTING AS ANORECTAL ABSCESS
   OR FISTULA-IN-ANO
   In women:
      Pelvic inflammatory disease
      Bartholin gland abscess
   In men:
      Infections of a Cowper gland (small periurethral glands)
      Pilonidal sinus (occasionally occurs in females)
FOREIGN BODY (*e.g.*, an ingested bone or a penetrating
   wooden splinter)
TRAUMA
   Surgery (*e.g.*, hemorrhoidectomy or prostatectomy)
   Radiation
   Laceration (*e.g.*, from an enema)
ABNORMALITIES OF HOST DEFENSE (*e.g.*, bone marrow
   aplasia, leukemia or lymphoma, diabetes)
CARCINOMA OF ANUS OR RECTUM

temic symptoms are frequently present and include malaise, chills, and fever. Most patients will have a marked leukocytosis. If the abscess has opened, the patient may complain of a mucopurulent discharge and/or a small amount of blood staining the stool and toilet paper.

An uncomplicated anal fistula may create only minor complaints. The most common symptom is painful perianal swelling. The swelling is frequently intermittent, and intensity of the discomfort is variable. Often the patient complains of purulent anal discharge. A high intramuscular fistula can cause tenesmus or pain during defecation. An anterior fistula in a female can cause dyspareunia.

Rectal Examination

A perianal abscess is easily recognized as a warm, tender, subcutaneous swelling located adjacent to the anus. An ischiorectal abscess may be identified by fluctuation in the ischiorectal fossa felt only on digital rectal examination. Often there is only tenderness detected by pressure to the skin overlying the ischiorectal fossa or the lateral wall of the anal canal during a rectal examination. Higher anorectal abscesses may present few or no findings on perianal examination. However, many of these individuals will complain of severe pain, pyrexia, and exhibit a marked leukocytosis. Under such circumstances, digital examination of the anal canal usually reveals a high, exquisitely tender, posterior rectal wall mass.

The diagnosis of an anorectal fistula is established by inspection and palpation of the perianal area and performance of a digital rectal examination. Frequently the external opening of the fistula in the perianal area can be seen. Digital examination of the rectum may enable identification of the indurated tract of the fistula as it transverses to its internal opening. Anoscopy is required to identify the internal opening.

Treatment

Identification or suspicion of an anorectal abscess with or without a fistula-in-ano should lead to urgent referral to a surgeon. If there is a history of inflammatory bowel disease, a gastroenterologist should also be consulted.

Without adequate drainage an abscess will progress, cause systemic infection, and can rupture spontaneously either externally or internally into deeper areas of the pelvis. An anorectal abscess may also be associated with a rapidly spreading necrotizing infection, destroying large areas of skin, subcutaneous tissue, and fascia. Patients with coincident diabetes mellitus are particularly vulnerable to complicated extensive perirectal involvement.

If possible, the surgeon will open and remove the fistulous tract during the drainage procedure. If simple incision and drainage of an anorectal abscess are performed, greater than 50% of patients will present postoperatively with a fistula-in-ano. If a fistulectomy is performed at the time of drainage, recurrence is uncommon. In the unusual event of a recurrence, referral to the surgeon is again appropriate. Most fistulas require excision. Both internal and external openings must be excised and the tract must be converted into an open wound and the granulation tissue excised or curetted. However, the wound can take 5 to 12 weeks to heal.

PROCTALGIA FUGAX

Occasionally healthy young adults develop the sudden onset of severe rectal pain, variably intermittent and generally lasting less than 30 minutes to 1 hour—proctalgia fugax. It frequently will awaken a patient at night. In women it can occur after sexual intercourse. The pain is described usually as a spasm or a cramp. The problem is not associated with systemic illness and the etiology is uncertain. Proctalgia fugax is thought to result from spasm of a portion of the levator ani muscle. Patients with proctalgia fugax may obtain relief by taking a hot sitz bath or by applying pressure in the perianal area near the site of the discomfort. Occasionally if the attacks are severe and frequent, the patient may find relief by the use of sublingual or cutaneous nitrates. The problem usually persists for many years but then disappears in later life.

RECTAL PROLAPSE

Definition

This problem is occasionally encountered by the general physician who should be able to recognize it and evaluate the need for referral to a surgeon. Prolapse is a protrusion of the rectum through the anus. The protrusion may contain only mucosa, a mucosal prolapse, or it may contain all layers of the bowel wall, a full thickness prolapse (procidentia).

Etiology

Prolapse is more prevalent in women (approximately 80% of the cases) with a peak incidence between the ages of 60 and 80. In men the peak incidence occurs at about the age of 40. The exact pathogenic mechanism of this disease is not known. Factors that are associated with this disease are multiple. Weakening of fascial attachments of the rectum, attenuated muscles in the perirectal area and pelvic diaphragm, straining due to chronic constipation, and even congential fascial defects all lead to the development of rectal prolapse. Prolapse is often observed after severe chronic diarrhea.

Diagnosis

History

Patients have variable symptoms, depending upon the degree of prolapse. There is always some incontinence; at first it is intermittent and consists only of liquid stool. Incontinence is associated with increased intra-abdominal pressure associated with coughing or sneezing. Prolapse will always progress and eventually the incontinence will become continuous. The patient may complain of a sensation of displaced tissue at the time of defecation. Since prolapse is often intermittent, most patients learn to reduce the prolapsed tissues. The patient often may complain of a sensation of inadequate evacuation of the bowel. With more profound prolapse the patient may complain of tenesmus and also develop a continuous mucous discharge. The prolapsed rectum will almost always become excoriated and ulcerated, leading many patients to complain of bleeding. In instances of advanced degree of prolapse the patient may suffer urinary incontinence and in the female there may be associated uterine prolapse. Patients with increasing degrees of prolapse suffer from considerable embarrassment and subsequently will avoid social contact.

Examination

The physician will best recognize rectal prolapse by inspecting the anus when the patient strains in a squatting position. It is usually best to anticipate incontinence with this maneuver. If the prolapse is full thickness (procidentia), concentric folds of the rectal mucosa will be seen, while if there is only mucosal prolapse, only radial folds are seen. Digital examination will almost always reveal a patulous and relaxed anal sphincter that often will admit two to four fingers. Palpation of the protruding tissue between the examiner's finger will provide the sensation of only mucosa in mucosal prolapse and a double layer of bowel wall in full thickness prolapse. The rectal examination in patients with prolapse is usually associated with minimal if any discomfort.

Occasionally prolapsed hemorrhoids may be confused with rectal prolapse, but absence of concentric or radial folds of mucosa and the prominent location of prolapsed hemorrhoids in the left lateral or right anterior or right posterior edges of the anus suggest the proper diagnosis (Fig. 92.3). On occasion, a prolapse may be associated with a rectal tumor. For that reason a sigmoidoscopic examination should be performed on any patient with rectal prolapse.

Treatment

When the prolapse is small and limited to the mucosa, the patient may benefit from the use of stool softeners and by use of an irritant rectal suppository (see Chapter 38) to initiate defecation and thereby avboid straining at stool. If prolapse progresses despite this treatment or if extensive mucosal prolapse is noted, it is appropriate to refer the patient to a surgeon. Redundant tissue may be treated either by banding or sclerosis. Both procedures can usually be performed in the surgeon's office under local anesthesia and are usually successful in preventing progressive degrees of rectal mucosal prolapse.

When procidentia (full thickness prolapse) is present, only operative treatment will be effective. Several procedures are available for restoration of anal continence and reduction of prolapse. Most surgical procedures require hospitalization and general anesthesia, although increasingly, in selected patients, ambulatory surgery is performed. All procedures are successful, with a recurrence rate of less than 4%. One important factor to consider before operation is whether incontinence will be improved. In some centers rectal manometric studies are advocated before surgical intervention. In most instances where the gastroenterologist and surgeon feel that incontinence will not be improved, it may be best to provide the patient with an end colostomy rather than to perform an abdominal proctopexy. All operative procedures for full thickness rectal prolapse require an abdominal proctopexy in which the rectum is secured to presacral fascia either by primary suture or by the use of synthetic mesh. Complications associated with surgical repair of prolapse are those of fecal impaction, presacral hemorrhage, stricture, infection, fistula formation, pelvic abscesses, and intestinal obstruction. The complication rate is less than 1 to 3%. Fecal impaction, however, can occur in up to 6 to 10% of the patients after operative repair. It is important to follow the patient carefully during this period so that this problem may be recognized early and treated appropriately.

General References

Lieberman DA: Common anorectal disorders. *Ann Intern Med* 101:837,1984.
    A well referenced review article.
Thompson JP, Nicholls RJ, Williams CB: *Colorectal Disease.* New York, Appleton-Century-Crofts, 1981.
    An excellent monograph.

Specific References

1. Lewis AAM, Rogers HS, Leighton M: Trial of maximal and dilatation, cryotherapy and elastic band ligation as alternatives to haemorrhoidectomy in the treatment of large prolapsing haemorrhoids. *Br J Surg* 70:54, 1983.
2. Murie AJ, Sim AJW, Mackenzie I: Rubber band ligation *versus* haemorrhoidectomy for prolapsing haemorrhoids: a long term prospective clinical trial. *Br J Surg* 69:536, 1982.
3. Nivatvongs S, Goldberg SM: An improved technique of rubber band ligation of hemorrhoids. *Am J Surg* 144:379, 1982.
4. Quinn TC: Gay bowel syndrome. The broadened spectrum of nongenital infection. *Postgrad Med* 76:197, 1984.
5. *Medical Letter*, vol 17, 1975.
6. Thomson HJ: Rectal disease. Nonsurgical treatment of haemorrhoids. *Br J Hosp Med* 24:298, 1980.

SECTION 13

Gynecological Problems

CHAPTER NINETY-THREE

Birth Control

J. COURTLAND ROBINSON, M.D., M.P.H.

INTRODUCTION

The avoidance of an unplanned or unwanted pregnancy is the decision of the patient and of her partner. In consultation with the physician, she (or they) acquires knowledge of the available contraceptive methods and then is helped in carrying out a satisfactory program.

There are many contraceptive methods. It is important for the physician to understand the limits and risks of all of them to be able to educate his patient fully about her options. The physician must be prepared to deal with patients who have varying knowledge and experience about contraception. Table 93.1 lists the current percentage distribution of use of contraceptive methods by married women in the United States.

Figure 93.1 shows the risks of using various methods of contraception. The figure is similar to that inserted in all oral contraceptive packages that are sold to patients. There is a low mortality rate associated with all methods in patients under 30 so that younger women have a wide choice. On the other hand, a patient who is over 35 years of age has a greater risk with some contraceptives, and the physician must inform his patients of these risks.

The theoretical and actual effectiveness of various methods of contraception is shown in Table 93.2. *Theoretical effectiveness* is determined in very carefully controlled studies in which a method is used exactly as it was designed to be used. *Actual effectiveness* is a measure of what is found when a method is used by large numbers of people in a less controlled manner. Clearly there is very little difference between the theoretical and actual effectiveness of some methods, while others show a considerable difference. This information should be used in helping to educate the patient.

In the physician's office, most often the discussion concerning fertility control will be initiated by the patient, and often it will be the main reason for the visit. However, the physician, as part of a routine health plan, should inquire about the method of contraception that the patient uses, and should offer help in understanding it and in monitoring any possible side effects. While pregnant patients with every kind of serious health condition have been carried successfully to term, there may be an increased risk (19) for the patient or the fetus. Therefore, the physician is responsible for ascertaining that patients who, because of an underlying health problem, do not want the added risk of pregnancy are educated about the various options for birth control.

Once it is established that fertility regulation is desired by the patient, a careful medical history should be obtained, including information about past pregnancies, menstruation, smoking, and family history which might suggest a contraindication to her getting pregnant (see below, "Risks"). A physical examination with special emphasis on the pelvic examination is important. A cancer detection smear and, if indicated (e.g., a patient with multiple sexual partners), a gonococcus culture and a *Chlamydia* smear (see Chapter 94) of the endocervix are suggested. After this evaluation, the physician and patient are ready to discuss the various contraceptive methods and to develop a satisfactory plan.

Although fertility declines with increasing age and eventually is lost, protection is necessary until

Table 93.1.
Contraceptive Use among Married Women at Risk[a,b]

Contraceptive Status	US Women Aged 15–44 (N = 6755)
TYPE USED	92
Oral contraceptive	27
IUD	6
Female sterilization	19
Male sterilization	13
Condom	12
Withdrawal	3
Diaphragm/cap	5
Rhythm	2
Other	5
NONE USED	8
TOTAL	100.0

[a] Adapted from Forrest JD, Henshaw SK: What U.S. women think and do about contraception. *Fam Plan Perspect* 15:157, 1983.
[b] Percentage distribution of contraceptive use among married women at risk of pregnancy (including the contraceptively sterilized), arranged by method, United States, 1982.

menopause (see Chapter 77). The uncertainty about pregnancy is further compounded by the increasing rate of abnormal menstrual cycles, and, in particular, episodes of amenorrhea, as a woman gets older. Missing a period is very disturbing to a woman in the perimenopause unless a very reliable method of contraception is being used.

The *postpartum patient* needs help in getting back on a contraceptive program, and usually her obstetrician will have given her advice in this regard. In general, all methods are suitable for the healthy patient except for the breast-feeding mother, who should avoid the oral contraceptives. Also, the patient wishing to use an intrauterine device (IUD) will need to wait for involution of the uterus—which is usually 4 to 6 weeks postpartum—and, therefore, is at risk for pregnancy until the IUD is inserted.

THE ORAL CONTRACEPTIVE

Mechanism of Action

Oral contraceptives prevent ovulation by inhibition of gonadotropin-releasing factors in the hypothalamus. The principal effect of this inhibition appears to be suppression of the surge in activity of luteinizing hormone at midcycle, thereby removing a major stimulus to ovulation. In addition, oral contraceptives make cervical mucus more viscid and therefore less easily traversed by sperm and have a direct effect on endometrial development, making the uterus less receptive to implantation of the fertilized ovum (3).

Preparations and Dosage Schedules

There are three basic types of preparations of oral contraceptives currently available: a *progestogen only* and either a *fixed or variable combination of estrogen and progestogen*. The progestogen only is taken every day without a break while the combination estrogen-progestogen preparations are taken from day 5 to day 26 of each cycle. The preparations containing either fixed or variable combinations are used far more commonly and should be recommended by the practitioner to most patients wishing hormonal contraception. The biphasic or triphasic variable combinations have been recently introduced into the United States. The biphasic combinations have a constant or near constant amount of estrogen with two sequential doses of progestogen; the triphasics have a constant low level of estrogen and three sequential doses of progestogen. The aim of the bi- and triphasic variability is to minimize side effects (see below), especially the lipid abnormalities. The progestogen-only preparations do not inhibit ovulation, and unwanted pregnancy is 3 to 5 times more likely than it is with the oral contraceptives which contain estrogen and progestogen. They should be prescribed, therefore, only for patients who cannot be given estrogen (e.g., those with a history of thromboembolism) and who prefer an oral hormone to another method of birth control. Many of the currently available oral contraceptive preparations are listed in Table 93.3. Because lower doses of estrogen are associated with fewer side effects, a combination preparation containing the lowest content of estrogen should be the first choice. Currently, a triphasic preparation (e.g., Ortho-Novum 7/7/7 or Tri-Norinyl) is recommended if there is no contraindication (see below); occasionally it will be necessary to change to a higher dose level of estrogen in order to control breakthrough bleeding (see below). However, preparations containing greater than 50 μg of an estrogen should be used only for a short period of time (e.g., two or three menstrual cycles). If higher doses seem necessary because there is no withdrawal bleeding or there continues to be breakthrough bleeding, consultation with an obstetrician-gynecologist is suggested.

In order to suppress ovulation and yet allow periodic bleeding the combination tablet is taken every day for 3 weeks beginning before the development in the ovary of the next follicle. This cycle is accomplished by packaging the tablets for use during either a 21 or 28-day period and having the patient start the medication on the fifth day of her cycle, counting the first day of menstrual bleeding as day 1. An alternative is to start it on the first Sunday which occurs after the onset of a menstrual period. This latter practice allows the packaging of the tablets to provide for the user a minicalendar which minimizes missing a dose. The tablets are arranged in either circles or rows making it easier to use them regularly. The 21-day formulation and the 28-day formulation are packaging techniques to improve compliance. In all 28-day preparations the last 7 tablets have no hormonal effect and are there only

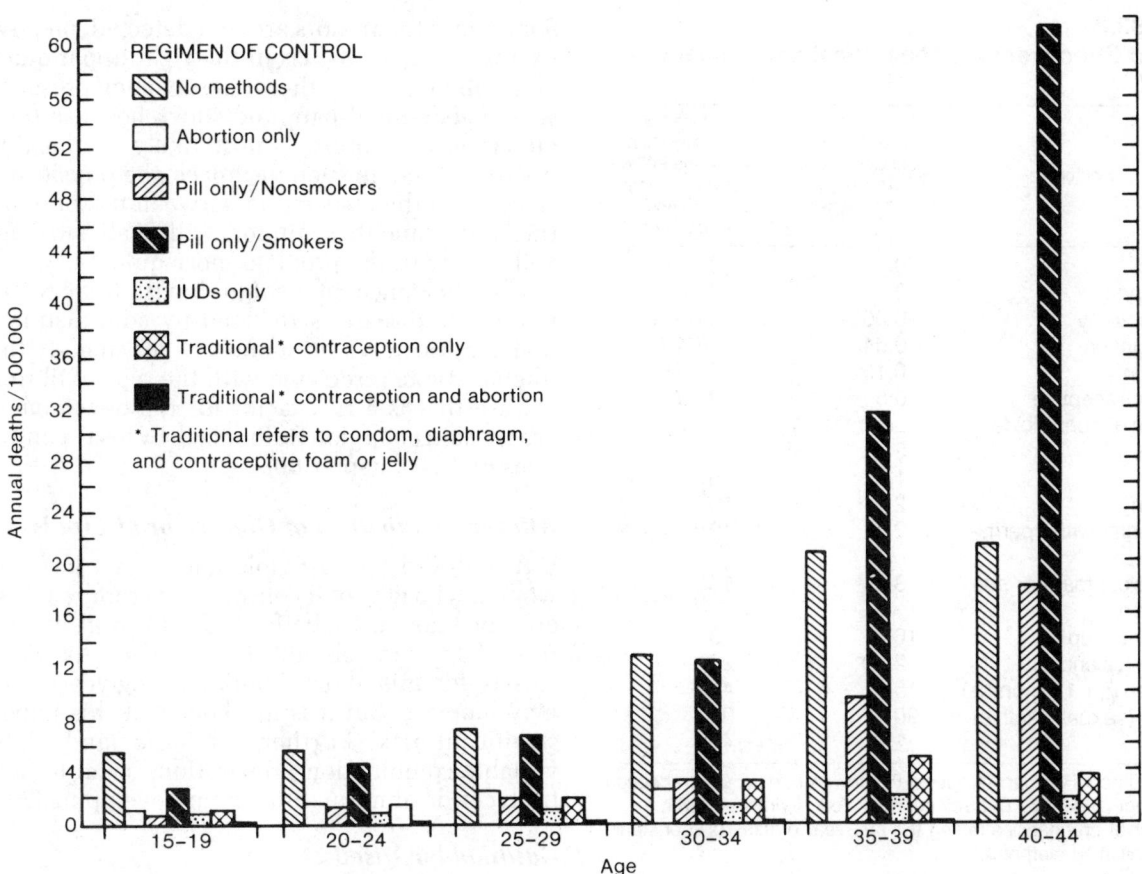

Figure 93.1. Death risk of various methods of contraception. (Data from Tietze C, Lewit S: Life risks associated with reversible methods of fertility regulation. *Int J Gynaecol Obstet* 16:456, 1979.)

to keep the patient on schedule. The drop in hormone level after 21 days produces withdrawal bleeding just as it does normally when fertilization has not taken place.

When a postpartum woman selects an oral contraceptive for contraception, it is initiated within a few days after parturition. Patients who have had a spontaneous or therapeutic abortion may start taking the drug on the first Sunday following the event. However, oral contraceptives are usually avoided in women who are breast-feeding as the medication appears in the milk; also, full time breast-feeding delays onset of ovulation.

Benefits

Oral contraceptives, used correctly, are very effective methods of contraception (Table 93.2). The ability to maintain effectiveness at the newer lower doses has improved the risk-benefit ratio. Reduction of benign breast disease, regular menses, less dysmenorrhea, less menstrual blood loss, and consequently less anemia are well established benefits. Also, patients taking oral contraceptives have a reduced incidence of ovarian cysts and ovarian cancer as well as endometrial cancer and a diminished

incidence of pelvic inflammatory disease (11, 12, 15).

Risks

Oral contraceptives should not be used by women with any of the conditions listed in Table 93.4.

Thromboembolic Disease

There is an increased risk of both venous and arterial thrombosis (and of hemorrhagic stroke) in women taking oral contraceptives (14). The magnitude of the risk is approximately 5 to 10 times that of the general population. The risk is even greater after the age of 35 and is compounded further by the smoking of cigarettes (7). Women who are over 40 or who smoke more than 15 cigarettes a day should be strongly advised to use another contraceptive method. A history of venous or arterial thrombosis or evidence on examination of thrombotic disease is an absolute contraindication to the administration of oral contraceptives. Also, because of the risk of thromboembolism, it is wise to discontinue the use of oral contraceptives for 1 to 2 months before elective surgery and in any patients immobilized for prolonged periods of time (for example,

Table 93.2.
Method Effectiveness: Theoretical and Actual Use Rates[a,b]

Method	Used Correctly and Consistently: Theoretical Effectiveness	Average US Experience among 100 Women Who Wanted No More Children: Actual Effectiveness
Abortion	0	0+
Abstinence	0	?
Hysterectomy	0.0001	0.0001
Tubal ligation	0.04	0.04
Vasectomy	0.15	0.15
Oral contraceptive	0.5	2
Condom + spermicide	Less than 1	5
Sponge	2	10
IUD	1.5	5
Condom	2	10
Diaphragm (with spermicide)	2	19
Spermicidal foam or suppository	3–5	18
Coitus interruptus	16	23
Rhythm (calendar)	2.20	24
Lactation (for 12 months)	15	40
Chance (sexually active)	90	90
Douche	?	40

[a] Adapted from Hatcher RA, Guest F, Stewart F, et al: Contraception Technology 1984–85, 12th rev ed. New York, Irvington, 1984.
[b] Number of pregnancies during the first year of use/100 nonsterile women initiating method.

patients in long leg casts). In such cases an alternate contraceptive method should be recommended.

Hypertension

The risk of developing high blood pressure is increased in women who use oral contraceptives, especially after several years of use. At the end of 5 years it has been shown that the prevalence of hypertension is 3 times that shown after initial exposure. Women with pre-existing hypertension or with a family or personal history of hypertension are probably more likely to develop high blood pressure when they take oral contraceptive hormones. Nevertheless, oral contraceptives can be used by these patients who are at greater risk if their physician measures their blood pressure (or teaches them to do so) every few months. If hypertension increases or develops, it is best to find another contraceptive method (see Chapter 62)

Neoplasia

There is no evidence that cancer is more common in women who use an oral contraceptive preparation. On the contrary, the careful monitoring of women who use this method of contraception may have resulted in earlier detection and easier management of cervical and uterine cancer.

Benign hepatic adenomas have been reported rarely in patients using oral contraceptives (4).

Sometimes the tumors are first detected, on physical examination, as masses in the right upper quadrant of the abdomen. At other times, women present with severe abdominal pain and shock because the adenomas have ruptured (most likely at the time of menstruation). In such instances, the physician who is aware of the association between use of oral contraceptives and these tumors will be able to diagnose and deal with the problem more quickly.

The incidence of benign breast tumors and of fibrocystic disease is reduced by administration of oral contraceptive hormones. Unfortunately the epithelial atypia associated with the type of fibrocystic disease that is a risk factor for the development of breast cancer is not influenced by oral contraceptives (9) (see Chapter 89).

Altered Metabolism of Glucose or of Lipids

A reduced glucose tolerance may be seen in women who take oral contraceptives for reasons that are not known. Diabetics may use oral contraceptives but they should be followed particularly closely for this effect. Similarly, triglyceride levels may increase, but it is unlikely that this imposes a significant risk. Further, triphasic (and biphasic) variable combination preparations seem to prevent triglyceride abnormalities from developing (20).

Gallbladder Disease

There is a 2-fold increase in the incidence of gallbladder disease requiring surgery within the first 1 to 2 years of oral contraceptive use. An estrogen-associated increase in the concentration of cholesterol in the bile has been demonstrated.

Headaches

Headaches, especially migraine headaches, are more common in women who use oral contraceptives. The development of severe recurrent headaches is a reason for the physician to recommend another contraceptive method.

Birth Defects

It has been believed that there is an increased risk of congenital abnormalities in fetuses exposed to exogenous estrogen or progesterone, but this topic is controversial (8). Nevertheless, until the controversy is resolved it would be prudent for the physician to advise patients who comtemplate pregnancy after having taken oral contraceptive hormones to use a barrier form of contraception for 2 to 3 months after discontinuing the oral contraceptive before attempting to become pregnant. This would prevent any risk of congenital abnormality as the result of having taken oral contraceptive agents.

Other Side Effects

In general, minor side effects occur early in the course of taking oral contraceptives and may be

Table 93.3.
Some Common Oral Contraceptives Currently Marketed in the United States[a]

Trade Name	Estrogen	Dose (μg)	Progestogen	Dose (mg)
Ovcon 35	Ethinyl estradiol	35	Norethindrone	0.4
Ovcon 50	Ethinyl estradiol	50	Norethindrone	1.0
Ortho-Novum 7/7/7	Ethinyl estradiol	35	Norethindrone	0.5
	Ethinyl estradiol	35	Norethindrone	0.75
	Ethinyl estradiol	35	Norethindrone	1.0
Ortho-Novum 10/11	Ethinyl estradiol	35	Norethindrone	0.5
	Ethinyl estradiol	35	Norethindrone	1.0
Ortho-Novum 1/35	Ethinyl estradiol	35	Norethindrone	1.0
Ortho-Novum 1/50	Mestranol	50	Norethindrone	1.0
Ortho-Novum 1/80	Mestranol	80	Norethindrone	1.0
Loestrin 1/20	Ethinyl estradiol	20	Norethindrone acetate	1.0
Loestrin 1.5/30	Ethinyl estradiol	30	Norethindrone acetate	1.5
Norlestrin 1/50	Ethinyl estradiol	50	Norethindrone acetate	1.0
Norlestrin 2.5/50	Ethinyl estradiol	50	Norethindrone acetate	2.5
Demulen 1/35	Ethinyl estradiol	35	Ethynodiol diacetate	1.0
Demulen	Ethinyl estradiol	50	Ethynodiol diacetate	1.0
Brevicon	Ethinyl estradiol	35	Norethindrone	0.5
Tri-Norinyl	Ethinyl estradiol	35	Norethindrone	0.5
	Ethinyl estradiol	35	Norethindrone	1.0
	Ethinyl estradiol	35	Norethindrone	0.5
Norinyl 1+35	Ethinyl estradiol	35	Norethindrone	1.0
Norinyl 1+50	Mestranol	50	Norethindrone	1.0
Norinyl 1+80	Mestranol	80	Norethindrone	1.0
Nordette	Ethinyl estradiol	30	Levonorgestrel	0.15
Lo-Ovral	Ethinyl estradiol	30	Norgestrel	0.3
Ovral	Ethinyl estradiol	50	Norgestrel	0.5
Progestogen Only Oral Contraceptives				
Micronor			Norethindrone	0.35
Nor-Q.-D.			Norethindrone	0.35
Ovrette			d-l-Norgestrel	0.075

[a] Adapted from Planned Parenthood Federation of America, 810 Seventh Ave, New York, NY 10019. Published in the *Manual of Medical Standards and Guidelines.*

Table 93.4.
Absolute Contraindications to Oral Contraceptives

Thrombophlebitis or thromboembolic disorders (current or remote)
Cerebral vascular or coronary artery disease (current or remote)
Known or suspected carcinoma of the breast
Known or suspected estrogen-dependent neoplasia
Undiagnosed, abnormal genital bleeding
Known or suspected pregnancy

transient. Thorough education by the physician will increase the likelihood that the patient will tolerate these effects and will continue taking the medication.

Nausea

Nausea occurs in approximately 5% of patients but can almost always be eliminated by taking the contraceptive at bedtime.

Fatigue

Increased fatigability is occasionally described by patients but usually is of short duration.

Change in Menstrual Flow

The most typical pattern is a reduction in the amount and duration of menstrual flow, and this is usually welcomed by the patient. On occaison, there will be no bleeding; and if the patient has taken the oral contraceptive regularly (so that pregnancy is not likely), she can be advised to continue it for another cycle. If she is again amenorrheic, a pregnancy test (see below) should be done. Whether positive or negative, an obstetrician/gynecologist should then be consulted, at least by telephone. If pregnancy is ruled out the patient can either select another contraceptive method or can be placed temporarily on a preparation with a slightly higher estrogen content which results in more menstrual bleeding.

Breakthrough Bleeding

Breakthrough bleeding is most common in the early cycles after initiation of an oral contraceptive. It is of no concern as long as the patient has not missed a dose. Failure to take daily doses increases the chance of breakthrough bleeding, particularly in the early part of the cycle. If a dose or two has been forgotten early in the cycle, the patient should catch up and continue the normal regimen together with temporary use of a barrier form of protection. If breakthrough bleeding continues for several cycles, referral to a gynecologist is indicated to rule out an organic cause and to consider using a higher dose of estrogen.

Weight Gain

About 5% of patients will show some weight gain, sometimes associated with fluid retention.

Vaginitis

It has been difficult to document a close relationship between oral contraceptives and vaginitis. The hormones do alter the vaginal milieu, but vaginitis will develop in only a small proportion of patients. Standard diagnostic methods and subsequent therapy (see Chapter 94) will allow the vast majority of patients to continue to use the oral contraceptive.

Skin Changes

Some patients, especially dark-skinned individuals, will note chloasma (yellowish-brown discoloration of the skin) and a change in hair texture. Chloasma is unlikely to resolve with continued administration of the oral contraceptive and is, therefore, a reason to discontinue it if the cosmetic effect is unacceptable.

Emotional Changes

Some women have become depressed while taking oral contraceptives. Therefore, patients who have a history of depression should be followed especially carefully. If depression develops, the medication should be discontinued.

Effects on Laboratory Tests

Oral contraceptives can alter the results of a number of laboratory tests (16). The alterations reflect physiological changes in the patient in most instances but rarely signify clinically significant disease. Table 93.5 lists alteration in selected laboratory tests.

Drug Interactions

Oral contraceptives may alter the effectiveness of a number of other drugs; and, conversely, a number of other drugs may alter the effectiveness of oral contraceptives. Physicians should investigate the possibility of drug interaction before prescribing any other medication to a patient using an oral contraceptive preparation. Table 93.6 lists drugs which may interact with oral contraceptives (21).

A patient taking oral contraceptives should see a physician twice a year for an interim history (including a menstrual history), an interim physical examination, and any tests warranted by this evaluation. Any possible change in family planning

should be discussed at that time. Once a year a pelvic examination should be done, which should include a cervical smear for cytology (at an appropriate interval, see Chapter 95). Sexually transmitted diseases (see Chapter 94) may need to be screened for if there are multiple sexual partners. Oral contraceptives may be discontinued at any time if pregnancy is desired or another method of contraception is planned. The first few menstrual periods after withdrawal may be heavier than during the time oral contraceptives were used. There is no change in fertility after a course of oral contraceptives compared to the time before their administration.

THE INTRAUTERINE DEVICE

The mechanism of action of the intrauterine device (IUD) is not known, but it is thought to cause a local inflammatory reaction and, in essence, to prevent uterine implantation of the ovum in the uterus (17). The device may also interfere with sperm and/or ovum transport. Devices which contain copper or progesterone are more effective in interfering with implantation.

The IUD is 95 ot 99% effective when properly inserted and monitored.

Types

The Lippes Loop is the most popular IUD in current use. It is a plastic device which straightens out for insertion. With careful monitoring (annual examination, no significant complications, (see below) and continued patient satisfaction) the Lippes Loop may remain in place until another form of contraception is desired or needed or the patient wishes to become pregnant. With proper surveillance it may stay in place for several years (occasionally even 8 to 12). The Cu 7 and Copper T are IUDs containing plastic and copper; they are smaller than the Lippes Loop, but the copper increases their effectiveness. They must, however, be replaced every 3 years. The progesterone-containing IUDs have been withdrawn from the market.

Use and Insertion

If the physician is not experienced in IUD insertion, it is wise to refer the patient to a gynecologist. The IUD is best inserted at the time of a menstrual period (the usual small amount of bleeding associated with insertion becomes a part of the normal menstrual flow; that way, it is assured that the patient is not pregnant; it is easier to insert because the cervix is slightly dilated; and the endometrium is not so hyperplastic as it would be later in the cycle, and therefore bleeding is lessened. The patient thereafter will usually notice some increased

Table 93.5.
Effects of Oral Contraceptives on Selected Laboratory Tests[a]

Laboratory Test	Effects	Probable Mechanism
SERUM, PLASMA, BLOOD		
Albumin	Slightly decreased	Decreased hepatic synthesis
Aldosterone	Increased	Activates renin-angiotensin system
Amylase	Slightly increased (common)	Not established
	Markedly increased (rare)	Pancreatitis
Antinuclear antibodies	Become detectable	Not established
Bilirubin	Increased (rare)	Reduced secretion into bile
Coagulation factors	Increased II, VII, IX, X	Increased synthesis
Cortisol	Increased	Increased cortisol-binding globulin
		Urinary free cortisol unchanged
Folate	Decreased or no change	Decreased folate absorption
Haptoglobin	Decreased	Decreased hepatic synthesis
High density lipoprotein cholesterol	Increased with estrogens and decreased with progestins	Not established
Iron-binding capacity	Increased	Increased transferrin levels
Magnesium	Decreased or no change	Decreased bone resorption
Phosphatase, alkaline	Increased (rare)	Altered secretion in bile
Platelets	Slightly increased	Not established
Prolactin	Increased	Not established
Renin activity	Increased	Increased synthesis of renin substrate
Thyroxine (total)	Increased	Increased thyroxine-binding globulin
Transaminases	Slightly increased	Not established
Triiodothyronine resin uptake	Decreased	Increased thyroxine-binding globulin
Vitamin B_{12}	Decreased	Not established
URINE		
δ-Aminolevulinic acid	Increased	Increased hepatic synthesis
Calcium	Decreased	Decreased bone resorption
Porphyrins	Increased (may precipitate porphyria in susceptible patients)	Increased δ-aminolevulinic acid synthetase
17-Hydroxycorticosteroids	Slightly decreased or no change	Increased binding proteins
17-Ketosteroids	Slightly decreased or no change	Increased binding proteins

[a] Adapted from *Med Lett Drugs Ther* 21:54, 1979.

bleeding with her periods, possibly some increased cramping, and a certain amount of vaginal discharge.

Patient experience. Most often the patient experiences minimal or no discomfort when the IUD is inserted. However, occasionally some cramps are experienced; which often subside in a few hours or days but which rarely may be so severe as to necessitate removal of the device.

The effectiveness of the IUD will be increased if the patient learns to feel for the string that protudes from the cervix and to report when she cannot feel it.

Benefits

The IUD is highly effective in preventing pregnancy. In contrast to oral contraceptives it has no systemic effects and requires relatively little partic-

ipation on the part of the user. It is therefore a preferred option for the woman with a single sexual partner who has completed her childbearing but is not willing to be sterilized.

Risks

Absolute and relative contraindications to the use of an IUD are shown in Tables 93.7 and 93.8. The most common serious side effect is the 2-fold increased incidence of *pelvic inflammatory disease* (1). The patient must be instructed to report any fever, pelvic pain, or discomfort promptly. She must also report any missed menstrual periods since they will indicate that she must be evaluated for pregnancy. Removing the IUD from a pregnant woman will result in an *abortion* in about 25% of patients. If the IUD is in place throughout pregnancy, an abortion

Table 93.6.
Selected Drugs Which May Interact with Oral Contraceptive Preparations (OCPs)

Drugs which may decrease the effectiveness of OCPs resulting in breakthrough bleeding, pregnancy, or both:
A. Well established, relatively commonly occurring drug interactions
1. *Anticonvulsants*—Barbiturates, phenytoin (Dilantin), or primidone (Mysoline)
2. *Antimicrobials*—Rifampicin
B. Reported instances of possible drug interactions
1. *Antimicrobials*
a. (Breakthrough bleeding only)—Neomycin, nitrofurantoin, phenoxymethylpenicillin (penicillin V)
b. (Breakthrough bleeding and pregnancy)—Ampicillin, chloramphenicol, sulfamethoxypridazine (Kynex, Midicel)
2. Others—Chlordiazepoxide (Librium), meprobamate, phenacetin, and phenylbutazone (Butazolidin)
Drugs whose effectiveness may be altered by OCPs:
A. *Anticoagulants*—The effect of anticoagulants may be reduced by the simultaneous administration of OCPs.
B. *Clofibrate (Atromid-S)*—Control of cholesterol and triglyceride levels may be lost when OCPs are simultaneously administered with clofibrate.
C. *Thyroid hormone in patients without functioning thyroid gland*—Mostly a theoretical concern; however, there may be a need for an increased dose of thyroid hormone in patients without a functioning thyroid gland.
D. *Tricyclic antidepressants*—Higher doses of estrogen may inhibit effect of antidepressants, and tricyclic toxicity may be increased.
E. *Caffeine*—There may be decreased metabolism of caffeine induced by OCPs. Patients who take large amounts of caffeine (e.g., 4–8 cups of coffee/day) should be cautioned regarding symptoms of caffeinism.

will occur in about 50% of patients; also, there is an increased risk of septic abortion in this population. The patient who has missed a menstrual period must be evaluated also for *ectopic pregnancy* since the IUD prevents only intrauterine pregnancy. *Uterine perforation*, a rare complication, is most likely to occur at the time of insertion. Finally, the use of the intrauterine device by a young nulliparous patient who has multiple sex partners is associated with an increased incidence of uterine infection.

Monitoring

There should be an annual follow-up at which time there should be a review of any problems, a pelvic examination including a cervical cancer smear, a gonorrhea culture, and detection of the device. The follow-up is best done by a gynecologist if the general physician is not experienced in managing patients with an IUD.

The IUD is easily removed by gentle traction on the string at or around the time of a menstrual period. Removal at this time allows the bleeding associated with removal to be part of the menstrual period. Also, it is easier to remove during menstruation than later in the cycle (see above).

As with oral contraceptives, if a patient terminates this form of contraception other than to attempt

pregnancy, she will need help in choosing another form of contraception.

THE SPONGE

The sponge is a barrier contraceptive device that has recently been approved for over-the-counter purchase. It is a small, donut-shaped, polyurethane plastic device filled with nonoxynol-9 (a spermicidal agent) that is placed high in the vagina prior to intercourse. Unlike the diaphragm (see below), it comes in one size. Studies have suggested 95% effectiveness where there is reasonable care on the part of the user. It may remain in the vagina for only 24 hours but must not be removed before 6 hours after intercourse. It is discarded after removal. If left in place longer than 24 hours, irritation may result. The chief advantage of the sponge is that it is available over the counter, that it may be inserted well ahead of need, and that intercourse may be repeated without further preparation. It is suggested for women having infrequent sexual intercourse, for postpartum patients, and for young women just starting to have intercourse for whom the diaphragm may be too complicated (6). Rare users of the sponge have developed the toxic shock syndrome (see Chapter 94), usually after the device has been used improperly.

THE DIAPHRAGM

The diaphragm is a dome-shaped rubber device which is held open by a metallic band or spring. It is filled with a spermicidal cream or jelly before each use and placed in the vagina over the cervix to prevent sperm deposited during ejaculation from reaching the cervical os. As seen in Table 93.2, the

Table 93.7.
Absolute Contraindications to the IUD

Acute or subacute pelvic inflammatory disease
Abnormal cancer detection smear
Recurrent pelvic infection
Acute cervicitis
Pregnancy
History of ectopic pregnancy
A single episode of pelvic inflammatory disease in a patient who has not had a child

Table 93.8.
Relative Contraindications to the IUD

Patients with severe dysmenorrhea (In the case of dysmenorrhea and mild hyperplasia the progestin-containing IUD has been thought to have a beneficial effect.)
Patients with heavy menstrual flow
Patients with dysfunctional uterine bleeding
Congenital anomalies of the uterus, such as bicornate uterus
Patients with a history of endometrial hyperplasia

theoretical effectiveness is much better than actual effectiveness, as is true of all barrier methods.

The diaphragm is fitted by a physician or his assistant. The device fits in the posterior fornix and tucks up behind the symphysis. The largest device which is comfortable is the proper one to use. The manufacturers of diaphragms have excellent booklets which are useful in helping a patient acquire the skill necessary for comfortable use of this form of contraception. For better effectiveness, the patient should be asked to insert the diaphragm and have the physician or assistant check its placement.

The patient will apply the spermicidal jelly to the inside of the dome and insert it in the vagina. She may insert it as long as 4 hours before intercourse. She should check for position with her finger and allow the device to remain in place for at least 6 to 8 hours following coitus. Repeat intercourse within 6 to 8 hours requires additional jelly without removal. The failure rate increases rapidly when an attempt is made to combine the diaphragm with the rhythm method of contraception.

With care a diaphragm should last 2 years. The patient will need a new fitting if she gains or loses significant weight, has a baby, or has pelvic surgery.

Benefits

The diaphragm is a low cost device that has no major risks other than the higher risk of unwanted pregnancy compared to oral contraceptives or to the IUD.

Risks

Contraindications to the use of the diaphragm are sensitivity to the rubber or to the spermicidal material. Alterations in pelvic shape may also preclude the proper fitting of the different diaphragms available. It is not suited for individuals who will not or cannot touch their vagina as, for example, in patients who are very obese or who have a musculoskeletal disorder.

Some women may report discomfort during the time the diaphragm is in place. This discomfort is most often related to a wrong design or to improper fitting, and re-evaluation usually resolves the problem.

THE CONDOM

The condom is a latex rubber sheath which is phallus shaped and is placed over the erect penis and thus prevents the sperm from remaining in the vagina after intercourse. Its effectiveness can be enhanced if it is combined with application of spermicidal jelly or foam in the vagina. Some care is needed when the penis is withdrawn as the condom may come off. The condom is available in a number of different colors and shapes, and it is the only device advocated as a way of increasing sexual

pleasure for the female partner. Its only side effect is a rare instance of sensitivity to the material. It requires male involvement and so is a good choice for couples who wish to share the responsibility of avoiding a pregnancy. It also is effective in reducing the spread of sexually transmitted disease. Condoms are available at most pharmacies.

BARRIER FOAM OR JELLY

A number of preparations are readily available without prescription which contain a spermicidal material combined with either a cream, jelly, or aerosol (18). The cream or jelly is inserted with an applicator just before intercourse and creates a barrier around the cervical os which theoretically prevents the sperm from entering. The foam material is more likely to remain dispersed and thus to provide better protection.

VAGINAL SUPPOSITORIES

Vaginal spermicidal suppositories are put in place at least 10 to 15 minutes before intercourse (18). This form of contraception may be obtained without a prescription and is especially useful when additional protection is desired at midcycle with the condom or to increase the effectiveness of the diaphragm when repeated intercourse occurs. It is also useful as a temporary aid to contraception when an IUD string is noted to be missing or when the patient is postpartum or has discontinued oral contraceptives. The only problems with its use are sensitivity to the material and a somewhat lower theoretical effectiveness.

RHYTHM

With the discovery of the point of ovulation in the menstrual cycle and the knowledge that sperm have a limited life expectancy, the development of a method of contraception that avoids intercourse at the fertile time was logical. Three methods have been developed:

1. The *calendar method* attempts to establish that portion of the cycle when intercourse is safe. The patient keeps a careful record of the duration of each cycle and then subtracts 18 days from the shortest cycle and 11 days from the longest cycle. This will then give her the beginning and the end of the fertile time. Obviously, the more regular she is, the shorter will be this interval and the better the protection. For example, if the shortest cycle is 27 days; and the longest is 33 days, then she is possibly fertile from day 9 until day 22, or an interval of 12 days. On the other hand, if she is very regular and bleeds every 28 days, her fertile period will be 7 days in duration.

2. The *basal body temperature method* takes advantage of the slight drop in body temperature as-

sociated with ovulation, followed by a rise in temperature of approximately 1°F (0.5°C). The woman takes her temperature each morning from day 3 of the cycle until it has remained elevated to approximately 98.6 to 99°F (36.8–37.2°C) for 72 hours, indicating that she is postovulatory and can resume coitus (the ovum must be fertilized within 24 or 48 hours).

3. The *cervical mucus method* requires the patient to learn, over a number of cycles, those changes which indicate ovulation. She is taught to examine her cervical mucus for clarity. She learns to identify abdominal discomfort associated with ovulation and then to use this information to avoid intercourse when conception is possible. This method requires effort and regular cycles but has been used effectively by many women.

The rhythm method is the only method of birth control approved by the Roman Catholic Church and other religious organizations who oppose contraception. The risk of pregnancy in women who use this method of contraception is relatively high (Table 93.2).

STERILIZATION

Simple methods of permanent contraception are available to both men and women (5, 13). At present in the United States sterilization is the most popular method of contraception in persons over 30. The total number of sterilizations is rising, and at present the rate of elective sterilization is about equal for both sexes.

Patients considering sterilization need very careful education so that they understand its nature and risks. Informed consent is required for these procedures.

Vasectomy

For the male, *vasectomy* is the most popular method and when properly performed has a failure rate of only 1/1000. The complication rate is approximately 4/1000; and, for the most part, complications are minor. They include infection, hematoma, epididymitis, and granuloma formation. Long term serious side effects have not been reported among the very large numbers of men who have had the procedure performed. There was a transient concern, now known to be unwarranted (10), that antibodies to sperm which develop in some men following vasectomy predispose to atherosclerosis.

Patient experience. This procedure is done under local anesthesia and there is minimal operative discomfort. Postoperatively there may be some discomfort, but this is controlled by the use of a mild analgesic, such as acetaminophen. Vigorous physical activity and sexual activity are restricted for 5 to 7 days until the wound has healed. Follow-up visits are necessary so that sperm counts can be performed, and it is usual to require 4 to 6 weeks for the ejaculate to become free of sperm before other methods of contraception can be abandoned.

Reanastomosis of the vas deferens may be accomplished surgically and results in potency in approximately 60% of patients. Vasectomy should, nevertheless, not be undertaken unless the patient genuinely wants permanent sterilization.

Tubal Ligation

For the female *tubal ligation* by either the mini-laparotomy or with the laparoscope is the method of choice (hysterectomy has too high a risk/benefit ratio to make it a satisfactory contraceptive method). The procedure in the female may be carried out either in the immediate postpartum period or at some later time. The overall failure rate is approximately 2 to 3/1000 and is largely a function of the experience of the surgeon. The complications are bleeding, infection, and the additional risk of general anesthesia. Laparoscopy and/or mini-laparotomy under local anesthesia is usually a completely satisfactory way to perform tubal ligation.

Patient expereince. Uncomplicated tubal ligation is generally very well tolerated. Mild abdominal discomfort, when present, lasts usually only for a few days and rarely for a few weeks. Mild analgesics, such as acetaminophen, provide relief. Sterilization is immediate and intercourse is permitted as soon as the wound is no longer painful. Tubal ligation is performed in the first half of the hormonal cycle before ovulation has occurred. This avoids the possibility of fertilization of an ovum occurring a day or two before the surgical procedure. If the woman is using effective contraception, tubal ligation may be performed at any time.

Reanastomosis of the fallopian tubes can be accomplished surgically and results in a significant chance of fertility. The success of reanastomosis depends primarily upon the type and extent of the initial ligation and is not related to the time betwen ligation and anastomosis. Nevertheless, a woman should not undergo tubal ligation unless she genuinely desires premanent sterilization.

The existence of a post-tubal syndrome has now been unequivocally refuted (2). The syndrome was said to be characterized by heavier menstrual bleeding, more pelvic pain, and more discomfort than found in the unsterilized population. Nevertheless, patients should be properly counseled about tubal ligation and if they are, they are almost always satisfied with the results of the procedure.

DIAGNOSING PREGNANCY

For the patient who on the basis of a history and/or examination is suspected to be pregnant, confirmation within a few minutes in the office can be done utilizing one of several urine slide immunological tests for the presence of human chorionic gonadotropin (for example, the Pregnosticon Dri-Dot Test). Six weeks after the first day of the last menstrual period (*i.e.*, 4 weeks after the onset of pregnancy) these tests are highly reliable. Chorionic gonadotropin in urine specimens can also be measured in the office by more sensitive tube tests (*e.g.*, Sensi-Tex) but they require more time (approximately 90 to 120 minutes). They may be used when early pregnancy is suspected and the slide test is negative. These more sensitive tests have been positive as early as 9 days after ovulation. Both the slide and tube test kits are supplied with detailed instructions as well as with a description of any limits of the test. In addition, highly sensitive and highly specific serum radioimmunoassay tests for measuring chorionic gonadotropin are available from many commerical laboratories. These tests may be used if a physician does not have an office kit, if delay for a day or two in obtaining results is not a concern, or if there is some concern about the validity of the urine test kit (*e.g.*, proteinuria is present). Also, sonographic evaluation is without risk and highly accurate provided the pregnancy is of 6 weeks' duration; it is of no value if done before 5 or 6 weeks.

General Reference

Hatcher RA, Guest F, Stewart F, *et al*: *Contraception Technology 1984–85*, 12th rev ed. New York, Irvington, 1984.

> A regularly updated text covering all aspects of contraception. It is highly recommended.

Specific References

1. Burkman RT, The Woman's Health Study: Association between intrauterine device and pelvic inflammatory disease. *Obstet Gynecol* 57:269, 1981.
2. DeStefano F, Huezo CM, Tererson HB, *et al*: Menstrual changes after tubal sterilization. *Obstet Gynecol* 62:673, 1983.
3. Durand JL, Bressler R: Clinical pharmacology of the steroidal oral contraceptives. *Adv Intern Med* 24:97, 1979.
4. Edmondson HA, Henderson B, Benton B: Liver-cell adenomas associated with use of oral contraceptives. *N Engl J Med* 294:470, 1976.
5. Hulka JF: Current status of elective sterilization in the United States. *Fertil Steril* 28:515, 1977.
6. Kafka D, Gold RB: Food and Drug Administration approves contraceptive sponge. *Fam Plan Pers* 15:146, 1983.
7. Layde PM, McCarthy PS, Lord JAH, Smith CFC: Incidence of arterial disease among oral contraceptive users: Royal College of General Practitioners Oral Contraceptive Study. *JR Coll Gen Pract* 33:75, 1983.
8. Linn S, Schoenbaum SC, Monson RR, *et al*: Lack of association between contraceptive usage and congenital malformation of offspring. *Am J Obstet Gynecol* 147:923, 1983.
9. LiVolsi VA, Stadel BV, Kelsey JL, *et al*: Fibrocystic breast disease in oral-contraceptive users. *N Engl J Med* 299:381, 1978.
10. Massey FJ Jr, Bernstein GS, O'Fallon WN, *et al*: Vasectomy and health. Results from a large cohort study. *JAMA* 252:1023, 1984.
11. Ory HW, Forrest JD, Lincoln R: Making choices, evaluating health risks and benefits of birth control methods. New York, The Alan Guttmacher Institute, 1983 (360 Park Ave, NY 10010).
12. Rosenberg L, Shapiro S, Sloane D, *et al*: Epithelial ovarian cancer and combination oral contraceptives. *JAMA* 247:3210, 1982.
13. Seiler JS: The evolution of tubal sterilization. *Obstet Gynecol Surv* 39:177, 1984.
14. Stadel BV: Oral contraceptives and cardiovascular disease (two parts). *N Engl J Med* 305:612, 672, 1981.
15. The Centers for Disease Control. Cancer and Steroid Hormone Study: Oral contraceptive use and ovarian cancer. *JAMA* 249:1596, 1983.
16. *The Medical Letter on Drugs and Therapeutics* 21:54, 1979.
17. *The Medical Letter on Drugs and Therapeutics* 22:86, 1980.
18. *The Medical Letter on Drugs and Therapeutics* 22:90, 1980.
19. Tyson LE (guest ed): Symposium on pregnancy. *Med Clin North Am* 61:1, 1977.
20. Wahl P, Walden C, Knopp R, *et al*: Effect on estrogen/progestin potency on lipid/lipoprotein cholesterol. *N Engl J Med* 308:862, 1983.
21. Westerholm B: Hormonal contraceptives. In Dukes MN (ed): *Meyler's Side Effects of Drugs*, ed 9. Amsterdam, Excerpta Medica, 1980.

CHAPTER NINETY-FOUR

Benign Vulvovaginal Disorders

J. COURTLAND ROBINSON, M.D., M.P.H., AND JOHN R. BURTON, M.D.

INTRODUCTION

Vulvovaginal complaints are very common. The probable anatomical location of the problems underlying these complaints can be appreciated from the report from one facility that of 1000 consecutive patients with vulvovaginal problems, 78% had a cutaneous vulvar disorder, 19% had a significant vaginal component (vulvovaginitis), and less than 3% could not be classified (13) (see Table 94.1).

Anatomy and Physiology (See Fig. 94.1)

The *vulva*, sometimes called the pudendum, consists of the labia majora, labia minora, clitoris, mons, perineal body, and prepuce. Bartholin's glands, vestigial lubricating organs, are located bilaterally on the posterior portion of the fourchette. With certain exceptions, the vulva is really specialized skin. It differs from ordinary integument in that it has an increased concentration of sweat and sebaceous glands and of hair follicles. It has a rich blood supply and an extensive venous plexus; this vasculature engorges the vulva under sexual stimulation. Along with this vascular supply there is also an abundant criss-crossing lymphatic system which provides a rational explanation for the finding that diseases which affect the vulva are almost always bilateral. There is also an extensive nerve plexus which has abundant sensory as well as sympathetic endings, and accounts for the increased sensitivity of the area.

The *vaginal mucosa* is composed of a stratified epithelium, the morphology of which changes when stimulated by estrogen. Determining the ratio of mature cells to less mature cells and the ratio of less mature to basal cells gives a reasonably accurate indication of the amount of estrogen present (see discussion of the maturation index, page 1347). The vaginal mucosa contains no secretory glands but under stimulation by estrogen increases the amount of material that is desquamated which then will allow leukocytes to pass and thus produce a normal vaginal "secretion." The cervix and its glands also contribute to the production of this "secretion."

Bacteriology

The vulva, vagina, and cervix are exposed to the external environment. The cervical canal is the main barrier of the female reproductive system to

Table 94.1.
Causes of Vulvovaginal Problems[a,b]

CUTANEOUS VULVAR DISORDERS (78%)
  Primary cutaneous disorders (70.3%)
  1. Inflammation (10.5%)
     Intertrigo, contact dermatitis, neurotic excoriation, *etc*
  2. Infection (35.3%)
     Bacterial, viral, mycotic, and parasitic
  3. Disorders of pigmentation (3.8%)
  4. Vulvar dystrophy (22.3%)
  5. Neoplasms (28.2%)
  Secondary cutaneous vulvar disorders (7.7%)
  Generalized skin inflammation or infections
VULVOVAGINAL DISORDERS (19.4%)
  Nonspecific vaginitis, candidiasis, trichomoniasis, and senescent vaginitis
UNDETERMINED DISORDERS (2.6%)

[a] Adapted from Tovell HM, Young HJ Jr: Classification of vulvar diseases. *Obstet Gynecol* 21:955, 1978.
[b] Based on experience with 1000 consecutive patients.

the external environment. Above this point, the organs are normally sterile. In the vagina, there are on the average four to five aerobic and a similar number of anaerobic species of bacteria. No organisms are consistently present, except for Döderlein bacilli, which are almost always found (5) and which seem to have a role in maintaining the normal low vaginal pH. Occasionally, even pathogenic organisms, such as *Clostridium welchii*, are present in healthy women, and the healthy vagina will occasionally also be found to contain fungi.

APPROACH TO DISORDERS OF THE VULVOVAGINAL AREA

General Considerations

It is important that the physician educate his patients about the normal variations in the vulvo-

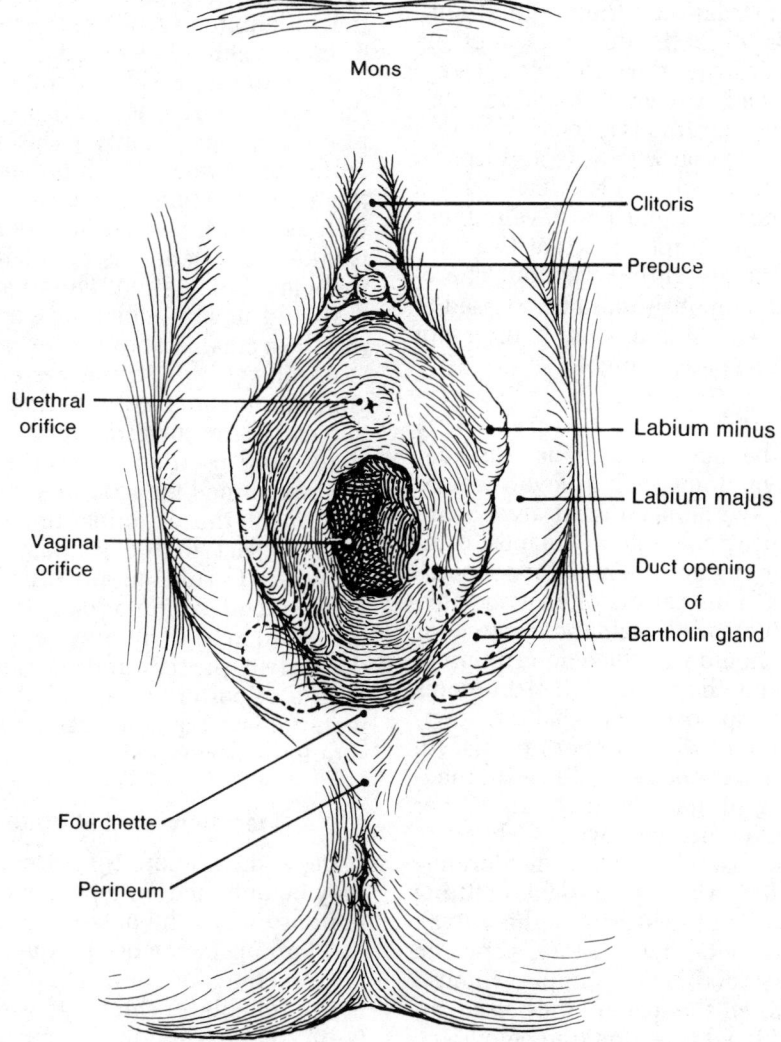

Mons

Clitoris

Prepuce

Urethral orifice

Labium minus

Labium majus

Vaginal orifice

Duct opening of Bartholin gland

Fourchette

Perineum

Figure 94.1. Anatomy of vulva.

vaginal "secretions," the consistency and amount of which will be influenced by menstrual flow, oral contraceptive hormones, antibiotics, and even clothing. Otherwise women may become needlessly concerned about changes that have no real significance.

Hygiene

Cleansing during a bath or a shower is all that is needed to maintain proper hygiene of the vulva. There is no evidence that swimming or tub bathing allows water to enter the vagina and reach the cervix. Routine douching of the vagina is unnecessary; however, some women will wish to douche after intercourse or menstruation. In such circumstances a tepid solution of vinegar (2 tablespoons of white vinegar to 1 quart of water) should be used. Many preparations are available at pharmacies also, but they offer no real advantage. Women should be especially cautioned about excessive douching because this usually results in increased irritation and increased vaginal discharge.

Menstruation

At the time of menstruation either vaginal tampons, absorbent pads, or both provide acceptable ways to absorb the menstrual flow. However, a rare "toxic shock" syndrome has been observed in menstruating women; the syndrome is associated with a pyrogenic exotoxin associated with a staphylococcal infection (2). There is a correlation between the use of highly absorbent tampons and the development of this syndrome. The assumption is that the tampons favor the development of the infection. Therefore, women who use tampons should be advised to change them at least every 8 hours and to interrupt their use by substituting pads at night.

History

A patient with a benign vulvovaginal disorder rarely has systemic symptoms such as fever, weight loss, or malaise. The symptoms almost always are restricted to the vulvovaginal region. The most common complaints reflecting an inflammatory process are itching or burning of the region, often associated with a bad odor, an increased vaginal discharge, or dysuria. The history should include a description of the onset, duration, and character of the symptoms and of their relationship to bowel, bladder, menstrual, and sexual activity. It is important also to question the patient about her general health, medications she is taking or has recently taken, her method of contraception, her vulvovaginal hygiene (frequency of bathing, use of douches, deodorants, tampons, etc), and her wearing of tight clothing (jeans, for example, which might irritate the vulva). If a physician is precise in taking a history, a specific etiology may be suggested. For example, intense itching that began after the patient has used an antibiotic suggests a fungal infection (see below).

Physical Examination

The extent of the general physical examination of a patient with vulvovaginal symptoms depends on the nature of the complaints and on the time that has passed since the last comprehensive evaluation. However, the *abdomen* should always be examined to assess especially the presence or absence of tenderness or of a suprapubic mass. During this phase of the examination, the inguinal nodes should also be evaluated.

Pelvic Examination

The patient is assisted to the lithotomy position and properly draped. A careful *inspection* of the vulva under a good light (such as a gooseneck lamp with a 100-watt bulb) is performed first. The labia are then gently separated to allow a complete examination. It is important to inspect the pubic hair for evidence of folliculitis, not uncommonly restricted to one follicle. The physician should note whether the vulva appears inflamed—more red than normal, tender, edematous, denuded, or excoriated—and the distribution (local or bilateral) of the inflammatory process. The appearance of any discharge should be noted.

After the external examination, the next step is the insertion of a dry, warm *speculum*. If the speculum does not readily pass, it may be moistened with warm water, but lubricant will interfere with the interpretation of a cancer detection smear as well as with growth of microorganisms if a culture is taken. Gentleness is mandatory, especially when there is inflammation. The vaginal wall is inspected; it should have a moist pink appearance, and there may be a small amount of "secretion" present which is usually pooled in the posterior fornix of the vagina. A bimanual examination is then carried out to determine the consistency of the cervix and the size, shape, and position of the uterus. The adnexa are next examined for size, shape, and tenderness. This portion of the examination is usually less useful with respect to the primary complaint, but it is necessary to rule out any other problem.

The *rectal examination* is last; the anus should be inspected to be certain there is no involvement from the vulvar process and palpated to determine the degree of posterior vaginal wall relaxation. If fecal material is present, a screening test for occult blood should be performed.

Specimens for Laboratory Examination

Depending upon the circumstances, specimens may be obtained for a number of laboratory examinations during the pelvic examination:

A *Pap smear* can be obtained at this time if needed for screening for cervical cancer (see Chapter 95); it is not reliable in the diagnosis of specific infection (with the exception of herpes simplex infection where the finding of multinucleated giant cells may be helpful (see below).

A *gonococcal culture* should be obtained routinely in sexually active women at risk for venereal disease (e.g., those with multiple sexual partners or those with known exposures) since gonorrhea is often asymptomatic or is associated with a nonspecific vaginal discharge. The culture should be obtained from the cervical os after removal of the mucus plug, if one is present. The swab should be placed in the end of the cervical canal (leaving the swab in the canal for a moment to absorb bacteria) and immediately plated (by rolling the swab) on a warmed gonococcal transport medium (Transgrow). The medium may be warmed to approximate body temperature by holding the container for several minutes in the hand or axilla. The transport medium supports the gonococcus for at least 48 hours, and transportation to the bacteriological laboratory should be accomplished within this time. A single culture obtained under ideal circumstances will be accurate 90% of the time (1). If gonorrhea is strongly suspected, the diagnostic accuracy will be even greater if a rectal gonococcal culture is obtained at the same time. The swab should be introduced approximately 2 to 3 cm into the anal opening; if the swab, when withdrawn, is visibly contaminated with feces it must be discarded and the test repeated.

A *Chlamydia* smear or a culture also must be obtained at this time if indicated (see below). The directions for both must be followed carefully. The culture is considerably more expensive than is the gonococcal culture and is therefore not obtained routinely, although *Chlamydia* infection appears to be more prevalent than is gonococcal infection.

Following the culture or smear, a specimen of the secretion from the posterior fornix should be obtained and placed on a slide containing a drop of physiological saline and on another slide containing a drop of 10% potassium hydroxide (KOH). When the material is dropped on the KOH slide the presence or absence of a "fishy" odor should be noted; this odor suggests nonspecific vaginitis (see below). After the completion of the pelvic examination the slides should be examined microscopically for *Trichomonas* and *Gardnerella vaginalis* (physiological saline) and *Candida* (KOH). After the "secretions" have been obtained, the cervix is inspected for evidence of inflammation, nodularity, *etc.* Determination of the pH of the secretion using pH tape is helpful, especially in the diagnosis of "nonspecific vaginitis" (see below).

Cultures of the cervical or vaginal "secretions," except for gonorrhea and *Chlamydia*, are not very satisfactory since various bacterial species (such as *G. vaginalis*) may be normal inhabitants of the region; finding them on culture is not proof that they are the cause of inflammation. Culture for herpes simplex, type II, is important in the pregnant patient

(where the disease is more severe and may affect the neonate); but in the nonpregnant patient, the signs and symptoms are usually sufficient to establish the diagnosis (see below).

HERPES SIMPLEX

Manifestations

Herpetic infection is probably the most common of the vulvovaginal disorders. It is sexually transmitted and is associated with significant pain and tenderness of the vulva area. Occasionally, the patient may develop urinary retention because of the intense pain she experiences when she voids and the urine passes over the lesions.

Herpes simplex infection is characterized by single or multiple vesicles, 1 to 10 mm in size and approximately 1 mm deep. Vesicles are most commonly found on the labia minora and the labia majora and around the clitoris. The lesions may be in clumps or, on occasion, they may be linear; in this instance they are diagnostic (Fig. 94.2). With extensive disease the entire vulvovaginal area and cervix may be involved. When there is vaginal and cervical involvement, a white thick exudate may be present that may mimic gonorrhea. Mucosal vesicles ulcerate early; those on the skin remain intact longer

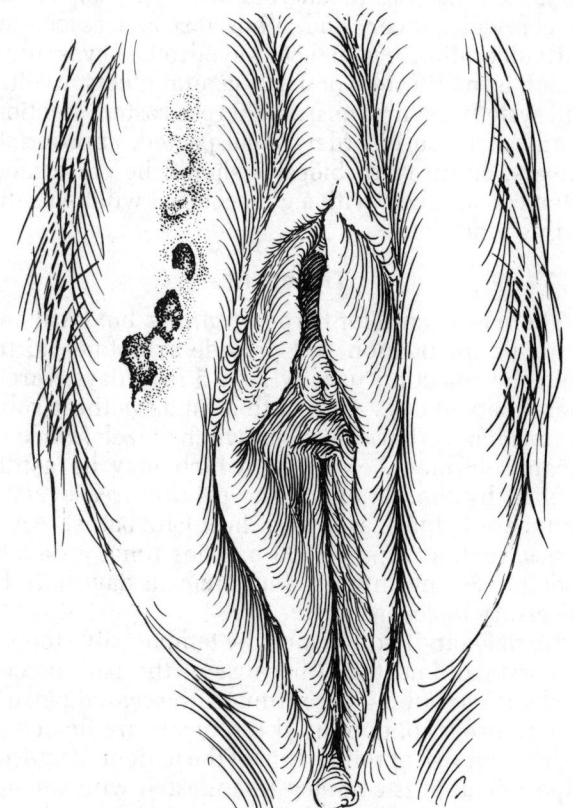

Figure 94.2. Herpes simplex.

but eventually break and become secondarily infected. Often, in patients who are infected for the first time and who have no protective antiviral antibodies, there is an intense inflammatory reaction with vulvar edema, lymphadenopathy, and, rarely, fever. Patients with recurrent disease, who have developed antibodies to the virus, usually have less inflammation and consequently are less symptomatic.

This infection is due to type II herpes simplex virus in 95% of cases; occasionally type I virus, ordinarily found in the mouth, may be incriminated because the patient has participated in oral-genital sexual activity. However, it is rarely possible or necessary for the general physician to arrange for viral cultures in his office so that the diagnosis of herpetic infection is almost always established by the appearance of the lesions and by cytology. In this regard a Pap smear of the vaginal wall, and also of the base of an ulcer, often reveals changes characteristic of herpes simplex (multinucleated giant cells and eosinophilic intranuclear inclusions); and the cytologist, therefore, should be alerted to the possibility of the diagnosis. The measurement of titers of serum antibodies to herpes virus is generally not helpful in diagnosing herpetic infection because of the lack of specificity of the findings.

The *differential diagnosis* in patients who present with herpetic vulvovaginitis includes other sexually transitted diseases (chancroid and syphilis), vulvar or cervical cancer, and other diseases associated with ulceration, e.g., Behçet's syndrome (a vasculitis which is manifest by oral and genital ulcers, uveitis, and systemic symptoms) and herpes zoster infection. If any of these disorders is suspected, appropriate smears, cultures, or biopsies should be performed; often consultation with a gynecologist will be useful at this juncture.

Treatment

There is no cure for herpes vaginitis, but local and systemic medication will provide symptomatic relief. The infection usually lasts 5 or 6 days, rarely more than 10 days. During that time, soothing solutions such as boric acid or witch hazel (Tucks—cream, ointment, or wipes) which may be gently applied by the patient to the painful area every 4 hours are helpful, as is local heat (sitz baths). Analgesics, such as aspirin, 600 mg four times a day, or codeine, 30 mg three to four times a day, may be necessary to control pain.

Sexual activity often must be temporarily stopped or drastically curtailed because of the pain associated with it; but if it is continued, the sexual partner should use a condom until the ulcers are healed to reduce the risk of reinfection of the patient. Bacterial superinfection is common (manifested with the appearance of exudate and crusting of the ulcers), and if it occurs, the application of an antibiotic cream such as Neosporin or Chloromycetin 1% applied three or four times a day will control the secondary infection. Dysuria is frequently improved by the use of sitz baths or by phenazopyridine (Pyridium), 100 to 200 mg three to four times a day for 3 or 4 days.

Acylovir, a topical antiviral agent approved in 1982, is now available in an oral preparation. Oral acylovir can significantly shorten the duration of initial genital herpes infection but is only marginally effective for treatment of recurrent episodes, and therefore in the latter instance should be restricted to patients with frequent severe recurrences (12a). For individuals with severe frequent recurrences acylovir must be patient initiated at the first sign of a recurrence. The dose of acyclovir (Zovirax) for the treatment of genital herpes simplex infections is one 200-mg capsule orally every 4 hours for a total of five capsules/day for 10 days (or 5 days for recurrent disease). Serious side effects have not been reported when used as suggested. The minor side effects of headache, diarrhea, nausea, vomiting, arthralgias, and vertigo are uncommon. Oral acylovir, 200 mg two to five times a day (frequency depends on control of symptoms), is also effective for the *suppression of recurrences* of genital herpes during the period the drug is taken (8). It should not be used beyond 6 months since the long term safety is unknown. Also once the drug is discontinued recurrences return to their pretreatment frequency, and some patients have experienced particularly severe symptoms with the first post-treatment episode. Acylovir does not eliminate the virus and, therefore, is not recommended for continuous suppression except where there are very severe and frequent recurrences; in that instance a gynecological consultation is suggested.

Prognosis

Recurrent infections are common and they seem to be milder than the initial infection (see above). They generally become less frequent as time goes on. However, after 1 year some patients still have recurrent problems and, in these situations, a gynecological consultation is suggested. It has been suggested that herpes simplex virus is associated with the development of cervical cancer. This possibility is currently under debate (6). However, there is no reason to perform more frequent Pap smears for early cancer detection (see Chapter 95) in patients who have had herpetic vulvovaginitis unless the smears show equivocal changes.

MOLLUSCUM CONTAGIOSUM

This benign lesion is probably caused by a pox virus and transmitted by contact, including sexual intercourse. The patient characteristically sees a physician because of a painless new growth in the vulva, perineal area, or thighs. The lesions have a typical appearance, permitting diagnosis by inspection in most instances (Fig. 94.3). The individual lesions are wart-like papules varying from 1 to 10 mm in size. They have a smooth surface and a central umbilical depression which contains a mass of keratin. There may be as many as 20 separate lesions; but, occasionally, the lesions will coalesce. If there is any doubt about the diagnosis, the central cheese-like core may be expressed onto a slide and examined under a microscope using the low power objective. Characteristically large inclusion bodies, which occupy most of the cytoplasm of the cells, will be identified. Occasionally, the lesion resembles bacterial infection, such as folliculitis or furunculosis; but in these instances, the expression of pus from the lesion permits differentiation. If doubt remains regarding the diagnosis, the patient should be referred to a dermatologist or a gynecologist for confirmation or for consideration of a biopsy of the lesion.

The disease is contagious, and because resolution may take many months or even 2 or 3 years, treatment should be given. *Therapy*, which accelerates healing, consists of scraping open the papule (with a scalpel blade), evacuating its contents, and curetting the base. It is *not* necessary to apply irritating chemicals to the lesions (large lesions may need to be anaesthetized before they are opened or curetted). The patient should be seen in 1 week for retreatment of any resistant or new lesions and should be reassured that healing is inevitable. Also the patient should be evaluated for new presence of

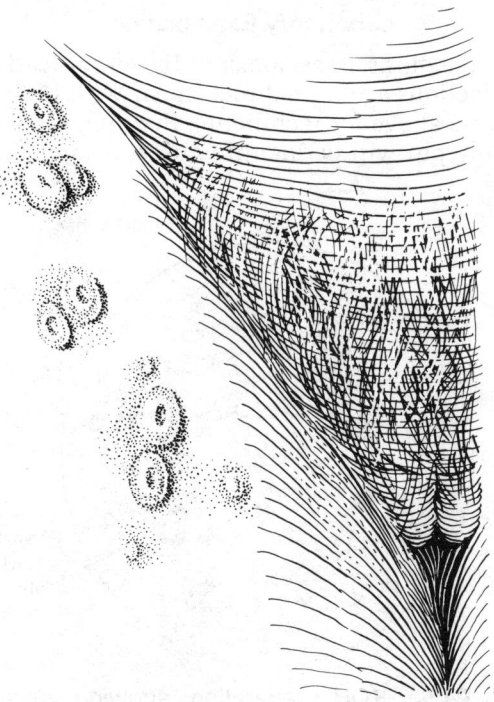

Figure 94.3. Molluscum contagiosum.

another venereal disease that may have been acquired simultaneously. Even if another venereal disease is not found, a culture for gonococcal infection (see above) and a serologic test for syphilis should be obtained and the latter repeated in 1 month if initially negative. The patient's sexual partner should be evaluated, if possible, as occasionally lesions of molluscum contagosium are found on the penis, or evidence of another venereal disease may be found.

CONDYLOMATA ACUMINATA (VENEREAL WARTS)

This common disorder is caused by a papovavirus and is transmitted sexually. This viral infection appears to be more prevalent now, and, importantly, it may be related to the subsequent development of cervical dysplasia (see Chapter 95) (12). It occurs usually during the reproductive years and is most commonly seen in association with other vulvovaginal infections (including candidiasis, trichomoniasis, *G. vaginalis* infection, gonorrhea, or syphilis). It occurs more frequently in pregnancy and has a more active course in pregnant women.

The patient most often complains of a new growth on her vulva, perineum, or anus; and there is often associated itching and a vaginal discharge. These symptoms may be part of an associated vaginal infection or may represent infection in the crevices of the wart. Often there will be a history of warts on the penis of the sexual partner, who should also be evaluated.

The examination is characteristic and is almost always diagnostic. A wart of 1 to 2 cm usually first appears on the labia, frequently about the posterior introitus, but then spreads, with discrete or congruent lesions appearing on the perineum, anus, vagina, and cervix. They may coalesce into a cauliflower-like lesion which may become huge (Fig. 94.4).

Treatment

Treatment of the warts is best accomplished by painting them carefully with a 20% tincture of podophyllum. This solution is very irritating: it commonly causes transient discomfort and will burn normal skin if applied to it. If such contamination does occur, the skin should be washed promptly with alcohol and then with water. The podophyllum should be left on the warts for 8 to 12 hours and then removed with soap and water. During that time, the patient should not engage in sexual intercourse. The patient should be seen every 5 to 7 days for retreatment until healing occurs. If her sexual partner has warts, he should be treated also and he should use a condom during intercourse until healing is complete.

Podophyllin is not suitable for eradication of large

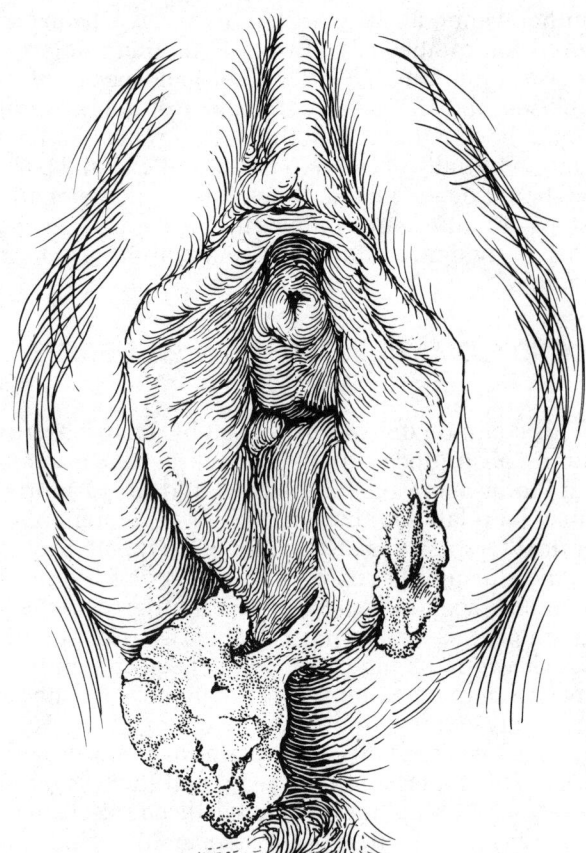

Figure 94.4. Condylomata acuminata.

warts (greater than 2 to 2.5 cm) on the cervix or vagina. Also, podophyllin has been reported to cause fetal abnormalities and should not be used during pregnancy. In these instances, referral to a dermatologist or a gynecologist is suggested for evaluation and for consideration of treatment using other modalities, such as cryosurgery, laser surgery, electrodesiccation, or simple surgical excision.

CANDIDIASIS ("MONILIASIS")

Candidiasis is a common vulvovaginal fungal infection that is seen more commonly in women who are in their reproductive years as well as in women with diabetes and/or immunological deficiencies (such as patients receiving corticosteroids or cytotoxic chemotherapy). The infection is caused by the yeast *Candida albicans* which has no true mycelial form; because of this, it is properly referred to as candidiasis rather than moniliasis, which implies infection by true mycelia. The incidence of candidiasis approaches 8% of women in the reproductive period, but as many as 25% of infected women are asymptomatic (3, 10).

The sources of the organism are not precisely known. It is likely that most organisms derive from the gastrointestinal tract where they are normal inhabitants. The organism very often may be cultured from the feces if the patient has been taking broad spectrum antibiotics. During intercourse, infection may be passed to the male, who may harbor it asymptomatically and thus may reinfect his partner or other women with whom he is sexually intimate.

While infection may occur *de novo*, there is a predisposition to infection in women who are being treated with broad spectrum antimicrobials (especially tetracycline), corticosteroids, those who are pregnant, or, as above, those who have diabetes mellitus—all of which change the vaginal milieu.

Symptoms

Patients complain typically of vaginal burning and itching, and of a thick vaginal discharge that, however, may be less voluminous than it is in *Trichomonas* infection (see below). Painful intercourse may be particularly disturbing.

Physical Examination

Examination may reveal an inflamed vulva, especially in older individuals. When vulvitis is present, red vesicular lesions spreading out from the vulva may also be seen, sometimes resembling intertrigo, from which they must be differentiated. (see Chapter 100). The vaginal walls are often intensely inflamed and covered with a curd-like, thick adhesive material. Occasionally, the actual discharge may be thin, but the thick curd-like material will be seen adhering to the intensely inflamed vaginal wall.

Laboratory Examination

The diagnosis is established by identification of the infectious agent on direct smear with the use of KOH (see above for technique). Budding spores and pseudohyphi will be identified (Fig. 94.5). Cultures

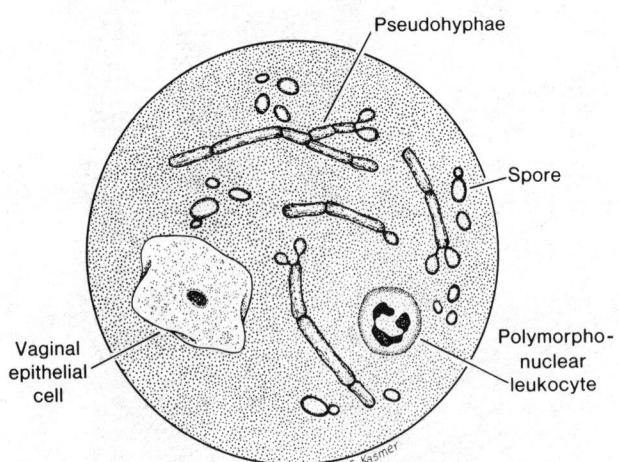

Figure 94.5. KOH preparation, showing yeast and pseudohyphi.

are not usually necessary and will not differentiate between pathogenic and nonpathogenic species of fungi.

Treatment

Treatment is aimed at eradication of the infection and requires attention to predisposing factors. Antimicrobials may have to be stopped or changed to an agent with a less broad spectrum; diabetes mellitus should be controlled (see Chapter 72); and glucocorticosteroids may need to be withdrawn or reduced in dose if possible. When vaginal candidiasis occurs in pregnancy, an obstetrician/gynecologist should be consulted. If there are no predisposing factors or if these are factors that cannot be controlled, specific antifungal agents are usually very effective.

The patient is instructed to administer the contents of one vaginal applicator or one vaginal suppository of miconazole nitrate (Monistat) daily at bedtime for 7 days. Monistat is very effective (4). Clotrimozole (Gyne-Lotrimin), one applicator of cream or a vaginal tablet used daily at bedtime for 3 to 7 days, is an effective alternative. In general, the creams are more effective for severe disease especially when the vulva is involved; the tablets or suppositories are easier to use and are satisfactory for milder forms. Nystatin (e.g., Mycostatin or Nilstat) vaginal tablets, one tablet twice daily, are also effective but require 2 weeks of use. Combination preparations containing an antifungal, an antibacterial, and a steroid agent (such as Mycolog) are not recommended; in fact, the application of any potent steroid in areas of skin folds may lead to serious cutaneous atrophy.

If there is a great deal of pain or if pruritus is intense, nonspecific therapy to control these symptoms is an important part of the initial treatment. The patient may benefit from tepid baths or from compresses of water and oatmeal (e.g., Aveeno) or of witch hazel. The use of daily vaginal douches with vinegar water (see page 1338) and the application of plain talc (e.g., Johnson's Baby Powder) may help also. If pain and itching are not controlled, excoriation and secondary bacterial infection may seriously complicate the situation. The patient should avoid the use of moisture-retaining underwear, such as nylon, and use more porous cotton materials. The sexual partner should use a condom until the infection is eradicated so that he does not become an asymptomatic reservoir for reinfection of the patient.

Because of the significant amount of itching associated with candidiasis, most patients will telephone their physician immediately if the condition recurs to ask for a renewal of the prescription for antifungal medication. A single renewal in this manner is acceptable; but if symptoms again recur, the patient should be seen by the physician and evaluated. The frequent use of vaginal antifungal agents may result in a secondary irritative vaginitis. Resistance to eradication should raise suspicion of diabetes mellitus, and a fasting blood sugar should be obtained. Furthermore, the patient may have become reinfected either from her sexual partner or from her gut or urinary tract, or both. Since it is difficult to prove any of these situations, a reasonable approach in resistant cases is to treat both the patient and her sexual partner with oral nystatin (such as Mycostatin) suspension or tablets, 500,000 units three times a day until the infection has been eradicated, which may require 2 to 3 weeks. Sometimes resistance to treatment results because of a mixed infection; this occurs most often when trichomoniasis (see below) emerges after control of candidiasis (which frequently overgrows and camouflages *Trichomonas* infection initially).

If a *Candida* infection cannot be eradicated, referral to a gynecologist is recommended. If the gynecologist confirms the diagnosis, he may consider the application of 1% gentian violet solution, which is very effective but causes considerable staining and requires some experience in application.

TRICHOMONIASIS

Trichomoniasis is an extremely common infection, second only to herpetic infection as a cause of vulvovaginitis; it is the most common vulvovaginal infection associated with a discharge. The protozoan flagellate, *Trichomonas vaginalis*, grows best in an environment which is slightly more alkaline than the normal vagina, but it will grow sometimes at a lower pH. The source of infection is not clear. The organism can exist in the vagina without causing symptoms; when the vaginal environment favors its growth, it multiplies and produces the discomfort which brings the patient to the physician. Men can harbor the organism, and treatment of the sexual partner is, therefore, important. The trichomonad has been implicated as a factor in the development of cervical dysplasia, but the significance of this is unknown.

Symptoms

The patient complains usually of a copious discharge, vaginal burning, discomfort, and, often, a musty odor. Itching is less common than it is in patients with candidiasis. Occasionally, minor vaginal bleeding will occur. Some patients will describe symptoms of urethral irritation—dysuria, frequency, and urgency—while others will experience pelvic discomfort. Dyspareunia is very common.

Physical Examination

Examination of the patient reveals a vaginal discharge which may be very profuse and may have a slightly dry musty odor. The discharge is usually greenish and frothy, but there is a wide variation. The mucosal surfaces appear moist but are only moderately inflamed. The cervix, in about 10% of patients, will show a pathognomonic "strawberry" pattern (reddish coloration with punctation).

A sample of the discharge should be examined under the microscope with physiological saline as a diluent; the motile protozoan will be identified under a lower power objective (Fig. 94.6). The preparation should be thin so that the pathogens are not obscured. It is important to use saline rather than water as a diluent as water causes swelling and immobilization of the organism, making diagnosis very difficult. Also, if the saline is too cold, it may inhibit the motility of the organisms. Staining of the slides is of little use, and a culture (using special media) also is rarely necessary and is probably best left to a gynecologist. Dead trichomonads can be seen on a Pap smear, but such a finding does not correlate very well with clinical symptoms.

Treatment

The therapy for this condition is metronidazole (Flagyl). This compound is readily absorbed from the intestinal tract. Its use topically in the vagina is not very effective and is not recommended. There have been disturbing reports of carcinogenic and mutagenic activity of Flagyl in animal and bacterial models. The use of the drug in pregnant women is, therefore, controversial; it is definitely contraindicated in the first 12 to 14 weeks of pregnancy. However, after 30 weeks, if there is significant discomfort and because of a suspected role of trichomonad in premature rupture of membranes, it is reasonable to prescribe Flagyl in consultation with the gynecologist-obstetrician.

Flagyl is given in a dose of either 2 g once by mouth or 250 mg three times a day for 7 days, along with a similar regimen for the sexual partner. Patients are to be cautioned to avoid alcohol because the combination frequently results in nausea and vomiting. The response to Flagyl is dramatic and often is permanent. The patient should avoid synthetic underwear that results in a more moist vulvar environment and should use cotton materials. The sexual partner should use a condom during sexual intercourse until the infection has been eradicated.

Initial symptomatic relief can be obtained with acid douches twice daily for 2 or 3 days (2 tablespoons of white vinegar in 1 quart of warm water). Commercial douches are more expensive, may be more irritating, and are not recommended.

Since no immunity develops, *recurrences* are common, especially in women with multiple sexual partners. When there is inadequate initial response to treatment (10% of patients do not respond to Flagyl) or when there is reinfection and only a single sexual partner, there may be an associated nonspecific vaginitis which sould be confirmed and treated.

"NONSPECIFIC VAGINITIS" (GARDNERELLA VAGINALIS)

Evidence over the past several years has accumulated indicating that *Gardnerella vaginalis* (formally called *Haemophilus vaginalis* or *Corynebacterium vaginale*) in combination with an anaerobic organism causes most, if not all, cases of "nonspecific vaginitis" (11). *G. vaginalis* is a very small, nonmotile, Gram-negative rod. The infectious agent may be transmitted by contact with contaminated objects, such as towels or toilet seats, but the major route is by sexual intercourse. To flourish, the organism requires an estrogen-enriched vaginal environment; for this reason, infection is seen almost exclusively in women who are in their reproductive years.

Infection with *G. vaginalis* is found in up to 20% of women in the reproductive period, but less than 25% of these individuals have symptoms.

The infection is limited to the vaginal surface, and *symptoms* are usually less prominent than they are in candidiasis or trichomoniasis. The patient may describe slight burning and pruritus, but usually the major complaint is of a discharge which characteristically is grayish and has an unpleasant odor.

Examination may show redness and/or some tenderness of the vagina, but often no abnormalities are seen. The discharge may be minimal or may be a sticky flour-like paste, adhering to the vaginal wall.

The *diagnosis* is made by finding a constellation of manifestations and by ruling out other infections. The clinician should first prepare and examine saline wet mounts and KOH preparations. Candidiasis and trichomoniasis will be ruled out by this method, and the saline preparation may show the short rods. In addition, under the low power objective and with

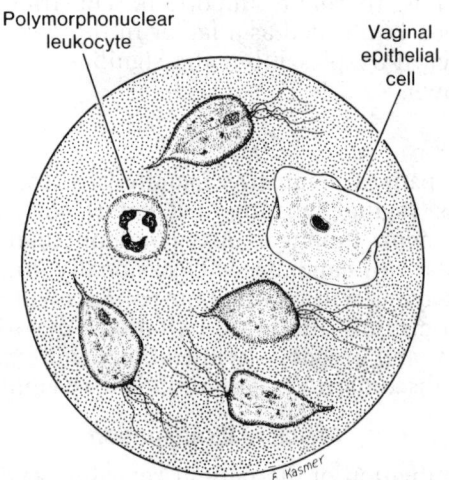

Figure 94.6. Saline preparation showing trichomonads.

Polymorphonuclear leukocyte

Vaginal epithelial cell

reduced light, *clue cells* (stippled epithelial cells) may be seen (Fig. 94.7); they are due to the bacteria adhering to the cell surface. A Gram stain is not usually very helpful. Culture is usually not necessary.

The application of KOH will often intensify the "fishy" odor of the secretions. Also, the pH of the vaginal secretions is always greater than 5.0 in *G. vaginalis* infection, but this finding is not specific.

Treatment

Treatment (when the diagnosis is confirmed by clinical and microscopic criteria) is best accomplished with metronidazole (Flagyl), 250 mg three times daily for 5 days (7). The patient should use cotton underwear. A gentle douche with vinegar (2 tablespoons of white vinegar in 1 quart of warm water) once or twice a day for 1 to 2 days will help to control symptoms if they are particularly uncomfortable. The sexual partner should use a condom during sexual intercourse until the infection has been eradicated. If there is recurrent infection the partner should be treated with metronidazole (Flagyl), but that is not necessary at the time of the initial episode.

As with other vaginal infections it takes time for complete healing to occur. Symptoms suggesting recurrent infection should be evaluated before treating as metronidazole will occasionally cause a superinfection with *Candida*. If this occurs, local treatment for candidiasis is indicated (see above). Vinegar douching will help to maintain a normal bacterial flora while healing is occurring.

Occasionally the physician will suspect (after ruling out trichomoniasis and candidiasis) "nonspecific vaginitis" but is unable to establish the diagnosis (see above). In this situation, the discharge may be *increased normal "secretion"* and there is a danger of inappropriate treatment. The patient should, in such circumstances, be reassured that there is no true infection and advised to use cleansing douches

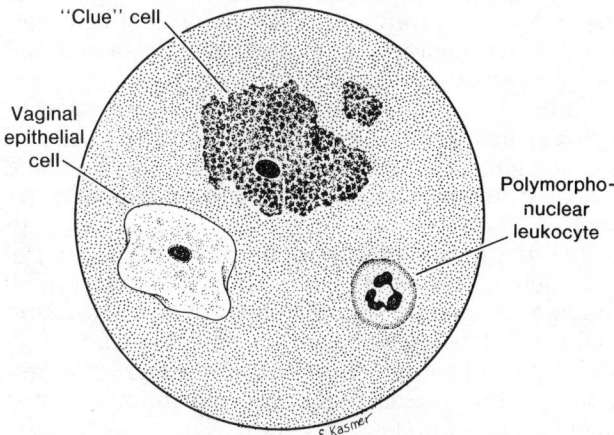

Figure 94.7. "Clue" cells.

(see above) daily for 2 or 3 days if the discharge is distressing. If symptoms do not improve, consultation with a gynecologist should be requested.

GONOCOCCAL INFECTION

Gonococcal infection is quite common in women, particularly those with multiple sexual partners. Infected patients may have no symptoms, symptoms due to direct inoculation of organisms (vaginal, rectal, or pharyngeal), or symptoms due to local or distant spread of infection. Transmission of gonorrhea from infected men to uninfected women or to other men (homosexuals) is efficient and occurs in 90% of exposures; transmission from infected women to uninfected men is somewhat less efficient, occurring in about 20 to 50% of exposures (the diagnosis and management of gonorrhea in male patients are discussed in Chapter 27).

In the majority of women the infection remains asymptomatic, so that routine screening for women who are at risk (see above) is important. In some 10 to 20% of injected women, for unknown reasons, the organism spreads, usually after a menstrual period, to the fallopian tubes and initiates acute salpingitis and acute pelvic inflammatory disease (PID). Early consultation and prompt therapy will significantly reduce the serious sequelae of this condition, *i.e.*, ectopic pregnancy and sterility. A single mild episode of acute salpingitis will cause infertility in approximately 5% of patients. This figure rises to almost 100% with severe and/or repeated episodes of PID. Other forms of dissemination (arthritis-dermatitis, endocarditis) are uncommon.

Clinical Manifestations

Clinical manifestations include vaginal symptoms (onset or increase in vaginal discharge, vaginal itching, dyspareunia, dysuria, vague lower abdominal pain), anorectal symptoms (pruritus, painful defecation, rectal fullness), and pharyngeal symptoms (see description of this entity, Chapter 28). PID usually begins shortly after a menstrual period and is characterized by fever, nausea, abdominal pain and tenderness, and marked tenderness of the pelvic organs to touch or motion. In addition, there may be a cervical discharge, alteration in the menstrual pattern, elevation of the white blood cell count, and evidence of enlarged adnexa. Symptoms and signs of the arthritis-dermatitis syndrome (polyarthralgia, tenosynovitis of elbows, wrists, or knees; skin lesions which begin as tiny red papules or petechiae, then either disappear or evolve through vesicular and pustular stages to develop a gray necrotic center; and, occasionally, purulent monarthritis) usually develop 1 or more weeks after the initial infection.

Diagnosis

Cervical culture for gonorrhea should be obtained as described above in all women at risk for venereal infection with or without symptoms. When the disease is suspected strongly because of new symptoms, the addition of a rectal culture will increase detection by about 10%. The value of routine culture of the rectum in asymptomatic patients is less certain. Gram stain of the cervical material, when properly done, is highly reliable and may be used as a basis for diagnosis and treatment before the results of culture are obtained. In most states the physician is required to report to the local health department a positive smear even if the culture is negative. Pharyngeal cultures are indicated in those who give a history of oral-genital sexual activity.

Management

The management plans appropriate for the various forms of gonococcal infection are summarized in Table 94.2. Follow-up cultures should be done 1 week after treatment is completed. Women being treated for gonorrhea should either abstain from sexual intercourse or assure that their partner(s) uses a condom until the result of the 1-week "proof of cure" culture is known. Furthermore, the partner(s) should be treated for presumed infection (see Chapter 27 for treatment of male partners).

Whenever gonorrhea is confirmed, the patient should be reported to the local health department so that sexual contacts will receive appropriate evaluation and treatment.

CHLAMYDIA TRACHOMATIS INFECTION

In recent years the role of *Chlamydia trachomatis* in the production of genitourinary infections has been clarified (9). Although the incidence of such infections is not known precisely, it is thought to be 2 to 3 times that of gonorrhea. Like gonorrhea, women with multiple sexual partners are more likely to be infected.

Lower genital tract infection is more indolent than is gonorrhea but symptoms are similar in both conditions: lower abdominal pain, dysuria, increased vaginal discharge, and rarely fever. On examination the cervix appears red and edematous and often bleeds when a Pap smear is done. The cervical discharge is less profuse than it is in patients with gonorrhea. Unlike gonorrhea, spread of the infection beyond the genitourinary tract does not seem to occur.

Chlamydial infection has been diagnosed with absolute certainty only by culture, but the media are expensive and the growth is slow, so culture is not recommended unless the patient does not respond to initial therapy. However, commercial laboratories increasingly have available diagnostic methods of detecting *Chlamydia trachomatis* in urogenital swab specimens. A *fluorescent antibody staining technique* and an *ezyme immunoassay* are the two methods currently available; both are quite accurate and relatively inexpensive. The laboratory should be consulted regarding the method of specimen collection and handling. When chlamydial infection is diagnosed or suspected (or if it is uncertain whether gonorrhea (see above) may be present in a patient with lower genital tract infection), a tetracycline is the drug of choice. Tetracycline or doxycycline for 7 days, to which both gonococci and *Chlamydia* are sensitive, are adequate (see Table 94.2). *Chlamydia* are not sensitive to penicillin so that that drug is best used in patients who almost certainly have gonorrhea (abrupt onset with relatively severe symptoms, positive cervical smear, or evidence of disseminated disease). Pregnant women should be treated with a sulfonamide (e.g., sulfisoxazole 0.5 g four times a day), but otherwise a tetracycline is preferred because other organisms that cause lower genital tract infection (e.g., *Ureaplasma urealyticum*) are sensitive to it. Because the male sexual partner is often infected as well (see Chapter 27), he should be treated also.

FOREIGN BODY

Another occasional cause of vaginal dicharge in adults, although it is much more common in children, is a foreign body. Lost tampons, forgotten diaphragms, and other smaller objects will be easily found by examination. Symptoms will improve after removal of the foreign body and, because secondary bacterial infection is also present, a triple sulfa cream (Sultrin), twice daily for 3 to 4 days, or povidone (such as Betadine or Femidine) douch, once daily for 3 to 4 days, may accelerate healing.

ATROPHIC VAGINITIS

This condition is very common and is caused by estrogen lack. It is primarily a problem of older, postmenopausal women, but may be seen in younger women who are postoophorectomy or who have been breast-feeding for a long period.

Estrogen deficiency results in a thinning of the vaginal vulvar epithelium, a loss of capillary network, and a decrease or loss of vaginal "secretions" as well as a rise in the pH of the vagina.

Patients with this problem complain of dyspareunia, dryness of their genitalia, and occasionally of some vaginal mucoid discharge which may be blood streaked. Symptoms are more prominent than are signs.

Examination reveals atrophy of the vulva and of the vagina, loss of the subcutaneous fat, and a reduction in the size of the clitoris. The vulvar skin and vaginal mucosa appear dry and pale, and adhesions may develop. There may be superficial erosions on the vaginal wall, and uterine atrophy is noted on bimanual examination.

The *diagnosis* is established by the history and

Table 94.2.
Management of Gonococcal and *Chlamydia* Infections

UNCOMPLICATED INFECTION (asymptomatic, cervicovaginal, or anorectal symptoms; pharyngitis)
1. a. Procaine penicillin, 4.8 million units IM plus 1.0 g of probenecid 30 minutes before injection,
      or
   b. Ampicillin, 3.5 g orally in a single dose plus 1.0 g of probenecid orally,
      or
   c. Amoxicillin, 3.0 g orally in a single dose plus 1.0 g of probenecid orally,
      or
   d. Spectinomycin, 2.0 g IM (single dose) for penicillin-resistant gonococci, or for patients allergic to penicillin who are pregnant or are intolerant of tetracycline.
2. Treat partner(s) appropriately.
3. Follow-up culture 1 week after completing treatment.
4. Report to local health department.

POSSIBLE GONORRHEA OR *CHLAMYDIA* INFECTION (a common situation with manifestations of infection present but without culture confirmation)
1. a. Tetracycline 500 mg orally 4 times a day for 7 days,
      or
   b. Doxycycline, 100 mg twice a day for 7 days.
2. Treat partner(s) appropriately.
3. Follow-up culture for gonorrhea or smear for *Chlamydia* 1 week after completing treatment (*Chlamydia* culture is much more expensive and time consuming than gonorrhea culture and is therefore probably not appropriate to obtain routinely).
4. Report to local health department

PELVIC INFLAMMATORY DISEASE (gonorrhea or *Chlamydia* or both may be cause)
1. Ambulatory treatment[a]
   a. Cefoxitin (Mefoxin), 2 g IM once
      and
      Probenecid, 1 g orally once followed by
      Doxycycline, 100 mg orally twice a day for 10 days
      or
   b. Tetracycline, 500 mg orally 4 times a day for 10 days.
   c. Daily contact or observation to assure improvement.
2. Indications for hospitalization
   a. Diagnosis uncertain (to exclude appendicitis, ectopic pregnancy, nongonococcal pelvic inflammatory disease, pelvic abscess).
   b. When an intrauterine device is present, in which case the addition of metronidazole (Flagyl) is recommended.
   c. Diagnosis is certain but patient is toxic or unable to follow ambulatory treatment reliably.
   d. Patient does not respond promptly to ambulatory treatment.

ARTHRITIS-DERMATITIS SYNDROME
1. In patients without known allergy to penicillin or probenecid.
   a. Hospitalize: Aqueous crystalline penicillin G, 10 million units IV/day for 3 days or until there is significant clinical improvement. This may be followed with ampicillin, 500 mg 4 times a day orally to complete 7 days of antibiotic treatment,
      or
   b. Hospital or ambulatory treatment: Ampicillin, 3.5 g orally, plus probenecid 1 g, followed by ampicillin, 500 mg 4 times a day orally for at least 7 days (may be given to an ambulatory patient who is not toxic, is reliable, and is contacted/examined daily).
2. In patients allergic to penicillin and/or probenecid.
   a. Tetracycline, 500 mg 4 times a day orally for at least 7 days (avoid in pregnancy, see below),
      or
   b. Erythromycin, 500 mg orally 4 times a day for 7 days,
      or
      Spectinomycin, 2.0 g IM twice a day for 3 days.

[a] Adapted from *Med Lett* 25:5, 1984.

physical examination and by ruling out an associated infection (if a discharge is prominent) by obtaining a wet mount and a KOH preparation. If there is some doubt about the diagnosis, determination of the *maturation index* may be helpful in confirming it. This technique takes advantage of the effect of estrogens and progesterone on the vaginal epithelium and is an index of the percentage of basal, intermediate, and superficial cells. A scraping of the vaginal wall is fixed on a slide with Pap smear fixative and sent to a cytologist. In atrophic vaginitis a typical report would be approximately 80-20-0, respectively, of basal-intermediate-superficial cells; in contrast, a well estrogenized vagina would show the percentage of cells as approximately 0-20-80.

Treatment

Atrophic vaginitis is treated with vaginal estrogens to improve vaginal epithelization. An estrogen-containing cream (such as Dienestrol or Premarin) should be prescribed, one or two applicators full every night for 2 to 3 weeks until symptoms have improved, and then the dose is gradually tapered, omitting one dose/week every 1 or 2 weeks until the patient is administering only one dose/week. Treatment should thereafter be continued as long as is necessary (usually as long as sexual activity continues); but the need for it should be reassessed every 3 to 6 months. A maturation index may be helpful when the patient reports no improvement, for evidence of estrogenization suggests the existence of another problem. The estrogen present in vaginal creams is readily absorbed into the circulation; therefore, precautions should be taken just as they are with the continued use of oral estrogens (see Chapter 77).

If the problem is mild the patient may be able to relieve dyspareunia by using a water-soluble lubricant such as K-Y jelly, available at pharmacies, just before sexual intercourse.

URETHRAL SYNDROME

This syndrome includes dysuria, frequency, and urgency, but "significant" bacterial infection is not identified. It has many causes, but vulvar, vaginal, or cervical inflammation accounts for a significant proportion of cases. This syndrome is discussed fully in Chapter 27.

CUTANEOUS VULVAR LESIONS

There are a large number of cutaneous vulvar lesions which may cause the patient to seek medical advice. In these situations, the *history* is very informative. There is usually a variable degree of itching, and often the patient says she has a feeling that her genitalia feel "different."

The history should include information about perineal hygiene, the use of perineal perfumes or recently acquired undergarments, medications, and general health. The *objective data base is developed* by a careful examination of the pelvis, cancer smears when needed, and in certain cases, biopsies of suspicious lesions (performed by the general physician if he is experienced or, if not, by a gynecologist or a dermatologist).

Cutaneous vulvar lesions can best be divided into

five primary disorders on the basis of their etiology (Table 94.1, page 1337): inflammation, infection, neoplasia, dystrophy and altered pigmentation (13). Molluscum contagiosum and condylomata acuminata are discussed on pages 1340 and 1341, respectively.

Inflammation

Intertrigo and contact dermatitis are the most common noninfectious problems of the vulva that are associated with inflammation.

Intertrigo

Intertrigo is an eruption that occurs on body surfaces where the skin rubs together. It is especially common in the vulva and inguinal area of obese patients. It appears as an erythematous sharply defined area, often with secondary excoriations. Infectious diseases such as candidiasis which may also have satellite lesions, tinea, or erythrasma should be ruled out by scraping the margin of the lesion and making a KOH preparation for the microscopic diagnosis of fungal infection or by showing coral red fluorescence using a Wood's lamp (an inexpensive lamp available from physician supply stores) for the diagnosis of erythrasma (caused by a *Corynebacterium* species) as discussed in Chapter 100.

Noninfectious causes of intertrigo, such as psoriasis and seborrheic dermatitis, also should be considered, and a search for other areas of involvement should be made (see Chapter 100). If there remains doubt about the diagnosis, a dermatologist should be consulted.

The treatment of various forms of intertrigo is discussed in detail in Chapter 100.

Contact Dermatitis

Contact dermatitis located in the vulva and perineum is quite common and may be either primary irritant or allergic in type. Soaps and deodorants are common irritants; and perfumes (such as in sprays, soaps, toilet tissue, pads, and tampons), dyes, rubber (in clothing), and drugs (both topical and systemic) are common allergens.

In acute contact dermatitis the eruption begins in the area of contact and is characterized by erythema, edema, and the formation of vesicles or bullae. Often, secondary excoriations and infections are present. In chronic cases, the diagnosis is more difficult and the changes are more indurated and less vesicular and edematous.

The management of contact dermatitis is discussed in Chapter 100.

Infection/Infestations

Vulvovaginal infections are sometimes limited to the cutaneous vulvar area; but they are managed in the same way as the more widespread vulvovaginal infections discussed above. In addition to the causative agents already discussed, parasitic infestation should be considered. Pediculosis and scabies are common and are usually associated with severe pruritus, and often the former simultaneously involves the umbilicus and breast. The diagnosis and management of these parasitic infestations are discussed fully in Chapter 100.

Miscellaneous Conditions

Bartholin Cysts

These are common swellings of the vulva. The Bartholin glands are located posteriorly on either side of the fourchette (see Fig. 94.1) and open onto the vaginal wall. They may become infected with a variety of organisms including *E. coli*, gonococcus, and *Trichomonas*, as well as staphylococci and streptococci. Where there is intense infection or abscess formation, the patient should be referred urgently to a gynecologist for evaluation and possibly marsupialization of the abscess under local anesthesia. The gynecologist will probably use systemic antimicrobials. If the patient is seen after resolution of the acute inflammation, the symptoms are not dramatic and often the swelling is episodic. The location of the lesion is diagnostic. Sitz baths several times a day may provide temporary relief, but recurrence is likely; when the cyst is large, the patient should be referred to a gynecologist for consideration of marsupialization or removal.

Sebaceous Cysts, Lipomata, and Fibromata

All of these conditions may occur in the vulvar area. When they are distressing to the patient or when there is doubt about their nature, referral to a gynecologist or a dermatologist for evaluation and consideration for removal is suggested.

Malignant disease of the vulvar area is rare and affects primarily postmenopausal women. Nevertheless, early detection may remarkably improve survival. Since vulvar malignancies have a precancerous phase, early detection is the responsibility of the physician performing the annual health maintenance assessment (see Chapter 95). Any abnormal appearing tissues, such as leukoplakia or Bowen's disease (which is observed as a superficially ulcerating red plaque which often appears granular and occasionally is secondarily infected), should raise concern, and the patient should be referred to a gynecologist for evaluation and, usually, biopsy.

Vulvar Dystrophy

Vulvar dystrophy is a condition best managed by a gynecologist or a dermatologist because it is chronic and very difficult to eradicate. Patients are older and usually complain of persistent itching and soreness; examination reveals whitish, thickened skin and excoriated, often atrophic areas.

A biopsy of these lesions is necessary for proper classification.

PSYCHOSEXUAL ASPECTS OF VULVOVAGINAL COMPLAINTS

Because of the normal variation in vaginal "secretions" and the normal physiological variations in the vulvovaginal region, a physician should not suggest treatment for an organic vulvovaginal disorder unless its diagnosis is confirmed. The vulvovaginal region is often the focus of symptoms of an emotional disorder. For example, sexual contact with a new partner often produces vulvovaginal symptoms in which the findings are normal and a sense of guilt is the real etiology. Also patients may develop persistent symptoms due to an unverbalized desire to avoid sexual intercourse. A psychological problem may affect a woman of any age; the diagnosis should be considered when the patient seeks appointments with the physician and no organic cause can be identified. The psychiatric section (Section 2) of this book deals in detail with diagnosis and management of psychological disorders.

General References

Gardner L, Kauman RH: *Benign Diseases of the Vulva and Vagina.* ed 2. Boston, GK Hall, 1981.
> This extensively illustrated textbook is a valuable resource covering diagnosis and treatment of common disorders of the vulva and vagina.

Friedrich EG Jr: Vulvar diseases. In Friedman EA (ed): *Major Problems in Obstetrics and Gynecology.* ed 2. Philadelphia, WB Saunders, 1983.
> An excellent monograph.

Specific References

1. Caldwell JG, et al: Sensitivity and reproducibility of Thayer Martin culture media in diagnosing gonorrhea in women. *Am J Obstet Gynecol* 109:463, 1971.
2. Chesney PJ, Davis JP, Pordy WK, et al: Clinical manifestations of toxic shock syndrome. *JAMA* 246:741, 1981.
3. Davis BA: Vaginal moniliasis in private practice. *Obstet Gynecol* 34:40, 1969.
4. Eliot BW, Howat RC, Mack AE: Comparison between effects of nystatin, clotrimazole and miconazole on vaginal candidiasis. *Br J Obstet Gynaecol* 86:573, 1979.
5. Larsen B, Galask RP: Vaginal microbial flora: practical and theoretic relevance. *Obstet Gynecol* 55:1005, 1980.
6. Lauke A: Herpes virus—cancer of the cervix. In LA Phillips (ed): *Viruses Associated with Human Cancer*, New York, Marcell-Decker, 1982.
7. Pheifer TA, Forsyth PS, Durfee MA, et al: Nonspecific vaginitis: role of *Haemophilus vaginalis* and treatment with metronidazole. *N Engl J Med* 298:1429, 1978.
8. Reichman RC, Badger GJ, Mertz GJ, et al: Treatment of recurrent genital herpes simplex infections with oral Acyclovir. *JAMA* 251:2103, 1984.
9. Schachter J: *Chlamydia* infections. *N Engl J Med* 298:428, 490, 540, 1978.
10. Sobel JD: Vulvovaginal candidiasis—what we do and do not

know. *Ann Intern Med* 106:390, 1984.

11. Spiegel CA, Amsel R, Eschenbach D, *et al*: An aerobic bacteria in nonspecific vaginitis. *N Engl J Med* 303:601, 1980.

12. Syrjanen, KJ: Current concepts of human papillomavirus infections in the genital tract and their relationship to intra-

epithelial neoplasia and squamous cell carcinoma. *Obstet Gynecol Surv* 39:252, 1984.

12a. *The Medical Letter on Drugs and Therapeutics* 27:41, 1985.

13. Tovell HM, Young HJ Jr: Classification of vulvar diseases. *Clin Obstet Gynecol* 21:955, 1978.

CHAPTER NINETY-FIVE

Early Detection of Gynecological Malignancy

J. COURTLAND ROBINSON, M.D., M.P.H.

PREVENTIVE GYNECOLOGY

The benefits of preventive medicine are especially applicable in office gynecology. Ambulatory care provides an ideal setting in which preventive measures can be carried out, particularly with respect to the early detection of cancer of the organs of reproduction.

The female organs of reproduction are important sites for the development of malignancies. Twenty percent of cancers found in women involve the genital organs (8). Overall 5-year cure rates are in the range of 55 to 60% and are related to the stage of the disease upon discovery. A most impressive event in the past 30 years has been the decline in mortality of cancer of the cervix and uterus, attributable primarily to earlier detection (7). As with the breast, having the patient herself take responsibility for looking for abnormalities in a regular and systematic manner and, equally important, the regular examination by a trained person, have resulted in the diagnosis of a higher proportion of lesions at early stages, at which time cures are much more likely (3).

DETECTION OF VULVAR LESIONS

The vulva, like the skin, has a premalignant phase in the development of epidermal carcinoma. Lesions of the vulva represent about 4% of all cancers of the pelvic organs. The invasive stage is seen primarily, but not exclusively, in postmenopausal women. *Intraepithelial carcinoma of the vulva* is the term now used to include diseases that were once called Bowen's disease, erythroplasia of Queyrat, squamous cell carcinoma *in situ*, and Paget's disease. While intraepithelial lesions can be distinguished by microscopic examination, they often appear to the physician to be well defined innocent lesions of the vulva or mucous membranes. They may be red, raised, granular, or velvety lesions, or simple white patches, or a mixture of these, with or without superimposed ulceration and crusting. The lesions are often asymptomatic but may be associated with itching or soreness. The physician should be suspicious when anything is seen other than well developed intact skin and mucous membrane and especially if the lesions are chronic and unresponsive to topical treatment. Biopsy should be performed by the general physician if he is familiar with the technique. Often the application of 1% toluidine blue to the lesions helps to localize the more active areas for biopsy. If the physician is unfamiliar with the biopsy technique, he should refer the patient to a gynecologist for consultation, biopsy, and treatment. Intraepithelial lesions are best managed by a gynecologist; either local surgery and/or a topical antineoplastic drug (such as 5-fluorouracil) will be used. Continued follow-up is necessary to detect recurrence.

Prevention of advanced disease requires that the patient be taught to examine her vulva periodically by use of a mirror, and to report to her physician any changes in the external genitalia. It is important that the physician examine the patient promptly if a change is noted and that periodic examination be performed when there are no complaints. Special care must be taken in older women who are often reluctant to complain of a vaginal or vulvar problem. Examination by both patient and physician requires a good light and separation of the labia majora and labia minora.

DETECTION OF CERVICAL LESIONS

Invasive *epidermoid carcinoma* of the cervix is the second most common malignancy of the reproductive organs (endometrial cancer is the first) (8); there are 16,000 new cases in the United States every year. Significant reduction in mortality and morbidity has been achieved by vigorous promotion and acceptance of the annual pelvic examination in combination with the cancer detection smear (Pap smear) (7).

The incidence of *preinvasive cervical cancer* (i.e., *in situ* cancer) seems to be increasing among younger patients (1). The etiology of this condition is still not settled, but at present, sexually transmitted diseases, particularly herpes simplex and human papilloma virus, along with trauma and/or irritation of the squamocolumnar junction are thought to be factors. The major risk factors are onset of sexual activity at a young age, early childbearing, and multiple sexual partners. The malignancy involves the squamocolumnar junction which is exposed in the young patient to an acid milieu resulting from estrogen stimulation, to foreign material secondary to intercourse, and to the trauma of childbearing (1). All of these are common events for most women; therefore, the reason why less than 1% of women develop invasive neoplasia of the cervix is still a mystery. *Metaplasia* in the cervix is a normal response; but in 2 to 6% of women *dysplasia* occurs; and it is in this group with a dysplastic cellular process that neoplasia may arise. It is in this situation that cytological screening becomes important since the changes are not visible to the naked eye.

The cancer detection smear, when properly obtained, is from 80 to 90% effective in identifying a problem (1). Proper technique requires an appropriately shaped plastic or wooden stick which abuts the cervical os and permits the squamocolumnar junction to be scraped. The anatomical relationship of this junction varies in the adolescent, the sexually

active woman, and the postmenopausal woman (see Fig. 95.1). When the junction is not seen (e.g., in an atrophic cervix), a cotton-tipped stick should be used. If no inflammation is present, secretion in the posterior fornix may be submitted along with the material from the squamocolumnar junction. Vaginal bleeding within 24 hours, douching, and vaginal medication are relative contraindications to obtaining a Pap smear since the vast majority will be technically unsatisfactory and will necessitate a repeat examination. Also, since lubricant will interfere with the reading of the smear, its use should be avoided, if possible. In patients with atrophic vaginitis, where lubricant may be necessary, it should be used sparingly to avoid contaminating the smear. The physician should select a cytology laboratory that has satisfactory quality control, use the proper fixative techniques required by the laboratory, and learn the systems of reporting. It is important for the physician to provide the laboratory the patient's age, the date of her last menstrual period, and to comment on the presence or absence of infection. The laboratory report should state whether the sample was satisfactory or unsatisfactory. An unsatisfactory slide must be repeated.

The cytologist's report usually will describe the results as negative (with or without inflammation) or as showing atypia, dysplasia, or changes suggestive of cancer; these findings may be quantitated as mild, moderate, or severe. Some laboratories are now using the cervical intraepithelial neoplasia (CIN) classification. The previous four-level classification (mild, moderate, severe, and intraepithelial carcinoma) is now replaced by CIN I, CIN II, and CIN III.

Patients with *significant dysplasia* (CIN II or greater) or with *moderate or severe atypia* should be referred for further evaluation of the cervix. The *colposcope* (Fig. 95.2) is an optical system which permits the magnification by 10 to 20 times of the appearance of the cervix and the squamocolumnar junction (Fig. 95.3) During colposcopy the woman is in the lithotomy position with a vaginal speculum in place; the procedure requires 5 to 10 minutes. Colposcopy is very important in helping the gynecologist to decide the site from which abnormal cells have arisen and to guide the location of a cervical biopsy.

Patients with *minimal dysplasia* (CIN I) or with inflammation (such as trichomoniasis) can be managed by local treatment of the infection (see Chapter 94), and a follow-up smear should be taken in 3 to 4 months. If the follow-up report is negative, the patient may return to annual examinations. If on follow-up examination the smear continues to show persistent mild dysplasia or mild atypia, the patient should be referred to a gynecologist for colposcopic examination. Patients in whom the report indicates

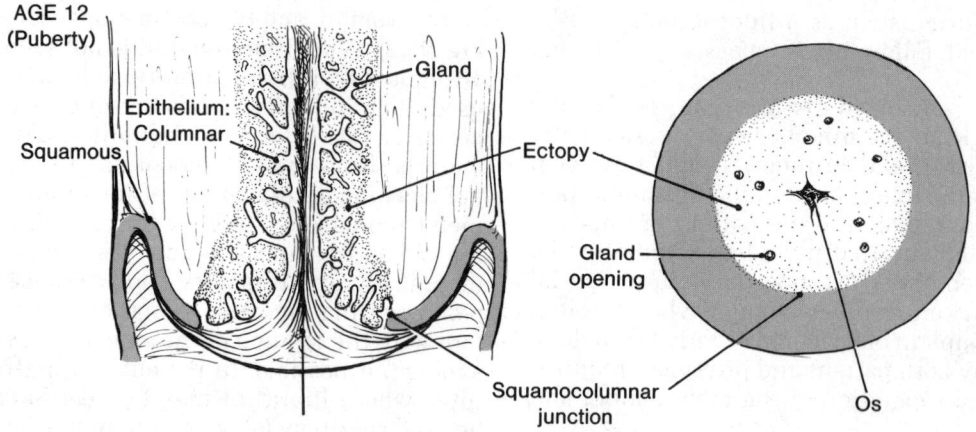

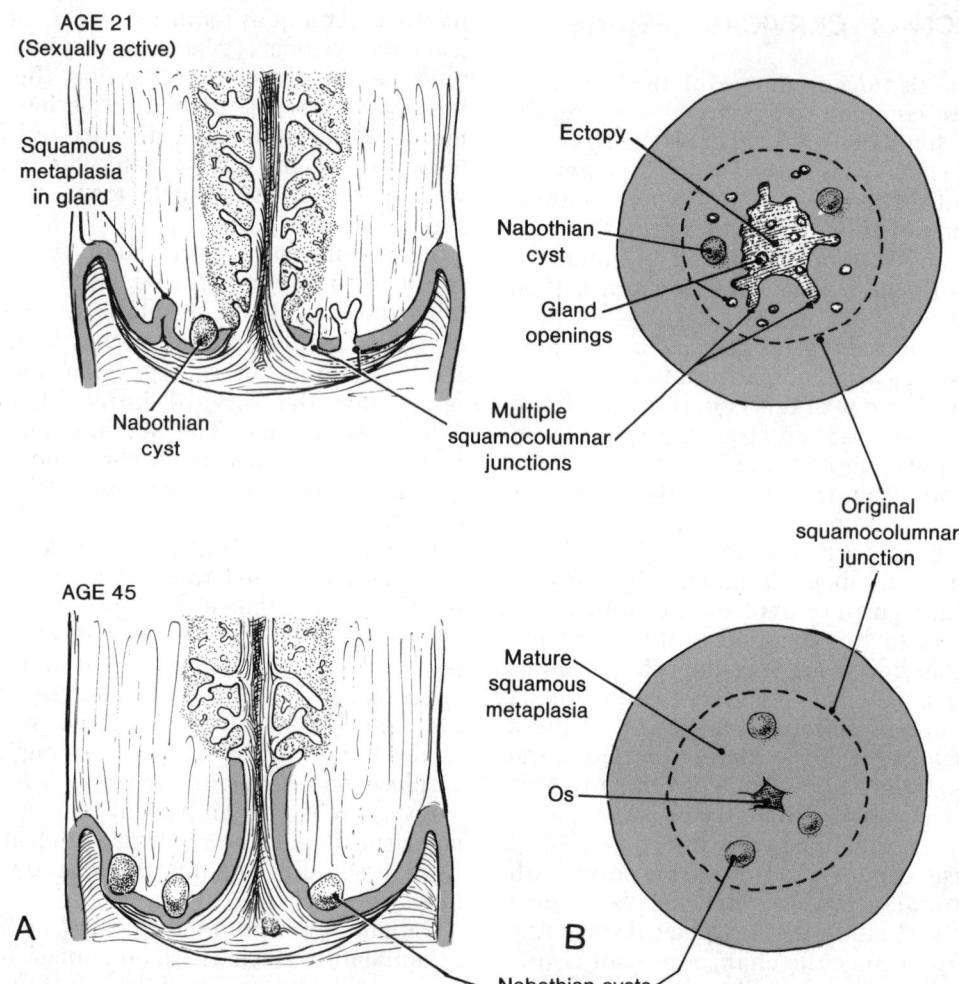

Figure 95.1. The uterine cervix in women of various ages. *A.* Coronal section of the cervix and vaginal vault. *B.* Vaginal view of the cervix. (Redrawn from Briggs RM: Dysplasia and early neoplasia of the uterine cervix. A review. *Obstet Gynecol Surv* 34:70, 1980.)

only inflammation with no reference to dysplastic cells do not need colposcopic examination. Also, asymptomatic patients with a report indicating the presence of a few yeast or trichomonad cells do not require therapy.

The suggested *frequency* of obtaining a cancer detection smear is controversial (2,6); it depends in part on the patient's virginity and age. Pap smears are not necessary until sexual activity beings (except for adolescent and young women who have been

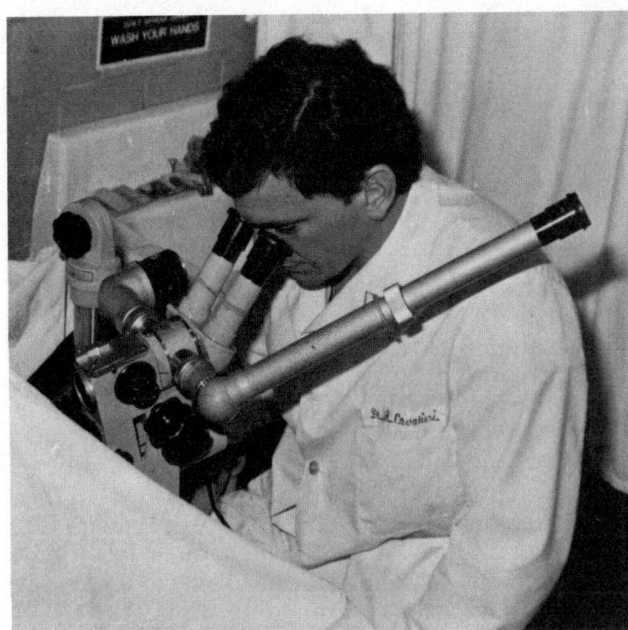

Figure 95.2. Use of the colposcope in examination of the cervix.

exposed to diethylstilbestrol *in utero*). Also, a woman who has had three negative smears taken at least a year apart after the age of 60 is at a very low risk of developing invasive cancer of the cervix and need not have routine smears obtained thereafter.

The appropriate frequency of Pap smears in women who are in their reproductive years is uncertain. Many argue that the current decline in the incidence of invasive cervical cancer is a direct result of the practice of yearly monitoring, and that that practice should be continued. Others point out that invasive neoplastic changes in the cervix take years to develop; they argue that smears at 5-year intervals are adequate and that the cost of more frequent Pap smears is not justified. Perhaps a reasonable compromise is to obtain a smear at 2–year intervals in women in the reproductive years if all reported are negative for dysplasia unless the patient feels more secure having an annual smear. Since an annual pelvic examination is designed to detect other lesions, such as gonorrhea or ovarian cancer, the additional cost of the Pap smear at the time of the pelvic examination is relatively low. Also, if a woman has had a total hysterectomy (cervix removed) there is no need for a Pap smear unless the surgery was for cervical dysplasia or cancer, in which case a regular smear from the apex of the vagina should be obtained every year.

DETECTION OF ENDOMETRIAL LESIONS

Adenocarcinoma of the endometrium is the most common cancer of the genital organs; there are 38,000 new cases in the United States every year. The disease is associated with a relative excess of estrogen and a lack of progesterone. This hormone pattern is found in the postmenopausal period, when 75% of these cancers occur (8). There is an increased risk of endometrial cancer in infertile patients, obese patients, patients with dysfunctional bleeding, women with a history of prolonged estrogen therapy, patients who do not ovulate regularly, patients with a history of adenomatous hyperplasia, and possibly patients with diabetes mellitus. Long term users of oral contraceptives appear to be at reduced risk for endometrial cancer (9). Bleeding is the major symptom, and early detection requires patients to be educated to report abnormal bleeding when they are approaching the perimenopausal period and when they are postmenopausal (see Chapter 77). With abnormal bleeding at these times, the physician should strongly suspect endometrial cancer and refer the patient to a gynecologist for endometrial biopsy and/or for dilation and curettage. A pelvic examination is not helpful in the early detection of malignancy of the endometrium.

The cancer detection smear is of use only in detecting endometrial cancer when, by chance, malignant cells from the endometrium have passed into the vaginal pool.

Therefore, attempts have been made to design a method of obtaining cells from the endometrium by uterine cytology. Recent studies suggest that there may be a role for periodic uterine cytology (4, 7). This technique requires that the physician swab the endometrial cavity and prepare a slide as in a Pap smear. The procedure is easy for the physician to learn and results in only slightly more discomfort for the patient than a cervical Pap smear. There are two major problems with this technique: there are

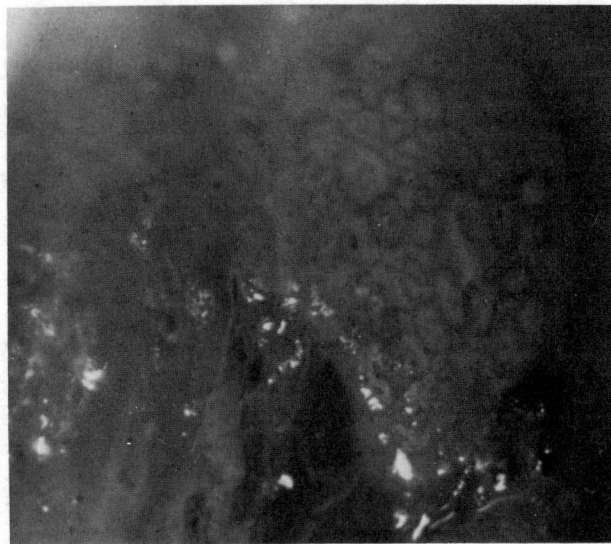

Figure 95.3. Photograph taken through the colposcope showing the mosaic pattern associated with dysplasia of the cervix. (From the files of the late Dr. Rafael Garcia-Bunuel.)

not yet agreed upon standards of cytological interpretation and large scale screening programs have not yet established its validity in improved endometrial cancer survival. Therefore it cannot yet be advised for routine use.

Most lesions which are precursors of endometrial carcinoma are present during the perimenopausal period, and they are recognizable by examination of material from an aspirational biopsy (as opposed to cytology, see above), an office procedure usually done by a gynecologist and which results in minimal discomfort to the patient. Therefore, it is reasonable that patients who have an increased risk of endometrial cancer (see above) and who are at the menopause be referred to a gynecologist for suction endometrial biopsy (5); the benefit of this approach to early detection will require time to confirm.

DETECTION OF OVARIAN CANCER

Malignancies of the ovary are silent until they are sufficiently large to produce symptoms or until they have spread to other organs. Early detection depends upon the annual pelvic and rectal examination; unfortunately, most ovarian cancers are advanced when diagnosed, and the cure rate is low (8, 10). On very rare occasions, a malignant ovarian tumor will be found in the premenarchal patient; but it is important to remember that most patients are postmenopausal and that the incidence increases with age. The risk factors for ovarian cancer are unknown, and little progress has been made in early detection (there is no evidence that periodic sonography has any value in detecting ovarian cancer) or in improving the survival rate (6).

Except for the relatively uncommon functioning ovarian tumors, symptoms from cancer of the ovary are minimal in the early stages, and the symptoms which develop later are largely a function of the size and location of the tumor. Symptoms of abdominal enlargement, a sense of fullness in the pelvis, changes in bowel function, or evidence in the lower extremities of venous or lymphatic obstruction all occur late. Sudden discomfort raising suspicion of an acute abdominal catastrophe may be experienced if a tumor undergoes torsion, necrosis, hemorrhage, rupture, or infection. Signs of ascites, nodules in the cul-de-sac, and either venous or lymphatic obstruction all suggest that a malignant disease is present.

The examination of the patient with ovarian cancer reveals that the ovary is enlarged, but it must be remembered that during the reproductive years some enlargement may be physiological. The normal ovary is about 1 × 2 × 3 cm in size and is found lateral to the dome of the uterus. When the uterus is retroverted, the ovaries may not be palpable. When the ovaries are compressed by the examining finger an uncomfortable sensation is noted by the patient. Functional ovarian (follicle or corpus luteum) cysts are common; they may enlarge up to 4 to 5 cm and may be detected during a pelvic examination. Functional cysts should be soft, cystic, and no larger than 4 to 5 cm in diameter; and after an observation period of 8 to 10 weeks, they should disappear. If there is any doubt about the nature of the cyst and follow-up of 8 to 10 weeks is not desired, physiological cysts may be shown to be functional by suppressing the pituitary hormones; this can accomplished by prescribing an oral contraceptive preparation such as Demulin. Norlestrin 1/50, or Ortho-Novum 1/50 daily for 6 weeks. Functional cysts regress, but tumors do not. When there is question about the presence of a cyst, a sonographic study of the pelvis may be helpful, especially in obese patients. A sonogram can detect a cyst which is 1 to 4 cm or greater in diameter; cysts that are less than 4 cm in the ovulating woman are usually functional and can be followed (see above). All patients found to have hard or firm adnexal masses and all cystic tumors larger than 4 to 5 cm regardless of the age of the patient should be evaluated by a gynecologist.

Based on the idea that the ovary shrinks in the menopause, there are those who feel that any ovary which can be felt in a postmenopausal women should be investigated. While there is some controversy about this, it is reasonable to refer for evaluation any postmenopausal patient in whom an adnexal mass is noted during the annual examination. This is mandatory if the mass was not detected on a previous examination.

General Reference

Jones HW, Jr, Jones GS (ed): *Novak's Textbook of Gynecology*, ed 10. Baltimore, Williams & Wilkins, 1981.

>This text is a valuable resource to the general physician and covers all aspects of pertinent gynecology. It is heavily illustrated and very readable.   •

Specific References

1. Briggs RM: Dysplasia and early neoplasia of the uterine cervix. A review. *Obstet Gynecol Surv* 34:70, 1980.
2. Consensus—more of less—on the Pap smear: *Science* 209:672, 1980.
3. Cramer DW: The role of cervical cytology in the declining morbidity and mortality of cervical cancer. *Cancer* 34:2018, 1974.
4. Ferenczy, A, Gelfand MM: Outpatient endometrial sampling with Endocyte: Comparative study of its effectiveness with endometrial biopsy. *Obstet Gynecol* 63:295, 1984.
5. Gusberg SB: An approach to the control of carcinoma of the endometrium. *CA* 30:16, 1980.
6. Guidelines for the cancer-related check-up. *CA* 30:194, 1980.
7. Koss LG, Schreiber K, Oberlander SG: Screening of asymptomatic woman for endometrial cancer. *Obstet Gynecol* 57:681, 1981.
8. Silverberg E: Cancer statistics, 1980. *CA* 30:23, 1980.
9. Weiss NS, Sayvetz TA: Incidence of endometrial cancer and oral contraceptive agents. *N Engl J Med* 301:551, 1980.
10. Woodruff D: The pathogenesis of ovarian neoplasia. *Johns Hopkins Med J* 144:117, 1979.

SECTION 14

Problems of the Eyes and Ears

CHAPTER NINETY-SIX

Hearing Loss and Associated Ear Problems

WARREN ROTHMAN, M.D., AND L. RANDOL BARKER, M.D.

A 1971 report from the National Health Survey estimated that 13.2 million persons in the United States had significant bilateral hearing impairment. Of these, 5.5 million were over 65 years of age (1). The survey also indicated that a large proportion of symptomatic adults go directly to a hearing aid dealer rather than to a physician and/or audiologist for initial evaluation. Many patients, however, will present the problem of hearing loss to their physician. This chapter provides an approach to hearing loss and associated ear problems that is appropriate in an ambulatory setting.

EAR STRUCTURE AND FUNCTION

In order to classify the mechanism of hearing impairment (conductive or sensorineural), the structure and function of the components of the ear must be understood (see Fig. 96.1).

The *external ear* is composed of the auricle, the auditory meatus, and the external auditory canal. The outer portion of the canal is cartilaginous and is covered by thick skin that contains hair follicles and the cerumen-secreting glands. Cerumen protects the epithelium and captures foreign particles entering the canal. The inner portion of the canal is bony and is covered by thin skin without hair follicles or cerumen glands.

The *middle ear* consists of the tympanic membrane, the air space behind it, and the three linked ossicles (malleus, incus, and stapes). The malleus is attached to the tympanic membrane, while the stapes makes contact with the inner ear *via* the bony stapes footplate at the oval window. The landmarks seen on inspection of the tympanic membrane are shown in Figure 96.2. The lining of the middle ear is a mucus-secreting epithelium similar to that which lines the nose. The middle ear communicates with the nose *via* the eustachian tube, which enters the lateral nasopharynx. Patency of the eustachian tube assures equal pressure on either side of the tympanic membrane, which facilitates the transmission of sound from the tympanic membrane to the oval window.

The *inner ear* is encased in very hard bone (the otic capsule) and is fluid filled. It consists of a sensory organ for hearing (cochlea) and the sensory organ for balance (labyrinth). Nerves from the cochlea and labyrinth unite to form the acoustic nerve (VIII), which runs through the bony internal auditory canal in the temporal bone to the brainstem.

EXTERNAL EAR | MIDDLE EAR | INNER EAR

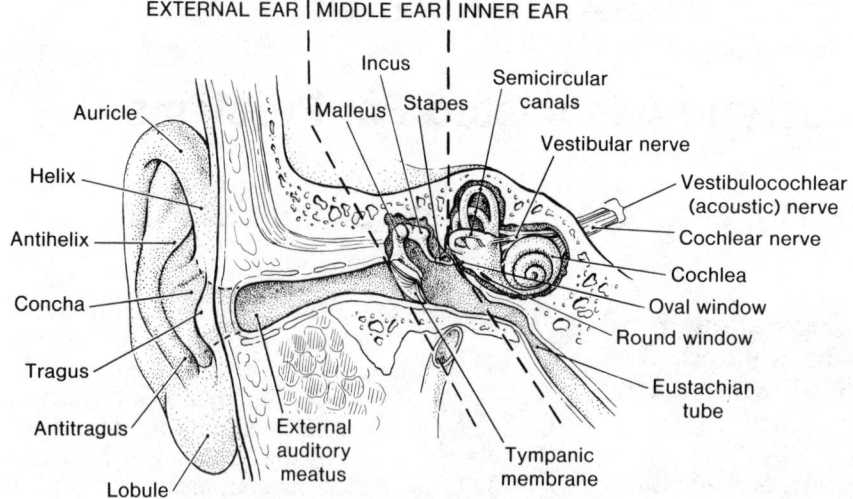

Figure 96.1.   Normal structures of the ear.

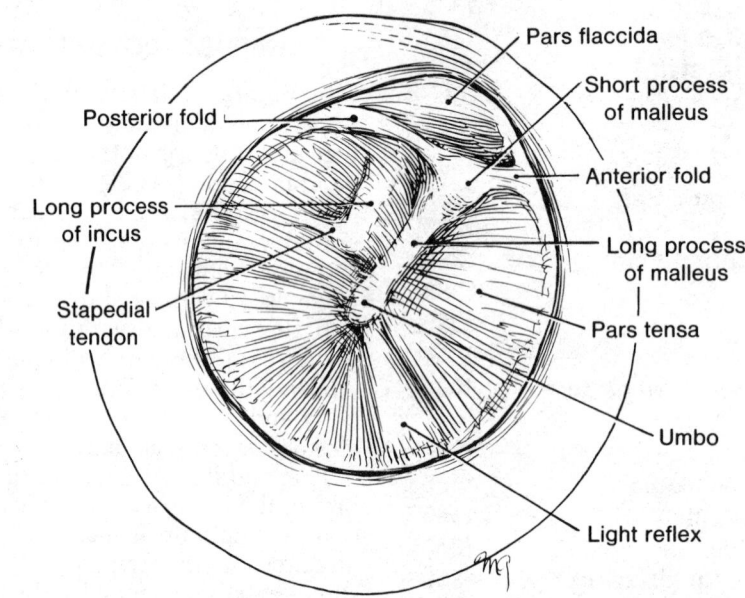

Figure 96.2.   Right tympanic membrane, showing important landmarks.

The *conductive system* of the ear includes the external auditory canal, the tympanic membrane, the middle ear, and the ossicles. Hearing loss due to defects in this portion of the ear is termed *conductive hearing loss*. The *sensorineural system* of the ear consists of the cochlea, the auditory nerve, and the brainstem auditory pathways projecting to the auditory cortex. In these structures, sound waves delivered by the conductive system are transformed into nerve impulses. Hearing loss due to defects in this portion of the ear is termed *sensorineural hearing loss*, which may be localized as cochlear or retrocochlear.

DETERMINING SEVERITY AND MECHANISM OF HEARING LOSS

Office Testing

Regardless of the specific cause of hearing loss, the severity of the impairment and the probable mechanism conductive or sensorineural) can be determined in the office. This determination can be made from a combination of the history, the patient's ability to hear the spoken voice in the office, and testing with a tuning fork and a ticking watch.

A practical method for evaluating the *severity of hearing impairment* includes an estimate of the social problems that have occurred due to difficulty in hearing and an assessment of response to voice testing in the office; these two findings can be equated with various levels of abnormality in the audiogram (see Table 96.1). *Slight* impairment indicates difficulty in hearing long distance speech—for example, at small group meetings, social gatherings, or the theater. *Moderate* impairment includes some difficulty with short distance speech and conversation. *Severe* impairment indicates no understanding of the conversational voice but understanding of the amplified voice. Amplification may be achieved by raising the voice or electronically by use of a hearing aid (see below). *Profound* (or total) impairment indicates inability to hear and understand the spoken voice despite maximum amplification.

In the patient with significant hearing impairment, the *frequency range* which is involved can also be approximated in the office by testing recognition of words containing the sound "ah" (low frequency, vowel sound), such as apple, hot dog, airplane, and the sound "ss" (high frequency, consonant), such as icecream, stairway, baseball, sunset, when these words are spoken about 2 feet behind the ear being tested, with the other ear covered. A ticking watch held 2 to 3 inches from the ear also tests hearing at high frequencies, while tuning forks test relatively low frequency hearing.

The *mechanism* of hearing impairment can be classified tentatively as conductive or sensorineural by the use of *tunning fork tests* (Rinne and Weber). A 256-Hertz tuning fork should be used. The fork should be struck lightly for the Rinne test to avoid overtones. The interpretation of tuning fork tests is summarized in Table 96.2.

Rinne Test

This test is used to evaluate hearing loss in one ear. It is important to mask the hearing in the other ear by rubbing crumpled paper over that ear to create a rustling sound. The tuning fork is struck gently against a firm surface. It is then held against the mastoid bone until the patient no longer hears the sound; then it is held about 1 inch from the canal. The patient with normal hearing should hear the sound longer by air than by bone conduction. A

modified Rinne is simply to have the patient compare the loudness of bone and air conduction. Air conduction should be louder than bone conduction in a patient with a normal ear.

Weber Test

This test is performed by placing the tuning fork on the forehead and asking the patient if the sound is louder on one side. Alternatively, the fork may be held between the teeth. The reason for lateralization to the side with conductive loss is that environmental noise is masked on this side, increasing the efficiency of cochlear detection of sound created by stimulating adjacent bone.

Audiometry

When the patient is referred to an otolaryngologist for evaluation of hearing loss, *puretone audiometry* is utilized to characterize the extent of impairment. Both air-conduction and bone-conduction measurements are made for sounds of varying intensity (decibels) and frequency (cps). The usual frequencies tested are 250, 500, 1000, 2000, 3000, 4000, 6000,

Table 96.2.
Classification of Probable Mechanism of Hearing Loss Using Tuning Fork Tests

Classification	Rinne Test	Weber Test
NORMAL HEARING		
Both ears	AC > BC[a]	Not lateralized
CONDUCTIVE LOSS[b]		
Right ear	Right ear—BC > AC	Lateralized to
	Left ear—AC > BC	right ear
Left ear	Right ear—AC > BC	Lateralized to
	Left ear—BC > AC	left ear
Both ears	Right ear—BC > AC	Lateralized to
	Left ear—BC > AC	poorer ear
SENSORINEURAL LOSS		
Right ear	AC > BC bilaterally	Lateralized to
		left ear
Left ear	AC > BC bilaterally	Lateralized to
		right ear
Both ears	AC > BC bilaterally	Lateralized to
		better ear

[a] AC, air conduction; BC, bone conduction,
[b] Because sound transmission by air is much more efficient than by bone, air conduction may remain greater than bone conduction in early or minimal conductive hearing loss.

Table 96.1.
A Practical Method for Assessing Severity of Hearing Loss in the Office[a]

Severity of Hearing Loss	Social Difficulty	Office Voice Test	Puretone Audiogram
Normal hearing	None	18 ft or more using normal voice	No loss over 10 dB[b]
Slight hearing loss	Long distance speech	Not over 12 ft using normal voice	10–30 dB loss
Moderate hearing loss	Short distance speech	Not over 3 ft using normal voice	Up to 60 dB loss
Severe hearing loss	All unamplified voices	Raised voice at meatus	Over 60 dB loss
Profound hearing loss	Voices never heard	All speech and sound	Over 90 dB loss

[a] Adapted from Mawson SR: *Diseases of the Ear.* Baltimore, Williams & Wilkins, 1974.
[b] dB, decibel.

and 8000 cps. The results are plotted on a graph called an audiogram. The vertical axis shows hearing loss in decibels and the horizontal axis shows the frequency of the stimulus in Hertz. Examples of audiograms showing normal hearing, conductive hearing loss, and sensorineural hearing loss are reproduced in Figure 96.3. Speech audiometry, which measures the subject's ability to hear *and* understand the spoken voice, is also done as part of a formal hearing evaluation.

GENERAL APPROACH TO CHRONIC HEARING LOSS

Assessment and care for moderate or severe chronic hearing loss usually require the assistance of a consulting otolaryngologist. For many patients, little can be done to reverse the primary process, and care consists of compensating for existing hearing loss and preventing further loss.

Communication

Counseling of the family and others who speak to the patient with moderate to severe hearing loss should emphasize two principles:

1. Facilitate communication by consistently using the following adjuncts to speech: face the patient; obtain his attention before speaking; speak slowly; utilize gestures; and speak louder or move closer if the patient says that it helps.

2. Expect some difficulty in discriminating consonants (the high frequency hearing loss typical of most sensorineural deafness particularly affects this type of discrimination; for example, the word "yes" may be understood as "yet, get, less, mess," *etc*).

For the patient with *profound or total hearing loss*, the principle governing all communication is that the message must be *seen* by the patient. Most pa-tients, will let the physician know the mode of communication they prefer: lipreading or writing. Whenever there is any question about the effectiveness of lipreading, written exchange of information should be utilized. This can be facilitated by assuring that paper and a pen or pencil are always available to the patient. In large communities, a translator who can communicate in American Sign Language may be available to assist patients who know sign language. Also videos are now available which make it possible for totally deaf persons to receive telephone calls (messages are entered by the sender in code on a touch-tone unit and displayed visually for the deaf receiver) and to follow television programs.

Hearing Aids (5)

Hearing aids (miniature microphone-amplifier-loudspeaker units) can assist the patient with sensorineural hearing loss (and some patients with irreversible conductive loss). These aids can increase the intensity of a sound by up to 70 dB. Thus, a sound of about 60 dB (the level of average conversational speech) passing through an aid may enter the ear at a level of 130 dB. This represents the maximum usable gain of an aid since sounds above this level become painful. Only trial and adjustment will determine whether an individual patient will benefit from a hearing aid. The cost to the patient is usually between $350.00 and $550.00. Most hearing aid dealers will allow a 30-day trial period for a rental fee.

A patient may mention certain specific *problems with the hearing aid* to his personal physician. There may be irritation of the conchal cartilage or even infection in the external canal. A poorly fitted hearing aid mold can cause pressure sores on the external ear (a particular hazard in the diabetic). Patients may also note an increase in cerumen accumulation

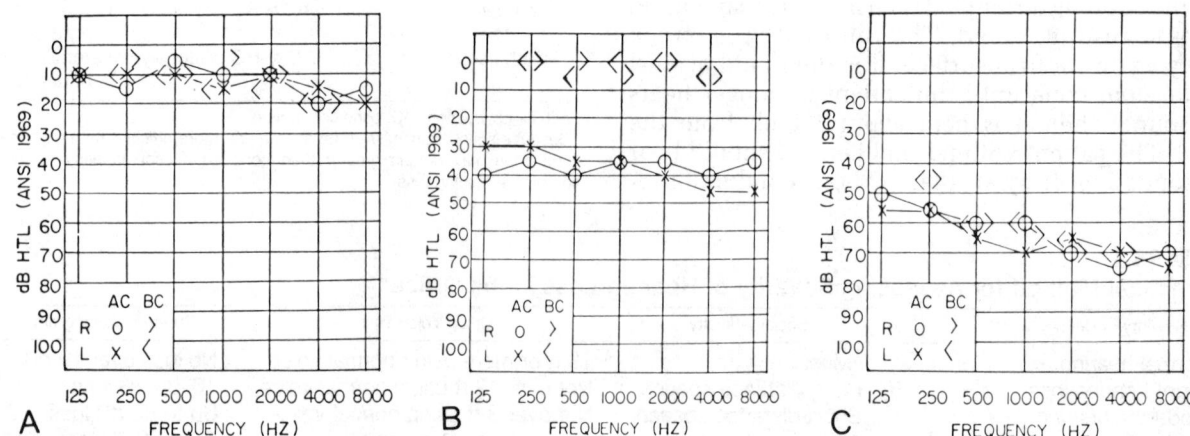

Figure 96.3. Examples of audiograms. *A.* Audiogram in a person with normal hearing. *B.* Bilateral conductive hearing loss (moderate). *C.* Bilateral sensorineural hearing loss (severe). (From Price L, Snider R: The geriatric patient: ear, nose and throat problems. In Reichel W (ed): *Clinical Aspects of Aging.* Baltimore, Williams & Wilkins, 1978, p 489.)

in the aided ear. In each of these situations use of the aid should be discontinued until the process resolves. A better fitting mold will be needed to avoid recurrence in some patients. Others may do well by removing the aid periodically during the day.

CAUSES OF HEARING LOSS

The major causes of hearing loss in adults are listed in Table 96.3. For each condition, the table indicates mechanism, onset (rapid or gradual), and whether the condition is unilateral or bilateral. The guidelines that follow will enable the general physician to reach a working diagnosis in most instances and to choose between primary treatment and referral for care by a specialist.

CONDITIONS OF THE EXTERNAL AUDITORY CANAL

A number of conditions may cause hearing impairment by blocking the external canal.

Cerumen Impaction

The patient will usually complain of intermittent fullness and hearing impairment on the affected side and may give a history of prior episodes. These symptoms may increase after showering, as moisture may cause cerumen to swell. Diagnosis is made by otoscopy.

If the cerumen appears to be soft, it may be removed by irrigation with use of a rubber-bulb syringe and warm tap water (close to body temperature), directing the water upwards and backwards against the wall of the canal. If the cerumen is impacted and difficult to remove, a few drops of hydrogen peroxide (or carbamide peroxide, Debrox) should be instilled twice daily for 1 week before removal. Alternatively, a cerumenolytic agent (Cerumenex) may be utilized. In general, cerumenolytic agents should be used only in the office, as casual use by the patient at home increases the risk of allergic dermatitis (seen in about 1% of users). The following steps are taken: With the patient's head tilted laterally at 45° the ear is filled with cerumenolytic drops: a cotton plug is inserted for 15 to 20

Table 96.3.
Major Causes of Hearing Loss in Adults

Causes	Mechanism[a]	Onset Rapid (Hours to Days) or Gradual (Months to Years)	Bilateral or Unilateral
EXTERNAL AUDITORY CANAL			
Cerumen impaction	C	Either	Usually unilateral
Foreign body	C	Rapid	Unilateral
Otitis externa	C	Rapid	Unilateral
New growth	C	Gradual	Unilateral
MIDDLE EAR			
Serous otitis media	C	Either	Either
Acute otitis media	C	Rapid	Unilateral
Barotrauma	C or SN	Rapid	Unilateral
Traumatic perforation of tympanic membrane	C	Rapid	Unilateral
Chronic otitis media	C	Gradual	Unilateral
Ossicular chain problems:			
Adhesive otitis media	C	Gradual	Unilateral
Tympanosclerosis	C	Gradual	Either
Traumatic injury	C or SN	Rapid	Unilateral
Otosclerosis	C and/or SN	Gradual	Bilateral
New growths	C or SN	Gradual	Unilateral
INNER EAR			
Presbycusis	SN	Gradual	Bilateral
Acoustic trauma	SN	Gradual	Bilateral
Drug-induced	SN	Either	Bilateral
Ménière's syndrome	SN	Rapid	Usually unilateral
Central nervous system infection:			
Meningitis	SN	Rapid	Either
Syphilis	SN	Either	Either
Tuberculosis	SN	Either	Either
Acoustic neurinoma	SN	Gradual	Unilateral
Mumps	SN	Rapid	Unilateral
ATRAUMATIC SUDDEN SENSORINEURAL HEARING LOSS	SN	Rapid	Unilateral

[a] C, conductive; SN, sensorineural.

minutes; the ear is then irrigated with lukewarm water and use of a soft rubber syringe. After irrigation, the tympanic membrane will usually show some injection around the handle of the malleus. In certain situations, cerumen removal should be done by an otolaryngologist: (a) in the patient with a known tympanic membrane perforation or a history of mastoidectomy, irrigation is contraindicated because water may transport bacteria to the middle ear or mastoid and thereby initiate an infection; wax removal should be done by suction-tip aspiration; (b) in the occasional patient with an impaction that does not respond to the usual measures described above; in this instance, removal of cerumen is accomplished by aspiration or by the use of an operating microscope. Hearing impairment will usually be relieved immediately after removal of cerumen.

An impaction often follows vigorous efforts by the patient to remove wax with a cotton-tipped applicator. The patient should be reminded that ear wax is secreted to protect the lining of the canal and that the applicator should be used only to remove cerumen in the outer portion of the canal, for cosmetic purposes. Patients who have had recurrent impactions, often due to excess secretion of cerumen, may prevent recurrences by gently syringing their ears once or twice monthly, by using a soft rubber bulb and warm water. Also, instillation of baby oil drops weekly will help to keep the wax soft.

Foreign Body

Usually the history discloses accidental insertion of a foreign body or entrance of an insect, which is followed by fullness and hearing impairment. Foreign bodies can be removed by use of fine forceps or a wax spoon. Removal by irrigation should be avoided if the foreign body is a vegetable, as water will cause further swelling. Insects should first be killed by instillation of mineral oil. Hearing impairment resolves promptly after removal of a foreign body.

Otitis Externa (Swimmer's Ear)

This condition is most common in the summer months, when heat and humidity, plus moisture introduced by swimming or perspiration, promote swelling and maceration of the stratum corneum of the skin. In the external canal, this process may at first cause pruritus. The patient will give a history of having scratched his ear for a few days, which is followed by exudation and pain. The pain is aggravated by movement of the external ear and sometimes the jaw. Hearing impairment will occur in those patients who present with swelling or debris that occludes the canal. The characteristics of the skin of the canal and of the exudate usually provide adequate clues to etiology, and cultures are needed only for patients who do not respond promptly to topical treatment. Copious or greenish exudate sug-

gests *Pseudomonas*, the bacteria most frequently seen in otitis externa. Yellow crusting in the midst of a purulent exudate suggests *Staphylococcus aureus*. Canal skin that is scaling, cracked, and weeping indicates eczema (the history usually indicates that the condition is chronic). Fluffy material resembling bread mold, varying color from white to black, suggests a fungal etiology (*Aspergillus* or *Candida*).

There are two general *principles of treatment* for all types of otitis externa: removal of all infected debris (with a cotton applicator with a tightly rolled fresh cotton bud and with a suction cannula if available) and instillation of an appropriate topical medication: for bacterial infections—an antimicrobial-corticosteroid combination, 3 or 4 drops, three to four times daily (e.g., Cortisporin Otic Suspension, containing polymyxin B-neomycin-hydrocortisone). For fungal infections, the canal should be thoroughly cleaned out and a light dusting of sulfanilamide powder should be applied, in the office. A dispenser containing sulfanilamide powder for this use can be obtained from any pharmacy. The fungal infection usually resolves after a single dusting with this powder. Liquid preparations for fungal otitis externa are not satisfactory because they maintain moist conditions, which support the infection.

For eczema without superimposed infection, a topical steroid cream or solution is applied three to four times daily (e.g., triamcinolone 0.1%).

In some patients, the canal may be so swollen that topical medication does not enter the canal efficiently. In this case, a cylindrical cotton wick (or a commercially available sponge wick, such as Otowick), approximately the length of the ear canal (1 inch in adults), should be saturated with the desired medication and worked by gentle twisting into the canal until only the end is visible. The patient may then apply several drops of the medication to the wick three to four times daily, and the wick will carry it into the canal. The wick can usually be removed after 48 to 72 hours, and treatment can be completed as stated above.

Most episodes of otitis externa resolve completely after 5 to 7 days, and it is important to terminate topical treatment at this time. The ear cannot return to a normal physiological state as long as a foreign substance (topical medicine) is constantly introduced into it; persistent treatment may lead to dermatitis medicamentosa. As a precaution against overtreatment, the prescription for eardrops should be nonrefillable, and only a small amount (10 ml) should be dispensed.

During treatment of otitis externa, moisture should be strictly avoided. During bathing, the ear should be plugged with cotton impregnated with petroleum jelly. To prevent recurrence, the patient should be warned against meddling with the ear (particularly frequent cleansing with cotton-tipped applicators, a common inciting cause).

Hearing impairment due to otitis externa should resolve promply when swelling recedes.

In the following two situations the patient with otitis externa requires prompt referral to an otolaryngologist: (a) patients whose findings suggest mastoiditis (these include slow response of the otitis externa to treatment plus tenderness over the mastoid process); and (b) patients with the findings of "malignant otitis externa," usually diabetics or severely debilitated patients. This process is actually an osteitis of the bone underlying the external auditory canal caused by Pseudomonas. The distinguishing features are fever, excruciating pain, and the presence of friable granulation tissue in the area of apparent otitis externa. Because of the propensity for rapid spread to contiguous structures, this condition is an emergency, requiring hospital admission for debridement and intravenous antibiotics.

New Growth

Occasionally, unilateral, gradual onset hearing impairment may be due to a benign or malignant growth seen in the canal. Such patients must be referred for diagnosis and surgical excision of the growth.

CONDITIONS OF THE MIDDLE EAR

Most conductive hearing loss is due to conditions within the middle ear. In addition to history, evaluation of the middle ear includes assessment of eustachian tube function by air insufflation (pneumatic otoscopy), inspection for signs of acute inflammation (erythema, discharge, or bulging of the tympanic membrane), and inspection for changes in the tympanic membrane not due to acute inflammation (fluid level, retraction, scarring, distortion of normal structures, perforation).

Serous Otitis Media

This problem is very common in childhood and relatively common in adults. The patient usually complains of fullness and decreased hearing in one or both ears with minimal or no pain. There is often a history of recent viral upper respiratory infection (see Chapter 28) or exacerbation of allergic or vasomotor rhinitis (see Chapter 23). Rarely, serous otitis media may be due to nasopharyngeal carcinoma. On physical examination the patient is afebrile, and there may be evidence of eustachian tube closure—retraction of the tympanic membrane, failure of the membrane to move on pneumatic otoscopy (a crude test of eustachian tube patency, not always abnormal in serous otitis), or a fluid level behind the membrane. Even when none of these signs is present, the presumptive diagnosis of serous otitis can be made in patients with typical symptoms and conductive hearing loss.

The objective of medical treatment is to relieve obstruction of the eustachian tube. This is accomplished by the use of topical decongestants. Systemic decongestants (e.g., pseudoephedrine) are not thought to be helpful (3, 4). Nasal sprays containing the decongestant phenylephrine (Neo-Synephrine Nasal Spay 0.25% or 0.50% or other over-the-counter preparations) are the simplest to use. The patient administers two puffs to each nostril followed 5 to 10 minutes later by two more puffs, four times daily. Alternatively, a phenylephrine-containing nasal solution (Neo-Synephrine 0.25% or 0.50%, also over-the-counter) can be instilled by dropper four times daily. The head is hyperextended, 3 or 4 drops are instilled in each nostril to open the nasal passages; the head is then turned to the lateral position with the involved ear down, and 3 to 4 more drops are instilled into the nostril. After 3 or 4 days of topical treatment, rebound nasal mucosal hyperemia may occur. Therefore, the patient should be explicitly instructed to discontinue spray (or drops) after 3 days.

If a patient with serous otitis media has a history of allergic rhinitis, an antihistamine may be helpful (see Chapter 23). In addition to medications, patients should be instructed to promote eustachian tube patency by blowing the nose against closed nostrils with the mouth closed (Valsalva maneuver) every few hours during the day. This should not be recommended to the patient with a purulent nasal discharge.

All patients should be re-evaluated after 4 to 6 weeks of continuous medical therapy. If conductive hearing loss persists beyond 6 weeks, the patient should be referred to an otolaryngologist. He will confirm and quantify the degree of conductive hearing loss, using an instrument known as an impedance audiometer. He will also examine the nasopharynx for a tumor or other mass lesion obstructing the eustachian tube and will examine the nose for anatomical derangements. Some patients will require myringotomy with aspiration of fluid from the middle ear to restore hearing and insertion of a ventilation tube.

Even with optimal treatment serous otitis media may recur in susceptible individuals. Gantrisin, 250–500 mg twice/day, may be used for prophylaxis in infection-prone children (8).

Acute Otitis Media

All patients with this condition will complain of marked pain in the inner ear; most will give a history of a recent upper respiratory infection with or without drainage of purulent material from the ear (indicating tympanic membrane perforation); some will describe unilateral hearing impairment. On examination, there is injection and loss of luster of the tympanic membrane, grayish-pink coloration of the entire membrane, and, eventually, bulging of the membrane and loss of landmarks. Some patients will have a conducted hearing loss demonstrated by tuning fork tests. There may be tenderness to palpation of the mastoid bone, since the mucosa lining the mastoid cells is continuous with that of the middle ear. Evidence of otitis externa is usually not present. The most common etiological agents are *Streptococcus pneumoniae* (pneumococcus), *Haemophilus influenzae, Staphylococcus aureus,* and β-hemolytic streptococcus. An unknown proportion of cases are due to viral pathogens. Since clinical distinction of these cases from those with bacterial infection is not possible, treatment should be the same for all patients with acute otitis media.

Medical treatment consists of systemic antimicrobials for 10 days. Amoxicillin, 500 mg three times daily, is the best regimen. For penicillin-allergic persons, trimethoprim-sulfamethoxazole, 2 tablets every 12 hours, is appropriate. Aspirin or acetaminophen every 4 to 6 hours should be recommended for pain. If needed, codeine, 30 mg, can be given with the aspirin.

If perforation with purulent discharge occurs, Cortisporin otic suspension, 4 drops three times daily for 1 week, may be used to eliminate the infection. If the tympanic membrane is bulging with pus and pain is very severe, myringotomy by an otolaryngologist is indicated.

Recovery from the pain of acute otitis media is usually prompt. Within 1 to 4 weeks, hearing impairment resolves, and the tympanic membrane returns to normal appearance. Serous otitis may be present after other signs or symptoms of acute otitis have resolved.

In the patient who is worse after several days of treatment or who is not well after 10 days, subacute mastoiditis may be present, and referral to an otolaryngologist is therefore indicated. Failure of serous otitis to resolve, persistence of a tympanic membrane perforation, and significant persistent hearing loss after 3 weeks are also indications for referral.

Barotrauma

Barotrauma refers to symptoms and signs produced by a sudden pressure differential between the middle ear and the surrounding atmosphere. The patient gives a history of fullness, pain, and decreased hearing in one or both ears, usually associated with flying or scuba diving. All patients with symptoms that are severe or that persist for more than a day should be examined. The findings on otoscopy vary from mild tympanic membrane retraction to hemotympanum with or without perforation. There may be conductive or neurosensory hearing loss. Any patient with moderate or severe unilateral hearing loss should be referred to an otolaryngologist because of the possibility of a surgically treatable fistula of the round or oval windows.

For patients with mild symptoms, treatment and outcome are similar to those described above for serous otitis media.

Prophylaxis against barotrauma consists of use of the Valsalva maneuver and swallowing or chewing of gum during descent in airplanes.

Traumatic Perforation of Tympanic Membrane

Traumatic rupture, affecting the pars tensa of the tympanic membrane (see Fig. 96.2), may be caused by solids (deliberate introduction of cotton-tipped applicator or other object for removing wax, foreign bodies entering during an accident, *etc*); liquids (forcefully directed jet of water used in syringing the ear); and air (blast waves resulting from detonation of high explosives). Symptoms are decreased hearing, tinnitus, pain, and at times, bleeding.

The *objective of treatment* is the prevention of infection. Most linear tears and small perforations of the membrane will heal spontaneously within 4 weeks without any residual loss of function. Large perforations may require fascia grafting by an otolaryngologist (myringoplasty). If there is a strong possibility that the middle ear has been contaminated at the time of injury (*i.e.,* by syringing), antibiotics (ampicillin or erythromycin, 250 mg four times daily for 1 week) are indicated. In addition, it is essential to guard against the subsequent entry of organisms as long as the perforation persists. Thus the patient should prevent water or other contaminants from entering the ear. Before bathing, the patient should insert a petroleum jelly-covered cotton plug. Swimming should be avoided altogether. Patients whose perforation was self-inflicted should be warned against future syringing and probing to remove cerumen.

After spontaneous closure (takes 2 to 4 weeks) or myringoplasty, the hearing loss due to perforation usually resolves completely.

Chronic Otitis Media

Chronic otitis media implies discharge from the middle ear, either persistent or recurrent, with perforation of the tympanic membrane and usually some degree of conductive hearing loss. The management of this problem has two objectives: eradication of infection and restoration of hearing. When chronic otitis media is initially recognized, the patient should be referred to an otolaryngologist for evaluation. An appreciation of the major clinical characteristics, the treatment principles, and the long term expectations for these patients is, however, important to the patient's primary physician.

Chronic otitis media can be divided into *two major subgroups, benign and dangerous.* The clinical characteristics of these two groups are summarized in Table 96.4. The fundamental difference in the dangerous subgroup is the presence of, or potential for, bone destruction due to invasion by squamous epithelium known as "cholesteatoma". Cholesteatoma occurs either when the squamous epithelium of the auditory canal invades the middle ear through a pre-existing perforation (secondary acquired choles-

Table 96.4.
Chronic Otitis Media: Features Distinguishing Benign and Dangerous Forms

Feature	Benign	Dangerous (Cholesteatoma)
Discharge	Mucoid or mucopurulent	Purulent, foul
Location of pathology	Middle ear; eustachian tube	Middle ear, attic, antrum, any part of temporal bone
Tympanic membrane perforation	Pars tensa (central)[a]	Pars flaccida[a] or marginal
Middle ear mucosa	Mucous membrane	Stratified squamous epithelium
X-rays	Normal; clouding of mastoid cells	Underdevelopment and sclerosis of mastoid cells; bone destruction
Cholesteatoma formation	No	Yes
Bone erosion	No	Yes
Treatment of infection	Medical/surgical (surgery if the perforation fails to heal spontaneously)	Surgical

[a] See Figure 96.2.

teatoma) or when squamous epithelium spontaneously replaces the columnar epithelium of the middle ear, leading to perforation (primary acquired cholesteatoma). The cholesteatoma is the mass of whitish debris which accumulates at the site of invasion of squamous epithelium. As this mass enlarges, it has the potential to erode bone and promote chronic infection.

The commonly performed surgical procedures for chronic otitis media are the following:

Simple mastoidectomy. This procedure removes the mastoid cells and cholesteatoma, usually through a postauricular incision. The canal wall remains intact.

Modified radical mastoidectomy. In this operation, the mastoid cells are exteriorized so that they form a common cavity with the external auditory canal, draining and eradicating infection due to cholesteatoma.

Mastoid obliteration. After infection is eradicated by mastoidectomy, the cavity which has been created is obliterated with the use of muscle or other tissue graft. The purpose of this procedure is to restore normal anatomical contour and to avoid the aftercare which a mastoid cavity requires.

Myringoplasty. The tympanic membrane perforation is closed by use of a tissue graft.

Tympanoplasty. The conduction mechanism, including tympanic membrane perforation and ossicular disruptions is repaired.

Complications of Otitis Media

Acute or chronic suppurative otitis media may become complicated by extension of infection beyond the confines of the middle ear into bone and other surrounding structures. The patient's primary physician should be aware that *symptoms not attributable to the typical course* of acute or chronic otitis media may signify the presence of one of these complications. They are uncommon and usually occur in compromised hosts (diabetics, immunosuppressed patients, *etc*) and in patients with untreated acute or chronic otitis media. All require immediate referral and hospitalization. The complications are mastoiditis, facial nerve paralysis, petrositis (inflammation of petrous portion of the sphenoid with diplopia, pain around the eye and persistent otorrhea), labyrinthitis, brain abscess, extradural abscess, subdural abscess, lateral sinus thrombophlebitis, meningitis, and otitic hydrocephalus.

Ossicular Chain Problems

A number of chronic conditions affect the ossicular chain. These may be recognized by the combination of conductive hearing loss (usually chronic, either unilateral or bilateral), the absence of evidence for active otitis media, and, in some cases, typical findings on otoscopy. Each of these conditions requires referral to an otolaryngologist for consideration of surgical management.

Adhesive Otitis Media

There is a history of prior ear infection, and the tympanic membrane is retracted and atrophic in areas of healed perforations. The eardrum is usually draped over the promontory and incudostapedial complex. Adhesive otitis media is usually a late complication seen in patients who have been inadequately followed up after treatment for repeated acute otitis or serous otitis and who have had persistent middle ear inflammation. Hearing loss is usually mild, though some patients may need a hearing aid. Surgical treatment is normally not necessary.

Tympanosclerosis

There is a history of prior infection, often bilateral. There is usually, but not always, a tympanic membrane perforation and discrete plaques of whittish material consisting of dense collagen at times replaced with calcified hyaline may be seen in the middle ear. In selected patients, surgical removal of the plaques restores lost hearing. In others, ossicular reconstruction is necessary to improve hearing.

Traumatic Ossicular Injury

There is a history of external trauma (such as basal skull fracture and those causes of traumatic perforation listed above) followed by unilateral hearing loss which may be conductive or mixed. A hemotympanum (blood behind the eardrum) is usually seen, although occasionally the tympanic membrane is normal. Hearing status after surgery depends upon the type of injury found at surgery.

Otosclerosis

This is a disease of the labyrinthine capsule in which a vascular type of spongy bone is laid down, causing fixation of the stapes and conductive hearing loss, usually bilateral. The history discloses slowly progressive hearing loss beginning in the second or third decade, usually bilateral, more commonly in females, and frequently accelerated after pregnancy. Also the use of oral contraceptive pills may induce or aggravate this disease. Examination of the tympanic membrane is usually normal. This is the most common cause of progressive conductive hearing loss in young adults. Since the results of surgery, consisting of stapedectomy or stapedotomy, and prosthetic replacement, are excellent, it is particularly important to detect and refer these patients. Sensorineural hearing loss is common as the disease progresses.

New Growths of Middle Ear

A number of benign and malignant growths may be seen on inspection of the tympanic membrane of patients with progressive unilateral conductive hearing loss. Malignant tumors most commonly present with a history of chronic discharge, occasionally bloody.

CHRONIC SENSORINEURAL HEARING LOSS

Presbycusis ("the Hearing of the Old")

A certain amount of hearing loss, beginning in the high frequency range, is virtually universal among elderly people. Approximately one in five people over 65 will develop moderate to severe hearing loss. The majority do not complain of deafness, and often a family member mentions the problem to the patient's physician. When hearing deficits are objectively evaluated in older persons, the deficits of the "complainers" and "noncomplainers" overlap considerably (9). Clearly, social and psychological factors are important in determining the seriousness of hearing loss reported by the individual patient.

Periodically, the primary physician should make a practical assessment of the hearing status of each of his patients over 65 (see Table 96.1). When an older patient is first found to have hearing loss, the patient and his family should be counseled as outlined above (page 1360), and the patient should be offered a referral for evaluation by an otolaryngologist.

Acoustic Trauma

This form of sensorineural hearing loss is found commonly in individuals employed in high noise industries or exposed to extremely loud, electrically amplified music. Like presbycusis, it is initially a high frequency hearing loss, eventually spreading to lower frequencies. Personal prevention by wearing earplugs in high noise settings and environmental prevention by reducing noise level are the best ways to prevent acoustic trauma. Established hearing loss due to noise is usually irreversible, but progressive hearing loss can be prevented. Acute hearing loss due to an acute episode of acoustic trauma; i.e., gunfire or cordless telephone ringer accidents is frequently reversible; this is also referred to as "temporary threshold shift."

Drug-Induced Hearing Loss

A number of drugs may produce bilateral sensorineural hearing loss (Table 96.5), and the patient's personal physician will often be the first to learn of this problem. (Example: a patient will be seen in the office following hospitalization for an illness that was treated with aminoglycoside antibiotics or with intravenous diuretics and will complain of hearing loss.) For most drugs, ototoxicity is dose related; however, hearing impairment may occur even at therapeutic doses. A recent study showed that objective mild hearing loss (15 to 30 dB at high frequencies) occurs in as many as 10% of individuals whose serum levels of gentamycin and tobramycin are maintained within the therapeutic range (10).

The prognosis for drug-induced hearing loss varies according to the drug. Salicylates and quinine usually produce temporary, high frequency deafness; but permanent deafness has been reported in patients surviving salicylate poisoning and in infants of mothers who received quinine during pregnancy. Aminoglycoside ototoxicity may occur suddenly after a few doses, may be permanent, and may progress after discontinuation of the drug. Diuretic-induced ototoxicity may be seen after extremely high doses, usually in patients with renal insufficiency. Its onset may be sudden, following intravenous or (in a few reported cases) oral administration, and the hearing deficit may be permanent. Fortunately, this complication is rare with ethacrynic acid, very rare with furosemide, and may not occur at all with bumetanide.

Ménière's Syndrome

This benign but temporarily disabling condition will be seen one or more times per year in a typical practice. It is present in any age group, but is most common in the fourth to sixth decade. Symptoms

Table 96.5.
Drugs Which May Cause Hearing Loss

ANTIBIOTICS	DIURETICS
Streptomycin	Ethacrynic acid
Neomycin	Furosemide
Gentamycin	
Tobramycin	OTHER DRUGS
Kanamycin	Salicylates
Chloramphenicol	Quinidine
Vancomycin	Quinine
Polymixin B	Cisplatin

are due to endolymphatic hydrops (excess fluid and pressure in the cochlea and the labyrinth).

The individual attack consists of a sudden temporary disturbance of vestibular function (vertigo) combined with fluctuating hearing loss, tinnitus, aural pressure, and nausea. An attack usually lasts for several hours. During the attack, spontaneous nystagmus will be present. The nystagmus will not be affected by position change. Between attacks, tinnitus and sensorineural hearing loss may persist. Symptoms are unilateral (2) in approximately 70% of cases. In about half of the cases vestibular and cochlear symptoms appear at the same time; in approximately 25%, deafness and/or tinnitus precedes the onset of vertigo; and in 25% vertigo precedes deafness (6). The vertigo is accompanied by nausea and vomiting, probably due to a spread of nervous impulses from the vestibular nerve to the vagal nuclei in the brainstem. In severe cases, other vagal symptoms may occur (abdominal pain, bradycardia, pallor, and sweating). Audiometry demonstrates sensorineural hearing loss, greater for lower frequencies in the early stage of the disease.

An attack may occur spontaneously at any time. Attacks may occur singly, with an interval of months or years between, or there may be a series of attacks over a period of weeks, followed by a long period of complete remission.

The *differential diagnosis* of Ménière's syndrome includes a number of conditions which may present with hearing loss and vertigo unrelated to position change: viral labyrinthitis, acoustic neurinoma, syphilitic vertigo, labyrinthine fistula, vestibular granuloma, temporal bone fracture, or multiple sclerosis. Additional information regarding the assessment of the patient with vertigo is found in Chapter 81.

Treatment. Patients with suspected Ménière's syndrome should be referred promptly to an otolaryngologist to confirm the diagnosis and to initiate treatment. All patients will be treated with diuretics (25 to 50 mg of hydrochlorothiazide daily or its equivalent). Bed rest is recommended when the patient is having recurrent severe symptoms; bed rest does not prevent the periodic vertigo but prevents exacerbation due to position change. The antihistamine meclizine (Antivert or Bonine) can be tried in a dose of 25 mg three to four times daily. For nausea, the patient should take the antiemetic prochlorperazine (Compazine) either as a 5- or 10-mg capsule four times daily, or as a 25-mg suppository twice daily. After the acute attack has subsided, the patient should continue diuretic treatment; after 1 year without recurrence, diuretic treatment can be stopped. For the occasional patient with severe recurrent Ménière's syndrome refractory to medical treatment, one of a number of surgical procedures can be performed, selectively decompressing, destroying the vestibular labyrinth or sectioning the vestibular nerve.

Acoustic Neurinoma

This uncommon, benign tumor usually arises from the vestibular fibers of the 8th cranial nerve. Rarely it may arise from the 7th cranial nerve. It grows slowly, expanding within the internal auditory meatus until large enough to extend into the posterior fossa and to cause damage to adjacent structures. Onset of symptoms is generally between the ages of 30 and 50. Essentially all patients will present with symptoms of 8th nerve impairment: unilateral hearing loss is found in the majority of patients and chronic, usually mild, positional vertigo or sense of imbalance occurs in many patients. Audiometry usually demonstrates significant sensorineural hearing loss with poor discrimination. Neurological examination shows involvement of the following neurological structures, in decreasing order of frequency: nerve VII, nerve V, nerve VI, and cerebellum (ataxia, with a tendency to fall toward the side of the lesion).

Referral to an otolaryngologist for evaluation is essential whenever unilateral sensorineural hearing loss is initially found. Diagnosis of acoustic neurinoma is based on a characteristic audiogram and on computerized tomography. The results of surgical treatment generally permit the patient to resume his or her usual activity, but usually with permanent unilateral hearing loss (7). In a few patients with good hearing preoperatively it may be possible to preserve the hearing.

SUDDEN SENSORINEURAL HEARING LOSS

This condition, usually unilateral, is an otological emergency. The etiology is often difficult to ascertain and includes viral cochleitis, and artery occlusion (in patients with other evidence of arterial occlusive disease, such as embolic transient ischemic attacks), inner ear fistula, sudden expansion of a cerebellopontine angle tumor, temporal bone fracture, and noise trauma (gunshot, for example). The symptom, which occurs over a matter of minutes to hours, is either tinnitus or hearing loss. After prompt evaluation for conductive hearing loss (including simple cerumen impaction), these patients should be referred immediately for evaluation by an otolaryngologist. A number of empirical medical therapies have been tried. For patients with inner ear fistulas, surgical closure is possible.

The majority of patients will have permanent, severe unilateral hearing loss, and they and their families should be instructed regarding hearing safety (adequate noise protection for the other ear, preferential seating for optimal use of the good ear, precautions when driving in heavy traffic).

TINNITUS

Tinnitus ("ringing") refers to the perception of sounds in the absence of a normal external stimulus.

Subjective Tinnitus

The term *subjective tinnitus* is used when the subject complains of noises which cannot be heard by the observer. Subjective tinnitus may be subdivided into two types:

Tympanic. This usually arises as a result of a conductive lesion (all of the causes of conductive hearing loss). It is thought to be due to removal of the normal masking effect of ambient noise, with emergence of otherwise subaudible tympanic, vascular, and muscular noises. The patient will often describe the tinnitus as pulsating.

Petrous. This is due to conditions affecting the cochlea or 8th nerve (all of the conditions leading to sensorineural hearing loss). It is attributed to cerebral recognition of auditory stimuli produced by mechanical cochlear deformation or by hyperirritability of the acoustic nerve. It may be intermittent or continuous with varying intensity.

After the patient's primary otological problem has been defined, the most important requirement in dealing with tinnitus is reassurance (many patients believe that their tinnitus signifies the presence of a serious intracranial condition). Bedtime sedation to assure adequate sleep is important. Some patients will also find that the sound of a radio helps them to get to sleep by competing with the more distressing sound due to tinnitus. For patients with severe tinnitus, masking treatment by the consulting otolaryngologist may be helpful.

Objective Tinnitus

This is a noise audible to the examiner, sometimes inaudible to the patient, and originating from the region of the patient's ear. Causes include aneurysm of the internal carotid artery, temporomandibular joint problems, and myoclonus of palatal muscles. These patients should be referred to an otolaryngologist for a diagnostic workup.

VERTIGO

The problem of vertigo is discussed in depth in Chapter 81.

General Reference

Paparella MM, Shumrick DA: *Otolaryngology*. Vol 2: *Ear*. Philadelphia, WB Saunders, 1980.
   Exhaustive textbook.

Specific References

1. Bailey HAT Jr, Pappas JJ, Graham S, Winston ME: Total hearing rehabilitation. *Arch Otolaryngol* 102:323, 1976.
2. Balkany TJ, Kires B, Arenberg IK: Bilateral aspects of Ménière's disease: *Otolaryngol Clin North Am* 31:4, 1980.
3. Bluestone CD, Mandel EM, Canterin EI, et al: Evaluation of decongestant antihistamine therapy for otitis media with effusion. Ann *Otol Rhinol Laryngol* 92:6, 35, 1983.
4. Cantekin, et al: Lack of efficacy of a decongestant antihistamine combination for otitis media with effusion in children. *N Engl J Med* 308:295, 1983.
5. Department of Health, Education and Welfare: A report on hearing aid health care. Washington, DC, US Government Printing Office, 1974.
6. Mawson ST: *Diseases of the Ear*. Baltimore, Williams & Wilkins, 1974, chap 17.
7. Ojemann RG, Montgomery WW, Weiss AD: Evaluation and surgical treatment of acoustic neuroma. *N Engl J Med* 287:895, 1972.
8. Paradise JL: Antimicrobial prophylaxis for recurrent acute otitis media. *Ann Otol Rhinol Laryngol* 90:53, 1984.
9. Price LL, Snider RM: The geriatric patient; ear, nose and throat problems. In Reichel W (ed): *Clinical Aspects of Aging*. Williams & Wilkins, Baltimore, 1978, p 489.
10. Smith CR, Lipsky JJ, Laskin OL, et al: Double-blind comparison of the nephrotoxicity and auditory toxicity of gentamicin and tobramycin. *N Engl J Med* 302:1106, 1980.

CHAPTER NINETY-SEVEN

Cataracts

EARL D. R. KIDWELL, Jr., M.D., AND JOHN R. BURTON, M.D.

A cataract is an opacification of the lens of the eye or of its capsule. Ninety-six percent of individuals over 60 years of age will have some opacification of the lens, but most often these opacities are of no importance. *A significant cataract* results in interference with visual acuity. In the United States cataracts are a very common cause of diminished vision and may result in blindness. The incidence of diminished visual acuity from cataracts increases steadily after age 50, reaching nearly 50% of individuals over the age of 75. Cataracts are usually bilateral, and the progression is slow and may vary between eyes. The rate of progression is not individually predictable, and there is no treatment that will retard the progression. When the cataract is advanced the only therapy is surgery.

This chapter will provide a review of the anatomy and physiology of the lens as well as a review of cataracts to help the general physician advise and follow his patients appropriately.

ANATOMY AND PHYSIOLOGY

The lens is derived entirely from the evagination of surface ectoderm in the fetus. It is located immediately posterior to the iris and is suspended there by radially attached zonular fibers from the ciliary body (see Fig. 98.1 in Chapter 98). It is a biconvex uniquely transparent structure with an elastic capsule whose shape may be altered by ciliary body contraction permitting images to be brought into sharp focus on the retina. The lens is acellular and avascular and lacks innervation. Nourishment is provided from the surrounding aqueous and vitreous humor, and metabolic by-products are removed by diffusion into the aqueous humor. The continued transparency of the lens requires the active metabolism of the elastic capsular epithelium so that any insult to the epithelium may result in lenticular opacities. Also, new lenticular fibers are produced throughout life; and, since none are lost, increasing density of the fibers of the lens develops with age, which contributes to cataract formation.

ETIOLOGY

There are many causes of cataracts (Table 97.1). While senescent cataracts—the result of the aging phenomena described above—account for the vast majority of cataracts, the general physician will occasionally see patients with congenital or traumatic lens opacities as well. The mechanism of opacification in all of these instances is thought to be due to interference with the metabolic activity of the capsular epithelium and with continued fiber production.

Many of these various types of cataracts have a distinctive appearance. The ophthalmologist may therefore suggest to the general physician the possibility of an underlying disorder such as hypoparathyroidism (punctate opacities in anterior and posterior lens cortex) or Wilson's disease ("sunflower" cataract).

SYMPTOMS AND EXAMINATION

The primary symptom of cataract is impaired vision; usually patients describe a constant fog over the eye. They may also see rings or halos around lights and objects. The color that objects appear change, particularly, toward blue and yellow. Not infrequently, with immature cataract formation, distant vision is impaired and near vision is preserved.

The location of the cataract within the lens determines the extent of the visual loss. Central opacities cause noticeable loss of vision and a distinct glare when the patient is in bright light, which will constrict the pupil so that the dense portion of the lens occludes and diffuses light. For this reason the patient who has central opacities finds his vision is better in low light when his pupil is open. Peripheral opacities will cause noticeable loss of vision only late in the development of the cataract.

Cataracts are easily identified by illuminating the lens with a slitlamp, but most general physicians will find that they can see a cataract easily through

Table 97.1.
Etiology of Cataracts

CONGENITAL
    Autosomal dominant inheritance—25% of congenital cataracts
    Maternal malnutrition
    Maternal infections—*e.g.*, rubella, syphilis
    Maternal metabolic disease—*e.g.*, diabetes mellitus
    Maternal medication—corticosteroids
    Prematurity
TRAUMATIC
SENESCENT
SECONDARY (Examples)
    Drug therapy—corticosteroids
    Degenerative eye disease—severe myopia
    Retinal dystrophy
    Essential iris atrophy
    Retinal detachment
    Glaucoma
    Intraocular neoplasia
    Ocular ischemia (*e.g.*, Takayasu's disease)
ASSOCIATED WITH METABOLIC DISEASE
    Diabetes mellitus
    Wilson's disease
    Hypoparathyrodism

the plus 4–10 lens of their direct ophthalmoscope. The lens appears cloudy. Similarly, a light from a small flashlight may be reflected off the opacity in the lens. Visual acuity should be tested in both eyes when cataracts are suspected. If the patient describes any visual symptoms or if the physician measures an impairment in visual acuity, the patient should be referred to an ophthalmologist. In individuals who are over 60 years of age, screening for cataracts is best done by a visual acuity examination with use of a Snellen chart.

CATARACT SURGERY

Indications

Even before surgery is indicated, glasses may improve the vision of patients with cataracts. Also, visual aids, such as magnifying lenses and large print materials, may be helpful (see below, "Advice for the Visually Impaired"). The decision to remove a cataract is determined by the visual needs of the patient, as well as by the degree of capsular involvement and of any other ocular abnormalities. The ophthalmologist will perform a complete ocular assessment (see Chapter 98) before advising the patient about surgery.

Each patient must determine his own visual need based on his daily activities. The ability to read, drive, cross streets safely, and perform a daily routine is clearly of prime importance. For example, a patient usually requires visual acuity of at least 20/40 in the better eye to operate a motor vehicle safely or to continue moderately active daily life.

Surgery

Cataract surgery should not be done without considerable deliberation as there are a number of complications which might occur (see below), and vision after cataract extraction may be a major problem (see below). The general physician and the ophthalmologist should plan cataract surgery together. Cataract extraction is an elective procedure, and the patient should be in the best possible condition at the time of operation.

Approximately 600,000 cataract extractions are performed in the United States every year, and cataract surgery is the most commonly performed major surgical procedure done in the elderly in this country. Surgery involves the removal of the opacified lens from the eye. The extraction may be intracapsular, involving complete removal of the lens, or extracapsular, leaving the posterior capsule of the lens intact. Microsurgical techniques have greatly improved the immediate outcome of surgery and have significantly shortened the period of disability. Extracapsular extraction is most commonly performed because it leaves the posterior capsule intact, permits easier lens implantation (see below), and is associated with fewer postoperative complications. Both eyes usually require operation, but normally only one lens is extracted at a time so that the patient will have vision in the nonoperated side when the eye that has been operated upon is covered by a patch for a few days after surgery.

Patient experience. Cataract surgery is performed most often by use of local anesthesia supplemented with intravenous analgesia and sedation. Surgery is usually done as an outpatient procedure. The patient experiences moderate discomfort, but it lasts only a day or so and is controlled with analgesics. A hyperosmotic agent (such as glycerin or mannitol) may be employed to dehydrate and to soften the eye in preparation for surgery.

After discharge from the surgical unit a patient must restrict his activities for several weeks to avoid complications. These restrictions are listed in Table 97.2. There are no permanent restrictions; however, caution with steps or when walking and working with machinery may be necessary if perception is seriously altered using aphakic spectacles (see below).

Complications

Complications occur in approximately 5% of patients who have had cataract extraction, and 1 of every 5000 eyes operated upon is lost because of complications. Knowledge of the possible complications following cataract surgery will aid the general physician in educating his patients. Because of the potential for complications, the general physician must be sure that the patient keeps his scheduled postoperative appointments with the ophthalmologist.

Table 97.2.
Temporary Restrictions following Cataract Surgery[a]

Wear eye shield during sleep and wear glasses at other times—shields are usually worn for 1 month and then discontinued.

Absolutely no bending or stooping for 3 or 4 weeks.

Do not sleep on side of operated eye for 3 or 4 weeks.

Do not wash hair for 2 weeks.

No showers for 2 weeks, although a bath is allowed (but with assistance to prevent a fall).

No strenuous or excessive physical activity for 4 weeks and then only after approval of the ophthalmologist.

Do not lift objects that weigh over 5 pounds for 3 or 4 weeks.

[a] These are suggested to prevent inadvertent injury to the eye, to diminish disruptive pressure on the wound, to avoid sudden rise in ocular pressure, and to diminish the chance of infection.

Glaucoma (See Chapter 98)

This secondary form of glaucoma is due to several factors leading to angle closure: the effect of the proteolytic agent, chymotrypsin, on the angular structures at the time of operation; scarring due to postoperative inflammation; or the misdirection into and subsequent trapping of the aqueous in the vitreous gel (Fig. 98.1). Glaucoma may develop within a few days of surgery and may occur in as many as 20% of patients depending on the technique and whether chymotrypsin is used. Early glaucoma is usually transient, but it may become chronic. Also, glaucoma may appear as late as 1 to 2 years after surgery in 0.6 to 5% of patients depending on the type of surgery. The patient who has developed secondary glaucoma will usually complain of redness, tenderness, and pain in the eye. Further, if the patient has been fitted with a temporary spectacle, he will notice decreased visual acuity due to corneal edema. A postoperative patient suspected of having glaucoma should be seen by an ophthalmologist immediately.

Inflammation and Infection

All postoperative patients have some degree of traumatic intraocular inflammation. This is usually controlled effectively with topical corticosteroids. Bacterial endophthalmitis is a dangerous postoperative inflammation that must be recognized early before it devastates the eye. If a patient complains of pain, discharge, and redness, endophthalmitis may be present and the patient should be seen immediately by an ophthalmologist. Most infections occur within a few days of surgery; however, an operated eye is predisposed to infection from systemic infection, and therefore a patient with an acute red eye occurring at any time after eye surgery should be seen urgently by an ophthalmologist.

Hemorrhage

The sudden occurrence of hemorrhage in the uveal tract (the iris, the ciliary body, and the cho-

roid) can adversely influence the final visual outcome. Although this complication is usually seen intraoperatively, rarely it may occur postoperatively. The event is characterized by a painless but precipitous change in visual acuity. Postoperative hemorrhage from the iris or from an inadequately closed scleral wound is, however, more common than is vitreous hemorrhage. In all instances of hemorrhage, urgent referral to an ophthalmologist is indicated.

Retinal Detachment

The incidence of retinal detachment following cataract surgery is approximately 1 to 3%. Retinal detachment is characterized by suddenly decreased visual acuity, flashes of light, and the development of floaters, veils, and/or curtains in the visual field. These patients should be seen immediately by an ophthalmologist so that surgical reattachment of the retina may be accomplished. The success of reattachment is excellent provided that it can be done expeditiously.

Delayed Opacification of the Posterior Capsule

The new technique of extracapsular extraction is most commonly performed since it is associated with fewer complications (as compared to intracapsular extraction). However, 20 to 50% of patients experience a gradual decrease in vision in the first few years after this technique due to opacification of the posterior capsule. This complication can now be treated highly effectively by a special laser instrument (YAG, yttrium aluminum garnet) that opens the posterior capsule without surgery.

OPTICAL CORRECTION AFTER CATARACT EXTRACTION

The removal of a cataract improves the transmission of light to the retina, but vision remains blurred without corrective lenses, which may be one of three types: aphakic spectacles, contact lenses, or intraocular lenses.

With *aphakic spectacles* there is a narrower field of vision, as well as considerable distortion of images, which appear rounded and 3 to 5 times larger than when the lens is present in the eye. Also, there are peripheral ring scotomata and loss of some depth perception. Even modern aphakic spectacles are heavy and thick so that a patient frequently will have considerable initial difficulty adjusting to them and will need support, understanding, and encouragement from family members. With experience, however, most patients will be able to function acceptably and perform all of their necessary daily activities.

A unilateral cataract extraction results in a pronounced disparity in image size if an aphakic spectacle is used postoperatively; therefore, unilateral surgery is generally not advised unless the patient will be able to use a contact lens or is a candidate for an intraocular lens implantation (see below). Under certain circumstances, however (such as when glaucoma or diabetic retinopathy is present in addition to cataract), monolenticular extraction may be indicated to permit the ophthalmologist to follow the course of these ocular diseases.

The use of *contact lenses* after cataract extraction provides considerable improvement over spectacles. There is, especially, improvement in distortion and expansion of the field of vision. The patient, however, must be motivated to use contact lenses, and this motivation must be considered before surgery is undertaken. Often elderly patients are concerned about being agile enough to insert contact lenses. The patient must also be fitted with a pair of spectacles with one lens missing so that he may see to place one contact lens. A regular set of aphakic spectacles is also necessary as a backup to the contact lens.

Because of the visual handicap experienced after cataract extraction, *plastic lenses* are inserted at the time of surgery in nearly 85 to 95% of patients undergoing cataract extraction. Long term survival of these inert prostheses is very good. The insertion of intraocular implants adds approximately 15 to 20 minutes to the operative time beyond that required for lens extraction. Utilizing this technique more than 90% of patients will experience an improvement in vision to 20/40 or better.

ADVICE FOR THE VISUALLY IMPAIRED

When vision cannot be improved or maintained at an acceptable level, it is important for the physician to aid the patient in finding resources that might provide some help in lessening the ever increasing isolation and loss of mobility resulting from blindness. Dr. DeWitt Stetten (see "General References") wrote an essay describing his experience with progressive blindness and outlined in that essay a number of useful aids that he identified. He described the increasingly available large print books, journals, and newsprint (*e.g.*, *The New York Times*). There are also many books available on tape from the *Talking Books Program* of the Library of Congress. Most local libraries will be able to provide information on the availability of these tapes. Some journals may be obtained on tapes from *Recorded Periodicals* (919 Walnut St, Philadelphia, PA 19107). *Newsweek* magazine is available on disposable phonographic records (Newsweek, PO Box 6435, 1839 Frankfort Ave., Louisville, KY 40206). A variety of aids for the blind may be ordered from the catalog of SFB Products (Box 385, Wayne, PA 19087). A portable cassette tape recorder designed for the blind can be purchased through the American Printing House for the Blind, Inc (General Office, PO Box 6085, Louisville, KY 40206). Talking clocks and Braille time pieces may be very useful, and information concerning these and other aids may be available from the National Institutes of Health (Volunteers for the Visually Handicapped, 4405 East-West Hwy, Bethesda, MD 20814). Several reading machines or magnifying devices are also available, although these are expensive (see Stetten, "General References").

Visual Foundation, Inc (770 Center St, Newton, MA 02158) is a self-help organization that was developed by people losing their sight. They have published a handbook, *Coping with Sight Loss*, which provides for the visually impaired information on visual aids, devices, recreation, tax benefits, reading materials, and referral sources. The handbook is published in large print and on cassette tapes and will be a useful resource for the patient experiencing loss of vision as well as for physicians caring for these patients.

General References

Liesegang TJ: Cataracts and cataract operations—two parts. *Mayo Clin Proc* 59:556, 622, 1984.
> Concise, well illustrated, and well referenced review.

Stetten D Jr: Coping with blindness. *N Engl J Med* 305:458, 1981.
> A concise description of aids to help cope with blindness written by Dr. Stetten as he experienced progressive loss of vision.

Straatsma BR, Foos RY, Horwitz J, *et al*: Aging-related cataract: laboratory investigation and clinical management. *Ann Intern Med* 102:82, 1985.
> This UCLA conference reviews all aspects of senescent cataracts and contains superb color photographs of a variety of common cataract patterns.

CHAPTER NINETY-EIGHT

Glaucoma

EARL D. R. KIDWELL, JR., M.D.

Glaucoma is a common disorder characterized by an increase in intraocular pressure sufficient to cause damage to the optic nerve and retina. The glaucomas are classified into primary and secondary groups (Table 98.1). The primary group accounts for 95% of all patients with glaucoma in the United States.

Patients with glaucoma will usually be followed by an ophthalmologist. However, the general physician will need to be familiar with the techniques of screening for and diagnosing glaucoma and with the long term care of patients who are found to have glaucoma.

ANATOMY AND PHYSIOLOGY (Fig. 98.1)

The aqueous humor maintains the shape of the eye and the correct relationship among the refractile elements of the eye; it provides also the nutrition of the avascular intraocular structures such as the lens. There is continuous production and removal of the aqueous humor. In most cases of glaucoma, an obstruction to the outflow of aqueous humor appears to be the basis for the increased intraocular pressure.

The aqueous humor is a clear ultrafiltrate of the blood and occupies part of the posterior and anterior chambers of the eye. It is produced by the ciliary epithelium of the ciliary body, which is a portion of the uveal tract of the eye. It appears most likely that the aqueous is formed partially by secretion and partially by a process of ultrafiltration. At least two enzymes have been implicated in aqueous formation: sodium/potassium-activated ATPase and carbonic anhydrase. Antagonists of these enzymes reduce the rate of aqueous formation and thereby lower intraocular pressure. Acetazolamide (Diamox), a carbonic anhydrase inhibitor, has in this manner proved clinically important in the treatment of glaucoma. Once reproduced, the aqueous humor circulates from the posterior chamber into the anterior chamber of the eye. The trabecular meshwork, an intricate system of connective tissue fibers,

is located in the periphery of the anterior chamber. The aqueous percolates through this meshwork to be reunited with the venous blood *via* Schlemm's canal.

TYPES OF GLAUCOMA

Table 98.1 outlines the major types and causes of glaucoma. However, only primary open-angle and primary angle-closure are discussed in this chapter since they are the only types of glaucoma likely to be seen with any frequency by the general physician. Open-angle glaucoma takes its name from the relatively normal appearing anterior chamber angle as shown in Figure 98.2, a contrast to the narrow angle of angle-closure glaucoma.

Primary Open-Angle Glaucoma

Prevalence and Risk Factors

This form of glaucoma is by far the most common cause of glaucoma in the United States; the prevalence increases after the age of 40 years and approaches 3% of individuals over 75 years of age. Primary open-angle glaucoma causes 15 to 20% of all blindness in this country (see Chapter 97 for a discussion of blindness). Men and women are affected equally; but blacks are affected at an earlier age, and open-angle glaucoma is the leading cause of blindness in black Americans. Open-angle glaucoma is familial, but the pattern of inheritance is not yet known with certainty. In patients who have a positive family history of glaucoma, there is an association between glaucoma and leukocyte antigen HLA B12. It has been proposed that there is an

Table 98.1.
Types of Glaucoma

PRIMARY
    Open-angle—90% of patients
    Angle-closure—5% of patients
    Congenital—Infant and juvenile onset
SECONDARY
    Open-angle—Results from topical or systemic steroids, ocular inflammation, or obstructed venous return from the eye (*e.g.*, carotid cavernous sinus fistula)
    Angle-closure—Results from trauma, neovascular change of the iris postoperatively, ocular neoplasia, cataracts, and iris degenerations from various causes

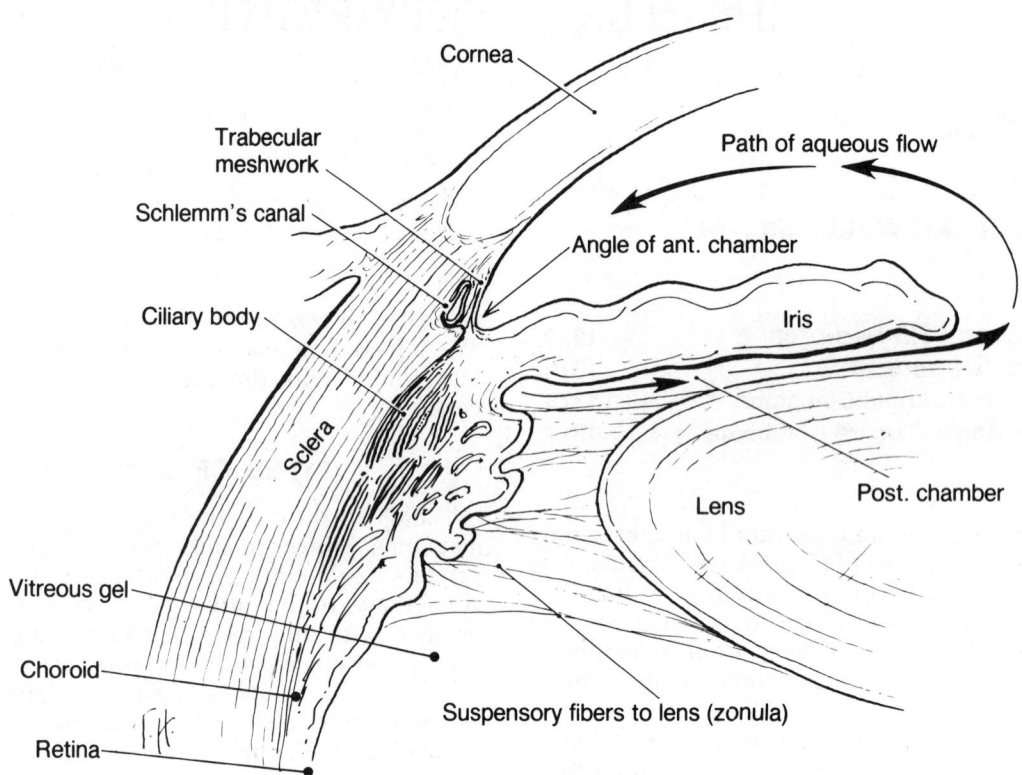

Figure 98.1. Anatomy of eye. (From Basmajian JV: *Grant's Method of Anatomy*, ed 8. Baltimore, Williams & Wilkins, 1971, p 543.)

association between open-angle glaucoma and both diabetes mellitus and elevated blood pressure, but these hypotheses are controversial and more research will be necessary to define or negate such relationships. Patients who have high degrees of myopia (defective distant vision) are often said to have a higher risk of open-angle glaucoma, but there remains more controversy about this hypothesis as well.

Diagnosis

In primary open-angle glaucoma, ocular hypertension results from resistance in the trabecular meshwork to aqueous outflow. The elevation of the intraocular pressure is roughly related to the degree of obstruction. The disease has no associated symptoms in its early stages. When symptoms do occur, neural damage is present and may be substantial. Macular (central) vision and the ability to recognize forms on a vision test chart are preserved until very late. For this reason testing of visual acuity is not a reliable method to screen for glaucoma. Occasionally a patient with open-angle glaucoma may notice halos around lights and blurring of vision if there is a sudden rise in intraocular pressure such as might occur with rapid ingestion of a large quantity of fluid (e.g., 1 liter). Patients with this history should be referred urgently to an ophthalmologist regardless

of the intraocular pressure. Patients only rarely complain of headache that can be attributed to increased intraocular pressure. The ocular pressure may be elevated for years, however, before any change in the optic disc is noted. The change will be revealed by increasing excavation of the central physiological disc cup, visible on funduscopic examination (Fig. 98.3). This is most easily seen by use of the red filter of the direct ophthalmoscope. Over years the pink color of the disc fades and becomes pale, and vessels coursing over the disc show a sharp bend at the rim.

In evaluating the patient with increased intraocular pressure the opthalmologist will perform tonometry, gonioscopy (see below), funduscopy, and visual field examinations. Characteristic visual field changes called "nerve fiber bundle defects" are seen in glaucoma.

Screening for Open-Angle Glaucoma

Screening for primary open-angle glaucoma is warranted for several reasons: (a) the disease is silent until permanent ocular damage has occurred, (b) screening is relatively simple and without significant risk, (c) treatment can prevent eye damage, and (d) this form of glaucoma is common, especially in older individuals. Screening in theory could be accomplished in one or more of three ways: tonometry, funduscopic assessment of the optic cup, and

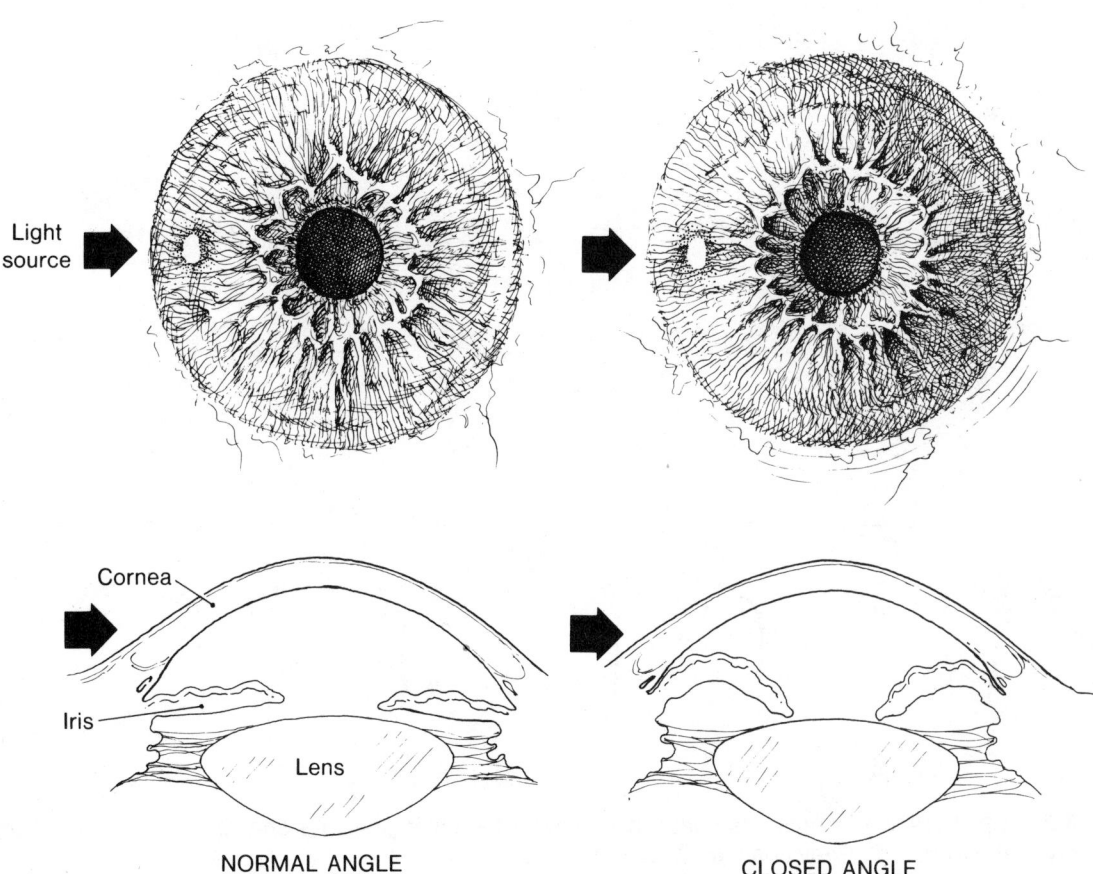

Light source

Cornea

Iris

Lens

NORMAL ANGLE

CLOSED ANGLE

Figure 98.2. Illustration showing a shadow cast on the iris resultant from the bowed iris in angle-closure glaucoma. In open-angle glaucoma, the iris is not bowed and the shadow, therefore, is not cast.

visual field assessment. Ophthalmologists generally do all three evaluations, but this is not practical for the general physician. While there are advocates for each of these three techniques, the most practical and reliable screening method for the general physician is tonometry with the use of the Schiötz tonometer (Fig. 98.4).

This tonometer measures the weight required to indent the anesthetized cornea of the eye. If the ocular pressure is elevated, an increased weight is necessary to cause indentation. The ocular pressure is less than 20 mm Hg in 95% of normal individuals. Patients found to have pressures in one or both eyes equal to or greater than 20 mm Hg should be referred to an ophthalmologist. Should the physician also notice an enlarged physiological cup (greater than 30% of the disc diameter, see Fig. 98.3), prompt referral to an ophthalmologist is indicated. Complications of tonometry include corneal abrasion, sensitivity reaction to the anesthetic, or infection. These complications are all quite rare and occur in less than 1% of examinations.

With practice, the general physician can perform ocular tonometry in 2 minutes. This, therefore, can be done at the time of a general physical examina-

tion or at the time of periodic health assessment. Tonometry can be performed with accuracy by technicians and office personnel under a physician's supervision. If the physician is unfamiliar with the use of the Schiötz tonometer or is unable to take the time to perform the test, patients should be encourated to have periodic glaucoma screening by an ophthalmologist.

Since open-angle glaucoma is a disease of older individuals, routine tonometry should be performed in individuals over 45 years of age. An initial assessment at the time of a general physician examination in these individuals is appropriate, with periodic follow-up at 5-year intervals until age 75 when the frequency of assessment should be increased to 1-year intervals in parallel with the increasing incidence of glaucoma.

Patients referred to an ophthalmologist because their intraocular pressure is equal to or greater than 20 mm Hg will generally have an evaluation consisting of several observations: *repeat assessment of the intraocular pressure by applanation tonometry,* by use of a complex piece of equipment and requiring only a drop of topical anesthetic; *funduscopic assessment of the optic disc and retina; formal visual*

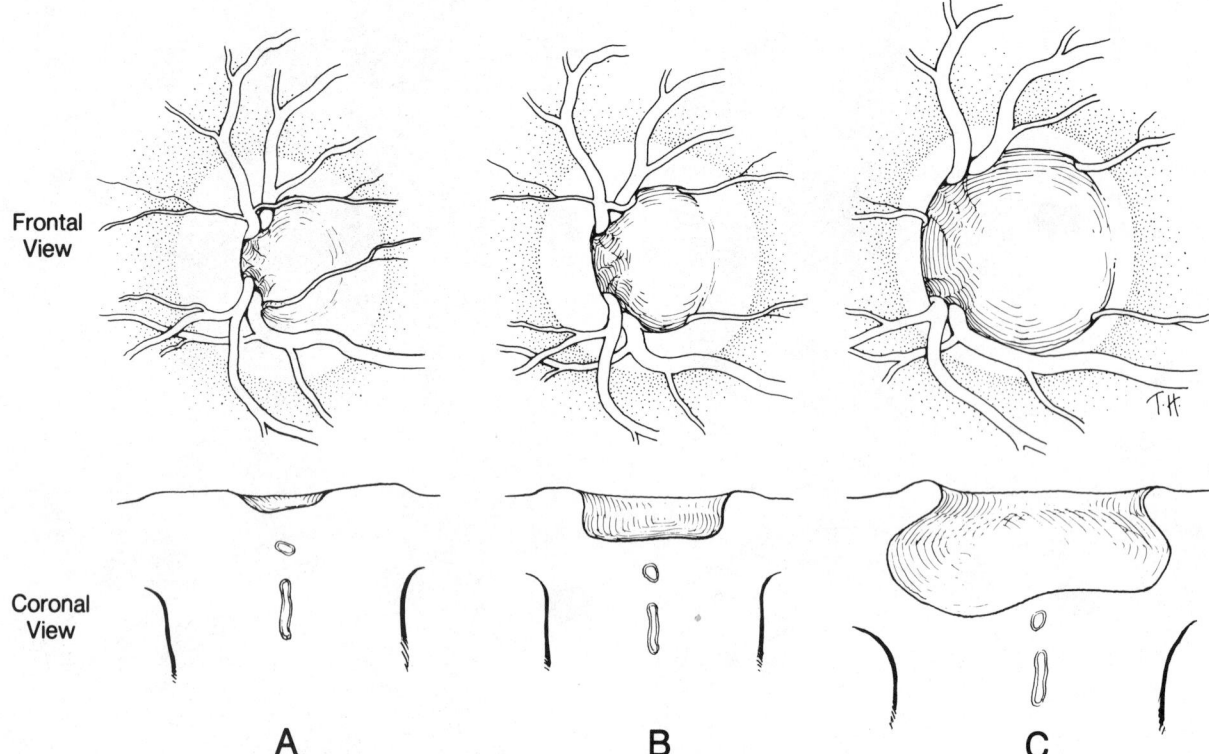

Frontal
View

Coronal
View

A   B   C

Figure 98.3.   Changes in the optic disc with increasing intraocular pressure showing on both the frontal and coronal views: *A.* Normal. *B.* Early change. *C.* Late change.

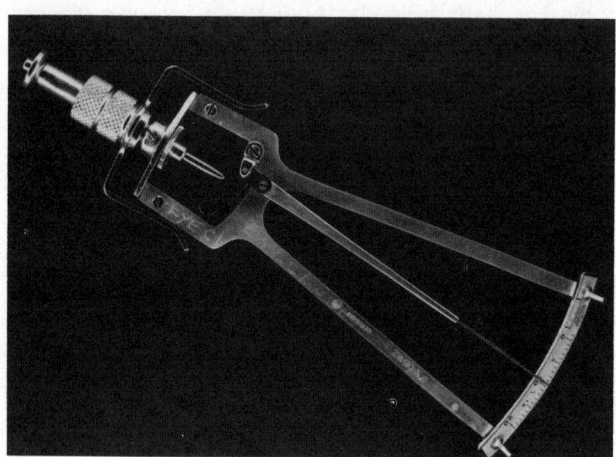

Figure 98.4.   Schiötz tonometer.

field assessment; and *gonioscopic examination,* which permits the ophthalmologist to visualize the angle of the anterior chamber by using an instrument containing a contact lens and mirror. The patient usually experiences minimal or no discomfort during any of these procedures.

Approximately one-third of patients referred to an ophthalmologist because of the finding of asymptomatic increased intraocular pressure will be found to have glaucoma. Approximately 30% may be found

not to have elevated pressures on reassessment, while about 25% will have ocular hypertension without glaucoma. This latter group should be followed yearly by the ophthalmologist; some of these patients may, over a period of time, develop glaucoma.

Rarely, patients may have normal pressure glaucoma, but the general physician will not be able to detect these patients unless an enlarged physiological optic cup is noticed, after which an ophthalmological consultation is indicated.

Treatment

When the opthalmologist establishes the diagnosis of open-angle glaucoma, he will prescribe treatment based on the level of intraocular pressure (although a pressure of greater than 30 mm Hg is an absolute indication for treatment), the degree of visual field loss, and the amount of optic nerve damage.

The treatment of open-angle glaucoma is largely medical, with use of agents that facilitate the outflow (e.g., miotics) or reduce the amount of production (e.g., β-blockers) of aqueous humor. The aim of therapy is to maintain the intraocular pressure below 20 mm Hg. Patients are usually prescribed a mild miotic, such as carbachol or pilocarpine. Other agents, such as carbonic anhydrase inhibitors and stronger miotics, are added or replace the milder agents as necessary. Also the β-adrenergic receptor blocking agent timolol maleate (e.g., Timoptic Ophthalmic Solution) will reduce ocular pressure and has the advantage of producing little or no effect on pupil size or visual acuity. For this reason decreased, blurred, or impaired night vision is not the problem with timolol that it is with miotic agents. However, systemic effects of the β-blocker may occur.

Frequently, early in the course, treatment may need to be changed by the ophthalmologist since tolerance is common and side effects may occur. Once the decreased ocular pressure has been attained, the ophthalmologist will usually examine the patient approximately three times/year for assessment of visual fields, measurement of intraocular pressure, funduscopic examination, and gonioscopy.

Argon laser trabeculoplasty may be used by the ophthalmologist to open a canal in the trabecular meshwork in order to lower ocular pressure when medical therapy is unsatisfactory. This office procedure requires only topical anesthesia and can result in a significant reduction in ocular pressure in nearly two-thirds of patients. Most patients, however, will continue to require the continued use of medications.

Surgery in primary open-angle glaucoma is designed to construct outflow channels for the aqueous humor or to freeze the ciliary body and destroy the site of aqueous production. This surgical procedure is reserved for patients in whom medical management fails. Medications may still be required after surgery.

Monitoring

The primary physician should ensure that the patient with diagnosed open-angle glaucoma is receiving regular ophthalmological follow-up. Further, he should be alert to any side effects from the drugs prescribed by the ophthalmologist.

There has been particular concern about systemic medications that have anticholinergic (atropine-like), adrenergic, vasodilator, or corticosteroid properties and that may adversely affect ocular pressure. However, there are few data that would contraindicate the use of these agents in patients with open-angle glaucoma. Only if an anticholinergic drug paralyzes accommodation (noticeable as blurriness when the eyes are used for close work as in reading) should there be concern about it causing increased ocular pressure, in which situation the drug should be withdrawn; or if its use is mandatory, an ophthalmologist should be consulted. Systemic corticosteroids and, in particular, corticosteroids applied to the eye in the absence of intraocular inflammation may make the control of open-angle glaucoma more difficult. There is no evidence that vasodilator or adrenergic drugs affect the course of glaucoma.

Primary Angle-Closure Glaucoma

While this form of glaucoma is far less common than open-angle glaucoma it is important that the general physician be aware of it because an attack may be precipitated by the use of mydriatics, and if this occurs, urgent recognition and treatment are mandatory to prevent damage to the eye. Patients frequently have a positive family history and women are affected more than men.

The basic defect in primary angle-closure glaucoma is the inability of aqueous humor to reach the filtration apparatus. There is a blockage of the trabecular meshwork by the peripheral iris. When the pupil is mid-dilated, the iris is bowed forward, which blocks the outflow of aqueous humor (Fig. 98.2).

Individuals who have narrow anterior ocular chambers are predisposed to primary angle-closure glaucoma. Moreover, the lens may be of such size that there is encroachment of the aqueous-filtering trabecular meshwork. Individuals with these predispositions often have acute attacks of increased intraocular pressure when the eye is dilated, occluding outflow, as might occur in the dark or when mydriatic is placed in the eye for funduscopic examination.

Diagnosis

Early diagnosis of this problem is critical because virtually every case is surgically curable. Cure is increasingly less likely if repeated attacks have occurred and have resulted in scarring of the trabecular meshwork at the angle of the anterior chamber. The acute attack frequently is unilateral and often is precipitated by emotion (from associated pupillary dilation). The classical symptoms are episodes of ocular pain (usually located in the periocular or supraocular region), episodes of blurred vision, and halos around lights at night. These symptoms occur because of corneal epithelial edema which has developed as a result of the increased intraocular pressure. Often patients find relief in well lighted rooms or out of doors where daylight causes constriction of the pupil and opening of the angle of the anterior chamber.

Examination during an acute attack usually reveals marked elevation of intraocular pressure, to 60 to 90 mm Hg. However, chronic obstruction may compromise the circulation of the ciliary body and result in a fall in aqueous production and subsequently reduce ocular pressure. However, there is considerable individual tolerance of the vascular supply of the ciliary body to the increased pressure.

In patients predisposed to angle-closure glaucoma, the anterior chamber is shallow. This may be seen by illuminating the eye with a flashlight from the side and showing a shadow resulting from the bowed iris over the nasal portion of the eye (Fig. 98.2).

Ophthalmoscopic examination may reveal scarring of the trabecular meshwork—peripheral anterior synechia. Corneal edema will be present during an acute attack, and the anterior chamber may appear cloudy due to inflammation.

If the diagnosis of acute angle-closure glaucoma is suspected, immediate administration of acetazolamide (Diamox), 250 mg orally, and instillation of 2 drops of a miotic—such as pilocarpine (Pilocar), 4% every 15 minutes—are indicated, and the patient should see an ophthalmologist within 6 hours. In severe cases, the ingesting of hyperosmotic glycerol—1 ml/kg mixed as a 50% solution with chilled juice—almost always will interrupt an acute attack. Physicians who use mydriatics for funduscopic examination or patients who have narrow anterior ocular chambers and who do not have immediate access to an ophthalmologist should have an "angle-closure kit" consisting of pilocarpine (Pilocar, 4%), glycerol (glycerin—available as generic), and acetazolamide (Diamox) for use during an acute attack. Patients found to have a shallow anterior chamber even if they have not had a symptomatic attack of glaucoma should be referred to an ophthalmologist for evaluation, for education regarding specific manifestations of an acute attack, and for their initial treatment as well as for consideration for prophylactic iridectomy.

Differential Diagnosis

The patient who has acute angle-closure glaucoma may come with an acute red eye to a general physician. Initially the physician will want to differentiate angle-closure glaucoma from acute iritis, acute conjunctivitis, and iridocyclitis. Chapter 99 discusses this differential diagnosis.

Course without Treatment

Severe attacks of angle-closure glaucoma may cause blindness in 2 to 3 days depending on the level of intraocular pressure and on the sensitivity of the ciliary body and optic nerve to ischemia. In some instances, ciliary ischemia stops aqueous production before blindness occurs; but repeated attacks are the rule, and these will eventually result in scarring of the trabecular meshwork. The frequency and rapidity of recurrences are unpredictable. An examination between attacks usually will reveal only a shallow anterior chamber (Fig. 98.2) and normal intraocular pressure. Peripheral anterior synechiae and segmental iris atrophy may be seen depending on the frequency and severity of previous attacks. A history of an acute attack, an actual acute attack, or the demonstration of a shallow anterior chamber should lead to an ophthalmological consultation.

Treatment

The treatment of primary angle-closure glaucoma is essentially surgical. If the diagnosis is made early enough in the course of the disease, a peripheral iridectomy can be done to prevent the attacks of increased intraocular pressure and the development of scarring. Surgical peripheral iridectomy under local anesthesia has little risk and results in cure. Iridectomy may also be done by using a laser beam. The eye involved in an acute attack is operated upon as soon as the attack is controlled (see above). Generally, the other eye is operated upon prophylactically a week or so later. Follow-up care by the ophthalmologist after surgery is necessary. If pressure control has not been achieved, medical therapy (see above) may be necessary. This, however, is unusual if surgery is performed early.

When the physician is aware that a patient has a narrow anterior chamber or is under treatment for angle-closure glaucoma, there should be concern about the use of certain medications. Systemic anticholinergics or adrenegic drugs may precipitate an acute attack by causing dilation of the pupils. Corticosteroids or vasodilating drugs are not contraindicated in patients with angle-closure glaucoma.

General References

Editorial: Intraocular pressure control in glaucoma. *Lancet* 2:81, 1984.
> A brief overview of current therapy of elevated intraocular pressure with pertinent references.

Fraunfelder FT, Roy FN: *Current Ocular Therapy*, ed 2. Philadelphia, WB Saunders, 1985.
> This text provides a brief definitive review of many common eye problems. It gives excellent therapeutic guidelines and has some pertinent references.

Havener WH: *Synopsis of Ophthalmology*, ed 6. St Louis, CV Mosby, 1984.
> A well written short textbook covering general ophthalmology with an excellent chapter on glaucoma.

Leske MC, Rosenthal J: Epidemiological aspects of open angle glaucoma. *Am J Epidemiol* 109:250, 1979
> A critical review of the prevalence.

Remis LL, Epstein DL: Treatment of glaucoma. *Annu Rev Med* 35:195, 1984.
> A well referenced review of the treatment of glaucoma.

Schwartz B: Current concepts in ophthalmology. The glaucomas. *N Engl J Med* 299:182, 1978.
> A brief, helpful review of the glaucomas.

CHAPTER NINETY-NINE

The Red Eye

EARL D. R. KIDWELL, Jr., M.D.

A patient who has developed a red eye is encountered frequently in an ambulatory practice. The problem is usually caused by an infection and most often is self-limited; however, there are serious considerations in the differential diagnosis that the general physician must recognize so that he can initiate urgent ophthalmological consultation if necessary. This chapter provides a framework for recognizing conditions that require consultation and provides a discussion of conditions that may be managed by the general physician. Figure 99.1 illustrates the important structures and landmarks of the external eye.

DIFFERENTIAL DIAGNOSIS (Table 99.1)

Conditions That Require Referral

The conditions requiring urgent ophthalmological consultation can be recognized by the general physician if he pays attention to several important fea-

tures of the history and physical examination. The patient should be asked specifically whether he has been treated for an *ocular disorder* or whether he has recently experienced *pain* in one or both of his eyes. When the eyes are examined, it is essential to evaluate the following features: visual acuity, the nature of the discharge, the appearance of the cornea, the size and reactivity of the pupil, and the extent of the redness. In selected patients special tests, such as measurement of ocular tension or inspection of the eye after fluorescein staining, are necessary. Table 99.2 shows how this information may suggest a specific diagnosis.

Specific Conditions

Acute glaucoma is discussed in Chapter 98.

Iritis may be due to a specific problem such as trauma or infection, but often a specific etiology cannot be identified. In this condition failure to initiate proper treatment may result in permanent scarring, which will affect pupillary movement and may cause glaucoma.

Iritis can usually be recognized by the general physician because it is a painful condition that characteristically is acute in onset and is associated with photophobia. Often vision is blurred as well. Occasionally, the pupil of the involved eye is small and fixed compared to the contralateral one. Typically the redness in iritis surrounds the cornea.

Corneal injury is usually recognized easily because of intense pain localized to the cornea following an injury and because of identification of a corneal lesion. If the injury is secondary to minor trauma (corneal abrasion) from a foreign body, the eye may be irrigated with a sterile eyewash (such as Collyrium) and a patch placed over it for 24 hours (see below, "Foreign Body"). If, on the other hand, an extensive epithelial defect (as revealed by fluorescein staining) is present, urgent ophthalmological referral is indicated.

Fluorescein staining is easily accomplished by moistening a sterile fluorescein strip in the lower conjunctival sac and waiting a moment for the fluorescein to diffuse into the tears. The eye is then irrigated with physiological saline or eyewash, and the epithelial defect will remain stained a brillant green. A corneal ulcer will also stain with fluorescein, but staining will appear to be deeper, indicating

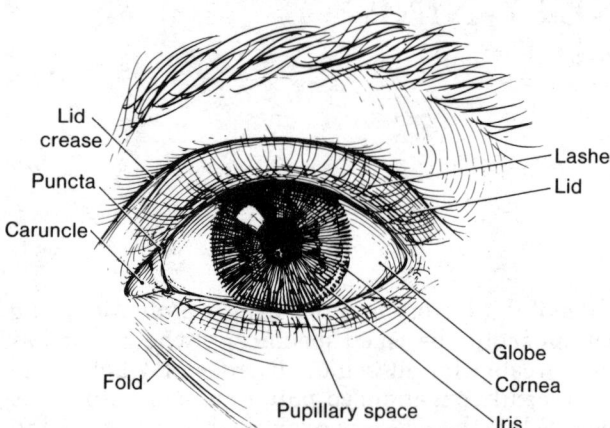

Figure 99.1. External landmarks of the eye.

Table 99.1.
Major Causes of a Red Eye

CONDITIONS THAT REQUIRE REFERRAL
  Acute glaucoma
  Acute iritis
  Acute corneal tear or infection
  Acute scleritis and/or episcleritis
CONDITIONS THAT USUALLY CAN BE MANAGED BY
    THE GENERAL PHYSICIAN
  Bacterial conjunctivitis—hyperacute, acute, and chronic
  Viral conjunctivitis
  Inclusion conjunctivitis
  Allergic conjunctivitis
  Chemical conjunctivitis
  Foreign body
  Subconjunctival hemorrhage

subepithelial corneal involvement. Patients with this latter problem should see an ophthalmologist urgently.

Scleritis usually is seen in association with a systemic disorder (such as rheumatoid arthritis). The deep vessels of the sclera are dilated; this may be demonstrated by the instillation of a drop of Neo-Synephrine 5 or 10%, which will constrict the superficial, but not the deep vessels. This mydriatic should be avoided in patients with a history of narrow-angle glaucoma (Chapter 98). The patient usually complains of a discomfort in the eye, and sometimes of severe pain, which is intensified if the eye is moved. Scleritis is often associated with iritis (see above).

Episcleritis is a relatively common problem characterized by pain caused by a characteristically sharply localized area of inflammation of the superficial layer of the sclera. The etiology is unknown, but it is occasionally associated with a systemic disorder such as rheumatoid arthritis or a specific infection such as herpes zoster or tuberculosis. A few patients will have an associated iritis (see above), which is usually mild. The palpebral con-

junctiva (*i.e.,* that lining the eyelid) is not involved and there is no discharge; these two observations help to differentiate this problem from conjunctivitis. Episcleritis is short lived but is frequently recurrent; for this reason, ophthalmological consultation is indicated.

Conditions That Usually Can Be Managed by the General Physician

Conjunctival infections, allergies, eyelid inflammation, and irritation are the commonest causes of red or irritated eyes and are discussed in detail below. Almost always a general physician can manage these problems without consulting with an ophthalmologist.

CONJUNCTIVITIS

General Considerations

The diagnosis and management of conjunctivitis can be confusing, considering the variety of ocular infections. Most cases are not absolute emergencies, and, frequently, they are self-limited. Conjunctivitis may, however, cause serious complications such as corneal scarring, lid damage, or, in cases in which the patient has had antecedent intraocular surgery, endophthalmitis.

Conjunctival Flora

Under normal conditions the conjunctival sac has a bacterial flora composed of several species. The most commonly encountered organism is *Staphylococcus albus*, followed by corynebacteria, *Staphylococcus aureus*, and *Streptococcus* species. This complex flora complicates the establishment of a specific etiology in a patient with infectious conjunctivitis.

Presentation

Conjunctivitis is usually not painful, but often there is mild discomfort, burning, discharge, tearing, itching, and lid swelling. Vision is well preserved. Most often, infectious conjunctivitis is bilateral.

Laboratory Diagnosis

Whenever there is doubt about the diagnosis, a simple culture and/or staining of the conjunctival material will help in determining the cause and subsequent management of the condition. Most often, however, an adequate diagnosis can be made from the appearance of the conjunctiva, and a culture is not necessary.

Culture

Specimens for culture should be obtained with a sterile cotton swab by everting the eyelid and wiping the conjunctival sac. This material must be obtained without topical anesthesia because the preservatives in the anesthetic solution might inhibit the growth

Table 99.2.
Important Observations in Evaluation of a Patient with a Red Eye

	Glaucoma	Iritis	Corneal Injury	Scleritis	Episcleritis	Bacterial Conjunctivitis	Inclusion Conjunctivitis	Viral Conjunctivitis
History of previous ocular disorder or condition predisposing to an ocular disorder	+	+/−	−	+	−	−	−	−
Pain	+	+ Photophobia	+	+	+	Mild discomfort or burning	Mild discomfort or burning	Mild discomfort or burning
Visual acuity	Diminished and blurred	Blurred	Usually diminished	Normal	Normal	Normal	Occasionally blurred, if chronic	Normal
Discharge	None	None	Usually some	None	None	Present: thick or thin	None or mucopurulent	None
Appearance of cornea	May be hazy	Normal	May be streaky	Normal	Normal	Normal	Normal except when superior dots or streaking may be seen	Normal
Pupil	Often dilated, mid-dilated, or fixed	Small and different from opposite side	Normal	Normal	Normal	Normal	Normal except if late when it may be small and different from other side	Normal
Redness	Around cornea	Around cornea	Localized or diffuse	Localized or diffuse	Localized	Diffuse	Diffuse (variable)	Segmental or diffuse
Selected evaluations	Ocular pressure in eye is high (see Chapter 98)[a]	Normal	Fluorescein stain[b] shows epithelial defect as brilliant green	A drop of Neo-Synephrine 5 or 10% in conjunctiva will constrict superficial but not deep vessels (see the text)	None	None	None	None

[a] Should not be measured if a discharge is present or if a corneal ulceration is seen.
[b] Use individually packaged sterile fluorescein strips.

**Table 99.3.
Diagnosis Based on Cells in Material Scraped from Conjunctiva**

Cells	Significance
Polymorphonuclear leukocytes	Bacterial, fungus, *Chlamydia* (inclusion conjunctivitis), trachoma, Stevens-Johnson syndrome
Mononuclear cells	Viral
Eosinophils	Allergy, ocular pemphigoid
Epithelial metaplasia (atypical, large cells)	*Chlamydia*, herpes simplex

of organisms. The specimen must be transferred immediately into transport media or delivered immediately to the laboratory for culturing. Whenever a culture is considered necessary, both eyes could be cultured separately, even if there is only monocular involvement, so that the apparently uninfected eye will provide information about the nature of the normal flora.

Scraping

Following culture, a topical anesthetic (such as Ophthaine) should be instilled, and scrapings of the conjunctiva, well away from the cornea, should be obtained. A sterile platinum *spatula* (available from physician supply stores) or the dull side of a sterile scalpel *blade* can be used to scrape the conjunctiva. The material obtained by this method is smeared on a glass slide and is stained with Gram stain and/or Giemsa stain. The appearance of the cells found in these scrapings is helpful in determining the diagnosis and, therefore, scraping is recommended in the evaluation of patients with conjunctivitis when the diagnosis is uncertain. The differential findings are discussed below and listed in Table 99.3.

Specific Types

Hyperacute Bacterial Conjunctivitis

The name of this condition reflects its onset and the very thick exudate associated with it (Fig. 99.2, page 1383). Typically, the discharge is so copious that it accumulates in the lashes or runs down the patient's cheek. One eye is usually involved before the other, but within several days the second eye becomes involved through autoinoculation. The infection quickly involves the surrounding structures and is associated with aching discomfort, swelling of the lid, and tenderness of the eye. Enlarged preauricular lymph nodes are often present. Early in the infection the cornea is not involved, but as the conjunctival swelling and reaction increase, a peripheral corneal ring ulcer may develop due to the compression of the peripheral corneal circulation.

Neisseria gonorrhoeae or *Niesseria meningitidis* is usually implicated in this infection. Inoculation is a result of fomite spread or through autoinoculation

from infected genitalia. The gonococcus has the ability to penetrate the intact corneal epithelium so that central corneal ulceration and endophthalmitis also may occur. Meningococcal conjunctivitis is indistinguishable from gonococcal conjunctivitis, although the former occurs more frequently in younger individuals, may be bilateral at the onset, and can proceed to metastatic meningitis or meningococcemia.

Conjunctival scrapings reveal an overwhelming number of polymorphonuclear leukocytes and intracellular Gram-negative diplococci. Culture should be obtained on Thayer-Martin selective medium or be sent to the laboratory on Transgrow medium. The differentiation between gonococcus and meningococcus requires special bacteriological studies.

Therapy of hyperacute conjunctivitis must be prompt to avoid corneal damage or systemic spread and should include the administration of both systemic and topical antibiotics (Table 99.4). Institution of appropriate antibiotics should result in the disappearance of the discharge within 24 to 48 hours, although lid swelling and conjunctival reaction do not abate for several days. If a corneal ulcer occurs, it is slow to heal; and if the cornea has been scarred or if endophthalmitis has developed, visual acuity may be affected. Therefore, whenever there is evidence of impaired vision, an ophthalmologist should be consulted immediately.

Acute Bacterial Conjunctivitis

This condition, like hyperacute bacterial conjunctivitis, has an abrupt onset but is characterized by a less thick, often mucopurulent, discharge. This form of conjunctivitis is often called *catarrhal or pink eye* (Fig. 99.3, page 1383); it is seen at all ages and at any time of year. The most common cause of the condition is *Staphylococcus aureus* infection. *Pneumococcus* and *Haemophilus* species also cause the problem, but infections with these organisms have a more restricted geographic distribution than do staphylococcal infections; pneumococcal infections occur primarily in the northern states during the colder months, and *Haemophilus* infections occur more commonly in the warmer regions of the United States throughout the year. Also, pneumococcal or *Haemophilus* conjunctivitis is more common in younger individuals than is staphylococcal conjunctivitis. Rarely, other bacteria, such as *Moraxella lacunata*, *Escherichia coli*, or *Proteus* species, cause this form of conjunctivitis.

Patients complain of eye irritation and watering and typically the eyelids stick together after sleep. The infection starts unilaterally; but very often, because of autoinoculation, the contralateral eye becomes involved in 1 or 2 days. Examination reveals hyperemia of the palpebra; bulbar conjunctival petechiae, characteristic of *Haemophilus* infection, may be seen.

These infections are self-limited and generally last

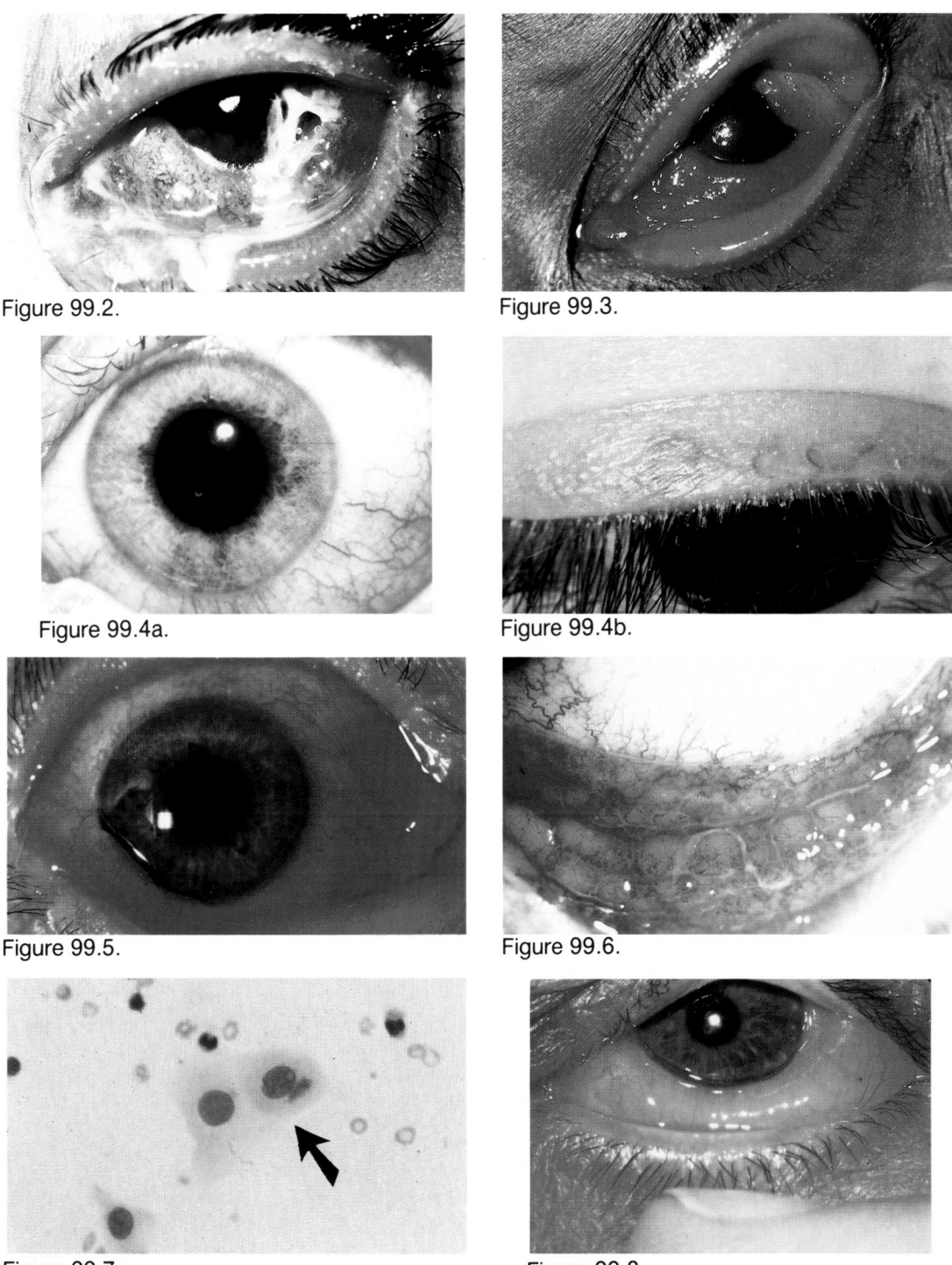

Figure 99.2.

Figure 99.3.

Figure 99.4a.

Figure 99.4b.

Figure 99.5.

Figure 99.6.

Figure 99.7.

Figure 99.8.

Figure 99.2. Hyperacute bacterial conjunctivitis. Note the severe degree of infection, swelling, and pustular discharge.

Figure 99.3. Acute bacterial conjunctivits. Note the severe erythema and edema.

Figure 99.4. Chronic bacterial conjunctivitis. *a.* Injected conjunctiva and erythema of lid margins. *b.* Telangiectasia of upper lid and debris in the lashes.

Figure 99.5. Viral conjunctivitis. Note the redness as well as the edema of the lid and conjunctiva.

Figure 99.6. Inclusion conjunctivitis. Note the redness as well as the edema of the lid and conjunctiva.

Figure 99.7. Scraping of conjunctiva from a patient with inclusion conjunctivitis showing inclusion body (*arrow*) (Giemsa stain).

Figure 99.8. Allergic conjunctivitis. Note the conjunctival edema.

Table 99.4.
Antimicrobials That May Be Used in Treatment of Hyperacute Conjunctivitis (Both a Systemic and Topical Agent Should Be Used)

SYSTEMIC

Procaine penicillin G, 4.8 million units intramuscularly preceded by 1 g of probenicid administered orally
or

Ampicillin, 3.5 g and probenicid 1 g administered orally, simultaneously
or, if penicillin-sensitive:

Spectinomycin, 4 g intramuscularly at initial visit given in 2 injections
or

Tetracycline 1.5 g orally as an initial dose followed by 0.5 g, 4 times a day for 4 days

TOPICAL

Gentamicin ophthalmic in the involved eye every 2 hours for 5 days, then 4 times a day for 7–10 days
or

Chloramphenicol, 0.5% ophthalmic in the involved eye every 2 hours for 2 days, then 4 times a day for 7–10 days
or

Bacitracin ointment, 500 units/g in the involved eye every 2 hours for 2 days, then 4 times a day for 7–10 days

---

7 to 14 days, although *Haemophilus* infections may last somewhat longer.

The diagnosis is suspected by the examination; however, wherever there is doubt, diagnosis should be confirmed by examination of the scrapings of the conjunctiva and by culturing the exudate.

Topical treatment usually results in the resolution of symptoms in a day or two. The preferred therapy is with sodium sulfacetamide (Sulamyd-10%)—either the solution, 2 drops in the eye every 3 hours while awake, or the ointment, a small amount applied to the lower conjunctival sac four times a day and at bedtime. If there is an allergy to sulfa drugs, a 1% chloramphenicol ointment (Chloromycetin ophthalmic ointment), four times a day and at bedtime, may be used. This agent is particularly efficacious against *Haemophilus* and *Moraxella*.

Chronic Bacterial Conjunctivitis

Staphylococcus aureus causes most cases of chronic bacterial conjunctivitis; but occasionally it is caused by other agents, such as *Staphylococcus epidermidis, Moraxella lacunata, Corynebacterium diphtheriae*, or *Streptococcus pyogenes. S. aureus* colonizes the margin of the eyelid and the follicles containing the eyelashes. Both *S. aureus* and *S. epidermidis* elaborate an exotoxin which injures the conjunctiva and cornea, and it is this toxin that is responsible for the chronic inflammation.

Patients with this problem complain of a sensation of a foreign body in the eye as well as of redness and itching; frequently eyelids stick together after sleep.

There is often a history of recurrent styles and of loss of eyelashes. Examination shows erythema of the lid margin and, sometimes, a minimal exudate is present. Occasionally, mucous strands may be found in the conjunctival fornices, and the eyelids may appear thickened and red (Fig. 99.4, page 1383).

The lid margins, surrounding skin, conjunctiva, and cornea may be involved singly or collectively. The skin may also show changes of seborrheic dermatitis or it may be excoriated and macerated, especially at the lateral canthal margin. Crusting is noted at the bases of the eyelashes. The conjunctiva may show changes of papillar hyperplasia (multiple conjunctival mounds with a central single vessel). Corneal changes occur after months of inflammation and are manifest as fine discrete inferior defects. There may also be ulceration, clouding, and vascularization of the margins of the cornea.

The diagnosis is made by examination and, in cases in doubt, by scraping the conjunctivae as well as the margins of the eyelids and by culturing the exudate.

Usually, gentamicin solution or ointment (Garamycin ophthalmic drops or ointment), 1 or 2 drops or a small amount of ointment every 4 hours while awake, or erythromycin ointment (Ilotycin ophthalmic ointment), every 4 hours while awake, will be effective. Treatment should be continued for 2 weeks. Daily cleansing of the eyelashes with a neutral soap (such as Johnson's Baby Shampoo) followed by the application of an antibiotic ointment (such as gentamicin or erythromycin) to the eyelashes four times a day for several weeks will reduce the bacterial count, cleanse the lids, and prevent recurrences.

Viral Conjunctivitis

Viral conjunctivitis is also known as *acute follicular conjunctivitis* and it quite common. It is caused by a variety of viral agents. The onset is abrupt and unilateral, but contralateral involvement from autoinoculation is frequent in a day or two. Excessive tearing is often a major complaint, but there is no purulent discharge. The conjunctiva nearly always shows hyperemia, which may be diffuse or segmental (see Fig. 99.5, page 1383). Viral conjunctivitis may be accompanied by tender preauricular lymphadenopathy. Frequently, the lymphoid tissue of the eyelid enlarges in response to the infection and may appear as elevated palpebral as well as bulbar conjunctival lesions (Fig. 99.5). In cases where there is doubt about the diagnosis, examination of the conjunctival scrapings shows mononuclear cells.

The disease is self-limited, lasting only a few days; and treatment is therefore supportive. Astringent drops containing naphazoline (such as over-the-counter agents—Albalon, Naphcon-A, or Vasocon-A) are very helpful in relieving conjunctival congestion and hyperemia, and cool compresses also provide relief. Sulfacetamide (Sulamyd) or erythromycin (Ilotycin), as described above, may be used if symptoms have not been controlled in 1 or 2 days with astringent drops, in this instance bacterial conjunctivitis may have developed.

Rarely, corneal inflammation may develop and cause an opacity in the cornea. When this complication is noted, an ophthalmologist should be consulted urgently because loss of vision may occur.

Inclusion Conjunctivitis (Inclusion Blennorrhea)

This problem is seen frequently in sexually active young adults. The disease is caused by a species of *Chlamydia* and is a result of contamination of the eye from the urethra after a sexual contact.

The problem is characterized, usually, by the abrupt onset of eye discomfort with varying degrees of diffuse conjunctival hyperemia and sometimes with mucopurulent discharge, which may result in matting of the eyelashes. The eyelids appear swollen and inspection of the palpebral conjunctiva, especially of the lower lid, shows many small follicles (raised pale mounts of varying size (Fig. 99.6, page 1383). Occasionally, preauricular lymphadenopathy develops. Without treatment, the disease becomes chronic and remitting and, in 2 or 3 weeks, a superficial corneal inflammation (keratitis) may appear. This may be identified with the naked eye as dots or cloudy streaks on the superior portion of the cornea. Also at this stage, there may be an associated iritis manifest by photophobia and blurring of vision.

This syndrome may occur in association with urethritis in the male or cervicitis and a vaginal discharge in the female. Most often, however, there are no genitourinary symptoms, although *Chlamydia* species can be cultured from the urethra in men or the endocervical canal in women. The culture is time consuming and expensive, however. Increasingly available commercially are two highly specific and sensitive direct slide tests for the detection of *Chlamydia* (see Chapter 27) and these appear to be diagnostic in patients with conjunctivitis. In some cases, Reiter's syndrome will be present (see Chapter 71).

The diagnosis is suggested by the history and appearance but, if there is doubt, it may be confirmed by the direct slide test (see above) of the conjunctiva or by examination of the material obtained from conjunctival scraping. This material when stained with Giemsa stain shows large basophilic cytoplasmic inclusion bodies (Fig. 99.7, page 1383). Gram stain will not reveal these bodies but will show many polymorphonuclear leukocytes.

Therapy is effective but must be systemic. Oral tetracycline, 250 mg four times daily for 21 days, is the preferable regimen; but where tetracycline cannot be given, good results will be achieved with erythromycin, 250 mg, four times a day for 21 days or sulfamethoxazole-trimethoprim (e.g., Bactrim DS or Septra DS), one twice a day for 21 days. It may take several months for the follicular hyperplasia to resolve, but the patient should experience symptomatic improvement within several days. The application of cool compresses for 20 minutes several times a day will also provide comfort in the first few days of treatment.

Since the disease must be assumed to be sexually transmitted, the sexual partner should be similarly treated; other venereal diseases should be looked for, and the male should use a condom until therapy has been completed.

Allergic Conjunctivitis

This is a common and mild conjunctivitis frequently encountered in patients with allergic rhinitis (see Chapter 23). Often the patient describes a history of allergy to grasses and pollens as well as to other agents and usually complains of itching and tearing. Frequently, there is marked swelling of the conjunctiva (Fig. 99.8, page 1383) and slight to moderate redness of the eye, and at times there is serous crusting in the morning.

Whenever there is doubt about the diagnosis, conjunctival scrapings may be examined. A finding of many esoinophils is diagnostic. When conjunctivitis is associated with allergic rhinitis, it usually parallels the rhinitis in severity and duration. When it occurs as an isolated problem, it is short lived, and treatment is symptomatic. An over-the-counter topical astringent solution (Albalon, Naphcon-A, or Vasocon-A) and cool compresses are very effective. Occasionally, symptoms are severe, and oral antihistamines may relieve itching.

Corticosteroid eyedrops are very effective for this condition, but they must be used cautiously because their use is associated with corneal ulceration and perforation in the presence of herpes simplex infection, the development of fungal infection, and when used chronically, with the development in some individuals of open-angle glaucoma and, rarely, cataract formation. For these reasons, topical corticosteroids are not recommended.

Chemical Conjunctivitis

Many agents may enter the conjunctiva and produce inflammation. Irritation from such agents as smoke, smog, sprays, chlorinated water, hair spray, makeup, or industrial dust occurs frequently. It is the history of the exposure that makes the diagnosis obvious. The patient should thoroughly rinse the conjunctival sac with water as soon as contamination with a chemical has occurred. The patient will also benefit from cool compresses for 15 to 20 minutes several times a day, and occasionally the use of an over-the-counter topical astringent solution (Albalon, Naphcon-A, or Vasocon-A) will be necessary.

In the case of an injury from an acid or alkali, serious permanent damage may occur and this problem is a true ophthalmological emergency. Patients should be advised to irrigate the conjunctival sac with copious amounts of water and to see an ophthalmologist immediately.

Foreign Body

Foreign bodies frequently lodge in the conjunctiva or cornea. Most often they can be visualized with the naked eye; but, if not, sterile fluorescein staining (see above) will outline the area of epithelial damage. Foreign bodies may be removed by irrigation of the conjunctival sac with a sterile solution of physiological saline or eyewash. If they are not rinsed away, mechanical removal is indicated. This may be accomplished, when the object is in the cornea, by placing in the eye a drop of topical anesthetic (such as Ophthaine) and removing the foreign body with a sterile needle held carefully with the physician's arm braced. A cotton swab should not be used to remove a foreign body from the cornea since frequently it is very irritating to the structure and thus delays healing. If the foreign body is not on the cornea, removal is easier and usually does not require anesthesia. After removal, it is wise to instill a drop of antibiotic (such as Sulamyd or Bacitracin) and the eye should be covered by a patch for 24 hours. The *eyepatch* should be applied tightly enough to prevent the eyelids from moving. If the patch falls off before the 24-hour period is up, the patient should not try to reapply it, as often this may cause more irritation.

If the offending material is a piece of metal, rust rings surrounding the area of the epithelial defect may be observed. These rings are not harmful *per se* and only the foreign body should be removed.

In any instance where the foreign body is not easily removed, an ophthalmologist should see the patient urgently.

Subconjunctival Hemorrhage

Subconjunctival hemorrhage is a common condition that very often is alarming to the patient. A small blood vessel ruptures in the conjunctival tissue after the patient coughs or strains and a painless wedge-shaped hemorrhage develops. Often the patient will have no memory of the coughing or straining, but incidentally notices the red eye. Occasionally, viral conjunctivitis may be manifest only by the appearance of a subconjunctival hemorrhage (Fig. 99.5, page 1383). Isolated subconjunctival hemorrhage requires no treatment and should resolve within several days. If the problem becomes recurrent and/or multiple, an abnormality of hemostasis should be considered.

EYELID CONDITIONS

Several conditions that affect the eyelid are commonly seen in ambulatory practice, and these may mimic a red eye. These conditions are usually readily diagnosed by their appearance and may be treated easily without an ophthalmological consultation.

Hordeolum

A hordeolum is a very common infection in the glands of the eyelid caused by *Staphyloccus aureus*. It is characterized by the sudden onset of localized pain, swelling, redness, and often purulent discharge. The infected gland may be a meibomian gland just under the conjunctival side of the eyelid: an *internal hordeolum*. This infection may be quite large and may point to either the skin or conjunctival side of the lid. Also, a smaller gland associated with an eyelash follicle under the skin side of the lid may be infected: an *external hordeolum or sty*. A sty usually is smaller than in internal hordeolum and always points to the skin side of the lid.

Both types of hordeolum may be treated without obtaining a culture. Treatment is tripartite: hot compresses applied for 15 to 20 minutes several times a day will provide comfort and establish drainage of the infected gland; the lid should be scrubbed with a neutral soap (e.g., Ivory) each morning; and the institution into the conjunctival sac every 3 to 4 hours for a few days of a topical antimicrobial, such as a sulfonamide (e.g., Sulamyd 10%) or gentamicin (Garamycin), helps to prevent the development of an associated cellulitis or metastatic eye infection. If the hordeolum has not begun to respond to treatment in a day or two, it may need to be incised; referral to an ophthalmologist is indicated in that situation if the physician is not familiar with the proper technique.

Blepharitis

Marginal blepharitis is a very common chronic bilateral inflammation of the lid margins usually associated with seborrhea or a contact dermatitis, e.g., from mascara. Marginal blepharitis is discussed in Chapter 100, Common Problems of the Skin. Blepharitis also may be associated with chronic bacterial infection (see above, "Chronic Bacterial Conjunctivitis").

Chalazion

A chalazion is a lipogranulomatous inflammation of the meibomian gland secondary to chronic inflammation and it may follow a hordeolum. It presents as a swelling similar to an internal hordeolum (see above) except that it is chronic and usually does not manifest change of acute inflammation. Usually a chalazion will not spontaneously resolve, and therefore referral to an ophthalmologist for excision is indicated.

General References

Fraunfelder FT: *Drug Induced Ocular Side Effects and Drug Interactions*, ed 2. Philadelphia, Lea & Febiger, 1982.

A useful text that provides a resource for possible drug-induced eye problems, including conjunctivitis, iritis, cataracts, and many other problems.

Havener WH: *Synopsis of Ophthalmology*, ed 6. St Louis, CV Mosby, 1984.

A very well written short textbook which provides an overview of many eye problems, including the differential diagnosis of the red eye and of the different forms of conjunctivitis.

Schachat AP, Cruess AF: *Ophthalmology*. Baltimore, Williams & Wilkins, 1984.

This short paperback text provides a useful overview and general approach to many common problems, including the red eye.

SECTION 15

Miscellaneous Problems

CHAPTER ONE-HUNDRED

Common Problems of the Skin

STANFORD I. LAMBERG, M.D.

One-third of all patients with a primary dermatological complaint consult a general physician or an internist rather than a dermatologist, according to a survey conducted by the American Academy of Dermatology (14).

This chapter provides assistance in diagnosing and managing the common dermatological problems that are likely to be encountered in the general practice of internal medicine.

ACNE

Definition

Acne vulgaris is a chronic disorder of the sebaceous glands, particularly those on the face, chest, and back, where the glands are the largest and most dense. Sebum from these glands reaches the surface by emptying into the hair follicle and flowing along the hair shaft, the two skin appendages forming the pilosebaceous unit. The earliest lesion of acne is the *comedone*, a plug formed by impaction of the opening of the pilosebaceous duct by horny material and dried sebum. The plugs are visible as closed comedones ("whiteheads") and, if the surface is darkened, open comedones ("blackheads"), black, not due to dirt, but to oxidation of melanin and sebum in the plugs. Comedones become inflamed as nonpathogenic bacteria, normal residents within the duct and gland, especially *Staphylococcus epidermidis* and an anaerobic diphtheroid, *Corynebacterium acnes*, proliferate within the obstructed glands and produce erythematous tender papules. As inflammation progresses, these papules may become pustular and, in severe cases, cystic, Cysts are presumed to be due to abscess formation deep in the dermis. Various manifestations of the disorder usually are present in the same patient.

Epidemiology

Acne occurs primarily in adolescents; there is an equal incidence in males and females, although the eruption often is worse in males. Almost all teenagers have acne to some degree, but only a minority require treatment. In most, the lesions resolve by age 20. Sometimes acne persists into adulthood or develops for the first time in adults, especially women, who use cosmetics (so-called acne cosmetica).

Acne can be produced or exacerbated by drugs, including corticosteroids, androgenic steroids, phenytoin, iodides, and lithium, and by external irritants, such as creosote, tar, and industrial cutting oils (chloracne). Pomade acne is acne near the hair line, especially common in blacks, caused by the use of hair pomades.

Pathogenesis

The underlying cause of acne is unclear, but several events participate in its development. These included proliferation of sebaceous glands and increased production of sebum by sebaceous glands under the stimulation of androgens as puberty occurs; obstruction of the sebaceous glands with proliferation of bacteria, followed by the development of inflammation and characteristic lesions of acne. The precise reasons why some individuals develop severe disease while most have mild disease is not known, although severe acne often is hereditary.

Evaluation

The following information should be recorded before planning therapy:

1. *Topical medications used*, past and present, including prescription and nonprescription prepara-

tions. Many of the patients will have initiated therapy themselves and the preparations they have used may be irritating. Response or failure to previously used antibiotics is particularly important information.

2. *Face care*, including soap used, scrubbing technique, use of skin machine, and cosmetics (brand and type). Information about the use of foundations, cold creams, and astringents also is important. These preparations or techniques may be irritating or actually acnegenic.

3. *Factors that improve or worsen the acne*, including menses, diet, and stress, should be explored. Diet is not an important factor, although patients who believe that certain foods lead to flare-ups may avoid those foods.

4. *Other medical conditions and current medications*, including oral contraceptive agents, corticosteroids, *etc* (see above).

A table should be entered into the patient's record for use in selecting and following therapy (Table 100.1). These data allow the physician to evaluate progress objectively.

Therapy

No single treatment is effective for all patients with acne. The overall goal is to reverse and prevent plugging of the sebaceous ducts as well as to reduce and prevent inflammation of the sebaceous glands and surrounding tissue (11). General instructions include: STOP hard scrubbing, including the use of skin machines; STOP use of antibacterial soaps because nonpathogenic bacteria are reduced and replaced by pathogens. Instead, substitute a plain soap such as Ivory, Camay, Purpose, or Basis; STOP use of oil-based cosmetics (ingredients of cosmetics are listed on the labels) as they obstruct the sebaceous duct. Water-based and oil-free makeup may be safe for some, but it is best to avoid all foundations. Blusher and eye shadow do not seem to aggravate acne. Improvement following exposure to large doses of summer sun does occur, probably from ultraviolet light entering the skin and damaging the sebaceous glands or ducts, but the improvement is

Table 100.1.
Data to Be Recorded in Evaluation and Follow-up of Patients with Acne

	Face	Back	Chest
Comedones	( )	( )	( )
Papules	( )	( )	( )
Pustules	( )	( )	( )
Cysts	( )	( )	( )

0 = none
1+ = few
2+ = moderate
3+ = many
4+ = extensive

temporary, while the actinic damage is long term. There is no justification for artificial ultraviolet exposure in acne. Patients should be told that a delay of 4 to 8 weeks before obvious improvement is common with any treatment of acne. If there is no improvement after 2 to 3 months or if lesions are cystic or deep and inflammatory with scarring, referral to a dermatologist is appropriate.

Comedones

If only comedones are present, a desquamating agent such as 5% benzoyl peroxide lotion, gel, or cream (such as Desquam-X 5 Gel, Oxy-5 lotion, Persadox lotion or cream, Xerac BP5 gel) should be prescribed. Initially the agent should be applied only at bedtime as it may cause intense inflammation if used excessively. After a few weeks, if treatment is tolerated, the end point being slight erythema and dryness, the frequency of use may be increased to twice a day and then the concentration increased to 10% (such as Desquam-X 10 Gel, Oxy-10 lotion, Persadox HP cream or lotion, or Xerac BP10 gel). Some of these agents are available without prescription such as Oxy-5, Oxy-10, Persadox, and Persadox HP.

Patients who do not respond to benzoyl peroxide within 4 to 8 weeks should be given topical vitamin A acid. The 0.01% gel (Retin-A gel, requires a prescription) seems to be least irritating and easiest to use. This agent appears to interfere with keratinization of the follicular duct, thereby decreasing the comedone plug. Because vitamin A acid is quite irritating, it too should be started at a low concentration at bedtime, applied to the entire face, increasing the dose to 0.025% gel gradually over 2 to 3 months. The patient need not experience discomfort and peeling for the drug to be effective. The drug should be avoided in blacks as it may darken their skin. Experiments in mice have shown an increased incidence of skin cancer when vitamin A acid was used with high doses of ultraviolet light. Therefore, patients should be told to stop using the medication if they intend to be in the sun extensively.

Inflammatory Lesions (Papules or Pustules)

If inflammatory lesions are present, the initial therapy differs depending on the sex of the patient (1, 20).

Females

(a) Topical clindamycin (Cleocin-T) should be applied to the entire face morning and afternoon after washing with plain soap (such as Ivory, Camay, Purpose, or Basis). This should be continued for 2 months before alternative topical antibiotics, such as topical erythromycin (A/T/S), EryDerm, or Staticin), or a systemic antibiotic is prescribed. Oral tetracycline (see below) generally should be avoided in women because of the common complication of vaginitis. However, if the lesions are pustular or cystic, systemic antibiotics will be necessary, at least initially. The dose schedule given for males (see below) may be followed. Tetracycline must not be used if the patient is pregnant because it may damage the bones and teeth of the fetus. (b) In addition to the antibiotic, a topical desquamating agent will be needed. Benzoyl peroxide or vitamin A acid should be used as for comedone acne (see above).

Males

(a) The physician should prescribe oral tetracycline, 250 mg three times daily. However, if the acne is severe, up to 2 g/day may be used. The medication should be taken 1 to 2 hours before or after meals to maximize absorption. The starting dose should be continued for 6 weeks or until there is clear improvement, then slowly decreased by 1 capsule daily each month. At the point that the acne recurs or flares up, the dose should be increased to the level that had maintained clearing and left at that level for several months. The lowest dose that is effective should be used. The usual maintenance level of tetracycline is 250 mg twice a day. (b) In addition to the antibiotics, a topical desquamating agent will be needed. Benzoyl peroxide or vitamin A acid should be used as for comedone acne (see above).

Both men and women should wash their hair frequently and should not apply oil to the scalp.

Cystic Acne

A new therapy, 13-cis-retinoic acid (isotretinoin, Accutane, 10, 20 and 40 mg, orally by prescription) cures or greatly improves nearly all cases of cystic acne. However, side effects are universal and include cheilitis, dry skin, and conjunctivitis, and, less commonly, musculoskeletal tenderness, hair thinning, and headache. It also is teratogenic, and women must take adequate birth control measures, have a negative pregnancy test, and be informed of the danger before starting the drug. Some patients develop elevated trigyceride levels but the significance of this is unknown. Nevertheless, it is suggested that a baseline triglyceride level be obtained before starting the drug and then repeated in 30 days (most who will develop elevated triglyceride levels from this drug will have done so in this time). Should the level become elevated dietary counseling usually results in improvement (see also Chapter 75). The usual dosage is 1 to 2 mg/kg divided in two daily doses for 2 to 4 months. The medication is expensive, costing about $150/month, and has not been approved for use in milder forms of acne. Patients with cystic acne generally should be followed by a dermatologist.

Prognosis

Acne in the adolescent may require treatment until age 20 or so. Good results from the treatment outlined above can be anticipated in 80%. About 15% will require alternative therapies, such as high doses of alternative antibiotics or such specialized techniques as cryotherapy, intradermal corticosteroid injections, or acne surgery performed by a dermatologist. The remaining 5% will not respond well to any therapy. Dermabrasion, the superficial abrasion of the skin to reduce scars, may be useful for some patients, although most scars flatten and become less noticeable with time. Persistent acne in middle-aged women usually is due to excessive use of occlusive cosmetics and moisturizers. Clearing will not occur until use of such cosmetics is stopped.

ATOPIC DERMATITIS (ATOPIC ECZEMA)

Atopic dermatitis is a chronic, pruritic inflammation of the skin that has a characteristic course and pattern and that is usually associated with a personal and family history of allergy (9).

Etiology

Although still debated, the cause appears to be immunological with both cellular and humoral mechanisms playing a role (see Chapter 23). Patients with severe atopy often have an elevated serum IgE level and about 30% have a personal history of allergic rhinitis or asthma. In addition, 60% have a family history of atopy with cutaneous and/or respiratory symptoms. However, more than the immune system may be involved as signs of decreased production of eccrine sweat and increased vasoconstriction of small blood vessels are often evident also.

Presentation

Onset may be as early as the second month after birth but almost always before age 10 years. The major distress is due to the chronic and pruritic nature of the condition. Sleep is difficult; the discomfort may make the individual appear nervous and demanding. Other manifestations of atopy, or hypersensitivity, also may develop, including hay fever, rhinitis, or asthma. Early cataracts are a complication in a small percentage of severe cases, but general health is otherwise unaffected. A parent with atopic dermatitis may need to be told that the disorder is inherited and that about half of his or her children are likely to be affected to some degree.

Although the entire skin seems "dry" with fine flaky scaling, dermatitis, with eczematous lichenified plaque, tend to involve certain regions and the distribution depends on age. During infancy, the disorder involves the extensor and exposed parts, and only later does it take on the adult distribution in flexoral folds including the antecubital, popliteals, wrists, and sides of the neck (Fig. 100.1). Itching is generalized but worse in the lichenified plaques,

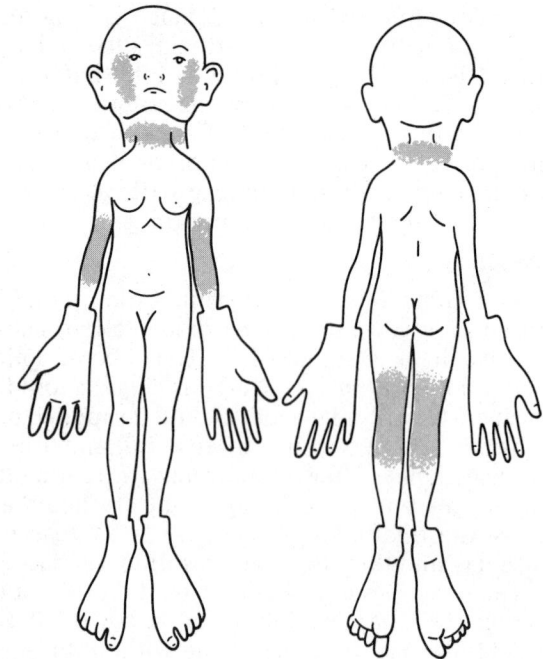

Figure 100.1.   Lichenified pruritic areas in flexual regions and on the face are typical locations for adult atopic dermatitis.

which sometimes become superinfected. Many patients will have an extra crease below the margin of the lower eyelids (Dennie or Morgan fold).

Itching may be triggered by low humidity, high temperature, sweating, environmental allergens such as irritating or occlusive medications, wool clothing, greases, and detergents. Dietary factors may be important, and control sometimes can be partially achieved through manipulation of the diet (see below). Many cases improve during infancy and about half the cases have cleared by puberty. Some will remain clear but in many the dermatitis will recur. Many atopic patients have exacerbations throughout life, often when under physical or emotional stress. In most cases itching improves during the summer although skin infections may be more common then.

Differential Diagnosis

Seborrheic dermatitis, psoriasis, and contact dermatitis may be confused with atopic dermatitis (see below).

Therapy

Bathing and Lubrication

The patient should reduce the frequency of hot water bathing and the use of soap; both remove lipids and topical medications and increase water loss from the skin and result in itching. In general the patient should not bathe more than twice a week. The house should be humidified (see Chapter 23) during the winter. For additional details see "Bathing Instructions for Dry or Irritated Skin" (page 1423).

Topical Corticosteroids

Corticosteroids are the mainstay of topical therapy and will control most cases. The cream should be used when the eruption is subacute with oozing; however, the ointment is better absorbed than the cream and is less drying in chronic dermatitis. For the details of preparations, techniques of use, and complications, see "Corticosteroids," page 1424.

Because potent topical corticosteroids can induce vascular dilatation, which may become permanent, nothing stronger than 1% hydrocortisone cream should be used on the face.

Systemic

Recent studies have confirmed that some children are helped by elimination of certain foods from the diet, most commonly citrus fruits, wheat, eggs, and nuts. Two-week trials with elimination of different food groups may be worth attempting if the patient is sufficiently cooperative. Systemic antibiotics should be prescribed at the first sign of pyoderma—oozing, crusting, and odor. Erythromycin, 250 mg four times daily for 10 days for an adult, usually is sufficient. Dicloxacillin, 500 mg twice daily may be used as an alternative. Cultures generally are not needed unless abscesses develop.

A rare complication, but a serious one, is infection with herpex simplex, particularly at the site of active dermatitis. This is called *eczema herpeticum*. Those affected are toxic, and the complication is life threatening. Hospitalization usually is required.

There is still a debate about whether antihistamines help beyond the side effect of sedation that normally accompanies their use. A trial for a week with 50 mg three times a day of diphenhydramine (Benadryl), 10 mg three times a day of hydroxyzine (Atarax, Cartrax, Vistrax), or an equivalent dose of other antihistamines (see Chapter 23) may be appropriate if the patient has marked pruritus and is restless. The dose may be increased at bedtime to help with sleep.

Therapy for Resistant Cases

Systemic corticosteroids occasionally are necessary for severe flare-ups of atopic dermatitis. A suggested starting schedule in an adult is 40 mg of prednisone in a single daily morning dose, reduced by 5 to 10 mg a day as soon as improvement is seen and tapered off completely within 2 to 3 weeks. Patients may obtain such relief from the systemic corticosteroids that the physician may not be able to persuade them to stop the drug; however, since atopic dermatitis may be lifelong, eventual difficul-

ties from continuous systemic corticosteroids are bound to ensue. Occasionally, hospitalization is necessary.

CONTACT DERMATITIS

Definition

Contact dermatitis is a cutaneous reaction to an external substance and may be either an irritant or an allergic reaction. An irritant reaction affects most individuals exposed and generally produces discomfort immediately after exposure. Allergic contact dermatitis affects only individuals previously sensitized to the contactant. The reaction is delayed until the cascade of cellular immunity is completed, requiring up to several hours. Both in industry and in the home, irritant reactions are more frequent than are allergic reactions (8).

Irritant contact dermatitis is due to direct injury of the skin as, for example, that caused by detergents, solvents, or alkaline abrasives, including cement. If the irritant is a mild one, repeated or prolonged exposure, or exposure combined with abrasion may be necessary to produce a reaction. In *allergic contact dermatitis*, lymphocytes, previously exposed to antigen that has been processed through the macrophage or Langerhan's cell system, react selectively to subsequent exposure with initiation of inflammation. Genetic predisposition, frequency of exposure to the antigen, and coexisting dermatitis are among the factors that affect the development of sensitization. Allergic sensitivity is usually a more difficult problem than irritation because sensitized individuals may respond to only minute quantities of the offending substance.

Characteristics

An eruption with an asymmetric or restricted distribution, such as a rash limited to the axillae or earlobes, or a rash only in exposed areas, such as the face, "V" of the neck, lower arms, and hands, probably is contact in origin. The deeper skinfolds protected from external contactants tend to remain clear, while an intrinsic dermatitis, such as seborrheic dermatitis, will involve the entire area, including the skinfolds. Involvement of the palms or soles or of the mucous membranes, ordinarily resistant to chemicals, is evidence against a contactant. Irritant and allergic dermatitides may be identical in appearance; distinction depends upon the history of exposure and the response to patch testing.

Allergic reactions to systemic medications are usually central and are worse on the trunk than on exposed peripheral parts. The major exceptions are reactions to drugs that induce *photosensitization* to ultraviolet light. Tetracycline, sulfonamides, and thiazides are known photosensitizers, leading to exaggerated sunburn reaction or eczematous dermatitis.

Common Contactants

Plant Dermatitis

Poison ivy, oak, and sumac, the most common of the plant contactants, produce eczematous or even blistering eruptions, usually restricted to exposed parts and often characterized by bizarrely shaped angular lesions, the result of contact with a plant resin (oleoresin). Contrary to popular belief, leakage of blister fluid does not "spread" the rash to other sites; however, lesions often are delayed in appearance because of the continuing unintentional exposure to the resin which may persist on the patient's clothing, tools, or sports equipment or on the fur of the family pet. Sensitive individuals will continue to develop new lesions for up to the 3 weeks that is required for the resin to evaporate.

Metal Allergy

Nickel contact allergy is common, particularly in women, where it may be seen near hooks, zippers, or jewelry, such as on the earlobe and the wrist. Dermatitis under a gold ring could be due to metal allergy but is more often due to irritating soap residue. The eruption of metal allergy tends to be mild and chronic with scaling, pigmentation, and pruritus. A simple and convincing patch test can be performed to confirm the diagnosis of nickel allergy: a moistened 5-cent piece should be taped to the upper inner arm with an occlusive tape (such as Blenderm) and left on for 48 hours. The patient should remove the patch earlier if itching develops. Individuals allergic to nickel will develop dermatitis under the coin; the area should be examined by the patient for several days, as a reaction occasionally may be delayed.

Topical Medications

Allergy to topical medications is frequent, probably due to the loss of the protective barrier of dermatitic skin. Common culprits include neomycin, anesthetics (such as benzocaine or tetracaine), and preservatives, such as parabens and merthiolate. The original eruption may appear to persist, but the difficulty may be due to the imposition of a new contact allergy from the medication. The situation becomes even more confusing if corticosteroids are in the medication, thus partly masking the dermatitis.

Cosmetics

Following Food and Drug Administration guidelines, ingredients of cosmetics are listed on the label. Manufacturers will make these substances available to the physician for patch testing. However, perhaps 40% of the reactions to cosmetics are caused by the perfume; the chemical composition of perfumes may not be known, even to the manufacturer. The physician should suggest discontinuing the cosmetic, a step the patient probably would have taken on her own. One percent hydrocortisone cream should be used sparingly until the reaction subsides. More potent topical corticosteroids are to be avoided on the face, since long use may lead to telangiectasis. The cosmetic should be discontinued for at least 2 weeks and during that time another brand should not be substituted; most cosmetics, used for the same purpose, have the same or similar ingredients. It should be recognized that cosmetic reactions may take weeks to regress. If after 2 weeks, the eruption has not cleared or if it recurs when a different brand is started, referral to a dermatologist is appropriate since patch testing may be necessary to identify the allergen; alternatively, another dermatitis, such as seborrheic dermatitis, may be present.

Therapy

Plant Dermatitis

Immediately after exposure, the patient should wash the exposed parts thoroughly and wash or clean items that were in contact with the irritant or allergen. If the item is not washable, it should be isolated in a ventilated area for 3 weeks. The family pet should be bathed if it could have come into contact with suspect plants.

If acute dermatitis does develop, the patient should start cooling compresses with saline (1 teaspoon of salt/pint of tap water) or Burow's solution (1 tablet or packet/pint of tap water) for 20 minutes every 2 or 3 hours. An antihistamine, such as diphenhydramine (Benadryl) 50 mg, or chlorpheniramine (Chlor-Trimeton), 4 mg every 4 to 6 hours, as well as a topical lotion, such as calamine, or a corticosteroid cream, such as triamcinolone 0.1%, may be used. If the reaction is particularly extensive, or is located on the face and is acute with edema and blisters, or if the patient is known to have had severe reactions to the same antigen in the past, systemic corticosteroids are helpful. A substantial dose of prednisone is needed to suppress acute contact dermatitis; low doses are not effective. The average sized adult patient should start with 60 mg each day in three divided doses until relief is produced, and continue for a total of 2 or 3 weeks, decreasing the dosage as the condition subsides. It should be kept in mind that systemic corticosteroids will reduce the dermatitis only partially if the irritant or antigen remains in the environment. Secondary bacterial infection is uncommon but, if present, requires treatment with systemic antibiotics, such as erythromycin, 250 mg four times a day for a week. Currently available preparations for hyposensitization treatment of poison ivy, oak, or sumac cannot be recommended except in unusual situations (such as a sensitive forestry worker), and in these situations referral to a dermatologist or allergist is appropriate.

Other Contactants

To be effective, therapy must include the identification and elimination of the irritant or allergen. If the contactant cannot be eliminated from the environment, protection may suffice. For dermatitis of the hands, vinyl gloves, best worn with separate thin white cotton liners that can be removed and washed when needed, provide protection. Low grade exposure may be kept under control with topical corticosteroid ointments, such as triamcinolone 0.1% or fluocinonide (Lidex, Topsyn), while the source of antigen is being investigated.

In the case of jewelry (nickel) sensitivity, the patient may still be able to use the jewelry provided that it is painted with a clear acrylic paint or colorless nail polish to prevent the metal from coming into contact with the skin.

After the dermatitis has subsided and suspicious irritants and antigens have been removed from the patient's environment, it is important to prove that the patient did have a specific allergy or irritant so that the substance can be avoided in the future. The relationship is proven with patch tests. A kit to perform patch tests may be obtained from the American Academy of Dermatology (820 Davis Street, Evanston, IL 60201). However, patch testing is time consuming, and experience is needed to interpret the test results properly; therefore, patients are usually referred to a dermatologist or an allergist for this testing. In the case of a possible cosmetic contact dermatitis, extensive investigation may be necessary before the cause can be determined; it is estimated that the average women applies 13 cosmetic products, including deodorants and shampoos, to herself each day and that Americans are exposed 30,000 chemicals during the year.

DRUG REACTIONS

Cutaneous eruptions from drugs take many forms ranging from a pink, evanescent, nonscaly rash to hives, blisters, pustules, erythema multiforme, purpura, or serum sickness.

The mechanism of drug eruptions may be allergic, toxic, or idiosyncratic. Allergic reactions may be IgE-mediated or non-IgE-mediated; IgE-mediated allergic drug reactions generally present with urticaria, angioedema, or anaphylaxis, while non-IgE reactions generally are macular, papular, petechial, or blistering. The only practical test for allergic reactions to an IgE-mediated sensitivity is the skin test to penicillin (Pre-Pen), but there are no laboratory tests to prove the cause of any of the non-IgE-mediated drug eruptions.

Drug eruptions usually improve or clear within 48 hours after the offending drug is discontinued, but occasionally they last for days or weeks, depending on the rate of clearance of the medication.

Table 100.2.
Drugs That Are Associated with the Highest Frequency of Skin Reaction[a]

Drug	Reactions/1000 Recipients
Trimethoprim-sulfamethoxazole	59
Ampicillin	52
Penicillin, semisynthetic	36
Corticotropin	38
Erythromycin	23
Sulfisoxazole	17
Gentamicin sulfate	16
Penicillin G	16
Practolol (Eradin)	16
Cephalosporins	13
Nitrofurantoin	9
Heparin	8
Chloramphenicol	7
Phenazopyridine HCl (Azo-Gantrisin)	7
Cyancobalamin (B$_{12}$)	6
Methenamine mandelate (Mandelamine)	6
Nitrazapam (Mogadon)	6
Barbiturates	5
Glutethimide (Doriden)	5
Chlordiazepoxide (Librium)	4
Diazepam (Valium)	4
Indomethacin	4
Metoclopramide HCl (Reglan)	4
Furosemide (Lasix)	3
Guaifenesin and theophylline (Tedral)	3
Nystatin	3
Propoxyphene (Darvon)	3
Phytonadione (Aqua-Mephyton)	1
Flurazepam HCl (Dalmane)	0.5
Chloral hydrate	0.2

[a] Modified from Arndt KA, Jick H: Rates of cutaneous reactions to drugs. A report from the Boston Collaborative Drug Surveillance Program. *JAMA* 235:918, 1976.

The drugs that are associated with the highest frequency of skin reactions are listed in Table 100.2.

When a cutaneous drug reaction is considered, elimination or change of *all* of the drugs suspected by causing the reaction is prudent; serious systemic reactions may develop if an attempt is made to suppress the reaction with antihistamines or systemic corticosteroids while continuing the drug. However, both of these agents relieve discomfort and help to speed resolution of an eruption once the offending agents have been stopped.

FOOT DERMATITIS

The most common dermatological disorders of the feet are: (*a*) tinea infection, (*b*) dyshidrosis, (*c*) contact allergy, (*d*) essential hyperhidrosis, and (*e*) ery-

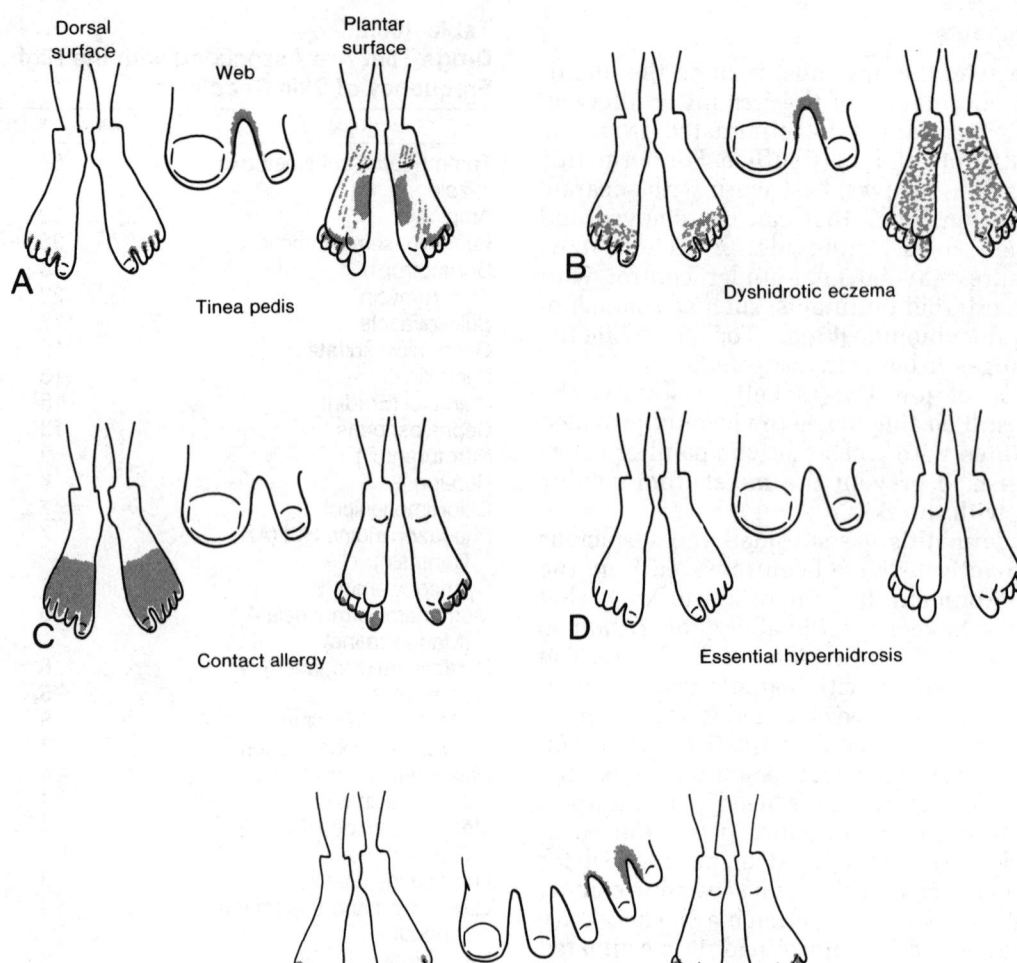

Figure 100.2. Distribution of lesions is useful to distinguish among causes of dermatitis of the feet. *A.* Tinea pedis—moisture, scale, and pruritus confined to the plantar surface (especially the instep) and between the toes. *B.* Dyshidrotic eczema—vesicles and severe pruritus on the plantar as well as the dorsal surface and between the toes. *C.* Contact allergy—the dorsum of the feet and underside of toes may be involved while the plantar surface and webs are clear. *D.* Essential hyperhidrosis—sodden soles but no dermatitis. *E.* Erythrasma—mild erythema and scale limited to the toe webs, especially the fourth to fifth.

thrasma. The most important diagnostic clues are location (Fig. 100.2) and appearance; all of these disorders, except hyperhidrosis, are pruritic.

Tinea

Presentation

Tinea pedis, or superficial fungal infection of the feet, occurs in about 20% of the population, a problem related to the common use of closed shoes which retain generated heat and moisture, conditions perfect for fungal growth. Summer exacerbations are typical. This infection presents as scales, itching,

and slight redness between the toes and on the soles. In acute stages, blistering can develop, usually involving the instep rather than the thick keratin on the balls of the feet. Secondary infection and lymphangitis may be superimposed in tinea pedis. Yellow crumbly toenails infected with fungi, onychomycosis, often are associated with chronic tinea pedis and serve as a source of continuing reinfection. A scraping of the scale or debris under the nail incubated on a slide with KOH for 10 minutes will reveal hyphae (see "Potassium Hydroxide (KOH) Preparation," page 1400). Culture usually is not necessary.

Therapy

The patient should be instructed to dry the toe webs thoroughly after bathing and to use talc freely. Footwear should be nonocclusive (ventilated leather shoes or sandals are best; vinyl footwear or sneakers should be avoided). The patient should use cotton socks (dark or light) and avoid wool and synthetic fibers which absorb moisture poorly. If the lesions are dry and pruritic, the physician should prescribe a topical antifungal agent such as miconazole cream (Monistat-Derm), haloprogin cream (Halotex), or clotrimazole cream (Lotrimin, Mycelex) to be applied to the feet sparingly each morning and evening. The patient should continue with the topical antifungals at bedtime until clear, then continue them for an additional month and reinstitute the therapy only upon recurrence. For additional details, see "Topical Antifungal Agents," page 1425. When the feet are particularly scaly and sweaty, a keratolytic is an insoluble ointment base (half-strength Whitfield's ointment, available without prescription) applied each morning, alternating with an antifungal cream at bedtime may be needed. If the lesions are moist and acute, they should be treated with compresses of Burow's solution for 3 days before starting topical antifungals. For additional details, see "Compresses," page 1423.

If initial therapy does not work, a 30-day course of griseofulvin, ultrafine (generic, by prescription), 250 mg three times a day with meals, usually will be effective. The topical antifungals should be continued after the griseofulvin is discontinued, to maintain clearing. If accompanied by hyperhidrosis (see below), 6% aluminum chloride in absolute ethanol (Xerac-AC, requires a prescription) applied to the feet each morning will induce dryness.

Onychomycosis of the toenails responds poorly to any therapy, including griseofulvin.

Dyshidrosis

Presentation

Dyshidrosis is the second most common dermatosis of the feet and the most difficult of the common disorders to diagnose and treat. It affects both sexes with equal frequency. The cause of dyshidrosis is uncertain but many patients have flare-ups following nonspecific irritation. The physician should inquire about causes, including contact allergens, especially from shoes, occupational sources, exposures to nonspecific irritants, and a history of atopy. The eruption also occurs on the hands where it is particularly common in persons whose hands frequently are wet—cooks, beauticians, and housewives. Dyshidrosis starts as minute, deep blisters on the sides of the palms and/or soles and between the fingers and/or toes. Scale and erythema accompanied by severe pruritus usually are present. Unlike tinea pedis, involvement of the dorsum of the foot is common. Dyshidrosis frequently is accompanied by hyperhidrosis (see below), but there is no disorder of the sweat glands, despite its name. Recurrences are typical. The KOH examination will be negative.

Therapy

Dyshidrosis is notoriously difficult to treat. During the blistering phase, the patient should compress for 20 minutes three times a day with Burow's solution (Domeboro, available without prescription), made with 1 packet or tablet dissolved in a pint of lukewarm water, followed by any high potency topical corticosteroid cream. For additional details, see "Corticosteroids," page 1424. At bedtime, in order to absorb serous fluid, a thick coating of zinc oxide paste, USP (available without prescription) should be applied and cotton socks used to keep the paste in place. In the morning, the patient should wipe off the paste with mineral oil on cotton balls and reapply the steroid. During the acute phase, an antihistamine (such as Benadryl, 25 or 50 mg three to four times a day) for sedation will be useful. As the dermatitis becomes less acute, the compressing should be stopped and a corticosteroid ointment, instead of cream, used three times a day.

If initial therapy does not work within 2 weeks, a short course of systemic steroids may be necessary. Prednisone, 40 mg/day for the average adult, is prescribed, continued until relief is obtained, and then tapered by giving 20 mg/day for a week and then 10 mg/day for an additional 2 weeks, after which it is discontinued. The dermatologist or allergist may help by performing contact allergy patch tests.

Contact Allergy

Presentation

Contact dermatitis of the feet is an allergic reaction to a footwear product, usually leather, tanning compounds, metals, dyes, adhesives, or foot medications (see also "Contact Dermatitis" above). It is less common than tinea pedis or dyshidrosis but should be considered when the dorsum of the feet and toes rather than the interdigital areas are involved with erythema, scale, and pruritus. If severe, even blisters may appear. Unlike tinea pedis, the toe webs, protected from direct exposure, and the soles, protected by thick keratin, do not become involved.

Therapy

Topical or even systemic corticosteroids do not fully suppress contact dermatitis if exposure to the antigen continues. If the dermatitis is severe, bed rest, compresses, and systemic antibiotics may be needed, while efforts to locate the source of the allergy are initiated. Referral to an allergist or dermatologist is suggested, as either will have access to specialized patch-testing materials as well as knowledge of sock and shoe components, and sources of less antigenic substitutes.

Hyperhidrosis

Presentation

This is a common disorder of excessive sweating of the soles, frequently accompanied by excess palmar sweating (5). It can be severe, with sweat dripping from the fingers and toes, interfering with the patient's occupation and social life. Pruritus or scale is not present. The increased moisture on the feet may lead to fissuring and infection and an objectionable odor.

Therapy

Six percent aluminum chloride solution (Xerac-AC or Drysol requires a prescription), applied nightly until the condition has improved (usually by 48 hours) and then as needed, often is effective. It appears to work by causing the sweat duct to leak sweat back into the dermis rather than transporting it to the surface. In severe cases, surgical sympathectomy has been used with fair success.

Erythrasma

Presentation

Erythrasma is a superficial skin infection with scale and erythema, particularly between the fourth and fifth toes. It is due to a bacterium, *Corynebacterium minutissimum*, which produces a porphyrin, recognized by a salmon-red fluorescence on exposure to Wood's light (see below). Although not a common cause of foot dermatitis, erythrasma should be considered when a scaly foot dermatitis does not respond to topical antifungal medications. A KOH examination (see below) will be negative.

Therapy

Erythrasma is successfully treated with erythromycin, 250 mg three times daily for 2 weeks, or with 2% erythromycin, topically for 2 weeks. Recurrences are frequent, but the infection generally is not passed among family members.

GROIN DERMATITIS

General Considerations

Rashes in the groin are common and most are due to one of four causes: candidiasis, tinea infections, intertrigo, and erythrasma. Less common causes of groin dermatitis are contact dermatitis, psoriasis, and seborrheic dermatitis. Rarely Bowen's disease and extramammary Paget's disease, forms of squamous cell carcinomas, must be considered, particularly if the lesions do not respond to topical therapy.

Table 100.3.
Diagnostic Criteria for Four Major Causes of Groin Dermatitis

	Moist	Sharp Border	Pustules at Edge	KOH[a]	Wood's light[a]	More Pain than Itch	More Itch than Pain
Candidiasis	Yes	No	Yes	+	–	Yes	
Tinea cruris	No	Yes	No	+	–		Yes
Intertrigo	Yes	No	Maybe	–	–	Yes	
Erythrasma	No	Yes	No	–	+		Yes

[a] See the text for description.

Because of the moist environment, dermatitides of the groin have some similarities in appearance regardless of cause. Most cases show erythema, scale, and oozing (if severe) and manifest some degree of pruritus. Table 100.3 provides criteria for the diagnosis of the four major causes of groin dermatitis. The proper evaluation of groin dermatitis requires a KOH preparation and an inspection with use of a Wood's lamp; both are easily performed.

Potassium Hydroxide (KOH) Preparation

The lesion should be scraped with a sterile no. 10 or 15 scalpel blade, and the scale should be transferred to a microscope slide. If the skin is moistened with a drop of water the scales will adhere, which will make collection easier. A drop or two of 15% KOH should be placed on the slide with the scale, a coverslip applied, and the slide should be heated to dissolve epidermoid cells. KOH does not dissolve fungal hyphae. Boiling may "bubble" the scales off the slide and should be avoided. The preparation should be examined with the low power (×10) objective with the light turned low and the condenser racked down to increase contrast between hyphae and cell borders. Hyphae are thin, branching, double-walled filaments that can be distinguished from cell borders by their double-walled smooth appearance often several cell diameters long (Fig. 100.3). The high dry (×40) objective can be used to confirm the observation.

Wood's Light Examination

An inexpensive "black light" can be obtained from physician supply stores or hobby shops. The examining room must be completely dark and the light placed close to the patient's skin since the light output is low. The physician should look for the coral-red or salmon-colored fluorescence of erythrasma. The light also will be useful for examination of patients with tinea versicolor and vitiligo (see below).

Candidiasis

Definition

Candidiasis is a yeast infection that is generally restricted to mucous surfaces and moist intertriginous areas of the skin (17).

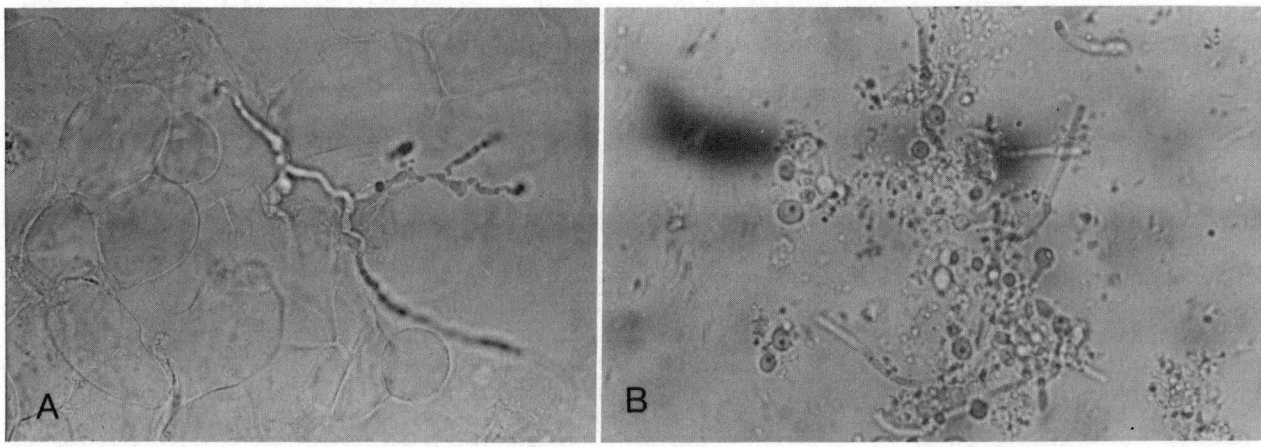

Figure 100.3. *A.* Hyphae of tinea (KOH preparation, ×400). *B.* Pseudohyphae of *Candida* (KOH preparation, ×400; photograph *B* courtesy of William G. Merz, Ph.D.).

Therapy

For inflammation with oozing and discomfort often associated with candidiasis, the patient should apply cool compresses of either saline (1 teaspoon of salt/pint of water) or Burow's solution (1 tablet or packet/pint of water) for 20 minutes three times daily. For details, see "Compresses," page 1423. The patient should, after compressing, thoroughly dry the area of dermatitis with a towel or fan and apply topical nystatin (Mycostatin) cream or a broad spectrum antifungal agent, such as clotrimazole (Lotrimin or Mycelex, requires a prescription) or Miconazole (Monistat-Derm, available without prescription). For additional detail, see Topical Antifungal Agents," page 1425.

In severe cases, where there is considerable oozing, the patient may layer zinc oxide paste (available without a prescription) thickly over the area at bedtime, to be removed with mineral oil-soaked cotton balls in the morning. Compresses usually are not needed for longer than 3 days. The antifungal agent, however, will need to be continued for 2 weeks. Distinct improvement should be apparent within 7 days of initiating therapy.

Evaluation and Therapy for Resistant Cases

A number of factors account for apparent clinical resistance, and these need to be considered if there has been no improvement within 7 days of initiating therapy. Local factors, such as polyester clothing that encourages sweat retention and maintains the infection, should be modified; loose, nonocclusive cotton clothes are preferred. Other skinfolds, such as the axilla, under the breasts, and about the neck and abdomen, should be examined for candidiasis. Candidiasis is likely to be present in the vagina and in the gut; organisms from these sites may be reinfecting the area (see Chapter 94). Reinfection is common, and the sexual partner should be examined for the presence of candidiasis. A KOH smear to search for pseudohyphae and spores is more practical than culture as results are immediate and are not invalidated by overgrowth of contaminants (Fig 100.3*B*). Among the *Candida* species, only *C. albicans* is a common pathogen.

In resistant cases in women, the physician should prescribe miconazole vaginal cream (Monostat 7), clotrimazole vaginal cream or tablets (Gyne-Lotrimin or Mycelex-G), or nystatin (Mycostatin) vaginal suppositories to be used daily for 2 weeks to control the vaginal candidiasis. Also for women with resistant cases, the gut may be the source of reinfection and a 3-day course of oral nystatin suspension (100,000 units/ml) at a dose of 5 ml (1 teaspoon) four times a day should be prescribed. Furthermore, diabetes mellitus predisposes patients to candidiasis; however, if diabetes mellitus is a true causal factor, glycosuria will be present.

Tinea Cruris

Definition

Tinea cruris, as the name defines, is a fungal infection of the groin. Tinea cruris is common in males and uncommon in females and does not occur in childhood. It tends to recur during the summer months (17).

Therapy

A topical antifungal agent (see "Topical Antifungal Agents," page 1425) (Monistat-Derm) should be applied to the rash sparingly twice a day for 3 weeks. The patient should try to decrease moisture in the area of the rash by using plain talc (such as Johnson's Baby Powder) and cotton underwear. If acute with oozing and discomfort, compresses for 2 or 3 days (see above) followed by the short term application (e.g., 1 week) of a topical corticosteroid (such as triamcinolone cream 0.1%) may be necessary before topical antifungal medications are begun.

If the lesions are extensive or involve other parts of the body as well, oral griseofulvin-UF (generic by prescription), 250 mg three times daily for 30 days taken with food, should be given. On occasion, griseofulvin may be the initial therapy with topical antifungal agents used to maintain the clearing. Griseofulvin generally is devoid of serious side effects; headaches and gastrointestinal distress develop when high doses are used and, rarely, photosensitivity can occur. Griseofulvin can reduce the effects of anticoagulants by increasing the rate of their metabolism by the liver.

Intertrigo

Definition

Intertrigo is a moist, brightly erythematous and irritating dermatitis occurring in occluded body folds, generally in obese individuals. Excessive moisture, heat, and maceration produce conditions conducive to superficial infection with mixed bacterial flora.

Therapy

Therapy is directed at reducing heat and maceration by wearing light absorbent clothing (*i.e.*, cotton rather than polyester), by frequent drying of the skin, and by the frequent use of plain talc (such as Johnson's Baby Powder). Cornstarch, which may encourage fungal and bacterial growth, should be avoided. Following the drying measures, a corticosteroid-containing cream (such as Vioform hydrocortisone cream) should be applied three times daily. Vioform is mildly antibacterial and antifungal. The patient should be warned that Vioform may permanently stain white clothing slightly yellow. Plain talc should be used over the cream during the day, and a thick layer of zinc oxide paste can be applied at bedtime, as with candidiasis, to absorb moisture. Improvement should be evident within a few days.

Treatment of obesity is important to prevent recurrences (see Chapter 76).

Erythrasma

Definition

Erythrasma is a dry, slightly scaly, mildly inflammatory dermatitis in the intertriginous areas and can easily be mistaken for tinea infection (13). Moisture and maceration are frequent underlying conditions. It is due to an infection by a bacteria, *Corynebacterium minutissimum*. The bacteria produce prophyrins which fluoresce a salmon-red color when exposed to a Wood's light (see above).

Therapy

Treatment with erythromycin, 250 mg three times daily for 2 weeks, or 2% erythromycin, topically for 2 weeks, generally is successful. Recurrences are frequent, but the disease generally is not transmissible.

HAIR

The social and sexual significance of hair is so great that the mention of hair loss should be received sympathetically and informed advice should be provided. Hair density varies considerably among individuals, and a substantial amount of hair, perhaps 20%, can be lost before the person notices the change; about 50% of the hair is lost before others notice thinning as well. Therefore the patient's estimate is more critical than the physician's assessment of hair loss.

Pathophysiology

The change from immature vellus hair of children to the coarse dark terminal hair of adults is induced by androgens, but is modified by genetic factors. Hair growth in man is cyclical, not continuous. The period of active growth is called anagen, and the resting phase is telogen. Growing and resting hairs are intermingled and not synchronized so that, unlike molting in animals, no obvious thickening and thinning cycle occurs. At any one time about 80% of the scalp hairs are in anagen and 20% are in telogen. Once hairs have entered telogen they do not restart their growth. Instead, as the hair follicle re-enters the growing phase, a new hair forms below the resting hair and eventually the resting hair is pushed up and out and is shed (much like the shedding of primary teeth). It takes about 3 months for hair to enter the resting phase and be shed by newly formed hair from below. Shedding is quite normal and involves 25 to 100 hairs every day. A very high level of metabolic activity is maintained in anagen hair follicles. About 1 cm of hair emerges every month from a follicular base that is no thicker than this page.

Patterns of Hair Loss

The physician must first decide whether the hair loss is diffuse or patchy (thinned in regions). For example, the usual male pattern balding is patchy. The second important observation which will be useful in the classification of alopecia is the appearance of the scalp (12).

Diffuse Alopecia with Normal Appearing Scalp

It is important to determine whether the hair loss has been recent (weeks or months). If so, the cause was usually a precipitating event that took place within 3 months of the time hair began to fall out. Events associated with such hair loss include the use of many drugs (most frequently oral contraceptives, see below), pregnancy, or traumatic events, such as surgery, crash diets, severe accidents, a high fever, or severe illness. Hair follicles are susceptible to conversion from anagen to telogen from such events and, when the hair follicle restarts its growth, the resting telogen hairs are shed in larger than normal numbers.

This hair loss is not seen at the time of the reversion from anagen to telogen but rather when growth resumes, generally 1 to 3 months later. This type of hair loss is called *telogen effluvium*. The hair eventually returns to its previous appearance. However, occasionally the thinned hair is not restored. In such individuals, mostly women, the hair loss apparently triggers a form of balding, female pattern baldness, that would have been delayed until a later age. Female pattern baldness is no more reversible than is male pattern baldness.

Drug-Induced Hair Loss

Hair thinning has been associated with numerous medications; the mechanism generally is that of telogen effluvium with excessive conversion of anagen hair follicles into telogen. Thinning of hair on the scalp is noticed anytime between about 3 months after beginning the drug and about 3 months after stopping it. Besides oral contraceptive preparations, other medications that may produce this effect include heparin, coumarin, high dose vitamin A, allopurinol, amphetamines, β-blockers, iodine, thiouracil, and trimethadione.

Cytotoxic medications cause another type of hair thinning which is usually more dramatic. The cytotoxic drugs have their greatest effect on rapidly growing cells; therefore, the disturbance is in the anagen rather than in the telogen phase follicle. It is easy to understand why the hair loss is dramatic—80% of hairs are in anagen and all of these may be damaged simultaneously. The result is a hair fall that is sudden and extensive. Fortunately, hair almost always regrows normally when treatment is concluded; in some patients hair grows back more profusely and darker than it was. The hair loss can be reduced in some instances by temporary reduction of the circulation to the scalp with a tight tourniquet about the head or cooling the scalp with icebags. This is practical only if perfusion of the scalp is not necessary for therapy and when the drug is given intravenously and has a short half-life in the circulation.

General debility due to any severe endocrine, nutritional, or other systemic disorder also can lead to hair loss, developing gradually over weeks, months, or even years. The scalp usually does not appear abnormal or inflamed. If caused by a systemic medical disorder, the hair is usually a minor sign with the medical problem overwhelming the picture. However, either hypo- or hyperthyroidism and iron deficiency anemia may present as hair loss without obvious signs or symptoms; both should be ruled out by appropriate laboratory tests (see Chapters 49 and 73).

Intrinsic Hair Shaft Disorders

Intrinsic disorders of the hair shaft usually develop over months or years. These disorders can be congenital, with scalp hair never having grown normally, or, more commonly, they are acquired. Acquired forms are usually due to trauma, such as harsh chemicals or excessive brushing. The diagnosis may be evident on low power (×10) microscopic examination of the hair shaft. The most common intrinsic hair shaft weakness developing in adulthood is *trichorrhexis nodosa*. In this disorder, the hair grows at a normal rate but breaks easily due to the development of clumps or nodes along the hair shaft, appearing as bristles under the microscope.

Diffuse Alopecia with Inflamed and/or Scaly Scalp

The most common dermatitic conditions of the scalp are psoriasis and seborrheic dermatitis, but these, by themselves, do not cause hair thinning. However, trauma from intense scratching or harsh "treatment" may break the hair and produce temporary and partial alopecia. Psoriasis tends to be restricted to the scalp, up to the margins, like a helmet, while seborrheic dermatitis tends to extend over the ears, forehead, and central part of the face. Seborrheic dermatitis and psoriasis of the scalp are best diagnosed by finding the condition elsewhere on the body (see pages 1413 and 1410). Psoriasis may be limited to the scalp and in those cases the diagnosis is more difficult. Dermatologists distinguish between dandruff and seborrheic dermatitis; dandruff has scale and mild itching but lacks the inflamed and erythematous component of seborrheic dermatitis.

Treatment

The physician should follow the treatment outlined for psoriasis and seborrheic dermatitis of the scalp (see below). If unresponsive after 1 or 2 months of care, the patient should be referred to a dermatologist.

Patchy Alopecia with a Normal Appearing Scalp

The usual cause is *alopecia areata*, particularly if the patches appeared during the previous few days or weeks or have been recurrent. The patches of hair loss in alopecia areata are sharply demarcated from the surrounding normal scalp and are nearly or entirely devoid of hair. The patches may be single or multiple. A striking feature is the lack of inflammation; the scalp is not reddened or scaly. A history of severe emotional or physical trauma preceding the hair loss is common, but the underlying cause of alopecia areata is not known. Currently, the suspicion is that the fault is immunological since anti-epithelial and antithyroid antibodies have been found in many of the cases studied. *Trichotillomania*, compulsive hair pulling, is an important diagnostic alternative, but patches in this disorder are not completely bald; the patient cannot pull short hairs out until they regrow and are long enough to grab again.

Spontaneous resolution of alopecia areata is the rule. Most patients will have regrowth of all hair within several months and almost all will resolve within 2 years. Alopecia areata does not cause scarring, and the potential for hair regrowth always remains. Unfortunately, one-third of the patients have recurrences. A severe course with recurrences is more likely if the patches appear at the nuchal hairline, are multiple, or if they began appearing in childhood.

Treatment

Moderate tugging of the hair at the margins of the patch with the fingertips is a useful test of activity of the process. If the hairs come out easily, the process is still active and the patch is going to continue to expand. Topical corticosteroids may slow or reverse progression. High potency topical steroids such as those used for acne keloid (see below) may be gently rubbed into the bald patch three times a day. Absorption can be increased by asking the patient to wear a plastic shower cap to bed. If hair does not appear in 1 month, intradermal injections of long acting repository corticosteroids, such as triamcinolone acetonide 10 mg/ml (Kenalog-10), may be tried. For details, see "Intralesional Corticosteroids," page 1425. Monthly repeated injections may be needed. In most cases, hair regrowth will be stimulated at the injection sites, although several weeks will pass before new hair growth becomes visible. The newly appearing hair often is light in color but it will eventually darken to the patient's normal hair color. The hair produced by the injections usually is retained.

Patchy Alopecia with Sore, Inflamed, Scaly, and/or Lumpy Scalp

This is most often caused by an infection, either fungal or bacterial.

Fungal Infection

Preadolescents with an infection of the scalp most frequently have a fungal ("ringworm") infection, due to either *Microsporum* or *Trichophyton* species. Infections of scalp hair due to *Microsporum* species are not usually inflammatory or symptomatic and show a typical apple-green fluorescence when viewed with a Wood's lamp (see above). However, infections due to *Trichophyton* infections are now far more common. Hence, inflammation often is severe with pustulation and discomfort. If the inflammation becomes sufficiently severe, a boggy swelling, a *kerion*, will develop which can lead to scarring of hair follicles and permanent hair loss. To diagnose a fungal infection, several hairs should be plucked, allowed to soak for 15 minutes in a drop of

KOH on a microscope slide, and examined with the high dry objective to look for spores and hyphae in and on the hair shaft. Hair also should be submitted for fungal culture. The physician should submit hair or scale in a sterile tube without medium; fungi withstand transport well and the laboratory personnel can choose appropriate media depending upon the site and clinical diagnosis.

Treatment

If it seems likely that a fungal infection is present, ultrafine griseofulvin (generic by prescription) using 5 mg/kg/day in two or three divided doses, should be started, generally before the species has been identified by culture, which may take weeks. The drug is best absorbed when taken with food. It is best to treat *Microsporum* species for 3 weeks and *Trichophyton* species for 6 weeks and then to continue griseofulvin in both for 4 additional weeks after apparent cure.

Bacterial Infection

The scalp is generally resistant to bacterial infection because of its rich blood supply, but pyodermas, with pustules and bogginess of the scalp and with discomfort and adenopathy, can develop, usually secondary to an underlying dermatitis. It is important to look carefully for associated pediculosis capitis (head lice). The larvae and nits of *Pediculus humanus* var. *capitis* are sometimes difficult to find if bacterial superinfection has overshadowed the evidence of infestation (see full discussion, page 1409).

Treatment

As for other cutaneous pyodermas, erythromycin, 250 mg four times a day for a week, usually is sufficient. It is best to obtain a culture at the time the erythromycin is begun so that an alternative, such as dicloxacillin, can be chosen if insensitivity is found and if the scalp pyoderma proves unresponsive to erythromycin. The scalp should be cleansed by shampooing with a mild soap (such as Johnson's Baby Shampoo) up to four times a day.

Pediculosis should be treated with Kwell Shampoo, leaving the shampoo on for 5 minutes and then combing out the nits with a fine-toothed comb (see below). The shampoo treatment should be repeated 1 week later.

Acne Keloid

Acne keloid resembles a bacterial infection of the scalp with pustules and abscesses scattered among firm papules, but the condition is limited to the occipital part of the scalp and the back of the neck and is seen primarily in black males. It is a granulomatous and inflammatory foreign body reaction due to disordered and incurving ingrown hairs, perhaps first induced by barber clipping. Permanent hair loss can result from the scarring that develops.

TREATMENT

Therapy tends to be disappointing. However, partial relief may be achieved by courses of systemic antibiotics, such as tetracycline or erythromycin, 250 mg three times a day for 2 months; or topical high potency corticosteroids such as triamcinolone cream 0.5% (Kenalog-HP), betamethasone cream (Valisone), or fluocinonide cream (Lidex, Topsyn). Intradermal injections of long acting steroids, such as triamcinolone acetonide (Kenalog-10), may be tried next if a satisfactory response has not been achieved. For details, see "Intralesional Corticosteroids," page 1425. The patient usually gets relief which may last for 1 or 2 months from this treatment.

Patchy Alopecia with Lumps and without Dermatitis

In this instance the hair loss is restricted to the scalp over the lumps. Nodules such as epidermal inclusion cysts, or tumors, benign or malignant, may lead to hair loss from either excessive underlying pressure or from infiltration of hair-bearing skin by tumor. These primary nodular conditions are described below.

Patchy "Pattern" Alopecia Progressive over Years without Dermatitis

The normal rate of scalp hair growth may slow and then stop due to androgen stimulation of hair follicles. The thinning and baldness usually accompanying aging are called *pattern baldness* because a stereotyped course and distribution are followed. If plugs of scalp containing viable hairs are transplanted into bald regions of the scalp, the newly planted hairs will follow the intrinsic growth pattern of the area the plugs came from rather than the bald area to which the plugs are placed. The hair follicles seem to have an intrinsic "clock." Underlying scalp vasculature has nothing to do with this clock; scalp massage cannot decrease baldness. Only the absence of hormones before puberty prevents the clock from being set, as in the case of male eunuchs castrated before puberty who never become bald. Graying of the hair also is dependent on this "clock," which, like balding, is modified by family inheritance patterns. The cause of graying is unknown.

The onset and rate of thinning vary with each individual due to complex genetic factors. It is often not appreciated that women as well as men develop thinning. The pattern in most women who develop thinning is not that seen in men but is rather a diffuse thinning over the crown. The balding process starts earlier in men than in women.

TREATMENT

There is no medical treatment for balding. No product sold to cure or treat balding is of any proven benefit and some may do harm. However, studies are under way to determine if topical minoxidil can induce hair growth, a side effect of systemic use of this antihypertensive. Until proven safe and effective, the use of this medication is not warranted. It is important to treat underlying inflammatory scalp conditions (see below, "Psoriasis" and "Seborrheic Dermatitis").

The portion of the scalp at the back of the head is likely to retain hair into very old age. Surgical procedures that involve the transplantation of plugs or strips of hair from that region to bald areas do work and are of value; however, hundreds of plugs may be needed for good coverage and many months may be necessary for placement; the process is painful and expensive.

The physician should advise against implantation of artificial hair into the scalp; the technique simply does not work; the fibers act like foreign bodies and their rejection is accompanied with infection and pain.

Most men learn to accept their appearance but, for those sufficiently motivated, referral to a dermatological surgeon or plastic surgeon may be justified for consideration of hair transplants.

HERPES SIMPLEX

General Considerations

Herpex simplex, caused by *Herpesvirus hominis*, is of two subtypes. One type appears in extragenital sites (most commonly about the mouth) and is caused by type 1 virus, while the type 2 strain causes most genital herpes infections. The initial or primary herpes simplex infection, due to type 1, usually occurs in childhood, while type 2 is spread by sexual contact, with most primary infections involving persons beyond the age of puberty. On occasion, type 1 virus causes genital herpes and type 2 causes extragenital infection usually due to sexual contact.

After primary infection, the virus remains latent within regional nerve root ganglia. Patients who suffer recurrent blisters do so because of periodic reactivation of the virus, which reaches the skin *via* nerve fibers and replicates.

Presentation

Cutaneous herpes simplex infection in the adult most commonly presents as a localized group of pinhead- to rice grain-sized blisters usually recurring at intervals and at the same site.

Primary infection, particularly type 1, usually occurs in young children and is associated with severe systemic symptoms including fever, malaise, and localized tender adenopathy. The primary infection resolves in 1 to 3 weeks without a scar. Primary herpes simplex infections of neonates are serious and may be fatal; therefore, a pregnant woman with active vaginal or vulvar herpes should be delivered by cesarean section. Primary ophthalmic herpes simplex is quite painful and may lead to corneal ulcerations, scarring, and blindness. Patients should be urgently referred to an ophthalmologist for diagnosis and therapy.

Patients with atopic dermatitis may develop a generalized herpes infection, *eczema herpeticum*, with the worst lesions in the areas of pre-existing dermatitis. Patients who are immunosuppressed, either due to an inherited disorder or acquired due to malignancy or drug therapy, may become seriously ill from herpes simplex, and fatalities may occur.

More frequent and quite troublesome are recurrent lesions, particularly if recurrences are frequent. Recurrent lesions usually are preceded by several hours to a day of a prodrome consisting of local burning or tingling. This is followed by the appearance of multiple small vesicles appearing at or near the site of previous episodes. The most common location for type 1 recurrences is about the mouth and is the usual cause of the "cold sore." The genitals and buttocks are the sites where type 2 infections appear.

The episode lasts 3 to 7 days and may recur almost immediately or not for a year or more. However, recurrence every month to every few months is more typical. Eventually the tendency for recurrence diminishes. The lesions are not scarring. Recurrences are more likely to develop following febrile episodes, systemic illness, or local trauma, such as sunburn or intercourse (16).

The diagnosis of a herpes infection can be confirmed with a Tzanck smear, or the finding of rising levels of viral antibodies, or a positive viral culture, if the latter two specialized techniques are available.

Tzanck (Cytology) Smear

The purpose of a Tzanck smear is to identify multinucleated giant cells and intranuclear inclusion bodies that suggest herpes or varicella virus infection in cells obtained from the base of the blister. For the smear to be reliable, an early intact blister must be examined. The technique involves removing the blister roof with a scalpel or scissors and gently scraping the floor of the vesicle with a no. 10 or no. 15 surgical blade to obtain cells. The examiner should make a thin smear on a glass slide, immerse the slide in methanol or 95% ethanol for 1 minute, air dry, stain with Wright's or Giemsa as for blood smears, and examine for abnormal large multinucleated cells (Fig. 100.4).

Differential Diagnosis

Primary herpes simplex, particularly in an unusual location, may be misdiagnosed as cellulitis or acute contact dermatitis. Herpetic whitlow resembles bacterial paronychia but is a herpes infection of the fingertip, perhaps acquired by a nurse while providing mouth care to a patient. As herpes type 2 generally is acquired through sexual contact, other

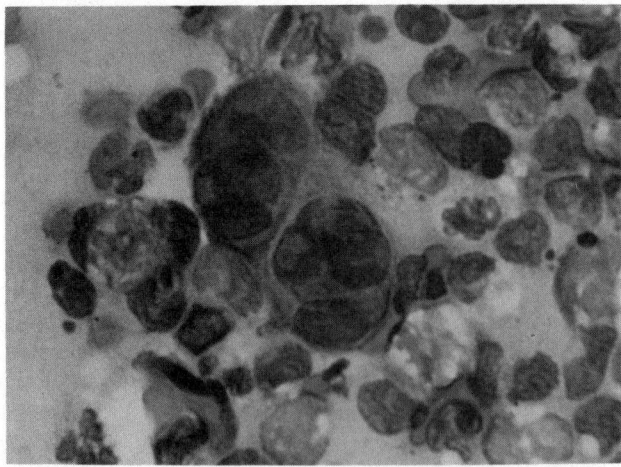

Figure 100.4. Tzanck smear: gentle scraping from the base of a vesicle and stained with Wright's or Giemsa stain. Multinucleated cells from herpes simplex are shown (×400).

venereal diseases may have been transmitted at the same time and should be considered. A urethral or vaginal smear and culture for gonorrhea, a serological test for syphilis (STS), and a slide test for *Chlamydia* (see Chapter 27) at the initial examination, with the STS repeated 2 months later, are advisable.

The grouped vesicles seen in recurrent herpes zoster closely resemble those of herpes simplex, but the two conditions can usually be distinguished by the tendency for herpes zoster to involve a more extensive area and to follow a dermatomal distribution. Zoster is only rarely recurrent so that the history of repeated episodes of blisters, particularly if they are at the same site, also strongly favors a diagnosis of herpes simplex. The Tzanck smear will be useful to rule out other blistering disorders including impetigo, erythema multiforme, and pemphigus.

Erythema multiforme, an acute blistering eruption with target-like lesions and mucosal erosions, appears to be a hypersensitivity reaction and may resemble herpes simplex, particularly as patients frequently give a history of an antecedent "cold sore." Erythema multiforme often follows herpes simplex infections, although it also follows drug and bacterial or nonsimplex viral exposure (see also Chapter 101).

Therapy

Therapy of the primary infection is aimed at relieving the discomfort by using analgesia, both systemic, with salicylates or mild opiates, and topical (Dyclone, Xylocaine), especially needed if mucosal surfaces are involved. The area should be kept cleansed. If oral lesions are extensive, the patient may need to be hospitalized for fluid replacement.

Some patients seem to have a decrease in the severity and length of recurrences with topical idoxuridine solution (Herplex, Stoxil), an analog of thymidine available as an ophthalmic solution by prescription. A drop should be applied to the site hourly during the first 12 hours of a prodrome. There is no apparent benefit after vesicles have appeared.

Acyclovir ointment (Zovirax, 15 g, by prescription) is approved for use in patients with primary genital herpes or in immunocompromised patients. The drug decreases pain and viral shedding and speeds healing. It is used every 3 to 4 hours during the day for up to 7 days. It does not prevent recurrent herpes. Oral acyclovir (200 mg), now available for genital herpes, also decreases viral shedding and shortens healing time, and, in addition, reduces systemic symptoms and complications. For primary infection, it should be given five times a day for 10 days. Unfortunately it does not reduce the frequency or severity of subsequent recurrences. For treatment of infrequent recurrences, healing time is reduced if oral acyclovir is started at the time of the prodrome (five times a day for 5 days). Frequent (more than five times/year) and severe recurrences may be suppressed with continuous acyclovir (two to five times a day for up to 6 months; see page 1340), but the drug is expensive (about $50/month) and acyclovir-resistant herpesvirus can arise. The use of acyclovir for the treatment of primary or recurrent oral herpes is under current investigation and is not yet recommended. A vaccine to prevent herpes simplex is being developed.

Corticosteroids applied to the skin may decrease inflammation after vesicles have developed. Any full strength cream, such as triamcinolone 0.1%, may be used, four times a day, but the periorbital region should be avoided to prevent steroids from entering the eye. Secondary bacterial infection of herpes lesions is not common, and lesions heal at the same rate whether antibiotics are used or not.

The contagious nature of the infection must be stressed to the patient. Herpes simplex can be transmitted from either primary or recurrent lesions, and crusts as well as blister fluid contain infectious virus.

HERPES ZOSTER (SHINGLES)

General Considerations

Two weeks following primary infection with zoster-varicella virus, clinical lesions of chickenpox appear and, in most patients, clear without complication during the next 2 weeks. However, in many or perhaps all individuals who have had chickenpox, the virus continues to reside in a latent state within dorsal root or cranial nerve ganglia. Latent virus does not replicate and can only be identified with specialized culture or antibody techniques. The clinical signs of zoster are due to the reactivation of the virus and its emanation from the ganglia to peripheral nerve endings. In support of the premise that reactivation of virus rather than new infection is the cause of zoster, epidemiological studies have shown that patients with zoster have not been exposed to recent active cases of chickenpox and do not have an increased likelihood of acquiring zoster during epidemics of chickenpox.

Zoster is more likely to appear when mechanisms limiting reactivation of the virus are blunted. Conditions associated with reactivation include old age, acute systemic illness, injuries to or neoplasia of cranial nerves or the spinal column, and disorders associated with diminished immunocompetency, including lymphoma-leukemia and immunosuppressive therapy.

Presentation

A prodrome of 1 to 4 days, but occasionally up to 10 days, is characterized by tingling, tenderness, or itch restricted to the nerve segment involved. Patients with a severe prodrome may present with acute chest or abdominal pain or acute sciatica or joint pain. Before lesions are visible, hypesthesia, dysesthesia, or, more commonly, hyperesthesia will be evident in the dermatome so that a sensory neurological examination of the area may provide early confirmation of the diagnosis.

Very occasionally, zoster manifests only with localized pain, in which case establishing the diagnosis requires the demonstration of a rising antibody titer. Usually, however, there is a typical skin lesion: a patch of grouped vesicles on an erythematous base, each vesicle having a central dell. The eruption is almost always strikingly demarcated at the midline. However, the earliest lesions will present closest to the ganglia, and the dermatomal distribution may not be obvious. A Tzanck test may be performed (see above for technique) to confirm the presence of multinucleated giant cells and of intranuclear inclusions. Like herpes simplex and varicella, zoster can present a serious danger to immunosuppressed patients who may get severe chickenpox and varicella pneumonia; patients with zoster must be isolated.

Differential Diagnosis

Difficulties with diagnosis are more likely in the early stages before the blistering becomes evident. Patients may be considered to have cellulitis, contact dermatitis, neuralgia, arthritis, or a chest or abdominal disorder. Herpes simplex may present in a linear pattern but usually causes less local discomfort and dysesthesia than zoster.

There is no increased risk of subsequent cancer following the diagnosis of herpes zoster, whether the zoster is localized or disseminated.

Therapy

For most patients treatment is symptomatic. The pain may be excruciating and often requires mild opiates such as codeine at the dose of 30 to 60 mg every 3 or 4 hours as well as nighttime sedation such as with diphenhydramine (Benadryl), 50 to 100 mg. A thick coat of zinc oxide paste (available without prescription) or an antibacterial cream, 1% silver sulfadiazine (Silvadene, requires a prescription) one to two times a day, reduces the tendency of serum from the denuded blisters to stick to clothing and decreases discomfort by providing an air-tissue barrier. The zinc oxide may be removed with cotton balls moistened with mineral oil and reapplied morning and bedtime. Silvadene washes off with water. An alternative is to have the patient apply compresses (such as Domboros solution) several times a day.

Controlled studies support the use of systemic corticosteroids during the acute phase to reduce postherpetic neuralgia, a severe and persistent pain in the involved nerve root and dermatome that may continue for years, particularly common and severe in the elderly (6). The mechanism of the pain probably is fibrosis and scarring of the nerve, a complication that may be reduced by corticosteroids. The steroids should be started during the acute phase, but administration may safely be delayed until new blisters are no longer appearing. The dose is 60 mg of prednisone in a single morning dose daily for 1 week, 30 mg daily for the second week, and 15 mg for the third. Corticosteroids should not be used if there is an overriding medical contraindication, such as bacterial infection, tuberculosis, or active peptic ulceration.

If the eye is involved, urgent ophthalmological consultation is necessary. High risk patients, such as those with leukemia-lymphoma or who are immunosuppressed, and who have had an exposure to varicella or zoster within the previous 72 hours, should receive varicella-zoster-immune globulin, obtainable commercially through local blood blanks or the Red Cross. The place for acyclovir in zoster is being assessed. Varicella vaccines have been developed but are not yet available.

HIDRADENITIS SUPPURATIVA

Single occasional abscesses or inflamed cysts on the trunk or intertriginous areas are common. If, however, there are frequent recurrences in the axillae, groin, and/or perianal regions that heal leaving fibrotic scars, hidradenitis suppurativa should be considered. Patients with this disorder also may develop abscesses on the buttocks and, in women, about or under the breasts. Patients also tend to have active acne vulgaris or old acne scars and develop epidermal inclusion cysts.

Hidradenitis suppurativa, an infection of apocrine sweat glands, does not appear until apocrine glands develop at puberty. Although bacteria are not the underlying cause of hidradenitis, they participate in the process. The course is chronic, leading, if severe, to fistulae, lymphedema, and even restriction of arm or leg movement. The painful, draining abscesses and accompanying odor often produce considerable occupational and social disability. Figure 100.20 (page 1421) shows an example of hidradenitis suppurativa.

Therapy

Acute and fluctuant lesions may be incised and drained, just like any bacterial abscess. A bacterial culture for antibiotic sensitivities from a fresh, non-draining lesion should be obtained when the disorder flares. Systemic antibiotics, selected on the basis of sensitivity testing, help to resolve acute flares. Generally, erythromycin (250 mg four times a day) or dicloxacillin (125 mg every 6 hours) for 10 to 14 days generally is adequate. Long term tetracycline (250 to 500 mg two to three times a day for months) may partially suppress the disorder. Between episodes, recurrences sometimes can be reduced with twice daily washing with hexachlorophene soap (PhisoHex, available with a prescription) or a quaternary iodine scrub (Betadine or Povidone, available without a prescription).

Permanent cure can be obtained by excision of the affected area, removing the apocrine glands, scars, and sinus tracts. This radical treatment is justified in severe cases. If the onset is recent and confined to one region, other causes of infection should be considered, such as tuberculosis, actinomycosis, cat-scratch disease, and, in the groin, granuloma inguinale.

MILIARIA (PRICKLY HEAT)

This common eruption is troublesome because of the prickling and itchy symptoms that accompany it. The eruption develops on occluded or rubbing skin surfaces when the skin temperature is abnormally hot. It usually consists of minute red papules, called *miliaria rubra*, but it sometimes presents as a myriad of pinhead-sized clear vesicles resembling water droplets, *miliaria crystallina*. The disorder is caused by occlusion of eccrine sweat ducts with rupture or leakage of the sweat into the surrounding tissue, with the specific type of miliaria depending on the depth of the obstruction within the duct.

Miliaria may develop in persons who work or exercise daily in a hot, humid environment as well as in patients who are wrapped with occlusive bandages, who are lying on plastic undersheets, or who have a high fever. The eruption clears when the skin is cooled and ventilated. Spending 8 hours in an air-conditioned sleeping room prevents the development of miliaria. Propylene glycol in water (50%) (available by prescription from most pharmacies), applied two times a day, may also help to clear the sweat duct blockage.

PEDICULOSIS CAPITIS (HEAD LICE)

Persistent itching of the scalp and crusting and oozing suggestive of a bacterial infection are the typical manifestations of pediculosis. Cervical lymph nodes frequently are enlarged and may be tender. The lice resemble grains of wild rice, in that they are brown and longer than they are wide (Fig. 100.5). They are attached to the scalp or loosely adherent in the hair. If the infestation has been prolonged, nits (egg cases) should be visible along the hair shaft as white granules, smaller than a pinhead. Since the eggs are deposited at scalp level, the duration of the infestation can be estimated by the distance of the nits from the scalp, each centimeter representing about 1 month of infestation.

Spread of pediculosis capitis requires close personal contact, such as may occur in children sleeping at one another's house or sharing the same towels and combs; ordinary contact between school children does not transfer the infestation.

Therapy

Treatment with lindane (also called gamma benzene hexachloride) (Kwell, available by prescription) shampoo is convenient and highly effective, but is potentially neurotoxic and should not be used in pregnant or lactating women; pyrethrin with pi-peronyl butoxide (Rid, 60 and 120 ml, available without prescription) may be safer for women in these groups. One tablespoon of the medication is shampooed thoroughly into the hair for 5 minutes. Nits should be removed with a fine-toothed comb and the shampooing repeated in 1 week. Combs and brushes should be submerged in boiling water, which quickly kills nits. Bed linens, towels, and clothing should be washed in hot water and dried at a high temperature or dry cleaned.

PITYRIASIS ROSEA

Pityriasis rosea (PR) is common, particularly during ages 15 to 35. Although the cause is not known, PR acts like an infectious disease as second episodes are uncommon and there are seasonal increases and mini-epidemics (3). Efforts to isolate an agent have been unsuccessful. There is no specific histopathology or blood test.

Presentation

The initial lesion, the "herald patch," is a 2- to 6-cm, round, scaly plaque that, in about half the patients, appears on the trunk. Several days later, 1- to 2-cm, pale, red, round to oval macular and papular scaly lesions appear on the trunk and proximal parts of the extremities, forming a fern-like

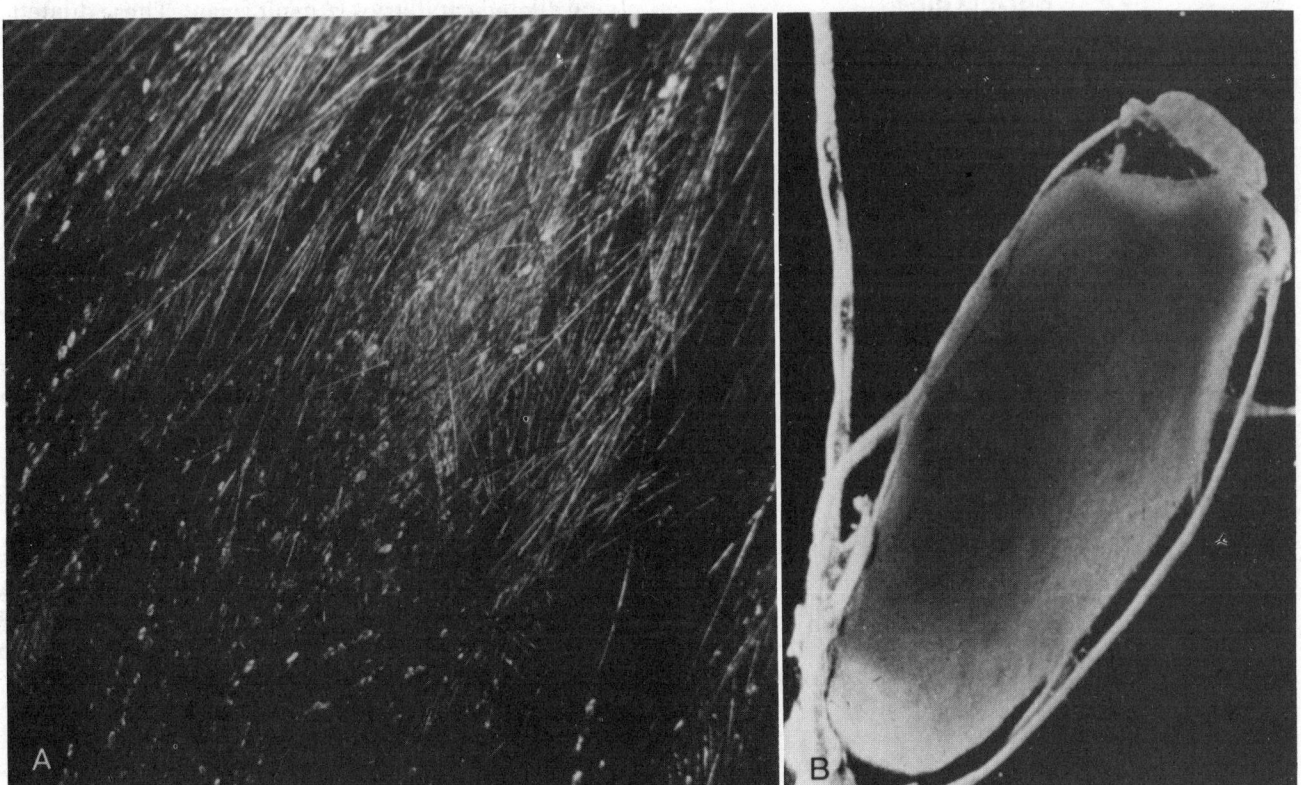

Figure 100.5. *Pediculus humanus var. capitis* (head louse). *A.* Gross appearance of nits on the hair shaft. *B.* Microscopic appearance (×100; photograph *B* courtesy of Reed and Carnrick, Kenilworth, NJ).

pattern (Fig. 100.6). New lesions develop on more distal parts, while others clear centrally. The face is involved infrequently and less often in whites than in blacks. The eruption usually is pruritic and, at times, intensely so, but it may be asymptomatic. PR runs its course in 6 to 8 weeks.

The eruption mimics secondary syphilis; an STS should be obtained in all sexually active patients suspected of having PR. The STS is always positive in secondary syphilis.

Therapy

If the lesions are not itchy, no treatment is needed. It is important, however, for the physician to explain the disease and to describe the anticipated course. If pruritus is mild, diphenhydramine (Benadryl), 25 to 50 mg three times a day, and a topical antipruritic suspension, such as calamine lotion with menthol or phenol added, may be prescribed.

Occasionally, pruritus is so severe that the patient cannot work or sleep. In that case, prednisone may be necessary to control the symptoms. The physician should prescribe 40 mg daily in divided doses until the patient is comfortable, usually a few days, then taper the prednisone over a 3-week period by prescribing 1 tablet less every third day. The patient does not require isolation and may attend school or work.

PSORIASIS

This probably genetic and usually lifelong disease affects 1 to 3% of the population. Psoriasis may first appear in childhood, especially in severe cases, but usually begins during the third decade. In most instances, it remains throughout adulthood, often improving in the summer and during pregnancies. The disease affects males and females equally. Most patients have only mild pruritus but the scaly patches are unsightly and may interfere with work, social relationships, and self-image.

Certain histocompatibility antigens (HLA) are associated with the disorder and over one-third of patients have another family member with psoriasis, supporting the theory that psoriasis is inherited, but the underlying cause of the disease still is unknown. Vastly increased epidermal proliferation explains the histological alterations of elongation of epidermal ridges and increased numbers of mitotic cells; epidermal turnover rates may be increased up to 10-fold over normal. This epidermal proliferation is reflected clinically as overproduction of scale, the characteristic sign of the disease.

Presentation

The typical lesion is an erythematous, circumscribed plaque covered by loosely adherent, silvery scales appearing most often on the elbows, knees, and scalp; the external genitalia, the umbulicus, and the gluteal fold frequently are involved as well (Fig. 100.7). Peeling of the scale often produces minute bleeding points that reflect the proximity of underlying dilated capillaries (Auspitz sign). These dilated capillaries, rather than inflammation, are the cause of the plaque's redness. Nails may show pitting (Fig. 100.8) or, when more severely involved, a large

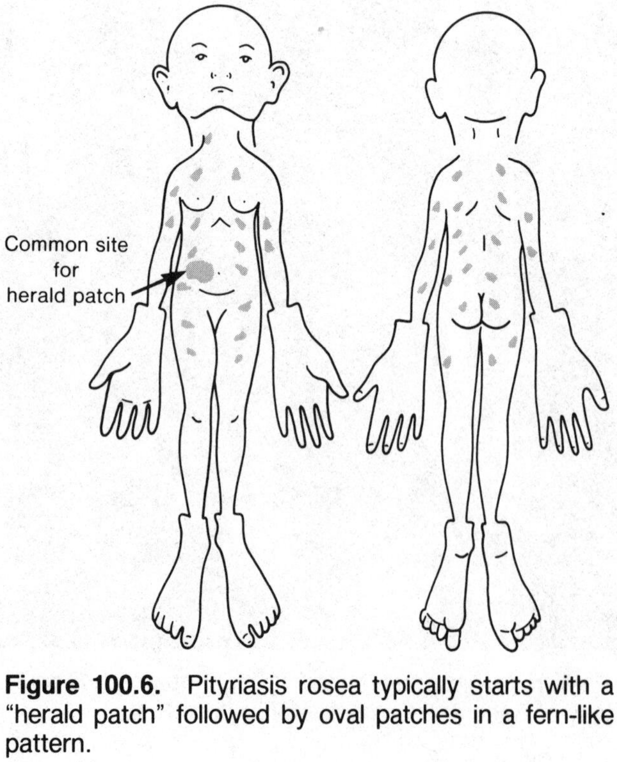

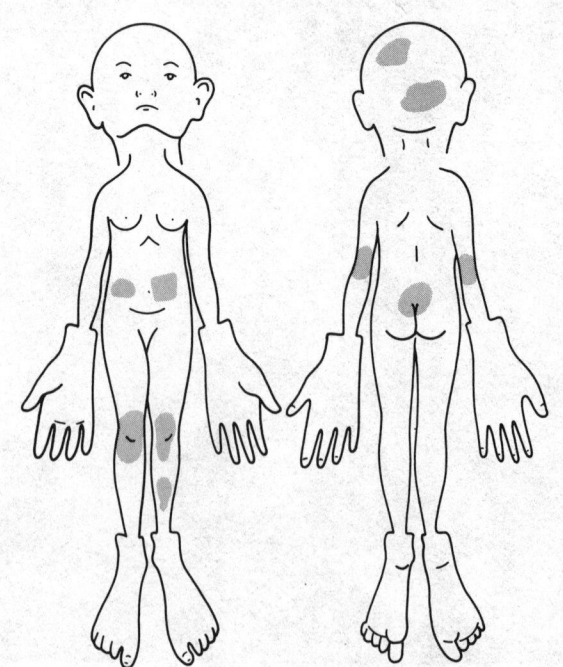

Figure 100.6. Pityriasis rosea typically starts with a "herald patch" followed by oval patches in a fern-like pattern.

Figure 100.7. Psoriasis tends to be found on extensor surfaces and areas of repeated trauma, such as the waistline.

Common site for herald patch

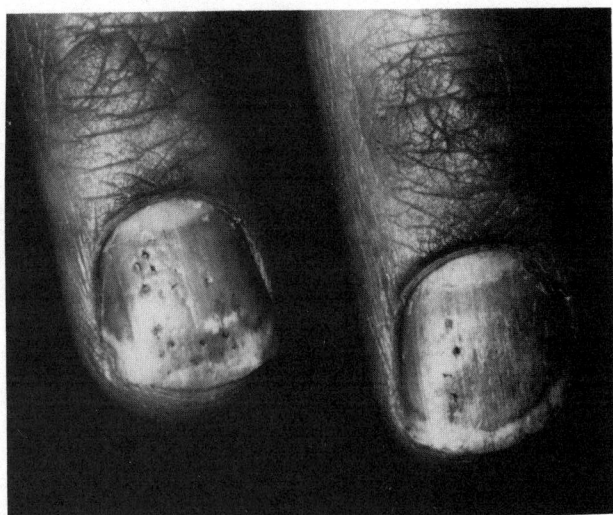

Figure 100.8. Minute pits are commonly seen on the surface of nails in patients with psoriasis.

volume of subungual keratotic debris leading to separation of the nail from the nail bed.

The diagnosis is not always obvious; the patient may present with severe "dandruff," with nail dystrophy, an apparent drug eruption, or arthritis and a rash. Seborrheic dermatitis (see below), fungal infection (see above), a psoriasiform drug eruption, or even a contact dermatitis to the therapy being used to treat the psoriasis must be considered.

There are several variants of psoriasis that are particularly virulent: *psoriatic erythroderma*, a generalized exfoliative dermatitis characterized by diffuse erythema and scaling and by systemic toxicity including chills and fever; and generalized *pustular psoriasis*, characterized by a diffuse pustular eruption and also by systemic toxicity.

The association between arthritis and psoriasis is still not precisely defined; some patients appear to have a typical seropositive rheumatoid arthritis, probably not related to the dermatological condition; others have a destructive arthritis, characteristically involving the terminal interphalangeal joints, that appears to be part of the psoriatic syndrome.

Therapy

Skin

Because topical fluorinated corticosteroids are clean, odorless, and rapidly suppress scale and pruritus, they are the first step in the topical therapy of psoriasis (4). However, topical steroids do not produce complete remissions and within a few days of discontinuing the medication, psoriasis returns to its pretreatment appearance. For additional details, see "Corticosteroids," page 1424.

The effectiveness of topical corticosteroids can be increased by applying them at bedtime and then wrapping the area with any kitchen plastic wrap

(Glad, Saran, *etc*) For additional details, see "Occlusion" under "Corticosteroids," page 1424.

Long term relief for psoriasis of the glabrous (hairless) skin often can be achieved through the addition of tar preparations including Alphosyl, Estar Tar Gel, or Psorigel—all of which are available without prescription. All of these have a slight tar odor and tint; they should be applied sparingly, only to the patch, and generally only at bedtime. If corticosteroids with occlusion by wrapping are being used at bedtime (see above), the two therapies can be used on alternate nights.

Further benefits may result from the use at home of ultraviolet (UV) light. The patient should choose a floor model (if the unit is too small the patient will become frustrated by the long time that the therapy requires) with a timer (an absolute necessity) and can expect to pay approximately $150 for it. The patient should follow the instructions with the unit to determine the initial exposure, as this time will vary among models. Treatments should be every other day, with increasing exposure each time until slight redness is still visible 24 hours after the UV light exposure. The patient can increase the dose when the persistent erythema no longer develops. Tanning will deepen after several weeks of UV light. The morning following the nighttime application of a tar preparation is the best time to use UV light, but the tar appears to be effective if left on for as short a time as 2 hours prior to the light. The psoriasis-suppressing effect of natural sunlight appears to be more effective than artificial UV light and should be utilized when it is available. Little evidence for late developing skin cancers has ever appeared in psoriatics exposed to UV light and tars.

Scalp

The patient should shampoo every day or two. Frequent shampooing may be all that is needed in mild cases. Although a number of shampoos containing tars (Ionil T, Sebutone, Zetar), selenium sulfate (Exsel, Iosel, Selsun), and zinc compounds (Danex, Head and Shoulders, Zincon) often are prescribed, very little medication will be left on the scalp after shampooing, so that medicated shampoos alone will help only those patients with minimal involvement.

If shampooing is not sufficient, the physician may prescribe a topical corticosteroid solution or lotion (Diprosone lotion, Lidex solution, Valisone lotion, Synalar solution) rubbed into the scaly plaques with the fingertips immediately following shampooing while the scalp is still moist. Ointments and creams are difficult to use in hairy parts. If scales are too thick to be loosened by shampoos alone, the patient may apply phenol/saline lotion (Bakers P&S liquid, available without prescription) to the scalp at bedtime before the morning shampooing. A stronger, but messier, preparation is a mixture of sulfur, salicylic acid, and tar (Pragmatar cream, available without prescription), which may be used if the phenol/saline lotion does not produce resolution of the thick scale within a month of use. Both preparations are used in the same way. Wearing a showercap at night may be advised to protect bed linens.

Nails

No consistently effective and easy treatment exists. On occasion, dermatologists inject nailfolds with steroids, but the treatment is painful and relief is temporary.

Treatment used by a dermatologist for patients with extensive psoriasis include psoralen with long wave ultraviolet light (PUVA) and systemic antimetabolites (methotrexate, hydroxyurea) or tar and UV light treatment, the Goeckerman regimen.

SCABIES

Presentation

Scabies is an infestation caused by a mite, *Sarcoptes scabiei* var. *hominis*. Scabies seems to run in cycles; there has been a dramatic upswing in cases since the 1970s, now apparently leveling off. Most of the signs and symptoms of scabies are due to sensitization to the mite and mite products rather than to the physical effects of the mite itself. Hence, there is delayed appearance of the rash until approximately 14 days after exposure, and there is delayed clearing following effective therapy. Because of the sensitization, symptoms start sooner with recurrent infection. Only a few mites usually are present, generally fewer than 10, even though the signs and symptoms can be extensive. The distribution of the mite does not correspond closely with the distribution of the rash (Fig. 100.9). Untreated scabies continues to progress; it is not self-healing.

The overwhelming symptom is severe itching, typically worse at night. The lesions appear as excoriated, inflamed, rice- to pea-sized papules, some with a burrow. Sites most involved are the finger webs, wrists, antecubital fossae, elbows, areolae, umbilicus, lower abdomen, genitalia, and gluteal cleft. Superimposed excoriations and eczematous dermatitis are common. Findings may be minimal in scrupulously clean individuals. Family members and sexual partners almost invariably are involved and should be treated. Transmission requires close contact, such as sleeping in the same bed or living in the same house; scabies usually is not transmitted casually, as between schoolmates. If the patient is sexually active, it is important to look for other venereal diseases.

A diagnosis of scabies should be considered in any patient who has a pruritic eruption with excoriated papules, especially if family members or close friends also are experiencing itching. Scabies can be proven by finding the mite microscopically. This is accomplished by placing a drop of glycerol or min-

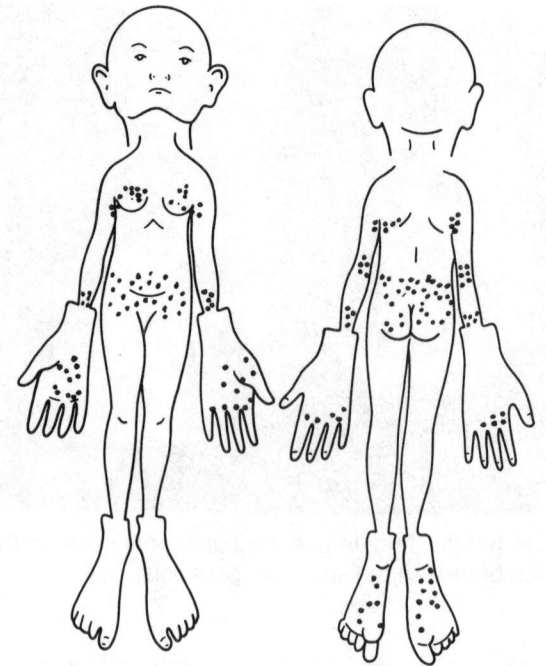

Figure 100.9. Pruritic papules are most prevalent about the waist, pelvis, elbows, and hands and feet in scabies.

eral oil, preferably sterile, on the papule to keep the scales and scrapings in place, and scraping through the oil with a blade or syringe needle to the point of just drawing blood. The mite or its eggs must be sought using the ×10 microscope objective. The mite is an ugly, bristled ectoparasite about 0.4 mm long with four pairs of legs. It is hard to find; even experts may be unable to confirm the diagnosis. Therefore, it is appropriate to treat on strong clinical suspicion.

Scabies is sometimes difficult to diagnose and may be confused, even by the experienced clinician, with a variety of cutaneous disorders. Atypical presentations account for delayed treatment and provide opportunities for spread. Further confusion is often generated by the use of topical corticosteroids that can partially suppress the eruption.

Therapy

Two topical scabicides are in general use, gamma benzene hexachloride (GBH), also called lindane (Kwell, available by prescription), and crotamiton (Eurax, available by prescription). Either is effective but GBH often is not used in children under 6 or in pregnant or lactating women because of neurotoxicity in children (19).

GBH

The patient should apply lotion to all crevices of the entire body from the chin down and leave it on for 8 to 12 hours, then remove it by thorough washing. It should be applied when the skin is dry, not immediately after bathing, because of the increased absorption through damp skin. Since GBH is not ovicidal, retreatment 1 week later is appropriate to destroy later hatching larvae. Recently used clothing should be thoroughly washed or dry cleaned, and linens and towels should be changed and laundered. For practical purposes, scabies is not transmissible after the first day of therapy. There is no need to suggest extermination procedures as the lifespan of the mite on clothing and bedding is short. All symptomatic family members should be treated at the same time. The physician should prescribe enough to apply 30 ml to each person for each of the two treatments and should not allow refills; extensive repeated use of GBH may cause irritation and pruritus, which may be confused with the original symptoms.

Crotamiton

Crotamiton is an alternative to GBH, but is not quite as effective. It is applied from the chin down and to all body folds and creases in the same way as GBH, but it is reapplied 24 hours later. Clothing and linen should be changed the first morning after treatment. The medication should be left on for a total of 72 hours, after which patients should take a cleansing bath. Crotamiton is antipruritic and appears to be safe for use in children and pregnant women.

Follow-up

If the initial therapy did not appear to work, there are several points to consider. First it must be kept in mind that itching often persists for 1 to 3 weeks following effective antiscabicide treatment, as a result of slow subsiding of the hypersensitivity reaction to the mite and mite products. An antihistamine, such as diphenhydramine (Benadryl, a 25- or 50-mg capsule three or four times a day) a topical corticosteroid ointment, such as triamcinolone 0.1%, or, if severe, systemic corticosteroids, such as prednisone, 30 mg/day in three divided doses and tapered over 2 weeks, may be needed to provide relief. Second, if symptoms persist beyond 2 weeks or recur when the antipruritics are stopped, the patient should be re-examined for persistent infestation or reinfestation. If there are signs of secondary infection, a 7-day course of an antibiotic, such as erythromycin, 250 mg four times a day, is indicated. The pruritic papules frequently accompanying scabies may require weeks to clear. Animal scabies is different from human scabies; therefore, pets are not a reservoir and do not have to be treated in order to control human infestation.

SEBORRHEIC DERMATITIS

Presentation

Seborrheic dermatitis takes its name because it is found in regions where sebaceous glands are in greatest density, i.e., the scalp, eyebrows, ear canals,

midface, and midchest area (Fig. 100.10). The main features are erythema and a yellow, greasy scaling. Itching is mild but troublesome. Typically, the severity fluctuates so that patients recall months of relative clearing and months of relative worsening.

Onset of seborrheic dermatitis is generally at puberty when it appears concomitantly with acne; the condition continues in its fluctuating course for years or decades without a decrease in old age. Both sexes are equally affected. Seborrheic dermatitis is worsened in patients with Parkinson's disease, syringomyelia, emotional stress, and at the time of an acute stroke or myocardial infarction.

Although occurring in regions of dense sebaceous glands and having a greasy appearance, seborrheic dermatitis does not appear to be a disorder of the sebaceous glands. Other possible causes of seborrheic dermatitis have been sought, including differences in bacteria and sebum, but none has been found (7).

Differential Diagnosis

The common scalp condition, dandruff, is distinguished from seborrheic dermatitis by the absence of erythema and the lack of involvement in other regions. The most frequent confusion is with psoriasis, as both conditions are erythematous, scaly, and chronic. Psoriasis, however, tends to involve the extensor surfaces, particularly the elbows and knees; a search for such lesions in patients with severe scalp dermatitis may be helpful. Psoriasis of the scalp often stops at the hairline, seborrheic dermatitis does not. The differential diagnosis also in-

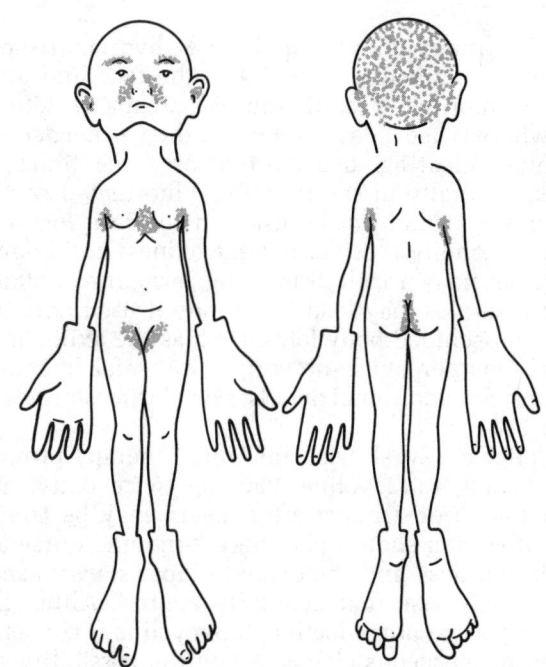

Figure 100.10. Usual location of erythema and scale in seborrheic dermatitis.

cludes contact dermatitis, a drug eruption, tinea corporis, and tinea versicolor. These alternative diagnostic possibilities should especially be considered when the response to therapy for seborrheic dermatitis is not satisfactory.

Therapy

The patient should understand that only relief, not cure, is possible. A fluctuating course is expected, and therapy will need to be modified with exacerbations. If the patient does not understand this, the result will be disappointing. The treatment depends on the site of involvement.

Scalp

If mild, control with shampoos (see above, "Psoriasis") may be sufficient. Frequent, even daily, shampooing is not harmful and does not cause hair loss.

If the condition is severe or is unresponsive to simple shampooing, the physician should prescribe a topical corticosteroid to be applied after shampooing, while the scalp is still damp. A lotion, such as betamethasone (Diprosone or Valisone lotion), a solution such as fluocinolone (Synalar solution), or a gel such as fluocinonide (Topsyn gel) must be used since creams and ointments are difficult to use in hairy parts. If the scales are thick, the phenol/saline or tar preparations (see above, "Psoriasis") may be used at bedtime, following by the steroid preparation after shampooing in the morning. If the condition still proves resistant to therapy, psoriasis is more likely to be the diagnosis than is seborrheic dermatitis.

Skin

The patient should apply 1% hydrocortisone cream (prescribed as generic) to the face and any potent fluorinated corticosteroid cream or lotion elsewhere twice a day until clear, then as needed to maintain clearing, usually two or three times a week, generally in the morning. Fluorinated corticosteroids should not be used on the face for *any* chronic condition as permanent redness and telangiectasias may result from long term use. Potent corticosteroids may lead to atrophy if used chronically in occluded body folds, such as the axilla and groin. One percent hydrocortisone is safer in those regions. For additional details, see "Corticosteroids," page 1424.

If, after a 3-week trial, the initial therapy proves insufficient, tetracycline, 250 mg twice daily, an hour before or 2 hours after meals, may be tried. The physician should plan on a 2-month course at the initial dose and then should taper slowly each month to a dose that maintains control. Although this may seem homeopathic, tetracycline is concentrated in sebaceous glands. Again the possibility of

psoriasis should be considered if the dermatitis is resistant to treatment.

Eyelids

Seborrheic marginal blepharitis is chronic scaling at the lid margins without signs of conjunctivitis or globe discomfort. It can be controlled by gentle scrubbing each morning with baby shampoo (e.g., Johnson's), diluted one to one with water, using a cotton-tipped applicator to cleanse the lids. If not sufficiently controlled, a mild topical corticosteroid such as 1% hydrocortisone cream twice daily may be used. However, long use of potent fluorinated topical corticosteroids can lead to glaucoma, is dangerous in the presence of herpes infection, and should not be used. Treatment should continue at this frequency only until the condition has cleared, after which the patient should decrease the frequency of application to two or three times a week for an additional 2 weeks and then should stop therapy. Like seborrheic dermatitis, the condition tends to recur; therapy can be restarted when needed.

Contact dermatitis to mascara or eye shadow can manifest as blepharitis, and both of these agents should be discontinued for at least a month to determine if either is causal. The patient should be referred to an ophthalmologist if unresponsive or if the rash is accompanied by conjunctivitis and/or cornea or globe discomfort.

SUNBURN

Symptoms and Consequences

The redness, pain, and tenderness from excessive sun exposure are maximal in 12 to 24 hours. When burning is severe, the skin may blister or peel 1 to several days later. Protective tanning also is induced; the increased pigment remains for months. Acute sunburn heals without scarring unless a secondary infection develops. Long term, chronic excessive sun exposure, especially in light-complexioned persons, eventually leads to fine wrinkling and sometimes actinic keratoses, basal cell and squamous cell carcinomas; it probably is a risk factor for malignant melanoma as well.

Sun Exposure

Most of the energy from the sun that reaches the earth's surface on a sunny day is in the long wave, UVA spectrum, the so-called "tanning" portion. About 10% of the energy is at the short wave, UVB end of the ultraviolet spectrum. These are the so-called "burning" rays. The proportion of UVB decreases if the sun is filtered by clouds or when the sun is low on the horizon. Nonetheless, because UVB is about 1000 times more potent than UVA in evoking the burning reaction, it is UVB that causes most solar-induced damage. "Suntan parlors" often advertise that they provide primarily UVA or "safe" exposure, but even UVA in sustained high doses is potentially harmful.

Except for inducing vitamin D, now incidental because of the widespread use of fortified foods, the effects of ultraviolet light are destructive. There is no "safe" ultraviolet light exposure. Tanning should be regarded as a response to injury; even tanning offers only partial protection, compared to the major protective value of melanin. The nearly universal frequency of skin cancers in albinos and the much decreased wrinkling and frequency of skin cancers in blacks attests to the protective value of melanin.

Therapy

A sunburn is like any other physical injury: the damage cannot be reversed and must be allowed to heal. Aspirin decreases the pain and perhaps lessens the inflammatory reaction by interfering with tissue prostaglandin metabolism. Large doses soon after exposure, 600 mg every 2 hours for six doses, seem beneficial. An extensive burn can be soothed with a 20-minute colloidal oatmeal bath, made by adding one-quarter cup of Aveeno Oatmeal, available without prescription, to lukewarm or cool bath water. If large blisters appear, they may be punctured with a sterile needle or surgical blade, but the roof should be left intact to serve as a pain-reducing biological dressing. Prophylactic antibiotics are not helpful.

Although the cause of sun exposure usually is obvious, some people develop an exaggerated response producing an unexpected "burn" or an unusual skin reaction, perhaps papules, hives, plaques, or a scaly dermatitis. An exaggerated sunburn reaction may be associated with a phototoxic or photoallergic drug reaction or a photosensitizing disorder. Systemic determination of the degree of photosensitivity and the separation of phototoxic and photoallergic responses require specialized equipment and the expertise of a dermatologist.

Prevention

Radiation from natural UVB is greatly reduced before 10 A.M. and after 2 P.M. because of filtration of the sun's rays through the atmosphere. Cosmetically acceptable and effective sunblockers are available, rated by their sun protection factor (SPF). The assigned number, which ranges from 3 to 15 or more, indicates the multiple by which the product extends the period of exposure. For example, if an individual would have developed a sunburn from a 30-minute exposure, a sunblock with SPF of 15 extends that time to 7.5 hours (0.5 hours × 15), obviously an effective level of protection for most purposes. Sunblocks should be applied 30 minutes prior to sun exposure. Most sunblocks are less effective in block-

ing UVA than UVB and most are washed away by sweat or water; the directions for use of each product should be followed.

TINEA VERSICOLOR

Presentation

Tinea versicolor is a common superficial fungal infection caused by *Malassezia furfur* (18). It appears as desquamating macular patches found primarily on the trunk, between the chin and the waist. The rash may be mildly itchy. The varied colors of the rash, from red to pink to brown, gives the eruption its name. Tinea versicolor is most common in hot, humid environments.

The fungus interferes with normal pigmentation, so that the patches become more noticeable during the summer when the skin under the patches does not tan as well as the rest of the skin. This effect is seen in blacks as well as whites. The infection does not seem to be contagious; marital partners usually are not both affected. However, individuals who have had tinea versicolor seem prone to have recurrences.

An examination with KOH shows short hyphae and spores ("spaghetti and meatballs") (Fig. 100.11). The physician should search under the high dry objective (×40); the low power objective (×10) is too low to reveal the fungal structures. A Wood's light examination (see page 1400) is useful as it reveals the extent of the infection better than does room light. The organism cannot be cultured on usual office media.

Differential Diagnosis

Because of the pigment disruption, vitiligo must be considered. However, vitiligo is never scaly and

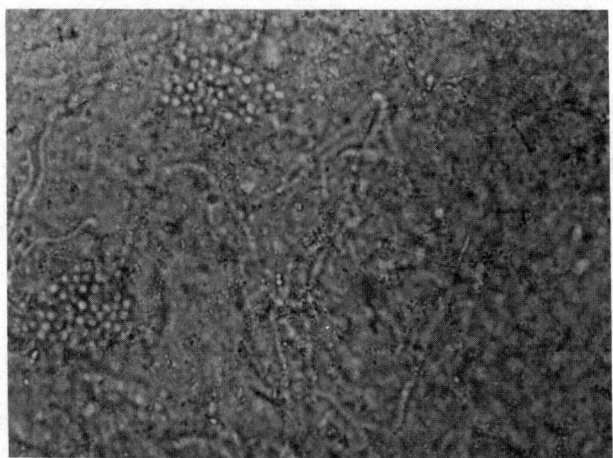

Figure 100.11. Short hyphae and spores of *Malassezia furfur* seen in tinea versicolor (KOH preparation, ×400).

a KOH examination will be negative. The pigment loss in tinea versicolor is partial; the pigment loss in vitiligo is complete. Other disorders to consider are seborrheic dermatitis (see above), pityriasis rosea (see above), and infection due to other tinea species. Seborrheic dermatitis most commonly involves the face and scalp, but tinea versicolor almost never goes above the chin; pityriasis rosea may be worse on the upper trunk but usually extends below the waist and the KOH examination will be negative; a KOH examination of the other tinea that affects man causing tinea cruris and corporis ("ringworm" of the groin and body) reveals long hyphae without spores, not short hyphae with spores.

Therapy

Numerous therapies work, but recurrences are common. An irritating soap applied at bedtime and showered off in the morning usually is sufficient. Selenium sulfide suspension (Exsel, 2.5%, requires a prescription; or Selsun Blue, 1%, available without prescription) or a peeling soap (Fostex cream, available without prescription) should be used for 4 consecutive nights or less if the skin shows irritation. The patient should apply the material from neck to wrists to waist, the areas most commonly affected. The use of 25% sodium thiosulfate (generic or Tinver, a prescription is required) twice a day for an additional 10 days assures resolution but should be used only after work and at bedtime as it has an unpleasant smell. Prescription antifungal agents, such as miconazole, clotrimazole, and haloprogin, are effective but too expensive to apply to the large surface area usually involved. Ketaconazol (Nizoral, 200-mg tablets, by prescription) is a newer, more convenient oral therapy and is effective in short courses, 200 mg each day for 5 days, repeated with 3 tablets at 2 additional monthly intervals (not an FDA-approved use). It probably is safe for short term use, but hepatitis has been associated with the medication.

After the initial therapy, the patient may expect the lesions to be cleared of fungi; a return visit is not needed. However, the patient must be warned that the lightened patches will remain until ultraviolet light-induced retanning occurs. Otherwise, the patient may consider the treatment to be a failure. Patients also should be told that recurrences are common and advised to repeat therapy if needed, generally in the following summer.

VITILIGO

Presentation

When melanocytes stop producing melanin and, later, completely disappear from the site, the skin turns nearly ivory in color, regardless of background racial coloration. The patches have sharp borders without erythema or inflammation. They are most frequent over bony prominences and around orifices such as the mouth and eyes (Fig. 100.12). The patches reflect light and appear bright white under a Wood's lamp (see page 1400), an examination which may be useful in revealing additional patches of vitiligo, especially if the patient is light complexioned. Vitiligo may be inherited, and its course is unpredictable.

Differential Diagnosis

The usual confusion is caused by postinflammatory hypopigmentation. In this case there is typically a history of a preceding inflammatory or traumatic condition as well as a persistence of at least some pigment, so that the patches are not ivory white as they are in vitiligo. Phenolic compounds, ingredients of some industrial janitorial products, may destroy melanocytes and lead to permanent depigmentation. The depigmentation may be indistinguishable from vitiligo, except by distribution, as the patches induced by phenol are restricted to the region of contact, notably the hands and arms.

Tinea versicolor also may be confused with vitiligo (see above). Vitiligo is more frequent in patients with thyroid disease, Addison's disease, pernicious anemia, and alopecia areata.

Therapy

There is no early medical therapy for vitiligo that will affect its course. Therefore, if new vitiliginous patches are appearing or extending, it is best to wait for the depigmentation to stabilize before beginning

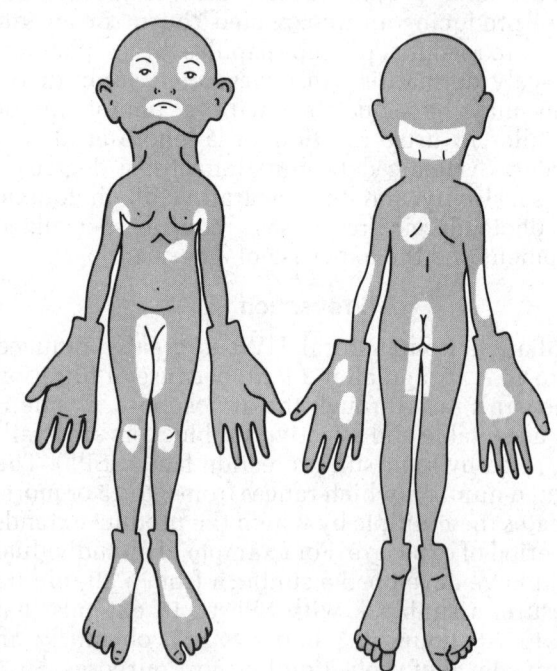

Figure 100.12. Depigmented macules of vitiligo occur most commonly at orifices, on extensor surfaces, and at areas of repeated trauma.

treatment. Several products are available that hide the lesions, with various degrees of success. They are either stains, including Dy-O-Derm and Vitadye, or cosmetics, such as Covermark, Dermablend, and Erase; all of these preparations are available without prescription at local department store or drug store cosmetic counters. The proper shading and use of Covermark needs to be taught; the Lydia O'Leary Co. (New York, NY 10022) will provide the names of local cosmetologists trained in the use of their products. One advantage of cosmetics over stains is that they provide a barrier to sunlight; the patches of vitiligo are easily sunburned since there are no melanocytes to produce tanning.

Patients with vitiligo should be advised always to use a sunblocker with an SPF of 15 or more before any sun exposure (see "Sunburn," above). Not only will sunburning of the patches of vitiligo be minimized but normal skin will tan less, thus minimizing the contrast between the light and dark areas.

When to Refer

Options used by a dermatologist include repigmentation with psoralen and long wave ultraviolet light (PUVA) or bleaching residual dark skin with hydroquinone. Both procedures generally are beyond the scope (and equipment) of the generalist; further, both are time consuming and potentially dangerous; PUVA can lead to severe ultraviolet light burns and perhaps, late skin cancer; and hydroquinone is irritating and a contact sensitizer. Only about half the patients will respond to PUVA and up to a year may be required for repigmentation to be "adequate." Bleaching residual dark skin to white will not be acceptable to all patients.

WARTS
Presentation

There are several types of warts, generally classified on the basis of their location or their appearance. These clinical types were once thought to be caused by the same virus, but each is known now to be due to a DNA papovavirus of a different antigenic subtype (15). Warts are all mildly contagious, venereal warts more than the others, and have an incubation period, after inoculation, of 1 to several months. They are frequent in immunosuppressed individuals in whom they may be nearly impossible to eradicate. However, in normal individuals, spontaneous involution is common; half will clear in 1 year.

The major types of warts are vulgaris, plantar, flat, and venereal.

Verruca Vulgaris (Common Wart)
Presentation

Common warts start as minute papules and grow over many weeks or months to raised, rough, cauli-flower-like papules. They are most common on the extremities but may be found on any part of the body in persons of all ages. The physician should consider that the patient may have become infected by a friend or family member. Should they be the source they will need to be treated also.

Differential Diagnosis

It is important to consider molluscum contagiosum (scattered small pearly umbilicated papules in the skin and caused by a virus, also discussed in Chapter 94) in children and young adults, and seborrheic keratoses or cutaneous horns in the elderly.

Therapy

Numerous methods to treat warts are used, some easier than others (Table 100.4). A most convenient, painless, and usually effective office treatment is salicylic acid and lactic acid in flexible collodion (Duofilm, requires a prescription), which works by softening the keratin in which the wart is growing, thereby allowing the wart to be pared away. It is particularly useful for warts around the nail as the medication seeps under the nail. The patient should follow the directions in the package insert, which suggests soaking the wart, at bedtime, in warm water for 5 minutes and then applying a small drop of medication to the wart with the applicator or a toothpick; the surrounding skin should be avoided to reduce irritation. The solution dries quickly. The patient should reapply 3 more drops, allowing each to dry before applying the next one. Excess dead tissue should be pared using a pumice stone or razor blade (if the patient is able) the next morning. The therapy should be stopped for a day or two if the area becomes sore. The patient should continue treatment for 5 days, after which the wart usually is tender; at that time the patient should stop treatment to allow the inflammation to subside, and should repeat the course every 2 weeks until clear. If the wart has not been eradicated after three courses, the patient should change the manner of Duofilm use. The patient should apply a single drop of Duofilm to each wart at bedtime, allow the medication to dry, then cover it overnight with an occlusive tape (such as Blenderm). The patient should pare (see above) the wart prior to the next nightly application of medication unless the area becomes tender.

Table 100.4.
Treatment of Warts in Order of Ease of Use

1. Salicylic acid/lactic acid in collodion (Duofilm) (podophyllin for venereal warts)
2. Liquid nitrogen
3. Electrodesiccation and curettage
4. Surgical excision

A common alternative initial therapy is liquid nitrogen. If liquid nitrogen is available, each wart should be frozen for 20 seconds by using a thick cotton swab pulled to a narrow point. The aim is to get full freezing of the wart as well as 2 to 3 mm beyond. It is important to avoid the lateral sides of the fingers as the digital nerves are subject to damage. The digital nerve is located at the tip of the crease made when the finger is flexed. Liquid nitrogen freezing is painful; the area will hurt for several hours. A blister usually develops 2 to 3 days later. If the blister becomes inconveniently large, the patient can be allowed to puncture it with a sterile needle to drain the contents, but it need not be deroofed. An 80% cure rate is usual. The patient should return in 1 month for retreatment if not clear. A large number of patients with warts must be treated to justify the expense of the material. Storage vessels are available (costing approximately $500) and only monthly replenishment (from a gas-medical supplier, listed as such in the telephone directory, costs about $80) is needed.

If initial therapy did not work and if facilities are available, the next best alternative is electrodesiccation and curretage; referral to a dermatologist may be appropriate at this point. The physician should consider underlying immunosuppression, such as Hodgkin's disease, diabetes mellitus, or drug abuse, if the warts are extensive and resistant.

Plantar Warts (See Also Chapter 102)

Presentation

Plantar warts can be troublesome in that they tend to be persistent and painful. They are not raised from the surface like other warts but extend into the horny layer. They may be distinguished from corns and calluses by paring them down with a scalpel blade. Warts show a speckled surface due to blood in dilated capillaries, while a shiny smooth surface is typical of corns. Corns and calluses are likely to be bilateral and over pressure points, especially the metatarsal heads, while warts may develop at any site.

Therapy

The goal of treatment is to destroy the wart without producing a scar, as such scars may be permanently painful. The best way to avoid scars is to avoid the use of surgical or electrodesiccation techniques in therapy. Surgical procedures may be justified if the wart proves untreatable by chemical means, but surgery is not appropriate initially. X-ray therapy is infrequently used as it also produces late scarring.

For initial therapy, the patient may use salicylic acid and lactic acid in flexible collodion (Duofilm) in the same way as suggested for verruca vulgaris. A single drop covered by an occlusive tape, as de-scribed, seems to work better than does the open technique. Salicylic acid plaster (such as Duke—available in rolls from a physician supply store or pharmacy or Scholls—available in individual plasters; both available without prescription) also may be used at bedtime under occlusive tape, followed by paring each morning (see above).

Freezing with liquid nitrogen does not work as well on the sole as elsewhere because of the thickness of the plantar surface.

Treatment of plantar warts can be frustrating; the physician may wish to refer a patient to a dermatologist or podiatrist if the warts are extensive or prove resistant.

Flat Warts

Presentation

Flat warts remain smaller than verruca vulgaris, usually only 2 to 3 mm in size, and are barely raised above the surface. Although always superficial, flat warts are troublesome because they usually are numerous and affect exposed parts, such as the face, neck, or legs. Flat warts often are spread by nicking the skin during shaving, with implanting of the virus.

Therapy

For a small number of flat warts, liquid nitrogen, salicylic acid/lactic acid in flexible collodion (Duofilm—see above), or gentle electrodesiccation may be satisfactory. Aggressive procedures should be avoided in order to prevent scarring. If numerous, the physician should prescribe 0.025% vitamin A acid gel (Retin-A gel, requires a prescription) once or twice daily. An electric razor or depilatory may be used to decrease spreading of the warts through nicks and autoinoculation. Spread to other family members is unlikely.

Flat warts take a long time to cure, perhaps months. Patients with flat warts usually are referred to a dermatologist.

Venereal Warts

Presentation

Also called moist warts, acuminate warts, or condyloma acuminatum, these primarily affect the anogenital area and usually are acquired through sexual contact. They seem to be more contagious than other types of warts. Patients may not be aware of intraurethral, anal, or intravaginal warts and must be properly examined. The physician should suspect homosexuality in a male with anal or perianal warts. All patients with venereal warts should be examined for other venereal diseases which may have been contracted. Venereal warts are also discussed in Chapter 94.

Differential Diagnosis

Condylomata of secondary syphilis (an STS always is positive in secondary syphilis) and malignancies, such as Bowen's disease or extramammary Paget's disease, must be considered (see Chapter 95).

Therapy

The mainstay of treatment is 20 to 25% podophyllin, an extract of the mandrake plant, in tincture of benzoin. Podophyllin is a poison and should never be dispensed to the patient. It works only for the moist verrucous warts, less well on dry warts located on the shaft of the penis or on the scrotum. Podophyllin should be applied carefully with a wooden stick just to the wart; it is quite irritating to normal skin. The benzoin should dry for a few minutes before the patient is allowed to dress. The medication should be thoroughly washed off in 4 hours. If this initial treatment has not been too irritating, the medication may be left on longer after the next application. It is important not to apply podophyllin to large areas at one time if the warts are extensive because it is quite irritating. The patient should return weekly for retreatment.

After several treatments, a nubbin of the wart may remain. As the wart is now dry, it may not resolve further with podophyllin; liquid nitrogen or electrodesiccation may be needed for final cure. Usually at least four treatments are necessary. Podophyllin should not be used in pregnant women as it is potentially cytotoxic to the fetus.

If the warts are vaginal or urethral, referral to a gynecologist or urologist is appropriate. If cutaneous warts recur or prove recalcitrant to therapy, a biopsy or referral to a dermatologist for diagnosis and further therapy is warranted.

XEROXIS (DRY SKIN)

Presentation

"Dry," itchy, and scaly skin is common increasing in frequency and degree in the elderly. Although usually generalized, xerosis is most frequent and severe on the legs. The cause is not fully understood, but there are diminished epidermal lipids, allowing loss of normally retained moisture from the stratum corneum. For that reason, dry skin is exacerbated by excessive soapy bathing and relieved somewhat by lubricating creams. Xerosis is worse in the winter when the humidity of warm air in the house is lowest.

Differential Diagnosis

A generalized itchy dermatitis, especially in the elderly, may be associated with underlying renal or hepatic insufficiency, diabetes mellitus, thyroid and other endocrine diseases, or lymphoma. Xerosis, to varying degrees, is present in all patients with atopic dermatitis. If present since an early age, the physician should consider congenital ichthyosis.

Therapy

The patient should reduce the frequency of hot water bathing generally to no more than twice a week and reduce the use of soap; both remove lipids and increase water loss and itching. For additional details, see "Bathing Instructions for Dry or Irritated Skin," page 1423.

Topical corticosteroids are not helpful. Antihistamines merely sedate and should be avoided for simple xerosis. The house or at least the sitting and sleeping rooms should be humidified. Successful treatment requires persistent care.

The patient should be much improved after the first course of treatment; if not relieved, the physician should consider underlying disease and obtain appropriate laboratory studies (see above).

BENIGN AND MALIGNANT GROWTHS

New growth on the skin are common, particularly in later life. It is important to be on the lookout for lesions during the physical examination and to distinguish benign from premalignant and/or malignant new growths. Two references (2, 10) provide resource information on skin tumors.

Cysts

Epidermal inclusion cysts are the most common newly appearing nodules in the skin. Their size ranges from 3 to 30 mm. Their surface is normal in color, but they may have a central, horny punctum. Most cysts start as dermal inclusions of epidermis and expand as horny material and sebum are produced within the cyst. About 10% of cysts, most on the scalp, are *pilar cysts*, composed of the expanded outer root sheath of a hair follicle.

Cysts are asymptomatic, except that they are annoying and unsightly, unless ruptured. If the wall of a cyst ruptures, their contents of keratin, hair, and sebum leak into the skin, and a brisk foreign body inflammatory reaction ensues. The reaction eventually subsides or drains, causing the cyst to shrink or disappear. If the cyst persists or reappears, it will be more bound in place. Cysts are not premalignant.

If the cyst is unsightly or irritating it may be excised or, if large, may be drained through a small incision and the sac pulled out through the opening with a hemostat. An inflamed cyst resolves more quickly after being injected with 0.2 to 0.5 ml of undiluted triamcinolone acetonide (Kenalog, 10 mg/ml).

A *milium* is a superficial 1- to 2-mm epidermal inclusion cyst that looks like a grain of rice embedded in the skin. Milia develop in adulthood, most commonly on the face and more frequently in women than men. They persist but remain small.

Milia can be removed by nicking the surface with a surgical blade and expressing the contents.

Fibroma

Any fleshy, skin-colored growth with a normal appearing, noneroded surface extending out from the skin is almost certainly benign and is most likely a fibroma or an intradermal nevus. *Skin tags* are small fibromas that appear at sites of friction, especially the neck, axilla, and groin. Skin tags can be easily snipped off with a scissors, often without anesthesia.

Keloid or Hypertrophic Scar

A keloid is a hyperplastic mass of fibrous connective tissue occurring in the dermis and originating from a scar. A keloid extends beyond the edge of the scar and involves normal skin, while a hypertrophic scar is restricted to the scar line. Keloids alone tend to recur if excised, but both conditions may be unsightly, and tenderness in the firmer lesions can interfere with wearing of clothing. Keloids are most common in blacks.

Both keloids and hypertrophic scars can be made softer and less tender by injecting them with undiluted triamcinolone acetonide (Kenalog, 10 mg/ml). The physician should use a 1-ml tuberculin syringe with no finer than a 25 gauge needle, as high pressure often is needed to inject the suspension into the growth. The injections are repeated at monthly intervals for 2 to 3 months, using enough material to make the keloid bulge out. If the keloid is treated by excision, postoperative intralesional injections of triamcinolone acetonide diminish the likelihood of recurrences. An injection at the time of surgery and at 2- to 3-week intervals for two to three injections after surgery should be used. Since the corticosteroid delays wound healing, the wound must be protected from dehiscence by adhesive taping. The patient should be advised not to repierce an ear which has had a keloid. Pressure garments (require referral to a physical therapist) have been used for large keloids or hypertropic scars and can produce excellent results, but 4 to 6 months of use may be required. They also may be used to decrease recurrence after keloids or hypertrophic scars are surgically removed.

Lipoma

Lipomas are soft lumps ranging in size from a bean to a fist or larger, located deep within the subcutaneous fat. The overlying skin may be elevated, but there are not surface changes. Usually only one or two are present, but some patients have multiple lipomas. Single lipomas are more common in women than men and are sporadic, while the multiple type usually occurs only in men and is hereditary. Lipomas develop during adulthood and persist indefi-

nitely. Lumps in the skin that become inflamed are more likely to be epidermal inclusion cysts. Malignant degeneration is rare; liposarcomas generally arise *de novo*, not in pre-existing lipomas.

Seborrheic Keratoses

These are common and practically universal, characterized by an irregular, rather than smooth, surface which feels waxy on being rubbed. These keratoses are superficial and they feel "stuck on" the skin rather than implanted or growing into the skin. They vary in color from beige or dark brown to black, occasionally resembling a malignant melanoma. Seborrheic keratoses never become malignant. Examples of seborrheic keratoses are shown in Figure 100.13 (page 1421).

The usual reason for their removal is bothersome irritation from clothing, belts, or straps or because their appearance is unacceptable to the patient. The simplest usually effective therapy for seborrheic keratoses is to paint them with trichloroacetic acid (obtainable from a pharmacy for office use but too caustic to be dispensed to the patient). The compound should be kept in the refrigerator. The keratoses should be lightly painted, taking care to avoid normal skin using a 50% solution on the face and 75% elsewhere. After about a minute the lesion will turn white and the patient will notice mild burning, which will subside shortly. A wet gauze sponge may be used to cool the skin and to remove excess acid. During the next week, the lesion will form a crust and fall away; however, thick lesions may require two or three monthly applications. One drop of trichloroacetic acid in the wrong place can cause great damage; therefore, the physician should take care not to hold the bottle or the applicator near the patient's eyes. If the lesions are thick or irritated, they may be lightly curetted after local anesthesia. Hemostasis may be obtained by fulguration or by application of Monsel's solution with a cotton-tipped applicator.

Cherry Angiomas

These common lesions are 1- to 3-mm bright red, cherry-colored, nonblanching, shiny papules usually located on the trunk (Fig. 100.14, page 1421). These are not premalignant. Because of their small size and lack of bleeding tendencies, therapy is not warranted.

Nevi

Although nevi usually are benign, each must be examined with care. If the patient believes the lesion recently has changed, or if the lesion has been bleeding, has irregular or dark pigment, or is large, removal is justified. However, less than half of all malignant melanomas come from pre-existing nevi and the average adult has 20 pigmented nevi; pro-

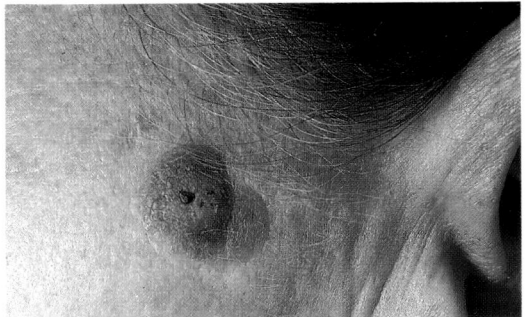
Figure 100.13a

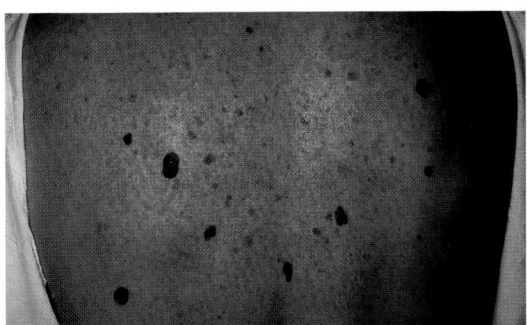
Figure 100.13b

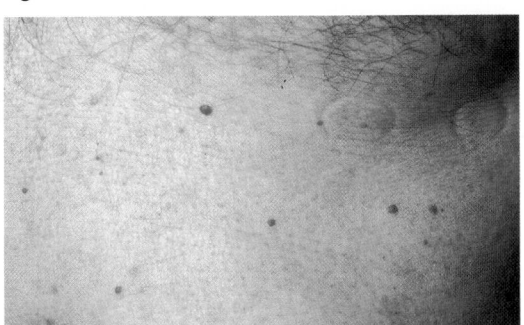
Figure 100.14

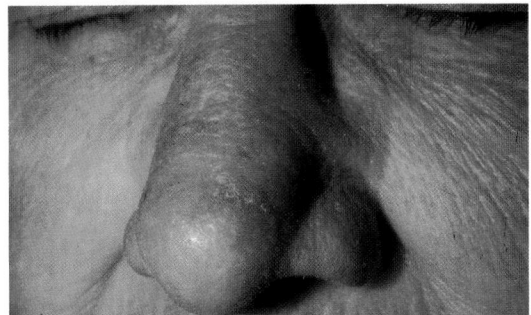
Figure 100.15

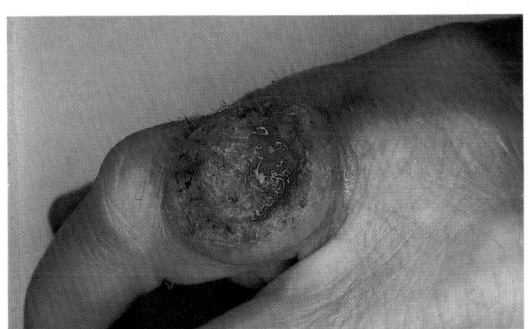
Figure 100.16

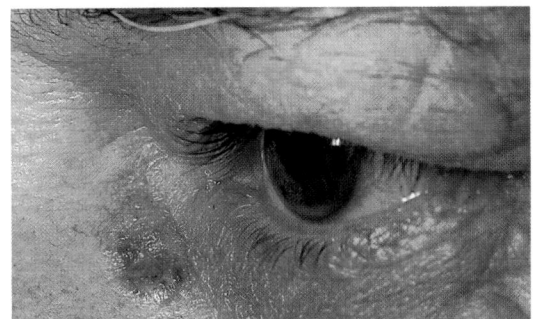
Figure 100.17

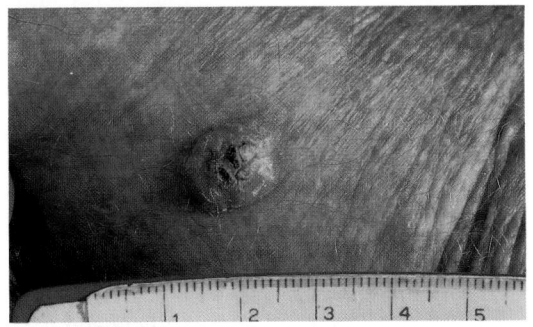
Figure 100.18

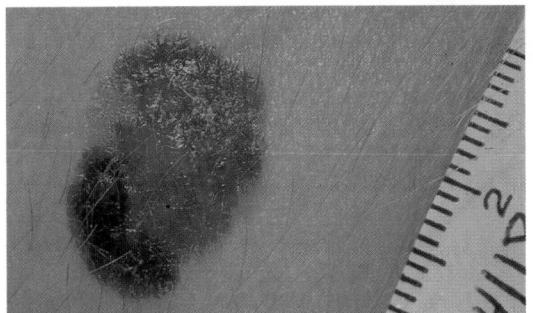
Figure 100.19

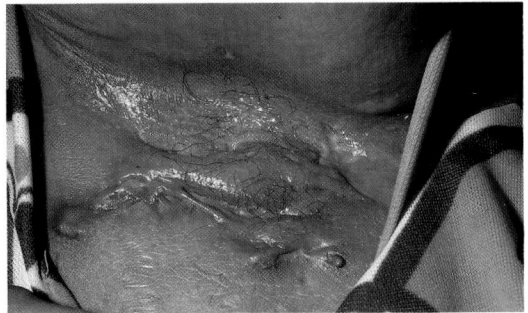
Figure 100.20

Figure 100.13. *a.* Seborrheic keratoses, face. *b.* Seborrheic keratoses, back.
Figure 100.14. Cherry angioma.
Figure 100.15. Actinic keratosis, face.
Figure 100.16. Keratoacanthoma.
Figure 100.17. Basal cell epithelioma.
Figure 100.18. Squamous cell epithelioma.
Figure 100.19. Malignant melanoma.
Figure 100.20. Hidradenitis suppurativa.

phylactic removal of all moles is practically impossible and certainly unjustified. If the primary reason for removal is cosmetic, without evidence of recent changes or suspicious signs, and if the mole is in a site visible to the patient, such as the face, the mole can be shaved with a scalpel blade to reduce it to the level of the skin surface. Hemostasis is achieved as with seborrheic keratosis removal (see above). The portion removed should be sent for pathological examination. The cosmetic result of this "shave removal" is better than with excision, and removal does not increase the likelihood that the nevus will evolve into a melanoma. On the other hand, if there have been recent changes or suspicious signs, the lesion should be excised in its entirety and with adequate margins. Malignant melanoma is discussed below.

Actinic Keratoses

These appear as red, scaly, nonhealing crusty lesions, predominantly restricted to light-exposed areas such as the face, nape and back of the hands (Fig. 100.15, page 1421). These keratoses are most common in light-complexioned individuals who have spent a lot of time in the sun. These lesions, are potentially malignant and should be destroyed using any one of several methods, usually desiccation and curettage, with local anesthesia or freezing with liquid nitrogen. 5-Fluorouracil (Fluoroplex, Efudex, requires prescription) is useful for patients with more than a dozen or so keratoses and has the advantage that early lesions will be destroyed as well. The medication is applied twice daily until irritation develops, normally in 2 weeks, and then continued for an additional 2 weeks. The patient should expect discomfort, redness, and peeling. A topical corticosteroid cream (such as triamcinolone 0.1%) can be applied four times a day for a week once the reaction has reached its peak. The keratoses will be cleared, but new ones will appear again in about 2 years as the tendency for their development remains. Any lesion still present after the course of topical therapy should be examined by biopsy or removed.

Individuals with actinic keratoses should be examined for recurrence twice yearly. Such patients are most often treated and followed by dermatologists.

Cutaneous Horn

A cutaneous horn is a single, hard, keratotic growth, resembling a wart. Its elevated hard center gives the lesion its name. While disordered keratin suggests disordered epidermis, most of these lesions are benign. However, they should be surgically removed for microscopic examination, since a few have a focus of squamous cell carcinoma at their base. Patients suspected of having this problem should be referred to a dermatologist or surgeon for removal.

Keratoacanthoma

A keratoacanthoma is a tumor that grows rapidly, usually within weeks, often becoming as large as a marble with a characteristic umbilicated hard keratotic center (Fig. 100.16, page 1421). Most patients are over the age of 50. Because most of the tumors occur in men and appear on the arms and hands, an occupational etiology has been suggested. These tumors also are more frequent in immunosuppressed patients.

Although technically benign, keratoacanthomas resemble squamous cell carcinoma and act aggressively. While it is safest to treat a keratoacanthoma by excision, wide excision is unnecessary. Left untreated, some have healed spontaneously in 4 to 12 months, generally leaving an unsightly scar. Although local surgery is curative, new tumors may appear elsewhere. Patients with a keratoacanthoma usually are referred to a dermatologist or surgeon.

Basal Cell Carcinoma

Basal cell carcinoma is a slowly spreading malignant growth that usually is single, shiny or pearly colored, with fine telangiectasias over the surface and a depressed center (Fig. 100.17, page 1421). Most appear on light-exposed parts of the skin, particularly the face, neck, or forearms. Basal cell carcinomas account for about 80% of skin cancers. If left untreated, they can invade deeply, but they rarely spread distantly; fewer than 100 cases of metastatic basal cell cancer have been reported.

Sunlight is the most obvious environmental inducer of basal cell cancers. These cancers are rare in blacks. After confirmation of the diagnosis by biopsy, the lesion can be destroyed by either desiccation and curettage or excision with about equal cure rates when performed by skilled practitioners. Because invasion tends to be deeper in the folds about the mouth, nose, and eyes, surgery in these areas needs to be more aggressive. Patients suspected of having a basal cell carcinoma should be referred to a dermatologist or surgeon.

Squamous Cell Carcinoma

A squamous cell carcinoma usually is firm and irregular with a scaly, keratotic, bleeding, and friable surface (Fig. 100.18, page 1421). Like basal cell cancers, squamous cell cancers occur most often on sun-exposed parts, but they also appear on covered areas or adjacent to chronic trauma, such as leg ulcers, burn scars, or sites of radiation therapy. Squamous cell cancers arising in trauma sites have a higher potential to metastasize than do those that arise in an actinic keratosis. The lower lip is a frequent location because of both chronic sun exposure and chronic irritation from heat and tobacco tar in smokers. Squamous cell cancers account for about 20% of skin cancers.

Patients suspected of having squamous cell carcinoma should be referred to a dermatologist or surgeon. Primary treatment is surgical. Electrosurgery, radiation, and cryosurgery are less definitive alternative techniques.

Melanoma

A *malignant melanoma* (Fig. 100.19, page 1421) (see above, "Nevi") usually is black or brown, but occasionally is of normal skin color. It tends to be irregular in outline, with outward spreading of pigment, may be itchy and, later, may bleed or ulcerate. Most cases occur in light-complexioned persons; they are rare in blacks. The incidence of melanoma has increased several-fold worldwide during the past few decades, perhaps due to increases in recreational sun exposure, decreasing ozone levels, or environmental toxins.

Although malignant melanomas have a high potential to recur, metastasize, and kill, the majority of patients with a melanoma can be cured; the present 5-year survival rate is 60 to 80%.

TOPICAL AND INTRALESIONAL THERAPY

Lubricants and Moisturizers

Lubricants and moisturizers slow evaporation of water from the horny layer of the corium, and their use improves suppleness and decreases dryness of the skin. Excessive dryness may be further improved by reducing the use of frequent long and hot soapy baths. Once or twice a week bathing is sufficient for the older person. Frequently used lubricating preparations are Aquaphor, Eucerin, Keri, Lubriderm, Nivea, and Shepard's.

Bathing Instructions for Dry or Irritated Skin

The patient must avoid soap on the inflamed areas of skin. If a shower/tub combination is available, the patient should first soap and shower areas needing most hygiene, such as axilla, groin, and buttocks, using a mild soap such as Ivory, Dove, Purpose, or Basis. The soapy water should be drained out and a few inches of lukewarm water drawn into the tub. The patient should add 15 to 30 ml of bath oil (such as Domol or Alpha-Keri) and use this water for sponge bathing. Unlike soap, the oil will cleanse but will not "dry out" the skin. The tub will be slippery and the patient should be careful. After the sponge bath and while the skin is still damp, a lubricating cream such as Eucerin, Aquaphor, or Shepard's should be applied and repeated as desired. Emollients with perfume should be avoided as they are potentially sensitizing.

Compresses (Wet Dressings)

Compresses applied to the eruption relieve swelling, oozing, and itching, are cooling, and provide gentle debridement. Compresses differ from soaks because compressing involves the repeated application of a moist dressing and transfer or debridement of the surface debris, while soaking is merely immersion and leads to maceration without crust removal, not useful in the treatment of dermatological problems.

Cool compresses should be used for acute inflammation with edema and itching, such as acute poison ivy dermatitis; warm compresses should be used to remove debris from chronic conditions, such as chronic leg ulcers.

The most convenient and least expensive solution for compressing is isotonic saline, prepared by dissolving 1 teaspoonful of table salt in 2 cups of tap water. Aluminum acetate (Burow's) solution is more drying. It is made by dissolving 1 packet or tablet (Bluboro or Domeboro, available without prescription) in 2 cups of lukewarm tap water (1:40 dilution). Ulcers contaminated with Gram-negative organisms, determined by culture of the surface, can be cleansed with 0.25% acetic acid made by adding 2 ounces of household white vinegar to 1 quart of lukewarm tap water.

To compress, the patient or the patient's helper should wet a soft cloth, squeeze out the excess solution, so that the cloth is not dripping wet, and apply the moistened cloth to the affected area. After 2 to 3 minutes, the cloth is removed, redipped, squeezed out again, and the process is repeated. Twenty minutes of compressing usually are sufficient, but the frequency should be adjusted to the degree of inflammation and crusting. If help is limited, "wet-to-dry" dressings may be used. Here the affected area is wrapped with a moist dressing which is covered with a dry dressing and left in place for an hour or two and replaced. Debridement is less efficient with this method.

Shake Lotions

Shake lotions are suspensions of powder that require shaking before use. They are soothing and cooling and are useful for pruritic lesions, such as poison ivy dermatitis, sunburn, acute drug eruptions, viral exanthems, and urticaria. The most commonly used shake lotion is calamine lotion, a suspension of zinc oxide and iron oxide with glycerin and calcium hydroxide. Phenolated or mentholated calamine improves the antipruritic properties of the lotion and is available in most pharmacies. Diphenhydramine in calamine lotion, such as Caladryl, should not be used because of the risk of sensitization to the antihistamine.

Pastes

Zinc oxide, as either paste or ointment (available without prescription), is used to provide protection and adsorption of serous drainage in acute and subacute oozing dermatitis, such as diaper dermatitis, intertrigo, pruritus ani (see Chapter 92), and acute dyshidrotic eczema. The paste is applied thickly, like icing on a cake, twice daily, and is easily removed with cotton balls moistened with mineral oil.

Corticosteroids

Topical corticosteroids are the most common topical anti-inflammatory agents prescribed. At least 20 brands are marketed, and most are available in various vehicles and in different strengths. A weak formulation with up to 0.5% hydrocortisone is available under several brand names without a prescription. The range of potency of preparations available by prescription is given in Table 100.5. Although a more potent preparation is occasionally needed for a recalcitrant eruption, the main difference between products is a difference in the speed of onset of improvement, differing by a day or two, rather than a difference in final outcome. The most common reason that a prescribed corticosteroid proved to be ineffective is that it was given for the wrong diagnosis or in too small an amount.

All topical corticosteroids are expensive, generally $5 to $10 an ounce. It is common for insufficient amounts to be prescribed because of this expense and because physicians generally underestimate the amount needed. About an ounce of any topical preparation is needed to cover the entire body once. As an example of the amount needed, consider treatment of both thighs and legs three times a day for 3

Table 100.5.
Some Topical Corticosteroids Grouped by Potency (within Potency Groups, Arranged Alphabetically)

VERY HIGH POTENCY
  Diprolene ointment
HIGH POTENCY
  Cyclocort ointment
  Diprosone cream and ointment
  Halog cream
  Lidex cream, ointment, and solution
  Topicort cream
  Topsyn gel
  Valisone ointment
INTERMEDIATE POTENCY
  Cordran cream, lotion, and ointment
  Cyclocort cream
  Synalar cream, ointment, and solution
  Triamcinolone cream, gel, lotion, and ointment
  Valisone cream and lotion
  Westcort cream and ointment
LOW POTENCY
  Desonide cream (nonfluorinated)
  Locorten cream (nonfluorinated)
  Hydrocortisone, dexamethasone, flumethasone, prednisolone, and methylprednisolone

weeks: Although only about a third of the total surface area is to be treated, about 1.5 pounds will be required (30 g × 0.33 × 3 times a day × 21 days = 630 g) which may cost $50 to $100. There are several ways to reduce the amount and costs of topical corticosteroid therapy. Creams can be spread further if applied when the skin is slightly damp, and the use of the corticosteroid should be limited to inflamed parts with only a moisturizer used elsewhere. (Patients may use the steroid preparation for lubrication unless instructed otherwise.) Also the corticosteroid may be used at bedtime with plastic wrap occlusion. The least expensive full strength topical corticosteroid is triamcinolone, which is available as a generic and in sizes up to 240 g.

Choice of Vehicle

Creams contain oils emulsified into water and appear white, while ointments are oils or oils into which water is emulsified and look and feel greasy, like petrolatum. Creams should be used for acute and subacute dermatitis where there is oozing because creams are miscible with serous fluids; ointments should be used for chronic dermatitis with scale and itching because they are better absorbed through intact skin. Corticosteroid solutions (Lidex or Synalar), lotions (Cordran or Valisone), or gels (triamcinolone, Benisone, or Tospyn) are useful in hairy or intertriginous regions or in the ear canals.

Occlusion

Absorption and effectiveness are increased by covering a corticosteroid cream with plastic film, such as plastic gloves or kitchen wrap (e.g., Glad or Saran) held in place by cotton gloves or socks. The plastic holds the preparation in place, interferes with scratching away the steroid, and improves absorption by hydrating the horny layer. A cream should be used for occlusion treatment rather than an ointment, which is more likely to induce miliaria and folliculitis. A convenient occlusive treatment for small areas is an occlusive tape, Cordran tape, available in 60- and 200-cm lengths by prescription, in which a corticosteroid has been incorporated in the adhesive. The tape can be left on for up to 36 hours and removed for 12 hours to prevent maceration.

Warnings

Potent topical corticosteroids may mask underlying skin infections, contact allergies, and even suppress inflammatory reactions to cutaneous tumors and lymphoma. Discrete lesions should be examined by biopsy, and referral to a dermatologist should be considered for any eruption that is persistent.

Local complications may follow the use of any topical corticosteroid but are most common following the use of those in the high and intermediate potency groups. Complications include persistent erythema and telangiectasias, an acneform eruption, interference with healing, atrophic striae, and easy bruising. Glaucoma and cataracts may develop after months of use near the eyes. Systemic effects from absorbed corticosteroids in adults do not develop unless more than half the body is treated with high potency corticosteroids under plastic occlusion for several months. When systemic effects occur, they include hypertension, glucose intolerance, glaucoma, salt and water retention, and depressed pituitary-adrenal responsiveness. However, growth retardation and hypertension have been reported in small children after using potent topical corticosteroids without occlusion.

Intralesional Corticosteroids

Long acting corticosteroids injected intralesionally often shrink epidermal inclusion cysts, inflammatory acne cysts, and hypertrophic scars and keloids. This therapy also may benefit other disorders, including lichen simplex chronicus, alopecia areata, granuloma annulare, psoriasis, and discoid lupus erythematosus. The most common preparation used is a suspension of triamcinolone acetonide (Kenalog, 10 mg/ml). The full strength concentration should be used only for scar reduction because that dose will induce skin atropy. For general use, the preparation may be injected after diluting it to about 3 mg/ml, because this level usually does not cause atrophy. The dilution is made by first drawing up two volumes of saline and, after thorough shaking of the stock, one volume of corticosteroid suspension.

Warnings

Complications of intralesional corticosteroid injections include atrophy or dimpling, local increase or decrease in pigmentation, and, rarely, telangiectasias or local infection. Atrophic dimpling usually resolves in 6 to 12 months. Patients with disorders requiring intralesional steroid injections usually are referred to a dermatologist.

Topical Antimicrobials

Topical antibiotics have only limited use, because infections superficial enough to respond to topical antibiotics also respond to simple cleansing and compresses. However, they have proven useful in mild inflammatory acne vulgaris. All have the potential to induce sensitization, allergic contact dermatitis, suggested by the appearance of redness, scale, and itching. For example, contact dermatitis is a common development during therapy of chronic leg ulcers. The reaction may be against the active agent or against a preservative or fragrance.

Topical Antifungal Agents

Common superficial fungal infections are caused either by dermatophytes or by a yeast, almost always *Candida albicans*. Infections may involve any body surface, but are most frequent in warm moist areas, such as the feet and groin.

Broad spectrum topical antifungal preparations (all require a prescription except as noted) effective against both dermatophytes and yeast, include ciclopirox (Loprox cream, 15/30 g), clotrimazole (Lotrimin cream, 15/30/45/90 g and solution, 10/30 ml, and Mycelex cream, 15/30/45 g and solution, 10/30 g), econazole (Spectazole, 15/30/85 g), and miconazole (Monistat-Derm cream, 15/30/90 g and lotion, 30/60 ml, available without prescription). Haloprogin (Halotex cream, 15/30 g and solution, 10/30 ml) and tolnaftate (Tinactin cream, solution, and powder, available without prescription) are useful for dermatophytes but not *Candida*. Nystatin (cream, ointment, or powder) is effective against candidal infections only. Nystatin oral preparations are poorly absorbed from the gastrointestinal tract and, therefore, have no effect on skin or systemic infections. However, oral nystatin may be needed if a groin infection recurs, as the gastrointestinal tract may be a reservoir for *Candida*. Oral nystatin is given as 1 teaspoon of the suspension (100,000 units/teaspoon) four times for 3 days for a total of 60 ml. Topical amphotericin B (Fungizone cream, 20 g, lotion, 30 ml and ointment, 20 g) also is effective against candidiasis, but it is more expensive and may stain the skin.

Topical antifungal agents are used twice daily, on arising and before bedtime, except for yeast infections in the diaper area which should be retreated with each diaper change. In addition to the topical agent, local heat and moisture must be decreased. Measures that increase ventilation and maintain dryness include the use of cotton underclothing or socks, open and leather shoes rather than vinyl or rubber boots or sneakers, and the liberal use of talcum powder. Although topical antifungal agents are believed to be safe when used during pregnancy, there are no adequate studies, and, therefore, the drugs should be used in pregnant women only if necessary.

General References

Arndt KA: *Manual of Dermatologic Therapeutics*, ed 3. Boston, Little, Brown, and Co, 1983.
    Handbook of therapy including details of usage, trade names, and prices.
Epstein E: *Common Skin Disorders*, ed 2. Oradell, NJ, Medical Economics Co, 1983.
    Practical advice including tear-sheets for the patient.
Fitzpatrick TB, Eisen AZ, Wolff K, *et al.*: *Dermatology in General Medicine*, ed 2. New York, McGraw-Hill, 1979.
    Complete reference for the specialist. It includes an exclusive discussion of pathophysiology of skin disease.
Lamberg SI: *Dermatology in Primary Care*. Philadelphia, WB Saunders, 1986.
    A practical, problem-oriented guide to dermatology.

Specific References

1. Ad Hoc Committee Report: Systemic antibiotics for the treatment of acne vulgaris. *Arch Dermatol* 111:1603, 1975.
2. Andrade R, Crumport S, Popkin L (eds): *Cancer of the Skin*. Philadelphia, WB Saunders, 1976.
3. Bjornberg A, Hellgren I: Pityriasis rosea. *Acta Derm Venereol* 42:1, 1962.

4. Cram OL: Psoriasis: current advances in etiology and treatment. *J Acad Dermatol* 14:2, 1981.

5. Cullen SI: Topical methenamine therapy for hyperhidrosis. *Arch Dermatol* 111:1158, 1975.

6. Eaglstein W, Katz R, Brown JA: The effects of early corticosteroid therapy in skin eruptions and pain in herpes zoster. *JAMA* 211:1681, 1970.

7. Editorial: Seborrheic dermatitis. *Br Med J* 1:436, 1973.

8. Fisher AA: *Contact Dermatitis*, ed 2. Philadelphia, Lea & Febiger, 1973.

9. Hanifin JM: Atopic dermatitis. *J Am Acad Dermatol* 16:1, 1982.

10. Lever WF, Schaumburg-Lever G: *Histopathology of the Skin*, ed 6. Philadelphia, Lippincott, 1983.

11. Melski JW, Arndt KA: Topical therapy for acne. *N Engl J Med* 302:503, 1980.

12. Muller SA: Alopecia; syndromes of genetic significance. *J Invest Dermatol* 60:475, 1973.

13. Noble WC (ed): Microbial skin disease. *Br J Dermatol* (suppl 8), 1972.

14. Odland GF, Kraning KK: Prevalence, morbidity and cost of dermatological diseases. *J Invest Dermatol* 73:395, 1979.

15. Pass F: Warts, biology and current therapy. *Minn Med* 57:844, 1974.

16. Raab B, Lorincz AL: Genital herpes simplex concepts and treatment. *J Am Acad Dermatol* 5:248, 1981.

17. Rippon JW: *Medical Mycology*, ed 2. Philadelphia, WB Saunders, 1982.

18. Roberts SOB: Tinea versicolor; a clinical and mycological investigation. *Br J Dermatol* 81:315, 1969.

19. Shacter B: Treatment of scabies and pediculosis with lindane preparations. An evaluation. *J Am Acad Dermatol* 5:517, 1981.

20. Stoughton RB: Topical antibiotics in acne vulgaris. *Arch Dermatol* 115:486, 1979.

CHAPTER ONE HUNDRED ONE

Common Problems of the Teeth and Oral Cavity

DOUGLAS K. MacLEOD, D.M.D.

The purpose of this chapter is 2-fold: first, to recognize, to treat, and to refer patients with acute dental and oral problems properly; and second, to increase the physician's awareness of chronic dental and oral problems which may require referral and treatment. These types of problems are often neglected by the patient because of fear or ignorance about possible corrective treatment, because of anticipated pain from the procedure, or because of the anticipated cost of treatment.

THE ORAL EXAMINATION

The clinician should examine the oral cavity in a systematic manner. The examination should include lips, cheeks (buccal mucosa), hard and soft palate, salivary ducts (parotid duct orifice in the buccal mucosa opposite the upper second molars and submandibular duct orifice beside the lingual frenulum), tonsillar area, tongue, floor of the mouth, gingiva, and teeth, noting the normal structures and any deviations from normal.

A dental examination includes an evaluation of the number (20 in the primary dentition and 32 in the permanent dentition—see Fig. 101.1), position, and arrangement of the teeth, and a check for caries (see below), erosions, abrasions, and fractures. It is important to examine the gingiva completely. The normal healthy gingiva is firm, pink, free of pain, and does not bleed on palpation. The parts of a tooth and its adjacent structures are shown in Figure 101.2, A and B.

ACUTE DENTAL AND ORAL PROBLEMS

Toothaches (Pulpitis)

Presentation

Patients with toothache present with a large carious lesion (see "Dental Caries", page 1435), a large restoration (filling), or a combination of both. In the early stages, there is inflammation involving a portion of the pulp tissue (the central portion of the tooth containing vital soft tissue—see Fig. 101.2A). There is relatively severe pain in response to thermal stimuli, particularly to cold, and this pain persists for longer than 15 seconds after the stimulus is removed. As the area of inflammation increases, the pain becomes more severe; it may radiate to the suborbital area, to the side of the face, or to the ear. When total necrosis of the pulp occurs, sensitivity to thermal stimuli is lost. If at this point the inflammatory exudate cannot escape into the oral cavity, the pressure is released via the root apex; and there is exquisite sensitivity to percussion of the crown of the tooth. The signs and symptoms of pulpitis may be confused with pericoronitis (painful wisdom teeth, see below) or periodontitis (see below), and without further diagnostic aids (i.e., dental radiographs) it may be difficult to differentiate between these conditions.

If pulpitis is not treated, *complications* may occur, ranging from a localized alveolar abscess (an abscess of the bony supporting structure of the teeth) to facial cellulitis. The rate and type of complication depend upon the location of the affected tooth, host resistance, and the virulence of the bacteria present.

Treatment

Depending upon the situation when the patient is seen, the physician has three options. For patients who are afebrile and have no extraoral swelling (a

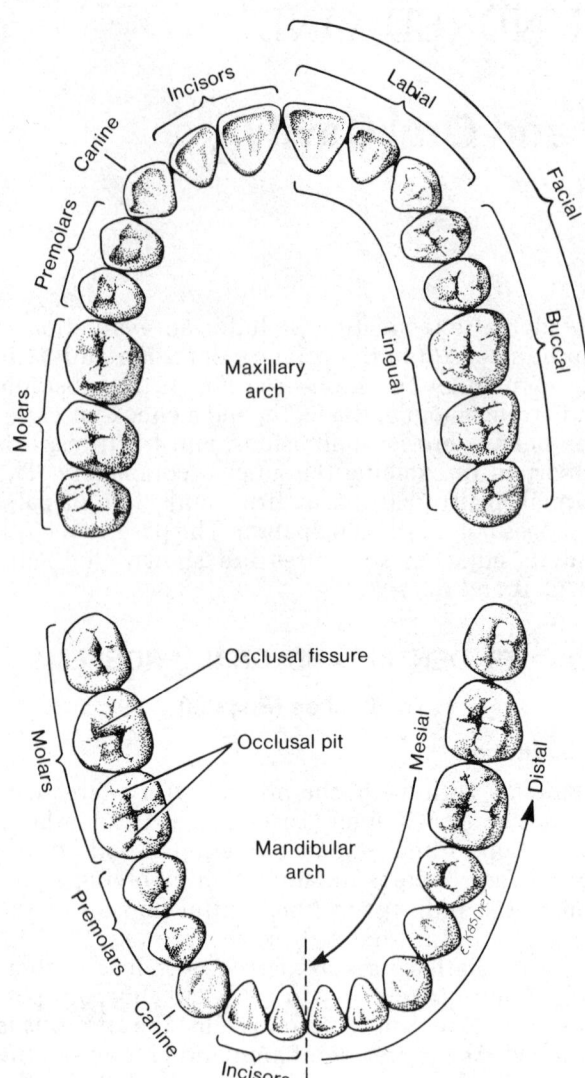

Figure 101.1.   Permanent dentition.

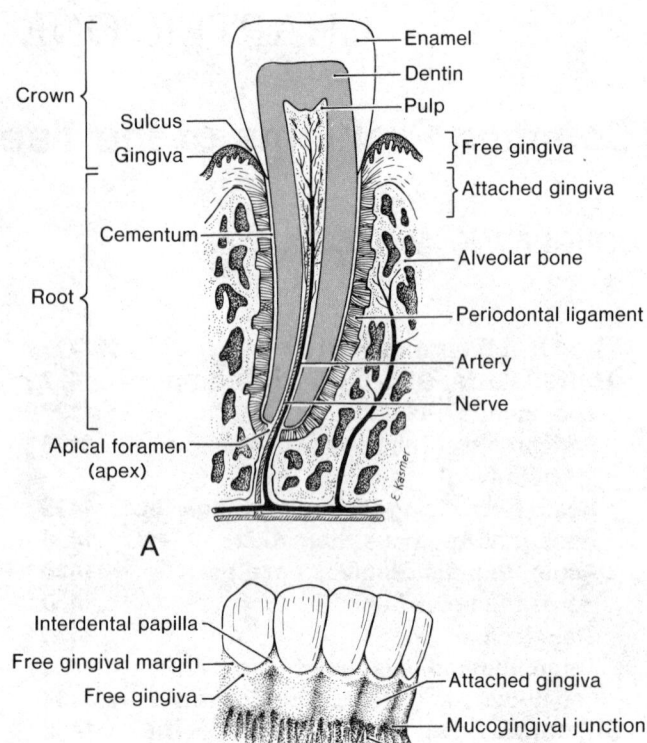

Figure 101.2.   Structure of normal teeth and gingiva. *A.* A tooth and its parts. *B.* Teeth and gingiva (shows lower incisors and canines).

swelling producing facial asymmetry) or intraoral swelling (swelling causing disruption of the supporting alveolar bone and soft tissue), analgesics (aspirin 600 mg and codeine 30 mg every 4 hours) and referral within 24 hours are indicated. When either slight extraoral or intraoral swelling or a low grade temperature elevation is present, antibiotics (penicillin V, 250 mg, or, for patients allergic to penicillin, erythromycin, 250 mg, every 6 hours) should be added, and the patient should be seen by a dentist within 12 to 24 hours. Patients with temperatures greater than 101°F (38.5°C) with intraoral and/or extraoral swelling causing facial asymmetry need immediate consultation and treatment by a dentist. Treatment of these types of problems varies from extraction of the affected tooth, root canal therapy (endodontics), or incision and drainage, to hospital admission for intravenous antibiotics for facial cellulitis.

Pericoronitis (Third Molar or Wisdom Tooth Pain)

Presentation

Pericoronitis is acute inflammation of the tissue around the crown of a partially erupted tooth. Patients presenting with pericoronitis are usually between the ages of 15 and 25 and may give a history of previous subacute episodes of pain of the gingiva, that partially covers the crown of an incompletely erupted tooth. The tooth most often affected is the mandibular third molar (wisdom tooth). The space between the crown of the tooth and the overlying gingival flap is an ideal area for the accumulation of food and bacteria; this leads to inflammation. The flap is traumatized by contact with the tooth in the opposing jaw, usually the maxillary third molar, and the inflammation is aggravated.

The patient describes pain that radiates to the ear, the throat, and the floor of the mouth. He complains of a foul taste, and there is swelling of the affected area so that he cannot close the jaw properly. In severe cases, pain spreading to the oropharynx and base of the tongue makes it difficult to swallow. The gingival tissue is markedly red, swollen and tender (Fig. 101.3*A*). Occasionally, tender lymphadenopathy and systemic manifestations (fever, leukocytosis, and malaise) are present. Peritonsillar abscess, cellulitis, and Ludwig's angina (cellulitis of the floor of the mouth) are possible complications.

Treatment

In afebrile patients the physician needs only to make a dental referral and to prescribe analgesics. Febrile patients should be treated with antibiotics (penicillin V, 250 mg, or, for patients allergic to penicillin, erythromycin, 250 mg, every 6 hours) and moderate analgesics (aspirin, 600 mg, and codeine, 30 mg, every 4 to 6 hours). All patients should be seen by a dentist within 24 hours. Depending upon many factors, the dentist will either excise or debride the flap or remove the partially erupted lower tooth. The preferred treatment for third molars which are erupting in a position that produces poor occlusion is to remove the traumatizing maxillary third molar tooth and to allow the infected flap to heal. The mandibular tooth is then removed 7 to 10 days later, after the acute infection has resolved. When pericoronitis involves eruption of third molars that are in good position for occlusion, the inflamed gingival flap is removed and the teeth are left in place.

Acute Necrotizing Ulcerative Gingivitis (ANUG, Vincent's Infection, Trench Mouth)

Acute necrotizing ulcerative gingivitis, or ANUG, may occur at any age, but is more common among young to middle-aged adults.

Presentation

ANUG has a sudden onset and is usually associated with a debilitating illness or an acute respiratory infection. Often there is a history of a change in the patient's life; for example, protracted work without rest or recent psychological stress. There is a fetid mouth odor and the patient describes a foul metallic taste, increased salivation, spontaneous gingival hemorrhage, and pronounced bleeding upon the slightest stimulation. The lesions are extremely sensitive to touch; pain is constant and gnawing and is intensified by hot or spicy foods. The oral findings are punched-out, crater-like depressions at the crest of the interdental papillae and/or marginal gingiva. The surface of the gingiva is covered by gray pseudomembranous slough which is demarcated from the gingiva by a pronounced linear erythema (Fig. 101.3B). Patients usually have submandibular lymphadenopathy and slight elevation in temperature; in severe cases, high fever, tachycardia, leukocytosis, loss of appetite, and malaise are seen.

Most investigators believe that ANUG is caused by two agents, which are normal oral flora; a fusiform bacillus and *Borrelia vincentii*, a spirochete. Histologically, the stratified squamous epithelium of the gingiva is ulcerated and replaced by a thick fibrinous exudate containing many polymorphonuclear leukocytes and microorganisms.

Complications include destruction of the gingiva and underlying supporting tissues. In rare cases, severe sequelae, such as noma (rapid spreading gan-

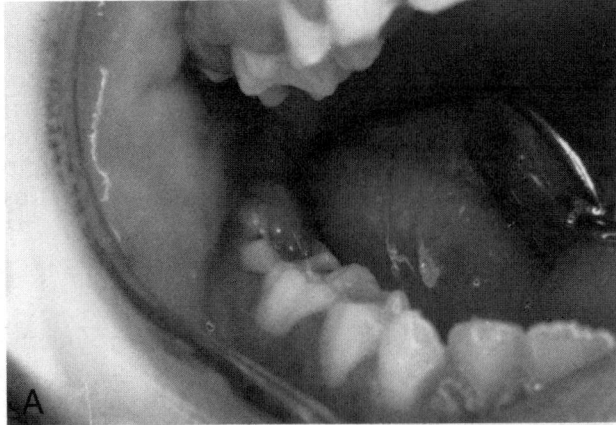
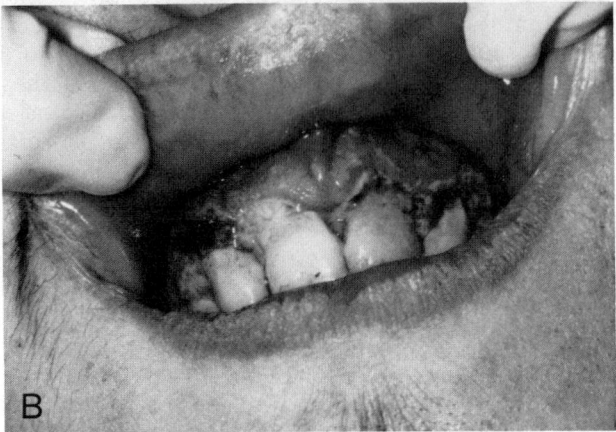

Figure 101.3. *A.* Pericoronitis of the mandibular third molar. *B.* Acute necrotizing ulcerative gingivitis.

grene of oral and facial tissue, which occurs in the debilitated and nutritionally deficient patient), fusospirochetal meningitis, peritonitis, pneumonia, bacteremia, and brain abscess, have been reported.

Treatment

Patients with severe ANUG need immediate hospital admission, intravenous antibiotics, and supportive care (analgesics, hydrogen peroxide mouthwashes) until systemic symptoms subside. Patients with less severe ANUG need immediate attention by a dentist. At this visit, after treatment with a topical anesthetic, a cotton pellet and glyoxide (an oxygenating and foaming agent) are used to remove the pseudomembrane and the surface debris. After irrigating with warm water, the superficial calculus is removed. Patients are instructed to avoid tobacco and alcohol, to rinse with warm water and 3% hydrogen peroxide every 2 hours, and to confine toothbrushing to the removal of surface debris. When these instructions are followed after effective removal of all irritants by the dentist, a patient usually improves markedly within 5 days. If after the acute phase the patient does not continue periodic dental care, ANUG may recur and lead to eventual tooth loss.

Recurrent Aphthous Stomatitis (RAS) (4)

Aphthous ulcers, also called *canker sores*, occur at some time in 20 to 50% of the adult population, are slightly more common in females, have familial tendencies, and occur most frequently during the winter and spring months. RAS was once thought to be a recurrent infection by the herpes simplex virus (HSV), but that is not the case; the cause of the condition is, in fact, still unknown.

Presentation

Aphthous stomatitis is characterized by superficial ulcerations on the mucous membranes of the lips, cheek, tongue, floor of the mouth, palate, and gingiva. This condition begins with a prodromal burning 1 to 48 hours before the appearance of discrete vesicles, which are approximately 2 to 5 mm in diameter and are painful. After 2 days, they rupture and form saucer-like ulcers which consist of a red or grayish-red central portion and an elevated rim-like periphery. There may be a single lesion or multiple ulcers; the etiology is unknown.

The lesions heal spontaneously within 7 to 10 days. As a rule the lesions are larger than those seen in acute herpetic gingivostomatitis (see below) and do not exhibit the diffuse gingival involvement or systemic symptoms seen in that condition.

RAS occurs in the following forms:

1. *Occasional aphthae* (a single lesion, at intervals from months to years, healing uneventfully).

2. *Acute multiple aphthae* (acute episode persisting for weeks, with lesions developing sequentially at different sites in the mouth, often associated with acute gastrointestinal disorders).

3. *Chronic recurrent aphthae* (one or more lesions always present for a period of years).

Treatment

Treatment of aphthae is symptomatic. A mouthwash containing equal parts of Benadryl suspension and Kaopectate (Benadryl 5 mg/ml mixed with an equal amount of Kaopectate, prepared by a pharmacist) is helpful in reducing the pain as is viscous Xylocaine applied by cotton-tip applicator to painful lesions. In more severe cases, tetracycline has been successful in decreasing pain and duration of the ulcers; the patient should be instructed to empty a 250-mg capsule in 50 ml of water and to use this as a rinse, which is then swallowed, three or four times a day for 5 to 7 days. The patient should be encouraged to take sufficient amounts of nonirritating liquids or soft food to maintain hydration and nutrition. Intake may be facilitated by using a straw to prevent contact with the painful ulcers.

Acute Herpetic Gingivostomatitis

Acute herpetic gingivostomatitis occurs most frequently in infants and children below the age of 6 years, and it is observed with equal frequency in males and females. It is caused by the herpes simplex virus (HSV), and most oral infections are due to HSV type 1. It occasionally occurs in adolescents and adults. Most adults have developed immunity to herpes simplex virus as a result of childhood infection, usually inapparent. Although recurrent acute herpetic gingivostomatitis has been reported, it does not usually recur unless immunity has been altered by a debilitating systemic disease.

Presentation

Acute herpetic gingivostomatitis appears as a diffuse, erythematous, shiny involvement of the gingiva and the adjacent oral mucosa with varying degrees of edema and gingival bleeding. In the initial stage it is characterized by the presence of discrete spherical gray vesicles which may occur in the gingiva, the labial and buccal mucosa, the soft palate, the pharynx, the sublingual mucosa, and the tonuge. Within 24 hours the vesicles rupture and form small painful ulcers with a red, elevated, halo-like margin and a depressed yellowish or grayish-white central portion. Regional lymphadenopathy, fever as high as 105°F (40.5°C), and generalized malaise are common. The course is limited to 7 to 10 days and the ulcers heal without scarring. It is differentiated from RAS by the diffuse gingival involvement and the systemic symptoms.

Treatment

There is no specific treatment for herpetic gingivostomatitis. The management is exactly the same as that for recurrent aphthous stomatitis (see above). Antibiotics are not helpful, and corticosteroids and contraindicated. Antiviral agents, such as idoxuridine (IUDR), have been used successfully in treating immunosuppressed patients with primary herpes infections, but because of toxicity their use should be limited to such patients, in consultation with a specialist in infectious disease. The role of oral acyclovir in herpetic gingivostomatitis in under investigation.

Herpes Simplex Labialis

Recurrent herpes simplex infections of the lips or perioral area occur in 20 to 40% of the adult population. Evidence suggests that recurrent herpes is not a reinfection but a reactivation of virus that remains latent in the nerve tissue.

Presentation

The natural history of this problem has been well delineated (8). Most affected subjects have several episodes during an average year. In approximately 60% of episodes, there is prodromal tingling for a number of hours before the appearance of the first vesicles. Pain is moderate to severe during the first 24 hours after appearance of vesicles and then rapidly diminishes. After 48 hours, vesicles are usually replaced by ulcer crusts. The process usually resolves after 7 to 9 days, but lesions may persist as long as 2 weeks.

The therapy of this condition is discussed in Chapter 100, Common Problems of the Skin.

Sialadenitis

Presentation

Sialadenitis is an inflammation of the salivary gland. Patients with sialadenitis present with pain and enlargement of the affected gland. In *bacterial* sialadenitis, the pain and swelling are not related to eating. The overlying skin may be red and tense; and the affected gland will yield a purulent discharge at the duct oriface. Bacterial sialadenitis is more common in children than in adults. *Obstructive* sialadenitis is more common than the bacterial condition and is associated with salivary stones or a mucous plug. It occurs most frequently in middle-aged males. The involved gland is enlarged and painful, and the symptoms are more prominent before, during, and soon after eating. The submandibular gland is most often affected (75% of cases), whereas the parotid (20% of cases) and major sublingual glands (5% of cases) are less often involved.

Treatment

Treatment of bacterial sialadenitis consists of heat application (external moist heat packs to affected gland for 15 to 20 minutes and intraoral warm rinses), analgesics (aspirin, 600 mg, and codeine, 30 mg, every 4 to 6 hours), antibiotics (penicillin V, 250 mg, or, for patients allergic to penicillin, erythromycin, 250 mg, every 6 hours for 10 days), and a liquid diet for the first 2 to 3 days.

The management of obstructive sialadenitis is more complex. When this diagnosis is suspected, the patient should be referred to a dentist or an otolaryngologist. In cases where the stone is lodged in the duct, the acute phase is managed in the same manner as is bacterial sialadenitis, after which a sialagram is obtained to determine the extent of the problem. Surgical removal of the stone from the duct is eventually performed to prevent recurrence. In chronic obstructive sialadenitis, surgical excision of the gland is often necessary. There is no knowledge regarding the likelihood of recurrence after the first episode.

Temporomandibular Joint Pain

Several studies of healthy populations have shown that symptoms of temporomandibular joint (TMJ) disorders are present at some time in 25 to 50% of people, but are not considered a serious problem by most patients (3). The vast majority (70 to 90%) of patients who present with these symptoms are women between the ages of 24 and 40. Multiple factors may lead to TMJ pain; there may be a history of emotional tension, bruxism (grinding of teeth), external blows to the jaws, or whiplash injury. TMJ pain may be present at some point in 20% of patients with rheumatoid arthritis (5). Patients with osteoarthritis of other joints may complain of TMJ clicking and snapping, but pain is usually absent.

Presentation

TMJ disorders are characterized by pain and tenderness in the muscles of mastication and in the TMJ, by crepitus when the joint is moved, and by a decrease in range of motion. In some severe cases there is a noticeable incoordination on the opening and closing of the jaw. This appears as a unilateral shift of the chin upon opening or closing the mouth. Examination may show malocclusion due to teeth that interfere with the normal movement of the mandible or to tenderness of the muscles of mastication.

Treatment

Patients with acute TMJ pain should be managed with moderate analgesics (aspirin, 600 mg, and codeine, 30 mg, every 4 to 6 hours) and referral to a dentist within 24 to 48 hours to begin therapy. The dentist's goal will be to make the patient aware of the etiology of his problem through education. Depending upon the severity of symptoms and the state of the patient's dentition, the dentist will prescribe one or a combination of the following: avoidance of excessive jaw motion; moist heat to affected muscles; soft diet; disengagement of upper and lower jaws with a night guard (a hard or soft appliance constructed by a dentist, used to separate the teeth); therapeutic exercises; and vapocoolant spray (ethylchloride to decrease muscle pain). In atypical cases, trigger point injections of Xylocaine may be utilized to distinguish TMJ symptoms from trigeminal neuralgia (see Chapter 79). Once the acute episode has subsided (in about 7 to 14 days) the dentist can detect and eliminate any occlusal interferences and rule out any degenerative joint disease that may have predisposed the patient to TMJ symptoms. In the past, injections of sclerosing agents into the TMJ and condylectomy were tried, but with very poor success.

In a 10-year study, 97 of 100 patients treated conservatively improved. Of these, 83 had permanent improvement. Of the 3 patients who had intractable, severe symptoms, 2 required prolonged psychotherapy and 1 developed systemic arteritis (1).

Local Alveolar Osteitis (dry socket)

Local alveolar osteitis (dry socket) is the most common complication of tooth extraction. It occurs in approximately 5% of all tooth extractions, but it is more common following the removal of an impacted third molar. This problem results from the loss of the blood clot located at the site of the extraction. Most often this occurs when the extraction has been difficult and has resulted in considerable trauma to the socket and gum.

Patients with this problem will describe intense localized pain 2 or 3 days following an extraction. This pain is caused by irritation of the sensory nerves in the dry exposed bony socket. Also there is often a foul odor emanating from the socket, but no suppuration is present.

The physician should control the pain the patient is experiencing with codeine, 30 mg every 3 to 4 hours, and aspirin, 600 mg three to four times/day. The patient should be referred promptly to a dentist for irrigation and for the placement of a dressing. The dentist will need to see the patient every day or two for approximately 10 days until the socket becomes re-epithelialized. There are no long term sequelae.

CHRONIC DENTAL AND ORAL PROBLEMS

Periodontal Disease (Pyorrhea) (Figs. 101.4 and 101.5)

Periodontal disease is a general term used to describe diseases which destroy the gingival and bony structures that support the teeth. Periodontal disease is usually subdivided into *gingivitis* and *periodontitis*. The major difference between the two is that in periodontitis there is loss of the supporting bony apparatus of the teeth.

Two-thirds of young adults, 80% of middle-aged adults, and 90% of people in the United States over 65 suffer from periodontal disease (10). Poor oral

hygiene, which permits plaque to accumulate on the teeth, is the major etiological factor. Most periodontal disease, and therefore most loss of teeth, is preventable. Prevention consists of routine plaque control (see below).

Gingivitis

Presentation

Gingivitis is usually seen in one of four forms: *acute*, a painful condition which has a rapid onset and is of short duration; *subacute*, which is less severe than the acute condition; *recurrent*, which reappears after being eliminated by treatment or after disappearing spontaneously; and *chronic*, the most common form, which has a slow onset, is of a long duration, and is usually painless unless complicated by acute exacerbations (see Fig. 101.5).

The early signs of inflammation of the gingiva, which precede frank gingivitis, are increased gingival fluid secretion and bleeding from the gingival sulcus upon gentle probing (7). Healthy gingiva is usually "coral pink," whereas in gingivitis the gingiva becomes "bright red" secondary to increased vascularity and a decrease in keratinization. These changes start in the interdental papillae and free gingiva and spread to the attached gingiva. Both acute and chronic forms produce changes in the normally firm, resilient consistency of the gingiva. In acute gingivitis the gingiva has a diffuse edematous appearance, whereas in the chronic form the tissue has a fibrous appearance that pits on pressure.

The development of gingivitis is a consequence of supragingival and subgingival *plaque formation* (see Fig. 101.4). Plaque is a transparent deposit that is composed primarily of bacteria and their by-products. Gram-positive filamentous rods,

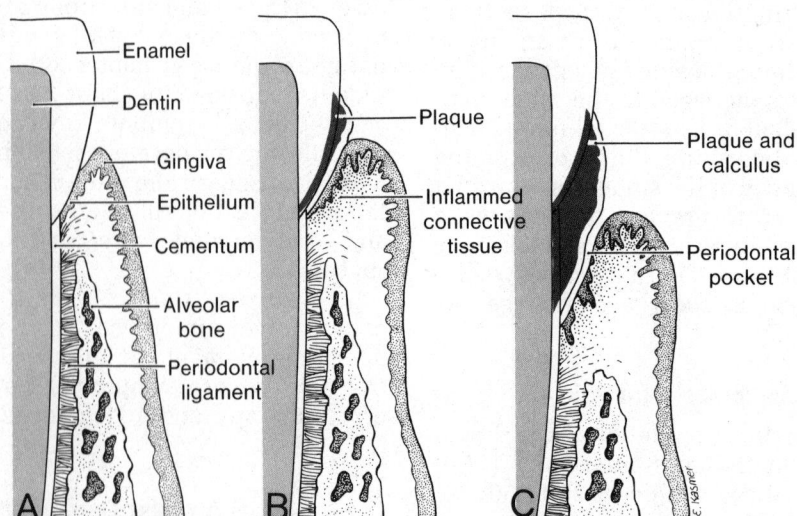

Figure 101.4. Dentogingival junction in health and plaque free (*A*), gingivitis resulting from plaque accumulation with inflammation of soft tissue (*B*), and peri- odontitis resulting from long-standing inflammation which has caused bone loss and tooth mobility (*C*).

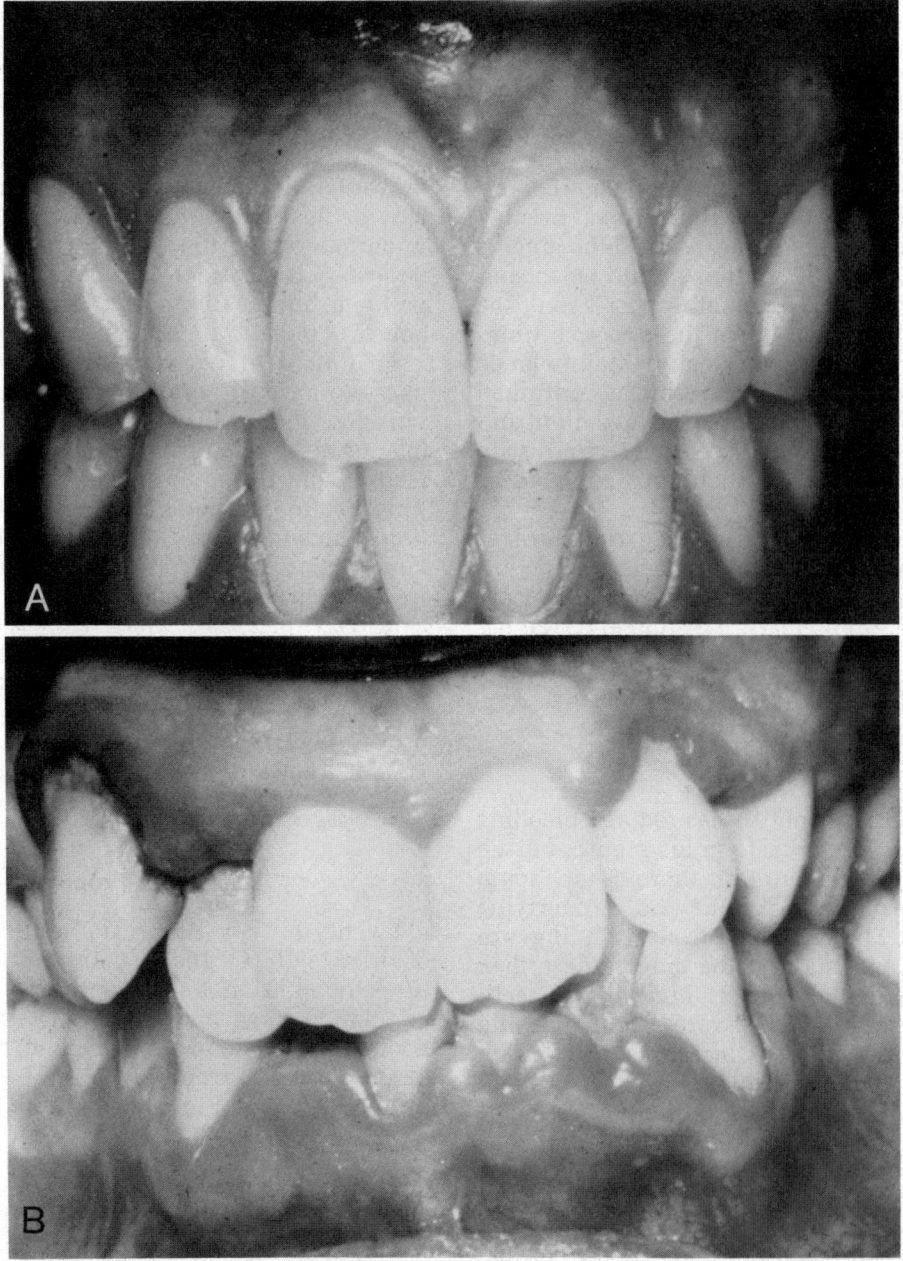

Figure 101.5. Normal gingiva (*A*) and chronic periodontal inflammation (*B*) showing swelling, blunting of interdental papillae, erythema, and bleeding.

mainly *Actinomyces*, appear to be of major significance. Small amounts of plaque are not visible unless they are stained. As plaque accumulates, it becomes visible as a mass that varies in color from gray to yellowish-gray to yellow. Measurable amounts of plaque may form within 1 hour after a thorough cleaning of the teeth with maximum accumulation in 30 days or less (9). Bacterial plaque, if left undisturbed, will mineralize and form *calculus* (tartar), as shown in Figure 101.4C. This process usually starts between the first and fourteenth day

after plaque formation. Calculus is always covered by plaque. When calculus is present, the gingival tissues are unhealthy by definition.

The major *complication* of untreated gingivitis is periodontitis, that is, the extension of the inflammation to the supporting bony structures of the teeth (see below and Fig. 101.4C).

Treatment

Patients presenting with any one of the four forms of gingivitis usually require one to three dental visits (spread over a 4-week period) for treatment. The mechanical removal of plaque and calculus from the affected areas of the teeth and gingiva is achieved with the appropriate instruments. After all of the plaque and calculus have been removed by the dentist, the disease process is explained to the patient, who is then instructed in proper *plaque control measures*, i.e., effective toothbrushing (a soft bristled toothbrush which facilitates cleansing of the gingiva and the teeth without laceration should be recommended) and effective flossing (the floss should be rubbed vertically up and down three to five times in each interdental space, once daily). Maintenance of the disease-free state is only possible by continued effective plaque control measures by the patient and by professional cleaning every 6 to 12 months (to remove plaque and calculus that may be missed by brushing and flossing).

Factors which usually result in recurrence are (a) incomplete removal of plaque and calculus, (b) inadequate plaque control because of insufficient patient instruction, (c) premature dismissal of the patient before he demonstrates competence, and (d) lack of patient cooperation.

Periodontitis (See Fig. 101.4C)

Presentation

A patient with periodontitis has red and bleeding gums and an unpleasant taste in his mouth, but he is usually free of pain unless there is an acute infection superimposed upon the underlying chronic process. The principal physical findings are the signs of inflammation of the gingiva described above and periodontal pockets around the teeth from which pus may often be expressed upon gentle pressure. As periodontitis advances, the teeth loosen and spread apart, creating unattractive spaces and exposing the roots of the teeth as the bony support is lost. Mastication is impaired, and spontaneous pain and acute abscess may occur.

The most important consequence of periodontitis is the destruction of the alveolar bone, which deprives the teeth of their support and is responsible for the loss of the teeth. The essential steps leading to destruction of bone are gingivitis, degeneration of collagen bundles of the periodontal ligament, and conversion of the shallow ($\leq$ 3 mm) physiological gingival sulcus to a deepened periodontal pocket (> 3 mm). As this pocket deepens, more debris accumulates in it. Inflammation progresses further inward, and the gums recede permanently. The apically progressing inflammation eventually reaches the alveolar crest, and bone resorption begins. This process continues, resulting in continued destruction of the alveolar bone.

Treatment

Most patients with periodontitis can be treated effectively, provided that the diagnosis is made be-

fore a significant amount of supporting alveolar bone is lost. The aims of treatment are to preserve the teeth by eliminating the disease, to restore effective function, and to prevent recurrence. When treated in the early stages, the major consequence of periodontitis (loss of bone support for the teeth) can be prevented. If proper treatment is postponed, there may be insufficient bone support once treatment is undertaken, and the natural teeth may eventually be lost. Some patients are not concerned with this problem, but are ultimately disappointed when their dentures do not function efficiently.

Treatment of periodontitis is divided into two phases. *Phase I* is similar to the treatment of gingivitis described above—i.e., removal of local irritant (plaque and calculus) and institution of effective plaque control (continual removal of the plaque). This treatment allows resolution of the inflammation. The success of this phase of therapy depends largely upon the patient's ability to maintain plaque-free teeth (see above under "Acute Necrotizing Ulcerative Gingivitis"). *Phase II* is the surgical phase in which the goal is to improve the gingival architecture which remains in spite of the disease. Experience has shown that patients have difficulty in preventing inflammation in periodontal pockets greater than 5 mm. Surgical treatment is therefore designed to decrease the depths of the pockets.

Denture Problems

Twenty million American adults are missing all of their teeth. Of these, many have obtained dentures. In addition, a large portion of the edentulous population have managed well without teeth, are content to remain as they are, and, regardless of the quality of dentures constructed, are unwilling and/or unable to adapt to using dentures.

Presentation

Often the physician will be confronted with a patient who, although he has had dentures for years, upon specific questioning by the physician indicates that the dentures are not as satisfactory as the patient would wish. The most common denture problems are looseness and discomfort. If the patient is followed at least yearly by his dentist, the physician can generally assume the present situation is the best that can be achieved. On the other hand, if the patient has tolerated the same set of loose or uncomfortable dentures without seeking help for a number of years, he should be encouraged to seek care promptly. Failure to remove dentures at night is the reason for denture problems in some patients. This practice can cause (a) bony erosion with loss of conformity of the dentures to the supporting structures, (b) mucosal ulceration, and (c) oral candidiasis.

Treatment

Depending upon the condition of the patient's oral cavity, the present dentures, and the edentulous ridges, a number of treatment modalities are available, including rebasing or relining the existing dentures (5 to 7 days), making a new set of dentures (2 to 5 weeks), and preprosthetic correction of soft and hard tissue (4 to 6 weeks healing), followed by relining, rebasing, or remaking of dentures.

Dental Caries

Dental caries is a disease of the calcified tissues of the teeth characterized by demineralization of the inorganic portion (enamel and dentin—see Fig. 101.2A of the tooth).

Dental caries is one of the most common diseases of man. It affects all persons regardless of race, location, or economic stratum, and it can occur at any age. Poor oral hygiene and a diet high in sugar promote caries, whereas routine oral hygiene and raw, coarse foods tend to reduce caries. Ingestion of fluorides in drinking water reduces susceptibility to caries. The form of the tooth affects caries, *i.e.*, the deep pits and fissures on molars and premolars especially predispose these teeth to the disorder.

Presentation

Dental caries usually presents as a nonpainful, white, brown, or black spot on the enamel of a tooth. The most common location is the biting surface in conjunction with the pits and fissures of the tooth. Other locations include the smooth surfaces where the teeth come into contact with each other. Without the aid of special equipment (radiographs and hand instruments) and expertise of dental personnel, the best indicator of dental caries is the presence of brown or black spots in areas associated with lost portions of the tooth.

When caries progresses rapidly to involve the pulp, as in children, the term *acute* caries is used. Slowly progressing caries seen in adults is referred to as *chronic* caries. Occasionally a carious lesion may cease to progress (*arrested* caries). This is due to breakage of enamel walls, thereby exposing the lesion to the cleaning action of the toothbrush, saliva, fluoride, and mastication. The term *recurrent* caries is used for carious lesions that begin around the margins of defective restorations.

A carious lesion usually develops after bacterial plaque (see above) forms on the tooth surface. The primary bacteria involved in this process are *Streptococcus mutans* and *Lactobacillus acidophilus*. These bacteria metabolize dietary fructose to produce lactic acid, which results in decalcification of the enamel. The rate of development of caries depends upon the susceptibility of the enamel.

Treatment

The treatment for most carious lesions is their removal, followed by a restoration (filling) which replaces the lost portions of the tooth. The goals are to remove the lesion, to protect the pulp from irritants, and to restore the tooth to function. In those cases when caries involves a tooth already significantly affected by peridontal disease, the tooth must be removed.

The major *complication* which results from delaying treatment is acute pulpitis and its complications (see above). In addition, delaying treatment may result in a more difficult restoration or possible loss of the involved tooth. In those cases where the existing decay process is very close to the pulp, the heat generated by the rotary instruments used to prepare the restoration may result in a transient pulpal inflammation. This inflammation results in a dull ache in the tooth for 2 to 3 days, which is usually relieved by aspirin. When the restoration process leaves only a paper-thin layer of dentin covering the pulp tissue, the transient pulpitis may be converted to acute pulpitis (irreversible), which then requires either tooth extraction or root canal therapy for relief of pain. Root canal therapy consists of three parts: the removal of the infected nerve tissue, the debridement and preparation of the nerve canal space, and obturation (filling) of the canal space with a biologically inert material.

Angular Cheilosis

Presentation

Angular cheilosis is characterized by a feeling of dryness and a burning sensation at the corners of the mouth. The epithelium at the commissures appears wrinkled and macerated. In time, the wrinkles deepen to fissures which appear ulcerated but do not bleed, although a crust may form. These lesions stop at the junction of the mucous membranes. They show a tendency for spontaneous improvement; only rarely do the lesions completely disappear.

There are several etiologies for cheilosis. A number of microorganisms may cause it in otherwise healthy people: *Candida albicans, staphylococci, and streptococci*. In addition, angular cheilosis due to overclosure of the jaws may be seen in edentulous patients. Overclosure causes a fold to be produced at the corners of the mouth in which saliva tends to collect, inviting the growth of microorganisms. Angular cheilosis is also seen in riboflavin deficiency, which usually occurs in patients with multiple vitamin deficiencies. The lips show fissures, painful cracks, and scaling; these changes become severe at the corners of the mouth and are similar in appearance to angular cheilosis due to overclosure of the mandible.

Treatment

Edentulous patients troubled by angular cheilosis should be referred to a dentist who will evaluate them for mandibular overclosure, as correction of this problem (making or remaking of dentures) may lead to remission. Treatment is otherwise symptomatic and consists of applying petrolatum-containing ointment (e.g., Vaseline, Chapstick) to the scaling area to minimize discomfort.

Thrush (Oral Candidiasis)

Presentation

The typical lesions of oral candidiasis are white, curd-like plaques on an erythematous mucosa (Fig. 101.6). These plaques are loosely attached and may be scraped off of the oral mucosa. They begin as pinpoint spots. Involvement may include the corners of the mouth, as noted in the previous section. The tongue is often reddened, and the patient describes a burning sensation.

Thrush may occur chronically in patients with poor oral hygiene and poor nutrition. It may also be brought on or exacerbated by debilitating systemic illness, antibiotic therapy, use of steroids or antimetabolites, or dental extraction. Thrush does not appear to be more common in diabetics.

The white plaques of thrush may suggest hyperkeratosis or leukoplakia. In these instances, a scraping will reveal hyphae and blastospores when the condition is candidiasis.

Treatment

The patient should be advised to practice good oral hygiene practices. Specific treatment consists of nystatin oral suspension, 4 to 6 ml held in the mouth for several minutes before swallowing, four times daily. Thrush usually resolves entirely after 1 to 2 weeks of treatment. Treatment should be continued for several days after visible lesions have disappeared.

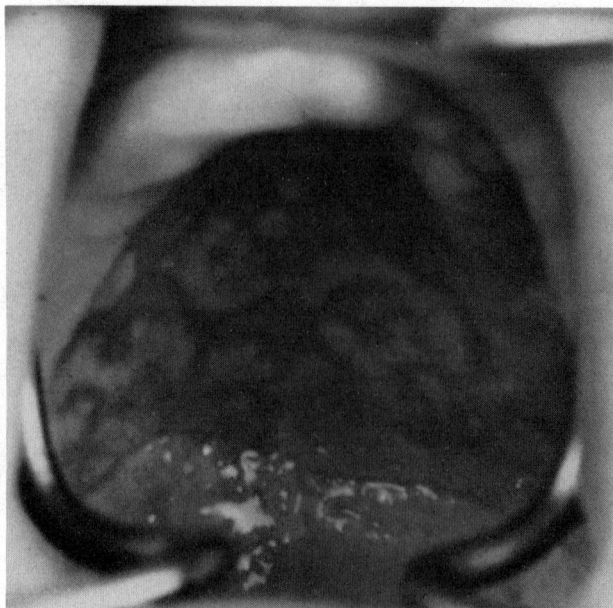

Figure 101.6. Candidiasis (thrush) of hard palate.

Halitosis

Presentation

Halitosis is a foul or offensive odor emanating from the oral cavity. Mouth odors originate from local or remote sites. The local causes can be retention of odoriferous food particles on or between the teeth, ANUG, caries, chronic periodontal disease, dentures, tobacco smoking, and healing of surgical or extraction wounds. Extraoral causes of halitosis include infection in adjacent structures (rhinitis, sinusitis, tonsillitis), pulmonary infections, alcoholic breath, the acetone odor of the diabetic, or the uremic breath associated with renal failure.

Treatment

Local causes of this condition are treated by improvement in oral hygiene and by specific treatment of the underlying conditions by a dentist. If these measures are unsuccessful, pleasant-smelling mouthwashes or breath fresheners used frequently (every 2 to 4 hours) may greatly reduce the problem. Halitosis due to remote factors may be masked with mouthwashes and fresheners until the remote problem has been resolved.

Xerostomia (Dry Mouth)

Presentation

Xerostomia or dry mouth results from a partial or complete lack of saliva. This defect results in cracking of the lips, difficulty in swallowing, and/or changes in the tongue texture. The patient often increases liquid consumption in order to eliminate the dryness. Xerostomia may be a secondary complication of salivary gland disease (e.g., Sjögren's syndrome) or radiation treatment, but medication is the commonest cause. Anticholinergic, decongestant, and antihistamine drugs are the most common offenders.

The loss of saliva results in a loss of the protective coating of the mucous membranes of the oral cavity. Infections, severe dental caries, and problems with dentures very commonly result from the loss of saliva.

Treatment

Treatment of xerostomia is symptomatic. Patients should be referred to a dentist for a complete dental evaluation and to eliminate any caries and for instruction in the use of daily topical fluoride to help prevent recurrence of caries. The dryness may be lessened if the patient regularly irrigates his mouth with topical methylcellulose, glycerin, or a saliva substitute (Oralube, Xerolube, or MOI-STIR—all available without prescription). The saliva substitutes also decrease somewhat the risk of caries because they contain sodium fluoride.

Common Tongue Conditions

Geographic Tongue

Benign migratory glossitis or geographic tongue is an asymptomatic inflammatory condition consisting of multiple areas of desquamation of the filiform papillae of the tongue in an irregular pattern (Fig. 101.7A). The central portion of an affected area is usually denuded, while the border may be outlined by a thin, yellowish-white line or band. The fungiform papillae persist in the desquamated area as small elevated red dots. The areas of desquamation remain for a short time in one location, then heal and reappear in other locations. The condition may persist for weeks or months and then regress, only to recur at a later date. Women are affected twice as often as men and there is no racial difference. Since the etiology is unknown and the condition is benign, management consists of reassurance. Large doses of vitamins are not effective.

Hairy Tongue

Hairy tongue is a condition characterized by hypertrophy of the filiform papillae of the tongue due to the lack of normal desquamation of the keratin layer (Fig. 101.7B). This results in a thick, matted layer on the dorsum of the tongue. The color of the papillae varies from yellowish-white to brown or even black depending upon their staining by extrinsic factors (tobacco, foods, or medications). The hypertrophied tissue may touch the palate and produce gagging in some patients. The majority of patients with hairy tongue are heavy smokers, but the etiology is unknown. Treatment of this benign condition is to brush the tongue with a tongue blade or toothbrush to promote desquamation and to remove debris.

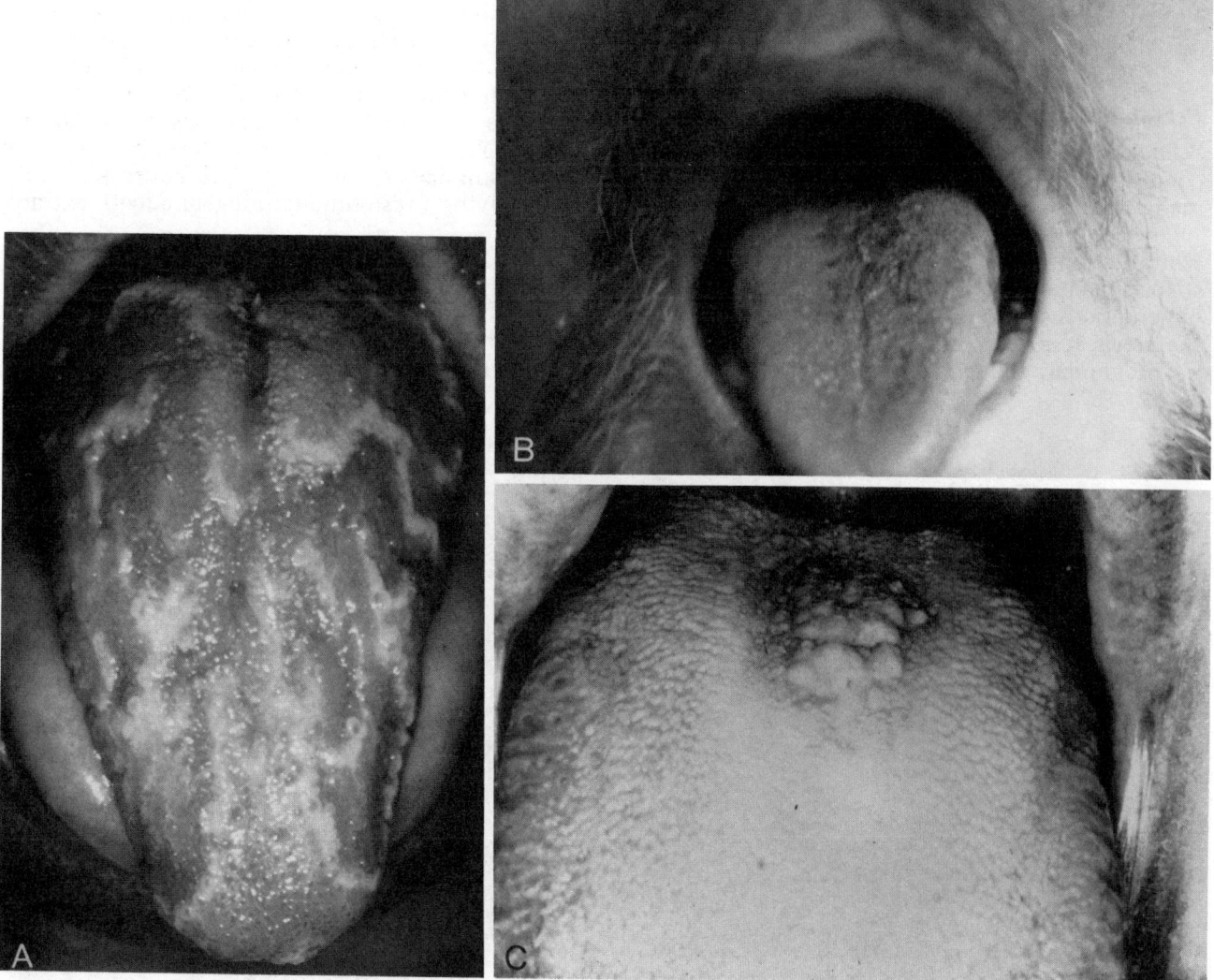

Figure 101.7. Common benign problems of the tongue. *A.* Geographic tongue. *B.* Hairy tongue. *C.* Median rhomboid glossitis.

Median Rhomboid Glossitis

Median rhomboid glossitis is a congenital abnormality of the tongue which appears clinically as an ovoid, diamond, or rhomboid-shaped reddish patch on the dorsal surface of the tongue. On examination, there is a slightly raised or flat area which is distinctive because there are no filiform papillae (Fig. 101.7C). Despite its name, this abnormality is not inflammatory; it is due to failure of the tuberculum impar to retract before fusion of the lateral halves of the tongue, so that a structure free of papillae is interposed. The prevalence of the abnormality is less than 1%, and there are no sex or racial differences. The only clinical significance of this innocuous condition is that it is occasionally mistaken for a carcinoma; differentiation from cancer is aided by a history of the presence of the lesion since childhood and by the fact that a carcinoma rarely develops on the dorsum of the tongue. If the physician is unsure of the diagnosis he should refer the patient to a dentist.

Leukoplakia and Erythroplakia

Presentation

Leukoplakia and erythroplakia are asymptomatic conditions of the oral mucosa that may become malignant.

Leukoplakia varies in appearance from a grayish-white flattened scaly lesion to a thick, irregularly shaped plaque (Fig. 101.8). Histologically, there is hyperkeratosis, acanthosis, and some degree of dyskeratosis. It is commonly associated with underlying inflammation due to a chronic irritant (tobacco, alcohol, poorly constructed dentures). Leukoplakia may be found anywhere in the oral cavity, but most frequently it is found in the buccal mucosa, followed, in descending order, by the alveolar mucosa, tongue, lip, hard and soft palates, floor of the mouth, and gingiva.

Erythroplakia refers to a lesion which is velvety red in appearance, small (2 cm or less), and with or without a hyperkeratotic component. It is found in the floor of the mouth, soft palate, and ventrolateral border of the tongue.

The significance of these lesions has been delineated in a longitudinal study of mucosal lesions (6). Of 200 white lesions examined by biopsy, only 4 were malignant. In the same study, an erythroplastic component was present in 90% of the 158 asymptomatic squamous cell carcinomas that were found, suggesting, but not proving, that erythroplakia may be an important precursor of squamous cell cancer.

Treatment

It is impossible to determine which lesion showing leukoplakia or erythroplakia will undergo malignant transformation. Discontinuance of chronic irritants is recommended, followed by a 14-day observation period to allow inflammatory lesions to heal. If the lesion persists, referral to a dental surgeon for a biopsy is indicated. The biopsy procedure is as simple as having a restoration (filling) or a tooth extraction.

Other conditions which may resemble leukoplakia or erythroplakia are lichen planus, chemical burns, moniliasis, psoriasis, lupus erythematosus, and syphilitic mucous patches. Each of these has characteristic histological features.

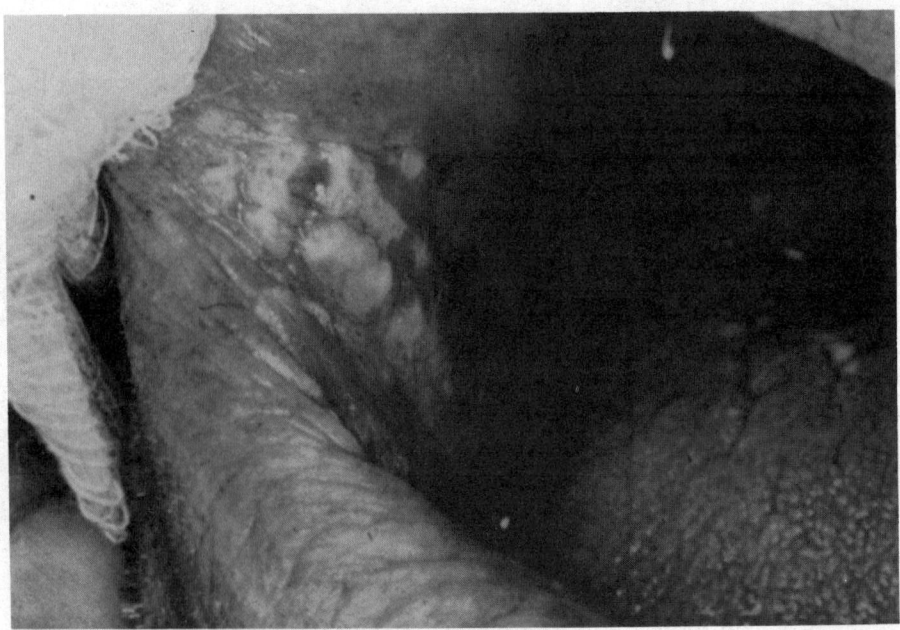

Figure 101.8. Leukoplakia showing early changes of epidermoid carcinoma.

Squamous Cell Carcinoma

Over 90% of all malignant tumors of the oral cavity are squamous cell carcinomas. It is 4 times more common in men than women and is most common after the fourth decade. In the United States oral cancer is the eighth most common form of cancer in men and the twelth in women. Fifteen thousand new cases are found each year, and about 7500 patients die of this disease annually. Of lip carcinomas, 95% occur on the lower lip and appear as an ulcer, wart, sore, or scale. This lesion is more frequent in fair-skinned individuals. Of the intraoral carcinomas, 50% occur on the tongue (usually ventrolateral border, Fig. 101.9) and 16% on the floor of the mouth; the remaining 34% are equally distributed between the gingival mucosa, palate, and buccal mucosa. Sixty percent of intraoral carcinomas present as ulcers, 30% as growths, and the remaining 10% as white lesions or other abnormalities of the mucosa (2). Carcinoma of the tongue and floor of the mouth metastasizes early and carries a very poor prognosis.

The etiology of oral carcinoma is unknown. Ill fitting dentures, actinic radiation, tobacco, jagged teeth, syphilitic glossitis, and alcoholism are believed to be risk factors.

Presentation and Evaluation

Patients usually give a history of knowledge of the lesion for 6 to 18 months when they first present; for many reasons they have not sought evaluation.

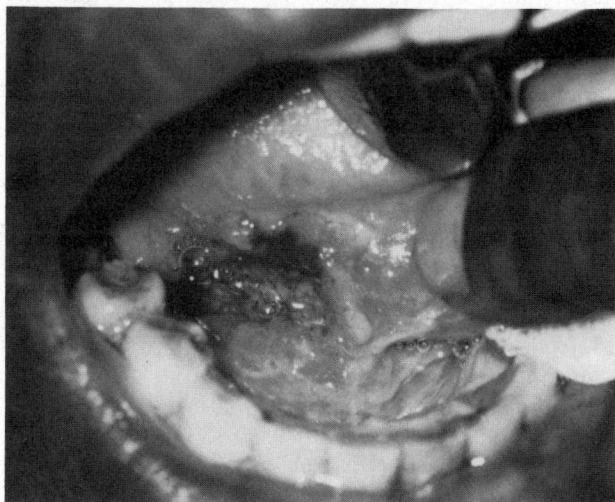

Figure 101.9. Squamous cell carcinoma of the floor of the mouth.

All patients with suspicious lesions should be referred promptly to a dental surgeon for biopsy. Biopsy is a simple procedure, not very different from having a restoration or tooth extraction; usually it is done under local anesthesia.

Treatment

Definitive surgery is a team effort between the otolaryngologist and the dentist. The dentist's role is to evaluate, for long term prognosis, any of the teeth which are *not* to be removed in the surgical field and to remove any of these teeth that are affected with untreatable periodontitis; this is done to avoid osteoradionecrosis, a condition seen in the postradiation patient in whom the socket of an extracted tooth fails to heal as the result of diminished blood supply. Lip tumors have the highest success rate (10-year cure rate between 80 and 92%), while only one-fifth of patients with tongue cancer live longer than 5 years.

General References

Carronza FA (ed): *Glickman's Clinical Periodontology*, ed 5. Philadelphia, WB Saunders, 1979.
Excellent text for discussion of periodontal disease and related problems.
Lynch MA (ed): *Bunket's Oral Medicine, Diagnosis and Treatment*, ed 8. Philadelphia, JB Lippincott, 1984.
Excellent reference.

Specific References

1. Apfelberg DB, Lavey E, Janetos G, *et al*: Temporomandibular joint disease: results of a ten year study. *Postgrad Med* 65:167, 1979.
2. Bhaskar SN: *Synopsis of Oral Pathology*, ed 4. St Louis, CV Mosby, 1973, p 463.
3. Franks AS: The social character of temporomandibular joint dysfunction. *Dent Pract Dent Rec* 15:94, 1964.
4. Graykowski EA, Barile MF, Lee WB, Stanley HR Jr: Recurrent aphthous stomatitis; clinical, therapeutic, histopathologic, and hypersensitivity aspects. *JAMA* 196:637, 1966.
5. Helkimo M: Epidemiological surveys of dysfunction of the mastication system. In Meicher AH, Zarb GA (eds): *Oral Sciences Reviews: Temporomandibular Joint Function and Dysfunction III*. Copenhagen, Munksgaard, 1976.
6. Mashberg A, Morrissey JB, Garfinkel L: A study of the appearance of early asymptomatic oral squamous cell carcinoma. *Cancer* 32:1436, 1973.
7. Mühlemann HR, Son S: Gingival sulcus bleeding—a leading symptom in initial gingivitis. *Helv Odontol Acta* 15:107, 1971.
8. Spruance SL, Overall JC, Kern ER, *et al*: The natural history of recurrent herpes simplex labialis: implications for antiviral therapy. *N Engl J Med* 297:69, 1977.
9. Thenard JC, Hefflin CM, Steinberg AI: Neuraminidase activity in mixed culture supernatant fluids of human oral bacteria. *J Bacteriol* 89:924, 1965.
10. United States Department of Health, Education and Welfare, Public Health Service: *Research Explores Pyorrhea and Other Gum Diseases: Periodontal Disease*, (PHS Publication 1482). Washington, DC, US Government Printing Office, 1970.

Common Problems of the Feet

BRUCE S. LEBOWITZ, D.P.M.

The internist or family physician is often called upon to treat patients who complain of problems with their feet, either as a primary care provider or in conjunction with a podiatrist. Although disorders of the feet are not life threatening, they should not be taken lightly. Any patient with a painful foot will attest that his pain can and does take the joy out of living.

STRUCTURE AND FUNCTION

The abnormal foot cannot be understood unless the structure of the foot and its function during gait are understood.

Normal Gait (See Fig. 102.1, *A* and *B*)

The bones and joints of the feet facilitate walking and running in an upright position. The foot and leg function together to allow a smooth, even transfer of weight as one extremity moves ahead of the other. During gait, the foot first adjusts to a variable terrain, and then acts to propel the body's weight forward.

In the *first stage of gait*, the heel strikes the ground and body weight begins to move distally over the lateral aspect of the foot. The foot is in a *pronated* position, meaning that the arch is relatively flattened. In effect, the foot resembles a "loose bag of bones" during this stage, permitting it to adapt to the terrain and to act as a shock absorber when body weight strikes the ground.

In the *second stage of gait*, as weight moves distally to the ball of the foot and the body is propelled forward, the foot must convert to a rigid lever. This conversion, or *supination*, takes place in the subtalar and midtarsal joints. Supination serves to heighten the arch, pushing the bones and joints of the foot together rigidly enough to propel body weight forward efficiently.

For the lower extremity to function normally, certain structural criteria must be met; if they are not met, compensation will occur. Ideally, the leg should be in a plane perpendicular to the foot and ground, as in a stick figure drawing. The forefoot should be in a plane parallel to the rearfoot; but various congenital factors may act to prevent this normal angulation. Varus (toward the midline or inverted) or valgus (away from the midline or everted) positions of the forefoot or hindfoot are the most common of these congenital factors.

Excessive Pronation

Excessive pronation (pronation extended through too much of the gait cycle) is the most common compensating mechanism when structural abnormalities are present. When the foot remains pronated during gait and does not resupinate in time, or at all, the condition known as "flatfoot" exists. The degree of this flatfoot position reflects the degree of pronation that is present. A number of problems may evolve from excessive pronation during gait—among them bunions, calluses, and hammertoes. As pointed out in the discussion of these conditions which follows, assessment of the mechanical basis for the condition is important in planning appropriate treatment for it.

Shoe Gear

Shoe gear clearly plays a role in the way feet function. Shoes protect feet from the elements, cushion the effect of walking on hard, flat surfaces, and provide some support to the bones and ligaments.

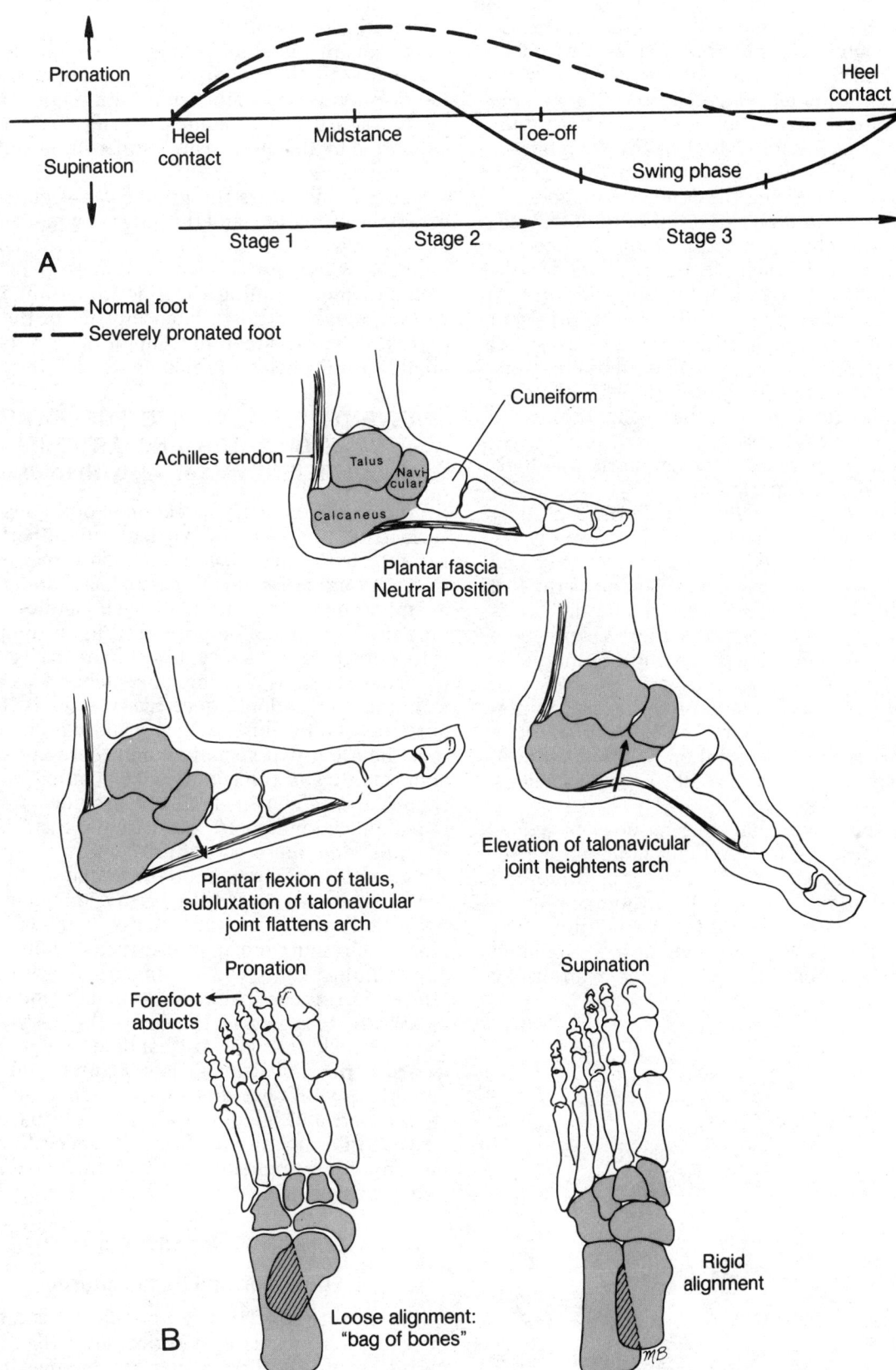

Figure 102.1.   *A*. Schematic representation of the gait cycle for a normal foot and for a foot with excessive pronation. *B*. Schematic illustration of foot structure during pronation and supination.

Unfortunately, many individuals favor short, narrow shoes, high heels, and pointed toes. Obviously, squeezing a basically rectangular foot into a triangular shoe with the feet elevated from 2 to 5 inches creates significant stress for the foot. Most of the disorders of the foot discussed in this chapter are intensified by these demands of fashion.

Most people, in fitting themselves for shoes, do not take into account the variations in their foot size throughout the day and the variation in shoe size from manufacturer to manufacturer. Therefore, the following advice is often helpful: buy shoes in the late afternoon when any swelling that might occur is already present; try to buy shoes in stores that also have an active trade in infant shoes, as shoe fitters for infants are experienced in fitting the shoe to the foot and not *vice versa*; lightweight shoes are preferable to heavy ones; and, finally, leather, because it is more porous, is preferable to synthetic materials in shoe construction.

Interest in *shoe gear related to sports*, especially to jogging and running, has escalated in recent years. Sneakers or running shoes should be well fitted and firm enough to prevent excessive splaying of the foot during activity. For shock absorption, the shoes should have studded soles; and there should be a raised, resilient heel wedge. The midsole should be flexible to help prevent Achilles tendon stress, and there should be a well molded Achilles pad to prevent irritation of the tendon. The tongue should be well padded to prevent irritation of the dorsum of the foot. These features are illustrated in Figure 102.2.

It is a misconception that wearing sneakers excessively will harm the feet. Actually, the better running shoes available today are so supportive and well padded that they may be recommended to patients for numerous painful foot conditions. For example, highly arched feet (which are supinated and may pronate only slightly) lack shock-absorbing

qualities; and constant impact on the ground can cause severe metatarsal, heel, and arch pain. For patients with this condition, the support and resiliency provided by a modern running shoe are ideal. Likewise, a flat or pronated foot may be very well supported by the built-in arch supports of well made running shoes.

Running magnifies the problems associated with excessive pronation, and the long term management of runners with this condition requires the selection of shoes which provide good support. The use of well designed running shoes is important in preventing most exercise-related injuries of the lower extremity as explained in Chapter 67, Exercise-Related Musculoskeletal Problems.

PREVENTIVE FOOT CARE FOR PATIENTS WITH DIABETES AND ARTERIAL INSUFFICIENCY (See Also Chapter 87)

Prevention and early detection of problems on the surface of the foot are particularly important in patients with these conditions. This requires periodic examination by the physician and routine examination by the patient. The single most important advice that can be impressed upon the patient is to look at his feet every day. When obesity or lack of visual acuity is a problem, someone else should examine the patient's feet every day. Irritations, abrasions, and calluses which usually produce pain must be identified visually when there are sensory abnormalities in the feet. Advice about selection of shoe gear (see above) should be provided routinely to patients with diabetes and vascular insufficiency. By following these procedures, most serious foot ulcers and infections can be prevented.

These patients should also be advised not to utilize over-the-counter corn and ingrown toenail remedies. Such commercial preparations include acids and tanning agents which can seriously injure the tender skin of these patients. Normal toenails should be allowed to grow past the end of the fleshy part of the toe; thick nails are best handled by a podiatrist, as are corns and calluses (see below). Soft cotton should be worn between toes which tend to rub each other, and talcum powder should be used to prevent interdigital moisture and maceration. Lanolin should be applied to dry and thickened skin to prevent fissuring.

BUNIONS (Fig. 102.3, *A* to *D*)

Definition and Pathogenesis

Bunion (literally "turnip") is a term used by laymen and physicians to describe the collective deformities of the first metatarsophalangeal joint. These deformities include enlargement of the medial, medial-dorsal, or dorsal aspect of the first metatarsophalangeal joint and lateral deviation of the

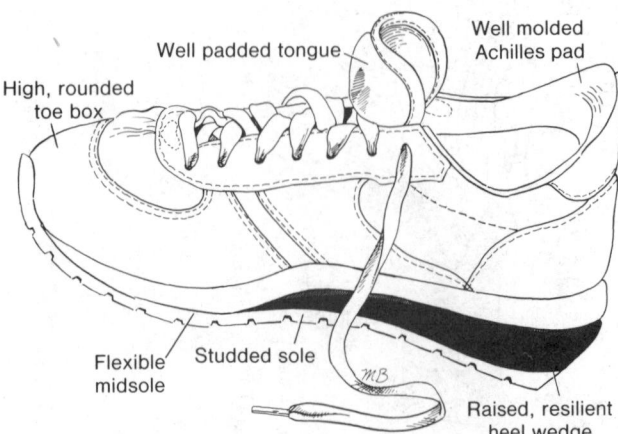

High, rounded toe box

Well padded tongue

Well molded Achilles pad

Flexible midsole

Studded sole

Raised, resilient heel wedge

Figure 102.2. Features of a well designed running shoe.

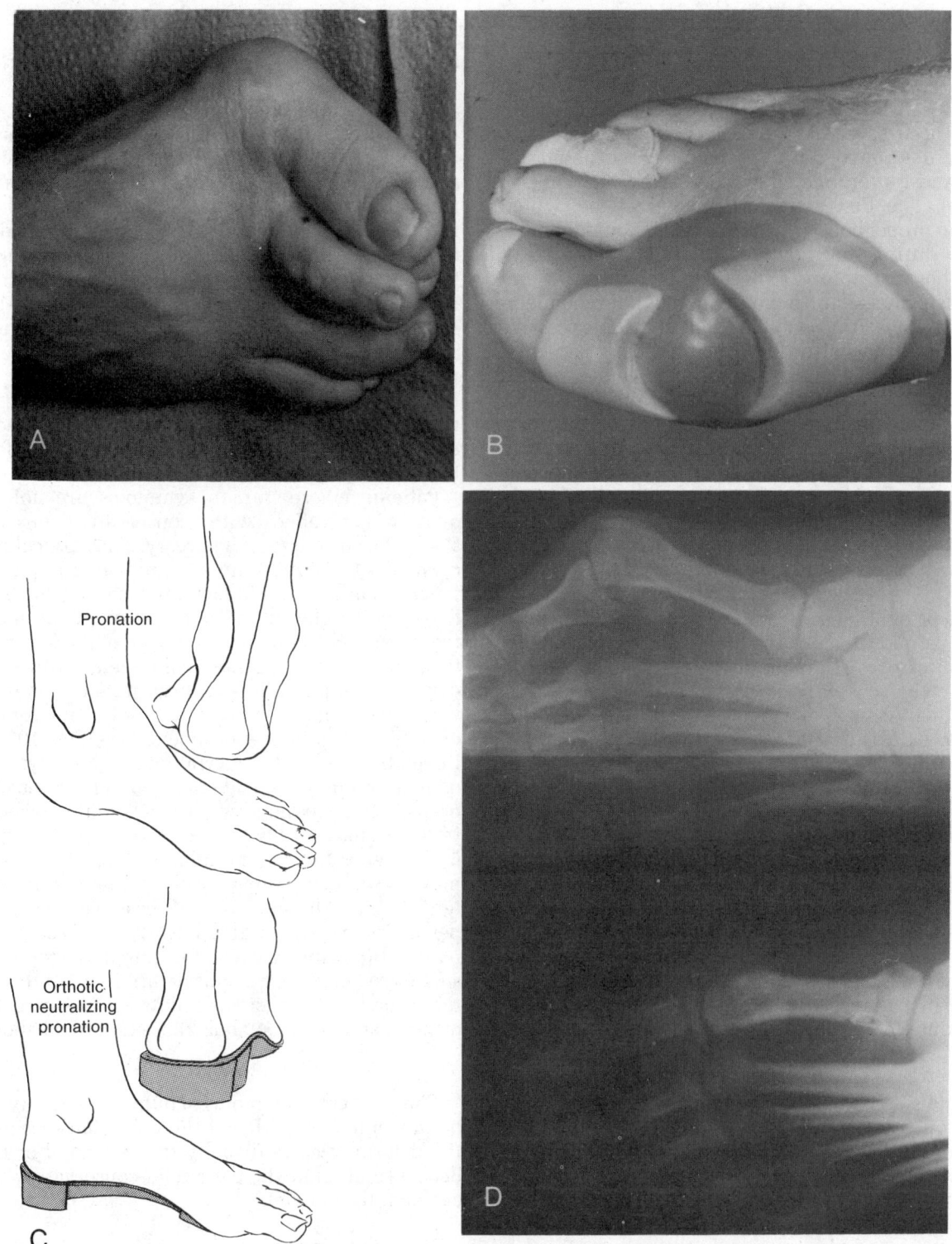

Labels within figure: Pronation; Orthotic neutralizing pronation; A; B; C; D

Figure 102.3. Bunions: appearance, orthotic compensation, and surgical repair. *A.* Bunion deformity. *B.* Bunion protected by latex shield. *C.* Leather orthotic arch support. *D.* Bunion deformity shown radiologically before and after surgical correction.

great toe. The enlargement of the joint may consist of bone or soft tissue or a combination of the two.

For many years, tight-fitting shoes were mistakenly considered to be the cause of bunions. It is known now that, while the pressure of tight shoes on an existing bunion can certainly result in pain which calls attention to the problem, bunions are not caused by poorly fitted shoes. The chief cause of the deformity is a hypermobile first metatarsal bone most often related to excessive pronation (see above). The first metatarsal and great toe, which help to propel body weight forward, should be quite stable during the final stage of gait when a tight, rigid bony structure is needed. The intrinsic and extrinsic musculature should help to hold the metatarsal tight at this point. When there is excessive pronation, the entire foot remains loose and relatively unstable. One result of such laxity in this stage of gait is the hypermobility of the first metatarsal and the "buckling" of the first toe: intrinsic and extrinsic muscles cause the first metatarsal to deviate medially and the great toe to deviate laterally. The combined deformity is called *hallux abducto valgus*. Eventually, arthritic hypertrophy of the head of the first metatarsal bone develops.

Symptoms

The presenting complaint of a patient with a bunion is pain localized to the first metatarsophalangeal joint. Pressure of the shoe on the enlarged metatarsal head, with or without pressure on adventitious bursa, can cause pain that is severe and even disabling; pain can also result from the joint motion itself. Often, crepitus can be felt within the joint. Sometimes the patient seeks help, not because of pain, but because he is unable to wear shoes as a result of the deformity.

In evaluating a patient, the physician must be certain that the symptoms are a result of the bunion alone. Gout (see Chapter 69) may not only produce acute pain in the first metatarsophalangeal joint, but may also aggravate a chronically painful joint. Therefore, gout should always be considered, especially in patients with bilateral bunion deformity and acute monarticular pain in a foot.

Management

Acute symptoms due to a bunion should be managed with rest, elimination of pressure on the bunion, soaks in warm water, and systemic anti-inflammatory medication (such as naproxen (Naprosyn), 250 mg every 6 to 8 hours, or piroxicam (Feldene), 10 to 20 mg every 24 hours; aspirin, 600 mg every 4 to 6 hours, may also be used, but the onset of action is slower). After the acute symptoms have subsided, the patient should be started on a program of long term management.

Conservative long term management of a bunion involves accommodating the deformity and attempting to arrest its progress. This is achieved by the use of molds and protective shields (see Fig. 102.3, B and C). A mold, usually referred to as an arch support, may be made from various types of materials to accommodate the plantar aspect of the foot. Protective shields are made of latex rubber.

Full foot molds or protective shields made by a podiatrist from a plaster impression are preferable to commercially made devices found in pharmacies and shoe stores. Commercial devices are manufactured to fit average shoe and foot sizes and do not take into account the shape of the individual patient's foot. The mold should be in place during the fitting of all new shoes. Occasionally, if the mold makes conventional shoes too tight, a specially built shoe, called an extra depth-inlay shoe, may be used. These enlarged shoes have a removable insole, for which one may substitute the patient's mold. The mold and shoes should minimize pressures against the bunion. In addition, the mold acts to reduce excessive pronation, thereby reducing the deforming forces in the forefoot.

Patients whose bunion symptoms are not adequately controlled with conservative measures should be considered for surgery. The *surgical management* of a bunion must be individually planned for each patient, and in fact, for each foot, to correct the specific deformity (3). Correction might involve resection of the bony protuberance of the first metatarsal head only. In occasional patients with severe degenerative joint disease surgical management involves removal of all or part of the joint and insertion of a Silastic joint replacement (see Fig. 102.3*D*). Depending on locale, referral for surgical correction of a bunion may be made to a general, orthopaedic, or podiatric surgeon. A patient should expect to return to most of his preoperative activities within 6 to 8 weeks following bunion surgery; the interval may be somewhat longer after bilateral surgery. A tendency for the foot to swell postoperatively may persist for many months, however. Excessive pronation, the primary cause for bunion, persists after surgery. Therefore, a major determinant of the long term results of surgery is follow-up foot care with orthotic appliances such as those described above.

Prevention

The annoying symptoms of bunion deformity may be prevented altogether if the physician recognizes the deformity early (usually in the second or third decade) and refers the patient for conservative management by a podiatrist.

CALLUSES AND CORNS (Fig. 102.4)

Definition and Pathogenesis

A *callus* is a thickening of the epidermis as a result of chronic intermittent trauma. When there is intermittent irritation of an area of skin, the initial re-

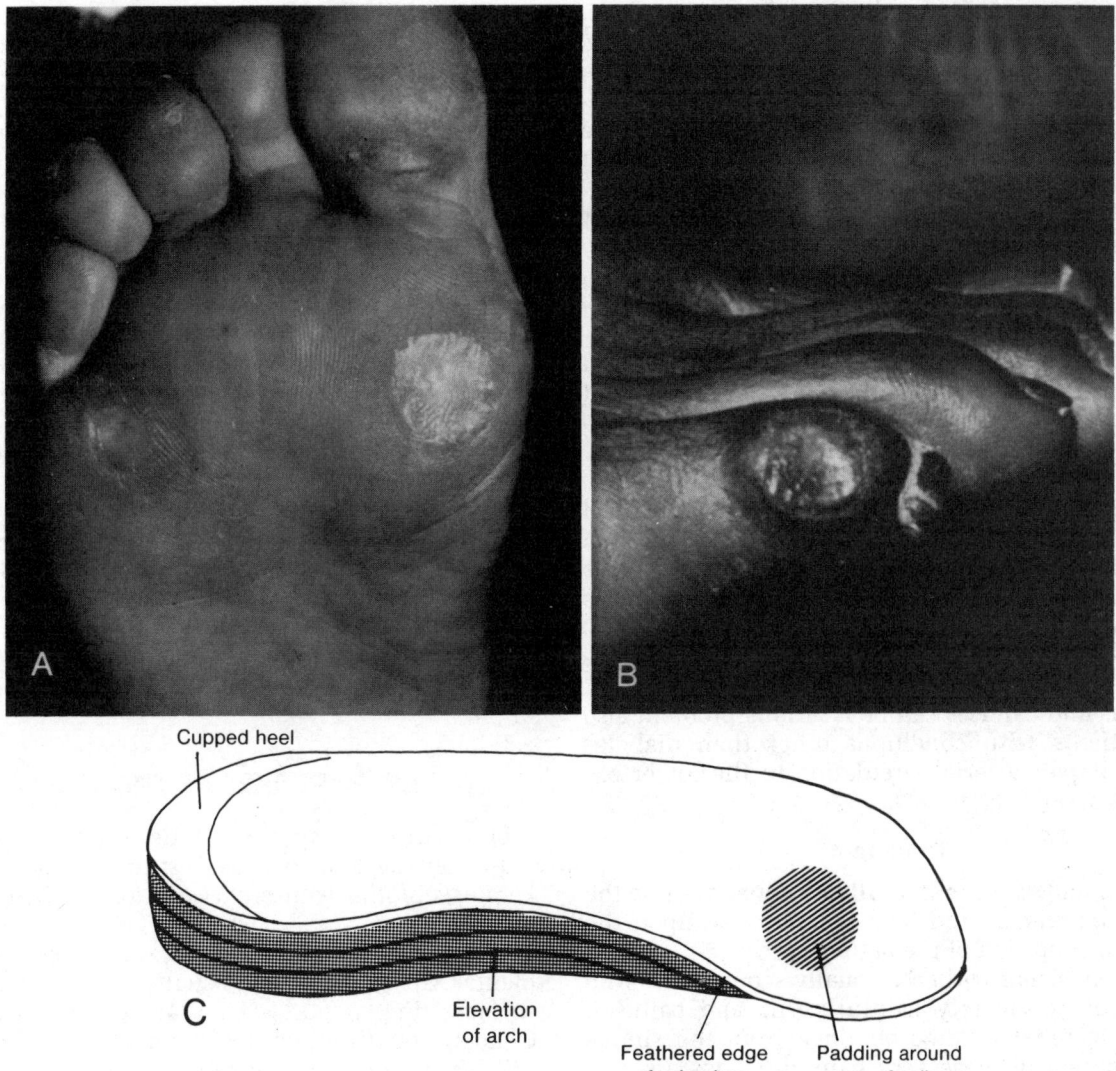

Figure 102.4. Calluses and corns. *A.* Typical plantar callus. *B.* Corn on the fifth digit. *C.* Orthotic device designed to shift weight from area of callus formation. (Photographs courtesy of Max Weisfeld, D.P.M.)

sponse is vasodilation; this is followed by increased production of corneum and hyperkeratosis. This process is normal and protective to skin and underlying tissue. When the process continues until there is buildup of excessive or highly concentrated callus, resulting in a *corn*, problems may develop. Skin lines may remain visible in callused tissue, but they usually do not pass through the highly concentrated center of a corn. Corns are most frequently located overlying the proximal interphalangeal joints of the lesser toes and centrally within plantar calluses. A number of processes not related to chronic trauma can produce focal calluses as well, namely *verruca plantaris* (plantar wart), foreign body granuloma, and *porokeratosis plantaris discreta*. These lesions are discussed below (page 1446).

The primary cause for most symptomatic calluses is excessive pronation (see above, page 1440) and

not restrictive shoes or walking on unyielding surfaces. During excessive pronation, the long flexor and extensor tendons pull on the distal phalanges, the toes appear to "hammer," and a retrograde force pushes down on the metatarsal heads, increasing pressure on the plantar skin. Other conditions which may promote this increased pressure are excessive supination (highly arched foot) and imbalance of the peroneal and tibial muscles due to weakness, arthritis, or other conditions affecting one or both legs.

Symptoms

Diffuse callus is usually asymptomatic and easily controlled by the patient with pumice stones and cleansing agents readily available in pharmacies. Both calluses and corns produce pain. Thick accumulation of callus tends to cause a burning sensation in the foot. A corn located within a plantar callus gives the sensation of walking on a sharp pebble. Corns which occur dorsolaterally on fifth toes (Fig. 102.4*B*) often cause exquisite pain, especially with tight-fitting shoes. Such corns often have adventitious bursae associated with them and may produce symptoms due both to bursitis and to the discomfort of the corn pressing down on subcutaneous tissues.

While corns and calluses can cause discomfort for the average person, they can cause serious morbidity in a *diabetic patient*. If hyperkeratotic lesions on an extremity are added to a diabetic's lowered resistance to infection, circulatory impairment, and decreased perception of pain, there is a clear potential for serious problems. A discrete lesion on the foot produces constant pressure on the underlying dermis. It is not unusual for this pressure, in a diabetic, to result in local breakdown of tissues, ulceration, and infection. Diabetics have the additional medical and mechanical problem of neurotrophic joints. In patients with the tendency to develop hammertoe and plantar-flexed metatarsal heads, these changes (and the calluses and corns which accompany them) may be accelerated by the loss of normal proprioception and pain sensation of a neurotrophic joint.

Corns and calluses can be a serious problem also for patients with conditions other than diabetes which impair arterial circulation to the lower extremities (see Chapter 87).

Treatment

Treatment of corns and calluses depends upon the location, severity, and type of lesion and upon the physical condition of the patient.

The physician will occasionally see patients who complain of severely painful corns and calluses. Dramatic relief may be obtained from the simple debridement of these very painful lesions, using a sterile no. 10 or no. 15 scalpel blade. If the blade is kept nearly parallel to the skin, injury to the underlying healthy dermis can be avoided. There is no need to debride the entire callus; any reduction in the thickness of the lesion will bring relief to the patient.

Conservative long term management of corns and calluses in the feet of otherwise healthy people requires the control of the source of the problem, namely excessive pronation. If excessive pronation is neutralized with orthotic devices (see above), foot function is improved, pathological forces are decreased, and lesions may regress. Lesions which have been present for a year or longer usually indicate that there have already been structural changes in the bones and joints, as well as histopathological changes in the skin.

For patients whose symptoms are not controlled with conservative treatment, *surgery* may be very helpful. A number of surgical procedures may be used to realign metatarsal heads or to reduce ham-

mertoe deformities. Often it is necessary to combine the surgical reconstruction of affected areas with control of pronation in order to achieve lasting resolution of symptoms. This may mean 6 to 8 weeks of convalescence (*i.e.*, non-weight bearing for several days then progression to partial, then full weight bearing usually by 6 weeks) after foot surgery and the continued use of orthotics in shoes. The end result, however, is greater foot health and comfort.

For the patient with *diabetes or peripheral vascular disease*, conservative treatment involves frequent debridement of the hyperkeratotic areas, padding for protection, and the fabrication of molds (by a podiatrist or orthopaedist) to shift weight away from problem areas and to accommodate deformities (see Fig. 102.4*C*). Extra depth shoes are often prescribed in conjunction with such appliances. When refractory infection or ulceration occurs despite conservative management, surgical procedures may be performed to eliminate a bony prominence. Surgery may return a bedridden patient to his feet or eliminate the need for future amputation. The management of this type of patient requires close collaboration between the patient's physician and the consultant.

OTHER HYPERKERATOTIC LESIONS

Other discrete hyperkeratotic lesions commonly found on the foot include *verruca plantaris, porokeratosis plantaris discreta, and foreign body granuloma*.

Verruca plantaris, or plantar warts, occur on the plantar aspect of the foot, usually on weight-bearing surfaces (Fig. 102.5*A*). They are discussed also in Chapter 100, Common Problems of the Skin, but a brief account is provided here because of the importance of differentiating them from corns, calluses, and other hyperkeratotic lesions. Plantar warts can by asymptomatic or extremely painful. They are caused by a papilloma virus for which there is no specific treatment or prevention. Because they are benign and often resolve spontaneously, aggressive or untried therapies should be avoided.

The appearance of a verrucous lesion is illustrated in Figure 102.5*A*. They may vary in size from 1 mm to 1 cm. The lesions can be differentiated from hyperkeratotic corns in several ways: warts usually have rough surfaces, are painful with the application of both surface and lateral pressure, and bleed upon debriding because of their capillary supply; corns are usually smooth surfaced, most painful with surface pressure, and do not bleed upon debridement.

The treatment of plantar warts is discussed in Chapter 100, Common Problems of the Skin.

A *porokeratotic lesion* is a circumscribed, discrete hyperkeratotic lesion on the plantar aspect of the foot which develops as a result of keratin occluding

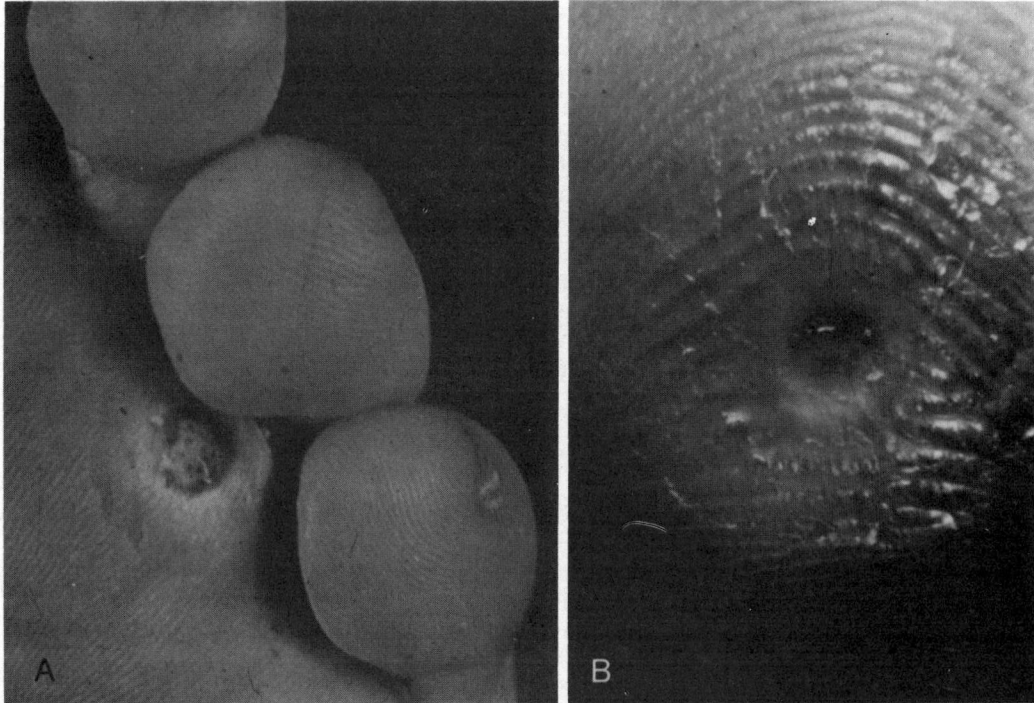

Figure 102.5. Hyperkeratotic lesions not due to chronic trauma. *A.* Plantar wart. *B.* Porokeratosis on plantar surface. (Photographs courtesy of Max Weisfeld, D.P.M.)

a sweat duct in the skin (see Fig. 102.5*B*). The obstruction and resultant backup create a reaction in the skin similar to a deep, large corn. This lesion need not be under a weight-bearing surface. It is usually very painful, and after debridement there is characteristically even more distress. Treatment by the dermatologist or podiatrist is usually by local curettage.

Foreign bodies in the plantar surface of the foot can generate a local inflammatory reaction and thus create a hyperkeratotic lesion. One of the most common offending substances is hair (animal or human). For example, a dog hair, trapped in a carpet long enough to have dried out, can penetrate the skin rather easily. This lesion, while grossly resembling a simple callus, will, upon examination with a magnifying glass, have a small aperture (entry wound) near the center. The local reaction may or may not include infection. Treatment is simple excision of the foreign body.

NAIL CONDITIONS

There are only two nail conditions which are frequently brought to medical attention: onychomycosis (fungal infection) and ingrown toenails, with or without concomitant inflammation (paronychia).

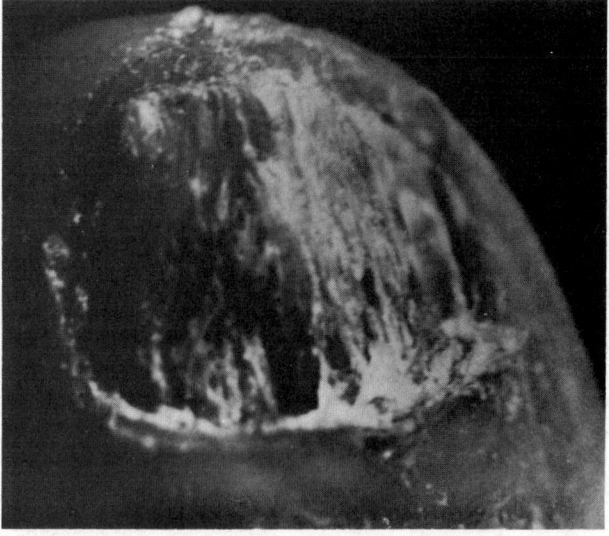

Figure 102.6. Mycotic toenail.

Onychomycosis (2) (Fig. 102.6)

Etiology and Findings

The typical fungal infection of a toenail begins distally at the tip of the toe and moves proximally, subungually, and through the nail plate itself. Etiological agents are *Trichophyton mentagrophytes,*

Trichophyton rubrum, or *Candida albicans.* The fungus produces yellowish discoloration and longitudinal striations in the nails and in the epidermis; the accompanying local inflammatory reaction stimulates hyperkeratosis under the nail. This hyperkeratotic accumulation tends to lift the nail up from the epidermis, facilitating further progression of the fungus. Eventually, the nail becomes brownish-yellow mottled, thickened, and powdery. Usually these infections are asymptomatic; patients are most concerned about the appearance of their nails, the possibility of spread of infection, and sometimes the inability to wear shoes when severe thickening of the nail plate is present.

Treatment

Fungus infections of toenails are difficult to eradicate medically. There are no topical medications that have been shown to be effective. Only the griseofulvin group of medications, taken orally, may eliminate the infection. Griseofulvin treatment is prolonged (1 to 2 years) and carries the small but real risk of bone marrow suppression. There is also the possibility that, following such a regimen, the infection will recur. Therefore, simple debridement or permanent removal of the nail is the treatment of choice for this problem.

When nail thickening is regarded as a problem by the patient, the process can be controlled by regular and thorough *debridement.* The debridement of mycotic or otherwise thickened toenails is a process generally performed by podiatrists. The debridement first involves soaking of the feet and cutting of the nails by heavy duty cutters. Finally, the nails are thoroughly filed down with an electrically powered, diamond-studded burr. These drills are fitted with vacuum extraction systems to protect the patient and podiatrist from breathing in the nail dust.

Another treatment is *permanent removal* of the nail, including matrixectomy. Since toenails serve no useful function, their absence causes no functional impairment. Surgical correction should be reserved, however, for those patients whose nails are painful or for whom the appearance of the feet is a significant factor. The most frequent type of surgical correction of toenails performed by dermatologists, podiatrists, or surgeons is nail excision, followed by chemical destruction of matrix tissue and nailbed with 88% phenol. After a sterile dressing is applied to the toe, the patient may continue his normal routine. He needs only to change bandages and soak his feet daily until healing is complete in 2 to 3 weeks. Skin formerly below the nail plate thickens. Women can disguise the fact that their nails have been removed by applying nail polish to this thickened skin.

Ingrown Toenails (Figs. 102.7 and 102.8)

Etiology and Findings

Ingrown toenail, a painful condition in which the medial or lateral border of a toenail penetrates the flesh, is a common problem. Ingrown toenails have been attributed to factors such as improper trimming, heredity, bony pathology, improper shoe fit, tight socks, obesity, and trauma. However, there is no clear-cut etiology, and there are probably many contributing causes. The nail of a great toe is almost always involved, and the problem can be identified by inspection and by the finding of point tenderness upon pressing the margin of the toenail.

Treatment

There is a popular misconception among many people that cutting a "V" in the center of a toenail will cause the lateral borders to grow toward the center, thereby relieving the ingrown condition. This belief has no basis in fact, since the nail plate is merely hornified keratin—nonliving, fixed tissue in which growth no longer occurs.

Initial treatment of ingrown toenail depends upon whether the patient's toe is infected (paronychia) or is chronically painful but not infected when the patient seeks care. The patient with an ingrown toenail will often seek help after attempting to excise the offending edge of toenail with whatever instruments are available; most of the nail edge may be

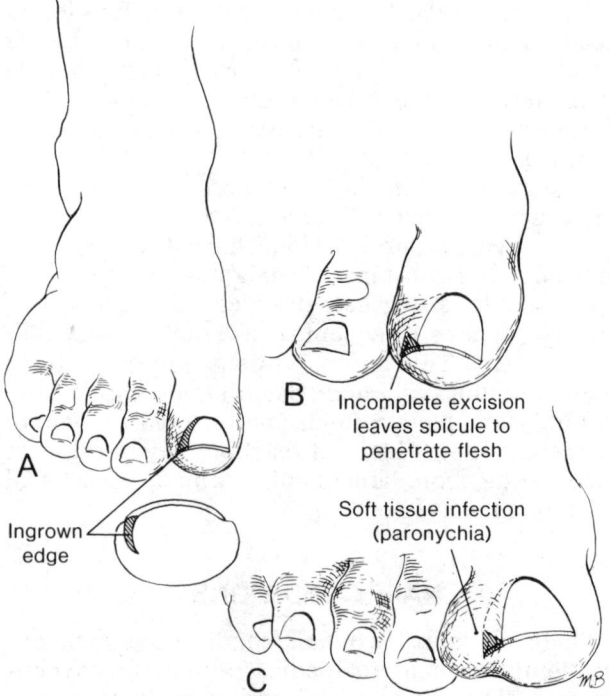

Figure 102.7. Schematic illustration of an ingrown toenail and complications which may occur.

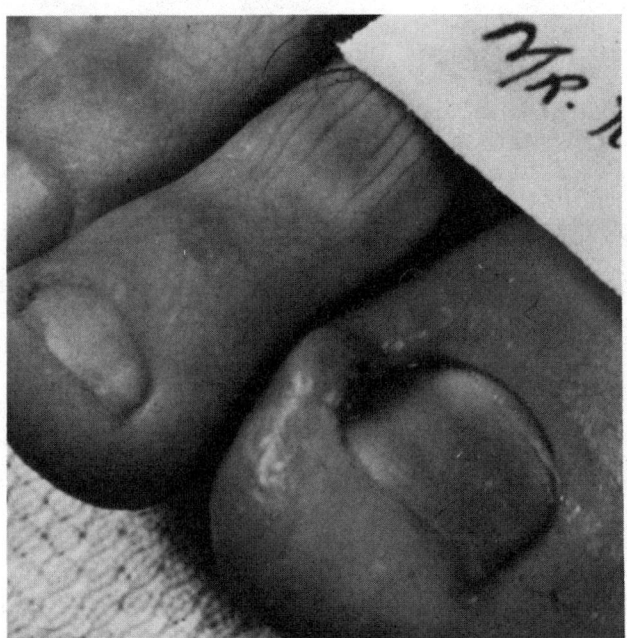

Figure 102.8. Infected ingrown toenail (paronychia).

removed in this way by the patient, but a small, sharp piece of nail usually remains (Fig. 102.8) which pierces the skin with each step and promotes infection: the toe becomes red, swollen, and exquisitely tender. The most vigorous soaking and the use of local and systemic antibiotics will not arrest such an infection as long as a nail spicule continues to penetrate the flesh. Therefore, the patient should be referred (to a dermatologist, podiatrist, or surgeon) for excision of the offending border of the nail; this procedure is done under local anesthesia and it is curative. However, approximately 10% of patients will have a recurrence, usually within 1 year. Systemic antimicrobials are rarely necessary.

Definitive treatment of the ingrown nail itself, varies according to the condition and needs of the patient.

For *otherwise healthy patients*, the procedure described above for removal of the entire toenail and for matrix destruction can also be utilized to eradicate permanently an ingrown border. Following local anesthesia, the offending edge of toenail is excised; then phenol and alcohol are applied to cauterize the matrix tissue. This procedure, followed by 2 to 3 weeks for complete healing, will usually eliminate permanently this painful and sometimes dangerous condition.

Management of *diabetics* and patients with arterial insufficiency must be conservative, as wound healing may be poor after surgical removal of the nail. In these patients, frequent and thorough debridement of ingrown borders is effective and safe. Treatment by a podiatrist or other practitioner who is skilled in this procedure may be needed every 3 to 4 weeks to prevent complicating soft tissue infection.

HEEL PAIN (1)

Heel pain is a common complaint. The most common pattern is pain that is localized to the medial plantar aspect of the heel. (Heel pain localized to the posterior aspect of the foot, the heel cord, is discussed in Chapter 67, and heel pain as a manifestation of the tarsal tunnel syndrome is discussed in Chapter 84.) Characteristically, the first step in the morning is particularly painful. After 5 to 10 minutes of walking the pain eases, but during the course of the day's activities it becomes progressively worse. The reason that these symptoms appear, disappear, and reappear is not understood.

Examination of the foot reveals a tender area of the heel approximately 4.5 cm from the posterior margin of the plantar surface, corresponding to the medial condyle of the calcaneus. X-rays frequently reveal a calcaneal exostosis or spur at the point of tenderness (Fig. 102.9). These spurs are commonly found on X-rays of asymptomatic heels, and they are not the cause of pain in symptomatic heels. Since the attachment of the plantar fascia coincides with the point of greatest tenderness, it is felt that pain is due to *plantar fasciitis*. One can picture the plantar fascia as an extension of the Achilles tendon, with the calcaneus acting as a fulcrum between fascia and tendon (see Fig. 102.1*B*). Any condition which increases stress on the Achilles tendon may also stress the plantar fascia, e.g., overuse in running or jogging (especially with shoes having inflexible mid-

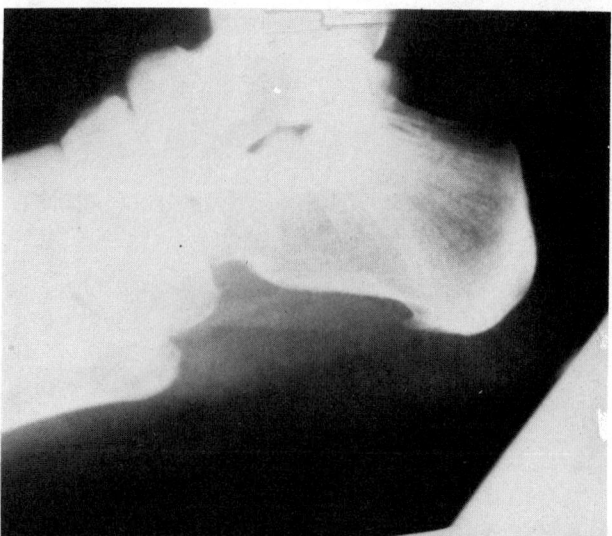

Figure 102.9. Radiological view of a calcaneal exostosis (spur). (Photograph courtesy of Max Weisfeld, D.P.M.)

soles), excessive pronation (see above), or a sudden change to flat shoes after wearing high heels for prolonged periods. Heel pain may also be a manifestation of gout or Reiter's syndrome, and these diagnoses should always be considered when evaluating such a patient (see Chapters 69 and 71).

Treatment

Treatment should be aimed at both the local inflammatory process and the underlying mechanical problem. Initial treatment includes use of an oral anti-inflammatory medication (such as naproxen (Naprosyn), 250 mg every 6 to 8 hours, or piroxicam (Feldene), 10 to 20 mg every 24 hours; aspirin, 600 mg every 4 to 6 hours may also be used but the onset of action is slower), rest, and soaking in warm water. An injection of a corticosteroid and Xylocaine (approximately 1 to 2 ml of a 1:3 dilution of the corticosteroid with Xylocaine) into the tender area from the medial aspect of the heel will usually bring dramatic relief from pain which has not responded to other measures.

Recurrent symptoms can be prevented by having the patient use a ¼-inch felt heel pad. When this is inserted into the shoes, it decreases tension on the Achilles tendon, and, consequently, tension on the plantar fascia is also reduced. The increased angulation of the foot shifts weight away from the heel to the forefoot. Felt—rather than foam, which is too compressible—is available from medical and surgical supply houses. When a simple heel pad is not sufficient, consultation with an orthopaedist or podiatrist is indicated. The consultant will fabricate an appropriate orthotic to minimize pronation, raise the heel, and protect the painful area. Rarely, a painful heel will require surgical fasciotomy and removal of the spur.

General References

Levin ME, O'Neal LW (eds): *The Diabetic Foot*, ed 3. St Louis, CV Mosby, 1983.
>A helpful and well illustrated guide to managing diabetic foot problems.

Samitz MH: *Cutaneous Lesions of the Lower Extremity.* Philadelphia, JB Lippincott, 1971.
>Well illustrated text covering dermatological conditions of the foot.

Weinstein F (ed): *Principles and Practices of Podiatry*, Philadelphia, Lea & Febiger, 1968.
>A useful text for basic understanding of podiatric medicine.

Specific References

1. Cailliet R: *Foot and Ankle Pain.* Philadelphia, FA Davis, 1968, p 108.
2. Lurdeen G: Onychomycosis: its classification, pathophysiology and etiology. *J Am Podiatry Assoc* 68:395, 1978.
3. Mercado OA: Surgical procedures. In Fielding M (ed): *The Surgical Treatment of Hallux Abducto Valgus.* Mt Kisco, NY, Futura, 1973, pp 39–71.

Index